Oxford Textbook of

Obstetrics and Gynaecology

Oxford Textbook of
Obstetrics and Gynaecology

Sabaratnam Arulkumaran

Foundation Professor of Obstetrics and Gynaecology, University of Nicosia, Nicosia, Cyprus
Professor Emeritus of Obstetrics and Gynaecology, St George's University of London,
London, UK
Visiting Professor, Institute of Global Health, Imperial College, London, UK

William Ledger

Professor of Obstetrics and Gynaecology, University of New South Wales, Sydney, Australia
Director of Reproductive Medicine, Royal Hospital for Women, Sydney, Australia

Lynette Denny

Professor: Special Projects, Department of Obstetrics and Gynaecology,
University of Cape Town/Groote Schuur Hospital, Cape Town, South Africa
Director, South African Medical Research Council, Gynaecological Cancer Research Centre, Cape Town,
South Africa

Stergios Doumouchtsis

Consultant Obstetrician Gynaecologist and Subspecialist Urogynaecologist, Epsom and St Helier
University Hospitals NHS Trust, London, UK
Honorary Reader, St George's University of London, London, UK
Visiting Professor, National and Kapodistrian University of Athens, School of Health Sciences,
Department of Medicine, Athens, Greece
Clinical Professor, Ross University, School of Medicine, Miramar, FL, USA
Associate Clinical Professor, American University of the Caribbean, School of Medicine, Cupecoy,
Sint Maarten

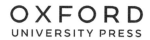
OXFORD
UNIVERSITY PRESS

OXFORD
UNIVERSITY PRESS

Great Clarendon Street, Oxford, OX2 6DP,
United Kingdom

Oxford University Press is a department of the University of Oxford.
It furthers the University's objective of excellence in research, scholarship,
and education by publishing worldwide. Oxford is a registered trade mark of
Oxford University Press in the UK and in certain other countries

First published 2020
First published in paperback 2023

Impression: 1

Published in the United States of America by Oxford University Press
198 Madison Avenue, New York, NY 10016, United States of America

British Library Cataloguing in Publication Data
Data available

Library of Congress Cataloging in Publication Data
Data available

ISBN 978–0–19–876636–0 (Hbk.)
ISBN 978–0–19–887482–9 (Pbk.)

Printed in the UK by
Ashford Colour Press Ltd, Gosport, Hampshire

Preface

This comprehensive text book of Obstetrics and Gynaecology consists of 72 chapters that spans over 900 pages. It has 12 subsections for easy navigation by the reader. The book covers all of the important aspects of the subject. Such comprehensive coverage was possible due to the International collaboration of hundreds of world renowned authors. We, as editors of the book, are most grateful to them. The authors are from various countries and have provided the knowledge based on available latest evidence in the literature and guidelines from well recognised National and International Professional organisations.

The editors have been selected to provide their expertise in the areas of feto-maternal medicine, reproductive medicine, uro and general gynaecology and gynaecological oncology. They are from the United Kingdom, Australia and South Africa and hold or have held responsible academic positions and have published extensively. They have contributed significantly to teaching, research and clinical practice. The editors have published books in their own rights and have written for and overseen the production of this book with the benefit of their vast experience. We have given the liberty to individual authors to interpret the evidence in their area of expertise and to provide opinions and advice where evidence is lacking.

The production of the book has been a huge undertaking, and has taken significant time from the submission of the manuscripts to final production. However our authors have been able to update their chapters to circumvent their content becoming out of date. The editors and the publishers are most grateful to them for their effort. This book will be the comprehensive text in Obstetrics and Gynaecology for consultants, postgraduates, midwives, nurses and allied health specialists. We would like to hear your comments and feedback so that we can correct or update the text in the reprint or the next edition.

Sabaratnam Arulkumaran
William Ledger
Lynette Denny
Stergios Doumouchtsis

September 2019

Contents

SECTION 9
Reproductive Medicine

SECTION 10
Sexual and Reproductive Care

SECTION 11
Urogynaecology and Pelvic Floor Disorders

SECTION 12
Gynaecological Oncology

Abbreviations

2D	two-dimensional	CHB	complete heart block
3D	three-dimensional	CHD	congenital heart disease
5-FU	5-fluorouracil	CI	confidence interval
ABC	airway, breathing, and circulation	CIN	cervical intraepithelial neoplasia
ABPM	ambulatory blood pressure monitoring	CIS	carcinoma *in situ*
AC	abdominal circumference	CKI	chronic kidney injury
ACA	anticardiolipin antibodies	CL	cervical length
ACE	angiotensin-converting enzyme	CNV	copy number variant
AChR	acetylcholine receptor	COC	combined oral contraceptive
ACOG	American College of Obstetrics and Gynecologists	COX	cyclooxygenase
ACTH	adrenocorticotropic hormone	CPD	cephalopelvic disproportion
ADPKD	autosomal dominant polycystic kidney disease	CPR	cardiopulmonary resuscitation
AED	antiepileptic drug	CRH	corticotropin-releasing hormone
AFC	antral follicle count	CRL	crown–rump length
AFLP	acute fatty liver of pregnancy	CSF	cerebrospinal fluid
aHUS	atypical haemolytic uraemic syndrome	CSP	cavum septum pellucidum
AI	aromatase inhibitor	CT	computed tomography
AIDS	acquired immunodeficiency syndrome	CTG	cardiotocography
AIP	abnormality invasive placenta	CTPA	computed tomography pulmonary angiography
AKI	acute kidney injury	CVS	chorionic villus sampling
ALT	alanine aminotransferase	CVT	cerebral venous thrombosis
AMH	anti-Mullerian hormone	D&E	dilatation and evacuation
AML	active management of labour	DFM	decreased fetal movement
aOR	adjusted odds ratio	DHEA	dehydroepiandrosterone
AP	anteroposterior	DIC	disseminated intravascular coagulation
APC	antigen-presenting cell	DSM-5	*Diagnostic and Statistical Manual of Mental Disorders*,
APH	antepartum haemorrhage		5th edition
APS	antiphospholipid syndrome	dVIN	differentiated vulval intraepithelial neoplasia
ARDS	acute respiratory distress syndrome	EC	emergency contraceptive
ARM	artificial rupture of membranes	ECG	electrocardiogram
ARV	assisted reproductive technology *or* antiretroviral therapy	ECV	external cephalic version
		EFI	Endometriosis Fertility Index
ASIS	anterior superior iliac spine	EFM	electronic fetal heart rate monitoring
ASRM	American Society of Reproductive Medicine	EFW	estimated fetal weight
ATP	adenosine triphosphate	EIN	endometrial intraepithelial neoplasia
AUB	abnormal uterine bleeding	EOC	epithelial ovarian cancer
AVP	arginine vasopressin	EOGBSD	early-onset neonatal group B *Streptococcus* disease
BMI	body mass index	EP	ectopic pregnancy
BP	blood pressure	EPAU	early pregnancy assessment unit
bpm	beats per minute	ER	oestrogen receptor
BV	bacterial vaginosis	ESHRE	European Society for Human Reproduction and Embryology
CAH	congenital adrenal hyperplasia		
CDC	Centers for Disease Control and Prevention	ESRD	end-stage renal disease
CDH	congenital diaphragmatic hernia	EVT	extravillous trophoblast
CFU	colony-forming unit	EXIT	ex utero intrapartum treatment
CGH	comparative genomic hybridization	FASP	Fetal Anomaly Screening Programme

FBS	fetal scalp blood sampling	HT	hydroxytryptamine *or* hormone therapy
FEV$_1$	forced expiratory volume in 1 second	HUS	haemolytic uraemic syndrome
FFN	fetal fibronectin	HyCoSys	hysterosalpingo contrast sonography
FGM/C	female genital mutilation/cutting	IADPSG	International Association of Diabetes and Pregnancy Study Groups
FGR	fetal growth restriction		
FHR	fetal heart rate	IARC	International Agency for Research on Cancer
FIGO	International Federation of Gynecology and Obstetrics	IBD	inflammatory bowel disease
		ICH	intracranial haemorrhage
FISH	fluorescence in situ hybridization	ICP	intrahepatic cholestasis of pregnancy
FMAIT	fetal alloimmune thrombocytopenia	ICS	International Continence Society
FRC	functional residual capacity	ICSI	intracytoplasmic sperm injection
FSAD	female sexual arousal disorder	Ig	immunoglobulin
FSD	female sexual dysfunction	IGRT	image-guided radiation therapy
FSH	follicle-stimulating hormone	IL	interleukin
FSIAD	female sexual interest and arousal disorder	ILT	interstitial laser therapy
FSIRS	fetal systemic inflammatory response syndrome	IM	intramuscular
		IMRT	intensity-modulated radiation therapy
FVL	factor V Leiden	ISSVD	International Society for the Study of Vulvovaginal Disease
G6PD	glucose-6-phosphate dehydrogenase		
GAS	group A *Streptococcus*	ISUOG	International Society of Ultrasound in Obstetrics and Gynecology
GBS	group B *Streptococcus*		
GDM	gestational diabetes mellitus	IUD	intrauterine device
GFR	glomerular filtration rate	IUFD	intrauterine fetal demise
GH	growth hormone	IUGA	International Urogynecological Association
GMC	General Medical Council	IUGR	intrauterine growth restriction
GnRH	gonadotropin-releasing hormone	IUI	intrauterine insemination
GOG	Gynecologic Oncology Group	IUT	intrauterine blood transfusion
GTD	gestational trophoblastic disease	IV	intravenous
GTN	gestational trophoblastic neoplasia	IVC	inferior vena cava
HAART	highly active antiretroviral therapy	IVF	*in vitro* fertilization
HbA1c	glycated haemoglobin	IVF-ET	*in vitro* fertilization with embryo transfer
HBPM	home blood pressure monitoring	IVH	intraventricular haemorrhage
HBV	hepatitis B virus	IVIG	intravenous immunoglobulin
HC	head circumference	JZ	junctional zone
hCG	human chorionic gonadotropin	LABA	long-acting beta-2-agonist
HCV	hepatitis C virus	LAC	lupus anticoagulant
HD	haemodialysis	LAM	lactational amenorrhoea method *or* levator ani muscle
HDP	hypertensive disorders of pregnancy		
HELLP	haemolysis, elevated liver enzymes, and low platelets	LARC	long-acting reversible contraception
		LAT	labour admission test
HFEA	Human Fertilization and Embryology Authority	LBW	low birth weight
		LEEP	loop electrosurgical excision procedure
HGESS	high-grade endometrial stromal sarcoma	LFCNT	lateral femoral cutaneous nerve of the thigh
HGSOC	high-grade serous ovarian cancer	LFT	liver function test
HIC	high-income country	LGA	large for gestational age
HIFU	high-intensity focused ultrasound	LGESS	low-grade endometrial stromal sarcoma
HIV	human immunodeficiency virus	LGSC	low-grade serous carcinoma
HLA	human leucocyte antigen	LH	luteinizing hormone
HMB	heavy menstrual bleeding	linac	linear accelerator
HNPCC	hereditary non-polyposis colorectal cancer	LLETZ	large loop excision of the transformation zone
HPA	human platelet antigen	LMIC	low- and middle-income countries
HPF	high power field(s)	LMP	last menstrual period
hPL	human placental lactogen	LMWH	low-molecular-weight heparin
HPO	hypothalamic–pituitary–ovarian	LNG-IUS	levonorgestrel-releasing intrauterine system
HPV	human papillomavirus		
HRAM	high-resolution anorectal manometry	LUNA	laparoscopic uterosacral nerve ablation
HRT	hormonal replacement therapy	LUTO	lower urinary tract obstruction
HSDD	hypoactive sexual desire disorder	LVSI	lymphovascular space invasion
HSG	hysterosalpingography	MAS	meconium aspiration syndrome
HSP	Henoch–Schönlein purpura		
HSV	herpes simplex virus		

MBP	mechanical bowel preparation	POI	premature ovarian insufficiency
MCDA	monochorionic diamniotic	POP	pelvic organ prolapse
MCM	major congenital malformation	PPH	postpartum haemorrhage
MCMA	monochorionic monoamniotic	PPROM	preterm prelabour rupture of membranes
MDG	Millennium Development Goal	PR	progesterone receptor
MEC	Medical Eligibility Criteria	PRES	posterior reversible encephalopathy syndrome
MFPR	multiple fetal pregnancy reduction	PSC	primary sclerosing cholangitis
MG	myasthenia gravis	PSN	presacral neurectomy
MHRA	Medicines Healthcare products Regulation Authority	PSTT	placental site trophoblastic tumour
MMC	myelomeningocoele	PTB	preterm birth
MMP	matrix metalloproteinase	PTSD	post-traumatic stress disorder
MOEWS	Modified Obstetric Early Warning Score	PUL	pregnancy of unknown location
MPA	medroxyprogesterone acetate	PVL	periventricular leucomalacia
MR	magnetic resonance	QI	quality improvement
MRgFUS	magnetic resonance-guided focused ultrasound surgery	RAS	renin–angiotensin system
		rASRM	revised American Society for Reproductive Medicine
MRI	magnetic resonance imaging	RCOG	Royal College of Obstetricians and Gynaecologists
MS	multiple sclerosis	RCT	randomized controlled trial
MSAF	meconium staining of the amniotic fluid	RCVS	reversible cerebral vasoconstriction syndrome
MSU	mid-stream urine	RDS	respiratory distress syndrome
MUI	mixed urinary incontinence	RFA	radiofrequency ablation
NAAT	nucleic acid amplification test	RLS	restless legs syndrome
NCCN	National Comprehensive Cancer Network	RM	recurrent miscarriage
NHS	National Health Service	RPL	recurrent pregnancy loss
NICE	National Institute for health and Care Excellence	RR	relative risk
NIH	National Institutes of Health	SCD	sickle cell disease
NIP	national immunization programme	SCENIHR	Scientific Committee on Emerging and Newly Identified Health Risks
NIPT	non-invasive prenatal testing		
NK	natural killer	SCT	sacrococcygeal teratoma
NSAID	non-steroidal anti-inflammatory drug	SDG	Sustainable Development Goal
NT	nuchal translucency	SET	single embryo transfer
OA	occipitoanterior	SGA	small for gestational age
OAB	overactive bladder	SHBG	sex hormone-binding globulin
OASIS	obstetric anal sphincter injuries	SIS	saline infusion sonography
OBGYN	obstetrics and gynaecology	sIUGR	selective intrauterine growth restriction
OHSS	ovarian hyperstimulation syndrome	SLE	systemic lupus erythematosus
OP	occipitoposterior	SNRI	serotonin noradrenaline reuptake inhibitor
OR	odds ratio	SPRM	selective progesterone receptor modulator
OT	occipitotransverse	sPTB	spontaneous preterm birth
OVD	operative vaginal delivery	SSRI	selective serotonin reuptake inhibitor
PAI	plasminogen activator inhibitor	STI	sexually transmitted infection
PAPP-A	pregnancy-associated plasma protein A	SUA	single umbilical artery
PARP	poly(ADP ribose) polymerase	SUI	stress urinary incontinence
PBC	primary biliary cholangitis	SVT	supraventricular tachycardia
PCOS	polycystic ovary syndrome	T_3	triiodothyronine
PCR	polymerase chain reaction or protein:creatinine ratio	T_4	tetraiodothyronine (thyroxine)
PD	peritoneal dialysis	TAUS	transabdominal ultrasound
PDE	phosphodiesterase	TBG	thyroxine-binding globulin
PE	pulmonary embolism	TCGA	The Cancer Genome Atlas
PEFR	peak expiratory flow rate	TCRE	transcervical resection of the endometrium
PET	pre-eclampsia/toxaemia	TKI	tyrosine kinase inhibitor
PFMT	pelvic floor muscle training	TMA	thrombotic microangiopathy
PFS	progression-free survival	TOLAC	trial of labour after caesarean
PGD	preimplantation genetic diagnosis	tPA	tissue plasminogen activator
PGM	prothrombin gene mutation	TRAP	twin reversed arterial perfusion
PGS	preimplantation genetic screening	TSG	tumour suppressor gene
PID	pelvic inflammatory disease	TTP	thrombotic thrombocytopenic purpura
PLD	pegylated liposomal doxorubicin	TTTS	twin-to-twin transfusion syndrome

TVUS	transvaginal ultrasound		VCI	velamentous insertion of the cord
TZ	transformation zone		VEGF	vascular endothelial growth factor
UAE	uterine artery embolization		VHD	valvular heart disease
UBA	urethral bulking agent		VIA	visual inspection with acetic acid
UCP	umbilical cord prolapse		VIN	vulval intraepithelial neoplasia
UDCA	ursodeoxycholic acid		VLDL	very low-density lipoprotein
UES	undifferentiated endometrial sarcoma		VP	ventriculoperitoneal
UFH	unfractionated heparin		VSCC	vulval squamous cell carcinoma
UI	urinary incontinence		VTE	venous thromboembolism
uPA	urokinase plasminogen activator		VUR	vesicoureteral reflux
USS	ultrasound screening		vWD	von Willebrand disease
UTI	urinary tract infection		vWF	von Willebrand factor
UUI	urgency urinary incontinence		VZIG	varicella zoster immunoglobulin
uVIN	usual-type vulval intraepithelial neoplasia		VZV	varicella zoster virus
V/Q	ventilation–perfusion		WHI	Women's Health Initiative
VAIN	vaginal intraepithelial neoplasia		WHO	World Health Organization
VAS	vesicoamniotic shunting		WwE	women with epilepsy
VBAC	vaginal birth after caesarean delivery			

Contributors

Jason A. Abbott Gynaecological Research and Clinical Evaluation (GRACE) Group, Royal Hospital for Women, Sydney; University of New South Wales, Sydney, Australia
47: Laparoscopy

Ganesh Adaikan Department of Obstetrics and Gynaecology, National University of Singapore, National University Health System, Singapore
60: Female sexual dysfunction

Anthony Addei Consultant Anaesthetist, St George's University Hospitals NHS Foundation Trust, London, UK
28: Obstetric analgesia and anaesthesia

Zarko Alfirevic Professor of Fetal and Maternal Medicine; Head of Department; Associate Pro-Vice-Chancellor (Clinical), Director of Harris-Wellbeing Preterm Birth Research Centre, University of Liverpool, Liverpool, UK
30: Preterm birth

Amanda Ali Consultant Obstetrician and Maternal Medicine Specialist, Kingston Hospital NHS Foundation Trust, UK
15: Haematological disorders in pregnancy

Stephanie S. Andriputri Gynaecological Research and Clinical Evaluation (GRACE) Group, Royal Hospital for Women, Sydney; University of New South Wales, Sydney, Australia
47: Laparoscopy

Mary Ann Lumsden Professor of Medical Education and Gynaecology, University of Glasgow Scotland, UK
46: Menopause

Sabaratnam Arulkumaran Foundation Professor of Obstetrics & Gynaecology, University of Nicosia, Cyprus Professor Emeritus of Obstetrics and Gynaecology, St George's University of London, London, UK; Visiting Professor, Institute of Global Health, Imperial College, London, UK
27: Fetal monitoring during labour

Sohail Bampoe Consultant Anaesthetist, University College London Hospital, London, UK
28: Obstetric analgesia and anaesthesia

Marina Berbic Conjoint Senior Lecturer, School of Women's and Children's Health, Department of Obstetrics and Gynaecology, Royal Hospital for Women and University of New South Wales, Sydney, Australia
41: Menstrual disorders, amenorrhea, and dysmenorrhoea

Smriti Bhatta Aberdeen Fertility Centre, Institute of Applied Health Sciences, University of Aberdeen, Aberdeen, UK
51: Infertility

Siladitya Bhattacharya Aberdeen Fertility Centre, Institute of Applied Health Sciences, University of Aberdeen, Aberdeen, UK
51: Infertility

Amarnath Bhide Consultant in Obstetrics and Fetal Medicine, St George's University Hospitals NHS Foundation Trust, London, UK
9: The placenta; 11: Prenatal diagnosis

Carmen Binding Postgraduate Medical Resident, Department of Obstetrics & Gynaecology, University of British Columbia, Vancouver, Canada
6: Preconceptional medicine

Dustin Boothe Department of Radiation Oncology, Huntsman Cancer Hospital, University of Utah, Salt Lake City, UT, USA
68: Radiation therapy in the management of gynaecological cancer

Matthys Hendrik Botha Associate Professor and Head of Obstetrics and Gynaecology, Stellenbosch University and Tygerberg Hospital, South Africa
72: Cancer in pregnancy

Graham J. Burton The Centre for Trophoblast Research, Department of Physiology, Development and Neuroscience, University of Cambridge, Cambridge, UK
9: The placenta

Joanna M. Cain Professor of Obstetrics & Gynecology and Radiation Oncology; Vice Chair, Department of Obstetrics and Gynecology, University of Massachusetts Medical School, Worcester, MA, USA
69: Palliative care

Angharad Care Clinical PTB Research Fellow, Harris-Wellbeing Research Centre for Preterm Birth, University of Liverpool, Liverpool, UK
30: Preterm birth

Marco Carlone Radiation Medicine Program, Princess Margaret Cancer Centre, and Department of Radiation Oncology, University of Toronto, Toronto, Canada
68: Radiation therapy in the management of gynaecological cancer

Ana Piñas Carrillo Consultant Obstetrician, St George's University Hospitals NHS Foundation Trust, London, UK
11: Prenatal diagnosis

Manas Chakrabarti Gynaecological Oncologist, Columbia Asia Hospital, Kolkata, India
71: Premalignant disease of the genital tract in pregnancy

Karen K.L. Chan Department of Obstetrics & Gynaecology, University of Hong Kong, Queen Mary Hospital, Hong Kong
66: Gestational trophoblastic disease

Yvonne Kwun Yue Cheng Assistant Professor, Department of Obstetrics & Gynaecology, The Chinese University of Hong Kong, Hong Kong
33: Obstetric procedures

Frank A. Chervenak Zucker School of Medicine at Hofstra/Northwell and Lenox Hill Hospital, New York, USA
2: Ethics in obstetrics and gynaecology

Jacqueline PuiWah Chung Assistant Professor, Department of Obstetrics and Gynaecology, Prince of Wales Hospital, The Chinese University of Hong Kong, Hong Kong
44: Chronic pelvic pain

Tim Craig Assistant Professor, Princess Margaret Cancer Centre, and Department of Radiation Oncology, University of Toronto, Toronto, Canada
68: Radiation therapy in the management of gynaecological cancer

Hilary O.D. Critchley MRC Centre for Reproductive Health, The University of Edinburgh, The Queen's Medical Research Institute, Edinburgh, UK
40: The menstrual cycle

Thomas D'Hooghe Lab of Experimental Gynaecology, G-PURE Research Group, Department of Development and Regeneration, Leuven University, Belgium
45: Endometriosis

Gillian Dean Consultant HIV & Sexual Health, Brighton & Sussex University Hospitals NHS Trust, Brighton & Hove, UK
43: Pelvic inflammatory disease

Lynette Denny Professor and Chair, Department of Obstetrics & Gynaecology, University of Cape Town/Groote Schuur Hospital, Cape Town, South Africa; Director, South African Medical Research Council, Gynaecological Cancer Research Centre
61: Cancer screening and prevention in gynaecology

Arianna Di Florio Clinical Senior Lecturer, Division of Psychological Medicine and Clinical Neurosciences, Cardiff University, Cardiff, UK
18: Psychiatric disorders in pregnancy and the postpartum

Stergios Doumouchtsis Consultant Obstetrician Gynaecologist and Urogynaecologist, Epsom and St Helier University Hospitals NHS Trust, UK, Honorary Senior Lecturer, St George's University of London, Visiting Professor, University of Athens, School of Health Sciences, Department of Medicine, Associate Clinical Professor, American University of the Caribbean, School of Medicine
1: Basic science in obstetrics and gynaecology;
59: Childbirth trauma

Tim Draycott Consultant Obstetrician, Department of Women's Health, North Bristol NHS Trust, Bristol, Avon, UK
29: Obstetric emergencies

Anupreet Dua Consultant in Obstetrics & Gynaecology and Sub-specialist Urogynaecologist, University Hospitals Plymouth NHS Trust, Plymouth, UK
56: Pelvic organ prolapse

Leroy C. Edozien Consultant in Obstetrics and Gynaecology, Manchester Academic Health Science Centre, St Mary's Hospital, Manchester, UK
5: Clinical governance

David A. Ellwood Professor of Obstetrics & Gynaecology, Griffith University, Queensland; Director of Maternal-Fetal Medicine, Gold Coast University Hospital, Southport, Australia
34: Stillbirth

Vicki Flenady Director of the Centre of Research Excellence in Stillbirth (Stillbirth CRE), Mater Research Institute, Mater Hospital, Brisbane; Honorary Professor, University of Queensland, Brisbane, Australia
34: Stillbirth

Christina Fotopoulou Consultant Gynaecological Oncologist, Faculty of Medicine, Department of Surgery and Cancer, Imperial College, London, UK
64: Ovarian, fallopian tube, and peritoneal cancer

Ian S. Fraser Conjoint Professor, School of Women's and Children's Health, Department of Obstetrics and Gynaecology, Royal Hospital for Women and University of New South Wales, Sydney, Australia
41: Menstrual disorders, amenorrhea, and dysmenorrhoea

Robert Freeman Consultant in Urogynaecology, University Hospitals, Plymouth and Hon Professor Plymouth University Peninsula Schools of Medicine and Dentistry, Urogynaecology, Plymouth, Devon, UK
56: Pelvic organ prolapse

Anthony Fyles Professor, Department of Radiation Oncology, Princess Margaret Hospital, Toronto, Canada
68: Radiation therapy in the management of gynaecological cancer

David Gaffney Academic Program Manager, Radiation Oncology, Huntsman Cancer Hospital, University of Utah, Salt Lake City, UT, USA
68: Radiation therapy in the management of gynaecological cancer

Kiren Ghag Obstetrics Clinical Research Fellow, Department of Women's Health, Southmead Hospital, Bristol, UK
29: Obstetric emergencies

Ian A. Greer President and Vice Chancellor of Queen's University Belfast, Belfast, UK
16: Thrombosis and embolism in pregnancy

Sahana Gupta Consultant in Obstetrics and Gynaecology, Northwick Park Hospital, Harrow, Middlesex, UK
49: Benign disease of the uterus

Jane E. Hirst Senior Fellow in Perinatal Health, Nuffield Department of Women's & Reproductive Health, University of Oxford, Level 3, Women's Centre, John Radcliffe Hospital, Oxford, UK
10: Fetal growth

Pak Chung Ho Emeritus Professor and Honorary Consultant, Obstetrics & Gynaecology, The University of Hong Kong, Hong Kong, People's Republic of China
54: Termination of pregnancy

Andrew W. Horne Professor of Gynaecology and Reproductive Sciences, MRC Centre for Reproductive Health, University of Edinburgh, Edinburgh, UK
39: Ectopic pregnancy

Zhongwei Huang Deputy Director, Undergraduate Medication Education for Obstetrics and Gynaecology, Associate Consultant, Department of Obstetrics and Gynaecology, National University Singapore, National University Health Systems, Singapore
42: Polycystic ovary syndrome

Thomas Ind Gynaecological Surgeon, Royal Marsden and St George's Hospital, London, UK
3: Clinical anatomy of the pelvis and the reproductive organs

Adonis Ioannides Professor of Clinical Genetics, University of Nicosia Medical School, Nicosia, Cyprus
4: Genetics for the obstetrician and gynaecologist

Jay Iyer Consultant and Senior Lecturer, Advanced Laparoscopic and Pelvic Floor Surgeon, Director AGES Advanced Laparoscopic Fellowship Program, Obstetrics and Gynaecology, The Townsville and Mater Hospitals, Townsville, Queensland, Australia
57: Urinary incontinence

Eric Jauniaux UCL EGA Institute for Women's Health, University College London, London, UK
9: The placenta

Anuja Jhingran Professor, Anderson Cancer Center, Houston, TX, USA
68: Radiation therapy in the management of gynaecological cancer

Ian Jones Professor of Psychiatry, Division of Psychological Medicine and Clinical Neurosciences, Cardiff University, Cardiff, UK
18: Psychiatric disorders in pregnancy and the postpartum

Devendra Kanagalingam Senior Consultant Obstetrician & Gynaecologist, Singapore General Hospital, Singapore
26: The management of labour

Mahantesh Karoshi Consultant Obstetrician & Gynaecologist, Royal Free London Hospital NHS Foundation Trust, London, UK
6: Preconceptional medicine

Shelley M. Kibel Medical Director, St Luke's Hospice, Kenilworth, South Africa (until Jan 2017) Now in Private Palliative Care Practice, Cape Town, South Africa
69: Palliative care

Justin C. Konje Professor of Obstetrics and Gynaecology Weill Cornell Medical College, Qatar; Executive Chair, Department of Obstetrics and Gynaecology, Sidra Medical and Research Centre, Doha, Qatar
22: Antepartum haemorrhage

Stephen Lapinsky Professor of Medicine, Division of Respirology, University of Toronto, Toronto, Canada
25: Respiratory diseases in pregnancy

Jonathan A. Ledermann Professor of Medical Oncology, UCL Cancer Institute; Director of Cancer Research UK and UCL Cancer Trials Centre, London, UK
64: Ovarian, fallopian tube, and peritoneal cancer

William Ledger Professor of Obstetrics and Gynaecology, University of New South Wales, Director of Reproductive Medicine, Royal Hospital for Women, Sydney, Australia
52: Assisted reproduction

Tak Yeung Leung Professor, Department of Obstetrics & Gynaecology, The Chinese University of Hong Kong, Hong Kong
33: Obstetric procedures

Stephanie Lheureux Assistant Professor, University of Toronto; Clinician Investigator, Gynecology, Drug Development Program, Princess Margaret Cancer Centre, Toronto, Canada
67: Chemotherapy and biological, targeted, and immune therapies in gynaecological cancers

Hang Wun Raymond Li Associate Professor, Department of Obstetrics and Gynaecology, The University of Hong Kong, Hong Kong
54: Termination of pregnancy

Tin Chiu Li Department of Obstetrics and Gynaecology, Prince of Wales Hospital, The Chinese University of Hong Kong, Hong Kong
44: Chronic pelvic pain

Stephen Lindow Hon Associate Professor of Obstetrics and Gynaecology, University of Cape Town, Groote Schuur Hospital, Cape Town, South Africa
55: Violence against women and girls

Stephen D. Lyons Gynaecological Research and Clinical Evaluation (GRACE) Group, Royal Hospital for Women, Sydney; University of New South Wales, Sydney, Australia
47: Laparoscopy

Mayank Madhra Fellow in Laparoscopic Surgery, Simpson Centre For Reproductive Health, Royal Infirmary of Edinburgh, Edinburgh, UK
39: Ectopic pregnancy

Laura A. Magee Professor of Women's Health, Department of Women and Children's Health, King's College London, Greater London, UK
21: Hypertension

Tahir Mahmood Consultant Obstetrician & Gynaecologist, Victoria Hospital, Kirkcaldy; Clinical Senior Lecturer, School of Medicine, University of St Andrews, St Andrews, UK
7: Obesity in obstetric and gynaecological practice

Isaac Manyonda Professor and Consultant in Obstetrics and Gynaecology, St George's University of London; St George's University Hospitals NHS Foundation Trust, London, UK
49: Benign disease of the uterus

Mushi Matjila Associate Professor and Consultant, Department of Obstetrics & Gynaecology, University of Cape Town/Groote Schuur Hospital, Cape Town, South Africa
38: Miscarriage and recurrent miscarriage

Jacqueline A. Maybin MRC Centre for Reproductive Health, The University of Edinburgh, The Queen's Medical Research Institute, Edinburgh, UK
40: The menstrual cycle

Nomonde H. Mbatani Gynaecological Oncology Unit, Department of Obstetrics and Gynaecology, University of Cape Town; Groote Schuur Hospital, Cape Town, South Africa
63: Uterine cancer

Laurence B. McCullough Zucker School of Medicine at Hofstra/Northwell and Lenox Hill Hospital, New York, USA
2: Ethics in obstetrics and gynaecology

Neena Modi Professor of Neonatal Medicine, Faculty of Medicine, Imperial College London and Chelsea London, UK

Caitriona Monaghan Consultant Obstetrician and Gynaecologist, Subspecialist Maternal and Fetal Medicine, Royal Maternity Hospital, Belfast, Northern Ireland; Professor of Neonatal Medicine, Consultant Neonatologist, Imperial College London and Chelsea and Westminster NHS Foundation Trust, London, UK
37: Neonatal care and neonatal problems

Caitriona Monaghan Consultant Obstetrician, Subspecialist Maternal and Fetal Medicine, Fetal Medicine, Royal Maternity Hospital, Belfast, County Antrim, Northern Ireland
19: Fetal therapy

Deirdre J. Murphy Professor of Obstetrics and Head of Department, Trinity College, University of Dublin; Coombe Women & Infants University Hospital, Dublin, Ireland
32: Malpresentation, malposition, and cephalopelvic disproportion

Surabhi Nanda Consultant in Maternal Fetal Medicine, Honorary Senior Lecturer, Women's Services, Guy's and St Thomas' NHS Foundation Trust, King's College, London, UK
20: Multiple pregnancy

James P. Neilson Emeritus Professor of Obstetrics & Gynaecology, University of Liverpool, Liverpool, UK
20: Multiple pregnancy

Catherine Nelson-Piercy Professor of Obstetric Medicine, Women's Academic Health Centre, King's Health Partners, London, UK
25: Respiratory diseases in pregnancy

Hextan Y.S. Ngan Department of Obstetrics & Gynaecology, University of Hong Kong, Queen Mary Hospital, Hong Kong
66: Gestational trophoblastic disease

Siew-Fei Ngu Department of Obstetrics & Gynaecology, University of Hong Kong, Queen Mary Hospital, Hong Kong
66: Gestational trophoblastic disease

Andy Nordin Gynaecological Oncologist and Lead Clinician for Cancer, East Kent Hospitals University Foundation NHS Trust, Margate, UK
71: Premalignant disease of the genital tract in pregnancy

Karen Nugent Senior Lecturer, Surgery, University of Southampton, Southampton, Hampshire, UK
58: Faecal incontinence and anorectal dysfunction

David Nunns Consultant Gynaecological Oncologist, Department of Obstetrics and Gynaecology, Nottingham University Hospitals, Nottingham, UK
50: Benign disease of the vulva

Gbemisola Okunoye Assistant Professor of Obstetrics and Gynaecology and Senior Attending Physician, Weill Cornell Medical College, Qatar; Sidra Medical and Research Centre, Doha, Qatar
22: Antepartum haemorrhage

Maaike Oonk Gynaecological Oncologist, Department of Obstetrics and Gynaecology, University Medical Center Groningen, University of Groningen, Groningen, The Netherlands
65: Premalignant and malignant disease of the vulva and vagina

Amit M. Oza Professor, University of Toronto; Co-Director, Drug Development Program, Princess Margaret Cancer Centre, Toronto, Canada
67: Chemotherapy and biological, targeted, and immune therapies in gynaecological cancers

Aris T. Papageorghiou Professor in Fetal Medicine and Obstetrics, St George's University Hospitals NHS Foundation Trust, Blacskhaw Road, London and Nuffield Department of Women's & Reproductive Health, University of Oxford, Level 3, Women's Centre, John Radcliffe Hospital, Oxford, UK
10: Fetal growth

Michael Permezel Emeritus Professor of Obstetrics and Gynaecology, Mercy Hospital for Women, University of Melbourne, Heidelberg, Victoria, Australia
13: Diabetes in pregnancy

Julia P. Polk Consultant Obstetrician Gynaecologist, The Permanente Medical Group (Kaiser Permanente), Walnut Creek, California, USA
36: Induction of labour

Jaime Prat Emeritus Professor, Department of Pathology, Hospital de la Santa Creu i Sant Pau, Autonomous University of Barcelona, Barcelona, Spain
70: Pathology of tumours of the female genital tract

Walter Prendiville Professor/ Consultant Gynaecologist & Director of Screening, University of Pittsburgh Medical Centre (UPMC), Beacon Hospital, Dublin, Republic of Ireland
62: Premalignant and malignant disease of the cervix

Suneetha Rachaneni Consultant in Gynaecology and Subspecialist in Urogynaecology, Gynaecology, Shrewsbury and Telford Hospitals NHS Trust, Shropshire, West Midlands, UK
56: Pelvic organ prolapse

Ajay Rane Professor and Head, Obstetrics and Gynaecology, James Cook University, Townsville, Queensland, Australia
57: Urinary incontinence

Dominic G.D. Richards Gynaecological Oncology Unit, Department of Obstetrics and Gynaecology, University of Cape Town; Groote Schuur Hospital, Cape Town, South Africa
63: Uterine cancer

Stephen J. Robson President, Royal Australian and New Zealand College of Obstetricians and Gynaecologists; Professor of Obstetrics and Gynaecology, Australian National University Medical School, Canberra, Australia
35: Postpartum care and problems in the puerperium

Linda Rogers Department of Obstetrics and Gynaecology, University of Cape Town/ Groote Schuur Hospital, Cape Town; SAMRC Gynaecology Cancer Research Centre, University of Cape Town, Cape Town, South Africa
65: Premalignant and malignant disease of the vulva and vagina

Jonathan Ross Professor of Sexual Health and HIV, University Hospital Birmingham NHS Foundation Trust, Birmingham, UK
43: Pelvic inflammatory disease

Sukhwinder Sahota Specialist Registrar, Edinburgh Royal Infirmary, Edinburgh, UK
7: Obesity in obstetric and gynaecological practice

Rengaswamy Sankaranarayan Screening Group, International Agency for Research on Cancer, Lyon, France
61: Cancer screening and prevention in gynaecology

Jenifer Sassarini Consultant Obstetrician and Gynaecologist, Glasgow Royal Infirmary, Glasgow, Scotland, UK
46: Menopause

Hassan Shehata Consultant Obstetric Physician and Honorary Senior Lecturer, Women's Health, Epsom & St Helier University Hospitals NHS Trust & St George's Medical School, London, UK
15: Haematological disorders in pregnancy

Andrew H. Shennan Department of Women and Children's Health, School of Life Course Sciences, Faculty of Life Sciences & Medicine, Kings College, London, UK
8: Maternal physiology

Alexis Shub Department of Obstetrics and Gynecology, University of Melbourne, Melbourne, Australia
13: Diabetes in pregnancy

Rosalind Simpson Clinical Research Fellow, Centre of Evidence Based Dermatology, University of Nottingham, Nottingham, UK
50: Benign disease of the vulva

Karolina Skorupskaite MRC Centre for Reproductive Health, The University of Edinburgh, The Queen's Medical Research Institute, Edinburgh, UK
40: The menstrual cycle

Philip Steer Emeritus Professor, Division of Surgery and Cancer, Faculty of Medicine, Imperial College London; Academic Department of Obstetrics and Gynaecology, Chelsea and Westminster Hospital, London, UK
12: Cardiac disease in pregnancy

Petrus S. Steyn Honorary Associate Professor, Department of Obstetrics and Gynaecology, Faculty of Health Sciences, University of Cape Town/Groote Schuur Hospital, Cape Town, South Africa
53: Contraception

Vikram Sinai Talaulikar Associate Specialist, Reproductive Medicine Unit, University College London Hospital, London, UK
27: Fetal monitoring during labour;
38: Miscarriage and recurrent miscarriage

Basky Thilaganathan Consultant and Director, Fetal Medicine Unit, St George's University Hospitals NHS Foundation Trust; Molecular & Clinical Sciences Research Institute, St George's University of London, UK
19: Fetal therapy

Jim G. Thornton Professor of Obstetrics and Gynaecology, Division of Child Health, Obstetrics and Gynaecology, School of Medicine, University of Nottingham, Nottingham City Hospital, Nottingham University Hospitals NHS Trust, Nottingham, UK
31: Prolonged pregnancy

Austin Ugwumadu Consultant Obstetrician & Gynaecologist / Clinical Director of Women's Health, Obstetrics & Gynaecology, St George's University Hospitals, London, UK
17: General and specific infections in pregnancy including immunization

Zephne M. van der Spuy Emeritus Professor/ Senior Scholar, Department of Obstetrics and Gynaecology, Faculty of Health Sciences, University of Cape Town/Groote Schuur Hospital, Cape Town, South Africa
53: Contraception

Ate van der Zee Professor of Gynecological Oncology, Vice President Board of Directors University Medical Center Gronigen, University of Gronigen, Faculty of Medical Sciences, Antonius Deusinglaan, The Netherlands
65: Premalignant and malignant disease of the vulva and vagina

Arne Vanhie Leuven University Fertility Center, Department of Obstetrics and Gynaecology, University Hospital Leuven, Belgium; Lab of Experimental Gynaecology, G-PURE Research Group, Department of Development and Regeneration, Leuven University, Belgium
45: Endometriosis

Vimal Vasu Consultant in Neonatal Medicine, East Kent Hospitals University NHS Foundation Trust, UK
37: Neonatal care and neonatal problems

Peter von Dadelszen Professor of Global Women's Health, Department of Women and Children's Health, King's College London, Greater London, UK
21: Hypertension

Tim J. von Oertzen Neurologist and Head of Department, Department of Neurology 1, Neuromed Campus, Kepler Universitätsklinik, Linz, Austria
24: Neurological disorders in pregnancy

Nicola Vousden Department of Women and Children's Health, School of Life Course Sciences, Faculty of Life Sciences & Medicine, Kings College, London, UK
8: Maternal physiology

Judith N. Wagner Neurologist, Department of Neurology 1, Neuromed Campus, Kepler Universitätsklinik, Linz, Austria
24: Neurological disorders in pregnancy

Kate F. Walker Clinical Assistant Professor in Obstetrics and Gynaecology, Division of Child Health, Obstetrics and Gynaecology, School of Medicine, University of Nottingham, Queen's Medical Centre, Nottingham University Hospitals NHS Trust, Nottingham, UK
31: Prolonged pregnancy

Andrew Weeks Professor of International Maternal Health, Women's and Children's Health, University of Liverpool, Liverpool, Merseyside, UK
36: Induction of labour

Lucy H.R. Whitaker MRC Centre for Reproductive Health, The University of Edinburgh, The Queen's Medical Research Institute, Edinburgh, UK
40: The menstrual cycle

David Williams Obstetric Physician, UCL EGA Institute for Women's Health, University College London Hospital, London, UK
14: Renal disease in pregnancy

Catherine Williamson Professor of Women's Health, King's College London, London, UK
23: Liver and endocrine diseases in pregnancy

Cathy Winter Senior Research Midwife, Women and Children's Health, North Bristol NHS Trust & PROMPT Maternity Foundation, Bristol, UK
29: Obstetric emergencies

Tonye Wokoma Consultant Sexual and Reproductive Health, Community Gynaecology, Sexual and Reproductive Health, Conifer House, City Healthcare Partnership, Hull, UK
55: Violence against women and girls

Eu Leong Yong Professor, Senior Consultant, Department of Obstetrics and Gynaecology, National University Singapore, National University Health Systems, Singapore
42: Polycystic ovary syndrome

Peter J. O'Donovan Consultant Gynaecologist, Yorkshire Clinic, West Yorkshire, UK
48: Hysteroscopy

O.A. O'Donovan GP Trainee, Airedale General Hospital, West Yorkshire, UK
48: Hysteroscopy

SECTION 1
Basics in Obstetrics and Gynaecology

1

Basic sciences in obstetrics and gynaecology

Stergios Doumouchtsis

Structure and function of the genome

Chromosomes

The normal human genome is diploid and consists of 46 human chromosomes in 23 pairs. Chromosome abnormalities may be related to the number (aneuploidy) or structure of chromosomes. A karyotype describes the number of chromosomes and major structural abnormalities such as deletions, duplications, or translocations.

Meiosis is the cell division process in germline cells, resulting in the production of haploid gametes (ova and sperm). The process of meiosis generates four haploid cells, which can participate in fertilization. *Mitosis* is a process of the cell cycle in somatic cells resulting in the formation of two diploid daughter cells with identical genomes to that of the parental cell.

Genes and gene expression

A *gene* is a sequence of nucleotides in deoxyribonucleic acid (DNA) which codes for a protein. The sequence of nucleotides determines the amino acid sequence of the protein and its function. Each gene is represented twice (alleles) in the complement of genes known as the genome. Genes contain information that determines phenotype.

Genes are made up of exons and introns. Exons code for the protein and introns are spliced out during processing to messenger ribonucleic acid (mRNA). The length of the introns is far greater than that of the exons. The exact function of the introns is unclear. Although the exon sequence is highly conserved between individuals, the intron sequence is not.

Gene expression is the process by which information from a gene is used in the synthesis of a protein or another gene product such as transfer RNA (tRNA) or functional RNA. This process involves transcription of RNA from a DNA template and translation of mRNA into protein.

Although all cells in an organism have the same information in their DNA, only 3–5% of genes are active in a cell. Most of the genome is suppressed, a characteristic of gene expression.

Changes in gene regulation result in the expression of various gene products and the suppression of others. Methods for measuring RNA to evaluate gene expression include northern blot, ribonuclease protection assay, *in situ* hybridization, reverse-transcription quantitative polymerase chain reaction (PCR), and spotted complementary DNA arrays. Genome-wide methods for profiling gene expression include oligonucleotide arrays (microarrays) and transcriptome sequencing.

Epigenetics

Epigenetics is the study of heritable genome modifications in gene expression that are not due to alterations in DNA sequences. DNA methylation and histone modification (acetylation, methylation) are common epigenetic changes and can affect the process of transcription or silencing of gene expression.

Other epigenetic changes include modifications in non-coding RNAs and telomere length. Influences of environmental factors and epigenetic changes in the development of diseases such as cancer have been investigated in recent years. Such factors may include drugs, ultraviolet light, infection, and diet. Geographic differences in the incidence of autoimmune diseases have also been studied (1). Ageing and development of disease is another area of epigenetics involvement.

Molecular biology techniques

Molecular diagnostic tools in clinical genetics are applied for genotyping, detection of mutations, and assessment of chromosomal structural variants.

PCR technology is used to identify mutations. It requires prior knowledge of the DNA sequence of the fragment to be amplified. Real-time PCR allows the simultaneous detection and quantification of a DNA molecule and selection of mutant DNA. Deletion and insertion mutations can be identified using this technique.

PCR can detect organisms such as human immunodeficiency virus (HIV), methicillin-resistant *Staphylococcus aureus*, as well as chromosomal translocations associated with cancers.

Cytogenetic karyotype analysis by chromosomal banding, fluorescence *in situ* hybridization (FISH) on metaphase or interphase nuclei, or array comparative genomic hybridization (CGH) can identify structural variations. The resolution improves from karyotyping to interphase FISH and to array CGH. New sequence variants continue to be discovered with methods that allow analysis of entire genes or genomes.

Ovulation and ovarian function

Control of the hypothalamic–pituitary axis

The hypothalamus is part of the diencephalon. It is separated from the thalamus by the hypothalamic sulcus. Its external boundaries are rostrally the optic chiasm, laterally the optic tract, and posteriorly the mammillary bodies.

Its rostral boundary is a line through the optic chiasm, lamina terminalis, and anterior commissure and the caudal boundary extends from the posterior commissure to the caudal limit of the mammillary body. Dorsolaterally, the hypothalamus extends to the medial edge of the internal capsule (**Figure 1.1**) (2). The hypothalamus is associated with visceral, endocrine, autonomic, affective, and emotional behaviour.

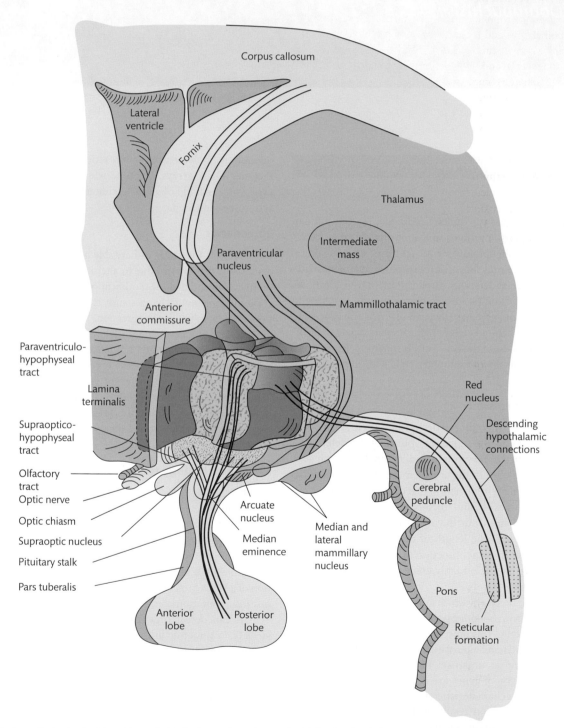

Figure 1.1 The hypothalamic nuclei and hypothalamic–hypophyseal tracts in relation to the thalamus, ventricular system, and brainstem.

Reproduced from Ignacio Bernabeu, Monica Marazuela, and Felipe F. Casanueva, General concepts of hypothalamus-pituitary anatomy, in: *Oxford Textbook of Endocrinology and Diabetes* 2e (eds: John Wass et al.), Oxford University Press, 2011, with permission from Oxford University Press.

The anterior pituitary is connected to the hypothalamus through a portal system. Hormones synthesized in the hypothalamus are transported to the nerve terminals on the hypophyseal portal capillaries. Hormones released into the hypophyseal portal system are transported to the anterior lobe of the pituitary. The posterior lobe of the pituitary consists of nerve terminals which lie in the supraoptic and paraventricular nuclei of the hypothalamus. Oxytocin and vasopressin are synthesized by the posterior pituitary.

Actions of pituitary and ovarian hormones

Gonadotropin-releasing hormone (GnRH) is synthesized in the preoptic area of the hypothalamus and is transported via portal vessels to the anterior pituitary where it stimulates the gonadotrophs to release luteinizing hormone (LH) and follicle-stimulating hormone (FSH). These glycoproteins share a common alpha-subunit and a specific beta-subunit. They control the steroid synthesis of the testes and ovaries.

Oestrogen and progesterone are the major hormones secreted by the ovarian follicles and the corpus luteum (**Figure 1.2**).

Ovulation

A rise in FSH secretion stimulates the growth and differentiation of preantral and antral follicles, which in turn stimulates oestrogen secretion with a peak approximately 1 day before ovulation. Then, the mid-cycle surge occurs (3) and is associated with a change from negative feedback control of LH secretion by ovarian hormones to

a positive feedback, resulting in a tenfold rise in serum LH and a smaller increase in FSH concentrations. The LH surge leads to substantial changes in the ovary. The oocyte in the dominant follicle completes its first meiotic division. The oocyte is subsequently released from the follicle at the surface of the ovary (4).

Before the release of the oocyte, the surrounding granulosa cells luteinize and produce progesterone. As a result, LH pulses become less frequent by the end of the surge (**Figure 1.3**).

The increasing serum progesterone concentrations have an effect on the endometrium, leading to cessation of mitoses and 'organization' of the glands.

Endometrial cycle

The average duration of the adult menstrual cycle is 28–35 days. The first day of menses represents the first day of the cycle. The cycle is then divided into two phases: follicular and luteal. The follicular

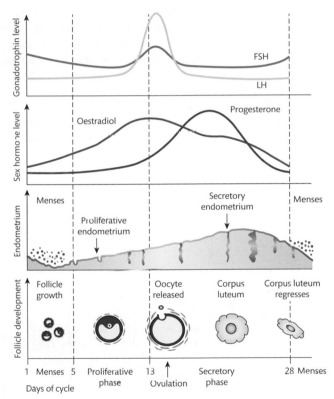

Figure 1.3 The hormonal and endometrial axis of the human menstrual cycle. After menstruation, rising levels of oestrogen exert a negative feedback, reducing follicle-stimulating hormone (FSH) release. Towards mid cycle, still higher levels of oestrogen then exert a positive feedback, causing a sudden peak release of luteinizing hormone (LH), which induces ovulation. An increased level in FSH also occurs. The endometrium during this phase has a thin surface epithelium and the glands are straight, short, and narrow (proliferative/follicular). In the luteal phase, LH levels maintain the corpus luteum, the source of progesterone. The endometrial glands become more tortuous during this phase (secretory/luteal) with secretion in the lumen and increasing fluid separating the stromal cells. If an embryo fails to implant, the corpus luteum deteriorates after about 7 days, with a resulting fall in progesterone and oestrogen concentrations.

Reproduced from S. Arulkumaran, Menstrual disorders, in: *Training in Obstetrics and Gynaecology* (eds. Ippokratis Sarris, Susan Bewley and Sangeeta Agnihotri), Oxford University Press, 2009, with permission from Oxford University Press.

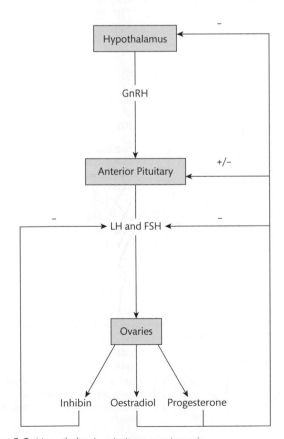

Figure 1.2 Hypothalamic–pituitary–ovarian axis.

Reproduced from S. Arulkumaran, Menstrual disorders, in: *Training in Obstetrics and Gynaecology* (eds. Ippokratis Sarris, Susan Bewley and Sangeeta Agnihotri), Oxford University Press, 2009, with permission from Oxford University Press.

phase begins with the onset of menses and ends on the day before the LH surge. The luteal phase begins on the day of the LH surge and ends at the onset of the next menses. The follicular phase lasts approximately 14–21 days and the luteal phase 14 days. Changes in the intermenstrual interval are primarily due to changes in the follicular phase. The luteal phase remains relatively stable. There is significantly more cycle variability during the first years after menarche and the 10 years before menopause. Menstrual cycle length peaks at the age of 25–30 years and then gradually declines. Between the ages of 20 and 40 years, there is relatively little cycle variability. Women in their 40s may have slightly shorter cycles (5).

During the menstrual cycle, endometrial changes include a proliferative phase and a secretory phase. The proliferative phase is characterized by an increased rate of mitotic division of endometrial glandular cells under the influence of oestradiol, leading to proliferation. The secretory phase is characterized by secretory activity following further proliferation under the influence of oestradiol and progesterone.

Luteinization of corpus luteum occurs 14 days after ovulation in the absence of conception. A rise in FSH is induced by the loss of negative feedback from oestradiol and progesterone, resulting in the start of another cycle. If, however, conception occurs, luteinization does not occur and the corpus luteum is maintained by human chorionic gonadotropin.

Puberty and menopause

Puberty is a process of physical and hormonal changes resulting in sexual maturity and capability of sexual reproduction. The two main physiological events include *gonadarche*, which is the activation of gonadal sex steroid production by the pituitary hormones FSH and LH, and *adrenarche*, which involves the increase in production of androgens by the adrenal cortex.

Thelarche is the appearance of breast tissue. *Menarche* is the onset of menstrual cycles. This is caused by the action of oestradiol on the endometrium and usually is not associated with ovulation. *Spermarche* is the onset of sperm production. *Pubarche* is the appearance of pubic hair, primarily due to the effects of androgens from the adrenal gland. The term also refers to the appearance of axillary hair (**Figure 1.4**).

In puberty, the increased frequency and amplitude of GnRH pulses stimulates secretion of FSH and LH and activates gonadal steroidogenesis.

Leptin is secreted by adipose tissues and along with kisspeptin plays a role in the onset of puberty. *Menopause* is defined as the permanent cessation of menstruation. It is an oestrogen- and progesterone-deficient state with an increase in the secretion of FSH and LH. The cessation of menstrual periods occurs as the ovary no longer contains follicles which are responsive to FSH. It is diagnosed retrospectively after 12 months of amenorrhea without any other cause (**Figure 1.5**).

Lack of oestrogen causes vasomotor symptoms including hot flushes and night sweats as well as mood swings and depression. Long-term effects include lower genital tract atrophy, osteoporosis, changes in lipid metabolism, and an increased risk of cardiovascular disease (6). Menopause usually occurs between 45 and 55 years of

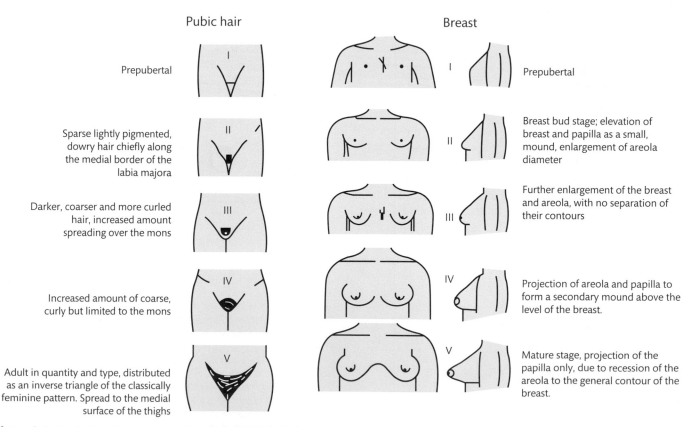

Figure 1.4 Marshall and Tanner stages of breast and pubic hair development.

Reproduced from McVeigh E, Homburg R, and Guillebaud J. *Oxford Handbook of Reproductive Medicine and Family Planning*, Oxford University Press, 2008, with permission from Oxford University Press.

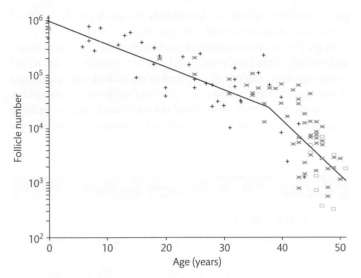

Figure 1.5 Decline in primordial follicle number with age.
Reproduced from Faddy MJ, Gosden RG. A mathematical model of follicle dynamics in the human ovary. *Hum Reprod.* 1995; 10: 770–5 with permission from Oxford University Press.

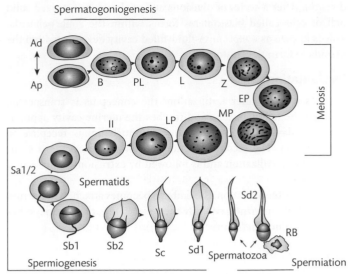

Figure 1.6 Schematic representation of the germ cell types and their development path during human spermatogenic process. Ad, A dark-spermatogonium; Ap, A pale-spermatogonium; B, B-spermatogonium; EP (early), MP (mid), and LP (late), pachytene spermatocyte; II, secondary spermatocyte; L, leptotene spermatocytes; M, mitochondria; PL, preleptotene spermatocytes; RB, residual body; Sa–Sd2, steps of spermatid differentiation (Sd2 spermatids are the mature testicular sperm). The developmental process from spermatogonium to formation of testicular sperm is considered to require at least 64 days (33–35).
Reproduced from C. Marc Luetjens and Gerhard F. Weinbauer, The male gamete: spermatogenesis, maturation, function, in: *Oxford Textbook of Endocrinology and Diabetes* 2e (eds: John Wass et al.), Oxford University Press, 2011, with permission from Oxford University Press.

age. In the United Kingdom, the average age of menopause is 51. Menopause before the age of 40 years is considered abnormal and is referred to as primary ovarian insufficiency (premature ovarian failure).

The transition to menopause, or perimenopause, is characterized by irregular menstrual cycles (7) and hormonal fluctuations, and a variable frequency and severity of symptoms such as hot flashes, sleep disturbances (8), mood changes, and vaginal dryness. It begins on average 4 years before the final menstrual period (9).

Fertilization and implantation

Gametogenesis

The full maturation of spermatozoa takes approximately 64–70 days. FSH causes stimulation of spermatogenesis and LH is responsible for stimulation of Leydig cells and testosterone production.

A large number of spermatogonia are produced by mitosis after puberty and are converted to spermatocytes in the testis. Following the first meiotic division, spermatozoa are released into the seminiferous tubules and then into the vas deferens. The second meiotic division is then completed (**Figure 1.6**).

Follicular development is characterized by enlargement of the ovum with aggregation of stromal cells to form the thecal cells. When a dominant follicle is selected, the innermost layers of granulosa cells become adherent to the ovum and form the *corona radiata*. A layer of gelatinous material around the ovum forms the *zona pellucida*. The follicle enlarges and bulges through the surface of the ovary and is released at the time of ovulation. The granulosa and the theca internal cells undergo luteinization. Formation of the *corpus luteum* occurs approximately 7 days after ovulation. Unless implantation occurs, it subsequently regresses.

Sperm transport

Once sperms arrive near the cervical os, sperm migration into the cervical mucous occurs with a rate normally of 6 mm/min. Motile

spermatozoa reach the uterine cavity and subsequently the fimbrial end of the fallopian tube.

Capacitation and fertilization

Capacitation is the functional maturation of the spermatozoon. It takes place once sperm passes through the epididymis and seminal vesicles. This process continues in the uterus or fallopian tube. Capacitation allows penetration of the zona pellucida by the sperm. Enzymes such as beta-amylase or beta-glucuronidase may act on the membranes of spermatozoa and facilitate sperm penetration. The capacitation process also involves modifications of membrane lipids, loss of cholesterol from plasma membrane, activation of the cyclic adenosine monophosphate/protein kinase A (cAMP/PKA) pathway, increases in calcium (Ca^{2+}) uptake and pH, hyperpolarization of membrane potential, and tyrosine phosphorylation (10).

The process of *fertilization* involves the union of the ovum and spermatozoon. When a spermatozoon reaches the cumulus around the ovum, the acrosome reaction is initiated. The outer acrosomal membrane fuses with the plasma membrane surrounding the spermatozoon and lytic enzymes are released. This facilitates the penetration of the oocyte membrane. The sperm head fuses with the oocyte plasma membrane and by phagocytosis the sperm head and mid piece are engulfed into the oocyte. The tail piece is left outside the cell membrane of the oocyte.

The sperm head forms the male pronucleus and with the female pronucleus they form the zygote. After disintegration of the membranes of the pronuclei, fusion of the male and female chromosomes occurs. This is called *syngamy* and is followed by the first cleavage division. After a series of divisions and at the 16-cell stage, a solid ball of cells called blastomeres forms within the zona pellucida. This is known as a *morula*. A fluid-filled cavity develops within the morula to form the blastocyst.

Implantation

Thirty-six hours after fertilization, the conceptus is transported through the fallopian tube and reaches the uterine cavity approximately 4 days later. The secretory endometrium is receptive to implantation. The second mitotic division of the oocyte is completed after fertilization and is followed by extrusion of the second polar body.

Six days after ovulation, the embryo becomes attached to the mid portion of the uterine cavity. By the seventh day, the blastocyst lies deep in the endometrium.

Physiology of coitus

The sexual response cycle described by Masters and Johnson has four phases in males and females. These phases are excitation, plateau, orgasmic, and resolution (**Figure 1.7**) (11, 12).

In the male, the excitation phase is associated with increased blood flow to the genitals and compression of venous channels of the penis resulting in erection. In the plateau phase, the penis remains in erection and the testes increase in size. Secretion of clear fluid may appear at the urethral meatus. In the orgasmic phase, reflex contractions of the bulbospongiosus (formerly bulbocavernosus) and ischiocavernosus muscles are followed by ejaculation of semen in spurts. During the resolution phase,

penile erection subsides. During this phase, the male becomes refractory to further stimulation.

In the female, the excitation phase involves erection of the clitoris and swelling of the labia minora and vagina, vaginal lubrication, and nipple erection. The orgasmic phase is associated with narrowing of the vaginal introitus and contractions of the pelvic floor muscles. The plateau phase may be sustained in females and result in multiple orgasms. Following orgasm, congestion of the pelvic organs resolves rapidly.

Embryology

Early embryo development

Cells differentiate into an outer layer, the *trophoblast*, and an *inner cell mass*, which will give rise to the *embryo proper*, the *amnion, yolk sac*, and *allantois*. Only two layers of cells intervene between the amniotic sac and yolk sac (**Figure 1.8**).

The layers of cells adjacent to the amniotic sac form the embryonic *ectoderm*. Ectodermal tissues of the fetus develop from these cells including skin, its appendages, neural tube, and its derivatives (brain, spinal cord, autonomic ganglia, and adrenal medulla). Cells adjacent to the yolk sac form the embryonic *endoderm*. Endodermal tissues include lining of the gut, epithelial cells of thyroid, parathyroid, trachea, lungs, liver, and pancreas. Between ectoderm and endoderm, a third layer of cells develops mainly from ectodermal proliferation. This middle layer forms the *mesoderm*. Mesodermal tissues are bones, muscles, cartilage, and subcutaneous tissues of the skin.

Organogenesis

Ectoderm, mesoderm, and endoderm initially take the form of a circular sandwich. Disproportionate growth of ectoderm results in elongation of the embryonic plate into an oval form. Each end of this plate curves, forming the head and tail folds. The amniotic sac enlarges and completely surrounds the developing embryo and the yolk sac. On the dorsal aspect of the ectoderm, a groove appears from the middle of the head to the tail and changes into the neural tube from which the nervous system develops.

Mesoderm starts to grow laterally and gives rise to the paraxial mesoderm, the intermediate cell mass, and the lateral plate mesoderm (**Figure 1.9**).

Endoderm grows first laterally and then ventrally to form the gut.

The lateral plate of the mesoderm divides into somatopleure, which remains adjacent to ectoderm, and the splanchnopleure, which grows around the developing gut. The space between the somatopleure and splanchnopleure form the coelomic cavity. This later becomes the pleural and peritoneal cavities.

The paraxial mesoderm develops into vertebrae, dura matter, and muscles of the body wall. The intermediate cell mass grows ventrally into the coelomic cavity and forms the urogenital system. See **Figure 1.10**.

Development of the genital organs

Genital and urinary systems arise from the intermediate mesoderm. The pronephros appears first and quickly disintegrates. At the caudal end of pronephros, the mesonephric duct (Wolffian duct) develops

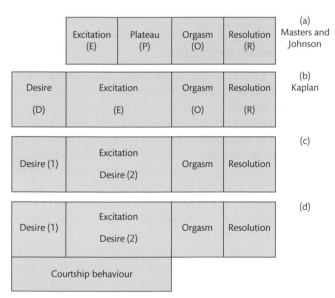

Figure 1.7 The development of the human sexual response model from (a) the original excitation, plateau, orgasmic, and resolution model of Masters and Johnson (11) through (b) the desire, excitation, orgasmic, and resolution model of Kaplan (12) to (c) the proposed modification with desire phase 1 (before initiation of the excitation phase and desire phase 2 during excitation phase) and finally (d) with added courtship behaviour.

Reproduced from Roy J. Levin, Normal sexual function, in: *New Oxford Textbook of Psychiatry* (eds. Michael Gelder, Nancy Andreasen, Juan Lopez-Ibor, and John Geddes), Oxford University Press 2012, with permission of Oxford University Press.

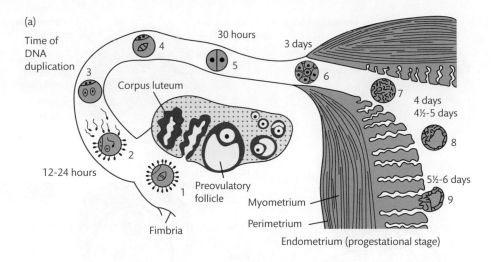

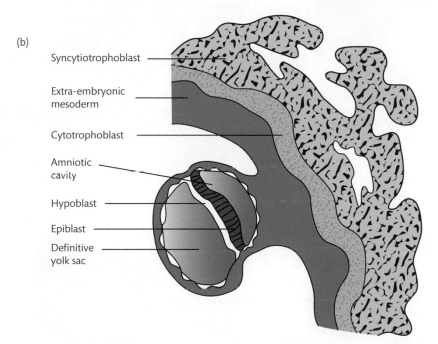

Figure 1.8 (a) Events of the first 6 days of development of a human embryo. 1: oocyte immediately after ovulation; 2: fertilization 12–24 h later results in the zygote; 3: zygote contains male and female pronuclei; 4: first mitotic division; 5: two-cell stage; 6: 3-day morula made up of up to 16 blastomeres; 7: morula stage (16–32 blastomeres) reaches the uterine lining; 8: early blastocyst; 9: implantation occurs at around day 6. (b) The site of implantation at the end of the second week.

Reproduced from Robert Wilkins, Simon Cross, Ian Megson, and David Meredith, Reproduction and development, *Oxford Handbook of Medical Sciences*, 2011, with permission from Oxford University Press.

and passes down the body to reach the cloaca. The mesonephros develops as a bulge in the dorsal wall of the coelom in the thoracic and lumbar regions. Two important structures appear on the coelomic surface of the mesonephros: (a) the genital ridge from which the gonad will form and (b) the paramesonephric (Mullerian) duct. The paramesonephric duct appears as a groove on the lateral aspect of the coelom and then becomes a tube. See **Figures 1.11–1.14**.

Placental development

Following implantation, the trophoblast completely surrounds the embryo in the form of proliferating cytotrophoblast and a syncytial layer. During the first trimester, a subset of trophoblast cells, the extravillous trophoblast (EVT) cells, become invasive and grow through the outer syncytium into the decidua where they invade maternal spiral arterioles. The trophoblast shell begins to break open, allowing maternal blood to enter the primitive intervillous space where it is utilized by the developing villous placenta and fetus. See **Figure 1.15**.

Development of membranes and amniotic fluid

The embryonic disc lies between the amniotic cavity and the primary yolk sac. The amniotic cavity develops between the embryonic ectoderm and cytotrophoblast. By the 12th postovulatory day, the base of this cavity is formed by embryonic ectoderm and the walls and roof are formed by the cytotrophoblast. Amniotic fluid is initially formed from the primitive cells around the amniotic vesicle.

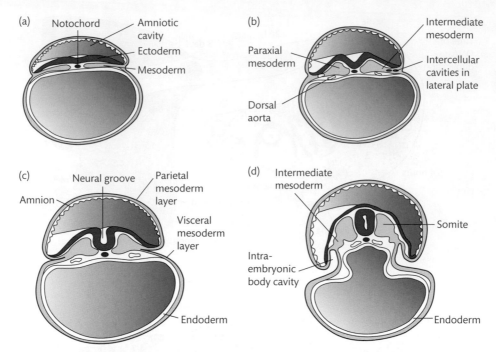

Figure 1.9 Transverse sections showing development of the mesodermal germ layer at days 17 (a), 19 (b), 20 (c), and 21 (d). The thin mesodermal sheet gives rise to paraxial mesoderm (future somites), intermediate mesoderm (future excretory units), and lateral plate, which is split into parietal and visceral mesoderm layers lining the intraembryonic cavity.

Reproduced from Robert Wilkins, Simon Cross, Ian Megson, and David Meredith, Reproduction and development, *Oxford Handbook of Medical Sciences*, 2011, with permission from Oxford University Press.

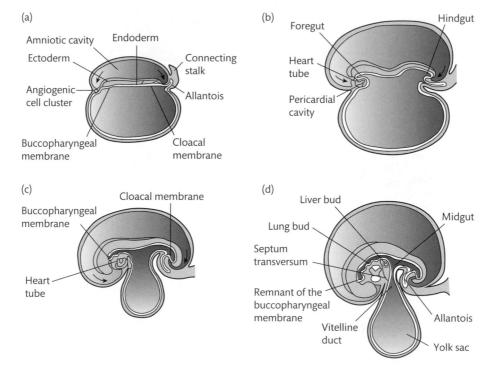

Figure 1.10 Sagittal midline sections of embryos at various stages of development demonstrating cephalocaudal folding and its effect on position of the endoderm-lined cavity. Presomite embryo (a), seven-somite embryo (b), 14-somite embryo (c), and 1-month embryo (d). Note the position of the angiogenic cell clusters in relation to the buccopharyngeal membrane.

Reproduced from Robert Wilkins, Simon Cross, Ian Megson, and David Meredith, Reproduction and development, *Oxford Handbook of Medical Sciences*, 2011, with permission from Oxford University Press.

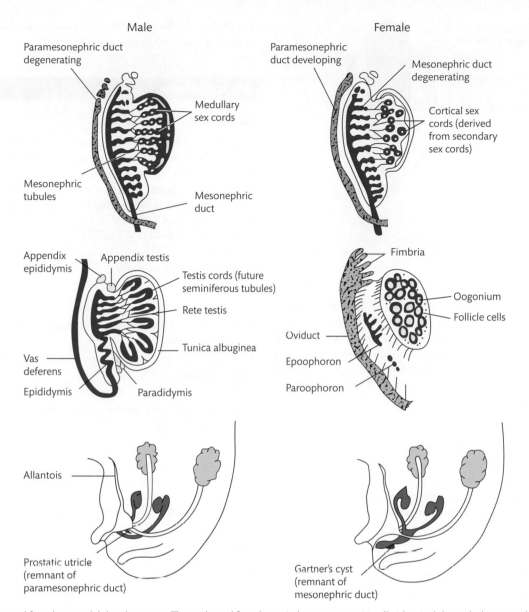

Figure 1.11 Male and female gonadal development. The male and female genital systems are virtually identical through the seventh week. In the male, SRY protein produced by the pre-Sertoli cells causes the medullary sex cords to develop into presumptive seminiferous tubules and rete testis tubules and causes the cortical sex cords to regress. Anti-Müllerian hormone produced by the Sertoli cells then causes the paramesonephric ducts to regress and Leydig cells also develop, which in turn produce testosterone, the hormone that stimulates development of the male genital duct system, including the vas deferens and the presumptive efferent ductules.

Reproduced from Robert Wilkins, Simon Cross, Ian Megson, and David Meredith, Reproduction and development, *Oxford Handbook of Medical Sciences*, 2011, with permission from Oxford University Press.

Later on, fetal extracellular fluid (ECF) is passed through the fetal skin and umbilical cord.

Pathology

Response to tissue injury

Tissue injury is associated with reversible and irreversible changes of the cell membrane. Potassium is transferred out of the cell and sodium is transferred in accompanied by water. This leads to cellular oedema and a reduction in protein synthesis. There is a switch to anaerobic metabolism. Glycogen is used for energy resulting in lactate production and a drop in pH.

Intracellular enzymes including lactate dehydrogenase, troponins, and creatinine phosphokinase become activated in association with mitochondrial damage. Lysosomal rupture results in release of lysosomal enzymes and autolysis followed by nuclear death.

Tissue growth and differentiation

Growth and differentiation aim to maintain the normal structure of a particular tissue. In tissues with continuous cell loss (blood, skin, mucosa), lost cells are continuously replaced. Stem cells frequently differentiate into a mature form during this process. In the skin, as superficial keratinized cells are shed, basal cells proliferate to replace them. The newly produced basal cells differentiate into squamous cells. When the cell turnover rate is normal,

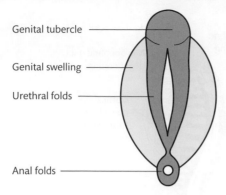

Figure 1.12 Indifferent stages of the external genitalia, approximately 6 weeks.

Reproduced from Robert Wilkins, Simon Cross, Ian Megson, and David Meredith, Reproduction and development, *Oxford Handbook of Medical Sciences*, 2011, with permission from Oxford University Press.

the skin appears histologically normal but if the rate is greatly increased, cells do not fully mature, and abnormalities are seen both on physical examination and histologically. The rate of cell proliferation is determined by the cell cycle and controlled by a variety of growth factors and receptors, and regulated by growth control genes. Many of the cellular proto-oncogenes encode for growth factors for receptors.

Placental pathology

The placental involvement in the pathogenesis of pre-eclampsia and particularly the link between pre-eclampsia and reduced placental perfusion has long been recognized (13).

The main defect seems to be related to endovascular trophoblast invasion. In pre-eclampsia, myometrial arteries fail to adapt to physiological change. Trophoblast invasion is impaired. Acute atherosis is common. Blood flow into the intervillous space is therefore decreased in pre-eclampsia.

Fetal growth restriction is associated with reduced uteroplacental blood flow, which in turn can be secondary to defective placentation.

Morphological abnormalities of the uterine arteries can be present in cases of fetal growth restriction.

Microbiology

Bacteriology

Bacteria are single-cell prokaryotic microorganisms. They have a single chromosome that is not enclosed in a nuclear membrane. They can have four shapes: cocci (spheres), bacilli (rods), spirilla (spirals), and vibrios (comma-shaped). Genetic information is encoded in the cell DNA. There are two types: chromosomal DNA and extrachromosomal DNA.

Bacterial metabolism is a balance between anabolic and catabolic functions. Their ability to utilize carbohydrates and convert them to glucose as well as oxygen requirement is used to characterize bacteria:

- Obligate anaerobes: oxygen is toxic.
- Aerotolerant anaerobes: anaerobic metabolism, but tolerant to the presence of oxygen.
- Facultative anaerobes: can grow in both anaerobic as well as aerobic conditions.
- Obligate aerobes: require oxygen to grow.
- Microaerophilic organisms: require low oxygen levels only; high levels may be inhibitory.

Bacteria can be Gram positive or Gram negative (**Figure 1.16**). Some bacteria can suspend growth and metabolism in adverse conditions and form resistant spores. Optimum temperature range is between 20°C and 40°C.

Bacteria have four phases of growth:

1. Initial lag phase
2. Exponential growth phase
3. Static phase
4. Death phase.

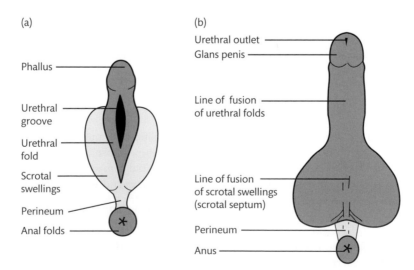

Figure 1.13 Development of the external genitalia in the male at (a) 10 weeks and (b) in the newborn. Genital tubercle extends rapidly to form the phallus, later the penis. Urethral folds close the urogenital sinus and genital swellings become scrotal swellings.

Reproduced from Robert Wilkins, Simon Cross, Ian Megson, and David Meredith, Reproduction and development, *Oxford Handbook of Medical Sciences*, 2011, with permission from Oxford University Press.

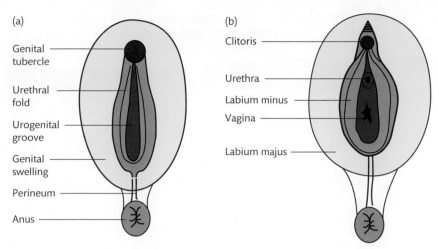

Figure 1.14 Development of the external genitalia in the female at (a) 5 months and (b) in the newborn. Genital tubercle elongates slightly, forming the clitoris. Urethral folds become labia minora and the urogenital sinus remains open. Genital swellings form the major labia.

Reproduced from Robert Wilkins, Simon Cross, Ian Megson, and David Meredith, Reproduction and development, *Oxford Handbook of Medical Sciences*, 2011, with permission from Oxford University Press.

Diagnosis of bacterial infection: bacteria are visible under direct microscopy. On a culture they are grown on solid agar or in liquid media and form visible colonies.

Control of infection

Antibiotics, also known as antibacterials, are used in the treatment and prevention of bacterial infections. They act by killing bacteria or inhibiting their growth. Different types of antibiotics have differences in chemical structure, mode of action, or spectrum of effect. Broad-spectrum antibiotics target a wide range of bacteria whereas narrow-spectrum ones target specific types. Antibiotics with bactericidal activities act on the bacterial cell wall (beta-lactam antibiotics: penicillins and cephalosporins as well as vancomycin and teicoplanin) or the cell membrane (polymyxins). Other bactericidal antibiotics target essential bacterial enzymes (rifamycins, lipiarmycin, quinolones, and sulphonamides). Bacteriostatic antibiotics inhibit protein synthesis (macrolides, lincosamides, and tetracyclines).

Sterilization is a process of eradication of microorganisms including the spores.

Disinfection is the removal of all actively dividing organisms. Components of disinfection include cleaning, heat, and chemicals.

Virology

A virus contains a nucleic acid (DNA or RNA) and is surrounded by a protein coat. There is no cytoplasm. Viruses must enter the host cell by endocytosis for their own replication. The virus first adheres to the host cell by binding to a specific receptor molecule.

A viral infection (**Table 1.1**) (14, p. 152) can cause cell death but can also cause a latent infection remaining in the host cell for many years in a dormant state.

Parasitology

Parasites are unicellular eukaryotic organisms. They can reproduce by simple asexual binary fission or a complex sexual cycle. The protozoa are larger than bacteria.

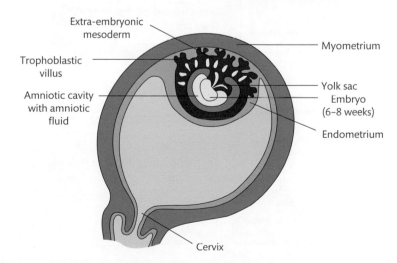

Figure 1.15 The placenta in relation to adjacent structures during early pregnancy.

Reproduced from Robert Wilkins, Simon Cross, Ian Megson, and David Meredith, Reproduction and development, *Oxford Handbook of Medical Sciences*, 2011, with permission from Oxford University Press.

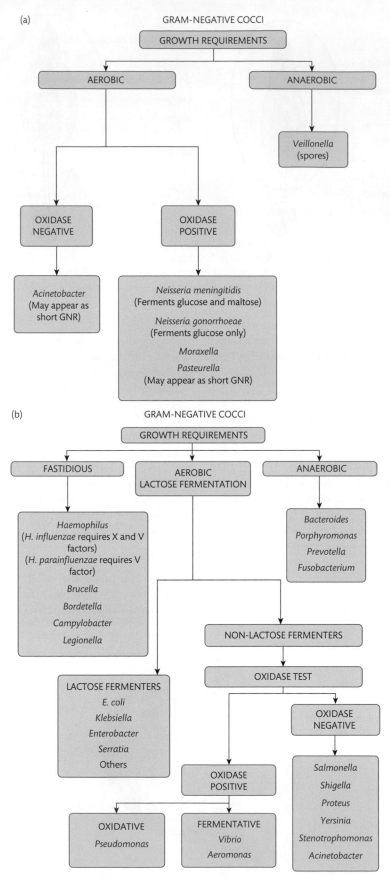

Figure 1.16 (a) Identification of Gram-negative cocci. (b) Identification of Gram-negative rods. (c) Identification of Gram-positive cocci. (d) Identification of Gram-positive rods. GNR, Gram-negative rods.

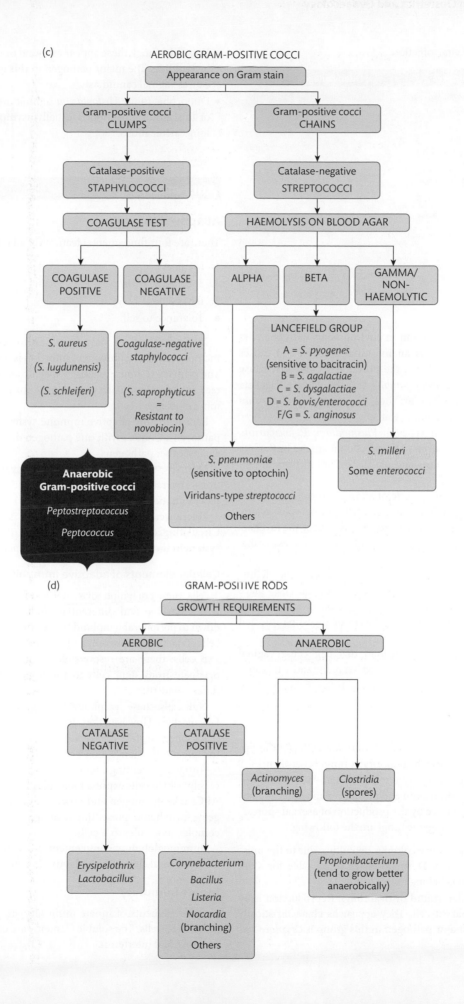

Table 1.1 Diagnosis of viral infection

Technique	Advantages	Disadvantages
Electron microscopy	Can see if any virus present	Expensive, time-consuming, requirement for complex equipment
Tissue culture	Virus cultures can be made available for further analysis	Slow, expensive
Enzyme immunoassay	Quick, automated, immunoglobulin M assays can diagnose recent infection	Not appropriate for all viruses
Fluorescence microscopy	Mainly for respiratory infections	Expensive
Polymerase chain reaction	Quick, highly sensitive, can be automated	Expensive DNA extraction can be difficult

Intestinal protozoa are common in environments with poor hygiene. *Entamoeba histolytica* is an intestinal amoeba and causes amoebic dysentery. It spreads via the portal veins and may cause amoebic liver abscess. *Giardia lamblia* is a binucleate flagellate protozoan. It causes chronic diarrhoea. *Cryptosporidium parvum* spreads via contaminated drinking water.

Malaria is caused by four types of *Plasmodium: P. falciparum, P. vivax, P. ovale,* and *P. malariae.* The infection is spread by the bite of female *Anopheles* mosquitos and usually occurs in tropical and subtropical areas.

Trypanosoma is spread by the bite of an infected tsetse fly and is prevalent in tropical Africa. It can enter red cells, the nervous system, and the reticuloendothelial system and can also affect the myocardium. Clinical symptoms and signs include fever, drowsiness, coma, and hepatosplenomegaly.

Toxoplasma gondii is the cause of toxoplasmosis. The definitive host of the trophozoites is the cat. Reproduction takes place in its gastrointestinal tract. Humans can become infected either by handling soil contaminated by cat faeces or ingesting infected undercooked meat.

Trichomonas vaginalis is a protozoan that can cause vaginal and urethral infections. It is transmitted sexually and can cause vulvovaginal irritation with a yellow or green, frothy, 'fishy'-smelling discharge.

Mycology

Fungi are eukaryotic organisms, commonly multicellular. The optimal growth temperature for the majority of fungi is between 25°C and 35°C. They are predominantly aerobic but many yeasts can produce alcohol by fermentation as an end product of anaerobic metabolism. They mainly reproduce by the production of asexual spores.

The main groups of pathogenic fungi are the following:

- Moulds: these form powdery colonies on culture due to the presence of abundant spores. Dermatophytes responsible for skin, hair, and nail infections belong to this group.
- True yeasts: unicellular, round or oval fungi. Reproduction is by budding from the parent cell. They appear as characteristically creamy colonies. A major pathogen in this group is *Cryptococcus neoformans.*

- Yeast-like fungi: these appear as round or oval cells and reproduce by budding. The major pathogen in this group is *Candida,* which causes vaginal candidiasis.
- Dimorphic fungi: *Histoplasma capsulatum* is a common member of this group. Infection is usually asymptomatic but may cause lung calcifications.

Immunology

Adaptive immunity

There are four fundamental features of adaptive immunity:

1. Memory
2. Specificity
3. Diversity
4. Tolerance to self.

Memory: the first contact with an infectious agent imparts the memory and then subsequent infection is repelled (i.e. chickenpox). The primary response against a specific antigen occurs on first contact, is slower, and is less vigorous. Future responses are rapid and more efficient.

Specificity: the adaptive immune system is specific to particular pathogens. Contact with one pathogen does not provide protection against other pathogens.

Diversity: this feature adds to the ability to combat different infections. Diversity is partly genetically encoded, but is also the result of recombination between gene segments (15) (**Figure 1.17**).

Tolerance: tolerance to self-antigens is established in early life. Circulating components, which reach the developing lymphoid system in the perinatal period, induce a permanent self-tolerance.

Cellular elements of adaptive immunity

T cells: these are lymphocytes derived from bone marrow stem cells which develop and differentiate in the thymus before travelling down to peripheral lymphoid tissue. There are three main types of T cells: T-helper, suppressor, and cytotoxic cells.

B cells: these are responsible for antibody production. B cells originate from stem cells in the bone marrow and develop and differentiate there.

Null cells: these lymphocytes express neither T- nor B-cell surface markers. However, they do express a mixture of lymphocyte and macrophage surface markers. They bind via the Fc receptor and kill the target cells. Hence, they are also called killer cells.

Antigen-presenting cells (APCs): antigen presentation is the process by which cells express molecules recognizable by T cells. These APCs take up antigen and process and modify it into an immunogenic form before presenting it along with major histocompatibility complex molecules to T cells.

Immunoglobulins, complement, and cytokines are the three principal humoral elements of adaptive immunity.

Innate immunity

Cellular elements of innate immunity are phagocytes and natural killer (NK) cells. The soluble elements are complement, acute phase proteins, and interferon.

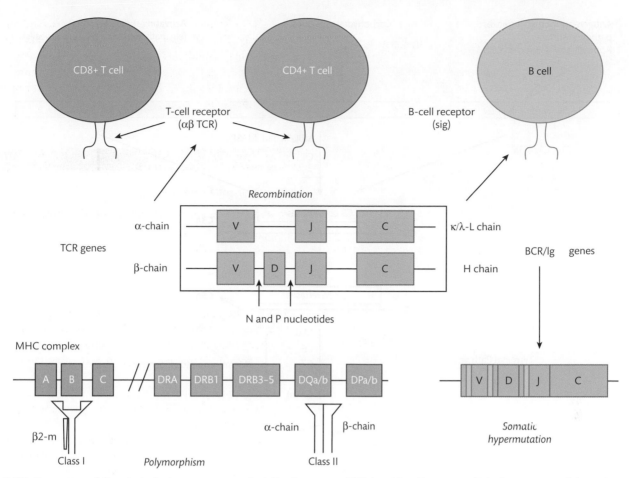

Figure 1.17 Generation of diversity in the immune system. Both T-cell receptors (TCRs) and B-cell receptors (BCRs) are generated through recombination. For immunoglobulin (Ig)-H chains there are 65, 27, and 8, variable (V), diversity (D), and joining (J) genes encoded in the germ line respectively. Somatic hypermutation occurs only in B cells. The major histocompatibility complex (MHC) complex is highly polymorphic—the class II genes actually lie upstream of the class I genes on chromosome 6. *DRA* encodes the α chain which is conserved and pairs with polymorphic β chains from the *DRB1* locus.

Reproduced from Paul Klenerman, Adaptive immunity, in: *Oxford Textbook of Medicine* 5e (eds. David Warrell, John Firth, Timothy Cox). Oxford University Press 2010, with permission from Oxford University Press.

Phagocytes are immune cells that phagocytose pathogens by engulfing, destroying, and processing before presenting to cells of the adaptive immunity. They are derived from bone marrow stem cells.

NK cells: these leucocytes destroy compromised host cells. They recognize cell surface changes on tumour cells or virus-infected cells. They engage and kill these cells.

Complement: this is an essential component of the innate immune system and consists of more than 30 interacting proteins and receptors. It can be activated by antigen–antibody interactions or by microorganisms. There are various mechanisms of function: some adhere to pathogens and promote phagocytosis, some attract phagocytes to the site of the reaction (chemotaxis), and some lyse the cell membranes of bacteria.

Pathways of complement activation include the classical pathway, the alternative pathway, the lectin pathway, and the terminal pathway (Figure 1.18).

Regulation of the immune system

Antigens taken up by APCs are presented to T-helper cells. The APCs release cytokines, which stimulate T cells and interleukin-2 receptor expression on the cells. T-helper cells help B cells to produce antibodies, which can neutralize the antigens. The antibodies can also promote the ingestion of antigens by macrophages. Cells infected by viruses can also be attacked by cytotoxic T cells, macrophages, or NK cells. The level of response is regulated by antibodies, suppressor T cells, APCs, and helper T cells. The primary purpose of such responses is to minimize damage caused by pathogens, eliminate pathogens, and establish future memory.

Pregnancy and immunity

The fetus contains antigens of both maternal and paternal origin and yet is not rejected by the mother. It is now clear that the fetus is antigenically mature from an early stage and that immunocompetence begins to develop in the first trimester of pregnancy. The uterus is not immunologically privileged. It has an extensive lymphatic and vascular network especially prominent during pregnancy.

There is ample evidence for a decrease in the maternal immune response in pregnancy. However, pregnant women are still sufficiently immunocompetent to remain healthy. This effect occurs from the time of implantation when the endometrium decidualizes. Only two types of fetoplacental tissue come into direct contact with maternal tissues: the villous trophoblast and EVT. There are

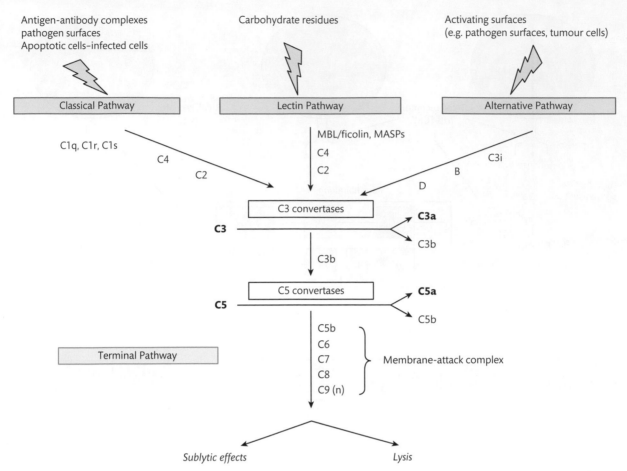

Figure 1.18 Simplified overview of the complement system showing the three main activation pathways and the terminal pathway culminating in the formation of C5b–9.

Reproduced from Marina Botto and Mark J. Walport, The complement system, in: *Oxford Textbook of Medicine* 5e (eds. David Warrell, John Firth, Timothy Cox). Oxford University Press 2010, with permission from Oxford University Press.

effectively no systemic maternal T- and B-cell responses to trophoblast cells in humans. The villous trophoblast, bathed by maternal blood, seems to be immunologically inert. It never expresses human leucocyte antigen (HLA) class I or class II molecules. EVT, which is directly in contact with maternal decidual tissues, does not express the major T-cell ligands, HLA-A or HLA-B, but does express the HLA class I trophoblast-specific HLA-G, which is strongly immunosuppressive.

A population of NK-derived, CD56 granulated lymphocytes is found in the first trimester. They release transforming growth factor beta-2, which also has immunosuppressive activity.

Biochemistry

Metabolism

Several sources of energy are metabolized to produce adenosine triphosphate (ATP), which is essential for protein synthesis and transport and maintenance of ionic ingredients across the plasma membrane.

Sugars, fatty acids, and amino acids are metabolized to produce acetyl coenzyme A (acetyl-CoA). The acetyl-CoA then enters the tricarboxylic acid (TCA) cycle, also known as the citric acid cycle or Krebs cycle. This cycle leads to products such as carbon dioxide and hydrogen in the form of nicotinamide adenine dinucleotide (NADH). The NADH feeds into the respiratory chain inside the mitochondrion and the energy of the NADH is used for oxidative phosphorylation to produce ATP.

Glycolysis: this pathway converts a molecule of glucose that contains six carbon atoms to two molecules of pyruvic acid, each containing three carbon atoms (**Figure 1.19**). There is a net production of two molecules of ATP. This pathway does not require oxygen and cells can survive for short periods by generating ATP via glycolysis.

Citric acid cycle: the enzymes involved in the cycle are mainly located inside the mitochondria. Pyruvate ions diffuse into the mitochondrion and become attached to CoA, which acts as a carrier. Nicotinamide adenine dinucleotide (NAD^+) plays a role in these reactions. During the citric acid, as a part of an enzymic reaction, a hydrogen ion is transferred to NAD^+ and a proton is released. NADH feeds into the respiratory chain and in the presence of oxygen provides energy for production of most of the ATP (**Figure 1.20**).

Respiratory chain: this electron transport chain resides in the mitochondria. A single molecule of NADH has sufficient energy to generate three ATP molecules from ADP. The chain consists of a series of electron carriers, which can accept and then donate

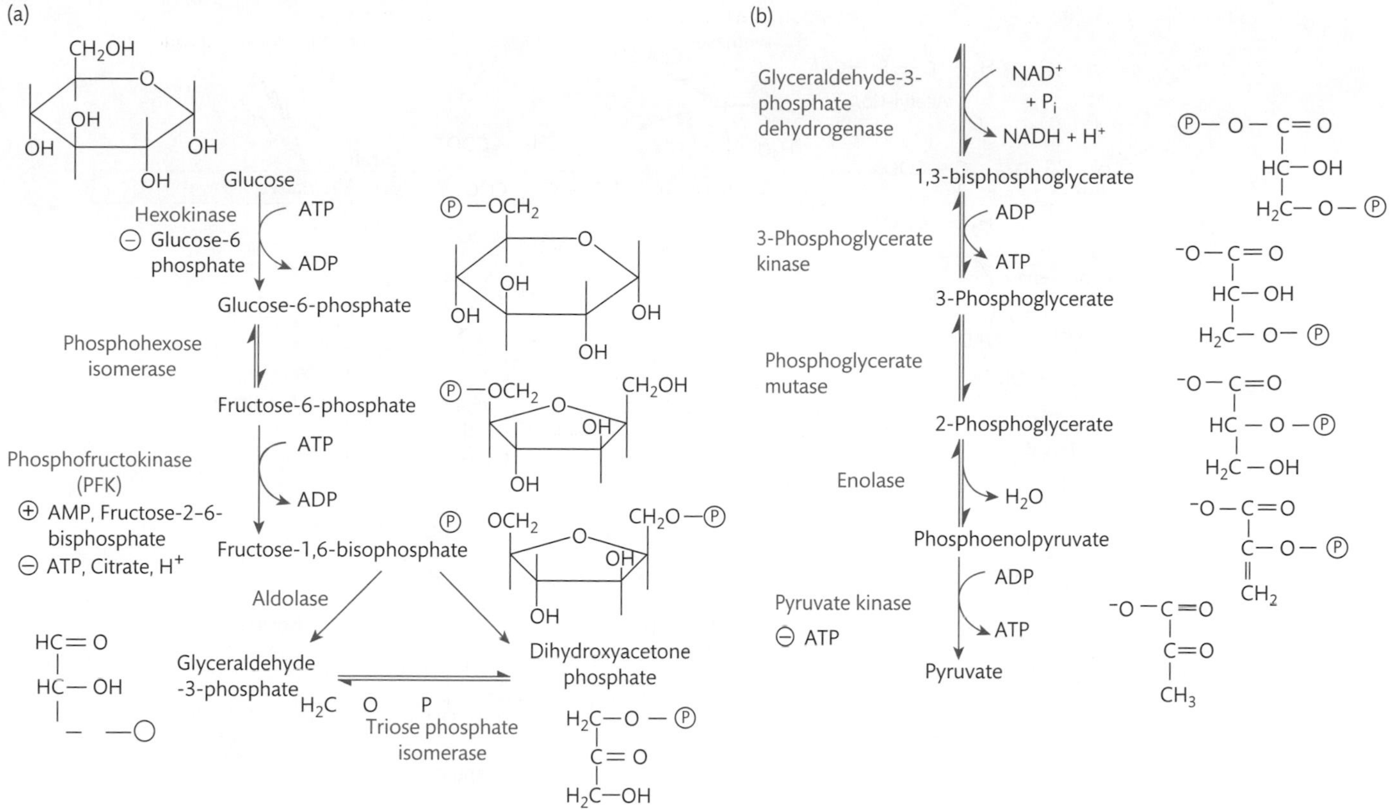

Figure 1.19 The glycolytic pathway. (a) The energy-investment phase. (b) The energy-generation phase, which only glyceraldehyde-3-phosphate can enter.

Reproduced from Neil Herring and Robert Wilkins, Biochemistry and metabolism, in: *Basic Science for Core Medical Training and the MRCP*, Oxford University Press (2015) with permission from Oxford University Press.

electrons. This results in the production of energy, which is used to stimulate the formation of ATP.

Fatty acid oxidation: this is a process whereby tissues produce energy by oxidation of fatty acids (**Figure 1.21**).

Triglycerides are stored in adipose tissue and in response to a variety of signals, a lipase enzyme becomes activated that cleaves fatty acids from glycerol. The free fatty acids are insoluble in water and are transported by albumin. Once a free fatty acid reaches the cell, it is subjected to pathway called beta-oxidation (**Figure 1.22**).

Catabolism

Haemoglobin: erythrocytes are degraded in spleen; the haemoglobin (Hb) is also catabolized. The globin chains of Hb are degraded to amino acids, which are reutilized. Haem is catabolized through various enzyme steps and finally converted to bilirubin. Bilirubin is then transferred to the liver where it is solubilized by the coupling of two glucuronic acid residues. The conjugated bilirubin is then excreted into the bile.

Urea cycle: this is an efficient detoxification process, which results in the excretion of more than 95% of the nitrogen via the urine in the form of urea. Most amino acid detoxification occurs in the liver. The first few reactions initiate in mitochondria and the latter part of the cycle takes place in the cytoplasm. Urea diffuses out of the liver into the circulation and gets filtered through the glomerulus of the kidney and passes into the urine (**Figure 1.23**).

Enzymes: these are proteins and mainly act as catalysts. The three-dimensional structure is crucial to their activity. A change of structure and loss of activity is called denaturation. Heating an enzyme usually results in complete loss of activity. Most enzymes are destroyed at 50–60°C. Organic solvents will also destroy their activity. Changes in pH affect the interactions between the amino acids and result in denaturation.

Cell signalling

Cells communicate by secreting chemicals that act at a distance by forming gap junctions, which join the cytoplasm of the cells, or by expression of plasma membrane-bound molecules, which can affect other cells. Endocrine cells secrete hormones, which can travel throughout the body or can have local effects (paracrine effects). Some secrete hormones, which bind back to the same cell's surface receptors (autocrine effects).

Nerve cells form specialized junctions known as synapses and secrete neurotransmitters.

Eicosanoids: these are signalling molecules that are made in the plasma membrane. They include prostaglandins, prostacyclins, thromboxanes, leukotrienes, and hydroxy-eicosanoic acids. They are all derived from arachidonic acid by the action of cyclooxygenase and lipoxygenase in the presence of oxygen (**Figure 1.24**).

Nitric oxide is also an important cellular signalling molecule involved in several physiological and pathological processes.

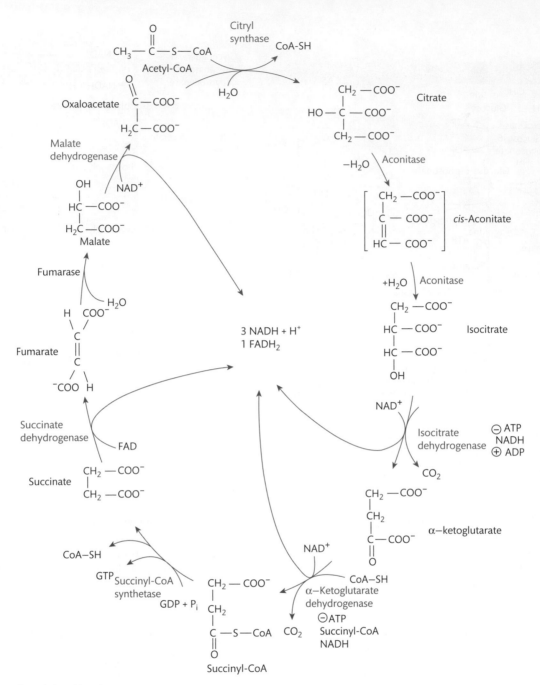

Figure 1.20 Complete citric acid cycle.

Reproduced from Neil Herring and Robert Wilkins, Biochemistry and metabolism, in: *Basic Science for Core Medical Training and the MRCP*, Oxford University Press (2015) with permission from Oxford University Press.

Calcium is an important intracellular messenger. Intracellular calcium is involved in the transmission of extracellular signals across the plasma membrane.

Physiology

Water and electrolyte balance

The total body water has two main compartments: the extracellular fluid (ECF) and the intracellular fluid, which are separated by the cell membrane (16–18) (**Figure 1.25**).

The cell membranes are freely permeable to water but not to electrolytes and maintain the different solute composition of the two compartments. Sodium (Na^+), chloride (Cl^-), potassium (K^+), phosphate (HPO_4^{2-}) calcium (Ca^{2+}), sulphate (SO_4^{2-}), magnesium (Mg^{2+}), and bicarbonate (HCO_3^-) ions are the main electrolytes in the human body. Interstitial fluid and blood plasma are similar in electrolyte composition, Na^+ and Cl^- being the major electrolytes. In the intracellular fluid, K^+ and HPO_4^- are the major electrolytes (**Table 1.2**) (19).

ECF volume: this constitutes approximately 33–40% of the body water. The ECF volume is regulated by urinary sodium excretion

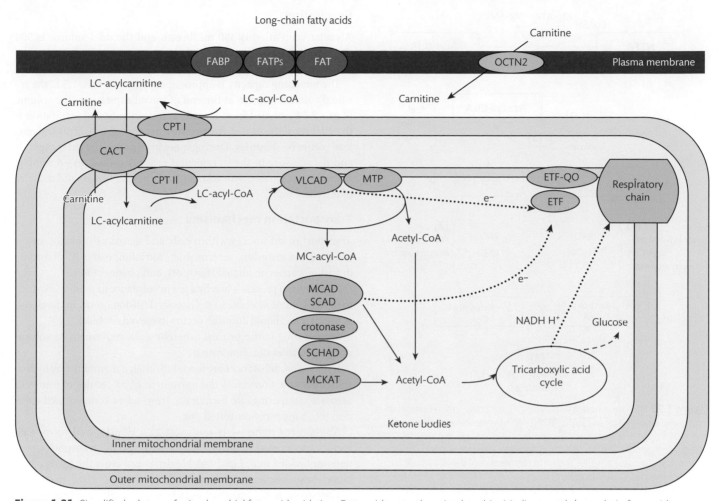

Figure 1.21 Simplified scheme of mitochondrial fatty acid oxidation. Fatty acids enter the mitochondria. Medium- and short-chain fatty acids enter independently of carnitine, but long-chain fatty acids need to be activated to coenzyme A and transferred to carnitine (CPT1) in order to cross the inner mitochondrial membrane (CACT). They are then transferred back to CoA esters in the mitochondrial matrix (CPT2). Beta-oxidation is catalysed by enzymes of different fatty acid chain length specificity (VLCAD, MTP, MCAD, SCAD, crotonase, SCHAD, and MCKAT). Electrons (e⁻) are passed to the respiratory chain either directly or via transfer proteins (ETF, FTF-QO). Acetyl CoA can be oxidized in the tricarboxylic acid (Krebs) cycle or, in the liver, used to synthesize ketone bodies. CACT, carnitine acylcarnitine translocase; CPT1, carnitine palmitoyltransferase 1; CPT2, carnitine palmitoyltransferase 2; ETF, electron transfer flavoprotein; ETF-QO, electron transfer flavoprotein ubiquinone oxidoreductase; FATPs, fatty acid transport proteins; FABP, plasma membrane fatty acid-binding protein; FAT, fatty acid translocase; LC-acyl-CoA, long-chain acyl-CoA; MCAD, medium-chain acyl-CoA dehydrogenase; MC-acyl-CoA, medium-chain acyl-CoA; MKAT, medium-chain acyl-CoA thiolase; MTP, mitochondrial trifunctional protein; OCTN2, high-affinity sodium-dependent carnitine transporter; SCAD, short-chain acyl-CoA dehydrogenase; SCHAD, short-chain 3-hydroxyacyl-CoA dehydrogenase; SC-thiolase, short-chain acyl-CoA thiolase; VLCAD, very-long-chain acyl-CoA dehydrogenase.

Reproduced from Elaine Murphy, Yann Nadjar, and Christine Vianey-Saban, Fatty Acid Oxidation, Electron Transfer and Riboflavin Metabolism Defects, in: *Inherited Metabolic Disease in Adults: A Clinical Guide* (eds. Carla E. M. Hollak and Robin Lachmann) Oxford University Press (2016) with permission from Oxford University Press.

primarily mediated by the renin–angiotensin–aldosterone and sympathetic nervous systems, which promote sodium retention, and the secretion of natriuretic peptides, which promotes sodium excretion.

Intracellular fluid volume: in normal adults, the intracellular fluid volume constitutes approximately 60–67% of the total body water. Potassium salts are the main intracellular solutes. The main regulating factor is the relative osmolarity of the interstitial fluid, which is determined by the balance between water intake and excretion (20).

Acid–base balance

pH is the negative of the base 10 logarithm of the hydrogen ion concentration. A low pH indicates a high hydrogen ion concentration (i.e. an acidic solution). A high pH represents lower hydrogen ion concentrations (i.e. alkaline solutions). The normal pH in human

tissues is 7.36–7.44. A pH value of 7.4 represents a hydrogen ion concentration of 0.00004 mmol/L.

The Henderson–Hasselbalch equation describes the relationship of hydrogen ion, bicarbonate, and carbonic acid concentrations. The partial pressure of carbon dioxide (PCO_2) is controlled by respiration. Short-term changes of pH may be controlled by changing the depth of respiration. The bicarbonate concentration can be altered by the kidneys.

Buffers: a buffer solution is one to which hydrogen or hydroxyl ions can be added with little change in the pH. A simple buffering system is the equilibrium between carbonic acid and bicarbonate ions in the blood (**Figure 1.26**). A major buffering system of the blood involves amino acids with different chemical side chains, and which ionize at different pH values (**Figure 1.27**). Haemoglobin has

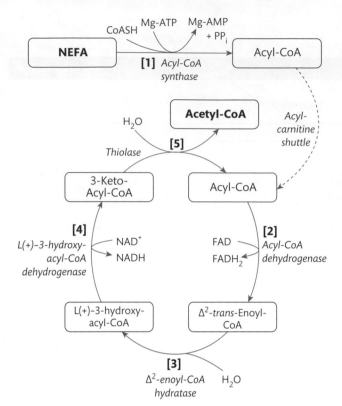

Figure 1.22 The beta -oxidation cycle of fatty acids. In the first instance, a cytosolic non-esterified fatty acid (NEFA), liberated from triglyceride stores by lipolysis, is esterified to coenzyme A (CoASH) to form an acyl-CoA molecule that can be imported into the mitochondrial matrix via the acyl-carnitine shuttle. The initial formation of the acyl-CoA complex requires the hydrolysis of magnesium (Mg)-ATP to Mg-AMP and pyrophosphate (PPi), where the spontaneous decay of the PPi to two inorganic phosphate (Pi) molecules prevents the acyl-CoA synthase reaction from reaching equilibrium.

Reproduced from Austin Ugwumadu, Biochemistry, in: *Basic Sciences for Obstetrics and Gynaecology*, Oxford University Press (2014) with permission from Oxford University Press.

a high buffering value and is found in higher concentrations than the plasma proteins.

Calcium homeostasis

Calcium is essential for several biological functions in the human body. Calcium is distributed in bones (99%), intracellular fluids (1%), and ECF (0.1%). The overall body Ca^{2+} balance is maintained through the intestinal absorption, renal reabsorption, and bone metabolism (**Figure 1.28**).

The ionized calcium concentration of ECF is closely regulated by the parathyroid hormone–vitamin D system acting on the kidneys, intestine, and bone. ECF Ca^{2+} is required for blood coagulation and maintenance of plasma membranes. It is also an important source of intracellular Ca^{2+}, which is required for several cellular functions. Channels control the transport of Ca^{2+} in and out of cells. Parathyroid cells respond to alterations in ECF Ca^{2+} levels with parathyroid hormone secretions having an effect on Ca^{2+} transport in kidney and bone. Homeostasis is also maintained through the renal production of 1,25-dihydroxy vitamin D, which modulates Ca^{2+} transport in intestine and bone.

Respiration

Alveolar ventilation is 350 mL/breath and the tidal volume is 500 mL/breath. The difference, 150 mL, is the anatomical dead space (**Figure 1.29**).

The total lung capacity is approximately 5 L. Of this, 1.5 L, the residual volume, remains at the end of forced expiration. The volume of gas, 3.5 L, inhaled from forced expiration to forced inspiration is the vital capacity. At rest, the pressure between the visceral and parietal pleura is –3 mmHg. During quiet inspiration, the chest expands and the pressure in the intrapleural space decreases to –6 mmHg. Expiration is passive with relaxation of the diaphragm and muscles of the chest wall.

Transportation mechanisms

Transport of substances within cells and across cell membranes is achieved via diffusion, solvent drag, filtration, osmosis, non-ionic diffusion, carrier-mediated transport, and phagocytosis.

Diffusion is a process whereby a gas or substance in solution expands to fill the volume available to it. Gaseous diffusion occurs in the alveoli of the lung and liquid diffusion occurs in the renal tubules.

Solvent drag is the process whereby bulk movement of solvent drags molecules of solute with it.

In *filtration*, substances are forced through a membrane by hydrostatic pressure. *Osmosis* is the movement of molecules of a solvent across a semipermeable membrane from a less concentrated solution into a more concentrated one.

Non-ionized diffusion is transport in a non-ionized form. Cell membranes consist of a lipid bilayer with specific transporter proteins embedded in it. Lipid-soluble drugs can cross the lipids of the blood–brain barrier or placenta by this process.

Carrier-mediated transport occurs across a cell membrane using a specific carrier. If the transport is down a concentration gradient, this is known as *facilitated transport*. If the carrier-mediated transport is up a concentration gradient, this is known as *active transport*.

Phagocytosis involves the incorporation of solid and liquid substances by the cell wall engulfing them. The cell appears to 'swallow' these substances.

Endocrinology

Mechanisms of actions of hormones

Cell surface receptors: hormones act in an autocrine, paracrine, or endocrine manner. Certain hormones (steroids, insulin-related growth factors, thyroid hormones) are bound to carrier proteins. Only free hormone is active and can bind to specific receptors and have an effect. Neurotransmitters and peptide hormones act mainly through cell surface receptors.

Steroid hormones, thyroid hormones, retinoic acid, and vitamin D act through nuclear receptors. Some of the receptors exist in the cytoplasm and some in the nucleus. Once these hormones bind to their receptors, they all act in the nucleus to alter gene expression.

Hypothalamus and pituitary

Embryologically, both the thalamus and the hypothalamus develop in the lateral walls of the diencephalon and the cavity becomes the

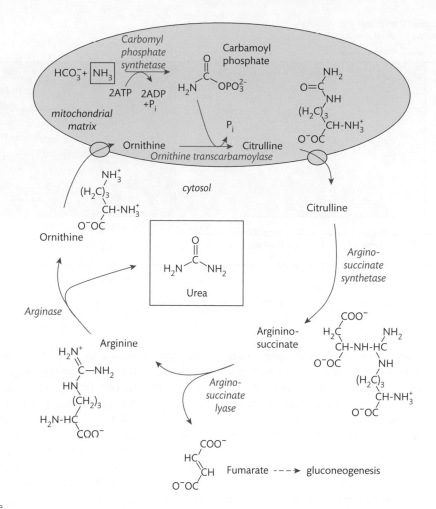

Figure 1.23 The urea cycle.

Reproduced from Neil Herring and Robert Wilkins, Biochemistry and metabolism, in: *Basic Science for Core Medical Training and the MRCP*, Oxford University Press (2015) with permission from Oxford University Press.

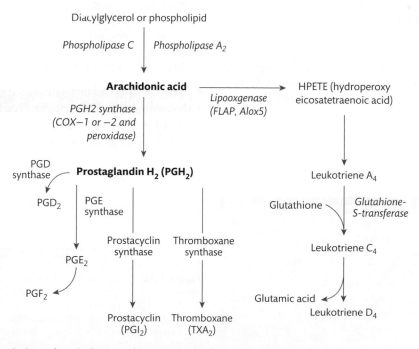

Figure 1.24 Pathways for metabolism of arachidonic acid into prostaglandins and leukotrienes.

Reproduced from Gary A. Rosenberg, Glucose, Amino Acid, and Lipid Metabolism, in: *Molecular Physiology and Metabolism of the Nervous System: A Clinical Perspective*, Oxford University Press, (2012) with permission from Oxford University Press.

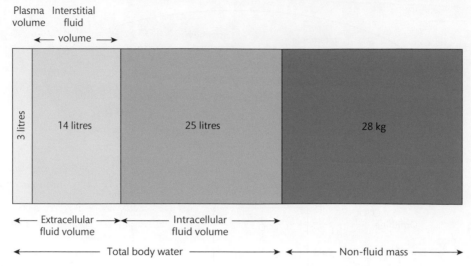

Figure 1.25 Body fluid compartments.

Reproduced from Anthony Delaney, Physiology of body fluids, in: *Oxford Textbook of Critical Care* (eds. Andrew Webb, Derek Angus, Simon Finfer, Luciano Gattinoni, and Mervyn Singer) Oxford University Press (2016), with permission from Oxford University Press.

third ventricle. The pituitary develops in close association and is made up of two parts: adenohypophysis, the anterior pituitary, and neurohypophysis, the posterior pituitary. The anterior pituitary develops from the ventral ridges of primitive neural tube, which are pushed forward by the developing Rathke's pouch. By 7 weeks of gestation, the sella floor has formed and the pituitary starts to form under the influence of the hypothalamus. The posterior pituitary is in contact with the hypothalamus while the anterior pituitary is connected to the hypothalamus via a portal system. The hypothalamus, pituitary stalk, and pituitary are supplied by carotid arteries via the superior and inferior hypophyseal arteries (**Figure 1.30**).

The posterior pituitary is a ventral extension of the central nervous system, where the hypothalamic hormones oxytocin and vasopressin are released (**Boxes 1.1 and 1.2**).

Thyroid

Embryologically, this is the first endocrine gland to develop. Its development starts 24 days after fertilization. It develops from the floor of the primitive pharynx as 'thyroid diverticulum'. Thyroid hormone secretion starts at about 11 weeks of pregnancy.

Table 1.2 Average electrolyte composition of body fluid compartments

Electrolyte	ICF (mmol/L)	ECF (mmol/L)	Plasma interstitial
Sodium	10	140	145
Potassium	155	3.7	3.8
Chloride	3	102	115
Bicarbonate	10	28	30
Calcium (ionized)	<0.01	1.2	1.2
Magnesium	10	0.8	0.8
Phosphate	105	1.1	1.0

ECF, extracellular fluid compartment; ICF, intracellular fluid compartment.

Source data from Delaney A. Physiology of body fluids. In: *Oxford Textbook of Critical Care* (2 ed.). Oxford University Press, 2016.

Thyroid hormones are iodinated metabolites of tyrosine. Their synthesis involves the following steps. Iodide is actively taken up into follicular cells by the iodide pump against the concentration gradient and is converted to iodine. Tyrosine is incorporated to form monoiodotyrosine and diiodotyrosine. Coupling of these iodotyrosines results in the formation of triiodothyronine (T_3) or tetraiodothyronine (thyroxine, T_4).

Once in circulation thyroid hormones are bound either to thyroxine-binding globulin, pre-albumin, or albumin. Only the free portion is active.

Thyroid-stimulating hormone is released from the anterior pituitary in response to thyrotropin-releasing hormone. Thyroid-stimulating hormone increases the size of thyroid, vascularity, iodine uptake, protein synthesis, storage of colloid, and the secretion of T_3 and T_4. Thyroid hormones feed back to both the hypothalamus and the pituitary (**Figure 1.31**).

Physiological actions of thyroid hormones include:

- stimulation of basal metabolic rate
- chronotropic and inotropic effects on the heart
- normal brain development
- anabolic actions, required for synthesis and secretion of growth hormone
- increased gut motility.

$$H_2O + CO_2 \rightleftharpoons H_2CO_3 \rightleftharpoons H^+ + HCO_3^-$$

Figure 1.26 The carbonic acid–bicarbonate equilibrium. Carbon dioxide (CO_2) generated by the oxidation of respiratory substrates combines with water in extracellular fluid and plasma to form carbonic acid (H_2CO_3), which can then dissociate into bicarbonate ions (HCO_3^-) and free protons (H^+), so lowering the pH of the extracellular fluid or plasma.

Reproduced from Austin Ugwumadu, Biochemistry, in: *Basic Sciences for Obstetrics and Gynaecology*, Oxford University Press (2014) with permission from Oxford University Press.

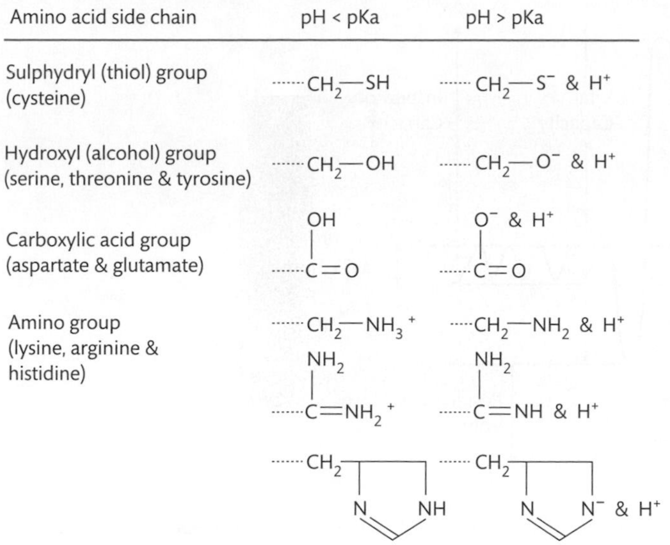

Amino acid side chain
pH < pKa
pH > pKa
Sulphydryl (thiol) group (cysteine)
CH2—SH
CH2—S− & H+
Hydroxyl (alcohol) group (serine, threonine & tyrosine)
CH2—OH
CH2—O− & H+
Carboxylic acid group (aspartate & glutamate)
OH
C=O
O− & H+
C=O
Amino group (lysine, arginine & histidine)
CH2—NH3+
CH2—NH2 & H+
NH2
C=NH2+
NH2
C=NH & H+
CH2
N
NH
CH2
N
N− & H+

Figure 1.27 The buffering capacity of amino acid side chains. At plasma pH values below the pKa for the relevant side chain (i.e. when the concentration of free protons exceeds the pKa), the side chains will exist in the protonated state (as polar SH/OH/NH groups, or protonated amino groups), but when the plasma pH value exceeds the pKa for the relevant side chain (i.e. when the concentration of free protons falls below the pKa), the side chains will release their proton (and so will exist as deprotonated $S^-/O^-/N^-$ groups, or as deprotonated NH_2/NH groups). When the plasma pH is exactly equal to the pKa value, the probability of any given side chain being in the protonated state will be exactly equal to the probability of that side chain being in the deprotonated state (i.e. half of those specific side chains will be protonated and half will be deprotonated).

Reproduced from Austin Ugwumadu, Biochemistry, in: *Basic Sciences for Obstetrics and Gynaecology*, Oxford University Press (2014) with permission from Oxford University Press.

Adrenal

The fetal adrenal cortex develops from coelomic mesoderm while the adrenal medulla is formed from an adjacent sympathetic ganglion derived from neural crest cells. Differentiation of the cortex begins in late fetal life. At birth, the adrenal cortex is large and regresses over the first year. The adrenal cortex produces three major classes of steroids:

- Aldosterone
- Cortisol
- Androgens: mainly dehydroepiandrosterone (DHEA) and its sulphated form (DHEAS) and androstenedione.

All adrenal steroids are derived from cholesterol (**Figure 1.32**).

Aldosterone secretion is regulated by angiotensin II and by potassium. Cortisol is a stress hormone. The synthesis of cortisol is controlled by adrenocorticotropic hormone (ACTH), which in turn is stimulated by corticotropin-releasing hormone (CRH) from the hypothalamus. Vasopressin neurosecretory cells can also potentiate the action of CRH on the corticotrophs of the anterior pituitary. ACTH secretion is controlled by the negative feedback of circulating cortisol both at the level of the hypothalamus and the pituitary. ACTH is released in a circadian rhythm. Cortisol is lowest in the evening and highest in the early hours of the morning. Once released, cortisol is bound to cortisol-binding globulin with a small fraction (<5%) entering target cells and initiatating glucocorticoid effects.

Cortisol's overall effect is anabolic in the liver and catabolic in muscle and adipose tissue, leading to raised circulating levels of blood glucose and fatty acids. Glucagon requires cortisol for glycogenolysis in the liver. Glucocorticoids also have effects on multiple organs including brain, bones, cardiovascular system, kidneys, skin, connective tissue, and the fetus.

Diet
1000mg
Intestine
500mg
325mg
ECF
Filtration
10,000mg
Reabsorption
9825mg
Kidney
Bone Formation
280mg
Resorption
280mg
Feces
825mg
Bone
Urine
175mg

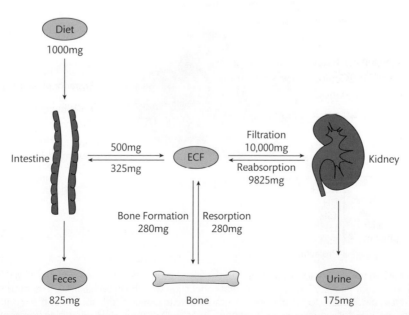

Figure 1.28 Daily Ca^{2+} balance in human. 175 mg Ca^{2+} is absorbed each day in the intestine, and the same amount of Ca^{2+} is excreted into the urine. Total body Ca^{2+} balance is maintained through the coordination of intestinal absorption, renal reabsorption, and bone metabolism.

Reproduced from Yoshiro Suzuki, Marc Bürzle, and Matthias A. Hediger, Physiology and pathology of calcium and magnesium transport, in: *The Spectrum of Mineral and Bone Disorders in Chronic Kidney Disease* (eds. Klaus Olgaard, Isidro B. Salusky, and Justin Silver) Oxford University Press (2010), with permission from Oxford University Press.

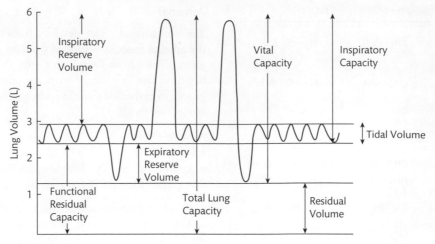

Figure 1.29 Lung volumes and capacities.

Reproduced from Mark Harrison, Respiratory physiology, in: *Revision Notes for the FRCEM Primary*, Oxford University Press (2017) with permission from Oxford University Press.

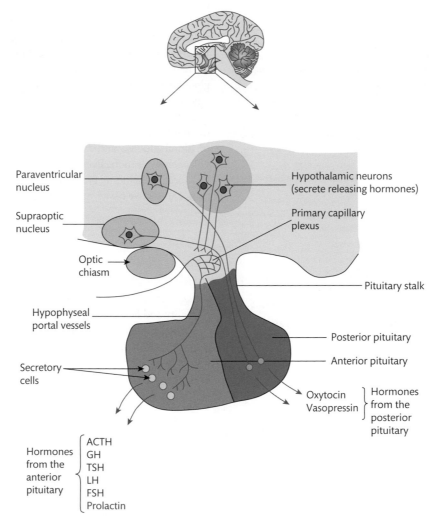

Figure 1.30 The relationship between the hypothalamus and the pituitary gland. Note the prominent portal system that links the hypothalamus to the anterior pituitary gland. The anterior pituitary has no direct neural connection with the hypothalamus. In contrast, nerve fibres from the paraventricular and supraoptic nuclei pass directly to the posterior pituitary where they secrete the hormones they contain into the bloodstream. ACTH, adrenocorticotropic hormone; FSH, follicle-stimulating hormone; GH, growth hormone; LH, luteinizing hormone; TSH, thyroid-stimulating hormone.

Reproduced from Neil Herring and Robert Wilkins, Endocrinology, in: *Basic Science for Core Medical Training and the MRCP*, Oxford University Press (2015) with permission from Oxford University Press.

Box 1.1 Hypothalamic hormones

- Gonadotropin-releasing hormone
- Corticotropin-releasing hormone
- Thyrotropin-releasing hormone
- Dopamine
- Growth hormone-releasing hormone
- Somatostatin

Excess cortisol secretion (Cushing syndrome) results in proximal myopathy, bruising, scarring, and purple striae of the abdomen, loss of bone mass, hypertension, and depression.

Primary adrenocortical deficiency (Addison's disease) causes low systolic blood pressure, weight loss due to reduced appetite, and skin pigmentation due to excess ACTH (reduction of negative feedback), which interacts with melanocortin receptors in the skin (21, p. 112).

Effects of pregnancy and lactation

The placenta can synthesize and secrete proteins but cannot synthesize steroids. Several maternal serum hormone changes occur during pregnancy (**Figure 1.33**).

Placental proteins: human chorionic gonadotropin (hCG) peaks at 10 weeks. Human placental lactogen (hPL) rises with placental weight. It induces insulin resistance. Oestrogens (oestradiol, oestriol, and oestrone) are synthesized in the placenta from DHEA produced by the fetus and increase to term. Androgens are derived from the fetoplacental unit and testosterone levels rise tenfold. Progesterone is mainly synthesized by the corpus luteum in the first 2–3 months of pregnancy. Levels rise up to term.

Pituitary hormones: LH and FSH decline while prolactin rises to term. Thyroid hormones (total T_4 and T_3) rise during the first trimester and then plateau. Cortisol increases to three times prepregnancy values and aldosterone plateaus at 34 weeks.

Several hormones during pregnancy stimulate breast growth (oestrogen, progesterone, hPL, prolactin, cortisol, and insulin). High concentrations of oestrogens inhibit lactation. After delivery, when the oestrogen levels fall, lactation is initiated by prolactin. Prolactin promotes milk formation and is released from the anterior pituitary. Prolactin is also released in response to suckling.

Box 1.2 Pituitary hormones

- Luteinizing hormone
- Follicle-stimulating hormone
- Proopiomelanocortin (POMC)
- Adrenocorticotropin
- Beta-endorphin
- Melanocyte-stimulating hormone (MSH)
- Thyrotropin
- Prolactin
- Growth hormone

Pharmacology

Pharmacokinetics

Pharmacokinetics refers to how a drug moves through an individual's body (22). A drug's pharmacokinetics includes absorption, distribution, metabolism, and elimination, which affect the drug's concentration at the site of action and its effect.

Clearance is the volume of blood from which a drug is completely eliminated in a period of time. It depends on liver metabolism or renal blood flow. *Volume of distribution* is the volume of fluid into which a drug distributes. It depends on protein binding and liquid solubility. *Half-life* is the time taken for the concentration of drug in blood to fall by half. *Bioavailability* is the proportion of drug, which reaches the systemic circulation unchanged. *First-pass metabolism* involves the metabolic breakdown of a drug during its first pass through the liver. In *steady-state concentration*, the peak and the trough blood concentrations of the drug remain the same with repeated equal doses.

Pharmacodynamics

Pharmacodynamics refers to an individual's therapeutic response to a drug and is determined by the drug's affinity and activity at its site of action.

Drugs mainly act on four different targets:

1. Receptors
2. Enzymes
3. Membrane ionic channels
4. Metabolic processes such as DNA synthesis.

Drug metabolism

Most drugs are metabolized in the liver. Water-soluble drugs are excreted by the kidneys. Lipid soluble ones pass across the cell membrane of the hepatocytes and then access microsomal P450 enzymes.

Drug metabolism in the liver involves simple oxidation, which creates hydroxyl groups and conjugation of these with various sulphate, acetyl, methyl, and glycyl groups. These processes increase solubility and facilitate renal excretion.

The mechanisms involved in renal excretion are filtration at the glomerulus, transport through the epithelium of the kidney tubules, and diffusion. Renal clearance is important as it affects the plasma concentration of the drug.

Drug interactions

Drugs can interact with each other. Enzyme inducers and enzyme inhibitors are common examples of such interactions.

Enzyme inducers: carbamazepine, phenobarbitone, phenytoin, griseofulvin, and rifampicin belong to this category. These drugs increase the activity of enzyme systems. Drugs metabolized by the same enzymes are metabolized and eliminated more rapidly. As a result, their plasma concentrations will fall with possible clinical implications. Efficacy of oral contraceptives is reduced by enzyme inducers.

Enzyme inhibition: drugs such as erythromycin, metronidazole, sulphonamides, and cimetidine have the potential to increase

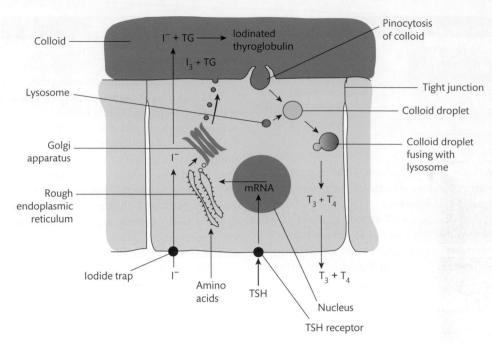

Figure 1.31 The cellular processes involved in the synthesis and subsequent release of the thyroid hormones. Note that thyroid-stimulating hormone (TSH) stimulates both the synthesis of thyroglobulin (TG) and the secretion of triiodothyronine (T_3) and thyroxine (T_4).

Reproduced from Neil Herring and Robert Wilkins, Endocrinology, in: *Basic Science for Core Medical Training and the MRCP*, Oxford University Press (2015) with permission from Oxford University Press.

the efficacy of other drugs by enzyme inhibition. For example, sulphonamides can lead to phenytoin toxicity.

Effect of pregnancy and breastfeeding on drug metabolism

Drugs can affect the developing fetus by direct action on the fetus causing birth defects, by affecting the placenta and limiting the supply of nutrients and oxygen to the fetus, and by causing premature labour (Table 1.3) (23). Drugs that do not cross the placenta are heparin, insulin, and curare.

Fluid retention and decreased protein concentrations tend to increase the volume of distribution, which in turn causes a decrease in the plasma concentration of the drug. In pregnancy, renal blood flow increases and liver metabolic pathways get induced. Anticonvulsants such as phenytoin and carbamazepine undergo increased drug clearance. Plasma levels fall significantly. Lithium and ampicillin are both eliminated by the kidney and their clearance increases by 100% during pregnancy, requiring increased doses.

Commonly used drugs, which can be safely administered to a breastfeeding mother, are non-narcotic analgesics, penicillins, cephalosporins, methyl-dopa, beta-blockers, phenytoin, carbamazepine, and sodium valproate.

Drugs which should be avoided during breastfeeding include:

- laxatives: can cause diarrhoea in neonates
- amiodarone: may affect the neonatal thyroid
- barbiturates: can cause drowsiness
- benzodiazepines can cause drowsiness and failure to thrive
- lithium: can cause hypotonia and cyanosis
- carbimazole and methimazole: can suppress the neonatal thyroid.

Teratogens and organogenesis

Drugs that are commonly implicated in fetal malformations include:

- cytotoxic anticancer drugs
- antiepileptic drugs
- some antirheumatic drugs
- antibiotics
- oral hypoglycaemic agents
- some antihypertensives
- tranquilizers.

Retinoic acids are vitamin A analogues, which are used in the treatment of acne. These drugs can cause major malformations including craniofacial, cardiac, thymic, and central nervous system defects.

Cytotoxic anticancer drugs: these inhibit rapid cell growth and are detrimental to fetal growth. Methotrexate and antifolate drugs may cause cleft palate and other abnormalities. Thalidomide should also be avoided in pregnancy.

Phenytoin causes a variety of abnormalities including cleft lip/palate, microcephaly, hypertelorism, and fingernail hyperplasia as well as growth deficiency. Sodium valproate is associated with neural tube defects. Carbamazepine causes similar defects as phenytoin. The incidence of fetal abnormality is around 10% with the anticonvulsants.

Aspirin is not the analgesic of choice but may still be used in pregnancy (24, 25). However, doses higher than 500 mg/day are contraindicated after 24 weeks of gestation. Aspirin administration during the last weeks of pregnancy may be associated with postpartum haemorrhage and intracranial bleeding of the newborn. Cyclooxygenase-2 inhibitors should be avoided during pregnancy.

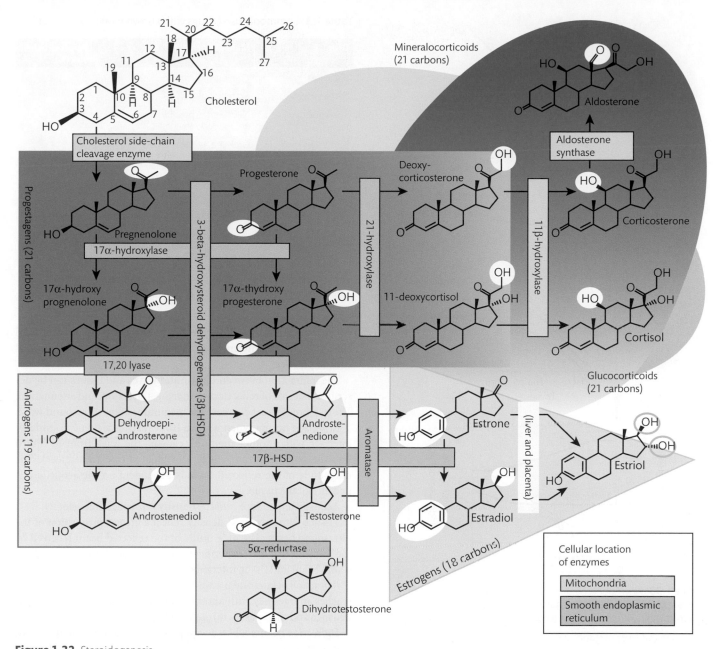

Figure 1.32 Steroidogenesis.

Reproduced from Neil Herring and Robert Wilkins, Endocrinology, in: *Basic Science for Core Medical Training and the MRCP*, Oxford University Press (2015) with permission from Oxford University Press.

The use of non-steroidal anti-inflammatory drugs is contraindicated as it may cause closure of the ductus arteriosus *in utero*, prolonged pregnancy, and postpartum haemorrhage.

Lithium can cause cardiac abnormalities when given in the first trimester, such as Ebstein's anomaly. The antiviral agent ribavirin is contraindicated in pregnancy and ciprofloxacin is not recommended. The antibiotics streptomycin, kanamycin, and gentamicin may cause deafness in the fetus. Tetracyclines may damage tooth growth in children under the age of 8. They may also lodge in the bone and should be avoided in pregnancy. Statins are not recommended in pregnancy. Angiotensin-converting enzyme inhibitors can damage the fetal kidney and cause oligohydramnios and neonatal anuria. Warfarin is a coumarin anticoagulant. Fetal warfarin

syndrome has been associated with warfarin exposure in pregnancy, with the highest risk between 6 and 12 weeks of gestation. Warfarin is associated with chondrodysplasia punctata, central nervous system defects, intracerebral haemorrhage, intellectual disability, and eye anomalies (optic atrophy).

In summary, the following rules should be considered when prescribing in pregnancy or lactation (26, 27):

- Prescribe only when absolutely necessary.
- Do not prescribe lower or higher doses than necessary.
- Avoid medications known to be contraindicated or newly released medications.
- Choose drugs that do not cross the placenta.

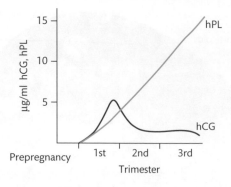

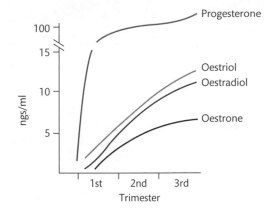

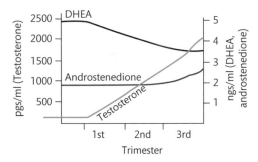

Figure 1.33 Hormonal changes during the three trimesters of pregnancy. DHEA, dehydroepiandrosterone; hCG, human chorionic gonadotrophin; hPL, human placental lactogen.

Reproduced from Austin Ugwumadu, Endocrinology, in: *Basic Sciences for Obstetrics and Gynaecology*, Oxford University Press (2014) with permission from Oxford University Press.

Physics

Ultrasound

Ultrasound imaging has been used for medical purposes for several decades. Ultrasound refers to sound waves greater than 20,000 cycles/sec, a frequency greater than that which the human ear can appreciate. In obstetrics and gynaecology, frequencies of 2–12 million cycles/sec (MHz) are used. The ultrasound probe consists of two elements: a transducer and a receiver.

Understanding the physical principles underlying ultrasound technology can help optimize image quality, and improve diagnostic capabilities. This information is also essential for ensuring this technology remains safe for the woman and the fetus.

Sound waves are described in terms of frequency, which is the number of repetitions (i.e. cycles) per second. The unit for measuring them is the Hertz (Hz). Another characteristic is wavelength.

Table 1.3 Commonly used drugs with known teratogenic effect

Drug	Main abnormality	Approximate risk (%)
Phenytoin	Craniofacial, cardiac	4
Carbamazepine	Craniofacial, limb	2
Sodium valproate	Neural tube, possible neurodevelopmental	6
Lamotrigine	Oral cleft, possibly others	3
Warfarin	Chondrodysplasia punctata	Up to 25
	Facial anomalies	
	Central nervous system anomalies	
Lithium	Cardiac (Ebstein's complex)	2
Danazol	Virilization of female fetus	Uncertain
Retinoids	Multiple defects	High

Source data from Rubin P. Prescribing in pregnancy. In: Warrell DA, Cox TM, Firth JD (eds) *Oxford Textbook of Medicine*. Oxford: Oxford University Press; 2010.

Ultrasound is an ideal means for imaging soft tissues and fluid collections commonly encountered in obstetric and gynaecological clinical practice.

The interaction between ultrasound waves and tissues can be described in terms of reflection, scattering, refraction, and attenuation. The last three factors decrease the magnitude of the ultrasound wave.

Reflection occurs when a wave front reaches a tissue boundary/interface with another medium, causing the wave front to return into the medium from which it originated (the transducer). The magnitude of the reflected wave is dependent on the acoustic impedance of the tissue:

Acoustic impedance = tissue density × propagation velocity

Tissues with increased density reflect a greater proportion of the ultrasound beam. The magnitude of the reflected beam received by the transducer is also dependent upon the angle between the ultrasound beam and tissue interface.

Refraction occurs when a wave front travelling through a medium reaches an interface with another medium of different acoustic impedance and then passes through it (**Figure 1.34**).

Diffraction occurs when a wave encounters an obstacle that has a diameter comparable to its wavelength. There is bending of waves around small obstacles and spreading out of the waves as they pass through small openings (**Figure 1.35**).

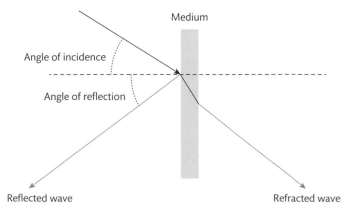

Figure 1.34 Wave front reflection and refraction.

Reproduced from Austin Ugwumadu, Medical Physics, in: *Basic Sciences for Obstetrics and Gynaecology*, Oxford University Press (2014) with permission from Oxford University Press.

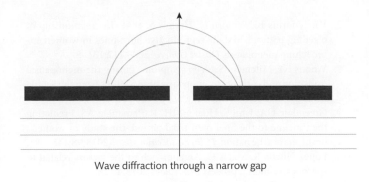

Wave diffraction through a narrow gap

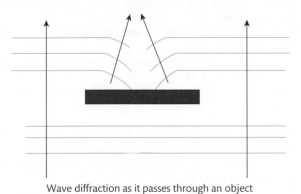

Wave diffraction as it passes through an object

Figure 1.35 Wave diffraction.
Reproduced from Austin Ugwumadu, Medical Physics, in: *Basic Sciences for Obstetrics and Gynaecology*, Oxford University Press (2014) with permission from Oxford University Press.

Scatter is the combination of irregular reflection, refraction, and diffraction of a wave in multiple directions.

Absorption is the conversion of sound energy into heat as it travels through a medium.

Attenuation is a process whereby ultrasound signal strength is progressively reduced during transmission due to absorption of the ultrasound energy by conversion to heat. Attenuation is frequency and wavelength dependent.

Ultrasound uses the pulse echo principle. This is where a pulse of known speed is emitted and the time taken for the reflected echo to return is measured.

Artefacts: some images vary due to artefacts of ultrasound imaging. Examples of common artefacts encountered in obstetric and gynaecological ultrasound include the following:

- *Shadowing* occurs when there is strong reflection or attenuation leading to a diminished ultrasound beam with loss of imaging data distal to the reflector or attenuator.
- Increased *through transmission* is associated with lower attenuation than surrounding tissues, typically due to a fluid-filled structure such as a cyst.
- *Reverberation* artefacts occur when two or more intensely reflective interfaces cause the ultrasound beam to echo, resulting in echoes in cystic structures, appearing as solid elements.
- *Refraction* artefacts are caused by non-linear bending of the sound waves when there is a change in the tissue.

Radioactivity and X-rays

Radiation is broadly divided into ionizing and non-ionizing radiation. *Ionization* is a process whereby an atom or molecule is converted into an ion by adding or removing charged particles. *Radioactive decay* is the process by which an unstable atomic nucleus spontaneously loses energy by emitting ionizing particles and radiation. Ionizing radiation produced by radioactive decay includes:

- alpha radiation
- beta radiation
- gamma radiation.

Alpha particles are emitted from the nucleus of an atom. They consist of two neutrons and protons. They have a high mass and high energy but low depth of penetration. They are heavily ionizing.

Beta particles are divided into β⁻ and β⁺ particles. The former is an electron that arises from beta minus decay of a neutron and the latter is a high-energy positron.

Gamma rays are high-frequency electromagnetic waves. They have a short wavelength. They are used for sterilization of medical equipment, gamma knife surgery, and in nuclear medicine.

X-rays are a form of electromagnetic radiation emitted by electrons with a wavelength in the range of 10 to 0.01 nm.

Ionizing radiation can be used for management of both malignant and non- malignant conditions in the form of radiation therapy. Radiation causes DNA damage by direct and indirect ionization of the atoms, which make up the DNA chain. Ionizing radiation is also used in the field of nuclear medicine where radioactive isotopes are administered internally. These radionuclides are atoms with an unstable nucleus and their radioactive decay emits ionizing radiation which is captured by a gamma camera. This is useful for both imaging and for treatment.

Magnetic resonance imaging

Magnetic resonance imaging (MRI) is an imaging technology using non-ionizing radiofrequency radiation inside a strong, constant, spatially homogeneous magnetic field. This process involves induction of protons by a magnetic field, followed by excitation with radiofrequency pulses and subsequent readout with receiver coils. Tesla (T) is the unit used in the International System of Units (SI) for magnetic fields. Most magnets in medical MRI produce a magnetic field of 0.5–3 T. Small differences in the microenvironment of different tissues can be detected by pulse sequences. The presence of multiple magnetic resonance properties of tissue leads to great flexibility in determining tissue contrast. This capability is superior to computed tomography (CT).

Limitations in the use of MRI include contraindications posed by metallic implants, and claustrophobia. Open MRI scanners and short-bore conventional scanners can address the issue of claustrophobia.

Intravenous contrast agents are often used to improve contrast between pathological and normal tissues or to perform angiography. Contrast agents carry a risk of inducing nephrogenic systemic fibrosis in patients with renal failure.

Lasers

Lasers are devices that emit electromagnetic radiation used to cut, coagulate, or ablate tissue in different clinical applications. Lasers are commonly used superficially for cutaneous and ocular applications, as well as for minimally invasive procedures. The safe and appropriate use of lasers requires knowledge of laser delivery systems and laser–tissue interactions to achieve the desired clinical effect while minimizing complications.

In the unexcited state, electrons orbit the nucleus at their lowest energy level, occupying orbits closer to the nucleus. Absorption of energy causes the electrons to become excited, moving to a higher orbit. As the electrons return from the excited state back to the ground state, they spontaneously emit photons of energy (electromagnetic radiation).

Laser devices produce a single, coherent wavelength within the ultraviolet, visible, or infrared portion of the electromagnetic spectrum. A laser beam can be continuous, pulsed, or quasi-continuous.

Concentration of energy into a small area in a very brief pulse causes production of high local temperatures and this in turn causes vaporization of tissues as well as cauterization action, which reduces blood loss.

Lasers are used predominantly as a source of energy to effect tissue destruction but also provide a coherent energy source for phototherapy or confocal microscopy, which allows for real-time imaging of tissues. Lasers destroy tissue through production of heat (photothermal), disruption of chemical bonds (photoablative), or reactions with a photosensitizer (photochemical). The interaction between the laser and tissue depends upon the wavelength, power, duration of exposure, and properties of the target tissue.

Gas lasers use noble gases (e.g. argon, helium) and other types of gases (e.g. CO_2).

The CO_2 laser is excellent as a cutting instrument because scattering is minimal, absorption in water is excellent, soft tissue vaporization is rapid, and the surrounding tissue damage is negligible. The CO_2 laser permits coagulation of blood vessels smaller than 0.5 mm in diameter.

Neodymium-doped yttrium aluminium garnet (Nd:YAG) lasers emit light at mid-infrared wavelengths with pulse durations in the millisecond range. The longer wavelength of the Nd:YAG laser penetrates deeper into the tissue and can cause collateral thermal damage.

The eye and skin are the organs most susceptible to damage by laser radiation.

REFERENCES

1. Renaudineau Y, Youinou P. Epigenetics and autoimmunity, with special emphasis on methylation. *Keio J Med* 2011;**60**:10–16.
2. Couce M, Dieguez C, Casanueva FF. Pituitary anatomy and physiology. In: Wass JAH, Shalet SM (eds), *Oxford Textbook of Endocrinology and Diabetes*, pp. 75–85. Oxford: Oxford University Press; 2002.
3. Adams JM, Taylor AE, Schoenfeld DA, et al. The midcycle gonadotropin surge in normal women occurs in the face of an unchanging gonadotropin-releasing hormone pulse frequency. *J Clin Endocrinol Metab* 1994;**79**:858–64.
4. Hillier SG. Current concepts of the roles of follicle stimulating hormone and luteinizing hormone in folliculogenesis. *Hum Reprod* 1994;**9**:188–91.
5. Sherman BM, West JH, Korenman SG. The menopausal transition: analysis of LH, FSH, estradiol, and progesterone concentrations during menstrual cycles of older women. *J Clin Endocrinol Metab* 1976;**42**:629–36.
6. Neer RM, SWAN Investigators. Bone loss across the menopausal transition. *Ann N Y Acad Sci* 2010;**1192**:66–71.
7. Van Voorhis BJ, Santoro N, Harlow S, et al. The relationship of bleeding patterns to daily reproductive hormones in women approaching menopause. *Obstet Gynecol* 2008;**112**:101–8.
8. Woods NF, Mitchell ES. Sleep symptoms during the menopausal transition and early postmenopause: observations from the Seattle Midlife Women's Health Study. *Sleep* 2010;**33**:539–49.
9. Greendale GA, Ishii S, Huang MH, Karlamangla AS. Predicting the timeline to the final menstrual period: the study of women's health across the nation. *J Clin Endocrinol Metab* 2013;**98**:1483–91.
10. López-Úbeda R, Matás C. An approach to the factors related to sperm capacitation process. *Andrology* 2015;**4**:128.
11. Masters WH, Johnson VE. *Human Sexual Response*. Boston, MA: Little, Brown; 1966.
12. Kaplan H. *Disorders of Sexual Desire*. New York: Simon and Schuster; 1979.
13. Roberts JM, Escudero C. The placenta in preeclampsia. *Pregnancy Hypertens* 2012;**2**:72–83.
14. Ugwumadu A. Medical microbiology. In: *Basic sciences for Obstetrics and Gynaecology*, pp. 141–60. Oxford: Oxford University Press; 2014.
15. Horton R, Wilming L, Rand V, et al. Gene map of the extended human MHC. *Nat Rev Genet* 2004;**5**:889–99.
16. Schoeller DA. Changes in total body water with age. *Am J Clin Nutr* 1989;**50** Suppl 5;1176–81.
17. Chumlea WC, Guo SS, Zeller CM, et al. Total body water reference values and prediction equations for adults. *Kidney Int* 2001;**59**:2250–8.
18. Ritz P, Vol S, Berrut G, Tack I, Arnaud MJ, Tichet J. Influence of gender and body composition on hydration and body water spaces. *Clin Nutr* 2008;**27**:740–6.
19. Delaney A. Physiology of body fluids. In: Webb A, Angus D, Finfer F, Gattinoni L, Singer M (eds), *Oxford Textbook of Critical Care*, 2nd edn, pp. 304–7. Oxford: Oxford University Press; 2016.
20. Ball SG. Vasopressin and disorders of water balance: the physiology and pathophysiology of vasopressin. *Ann Clin Biochem* 2007;**44**:417–31.
21. Ugwumadu A. Endocrinology. In: *Basic sciences for Obstetrics and Gynaecology*, pp. 103–20. Oxford: Oxford University Press; 2014.
22. Preskorn SH, Hatt CR. How pharmacogenomics (PG) are changing practice: implications for prescribers, their patients, and the healthcare system (PG series part I). *J Psychiatr Pract* 2013;**19**: 142–9.
23. Rubin P. Prescribing in pregnancy. In: Warrell DA, Cox TM, Firth JD (eds) *Oxford Textbook of Medicine*, 5th edn, pp. 2186–90. Oxford: Oxford University Press; 2010.
24. CLASP Collaborative Group. Low dose aspirin in pregnancy and early childhood development: follow up of the collaborative low dose aspirin study in pregnancy. *Br J Obstet Gynaecol* 1995;**102**:861–8.
25. CLASP (Collaborative Low-dose Aspirin Study in Pregnancy) Collaborative Group. CLASP: a randomised trial of low-dose aspirin for the prevention and treatment of pre-eclampsia among 9364 pregnant women. *Lancet* 1994;**343**:619–29.
26. Buhimschi CS, Weiner CP. Medications in pregnancy and lactation: part 1. Teratology. *Obstet Gynecol* 2009;**113**:166–88.
27. Buhimschi CS, Weiner CP. Medications in pregnancy and lactation: part 2. Drugs with minimal or unknown human teratogenic effect. *Obstet Gynecol* 2009;**113**:417–32.

2

Ethics in obstetrics and gynaecology

Frank A. Chervenak and Laurence B. McCullough

Introduction

This chapter provides a concise overview of ethical dimensions of obstetrics and gynaecology, based on the professional responsibility model of ethics in obstetrics and gynaecology (1–3). We first describe this model. We then demonstrate its relevance to three especially timely domains of ethics in obstetrics and gynaecology of importance to all obstetrician-gynaecologists: clinical ethical topics in gynaecology, clinical ethical topics in obstetrics, and professionally responsible advocacy in obstetrics and gynaecology.

The professional responsibility model of ethics in obstetrics and gynaecology

The professional responsibility model of obstetrics and gynaecology invokes the professional virtues of physicians—self-effacement, self-sacrifice, compassion, and integrity—and clinically applicable ethical principles—beneficence, respect for autonomy, and healthcare justice (1–3). Some readers might assume that professional ethics in obstetrics and gynaecology, as a subset of professional ethics in medicine more generally, derive from ancient Greece and the writings known as the Hippocratic Corpus, especially the renowned Hippocratic Oath. Other readers might assume that these professional virtues and ethical principles have only been introduced in the past four decades, dating from the beginnings of bioethics in the United States and the United Kingdom and spreading around the world since that time. We take exception to both views.

Is there a Hippocratic tradition of professional medical ethics?

The origin and author of the Hippocratic Oath are unknown. The Oath itself appeals to two concepts (4). The first concept is *techné*, which is often—but erroneously—translated as the art of medicine that is somehow understood to be distinct from the science of medicine. For the physicians of the Hippocratic or Koan school of medicine—no surgeons were permitted—*techné* was understood to be the fixed, unchanging, and unchangeable fund of knowledge of health and disease, both of which were a function of the four humours and the clinical skills of very carefully deploying this fund of knowledge in clinical practice. The result is therapeutic minimalism, in which clinical observation is central, with only modest clinical interventions permitted and always deployed with preventing the physician from being blamed for the patient's death. *Techné* is a self-interested, antiscientific basis for clinical practice, wholly antithetical to modern science as the basis of clinical practice.

The second concept is reputation—what others think about one. Other physicians will think well of one when one adheres to the requirements of *techné*, especially, as called for in the Oath, by keeping *techné* 'pure and holy', that is, uncorrupted by change (which does not define the modern science of medicine). One keeps *techné*, now understood as a set of trade secrets, 'pure and holy' by not sharing trade secrets with physicians who have not sworn the Oath as a written covenant with colleagues, that is, as a guild Oath. When reputation prioritizes individual and guild self-interest rather than excellent patient care, reputation becomes wholly antithetical to the life of service to patients that should characterize medicine as a profession.

Even if, contrary to this interpretation of the Oath, it were a professional Oath worthy of the name, there is no unbroken tradition of taking the Oath that comes down to us from ancient Greece, what Baker has called the Hippocratic 'footnote' (5). Nutton (6) has shown that references to the Oath do not appear after the first several centuries of the Common Era. When the Oath comes back into favour in the early decades of the twentieth century, it is invoked in what Nutton calls a conservative fashion. By this, Nutton means that the purpose of the invocation was to validate medicine as a profession by appealing to the memory of a revered historical figure, a purpose to which the figure of Hippocrates has often been put in the history of medicine (7). This appeal to the figure of Hippocrates, Nutton adds, was used an antidote to the fragile social standing of medicine at that time. The idea that there was a Hippocratic tradition of professional medical ethics turns out to be a twentieth-century creation, out of whole cloth.

Ahistorical bioethics

The field of bioethics, especially in the United States, was taken by many of its founders to be engaging new and unprecedented ethical challenges in medical science and practice to which the tools of contemporary philosophical ethics should be brought to bear (8). This occurred at a time—the late 1960s and early 1970s—when the dominant methods in philosophical ethics were, like the dominant methods of philosophy generally, ahistorical. The result was that that early bioethics was almost exclusively ahistorical. One important exception was the first edition of the *Encyclopedia of Bioethics*, the editor of which, Warren Reich, was historically minded and thus included a large section on the history of medical ethics (9). However, the self-understanding of bioethics as having a history that preceded it, the history of medical ethics, did not gain wide traction in the field. The consequence was the failure to recognize the transformative accomplishment of medical ethics in eighteenth-century Enlightenment Scotland and England.

The invention of professional medical ethics

Two remarkable physicians of these national enlightenments invented professional medical ethics, the physician-ethicists John Gregory (10) (1724–1773) of Scotland and Thomas Percival (11) (1740–1804) of England (12, 13). They did so in response to the corrosive distrust of physicians, surgeons, midwives, apothecaries, and 'unorthodox' practitioners (less kindly, 'quacks') who competed fiercely with each other for the small private-practice market. Private medical care was purchased by the well-to-do and provided for them in their homes. There were almost as many concepts of health and disease and remedies as there were practitioners. Dorothy Porter and Roy Porter have provided compelling documentation of widespread distrust of the sick towards practitioners (14). The sick did not think that practitioners, including physicians and surgeons who had been admitted to the ranks of the royal colleges in London and Edinburgh, knew what they were doing. The sick thought that the primary motivation of practitioners was self-interest in money and reputation. Gregory and Percival thought that this rampant distrust made becoming sick or injured even more of a trial than it already was. They also thought that practising medicine and surgery—they were among the first to call for physicians and surgeons to work together for the benefit of patients—in such a corrosive context was antithetical to what the life of service to patients should be. They set out to change medicine by using the tools of science and ethics.

The scientific tool that they both invoked was the philosophy of medicine of Francis Bacon (1561–1626) (12). Bacon called for medicine to be based on what he called 'experience'. By this, he emphatically did not mean the individual, personal experiences of physicians and surgeons, because this was (and still is) a hopelessly biased source of knowledge. Instead, 'experience' meant the carefully observed results of natural and controlled experiments. The Baconian physicians of Edinburgh, where Gregory was both a student and professor and where Percival was a student, introduced a nascent form of what has become evidence-based medicine.

The ethics tool was the 'science of man' and the 'science of morals' in the work of David Hume (1711–1776) for Gregory and the lesser known but still very important Richard Price (1723–1791) for Percival (12, 13). Both based ethical reasoning on scientific discoveries about human nature and eschewed 'speculative philosophy', that is, philosophy disconnected from Baconian experience. Hume and Price both emphasized that human nature is defined by relationships among individuals. We are, by our nature, directed to the protection and promotion of the interests of others, provided that this natural capacity is supported by requisite virtues (traits or habits of character that blunt self-interest in favour of the life of service to others).

In their enormously influential medical ethics writings, Gregory and Percival invented the ethical concept of medicine. Becoming a physician requires three sustained commitments:

1. The physician or surgeon should commit to becoming and remaining scientifically and clinically competent by engaging in evidence-based practice and research.
2. The physician or surgeon should commit to using scientific clinical competence primarily to protect and promote the health-related interests of each patient, keeping self-interest systematically secondary.
3. Physicians and surgeons should commit to sustaining medicine as what Percival called a 'public trust' rather than a self-interested merchant guild. As a public trust, medicine belongs both to current and future physicians, surgeons, patients, and society (1, 3, 13).

Four professional virtues and three ethical principles

The implications of these three commitments for clinical practice, research, and health policy can be expressed in the language of four professional virtues and three ethical principles. The professional virtue of self-effacement calls for the doctor to put aside and not be influenced by sources of bias that might distort the commitment to scientific and clinical competence or the second commitment to putting the patient's interests first. The professional virtue of self-sacrifice requires the doctor to accept reasonable limits on individual self-interest in order to fulfil the second commitment and to accept limits on group self-interest in order to fulfil the third commitment. The professional virtue of compassion requires the doctor to be alert to, prevent, and appropriately manage pain, distress, and suffering of patients.

The professional virtue of integrity is the bedrock professional virtue. It requires the doctor to provide clinical care, conduct research, and teach to standards of intellectual and moral excellence. Intellectual excellence requires the doctor to base clinical care and research on deliberative—evidence-based, rigorous, transparent, and accountable—clinical judgement. Deliberative clinical judgement is essential for the task of responsibly reducing variation in the processes of patient care and thereby improving quality and safety. Moral excellence requires the doctor to focus primarily on the protection and promotion of the patient's health-related interests and keep individual and group self-interest systematically secondary.

Ethical principles provide guidance on how to protect and promote the health-related interests of the patient. The ethical principle of beneficence has ancient roots and the word, 'beneficence', was first used in Percival's *Medical Ethics* of 1803 (11). This ethical principle requires the physician to identify and provide clinical care that is reliably expected in deliberative clinical judgement to result in net clinical benefit for the patient. The ethical principle of beneficence supports the clinical concept of medically reasonable: a form of clinical management is medically reasonable when it is technically possible and in deliberative clinical judgement is expected to result in net clinical benefit. The ethical principle of beneficence subsumes the well-known admonition to 'first do no harm', which is known as the ethical principle of non-maleficence. It is not well appreciated that the Hippocratic text *Epidemics* does not say 'first do no harm' but 'As to diseases, make a habit of two things –to help, or at least to do no harm' (15). This means that the doctor should first aim to benefit the patient and then, when the limits of medicine to alter the course of disease or injury are being approached, to proceed with caution to prevent net iatrogenic clinical harm to the patient. This beautifully captures the relationship between beneficence and non-maleficence: the latter should guide deliberative clinical judgement when the limits of clinical care to benefit the patient are being approached or have been exceeded. Beneficence is thus the more comprehensive and clinically useful of the two principles.

The ethical principle of respect for autonomy requires the doctor (a) to empower the patient with information about the nature, benefits, and risks of the medically reasonable alternatives for the management of the patient's condition, disability, disease, or injury; (b) to support the patient as she undertakes to understand and evaluate this information and set her priorities; and (c) to take reasonable measures to ensure that the patient's decision-making process is voluntary (1–3), that is, free from controlling internal influences such as uncontrolled anxiety or fear and external influences such as the attempts of family members to dominate or take over the decision-making process (16).

The ethical principle of healthcare justice applies to health policy regarding populations of patients (3). For obstetrician-gynaecologists, these are female, pregnant, fetal, and neonatal patients. In general, the ethical principle of justice requires that all like cases be treated alike. This very general formulation is too abstract to provide clinical guidance. However, when specified to the healthcare setting, healthcare justice does provide guidance. In the specific context of healthcare, cases are alike on the basis of deliberative clinical judgement about diagnosis and clinical management. Healthcare justice therefore requires the doctor to manage each diagnosis on the basis of deliberative clinical judgement about the medically reasonable alternatives for managing that diagnosis. The ethical principles of healthcare justice and beneficence are thus closely related.

Obligations of doctors and rights of patients

Ethical principles are essential for understanding the key ethical concepts of rights and obligations. A right is a justified claim to be treated in a specified way. A right can be a negative right, that is, a claim to non-interference. For example, the first and second components of the ethical principle of respect of autonomy justify the patient's right to make an informed decision and its third component justifies the patient's right to make a voluntary decision. A right can be a positive right, that is, a claim to the time, energy, and resources of others to protect and promote one's interests. The right to healthcare is a positive right. The ethical principle of healthcare justice supports a positive right to effective healthcare, that is, clinical care that is supported in deliberative clinical judgement. A right can also be a combination of a negative and positive right, for example, when a patient refuses all medically reasonable alternatives but remains a patient. For instance, a patient with well-documented, intrapartum placenta previa may refuse caesarean delivery but remain a patient, in effect exercising a positive right to vaginal delivery.

Rights generate obligations or duties of doctors, two words that can be used interchangeably. We will use 'obligation' in this chapter. In the professional responsibility model, the relationship between the doctor and the patient is asymmetrical. The doctor's relationship to the patient is based on the four professional virtues and three ethical principles and the obligations that they generate. The patient's relationship to the doctor is based on rights. A very important feature of the professional responsibility model is that professional obligations can sometimes justifiably limit patients' rights, especially positive rights and combined negative and positive rights.

Informed decision-making

The professional virtue of integrity and the ethical principles of beneficence and respect for autonomy shape the informed decision-making process with the patient who has decision-making capacity or the surrogate of the patient who does not have decision-making capacity. This process begins with the doctor identifying, on the basis of deliberative clinical judgement, the medically reasonable alternatives for managing the patient's condition, disease, disability, or injury. To repeat, that a form of clinical management is technically possible is not sufficient for considering it to be medically reasonable. The doctor should then present the medically reasonable alternatives to the decision maker, patient or surrogate, and provide in lay terms the nature of each alternative along with the clinical benefits and clinical risks of each. This disclosure does not include theoretical benefits and risks. The determination that a form of clinical management is medically reasonable is an expert clinical judgement and therefore not a lay judgement. The doctor should then support the decision maker, alert to deficits in paying attention, memory, and recall, reasoning from present events to their expected consequences (cognitive understanding), believing that those consequences could happen to the patient (appreciation), and evaluating those consequences (evaluative understanding) (17). The point of this is that the doctor's role in the informed decision-making process should not be at 'arm's length' but engaged and supportive.

There are two clinical contexts in which the doctor should be directive. The first is when there is only one medically reasonable alternative, which the doctor should recommend. The second is when, among two or more medically reasonable alternatives, one is clinically superior in deliberative clinical judgement, which the doctor should recommend.

Sometimes, among medically reasonable alternatives, no one stands out as superior in deliberative clinical judgement. In this clinical context, the doctor should be cautious in making a recommendation and explain the basis for doing so, for example, that one form of medically reasonable care is well supported by the doctor's clinical experience.

It sometimes occurs that a form of clinical management that was justifiably considered medically reasonable and therefore was initiated should later be considered to no longer result in net clinical benefit, for example, failure to progress in labour or the progression of a critically ill female patient to the end stage of gynaecological cancer. In such clinical circumstances, the doctor should explain that the clinical management is no longer medically reasonable and recommend that it be discontinued in favour of a medically reasonable alternative, for example, caesarean delivery for failure to progress in labour and comfort care when a patient has end-stage, terminal gynaecological cancer. We emphasize that making recommendations of the kinds we have described here is not disrespectful of patient autonomy or inconsistent with shared decision-making, because such recommendations empower the decision maker with the valued input of the doctor's professional clinical judgement.

The decision maker considers the information that has been provided, with the goal of achieving adequate cognitive understanding, appreciation, and evaluative understanding. The decision maker then expresses a preference, which should be based on cognitive understanding, appreciation, and evaluative understanding.

Responding to refusal of medically reasonable clinical management

There are two outcomes of the informed decision-making process. The most common, by far, is that the decision maker authorizes medically reasonable clinical management. In rare circumstances, however, the decision maker may reject all medically reasonable alternatives. If the patient dismisses the doctor, refusal should be understood as the exercise of a negative right. If the patient remains a patient, refusal should be understood as a negative right combined with a positive right to clinical management that is not medically reasonable.

Doctors should not take refusal personally, because doing so interferes with an ethically justified approach. Responding to such refusals should begin by ruling out inadvertent miscommunication, which can sometimes occur when the patient is being attended by multiple clinicians. The patient should be provided with accurate information and the informed decision-making process recycled. If this fails, the doctor should be alert to deficits in decision-making capacity of the patient and address them, with the assistance of mental health professionals as needed. The goal should be reversing these deficits so that the patient can exercise her autonomy. This is known as assisted decision-making (17). If this fails, then the patient should be evaluated for irreversible deficits of decision-making and a surrogate decision maker identified on the basis of applicable law. The surrogate decision maker should be guided by the substituted judgement, that is, making a decision on the basis of the reliably identifiable patient's values and beliefs (18). If this standard cannot be met, the surrogate should be guided by the best interests standard, which is beneficence based (18).

Sometimes a patient who refuses all medically reasonable forms of clinical management has intact decision-making capacity. In all cases, the doctor should fulfil his or her obligation of informed refusal: explain in detail the risks that the patient is taking; document this disclosure in the record; and ask her to reconsider. If the patient does not do so and dismisses the doctor, this should not be taken personally and the patient should be informed that she is welcome to return for care, especially if her condition worsens. If the patient does not reconsider but wants to remain a patient, then the patient is in effect exercising a positive right to non-beneficial clinical management. The provision of non-beneficial clinical management, especially when it is clinically harmful, is not consistent with professional integrity, beneficence, or non-maleficence (19, 20). There is therefore no ethical obligation to provide such care.

Responding to requests for non-beneficial clinical management

Sometimes patients will make an unprompted request for non-beneficial clinical management. The doctor should be guided by Gregory's advice, based on what he called the professional virtue of candour (10): assess the patient's request to determine whether it is medically reasonable. If her request passes muster, it is consistent with the professional responsibility model to include consideration of it in the informed decision-making process. If it does not pass muster, then it is ethically impermissible to implement it. The doctor should recommend against it and explain the basis in deliberative clinical judgement for this recommendation. Despite being importuned, the doctor should repeat the recommendation and its explanation and explain that the request will not be fulfilled.

Clinical ethical topics in gynaecology

Contraception and sterilization

There are rarely in deliberative clinical judgement beneficence-based clinical indications for the prevention of pregnancy, secondary to severe medical illness, such as end-stage heart failure. Contraception and sterilization are the only medically reasonable alternatives and should be recommended. The patient or the patient's surrogate is free to authorize either, on the basis of the patient's values and beliefs.

Much more commonly, women without such medical indications wish to prevent pregnancy. So long as there are no medical contraindications, the doctor should engage in shared decision-making by presenting all medically reasonable options without making a recommendation and supporting the patient or surrogate in making a well-informed decision. The doctor should emphasize the irreversibility of sterilization and the distinction between self-administered and implantable contraception. In some cases, counselling by a mental health professional may be needed, for example, when the doctor has clinical concern about impairments of the patient's decision-making capacity. In some cases, counselling should depart from shared decision-making and become directive, for example, when a 20-year-old nulliparous patient who wishes to prevent pregnancy asks for sterilization before all of the options to prevent pregnancy have been considered. Respect for autonomy calls for empowering such a patient with the information that she needs, to prevent an inadequately informed, precipitous decision, rather than simply acquiescing. The professional responsibility model supports the obligation to protect such a patient from herself by directive counselling aimed at the informed exercise of her positive right to request sterilization.

Assisted reproduction

The ethics of assisted reproduction has one of the most extensive literatures. Clinically and ethically sophisticated guidance has been provided by professional associations such as the Society for Assisted Reproduction (21) in the United States and the Royal College of Obstetricians and Gynaecologists (22) in the United Kingdom, as well as government agencies such as Human Embryo and Fertilisation Authority (23) in the United Kingdom.

We therefore focus only on the obligations of doctors who provide primary gynaecological care for women with limitations on fertility. Professional integrity and beneficence both require the doctor to provide a comprehensive workup of the patient, including referral to fertility specialists when indicated. This workup should also aim to identify risks of assisted reproduction and pregnancy for the patient, so that she can be provided with this clinically significant information. Respect for patient autonomy then requires the doctor to present the results of this evaluation to the female patient and assist her in understanding and evaluating the medically reasonable alternatives for managing it. The doctor should also offer to assist the patient to think through fundamental, related questions: How important is it to you to attempt to bear a child? How do you assess the biopsychosocial benefits and risks of assisted reproduction? Are you prepared for what could be considerable out-of-pocket (depending on scope of insurance, co-payments, and deductibles) financial costs? Are you prepared for the biopsychosocial benefits and risks of a multiple pregnancy that can result when more than one embryo is transferred? The doctor should offer to include the patient's partner or others, as the patient agrees, as she addresses these questions. Some women will accept limitations on their fertility and elect not to proceed with reproductive medical service. Some women will not accept such limitations. For such patients, the doctor should make a referral to a centre of excellence and prepare for the management of a subsequent pregnancy should one result.

Ectopic pregnancy

The standard of care for ectopic pregnancy may be so obvious that ethical justification is obvious. It is always good ethical practice in ethics to spell out the obvious. Ectopic pregnancy, with the very rare exception of some abdominal pregnancies, will not result in a livebirth. Clinical maintenance of such pregnancies is therefore physiologically futile. Provision of such clinical maintenance violates both professional integrity and beneficence. Moreover, such pregnancies pose a threat to the woman's health and life, risks that are not offset by the benefit of livebirth. This reinforces the violation of professional integrity and beneficence. There is therefore only one medically reasonable alternative, ending the pregnancy promptly, and it should therefore be strongly recommended.

In very rare circumstance, a patient may refuse the recommendation on religious grounds. Including appropriately trained and experienced colleagues from pastoral care could be invaluable in persuading the woman to accept the physiologically futile nature of the pregnancy and that the risks to her will not have the benefit of a live-born child. The woman's right to a voluntary decision becomes unjustifiably violated when she is being subjected to potentially controlling influences, for example, insistence by a partner or family member that she refuse ending of the pregnancy. These individuals should be informed that their role is to respect and support the patient's exercise of her autonomy in the decision-making process and not usurp it.

Gynaecological cancers

There is a strict beneficence-based obligation of the primary doctor to make a timely and effective referral whenever gynaecological cancer is detected. Doctors who specialize in the management of gynaecological cancers have distinctive ethical obligations to patients referred to them. As the clinical management of the various gynaecological cancers continues to evolve, the range of medically reasonable alternatives will expand. It is therefore incumbent upon the gynaecological oncologist to become well informed about all of the medically reasonable alternatives for a newly diagnosed patient and inform the patient about them. The professional virtue of self-sacrifice requires that this disclosure should not be limited by self-interest originating in such considerations as lack of experience or comfort with new approaches with newer modalities, financial gain for one's practice, or limited resources.

Gynaecological oncologists have an indispensable role to play in preparing patients whose disease is not responding to treatment for decision-making about the management of end-stage disease. The oncologist should explain the concept that, while current treatment remains medically reasonable, it should be expected to become no longer medically reasonable in the end stages of disease. The oncologist should add that, when deliberative clinical judgement supports this view, the oncologist will recommend cessation of treatment and redirection of the goals of care to comfort and a dignified dying process, including hospice care where it is available. The patient should be supported to achieve cognitive understanding, appreciation, and evaluation of the clinical reality of the limits of medicine to alter end-stage disease. Her preferences should be elicited and documented in the patient's record. She should be encouraged to communicate her preferences, to prevent provision of life-sustaining treatment by default (24).

Where supported by law and health policy, the patient should be encouraged to document her preferences in an advance directive. A directive to physicians, or living will, communicates preferences directly to the care team and takes effect when the patient has a terminal or irreversible condition as defined in applicable law and has lost decision-making capacity. A medical power of attorney, or durable power of attorney for healthcare, allows the patient to appoint an agent to act as her surrogate decision maker when the patient has lost decision-making capacity. Patients completing a medical power of attorney should be strongly encouraged to write down their preferences in the document and to communicate them both to the agent and to family members.

Decision-making with adolescent patients

There is ethically justified, practical guidance from the American Academy of Paediatrics regarding the professional responsibility of doctors to include paediatric patients, especially adolescents who are legal minors, in the decision-making process about their clinical care (25). The Academy invokes a concept based on respect for autonomy: paediatric assent. This concept calls for adolescent patients to be involved in a developmentally appropriate way in the decision-making process about their clinical care. Paediatric assent is to be implemented in clinical practice in four steps:

1. Helping the patient achieve a developmentally appropriate awareness of the nature of his or her condition.
2. Telling the patient what he or she can expect with tests and treatment(s).
3. Making a clinical assessment of the patient's understanding of the situation and the factors influencing how he or she is responding (including whether there is inappropriate pressure to accept testing or therapy).
4. Soliciting an expression of the patient's willingness to accept the proposed care (25).

The ethical concept of paediatric assent requires the gynaecologist to respond to parental requests not to inform the patient by explaining the concept of paediatric assent and its implication: the child should be informed and involved in a developmentally appropriate way. The child and her parents should be supported as they adjust to this change.

Multicultural challenges

One of the distinctive features of life in modern nation-states is their cultural pluralism. Patients also travel from their home countries for obstetric or gynaecological care. Finally, some women are involuntarily displaced by conflict or famine or forced migration. As a consequence, a doctor's patients will present from backgrounds that are remarkably diverse in their values and beliefs, including values and beliefs about the roles and prerogatives of women. Some female patients may accept these values and beliefs and others may not.

Managing the challenges of multiculturalism in a professionally responsible way should be guided by two ethical considerations: (a) adherence to the obligations generated by the professional virtues and ethical principles, and (b) respect for the values and traditions of the cultures from which patients come.

In some cultures, patients with serious diagnoses, such as gynaecological cancers, are not to be told their diagnosis and others in the family are expected to make decisions for them. Freedman provides guidance for the management of such cultural practices (26). The professional virtue of integrity and the ethical principle of respect for autonomy are clear: patients who have decision-making capacity have the right to participate in the decision-making process about their clinical care. This includes the right to opt out of this role, if the patient wishes. Moreover, some women may not accept the passive role that is expected of them by their culture and respect for autonomy requires that the preferred role of such patients be identified and implemented. Freedman introduced the concept of 'offering truth' to address culturally based requests that a patient with decision-making capacity not be told the diagnosis or make decisions about its clinical management. The family should be informed that the patient has the right to determine her decision-making role and that she will be informed by her doctor that her family is making decisions for her and asked if this is acceptable to her. This approach risks some psychosocial disruption in the family but this disruption should be assumed to be temporary and therefore manageable.

There is an additional, practical reason why requests not to inform patients—adult and minor adolescent alike—about their diagnoses and treatment should not be implemented. In the modern hospital, care is delivered in multidisciplinary teams, the membership of which changes over time. It is inevitable that the patient will be informed, because some team members will fulfil their professional responsibility to inform patients, which the physician in charge will not be able to control. Patients talk to each other and overhear conversations. The promise not to inform the patient cannot as a practical reality be kept. The patient will learn her diagnosis. It is far better that she learn it in a way structured by the informed decision-making process or in the paediatric assent process.

In some cultures there is an expectation that women who marry for the first time are virgins. In some cultures there is also a practice of vaginal cutting. Vaginal cutting, that is, female genital mutilation, is illegal in many countries, including the United Kingdom and the United States. It also violates women's human rights. Ethically and legally, genital mutilation is completely incompatible with professional integrity. It follows that there is no ethical justification in the professional responsibility model for these practices. Doctors are therefore ethically prohibited from performing a physical examination to determine whether a female patient's hymen is intact or from surgically altering female genitalia (27). In cultural contexts in which non-adherence by the woman with the culture's expectations may put her life in danger, the doctor should report this danger to law enforcement.

Clinical ethical topics in obstetrics

The professional responsibility model of obstetric ethics is based on the ethical concept of the fetus as a patient and respect for the pregnant patient's autonomy. The concept of being a patient is beneficence based, creating an obligation to protect the health and life of the fetus. The authors have argued elsewhere that the viable (approximately 24 completed weeks of gestation) fetus is a patient and that the previable fetus is a patient as a function of the pregnant woman's autonomous decision to confer this moral status on the fetus (1–3). In the professional responsibility model, when the fetus is a patient, the doctor has three ethical obligations, all of which must be considered in all cases: (a) beneficence-based obligations to the pregnant patient, (b) autonomy-based obligations to the pregnant patient, and (c) beneficence-based obligations to the fetal patient. In clinical obstetrics, almost always these obligations are in concert. When these obligations are incompatible, none automatically takes precedence over the others; the priority among them must be established by reasoned argument.

In this respect, the professional responsibility model differs from two other approaches in the literature. Both appeal to rights and treat rights as absolute, that is, admitting of no exceptions. One approach we call maternal rights-based reductionism and the other, fetal rights-based reductionism (1, 3). Both are ethically and clinically simplistic but inadequate for the complexities of obstetric practice.

Offering induced abortion or feticide

The ethical justification for offering feticide after viability requires the reliable diagnosis of a severe fetal anomaly: a certain or near-certain diagnosis of an anomaly that is reliably expected either to result in death, even with aggressive obstetric and neonatal intervention, or short-term survival with severe and irreversible deficit of cognitive developmental capacity (28, 29). The beneficence-based obligation to protect the life of a fetus that has been diagnosed with a severe anomaly has reached its limits, because the outcomes of death or of short-term survival with severe and irreversible deficit of cognitive developmental capacity cannot be prevented (28, 29). When a viable fetus has a severe anomaly, offering feticide followed by termination of pregnancy is ethically appropriate. It is ethically impermissible to offer feticide for viable fetuses without anomalies or with less-than-severe anomalies, such as Down syndrome or achondroplasia. This is because less-than-severe anomalies do not involve a high probability of death or a high probability of the absence or virtual absence of cognitive developmental capacity (28, 29).

There are ethical justifications for offering induced abortion before viability. The first is based on a deliberative clinical judgement that continuing pregnancy poses a threat to the health or life of the pregnant woman. When deliberative clinical judgement is that continuing pregnancy poses a risk to the pregnant woman's health or life, she should be informed about this matter and offered the alternative of induced abortion. Some women, because of moral convictions about the general moral status of the fetus, will refuse this offer. They should be informed that their refusal increases the risk that their health could be severely compromised and that they could die. The final decision to remain pregnant or to elect induced abortion is ultimately a function of the pregnant woman's autonomy and should be respected by the physician.

The second justification for offering feticide before viability is based on the deliberative clinical judgement that continuing pregnancy poses a threat to the life or health of coexistent fetuses. This can occur in higher-order pregnancies and twin pregnancies in which the continued existence of the anomalous fetus that is causing hydramnios poses a threat to the health or life of the other fetus. Current evidence supports the clinical judgement that these risks can be reduced by selective feticide (30). When deliberative clinical judgement is that continuing multifetal, previable pregnancy poses a risk to the health or life of the other fetus or fetuses, the pregnant woman should be informed about this matter and offered the alternative of selective feticide. Some women, because of moral convictions about the general moral status of the fetus, will refuse this offer. They should be informed that their refusal increases the risk that the pregnancy will end before viability without any surviving fetuses or end prematurely after viability with increased risk of infant mortality and morbidity. The decision to remain pregnant, to elect induced abortion, or to elect selective feticide is ultimately a function of the pregnant woman's autonomy and should be respected by the physician.

When deliberative clinical judgement is that continuing a previable pregnancy does not pose an increased risk to the health or life of the pregnant woman or fetuses, the only remaining justification for offering induced abortion or feticide is autonomy based. Some pregnant women will request an induced abortion. For others, a previable pregnancy will be diagnosed with an anomaly or a viable pregnancy will be diagnosed with a severe anomaly. For some women, a complication occurs that threatens the successful continuation of a previable pregnancy, such as preterm premature rupture of membranes. Some pregnant women will directly or indirectly express concern about remaining pregnant or will be concerned about a multiple birth and will prefer for economic or other personal reasons to have a singleton pregnancy. Physicians should respond to these women by discussing the option of induced abortion and, when appropriate, explaining time limitations created by applicable law.

In response to the offer of induced abortion, physicians should plan for pregnant women to sort themselves into three subgroups (31). Some women will want to continue pregnancy because they decide to accept whatever child results. Some will not want to remain pregnant and will elect induced abortion. Some will be uncertain about whether to continue the pregnancy. Respecting the autonomy of pregnant women requires doctors to respect this self-sorting, by limiting their role to providing information in a nondirective fashion in a shared decision-making process (offering but not recommending induced abortion) that these women can use to address and resolve their uncertainty.

Shared decision-making should guide physicians in discussing induced abortion with women with previable pregnancies who remain uncertain. Physicians should refrain from making, suggesting, or implying a recommendation about continuation or termination of a previable pregnancy. Directive counselling towards continuation of a previable pregnancy based on alleged benefit to the pregnant woman of providing information about fetal development or showing images of fetal development, to prevent remorse or regret, lacks an evidence base. Such directive counselling is an ethically impermissible distortion of the physician's professional role in the informed consent process (3). All women should be informed

that their decision about termination is time-limited, given the legal availability of induced abortion. In addition, in order to respect autonomy, the doctor should provide frank, evidence-based information about maternal or fetal conditions, even if it is emotionally distressing. Doctors need to make the time available for the sometimes extensive discussions required to disclose the medical facts and assist the woman to assimilate those medical facts into her decision-making process.

Individual conscience concerns the values and beliefs of a doctor that arise from sources outside the ethical concept of medicine as a profession, such as upbringing and religion. Individual conscience does not justifiably place limits on the ethics of offering induced abortion or feticide after and before viability, when the earlier mentioned ethical justifications apply. This is because every doctor's obligation to provide appropriate information in the informed consent process is a matter of professional responsibility, not individual conscience. Moreover, one cannot predict how women will sort themselves in response to offering induced abortion or feticide. Subsequent decisions are a function ultimately of the pregnant woman's autonomy. It is a mistake to think that offering induced abortion or feticide makes the doctor somehow responsible for the informed, deliberative, and voluntary decisions of a pregnant patient that may not be consistent with the doctor's individual conscience, because the offer does not control the pregnant woman's decision-making process: she controls it (32).

Performing induced abortion and feticide

Before viability, it is ethically permissible in the professional responsibility model to perform an induced abortion. This is because the pregnant woman is free to withhold or withdraw the moral status of being a patient from the previable fetus at her discretion. Induced abortion of the previable fetus in such circumstances therefore does not involve the killing of a patient (2, 3). For the same reason, performing feticide in a previable pregnancy is ethically permissible.

Pregnant women should not be presumed to understand that expelling the near-viable fetus with a severe anomaly from the uterus could result in a live birth and that feticide can prevent this outcome. In such circumstances, live birth creates an increased risk of preventable neonatal morbidity. There is a beneficence-based obligation to prevent this risk. Refusal of feticide can also be seen as contradictory because election of termination of pregnancy means that the pregnant woman does not wish to have a live-born child issue from her current pregnancy. Such contradictory thinking is evidence of significant impairment of the capacity for autonomous decision-making. It is therefore reasonable for the doctor to require that the pregnant woman accept feticide as a condition for performing termination of her pregnancy. Performing feticide in this setting protects the doctor from being accused of performing a so-called partial-birth abortion. The correct account is that the doctor is evacuating the uterus after ethically justified iatrogenic fetal demise.

Some doctors may have objections in individual conscience to participation in induced abortion or feticide. Respecting individual conscience means that such doctors should be free to refuse to perform induced abortion or feticide. An important implication of this analysis of individual conscience is that a requirement of residents or fellows to participate in induced abortion or feticide is ethically impermissible. However, a requirement that trainees have an appropriate fund of knowledge about these procedures and an appropriate fund of knowledge and clinical skills in managing their complications is consistent with individual conscience and a matter of professional obligation (2, 3).

Doctors with individual conscience-based objections to induced abortion or feticide must keep in mind, when they refuse to perform the procedure, that individual conscience does *not* govern the doctor's professional role. It is therefore impermissible for the doctor to invoke individual conscience to justify expression of judgements about the morality of a woman's election of induced abortion or feticide or of colleagues who perform these procedures (2, 3).

Referring for induced abortion or feticide

The ethics of referral for induced abortion or feticide is straightforward for physicians who do not have conscience-based objections to induced abortion. They can make what we call direct referrals (33). The referring physician sees to it that the patient will be seen by a colleague competent and willing to perform the procedure with the patient's informed consent.

Direct referral appears not to be an option for doctors with a conscience-based objection to induced abortion or feticide, because of the explicit involvement of the physician in the subsequent termination of a pregnancy. To concomitantly respect the pregnant woman's autonomy and the individual conscience of doctors, an indirect referral for termination of pregnancy should be made. Indirect referral is both autonomy based and beneficence based. When it is obligatory to offer induced abortion or feticide, respect for the pregnant woman's autonomy in previable pregnancies requires the doctor to inform her that induced abortion or feticide is an option. Beneficence requires the doctor to provide information about clinics or agencies, such as Planned Parenthood in the United States, that provide competent and safe induced abortion or feticide. The doctor's individual conscience is not violated, because whether an induced abortion or feticide subsequently occurs is solely a function of the pregnant woman's subsequent exercise of her autonomy. The referring doctor is therefore not responsible for her subsequent decision: the woman is. Direct referral for induced abortion or feticide is not ethically required but is ethically permissible. Conscience-based objections to direct referral for induced abortion or feticide have merit; conscience-based objections to indirect referral do not (33).

Intrapartum management

Sometimes, caesarean delivery is well supported and vaginal delivery is not supported in beneficence-based deliberative clinical judgement. For example, when there is a previous classical incision on the uterus, caesarean delivery is clearly preferable to vaginal delivery because caesarean delivery prevents the fetal and maternal risk of a ruptured classical incision in the uterus (34). Vaginal delivery in these circumstances would result in a substantial increase in preventable maternal–fetal morbidity and mortality. No well-founded beneficence-based clinical judgement could support offering vaginal delivery to women with a previous classical uterine incision. The professional responsibility model therefore requires that caesarean delivery should be recommended to such patients. With the patient's consent, it should then be performed.

Sometimes, caesarean delivery and vaginal delivery are both well supported in beneficence-based deliberative clinical judgement. In some clinical circumstances there is scientific controversy as to whether caesarean delivery or vaginal delivery is the better alternative. Competing well-founded, beneficence-based, deliberative clinical judgements regarding how to balance the fetal benefit of preventing harm against the maternal risk of caesarean delivery generate these controversies. Whenever two management strategies are well supported in beneficence-based, deliberative clinical judgement, both should be offered to the pregnant woman so that she can exercise her autonomy in a shared decision-making process.

Trial of labour after a low transverse caesarean delivery (TOLAC), or vaginal birth after caesarean delivery (VBAC), illustrates this category. In 2010, both the United States National Institutes of Health (NIH) Consensus Panel (35) and American College of Obstetricians and Gynecologists (ACOG) (36) issued updated statements on VBAC. In the United Kingdom, the National Institute for Health and Care Excellence (NICE) report provides a thorough review of the clinical benefits and risks to both pregnant and fetal patients and calls for an evidence-based approach to the informed consent process (37). Both agree that there should be an evidence-based informed consent process in which pregnant women with a prior caesarean delivery be counselled concerning VBAC. Here we provide an ethically justified, practical to the informed consent process for TOLAC.

When both repeat caesarean and TOLAC are supported in evidence-based, beneficence-based, deliberative clinical judgement, both should be offered in clinical settings where TOLAC can be performed safely. The NIH Consensus Panel (35) and ACOG (36) statements are in consensus that TOLAC after a previous single low transverse uterine incision is medically reasonable and should be offered when there has been one previous low transverse incision. Current evidence supports the beneficence-based clinical judgement that the clinical risks of TOLAC to both pregnant and fetal patients are acceptable when there has been one previous low transverse incision. Planned repeat caesarean delivery also has acceptable risks to both pregnant and fetal patients. Both therefore should be offered in the decision-making consent process to the pregnant woman with one previous low transverse incision, because both are medically reasonable in this clinical circumstance. Counselling about these alternatives should be non-directive in a shared decision-making process.

There is controversy concerning TOLAC after two low transverse incisions. The ACOG statement, on the basis of level B evidence, states: 'Women with two previous low transverse incisions may be considered candidates for TOLAC' (36). The NIH Consensus Panel was silent on this topic (35). Level B evidence is inherently controversial in beneficence-based clinical judgement. As a result, doctors should responsibly manage competing evidence-based, beneficence clinical judgement about the safety for pregnant and fetal patients of TOLAC when the pregnant woman has had two previous low transverse incisions. In the informed consent process, responsible management is achieved by offering TOLAC but only when the doctor explains the uncertainties of the current state of the evidence in this clinical circumstance.

For women with one previous low transverse incision, both TOLAC and planned repeat caesarean delivery should be offered. TOLAC should be offered only in clinical settings properly equipped and staffed to do so. Doctors should recommend against TOLAC when the pregnant woman has had a previous classical incision. TOLAC after two previous low transverse incisions may be offered provided that the informed consent process presents the uncertainties of the evidence.

Sometimes vaginal delivery is well supported in beneficence-based clinical judgement and caesarean delivery is not supported in beneficence-based deliberative clinical judgement. When deliberative beneficence-based clinical judgement concludes that vaginal delivery is the only medically reasonable alternative, it should be recommended. Caesarean delivery involves a clinically significant increased risk of unnecessary and preventable maternal morbidity and mortality (38). The unnecessary and preventable nature of the risks of caesarean delivery loom large in this beneficence-based deliberative clinical judgement. As a consequence, the professional responsibility model prohibits the offering of caesarean delivery; only vaginal delivery should be recommended.

Some women will, unprompted, request non-indicated caesarean delivery. This is known as patient-choice caesarean delivery, maternal-choice caesarean delivery, or caesarean delivery on demand. One review reported a range from 2% of patient-choice caesarean deliveries in Canada to 17% in Australia and perhaps as high as 80% in Brazil (39).

How to respond to such requests has become controversial throughout the world. In the United States, for example, the ACOG stated in a committee opinion in 2003 that, while the right of patients to refuse unwanted surgery is well known, less clear is the right of patients to have a surgical procedure when scientific evidence supporting it is incomplete, of poor quality, or totally lacking (40). The Committee concluded that the evidence to support the benefit of caesarean delivery remains incomplete and that there are insufficient morbidity and mortality data to compare caesarean delivery with planned vaginal delivery. In addition, the United States NIH convened a 2006 conference regarding this issue that concluded that there is insufficient evidence to evaluate fully the benefits and risks of primary caesarean delivery as compared to vaginal delivery, and that more research is needed (41). The NIH conference concluded: 'The magnitude of caesarean delivery on maternal request is difficult to quantify. There is insufficient evidence to evaluate fully the benefits and risks of caesarean delivery on maternal request compared with planned vaginal delivery. Any decision to perform a caesarean delivery on maternal request should be carefully individualized and consistent with ethical principles' (20).

In the United Kingdom, the NICE 2011 report notes the increasing rates of 'maternal request for caesarean delivery' and that a common reason for such requests is the pregnant woman's concern for the safety of her baby. The report also notes that obstetricians implement as much as half of the requests that they receive. The report provides guidance for obstetricians in response to maternal request for caesarean delivery: 'When a woman requests a CS [caesarean section] the first response should be to determine the reason for the request and the factors that are contributing to the request. This can then be followed by the provision of information that compares the risks and benefits of planned CS and vaginal birth' (37). The report makes the following recommendation: 'For women requesting a CS, if after discussion and offer of support (including perinatal mental health support for women with anxiety about childbirth), a vaginal birth is still not an acceptable option, offer a planned CS' (37). Obstetricians unwilling to perform caesarean delivery on maternal request 'should refer the woman to an obstetrician who will perform CS' (37).

Currently, beneficence-based deliberative clinical judgement favours vaginal delivery (2). Hence, counselling should be directive, as opposed to non-directive counselling, in response to requests for non-indicated caesarean delivery: the obstetrician should clearly recommend vaginal delivery. We therefore disagree with the NICE report's purely non-directive approach (37).

The obstetrician is expected to exercise professional, beneficence-based clinical judgement when making clinical recommendations and present the medically reasonable alternatives as well as the alternative of non-intervention. The patient can then exercise her rights to accept or refuse intervention. Respect for autonomy in informed decision-making does not warrant routine offering of caesarean delivery, because doing so is not supported in beneficence-based clinical judgement. Routinely offering caesarean delivery does not empower pregnant women.

Considering beneficence-based and autonomy-based obligations to the pregnant woman together, there is no ethical obligation to offer non-indicated caesarean delivery to all pregnant women. Offering caesarean delivery to all patients does not promote their health-related interests. Obstetricians must rigorously adhere to the requirments of professional integrity, to prevent potential bias from influencing the physician's discussion with the patient introduced by economic gain or other forms of self-interest. The NICE report's indications for offering planned caesarean delivery do not include routine offering of caesarean delivery (37) and therefore reflect this ethical position.

Professionally responsible advocacy in obstetrics and gynaecology

'Women and children first' is certainly a familiar phrase but its origin is less well known (42, 43). In 1852, the HMS Birkenhead, with more than 600 sailors, troops, and civilians aboard, was evacuating the civilians from Cape Town, South Africa, during the Cape Frontier War (1850–1853). At 2 am on the morning of 26 February she struck unchartered rocks near Danger Point and began to take on water and sink. The number of lifeboats was not sufficient to convey all safely off the doomed ship. Many of the troops on board drowned in their berths as the ship foundered. The remaining men and officers of the 74th Regiment of Foot were mustered on deck by their commanding officer, Lt. Colonel Seton. He realized the nature of the situation and ordered his men to stand fast while the women and children were boarded onto the lifeboats. His soldiers obeyed and went down with the ship (44). While it is not known whether Lt. Colonel Seton used the phrase, 'women and children first', he is credited with being among the first to put it into practice. His heroism and that of his men allowed the women and children on board to be saved.

The Birkenhead incident occurred during a period of British imperialism and colonialism. Any incident from such a time would seem to be out of place as an exemplar for the ethics of women's health policy today. We think otherwise: making 'women and children first' was a defining moment in the history of world civilizations and therefore has direct relevance for healthcare today.

The reality is that women and children are not first in our world; indeed, they are often last. This is especially the case in low-resource regions, which often do not provide adequate healthcare for women and children, as reflected in perinatal mortality rates (45). International organizations, such as UNICEF (45), the World Health Organization (46), and the World Bank (47), and international associations of physicians, such as the International Federation of Gynecology and Obstetrics (FIGO) (48), Matres Mundi (49), and the World Association of Perinatal Medicine (50), have led major efforts to identify problems in obstetric and neonatal care in developing countries and have advocated for improvement. The International Academy of Perinatal Medicine has added its voice to these advocacy efforts, with its 'New York Declaration' on 'Woman and Children First', which was presented at the United Nations on 7 July 2008. The Declaration defined sources of bias against the just allocation of healthcare resources for women and children in low-resource regions (42, 43).

The lack of prioritization for healthcare for women and children is not confined to low-resource regions. This can also be a problem in the United States and other high-resource regions. This is not compatible with the ethical principle of healthcare justice, which requires that all pregnant patients receive treatment based on deliberative clinical judgement about the clinical management of pregnancy.

Challenges to healthcare justice in the care of pregnant, fetal, and neonatal patients arise from the self-interest of adults, age bias, and economic bias, as well as economic bias against pregnant, fetal, and neonatal patients and obstetric services.

Obstetricians' advocacy for healthcare justice for pregnant, fetal, and neonatal patients should begin with identifying and exposing allocations of healthcare resources based on these biases. Obstetricians should then advocate for highly efficient, cost-conscious obstetric care that seeks to continuously improve its quality and safety.

There is a tendency in all healthcare systems for economic values to trump or automatically override all other considerations, especially including professional integrity. By getting their own financial houses in order, and advocating for the equal importance of pregnant, fetal, and neonatal patients, obstetricians will be in a position to talk back, countering the trumping power of economic considerations.

Obstetricians are in a unique position to assume an advocacy role because they have expert scientific and clinical knowledge about how to identify and protect the health-related interests of fetal, neonatal, and pregnant patients (9). On this basis, obstetricians should advocate for healthcare priorities that create resources to support the development and global implementation of evidence-based medical care for fetal, neonatal, and pregnant patients, so that their interests are taken into account in a scientific, unbiased fashion. The goal should be the elimination, to the greatest extent possible, of national and wide area variation in the processes and outcomes of obstetric care. Ideally, where a patient lives should not make a difference to the quality of medical care that an individual receives.

Conclusion

Ethics is an essential dimension of the professionally responsible clinical practice of obstetrics and gynaecology. Our goal in this chapter has been to provide ethical guidance, based on the professional responsibility model of ethics in obstetrics and gynaecology, for commonly encountered ethical challenges in clinical practice. This model emphasizes both the professional virtues of doctors and ethical

principles. Together, these virtues and principles generate the ethical obligations of obstetrician-gynaecologists to their patients. The result is a model for ethics in obstetrics and gynaecology that is ethically sound and clinically actionable, comprehensive, and practical.

REFERENCES

1. Chervenak FA, McCullough LB, Brent RL. The professional responsibility model of obstetric ethics: avoiding the perils of clashing rights. *Am J Obstet Gynecol* 2011;**205**:315.e1–5.
2. McCullough LB, Chervenak FA. *Ethics in Obstetrics and Gynecology*. New York: Oxford University Press; 1994.
3. Chervenak FA, McCullough LB. *The Professional Responsibility Model of Perinatal Ethics*. Berlin: Walter de Gruyter; 2014.
4. von Staden H. 'In a pure and holy way:' personal and professional conduct in the Hippocratic Oath. *J Hist Med Allied Sci* 1996;**51**:404–37.
5. Baker RB. The eighteenth-century philosophical background. In: Baker RB, Porter D, Porter R (eds), *The Codification of Medical Morality: Historical and Philosophical Studies of the Formalization of Western Medical Morality in the Eighteenth and Nineteenth Centuries: Volume One: Medical Ethics and Etiquette in the Eighteenth Century*, pp. 93–8. Dordrecht: Kluwer Academic Publishers; 1993.
6. Nutton V. The discourses of European practitioners in the tradition of the Hippocratic texts. In: Baker RB, McCullough LB (eds), *The Cambridge World History of Medical Ethics*, pp. 359–62. New York: Cambridge University Press; 2009.
7. Gãlvao-Sobrinho CR. Hippocratic ideals, medical ethics, and the practice of medicine in the early middle ages: the legacy of the Hippocratic Oath. *J Hist Med Allied Sci* 1996;**51**:438–55.
8. Jonsen AR. *The Birth of Bioethics*. New York: Oxford University Press; 1998.
9. Reich WT (ed). *Encyclopedia of Bioethics*. New York: Macmillan; 1978.
10. Gregory J. Lectures on the Duties and Qualifications of a Physician. London: W. Strahan and T. Cadell, 1772. In: McCullough LB (ed), *John Gregory's Writings on Medical Ethics and Philosophy of Medicine*, pp. 161–248. Dordrecht: Kluwer Academic Publishers; 1998.
11. Percival T. *Medical Ethics, or a Code of Institutes and Precepts, Adapted to the Professional Conduct of Physicians and Surgeons*. London: Johnson & Bickerstaff; 1803.
12. McCullough LB. *John Gregory and the Invention of Professional Medical Ethics and the Profession of Medicine*. Dordrecht: Kluwer Academic Publishers; 1998.
13. McCullough LB. The ethical concept of medicine as a profession: its origins in modern medical ethics and implications for physicians. In: Kenny N, Shelton W (eds), *Lost Virtue: Professional Character Development in Medical Education*, pp. 17–27. New York: Elsevier; 2006.
14. Porter D, Porter R. *Patient's Progress: Doctors and Doctoring in Eighteenth Century England*. Cambridge: Cambridge University Press; 1989.
15. Hippocrates. Epidemics. In: Jones WHS (trans), *Hippocrates*, vol. **1**, p. 165. Cambridge, MA: Harvard University Press; 1923.
16. Faden RR, Beauchamp TL. *A History and Theory of Informed Consent*. New York: Oxford University Press; 1986.
17. McCullough LB, Coverdale JH, Chervenak FA. Ethical challenges of decision making with pregnant patients who have schizophrenia. *Am J Obstet Gynecol* 2002;**187**:696–702.

18. Buchanan AE, Brock DW. *Deciding for Others: The Ethics of Surrogate Decision Making*. Cambridge: Cambridge University Press; 1989.

19. Brett AS, McCullough LB. When patients request specific interventions: defining the limits of the physician's obligation. *N Engl J Med* 1986;**315**:1347–51.

20. Brett AS, McCullough LB. Addressing requests by patients for non-beneficial interventions. *JAMA* 2012;**307**:149–50.

21. American Society for Reproductive Medicine. Homepage. Available at: https://www.asrm.org/splash/splash.aspx (accessed 30 March 2016).

22. Royal College of Obstetricians and Gynaecologists. Homepage. Available at: https://www.rcog.org.uk/ (accessed 30 March 2016).

23. Human Embryo and Fertilisation Authority. Homepage. Available at: http://www.hfea.gov.uk/ (accessed 30 March 2016).

24. Braun UK, McCullough LB. Preventing pathways to life-sustaining treatment by default. *Ann Fam Med* 2011;**9**:250–6.

25. American Academy of Pediatrics, Committee on Bioethics. Informed consent, parental permission, and assent in pediatric practice. *Pediatrics* 1995;**95**:314–17.

26. Freedman B. Offering truth: one ethical approach to the uninformed cancer patient. *Arch Intern Med* 1993;**153**:572–6.

27. Moaddab A, McCullough LB, Chervenak FA, Dildy GA, Shamshirsaz AA. Virginity testing is unethical in professional obstetric and gynecologic ethics. *Lancet* 2016:**388**:98–100.

28. Chervenak FA, McCullough LB, Campbell S. Is third trimester abortion justified? *Br J Obstet Gynaecol* 1995;**102**:434–5.

29. Chervenak FA, McCullough LB, Campbell S. Third trimester abortion: is compassion enough? *Br J Obstet Gynæcol* 1999;**106**:293–6.

30. American College of Obstetricians and Gynecologists. Committee on Ethics. Multifetal Pregnancy Reduction. ACOG committee opinion number 369. *Obstet Gynecol* 2007;**109**:1511–15.

31. Chervenak FA, McCullough LB, Sharma G, Davis J, Gross S. Enhancing patient autonomy with risk assessment and invasive diagnosis: an ethical solution to a clinical challenge. *Am J Obstet Gynecol* 2008;**199**:19 e1–4.

32. Thorp JM, Wells SR, Bowes WA Jr, Cefalo RC. Integrity, abortion, and the pro-life perinatologist. *Hastings Cent Rep* 1995;**25**:27 8.

33. Chervenak FA, McCullough LB. The ethics of direct and indirect referral for termination of pregnancy. *Am J Obstet Gynecol* 2008;**199**:232.e1–3.

34. American College of Obstetricians and Gynecologists, Committee on Obstetric Practice. *Vaginal Delivery After a Previous Cesarean Birth. ACOG Committee Opinion No. 143*. Washington, DC: American College of Obstetricians and Gynecologists; 1994.

35. National Institutes of Health. National Institutes of Health Consensus Development Conference Statement: vaginal birth after cesarean: new insights March 8–10, 2010. *Semin Perinatal* 2010;**34**:351–65.

36. American College of Obstetricians and Gynecologists. ACOG Practice bulletin no. 115: vaginal birth after prior cesarean delivery. *Obstet Gynecol* 2010;**116**:450–63.

37. National Institute of Health and Care Excellence (NICE). *Caesarean Section*. Clinical guideline [CG132]. London: NICE; 2011.

38. American College of Obstetricians and Gynecologists and Society for Maternal-Fetal Medicine. Obstetric care consensus: safe prevention of the primary cesarean delivery. Number 1 March 2014. Available at: http://www.acog.org/Resources_And_Publications/Obstetric_Care_Consensus_Series/Safe_Prevention_of_the_Primary_Cesarean_Delivery (accessed 30 March 2016).

39. D'Souza R, Arulkumaran S. To 'C' or not to 'C' Cesarean delivery upon maternal request: a review of facts, figures and guidelines. *J Perinat Med* 2013;**41**:5–15.

40. American College of Obstetrics and Gynecology. ACOG Committee Opinion. Surgery and patient choice: the ethics of decision making. *Obstet Gynecol* 2003;**102**:1101–6.

41. [No authors listed]. NIH State-of-the Science Conference Statement on Cesarean Delivery on Maternal Request. *NIH Consens State Sci Statements* 2006;**23**:1–29.

42. Chervenak FA, McCullough LB, International Academy of Perinatal Medicine. Women and children first—or last? The New York Declaration. *Am J Obstet Gynecol* 2009;2001;**35**.

43. Chervenak FA, McCullough LB. Women and children first: transforming an historic defining moment into a contemporary ethical imperative. *Am J Obstet Gynecol* 2009;**201**:335.e1–5.

44. Historic UK.Com. 'Women and children first'—the silent heroes of the Birkenhead. Available at: http://www.historic-uk.com/CultureUK/WomenandChildrenFirst.htm (accessed 30 March 2016).

45. United Nations. UNICEF. Available at: http://www.unicef.org/ (accessed 30 March 2016).

46. World Health Organization. Homepage. Available at: http://www.who.int/en/ (accessed 30 March 2016).

47. The World Bank. Homepage. Available at: http://www.worlbdbank.org/ (accessed 30 March 2016).

48. International Federation of Gynecology and Obstetrics. Homepage. Available at: http://www.figo.org/ (accessed 30 March 2016).

49. Matres Mundi. Homepage. Available at: http://www.matres-mundi.org/ (accessed 30 March 2016).

50. World Association of Perinatal Medicine. Homepage. Available at: http://www.wapm.info/ (accessed 30 March 2016).

3

Clinical anatomy of the pelvis and the reproductive organs

Thomas Ind

Introduction

Proficient surgery requires good basic surgical skills and an understanding of the relevant anatomy. The time when a surgeon watched an operation, performed the same procedure, and then taught it has elapsed. Routine formulaic surgical procedures have become outdated and modern surgical practice is focused on individual patients and their specific needs. The main focus of surgery is now dedicated to the competent obtainment of skills and a complete understanding of human anatomy and its variations.

This chapter focuses on the main anatomical structures encountered during gynaecological surgery. The anatomy of the pelvis in relation to the fetal skull is also covered.

The abdominal wall

The anterior abdominal wall serves many functions (**Box 3.1**). Its primary role is to protect the viscera from injury and infection. It not only houses the viscera within the abdomen but also maintains visceral anatomical position against gravity. The muscles of the anterior wall also aid in increasing intra-abdominal pressure and assist with forceful expiration, pushing the abdominal viscera up high in the abdomen. It also assists with functions such as defecation, micturition, vomiting, and coughing.

The structures of the anterior abdominal wall are shown in **Figure 3.1**. They consist of skin, subcutaneous tissue, rectus sheath and associated muscles, rectus muscle, transversalis fascia, and peritoneum. The inferior epigastric vessels pass up the abdomen from their origin at the external iliac artery to travel in the transversalis fascia between the peritoneum and the rectus sheath and muscle (**Figure 3.1**).

The subcutaneous tissue differs above and below the umbilicus. Above the umbilicus it consists of a single sheet of fascia continuous with the other subcutaneous tissues of the body. Below the umbilicus it consists of two layers. The superficial fatty layer is called Camper's fascia and the deeper membranous layer is called Scarpa's fascia. It is between these two layers of fascia that nerves and vessels run.

There are two main groups of muscle within the anterior abdominal wall, which are the flat and the vertical muscles. The vertical muscles consist of the rectus abdominis (**Figure 3.1**) and pyramidalis. The two rectus abdominis muscles run either side of the midline and are split by the linea alba. Laterally the margin is called the linea semilunaris and the muscle is split by a number of tendinous intersections that give rise to the classical appearance of a muscular anterior abdominal wall (a 'six pack'). The pyramidalis is not always present. It is a small triangular-shaped muscle that is superficial to the rectus abdominis and superior to the pubis attached to the linea alba.

The three main flat muscles are the external oblique, internal oblique, and transversus abdominis muscles (**Figure 3.1**). These muscles have fibres that run perpendicular to each other thus reducing the risk of hernia and facilitating rotational abdominal movements. The muscles come together in the centre of the abdomen forming the rectus sheath. The rectus sheath passes superficial and deep to the rectus muscle. Superficially it is composed of the aponeurosis of the external oblique and half of the internal oblique with the other half passing posteriorly and joining with the fibres of the transversus abdominis. Below the umbilicus all the aponeuroses move superficial to the rectus abdominis. This area of transition between where the rectus sheath has a posterior wall and where it does not is called the arcuate line (**Figure 3.1**).

The posterior abdominal wall is of lesser importance to the gynaecological surgeon as the pelvis is rarely approached through it. The posterior borders of the abdomen include the ribs, vertebrae, psoas major and psoas minor, quadratus lumborum, and iliacus.

Clinical considerations

The anatomy of the anterior abdominal wall is important when considering surgical incisions. In a low transverse or Pfannenstiel incision as might be performed for a caesarean section, the surgeon passes through only one layer of rectus sheath as the incision is below the arcuate line. A midline incision crosses the arcuate line and passes through the linea alba. A McBurney ('grid iron') incision is commonly performed for an appendicectomy and is performed at McBurney's point, a third of the distance between the anterior superior iliac spine (ASIS) and the umbilicus. For this latter incision,

---

Box 3.1 Functions of the anterior abdominal wall

- Houses abdominal viscera
- Protects viscera from injury
- Protects viscera from infection
- Helps maintain position of the viscera
- Assists with increases of intra-abdominal pressure
- Forceful expiration
- Coughing
- Vomiting
- Defecation
- Micturition

Box 3.2 Structures of the external genitalia

- Mons pubis
- Labia majora
- Labia minora
- Clitoris
- Clitoral glans
- Clitoral hood
- Clitoral frenulum
- Vestibule
- Urethral opening
- Skene's glands and ducts
- Bartholin's glands and ducts
- Introitus
- Hymen
- Fourchette
- Perineum

---

the fibres of the oblique muscles are separated perpendicular to each other, reducing the risk of hernia. The risk of incisional hernia is greatest during a midline incision where only the midline structures are sutured. What is defined as 'mass closure' involving the peritoneum, sheath, and rectus muscles minimizes the risk of a subsequent hernia.

The presence of the epigastric vessels is also important during laparoscopic surgery. These can normally be visualized prior to the insertion of lateral ports, thus preventing them from being ruptured.

External genitalia

The external genitalia or vulva consists of the mons pubis, clitoris, urethral opening, vestibule, hymen, labia minora, labia majora, and Bartholin's glands (**Box 3.2**). The functions of the external genitalia are to provide a protective cushion during sexual intercourse, to help with lubrication during sexual intercourse, to provide a protective barrier to the internal genital organs, to provide an area for the excretion of urine, and to secrete pheromones.

The mons pubis is a rounded mound of fatty tissue that lies over the pubic bone (**Figure 3.2**). The two labia majora are the two most lateral structures and also consist of fatty mounds. During puberty,

the mons and labia majora enlarge, become hair bearing, and contain sebaceous glands.

The labia minora lie just inside the labia majora and surround the opening to the vagina and the urethra (**Figure 3.2**). During sexual stimulation, the blood vessels of the labia minora become engorged, making them more sensitive. The clitoris lies between the two labia minora at their upper pole and is a small protrusion that corresponds to the penis in the male. It consists of the clitoral glans, the clitoral hood which is a small covering of skin, and the clitoral frenulum. The clitoris can become erect like the penis and is very sensitive to sexual stimulation, resulting in orgasm.

The vulval vestibule is the area bordered by the labia minora laterally, clitoris superiorly, and the fourchette inferiorly (**Figure 3.2**). The sides of the vestibule are bordered by Hart's lines which are on the inside of the labia minora and are the transition between the vulval skin and the softer epidermis of the vestibule. The vestibule is the location for the opening of the vagina and Bartholin's glands as well as the opening of the urethra and Skene's ducts.

The vaginal opening is called the introitus (**Figure 3.2**). This serves to function as the entrance for the penis during sexual intercourse, an exit for menstrual blood during menstruation, and an opening for delivery of a baby. The entrance to the upper vagina is bordered by the hymen which is a membranous structure. Sexual intercourse and childbirth normally disrupt the hymen, leaving remnants called carunculae myrtiformis. Bartholin's glands lie either side, inferior and posterior to the introitus, just caudal to the hymen. They produce a thick secretion that functions as a lubricant for sexual intercourse.

The urethra opens into the vestibule inferior to the clitoris and superior to the hymen (**Figure 3.2**). Its function is to carry urine to the outside. It is bordered by two duct openings from Skene's glands (periurethral glands). These are homologous with the prostate in the male. The function is unknown and they may be an embryological remnant of no importance. The anatomical location is very variable. It has been postulated that the Skene's glands are the site of fluid production when female ejaculation occurs.

The area between the fourchette (posterior part of the introitus) and the anus is called the perineum (**Figure 3.2**). This area of skin is sensitive to stimulation and may play a role in sexual arousal. The

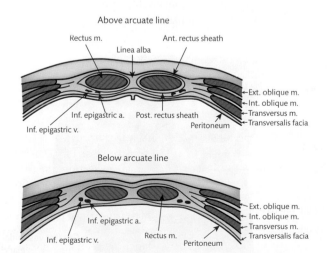

Figure 3.1 Anterior abdominal wall. a, artery; m, muscle; v, vein.

Female external genitalia

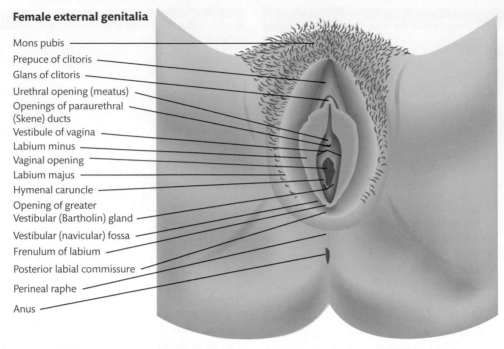

Mons pubis
Prepuce of clitoris
Glans of clitoris
Urethral opening (meatus)
Openings of paraurethral (Skene) ducts
Vestibule of vagina
Labium minus
Vaginal opening
Labium majus
Hymenal caruncle
Opening of greater Vestibular (Bartholin) gland
Vestibular (navicular) fossa
Frenulum of labium
Posterior labial commissure
Perineal raphe
Anus

Figure 3.2 Female external genitalia.

length varies from 0.5 to 2.5 cm and can be traumatized during childbirth.

Clinical considerations

The vulva surface is a skin similar to that in other parts of the body. For this reason, it is vulnerable to any dermatological condition that can occur in other locations such as neoplasia, infection, and dermatitis. Itching of this area is called pruritus vulvae, and pain is called vulvodynia (see Chapter XX).

Bartholin's ducts and Skene's ducts can become blocked resulting in cyst formation. If these cysts become infected, abscesses can form that might require intervention (see Chapter XX).

The labia minora vary in size immensely. Some are only a few millimetres long while others can be many centimetres. This has resulted in a fashion for cosmetic surgery to the labia minora to make them smaller. However, the term 'labial hyperplasia' is often incorrect and just describes normal organs that are larger than others and such surgery is usually unnecessary.

Internal genital organs

The internal genital organs consist of the ovaries, the Fallopian tubes, the uterus, and the vagina (**Figure 3.3**). These all lie in close proximity between the rectum posteriorly and the lower urinary tract anteriorly.

Ovaries

The ovaries are white, almond-shaped structures that are situated behind the broad ligaments on each side of the pelvis within a depression called the ovarian fossae. The superior pole is attached to a sheet of tissue containing vessels and nerves called the infundibulopelvic ligament. The inferior pole is attached to the uterus by the ovarian ligament. The medial surface lies free within the pelvic cavity and the

lateral surface is attached to the Fallopian tube by the mesosalpinx and suspensory ligament which contain further vessels and nerve fibres.

The blood supply to the ovaries is via the ovarian artery that arises from the aorta and descends into the pelvis within the infundibulopelvic ligament (also called the suspensory ligament). The venous drainage mirrors the arterial supply. On the right side, the vein drains into the inferior vena cava. On the left side, the vein drains into the renal vein. Anastomoses occur with branches from the uterine artery within the mesosalpinx. The lymphatic drainage is via lymph vessels associated with the ovarian artery to the para-aortic nodes, in addition to iliac nodes via lymphatics following the anastomoses with the uterine artery.

Fallopian tubes

The Fallopian tubes are 10–12 cm long and pass from the superior angle of the uterus alongside the ovary. The attachment to the ovary is called the mesosalpinx and contains blood vessels and nerves that supply the ovary and the Fallopian tube.

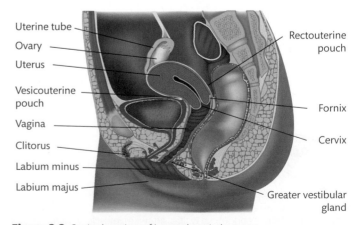

Uterine tube
Ovary
Uterus
Vesicouterine pouch
Vagina
Clitorus
Labium minus
Labium majus
Rectouterine pouch
Fornix
Cervix
Greater vestibular gland

Figure 3.3 Sagittal section of internal genital organs.

There are six main parts to the Fallopian tube. These are the ostium, interstitial portion, isthmus, ampulla, infundibulum, and fimbriae. The ostium is the opening of the tube into the uterine cavity. The interstitial portion is the part that lies within the myometrium of the uterus. The isthmus is the narrowest part of the Fallopian tube that connects with the interstitial portion. The tube is less narrow at the ampulla and connects with the isthmus with the opening near the ovary called the infundibulum. This contains a number of frond-like structures called fimbriae.

The blood supply to the Fallopian tubes is via branches from the ovarian and uterine arteries. The lymphatic drainage is to the internal and external iliac nodes and para-aortic nodes.

Uterus

The uterus is divided into the cervix and corpus. The corpus is the upper part of the uterus and is lined by endometrium that sheds during each menstrual cycle. The most superior part is called the fundus. Laterally, the Fallopian tubes extend from their ostia (opening) within the uterine cavity.

The cervix is the lower part of the uterus. The part of the cervix that projects into the vagina is called the portio vaginalis and the outside that can be seen within the vagina is the ectocervix. The cavity of the cervix (endocervix) starts from the external os within the vagina and extends to the internal os before entering the uterine cavity.

The blood supply to the uterus is via the uterine artery and ovarian artery. The uterine artery divides into a superior and inferior branch after it passes over the ureter. The superior branch passes upwards and anastomoses with branches from the ovarian artery. The inferior branch is the vaginal artery. The lymphatic drainage is to the obturator, internal iliac, and external iliac nodes and via the chain associated with the ovarian artery to the para-aortic nodes.

Vagina

The vagina is a tubular structure and extends from the cervix to the introitus. The walls of the vagina come together from anterior to posterior in the upper two-thirds and from left to right in the lower third. The arterial supply is from vaginal arteries from the uterine and internal iliac artery.

The lymphatic drainage in the upper two-thirds is via the obturator, internal iliac, and external iliac nodes. Lymphatics of the lower third of the vagina drain via the vulva to the femoral nodes.

Clinical considerations

The Fallopian tubes, uterus, cervix, and upper vagina develop *in utero* from the Müllerian ducts on both sides. A variety of malformations can occur when the two Müllerian ducts fail to join or the system fails. They range from uterine and vaginal agenesis to a bicornuate uterus and vagina and minor abnormalities of the uterine cavity. Müllerian malformations are frequently associated with abnormalities of the renal tract. This area is covered in Chapter XX.

Urinary tract

The anatomy of the urinary tract is important for gynaecological surgeons as the bladder and ureters are intimately related to the genital organs and can be damaged perioperatively.

Ureters

The ureters drain urine from the renal pelvises into the bladder. They descend into the pelvis retroperitoneally passing down on the psoas major muscle. When they reach the brim of the pelvis they turn posterioinferiorly, passing over the bifurcation of the common iliac arteries. They continue to pass into the pelvis attached to the lateral pelvic peritoneum and pass underneath the uterine artery before turning anteromedially into the bladder. The position in relation to the uterine artery is classically described as 'water under the bridge' with the ureters containing 'water' passing under the 'bridge' of the uterine arteries.

During radical hysterectomy, when the uterus is lifted out of the pelvis, the ureters appear to pass downwards before entering the bladder and this is often referred to as the 'genu'. As the ureter turns medially to enter the bladder, there are often vascular fibres between the bladder and the vagina that have to be divided during a radical hysterectomy for cancer. This area is often referred to as the 'ureteric tunnel'. At the entrance to the bladder, the ureters are surrounded by valves that prevent the backflow of urine. These are the ureterovesical valves.

The blood supply to the ureters varies along their course. The upper part is supplied by the renal arteries. The middle is supplied by branches from the aorta and common iliac artery. The lower part is supplied from braches of the internal iliac, uterine, and superior vesical arteries.

The innervation is from nerves from T12–L2. It is for this reason that ureteric pain may be referred to the back and sides of the abdomen as well as the labia majora.

The ureters are normally single on both sides. It is possible to have duplex (two) ureters that can be complete (involving the whole ureteric course) or partial (involving only part of the course). Another anomaly is that of a retrocaval ureter which is thought to be a developmental disorder of the vena cava. In this anomaly, the right ureter traces out an 'S' at the L4 level behind the vena cava.

Bladder and urethra

The bladder is divided into a fundus at the top and a trigone. The trigone is the triangular part of the bladder bordered by the two ureteric orifices and urethral opening. When empty, the posterior part of the bladder lies on the cervix and anterior vagina (**Figure 3.3**). The fundus is covered by peritoneum that is continuous with that over the uterus at the uterovesical fold. Similarly, the peritoneum is continuous with that of the abdominal wall anteriorly. Anteriorly and inferior to the abdominal wall fold of peritoneum there is an avascular space between the pubic bone and the bladder called the space of Retzius which is entered during some urogynaecological procedures. Either side of the space of Retzius are the paravesical spaces which are developed in some urogynaecological and gynaecological oncology procedures.

The blood supply is via the internal iliac artery that gives off an inferior vesical artery and several superior vesical branches. Some blood supply also comes from the obturator, uterine, and vaginal arteries. The lymphatic drainage is via the obturator, internal, and external iliac chains nodes.

When full, the bladder has a capacity of about 400 mL. The sensation to void occurs via general visceral afferent fibres that follow the sympathetic efferent nerves from the hypogastric plexus on the superior surface and the course of the parasympathetic efferent from the splanchnic nerves and inferior hypogastric plexus on the inferior portion. Urine is expelled through the urethra following a contraction of its main muscle (the detrusor muscle) with the opening of both the autonomically controlled internal urethral sphincter and voluntarily controlled external sphincter.

The female urethra is about 4 cm long and extends from the bladder neck and terminates at the vaginal vestibule. The urethra pierces the pelvic diaphragm and perineal membrane just posterior to the pubic symphysis. The opening can be seen on the external genitalia (**Figure 3.2**).

Clinical considerations

The hypogastric nerves can be damaged during some gynaecological oncology and urogynaecological surgical procedures. This can sometimes result in altered bladder function. Modern surgical techniques now involve attempts to identify these fibres and preserve them.

Damage to supporting muscles and connective tissue in the pelvic diaphragm (often from childbirth) can cause prolapse of the bladder and incontinence. This is described in more detail in Chapters 56 and 57.

Pelvic floor, rectum, and anus

Pelvic floor

The pelvic floor comprises three muscle layers: the superficial perineal layer, which is innervated by the pudendal nerve; the urogenital diaphragm layer, which is also innervated by the pudendal nerve; and the pelvic diaphragm, which is innervated by the nerve roots S3–S5 (**Box 3.3**). The position of these muscles is illustrated in **Figure 3.4**.

Rectum

The rectum begins at the rectosigmoid junction at the level of the third vertebra. The calibre is similar to that of the sigmoid colon but near its termination it becomes dilated forming the rectal ampulla. It terminates at the dentate line to become the anus. The rectum is

---

Box 3.3 The pelvic floor muscle layers

Superficial perineal layer
- Bulbospongiosus (formerly bulbocavernosus)
- Ischiocavernosus
- Superficial transverse perineal
- External anal sphincter

Deep urogenital diaphragm layer
- Compressor urethra
- Urethrovaginal sphincter
- Deep transverse perineal

Pelvic diaphragm
- Levator ani: pubococcygeus (pubovaginalis), puborectalis, and iliococcygeus
- Coccygeus/ischiococcygeus
- Piriformis
- Obturator internus

---

covered in its superior part by peritoneum. It lies posterior to the vagina, cervix, and corpus, forming a space called the pouch of Douglas. The pouch of Douglas is bordered by the rectum posteriorly, the vagina and cervix anteriorly, and the uterosacral ligaments on the lateral side. Distal to the fold of peritoneum in the pouch of Douglas, the rectum lies in close proximity to the vagina divided by a rectovaginal fascial plane. This plane corresponds to that named Denonvilliers' fascia in the male and sometimes this term is used to describe the rectovaginal fascia in women.

The superior rectal artery provides the chief blood supply to the rectum and is a continuation of the inferior mesenteric artery, which is a branch of the aorta. Venous drainage is via the superior rectal vein that drains into the inferior mesenteric vein and the middle rectal vein that drains into the internal iliac vein. Lymphatic drainage is to the internal and external iliac nodes, as well as para-aortic nodes via the inferior mesenteric chain. The nerve supply to the rectum is via the rectal plexus that derives from the posterior part of the inferior hypogastric plexus. This provides sympathetic fibres to the vascular smooth muscle of the rectum and parasympathetic fibres to the smooth muscle of the rectum.

Anus

The anal canal is the terminal part of the large intestine and extends from the rectum to the anal opening. The upper two-thirds of the anal canal are lined by columnar mucosa and contain longitudinal folds. The lower third is lined by squamous epithelium. Within this area is Hilton's white line, which marks the junction between keratinized stratified squamous epithelium and unkeratinized stratified squamous epithelium. The lower third is surrounded by folds, called anal valves. These valves converge at a line called the pectinate (dentate) line, which represents the embryological transition between the hindgut and the ectoderm, below which the mucosa becomes skin. This is subtly different to the 'anal verge' which is the term used to define the transition between the epithelium of the anal canal and the perianal skin.

The upper two-thirds of the anus receives its arterial supply from the superior rectal artery, a branch of the inferior mesenteric artery, and the inferior third receives its supply from the inferior rectal artery, a branch of the internal pudendal artery which is a branch of the anterior division of the internal iliac artery (**Box 3.4**). Lymphatic drainage is via the internal and para-aortic chain of nodes above the pectinate line and to the superficial inguinal nodes below this. The upper two-thirds of the rectum are supplied by branches from the inferior hypogastric plexus. In the lower third, the nerve supply is somatic, receiving its supply from the inferior rectal nerves, which are branches of the pudendal nerve. These are somatic and sensitive to temperature, touch, and pain.

The anus is surrounded by the internal and external anal sphincters, which are two muscle rings that control defecation. The internal sphincter is about 3–4 cm in length and surrounds the anus. It is entirely involuntary and in a state of continuous contraction. Its nervous supply is from sympathetic fibres from the superior rectal and hypogastric plexuses which stimulate contraction. Inhibition of contraction of the internal sphincter is by parasympathetic fibres. The external anal sphincter is about 8–10 cm long, elliptical in shape, and caudally lies close to the skin around the anus. It has a superficial and deep layer. The deep layer forms a complete circular sphincter

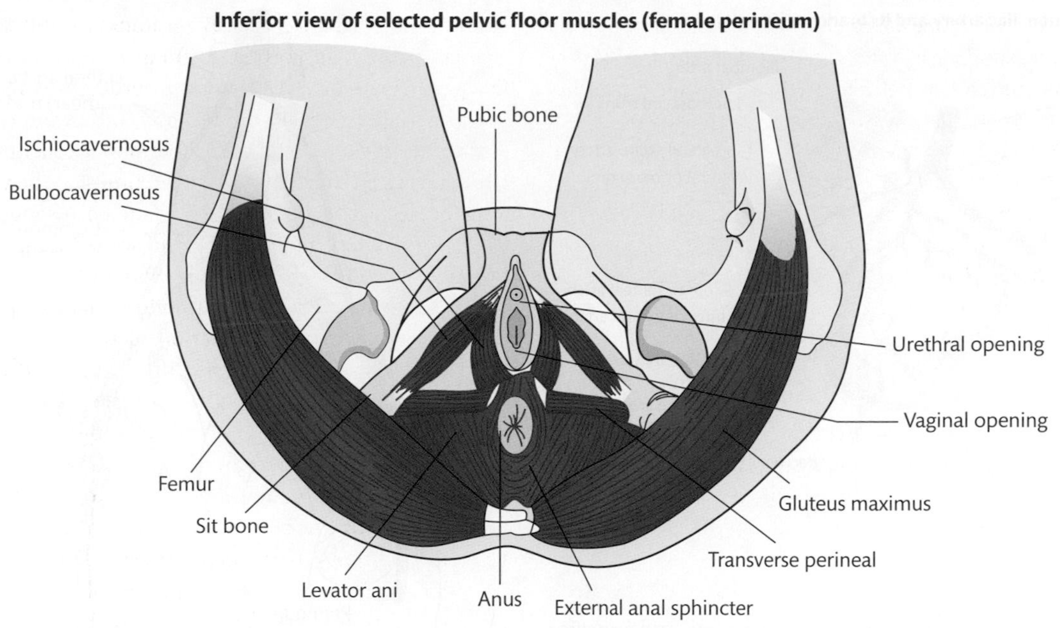

Inferior view of selected pelvic floor muscles (female perineum)

Figure 3.4 Anus and sphincter.

around the anus and lies next to the internal anal sphincter. Some fibres are shared with other muscles of the perineum. The superficial layer shares fibres with the transverse perineal, levator ani, and bulbospongiosus (formerly bulbocavernosus) muscles (**Figure 3.4**). Like the internal sphincter, the external sphincter is passively in a state of tonic contraction. It can be contracted further under the influence of the will, so as to further occlude the anus in expiratory efforts.

Clinical considerations

During radical hysterectomy, nerves from the hypogastric plexus are often divided. This can often leave the patient with permanent changes in bowel function. More recent techniques for performing radical hysterectomy are designed to try and preserve these nerve fibres by identifying them in a space deep to the uterosacral ligaments

called Kobayashi's space. Similar techniques have been employed to prevent damaging these nerves during sacrocolpopexy and other urogynaecological procedures.

Injury to the anal sphincters can occur during childbirth. Injury to the muscles of the sphincter are termed third-degree tears and those that enter the anus or rectum fourth-degree tears. These are described in more detail in Chapter 59.

Blood supply to the pelvis

The main blood supply to the pelvis comes from the aorta via the two common iliac arteries and the ovarian artery. There is a further supply to the rectum via the inferior mesenteric artery (a branch of the aorta).

The ovarian arteries emerge from the aorta below the renal arteries and descend into the pelvis entering the infundibulopelvic ligament. Branches are given off to the Fallopian tubes and anastomoses occur with the uterine blood supply originating from the internal iliac artery. Venous drainage from the ovary is also via a network of vessels, but predominantly through the ovarian vein that drains into the inferior vena cava on the right and renal vein on the left.

The common iliac arteries divide at the level of the pelvic brim into the external and internal iliac arteries (**Figure 3.5**). The external iliac artery passes down the brim of the pelvis above the external iliac vein and becomes the femoral artery once it passes under the inguinal ligament. Before this, it gives off two branches: the deep circumflex iliac artery that travels along the pelvic brim and the inferior epigastric artery that passes upwards on the anterior abdominal wall and anastomoses with the superior epigastric artery (**Box 3.4**). The first two branches supply the skin and muscles of the anterior abdominal wall and the femoral artery supplies the leg.

The internal iliac artery is classically described as having an anterior and posterior division (**Figure 3.5** and **Box 3.4**). The posterior division gives off three branches classically described in a mnemonic

---

Box 3.4 Arteries of the pelvis

External iliac artery
- Deep circumflex iliac artery
- Inferior epigastric artery
- Femoral artery

Internal iliac artery

Anterior division
- Inferior gluteal artery
- Middle rectal artery
- Obturator artery
- Inferior vesical artery
- Internal pudendal artery
- Uterine artery
- Umbilical artery

Posterior division
- Iliolumbar artery
- Lateral sacral artery
- Superior gluteal artery

Common iliac artery and its branches (female)

Common iliac artery
Internal iliac artery
External iliac artery
Umbilical artery
Obturator artery
Deep circumflex iliac artery
Inferior epigastric artery
Obliterated umbilical artery
Superior vesical arteries
Urinary bladder
Vagina

Iliombar artery
Lumbosacral trunk
Lateral sacral artery
Ventral primary rami:
S1
S2
S3
S4
Superior gluteal artery
Inferior gluteal artery
Internal pudendal artery
Uterine artery
Middle rectal artery
Rectum

Figure 3.5 Blood supply to the pelvis.

as PILS (Posterior division, Iliolumbar, Lateral sacral, and Superior gluteal) (**Box 3.4**). The iliolumbar artery has an iliac and lumbar branches and the lateral sacral often has a superior and inferior branch. There are multiple anastomoses between these vessels that supply the posterior compartment of the pelvis and gluteal muscles (**Figure 3.5** and **Box 3.4**). The anterior division gives off a number of branches that supply the uterus, vagina, bladder, and perineum (**Box 3.4**). The uterine artery passes over the ureter before dividing and providing a superior and inferior branch. This is classically described as 'water under the bridge' as the ureter passes under the uterine artery.

Blood vessels in the pelvis all have numerous anastomoses. The venous drainage often corresponds to the arterial supply but a large venous plexus of anastomoses exists in the pelvis, from which blood drains into named vessels.

Clinical considerations

The most important clinical considerations with relation to blood vessels in the pelvis involve surgical ligation and avoidance of non-intentional damage. Knowledge of the arterial supply and venous drainage allows a surgeon to resect structures (such as the uterus) without haemorrhage. The multiple anastomoses and venous plexuses mean that surgical haemorrhage can be quite profuse and numerous surgical techniques can be used to control unintentional bleeding. Ligating the internal iliac arteries often controls profuse bleeding from the uterus during a caesarean section. This is normally done at a level below the posterior division (see Chapter 29).

Individual arterial branches can be identified radiologically and embolized. This can be done to control haemorrhage or to devascularize a structure such as in uterine artery embolization for the management of fibroids (see Chapter 49).

Lymphatic drainage of the pelvis

The lymphatic drainage from the pelvis varies with each organ (**Figure 3.6**). However, there is a widespread network of lymph channels within the pelvis for lymph drainage to occur.

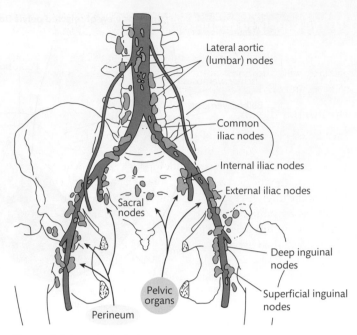

Lateral aortic (lumbar) nodes
Common iliac nodes
Internal iliac nodes
External iliac nodes
Sacral nodes
Pelvic organs
Perineum
Deep inguinal nodes
Superficial inguinal nodes

Figure 3.6 Lymphatic drainage.

From the vulva, the lymph drainage is reported to pass to the deep and superficial inguinal nodes passing up to the femoral nodes. These lymph channels continue up the major blood vessels of the pelvis (external iliac, and common iliac).

The lower third of the vagina has similar lymph drainage to the vulva with the upper two-thirds having a lymph drainage more similar to the cervix. The cervix has lymph channels that pass laterally from the uterine artery to the internal iliac chain, as well as to the obturator group and external iliac chain. Some lymph tracts pass to the presacral nodes and then on to the para-aortic nodes.

The corpus of the uterus is classically described as having lymph drainage to the obturator, internal iliac, external iliac, and presacral nodal groups as well as nodes in the uterine parametrium. Sometimes lymph spread can occur along the round ligament to the superficial inguinal nodes.

The lymph drainage of the ovaries is classically described as passing along the vessels of the infundibulopelvic ligament and ovarian arteries towards the para-aortic chain just below the renal vessels. However, there is considerable interlinking of pelvic lymphatics and therefore cancer lymphatic spread in ovarian cancer can follow these chains of nodes or those from the uterus via links in the mesosalpinx (see Chapter 64).

Clinical considerations

Gynaecological cancers can spread via the lymph nodes. For this reason, lymph nodes are often removed surgically during treatment for these cancers. When lymph nodes are removed, cysts of lymph fluid can collect called lymphocysts. If the channels are completely divided, this can result in a build-up of lymph tissue in the lower limbs and swelling of the legs called lymphoedema.

Modern-day strategies for the treatment of gynaecological cancers have therefore centred on more conservative approaches to the lymph glands with removal of the first (sentinel) lymph node identified after an injection of dye or selecting cases where no lymph nodes are removed at all.

Nerve supply to the pelvis

The nerve supply to the pelvis comes from the lumbar and sacral plexuses with additional autonomic supply from the hypogastric plexuses and pelvic splanchnic nerves.

The lumbar plexus

The lumbar plexus is a web of nerves in the lumbar region that arise from L1–L4 with contributing branches from T12. This plexus of nerves form the iliohypogastric, ilioinguinal, genitofemoral, femoral, and obturator nerves as well as the lateral femoral cutaneous nerve of the thigh (LFCNT). The ventral rami of the fourth lumbar plexus passes communicating branches to the sacral plexus (lumbar-sacral plexus) (**Box 3.5** and **Figure 3.7a**).

The ilioinguinal nerve passes around into the anterior abdominal wall entering 3–4 cm medial and inferior to the ASIS and terminates between the transversus abdominus muscle and the internal oblique about 2–3 cm lateral to the midline and superior to the pubis. The iliohypogastric nerve travels in a similar direction but enters the abdominal wall higher but still below the ASIS and terminates in a more lateral and superior position. The genitofemoral nerve travels inferiorly on the psoas muscle lateral to the external iliac vessels, while the femoral nerve travels within psoas, emerging at its lower and lateral border and passing under the inguinal ligament. The obturator nerve descends through the psoas muscle and emerges from its medial border at the level of the pelvic brim. It then passes behind the common iliac vessel leaving the pelvis through the obturator foramen. The LFCNT emerges from the lateral border of psoas and crosses the iliacus muscle and towards the ASIS, passing underneath the inguinal ligament.

Clinical considerations

Branches of the lumbar plexus are commonly cut during gynaecological surgery. Damage to the ilioinguinal and iliohypogastric nerves can occur during a Pfannenstiel incision or during laparoscopic surgery when ports are placed below the ASIS. Damage to these nerves can cause paraesthesia and burning pain to the lower abdomen, groin, labia, suprapubic area, and inner thigh.

The genitofemoral nerve appears like a piece of white cotton lying on the psoas muscle and can be seen and cut while performing an external iliac lymphadenectomy. Transection of the genitofemoral nerve can cause neuralgia and paraesthesia of the inner thigh and labia majora. The femoral nerve can be damaged by deep retractor blades pressing on the psoas muscle and can cause weakness of the quadriceps muscle, difficulty with ambulation, and severe pain.

The obturator nerve can be seen during an obturator lymphadenectomy. Great care is required to avoid transecting this nerve during this surgery. Transection of this nerve can cause

problems with hip adduction, unstable walking, and paraesthesia of the inner thigh and groin.

Damage to the LFCNT causes numbness of the skin of the outer thigh called meralgia paraesthetica. This can occur in obese patients while the nerve is stretched under the inguinal ligament by the weight of a panniculus hanging down. A similar injury can occur while placing a patient in surgical stirrups causing strain on the nerve as it passes under the inguinal ligament.

The sacral plexus

The sacral plexus derives from S1–S4 with additional nerves from L4 and L5 (**Box 3.6** and **Figure 3.7b**). Fibres run down on the posterior pelvic wall on top of pyriformis.

The superior gluteal nerve (L4–S1) passes through the greater sciatic foramen and innervates the gluteal muscles along with the inferior gluteal nerve (L5–S3). The sciatic nerve (L4–S3) is the largest nerve in the body and also passes through the greater sciatic foramen towards the gluteal area. The nerve to the quadratus femoris (L4–S1) also leaves the greater sciatic foramen and innervates the hip muscles along with the nerve to the obturator internus (L5–S2). The other muscles of the sacral plexus supply the muscles they refer to. The pelvic splanchnic nerves are part of the autonomic nervous supply.

Pelvic bones and fetal skull

Understanding of the anatomy of the fetal skull and pelvic bones is important to obstetricians, midwives, and all those involved in attending childbirth as it is the relationship between these two structures that defines the mechanics of normal and abnormal childbirth. From an obstetric view, the fetal skull is the largest and least compressible part of the fetus that has to pass through the birth canal and is usually the presenting part during labour. The pelvis supports the gravid uterus after the first trimester and is the canal through which a fetus must pass if labour is to be successful.

Fetal skull

This consists of the two parietal, frontal, and temporal bones. In addition, there is the occipital bone that is attached to the cervical vertebrae (**Figure 3.8**). In the fetus, the bones of the skull have not yet fused and are separated by spaces called sutures and fontanelles (**Figure 3.8**).

There are four named sutures of the skull. The frontal suture represents the space between the two frontal bones at the front of the head and the sagittal suture joins the two parietal bones (**Figure 3.8**). The coronal suture is the space between the frontal and parietal bones. The lambdoid suture is the space between the parietal and occipital bones.

The two areas where the sutures join are called fontanelles (**Figure 3.8**). The anterior fontanelle is the junction between the frontal, coronal, and sagittal sutures and is diamond shaped. It is also known as the *bregma*. The posterior fontanelle is the junction between the sagittal and lambdoid sutures and is triangular in shape. It is also known as the lambda.

Clinical considerations

Understanding the bones, fontanelles, and sutures of the fetal skull helps identify normal and abnormal presentation during labour (see Chapters 26 and 32).

Box 3.5 Nerves of the lumbar plexus

- T12–L1: iliohypogastric
- L1: ilioinguinal
- L1–L2: genitofemoral
- L2–L3: lateral femoral cutaneous nerve of the thigh (LFCNT)
- L2–L4: femoral
- L2–L4: obturator

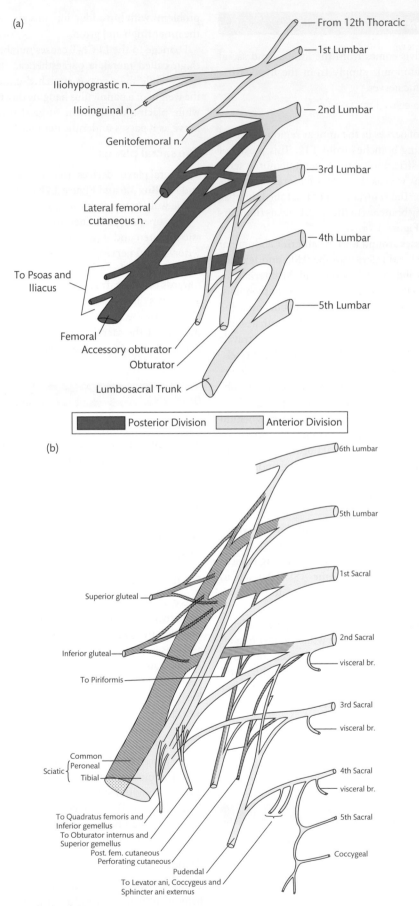

(a)

From 12th Thoracic

1st Lumbar

Iliohypograstic n.

Ilioinguinal n.

2nd Lumbar

Genitofemoral n.

3rd Lumbar

Lateral femoral
cutaneous n.

4th Lumbar

To Psoas and
Iliacus

5th Lumbar

Femoral
Accessory obturator
Obturator

Lumbosacral Trunk

| Posterior Division | Anterior Division |

(b)

6th Lumbar

5th Lumbar

1st Sacral

Superior gluteal

2nd Sacral

visceral br.

Inferior gluteal

To Piriformis

3rd Sacral

visceral br.

Common
Peroneal
Sciatic
Tibial

4th Sacral

visceral br.

5th Sacral

To Quadratus femoris and
Inferior gemellus
To Obturator internus and
Superior gemellus
Post. fem. cutaneous
Perforating cutaneous

Coccygeal

Pudendal

To Levator ani, Coccygeus and
Sphincter ani externus

Figure 3.7 Lumbar plexus. a, artery; br, branch.

The occiput is the area between the base of the skull and the posterior fontanelle. The brow is the area between the anterior fontanelle and the upper part of the orbits. The face extends from the orbits to the chin. An occipital, brow, or face presentation of the fetus during labour may cause failure to progress (see Chapter 32).

Pelvic bones

These consist of pairs of tightly fused bones (ilium, pubic bone, and ischium) (**Figure 3.9a**). These are joined together medially and posteriorly by the sacrum and anteriorly in the midline by the pubic symphysis (**Figure 3.9a**). The bony pelvis in a woman is different to that in the male to accommodate childbirth. The differences are detailed in **Box 3.7**. In summary, the female pelvis is wider compared to the male pelvis with smaller protuberances (e.g. ischial spines).

The ilium is the largest bone in the pelvis and consists of two parts, the ala and the body (**Figure 3.9a**). The ala is the large wing that forms part of the greater pelvis. The upper surface of the ala is called the iliac crest which has a spinous process at the front called the Anterior Superior Iliac Spine (ASIS). The two ASISs can be palpated as bony protuberances either side of the lower abdomen and are the lateral-most extremity of the inguinal ligaments on each side. The body of the ilium extends into the acetabulum of which it forms about two-fifths.

The ischium is the most inferior part of the pelvic bones and has a spine (ischial spine) that projects inwards (Figure 3.9a). This spine can be palpated on vaginal examination and is the constant position against which the descent of the fetal head is measured. The distance between the two ischial spines is the narrowest part of the pelvis through which a fetus must pass during normal labour.

The two pubic bones lie at the front and are joined together by the pubic symphysis, which is a cartilaginous joint (Figure 3.9a). During pregnancy, a hormone called relaxin is produced by the placenta. Relaxin helps loosen this joint, allowing some separation during labour.

Pelvic inlet

The pelvic inlet is also termed the pelvic brim. It is bounded posteriorly by the sacral promontory and anteriorly by the superior pubic rami and symphysis pubis. Laterally it is bounded by the iliopectineal lines. The transverse diameter is about 13.5 cm. The shortest diameter and the one most important clinically is that between the sacral promontory and symphysis pubis, which is about 11.5 cm. It is for this reason that, during labour, the fetal head normally passes

The normal presentation is the vertex, which is the area midway between the anterior and posterior fontanelles. This can be defined on vaginal examination in labour by palpating the fontanelles and bones. When the posterior fontanelle and occipital bones are anterior, this is defined as being 'occiput anterior'. When there is a malpresentation in the head may be rotated and the position be 'occiput posterior' with the anterior fontanelle in the anterior position (**Figure 3.8**) (see Chapter 32).

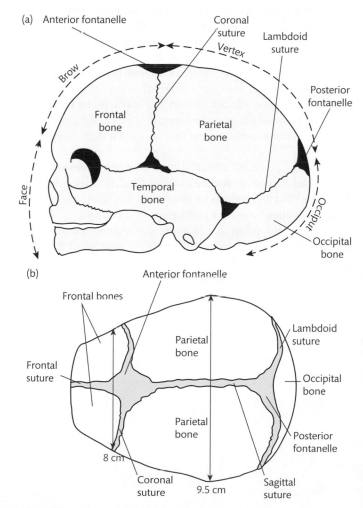

Figure 3.8 Fetal skull.

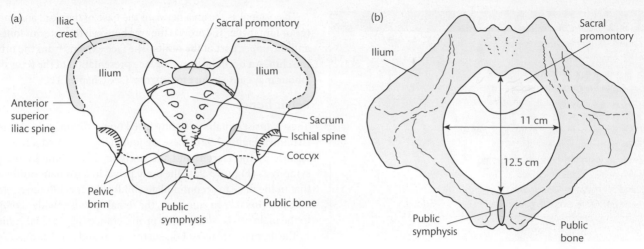

Figure 3.9 Female pelvis, pelvic inlet, and pelvic outlet.

through the pelvic inlet in a left or right occipitolateral position (see Chapter 32).

Pelvic cavity

The pelvic cavity is bounded superiorly by the zone of inlet (see Figure 3.9) and inferiorly by the outlet (see Figure 3.9). This contains the zone of cavity (plane of greatest dimensions) and the zone of mid pelvis (plane of least dimensions).

The zone of cavity has an anteroposterior and transverse diameter of about 13 cm and extends from the inlet to the junction of the second and third sacral vertebrae. It is within this cavity that the fetal head rotates from an occipitolateral to an occipitoanterior position.

The mid pelvis extends anteroposteriorly between the pubic symphysis and the bottom of the sacrum. The transverse diameter is that between the two ischial spines and this is the narrowest part of the pelvic space, measuring about 10 cm. During labour, the ischial spines are the anatomical position most likely to cause an obstruction. The presentation of the fetal head in relation to the ischial spines can be palpated vaginally during labour and is often used as a measure of progress.

Pelvic outlet

The pelvic outlet is diamond shaped with the tip of the sacrum and sacrotuberous ligaments posteriorly (Figure 3.9b) and the area under the pubic arch anteriorly. The anteroposterior diameter is about 12.5 cm (Figure 3.9b). The transverse diameter of the pelvic outlet is measured between the two ischial tuberosities and is about 11 cm. The narrower transverse diameter is the reason that during childbirth the baby is usually delivered through an occipitoanterior position (see Chapter 26).

Clinical variations

The typical female pelvis is described as *gynaecoid*. A gynaecoid pelvis has a round pelvic inlet, short ischial spines, and a shallow pelvic cavity that allows for rapid childbirth.

An *anthropoid* pelvis has an oval-shaped inlet and a smaller transverse diameter comparative to its anteroposterior diameter. It is for this reason that it favours an occiput-posterior position in labour that may lead to a failure to progress. An anthropoid pelvis is more common in African women, but is also found in a significant proportion of Caucasian women. It can be associated with an additional lumbar vertebra and this is called a high assimilation pelvis.

An *android* pelvis has a heart-shaped inlet and is narrower from front to back. This shape is more associated with the male pelvis than the female (**Box 3.7**) and it is for this reason that women with an android pelvis often have more problems with childbirth.

A *platypelloid* pelvis has a narrower anteroposterior diameter compared to its transverse. Due to the position of the sacral promontory, the inlet is slightly kidney shaped. This shape results in difficulty for a fetal head to engage but normally allows for easy childbirth thereafter.

4

Genetics for the obstetrician and gynaecologist

Adonis Ioannides

Introduction

There has been remarkable progress in the field of genetics over recent years and applications of genetic concepts are increasingly shaping clinical practice by informing the way we investigate, counsel, and treat our patients. Certain key milestones, such as the delineation of the human genome, have marked this progress as has the realization that the way genes function is far more complex than the information contained in the sequence of their DNA bases. The field of epigenetics is beginning to unravel the intricate ways in which gene function is influenced by factors external to the genes themselves.

Obstetric and gynaecological practice has been greatly influenced by the fast-moving developments in genetics. This is not surprising considering how closely linked genetic concepts are with patterns of inheritance, fertility, the development and function of the fetoplacental unit, the effect of genetic conditions both on the developing fetus and the pregnant woman, and the approaches to prenatal and perinatal diagnosis. Genetics also influences the way gynaecological conditions are diagnosed and treated and has shed new light on the aetiology of many common gynaecological cancers as well as revealed new targets for therapeutic intervention.

This chapter provides an overview of basic concepts in genetics and the evolution of key laboratory techniques and genetic testing. It introduces genetic aspects of the clinical consultation and the principles underlying genetic counselling, as well as their application in the preconception and prenatal periods, and reviews the genetics of preimplantation and prenatal diagnosis. Finally, the way oncogenetics is shaping our understanding of common gynaecological cancers is reviewed. In many of the clinical scenarios outlined in the subsequent sections, close collaboration with clinical genetics colleagues is indicated.

Basic genetic concepts in clinical practice

Our understanding of how genetic information is organized within cells, the way it underlies development and function by directing protein synthesis, and how it is transmitted from generation to generation has relied on our deciphering of chromosomes and genes. Within the field of human genetics, this broadly translates into the cytogenetic (chromosomes) and molecular genetic (genes) approaches. The DNA double helix is wound around histone molecules constituting the chromosomes that are visible on light microscopy under certain conditions whereas the study of the nucleotide sequence within genes themselves is beyond the resolution of the microscope and requires the use of specific molecular techniques. In some ways, the difference between cytogenetics and molecular genetics is one of scale: a deletion of a small chromosomal segment may lead to the loss of multiple genes whereas a point mutation only affects one gene. Recently, however, the distinction between these two disciplines has been increasingly blurred by the development of newer techniques and the emergence of the so-called molecular cytogenetics that has greatly augmented the resolution of traditional cytogenetic approaches (1, 2). Moreover, genetics has been revolutionized by the emergence of novel approaches such as next-generation sequencing and the evolution of these techniques has transformed the impact of genetics on clinical practice (3–7).

Genetic variation

The application of genetics in clinical medicine is largely based on the study of genetic variation. It is very important that terminology is used accurately and in the right context otherwise it can lead to confusion and misinterpretation. Changes in the sequence of bases within a gene do not necessarily cause problems and the term variant of unknown significance denotes genetic variation with an undetermined impact on gene function. The term polymorphism refers to genetic variants that are relatively common within specific populations, have no known detrimental impact, and are considered to be variations of normality. On the other hand, the term mutation or pathogenic mutation describes genetic variants that affect gene function and alter the phenotype. It is important to use these terms accurately and consistently and interpret them correctly when they appear in the reports of genetic tests.

When referring to individual genes, variants are categorized as substitutions, deletions, or insertions and can occur either within the coding sequences of genes or the non-coding regions (introns or regulatory elements). Though most clinically important mutations are located in the part of the genome that is translated into proteins, non-coding variants can affect gene function by disturbing transcription and post-transcriptional modification (8–10). Within the coding region, a single base substitution may not alter the corresponding amino acid based on the degeneracy of the genetic code (synonymous). On the other hand, substitutions may lead to the incorporation of a different amino acid in the polypeptide chain (missense) or the introduction of a stop signal in which case protein synthesis is terminated altogether (nonsense).

Variants of unknown significance within coding sequences are most likely to be of the missense variety. The impact of substituting one amino acid for another within a polypeptide chain will be determined by a number of factors including the physicochemical similarity between the two amino acids, the location of the substitution within the chain, and the functional role of that part of the protein and the segregation of the variant with the relevant phenotype in the family being investigated (11–14).

Deletions or insertions involve one or more nucleotides, exons, or the entire gene. When chromosomal regions are involved, many genes may be affected. Referring to smaller-scale variants, these can be described as either in-frame or out-of-frame depending on whether the number of deleted/inserted nucleotides is a multiple of three. If it is, the overall reading frame of the gene is maintained (as the code is read in triplets) and a protein is synthesized even though there will be loss or introduction of amino acids in the polypeptide chain. If it is not a multiple of three, the reading frame shifts and the process is deranged.

Epigenetic regulation

Epigenetics deals with influencing gene function without altering the gene's sequence of bases. Epigenetic mechanisms underlie the differential expression of genes in different tissues and, in doing so, underpin development and tissue specification (15). The pattern of selective silencing of certain genes and transcriptional activation of others is mediated by specific protein complexes and is stably inherited through mitotic divisions unless specifically erased and reprogrammed. Gametogenesis and early embryo development are particularly important periods in epigenetic programming. The main epigenetic mechanisms are DNA methylation which involves the transfer of a methyl group to the cytosine of a CpG dinucleotide, modification of histone molecules which results in genes becoming more or less accessible for transcription, and non-coding RNAs which are RNA molecules that do not get translated and play key regulatory roles at multiple steps including transcription, post-transcriptional modification, splicing, and translation (16–19).

Genomic imprinting is a well-described example of epigenetic modification and is the process, established during gametogenesis, which ensures monoallelic expression of specific genes in the zygote based on differential gene silencing according to the parent of origin (20–22). There is strong evidence that imprinted genes play an important role in the regulation of fetal growth, shedding new light on this key aspect of pregnancy (23, 24). Techniques of assisted reproduction have been associated with an increased risk of imprinting disorders such as Beckwith–Wiedemann syndrome and this has been attributed to a possible disturbance of the imprinting process

(25–27). However, it is not clear whether this is a result of the technique itself or the underlying aetiology of infertility (28, 29).

Applied cytogenetics

The technique of karyotyping, which allows the visualization of chromosomes of cultured cells that are arrested in metaphase, has been the mainstay of cytogenetic investigations. Chromosomes are stained to produce a characteristic banding pattern with Giemsa stain being widely used (G-banding) (30, 31). Apart from diagnosing numerical chromosomal abnormalities such as aneuploidy and triploidy, the technique can identify structural rearrangements such as translocations and ring chromosomes as well as segmental deletions, duplications, or inversions, and can pinpoint their position on specific chromosomes based on the bands involved (**Figure 4.1**). Its usefulness is limited by its sensitivity which depends on the size of the chromosomal segment involved and the skill of the operator. Though the technique has evolved and its resolution has improved over the years, it can still only detect abnormalities which are about 5 million base pairs (Mb) in length or greater.

The technique is particularly useful in identifying balanced chromosomal rearrangements such as translocations or inversions even if these rearrangements do not result in the net loss or gain of genetic material, an advantage over newer molecular techniques that rely on quantification rather than visualization. In the context of obstetric practice, the karyotype remains the basis of genetic assessment of a fetus following interventional prenatal techniques such as chorionic villous sampling and amniocentesis. It is also the technique of choice in investigating couples presenting with recurrent early pregnancy losses or who have had a baby diagnosed with a chromosomal abnormality based on its ability to detect balanced rearrangements that can themselves predispose to unbalanced chromosome complements in the offspring.

Smaller, submicroscopic deletions (microdeletions) cannot be identified using the routine karyotype. The technique of fluorescence *in situ* hybridization (FISH) uses fluorescently labelled DNA probes corresponding to specific DNA sequences which hybridize with the specific chromosomal segment and allow confirmation of the presence of this segment under the microscope (32) (**Figure 4.2**). In contrast to the karyotype, the clinician needs to ask the laboratory to carry out a targeted test using a specific probe, the implication being that this requires prior clinical suspicion. An example of this approach in prenatal diagnosis is the use of FISH to exclude 22q11.2 microdeletion syndrome in fetuses diagnosed with cardiac malformations (33). With the exception of chromosomal aneuploidies, this syndrome is one of the commonest causes of heart defects detected antenatally (34).

The need to identify even smaller chromosomal deletions/duplications was addressed by the development of a molecular cytogenetic technique known as array comparative genomic hybridization (array CGH) (35–37). It is based on differentially fluorescently labelling DNA from the individual to be tested and a reference DNA and then allowing both to competitively hybridize with an array of DNA segments representing the entire genome. Any missing or extra genetic material in the test DNA will disturb the comparative hybridization at the corresponding unbalanced regions resulting in a different fluorescent signal compared to the rest of the genome where test and reference DNA have no quantitative difference. The signal patterns are analysed by a computer which collates a genome-wide

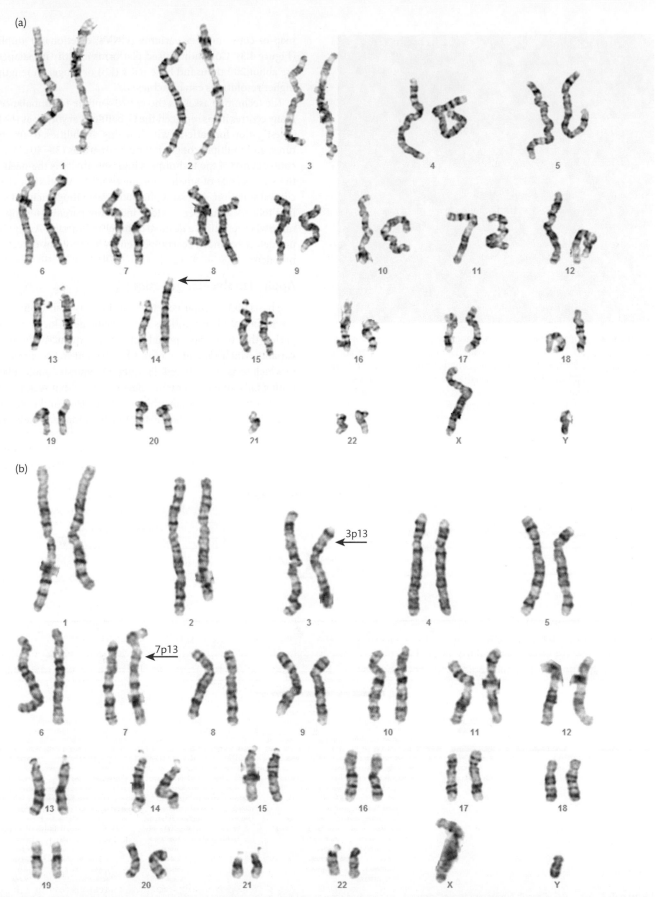

Figure 4.1 G-banded karyotyping showing a 14;21 Robertsonian translocation in (a) and a reciprocal translocation between chromosomes 3 and 7 in (b). The karyotype in (a) has 45 chromosomes as a result of fusion of the long arms of the acrocentric chromosomes 14 and 21 (arrow shows the derivative chromosome). In (b), there is an exchange between the short arms of one chromosome 3 and one chromosome 7. The arrows denote the derivative chromosomes and the break points at bands 3p13 and 7p13. Both chromosome complements can give rise to genetically unbalanced gametes.

Courtesy Dr Carolina Sismani, Cyprus Institute of Neurology & Genetics.

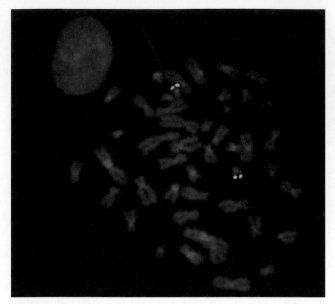

Figure 4.2 Fluorescent *in situ* hybridization showing a heterozygous 22q11.2 deletion. The chromosome with the deletion (arrow) exhibits the green signal for the chromosome 22 marker but lacks the red signal for the 22q11.2 locus which is seen on the homologous chromosome. The signals appear paired because chromosomes are in the form of duplicated chromatids at this stage of mitosis.

Courtesy Dr Carolina Sismani, Cyprus Institute of Neurology & Genetics.

map of copy number variants (CNVs; deletions or duplications) (**Figure 4.3**). Commonly used platforms identify imbalances which are about 200 thousand base pairs (kb) or longer in length though higher resolutions can be achieved.

The technique assesses the entire genome for imbalances and in many centres it has replaced the G-banded karyotype as the first-line investigation for patients with learning disabilities, dysmorphic features, and multiple congenital malformations (38–40). An inherent consequence of the technique's high sensitivity is the need to assess the significance of small imbalances in the context of the specific clinical situation. Assessing the potential pathogenicity of such findings follows a number of steps including parental testing to determine whether this is a *de novo* or inherited variant. Array CGH does not detect balanced rearrangements and may not detect low-level mosaicism.

Applied molecular genetics

The basis of molecular genetic techniques is their ability to identify the sequence of nucleotides at a specific gene locus and, by comparing this with the normal reference sequence, identify genetic variants which may or may not be relevant to the clinical context in which tests are initiated. Frequently requested molecular genetic testing falls under two main categories: tests that seek to determine whether variation exists within a specific gene, and in doing so aim to establish a genetic diagnosis, and tests that are more limited in

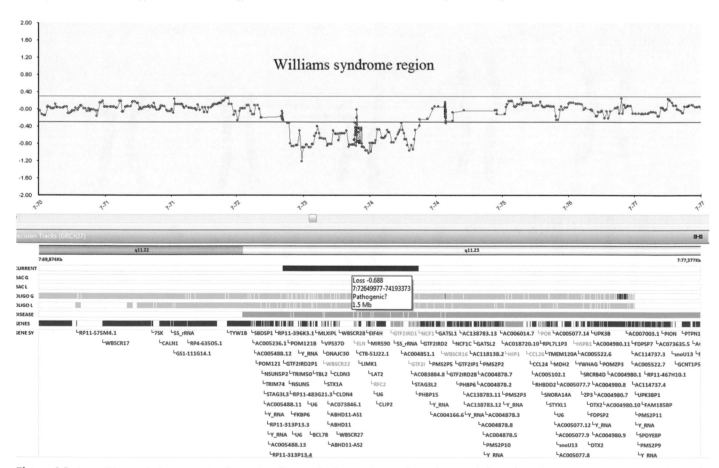

Figure 4.3 Array CGH result showing ratio of intensity of test and reference DNA in logarithmic scale (y axis) in relation to the genomic coordinates (x axis). In the logarithmic scale, deletions are represented by negative ratios. This result shows a deletion of approximately 1.5 Mb in length (thick red line) in the long arm of chromosome 7 which corresponds to the Williams syndrome critical region.

Courtesy Dr Carolina Sismani, Cyprus Institute of Neurology & Genetics.

scope, which aim to establish whether the individual being tested has inherited a specific mutation.

Gene sequencing is the centrepiece of modern molecular genetics with Sanger sequencing being considered as the gold standard (41). The technique uses DNA replication to determine the sequence of nucleotides in a single-stranded fragment of DNA. It relies on the introduction in the nucleotide mix (used in DNA replication) of additional modified nucleotides (containing the four bases) which lead to the termination of replication once they are introduced into the new chain (42). A computerized system determines the sequence of DNA bases by interpreting the position of this termination (**Figure 4.4**).

Sequencing techniques are not always best placed to detect specific types of mutations and partial or whole gene deletions/duplications require a different approach. A polymerase chain reaction (PCR)-based technique known as multiplex ligation-dependent probe amplification uses the concurrent amplification of different gene segments (43). The resulting amplified segments have, by

design, different sizes and can be separated by electrophoresis and visualized based on their fluorescent labels. The various signal peaks produced correspond to the different gene segments and a comparison with a reference sequence allows identification of parts of the gene that are either deleted, resulting in a reduced signal, or duplicated, resulting in an increased signal (**Figure 4.5**).

Sequencing techniques are also widely used to determine the presence of a specific mutation though this can also be achieved by techniques targeting the specific position within the gene. In PCR-based techniques, amplification is dependent on the presence of the mutation and can be detected using fluorescent labelling (44, 45).

While the techniques previously described continue to constitute the basis of molecular genetic investigations in many settings, the emergence of next-generation sequencing has revolutionized genetic testing (46–48). It relies on a technique known as massively parallel sequencing which is based on genome fragmentation and parallel sequencing of fragments using novel sequencing approaches that allow rapid identification of incorporated bases during replication of DNA templates. The sequence data is then contrasted against a library of reference sequences and discrepancies are noted. The efficiency of this technology has made the assessment of the entire exome and genome available for the investigation of disease and has led to the identification of the genetic basis of many monogenic disorders that had eluded molecular characterization (49, 50).

Genetic aspects of the clinical encounter

The assessment of the inheritance pattern of disorders and traits is by no means restricted to the work of clinical geneticists and a family history is an essential component of most clinical encounters. The relevant information is depicted in the genogram which can be updated as and when necessary and which underpins genetic interpretation. A number of computer programs allow genograms to be generated and updated electronically. However, in the author's experience, a well-constructed hand-written genogram is an efficient and effective way of recording this information. It conveys details on diagnoses, causes of death, and adverse pregnancy outcomes and is an accurate record of genetic relationships. Certain basic rules underlie reliable and reproducible genogram generation. It should record the date when first constructed as well as the dates of any updates, full names of affected family members and dates of birth (not ages as this will hinder interpretation), and a diagnostic index and should be based on the consistent use of established symbols (**Figure 4.6**).

The genogram helps establish modes of inheritance for genetic conditions, demonstrates risk patterns, and identifies clusters of events (such as recurrent early pregnancy loss) that are relevant to the consultation. In a woman with a new diagnosis of ovarian cancer, a careful record should be made of other cases of cancer, clustering of cases on either of the two sides of the woman's family, and the age at diagnosis. In addition to other cases of ovarian malignancy, particular attention is paid to cancers that point towards the possibility of an underlying cancer predisposition syndrome (breast, endometrial, colorectal).

The preconception interview

Genetic concepts frequently feature in clinical consultations and women (or couples) request counselling when planning to start or

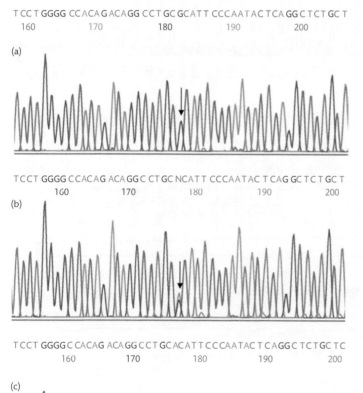

T CC T GGGG CC ACA G ACA GG CCT GC GCAT T CCCAATAC TCA GG C T CT GC T
160   170   180   190   200

(a)

T CC T GGGG C CAC AG ACA GG C CT GC NCAT T CCCAATAC T CAG GC T C T GC T
160   170   180   190   200

(b)

T CC T GGGG C CACA G ACA GG CCT GC ACAT T CCCAATAC T C AGGC TCTGC TC
160   170   180   190   200

(c)

Figure 4.4 Sanger sequencing chromatogram. The peaks represent the four bases, each labelled with a different fluorescent dye, with the control sequence represented in (a). Guanine is substituted by adenine in a heterozygous state in (b), where both peaks are seen, and in a homozygous state in (c). The software sequencing numbers shown in this chromatogram do not correspond to base positions and differ between alignments.

Courtesy Dr Maria Loizidou, Cyprus Institute of Neurology & Genetics.

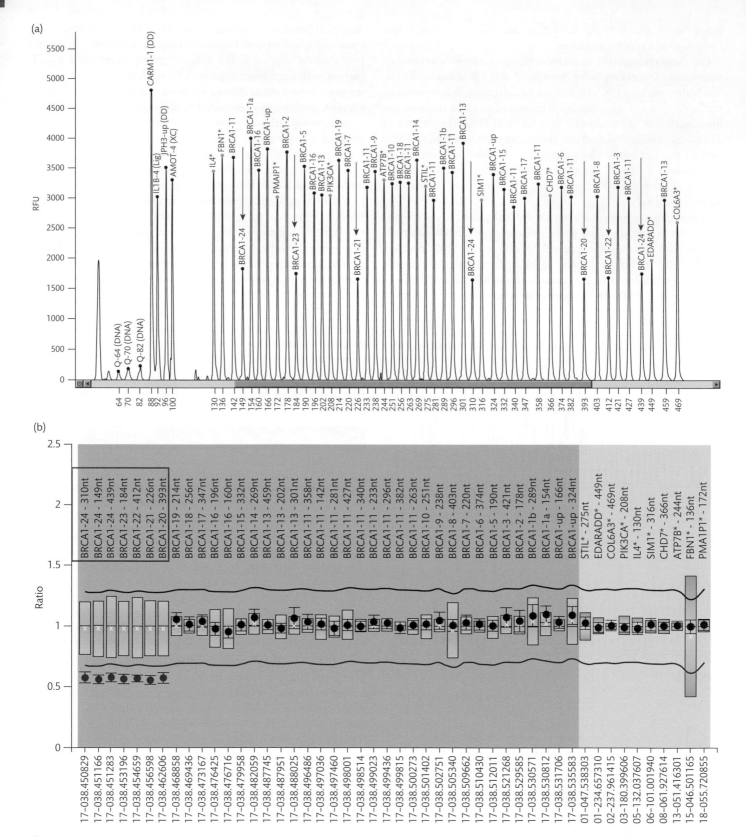

Figure 4.5 Multiplex ligation-dependent probe amplification electropherogram (a) and peak ratio plot (b) for the *BRCA1* gene. In (a), there are reduced relative fluorescent unit (RFU) peaks for exons 20 to 24 (arrows) and a halving of the ratio of the signal for those exons compared to the reference sequence as shown by the red dots in (b). This result is consistent with heterozygous deletion of exons 20 to 24 of the *BRCA1* gene.

Courtesy Dr Maria Loizidou, Cyprus Institute of Neurology & Genetics.

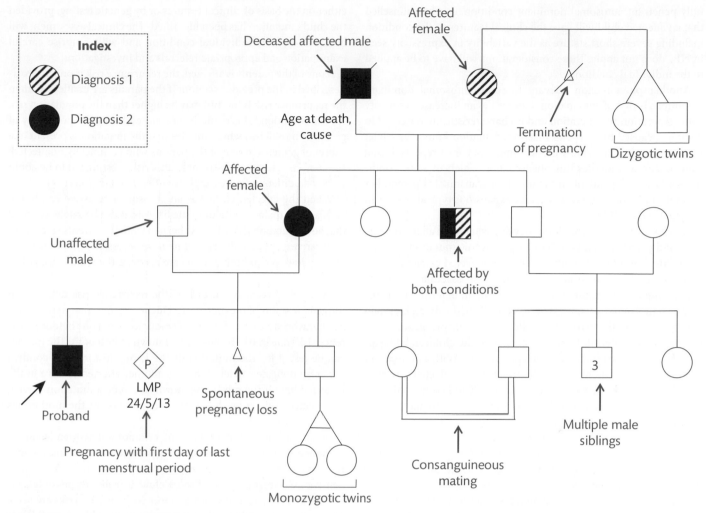

Figure 4.6 Symbols used in the construction of a genogram in conjunction with relevant information. Sample genogram drawn to illustrate use of the symbols.

extend their family or in an established pregnancy. Issues that feature in the preconception interview include infertility or subfertility, health-promotion advice, the impact of pregnancy on a pre-existing medical condition, and possible genetic risks to the baby. Discussion of most of these issues is beyond the scope of this chapter and the following subsections will concentrate on the approach to possible genetic implications in a future pregnancy.

The prospective parents may themselves be affected or concerns may be raised because of a previously affected child, a possible or confirmed genetic diagnosis in the family, a genetic condition that is prevalent in the specific population, the possible implications of consanguinity, and repeated losses of pregnancy or birth of babies with congenital malformations in the family. Whatever the specific concerns, a detailed family history should be taken and a genogram drawn capturing as many relevant details as possible. This will form the basis for subsequent discussion, planning, investigation, and relevant counselling.

Affected prospective parents

A distinction should be made between monogenic conditions, conditions with multifactorial aetiology and recognized genetic predisposition, and sporadic disease. The rest of the discussion will

concentrate on the scenario of prospective parents with single gene disorders.

A woman with a diagnosis of neurofibromatosis type 1 (NF1) needs to be counselled that, as this is an autosomal dominant condition, the baby in a future pregnancy will have a one in two chance of inheriting the responsible mutation in the *NF1* gene. Logical follow-up questions include whether inheritance of the mutation means that the child will develop the condition and if the child will be affected in the same way as the parent. These are key questions in genetics and relate to the concepts of penetrance and expressivity.

Penetrance is the percentage of individuals carrying a pathogenic dominant mutation known to cause a condition who will go on to develop the condition regardless of its severity. Expressivity describes the variation in severity of a genetic condition between affected individuals who carry the same mutation (parent and child, for example). NF1 is virtually fully penetrant and a child inheriting an *NF1* mutation is expected to develop the condition. On the other hand, this is a condition with very variable expressivity and a mildly affected parent with mostly cutaneous manifestations may have an affected child with complex plexiform neurofibromas or an optic glioma. In contrast, a parent affected by achondroplasia, another fully penetrant autosomal dominant condition, can be counselled that an affected child will have the clinical features of the condition including severe short stature as the variability in expressivity seen in NF1 does not apply. These considerations will have to be applied to the individual conditions.

Another phenomenon relevant to some autosomal dominant conditions is that of anticipation. It describes an increase in severity from generation to generation and is characteristically observed in disorders caused by a type of insertion mutation known as triplet repeat expansion. Instability of the number of triplet repeats during gametogenesis underlies this phenomenon which in some conditions is largely dependent on the sex of the transmitting parent. For example, in Huntington disease, large expansions typically occur in the paternal line (51).

Autosomal recessive conditions develop when both alleles (maternally and paternally inherited) carry pathogenic mutations and are exemplified by affected children born to unaffected carrier parents. In the case of a woman affected by beta thalassaemia requesting counselling about a future pregnancy, the main determinant is the carrier status of her partner. Whereas the affected woman is certain to pass on one of the two mutated alleles to her offspring, only if the partner is a carrier will there be a chance of the children being affected (a one in two chance for each pregnancy). With a non-carrier partner, there is certainty of the children being unaffected carriers.

In X-linked recessive conditions, such as X-linked hypohidrotic ectodermal dysplasia, affected fathers cannot pass the mutation to their sons but are certain to pass it on to their daughters who are obligate carriers and may exhibit mild clinical features. These specific considerations do not apply to disorders such as Duchenne muscular dystrophy where affected males do not reproduce because of the severity of the condition.

Whatever the mode of inheritance, there are certain key considerations at the preconception stage. Has the condition been diagnosed based only on clinical criteria or has it been confirmed by genetic testing? Identification of parental mutations is crucial to the planning for preimplantation genetic or prenatal diagnosis and a referral to the clinical genetics service at this stage is appropriate. Moreover, in the absence of genetic confirmation, the possibility of using antenatal sonographic markers needs to be explored. Examples include sonographic evaluation of fetuses for fractures or deformities in osteogenesis imperfecta or the tumours related to tuberous sclerosis. These features, however, are variable and mainly detectable in the latter stages of pregnancy (52–54).

Previous affected child

Providing counselling on recurrence risks is a frequent component of preconception consultations and a key task for clinical geneticists (55, 56). First, it must be established whether the affected child has a genetic diagnosis following a single gene inheritance pattern and whether laboratory confirmation has taken place.

A basic principle is that the recurrence risk depends on the genetic status of the parents. In autosomal dominant disorders, a pathogenic mutation in an affected child has either been inherited from one of the parents or has arisen as a new mutation (de novo) in the child. This will vary depending on the specific condition. In NF1, about 50% of cases are the result of de novo mutations and in achondroplasia about 80% of affected children are born to unaffected parents. Depending on the condition, the parental status can be established

either on the basis of clinical features or by genetic testing, provided the child's mutation has been identified. The clinical assessment will be tailored to the individual condition and will comprise careful examination and appropriate referrals and investigations.

If one of the parents is affected, the recurrence risk is one in two as described in the previous section. If the parents are unaffected, then the recurrence risk is low but may be higher than the population risk for the condition. This could be accounted for by the possibility of germline mosaicism which implies that the mutation is present in a subset of gametes in one of the parents who is clinically unaffected. In tuberous sclerosis, for example, this risk is estimated to be about 1–2% and different figures apply to different conditions (57).

When the affected child has an autosomal recessive condition, such as beta thalassaemia or cystic fibrosis, it can be safely assumed that both mutations have been inherited from the parents since, with very rare exceptions, the rate of de novo recessive mutations is extremely low. When both parents are carriers, the recurrence risk is one in four.

In X-linked recessive disorders, the recurrence risk depends on the genetic status of the mother. In Duchenne muscular dystrophy, a mother who is a carrier for a DMD mutation has a one in four recurrence risk (one in two if the baby is known to be a boy). The mother can be tested for the mutation or the family history may confirm her as an obligate carrier if there is another affected relative in the maternal line. If the mother is shown not to be a mutation carrier, the affected child either has a de novo mutation or the mother has germline mosaicism.

When dealing with conditions that do not follow Mendelian inheritance, such as many isolated congenital malformations, empiric risks based on observed recurrence data can be given. A comprehensive assessment of the affected child to rule out possible syndromic associations is necessary before such empiric risks are used. There are also occasions when it may not be possible to confidently distinguish between an undiagnosed single gene disorder that is recessively inherited and one that is the result of a de novo dominant mutation. Recurrence risks differ greatly in the two scenarios and clinical geneticists may use intermediate risk estimates based on the level of probability in the specific clinical context. If a recurrence does occur or if genetic testing subsequently confirms a single gene disorder, future advice will be adjusted accordingly.

Familial conditions

Women and their partners who are neither affected nor have affected children may raise the possibility of a genetic condition running in the family. The overall objective is to establish the likelihood of unaffected prospective parents being carriers for a genetic condition so that appropriate genetic testing can be offered or suggest that such testing may not be indicated.

Constructing a genogram is instrumental in helping the clinician understand and quantify any possible risks to a future pregnancy and counsel appropriately. The information needs to be as accurate and as comprehensive as possible and women are often asked to return to the clinic with additional details and clarifications in order to fill in any gaps and it may be necessary for consent to be obtained from family members in order to access details of a specific diagnosis.

When interpreting the genogram, the ratio of affected males to females, the severity in males compared to females, and any male-to-male transmission need to be assessed in evaluating the possibility of an X-linked disorder. Successive generations being affected may point towards autosomal dominant inheritance and the skipping of generations raises the possibility of reduced penetrance. Consanguinity supports autosomal recessive conditions and the lack of any transmission from males would be consistent with mitochondrial (non-Mendelian) inheritance. These considerations form the basis of genogram analysis which should be used in the context of the available clinical details. This interpretation may be hampered by the small number of affected individuals in a family. Moreover, there may be insufficient evidence to suggest a single gene disorder.

Risk in the absence of a familial diagnosis

It is also possible for women or couples to request genetic counselling even if there are no documented cases of possible genetic disorders in the family. A careful family history should be taken as this may reveal potentially relevant diagnoses. Counselling may be requested on the basis of parental consanguinity or the prevalence of a genetic disorder in a population.

If the prospective parents are related to each other, there is primarily an increased risk of the baby being affected by autosomal recessive conditions as a result of the parents sharing a proportion of their genome depending on the degree of relationship. It is estimated that humans carry about one to two harmful autosomal recessive alleles and consanguinity increases the chance that the same pathogenic allele will be inherited by a baby from both parents. Couples need to be counselled about this with the relevant level of estimated and empiric risk being conveyed (55, 58).

The couple's ethnic background may also identify genetic risks and targets for testing particularly in relation to the carrier state for autosomal recessive disorders. In Northern European populations, the carrier rate for cystic fibrosis is about 1 in 25 and it is possible that a couple may request carrier testing (59). The carrier rate for beta thalassaemia is very high in some Mediterranean countries (in Cyprus it is as high as one in seven) and it is very important that prospective parents are counselled appropriately and appropriate testing is offered (60).

Recurrent early pregnancy losses

About 15% of all recognized pregnancies miscarry and chromosomal abnormalities account for about half of these losses (61, 62). In recurrent miscarriage, affecting up to 5% of couples if defined as two or more losses, products of conception are analysed cytogenetically to establish a diagnosis and determine whether balanced rearrangements in the parents might be the underlying factor (62–64).

For example, women carrying a Robertsonian translocation involving chromosomes 14 and 21 have a 10–15% risk of having a baby with Down syndrome and preimplantation and prenatal options need to be discussed (65–67). When a parent is found to be a carrier of a balanced reciprocal translocation, the associated risk of a viable imbalance needs to be assessed and appropriate plans need to be made in a future pregnancy (68, 69).

Communication aspects of genetic counselling

One of the central pillars of genetic counselling is the element of non-directiveness. Clinical geneticists and other clinicians and professionals involved in genetic counselling have a responsibility to provide their patients with the necessary information in order for them to decide on their preferred course of action (55, 70, 71).

What needs to be thoroughly explored is a plan that is appropriate for the individuals involved in a particular context and at a particular moment in time. This principle is illustrated well in the context of a prenatal consultation. This is a period during which decisions need to be made regarding invasive prenatal tests and often about whether to continue with a pregnancy or proceed with termination.

Given the inherent uncertainty and complexity of many of these issues, it is not surprising that many women request guidance from their doctor in order to make a choice. In the author's opinion, clinicians would be most helpful by carefully exploring the various options with their patients with well-supported and constructive arguments on the advantages, disadvantages, and limitations of the various courses of action, empowering them to make informed choices. Moreover, directiveness in counselling can be problematic in situations, for example, where there are differing approaches among couples themselves. A good review of these issues is provided by Harper (55).

Preimplantation genetic diagnosis

The evolution of assisted reproduction has transformed the prospects for many infertile and subfertile couples. It has also made possible genetic scrutiny of the preimplantation embryos before these are returned to the uterus based on biopsy at the cleavage or blastocyst stage (72–74). This approach offers significant advantages for couples who have been identified at the preconception consultation as being at increased risk of having babies with genetic conditions.

There are two main categories of preimplantation genetic scrutiny: preimplantation genetic diagnosis (PGD) and preimplantation genetic screening (PGS). PGD is used to select unaffected embryos where there is high genetic risk for a specific disorder. The desire not to have children affected by a specific condition coupled with the unwillingness to consider prenatal diagnosis and possible termination of an established pregnancy is one of the main indications for considering PGD. The two main examples are inherited chromosomal disorders and monogenic diseases. The diagnosis of chromosomal abnormalities is based on FISH (75, 76) and of single gene disorders on PCR techniques (73, 77). The laboratory must have a validated preimplantation protocol for the specific diagnoses.

PGS is used to screen and select embryos free from chromosomal aneuploidy or other chromosomal imbalance, aiming to increase the chances of a successful pregnancy and take-home baby rates (78). Indications for PGS include advancing maternal age, recurrent early pregnancy loss, recurrent implantation failure, and severe male factor infertility and in these cases the parents do not have a known genetic risk or chromosomal rearrangement (79–82). The usefulness of PGS in improving pregnancy outcomes is under debate and may be limited by early embryo mosaicism and limitations of FISH techniques (83, 84). The use of array CGH and next-generation sequencing techniques may improve outcomes in this context (85, 86).

Prenatal testing

The monitoring and testing of a pregnancy known to be at genetic risk is usually planned at the preconception stage. Depending on the circumstances, it may involve invasive or non-invasive genetic testing, sonographic assessment, or a combination of these.

Mutation testing is still most commonly performed through invasive techniques: either a chorionic villous sampling, usually performed between 11 and 13 weeks of gestation, which tests the genetic material of placental tissue of fetal origin, or amniocentesis, usually performed between 15 and 20 weeks of gestation, which allows the examination of the genetic material of fetal cells suspended in the amniotic fluid. Both techniques are associated with a small, but not insignificant, risk of pregnancy loss of 0.5–1% (87). Another form of invasive testing, percutaneous umbilical cord sampling, is not commonly performed for genetic diagnosis and its use is largely restricted to haematological assessment of the fetus suspected to have severe anaemia and thrombocytopenia (88).

The demonstration of free fetal DNA in the maternal plasma has been the basis for developing alternative, non-invasive approaches to prenatal diagnosis (89, 90). An early application was the use of this free fetal DNA for the determination of the sex of the fetus. This is very important for pregnancies at risk of X-linked recessive disorders such as haemophilia A or Duchenne muscular dystrophy. As female fetuses are at most at risk of being carriers, this reduces the need for invasive procedures. The test, which is commonly performed after the eighth week of gestation, is based on the identification of male sex-determining region Y (*SRY*) sequences in the maternal plasma and the use of real-time PCR is associated with very high sensitivity and specificity (91–94). A fetal sonographic technique has also been developed which assesses the angle between the genital tubercle and the lumbosacral vertebral line (95). This is only feasible, however, after 11 weeks and its accuracy improves with increasing gestation (96). Some centres also advocate a combination of the two techniques (92, 97).

Non-invasive testing of free fetal DNA has also been used in the prenatal diagnosis of paternally inherited or *de novo* autosomal dominant conditions where mutations detected in the maternal plasma must be of fetal origin (98, 99). Moreover, it can be used to exclude inheritance of the paternal mutated allele in autosomal recessive cases where this is different from the maternal mutation (100, 101). The early techniques have been based on the use of PCR which requires prior knowledge of the mutation to be tested and its use in *de novo* diagnoses is limited to conditions such as achondroplasia where the vast majority of cases are caused by a single mutation. There is evidence that the application of next-generation sequencing techniques may improve the scope and accuracy of such testing in the future (102).

In pregnancies with no specific genetic risks identified in the preconception period, antenatal screening may identify risk factors for genetic diagnoses. Established aneuploidy screening programmes combine biochemical testing with sonographic markers to modify the age-related risk (103). When an invasive test is indicated in high-risk pregnancies, many laboratories use rapid aneuploidy testing such as interphase FISH (104, 105) or quantitative fluorescent PCR (106, 107) (**Figure 4.7**). There is a debate about the cost-effectiveness and additional diagnostic yield of routinely proceeding with a karyotype if these rapid tests are negative (108, 109). However, individual cases need to be evaluated based on the indications for the invasive test (such as sonographic abnormalities) and the possibility of missing other chromosomal abnormalities should be taken into account.

Recently, testing for fetal aneuploidy has been revolutionized by the introduction of non-invasive techniques using massively parallel sequencing which have a very high negative predictive value and have significantly reduced the need for invasive procedures, though invasive tests are still required to confirm a positive result (110–113). The wider clinical application of these techniques and their possible incorporation into national programmes are under consideration (114).

The fetus with sonographic abnormalities and a normal karyotype remains a diagnostic challenge. Recently, array CGH has been introduced to prenatal diagnosis based on its superior sensitivity for chromosomal imbalances (115–118). One of the main challenges of the use of array CGH in this setting is the potential difficulty in interpreting the significance of some CNVs (119, 120). It is particularly important in prenatal cases to discern between incidental findings and chromosomal variants that are relevant to the fetal abnormalities. In that context, cytogenetic laboratories have assumed a stepwise approach to evaluate these findings (121). Parental tests are used to establish whether the CNV has been inherited as its identification in an unaffected parent makes it less likely to be relevant. Moreover, the region of imbalance is assessed for the presence of relevant genes and databases, such as the Database of Genomic Variants, are assessed to determine whether it has been previously reported in association with a syndrome or specific phenotype or whether it has been reported as polymorphic.

Oncogenetics

Principles

'All cancer is genetic but some cancers are more genetic than others.' This paraphrase from George Orwell's *Animal Farm* conveys the essence of the genetic basis of malignancy. At the tissue level, all cancers are the result of the cumulative effect of environmental insults and genetic changes leading to dysregulated, uncontrolled growth of abnormal clones of cells. In a minority of cases, these tissue-specific genetic alterations leading to cancer are predisposed to by highly penetrant, inherited germline mutations (122). Sporadic cancers are the result of detrimental genetic dysregulation of growth in the affected organ whereas in the so-called inherited cancers, the underlying factors are genetic changes affecting all cells of the body. In reality, there exists a spectrum between true sporadic and 'inherited' disease with many cancers being the result of the cumulative effect of a number of lower-penetrance familial genetic alterations (123–126).

Genes in which mutations predispose to cancer are broadly classified under two categories: proto-oncogenes and tumour suppressor genes (TSGs). Genes of both categories fulfil important functions in the human body. Proto-oncogenes play important roles in regulated growth and proliferation and include growth factors and components of signal transduction pathways. Mutations can result in a proto-oncogene becoming an oncogene, driving uncontrolled growth and tumour formation. On the other hand, TSGs function as guards against unregulated growth either by controlling proliferation, promoting programmed cell death (apoptosis) of abnormally proliferating cell clones, or, at a more fundamental level, by repairing damage to DNA. This class of TSGs are known as DNA repair genes and mutations in them do not directly lead to tumorigenesis but increase the likelihood of mutations in other TSGs or proto-oncogenes.

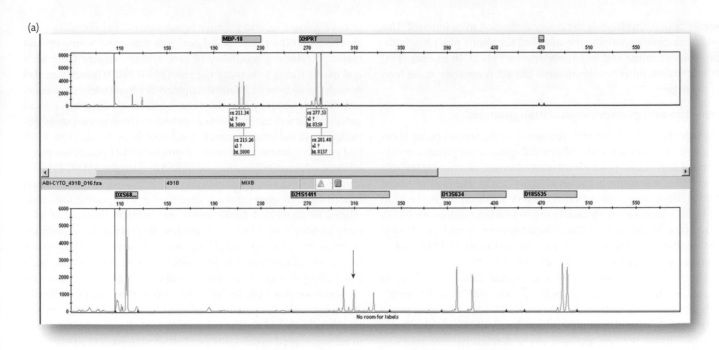

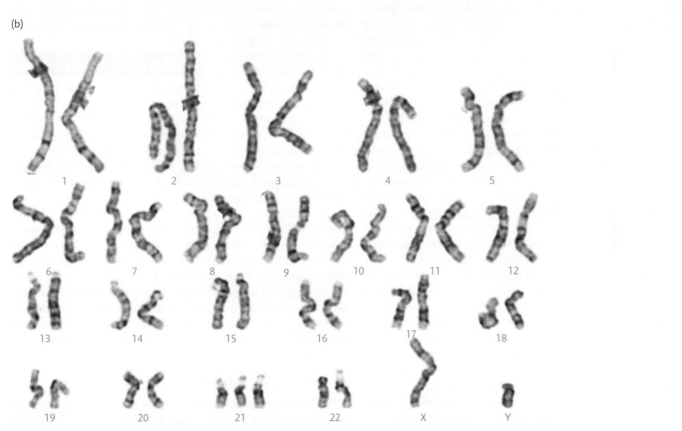

Figure 4.7 Quantitative fluorescent PCR electropherogram in (a) showing three copies of amplified markers specific for chromosome 21 as indicated by the three peaks (arrow). Trisomy 21 is confirmed by the G-banded karyotype in (b).
Courtesy Dr Carolina Sismani, Cyprus Institute of Neurology & Genetics.

Mutations in both proto-oncogenes and TSGs are linked to specific cancer predisposition syndromes which are most commonly inherited in an autosomal dominant manner. In the case of proto-oncogenes, gain-of-function mutations in the heterozygous state confer increased cancer susceptibility as the abnormal gene products of the mutated allele drive growth. On the other hand, both alleles of TSGs need to be altered at the tissue level for that specific tumour suppressor function to be deficient. So, the TSG mutations (and the resulting syndromes) are inherited in the heterozygous state but the inactivation of the second allele at the organ level is required for the sequence of events leading to tumour formation to be initiated. This is the principle underlying the so-called Knudson's two-hit hypothesis (one germline and one tissue-specific) (127). In essence, TSG mutations are inherited dominantly but act recessively at the level of the organs.

Genetics and gynaecological malignancies

Though the majority of gynaecological malignancies occur sporadically, both ovarian and endometrial cancers are prominent features of key cancer predisposition syndromes, illustrating the role of germline mutations in the aetiology of cancer. The lifetime risk of women developing ovarian cancer is very significantly increased in two of the most common cancer predisposition syndromes: BRCA hereditary breast and ovarian cancer syndrome and Lynch syndrome. Both syndromes are caused by mutations in TSGs and in both cases these are TSGs involved in DNA repair.

The BRCA hereditary breast and ovarian cancer syndrome is caused by mutations in the genes *BRCA1* and *BRCA2* which are involved in post-replication DNA repair (128–130). The gene products repair breaks following DNA replication and loss of this repair function leaves the cells exposed to the detrimental effects of uncorrected errors. It is the accumulation of such errors that eventually leads to tumorigenesis. The presence of *BRCA* mutations in the heterozygous state is not sufficient to disrupt the DNA repair ability of the cell. It is the loss of the functioning second allele that occurs through an independent event (second hit) at the tissue level that is the critical step. The syndrome is associated with a significant increase in breast and ovarian cancer risks as well as the risk of other malignancies including prostate and pancreas (131–134).

Lynch syndrome is caused by mutations in a family of genes involved in DNA repair known as mismatch repair genes (135–138). The function of the gene products is to correct errors in base-matching following DNA replication. As with *BRCA*, the presence of germline mutations in these genes confers susceptibility to cancer and it is the loss of the second, functioning allele that results in loss of the mismatch repair function and the subsequent sequence of events that leads to cancer development. The syndrome is associated with an increased risk of many cancers including colorectal, endometrial, gastric, and ovarian (139–141).

Oncogenetics in clinical practice

In assessing a woman diagnosed with a malignancy such as ovarian or endometrial cancer, a gynaecologist may consider the possibility that the disease developed in the context of a cancer predisposition syndrome. The woman's age, previous personal history of cancer, and relevant family history of malignant disease can be pointers to a possible genetic predisposition and the genogram is particularly useful in that context. A woman being diagnosed with ovarian cancer in her early 40s with a strong family history of breast cancer will need to be counselled for the possibility of an underlying *BRCA* mutation. In a woman diagnosed with endometrial cancer in her 50s who has a past history of colorectal cancer, the possibility of Lynch syndrome will need to be considered. Usually, a referral will be made to the clinical genetics service for consideration of genetic testing.

The identification of an underlying genetic predisposition is important and may influence the therapeutic options available and subsequent surveillance. For example, women with breast cancer and an underlying *BRCA* mutation have a significant lifetime risk

of developing a second primary breast cancer (142–145). This has an impact on the choice of surgical procedure and follow-up and may also raise the possibility of prophylactic surgery (contralateral mastectomy) to manage the risk (146–149). Women may also consider prophylactic bilateral salpingo-oophorectomy after completing their families to reduce the significant associated ovarian cancer risk as well as the breast cancer risk in the premenopausal period, though the latter is currently the subject of debate (150–153). In Lynch syndrome, the option of prophylactic hysterectomy and bilateral salpingo-oophorectomy should be discussed (154, 155).

A test for a cancer predisposition syndrome offered to a woman already affected from cancer is described as a diagnostic test. Tests offered to unaffected family members to establish whether they carry a known familial mutation are described as predictive. Women offered genetic testing should be counselled comprehensively about the nature of the tests and the implications of their results. Such counselling should address the complex medical, ethical, and psychosocial aspects that are inherent to this process (156–159). In diagnostic tests, the possibility of identifying variants of unknown significance should be discussed (160, 161). Beyond the relevance to management decisions, the psychological impact, at a time when a woman is dealing with her own diagnosis of cancer, should be explored, also taking into account the implications for other family members who are potentially at risk.

There are a number of considerations in relation to predictive tests. The ability to achieve prevention through close surveillance is one of the main indications and this relies on the availability of validated screening programmes for the relevant cancers. Examples include colonoscopy screening for Lynch syndrome (162, 163) and breast screening with magnetic resonance imaging in women with *BRCA* mutations (164, 165). Unaffected women also have the option of prophylactic surgery and the possibility of modifying risks through changes in lifestyle and avoidance of additional risk factors should also be explored.

The inheritance implications for existing or future children should be discussed. Some women may consider the option of prenatal (or preimplantation) genetic diagnosis though this is unusual because of the incomplete penetrance of many of the syndromes and the opportunities for prevention (166, 167). The potential impact on the ability of women to secure appropriate personal insurance once tested positive for a cancer predisposition syndrome needs to be part of pretest counselling though legislation has been passed in many countries to protect individuals from resulting discrimination (168, 169).

Novel therapeutic implications of oncogenetics

Establishing the molecular basis of cancer susceptibility has revealed new potential targets for treatment. Paradoxically, the chink in the armour of the cell's repair mechanisms may offer hope for novel therapeutic targeting of tumour cells (170). As described previously, loss of BRCA DNA-repair activity leaves cells vulnerable to other mutations and predisposes to oncogenesis. If manipulated, however, that disturbance in DNA repair ability can compromise the viability of tumour cells leading to cell death. One such manipulation is the use of poly ADP ribose polymerase (PARP) inhibitors which makes cells even more dependent on BRCA and has shown promising results in treating tumours which form part of the BRCA hereditary breast and ovarian cancer syndrome. PARP supports single-stranded

DNA repair and if its function is impaired, cells rely on more complex double-stranded repair mechanisms, such as homologous recombination and non-homologous end joining which are mediated by BRCA. If BRCA-mediated repair is itself deficient as a result of a germline mutation then PARP inhibition tips the balance towards genomic instability and cell death in these tumour cells (171–174).

REFERENCES

1. Speicher MR, Carter NP. The new cytogenetics: blurring the boundaries with molecular biology. *Nat Rev Genet* 2005;**6**:782–92.
2. Pinkel D, Segraves R, Sudar D, et al. High resolution analysis of DNA copy number variation using comparative genomic hybridization to microarrays. *Nat Genet* 1998;**20**:207–11.
3. Margulies M, Egholm M, Altman WE, et al. Genome sequencing in microfabricated high-density picolitre reactors. *Nature* 2005;**437**:376–80.
4. Fogel BL, Lee H, Strom SP, Deignan JL, Nelson SF. Clinical exome sequencing in neurogenetic and neuropsychiatric disorders. *Ann N Y Acad Sci* 2015;**1366**:49–60.
5. Shendure J, Porreca GJ, Reppas NB, et al. Accurate multiplex polony sequencing of an evolved bacterial genome. *Science* 2005;**309**:1728–32.
6. Xue Y, Ankala A, Wilcox WR, Hegde MR. Solving the molecular diagnostic testing conundrum for Mendelian disorders in the era of next-generation sequencing: single-gene, gene panel, or exome/genome sequencing. *Genet Med* 2015;**17**:444–51.
7. Gagan J, Van Allen EM. Next-generation sequencing to guide cancer therapy. *Genome Med* 2015;**7**:80.
8. Cooper DN, Chen JM, Ball EV, et al. Genes, mutations, and human inherited disease at the dawn of the age of personalized genomics. *Hum Mutat* 2010;**31**:631–55.
9. Benko S, Fantes JA, Amiel J, et al. Highly conserved non-coding elements on either side of SOX9 associated with Pierre Robin sequence. *Nat Genet* 2009;**41**:359–64.
10. Lettice LA, Heaney SJ, Purdie LA, et al. A long-range Shh enhancer regulates expression in the developing limb and fin and is associated with preaxial polydactyly. *Hum Mol Genet* 2003;**12**:1725–35.
11. Mirkovic N, Marti-Renom MA, Weber BL, Sali A, Monteiro AN. Structure-based assessment of missense mutations in human BRCA1: implications for breast and ovarian cancer predisposition. *Cancer Res* 2004;**64**:3790–97.
12. Ferrer-Costa C, Orozco M, de la Cruz X. Characterization of disease-associated single amino acid polymorphisms in terms of sequence and structure properties. *J Mol Biol* 2002;**315**:771–86.
13. Kanai K, Yoshida S, Hirose S, et al. Physicochemical property changes of amino acid residues that accompany missense mutations in SCN1A affect epilepsy phenotype severity. *J Med Genet* 2009;**46**:671–79.
14. Hofstra RM, Spurdle AB, Eccles D, et al. Tumor characteristics as an analytic tool for classifying genetic variants of uncertain clinical significance. *Hum Mutat* 2008;**29**:1292–303.
15. Inbar-Feigenberg M, Choufani S, Butcher DT, Roifman M, Weksberg R. Basic concepts of epigenetics. *Fertil Steril* 2013;**99**:607–15.
16. Cedar H, Bergman Y. Linking DNA methylation and histone modification: patterns and paradigms. *Nat Rev Genet* 2009;**10**:295–304.
17. Lande-Diner L, Zhang J, Ben-Porath I, et al. Role of DNA methylation in stable gene repression. *J Biol Chem* 2007;**282**:12194–200.
18. Gardner KE, Allis CD, Strahl BD. Operating on chromatin, a colorful language where context matters. *J Mol Biol* 2011;**409**:36–46.
19. Kaikkonen MU, Lam MT, Glass CK. Non-coding RNAs as regulators of gene expression and epigenetics. *Cardiovasc Res* 2011;**90**:430–40.
20. Barton SC, Surani MA, Norris ML. Role of paternal and maternal genomes in mouse development. *Nature* 1984;**311**:374–76.
21. McGrath J, Solter D. Completion of mouse embryogenesis requires both the maternal and paternal genomes. *Cell* 1984;**37**:179–83.
22. Ishida M, Moore GE. The role of imprinted genes in humans. *Mol Aspects Med* 2013;**34**:826–40.
23. Moore GE, Ishida M, Demetriou C, et al. The role and interaction of imprinted genes in human fetal growth. *Philos Trans R Soc Lond B Biol Sci* 2015;**370**:20140074.
24. Demetriou C, Abu-Amero S, Thomas AC. Paternally expressed, imprinted insulin-like growth factor-2 in chorionic villi correlates significantly with birth weight. *PLoS One* 2014;**9**:e85454.
25. Gicquel C, Gaston V, Mandelbaum J, Siffroi JP, Flahault A, Le Bouc Y. In vitro fertilization may increase the risk of Beckwith-Wiedemann syndrome related to the abnormal imprinting of the KCN1OT gene. *Am J Hum Genet* 2003;**72**:1338–41.
26. Hoeijmakers L, Kempe H, Verschure PJ. Epigenetic imprinting during assisted reproductive technologies: the effect of temporal and cumulative fluctuations in methionine cycling on the DNA methylation state. *Mol Reprod Dev* 2016;**83**:94–107.
27. Uyar A, Seli E. The impact of assisted reproductive technologies on genomic imprinting and imprinting disorders. *Curr Opin Obstet Gynecol* 2014;**26**:210–21.
28. Doornbos ME, Maas SM, McDonnell J, Vermeiden JP, Hennekam RC. Infertility, assisted reproduction technologies and imprinting disturbances: a Dutch study. *Hum Reprod* 2007;**22**:2476–80.
29. Houshdaran S, Cortessis VK, Siegmund K, Yang A, Laird PW, Sokol RZ. Widespread epigenetic abnormalities suggest a broad DNA methylation erasure defect in abnormal human sperm. *PLoS One* 2007;**2**:e1289.
30. Bickmore WA. Karyotype analysis and chromosome banding. In: *Encyclopedia of Life Sciences*, pp. 1–7. London: Nature Publishing Group; 2001.
31. Francke U. Digitized and differentially shaded human chromosome ideograms for genomic applications. *Cytogenet Cell Genet* 1994;**65**:206–18.
32. Pinkel D, Gray JW, Trask B, van den Engh G, Fuscoe J, van Dekken H. Cytogenetic analysis by in situ hybridization with fluorescently labeled nucleic acid probes. *Cold Spring Harb Symp Quant Biol* 1986;**51**:151–57.
33. Moore JW, Binder GA, Berry R. Prenatal diagnosis of aneuploidy and deletion 22q11.2 in fetuses with ultrasound detection of cardiac defects. *Am J Obstet Gynecol* 2004;**191**:2068–73.
34. Goldmuntz E, Clark BJ, Mitchell LE. Frequency of 22q11 deletions in patients with conotruncal defects. *J Am Coll Cardiol* 1998;**32**:492–98.
35. Pinkel D, Segraves R, Sudar D, et al. High resolution analysis of DNA copy number variation using comparative genomic hybridization to microarrays. *Nat Genet* 1998;**20**:207–11.
36. Pollack JR, Perou CM, Alizadeh AA, et al. Genome-wide analysis of DNA copy-number changes using cDNA microarrays. *Nat Genet* 1999;**23**:41–46.
37. Albertson DG, Ylstra B, Segraves R, et al. Quantitative mapping of amplicon structure by array CGH identifies CYP24 as a candidate oncogene. *Nat Genet* 2000;**25**:144–46.

38. Ahn JW, Bint S, Bergbaum A, Mann K, Hall RP, Ogilvie CM. Array CGH as a first line diagnostic test in place of karyotyping for post-natal referrals—results from four years' clinical application for over 8,700 patients. *Mol Cytogenet* 2013;**6**:16.

39. Miller DT, Adam MP, Aradhya S, et al. Consensus statement: chromosomal microarray is a first-tier clinical diagnostic test for individuals with developmental disabilities or congenital anomalies. *Am J Hum Genet* 2010;**86**:749–64.

40. Park SJ, Jung EH, Ryu RS, Kang HW, et al. Clinical implementation of whole-genome array CGH as a first-tier test in 5080 pre and postnatal cases. *Mol Cytogenet* 2011;**4**:12.

41. Sanger F, Nicklen S, Coulson AR. DNA sequencing with chain-terminating inhibitors. *Proc Natl Acad Sci U S A* 1977;**74**:5463–67.

42. Lee LG, Connell CR, Woo SL, et al. DNA sequencing with dye-labeled terminators and T7 DNA polymerase: effect of dyes and dNTPs on incorporation of dye-terminators and probability analysis of termination fragments. *Nucleic Acids Res* 1992;**20**:2471–83.

43. Schouten JP, McElgunn CJ, Waaijer R, Zwijnenburg D, Diepvens F, Pals G. Relative quantification of 40 nucleic acid sequences by multiplex ligation-dependent probe amplification. *Nucleic Acids Res* 2002;**30**:e57.

44. Aarskog NK, Vedeler CA. Real-time quantitative polymerase chain reaction. A new method that detects both the peripheral myelin protein 22 duplication in Charcot-Marie-Tooth type 1A disease and the peripheral myelin protein 22 deletion in hereditary neuropathy with liability to pressure palsies. *Hum Genet* 2000;**107**:494–98.

45. Horowitz M, Pasmanik-Chor M, Borochowitz Z, et al. Prevalence of glucocerebrosidase mutations in the Israeli Ashkenazi Jewish population. *Hum Mutat* 1998;**12**:240–44.

46. Campbell PJ, Stephens PJ, Pleasance ED, et al. Identification of somatically acquired rearrangements in cancer using genome-wide massively parallel paired-end sequencing. *Nat Genet* 2008;**40**:722–29.

47. Metzker ML. Sequencing technologies—the next generation. *Nat Rev Genet* 2010;**11**:31–46.

48. Koboldt DC, Steinberg KM, Larson DE, Wilson RK, Mardis ER. The next-generation sequencing revolution and its impact on genomics. *Cell* 2013;**155**:27–38.

49. Bamshad MJ, Ng SB, Bigham AW, et al. Exome sequencing as a tool for Mendelian disease gene discovery. *Nat Rev Genet* 2011;**12**:745–55.

50. Gilissen C, Hoischen A, Brunner HG, Veltman JA. Disease gene identification strategies for exome sequencing. *Eur J Hum Genet* 2012;**20**:490–97.

51. Trottier Y, Biancalana V, Mandel JL. Instability of CAG repeats in Huntington's disease: relation to parental transmission and age of onset. *J Med Genet* 1994;**31**:377–82.

52. Tsai PY, Chang CH, Yu CH, Cheng YC, Chang FM. Three-dimensional ultrasound in the prenatal diagnosis of osteogenesis imperfecta. *Taiwan J Obstet Gynecol* 2012;**51**:387–92.

53. Thompson EM. Non-invasive prenatal diagnosis of osteogenesis imperfecta. *Am J Med Genet* 1993;**45**:201–206

54. Gusman M, Servaes S, Feygin T, Degenhardt K, Epelman M. Multimodal imaging in the prenatal diagnosis of tuberous sclerosis complex. *Case Rep Pediatr* 2012;**2012**:925646.

55. Harper PS. *Practical Genetic Counselling*. Boca Raton, FL: CRC Press; 2010.

56. Young ID. *Introduction to Risk Calculation in Genetic Counselling*. New York: Oxford University Press; 2007.

57. Yates JR, van Bakel I, Sepp T, et al. Female germline mosaicism in tuberous sclerosis confirmed by molecular genetic analysis. *Hum Mol Genet* 1997;**6**:2265–69.

58. Bittles A. Consanguinity and its relevance to clinical genetics. *Clin Genet* 2001;**60**:89–98.

59. Massie J, Ioannou L, Delatycki M. Prenatal and preconception population carrier screening for cystic fibrosis in Australia: where are we up to? *Aust N Z J Obstet Gynaecol* 2014;**54**:503–509.

60. Cousens NE, Gaff CL, Metcalfe SA, Delatycki MB. Carrier screening for beta-thalassaemia: a review of international practice. *Eur J Hum Genet* 2010;**18**:1077–83.

61. Rai R, Regan L. Recurrent miscarriage. *Lancet* 2006;**368**:601–11.

62. Hogge WA, Byrnes AL, Lanasa MC, Surti U. The clinical use of karyotyping spontaneous abortions. *Am J Obstet Gynecol* 2003;**189**:397–400.

63. De Braekeleer M, Dao TN. Cytogenetic studies in couples experiencing repeated pregnancy losses. *Hum Reprod* 1990;**5**:519–28.

64. Goddijn M, Joosten JH, Knegt AC, et al. Clinical relevance of diagnosing structural chromosome abnormalities in couples with repeated miscarriage. *Hum Reprod* 2004;**19**:1013–17.

65. Munné S, Morrison L, Fung J, et al. Spontaneous abortions are reduced after preconception diagnosis of translocations. *J Assist Reprod Genet* 1998;**15**:290–96.

66. Munné S, Sandalinas M, Escudero T, Fung J, Gianaroli L, Cohen J. Outcome of preimplantation genetic diagnosis of translocations. *J Fertil Steril* 2000;**73**:1209–18.

67. Scriven PN, Flinter FA, Braude PR, Ogilvie CM. Robertsonian translocations-reproductive risks and indications for preimplantation genetic diagnosis. *Hum Reprod* 2001;**16**:2267–73.

68. Midro AT, Stengel-Rutkowski S, Stene J. Experiences with risk estimates for carriers of chromosomal reciprocal translocations. *Clin Genet* 1992;**41**:113–22.

69. Barisić I, Zergollern L, Muzinić D, Hitrec V. Risk estimates for balanced reciprocal translocation carriers—prenatal diagnosis experience. *Clin Genet* 1996;**49**:145–51.

70. Witmer JM, Wedl L, Black BJ. Genetic counseling: ethical and professional role implications. *Couns Dev* 1986;**64**:337–40.

71. Kessler S. Psychological aspects of genetic counseling. XIV. Nondirectiveness and counseling skills. *Genet Test* 2001;**5**:187–91.

72. Hardy K, Martin KL, Leese HJ, Winston RM, Handyside AH. Human preimplantation development in vitro is not adversely affected by biopsy at the 8-cell stage. *Hum Reprod* 1990;**5**:708–14.

73. Harper JC, Sengupta SB. Preimplantation genetic diagnosis: state of the art 2011. *Hum Genet* 2012;**131**:175–86.

74. Hanson C, Jakobsson AH, Sjögren A, et al. Preimplantation genetic diagnosis (PGD): the Gothenburg experience. *Acta Obstet Gynecol Scand* 2001;**80**:331–36.

75. Fridström M, Ahrlund-Richter L, Iwarsson, et al. Clinical outcome of treatment cycles using preimplantation genetic diagnosis for structural chromosomal abnormalities. *Prenat Diagn* 2001;**21**:781–87.

76. Mackie Ogilvie C, Scriven PN. Meiotic outcomes in reciprocal translocation carriers ascertained in 3-day human embryos. *Eur J Hum Genet* 2002;**10**:801–806.

77. Harton GL, De Rycke M, Fiorentino F, et al. ESHRE PGD consortium best practice guidelines for amplification-based PGD. *Hum Reprod* 2011;**26**:33–40.

78. Verlinsky Y, Cieslak J, Freidine M, et al. Pregnancies following pre-conception diagnosis of common aneuploidies by fluorescent in-situ hybridization. *Hum Reprod* 1995;**10**:1923–27.

79. Silber S, Escudero T, Lenahan K, Abdelhadi I, Kilani Z, Munné S. Chromosomal abnormalities in embryos derived from testicular sperm extraction. *Fertil Steril* 2003;**79**:30–38.

80. Wilding M, Forman R, Hogewind G, et al. Preimplantation genetic diagnosis for the treatment of failed in vitro fertilization-embryo transfer and habitual abortion. *Fertil Steril* 2004;**81**:1302–307.

81. Platteau P, Staessen C, Michiels A, Van Steirteghem A, Liebaers I, Devroey P. Preimplantation genetic diagnosis for aneuploidy screening in patients with unexplained recurrent miscarriages. *Fertil Steril* 2005;**83**:393–97.

82. Chen CK, Yu HT, Soong YK, Lee CL. New perspectives on preimplantation genetic diagnosis and preimplantation genetic screening. *Taiwan J Obstet Gynecol* 2014;**53**:146–50.

83. van Echten-Arends J, Mastenbroek S, Sikkema-Raddatz B, et al. Chromosomal mosaicism in human preimplantation embryos: a systematic review. *Hum Reprod Update* 2011;**17**:620–27.

84. Mastenbroek S, Twisk M, van Echten-Arends JN. In vitro fertilization with preimplantation genetic screening. *N Engl J Med* 2007;**357**:9–17.

85. Yang Z, Liu J, Collins GS, et al. Selection of single blastocysts for fresh transfer via standard morphology assessment alone and with array CGH for good prognosis IVF patients: results from a randomized pilot study. *Mol Cytogenet* 2012;**5**:24.

86. Wells D, Kaur K, Grifo J, et al. Clinical utilisation of a rapid low-pass whole genome sequencing technique for the diagnosis of aneuploidy in human embryos prior to implantation. *J Med Genet* 2014;**51**:553–62.

87. Tabor A, Alfirevic Z. Update on procedure-related risks for prenatal diagnosis techniques. *Fetal Diagn Ther* 2010;**27**:1–7.

88. Society for Maternal-Fetal Medicine (SMFM), Berry SM, Stone J, Norton ME, Johnson D, Berghella V. Fetal blood sampling. *Am J Obstet Gynecol* 2013;**209**:170–80.

89. Lo YM, Corbetta N, Chamberlain PF, et al. Presence of fetal DNA in maternal plasma and serum. *Lancet* 1997;**350**:485–87.

90. Lo YM. Fetal DNA in maternal plasma: biology and diagnostic applications. *Clin Chem* 2000;**46**:1903–906.

91. Rijnders RJ, Van Der Luijt RB, Peters ED, et al. Earliest gestational age for fetal sexing in cell-free maternal plasma. *Prenat Diagn* 2003;**23**:1042–44.

92. Hyett JA, Gardener G, Stojilkovic-Mikic T, et al. Reduction in diagnostic and therapeutic interventions by non-invasive determination of fetal sex in early pregnancy. *Prenat Diagn* 2005;**25**:1111–16.

93. Guibert J, Benachi A, Grebille AG, Ernault P, Zorn JR, Costa JM. Kinetics of SRY gene appearance in maternal serum: detection by real time PCR in early pregnancy after assisted reproductive technique. *Hum Reprod* 2003;**18**:1733–36.

94. Honda H, Miharu N, Ohashi Y, et al. Fetal gender determination in early pregnancy through qualitative and quantitative analysis of fetal DNA in maternal serum. *Hum Genet* 2002;**110**:75–79.

95. Elejalde BR, de Elejalde MM, Heitman T. Visualization of the fetal genitalia by ultrasonography: a review of the literature and analysis of its accuracy and ethical implications. *J Ultrasound Med* 1985;**4**:633–39.

96. Efrat Z, Akinfenwa OO, Nicolaides KH. First-trimester determination of fetal gender by ultrasound. *Ultrasound Obstet Gynecol* 1999;**13**:305–307.

97. Chi C, Hyett JA, Finning KM, Lee CA, Kadir RA. Non-invasive first trimester determination of fetal gender: a new approach for prenatal diagnosis of haemophilia. *BJOG* 2006;**113**:239–42.

98. Chitty LS, Griffin DR, Meaney C, et al. New aids for the non-invasive prenatal diagnosis of achondroplasia: dysmorphic features, charts of fetal size and molecular confirmation using cell-free fetal DNA in maternal plasma. *Ultrasound Obstet Gynecol* 2011;**37**:283–89.

99. Chitty LS, Khalil A, Barrett AN, Pajkrt E, Griffin DR, Cole TJ. Safe, accurate, prenatal diagnosis of thanatophoric dysplasia using ultrasound and free fetal DNA. *Prenat Diagn* 2013;**33**:416–23.

100. Bustamante-Aragones A, Gallego-Merlo J, Trujillo-Tiebas MJ, et al. New strategy for the prenatal detection/exclusion of paternal cystic fibrosis mutations in maternal plasma. *J Cyst Fibros* 2008;**7**:505–10.

101. Nasis O, Thompson S, Hong T, et al. Improvement in sensitivity of allele-specific PCR facilitates reliable noninvasive prenatal detection of cystic fibrosis. *Clin Chem* 2004;**50**:694–701.

102. Chitty LS, Mason S, Barrett AN, et al. Non-invasive prenatal diagnosis of achondroplasia and thanatophoric dysplasia: next-generation sequencing allows for a safer, more accurate, and comprehensive approach. *Prenat Diagn* 2015;**35**:656–62.

103. Nicolaides KH. Screening for fetal aneuploidies at 11 to 13 weeks. *Prenat Diagn* 2011;**31**:7–15.

104. Weremowicz S, Sandstrom DJ, Morton CC, Niedzwiecki CA, Sandstrom MM, Bieber FR. Fluorescence in situ hybridization (FISH) for rapid detection of aneuploidy: experience in 911 prenatal cases. *Prenat Diagn* 2001;**21**:262–69.

105. Klinger K, Landes G, Shook D, et al. Rapid detection of chromosome aneuploidies in uncultured amniocytes by using fluorescence in situ hybridization (FISH). *Am J Hum Genet* 1992;**51**:55–65.

106. Pertl B, Pieber D, Lercher-Hartlieb A, et al. Rapid prenatal diagnosis of aneuploidy by quantitative fluorescent PCR on fetal samples from mothers at high risk for chromosome disorders. *Mol Hum Reprod* 1999;**5**:1176–79.

107. Mansfield ES. Diagnosis of Down syndrome and other aneuploidies using quantitative polymerase chain reaction and small tandem repeat polymorphisms. *Hum Mol Genet* 1993;**2**:43–50.

108. Leung WC, Lao TT. Rapid aneuploidy testing, traditional karyotyping, or both? *Lancet* 2005;**366**:97–98.

109. Caine A, Maltby AE, Parkin CA, Waters JJ, Crolla JA; UK Association of Clinical Cytogeneticists (ACC). Prenatal detection of Down's syndrome by rapid aneuploidy testing for chromosomes 13, 18, and 21 by FISH or PCR without a full karyotype: a cytogenetic risk assessment. *Lancet* 2005;**366**:123–28.

110. Gil MM, Quezada MS, Revello R, Akolekar R, Nicolaides KH. Analysis of cell-free DNA in maternal blood in screening for fetal aneuploidies: updated meta-analysis. *Ultrasound Obstet Gynecol* 2015;**45**:249–66.

111. Gregg AR, Gross SJ, Best RG, et al. ACMG statement on non-invasive prenatal screening for fetal aneuploidy. *Genet Med* 2013;**15**:395–98.

112. Norton ME, Jacobsson B, Swamy GK, et al. Cell-free DNA analysis for noninvasive examination of trisomy. *N Engl J Med* 2015;**372**:1589–97.

113. Warsof SL, Larion S, Abuhamad AZ. Overview of the impact of noninvasive prenatal testing on diagnostic procedures. *Prenat Diagn* 2015;**35**:972–79.

114. Minear MA, Lewis C, Pradhan S, Chandrasekharan S. Global perspectives on clinical adoption of NIPT. *Prenat Diagn* 2015;**35**:959–67.

115. Kleeman L, Bianchi DW, Shaffer LG, et al. Use of array comparative genomic hybridization for prenatal diagnosis of fetuses with sonographic anomalies and normal metaphase karyotype. *Prenat Diagn* 2009;**29**:1213–17.

116. Van den Veyver IB, Patel A, Shaw CA, et al. Clinical use of array comparative genomic hybridization (aCGH) for prenatal diagnosis in 300 cases. *Prenat Diagn* 2009;**29**:29–39.

117. Le Caignec C, Boceno M, Saugier-Veber P, et al. Detection of genomic imbalances by array based comparative genomic hybridisation in fetuses with multiple malformations. *J Med Genet* 2005;**42**:121–28.

118. Tyreman M, Abbott KM, Willatt LR, et al. High resolution array analysis: diagnosing pregnancies with abnormal ultrasound findings. *J Med Genet* 2009;**46**:531–41.

119. Van den Veyver IB, Beaudet AL. Comparative genomic hybridization and prenatal diagnosis. *Curr Opin Obstet Gynecol* 2006;**18**:185–91.

120. D'Amours G, Kibar Z, Mathonnet G, et al. Whole-genome array CGH identifies pathogenic copy number variations in fetuses with major malformations and a normal karyotype. *Clin Genet* 2012;**81**:128–41.

121. Evangelidou P, Alexandrou A, Moutafi M, et al. Implementation of high resolution whole genome array CGH in the prenatal clinical setting: advantages, challenges, and review of the literature. *Biomed Res Int* 2013;**2013**:346762.

122. Beggs AD, Hodgson SV. Genomics and breast cancer: the different levels of inherited susceptibility. *Eur J Hum Genet* 2009;**17**:855–56.

123. Volgelstein B, Kinzler KW. *The Genetic Basis of Human Cancer*. London: McGraw-Hill; 2002.

124. Turnbull C, Hodgson S. Genetic predisposition to cancer. *Clin Med (Lond)* 2005;**5**:491–98.

125. Seal S, Thompson D, Renwick A, et al. Truncating mutations in the Fanconi anemia J gene BRIP1 are low-penetrance breast cancer susceptibility alleles. *Nat Genet* 2006;**38**:1239–41.

126. Ripperger T, Gadzicki D, Meindl A, Schlegelberger B. Breast cancer susceptibility: current knowledge and implications for genetic counselling. *Eur J Hum Genet* 2009;**17**:722–31.

127. Knudson AG. Mutation and cancer: statistical study of retinoblastoma. *Proc Natl. Acad Sci U S A* 1971;**68**:820–23.

128. Wooster R, Bignell G, Lancaster J, et al. Identification of the breast cancer susceptibility gene BRCA2. *Nature* 1995;**378**:789–92.

129. Scully R. Role of BRCA gene dysfunction in breast and ovarian cancer predisposition. *Breast Cancer Res* 2000;**2**:324–30.

130. Sowter HM, Ashworth A. BRCA1 and BRCA2 as ovarian cancer susceptibility genes. *Carcinogenesis* 2005;**26**:1651–56.

131. Hopper JL, Southey MC, Dite GS, et al. Population-based estimate of the average age-specific cumulative risk of breast cancer for a defined set of protein-truncating mutations in BRCA1 and BRCA2. Australian Breast Cancer Family Study. *Cancer Epidemiol Biomarkers Prev* 1999;**8**:741–47.

132. Thompson D, Easton DF; Breast Cancer Linkage Consortium. Cancer incidence in BRCA1 mutation carriers. *J Natl Cancer Inst* 2002;**94**:1358–65.

133. Kirchhoff T, Kauff ND, Mitra N, et al. BRCA mutations and risk of prostate cancer in Ashkenazi Jews. *Clin Cancer Res* 2004;**10**:2918–21.

134. Iqbal J, Ragone A, Lubinski J, et al. The incidence of pancreatic cancer in BRCA1 and BRCA2 mutation carriers. *Br J Cancer* 2012;**107**:2005–2009.

135. Boland CR. Recent discoveries in the molecular genetics of Lynch syndrome. *Fam Cancer* 2016;**15**:395–403.

136. Lynch HT, Lynch PM, Lanspa SJ, Snyder CL, Lynch JF, Boland CR. Review of the Lynch syndrome: history, molecular genetics, screening, differential diagnosis, and medicolegal ramifications. *Clin Genet* 2009;**76**:1–18.

137. Bronner CE, Baker SM, Morrison PT, et al. Mutation in the DNA mismatch repair gene homologue hMLH1 is associated with hereditary non-polyposis colon cancer. *Nature* 1994;**368**:258–61.

138. Papadopoulos N, Nicolaides NC, Wei YF, et al. Mutation of a mutL homolog in hereditary colon cancer. *Science* 1994;**263**:1625–29.

139. Stoffel E, Mukherjee B, Raymond VM, et al. Calculation of risk of colorectal and endometrial cancer among patients with Lynch syndrome. *Gastroenterology* 2009;**137**:1621–27.

140. Barrow E, Robinson L, Alduaij W, et al. Cumulative lifetime incidence of extracolonic cancers in Lynch syndrome: a report of 121 families with proven mutations. *Clin Genet* 2009;**75**:141–49.

141. Watson P, Vasen HF, Mecklin JP, et al. The risk of extra-colonic, extra-endometrial cancer in the Lynch syndrome. *Int J Cancer* 2008;**123**:444–49.

142. Metcalfe K, Gershman S, Lynch HT, et al. Predictors of contralateral breast cancer in BRCA1 and BRCA2 mutation carriers. *Br J Cancer* 2011;**104**:1384–92.

143. van der Kolk DM, de Bock GH, Leegte BK, et al. Penetrance of breast cancer, ovarian cancer and contralateral breast cancer in BRCA1 and BRCA2 families: high cancer incidence at older age. *Breast Cancer Res Treat* 2010;**124**:643–51.

144. Malone KE, Begg CB, Haile RW, et al. Population-based study of the risk of second primary contralateral breast cancer associated with carrying a mutation in BRCA1 or BRCA2. *J Clin Oncol* 2010;**28**:2404–10.

145. Graeser MK, Engel C, Rhiem K, et al. Contralateral breast cancer risk in BRCA1 and BRCA2 mutation carriers. *J Clin Oncol* 2009;**27**:5887–92.

146. Angelos P, Bedrosian I, Euhus DM, Herrmann VM, Katz SJ, Pusic A. Contralateral prophylactic mastectomy: challenging considerations for the surgeon. *Ann Surg Oncol* 2015;**22**:3208–12.

147. Pierce LJ, Phillips KA, Griffith KA, et al. Local therapy in BRCA1 and BRCA2 mutation carriers with operable breast cancer: comparison of breast conservation and mastectomy. *Breast Cancer Res Treat* 2010;**121**:389–98.

148. Smith KL, Isaacs C. BRCA mutation testing in determining breast cancer therapy. *Cancer J* 2011;**17**:492–99.

149. van Sprundel TC, Schmidt MK, Rookus MA, et al. Risk reduction of contralateral breast cancer and survival after contralateral prophylactic mastectomy in BRCA1 or BRCA2 mutation carriers. *Br J Cancer* 2005;**93**:287–92.

150. Finch A, Evans G, Narod SA. BRCA carriers, prophylactic salpingo-oophorectomy and menopause: clinical management considerations and recommendations. *Womens Health (Lond Engl)* 2012;**8**:543–55.

151. Rebbeck TR, Levin AM, Eisen A, et al. Breast cancer risk after bilateral prophylactic oophorectomy in BRCA1 mutation carriers. *J Natl Cancer Inst* 1999;**91**:1475–79.

152. Kauff ND, Satagopan JM, Robson ME, et al. Risk-reducing salpingo-oophorectomy in women with a BRCA1 or BRCA2 mutation. *N Engl J Med* 2002;**346**:1609–15.

153. Rebbeck TR, Kauff ND, Domchek SM. Meta-analysis of risk reduction estimates associated with risk-reducing salpingo-oophorectomy in BRCA1 or BRCA2 mutation carriers. *J Natl Cancer Inst* 2009;**101**:80–87.

154. Vasen HF, Blanco I, Aktan-Collan K, et al. Revised guidelines for the clinical management of Lynch syndrome (HNPCC):

recommendations by a group of European experts. *Gut* 2013;**62**:812–23.

155. Schmeler KM, Lynch HT, Chen LM, et al. Prophylactic surgery to reduce the risk of gynecologic cancers in the Lynch syndrome. *N Engl J Med* 2006;**354**:261–69.

156. Wevers MR, Ausems MG, Verhoef S, et al. Behavioral and psychosocial effects of rapid genetic counseling and testing in newly diagnosed breast cancer patients: design of a multicenter randomized clinical trial. *BMC Cancer* 2011;**11**:6.

157. Graves KD, Vegella P, Poggi EA, et al. Long-term psychosocial outcomes of BRCA1/BRCA2 testing: differences across affected status and risk-reducing surgery choice. *Cancer Epidemiol Biomarkers Prev* 2012;**21**:445–55.

158. Braithwaite D, Emery J, Walter F, Prevost AT, Sutton S. Psychological impact of genetic counseling for familial cancer: a systematic review and meta-analysis. *Fam Cancer* 2006;**5**:61–75.

159. Hesse-Biber S, An C. Genetic testing and post-testing decision making among BRCA-positive mutation women: a psychosocial approach. *J Genet Couns* 2016;**25**:978–92.

160. Cheon JY, Mozersky J, Cook-Deegan R. Variants of uncertain significance in BRCA: a harbinger of ethical and policy issues to come? *Genome Med* 2014;**6**:121.

161. Richter S, Haroun I, Graham TC, Eisen A, Kiss A, Warner E. Variants of unknown significance in BRCA testing: impact on risk perception, worry, prevention and counseling. *Ann Oncol* 2013;**24** Suppl 8:viii69–74.

162. Järvinen HJ, Mecklin JP, Sistonen P. Screening reduces colorectal cancer rate in families with hereditary nonpolyposis colorectal cancer. *Gastroenterology* 1995;**108**:1405–11.

163. Vasen HF, Abdirahman M, Brohet R, et al. One to 2-year surveillance intervals reduce risk of colorectal cancer in families with Lynch syndrome. *Gastroenterology* 2010;**138**:2300–306.

164. Passaperuma K, Warner F, Causer PA, et al. Long-term results of screening with magnetic resonance imaging in women with BRCA mutations. *Br J Cancer* 2012;**107**:24–30.

165. Warner E, Messersmith H, Causer P, Eisen A, Shumak R, Plewes D. Systematic review: using magnetic resonance imaging to screen women at high risk for breast cancer. *Ann Intern Med* 2008;**148**:671–79.

166. Donnelly LS, Watson M, Moynihan C, et al. Reproductive decision-making in young female carriers of a BRCA mutation. *Hum Reprod* 2013;**28**:1006–12.

167. Ormondroyd E, Donnelly L, Moynihan C, et al. Attitudes to reproductive genetic testing in women who had a positive BRCA test before having children: a qualitative analysis. *Eur J Hum Genet* 2012;**20**:4–10.

168. Lane M, Ngueng Feze I, Joly Y. Genetics and personal insurance: the perspectives of Canadian cancer genetic counselors. *J Genet Couns* 2015;**24**:1022–36.

169. Joly Y, Ngueng Feze I, Simard J. Genetic discrimination and life insurance: a systematic review of the evidence. *BMC Med* 2013;**11**:25.

170. Goyal G, Fan T, Silberstein PT. Hereditary cancer syndromes: utilizing DNA repair deficiency as therapeutic target. *Fam Cancer* 2016;**15**:359–66.

171. Ricks TK, Chiu HJ, Ison G, et al. Successes and challenges of PARP inhibitors in cancer therapy. *Front Oncol* 2015;**5**:222.

172. Bryant HE, Schultz N, Thomas HD, et al. Specific killing of BRCA2-deficient tumours with inhibitors of poly(ADP-ribose) polymerase. *Nature* 2005;**434**:913–17.

173. Farmer H, McCabe N, Lord CJ, et al. Targeting the DNA repair defect in BRCA mutant cells as a therapeutic strategy. *Nature* 2005;**434**:917–21.

174. Tutt AN, Lord CJ, McCabe N, et al. Exploiting the DNA repair defect in BRCA mutant cells in the design of new therapeutic strategies for cancer. *Cold Spring Harb Symp Quant Biol* 2005;**70**:139–48.

5

Clinical governance

Leroy C. Edozien

What is clinical governance?

Definition: what it is and what it isn't

Clinical governance is the totality of structures and processes that are in place to ensure that, as far as practicable, the right person receives the right treatment, in the right way, at the right time, in the right place, with the right outcome. This goal does not happen by chance; it has to be secured by conscious effort, and that effort—creating and sustaining the required structures and processes—has to be actively and efficiently managed. Further, this active management is not just at the level of the healthcare organization but also at the level of the individual practitioner, and it is not just the business of healthcare managers but is (or should be) at the core of clinical practice.

The value of clinical governance

Clinical governance is important for the benefit of service users, hospital staff, the healthcare organization, and the wider health economy. Recipients of healthcare expect to have the treatment that is tailored to their needs and circumstances, delivered in an appropriate and respectful manner, with the best possible prospects of achieving the right outcome. Their family and friends share this expectation and would like to be appropriately engaged by healthcare staff. The morale and productivity of staff is enhanced if their work environment is enabling, and if there is individual and collective accountability for the quality of care delivered. The productivity of the organization is similarly enhanced, as is its standing. The organization's resources are efficiently deployed. There is less wastage and less money is spent on iatrogenic complications, unnecessary investigations and treatment, and avoidable extensions of inpatient care—these all translate to a healthier population and better health economy.

The domains of clinical governance

To achieve the goals of clinical governance, the organization has to move from a 'fire-fighting' position to one of proactive management. Also, all of the pertinent domains have to be addressed.

The structures and processes that constitute clinical governance are encapsulated in the RADICAL framework: Raise awareness, Apply quality improvement (QI) methodology, Design for quality (including safety), Involve service users, Collect and Analyse data, and Learn from incidents—see **Figure 5.1**.

Implementation and monitoring of clinical governance

The RADICAL framework is an integrative tool for implementing and monitoring clinical governance. It develops and integrates the following activities:

Raising awareness—staff are kept abreast of the basic principles of clinical governance, the current developments, and emerging lessons. This task, and others relating to the coordination of activities, is usually undertaken by designated managers and committees at various levels in the organization. Educational activities and feedback loops are in this domain.

Applying QI methods—whether at an individual or at an organizational level, some change is usually required in order to achieve improvement. Such change has to be managed, using a structured approach. For this purpose, formal QI methods should be applied.

Designing for quality—healthcare should be purposefully designed to ensure that the highest possible level of quality is achieved. One mechanism for doing this is the concept of 'clinical effectiveness', discussed in a later section.

Involving service users—in all of these activities, from raising awareness to organizational learning, the service users should be constructively engaged.

Collecting and Analyse data on service quality—once we have designed the way healthcare should be delivered, we should continually check that care is actually delivered to the designated standards. This is done through clinical audit. Data is also collected and analysed as part of risk management.

Learning—data collection and analysis would be a mere paper exercise unless there is individual and organizational learning.

These clinical governance activities are discussed in the following sections.

Raising awareness

The implementation of clinical governance entails not only embedding *structures* and *processes* for promoting quality of care but also shaping the *thinking* and *behaviour* of staff and enhancing their knowledge of issues pertaining to quality.

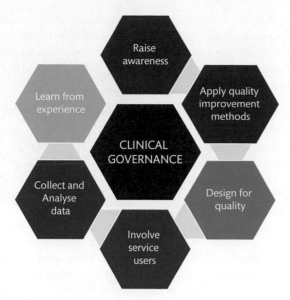

Figure 5.1 The domains of clinical governance.

Dimensions of quality

There are six dimensions of quality in healthcare and health systems (1, 2):

1. Effective—ensure that delivery of care is supported by evidence (see 'Clinical effectiveness').
2. Efficient—deliver healthcare in a manner that optimizes the use of available resources and avoids waste.
3. Accessible—delivery care in a timely manner and ensure that service users can physically access this service without difficulty.
4. Patient focused—deliver care in a manner that takes account of the preferences and aspirations of individual service users and their culture.
5. Equitable—ensure that care does not vary in quality because of personal characteristics such as gender, race, ethnicity, geographical location, or socioeconomic status.
6. Safe—in the delivery of healthcare, ensure that the risk of harm to service users is minimized.

These should not be treated as stand-alone silos but as pieces of a jigsaw that fit together to constitute one entity.

Raising awareness of patient safety

Historically, the individual clinician at the sharp end was blamed when a patient safety incident occurred—this was the 'person approach' to patient safety, which nurtured a culture of blame. With the emergence of risk management, there was a gradual shift from this approach to a 'systems approach' in which causation of patient safety incidents is attributed not to individuals but to loopholes in the organization's defences. It is arguable that while the systems approach shuns the blame culture, it could shy from holding individuals accountable for patient safety.

A 'bionomic' approach has been advocated as an alternative way of conceptualizing patient safety (3). This paradigm, which is adapted from ecosystems, places more emphasis on the relationships between the individual at the sharp end and other components of the system; the individual is seen as an intrinsic component of the system rather than an adjunct.

Conceptualizing patient safety in this way lays the foundation for a fuller appreciation of the importance of human factors, non-technical skills, and safety culture in the delivery of safer healthcare.

Human factors and non-technical skills

The systems approach to patient safety has its roots in engineering where the ultimate aim is to optimize standardization and minimize reliance on fallible human effort. Interventions designed on this basis include guidelines and protocols, perioperative safety checklist (to ensure that the correct person has the correct operation at the correct site) and other checklists. In the bionomic approach, the value of checklists and protocols is recognized but emphasis is placed on individual and group attributes of the clinical team such as communication skills, leadership, teamwork, and situational awareness. Situational awareness is the attribute of being aware of what is happening in the environment; understanding the importance of ongoing events and making projections based on this understanding. A range of factors including fatigue, task saturation, miscommunication, and loss of attention could compromise situational awareness. Situational awareness is particularly important in high-risk, dynamic environments such as the operating theatre and the delivery suite (4).

These cognitive, social, and personal attributes are referred to as non-technical skills: they complement technical proficiency and are just as important. The term 'human factors approach' is applied when these individual characteristics are combined with environmental, organizational, and task factors to understand, protect, and promote patient safety. An example of how this approach can be applied in obstetrics and gynaecology was described by Stanhope and colleagues (5).

Safety culture

An organization's safety culture is the totality of values, attitudes, competencies, and behaviours within the organization that reflect its commitment to the protection of patient safety. Clinicians should take it that they have a professional responsibility to nurture a culture of safety in their workplace. Tools and strategies have been developed for assessing and improving safety culture, but culture is a complex construct and the adoption of an integrated, multifaceted approach gives the best chances of success in shaping safety culture (6).

Resilience

Resilience is the ability of a team or organization to consistently maintain the quality of its performance in the face of evolving challenges and constraints. Policies, protocols, and guidelines have their use but resilience requires more than these (7). An organization that adopts the bionomic approach to quality, implements an integrated quality management programme (as facilitated by the RADICAL framework), and emphasizes organizational learning is likely to have a high degree of resilience.

Application of quality improvement methodology

Optimal results from QI initiatives do not just happen by chance or as a matter of course. QI is a science and an art, and appropriate methods have to be employed in order to secure the desired effects.

This was recognized decades ago in the manufacturing industry but only recently in the healthcare sector. Poorly planned initiatives often turn out to be mere tick-box exercises but well-designed interventions have been shown to produce demonstrable benefit in obstetrics (8, 9) and gynaecology (10).

A range of QI methodologies has been devised, researched, and refined in the industry. This includes continuous QI, Six Sigma, total quality management (TQM), Plan-Do-Study-Act (PDSA) cycles, statistical process control (SPC), Lean, and Lean Six Sigma. Systematic reviews showed that these methodologies potentially have significant effects on improving surgical care (11, 12).

A full discussion of QI methodologies is beyond the scope of this chapter. One methodology, the Model for Improvement (13), which is readily applicable in healthcare QI is briefly described. This methodology is based on three questions: (1) What are we trying to achieve? (2) How will we know that a change is an improvement? (3) What changes can we make that will result in an improvement? These questions require that a specific and measureable aim should be stated, that the right measures or measurements should be taken, and that collection of information should be purposeful and incremental. Changes are made using iterative Plan (planning what needs done), Do (running the test), Study (observing the results), Act (acting on what has been learned) cycles—better known as PDSA cycles. A test of change is performed in a small area with a small sample, and if there is demonstrable improvement, the test is extended to a broader area. An example of the use of PDSA cycles in gynaecology can be seen in a project which aimed to reduce the overuse of beta-human chorionic gonadotropin measurements in the emergency gynaecology clinic (14). The measure being assessed in a PDSA cycle may be a process measure (9, 14) or an outcome measure (8). It is helpful to also have a 'balancing measure' to check that the planned change has not had unintended consequences. For example, in implementing an enhanced recovery programme so that women with an uncomplicated caesarean delivery are discharged home the day after delivery, a balancing measure could be the number of readmissions or a measure of user satisfaction.

Designing for quality

Good practice in clinical governance requires that systems are continually being designed, monitored, and redesigned to ensure that QI is sustained. One approach to designing for safety is standardization of processes. This is usually achieved through policies, protocols, and guidelines. Another approach is the technological approach; this aims to promote automation and eliminate or reduce the human element, thus promoting quality (in particular, the safety dimension of quality). Both approaches have their foundations in systems engineering. They bring about first-order change, but second-order change (which involves change in attitudes and behaviour) is essential for sustained QI in healthcare.

Some examples of 'designing for quality' are briefly discussed in the following sections.

Handover

Handover is the transfer of responsibility and/or accountability for patient care from one provider or team of providers to another. Along with the transfer of responsibility goes transfer of clinical information. A handover between shifts is an opportunity to assess the resources available (staff, beds, cots, etc.), to plan contingencies, and to maintain team situational awareness. Each team should design its own handover procedures, using the available good practice guidance.

Recognizing and responding to clinical deterioration in acute care

One of the major causes of mortality or serious morbidity in healthcare globally is the failure to recognize the deteriorating condition of a patient or, if recognized, failure to respond appropriately to clinical deterioration (sometimes referred to as 'failure to rescue'). Failure to rescue is often due to loss of situational awareness.

To address the problem of recognition, scoring charts based on physiological parameters have been designed. A modified early obstetric warning score (MEOWS) chart was introduced for routine use in the care of all pregnant or postpartum women who become unwell. The United Kingdom Confidential Enquiry report recommends that care providers should use the charted observations in order to 'ensure confirmation of normality rather than presumption' (15). In other words, use of the chart should change behaviour such that clinicians constantly seek objective confirmation of normality, rather than presume normality and passively await any development that challenges this presumption. The report also states that 'it is the response to the abnormal score that will affect outcome not simply its documentation'—another pointer to the importance of clinician behaviour in the management of risk.

Prevention and management of sepsis

One aspect of clinical practice where an early warning score and/or other structured set of observations makes a big difference to clinical outcome is the prevention and management of sepsis. An initial evaluation showed that a scoring system designed specifically for an obstetric population can reliably identify women at high risk for admission to the intensive care unit (16).

Sepsis is a major cause of maternal death globally. In the United Kingdom, the National Institute for Health and Care Excellence (NICE) produced national guidelines on the management of sepsis in 2016, and these were updated in 2017 (17). The Royal College of Obstetricians and Gynaecologists has produced guidelines for the management of sepsis in pregnancy and a second edition is currently in development (18). National and local guidelines provide algorithms for the recognition and management of sepsis.

Critical to survival in cases of severe sepsis is the Sepsis Six bundle, which comprises three diagnostic and three therapeutic steps. This bundle—all of it—should be delivered within 1 hour of the initial diagnosis of sepsis. The components of this bundle are as follows:

- Deliver high-flow oxygen.
- Administer intravenous antibiotics.
- Commence intravenous fluids.
- Obtain blood cultures.
- Check serum lactate and perform a full blood count.
- Measure urine output.

The Sepsis Six could halve the number of deaths from sepsis but a national audit in the United Kingdom showed that its implementation was poor, with median implementation rates of 27–47% for individual components of the bundle (19). For implementation to be effective and sustainable, it has to draw from behavioural science (20). This provides another illustration of the value of a bionomic approach to quality in healthcare.

Safety in blood transfusion

Antenatal haemorrhage and postpartum haemorrhage are anticipated events in everyday obstetric practice. Obstetricians (and gynaecologists too) should be familiar with procedures and practices to minimize the risks associated with blood transfusion. These risks include infection, blood transfusion reactions, transfusion-associated circulatory overload, transfusion-related acute lung injury, and blood administration errors. Concern about these risks has led to the establishment of various mechanisms of haemovigilance at local, national, and international levels. Haemovigilance is the totality of surveillance procedures covering the whole transfusion chain from the donation of blood and its components to the follow-up of recipients. Information on adverse events is collected and used to improve the safety of blood transfusion.

The first step towards reducing complications of blood transfusion is to reduce the need for transfusion—for example, through optimization of antenatal and preoperative haemoglobin concentration and through the use of cell-salvage techniques. Decisions to transfuse should be made on the basis of the complete clinical picture and not just on the basis of the haemoglobin result. Transfusion should be avoided at night, unless there is a strong clinical indication for immediate transfusion. National and local protocols for massive haemorrhage and massive transfusion should be applied and a multidisciplinary team approach should be adopted (21–23). The protocols should be supported by training and regular drills.

Administration errors are not limited to red cell transfusion; the incidence of errors in administration of anti-D immunoglobulin is rising. Such errors include omission of anti-D and administration of anti-D immunoglobulin to a mother of a rhesus D negative baby, to a rhesus D-positive mother, or to the wrong woman. These highlight the need for anti-D prescription and administration to be as stringent as those of blood transfusion.

Medical devices, including new technologies

Clinical governance leads should implement procedures for ensuring that staff are familiar with the medical devices that they are expected to use, and individual practitioners should ordinarily not use devices that they are unfamiliar with.

The implementation of new approaches to management of acute conditions (e.g. non-surgical, outpatient management of ectopic pregnancy) introduces new risks, and these have to be identified and contained. Procedures for the safe introduction of new technology should be implemented.

Clinical effectiveness

Clinicians have a professional responsibility to ensure that the treatment they provide is treatment that can achieve the optimal outcome for the patient. To discharge this responsibility they are obliged to follow recognized best practice, based on the best available evidence.

In the spheres of research and evidence-supported practice, it is customary to grade evidence according to levels. Various modifications, including subclassification, have been made to the original grading but all variants conform approximately to the following simple hierarchy:

Level 1: random allocation trials, more widely known as 'randomized controlled trials', and systematic reviews of such trials.

Level 2: cohort studies and systematic reviews of cohort studies.

Level 3: case–control studies and systematic review of case-control studies.

Level 4: case-series.

Level 5: expert opinion.

NICE and the colleges of obstetrics and gynaecology in the United Kingdom, United States, Canada, and Australia produce evidence-based guidelines on a range of conditions and these are available on their websites. The guidelines will usually specify what level of evidence their recommendations are based on. The evidence from research is also used to produce local guidelines.

It is important to continually benchmark current practice against the guidelines in place. The mechanism for this is clinical audit (discussed in a later section).

Clinical effectiveness is not, however, just about plucking the evidence from the literature. The clinician has to determine how that evidence can be applied in the care of the particular woman he or she is about to treat, taking account of the woman's individual characteristics and preferences.

Involvement of service users

Taking account of the woman's preferences is an essential part of the involvement of service users in the delivery of care. In contemporary practice, the paternalistic doctor–patient relationship (whereby the patient was a passive recipient of whatever care the doctor decided was in her best interests) has given way to patient-centred care. Obstetricians and gynaecologists work in partnership with patients to determine the appropriate and acceptable treatment. In broader terms, patients and other service users (partners, families, and visitors) should be engaged in designing and delivering services and promoting quality of care. This sounds simple and sensible, but is not always easy and how best to achieve it is not always clear.

Guidance

The Scottish Health Council has published a document to guide health boards and managers in promoting service user involvement in maternity services (24). The recommendations in this guidance include the use of tools (such as questionnaires, comments cards, graffiti boards, kiosks, and hand-held patient devices) which encourage women to provide feedback during their hospital treatment, and the use of new technologies (such as Skype, Twitter, and social networking sites) to promote user involvement. Community groups, employment networks, and education networks could be used to engage maternity service users and to disseminate safety information.

Consent

No treatment (including physical examinations and diagnostic procedures) should be performed without the consent of the woman. Consent is not just the woman's assent to what the clinician proposes; it is the upholding of her right to self-determination, enabling her to make an informed choice. The protection of patient self-determination entails: (a) recognition of, and respect for, the patient's right to decide what treatment to have or not to have; (b) provision of an enabling climate for the patient to make self-determined choices (ensuring effective communication and building trust); and (c) having regard for the context (social, cultural, emotional, etc.) in which the patient has to make his/her decision (25).

For consent to be valid the following must apply:

1. The patient must have the capacity to make the decision.
2. There must be no undue influence.
3. The patient must have been given (or offered) sufficient information about the proposed treatment.

A woman who has capacity (the ability to understand information and use it to make a decision) may legally decline any treatment offered by her doctor, even if this means the death of the woman or her baby. This means, for example, that a caesarean delivery cannot be forced on a woman who has capacity. No one can give consent on behalf of an adult woman who has capacity. In maternity care, the husband cannot give a legally valid consent on behalf of his pregnant wife who does not lack capacity. Where the woman lacks capacity (e.g. due to unconsciousness or mental ill-health), the clinician should, in consultation with colleagues and the woman's family, provide treatment that is deemed to be in the best interests of the woman.

Consent is also not just about signing a form. Most clinicians are unaware that consent can be valid without a signed consent form. It is the patient's informed choice that constitutes consent, not the form. It is also not widely appreciated that consent can be invalid even though a consent form has been signed—if the patient has not made a self-determining, informed choice.

In obtaining consent to treatment, the clinician should provide the woman with clear, accurate information about both the benefits and the risks of the proposed treatment and of any reasonable alternative options (26). The clinician should check that the woman understands the information that has been given. Any risk that she is likely to consider as important should be disclosed, even if it is a remote risk.

Openness: the duty of candour

Doctors have an *ethical* duty to be open and honest with their patients, particularly in relation to patient safety incidents. This duty is stated by the United Kingdom General Medical Council (GMC) as follows:

> You must be open and honest with patients if things go wrong. If a patient under your care has suffered harm or distress, you should:
> put matters right (if that is possible)
> offer an apology
> explain fully and promptly what has happened and the likely short-term and long-term effects. (27)

The GMC advises that, in offering an apology, patients should be told what happened, what can be done to deal with any harm caused, and what will be done to prevent someone else being harmed.

An apology is not an admission of legal liability.

There is now also a *legal* duty to be open and honest—known as the duty of candour—which applies to all National Health Service (NHS) bodies and other care providers registered with the Care Quality Commission in the United Kingdom (28).

As soon as is reasonably practicable after a notifiable patient safety incident occurs, the organization must inform the patient (or their representative) about it in person, provide an apology, and give a full explanation. A notifiable patient safety incident is one where a patient has suffered (or could suffer) unintended harm that results in death, severe harm, moderate harm, or prolonged (>28 days) psychological harm. There is a statutory duty to provide reasonable support (such as emotional support) to the patient.

Complaints

The NHS Constitution (29) states the rights and responsibilities of persons receiving treatment in the NHS. These include the right to complain about the care she or he has received. Patients are encouraged to make informal complaints about matters that can be resolved readily by the clinician or manager at ward or clinic level. Such complaints may be made orally to the ward/clinic staff or to the Patient Advice and Liaison Service (PALS).

Formal complaints are mostly made in writing and may be made to the organization that has provided the care complained about or to the body that commissions the service. The complaint is handled according to local arrangements that comply with guidelines laid down by law (30). These arrangements include timescales, routes of communication, and an obligation to state any action that has been taken or will be taken in response to the complaint. Apart from PALS support, the complainant may also obtain support (such as being accompanied to meetings) from a local Independent Complaints Advocacy Service (ICAS) which is funded by the local government.

Collecting and analysing data on quality of care

Clinical governance seeks not just to maintain the status quo, but to promote continual improvement. For this purpose, appropriate data have to be collected and analysed, then applied in benchmarking and QI. The main sources of clinical governance data are clinical audit and risk management. These are usually operationalized as separate entities but in holistic clinical governance they should be integrated or, at least, inform each other. For example, if a clinical audit shows that an unacceptable proportion of rhesus D-negative women undergoing external cephalic version (ECV) do not receive anti-D prophylaxis at the time, this should be flagged as a risk management issue and managed accordingly in line with local protocols. In a similar vein, an incident of missed anti-D prophylaxis reported through the risk management system could trigger an audit of ECVs.

Clinical audit

What is healthcare audit?

Healthcare audit is the collection and analysis of healthcare data for the purposes of assessing quality of care, benchmarking, and improvement of performance. The term 'clinical audit' is used to describe this activity but it is important to appreciate that audits may look not only at clinical outcomes but also at other health outcomes, such as quality of life and user satisfaction.

Types of audit

Healthcare audit can take any of a number of forms such as criterion-based audit, normative audit, or case notes review.

Criterion-based audit is the type of audit commonly represented in the form of an audit cycle (or spiral) that includes standard setting, comparison of current practice with standard(s), implementation of change, and closure of the loop by re-audit—see **Figure 5.2**). Criterion-based audit starts off with evidence-based criteria and agreement on expected levels of performance, thus establishing both ownership and robust foundation at the outset. Criteria provide reference points against which current practice is compared. For each criterion, the standard prescribes the expected level of performance. An example of a criterion is the evidence-based statement 'Women undergoing caesarean section should have thromboembolism prophylaxis'. The corresponding standard could be '100% of women undergoing emergency caesarean section should have thromboembolism prophylaxis'. Criteria should be measurable and relevant to the clinical practice being audited. The value of criterion-based audit has been established not only in the Western world but also in low-income countries (31, 32).

Normative audit involves collection of data, usually on large numbers of patients, to identify trends, health outcomes, complications, readmission rates, or similar indices. By definition it may not start with criteria (as defined previously) but its findings could be used to set up local criterion-based audits. Examples of normative national audits include the audit to assess patient outcomes and experiences of care for women with heavy menstrual bleeding in England and Wales (33) and the National Pregnancy in Diabetes audit (34). The longest running national audit in the United Kingdom, the Confidential Enquiries into Maternal Deaths, is also a normative audit. At a local level, normative audits may be used to populate maternity dashboards (e.g. rates of third-degree perineal tear) or to monitor readmission rates or responses to early warning scores.

Case-notes (charts) review is a time-honoured type of audit in medical practice. A case record (in some cases, more than one) is reviewed and presented at a meeting, and judgements are made about the quality of care, based on implicit standards (i.e. standards defined by the personal experience and perspective of the assessors).

This is audit's equivalent to expert consensus in research's hierarchy of evidence.

From the purist's point of view, criterion-based audit is the highest form of audit. Indeed it is only this type of audit that fits the definition of 'clinical audit' endorsed by NICE: 'a quality improvement process that seeks to improve patient care and outcomes through systematic review of care against explicit criteria and the implementation of change'.

As outlined in the earlier section on clinical effectiveness, there is a hierarchy by which research evidence, and recommendations flowing from the evidence, are graded. This hierarchy can be represented as a pyramid, with random allocation trials at the top and case series and expert opinion at the bottom (the pyramid on the left in **Figure 5.3**). A similar pyramid can be devised for a healthcare audit, with criterion-based audit at the top and case-notes review at the bottom (the pyramid on the right in **Figure 5.3**). Criterion-based audit is, in hierarchical terms, audit's equivalent of the randomized controlled trial.

Figure 5.3 also illustrates the overlap between audit and research—some normative audits may be undertaken or presented in the context of research. For example, the Birthplace study (35) falls into the overlap between the two triangles, being a normative audit but also an observational research study.

The practicalities and challenges of clinical audit

There would be no purpose served if clinical audit does not lead to improvement and sustenance of clinical standards. This should be borne in mind when selecting a subject for audit. The chosen subject (a clinical condition or a process of care) should be pertinent to local practice, and one for which data can be collected readily.

When the subject/topic has been selected, the next step is to set out criteria and standards. A criterion is an evidence-based statement that can be used to assess the appropriateness of current practice. In an audit of perioperative care in caesarean section, for example, one of the criteria could be 'Women undergoing caesarean section should have thromboembolism prophylaxis'. The standard specifies

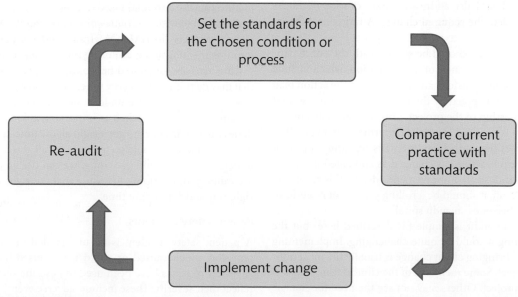

Figure 5.2 The clinical audit cycle.

[Re-audit] → [Set the standards for the chosen condition or process] → [Compare current practice with standards] → [Implement change] → [Re-audit]

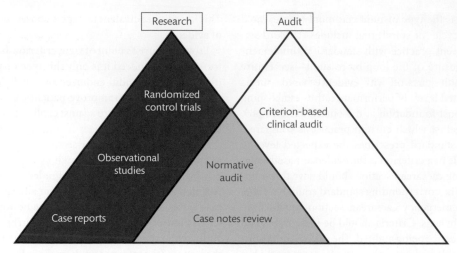

Figure 5.3 The research and audit hierarchies.

the expected level of performance for the corresponding criterion. This will commonly be 100% but in some cases, could be lower—for example, when local practice is being compared with a regional or national benchmark that falls below 100%. The criteria are usually derived from evidence-based guidelines or research findings. Where no guidelines exist, standards can be agreed by consensus locally.

A data collection pro forma is designed and tested on a handful of cases, and a final version is agreed by the audit team. The pro forma may be in paper and/or electronic form. The pro forma should protect the anonymity of patients and staff.

Data are then collected for a pre-agreed number of cases or period. The minimum number of cases required for criterion-based audit is usually modest in comparison with research where it is usually an advantage to have large numbers of cases. Descriptive statistics are usually adequate for audit but more complex statistical analysis may be required for larger audits.

Current practice is compared with the set standards and any deficiencies are identified, as well as possible explanations for the shortfall. A plan of action is devised to change/improve current practice. The plan should specify what needs to be done, by whom, and in what time frame. It should also address the issue of what resources may be needed to effect the required change. A target date for re-audit should be set.

The findings of the audit should be shared with the entire clinical team, using effective channels of dissemination, which include face-to-face presentations, posters, and newsletters. The action plan should be discussed and agreed by the entire clinical team, so that everyone takes ownership of the project. This will facilitate any behaviour change that is required in order to improve current practice.

The re-audit closes the audit loop. It entails repeating the audit cycle to see if current practice has changed as stipulated in the action plan and to demonstrate improvement. Ideally, this repetition should not be a one-off; it should be a rolling process of re-audit so that the audit cycle becomes an audit spiral.

The structure of an audit is simple (as described here) but the process of conducting it could be quite challenging. Implementing the action plan and bringing about change is usually the most difficult part of the project. Some members of the clinical team may feel threatened by the project. Others may not see the need for change.

Some may argue about the appropriateness, reliability, or applicability of the criteria or standards. There may be constraints of time, or the resources for implementing change may not all be available. The audit team should address these potential barriers proactively. Blame should be avoided and anonymity should be preserved when reporting audit findings. The focus should be on overall QI, not individual failings (31).

Risk management

What is risk management?

Risk management is the totality of structures, processes, and behaviours that are put in place to ensure that, as much as possible, clinicians do the right thing every time; to mitigate damage from error; and to learn from safety incidents. The structures include committee for overseeing the unit's risk management programme, data-gathering structures (e.g. electronic incident reporting system), and appointment of risk leads. The processes include formal mechanisms for identifying risk, investigating incidents, and sharing lessons learned. Behaviours reflect the safety culture of the unit and are best managed if the unit's approach to risk management is holistic, manifesting the attributes listed in **Box 5.1**. Risk is best managed not in isolation but within a framework that integrates all aspects of clinical governance. The RADICAL framework has been recommended for implementing and monitoring risk management (32).

Clinicians are, or should be, concerned primarily with ensuring that they do things right every time. Getting it right all the time does, however, require that we understand what could go wrong. In designing the way we work, it is important to know what should be done and how, in order to get it right all the time. It is also important to understand what could go wrong; after all, it is human to err. If we understand what could go wrong, we can design our care delivery accordingly, thus helping to ensure that the right thing is done the right way and at the right time.

Patient safety incidents

A patient safety incident is an unintended or unexpected act or omission which caused or could have caused harm to a patient. A variety of terms have been used to describe such incidents or to reflect their severity. These include 'adverse event', 'serious incident',

Box 5.1 Attributes of a good risk management programme

- Comprehensive (includes all domains of the RADICAL framework).
- Evidence-supported (incorporates best practice, user experience, and available resources).
- Takes account of human factors.
- Intrinsic to clinical practice (not a stand-alone activity but applied as part of clinical care).
- Applies across professional and disciplinary boundaries.
- Visibly fair to all and promotes a just culture.
- Tailored to local requirements.
- Responsive to evolving challenges (such as structural or staff changes, and new threats to patient safety).
- Integrated with clinical audit and other quality initiatives.

'serious, untoward event', and 'critical incident'. A 'near miss' is an event which had the potential to cause harm but the harm did not materialize. A 'never event' is a patient safety incident that is presumed to be wholly preventable; for example, the retention of a swab or instrument in the patient's body or an operation conducted on the wrong person or wrong site. In reality, no incident is wholly preventable, as human error or violation of rules will occur at some point.

It is important to report patient safety incidents as part of the process of managing risk. For some events there are external reporting requirements—for example, all maternal deaths in the NHS have to be reported to the local Clinical Commission Group.

Identifying risk

All clinical areas should have formal processes for identifying anything that might interfere with the delivery of a safe, good-quality service. Identifying risk is, put simply, finding answers to the question 'What could go wrong?' To answer this question, we could look back at patient safety incidents that have occurred and been reported in the department. The monitoring and analysis of reported patient safety incidents can reveal trends (upward or downward) and show areas of weakness or unsafe practice in the unit. Risk may also be identified from prospective risk assessments, patients' complaints, clinical audit, or concerns raised by staff. External sources of risk identification include national enquiries, national safety alerts, and findings of visitations by regulatory and monitoring agencies. Patients should be encouraged to report patient safety incidents, including near misses. Unfortunately, while this role of patients in reporting incidents is valued, robust mechanisms for promoting it have not been developed (36).

Risk assessment

This is a prospective and continual exercise to determine what risks lurk in the clinical area, the potential impact of these risks, and the effect of measures introduced to contain them. The potential impact is quantified by assigning a score derived from a risk matrix (**Figure 5.4**). The likelihood of the risk materializing is multiplied by the severity of harm that may be caused in the event that the risk materializes. The assessment is incomplete without an action plan designed to contain the risk.

Risk registers

The risk register is a log of ranked risks that facilitates the monitoring, review, and management of risks across the organization.

Evaluating risk

Severity \ Likelihood	1 Remote	2 Unlikely	3 Possible	4 Likely	5 Certain
1 Trivial	1	2	3	4	5
2 Minor	2	4	6	8	10
3 Lost time	3	6	9	12	15
4 Major	4	8	12	16	20
5 Fatal	5	10	15	20	25

Figure 5.4 Risk scoring matrix.

Each clinical area should have a risk register. The major risks are escalated to an organization-wide risk register. The register includes controls that have been put in place to contain each risk.

Investigation of patient safety incidents

To learn from patient safety incidents we need to undertake a structured analysis of what went wrong, what went well, what could have been done differently, and why events unfolded the way they did. This exercise is commonly referred to as 'root cause analysis'. There are reservations about this term because although it has its merits (taking us to the factors underlying the incident), it may give the impression that there is one 'root' cause and it fails to focus attention on systems improvement rather than finding of a cause. An alternative term used in the NHS, 'high-level investigation', is also unsatisfactory—as it sounds inquisitorial. A preferable term is 'system analysis'—an analysis aimed at unravelling the reasons why the system failed to deliver the quality care it was designed to deliver.

There are many approaches to the investigation of patient safety incidents. A widely used one is the London Protocol (or variants of it). This protocol offers a structured and systematic approach to the investigation of incidents (37). The key steps are as follows:

1. Identify incident and take decision to investigate.
2. Select members of the investigation team.
3. Gather data.
4. Outline the chronology of the incident.
5. Identify care and service delivery problems.
6. Identify contributory factors.
7. Devise an action plan.

The investigation team should have knowledge pertinent to the clinical issues being investigated and competence in conducting accident investigation. This competence can be achieved by attending a training course. Investigators must be familiar with mechanisms underlying error, particularly the role of the human factor.

Data are gathered from health records, written accounts provided by staff, interviews, protocols, site visits, and any other means considered useful by the investigating team.

Care delivery problems are proximal problems arising in the process of care, usually actions or omissions by members of staff, where care deviated beyond safe limits of practice and this deviation had at least a potential direct or indirect on the eventual adverse outcome. Service delivery problems are distal failures associated with organizational procedures and systems—for example, lack of supervision.

In analysing incidents, it is helpful to distinguish between 'active' and 'latent' failures. An active failure is the immediate cause of a patient safety incident, for example, misidentification of a patient or sample; while a latent failure is a more remote but important cause, such as the absence of protocols for checking and confirming identification. Care delivery problems are typically active failure while service delivery problems are latent failures.

Contributory factors are those thought to have some effect on the performance of individuals at the end of the error chain but are not directly causative of the incident. There is a wide range of internal and external factors that could be contributory to a patient safety incident. The Yorkshire Contributory Factors Framework, which covers 16 domains, is an evidence-based framework that could be used to analyse contributory factors when investigating an incident (38).

As with audit, the action plan following an investigation should state in specific terms what needs to be done, by whom, and in what timescales; resource implications should also be addressed.

It is important to engage service users and staff in the course of the investigation. As discussed previously, any patient involved in a patient safety incident should be informed of what happened, and be given an apology and explanations. The patient, and where relevant their family, should be kept informed of progress with the investigation, the findings, and the action plan. The staff involved in the incident should also be supported. They may suffer vicarious traumatization as a result of the incident, and this is more likely to happen if they have not had support from the hospital.

Unfortunately, evidence from multiple sources (15, 39–42) indicates that the quality and impact of incident investigations performed in the United Kingdom and elsewhere is generally of poor quality, and the 'blame culture' is still very much alive. There are many reasons for this, including the use of investigators who lack the appropriate training, insight, and competence required for incident investigation, the pressures of time, cultural barriers, and conflation of QI with litigation concerns. The first step in addressing this problem is for units to incorporate into their clinical governance the continuous structured quality assessment of their investigation reports, using external assessors where possible. At national level, a new United Kingdom safety investigation body, the Healthcare Safety Investigation Branch (HSIB), has been set up to act as 'an enabler, exemplar and catalyst for learning-oriented safety investigation' (43).

Learning: individual and organizational

The ultimate measure of clinical governance activities is the degree to which they contribute to organizational learning. Organizational learning occurs when the body of knowledge, competencies, and experiences within the organization is expanded. This body comprises the contributions of individuals and teams within the organization but it is greater than the sum of its building blocks. The way that organizations learn and disseminate learning is a complex matter but it is essentially a social process. From a clinical

governance perspective, learning is facilitated if a bionomic conception of quality is adopted. It is often said that learning is facilitated by systems thinking. This is true, but healthcare involves more than inanimate systems—it is highly dependent on human behaviour and relationships. For that reason, this author advocates a bionomic approach (3).

Bionomic means 'pertaining to ecology'. A bionomic approach to patient safety is based on principles and concepts of human ecology, and applies them to the healthcare system. The core attribute of an ecosystem is that of interdependence between living organisms and their environment, these constituent elements working together as a system; the individual organisms are in dynamic relationships with each other and with their surroundings. Interacting levels of organization range from the cellular level to the biosphere. Variety also exists within the ecosystem, but this biodiversity is strength rather than weakness.

The relevance of the bionomic approach to organizational learning is that it creates an environment in which relationships are valued and nurtured, experiences can be shared, ideas can flourish, new ideas are given a chance to germinate, and emphasis is placed on integration. Individuals take responsibility for quality of care and develop shared visions with other team members. Also, learning is transferred across teams, clinical areas, and institutions. A full account of organizational and individual learning is beyond the scope of this chapter but one example illustrates the transferability of learning. A 'maternity dashboard' was developed as a clinical governance tool for obstetric services and has been widely adopted in the United Kingdom (44). The concept of a dashboard has now been successfully adapted to emergency gynaecology where its implementation has been shown to generate improvements in patient management, service provision, and training (45).

Adoption and implementation of clinical governance as described in this chapter will create this learning environment. Lessons learned are shared with staff ('Raise awareness') and with service users ('Involve service users'). The lessons inform the delivery of services ('Design for quality') through quality improvement ('Apply QI methodology'). The 'Learning' is demonstrable by reference to quantitative and qualitative data ('Collect and Analyse data').

Conclusion

Clinical governance is at the heart of medical professionalism. The exhortation 'first, do no harm' should be understood in its broad meaning and context. Harm is not limited to physical injury; psychological injury is also important. In carrying out our professional duties, obstetricians and gynaecologists should aim not only for optimal clinical outcomes but also the best possible patient experience, and in so doing derive personal, professional, and occupational satisfaction. These lofty aims are best achieved if clinical governance is integral to clinical practice rather than being regarded as separate from everyday clinical activities.

REFERENCES

1. World Health Organization (WHO). *Quality of Care: A Process for Making Strategic Choices in Health Systems*. Geneva: WHO; 2006.

2. Institute of Medicine. *Crossing the Quality Chasm: A New Health System for the 21st century*. Washington DC, National Academy Press; 2001.

3. Edozien LC. The bionomic approach to patient safety and its application in gynaecological surgery. *Best Pract Res Clin Obstet Gynaecol* 2013;**27**:549–61.

4. Edozien LC. Situational awareness and its application in the delivery suite. *Obstet Gynecol* 2015;**125**:65–9.

5. Stanhope N, Vincent C, Taylor-Adams SE, O'Connor AM, Beard RW. Applying human factors methods to clinical risk management in obstetrics. *Br J Obstet Gynaecol* 1997;**104**:1225–32.

6. Morello RT, Lowthian JA, Barker AL, McGinnes R, Dunt D, Brand C. Strategies for improving patient safety culture in hospitals: a systematic review. *BMJ Qual Saf* 2013;**22**:11–18.

7. Braithwaite J, Wears RL, Hollnagel E. Resilient health care: turning patient safety on its head. *Int J Qual Health Care* 2015;**27**:418–20.

8. Witter FR, Lawson P, Ferrell J. Decreasing cesarean section surgical site infection: an ongoing comprehensive quality improvement program. *Am J Infect Control* 2014;**42**:429–31.

9. Srofenyoh EK, Kassebaum NJ, Goodman DM, Olufolabi AJ, Owen MD. Measuring the impact of a quality improvement collaboration to decrease maternal mortality in a Ghanaian regional hospital. *Int J Gynaecol Obstet* 2016;**134**:181–5.

10. Leung S, Leyland N, Murji A. Decreasing diagnostic hysteroscopy performed in the operating room: a quality improvement initiative. *J Obstet Gynaecol Can* 2016;**38**:351–6.

11. Nicolay CR, Purkayastha S, Greenhalgh A, et al. Systematic review of the application of quality improvement methodologies from the manufacturing industry to surgical healthcare. *Br J Surg* 2012;**99**:324–35.

12. Mason SE, Nicolay CR, Darzi A. The use of Lean and Six Sigma methodologies in surgery: a systematic review. *Surgeon* 2015;**13**:91–100.

13. The Health Foundation. *Quality Improvement Made Simple*, 2nd edn. London: Health Foundation; 2013.

14. Frost L. Reducing the overuse of βhCG measurements in the emergency gynaecology clinic. *BMJ Qual Improv Rep* 2016;**5**:u210039.w4218.

15. Knight M, Kenyon S, Brocklehurst P, et al. *Saving Lives, Improving Mothers' Care—Lessons Learned to Inform Future Maternity Care from the UK and Ireland Confidential Enquiries into Maternal Deaths and Morbidity 2009–12*. Oxford: National Perinatal Epidemiology Unit, University of Oxford; 2014.

16. Albright CM, Ali TN, Lopes V, Rouse DJ, Anderson BL. The Sepsis in Obstetrics Score: a model to identify risk of morbidity from sepsis in pregnancy. *Am J Obstet Gynecol* 2014;**211**:39.e1–8.

17. National Institute for Health and Care Excellence (NICE). *Sepsis: Recognition, Diagnosis and Early Management*. NICE guideline [NG51]. London: NICE; 2016.

18. Royal College of Obstetricians and Gynaecologists (RCOG). *Bacterial Sepsis in Pregnancy*. Green-top Guideline No. 64a. London: RCOG; 2012.

19. College of Emergency Medicine (CEM). *Clinical Audits 2011–2012: Severe Sepsis and Septic Shock*. London: CEM; 2012.

20. Steinmo S, Fuller C, Stone SP, Michie S. Characterising an implementation intervention in terms of behaviour change techniques and theory: the 'Sepsis Six' clinical care bundle. *Implement Sci* 2015;**10**:111.

21. Engelbrecht S, Wood EM, Cole-Sinclair MF. Clinical transfusion practice update: haemovigilance, complications, patient blood management and national standards. *Med J Aust* 2013;**199**:397.

22. Norfolk D (ed). Effective transfusion in obstetric practice. In: *Handbook of Transfusion Medicine*, 5th edn, pp. 105–12. Sheffield: UK Blood Services; 2013.

23. Royal College of Obstetricians and Gynaecologists (RCOG). *Blood Transfusion in Obstetrics*. Green-top Guideline No. 47. London: RCOG; 2015.

24. Scottish Health Council. *Good Practice in Service User Involvement in Maternity: Involving Women to Improve their Care*. Edinburgh: Scottish Health Council; 2011.

25. Edozien LC. Self-determination in childbirth: the law of consent. In O'Mahony D (ed), *Medical Negligence and Childbirth*. Dublin: Bloomsbury Professional; 2015.

26. General Medical Council (GMC). *Consent: Patients and Doctors Making Decisions Together*. London: GMC; 2008.

27. General Medical Council (GMC). *Good Medical Practice*. London: GMC; 2013. Available at: http://www.gmc-uk.org/gmp (accessed 12 June 2016).

28. Health and Social Care Act 2008 (Regulated Activities) Regulations 2014, Regulation 20.

29. Department of Health. The NHS Constitution for England. October 2015 Available at: https://www.gov.uk/government/publications/the-nhs-constitution-for-england/the-nhs-constitution-for-england (accessed 12 June 2016).

30. Local Authority Social Services and National Health Service Complaints (England) Regulations 2009.

31. The Royal College of Obstetricians and Gynaecologists (RCOG). *National Heavy Menstrual Bleeding Audit, Final Report*. London: RCOG; 2014.

32. Healthcare Quality Improvement Partnership (HQUIP). *National Pregnancy in Diabetes Audit Report, 2014: England, Wales and the Isle of Man*. London: HQUIP; 2014.

33. Birthplace in England Collaborative Group, Brocklehurst P, Hardy P, et al. Perinatal and maternal outcomes by planned place of birth for healthy women with low risk pregnancies: the Birthplace in England national prospective cohort study. *BMJ* 2011;**343**:d7400.

34. Johnston G, Crombie IK, Davies HT, Alder EM, Millard A. Reviewing audit: barriers and facilitating factors for effective clinical audit. *Qual Health Care* 2000;**9**:23–36.

35. Edozien LC. Mapping the patient safety footprint: the RADICAL framework. *Best Pract Res Clin Obstet Gynaecol* 2013;**27**:481–8.

36. Ward JK, Armitage G. Can patients report patient safety incidents in a hospital setting? A systematic review. *BMJ Qual Saf* 2012;**21**:685–99.

37. Taylor-Adams S, Vincent C. Systems analysis of clinical incidents: the London Protocol. *Clin Risk* 2004;**10**:211–20.

38. Lawton R, McEachan RR, Giles SJ, Sirriyeh R, Watt IS, Wright J. Development of an evidence-based framework of factors contributing to patient safety incidents in hospital settings: a systematic review. *BMJ Qual Saf* 2012;**21**:369–80.

39. Nicolini D, Waring J, Mengis J. Policy and practice in the use of root cause analysis to investigate clinical adverse events: mind the gap. *Soc Sci Med* 2011;**73**:217–25.

40. Taitz J, Genn K, Brooks V, et al. System-wide learning from root cause analysis: a report from the New South Wales Root Cause Analysis Review Committee. *Qual Saf Health Care* 2010;**19**:e63.

41. Parliamentary and Health Service Ombudsman. A review into the quality of NHS complaints investigations where serious or avoidable harm has been alleged. December 2015. Available at: https://www.ombudsman.org.uk/publications/review-quality-nhs-complaints-investigations-where-serious-or-avoidable-harm-has (accessed 5 April 2019).

42. Department of Health. *Learning not Blaming: The Government Response to the Freedom to Speak Up Consultation, the Public Administration Select Committee report 'Investigating Clinical Incidents in the NHS', and the Morecambe Bay Investigation.* London: Department of Health; 2015.

43. Department of Health. Report of the Expert Advisory Group. Healthcare Safety Investigation Branch. May 2016. Available at: https://www.gov.uk/government/publications/ improving-safety-investigations-in-healthcare (accessed 15 June 2016).

44. Royal College of Obstetricians and Gynaecologists (RCOG). *Maternity Dashboard: Clinical Performance and Governance Score Card (Good Practice No. 7).* London; RCOG; 2008.

45. Guha S, Hoo WP, Bottomley C. Introducing an acute gynaecology dashboard as a new clinical governance tool. *Clin Govern Int J* 2013;**18**:228–37.

6

Preconceptional medicine

Carmen Binding and Mahantesh Karoshi

Age and fertility

Advanced maternal age

The developed world has seen a gradual increase in child-bearing age of women throughout the last three decades. The term 'advanced maternal age' is used to define women age 35 or older at the time of delivery. There are specific factors that can negatively affect the desired outcome of a pregnancy that must be taken into account when discussing advanced maternal age, including ovarian ageing, declining fertility, miscarriage, risk of congenital cytogenic abnormalities, hypertensive complications, stillbirth, and maternal mortality.

Fertility, ovarian ageing, and chromosomal abnormalities

Although there are many factors that contribute to decreased fertility, a significant factor in age-associated infertility appears to be ovarian ageing and the diminishing ovarian follicle count. There appears to be less contribution from the uterine endometrium, as this has the capacity to maintain a pregnancy throughout a woman's reproductive years.

When a girl enters puberty, there are approximately 300,000–500,000 oocytes available in the ovaries, however only approximately 400–500 eventually undergo ovulation (1) (**Figure 6.1**). Due to a bi-exponential decline in the ovarian pool of follicles with advancing age, there is an accelerated loss of follicles from the age of 35 (2). For example, a woman at age 38 will have only approximately 25,000 follicles available, with a further decline to approximately 15,000 at age 40, and by 51, only a few hundred remain (2, 3).

Advanced maternal age increases the baseline risk of chromosomal abnormalities and Down syndrome (trisomy 21) (4, 5). The risk of having a baby with Down syndrome rises with maternal age, essentially doubling from approximately 1 in 1000 at age 30 to approximately 1 in 400 at age 35 (6). This risk continues to climb to approximately 1 in 30 at the maternal age of 45 years (6) (**Table 6.1**).

Biopanic

Although the average age of women conceiving is increasing, there remains a considerable societal pressure for women of this age group to achieve success in areas of life such as occupation, financial stability, and relationships. Many women find themselves feeling pressure to balance the desire to achieve successes in their profession, while expecting to conceive spontaneously, which has led to an emerging public health effect of 'biopanic'. As can be seen in **Figure 6.2**, the largest increase in conception rates has occurred in women age 35 and older, which unfortunately coincides with the same age at which there is an accelerated loss of follicles, and subsequent reduction in fertility (7).

Fertility techniques

This sense of 'biopanic', with the conflicting desire to achieve spontaneous conception has led to increased rates of women older than 35 years undergoing advanced fertility techniques, including *in vitro* fertilization and donor insemination, as can be seen in **Figure 6.3** (8).

Embryo cryopreservation is the process in which eggs are retrieved from a woman's ovaries, followed by fertilization with sperm either from a partner or donor, and then stored at freezing temperatures for a period of time.

Oocyte cryopreservation is the process in which eggs are retrieved from a woman's ovaries and stored at freezing temperatures for a period of time. While embryo cryopreservation is a technique of fertility preservation that has been used for decades, oocyte cryopreservation is a relatively new technique.

Societal changes have led to new developments and unique uses of fertility techniques for women in the workforce. Companies such as Apple and Facebook have been reported to offer their female employees fully-compensated oocyte cryopreservation (9). As can be seen in **Figure 6.4**, there is an increase in the percentage of women starting fertility treatments after age 35 since 1997 to 2009. However, in 2013, there appears to be a bimodal distribution of women's age less than 35 and greater than 35 at the time of starting treatment, which is likely contributed in part to women in the workforce starting this process earlier in their careers.

Obesity and preconceptional counselling

Almost a third of women entering pregnancy in the United States are obese (10). The challenge of obesity in pregnancy is multifaceted. While obesity is foremost associated with reduced fertility, there are many other factors that must be considered. Obesity in women of reproductive age is important both because of the risks of associated

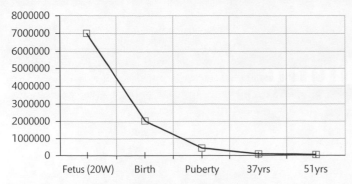

Figure 6.1 Number of follicles in the ovaries during a woman's life.
Reproduced with permission from Tarlatzis BC, Zepiridis L. Perimenopausal conception. *Ann N Y Acad Sci.* 2003;997:93–104 with permission from John Wiley and Sons.

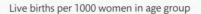

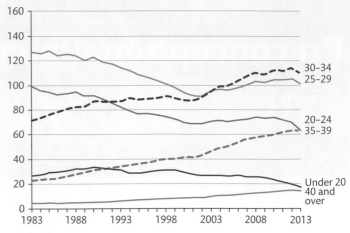

Figure 6.2 Maternal age groups at childbirth in England and Wales, 1983–2013.
Source data from Office for National Statistics, UK. *Statistical Bulletin for Births in England and Wales.* Retrieved from http://www.ons.gov.uk/ons/dcp171778_371129.pdf. 2013.

downstream diseases (including type 2 diabetes and cardiovascular disease) and because obesity is associated with poor outcomes for both the pregnant woman and the fetus. Such outcomes include fetal anomalies, gestational diabetes, pre-eclampsia, medically indicated preterm birth, caesarean delivery, and fetal macrosomia; longer-term risks for offspring include childhood obesity and the metabolic syndrome.

Physiology of obesity in preconception

Studies have shown that there is reduced fertility in obese patients, which is hypothesized to be a result of insulin resistance-induced oligo-ovulation and anovulation from hormonal and metabolic parameters (11, 12). Although polycystic ovarian syndrome is known to be a key contributor in ovulatory dysfunction, there is an independent contributing factor from obesity as well. Key hormonal effects include reduction of sex hormone-binding globulin, which effectively leads to functional hyperandrogenism, an increased production of oestrogen, and subsequent reduction in gonadotropin secretion (12). Additionally, there is evidence to show that leptin, an adipokine produced by adipose tissue, can directly inhibit ovarian function (12, 13).

Table 6.1 Rate of Down syndrome at live birth, according to maternal age

Maternal age at delivery (years)	Incidence of Down syndrome per 1000 live births
20	0.601
25	0.772
30	0.978
35	2.717
37	4.082
40	10.989
42	15.385
45	34.482

Source data from Chuckle HS, Wald NJ, Thompson SG. Estimating a woman's risk of having a pregnancy associated with Down's syndrome using her age and serum alpha-fetoprotein level. *Br J Obstet Gynaecol* 1987;94(5):387–402.

Pregnancy after bariatric surgery

Pregnancy following bariatric or weight loss surgery presents unique challenges and considerations. Bariatric surgery is an option for weight loss provided by the National Health Service for patients with a body mass index of at least 40 kg/m², or 35 kg/m² with significant comorbidities. During preconceptional counselling, topics including timing of conception, health of mother and baby, and fertility can be discussed. Bariatric surgery has the potential to reduce the risks of gestational diabetes and large-for-gestational-age neonates but is also associated with some risks in pregnancy.

There is currently limited evidence to show that women should wait a specific time prior to conceiving (14, 15); however, according to the recommendations from the American College of Obstetricians and Gynecologists, women should be advised to delay conceiving until 12–24 months after surgery, the period when the most rapid weight loss occurs (16). Due to the different absorption pattern of the gastrointestinal tract following bariatric surgery, nutritional deficiencies have been reported, and dietary supplementation should be considered in this specific population of women in the preconception period (17). Specific daily nutrient supplementation recommendations include greater than 65 mg of iron, greater than 400 mcg of folic acid, greater than 400 IU of vitamin D, and 350 mcg of vitamin B.

The pathophysiology that contributes to obesity and infertility appears to be multifactorial, with contributions primarily from insulin resistance and altered hormone profiles (18). Some women undergo bariatric surgery in attempts to reverse some of these effects, and there have been reports of successful increases in fertility following bariatric surgery (17, 19).

Diabetes mellitus

Preconceptional counselling is equally important for women with type 1 or type 2 diabetes mellitus. The main goals of preconceptional counselling around diabetes includes the following: optimizing

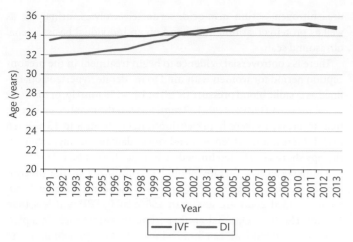

Figure 6.3 Average age of women undergoing *in vitro* fertilization (IVF) and donor insemination (DI) treatment using fresh eggs (1991–2013).

Source data from Human Fertilisation & Embryology Authority. Fertility Treatment in 2013. Retrieved from http://www.hfea.gov.uk/docs/HFEA_Fertility_Trends_and_Figures_2013.pdf. 2013.

preconceptional glycaemic control; risk management of adverse fetal and maternal outcomes; education around diabetes self-care; medication changes; and managing pre-existing complications and comorbidities associated with diabetes. Women of reproductive age with type 1 or 2 diabetes should be counselled to supplement with folic acid, 1.0 mg daily, beginning at least 3 months before conception.

One of the important factors in consideration of the health of the fetus in a mother with diabetes is the physiology of glucose and insulin in pregnancy. Glucose readily crosses the placenta via the GLUT1 transporter, while insulin does not. Because of this, optimization of glycaemic control is of utmost importance in the preconception period due to the teratogenic effects of hyperglycaemia on the fetus. There are increased risks of both adverse maternal

and fetal outcomes, including congenital malformations, miscarriage, preterm delivery, pre-eclampsia, macrosomia, and perinatal mortality (20–22). In the first trimester, hyperglycaemia is a known teratogen, resulting in neural tube defects and fetal heart malformations (23, 24). As can be seen in **Figure 6.5**, studies have shown that hyperglycaemia is the primary driver in these adverse events, and therefore tighter glycaemic control in the preconception period is critical.

Goals for glycaemic control in the preconception period are in line with the conception period, which is to optimize glycaemic control. The following parameters provide a framework for glycaemic control in the preconception period, with a goal of near-normal blood glucose while avoiding hypoglycaemia:

- Fasting glucose concentration of 5.3 mmol/L or lower.
- 1-hour postprandial glucose concentration of 7.8 mmol/L or lower, *or* 2-hour postprandial glucose concentration of 6.4 mmol/L or lower.
- Glycated haemoglobin level of less than 6.5% in the preconception period.

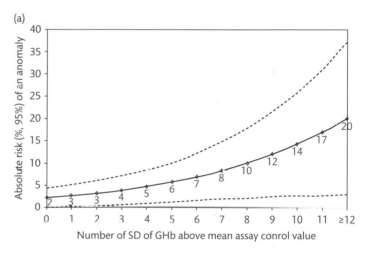

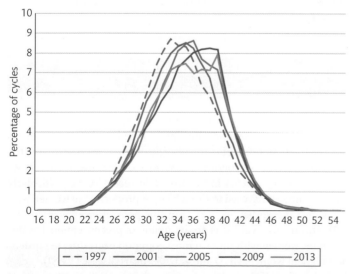

Figure 6.4 Percentage of cycles started by patients' age at start of treatment (1997–2013).

Source data from Human Fertilisation & Embryology Authority. Fertility Treatment in 2013. Retrieved from http://www.hfea.gov.uk/docs/HFEA_Fertility_Trends_and_Figures_2013.pdf. 2013.

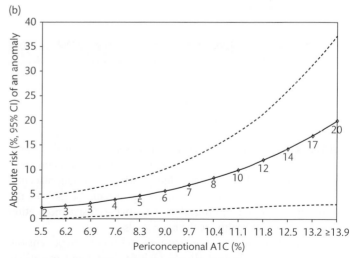

Figure 6.5 Risk of a major or minor anomaly according to periconceptional A1C.

Reproduced from Guerin A, Nisenbaum R, Ray JG. Use of maternal GHb concentration to estimate the risk of congenital anomalies in the offspring of women with prepregnancy diabetes. *Diabetes Care.* 2007;30(7):1920-5 with permission from American Diabetes Association.

- Avoid hypoglycaemia and maintain a capillary plasma glucose concentration of at least 4.0 mm/L.

Hypothyroidism and pregnancy

Thyroid physiology in pregnancy adapts to meet increased metabolic demands, and therefore women with pre-existing thyroid disease should be examined in the preconception period to optimize thyroid function. Some major changes in the function of the thyroid that are seen during pregnancy include stimulation of the thyroid-stimulating hormone (TSH) receptor by human chorionic gonadotropin (hCG), and an increase in serum thyroxine-binding globulin (TBG).

In response to the rise in oestrogen in pregnancy, a corresponding almost twofold rise in serum levels of TBG is seen. The rise in TBG is a direct result of increased TBG production from increased levels of oestrogen, as well as decreased TBG clearance. To maintain free thyroid hormone levels, serum total thyroxine (T_4) and triiodothyronine (T_3) concentrations also rise in the first half of pregnancy. Due to the homology of the beta-subunits of hCG and TSH, hCG contributes to thyroid stimulation through weak thyroid-stimulating activity.

Complications of maternal hypothyroidism include increased incidence of preterm labour, pre-eclampsia, placental abruption, perinatal morbidity and mortality, and neuropsychological and cognitive impairment (26–28). For these reasons, optimization of thyroid function in the preconception period is of utmost importance. In the preconception period, TSH should be optimized at less than 2.5 mU/L (29). Due to the changes seen in normal physiology in pregnancy, thyroid function tests should be interpreted with trimester-specific reference ranges, with lower acceptable ranges of TSH in the first trimester (2.5 mU/L), graduating to 3.0 mU/L in the second and third trimesters (29). Alternatively, another approach is to preconceptionally increase the dosing of levothyroxine; however, this should be done with close monitoring of TSH with goal TSH levels as described previously.

Preconceptional optimization of hypertension

The discussion of optimization of hypertension in pregnancy includes women with pre-existing or chronic hypertension, a history of gestational hypertension, and a history of pre-eclampsia or eclampsia. Many of the precautions and optimization of these conditions are similar in the preconceptional phase. Women with chronic hypertension are at increased risk for adverse obstetrical outcomes including preterm birth, intrauterine growth restriction, placental abruption, fetal death, and developing pre-eclampsia (30). In the preconception period, optimization of antihypertensive medication and cardiovascular health are the main goals.

For women with long-standing chronic hypertension, preconceptional evaluation should include assessment of cardiac and renal involvement, including baseline heart and kidney function tests. Depending on the chronicity and severity of the disease, baseline investigations may include an electrocardiogram, echocardiogram, serum creatinine, glomerular filtration rate, blood

urea nitrogen, serum uric acid, serum electrolytes, urinalysis, as well as protein:creatinine ratio, and on an individual basis, a renal ultrasound scan.

There is controversial evidence to begin treatment in the preconception period for women with mild to moderate hypertension, defined as systolic blood pressure (SBP) of 140–159 mmHg, or diastolic blood pressure (DBP) of 90–109 mmHg, with the number needed to treat to prevent severe hypertension ranging from 8 to 13 women (31). If there is any evidence of end-organ damage, antihypertensive therapy should be started immediately, regardless of blood pressure.

Antihypertensive therapy should be optimized in the preconception period. There is not a universal blood pressure goal, but recommended goals are less than 150 mmHg SBP and less than 100 mmHg DBP. Optimal antihypertensive agents include alpha-agonists (methyldopa), calcium channel blockers (nifedipine), and beta-blockers (labetalol). Angiotensin-converting enzyme (ACE) inhibitors should be avoided in the preconception period, as they have been shown to cause major congenital malformations with exposure in the first trimester (32).

Women should have a postpartum visit planned 6–8 weeks following delivery, with standard postpartum care including blood pressure monitoring and weight measurement, with the goal of obtaining preconceptional weight within 6 months following delivery.

Women with previous pre-eclampsia

Women with a previous history of pre-eclampsia require increased monitoring starting at 20 weeks gestational age. The United States Preventative Services Task Force recommends that women identified at high risk for pre-eclampsia take low-dose aspirin (81 mg daily) at 12 weeks gestational age as preventative medication (33). In this systematic evidence review, there was limited evidence of harms; however, an increased risk of placental abruption could not be ruled out (33). Although there was no evidence of increased risk of bleeding-related complications, including postpartum haemorrhage, maternal blood loss, or neonatal intracranial haemorrhage, it is generally recommended to discontinue aspirin 2 weeks prior to delivery.

Preconceptional evaluation of women with heart disease

Women of reproductive age with existing heart disease require evaluation in the preconception period, with unique implications for treatment options. Historically, rheumatic heart disease was the most prevalent heart condition in women of reproductive age; however, the advancements in healthcare in recent years, particularly cardiac surgery, have led to a much larger proportion of women with congenital heart disease (CHD) in this population of women (34, 35). This section will focus on discussion of preconceptional evaluation for women with the two most common heart disease burdens in pregnant women: CHD and valvular heart disease (VHD).

Although CHD is now the most prevalent heart disease for women in pregnancy, they also have relatively favourable outcomes in regards to maternal mortality, cardiac complications, preterm birth, low birth weight, and neonatal mortality (34). Interestingly, statistics show that caesarean delivery rates are still high in this population; however, in most cases of CHD, spontaneous vaginal delivery is recommended (36). There are specific cases in which caesarean section is recommended, including severe pulmonary stenosis and ventricular function deterioration, and discussion of this should be considered in the preconceptional period (36).

VHD is the second most prevalent heart disease among women of reproductive age. Unfortunately, many women with VHD are not aware of their diagnosis prior to conception, and therefore preconceptional counselling is often limited. In cases where VHD is diagnosed prior to conception, preconceptional evaluation is important to identify the modifiable risk factors that confer a poor outcome, including functional capacity of the individual, ventricular systolic function, and the presence of pulmonary hypertension. Preconceptional evaluation includes a baseline cardiovascular stress test and screening tests with electrocardiography and echocardiography in order to detect these modifiable risk factors. In cases where valvular surgery is indicated, preconceptional counselling is paramount regarding the timing of the surgery, as well as the resulting implications of treatment following the interventions of bioprosthetic versus mechanical valve replacement. Management of women in pregnancy with mechanical heart valves is exceedingly difficult and controversial, as they require long-term anticoagulation; however, there is no ideal regimen that balances the risks and benefits to both mother and fetus (37–39). The trade-off with bioprosthetic valves is the limited lifetime of the valve, often requiring replacement at least once in a patient's lifetime. In cases where valve replacement is indicated, there is no clear consensus on the recommendations, as the individual case should be discussed and managed by a cardiologist with specialties in management of pregnancy in conjunction with an obstetrician. The most common perinatal complication in women with VHD is heart failure, with an increased incidence of postpartum haemorrhage, most likely observed due to the increased use of anticoagulants in this population (34). However, despite the high rates of morbidity in pregnant women with VHD, mortality remains low (40).

Preconceptional counselling of women with inflammatory bowel disease

Preconceptional counselling for women of reproductive age with inflammatory bowel disease (IBD) includes education around the effects of IBD on fertility and pregnancy, the effect of pregnancy on the disease process of IBD, medication safety, and the potential effects of IBD on the fetus. Studies have shown increased risk of low birth weight, preterm delivery, and risk of antepartum haemorrhage (41, 42). There is controversial opinion regarding the risk of congenital fetal malformations for women with IBD; however, evidence suggests that there is no increased risk for women with IBD compared with controls (43, 44). The preconception period for women of reproductive age is paramount to optimize disease management, including discussion of nutritional requirements such as increased folic acid requirements of 1.0 mg daily in cases where medications can inhibit the absorption of folic acid, such as sulfasalazine (45).

The principles of IBD management in pregnancy begin with optimization of therapy in preconception in order to achieve remission prior to conception. A recent study showed that women who conceive in remission have a decreased risk of having active disease during pregnancy (46). Optimization of preconceptional management includes achieving monotherapy with oral aminosalicylate (5-ASA), thiopurines (azathioprine and mercaptopurine), or anti-tumour necrosis factor (anti-TNF), as these have been shown to be safe for use in pregnancy (47–50). If monotherapy is going to be considered, there is more evidence to suggest de-escalation to monotherapy with anti-TNF results in sustained remission (51). However discontinuation from combination anti-TNF and thiopurines to achieve monotherapy should be done 3–6 months preconceptionally, and only be considered in a select group of low-risk patients, including those in sustained remission for 12 months preconceptionally, with no history of anti-TNF medication failure, prior surgeries, or hospitalizations in the past 3 years (52). Despite the improved outcomes from quiescent disease in preconception, unfortunately approximately one-third of women still relapse in pregnancy, with most relapses occurring in the first trimester.

Optimization of therapy preconceptionally is also important to preserve fertility. Although there is no intrinsic infertility in the disease process of IBD, active disease can affect fertility from inflammation of the fallopian tubes and most commonly previous surgical intervention (53–56). An important, but often forgotten, discussion includes the effects of IBD on male fertility (57). This effect is related to both medication use as well as surgical intervention, and is a potentially reversible cause of infertility that should be addressed with couples in the preconception period (58, 59). The medication safety profile of pharmacological therapies for IBD should include discussion of both the female and male partner, as both fertility as well as teratogenic effects have been reported with specific medications, including infertility with male partners taking sulfasalazine and potent abortifacient effect and congenital malformations with methotrexate (59, 60).

The preconceptional counselling of women with IBD should include discussion around planning the mode of delivery. There are specific aspects of the IBD disease process that can affect vaginal delivery, in which case elective caesarean section should be planned. In women who have active perianal disease, or those who have undergone ileal pouch–anal anastomosis surgical procedure, an elective caesarean section is recommended (52). Although evidence is controversial, there is more evidence to show that the diagnosis of IBD alone is not sufficient to recommend delivery by caesarean section, with no difference in outcome for mother in exacerbations or neonatal outcomes when there is no active perianal disease (61–63).

Preconceptional optimization of women with neurological disorders

Many neurological conditions can affect women in the preconceptional period; this chapter will focus on two common conditions that affect women during pregnancy: epilepsy and multiple sclerosis (MS).

Epilepsy

Though more than 90% of women with epilepsy have a normal pregnancy, women with epilepsy have an increased risk of serious perinatal complications, including pre-eclampsia, preterm labour, and congenital malformations, and therefore should be discussed in the preconception period (64). Particular consideration should be taken regarding the management of epilepsy in relation to pregnancy, the effect of pregnancy on seizure frequency, the potential effects of epilepsy treatment on the fetus, the increased risks of obstetrical complications, and the preparation for the postpartum period.

Many women of childbearing age with epilepsy use antiepileptic drugs (AEDs) to control their condition. One of the principles of treatment with AEDs for women of reproductive age is optimization of AED therapy most appropriate for the seizure type at least 6 months in advance of the preconception period, and continuation of the same treatment regimen from the preconception period throughout pregnancy, as changes in AEDs during pregnancy are contraindicated (64). Although approximately 25% of women have increased seizures in pregnancy, there is evidence to show that if a woman has been seizure free for more than 9 months, there is a high likelihood (84–92%) of remaining seizure free during pregnancy (65).

The risk of major fetal structural malformations in the general population is 2–3%, which increases to 4–6% for women taking AEDs (65). Specific AEDs have higher rates of major fetal structural malformations, including divalproex sodium and valproic acid, and should therefore be avoided in women of reproductive age for initiation of AED therapy. Those women who are on a stable AED regimen with any of the previously mentioned AEDs, as well as carbamazepine, should have their alpha-fetoprotein levels measured at 14–16 weeks, with a structural ultrasound at 16–20 weeks for screening purposes. Similar to all women in the preconception period, it is strongly recommended that women taking AEDs also take folic acid supplementation of at least 1.0 mg in the preconception period for at least 3 months prior to conception, as many of the AEDs impair folic acid absorption, including phenytoin, carbamazepine, and barbiturates (66).

It is important to discuss some of the increased risk for obstetrical complications that women with epilepsy have. Historically, it was theorized that women with epilepsy are at increased risk of developing pre-eclampsia and eclampsia in pregnancy. However, recent studies have not shown evidence of an increased risk for development of pre-eclampsia, although these were insufficiently sensitive to rule out the increased risk (65). There is evidence to show that women with epilepsy have an increased risk of preterm labour, however recent studies demonstrate that smoking may be a confounder, as the risk is substantially higher in those women with epilepsy who also smoke (65).

In preparation for pregnancy and the postpartum period, counselling should be undertaken for women taking AEDs regarding the need for vitamin K supplementation in the third trimester, as well as transmission of AEDs through breast milk. Decreased levels of vitamin K in neonates born to women taking some enzyme-inducing AEDs have been reported, and therefore supplementation is indicated in the third trimester (67). Although breastfeeding is not contraindicated for women taking AEDs, for those taking sedating AEDs, special monitoring of the neonate for sedation is recommended (67).

Multiple sclerosis

The disease course of MS is variable in nature, typically characterized by relapse exacerbations and remissions of neurological deficits. This is particularly important in discussions of preconceptional health, as the disease has an increased prevalence in women of childbearing age (68, 69).

The disease course of MS in pregnancy is a controversial topic, however a meta-analysis published in 2011 reported a significant decrease in disease activity during pregnancy, and an overall increase in disease activity during the postpartum period (70). Although there is no net effect of overall increase in exacerbations during pregnancy and postpartum combined, the two reports of the PRIMS study in 1998 and 2004 demonstrate decreased incidence of disease exacerbation in the preconception, and pregnancy periods, and an increased relapse rate in the first 3 months postpartum (71, 72). These reports also demonstrate that pregnancy does not have an effect on the ultimate disease course of MS, specifically no effect on the disease progression overall (72).

In the preconception period, it is advised that women discontinue disease-modifying agents, as some of these are known to be teratogenic (methotrexate, teriflunomide). Current evidence suggests that women discontinue disease-modifying agents in the preconception period from 1 to 6 months prior to conception, depending on the drug, and this decision should be discussed with a neurologist (73). Similarly, women are cautioned against using disease-modifying agents in the postpartum period if breastfeeding, and this schedule should be discussed with a neurologist.

Preconceptional management strategies in women with thrombophilic disorders

The discussion of thrombophilic disorders in preconceptional management is important, as it is one of the leading causes of maternal morbidity and mortality, despite being a rare complication in pregnancy with a prevalence of only 0.06–0.1%. Although many women have no prior history of venous thromboembolism (VTE), those with thrombophilic disorders must take special precautions in the preconception period, as the risk of VTE increases fivefold for this population.

Pregnancy increases the risk of VTE through all avenues of Virchow's triad: including increased hypercoagulability through increased levels of fibrinogen, factors II, VII, VIII, X, and XII; venous stasis due to compressive forces from the gravid uterus; and endothelial injury in cases of caesarean section.

Thrombophilias can be categorized as inherited or acquired conditions. The most common inherited thrombophilias, with associated odds ratio (OR) for development of VTE during pregnancy, include factor V Leiden (OR 34.4) and prothrombin gene (G20210) mutation (OR 26.4), while the primary acquired thrombophilia is antiphospholipid antibody syndrome (OR 15.8) (74–77).

Women of child-bearing age with known thrombophilia, as well as those with a history of VTE, should undergo special surveillance and investigations in the preconception period to stratify the risk for VTE in pregnancy. Those with an unprovoked VTE event can be managed with surveillance alone, or surveillance in the antepartum period followed by thromboprophylaxis in the postpartum period, while those with hormonal-provoked VTE and known thrombophilia (inherited or acquired) should undergo thromboprophylaxis for VTE in pregnancy. Due to the difference in treatment, it is an important distinction to make in the preconception period, and accordingly, a prior history of VTE and thrombophilias should be screened for in the preconception period. Although screening should be completed in the preconception period, there is no indication for thromboprophylaxis in the preconception period, unless the condition itself requires this treatment. The recommended thromboprophylaxis in the antepartum period may include daily low-molecular-weight heparin administration, with the risks and benefits of treatment discussed on an individual basis with each woman.

Preconceptional optimization of couples with HIV infection

The preconceptional evaluation of couples with human immunodeficiency virus (HIV) includes many aspects of care including preconceptional health, mental health, antiretroviral (ARV) medications, transmission between partners, and perinatal transmission to the fetus. With the evolving nature of the prevalence of disease, advancements in treatment options, and evolution of the virus itself, the interpretation of research before the discovery of ARVs and recommendations must evolve as well. Historically, people living with HIV had significantly reduced life expectancy; however, with the introduction of highly successful ARVs, couples can now have the same life expectancy as the general population (78).

Preliminary preconceptional assessment of women with positive HIV infection must include assessment of overall health, discussion of prevention of infection to others, including the risk of horizontal and vertical transmission, and provision of support and close monitoring. Studies have shown that there is an association of an increased risk of perinatal transmission of HIV with certain behaviours including smoking, illicit drug use, and sexual intercourse with multiple partners (79, 80); however, caution should be taken with interpretation of potential confounding factors (81). Specific considerations that should be assessed at the initial preconception visit include general diet and weight, possible issues of smoking and/or substance use, obesity/diabetes, hypertension, possible cultural context, vaccination status, possible hepatitis C coinfection, and signs of immunosuppression including fevers and history of opportunistic infections. Careful physical examination should also include signs of immunosuppression, including signs of thrush, cachexia, genital ulcers, or vaginal discharge. Optimization of maternal health in the preconception period is paramount to a healthy pregnancy, and should include folic acid supplementation of 1 mg per day for at least 3 months preconceptionally, treatment of any active infections, evaluation of maternal psychosocial health, and counselling regarding smoking cessation, alcohol and drug use, and safe sex practices.

The initial evaluation of couples with HIV includes measuring levels of CD4 counts as well as HIV viral load. It is important to evaluate these levels in regards to the initiation of ARVs, and for a baseline assessment in the preconception period. Monitoring of CD4 counts and HIV viral load should be continued throughout pregnancy, in regard to the potential need for prophylaxis for opportunistic infections such as *Pneumocystis*, toxoplasmosis, or *Mycobacterium avium* complex. Mode of delivery can be affected by viral load, and therefore should be discussed during the preconception period (82, 83). In women with an undetectable viral load who have been compliant with ARV therapy, there is no contraindication to vaginal delivery, and caesarean section should be considered for obstetrical indications.

There is a risk of HIV transmission in HIV-discordant couples, as well as a risk of superinfection between concordant couples, and therefore discussion in the preconception period should include options for reducing the risk of horizontal HIV transmission during conception. Previously, naturally timed conception was inconceivable for discordant couples; however, with the advancement of ARVs, this is now a possible option (84). HIV-discordant couples in which the woman is HIV positive and the man is HIV negative should take precautions, as a study has shown that despite the effectiveness in ARVs demonstrating no detectable viral load, there can still be detectable viral shedding from the female genital tract (85). Couples should be counselled extensively regarding the risk of transmission, and provided with conception options including unprotected sex only during times of ovulation to reduce the number of times the HIV seronegative partner is exposed, as well as home insemination for HIV-discordant couples in which the woman is HIV positive and the man is HIV negative, and semen washing for HIV-discordant couples in which the man is HIV positive and the woman is HIV negative (86).

Previous fetal loss and future management considerations

The rate of fetal loss in the United Kingdom historically is approximately 1 in every 200 deliveries, which is a devastating experience for mothers and families (87). Fetal loss includes intrauterine fetal demise (IUFD), defined as the absence of life *in utero*, as well as stillbirth, defined as the death of a fetus after 24 weeks' gestation with absence of breath and signs of life (88, 89). In 2013, the rate of stillbirth was 4.6 per 1000 births, which was slightly decreased from 5.7 per 1000 in 2003 (87). Although there are identifiable risk factors for stillbirth and IUFD, unfortunately near 50% of fetal loss in the United Kingdom remains unexplained (87).

Counselling around fetal loss includes recognition of the psychosocial effects for the mother and family, and discussion about the risk of having another stillbirth or IUFD. There is controversial evidence regarding the relative risk of recurrence of stillbirth in low-risk women with previous unexplained fetal loss, with some studies showing no increased risk, and others finding a 3.5–6-fold increased risk relative to women who have previously had a live birth (90–92).

Identifiable causes of fetal loss can be broken down into categories of obstetrical complications, fetal complications, maternal complications, and unknown causes. Obstetrical causes include placental abruption, preterm premature rupture of membranes, cervical insufficiency, maternal–fetal haemorrhage, umbilical cord complications (including cord thrombosis, velamentous cord insertion, and cord accidents), amniotic band syndrome, and placental pathology (93–95). Many of these are either difficult to diagnose in early pregnancy, or non-modifiable, making counselling around these obstetrical complications difficult for future expectations. Although one study has suggested an increased risk of unexplained stillbirth at greater than 39 weeks' gestation, and highest at 41 weeks' gestation (96, 97), delivery should be guided by obstetrical indications, as there is no concrete recommendation for timing of delivery for previous unexplained fetal loss.

Fetal complications mainly include karyotype abnormalities, with the most common being trisomy 18 and 21 (98). Counselling regarding these fetal complications is presented at the time of diagnosis, usually prior to 20 weeks, and includes discussion of therapeutic termination of pregnancy in cases where karyotype abnormalities may lead to IUFD or stillbirth. One of the fetal complications that poses a modifiable intervention to reduce the risk of congenital malformations leading to fetal loss includes ensuring adequate counselling regarding maternal folic acid fortification (99).

Maternal causes include primarily pre-existing maternal disease, maternal trauma, and infection with syphilis, malaria, cytomegalovirus, and Coxsackie B virus as potential infections that contribute to fetal loss (93, 100). It is estimated that approximately 10–25% of stillbirths in high-income countries are the result of infection, which in some cases can be preventable (100). Counselling in this area should include discussion around vaccinations, including influenza vaccine, and to counsel women regarding foods to avoid including soft cheeses, and as well as some meats and seafood products (100). Maternal diabetes and hypertensive disorders are the two most common maternal complications that have identifiable and preventable risk factors (95). Counselling around these disorders begins with identification and subsequently preconceptional management to achieve maternal health prior to the woman's next pregnancy.

Counselling for couples with genetic abnormalities and inheritable conditions

Detection of genetic abnormalities in the antenatal period can significantly affect the outcome of a pregnancy. Congenital abnormalities as a cause of death in the perinatal period have decreased dramatically from 1960 to 2013 (101, 102). Infant deaths, postneonatal deaths, and neonatal deaths have decreased from 4.5, 1.7, and 2.8 per 1000 live births in 1959–1961 in England and Wales (102), respectively, to 1.1, 0.4, and 1.2 per 1000 live births in 2013 (101). This can be attributed, in part, to the higher rates of detection in the prenatal period, with medical advances in treatment options as well as subsequent selective termination.

New advances in genetic screening tests have made preconceptional carrier testing possible through genetic testing across single genes and more recently multiple genetic mutations with genome sequencing. Typically, carrier testing is performed on the maternal genes, followed by paternal testing if any genes of interest are identified. This can be offered to couples at high risk for specific inheritance, or for those who wish to pursue this testing through the private sector. Additionally, advancements in tests available during the conceptional period include non-invasive prenatal testing (NIPT), whereby cell-free fetal DNA can be measured with very precise relative quantification in the maternal circulating blood, and used for early diagnosis of genetic conditions in the first trimester. Although this is not the standard method of screening for chromosomal abnormalities, non-invasive testing is being used more commonly as a screening tool to diagnose several genetic conditions due to the high sensitivity and specificity that it offers.

During a preconceptional evaluation of couples with genetic abnormalities, specific factors should be discussed in detail, including personal and family history of known or suspected inheritable diseases, consanguinity, advanced maternal and paternal age, potential teratogen exposure, ethnic background with an increased prevalence of disease, and recurrent pregnancy loss. If any of these factors are of concern, genetic counselling referral with a geneticist is indicated and should be done preconceptionally if possible. A detailed family history, including first-, second-, and third-degree relatives, is important to identify any unexplained perinatal or infant deaths, intellectual disability, or congenital abnormalities that could otherwise be missed.

When an inheritable disease is identified, a couple should be informed regarding the likelihood of future offspring developing the condition, which may depend on the pattern of inheritance, including Mendelian versus di- or multigenic, as well as penetrance and variable expression. The burden of disease on both the inheriting individual as well as the family should be discussed, including the potential for requirement for chronic hospitalization or shortening of life span; cost of treatments; impact on future reproductive potential; and effects on physical and mental development, with special consideration of future ability to engage in activities of daily living independently.

In planning conception, it is important to discuss the expectations of a couple, including the types and sensitivity of genetic tests available, including amniocentesis, chorionic villus sampling, NIPT, and ultrasonography, and if the couple would wish to pursue investigations. Alternative options to modify the impact of disease for couples with known inheritable disease include artificial insemination by donor, ovum transfer from surrogate, as well as adoption.

Drugs to avoid preconceptionally

Women of reproductive age can be taking medications for chronic diseases, may start new medications during pregnancy, or require over-the-counter medications during the preconception period or during pregnancy. We will discuss medications taken commonly during pregnancy separately from those taken for chronic illness. For these chronic illnesses, most prescription drug regimens should be optimized in the preconception period, and medication changes avoided during pregnancy, unless indicated. For more detailed information regarding drugs used in the following chronic diseases, please see the appropriate section elsewhere in this chapter for the specific chronic disease category: diabetes mellitus, hypothyroidism, hypertension, heart disease, IBD, neurological disease, thrombophilic disorders, and HIV infection.

Many medications require a period of clearance from the maternal circulation, prior to conception. The following commonly used medications should be optimized in the preconception period, with the optimal period of clearance prior to conception dependent on the medication, if indicated:

Pain and fever

- Non-steroidal anti-inflammatory drugs (NSAIDs): safety profile varies with gestational age, however NSAIDs should generally be avoided during pregnancy. Limit use in months of preconception.

- Acetaminophen/paracetamol: generally regarded as safe in pregnancy. Long-term use is not advised, but it is the antipyretic and analgesic of choice in pregnancy if short-term medication is needed.
- Opioids: although not recommended for use in pregnancy, the balance of maternal pain control with the potential effects on the fetus must be considered. Studies have shown evidence of neonatal withdrawal syndrome; however, this is uncommon (103). First-line treatment for non-cancer chronic pain in pregnancy is initiation of methadone, and should be considered in the preconception period.

Antibiotics

Antibiotics deemed safe in pregnancy include the following, and can thus be used in the preconception period: penicillins, cephalosporins, azithromycin, clindamycin, and erythromycin.

Gastroesophageal reflex disease

- Antacids: considered generally safe in pregnancy, and can be used in the preconception period.
- H$_2$ receptor antagonists (e.g. ranitidine (104)): considered safe in pregnancy, and can be used in the preconception period. Caution should be used in breastfeeding.
- Proton pump inhibitors (e.g. pantoprazole) (105): considered generally safe in pregnancy, and can be used in the preconception period.

Headaches and migraine

Preferred agents include acetaminophen and metoclopramide, which are considered safe in pregnancy and thus recommended in the preconception period.

Vaccinations

For all women of reproductive age in the preconception period, immunization status should be checked annually and updated as indicated for the following: tetanus–diphtheria toxoid/diphtheria–tetanus–pertussis; measles, mumps, and rubella; and varicella.

- Tetanus–diphtheria toxoid/diphtheria–tetanus–pertussis: preferred immunity in the preconception period, however can be given in pregnancy after 20 weeks' gestation, and ideally after 28 weeks' gestation.
- Measles, mumps, and rubella: contraindicated in pregnancy, and therefore should be given 3 or more months prior to conception. If preconception immunization is not possible, then the vaccine should be given immediately postpartum.
- Varicella: contraindicated in pregnancy, and therefore should be given prior to conception. If preconception immunization is not possible, then the vaccine should be given immediately postpartum.
- Influenza: one dose in preconception or conception period, given annually.
- Hepatitis B: preferred immunity in the preconception period, however can be given in pregnancy if unvaccinated or at high risk of exposure.

- HPV: routine screening, with recommended subgroups vaccination as per regional health authority recommendations.

Antidepressants

Antidepressants are commonly used in pregnancy, in approximately 3% of women in Europe, and 8% of women in the United States. This class of medications crosses the placenta and the fetal blood–brain barrier, and should therefore be used with caution. In consideration of this class of drugs in the preconception period, a trial of taper can be tried 6 months in advance of conception, with the goal to have the medication regimen optimized 3 months prior to conception. When considering discontinuation of antidepressants, the balance between the maternal psychiatric condition and health of the fetus must be balanced, with an emphasis placed on maternal health in the preconception period. If multiple agents are used, then transition to a single agent in the preconception period is advised if possible.

Antihypertensives

- ACE inhibitors are contraindicated in pregnancy, and should be discontinued with an appropriate antihypertensive regiment established 2–3 months preconceptionally (32). Preferred agents include labetalol, nifedipine, and methyldopa.
- Angiotensin II receptor blockers, similar to ACE inhibitors, are contraindicated in pregnancy and should be discontinued with an appropriate antihypertensive regiment established 2–3 months preconceptionally (32).

Antiepileptic drugs (AEDs)

(See 'Epilepsy' for more detailed information.)

- Divalproex sodium and valproic acid are contraindicated in pregnancy, and should therefore be replaced with a different AED 6 months prior to conception. The benefits of switching AEDs should be balanced with the maternal seizure condition, with an emphasis placed on maternal health.

Immunosuppressive agents

(See 'Preconceptional counselling of women with inflammatory bowel disease' for more detailed information.)

- Methotrexate is contraindicated in pregnancy due to the potent abortifacient effect and congenital malformations, and should be replaced with a different monotherapy of anti-inflammatory or immunosuppressive therapy in discussion with a gastroenterologist (60). Discontinuation at least 4 months prior to conception, and 6 months if possible is recommended (106).

Treatment of thromboembolic disorders

(See 'Preconceptional management strategies in women with thrombophilic disorders' for more detailed information, including treatment course and timeline.)

- The recommended agent for treatment of VTE in pregnancy is low-molecular-weight heparin (e.g. dalteparin), and should therefore be considered as the first-line treatment in the preconception period.

- Warfarin (brand name: Coumadin) is contraindicated in pregnancy due to congenital malformations (37).

Antiretroviral therapy

- Considered safe in pregnancy, and should be continued throughout pregnancy. If not initiated prior to conception, and there is no urgent medical indication for ARV therapy, then initiation can be delayed until 14 weeks' gestation.
- Two ARV therapies, didanosine and efavirenz, are not recommended in pregnancy, and therefore should be avoided if alternatives are available, with transition to a different ARV. These have shown toxicity and an increased rate of fetal congenital malformations in human and/or animal studies, respectively.

In the United Kingdom, the *British National Formulary* provides an exhaustive reference guide for medications and their safety profile in pregnancy. Historically, the United States Food and Drug Administration (FDA) provided a five-letter categorization of drug safety profile in pregnancy (A, B, C, D, and X) that was commonly used to report the safety profile of medications (107). The FDA has recently published the Pregnancy and Lactation Labelling Rule, which changes the labelling system to provide more comprehensive information, and also provides an additional category of information for couples regarding contraception and infertility related to medications (108).

Preconceptional counselling of women with previous third- and fourth-degree perineal tears

Reports show that approximately 85% of women undergo perineal trauma during the second stage of labour, with 1.5% of those reported as third- or fourth-degree perineal tears (109). Perineal tears are classified as first, second, third, or fourth degree, depending on the anatomical depth of the tear. First- and second-degree tears involve the depth of the skin, and perineal muscles, respectively, with no involvement of the anal sphincter (110). When the anal sphincter is involved, this is considered a third-degree tear, with three levels of depth of involvement: 3a, less than 50% thickness of the external anal sphincter; 3b, more than 50% thickness of the external anal sphincter; and 3c, involvement extends to the internal anal sphincter (110). Fourth-degree tears penetrate to the depth of the anal mucosal layer, and are the most severe form of perineal tears (110). Classification of anal sphincter involvement, as in third- and fourth-degree tears, is classified as obstetrical anal sphincter injuries (OASIS), and can have significant morbidity for women, including perineal pain, dyspareunia, and anal incontinence (111, 112). The additional psychological impact should not be underestimated, as this can play a major role in preventing women from seeking medical attention for these symptoms (112).

During preconceptional counselling of women with previous OASIS, the risk factors should be discussed, both for future management decisions and to identify any modifiable risk factors that may be present. Obstetrical risk factors for OASIS include macrosomia

(>4500 g), operative vaginal delivery with forceps or vacuum assistance, and midline episiotomy, but not mediolateral episiotomy (113). Women with previous OASIS should be counselled regarding the modifiable risk factors if vaginal birth is planned, including location of episiotomy if indicated at the time. There is evidence to show that the fetal head position can affect the relative risk of OASIS, with occiput posterior position causing a sevenfold increase in the incidence of OASIS in one study (114). Unfortunately there is no conclusive evidence to recommend specific birthing positions or delayed second-stage pushing to influence the rate of third- and fourth-degree perineal tears.

Due to the physical and emotional trauma surrounding OASIS for many women, one of the pertinent questions to be addressed in the preconceptional period following previous third- and fourth-degree tears is the mode of delivery for a subsequent pregnancy. Evaluation of the risk of recurrence is an important factor to consider, as well as the emotional trauma surrounding the woman's previous experience. Studies have shown that there is an increased risk of subsequent sphincter laceration for woman with previous OASIS who deliver vaginally (115, 116). Specific risk factors for recurrent OASIS have been identified, including Asian ethnicity, forceps delivery, and birthweight more than 4 kg (110). For this reason, many women request an elective caesarean delivery, with evidence that shows even obstetricians themselves demonstrate a bias to choose elective caesarean with the primary reason being the potential risk of perineal trauma (117, 118).

REFERENCES

1. Hansen KR, Knowlton NS, Thyer AC, Charleston JS, Soules MR, Klein NA. A new model of reproductive aging: the decline in ovarian non-growing follicle number from birth to menopause. *Hum Reprod* 2008;**23**:699–708.
2. Faddy MJ, Gosden RG, Gougeon A, Richardson SJ, Nelson JF. Accelerated disappearance of ovarian follicles in mid-life: implications for forecasting menopause. *Hum Reprod* 1992;**7**:1342–46.
3. Tarlatzis BC, Zepiridis L. Perimenopausal conception. *Ann N Y Acad Sci* 2003;**997**:93–104.
4. Hook EB, Cross PK, Schreinemachers DM. Chromosomal abnormality rates at amniocentesis and in live-born infants. *JAMA* 1983;**249**:2034–48.
5. Loane M, Morris JK, Addor MC, Arriola L, Budd J, Doray B, et al. Twenty-year trends in the prevalence of Down syndrome and other trisomies in Europe: impact of maternal age and prenatal screening. *Eur J Hum Genet* 2013;**21**:27–33.
6. Cuckle HS, Wald NJ, Thompson SG. Estimating a woman's risk of having a pregnancy associated with Down's syndrome using her age and serum alpha-fetoprotein level. *Br J Obstet Gynaecol* 1987;**94**:387–402.
7. Office for National Statistics, UK. Statistical Bulletin for Births in England and Wales. 2013. Available at: http://www.ons.gov.uk/ons/dcp171778_371129.pdf.
8. Human Fertilisation and Embryology Authority. Fertility treatment in 2013. Available at: http://www.hfea.gov.uk/docs/HFEA_Fertility_Trends_and_Figures_2013.pdf.
9. Friedman D. Perk up: Facebook and Apple now pay for women to freeze eggs. NBC News; 2014. Available at: http://www.nbcnews.com/news/us-news/perk-facebook-apple-now-pay-women-freeze-eggs-n225011.

10. Kim SY, Dietz PM, England L, Morrow B, Callaghan WM. Trends in pre-pregnancy obesity in nine states, 1993–2003. *Obesity (Silver Spring)* 2007;**15**:986–93.

11. McCartney CR, Blank SK, Prendergast KA, et al. Obesity and sex steroid changes across puberty: evidence for marked hyperandrogenemia in pre- and early pubertal obese girls. *J Clin Endocrinol Metab* 2007;**92**:430–36.

12. Pasquali R, Pelusi C, Genghini S, Cacciari M, Gambineri A. Obesity and reproductive disorders in women. *Hum Reprod Update* 2003;**9**:359–72.

13. Greisen S, Ledet T, Møller N, et al. Effects of leptin on basal and FSH stimulated steroidogenesis in human granulosa luteal cells. *Acta Obstet Gynecol Scand* 2000;**79**:931–35.

14. Kjær MM, Nilas L. Timing of pregnancy after gastric bypass-a national register-based cohort study. *Obes Surg* 2013;**23**:1281–85.

15. Manning S, Finer N, Elkalaawy M, et al. Timing of pregnancy in obese women after bariatric surgery. *Pregnancy Hypertens* 2014;**4**:235.

16. American College of Obstetricians and Gynecologists. ACOG practice bulletin no. 105: bariatric surgery and pregnancy. *Obstet Gynecol* 2009;**113**:1405–13.

17. Magdaleno R, Pereira BG, Chaim EA, Turato ER. Pregnancy after bariatric surgery: a current view of maternal, obstetrical and perinatal challenges. *Arch Gynecol Obstet* 2012;**285**:559–66.

18. Shah DK, Ginsburg ES. Bariatric surgery and fertility. *Curr Opin Obstet Gynecol* 2010;**22**:248–54.

19. Marceau P, Kaufman D, Biron S, et al. Outcome of pregnancies after biliopancreatic diversion. *Obes Surg* 2004;**14**:318–24.

20. Kitzmiller JL, Wallerstein R, Correa A, Kwan S. Preconception care for women with diabetes and prevention of major congenital malformations. *Birth Defects Res A Clin Mol Teratol* 2010;**88**:791–803.

21. Evers IM, de Valk HW, Visser GH. Risk of complications of pregnancy in women with type 1 diabetes: nationwide prospective study in the Netherlands. *BMJ* 2004;**328**:915.

22. Persson M, Norman M, Hanson U. Obstetric and perinatal outcomes in type 1 diabetic pregnancies: a large, population-based study. *Diabetes Care* 2009;**32**:2005–2009.

23. Jensen DM, Korsholm L, Ovesen P, Beck-Nielsen H, Moelsted-Pedersen L, Westergaard JG, et al. Peri-conceptional A1C and risk of serious adverse pregnancy outcome in 933 women with type 1 diabetes. *Diabetes Care* 2009;**32**:1046–48.

24. Schaefer UM, Songster G, Xiang A, Berkowitz K, Buchanan TA, Kjos SL. Congenital malformations in offspring of women with hyperglycemia first detected during pregnancy. *Am J Obstet Gynecol* 1997;**177**:1165–71.

25. Guerin A, Nisenbaum R, Ray JG. Use of maternal GHb concentration to estimate the risk of congenital anomalies in the offspring of women with prepregnancy diabetes. *Diabetes Care* 2007;**30**:1920–25.

26. Casey BM, Dashe JS, Wells CE, et al. Subclinical hypothyroidism and pregnancy outcomes. *Obstet Gynecol* 2005;**105**:239–45.

27. Haddow JE, Palomaki GE, Allan WC, et al. Maternal thyroid deficiency during pregnancy and subsequent neuropsychological development of the child. *N Engl J Med* 1999;**341**:549–55.

28. Leung AS, Millar LK, Koonings PP, Montoro M, Mestman JH. Perinatal outcome in hypothyroid pregnancies. *Obstet Gynecol* 1993;**81**:349–53.

29. De Groot L, Abalovich M, Alexander EK, et al. Management of thyroid dysfunction during pregnancy and postpartum: an Endocrine Society clinical practice guideline. *J Clin Endocrinol Metab* 2012;**97**:2543–65.

30. Ferrer RL, Sibai BM, Mulrow CD, Chiquette E, Stevens KR, Cornell J. Management of mild chronic hypertension during pregnancy: a review. *Obstet Gynecol* 2000;**96**:849–60.

31. Abalos E, Duley L, Steyn DW. Antihypertensive drug therapy for mild to moderate hypertension during pregnancy. *Cochrane Database Syst Rev* 2014;**2**:CD002252.

32. Cooper WO, Hernandez-Diaz S, Arbogast PG, et al. Major congenital malformations after first-trimester exposure to ACE inhibitors. *N Engl J Med* 2006;**354**:2443–51.

33. Henderson JT, Whitlock EP, O'Connor E, Senger CA, Thompson JH, Rowland MG. Low-dose aspirin for prevention of morbidity and mortality from preeclampsia: a systematic evidence review for the U.S. Preventive Services Task Force. *Ann Intern Med* 2014;**160**:695–703.

34. Roos-Hesselink JW, Ruys TP, Stein JI, et al. Outcome of pregnancy in patients with structural or ischaemic heart disease: results of a registry of the European Society of Cardiology. *Eur Heart J* 2013;**34**:657–65.

35. Opotowsky AR, Siddiqi OK, D'Souza B, Webb GD, Fernandes SM, Landzberg MJ. Maternal cardiovascular events during childbirth among women with congenital heart disease. *Heart* 2012;**98**:145–51.

36. Regitz-Zagrosek V, Blomstrom Lundqvist C, Borghi C, et al. ESC Guidelines on the management of cardiovascular diseases during pregnancy: the Task Force on the Management of Cardiovascular Diseases during Pregnancy of the European Society of Cardiology (ESC). *Eur Heart J* 2011;**32**:3147–97.

37. Hall JG, Pauli RM, Wilson KM. Maternal and fetal sequelae of anticoagulation during pregnancy. *Am J Med* 1980;**68**:122–40.

38. Castellano JM, Narayan RL, Vaishnava P, Fuster V. Anticoagulation during pregnancy in patients with a prosthetic heart valve. *Nat Rev Cardiol* 2012;**9**:415–24.

39. Hung L, Rahimtoola SH. Prosthetic heart valves and pregnancy. *Circulation* 2003;**107**:1240–46.

40. Hameed A, Karaalp IS, Tummala PP, et al. The effect of valvular heart disease on maternal and fetal outcome of pregnancy. *J Am Coll Cardiol* 2001;**37**:893–99.

41. Elbaz G, Fich A, Levy A, Holcberg G, Sheiner E. Inflammatory bowel disease and preterm delivery. *Int J Gynaecol Obstet* 2005;**90**:193–97.

42. Bröms G, Granath F, Linder M, Stephansson O, Elmberg M, Kieler H. Complications from inflammatory bowel disease during pregnancy and delivery. *Clin Gastroenterol Hepatol* 2012;**10**:1246–52.

43. Dominitz JA, Young JC, Boyko EJ. Outcomes of infants born to mothers with inflammatory bowel disease: a population-based cohort study. *Am J Gastroenterol* 2002;**97**:641–48.

44. Bush MC, Patel S, Lapinski RH, Stone JL. Perinatal outcomes in inflammatory bowel disease. *J Matern Fetal Neonatal Med* 2004;**15**:237–41.

45. Van Assche G, Dignass A, Reinisch W, et al. The second European evidence-based Consensus on the diagnosis and management of Crohn's disease: special situations. *J Crohns Colitis* 2010;**4**:63–101.

46. Abhyankar A, Ham M, Moss AC. Meta-analysis: the impact of disease activity at conception on disease activity during pregnancy in patients with inflammatory bowel disease. *Aliment Pharmacol Ther* 2013;**38**:460–66.

47. Francella A, Dyan A, Bodian C, Rubin P, Chapman M, Present DH. The safety of 6-mercaptopurine for childbearing patients with inflammatory bowel disease: a retrospective cohort study. *Gastroenterology* 2003;**124**:9–17.

48. Alstead EM, Ritchie JK, Lennard-Jones JE, Farthing MJ, Clark ML. Safety of azathioprine in pregnancy in inflammatory bowel disease. *Gastroenterology* 1990;**99**:443–46.

49. Habal FM, Hui G, Greenberg GR. Oral 5-aminosalicylic acid for inflammatory bowel disease in pregnancy: safety and clinical course. *Gastroenterology* 1993;**105**:1057–60.

50. Schnitzler F, Fidder H, Ferrante M, et al. Outcome of pregnancy in women with inflammatory bowel disease treated with antitumor necrosis factor therapy. *Inflamm Bowel Dis* 2011;**17**:1846–54.

51. Torres J, Boyapati RK, Kennedy NA, Louis E, Colombel JF, Satsangi J. Systematic review of effects of withdrawal of immunomodulators or biologic agents from patients with inflammatory bowel disease. *Gastroenterology* 2015;**149**:1716–30.

52. Nguyen GC, Seow CH, Maxwell C, et al. The Toronto Consensus Statements for the management of inflammatory bowel disease in pregnancy. *Gastroenterology* 2016;**150**:734–57.

53. Hudson M, Flett G, Sinclair TS, Brunt PW, Templeton A, Mowat NA. Fertility and pregnancy in inflammatory bowel disease. *Int J Gynaecol Obstet* 1997;**58**:229–37.

54. Khosla R, Willoughby CP, Jewell DP. Crohn's disease and pregnancy. *Gut* 1984;**25**:52–56.

55. Ørding Olsen K, Juul S, Berndtsson I, Oresland T, Laurberg S. Ulcerative colitis: female fecundity before diagnosis, during disease, and after surgery compared with a population sample. *Gastroenterology* 2002;**122**:15–19.

56. Woolfson K, Cohen Z, McLeod RS. Crohn's disease and pregnancy. *Dis Colon Rectum* 1990;**33**:869–73.

57. Anderson BT, Ertle JT, Borum ML. Men with inflammatory bowel disease are rarely counseled regarding effects of immunosuppressive therapy on fertility and pregnancy. *J Crohns Colitis* 2013;**7**:e716.

58. Narendranathan M, Sandler RS, Suchindran CM, Savitz DA. Male infertility in inflammatory bowel disease. *J Clin Gastroenterol* 1989;**11**:403–406.

59. Toovey S, Hudson E, Hendry WF, Levi AJ. Sulphasalazine and male infertility: reversibility and possible mechanism. *Gut* 1981;**22**:445–51.

60. Powell HR, Ekert H. Methotrexate-induced congenital malformations. *Med J Aust* 1971;**2**:1076–77.

61. Bruce A, Black M, Bhattacharya S. Mode of delivery and risk of inflammatory bowel disease in the offspring: systematic review and meta-analysis of observational studies. *Inflamm Bowel Dis* 2014;**20**:1217–26.

62. Grouin A, Brochard C, Siproudhis L, et al. Perianal Crohn's disease results in fewer pregnancies but is not exacerbated by vaginal delivery. *Dig Liver Dis* 2015;**47**:1021–26.

63. Smink M, Lotgering FK, Albers L, de Jong DJ. Effect of childbirth on the course of Crohn's disease; results from a retrospective cohort study in the Netherlands. *BMC Gastroenterol* 2011;**11**:6.

64. Practice parameter: management issues for women with epilepsy (summary statement). Report of the Quality Standards Subcommittee of the American Academy of Neurology. *Neurology* 1998;**51**:944–48.

65. Harden CL, Meador KJ, Pennell PB, Hauser WA, Gronseth GS, French JA, et al. Practice Parameter update: Management issues for women with epilepsy—Focus on pregnancy (an evidence-based review): Teratogenesis and perinatal outcomes: Report of the Quality Standards Subcommittee and Therapeutics and Technology Assessment Subcommittee of the American Academy of Neurology and American Epilepsy Society. *Neurology* 2009;**73**:133–41.

66. Ogawa Y, Kaneko S, Otani K, Fukushima Y. Serum folic acid levels in epileptic mothers and their relationship to congenital malformations. *Epilepsy Res* 1991;**8**:75–78.

67. [No authors listed.] Appendix C: AAN summary of evidence-based guideline for clinicians: management issues for women with epilepsy-focus on pregnancy: vitamin k, folic acid, blood levels, and breastfeeding. *Continuum (Minneap Minn)* 2016;**22**:285–86.

68. Alonso A, Hernán MA. Temporal trends in the incidence of multiple sclerosis: a systematic review. *Neurology* 2008;**71**:129–35.

69. Ramagopalan SV, Sadovnick AD. Epidemiology of multiple sclerosis. *Neurol Clin* 2011;**29**:207–17.

70. Finkelsztejn A, Brooks JB, Paschoal FM, Fragoso YD. What can we really tell women with multiple sclerosis regarding pregnancy? A systematic review and meta-analysis of the literature. *BJOG* 2011;**118**:790–97.

71. Confavreux C, Hutchinson M, Hours MM, Cortinovis-Tourniaire P, Moreau T. Rate of pregnancy-related relapse in multiple sclerosis. Pregnancy in Multiple Sclerosis Group. *N Engl J Med* 1998;**339**:285–91.

72. Vukusic S, Hutchinson M, Hours M, et al. Pregnancy and multiple sclerosis (the PRIMS study): clinical predictors of postpartum relapse. *Brain* 2004;**127**:1353–60.

73. Coyle PK. Multiple sclerosis and pregnancy prescriptions. *Expert Opin Drug Saf* 2014;**13**:1565–68.

74. Lockwood CJ, Rand JH. The immunobiology and obstetrical consequences of antiphospholipid antibodies. *Obstet Gynecol Surv* 1994;**49**:432–41.

75. Lockwood CJ. Inherited thrombophilias in pregnant patients: detection and treatment paradigm. *Obstet Gynecol* 2002;**99**:333–41.

76. James AH, Jamison MG, Brancazio LR, Myers ER. Venous thromboembolism during pregnancy and the postpartum period: incidence, risk factors, and mortality. *Am J Obstet Gynecol* 2006;**194**:1311–15.

77. Robertson L, Wu O, Langhorne P, et al. Thrombophilia in pregnancy: a systematic review. *Br J Haematol* 2006;**132**:171–96.

78. Mocroft A, Ledergerber B, Katlama C, et al. Decline in the AIDS and death rates in the EuroSIDA study: an observational study. *Lancet* 2003;**362**:22–29.

79. Burns DN, Landesman S, Muenz LR, et al. Cigarette smoking, premature rupture of membranes, and vertical transmission of HIV-1 among women with low CD4+ levels. *J Acquir Immune Defic Syndr* 1994;**7**:718–26.

80. Turner BJ, Hauck WW, Fanning TR, Markson LE. Cigarette smoking and maternal-child HIV transmission. *J Acquir Immune Defic Syndr Hum Retrovirol* 1997;**14**:327–37.

81. Kalish LA, Boyer K, Brown G, et al. Cigarette smoking and maternal-child HIV transmission. Women and Infants Transmission Study Group. *J Acquir Immune Defic Syndr Hum Retrovirol* 1998;**18**:86–89.

82. Townsend CL, Cortina-Borja M, Peckham CS, de Ruiter A, Lyall H, Tookey PA. Low rates of mother-to-child transmission of HIV following effective pregnancy interventions in the United Kingdom and Ireland, 2000-2006. *AIDS* 2008;**22**:973–81.

83. Study EC. Mother-to-child transmission of HIV infection in the era of highly active antiretroviral therapy. *Clin Infect Dis* 2005;**40**:458–65.

84. Anglemyer A, Rutherford GW, Egger M, Siegfried N. Antiretroviral therapy for prevention of HIV transmission in HIV-discordant couples. *Cochrane Database Syst Rev* 2011;**8**:CD009153.

85. Fiore JR, Suligoi B, Saracino A, et al. Correlates of HIV-1 shedding in cervicovaginal secretions and effects of antiretroviral therapies. *AIDS* 2003;**17**:2169–76.

86. Semprini AE, Levi-Setti P, Bozzo M, et al. Insemination of HIV-negative women with processed semen of HIV-positive partners. *Lancet* 1992;**340**:1317–19.

87. Manktelow BN, Smith LK, Evans TAA, et al. *Perinatal Mortality Surveillance Report: UK Perinatal Deaths for Births from January to December 2013*. Leicester: The Infant Mortality and Morbidity Group, Department of Health Sciences, University of Leicester; 2015.

88. Royal College of Obstetricians and Gynaecologists (RCOG). *Registration of Stillbirths and Certification for Pregnancy Loss Before 24 Weeks of Gestation*. Good Practice Guideline No. 4. London: RCOG; 2005. Available at: https://www.rcog.org.uk/en/guidelines-research-services/guidelines/good-practice-4/.

89. Royal College of Obstetricians and Gynaecologists (RCOG). *Late Intrauterine Fetal Death and Stillbirth*. Green-top Guideline No. 55. London: RCOG; 2010. Available at: https://www.rcog.org.uk/en/guidelines-research-services/guidelines/gtg55/.

90. Black M, Shetty A, Bhattacharya S. Obstetric outcomes subsequent to intrauterine death in the first pregnancy. *BJOG* 2008;**115**:269–74.

91. Robson S, Chan A, Keane RJ, Luke CG. Subsequent birth outcomes after an unexplained stillbirth: preliminary population-based retrospective cohort study. *Aust N Z J Obstet Gynaecol* 2001;**41**:29–35.

92. Sharma PP, Salihu HM, Kirby RS. Stillbirth recurrence in a population of relatively low-risk mothers. *Paediatr Perinat Epidemiol* 2007;**21** Suppl 1:24–30.

93. Silver RM. Fetal death. *Obstet Gynecol* 2007;**109**:153–67.

94. Kortweg FJ, Erwich JJ, Holm JP, et al. Diverse placental pathologies as the main causes of fetal death. *Obstet Gynecol* 2009;**114**:809–17.

95. Group SCRNW. Causes of death among stillbirths. *JAMA* 2011;**306**:2459–68.

96. Yudkin PL, Wood L, Redman CW. Risk of unexplained stillbirth at different gestational ages. *Lancet* 1987;**1**:1192–94.

97. Caughey AB, Musci TJ. Complications of term pregnancies beyond 37 weeks of gestation. *Obstet Gynecol* 2004;**103**:57–62.

98. Won RH, Currier RJ, Lorey F, Towner DR. The timing of demise in fetuses with trisomy 21 and trisomy 18. *Prenat Diagn* 2005;**25**:608–11.

99. Bhutta ZA, Yakoob MY, Lawn JE, et al. Stillbirths: what difference can we make and at what cost? *Lancet* 2011;**377**:1523–38.

100. Goldenberg RL, McClure EM, Saleem S, Reddy UM. Infection-related stillbirths. *Lancet* 2010;**375**:1482–90.

101. Office for National Statistics. Childhood, infant and perinatal mortality in England and Wales, 2013. 2015. Available at: https://www.ons.gov.uk/peoplepopulationandcommunity/birthsdeathsandmarriages/deaths/bulletins/childhoodinfantandperinatalmortalityinenglandandwales/2015-03-10.

102. US Department of Health Education, and Welfare. *The United States and Six West European Countries*. Washington DC: National Centre for Health Statistics; 1967.

103. Sharpe C, Kuschel C. Outcomes of infants born to mothers receiving methadone for pain management in pregnancy. *Arch Dis Child Fetal Neonatal Ed* 2004;**89**:F33–6.

104. Larson JD, Patatanian E, Miner PB, Rayburn WF, Robinson MG. Double-blind, placebo-controlled study of ranitidine for gastroesophageal reflux symptoms during pregnancy. *Obstet Gynecol* 1997;**90**:83–87.

105. Gill SK, O'Brien L, Einarson TR, Koren G. The safety of proton pump inhibitors (PPIs) in pregnancy: a meta-analysis. *Am J Gastroenterol* 2009;**104**:1541–45.

106. Charache S, Condit PT, Humphreys SR. Studies on the folic acid vitamins. IV. The persistence of amethopterin in mammalian tissues. *Cancer* 1960;**13**:236–40.

107. Food and Drug Administration. Federal Register. Available at: https://www.federalregister.gov/index/2018/food-and-drug-administration.

108. Department of Health and Human Services, Food and Drug Administration. Content and format of labeling for human prescription drug and biological products; requirements for pregnancy and lactation labeling. 2014. Available at: https://www.fda.gov/downloads/aboutfda/reportsmanualsforms/reports/economicanalyses/ucm427798.pdf.

109. McCandlish R, Bowler U, van Asten H, et al. A randomised controlled trial of care of the perineum during second stage of normal labour. *Br J Obstet Gynaecol* 1998;**105**:1262–72.

110. Fernando RJ, Williams AA, Adams EJ. *The Management of Third and Fourth Degree Perineal Tears*. Green-top Guideline No. 29. London: RCOG; 2007.

111. Haadem K, Dahlstrom JA, Ling L, Ohrlander S. Anal sphincter function after delivery rupture. *Obstet Gynecol* 1987;**70**:53–56.

112. Haadem K, Ohrlander S, Lingman G. Long-term ailments due to anal sphincter rupture caused by delivery – a hidden problem. *Eur J Obstet Gynecol Reprod Biol* 1988;**27**:27–32.

113. Fenner DE, Genberg B, Brahma P, Marek L, DeLancey JO. Fecal and urinary incontinence after vaginal delivery with anal sphincter disruption in an obstetrics unit in the United States. *Am J Obstet Gynecol* 2003;**189**:1543–49.

114. Fitzpatrick M, McQuillan K, O'Herlihy C. Influence of persistent occiput posterior position on delivery outcome. *Obstet Gynecol* 2001;**98**:1027–31.

115. Ali A, Glennon K, Kirkham C, Yousif S, Eogan M. Delivery outcomes and events in subsequent pregnancies after previous anal sphincter injury. *Eur J Obstet Gynecol Reprod Biol* 2014;**174**:51–53.

116. Yogev Y, Hiersch L, Maresky L, Wasserberg N, Wiznitzer A, Melamed N. Third and fourth degree perineal tears – the risk of recurrence in subsequent pregnancy. *J Matern Fetal Neonatal Med* 2014;**27**:177–81.

117. Al-Mufti R, McCarthy A, Fisk NM. Obstetricians' personal choice and mode of delivery. *Lancet* 1996;**347**:544.

118. Al-Mufti R, McCarthy A, Fisk NM. Survey of obstetricians' personal preference and discretionary practice. *Eur J Obstet Gynecol Reprod Biol* 1997;**73**:1–4.

7

Obesity in obstetric and gynaecological practice

Sukhwinder Sahota and Tahir Mahmood

Introduction

Obesity is a complex multifactorial disorder, which has reached epidemic proportions worldwide. It affects all aspects of an individual's life: physical, social, emotional, and psychological. Although it is largely preventable, obesity is now a major public health issue, being associated with chronic illnesses such as type 2 diabetes, cardiovascular disease, depression, disability, and some cancers (1). Overweight and obese individuals now make up approximately one-third of the world's population (2). Obesity has been coined the 're-productive hurdle' as pregnancy in an obese woman is associated with multiple adverse outcomes such as congenital abnormalities, gestational diabetes, stillbirth, and higher caesarean section rates (3, 4). It also has far-reaching sequelae for the offspring as a consequence of being exposed to the *in utero* environment of an obese mother (5). Pregnant obese women have a higher incremental cost of antenatal and intrapartum care (6). It has been estimated that the toll of obesity on healthcare systems alone is between 2% and 7% of all healthcare spending in developed countries (7).

The classification of obesity is based on the body mass index (BMI) and is expressed as weight in kilograms over the height (in metres) squared (**Table 7.1**). The definitions, however, remain controversial. The current 'normal' BMI was a compromise reached by the World Health Organization (WHO) when it was recognized that in the United States, higher BMIs are considered 'normal' (8).

There are strong advocates of tightening the WHO classifications further according to the population assessed. A WHO Expert Consultation in 2004 assessed scientific data suggesting that Asian populations have different associations between health risk, BMI, and body fat percentage (9). This report concluded that Asians have a higher risk of comorbidities at lower BMI compared to Caucasians. They found that obesity-related disease, particularly type 2 diabetes and cardiovascular disease, occurred at a higher rate even at the normal BMI ($25\,\mathrm{kg/m^2}$) cut-off by the WHO standards. As a consequence, the report concluded that in these populations the normal BMI should be limited to 18.5–$22.9\,\mathrm{kg/m^2}$. In Japan, obesity is now defined as a BMI value greater than 25 and in China the bar is set at a BMI value of 28 (10, 11). For simplicity, the current BMI is calculated the same for men and women over the age of 18 years. In the under 18 years age group, sex- and BMI-specific measures are used. However, again the cut-offs are arbitrary.

Epidemiology

Although initially identified as an epidemic in the United States and Europe, obesity is not just an epidemic of the Western world. It is no longer associated only with affluence but occurs in lower socioeconomic groups and the developing world (12–14). In 2010, worldwide 11.5% of adults were obese compared with 13% in 2014 (15). An incremental rise in obesity since 1980 in all age groups irrespective of gross domestic product, especially among adolescents in both sex groups, has been reported by Ng et al. (16).

As defined earlier, obesity is more prevalent in women (14%) than in men (10%) although there is no difference at the overweight stage (17). In comparison to men, women also disproportionately represent the extreme obesity groups (BMI $\geq 35\,\mathrm{kg/m^2}$) regardless of age or ethnicity. Rural women in Europe are more likely to be obese whereas in Africa, women living in urban areas are more obese. The prevalence of obesity can be significantly different even within different parts of the same country (12).

There is concern that although the prevalence of adult obesity in developed countries is stabilizing to one in three, the prevalence among children and adolescents is rising (14). Obese children are at risk of chronic illness and mortality as obese adults, but worryingly, these also occur with premature onset or earlier in adulthood.

Factors contributing to female obesity

The aetiology of obesity is multifactorial. The prevailing cause is an excess of calories consumed with reduced calorie expenditure (mainly physical activity) resulting in a positive energy balance and thus excess body weight (14). It is therefore a largely preventable state. The factors contributing to this state of excess body weight are well known but their interaction is more complex in the development of obesity. There is evidence of genetic, biological, behavioural, psychological, and environmental factors contributing to obesity, which are confounded by economic, social, and cultural factors. Adding to the equation is evidence on the contribution of the *in utero* environment to the development of obesity in the future life of the unborn fetus (18).

There are clear gender differences with women having more class II and III obesity than men (19). This is more significant in

Table 7.1 The classification of obesity

Class	Category	BMI (kg/m²)
	Underweight	<18.5
	Normal	18.5–24.9
	Overweight	25–29.9
I	Obese	30–34.9
II	Very obese	35–39.9
III	Morbid obesity	≥40

Source data from World Health Organization (2000) *Obesity: Preventing and Managing the Global Epidemic.* WHO Obesity Technical Report Series 894: World Health Organization Geneva, Switzerland.

developing countries where women are three times more likely to be obese in comparison to men. Many of these women are from the higher socioeconomic classes in lower-middle-income countries but with economic progress, women of lower socioeconomic class are disproportionately affected. Unlike in higher-income countries, education in women is proportionately related to the prevalence of obesity in the lower-middle-income countries (20).

Geographical factors such as shortened distance to walk during activities of daily living in high-income countries and consequently reduced energy expenditure perpetuate the problem (18). This scenario is not confined to the Western world, individuals living in urban areas in Africa are significantly more likely to be overweight or obese compared to those living in rural areas (20). Urban areas are susceptible to the availability of food 24 hours a day and a cultural shift to a more sedentary lifestyle with computers and television, which also perpetuate the problem. Global markets saturated with high-calorie-density foods have led to a change in food consumption together with the fast-food marketplace allowing 24-hour access to food.

Interestingly in comparing body weight in women with men, the former sex is influenced more by nationality, race-ethnicity, and socioeconomic status in comparison to men. This suggests that a closer link exists between body weight and social and cultural roles in women in comparison to men (19).

Ethnicity

Ethnicity also tends to influence obesity. In the United States, non-Hispanic black women were more obese (53%) than Mexican American women (48%) but significantly more obese than non-Hispanic white women (36%). This ethnic influence was not seen in males of the same age group (40–59 years) (19). Where mean age- and BMI-matched women have been used to identify cardiovascular risk factors, it was noted that African women had higher systolic blood pressures and peripheral vascular resistance in comparison to Caucasians (20). In 2004 in the United Kingdom, it was noted that significantly more men and women from a Caribbean or Irish ethnicity were obese when compared to the general population (21). Women of Chinese and Bangladeshi descent had the lowest prevalence of obesity but black African women had some of the highest.

Genetics

There is evidence that obesity is more common in genetically susceptible individuals. However, monogenic and syndromic-related obesity conditions are relatively rare. Syndromes such as trisomy 21, Prader–Willi, and Beckwith–Wiedemann are relatively uncommon as a cause of obesity. Research into the aetiology of common obesity is fierce, however; genetic susceptibility is complicated by the ability of environmental change to alter gene expression by mechanisms such as methylation (22).

In the majority of individuals, the balance of calorific intake and energy expenditure (physical activity, basal metabolic rate, and thermogenesis) maintains a homeostatic BMI. The hypothalamus regulates energy homeostasis through integrating neural, hormonal, and metabolic signals from peripheral and central nervous systems, endocrine glands, including adipocytes, and blood metabolites such as glucose and fatty acids (23). Congenital or acquired causes of dysregulation in any of these pathways have the potential to cause the accumulation of excess energy as lipids. Linkage analysis has revealed single gene disorders as a cause for obesity with mutations in genes such as the leptin-encoding gene, the leptin receptor gene, and pro-opiomelanocortin. These mutations are rare causes of obesity (24).

In the more common form of obesity that we are seeing as an epidemic, research indicates that although there are around 60 genetic factors implicated, only approximately 32 are associated with less than 1.5% of BMI variation between individuals (22). This would mean an average difference of 7 kg between two individuals of similar height/ethnicity/age (14). Therefore for such a common condition, genetics cannot be the prevailing cause for the increasing waistline.

Effect of obesity in childhood and adolescence

There is increasing evidence to associate maternal prepregnancy obesity with an increased risk of obesity and cardiometabolic risk factors in the offspring (25). Prepregnancy maternal obesity is associated with a higher likelihood of obesity in children at the age of 3 years (26). It also confers a higher BMI and increased risk of diabetes in offspring during adolescence and adulthood (26, 27). This association is independent of genetic and environmental factors shared by mother and child (28). Maternal obesity is also associated with a risk of developmental delay and autism spectrum disorder in early childhood (29).

There is also emerging evidence that excessive pregnancy weight gain as defined by the American Institute of Medicine is associated in offspring with obesity and an adverse cardiometabolic profile (25, 30, 31). The latter measures included raised C-reactive protein, systolic blood pressure, and lower high-density lipoprotein level. The critical period is suggested to be excessive weight gain in early pregnancy. These adverse metabolic profiles together with an increased risk of obstructive sleep apnoea in obese adolescents are associated with an increased cardiovascular risk in adults (32).

The onset of puberty has lowered over the past 150 years from approximately 14 years of age to 11.5–12 years old in girls in the United Kingdom (33, 34). The factors influencing menarche are well characterized including genetic, hormonal, psychological, and socioeconomic factors. However, this drop in age in girls has also coincided with the rise in obesity seen in the Western world. Since body fat is closely related to pulsatile release of gonadotrophin-releasing hormone and therefore the onset of puberty, a link cannot be excluded.

In young boys, puberty may be delayed with obesity and although the reason is not currently clear as to why, it may be related to feedback inhibition of androgens by a rise in aromatized oestrogen levels by adipocytes (32).

Obesity is also associated with an increased risk of developing asthma. Other problems may be exacerbated in adolescence for obese children such as psychological depression, anxiety, body image disorder, and negative self-esteem, particularly in girls. Increasing BMI is also associated with ovulatory dysfunction, menstrual irregularity, and, later in life, increased time to conception (35).

Obesity is a common feature of polycystic ovarian syndrome (PCOS), but only 20% of obese women have PCOS. This disorder affects 5–10% of women and is commonly diagnosed with two of the following three parameters: hyperandrogenism, chronic anovulation, and polycystic ovaries on ultrasonography. The disorder is closely linked to insulin resistance, type 2 diabetes, infertility, endometrial cancer, and possibly an increased risk of cardiovascular disease. A comparison between normal healthy and PCOS adolescents showed an increased risk of hirsutism, total testosterone, and hyperinsulinaemia in the latter but not dyslipidaemia when adjusted for BMI or waist/waist to hip ratio (36).

Obesity and contraception

As previously stipulated, obesity presents a real challenge in pregnancy and therefore prepregnancy planning is imperative to optimize care antenatally. An important part of this planning is the use of contraceptives for reproductive control and also associated menstrual dysfunction. The safety and efficacy of contraceptives in overweight and obese patients is difficult to ascertain due to exclusion of such patient groups from many trials (37–39).

Metabolic changes in obesity are known and therefore they may affect pharmacokinetics of contraceptives, particularly steroid-based contraceptives. Oral contraceptives are associated with changes in lipid, fibrinogen, and glucose metabolism. Some effects are enhanced further in smokers (40). The effect of hormonal contraceptives in obese patients is largely unknown due to the exclusion of this population in studies, which is of concern since obesity itself causes metabolic changes to increase cardiovascular risks. A recent study has shown that very obese women (BMI >35 kg/m²) using the combined oral contraceptive pill are at an increased risk of venous thromboembolic disease in comparison to non-obese women (41). Obesity is a known independent risk factor for thromboembolic disease and this needs to be considered when prescribing hormonal contraceptives.

Another challenge is the actual ability to perform the necessary examination for the introduction of the contraceptive. For example, inserting of intrauterine devices or laparoscopic sterilization may be technically difficult particularly in the morbidly obese (42). In the United States, procedure-based methods (tubal ligation, implants, and intrauterine devices) have been shown to be favoured by women with increasing BMI with 50.5% of obese women but only 36.2% of normal weight women using these methods (35).

Weight gain is one of the commonest reasons for discontinuation of hormonal contraceptives. However, studies in women using the combined oral contraceptive pill have shown little evidence that this is true (38). Evidence of weight gain identified in patients using

depot medroxyprogesterone acetate (DMPA) is small (<2 kg) but, over time, is more likely to be associated with a natural tendency of weight gain with age.

The use of contraceptives in normal weight and overweight/obese women has been shown to be similar (35). Consequently, further research is necessary into the efficacy and safety of contraceptives in obese patients. Importantly, data on the sexual behaviour of obese adolescents is of concern: in comparison to white non-obese and black obese adolescent females, obese white adolescent girls are more likely to have had coitus before the age of 13, are at increased odds of having a partner 3 years older, and more than three sexual partners per year, and less likely to use condoms during their most recent sexual experience (43). Furthermore, changes in metabolism after bariatric surgery mean that research after such procedures is also necessary as pharmacokinetics of hormonal contraceptives are altered after such procedures (44).

The use of hormonal contraceptives is not limited to the reproductive cycle. The significant risk of endometrial hyperplasia and endometrial cancer in obese women suggests increasing use of the levonorgestrel intrauterine device for effective protection against these disorders in this cohort of women (35).

Obesity and pregnancy

Obesity in pregnancy is associated with poor pregnancy outcomes including miscarriage, gestational diabetes, pre-eclampsia, thromboembolism, prolonged labour, and postpartum haemorrhage (45). Fetal complications such as congenital anomalies, shoulder dystocia, stillbirth, and neonatal death are also increased in maternal obesity (46). The problems are not confined to the pathophysiological pathways but also technical difficulties. There is a higher risk of instrumental delivery and caesarean section in obese pregnant women (47, 48).

One-fifth of women from Scotland and one-third of American women entering pregnancy are obese (49, 50). The consequences of obesity in pregnancy extend beyond the immediate gestation as previously discussed. The maternal intrauterine environment impacts the fetal development and the lifetime health of the offspring. Therefore, effective screening policies in early pregnancy should be in place not only to identify high-risk pregnancies but also to put focused care in place (51).

Obesity and miscarriage

Overweight (BMI >25 kg/m²) and obese women are at significantly increased risk of miscarriage regardless of the mode of conception (48, 52, 53). Furthermore, they have a threefold increased risk of recurrent miscarriage (54, 55). These studies have shown obesity to be an independent risk factor for miscarriage and the single most modifiable risk factor in high-income countries (56). Lashen et al. (54) have reported an odds ratio (OR) of 1.2 (95% confidence interval (CI) 1.01–1.46) for miscarriage and an OR of 3.5 (CI 1.03–12.01) for recurrent miscarriage in obese women with a BMI greater than 30. The higher incidence of spontaneous pregnancy loss is directly linked to a rise in insulin levels. It has been proposed that treatment with insulin-sensitizing agents such as metformin may reduce miscarriage rates. A meta-analysis identified an increased risk of miscarriage after ovulation induction and even oocyte donation suggesting a generally adverse milieu for the fertilized egg in the obese woman (53).

Fetal abnormality risk

Once conception has occurred, there is a two- to threefold increased risk of birth defects associated with maternal preconception obesity including neural tube defects, cardiac anomalies (septal, tetralogy of Fallot, transposition of the great arteries), and diaphragmatic hernia (57). This increased risk is directly proportional to increasing maternal weight. The risk of gastroschisis is, however, reduced in obese mothers. A worrying consequence of obesity is the reduced sensitivity of ultrasonography as a screening test for fetal anomalies. It has been estimated that approximately 15% of normally visible structures will be suboptimally seen in women with a BMI above the 90th centile. The anatomical structures commonly less well seen with increasing BMI include the fetal heart, spine, kidneys, diaphragm, and umbilical cord (58). It has been recommended that obese mothers have increased folic acid (5 mg) periconceptually and antenatally, again highlighting the necessity of preconception care for such women (59).

Metabolic syndrome of pregnancy

Obesity is associated with a broad range of complications including diabetes, cardiovascular disease, dyslipidaemia, and hypertension, labelled as metabolic syndrome of pregnancy. Maternal obesity is related to metabolic complications, including the pregnancy-specific conditions of pre-eclampsia and gestational diabetes. Pregnancy-related endocrine changes favour lipogenesis and fat accumulation (60). All women increase maternal fat stores irrespective of prepregnancy adiposity to meet the fetoplacental and maternal demands of late gestation and lactation; the main increase is towards the end of the second trimester. In normal-weight women, the majority of fat is accumulated centrally in the subcutaneous compartment of the trunk and upper thighs. In later stages of pregnancy, there is an increase in both the thickness of pre-peritoneal fat (visceral) and the ratio of pre-peritoneal to subcutaneous fat as measured by ultrasonography. This pattern of fat deposition is relevant to increasing insulin resistance as accumulation of hepatic fat has been shown to be an important mediator of insulin resistance during pregnancy in the rat model (61). Visceral adiposity is more closely related to adverse metabolic outcomes, including insulin resistance, hyperinsulinaemia, dyslipidaemia, hypertension, and the metabolic syndrome. As obese women have more saturated subcutaneous fat stores, they tend to accumulate more centrally than lean women, an observation which may reflect their higher insulin resistance (60). Central obesity appears to be correlated more strongly with adverse metabolic outcomes in pregnancy including gestational diabetes mellitus (GDM), gestational hypertension, and pre-eclampsia (62).

Impaired glucose tolerance and gestational diabetes mellitus screening

The International Diabetes Federation estimates that one in six live births is to women with some form of hyperglycaemia in pregnancy. While 16% of these cases may be due to diabetes in pregnancy (either pre-existing diabetes (type 1 or type 2) which antedates pregnancy or is first identified in the index pregnancy), the majority (84%) is due to GDM (6). GDM is defined by the WHO as carbohydrate intolerance resulting in hyperglycaemia first recognized in pregnancy (63).

A meta-analysis of 20 studies showed that the unadjusted ORs for the development of GDM were 2.14 (95% CI 1.82–2.53), 3.56 (3.05–4.21), and 8.56 (5.07–16.04) in overweight, obese, and severely obese women respectively compared with normal-weight pregnant women (47).

However, in women who do not reach diabetes diagnostic criteria, there is mounting evidence that increasing BMI causes higher glucose levels, which in pregnancy are associated with adverse outcomes (49).

In 1954, Pedersen hypothesized that in diabetic mothers, high glucose levels were transferable to the fetus. In order to prevent hyperglycaemia, the fetus produces increased levels of insulin, which results in increased fetal growth (64). Later studies have shown that glucose levels need not reach diagnostic levels for diabetes in order to have similar outcomes. A study of over 1100 non-diabetic pregnant women given an oral glucose tolerance test showed that with resultant increasing glucose levels there was an increasing risk of large-for-gestational-age fetuses, preterm birth with a twofold increase in caesarean section, and clinical chorioamnionitis (64). In the latter case, with high glucose levels, chorioamnionitis was associated with a 12-fold increased risk of very preterm delivery. Later studies have corroborated the link between increasing prepregnancy BMI and neonatal adiposity (66). Fetal macrosomia is associated with an increased risk of caesarean section, birth trauma (vaginal tears, shoulder dystocia, and asphyxia), as well as transient hypoglycaemia (67).

Women who have developed gestational diabetes are at an added risk of then developing type 2 diabetes in later life. This is compounded by associated factors: high BMI, ethnicity, and a family history of type 2 diabetes as well as gestational glycaemic status (68). The gestational age of onset of GDM is linked to an increased risk of hypertensive disorders in pregnancy and preterm delivery, each of which are also associated with a raised BMI.

There remains controversy about the best way of screening women for GDM during pregnancy: should it be risk based? Or one-step screening or two-step screening (69)? In 2015, the European Board and College of Obstetrics and Gynaecology published its position statement on GDM screening in Europe (70). Later in the year, the International Federation of Gynecology and Obstetrics (FIGO) responded to this global challenge and published a report, entitled 'FIGO Initiative on Gestational Diabetes Mellitus: A pragmatic guide for diagnosis, management and care' (5). This report has advocated one-step GDM screening for all women during pregnancy and has made recommendations for the GDM screening adaptations in different resource settings.

Hypertensive disorders during pregnancy

There is a large body of evidence highlighting the increased risk of hypertension and pre-eclampsia/eclampsia when obese (71–73). Both prepregnancy BMI and adulthood weight gain is associated with an increasing risk of pre-eclampsia. An American prospective study of 1644 pregnant women identified an increased risk of pre-eclampsia with weight gain in adulthood from the age of 18 years (71). This translated as a 4% increased risk of pre-eclampsia for every 1 kg of adult weight gain after adjusting for maternal age, ethnicity/race, parity, educational attainment, and weight at age 18 (71).

A large United Kingdom study analysing over a quarter of a million singleton pregnancies (74) showed that the risk of adverse

Table 7.2 Adverse outcomes in pregnant women who are overweight or obese

Condition	Overweight mothers, odds ratio (confidence interval)	Obese mothers, odds ratio (confidence interval)
Gestational diabetes	1.68 (1.53–1.84)	3.6 (3.25–3.98)
Pre-eclampsia	1.44 (1.28–1.62)	2.14 (1.85–2.47)
Induction of labour	2.14 (1.85–2.47)	1.70 (1.64–1.76)
Emergency caesarean section delivery	1.30 (1.25–1.34)	1.83 (1.74–1.93)
Postpartum haemorrhage	1.16 (1.12–1.21)	1.39 (1.32–1.46)
Genital tract infection	1.24 (1.09–1.41)	1.30 (1.07–1.56)
Urinary tract infection	1.17 (1.04–1.33)	1.39 (1.18–1.63)
Wound infection	1.27 (1.09–1.48)	2.24 (1.91–2.64)
Birthweight >90th centile	1.57 (1.50–1.64)	2.36 (2.23–2.50)
Intrauterine death	1.10 (0.94–1.28)	1.40 (1.14–1.71)

Source data from Sebire NJ, Jolly M, Harris JP, Wadsworth J, Joffe M, Beard RW, Regan L, Robinson S. Maternal obesity and pregnancy outcome: a study of 287 213 pregnancies in London. *International Journal of Obesity & Related Metabolic Disorders* 2001;25(8):1175.

outcomes during pregnancy was not confined to the obese but also to the overweight group (BMI 25–30) (Table 7.2). Overweight pregnant women have an increased risk of conditions such as GDM and pre-eclampsia. During the intrapartum and postpartum periods, they are also at increased risk of delivery by emergency caesarean section, postpartum haemorrhage, and infection.

Obesity and risk of preterm rupture of membranes

There is mounting evidence that maternal obesity is associated with preterm rupture of membranes (PPROM) and induced preterm delivery (75, 76). In a systematic meta-analysis of over 1 million singleton births, there was evidence of an increased risk of spontaneous preterm birth in both overweight and obese women. An earlier study of over 250,000 singleton births in the United Kingdom did not find an increased risk of preterm delivery (<32 weeks) in overweight or obese women (74).

A large study analysing the risk of poor pregnancy outcomes with increasing BMI in non-donor oocyte *in vitro* fertilization cycles identified a significant increased relative risk of premature birth with obesity (78). Women with a BMI higher than 35 kg/m² fared worse with a relative risk of 2.6 of babies born before 28 weeks. This was for both singleton and twin pregnancies. A confounding factor in this work was that assisted reproductive technology pregnancies are associated with premature birth.

Thromboembolic disease

A large Danish study analysing the risk of venous thromboembolism with maternal smoking and obesity in pregnancy and the puerperium found a greater risk with obesity than with smoking (adjusted OR 5.3 (95% CI 2.1–13.5) compared with adjusted OR 2.7 (95% CI 1.5–4.9)). Interestingly, it was seen that obesity was associated with a higher risk of pulmonary embolism (adjusted OR 14.9; 95% CI 3.0–74.8) than of deep venous thrombosis (adjusted OR 4.4; 95% CI 1.6–11.9) (79). The Royal College of Obstetricians and Gynaecologists recommends a thromboprophylaxis policy for

overweight and obese women during pregnancy and postpartum whether delivered vaginally or by caesarean section (80).

Operative delivery risks

There are inherent risks associated with elective or emergency caesarean section in obese women, particularly the morbidly obese, such as surgical access into the abdomen, failed spinal analgesia, failed intubation, and maternal death (81). Maternal infection and sepsis is also increased in obese pregnant women. All of these problems are accentuated in extremely obese women (BMI ≥50 kg/m²) which in the United Kingdom in 2010 constituted 1 in 1000 maternities (82). The availability of basic equipment for such women's preliminary observations confounds morbidity and, advanced equipment requirements (e.g. bariatric chairs and beds) in such women adds to the demand on maternity health services. This incremental economic burden on health services needs special consideration when maternity services reorganization is being considered (83).

Stillbirth risk

Stillbirth or death of a fetus *in utero* after 24 weeks of gestation (or a birth weight >500 g) affects 1 in 200 births in the Western world (56). Yao et al. performed a retrospective cohort study of over 2 million singleton live births and stillbirths in the United States. This study identified the risk of stillbirth to be linearly related to increasing BMI and that 25% of term stillbirths were associated with obesity. Women with extreme obesity (BMI ≥50 kg/m²) were at 5.7 times greater risk of stillbirth than normal-weight women at 39 weeks' gestation and 13.6 times greater at 41 weeks' gestation of stillbirth. However, across all the obesity classes there was an increased risk of stillbirth after 39 weeks (84). The incidence of post-term pregnancy is increased in obese mothers and with the significant risk of stillbirth, induction of labour at term in this group has increased with a consequent rise in emergency caesarean section rates (85, 86).

Unfortunately, obese women are known to have slower labour progression and an increased requirement for labour augmentation (87). This group is also likely to have failed induction of labour, particularly in the morbidly obese where failure rate figures up to 80% have been documented (88).

Maternal morbidity and mortality risk

Obesity is a risk throughout the course of a woman's pregnancy. It increases the risk of gestational diabetes, thromboembolism, and pre-eclampsia (49). During peripartum, the risk of induction of labour increases in obese mothers with its associated complications and during intrapartum, there is further difficulty with an increased risk of operative delivery and postpartum haemorrhage. The burden of maternal morbidity in obese women continues through the postpartum and puerperium by the subsequent risk of infection (urinary tract, wound infection) and thromboembolism.

The Confidential Enquiries into Maternal Deaths in the United Kingdom (82) reported that almost one-third of women who died in the triennium reviewed were obese, and a disproportionate number of obese pregnant women had a BMI greater than 35. The grim statistics were not confined to obese patients. Overweight and obese women were more likely to die of thromboembolism (78%) or cardiac events (61%). Although overall maternal mortality in the United Kingdom has fallen, the most recent report covering

2011–2013 follows the same trend in that maternal mortality in obese women was 30% and 22% in overweight women. Obesity is independently associated with having higher odds of dying due to specific pregnancy-related complications. Of concern is that an earlier report indicated that in some deaths procedure-related difficulties in obese patients may have contributed to their death such as inappropriately sized sphygmomanometer cuffs for the measurement of blood pressure or logistical issues (e.g. transport of the obese pregnant woman) (89, 90).

There should be clearly defined standards of care for the management of obese pregnant women throughout the course of their pregnancy, including advise as regards pre-conceptual weight loss, antenatal screening strategy, GDM screening, care during labour and postnatally. Each unit should be encouraged to collect data to quality assure their performance (69, 91, 92).

Obesity and gynaecological practice

Obesity impacts a wide variety of situations in gynaecological practice. As discussed previously, obese adolescent girls are at risk of premature menarche and physical maturity in comparison to lean counterparts. Obesity in adolescence, a time of vulnerability, contributes to poor body image and self-esteem as well as adverse psychosocial and sexual behaviour.

Menstrual disorders

Obesity in adolescents is also associated with menstrual irregularities. Although obese adult women often present with menstrual irregularities, there is limited data describing the association between obesity and heavy menstrual bleeding (93).

Although obese women often present with menstrual disorders, such as oligomenorrhoea or amenorrhoea, there are limited data on the link between obesity and heavy menstrual bleeding (94). The prevalence of menstrual cycle irregularities was 8.4% in women who were 74% overweight compared to 2.6% in women who were less than 20% overweight. It has also been reported that the relative risk of oligomenorhoea in women with upper body fat predominance was 3.15 compared with lower body fat predominance (93). The investigation and treatment protocols should be the same as for women with normal weight but particular focus is required to rule out endometrial hyperplasia in obese women. The risk of developing endometrial cancer in women with PCO is three times higher than in women with a normal BMI. The medical treatment of menstrual disorders for obese women is similar to normal-weight women, their therapeutic effectiveness and adverse outcomes require careful consideration in the former group. It is known that BMI does not affect the efficacy of the combined oral contraceptive pill and therefore, the use of the combined oral contraceptive pill remains a viable option in this group of women with BMI of up to 35 (93). Although not all hormonal treatments, including progestogen-loaded intrauterine devices, may be as effective in obese women as in normal-weight women, they may still be beneficial as surgical risk can be avoided and fertility maintained. High-quality randomized controlled trials are required to provide evidence on the therapeutic benefits of various medical and surgical treatment options in obese women.

Polycystic ovarian syndrome

PCOS is common in obese women but not all women with PCOS are obese. Obesity may enhance the biochemical and hormonal changes observed in women with PCOS and this in turn has adverse effects on reproductive outcomes in these women (95, 96). The severity of hyperandrogenism seems to be amplified in obese women with PCOS and ovarian hyperandrogenism may arrest the development of antral follicles. Adipocyte conversion of androgens to oestrogens with consequent reduction in sex hormone-binding globulin disrupts the delicate milieu required for folliculogenesis. Obese women with PCOS exhibit a higher degree of insulin resistance and hyperinsulinaemia. It has been shown that insulin infusion decreases basal and gonadotropin-releasing hormone-induced luteinizing hormone (LH) secretion. Several substances produced by the adipose tissue including leptin, adiponectin, resistin, and visfatin may play a role in the pathophysiology of PCOS. Leptin plays an important role, as an inverse relationship between leptin and LH levels and LH pulse amplitude has been reported. When there is a short-term caloric restriction, leptin levels decline and there is an increase in LH pulse amplitude. Obesity also changes inflammatory markers (C-reactive protein, interleukin-6, and tumour necrosis factor alpha), coagulation, and fibrinolysis mechanisms (97). These aberrant changes may therefore interfere with the reproductive cycle to cause deleterious outcomes. Diet and lifestyle changes are recommended for the obese women before they attempt conception. For induction of ovulation, clomiphene citrate remains the first line therapy. Other modalities used are human gonadotrophin, insulin sensitizers (metformin), aromatase inhibitors, laparoscopic ovarian drilling, and *in vitro* fertilization.

Infertility

Infertility and reduced fecundity is demonstrated in obese women. Obesity in women is associated with anovulatory subfertility, altered oocyte quality, and endometrial receptivity (97). All modes of conception (natural, ovulation induction, *in vitro* fertilization, intracytoplasmic sperm injection, and ovum donation) in obese women are associated with poorer reproductive outcomes. The probability of conceiving naturally within one menstrual cycle is reduced by 18% in obese women compared to women with a normal BMI after adjusting for age, smoking, and race (98). Furthermore, in subfertile ovulatory women, each single-digit increase in BMI over 29 kg/m² was associated with an approximately 5% reduction in pregnancy rate comparable to a 1-year increase in female age-associated reduction in pregnancy rate.

Methods of assisted reproductive technology fare no better. When compared between obese and normal-weight young (<35 years) women undergoing egg recovery as part of assisted reproductive technology, obese women required higher doses of gonadotrophin and also had suboptimal oocytes recovered (52). The embryos were also of a substandard grade with less likelihood of being cryopreserved. The mitigating effect of egg donation is not encouraging in recipient obese women. Bellver et al. (99) showed that egg donation from women with a normal BMI to obese recipients resulted in lower implantation rates, clinical pregnancy rates, and singleton/twin pregnancy rates. The live birth rates were also reduced with increasing BMI with lean women (BMI <20 kg/m²) having a live birth rate of 38.6% compared with 27.7% in obese women. This study provides evidence of suboptimal receptivity of endometrium as an underlying factor in obese women (99).

Fertility issues in obese women are an important aspect of infertility care with various medical and surgical interventions having variable results in improving fertility rates. Two recent meta-analyses on the impact of lifestyle interventions have not demonstrated any effect of lifestyle on infertility outcomes such as pregnancy, ovulation, or menstrual regularity except a reduction in the risk of both pre-eclampsia and shoulder dystocia (100). Medical treatment for weight management in obese women have had limited success due to expression of safety concerns. However, bariatric surgery techniques have been reported to promote weight loss by decreasing gastric volume, reducing nutrient absorption, and thereby inducing an iatrogenic malabsorptive state. The nutritional deficiencies associated with bariatric surgery are of the greatest concern. Although bariatric surgery leads to significant weight loss, its role in improving fertility in obese women remains unclear.

Pelvic floor disorders

Urinary and faecal incontinence, uterovaginal prolapse, and sexual dysfunction are more prevalent in patients with obesity (101). Increasingly, BMI seems to have a direct effect on the severity of pelvic floor dysfunction by a chronic increase in intra-abdominal pressure, damage to pelvic musculature, nerve damage, and associated conduction abnormalities. Obesity-related comorbidities such as diabetic neuropathy and intervertebral disc herniation may also be contributory factors. Significant weight loss by surgical or non-surgical means leads to improvement in symptoms of incontinence. Stress incontinence surgery in obese women is equally effective as in normal-weight women. Unfortunately weight loss has not been shown to reverse the severity of symptoms due to pelvic organ prolapse. Weight loss may, however, alleviate the postsurgical morbidity associated with obesity and prolapse surgery. Faecal incontinence improves after surgical-induced weight loss. Therefore, the first line of management for such women in primary care settings should focus on lifestyle changes, weight management, and physiotherapy (102).

Post-reproductive symptoms

Western women now spend more than a third of their lifetime beyond the menopausal transition. Research has explored the impact of obesity on the timing of menopause and the effect of obesity on menopausal symptoms and reproductive hormones (103). It has shown no significant impact of obesity on the timing of menopause and the levels of oestrogens and follicle-stimulating hormone as compared with non-obese women. These studies did not identify why obese women suffer from exaggerated vasomotor symptoms. Vulvovaginal atrophy with its symptoms of vaginal dryness, itching, dyspareunia, and irritation is strongly and consistently linked to oestrogen deficiency and is highly prevalent in menopausal and perimenopausal women. Weight gain reported around the transition of menopause is mainly due to lack of activity rather than hormonal changes.

Risk of developing cancers

It has been estimated that obesity is associated with approximately 20% of cancers (104) and a 15–30% decrease in weight is associated with a reduced risk of cancer (105). Obesity increases the risk of endometrial cancer, oestrogen receptor-positive postmenopausal breast cancer, and, to a lesser extent, ovarian cancer. It is postulated that oestrogens, sex hormones, hyperinsulinaemia, adipokines, and inflammatory cytokines among other factors may be involved in the promotion of cancer in obese women. Although a high risk of cancer recurrence among obese women has been reported, it is most likely due to suboptimal treatment and/or comorbidities. Equally, adjuvant chemotherapy and radiation dosimetry in breast and ovarian cancer patients may be less effective in obese women. A meta-analysis of observational studies published in 2015 has also reported a strong association between type 2 diabetes mellitus and the risk of breast, intrahepatic cholangiocarcinoma, colorectal, and endometrial cancers (106).

Another meta-analysis from 2014 has shown an increased risk of endometrial cancer in overweight and obese women (107). The evidence pointed towards a strong association between rising BMI and endometrial cancer. Women with PCOS are known to have an increased risk of endometrial hyperplasia and a threefold increased risk of developing endometrial cancer and this is confounded by obesity in PCOS women (108).

Role of bariatric surgery in obese women

Developments in minimal access surgical techniques are now allowing an increasing number of more complex gynaecological procedures to be undertaken for women with complex comorbidities and obesity laparoscopically. This is largely to minimize difficulties confronted with open surgery in obese women.

Anaesthetic issues

Cardiac and respiratory responses are often altered in patients with an increased BMI, and they are predisposed to decreased functional reserve capacity (42, 109). Cardiorespiratory functions are further compromised with Trendelenburg positioning and raised intra-abdominal pressure following the creation of a pneumoperitoneum. Obesity also affects gastric functioning with delayed emptying time. These women are also at an increased risk of infection secondary to impaired immune surveillance. Prolonged surgery (> 4 hours) increases the risk to obese patients. Technical issues should be considered in order to reduce visceral and vascular injuries. The cumulative experience globally with the minimal-access approach to treat benign pelvic pathology and selected cases of gynaecological cancers for obese women has not reported higher complication rates compared to their non-obese counterparts, despite having prolonged operating time. Potential advantages include shortened hospital stay with shorter recovery time and lower infection rates.

Weight management

The best way to reduce the risk of medical and obstetric complications in obese women is for weight loss to occur prior to conception. There is limited maintained weight loss with dieting, exercise, behavioural therapy, and medical therapy. The average weight loss at 1 year is approximately 5 kg (110). A Cochrane review concluded that surgery was a more effective intervention in comparison to non-surgical methods in terms of weight loss outcomes (111). Bariatric surgery is therefore considered to be an effective treatment for morbid obesity, with long-term excess weight loss greater than 60%. A meta-analysis identified a 20–30 kg maintained weight loss over 10 years following bariatric surgery (112).

There are three main surgical approaches: restrictive, malabsorptive, and combined procedures. Restrictive procedures include gastric bands and sleeves whereas malabsorptive methods include biliopancreatic diversion and duodenal switch. The most commonly used procedure is the Roux en Y gastric bypass which is a combined restrictive and malabsorptive method. It involves bypassing the duodenum by creating a small gastric pouch and gastroenterostomy stoma.

Bariatric surgery has been shown to improve hormonal levels in obese women wishing to conceive. There are conflicting data on miscarriage rates following surgery. There is no difference after biliopancreatic diversion but restrictive procedures are associated with high rates of miscarriage despite weight loss (113). However there are improved maternal and neonatal outcomes in obese women who have had bariatric surgery. There is a reduction in the incidence of pregnancy-induced hypertension and pre-eclampsia but not always gestational diabetes (44, 113). There is a significant reduction in the number of large-for-gestational-age infants. Women who have had malabsorptive and combined bariatric procedures are at an increased risk of fetal growth restriction and prematurity compared with women who have had restrictive procedures.

It is recommended that women who have had bariatric surgery should delay conception and the American College of Obstetricians and Gynaecologists suggests a delay of approximately 12–24 months. The impact of pregnancy on the prior weight loss surgery can be dramatic. Band migration can lead to vomiting, dehydration, and band leakage. There is also a risk of intestinal obstruction secondary to adhesions, intestinal hernia, gastric ulcer, and strictures in the staple line. These are associated with a requirement for surgical intervention.

Summary

Obesity is a worldwide epidemic with a complex multifactorial aetiology. The commonest cause is an excess of calories that are not balanced by increased energy expenditure. Although genetic and biological pathways may contribute to the development of obesity, behavioural, psychological, and environmental factors are now the prevailing risk factors. As discussed, female obesity is more prevalent than male obesity and this is significantly increased at the higher classes of obesity (II and III). This places an unprecedented burden on the speciality of obstetrics and gynaecology. The prevailing evidence indicates that female obesity is associated with increased risks in all aspects of a woman's life; during adolescence, reproductive years, and post-reproductive years. Obese pregnant women are at an increased risk of gestational diabetes, thromboembolism, pre-eclampsia, operative delivery, and postpartum haemorrhage. Her child's health will bear the burden of their exposure in the obese *in utero* environment with an increased risk of shoulder dystocia, obesity, diabetes, and developmental delay. There is therefore an urgent need for effective screening policies in early pregnancy and these should identify high-risk pregnancies in order to then have a focused care plan in place.

Women who are obese are at an increased risk of gynaecological morbidity such as menstrual dysfunction, infertility, miscarriage, and urogynaecological disorders. Of concern is the increased risk of gynaecological cancers such as endometrial cancer, postmenopausal breast cancer, and, to a lesser degree, ovarian cancer in obese women. Their body habitus influences the choice of management options thereafter. Morbidly obese women are at an increased risk of surgical and postsurgical complications and therefore medical options have to be heavily considered, for example, in the management of endometrial cancer. The developments in minimal access surgical techniques are now allowing an increasing number of more complex gynaecological procedures to be undertaken laparoscopically for women with complex comorbidities and obesity.

Obesity is a considerable burden on an individual and on healthcare systems. It has had a significant impact in the practice of obstetrics and gynaecology. Its far-reaching sequelae mean that urgent action is required to educate the public with regard to healthy eating and lifestyle habits. It requires governments to acknowledge the current evidence and adjust policymaking accordingly, including regulation of advertising by the food industry, particularly towards children.

REFERENCES

1. Mahmood TA. Preface. *Best Pract Res Clin Obstet Gynaecol* 2015;**29**:285–88.
2. Stevens GA, Singh GM, Lu Y, et al. National, regional and global trends in adult overweight and obese prevalences. *Popul Health Metr* 2012;**10**:22.
3. Thanoon O, Gharaibeh A, Mahmood T. The implications of obesity on pregnancy outcome. *Obstet Gynaecol Reprod Med* 2015;**25**:102–105.
4. Mahmood TA. Obesity and pregnancy: an obstetrician's view. *Br J Diabetes Vasc Dis* 2009;**9**:19–22.
5. Hod M, Kapur A, Scaks DA, et al. The International Federation of Gynaecology and Obstetrics (FIGO) initiative on gestational diabetes mellitus: a pragmatic guide for diagnosis, management, and care. *Int J Gynaecol Obstet* 2015;**131** Suppl 3:S173–211.
6. Denison FC, Norwood P, Bhattacharya S, et al. Association between maternal body mass index during pregnancy, short term morbidity, and increased health service costs: a population based study. *BJOG* 2014;**121**:72–82.
7. Dobbs R, Sawers C, Thompson F, et al. *Overcoming Obesity: An Initial Economic Analysis*. Discussion paper. New York: The McKinsey Global Institute: McKinsey & Company; 2014.
8. World Health Organization (WHO). *Obesity: Preventing and Managing the Global Epidemic*. WHO Obesity Technical Report Series 894. Geneva: WHO; 2000.
9. WHO Expert Consultation. Appropriate body-mass index for Asian populations and its implications for policy and intervention strategies. *Lancet* 2004;**363**:157–63.
10. Bei-Fan Z, Cooperative Meta-analysis Group of Working Group on Obesity in China. Predictive values of body mass index and waist circumference for risk factors of certain related diseases in Chinese adults: study on optimal cut-off points of body mass index and waist circumference in Chinese adults. *Asia Pac J Clin Nutr* 2002;**11**:S685–93.
11. Kanazawa M, Yoshiike N, Osaka T, Numba Y, Zimmet P, Inoue S. Criteria and classification of obesity in Japan and Asia-Oceania. *Asia Pac J Clin Nutr* 2002;**11**:S732–37.
12. Devlieger R, Benhalima K, Damm P, et al. Maternal obesity in Europe: where do we stand and how to move forward? A scientific paper commissioned by the European Board and College

of Obstetrics and Gynaecology (EBCOG). *Eur J Obstet Gynecol Reprod Biol* 2016;**201**:203–208.

13. Benhalima K, Mathieu C, van Assche A, et al. Survey by the European Board and College of Obstetrics and Gynaecology on screening for gestational diabetes in Europe. *Eur J Obstet Gynecol Reprod Biol* 2016;**201**:197–202.

14. Hruby A, Hu F. The epidemiology of obesity: a big picture. *Pharmoeconomics* 2015;**33**:673–89.

15. Crosbie E, Berggren E, Marin-Hirsch P. Editors' choice. *BJOG* 2016;**123**:157–58.

16. Ng M, Fleming T, Robinson M, et al. Global, regional and national prevalence of overweight and obesity in children and adults during 1980-2013: a systematic analysis for the global burden of disease study 2013. *Lancet* 2014;**384**:766–81.

17. World Health Organization. Global Health Observatory (GHO) data: overweight and obesity. Available at: https://www.who.int/gho/ncd/risk_factors/overweight/en/.

18. Mitchell S, Shaw D. The worldwide epidemic of female obesity. *Best Pract Res Clin Obstet Gynaecol* 2015;**29**:289–99.

19. Ogden CL, Carroll MD, Kit BK, Flegal KM. Prevalence of childhood and adult obesity in the United States, 2011–2012. *JAMA* 2014;**311**:806–14.

20. Adeboye B, Bermano G, Rolland C. Obesity and its health impact in Africa: a systematic review. *Cardiovasc J Afr* 2012;**23**:512–21.

21. Canoy D, Buchan I. Challenges in obesity epidemiology. *Obes Rev* 2007;**8** Suppl 1:1–11.

22. Savona-Ventura C, Savona-Ventura S. The inheritance of obesity. *Best Pract Res Clin Obstet Gynaecol* 2015:**29**;300–308.

23. Hasan A, Mahmood T. Genetic and molecular basis of obesity. In: Mahmood TA, Arulkumaran S (eds), *Obesity: A Ticking Time Bomb for Reproductive Health*, pp. 23–34. London: Elsevier; 2013.

24. O'Rahilly S. Human genetics illuminates the paths to metabolic disease. *Nature* 2009;**462**:307–14.

25. Gaillard R, Welten M, Oddy WH, et al. Associations of maternal prepregnancy body mass index and gestational weight gain with cardio-metabolic risk factors in adolescent offspring: a prospective cohort study. *BJOG* 2016;**123**:207–16.

26. Olson CM, Strawderman MS, Dennison BA. Maternal weight gain during pregnancy and child weight at age 3 years. *Matern Child Health J* 2009;**13**:839–46.

27. Ma RCW, Gluckman PD, Hanson MA. Maternal obesity and developmental priming of risk of later disease. In: Mahmood TA, Arulkumaran S (eds), *Obesity: A Ticking Time Bomb for Reproductive Health*, pp. 193–212. London: Elsevier; 2013.

28. Catalano PM, Ehrenberg HM. The short- and long-term implications of maternal obesity on mother and her offspring. *BJOG* 2006;**113**:1126–33.

29. Furber CM, McGowan L, Bower P, Kontopantelis E, Quenby S, Lavender T. Antenatal interventions for reducing weight in obese women for improving pregnancy outcome. *Cochrane Database Syst Rev* 2013;**1**:CD009334.

30. Freedman DS, Dietz WH, Srinivasan SR, Berenson GS. The relation of overweight to cardiovascular risk factors among children and adolescents: the Bogalusa Heart Study. *Pediatrics* 1999;**103**:1175–82.

31. Fraser A, Tilling K, Macdonald-Wallis C, et al. Association of maternal weight gain in pregnancy with offspring obesity and metabolic and vascular traits in childhood. *Circulation* 2010;**121**:2557–64.

32. Busby G, Seif MW. Obesity in adolescence. In: Mahmood TA, Arulkumaran S (eds), *Obesity: A Ticking Time Bomb for Reproductive Health*, pp. 53–66. London: Elsevier; 2013.

33. Bellis MA, Downing J, Ashton JR. Adults at 12? Trends in puberty and their public health consequences. *J Epidemiol Community Health* 2006;**60**:910–11.

34. Edmonds DK. Gynaecological disorders of childhood and adolescence. In: Edmonds DK (ed), *Dewhurst's Textbook of Obstetrics and Gynaeology*, 7th edn, pp. 12–16. Oxford: Blackwell Publishing; 2007.

35. Simmons KB, Edelman AB. Contraception and sexual health in obese women. *Best Pract Res Clin Obstet Gynaecol* 2015;**29**:466–78.

36. Fulghesu A, Magnini R, Portoghese E, Angioni S, Minerba L, Melis GB. Obesity-related lipid profile and altered insulin incretion in adolescents with polycystic ovary syndrome. *J Adolesc Health* 2010;**46**:474–81.

37. Damodaran S, Swaminathan K, Mahmood T. Obesity and contraception. *Br J Sexual Med* 2008;**31**:12–14.

38. Damodaran S, Swaminathan K. Obesity and contraception. In: Mahmood TA, Arulkumaran S (eds), *Obesity: A Ticking Time Bomb for Reproductive Health*, pp. 67–90. London: Elsevier; 2013.

39. Alsharaydeh I, Gharaibeh A, Thanoon O, Mahmood TA. Contraception in patients with medical conditions. *Obstet Gynaecol Reprod Med* 2014;**24**:33–38.

40. Scarabin PY, Vissac AM, Kirzin JM, et al. Elevated plasma fibrinogen and increased fibrin turnover among healthy women who both smoke and use low-dose oral contraceptives—a preliminary report. *Thromb Haemost* 1999;**82**:1112–16.

41. Suchon P, Al Frouh F, Henneuse A, et al. Risk factors for venous thromboembolism in women under combined oral contraceptive. The PILl Genetic RIsk Monitoring (PILGRIM) Study. *Throm Haemostat* 2016;**115**:135–42.

42. Thanoon O, Dewart P, Mahmood T. Laparoscopy in the obese patient. In: Metwally M, Li TC (eds), *Reproductive Surgery in Assisted Conception*, pp. 135–41. London: Springer-Verlag; 2015.

43. Leech TG, Dias JJ. Risky sexual behaviour: a race-specific social consequence of obesity. *J Youth Adolesc* 2011;**41**:41–52.

44. Mahmood T, Thanoon O. The role of bariatric surgery on female reproductive health. *Obstet Gynaecol Reprod Med* 2016;**26**:155–57.

45. Lim CC, Mahmood T. Obesity in pregnancy. *Best Pract Res Clin Obstet Gynaecol* 2015;**29**:309–19.

46. Knight M, Kurinczuk JJ, Spark P, et al. Extreme obesity in pregnancy in the United Kingdom. *Obstet Gynecol* 2010;**115**:989–97.

47. Chu SY, Kim SY, Schmid CH, et al. Maternal obesity and risk of caesarean delivery: a meta-analysis. *Obes Rev* 2007;**8**:385–94.

48. Heslehurst N, Rankin J, Wilkinson JR, et al. A nationally representative study of maternal obesity in England, UK: trends in incidence and demographic inequalities in 619 323 births, 1989–2007. *Int J Obes* 2010;**34**:420–28.

49. Norman JE, Reynolds R. The consequences of obesity and excess weight gain in pregnancy. *Proc Nutrit Soc* 2011;**70**:450–56.

50. Edlow AG, Hui L, Wick HC, Fried I, Bianchi DW. Assessing the fetal effects of maternal obesity via transcriptomic analysis of cord blood: a prospective case-control study. *BJOG* 2016;**123**:180–89.

51. Overton C, Mahmood T. Access to early pregnancy care. In: Mahmood T, Owen P, Arulkumaran S, Dhillon C (eds), *Models of Care in Maternity Services*, pp. 34–47. London: RCOG Press; 2010.

52. Metwally M, Cutting R, Tipton A, et al. Effect of increased body mass index on oocyt and embryo quality in IVF patients. *Reprod Biomed Online* 2007;**15**:532–38.

53. Metwally M, Ong KJ, Ledger WL, Li TC. Does high body mass index increase the risk of miscarriage after spontaneous and assisted conception? A meta-analysis of the evidence. *Fert Steril* 2008;**90**:714–26.

54. Lashen H, Fear K, Sturdee DW. Obesity is associated with increased risk of first trimester and recurrent miscarriage: matched case–control study. *Hum Reprod* 2004;**19**:1644–46.

55. Lo W, Rai R, Hameed A, Brailsford SR, Al-Ghamdi AA, Regan L. The effect of body mass index on the outcome of pregnancy in women with recurrent miscarriage. *J Fam Community Med* 2012;**19**:167–71.

56. Flenady V, Koopmans L, Middleton P, et al. Major risk factors for stillbirth in high-income countries: a systematic review and meta-analysis. *Lancet* 2011;**377**:1331–40.

57. Stothard KJ, Tennant PW, Bell R, Rankin J. Maternal overweight and obesity and the risk of congenital anomalies: a systematic review and meta-analysis. *JAMA* 2009;**301**:636–50.

58. Hendler I, Blackwell SC, Bujold E, et al. Sub-optimal second trimester ultra-sonographic visualisation of the fetal heart in obese women: should we repeat the experiment? *J Ultrasound Med* 2005;**24**:1205–209.

59. Modder J, Fitzsimons KJ. *Joint CMACE/RCOG Guideline: Management of Women with Obesity in Pregnancy*. London: Royal College of Obstetricians and Gynaecologists; 2010.

60. Huda SS, Nelson SM. Pregnancy and metabolic syndrome of obesity. In: Mahmood TA, Arulkumaran S (eds), *Obesity: A Ticking Time Bomb for Reproductive Health*, pp. 299–314. London: Elsevier; 2013.

61. Einstein FH, Fishman S, Muzumdar RH, et al. Accretions of visceral fat and hepatic insulin resistance in pregnant rats. *Am J Physiol Endocrinol Metab* 2008;**294**:E451–55.

62. Sattar N, Clark P, Holmes A, et al. Antenatal waist circumference and hypertension risk. *Obstet Gynecol* 2001;**97**:268–71.

63. World Health Organization (WHO). *Diagnostic Criteria and Classification of Hyperglycaemia First Detected in Pregnancy*. Geneva: WHO; 2013. Available at: http://apps.who.int/iris/bitstream/10665/85975/1/WHO_NMH_MND_13.2_eng.pdf.

64. Pedersen J. Weight and length at birth of infants of diabetic mothers. *Acta Endocrinol* 1954;**16**:330–42.

65. Scholl TO, Sowers M, Chen X, et al. Maternal glucose concentration influences fetal growth, gestation, and pregnancy complications. *Am J Epidemiol* 2001;**154**:514–20.

66. Shapiro ALB, Schmiege SJ, Brinton JT, et al. Testing the fuel-mediated hypothesis: maternal insulin resistance and glucose mediate the association between maternal and neonatal adiposity, the Healthy Start study. *Diabetologia* 2015;**58**:937–41.

67. Kjos SL, Buchanan TA. Gestational diabetes mellitus. *N Engl J Med* 1999;**341**:1749–56.

68. Rayanagoudar G, Hashi AH, Zamora J, Khan KS, Hitman GA, Thangaratinam S. Quantification of the type II risk in women with gestational diabetes: a systematic review and meta-analysis of 95 750 women. *Diabetologia* 2016;**59**:1403–11.

69. Benhalima K, Damm P, Van Assche A, et al. Screening for gestational diabetes in Europe: where do we stand and how to move forward? A scientific paper commissioned by the European Board and College of Obstetrics and Gynaecology (EBCOG). *Eur J Obstet Gynecol Reprod Biol* 2016;**199**:192–96.

70. Benhalima K, Chantel M, Damm P, et al. A proposal for the use of uniform diagnostic criteria for gestational diabetes in Europe: an opinion paper by the European Board & College of Obstetrics and Gynaecology (EBCOG). *Diabetolgia* 2015;**58**:1422–29.

71. Frederick IO, Rudra CB, Miller RS, Foster JC, Williams MA. Adult weight change, weight cycling, and prepregnancy obesity in relation to risk of preeclampsia. *Epidemiology* 2006;**17**:428–34.

72. Villamor E, Cnattingius S. Interpregnancy weight change and risk of adverse pregnancy outcomes: a population-based study. *Lancet* 2006;**368**:1164–70.

73. Guelinckx I, Devlieger R, Beckers K, Vansant G. Maternal obesity: pregnancy complications, gestational weight gain and nutrition. *Obes Rev* 2008;**9**:140–50.

74. Sebire NJ, Jolly M, Harris JP, et al. Maternal obesity and pregnancy outcome: a study of 287 213 pregnancies in London. *Int J Obes Relat Metab Disord* 2001;**25**:1175–82.

75. Nohr EA, Bech BH, Vaeth M, Rasmussen KM, Henriksen TB, Olsen J. Obesity, gestational weight gain and preterm birth: a study within the Danish National Birth Cohort. *Paediatr Perinat Epidemiol* 2007;**21**:5–14.

76. McDonald SD, Han Z, Mulla S, Beyene J. Overweight and obesity in mothers and risk of preterm birth and low birth weight infants: systematic review and meta-analyses. *BMJ* 2010;**341**:c3428.

77. Dickey RP, Xiong X, Xie Y, Gee RE, Pridjian G. Effect of maternal height and weight on risk for preterm singleton and twin births resulting from IVF in the United States, 2008–2010. *Am J Obstet Gynecol* 2013;**209**:349.e1–6.

78. Mahmood TA, Hasan A. Deep vein thrombosis and pulmonary embolism. In: Chandraharan E, Arulkumaran S (eds), *Obstetric and Intrapartum Emergencies*, pp. 15–23. Cambridge: Cambridge University Press; 2012.

79. Larsen TB, Sørensen HT, Gislum M, Johnsen SP. Maternal smoking, obesity, and risk of venous thromboembolism during pregnancy and the puerperium: a population-based nested case-control study. *Thromb Res* 2007;**120**:505–509.

80. Royal College of Obstetricians and Gynaecologists. *Thromboprophylaxis during Pregnancy, Labour and after Vaginal Delivery*. RCOG Green-top Guideline No. 37. London: RCOG Press; 2004.

81. Malarselvi M, Quenby S. Obesity and prolonged pregnancy. In: Mahmood TA, Arulkumaran S (eds), *Obesity: A Ticking Time Bomb for Reproductive Health*, pp. 223–26. London: Elsevier; 2013.

82. Knight M, Tuffnell D, Kenyon S, et al. *Saving Lives, Improving Mothers' Care—Surveillance of Maternal Deaths in the UK 2011–13 and Lessons Learned to Inform Maternity Care from the UK and Ireland Confidential Enquiries into Maternal Deaths and Morbidity 2009–13*. Oxford: National Perinatal Epidemiology Unit, University of Oxford; 2015.

83. Jefferys A, Draycott T, Mahmood T. Planning for the future: maternity services in 2035. In: Mahmood TA, Arulkumaran S (eds), *Obesity: A Ticking Time Bomb for Reproductive Health*, pp. 607–22. London: Elsevier; 2013.

84. Yao R, Ananth CV, Park BY, Pereira L, Plante LA. Obesity and the risk of stillbirth: a population-based cohort study. Perinatal Research Consortium. *Am J Obstet Gynecol* 2014;**210**:457.e1–9.

85. Bhattacharya S, Campbell DM, Liston WA. Effect of body mass index on pregnancy outcomes in nulliparous women delivering singleton babies. *BMC Public Health* 2007;**7**:168.

86. El-Chaar D, Finkelstein SA, Tu X, et al. The impact of increasing obesity class on obstetrical outcomes. *J Obstet Gynaecol Can* 2013;**35**:224–33.

87. Tsai PJS, Marshall NE. Maternal obesity and pregnancy outcomes. *Obes Open Access* 2015;**1**. http://dx.doi.org/10.16966/2380-5528.113.

88. Wolfe KB, Rossi RA, Warshak CR. The effect of maternal obesity on the rate of failed induction of labor. *Am J Obstet Gynecol* 2011;**205**:128.e1–7.

89. Confidential Enquiry into Maternal and Child Health (CEMACH). *Saving Mothers' Lives. Reviewing Maternal Deaths to make Motherhood Safer: 2003–2005*. London: CEMACH; 2007.

90. Nair M, Kurinczuk JJ, Brocklehurst P, et al. Factors associated with maternal death from direct pregnancy complications: a UK national case-control study. *BJOG* 2015;**122**:653–62.

91. Churchill D, Forbes G, Mahmood T. Developing standards of care for obese women during pregnancy. In: Mahmood TA, Arulkumaran S (eds), *Obesity: A Ticking Time Bomb for Reproductive Health*, pp. 483–500. London: Elsevier; 2013.

92. Mahmood TA (Chair). Care of Obese Pregnant Women – Standard 9. In: *Obstetric and Neonatal Services 2014: Standards of Care for Women's Health in Europe*. Brussels: European Board and College of Obstetrics and Gynaecology (EBCOG); 2014.

93. Seif MW, Diamond K, Nickkho-Amiry M. Obesity and menstrual disorders. *Best Pract Res Clin Obstet Gynaecol* 2015;**29**:516–27.

94. Bano R, Datta S, Mahmood TA. Heavy menstrual bleeding. *Obstet Gynaecol Reprod Med* 2014;**26**:167–83.

95. Messinis IE, Messini CI, Anifandis G, Dafopoulos K. Polycystic ovaries and obesity. *Best Pract Res Clin Obstet Gynaecol* 2015;**29**:479–88.

96. Messinis IE, Messinis CI, Dafopoulos K. Obesity in PCOS and infertility. In: Mahmood TA, Arulkumaran S (eds), *Obesity: A Ticking Time Bomb for Reproductive Health*, pp. 99–116. London: Elsevier; 2013.

97. Talmor A, Dunphy B. Female obesity and infertility. *Best Prac Res Clin Obs Gynae* 2025;**29**:498–506.

98. van der Steeg JW, Steures P, Eijkemans MJ, et al. Obesity affects spontaneous pregnancy chances in subfertile, ovulatory women. *Hum Reprod* 2008;**23**:324–28.

99. Bellver J, Pellicer A, García-Velasco JA, Ballesteros A, Remohí J, Meseguer M. Obesity reduces uterine receptivity: clinical experience from 9,587 first cycles of ovum donation with normal weight donors. *Fertil Steril* 2013;**100**:1050–58.

100. Sharma A, Bahadursingh S, Ramsewak S, Teelucksingh S. Medical and surgical interventions to improve outcomes in obese women planning for pregnancy. *Best Prac Res Clin Obstet Gynaecol* 2015;**29**:565–76.

101. Ramalingam K, Monga A. Obesity and pelvic floor dysfunction. *Best Prac Res Clin Obstet Gynaecol* 2015;**29**:541–47.

102. Lim C, Mahmood T. Management of urinary incontinence in primary care. *BIDA J* 2014;**20**:8–9.

103. Al-Safi ZA, Polotsky AJ. Obesity and menopause. *Best Prac Res Clin Obstet Gynaecol* 2015;**29**:548–53.

104. Wolin KY, Carson K, Colditz GA. Obesity and cancer. *Oncologist* 2010;**15**:556–65.

105. Birks S, Peeters A, Backholer K, et al. A systematic review of the impact of weight loss on cancer incidence and mortality. *Obes Rev* 2012;**13**:868–91.

106. Tsilidis K, Kasimis JC, Lopez DS, et al. Type 2 diabetes and cancer: umbrella review of meta-analysis of observational studies. *BMJ* 2015;**350**:g7607.

107. Zhang Y, Liu Y, Yang S, Zhang, J, Qian, L, Chen X. Overweight, obesity and endometrial cancer risk: results from a systematic review and meta-analysis. *Int J Biol Markers* 2014;**29**:21–29.

108. Chittenden BG, Fullerton G, Maheshwari A, Bhattacharya S. Polycystic ovary syndrome and the risk of gynaecological cancer: a systematic review. *Reprod Biomed Online* 2009;**19**:398–405.

109. Afors K, Centini G, Murtada R, Castellano R, Meza C, Wattiez A. Obesity in laparoscopic surgery. *Best Prac Res Clin Obstet Gynaecol* 2015;**29**:554–64.

110. Li Z, Maglione M, Tu W, et al. Meta-analysis: pharmacologic treatment of obesity. *Ann Intern Med* 2005;**142**:532–46.

111. Colquitt JL, Pickett K, Loveman E, Frampton GK. Surgery for weight loss in adults. *Cochrane Database Syst Rev* 2014;**8**:CD003641.

112. Maggard MA, Shugarman LR, Suttorp M, et al. Meta-analysis: surgical treatment of obesity. *Ann Intern Med* 2005;**142**:547–59.

113. Kumari A, Nigam A. Bariatric surgery in women: a boon needs special care during pregnancy. *J Clin Diagn Res* 2015;**9**: QE01–05.

SECTION 2
Fetomaternal Medicine

8

Maternal physiology

Nicola Vousden and Andrew H. Shennan

Introduction

Pregnancy requires physiological adaptations. These are often initiated in the luteal phase of every ovulatory cycle. They are proactive and amplified if conception occurs. All physiological systems are affected to some extent in order to provide a suitable environment for the growth and development of the fetus, and to protect and prepare the mother for the process of labour and the postnatal period. This chapter gives an overview of the major changes.

Changes in the haematological and immune system

Blood volume includes both plasma volume and red cell mass. These are under different physiological control. Plasma volume increases by approximately 50% in pregnancy from 2600 mL prepregnancy to 3850 mL by 32–34 weeks' gestation where it plateaus (1, 2). In multiparous women this increase can be higher (up to 60%). Plasma volume is directly correlated to the growth of the baby (2) with multiple pregnancies associated with significantly increased plasma volumes (1). Impaired fetal growth is associated with a poor increase in plasma volume (3).

There is also a steady increase in the red cell mass in pregnancy. The circulating volume of red cells prior to pregnancy is approximately 1300 mL which increases by 20–30% in pregnancy (4). This change in mass is due to an increase in both red cell number and size. Women taking iron supplements and women with multiple pregnancies have a greater increase (5). Erythropoietin is increased in pregnancy by 50%, but less so with iron supplementation (25%) (6). This is thought to be stimulated by human placental lactogen (7).

Serum iron concentrations decrease in pregnancy despite the increase in absorption of iron from the gut. The increase in transferrin increases the iron-binding capacity. The increased renal clearance of folate towards the term pregnancy causes plasma folate concentrations to be halved.

The total white cell count increases during pregnancy due to an increase in neutrophil polymorphonuclear leucocytes which peaks at 30 weeks' gestation before plateauing. This increase in neutrophils is initiated at the time of the oestrogen peak in a normal menstrual cycle and then continues if conception occurs (8). A further fourfold increase in the number of polymorphs occurs during labour and immediately following delivery. Their phagocytic function increases during pregnancy. Eosinophil, basophil, and monocyte levels remain relatively constant during pregnancy until a significant reduction in eosinophils occurs at the time of labour and delivery. The lymphocyte count does not alter significantly during pregnancy and there is no change in the number of circulating T and B cells (9). However, their function is depressed in pregnancy, potentially due to the increased concentration of glycoprotein coating as stimulated by the high levels of oestrogen in pregnancy which reduce the response to stimuli (10). Human chorionic gonadotropin and prolactin are also known to supress lymphocyte function, but there is no reduction in humoral immunity or immunoglobulins.

In pregnancy, two types of fetal tissue are in direct contact with maternal tissues. Villous trophoblasts form a continuous syncytium that is bathed in maternal blood and extravillous trophoblasts contact maternal endometrial/decidual tissues. Both appear to be immunologically inert. Villous trophoblasts do not express human leucocyte antigen (HLA) class I or II molecules. Extravillous trophoblasts do not express HLA-A or HLA-B but do express trophoblast-specific HLA-G, HLA-C, and HLA-E. The main type of decidual lymphocyte is the decidual natural killer cells. These differ from systemic natural killer cells as they express surface killer immunoglobulin-like receptors (KIRs) which bind to HLA-G and HLA-C on the trophoblast. KIRs are highly polymorphic and HLA-C is also polymorphic, therefore there is a potentially very variable receptor–ligand system. The impact of this is that one receptor ligand combination, KIR AA and HLA-C2, is associated with an increased possibility of miscarriage or pre-eclampsia (11).

Platelets can decrease in number throughout a normal pregnancy and the platelet volume increases from 28 weeks' gestation due to an increase in large and immature platelets. This suggests that there is destruction of platelets in pregnancy. The reactivity of platelets is increased in the second and third trimester and returns to normal 12 weeks after delivery.

There are dramatic changes to the coagulation system in pregnancy with a mild coagulopathy throughout normal pregnancy. The end result of coagulation is formation of a fibrin clot from fibrinogen involving a complex interaction of clotting factors. There are changes in many clotting factors as summarized in **Figure 8.1**, which contribute to this coagulopathy. Factors VII, VIII, VIII:C, X,

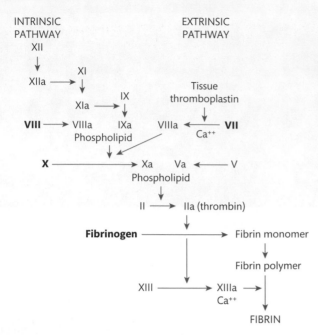

Figure 8.1 Alterations in the coagulation pathways associated with human pregnancy. Factors which increase during normal pregnancy are shown in colour.

Source data from Chamberlain G, Broughton Pipkin F (eds); *Clinical Physiology in Obstetrics*, 3rd edn. Oxford: Blackwell Science, 1998:71–110.

and IX are all increased in pregnancy and factors II and V remain constant. Factor XI and XIII both decrease in pregnancy by 60–70% and 50% respectively. Protein S, a cofactor of protein C which inactivates factors V and VIII, is reduced in the first two trimesters of pregnancy.

Plasma fibrinogen levels approximately double in pregnancy from 2.5–4 g/L to 6.0 g/L in late pregnancy. Concentrations of high-molecular-weight fibrin/fibrinogen complexes also increase in normal pregnancy. This increase in fibrinogen contributes to a rise in the erythrocyte sedimentation rate. An estimated 5–10% of all circulating fibrinogen is consumed at the time of placental separation. In contrast, plasma fibrinolytic activity is decreased in pregnancy and labour but quickly returns to non-pregnant values after delivery suggesting that mediators are derived from the placenta (12).

Clinical considerations

- The increase in plasma volume is greater than the increase in red cell mass, therefore the concentration of haematocrit, haemoglobin, and red cell count will reduce in pregnancy. This is termed physiological anaemia.
- Dramatic changes in the blood volume occur at delivery. Average blood loss can be tolerated without a significant decrease in haemoglobin concentrations. In the non-pregnant state, acute blood loss is associated with a subsequent increase in plasma volume causing a decrease in haematocrit over the following days. In pregnancy, there is gradual decrease in plasma volume due to diuresis following delivery and therefore haematocrit gradually increases.
- The activation of the clotting system during labour increases the risk of disseminated intravascular coagulation, which may be triggered by other stimulus, such as amniotic fluid embolus. In this

case, clotting factors and platelets are consumed resulting in massive haemorrhage. Fibrinolysis is stimulated and the fibrinogen degradation products interfere with clot formation, and potentially myometrial contraction, thus worsening the haemorrhage.
- Adolescents are at particular risk of iron deficiency in pregnancy. Even mild anaemia is associated with decreased birthweight therefore appropriate supplementation is key.
- Neutrophilia during labour and immediate puerperium should not be assumed to be due to infection as this is a normal physiological response.
- The increased coagulability increases the risk of thrombotic disease therefore all women should be assessed for their risk of venous thromboembolism and appropriate precautions taken if their risk is increased.

Changes in the cardiovascular system

The increase in plasma volume in pregnancy dramatically increases the cardiovascular preload. The most important changes in the cardiovascular system are the decrease in peripheral vascular resistance (affecting afterload) and the increase in cardiac output. These changes are a proactive process, initiated in anticipation of increased physiological demand. Indeed, some are initiated during each ovulatory menstrual cycle and then amplified by stimuli from the growing uterus and fetoplacental unit in the first 8 weeks of pregnancy (13).

Haemodynamic stimuli in pregnancy

The stimuli for the dramatic cardiovascular changes in early pregnancy are due to a number of vasoactive substances. The three major oestrogens in pregnancy—oestrone, oestriol, and oestradiol—all increase until term although different patterns of change are demonstrated. Oestrone and oestradiol show a gradual increase from conception throughout early pregnancy whereas oestriol levels remain undetectable until the ninth week of pregnancy. By term, oestrone and oestriol levels are increased by about 100-fold and oestradiol by 1000-fold (13). Extensive studies of the effect of exogenous oestrogen on the cardiovascular system conclude that oestrogen increases the stroke volume and reduces vascular resistance, thus increasing cardiac output (14). The pathways of action are complex including increased synthesis of nitric oxide, stimulating production of prostaglandins (15) as well as exerting structural effects by altering production of collagen in the vasculature (16). In contrast, the serum level of progesterone remains unchanged until after the tenth week of pregnancy. At this point it gradually increases until at term it is increased threefold. Progesterone is thought to exert a vasodilatory effect. Exogenous progesterone has been reported to reduce blood pressure in non-pregnant hypertensive people (17) and increase venous distensibility (18).

The renin–angiotensin system (RAS) also exerts significant effects on maternal cardiovascular function during pregnancy. During each ovulatory menstrual cycle there is a peak in both the precursors and the hormones of this system following ovulation. If conception occurs, this peak does not return to basal levels. During pregnancy, the peripheral concentration of active renin, angiotensinogen, and angiotensin II increases until the 30th week of gestation. The RAS regulates aldosterone release therefore aldosterone concentration is also raised in pregnancy. This counters the natriuretic effect of progesterone at the distal tubule and results in sodium retention and plasma volume expansion. Angiotensin II is primarily a vasoconstrictor. Despite its elevated levels in pregnancy, the blood pressure remains reduced in pregnancy due to reduced sensitivity to its vasopressor effects (19, 20). The only component of this system reported to be reduced in pregnancy is angiotensin-converting enzyme (21).

Cardiac output, stroke volume, and heart rate

In nulliparous women, the cardiac output is increased by approximately 35–40%, and by around 50% in multiparous women. This can rise by a further 33% during labour. The cardiac output remains high for 24 hours after delivery and then gradually declines over 2 weeks to prepregnancy levels (22, 23). The majority of the increase in cardiac output occurs in the first trimester. By 8 weeks' gestation, the cardiac output has increased by 13% compared to at 5 weeks' gestation; this is further increased in the second and third trimesters due to increases in stroke volume and heart rate. Nearly 90% of the increase in cardiac output in the first 5 weeks of pregnancy can be attributed to the increase in heart rate. The heart rate then continues to rise more slowly until 32 weeks' gestation. The average increase is 10–15 beats per minute although there is wide individual variation. The increase in stroke volume occurs slightly later, starting gradually by the fifth week of pregnancy and plateauing in the second trimester (23, 24).

Total peripheral resistance decreases significantly by just 6 weeks' gestation. This decrease continues until approximately 20 weeks' gestation when a 40% reduction in peripheral vascular resistance is observed. This decreased total peripheral resistance is due to the changes in hormonal vasodilator and vasoconstrictor functions, rather than sympathetic tone, in addition to circulating prostaglandins and locally synthesized nitric oxide. The reduction in afterload

causes an initial decrease in both the systolic and diastolic blood pressures in the first half of pregnancy with the diastolic blood pressure decrease exceeding the systolic. The most dramatic reduction in blood pressure (by 80–90%) occurs before 8 weeks of pregnancy where the mean arterial pressure is approximately 10 mmHg lower than during prepregnancy (23). Following this, the mean arterial pressure continues to decrease steadily, reaching a nadir at approximately 24 weeks (23). The reduction in blood pressure, in addition to increased levels of oestrogen and progesterone, trigger the renin–angiotensin–aldosterone system causing retention of sodium, an increase in total body water, and an increase in the plasma volume by about 50%. Thus in the latter half of pregnancy, the blood pressure then steadily increases in parallel with the increasing plasma volume and peripheral sympathetic activity. These changes are demonstrated in **Figure 8.2** and **Table 8.1**.

Systemic vascular resistance is calculated by the ratio of mean arterial pressure and cardiac output. As with blood pressure it decreases in the first weeks of pregnancy, reaching a nadir in mid pregnancy and gradually increasing towards term. Blood flow increases in the low impedance uteroplacental circulation. Renal blood flow also gradually increases during pregnancy until the third trimester when it is 60–80% higher than prepregnancy levels. These are a result of renal vasodilatation resulting in lower glomerular filtration rates (GFRs). The pulmonary resistance decreases in early pregnancy and remains fairly static throughout pregnancy. This is due to the capacity of the pulmonary circulation to absorb high rates of flow without an increase in pressure.

The physiological changes in preload and afterload are accompanied by remodelling of the atria and ventricles. The left ventricular end-diastolic diameter is increased between the 10th and 20th weeks of pregnancy and then plateaus at approximately 5% greater than the prepregnancy value (27, 28). This higher left ventricular end-diastolic

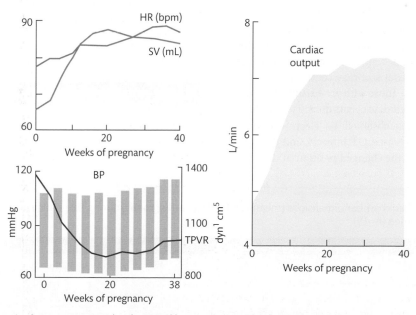

Figure 8.2 Major haemodynamic changes associated with normal human pregnancy. The marked augmentation of cardiac output results from asynchronous increases in both heart rate (HR) and stroke volume (SV). Despite the increase in cardiac output, blood pressure (BP) decreases for most of pregnancy. This implies a very substantial reduction in total peripheral vascular resistance (TPVR).

Reproduced from Broughton Pipkin F. Maternal physiology. In: Edmonds KD (ed); *Dewhurst's Textbook of Obstetrics & Gynaecology*, 8th edn: John Wiley & Sons; 2012: 5–15 with permission from Wiley.

Table 8.1 Percentage changes in key cardiovascular variables in pregnancy

	First trimester (%)	Second trimester (%)	Third trimester (%)
Heart rate (beats per minute)	+11	+13	+16
Stroke volume (mL)	+31	+29	+27
Cardiac output (L/min)	+45	+47	+48
Systolic blood pressure (mmHg)	−1	+1	+6
Diastolic blood pressure (mmHg)	−6	−3	+7
Mean pulmonary artery pressure (mmHg)	+6	+5	+5
Total peripheral resistance (resistance units)	−27	−27	−29

Mean pulmonary artery pressure data are derived from studies in which preconception values were determined. The mean values shown are those at the end of each trimester and are thus not necessarily the maxima.

Source data from Robson SC, Hunter S, Boys RJ, Dunlop W. Serial study of factors influencing changes in cardiac output during human pregnancy. *American Journal of Physiology - Heart and Circulatory Physiology.* 1989;256(4):H1060–65.

diameter is associated with a rise in preload. In addition, the left ventricular end-systolic diameter is reduced in the first trimester compared to prepregnancy in accordance with the increased heart rate and contractility. There are also changes in the right ventricle, right atrium, and left atrium as described in Table 8.2.

Clinical considerations

- In pregnancy, the heart is pushed upwards by the elevation of the diaphragm and rotated forwards. The volume of the heart is increased by about 12% in pregnancy (28). Small pericardial effusions are frequently found which resolve after delivery.
- The apex beat is moved upwards and laterally under the fourth rib. The first heart sound becomes louder and there is an exaggerated splitting of this sound as the mitral valve closes earlier.
- Most women remain in sinus rhythm throughout pregnancy although premature atrial and ventricular complexes are more frequent. Increases in the atrial size may contribute to atrial arrhythmias during pregnancy. Those with pre-existing arrhythmias are at higher risk of adverse cardiac events during pregnancy.
- The most common changes observed on electrocardiography are increased heart rate, increased QT interval, and deviation to the left electrical axis due to the changed position of the heart. In

many women the T wave becomes flattened or inverted in lead III (30, 31) and one-third of women show ST segment changes after exercise at the end of pregnancy (32, 33).

- In pregnancy, a special effort must be made to obtain accurate blood pressure measurements. Blood pressure is lowest when the woman is lying supine on her left side and is significantly different to when recorded sitting. Sequential measurements should be made in the same positon for comparable results.
- In addition, the difference between Korotkoff sounds IV (muffling of sound) and V (disappearance of sound) is increased in pregnancy. It is the current consensus that Korotkoff sound V is the most reliable in pregnancy.
- Many automatic devices are inaccurate in pre-eclampsia. Care should also be taken to ensure that blood pressure devices are validated in accordance with an established protocol.
- The vena cava is compressed by the uterus. This can result in a profound drop in blood pressure when the mother lies on her back. This is known as supine hypotension syndrome. Venous return from the lower limbs is restricted causing a drop in the stroke volume.
- The increased demand of pregnancy on the cardiovascular system may be detrimental to those with limited cardiac reserve. Despite the increased blood volume and the atrial and ventricular distension, cardiac filling pressures are not increased in women at term compared to postpartum because in pregnancy the normal heart compensates for these changes. Women with valve disease such as mitral stenosis or with dilated cardiomyopathy may not be able to compensate for the increased preload and are at risk of developing heart failure. In contrast, the increased preload and ventricular dimensions may improve the cardiovascular haemodynamics for women with hypertrophic cardiomyopathy. The increased cardiac work of pregnancy requires increased myocardial oxygen consumption. Therefore, women with coronary disease are at increased risk of ischaemia.
- Blood flow to the peripheries increases, resulting in warm hands and feet. Nasal congestion occurs due to increased blood flow to the nasal mucosa.

Changes in the respiratory system

The effect of pregnancy on the respiratory system is less than the effect on the cardiovascular system. Tidal volume is the volume of gas inspired or expired in each respiration; in the non-pregnant state this

Table 8.2 Cardiac chamber dimensions (measured by echocardiography) during pregnancy and postpartum in pregnant women (n=18)

Chamber	Weeks 8–12	Weeks 20–24	Weeks 30–34	Weeks 36–40	Puerperium	Control
LVd (mm)	41.1 ± 3.1	42.7 ± 2.2	43.0 ± 1.7	43.6 ± 2.5	41.8 ± 1.8	40.1 ± 3.0
RVd (mm)	30.1 ± 2.0	31.9 ± 2.1	35.5 ± 3.2	35.5 ± 2.3	31.1 ± 2.1	28.5 ± 3.0
LA (mm)	29.6 ± 2.1	31.5 ± 2.4	33.1 ± 2.4	32.8 ± 3.0	29.9 ± 3.1	27.9 ± 2.4
RA (mm)	42.8 ± 2.3	47.4 ± 2.4	50.8 ± 2.7	50.9 ± 2.8	46.6 ± 3.3	43.7 ± 4.4

LA, left atrial dimension; LVd, left ventricular diastolic dimension; RA, right atrial dimension; RVd, right ventricular diastolic dimension. Values represent the mean value ± standard deviation.

Reproduced from Campos O., Doppler Echocardiography During Pregnancy: Physiological and Abnormal Findings, *Echocardiography*, Vol 13, No 2, pp.135–146, 1996, with permission from John Wiley and Sons.

is approximately 500 mL, increasing to 700 mL in late pregnancy (34, 35). The inspiratory reserve volume is the maximum amount of air which can be inspired beyond normal tidal inspiration. Together these make the inspiratory capacity which in pregnancy progressively increases (by approximately 300 mL). Residual volume is the volume of gas remaining in the lungs at the end of maximal expiration. In pregnancy, this decreases by 300 mL. Its reduction means that the vital capacity, the maximum volume of gas that can be expired after maximum inspiration, is increased and gas mixing is improved (34, 35).

These changes are stimulated by progesterone which decreases the threshold and sensitizes the medulla oblongata to carbon dioxide. This causes overbreathing which begins in each luteal phase of the menstrual cycle and is maintained if conception occurs (36). Pregnancy does not change the resting respiratory rate, which remains constant at approximately 14–15 breaths per minute (34). Minute ventilation is a measure of tidal volume and respiratory rate which is increased in pregnancy by about 40% from 7.5 L/min to 10.5 L/min due to the increase in tidal volume. Therefore, the resting pregnant woman increases her ventilation by breathing more deeply and not more frequently.

Progesterone also increases erythrocyte carbonic anhydrase concentration in red cells causing carbon dioxide levels to be lower in pregnancy than non-pregnancy. Arterial pH remains constant due to an associated decrease in plasma bicarbonate concentration from 28 to 22 mmol/L (37). This contributes to a decrease in plasma osmolality. These changes are shown in **Table 8.3**. The low maternal carbon dioxide levels allow efficient placental transfer of fetal carbon dioxide which increases during the third trimester due to increased fetal metabolism.

Alveolar ventilation is increased which causes a 5% increase in maternal oxygen concentration. The increased levels of 2,3-diphosphoglycerate (DPG) in the red cells causes a rightward shift of the maternal oxyhaemoglobin dissociation curve. This facilitates oxygen transfer to the fetus which has a lower oxygen concentration than the mother. This lower sensitivity of fetal haemoglobin to 2,3-DPG causes a marked leftward shift of the oxyhaemoglobin dissociation curve. Oxygen consumption increases by about 16% from 220 to 255 mL/min in pregnancy due to the increased demands of fetal and maternal tissues. As the capacity of the blood to carry oxygen is increased by approximately 18%, the oxygen difference is actually reduced (13).

Forced expiratory volume (FEV_1) describes the volume of air that can be forcibly expired in 1 second. This is approximately 80–85% in non-pregnant adults and this is not changed in pregnancy. Peak expiratory flow rate is similarly unchanged (38, 39). This lack of

change is likely due to the net effect of bronchodilation in response to prostaglandin E and progesterone and bronchoconstriction due to prostaglandin $F_2\alpha$.

Clinical considerations

- Prostaglandin E is commonly used for induction of labour. Prostaglandin $F_2\alpha$ is commonly used for severe postpartum haemorrhage (e.g. carboprost); its effects on bronchoconstriction can be severe in women with asthma.
- Dyspnoea is a common symptom experienced in pregnancy. It cannot be attributed to airway restriction given resistance is actually reduced. It is therefore attributed to the level of effective reflex stimulation of overbreathing in the medulla.
- Spinal anaesthesia is commonly used for analgesia in labour and caesarean section. However, effective spinal anaesthesia is associated with a significant reduction in FEV_1, vital capacity, and peak flow and this is significantly greater in women with a body mass index (BMI) greater than 30 kg/m² (40).

Changes in uterine physiology

The uterus consists of bundles of smooth muscle cells which are spontaneously contractile. During pregnancy, rapid changes are required to prevent contractility, accommodate the growing fetus, and supply sufficient nutrients and oxygen. It is thought that during the first trimester the embryo gains nutrients from the glandular secretions of the endometrial glands that are rich in carbohydrates and lipids (41).

The muscle cells are arranged into three discrete layers separated by thin layers of connective tissue composed of collagen, elastic fibres, and fibroblasts. The innermost layer contains longitudinal fibres. The middle layer runs in all directions and contains the vascular supply and the outer layer has both circular and longitudinal fibres that are partly in continuation with the ligamentous support of the uterus (13). The prepregnancy uterus weighs 40–100 g. During pregnancy, this increases to 300–400 g at 20 weeks and 800–1000 g at term, a 20-fold increase. This growth is due to hypertrophy and elongation of the smooth muscle cells. Prior to pregnancy the smooth muscle cells are approximately 50 µm in length and this increases to between 200 and 600 µm by term (13). In later pregnancy, the enlargement is more prominent at the fundus, changing the shape of the uterus from the pear shape seen prior to pregnancy to an ovoid shape in the second and third trimesters. The isthmus is the junctional zone between the cervix and the body of the uterus. Regular contractions after 28 weeks' gestation cause the isthmus to stretch and thin. This is completed during labour to form the lower segment, a relatively avascular, thin part of the uterus. The cavity expands from 4 to 4000 mL by term. These changes are stimulated by the increasing levels of oestrogen and progesterone and the effect of the growing fetus.

The blood supply to the uterus prior to pregnancy is almost exclusively via the uterine arteries. In pregnancy, 20–30% is contributed via the ovarian vessel, and a small proportion by the superior vesical arteries. In pregnancy, all the vessels undergo massive hypertrophy, dilating to 50% larger diameters than the prepregnancy state. Uterine blood flow increases from 50 mL/min at 10 weeks of gestation to

Table 8.3 The influence of pregnancy on respiratory variables

	Non-pregnant	Pregnant–term
PO₂ (mmHg)	93 (12.5 kPa)	102 (13.6 kPa)
O₂ consumption (mL/min)	200	250
PCO₂ (mmHg)	35–40 (4.7–5.3 kPa)	30 (4.0 kPa)
Venous pH	7.35	7.38

PCO₂, partial pressure of carbon dioxide; PO₂, partial pressure of oxygen.

Source data from Broughton Pipkin F. Maternal physiology. In: Edmonds KD (ed), *Dewhurst's Textbook of Obstetrics & Gynaecology*, 8th edn, pp. 5–15. Chichester: John Wiley & Sons; 2012.

500–600 mL/min at term. The spiral arterioles are the final vessels that deliver blood into the intervillous space. Each radial artery gives rise to two or three spiral arterioles which supply a placental cotyledon. These undergo dramatic remodelling by extravillous trophoblasts in pregnancy. This reduces their tone and capacity to react to vasoconstrictor stimuli, thus ensuring maximal placental blood flow. This process is completed in the second trimester. The spiral arteriole remodelling that occurs in normal pregnancy is impaired in women with pre-eclampsia and normotensive growth restriction, reducing placental blood flow.

The innervation of the uterus is predominantly via the autonomic nervous system. The sympathetic supply from T12–L1 produces vasoconstriction and uterine contraction. The parasympathetic fibres from S2–S4 stimulate vasodilation and uterine relaxation (42). These effects are modulated by hormonal effects. The uterus also has afferent nerve supplies with the main sensory fibres of the cervix arising from S1–S2, and from the uterus from T11–T12. Ferguson's reflex describes the afferent pathway from the cervix to the hypothalamus whereby stretching of the cervix simulates release of oxytocin (43).

The pregnant human myometrium has spontaneous electrical activity which is generated from pacemaker cells then transmitted over the whole of the uterus (13). Gap junctions are low-resistance connections between two cells that allow rapid propagation of electrical activity allowing synchronous contraction across the myometrium (44). The continuation of successful pregnancy is dependent on myometrial quiescence until term. The myometrium in pregnancy has much greater compliance than non-pregnant myometrium. Therefore, despite the growing fetus distending the uterus, intra-uterine pressure does not increase until the maximal active tension is reached. This quiescence is promoted by a reduction in pacemaker activity, cell excitability, and cell connections. The exact mechanism for this remains to be elucidated. Nitric oxide is associated with uterine quiescence via cyclic guanosine monophosphate channels (45). In addition, a number of hormones such as prostacyclin, calcitonin gene-related peptide, and progesterone are thought to maintain quiescence by increasing the resting membrane potential and impairing conduction of electrical activity.

Uterine contractions are measurable as early as 7 weeks of gestation; although these are very high frequency (two per minute), they are very low intensity (1–1.5 kPa) (46). These continue until approximately 20 weeks' gestation before gradually increasing in frequency and amplitude until term (46). These are often felt by the mother as Braxton Hicks contractions. The sensitivity of the uterus to oxytocin is dependent on the gestational age (46, 47). Prior to 20 weeks' gestation the uterus is insensitive to oxytocin and following 30 weeks' gestation, sensitivity is markedly increased. Considerable individual variability exists and therefore oxytocin infusion rates can only be calculated based on the rates of uterine activity (47). In contrast, prostaglandins can induce contractions at any gestational age, by directly affecting myometrial cyclic adenosine monophosphate or calcium mobilization.

As uterine activity increases during pregnancy, the cervix softens and the canal dilates. In late gestation, the fetus continues to grow but the uterus stops growing, therefore tension across the uterine wall increases. This stimulates the expression of oxytocin and prostaglandin receptors, sodium channels, and gap junction proteins in preparation for labour. Downregulation of progesterone and the

other factors associated with uterine quiescence also occurs. Uterine involution occurs rapidly in the few days following delivery, reducing the total weight of the uterus by about 50% in 7 days.

Clinical considerations

- Cervical changes can be used to predict gestation of labour in prematurity but great individual variation does occur in low-risk women and therefore cervical changes are poor predictors of the gestation at which labour will start.
- The pain of labour is primarily due to cervical dilatation. While Braxton Hicks contractions can be high pressure and cause discomfort they are not normally associated with pain, and changes in the cervix are relied on to indicate possible labour.
- The stretched lower segment of the uterus is relatively avascular and thin which makes it the place of choice for incision at caesarean section as it recovers well and is less prone to rupture in future pregnancies. However, the lack of muscle fibres in this segment means that women with placenta praevia are at risk of excessive bleeding from the vascular placental bed as the lower segment struggles to contract adequately and constrict the vessels.
- Evidence that progesterone is involved in maintaining uterine quiescence during pregnancy is supported by several large trials and meta-analyses suggesting that progesterone may prevent or delay preterm labour in those at high risk (48, 49). In addition, progesterone antagonists such as mifepristone can induce labour.

Changes in the renal system

In pregnancy the renal parenchymal volume increases by 70% by the third trimester. Both the vascular volume and the interstitial space increases with the most dramatic anatomical changes in dilatation of the calyces, renal pelvis and ureter (50). These changes occur in the first trimester due to the hormonal changes in pregnancy. The changes are more prominent on the right side due to anatomical distribution. As pregnancy progresses the uterus may cause partial ureteric obstruction as it compresses the ureters at the pelvic brim. There is hypertrophy of the ureteric smooth muscle and hyperplasia of the connective tissue, ureteral peristalsis is unchanged.

Renal blood flow and GFR are both increased during a normal ovulatory menstrual cycle. If conception occurs these changes are maintained, thus renal blood flow increases by 50–80% in the first trimester (51, 52). This is maintained in the second trimester and decreases by 15% during the third trimester. GFR also increases in the first trimester and then is maintained until delivery although the extent of increase is less than that of renal blood flow. These changes are shown in **Figure 8.3**. Changes in the 24-hour creatinine clearance are a convenient method of assessing probable change in the GFR. By 4 weeks of gestation, the 24-hour creatinine clearance has increased by 25% and by 9 weeks, by 45% (51). During the third trimester there is a steady decrease towards non-pregnant values (53). A small increase in the GFR and creatinine clearance is seen in the initial few days following delivery (53).

The increase in plasma volume in pregnancy is secondary to water retention. Very early in pregnancy the plasma osmolality decreases to about 10 mOsm/kg less than prepregnancy (54). In the

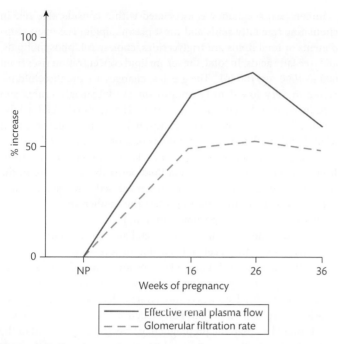

Figure 8.3 The changes in renal function during pregnancy are largely complete by the end of the first trimester and are thus proactive not reactive to the demands of pregnancy. The filtration fraction falls during the first trimester but begins to return to non-pregnant (NP) levels during the third trimester.

Reproduced from Chamberlain G & Broughton Pipkin F (eds); *Clinical Physiology In Obstetrics*; 3rd edn; Blackwell Science; 1998 with permission from Blackwell.

non-pregnant state, this reduction in plasma sodium and anions would inhibit antidiuretic hormone arginine vasopressin (AVP) release, therefore causing diuresis. However, in pregnancy the osmotic thresholds are reduced by 4–6 weeks of pregnancy, stimulating water intake and diluting bodily fluids (54). These changes are thought to be secondary to human chorionic gonadotropin. AVP continues to circulate at a sufficient concentration to stimulate water reabsorption from the renal medullary collecting ducts until the plasma osmolality decreases below the new threshold of pregnancy. Renal sodium handling is the prime determinant of volume haemostasis. In pregnancy, there is an accumulation of approximately 950 mmol of sodium in the fetus and the mother's extracellular volume. This retention occurs very gradually by just 3–4 mmol of sodium a day. It is thought to occur as a result of high circulating concentrations of progesterone acting at the distal tubule, increased natriuretic prostacyclin, atrial natriuretic peptide, and plasma prolactin. Despite this, plasma concentration of sodium is reduced by approximately 4–5 mmol/L in pregnancy due to the increase in plasma volume.

Clinical considerations

- Vesicoureteric reflux occurs in at least 3% of pregnant women due to the lateral displacement of the ureters and shortened intravesical portion. The presence of ureteric dilatation in combination with vesicoureteric reflux is associated with a high incidence of urinary stasis which may cause urinary tract infection in pregnancy.

- The normal kidney is increased in size by 1 cm in pregnancy. Dilatation of the ureters may persist until 16 weeks after delivery.
- The significant increase in GFR and plasma volume cause a reduction in the plasma concentration of solutes such as creatinine and urea. Interpretation of laboratory reports should always take this into consideration as using non-pregnant thresholds incorrectly during pregnancy may lead to failure to identify decreased renal function. Serum creatinine decreases from an average of 73 mmol/L to 65, 51, and 47 mmol/L in the successive trimesters of pregnancy (52).
- Renal tubular function also changes significantly during pregnancy. Uric acid filtration doubles and there is a decrease in net tubular reabsorption, thus serum uric acid concentrations decrease by 25% by mid pregnancy. At later gestations, less filtered uric acid is excreted so a rise in serum concentrations is normal (52). The normal pregnancy range of serum uric acid is 148–298 μmol/L.
- Glucose excretion increases during pregnancy by tenfold. Intermittent glycosuria is a normal feature of pregnancy and not helpful in the diagnosis of diabetes mellitus which requires assessment of blood glucose (52).
- The excretion of amino acids also increases although the pattern of excretion is not constant and differs for individual amino acids. This is due to inadequate tubular reabsorption to cope with the 50% increase in GFR.
- Excretion of total protein and albumin rises during pregnancy until at least 36 weeks. In late pregnancy, the upper limit of normal is 200 mg per 24 hours of urine collection (55).
- Despite increased reabsorption of calcium from the renal tubules, urinary calcium excretion is two- to threefold higher in normal pregnancy compared to prepregnancy. This is thought to be secondary to the increased concentrations of 1,25-dihydroxyvitamin D. Renal bicarbonate reabsorption and hydrogen ion excretion remain the same, therefore the urine is usually mildly alkaline in pregnancy.

Changes in the gastrointestinal and hepatic systems

Gastric emptying is delayed in pregnancy due to reduced gastric secretions and gastric motility. The reduced motility is experienced in both the small and large bowel and colonic absorption of water and sodium is increased, contributing to increased rates of constipation in pregnancy. The lower oesophageal sphincter may be displaced through the diaphragm and this combined with the increased intra-abdominal pressure can contribute to increased heartburn experienced in pregnancy. In addition, this increases the risk of aspiration of gastric contents during induction of anaesthesia.

The gallbladder increases in size and releases bile more slowly in pregnancy but the amount of bile excreted is unchanged. Increased progesterone concentrations reduce the levels of cholecystokinin and contractile response to cholecystokinin. Therefore, cholestasis is almost physiological in pregnancy but should not be high enough to cause jaundice.

Nutrition in pregnancy

The average weight gain in pregnancy in a woman of a normal BMI is 12.5 kg although this varies greatly between individuals. This increase in weight is due to increased blood volume and retention of water, the increased size of maternal tissues such as uterus and breasts, the products of conception, and greater maternal fat stores. The basal metabolic rate increases by approximately 5% by term in a woman of a normal BMI (56). Total fat deposited by the mother is between 2 and 6 kg. This is stored during the second trimester in preparation for the increased metabolic demands of late pregnancy and lactation (57). This process is regulated by the hormone leptin which alerts the brain to the extent of the fat stores. Recent studies suggest that the sensitivity of the brain to the effects of leptin is reduced in pregnancy, allowing the mother to deposit greater fat stores (58).

Following delivery there is immediate weight loss of 6 kg associated with delivery of the baby and other products of conception. Diuresis of the water retained in pregnancy occurs in the days following delivery. From day 3, body weight decreases by 0.3 kg a day until day 10. This stabilizes at 10 weeks after delivery where weight is approximately 2.3 kg greater than prepregnancy weight. The average weight gain at 6–18 months after delivery is 1–2 kg but in approximately 20% of women this is greater than 5 kg (59).

In pregnancy, the total protein concentration decreases by about 1 g/dL during the first trimester and then plateaus. This represents a reduction from 7 to 6 g/dL. Albumin concentration decreases more dramatically in the first and second trimester then more slowly until late pregnancy. Typically, this represents a reduction from 3.5 to 2.5 g/100 mL. It is this that causes the majority of the decrease in total protein content; the reason is unknown. The decrease in albumin concentration causes a reduction in total plasma calcium but unbound ionized calcium levels are unchanged. Increased synthesis of 1,25-dihydroxycholecalciferol promotes increased calcium absorption from the intestines. This is doubled by 24 weeks but then plateaus.

In contrast, pregnancy is associated with a considerable rise in circulating free fatty acids and most plasma lipids. The main components of total lipids are triglycerides, cholesterol, phospholipids, and free fatty acids. In total, the serum lipid concentration rises from 600 to 1000 mg/100 mL. The greatest changes are the threefold increase in very low-density lipoprotein (VLDL) triglycerides and 50% increase in VLDL cholesterol (60). The levels of VLDL triglyceride directly correlates to the birthweight and placental weight at term. Lipids undergo peroxidation as part of normal cellular function. Excess production of lipid peroxidases causes oxidative stress. In normal pregnancy, the plasma lipid peroxidases increase in the second trimester but there are also increased endogenous antioxidants which are thought to protect the mother and prevent the atherogenic effects of hyperlipidaemia (61).

Glucose is the main substrate for fetal growth and nutrition and it readily crosses the placenta. Fetal glucose levels are closely correlated with maternal levels but are 15–20% lower. Blood glucose levels in the mother are regulated by insulin which is increased in pregnancy. Longitudinal studies demonstrate a decrease in plasma glucose levels in pregnancy, a nadir is reached at 12 weeks of gestation at 0.5–1 mmol less than the prepregnancy level (62). By the end of the first trimester, the increase in blood glucose following a carbohydrate load is less than outside pregnancy (62). Increased resistance to the action of insulin develops from mid pregnancy and plasma glucose concentrations rise towards term, although normally remaining below that of non-pregnant levels—this is shown in **Figure 8.4**. This reduced sensitivity to insulin is thought to be driven by human placental lactogen or cortisol. As well as moving glucose into cells, transport of amino acids and free fatty acids is also increased.

Clinical considerations

Obesity is associated with pre-existing insulin resistance which increases under the influence of pregnancy hormones, therefore much higher insulin levels are required to prevent glucose levels

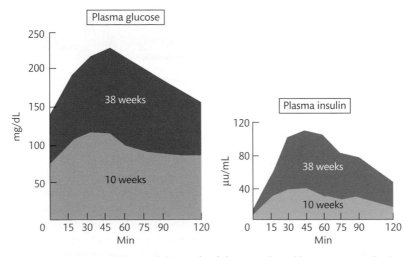

Figure 8.4 Responses in normal pregnant women to a 50 g oral glucose load during early and late pregnancy. During early pregnancy, there is a normal plasma insulin response with a relative reduction in plasma glucose concentration compared to the non-pregnant state. In contrast, during late pregnancy, plasma glucose concentrations reach higher levels after a delay despite a considerably enhanced insulin response, a pattern which could be explained by relative resistance to insulin.

from rising. More marked insulin resistance in pregnancy will cause chronically elevated blood glucose and be classified as gestational diabetes.

Physiology of the breasts

High concentrations of oestrogen, growth hormone, and glucocorticoids stimulate the breast ducts to proliferate during pregnancy. Progesterone and prolactin stimulate alveolar growth (63). From 3–4 months until the first 30 hours after delivery the breasts secrete a thick, protein-rich fluid called colostrum. This is stimulated by prolactin and placental lactogen. During pregnancy, the high levels of oestrogen and progesterone prevent alveolar transcription of alpha-lactalbumin, the protein contained in milk, thus preventing full lactation. Following delivery, the sudden decrease in progesterone and oestrogen levels allows prolactin to act directly on the alveolar cells to stimulate synthesis of milk (64). Suckling sends impulses to the hypothalamus which stimulates release of prolactin and oxytocin. By day 5 after delivery, milk production is at full flow of approximately 500–1000 ml/24 hours (65). This demands an additional 500 kcal intake per day of the mother. Oxytocin causes the myoepithelial cells to contract and milk to be ejected. This reflex may be inhibited by catecholamine release or adverse environmental or emotional factors (66).

Clinical considerations

- Dopamine antagonists such as bromocriptine act as prolactin antagonists and prevent milk production.

Endocrine changes in pregnancy

The placenta

There are significant changes in all maternal endocrine organs in pregnancy. These changes are dominated by the considerable production of sex steroids produced by the placenta. Human chorionic gonadotropin is the signal for pregnancy that stimulates physiological changes. High levels of oestrogen stimulate increased hepatic synthesis of binding globulins such as thyroid-binding globulin, which is doubled by the end of the first trimester, and cortisol-binding globulin, which is doubled by the end of pregnancy; these also impact the mother's wider endocrinological function.

Large amounts of oestrogen and progesterone are produced by the fetoplacental unit. These are important for uterine growth and quiescence. Oestrogens stimulate the synthesis of vascular endothelial growth factor and angiogenesis. This in turn interacts with angiopoietin-2 and other placentally derived hormones which are vital in the formation of the villous capillary bed in early pregnancy. The human villous and extravillous cytotrophoblasts express the peroxisome proliferator-activated receptor gamma. This is a nuclear receptor that binds eicosanoids, fatty acids, and oxidized low-density lipoproteins which is essential for placental development (67).

The hypothalamus and pituitary

The pituitary gland increases in weight by 30% in nulliparous women and by 50% in multiparous women. This increase is largely due to

changes in the anterior pituitary. The anterior pituitary produces three glycoproteins: luteinizing hormone (LH), follicular-stimulating hormone (FSH), and thyroid-stimulating hormone (TSH). It also produces three polypeptide and peptide hormones: growth hormone (GH), prolactin, and adrenocorticotropic hormone (ACTH). The elevated oestrogen levels in pregnancy cause an increase in the number of lactotrophs. Within a few days of conception, plasma prolactin concentrations begin to increase and this continues steadily until a surge at the time of delivery and subsequent decrease. By term, prolactin concentrations are increased 10–20 times compared to non-pregnancy (68). They remain raised above basal levels while breastfeeding. All other anterior pituitary hormones are either relatively constant or reduced. The high concentration of human chorionic gonadotropin suppresses secretion of FSH and LH thus inhibiting ovarian follicle development. TSH remains constant. ACTH concentrations rise but remain within the normal non-pregnant range. This rise is due to placental synthesis of ACTH and corticotropin-releasing hormone (CRH) which is normally produced in the hypothalamus. Therefore, ACTH does not respond to normal control mechanisms in pregnancy. Plasma levels of CRH increase in the third trimester and are thought to be a potential trigger for labour.

The posterior pituitary releases AVP and oxytocin. Renal clearance of AVP is increased (see 'Changes in the renal system'). Oxytocin concentrations are low during pregnancy and their effects on uterine contractility were described earlier in 'Changes in uterine physiology'.

The thyroid and parathyroids

The thyroid gland enlarges in up to 70% of pregnant women; this varies according to iodine intake. Iodine uptake by the thyroid is increased threefold, urine excretion increases, and iodothyronines are transferred to the fetus, thus plasma inorganic iodide levels in the mother decrease (69). Concentrations of thyroid-binding globulin double in pregnancy (70). Concentrations of total tri-iodothyronine (T_3) and thyroxine (T_4) are increased in very early pregnancy then decrease to the non-pregnant range. T_3, T_4, and TSH do not cross the placental barrier and therefore have no direct effect on fetal thyroid function.

Calcitonin, also produced in the thyroid, increases during the first trimester, peaks in the second, and then decreases. It may contribute to the regulation of 1,25-dihydroxyvitamin D. Parathyroid hormone (PTH), produced by the parathyroids, regulates synthesis of 1,25-dihydroxyvitamin D in the proximal convoluted tubule. During pregnancy, the placenta and the fetal parathyroid gland produce PTH-related protein which also affects calcium homeostasis by acting on PTH receptors.

Renal hormones

The RAS is activated from very early pregnancy as explored earlier in the cardiovascular section. Angiotensin II acts through directly opposing receptors. AT_1 receptors promote angiogenesis hypertrophy and vasoconstriction. AT_2 receptors promote apoptosis. It is thought that AT_2 expression dominates in early pregnancy implantation and vascular remodelling (71).

Adrenal hormones

In pregnancy, the rise in ACTH stimulates cortisol synthesis and there is a rise in total plasma cortisol concentrations from the end of the first trimester. Concentrations of cortisol-binding globulin double but despite this, the concentration of free cortisol also increases during pregnancy and the diurnal variation is lost (72). Excess glucocorticoid exposure to the growing fetus inhibits fetal growth. However, the normal placenta synthesizes 11β-hydroxysteroid dehydrogenase which inhibits the transfer of maternal cortisol to the fetus. High circulating oestrogen increases the production of sex hormone-binding globulin which in turn results in an increase in total testosterone levels (73). Plasma catecholamine concentrations decrease from the first to the third trimester.

Clinical considerations

- Most women are euthyroid in pregnancy.
- Grave's hyperthyroidism is often improved in pregnancy with a reduction in the antibody titre. Maternal thyroid disease usually does not directly affect the fetus. However, if this does not occur, antibodies will cross the placenta, stimulating the fetal thyroid. This can be evidenced by signs of fetal hyperthyroidism such as tachycardia, intrauterine growth restriction, and cardiac failure. In addition, iodine is required for fetal thyroid growth and antithyroid drugs do cross the placenta. The fetus can also be affected by the implications of autoimmune thyroid disease.
- Labour is associated with massive increases in adrenaline and noradrenaline as a result of stress and muscle activity.

REFERENCES

1. Hytten F. Blood volume changes in normal pregnancy. *Obstet Gynecol Surv* 1986;**41**:426–28.
2. Pirani BB, Campbell DM, MacGillivray I. Plasma volume in normal first pregnancy. *J Obstet Gynaecol Br Commonw* 1973;**80**:884–87.
3. Hays PM, Cruikshank DP, Dunn LJ. Plasma volume determination in normal and preeclamptic pregnancies. *Am J Obstet Gynecol* 1985;**151**:958–66.
4. Hytten FE, Leitch I. *The Physiology of Human Pregnancy*, 2nd edn. Oxford: Blackwell Scientific Publications Ltd; 1971.
5. Rovinsky JJ, Jaffin H. Cardiovascular hemodynamics in pregnancy. I. Blood and plasma volumes in multiple pregnancy. *Am J Obstet Gynecol* 1965;**93**:1–15.
6. Milman N, Agger AO, Nielsen OJ. Iron status markers and serum erythropoietin in 120 mothers and newborn infants. Effect of iron supplementation in normal pregnancy. *Acta Obstet Gynecol Scand* 1994;**73**:200–204.
7. Jepson JH, Friesen HG. The mechanism of action of human placental lactogen on erythropoiesis. *Br J Haematol* 1968;**15**:465–71.
8. Cruickshank JM, Morris R, Butt WR, Crooke AC. The relationship of total and differential leukocyte counts with urinary oestrogen and plasma cortisol levels. *J Obstet Gynaecol Br Commonw* 1970;**77**:634–39.
9. Brain P, Marston RH, Gordon J. Immunological responses in pregnancy. *Br Med J* 1972;**4**:488.
10. Hill CA, Finn R, Denye V. Depression of cellular immunity in pregnancy due to a serum factor. *Br Med J* 1973;**3**:513–14.
11. Moffett A, Hiby SE. How does the maternal immune system contribute to the development of pre-eclampsia? *Placenta* 2007;**28** Suppl A:S51–56.
12. Wiman B, Csemiczky G, Marsk L, Robbe H. The fast inhibitor of tissue plasminogen activator in plasma during pregnancy. *Thromb Haemost* 1984;**52**:124–26.
13. Chamberlain G, Broughton-Pipkin F. *Clinical Physiology in Obstetrics*, 3rd edn. Oxford: Blackwell Science; 1998.
14. Salerni S, Di Francescomarino S, Cadeddu C, Acquistapace F, Maffei S, Gallina S. The different role of sex hormones on female cardiovascular physiology and function: not only oestrogens. *Eur J Clin Invest* 2015;**45**:634–45.
15. Lieberman EH, Gerhard MD, Uehata A, et al. Estrogen improves endothelium-dependent, flow-mediated vasodilation in postmenopausal women. *Ann Intern Med* 1994;**121**:936–41.
16. Beldekas JC, Smith B, Gerstenfeld LC, Sonenshein GE, Franzblau C. Effects of 17 beta-estradiol on the biosynthesis of collagen in cultured bovine aortic smooth muscle cells. *Biochemistry* 1981;**20**:2162–67.
17. Rylance PB, Brincat M, Lafferty K, et al. Natural progesterone and antihypertensive action. *Br Med J (Clin Res Ed)* 1985;**290**:13–14.
18. Fawer R, Dettling A, Weihs D, Welti H, Schelling JL. Effect of the menstrual cycle, oral contraception and pregnancy on forearm blood flow, venous distensibility and clotting factors. *Eur J Clin Pharmacol* 1978;**13**:251–57.
19. Abdul-Karim R, Assalin S. Pressor response to angiotonin in pregnant and nonpregnant women. *Am J Obstet Gynecol* 1961;**82**:246–51.
20. Assali NS, Westersten A. Regional flow-pressure relationship in response to angiotensin in the intact dog and sheep. *Circ Res* 1961;**9**:189–93.
21. Merrill DC, Karoly M, Chen K, Ferrario CM, Brosnihan KB. Angiotensin-(1-7) in normal and preeclamptic pregnancy. *Endocrine* 2002;**18**:239–45.
22. Clark SL, Cotton DB, Lee W, et al. Central hemodynamic assessment of normal term pregnancy. *Am J Obstet Gynecol* 1989;**161**:1439–42.
23. Robson SC, Boys RJ, Hunter S, Dunlop W. Maternal hemodynamics after normal delivery and delivery complicated by postpartum hemorrhage. *Obstet Gynecol* 1989;**74**:234–39.
24. Hunter S, Robson SC. Adaptation of the maternal heart in pregnancy. *Br Heart J* 1992;**68**:540–43.
25. Edmonds DK, Dewhurst CJS (eds). *Dewhurst's Textbook of Obstetrics & Gynaecology*, 7th edn. Malden, MA: Blackwell; 2007.
26. Robson SC, Hunter S, Boys RJ, Dunlop W. Serial study of factors influencing changes in cardiac output during human pregnancy. *Am J Physiol* 1989;**256**:H1060–65.
27. Laird-Meeter K, van de Ley G, Bom TH, Wladimiroff JW, Roelandt J. Cardiocirculatory adjustments during pregnancy – an echocardiographic study. *Clin Cardiol* 1979;**2**:328–32.
28. Rubler S, Damani PM, Pinto ER. Cardiac size and performance during pregnancy estimated with echocardiography. *Am J Cardiol* 1977;**40**:534–40.
29. Campos O. Doppler echocardiography during pregnancy: physiological and abnormal findings. *Echocardiography* 1996;**13**:135–46.
30. Hollander AG, Crawford JH. Roentgenologic and electrocardiographic changes in the normal heart during pregnancy. *Am Heart J* 1943;**26**:364–76.
31. Greenhill JP. Cardiodynamic and electrocardiographic changes in normal pregnancy. *Am J Obstet Gynecol* 1938;**36**:353.
32. Asher UA, Ben-Shlomo I, Said M, Nabil H. The effects of exercise induced tachycardia on the maternal electrocardiogram. *Br J Obstet Gynaecol* 1993;**100**:41–45.
33. van Doorn MB, Lotgering FK, Struijk PC, Pool J, Wallenburg HC. Maternal and fetal cardiovascular responses to strenuous bicycle exercise. *Am J Obstet Gynecol* 1992;**166**:854–59.

34. Pernoll ML, Metcalfe J, Kovach PA, Wachtel R, Dunham MJ. Ventilation during rest and exercise in pregnancy and post-partum. *Respir Physiol* 1975;**25**:295–310.

35. Puranik BM, Kaore SB, Kurhade GA, et al. A longitudinal study of pulmonary function tests during pregnancy. *Indian J Physiol Pharmacol* 1994;**38**:129–32.

36. Machida H. Influence of progesterone on arterial blood and CSF acid-base balance in women. *J Appl Physiol Respir Environ Exerc Physiol* 1981;**51**:1433–36.

37. Lucius H, Gahlenbeck H, Kleine HO, Fabel H, Bartels H. Respiratory functions, buffer system, and electrolyte concentrations of blood during human pregnancy. *Respir Physiol* 1970;**9**:311–17.

38. Gazioglu K, Kaltreider NL, Rosen M, Yu PN. Pulmonary function during pregnancy in normal women and in patients with cardio-pulmonary disease. *Thorax* 1970;**25**:445–50.

39. Rubin A, Russo N, Goucher D. The effect of pregnancy upon pulmonary function in normal women. *Am J Obstet Gynecol* 1956;**72**:963–69.

40. Von Ungern-Sternberg BS, Regli A, Bucher E, Reber A, Schneider MC. Impact of spinal anaesthesia and obesity on maternal respiratory function during elective caesarean section. *Anaesthesia* 2004;**59**:743–49.

41. Burton GJ, Jauniaux E, Charnock-Jones DS. Human early placental development: potential roles of the endometrial glands. *Placenta* 2007;**28** Suppl:S64–S9.

42. Davies DV, Davies F (eds). *Gray's Anatomy*, 3rd edn. London: Longman; 1964.

43. Ferguson JKW. A study of the motility of the intact uterus at term. *Surg Gynaecol Obstet* 1941;**73**:359–66.

44. Bala GA, Thakur NR, Bleasdale JE. Characterization of the major phosphoinositide-specific phospholipase C of human amnion. *Biol Reprod* 1990;**43**:704–11.

45. Morris NH, Eaton BM, Dekker G. Nitric oxide, the endothelium, pregnancy and pre-eclampsia. *BJOG* 1996;**103**:4–15.

46. Csapo A, Sauvage J. The evolution of uterine activity during human pregnancy. *Acta Obstet Gynecol Scand* 1968;**47**:181–212.

47. Embrey MP. The effects of intravenous oxytocin on uterine contractility. *BJOG* 1962;**69**:910–17.

48. Romero R, Nicolaides K, Conde-Agudelo A, et al. Vaginal progesterone in women with an asymptomatic sonographic short cervix in the midtrimester decreases preterm delivery and neonatal morbidity: a systematic review and metaanalysis of individual patient data. *Am J Obstet Gynecol* **206**:124.e1–e19.

49. Dodd JM, Flenady VJ, Cincotta R, Crowther CA. Progesterone for the prevention of preterm birth: a systematic review. *Obstet Gynecol* 2008;**112**:127–34.

50. Fried AM. Hydronephrosis of pregnancy: ultrasonographic study and classification of asymptomatic women. *Am J Obstet Gynecol* 1979;**135**:1066–70.

51. Davison JM, Noble MCB. Serial changes in 24 hour creatinine clearance during normal menstrual cycles and the first trimester of pregnancy. *BJOG* 1981;**88**:10–17.

52. Sturgiss SN, Dunlop W, Davison JM. Renal haemodynamics and tubular function in human pregnancy. *Baillieres Clin Obstet Gynaecol* 1994;**8**:209–34.

53. Ezimokhai M, Davison JM, Philips PR, Dunlop W. Non-postural serial changes in renal function during the third trimester of normal human pregnancy. *BJOG* 1981;**88**:465–71.

54. Davison JM, Vallotton MB, Lindheimer MD. Plasma osmolality and urinary concentration and dilution during and after pregnancy: evidence that lateral recumbency inhibits maximal urinary concentrating ability. *Br J Obstet Gynaecol* 1981;**88**:472–79.

55. Symonds I, Arulkumaran S (eds). *Essential Obstetrics and Gynaecology*, 5th edn. Edinburgh: Churchill Livingstone; 2013.

56. Butte NF, King JC. Energy requirements during pregnancy and lactation. *Public Health Nutr* 2005;**8**:1010–27.

57. Kopp-Hoolihan LE, van Loan MD, Wong WW, King JC. Longitudinal assessment of energy balance in well-nourished, pregnant women. *Am J Clin Nutr* 1999;**69**:697–704.

58. Hauguel-de Mouzon S, Lepercq J, Catalano P. The known and unknown of leptin in pregnancy. *Am J Obstet Gynecol* 2006;**194**:1537–45.

59. Gunderson EP, Abrams B, Selvin S. Does the pattern of postpartum weight change differ according to pregravid body size? *Int J Obes Relat Metab Disord* 2001;**25**:853–62.

60. Herrera E, Ortega H, Alvino G, Giovannini N, Amusquivar E, Cetin I. Relationship between plasma fatty acid profile and antioxidant vitamins during normal pregnancy. *Eur J Clin Nutr* 2004;**58**:1231–38.

61. Poston L, Raijmakers MT. Trophoblast oxidative stress, antioxidants and pregnancy outcome – a review. *Placenta* 2004;**25** Suppl A:S72–78.

62. Lind T, Billewicz WZ, Brown G. A serial study of changes occurring in the oral glucose tolerance test during pregnancy. *BJOG* 1973;**80**:1033–39.

63. Ormandy CJ, Binart N, Kelly PA. Mammary gland development in prolactin receptor knockout mice. *J Mammary Gland Biol Neoplasia* 1997;**2**:355–64.

64. Kuhn NJ. Progesterone withdrawal as the lactogenic trigger in the rat. *J Endocrinol* 1969;**44**:39–54.

65. Neville MC, Allen JC, Archer PC, et al. Studies in human lactation: milk volume and nutrient composition during weaning and lactogenesis. *Am J Clin Nutr* 1991;**54**:81–92.

66. Chen DC, Nommsen-Rivers L, Dewey KG, Lönnerdal B. Stress during labor and delivery and early lactation performance. *Am J Clin Nutr* 1998;**68**:335–44.

67. Schaiff WT, Carlson MG, Smith SD, Levy R, Nelson DM, Sadovsky Y. Peroxisome proliferator-activated receptor-γ modulates differentiation of human trophoblast in a ligand-specific manner. *J Clin Endocrinol Metab* 2000;**85**:3874–81.

68. Rigg LA, Lein A, Yen SS. Pattern of increase in circulating prolactin levels during human gestation. *Am J Obstet Gynecol* 1977;**129**:454–56.

69. Aboul-Khair SA, Crooks J, Turnbull AC, Hytten FE. The physiological changes in thyroid function during pregnancy. *Clin Sci* 1964;**27**:195–207.

70. Man EB, Reid WA, Hellegers AE, Jones WS. Thyroid function in human pregnancy. 3. Serum thyroxine-binding prealbumin (TBPA) and thyroxine-binding globulin (TBG) of pregnant women aged 14 through 43 years. *Am J Obstet Gynecol* 1969;**103**:338–47.

71. Cooper AC, Robinson G, Vinson GP, Cheung WT, Broughton Pipkin F. The localization and expression of the renin–angiotensin system in the human placenta throughout pregnancy. *Placenta* 1999;**20**:467–74.

72. Carr BR, Parker CR Jr, Madden JD, MacDonald PC, Porter JC. Maternal plasma adrenocorticotropin and cortisol relationships throughout human pregnancy. *Am J Obstet Gynecol* 1981;**139**:416–22.

73. O'Leary P, Boyne P, Flett P, Beilby J, James I. Longitudinal assessment of changes in reproductive hormones during normal pregnancy. *Clin Chem* 1991;**37**:667–72.

9

The placenta

Eric Jauniaux, Amarnath Bhide, and Graham J. Burton

Introduction

The word 'placenta' comes from the Latin term for 'cake'. Historians and cultural anthropologists have explored cross-cultural beliefs and practices that invest the afterbirth with symbolic value, whether it is buried, burned, frozen, or eaten (1). The first known representation of a human placenta can be found on the Narmer Palette (**Figure 9.1**). Narmer was an Egyptian pharaoh of the Early Dynastic Period (31st century BC) and the ancient Egyptians believed the placenta to be the 'seat of the human soul'. The placenta was mummified immediately after the birth of the future pharaoh, used in dynastic processions, and buried in the tomb at the time of the pharaoh's death.

The development of a placenta is characteristic of those mammalian species called the 'placentals'. True placentals probably originated after the significant extinction horizon known as the Cretaceous–Paleogene event 66–65 million years ago (2). The majority of mammals are placentals, meaning that their fetus (or fetuses) is nourished by the placenta during the entire pregnancy and develops entirely inside the placental membranes. In most mammals, the yolk sac and chorion combine to form a choriovitelline placenta to support the early embryo, although a chorioallantoic placenta soon supplants this. Humans and haplorrhine primates follow a second pattern where precocious development of the extraembryonic mesoderm leads to formation of a secondary yolk sac within the exocoelom (3).

Scientific investigations of the development, structure, and function of the placenta can be traced to antiquity (4). An issue of importance that was only resolved in the late eighteenth century is that of the separate nature of the maternal and fetal placental circulations. The breakthrough came in 1754, when John Hunter (1728–1793), who is considered the father of modern surgery, injected coloured molten wax into the vessels of the umbilical cord and the uterine arteries and veins during autopsies of pregnant women (4). Assisted by Colin MacKenzie (died 1775), he demonstrated conclusively that the maternal and fetal circulations are separated, thus putting to rest a debate that had gripped anatomists for many centuries, including Galen (130–210), Leonardo Da Vinci (1452–1519), and Vesalius (1514–1564).

Twentieth-century researchers have established that the placenta in mammals is the essential interface between the maternal circulation carrying oxygen-rich blood and nutrients, and the fetal circulation. No organ can match the placenta for the diversity of its functions, since it performs the actions of all the major organ systems while these differentiate and mature in the fetus (5). During the course of a pregnancy, it acts as the lungs, gut, kidneys, and liver of the fetus. The placenta also has major endocrine actions that modulate maternal physiology and metabolism.

From the perspective of laypeople, the twentieth-century perception of the placental barrier that is most readily available is a simple one: 'we' once thought that the fetus was protected from external insult by the placenta (1). Recent changes in human environmental habitats caused by pollution, habits such as smoking, and the increased use of medical and recreational drugs have challenged the concept of a complete protective role of the placental barrier. The thalidomide and diethylstilbestrol teratogenic catastrophes tragically illustrate its limitations (1, 5). By contrast, recent data from metagenomic sequencing show that the placenta is frequently colonized with maternal commensal bacteria during pregnancy, and indicate the selective role of the placental barrier and indirectly its additional metabolic and immune contributions to the developing fetus (6).

Aberrations of placental function are widely recognized as having immediate consequences on the outcome of a pregnancy, and more recently for influencing the lifelong health of the offspring. It is notable, for example, that the placenta grows more slowly during the first trimester in pregnancies that subsequently go on to miscarry or are associated with fetal growth restriction (FGR) than in normal cases (7). Recent changes in human lifestyle, such as delayed childbirth and hypercaloric diets, may have increased the global incidence of placental-related disorders over the last decades. However, the fact that populations of hunter-gatherers still in existence today are affected by these pregnancy complications suggests that they are not a direct consequence of the modern human lifestyle, but are more likely to be due to an evolutionary step in human reproduction and development (8).

This chapter presents an overview of the normal and abnormal development of the human placenta, together with a description of the physiology of placental biological functions, an analysis of the pathophysiology of placental-related disorders, and the prenatal diagnosis and management of placental and cord anomalies.

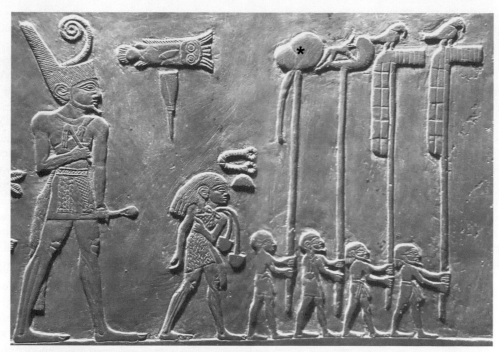

Figure 9.1 Photograph of the Narmer Palette (Early Dynastic Period; Egypt 31st century bc) showing the dynastic procession of the pharaoh Narmer preceded by a priest and four attendants, the first one carrying the placenta (star).

Placentation and normal placenta development

The development of the placenta starts from implantation, when the embryonic pole of the blastocyst enters into contact with the maternal uterine epithelium. Human placentation is almost unique amongst mammals in that it is highly invasive and the gestational sac embeds itself completely within the uterine endometrium and superficial myometrium (5, 8). Human placentation is also characterized by remodelling of the spiral arteries, during which the vessels lose their elastic lamina and smooth muscle coat, and consequently their responsiveness to circulating vasoactive compounds. At term, the spiral arteries that, in the non-pregnant state, transport just a few millilitres of blood per minute need to carry up to 600 mL per minute.

Implantation, decidualization, and anchoring

The formative stages of human placental development are largely unknown. The earliest events have never been studied *in vivo* for obvious ethical reasons (9). Implantation relies on the interaction of the trophectoderm cells forming the wall of the blastocyst with the cells of the uterine epithelium. On establishing contact, some of the trophectoderm cells undergo proliferation and fusion to form the multinucleated syncytiotrophoblast, whereas others remain as a deeper, progenitor population, the cytotrophoblast cells (10).

During the secretory phase of the menstrual cycle, the endometrium transforms into a well-vascularized receptive tissue, which is characterized by the proliferation and differentiation of the stromal cells into decidual cells, the infiltration of maternal immune cells, and vascular remodelling of the endometrial vessels (11, 12). Decidualized stromal cells are derived from the fibroblast-like cells within the endometrium. The uterine glands undergo characteristic hypersecretory morphological changes, the so-called Arias-Stella reaction under the influence of progesterone (13). Their cytoplasm contains abundant organelles and large accumulations of glycogen, an important source of nutrients for the early embryo. Their secretions are also rich in growth factors such as leukaemia inhibitory factor, vascular endothelial growth factor, epidermal growth factor, and transforming growth factor beta, which all play a role in placentation (14).

Soon after implantation, projections of syncytiotrophoblast (primitive villi) penetrate between the epithelial cells of the uterine decidua, while at the same time the endometrial stromal cells grow over and encapsulate the whole gestational sac. Strands of mononuclear cytotrophoblast start to proliferate at the fetal side of the implanted blastocyst wall (9, 10). The resulting cytotrophoblastic columns push themselves into the primitive syncytiotrophoblastic mass to form the secondary placental villi. The most distal cytotrophoblast cells break through the syncytium and spread laterally to form the cytotrophoblastic shell separating the placenta from the decidua. Cells on the outer surface of the shell differentiate into non-proliferative, cytotrophoblast cells that invade the decidual stroma, collectively called extravillous trophoblast (EVT). They differentiate primarily into interstitial and endovascular subpopulations that migrate through the decidual stroma and down the lumens of the spiral arteries respectively. The interstitial EVT invade the uterine wall as far as the inner third of the uterine myometrium, where they fuse to form multinucleated trophoblast giant cells (15). This area is known as the junctional zone.

Development of the uteroplacental circulation

The left and right uterine arteries are the main blood supply to the uterus. They ascend along the lateral aspects within the broad ligament and terminate by anastomosing with the corresponding ovarian artery. The uterine arteries give rise to arcuate arteries that pass medially and penetrate the myometrium and divide into anterior and posterior branches that run circumferentially between the outer and middle thirds of the myometrium, and anastomose freely with their counterparts from the opposite side in the midline (**Figure 9.2**). The arcuate arteries give rise to the radial arteries that are directed towards the lumen of the uterus. As they reach the junctional zone, each radial artery gives off lateral branches, the basal arteries that supply the myometrium and the deeper basalis parts of the endometrium, and continues as a spiral artery (16).

The spiral arteries are highly coiled within the decidua basalis and the deeper parts of the functionalis. As they approach the uterine cavity they rapidly narrow, and divide into several smaller branches that follow a straighter course before terminating in a capillary plexus just beneath the uterine epithelium. Each spiral artery also gives off small branches supplying the capillary plexus surrounding the

uterine glands. In the non-pregnant state, the walls of the spiral and radial arteries contain large quantities of smooth muscle equipped with a rich autonomic innervation. Hence, they are highly responsive to both exogenous and endogenous adrenergic stimuli (17).

The EVT cells penetrate the junctional zone via the action of their proteases on the intercellular ground substance, affecting its mechanical and electrophysiological properties, and changing the structure of the walls of the spiral arteries. EVT cells can first be found both within and around the spiral arteries in the central area of the placenta. They gradually extend laterally, reaching the periphery of the placenta around mid gestation. Depth-wise, the changes are maximal within the central region of the placental bed and the extent of invasion is progressively shallower towards the periphery.

The remodelling of the spiral arteries is characterized by the progressive loss of myocytes from their media and of their internal elastic laminae, which are replaced by fibrinoid material (10, 17). Consequently, these vessels lose their responsiveness to circulating

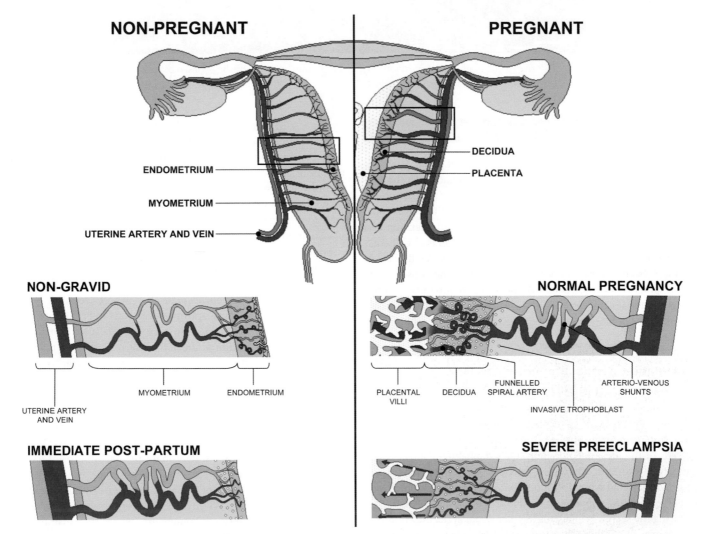

Figure 9.2 Diagrammatic representation of uterine and placental vasculature (red shading, arterial; blue shading, venous) in the non-pregnant, pregnant, and immediate postpartum state. Normal pregnancy is characterized by the formation of large arteriovenous shunts that persist in the immediate postpartum period. By contrast, pregnancies complicated by severe pre-eclampsia are characterized by minimal arteriovenous shunts and thus narrower uterine arteries. Extravillous cytotrophoblast invasion in normal pregnancy (diamonds) extends beyond the decidua into the inner myometrium resulting in the formation of funnels at the discharging tips of the spiral arteries. Contrast with severe pre-eclampsia.

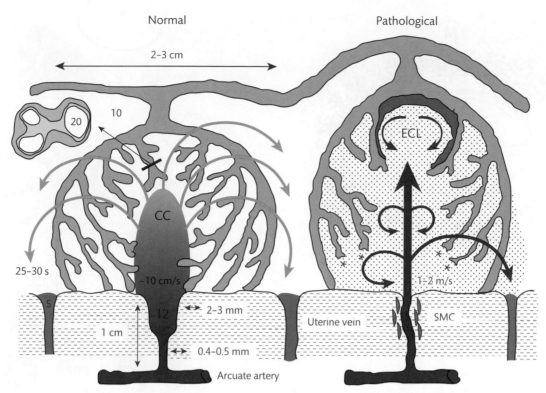

Figure 9.3 Diagrammatic representation (not to scale) of the effects of spiral artery conversion on the inflow of maternal blood into the intervillous space in normal pregnancy and in pregnancies complicated by insufficient transformation of the spiral arteries. The retention of smooth muscle cells (SMCs) around the spiral artery will increase the risk of spontaneous vasoconstriction and ischaemia–reperfusion injury CC, central cavity; ECL, echogenic cystic lesions.

Reproduced from Burton GJ, Woods AW, Jauniaux E, Kingdom JC. Rheological and physiological consequences of conversion of the maternal spiral arteries for uteroplacental blood flow during human pregnancy. *Placenta*. 2009;30:473–82 (https://creativecommons.org/licenses/by/3.0/).

vasoactive compounds and become a low-resistance network by dilatation. This transformation, termed 'physiological changes', results in the metamorphosis of small-calibre spiral vessels into flaccid distended arteries with a five- to tenfold dilation at the vessel mouth (**Figures 9.3** and **9.4**). Around 30–50 spiral arteries are transformed during the first trimester. In normal pregnancies, the transformation of spiral arteries into uteroplacental arteries is described as completed around mid gestation (17). These major anatomical changes are associated with a fall in resistance to blood flow in the uterine arterial circulation as observed by Doppler ultrasonography, and a reduction in the velocity and the pressure of the maternal blood entering the placenta (17–19). However, there is a gradient in the infiltration of the EVT along the spiral artery and even in normal pregnancies, not all spiral arteries are completely transformed (17).

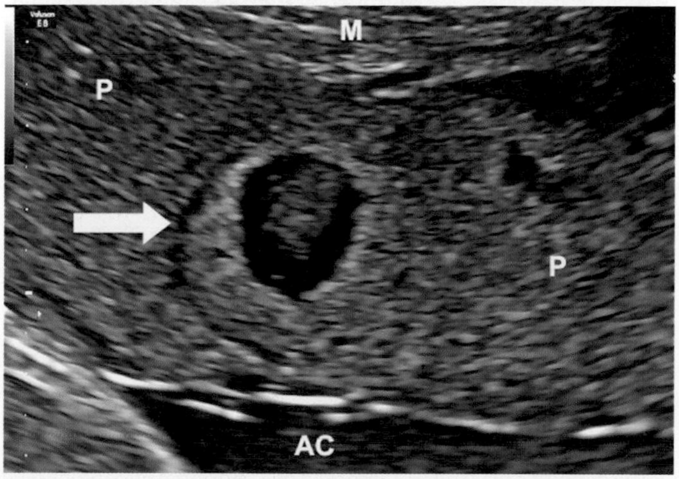

The early or primitive placenta

During the fifth week of pregnancy (third week after conception) fetal capillaries develop in the mesenchymal core of the secondary villi, transforming them into tertiary villi (20). By 6 weeks, the villous vasculature is connected with the primitive heart and the vascular plexus of the yolk sac via the vessels of the connecting stalk. The fetoplacental circulation is established from around 8 weeks of gestation but placental capillary formation will only be completed by mid gestation (20). These anatomical changes can explain the major changes in blood flow velocity waveforms obtained from the umbilical artery during that period (18). Lateral projections from the main stem villus branch repeatedly to form intermediate, and finally terminal, villi. Collectively, these are often referred to as floating villi as they are not attached to the decidua.

From the third week until about the second month of pregnancy, the entire chorion of the primitive placenta is covered with villus stems (20). Placental villi form initially over the entire surface of the chorionic sac, but starting towards the end of the first trimester the

Figure 9.4 Ultrasound view of an echogenic cystic lesion (arrow) in a pregnancy at 36 weeks complicated by late-onset pre-eclampsia. AC, amniotic cavity; M, myometrium; P, placenta.

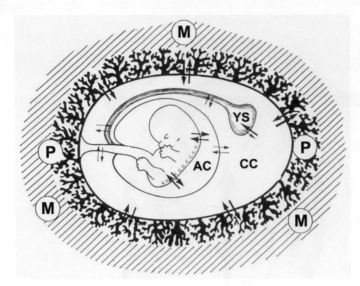

Figure 9.5 Diagram of a normal gestational sac at 8 weeks showing the outside to inside by the placental villi (P), the chorionic cavity (CC) containing the secondary yolk sac (YS), and the amniotic cavity (AC) containing the fetus. M, myometrium.

villi over the superficial pole regress, leaving the villi of definitive placenta to continue to grow. At 8 weeks, the typical normal gestational sac is composed from outside to inside by the placental villi, the extraembryonic coelom or chorionic cavity, which contains the secondary yolk sac, and the amniotic cavity, which contains the developing fetus (**Figure 9.5**). The secondary yolk sac is the first structure that can be detected ultrasonographically within the chorionic cavity. Its diameter increases slightly between 6 and 10 weeks of gestation, reaching a maximum of 6–7 mm after which it decreases (21).

Anatomically, *in vivo* and *in vitro* studies have shown that the EVT cells not only invade the uterine tissues and wall of the spiral arteries but also form a continuous cytotrophoblastic shell at the interface with the decidua. This shell and the trophoblastic plugs that extend from it into the mouths of the spiral arteries act like a labyrinthine interface that filters maternal blood, permitting a slow seepage of plasma, but no true blood flow, into the intervillous space (22, 23). This has led to the concept that human placentation is in fact not truly haemochorial in early pregnancy (**Figure 9.6**). During the period when there is no true maternal blood circulation entering the placenta, the uterine glands deliver nutrient-rich secretions through the shell directly into the intervillous space. These secretions are a heterogeneous mix of maternal proteins, carbohydrates, including glycogen, and lipid droplets, and are phagocytosed by the syncytiotrophoblast indicating a histotrophic nutrition process (24). They also contain a variety of growth factors, and so create a highly stimulatory microenvironment within the developing placenta.

During the 'plugging phase' of the spiral arteries, there is physiological hypoxia inside the gestational sac, which is essential for normal placental and fetal development to occur (25, 26). This paradox reflects the fact that organogenesis is characterized by cell lineage differentiation and morphogenetic events that are critical for the development of a healthy fetus. Disruption of signalling pathways or oxidative damage to the fetal DNA at this stage will have profound consequences, and so maintaining metabolism at a low level must be advantageous (27). This concept is consistent with our

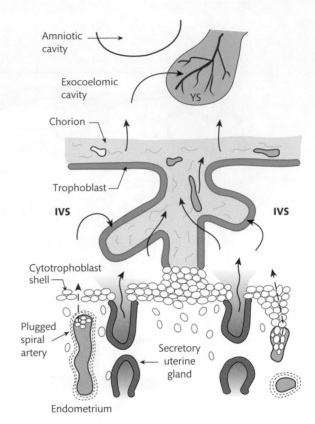

Figure 9.6 Diagram showing the histotrophic nutrition pathways in the first-trimester gestational sac. Note that there is no true maternal blood circulation entering the placenta and that the uterine glands deliver their secretions through the trophoblastic shell directly into the intervillous space (IVS). Nutrients are then transferred through the trophoblast of the placental villi into the exocoelomic cavity and into the secondary yolk sac (YS).

finding that during the first trimester placental metabolism is heavily dependent on phylogenetically ancient pathways that are less reliant on oxidative phosphorylation and so reduce the risk of generation of dangerous oxygen free radicals (27). The plugging of the spiral arteries also creates a uteroplacental oxygen gradient which exerts a regulatory effect on placental tissue development and function. In particular, it influences cytotrophoblast proliferation and differentiation along the invasive pathway, villous vasculogenesis, and the formation of the chorion laeve or free placental membranes (26, 27).

The definitive placenta

At the end of the first trimester, the EVT plugs of the cytotrophoblastic shell are progressively dislocated, allowing maternal blood to flow more freely and continuously within the intervillous space (22, 23). This transforms the placenta into a haemochorial organ. During this transitional phase, which takes place between 10 and 14 weeks of gestation, two-thirds of the primitive placenta disappears and the chorionic cavity is obliterated by the growth of the amniotic sac (26). These events bring the maternal erythrocytes closer to the fetal tissues, facilitating nutrient and gaseous exchange between the maternal and fetal circulations.

The definitive placenta is composed of a chorionic plate on its fetal aspect and a basal plate on the maternal aspect, and an intervening intervillous space containing villus stems with branches in contact with maternal blood. Towards the end of the first trimester, the villi begin to differentiate into their principal types. The connections to the chorionic plate become remodelled to form stem villi, which represent the supporting framework of each villus tree (20). These progressively develop a compact fibrous stroma, and contain branches of the chorionic arteries and accompanying veins. After several generations of branching, stem villi give rise to intermediate immature and mature villi. Mature intermediate villi provide a distributing framework, and terminal villi arise at intervals from their surface. The terminal villi are the main functional units of the villus tree. They are highly vascularized, but by capillaries alone, and are highly adapted for diffusional exchange. This differentiation of the villi coincides temporally with the development of the lobular architecture, and the two processes are most likely interlinked. Lobules can be first identified during the early second trimester, following onset of the maternal circulation when it is thought haemodynamic forces may shape the villus tree (17). Each lobule represents an individual maternofetal exchange unit.

At term, the human placenta is usually a discoid organ, 15–20 cm in diameter, approximately 3 cm thick at the centre, and weighing on average 450 g (20). Macroscopically, the organ consists of two surfaces or plates; the chorionic plate to which the umbilical cord is attached, and the basal plate that is attached the uterine wall. The placenta is incompletely divided into between 10 and 40 lobes by the presence of septa created by invaginations of the basal plate. The septa are thought to arise from differential resistance of the maternal tissues to trophoblast invasion, and may help to compartmentalize and hence direct maternal blood flow through the intervillous space (17). The maternal blood percolates through this network of channels, exchanging gases and nutrients with the fetal blood circulating within the villi, before draining through the basal plate into openings of the uterine veins.

Placental physiology

In the past, it was assumed that the principal function of the organ was transport. While maternofetal exchange through the placenta is undeniably highly important, the definition fails to recognize the organ's other facets. It is now well established that the placenta provides the fetus with all essential nutrients, water, and oxygen, and a route for clearance of fetal excretory products, but it also produces a vast array of protein and steroid hormones and factors necessary for the maintenance of pregnancy. Furthermore, transport is selective and in general the placenta either excludes or renders inactive maternal hormones and xenobiotics to allow the fetus to develop in a safe and independent milieu (28). The placenta is metabolically highly active. Placental oxygen consumption per unit mass of the tissue is three times higher than that of the developing fetus.

The transport pathways change with gestation. In particular, during most of the first trimester, the secondary yolk sac and the extraembryonic coelom play important roles as an additional transport route inside the gestational sac (29, 30). As described previously, the absence of a continuous maternal circulation inside most of the primitive placenta during the first trimester placenta is essential to control the oxygen level inside the gestational sac during organogenesis (**Figure 9.6**). It also adds to the natural defence of the fetus against parasites and viruses when at its most vulnerable. Once

maternal blood flow to the intervillous space begins at around 10 weeks' gestation, exchange across the barrier between the maternal and fetal circulations within the villi will become predominant.

During most of the first trimester, in addition to its absorptive role, the secondary yolk sac synthesizes several essential serum proteins such as alpha-fetoprotein, alpha-1-antitrypsin, albumin, pre-albumin, and transferrin until the fetal liver has reached its full metabolic capacity (30, 31). With rare exceptions, the secretion of most of these proteins is confined to the embryonic compartments. The uterine glands are also important in the early fetal and placental metabolic activities (24, 26). They are most prolific and active during the early weeks of pregnancy, with their contribution gradually waning during the first trimester. This would be consistent with a progressive switch from histotrophic to haemotrophic nutrition as the maternal arterial circulation to the placenta is established. Thus, the early, primitive human placenta may function physiologically as a choriovitelline placenta, in common with those of many mammalian species, although morphologically it never develops as such.

Placental exchanges mechanisms

Many of the transport mechanisms required to effect exchange are present in the primitive placenta and these may be up- or downregulated throughout the rest of pregnancy to meet the requirements of fetal growth and homeostasis. For a molecule to reach the fetal plasma from the maternal plasma, and vice versa, it must cross the syncytiotrophoblast, the villous mesenchyme, and the endothelium of the fetal capillary. There is also some limited transfer between maternal blood in the decidua and the fluid of the amniotic sac.

Exchange across the definitive placenta occurs by one of the four following mechanisms: bulk flow/solvent drag, diffusion, transporter-mediated mechanisms, and endocytosis/exocytosis (32–35). Water, and with it dissolved solutes, is transferred by bulk flow and is driven by differences in hydrostatic and osmotic pressures between the maternal and fetal circulations across the exchange barrier. The dissolved solutes are filtered as they move through the components of the villous barrier. Water movement may also be via paracellular channels or through pores in the plasma membranes.

Diffusion of any molecule occurs in both directions across the villous barrier. When there is a concentration gradient and/or, for charged species, an electrical gradient, one of these unidirectional fluxes (rates of transfer) is greater in one direction than it is in the other, so that there is a net flux in one direction. The rate of diffusion of an inert molecule is governed by Fick's law, and so is proportional to the surface area for exchange divided by the thickness of the tissue barrier. A large surface area will therefore facilitate exchange, and this is achieved by repeated branching of the villus trees. Small molecules such as oxygen diffuse rapidly whereas hydrophilic molecules such as glucose will not diffuse easily. Rates of diffusion of many molecules are flow limited, and thus may vary over gestation with changes in uteroplacental and fetoplacental blood flow. Changes in concentration and, for charged molecules, electrical gradients between maternal and fetal plasma will also affect rates of transfer.

Some amino acids and glucose are transported across the villous membrane at faster rates than they would occur by diffusion and down concentration gradients (35). Transporter proteins are a large and diverse group of molecules which are found most abundantly in the placenta in the microvillous, and basal plasma membranes of the syncytiotrophoblast. Large proteins such as immunoglobulin cross the placenta via endocytosis. These molecules are entrapped in invaginations of the microvillous plasma membrane of the syncytiotrophoblast which detach and pass across the intracellular compartment. They eventually fuse with the basal plasma membrane and undergo exocytosis, releasing their contents into the fetal circulation.

Placental endocrinology

As pregnancy advances, the relative number of trophoblastic cells increases and fetomaternal exchange begins to be dominated by the secretory function of the placenta (36). The placenta is a major endocrine organ, secreting over 100 peptide and steroid hormones that modulate maternal physiology. Placental hormones have profound effects on maternal metabolism, initially building up her energy reserves and then releasing these to support fetal growth in later pregnancy and lactation postnatally (28).

Human chorionic gonadotropin (hCG) is the major pregnancy glycoprotein hormone (37). It is mainly secreted by the villous syncytiotrophoblast into the maternal blood, where its concentration peaks around 8–10 weeks of gestation. It is detectable in maternal blood 2 days after implantation and behaves like an agonist of luteinizing hormone, stimulating progesterone secretion by the corpus luteum. hCG has also a role in inducing quiescence of the myometrium and local immune tolerance.

One of the essential roles of the human placenta is to produce the steroid hormone progesterone, which is required for the maintenance of pregnancy (15). Placental synthesis of progesterone begins with the conversion of cholesterol to pregnenolone, as in other steroid-secreting tissues. The rate-determining step of placental progesterone synthesis is the conversion of cholesterol to pregnenolone. The principal actions of the hormone are to maintain quiescence of the myometrium, and maintain the secretory activity of the endometrial glands. Progesterone acts as a negative regulator of trophoblast invasion by controlling matrix metalloproteinase activity (36). It may also be part of the compensatory mechanism that limits the inflammation-induced cytotoxic effects associated with an infection process during gestation (38).

Placental lactogens and growth hormone exert anti-insulin effects and promote lipolysis, boosting maternal glucose and free fatty acid concentrations for exchange to the fetus. Placental growth hormone induces maternal insulin resistance and thereby facilitates the mobilization of maternal nutrients for fetal growth. Human placental lactogen and prolactin increase maternal food intake by induction of central leptin resistance and promote maternal beta-cell expansion and insulin production to defend against the development of gestational diabetes (18). Pregnancy-associated protein A, which is mainly produced by the villous trophoblast, is a key regulator of insulin-like growth factor bioavailability essential for normal fetal development.

The transcriptional regulation of the P450arom gene has been shown to be oxygen responsive through a novel pathway involving the basic helix-loop-helix transcription factor Mash-2 (39). Changes in oxygenation that occur at the end of the first trimester when the intervillous circulation begins may modulate the synthesis of various trophoblastic proteins, such as oestrogens (39) and hCG (40). These findings illustrate the impact of the anatomical changes occurring during the transition from the primitive to the definitive placenta on trophoblastic hormonal synthesis.

Placental-related disorders of pregnancy

Placental-related disorders of pregnancy are almost unique to the human species. These disorders, which affect around a third of human pregnancies, primarily include miscarriages, pre-eclampsia, and FGR. In other mammalian species, the incidence of these disorders is extremely low. In humans, these disorders may relate to the fact that our invasive form of implantation, and subsequent haemochorial placentation, poses special haemodynamic challenges. These complications are often associated with abnormal maternal adaptations to pregnancy in the second trimester, including failure to gain weight, lack of blood pressure reduction, and persistent non-pregnant haematocrit levels (17).

There is mounting evidence that once organogenesis is complete, oxidative stress plays a major role in both the physiological changes associated with the remodelling of the human placenta and the pathophysiology of placental-related disorders of pregnancy (8, 41). Pathological oxidative stress arises when the production of reactive oxygen species overwhelms the intrinsic antioxidant defences, causing indiscriminate damage to biological molecules and leading to loss of function and cell death.

Miscarriages

First-trimester pregnancy losses are the consequence of an extreme disorder of placentation with rapid degeneration of the placental tissue, independently of the aetiology (8). In about two-thirds of first-trimester miscarriages there is anatomical evidence of defective placentation, which is mainly characterized by a thinner and fragmented trophoblastic shell, reduced cytotrophoblast invasion of the endometrium, and incomplete plugging of the lumen at the tips of the spiral arteries (42, 43). These deficiencies are associated with the absence of physiological changes in most of the spiral arteries, and lead to premature and disorganized onset of the maternal circulation throughout the entire placenta (**Figure 9.7**).

Independent of the cause of the miscarriage, the excessive entry of maternal blood into the intervillous space has two effects; a direct mechanical effect on the villous tissue, which becomes progressively enmeshed inside large intervillous blood thrombi, and widespread indirect oxygen-mediated trophoblastic oxidative damage, with increased apoptosis (44, 45). Overall, the consequences are placental degeneration with extensive loss of syncytiotrophoblast function and detachment of the placenta from the uterine wall. This mechanism is common to all miscarriages with the time at which it occurs dependent on the aetiology, aneuploidies being associated with early (5–9 weeks) and maternal antiphospholipid syndrome with late (10–14 weeks) placental degeneration (41).

Pre-eclampsia

There is increasing evidence that pre-eclampsia is a heterogeneous syndrome, and early- and late-onset forms are now recognized with a distinction of onset before or after 34 weeks of gestation (46). Early-onset pre-eclampsia stems from a similar, though lesser, defect in early trophoblast invasion as in spontaneous miscarriage, whereas

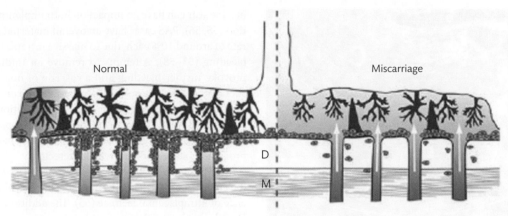

Figure 9.7 Diagrammatic representation of the trophoblast invasion in a normal pregnancy and a miscarriage. In miscarriages, the shallow invasion of the deciduas (D) and superficial myometrium (M) results in a deficient plugging of the spiral arteries and early onset of the intervillous circulation.

late-onset pre-eclampsia is thought to reflect maternal predisposition to cardiovascular disease.

In early-onset pre-eclampsia, while invasion is sufficient to anchor the gestational sac it is too shallow for complete transformation of the spiral arteries into low-resistance channels (47). As a consequence, the spiral arteries retain smooth muscle cells within their walls, particularly in their myometrial segments (**Figures 9.2** and **9.3**), and remain responsive to circulating vasoactive compounds. This may lead not only to diminished perfusion of the intervillous space, but more importantly to intermittent perfusion. Since the placenta and fetus continually extract oxygen it is expected that transient hypoxia will result, and that consequently the placenta suffers a chronic low-grade ischaemia–reperfusion type injury (48). By contrast to miscarriage where there is rapid and generalized degeneration of the placental tissue, in pre-eclampsia the damage is progressive and can be compensated for some time depending on the severity of the deficiency in both spiral arterial remodelling and placental intrinsic antioxidant capacity.

For many years, pre-eclampsia has been considered to be a two-stage disease. Pre-eclampsia is at least a three-stage disorder starting with the primary pathology being an excessive or atypical maternal immune response leading to insufficient placentation (8, 49). Dysfunctional perfusion of the intervillous space of the placenta leads to oxidative and haemodynamic stress. Chronic trophoblastic oxidative stress releases excessive proinflammatory and antiangiogenic factors into the maternal circulation leading to diffuse maternal endothelial cell dysfunction and the clinical symptoms of pre-eclampsia. Early-onset pre-eclampsia is therefore predictable from the beginning of the second trimester because of the major syncytiotrophoblast stress in early pregnancy and the corresponding changes in its biomarkers (50). By contrast, prediction of late-onset pre-eclampsia is poor because there is no early trophoblast pathology in these cases.

Placental insufficiency and fetal growth

FGR is a failure of the fetus to reach its full growth potential. The definition is conceptual but impossible to verify, because it is not possible to determine the exact growth potential of an individual fetus. In practice, smallness, with or without evidence of fetal response to undernutrition, is used to ascertain FGR. It can have many causes, but the majority of cases that have no genetic or infectious aetiology

are thought to arise from abnormal placentation. Pathological studies have demonstrated deficient physiological conversion of the arteries as in pre-eclampsia, but to a lesser degree, especially in the myometrial segment and a positive correlation between the birth weight and the degree of conversion (51).

The distinction between 'placental' and 'maternal' causation has been proposed, with 'placental' cases being more frequently associated with early-onset pre-eclampsia and FGR (52). In cases of isolated FGR, there is scanty evidence showing the level of stress is either similar to the normal control or intermediate between a normal control and an early-onset pre-eclamptic placenta. The fact there is morphological and molecular evidence of oxidative stress in most FGR placentas indicates a chronic low-level oxidative stress may occur from the time of onset of the maternal circulation onwards, and leads to a lower growth trajectory of the placenta. This is consistent with the reduced rate of growth of the placenta observed with serial ultrasound scans in these cases (50).

Prenatal screening, diagnosis, and management of common placental and cord anomalies

Before the development of ultrasound imaging, morphological examination of the placenta and the cord was only of epidemiological value and was therefore of little influence on pregnancy management. With modern ultrasound equipment, it is now possible to examine the placenta and the cord in detail from the beginning of the first trimester and screen for placental and umbilical cord structural anomalies that are associated with perinatal complications (53–61).

Anomalies of placentation

Placenta praevia is defined as implantation of the placenta fully or partially in the lower uterine segment. Determining placental location was the first aim of placental routine examination *in vivo*. Placenta praevia has a prevalence of 4–5 per 1000 pregnancies and is associated potentially with life-threatening complications for the mother, including severe ante- and postpartum bleeding, need for hysterectomy, blood transfusions, septicaemia, and thrombophlebitis, and adverse fetal and neonatal outcome including preterm

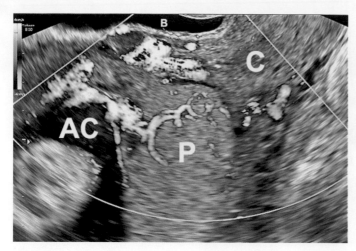

Figure 9.8 Transvaginal ultrasound image of the cervix (C) and placenta (P) at 32 weeks of gestation showing a major placenta praevia covering the cervix (grade IV). AC, amniotic cavity; B, bladder.

delivery and perinatal death (53). Placenta praevia is more common in multiple gestation pregnancy and in pregnancies following a caesarean section delivery (53, 54).

Placental location is usually reported during the routine anomaly scan at 20–22 weeks of gestation. If the placenta is found to be reaching, overlapping, or covering the internal cervical os, a follow-up scan should be scheduled at the beginning of the third trimester (28–30 weeks) before the lower uterine segment starts to form. Almost 90% of the placentas defined as low around mid gestation are found to be completely outside of the lower uterine segment later in gestation, and are entirely safe (53). Transvaginal ultrasound is the preferred technique for assessment of placental location, particularly in suspected low posterior placentas. The term 'placenta praevia' should only be used when the placental edge covers, overlaps, or is within 2 cm of the internal cervical os in the third trimester. If the placental edge is located further than 2 cm but within 3.5 cm from the internal cervical os, the placenta should be termed low lying. In the latter case, there is a good chance of a vaginal delivery but the incidence of postpartum haemorrhage remains high.

A placenta that covers the entire internal cervical os is classified as major placenta praevia (**Figure 9.8**) and always requires a caesarean delivery. Caesarean section for major placenta praevia is associated with a high risk of massive intra- and postpartum bleeding which will require blood transfusion and possible admission of the mother to intensive care. Additional surgical procedures including hysterectomy may be required in case of excessive bleeding during delivery, and thus caesarean sections for major placenta praevia should be planned to occur in a tertiary care centre with management by a multidisciplinary team.

Placenta accreta spectrum (PAS) is defined as an abnormally adherent or invasive placenta to the uterine wall (53). When the villi invade deeply into the myometrium it is described as increta and when the villi penetrate the entire thickness of the uterine wall and beyond it is reported as percreta. The vast majority of PAS are found in women with placenta praevia and also a previous caesarean section. Recent epidemiological studies have also found that the strongest risk factor for placenta praevia is a prior caesarean section suggesting that a failure of decidualization in the area of a previous

uterine scar can have an impact on both implantation and placentation (55, 56). PAS cases have an overall maternal and fetal mortality rate of around 10% each, due to massive intrapartum or postpartum bleeding (53–58). Attempts to remove an undiagnosed PAS may provoke further bleeding and a cascade of ongoing haemorrhage, shock, and coagulation disorders requiring complex clinical management. Thus prenatal diagnosis of this condition is pivotal to allow the surgical team to demarcate the areas of the placenta that require resection before surgery and/or to consent the patient for additional procedures such as a caesarean hysterectomy.

The most common sonographic finding associated with PAS is the enlargement of the underlying uterine vasculature with the presence of intraplacental lacunae (55). The addition of colour or power Doppler evaluation has been valuable in improving the diagnosis of of invasive PAS (55, 56). All women presenting with a history of previous caesarean delivery or uterine surgery and an anteriorly situated low-lying or placenta praevia at the anomaly scan require a detailed examination of the placenta and follow-up scan at 28 weeks for the identification of PAS (53). Women managed by a multidisciplinary care team are less likely to require large-volume blood transfusion, reoperation within 7 days of delivery for bleeding complications, and to experience prolonged maternal admission to the intensive care unit, large-volume blood transfusion, coagulopathy, and urethral injury than women managed by standard obstetric care (53, 58).

Vascular anomalies of the placenta

Thrombosis and infarcts are usually found during the third trimester of pregnancy and are often associated with placental-related disorders of placentation (51, 62). Placental thromboses are the result of focal coagulation of blood in the intervillous space and appear on ultrasound examination as large hypoechoic central areas of turbulent blood flow surrounded by an echogenic shell of villi embedded in fibrin. Extensive infarcts are found in pregnancies complicated by pre-eclampsia or essential hypertension, and are associated with an increase in perinatal mortality and intrauterine growth retardation. Sonographically, placental infarcts appear as large intraplacental areas, irregular and hyperechoic in the acute stage and isoechoic in a more advanced stage. In pre-eclampsia with FGR, infarcts are often associated with microscopic diffuse villitis and excessive fibrin deposition (51), which is probably secondary to major impairment of the uteroplacental circulation. These placental vascular lesions are more frequent in twins, and pre-eclampsia is associated with a higher incidence of placental infarctions and thrombosis in dichorionic twin placentas than in monochorionic twins and singletons (54).

Haematomas are the results of extravasation of maternal or fetal blood and may be subamniotic, subchorionic, or retroplacental (63, 64). A subchorionic or retroplacental haematoma reflects bleeding of maternal origin and is identified sonographically as a hypoechoic area between the chorion and uterine wall (**Figure 9.9**). Such lesions are seen in more than 1% of pregnancies, commonly in the first trimester. In very early pregnancy (<7 weeks), the risk of further complications after bleeding is small. After 7 weeks, vaginal bleeding with or without a haematoma on ultrasound examination is associated with a 10% risk of subsequent complete first-trimester miscarriage and with long-term adverse pregnancy outcomes, including preterm delivery, placental abruption, and low birthweight (65).

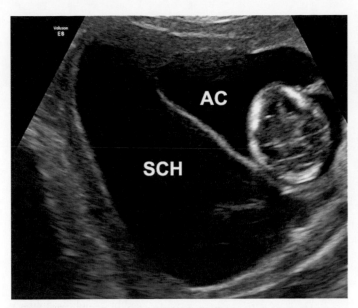

Figure 9.9 Ultrasound image of a large subchorionic haematoma (SCH) displacing the amniotic cavity (AC) membrane at 12 weeks of gestation. Note that the lesion is sonolucent, indicating an old haematoma.

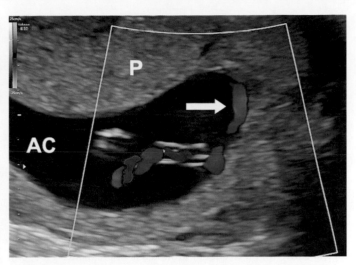

Figure 9.10 Longitudinal view of a velamentous umbilical cord with a vasa praevia (arrow) at 12 weeks of gestation. AC, amniotic cavity; P, placenta.

Placental tumours

Hydatidiform moles are gestational trophoblastic tumours which can affect the entire villous tissue or small groups of villi, and which can be associated with the development of a choriocarcinoma (66, 67). Complete or classical hydatidiform moles (CHMs) are described as a generalized swelling of the villous tissue, diffuse trophoblastic hyperplasia, and the absence of any embryonic or fetal tissue. Classically, patients with CHMs present with vaginal bleeding, uterine enlargement greater than expected for gestational age, and an abnormally high level of serum beta-hCG. Medical complications include severe pre-eclampsia, hyperthyroidism, hyperemesis, anaemia, and the development of ovarian theca lutein cysts. With earlier prenatal diagnosis, the incidence of these complications has decreased (66). The development of a CHM follows a well-defined pattern starting with a macroscopically normal gestation sac at 4 weeks, which transforms into a polypoid mass between 5 and 7 weeks of gestation. The hydropic changes of the villous tissue is progressive and rarely visible in utero on ultrasound before 8 weeks of gestation (66). From 9 weeks, the hydropic changes are visible in over 90% of the cases and appear multiple sonolucent ares of varying size and shape also called snow storm appearance on ultrasound (**Figure 9.10**).

Partial hydatidiform moles refer to the combination of a fetus with localized placental molar degenerations, characterized by focal swelling of the villous tissue, and focal trophoblastic hyperplasia (68). The abnormal villi are scattered within macroscopically normal placental tissue, which tends to retain its shape.

Before 13 weeks' gestation, some partial moles may present as an enlarged placenta with or without only a few vesicular changes (68, 69). From 16 weeks, almost all triploid fetuses have a least one measurement below the normal range, and more than 70% present with severe FGR. Structural fetal defects are observed antenatally in about 93% of the cases. The most common are abnormalities of the hands, bilateral cerebral ventriculomegaly, heart anomalies, and micrognathia.

Chorioangiomas are the most common benign tumour of the placenta with an incidence at delivery of 0.5–1% of placentas examined (70). Chorioangiomas are non-trophoblastic tumours of the placenta derived from excessive vascular proliferation within the stroma of chronic villi. The incidence of large chorioangiomas is lower and varies from 1 in 8000 to 1 in 50,000 pregnancies. These tumours are well circumscribed, have a different echogenicity from the rest of the placental tissue, and have often been documented sonographically from 16 weeks of gestation. Chorioangiomas can be complicated by fetal hydrops due to congestive heart failure and secondary to chronic shunting of large volumes of fetal blood through the tumour (70). Polyhydramnios is also a common complication of chorioangiomas and like hydrops is linked to its vascular nature of the tumour and not to size. Abnormal cardiovascular profile scores have recently been observed in 46% of chorioangiomas, and 39% of those cases show a poor neurodevelopmental outcome after birth (71). The fetal risk depends on the proportion of angiomatous versus mixoid tissue inside the chorioangioma, and thus prenatal identification of the vascularization of the tumour with colour Doppler imaging is essential for the management of this tumour. If the tumour is avascular, no specific complications should be expected (70). If the tumour is vascularized, and in particular if it contains numerous large vessels, serial ultrasound and Doppler examinations are warranted to detect polyhydramnios and fetal cardiovascular dysfunction.

Anomalies of the umbilical cord

A *single umbilical artery* (SUA) cord is the result of the absence of one of the two normal arteries, and is one of the most common congenital fetal malformations with an incidence of approximately 1% of all deliveries (72). SUA occurs three to four times more frequently in twins, and almost invariably accompanies the acardia malformation and sirenomelia or caudal regression syndrome (54, 72). There is also a sixfold increase of the incidence of marginal and velamentous insertion of the cord among SUA infants. Major fetal anatomical defects are largely responsible for the high fetal and neonatal loss from this pathology and can affect any organ system. The discovery of a SUA in the perinatal period justifies a detailed ultrasound examination of the neonate to exclude minor anomalies of internal organs, such as the kidney or heart. The incidence of FGR is significantly elevated among fetuses with a SUA and may be present without any other congenital anomalies in 15–20% of the cases (72). SUA twins are at higher risks of FGR and preterm delivery. Discordance for SUA in monochorionic twins can be present, and provides evidence against an exclusively genetic origin of this anomaly (54).

Vasa praevia are fetal vessels running through the membranes, over the cervix, and under the fetal presenting part, unprotected by the placental tissue or the umbilical cord (59, 60). This particular vascular arrangement is usually the result of a velamentous insertion of the umbilical cord in a single or bi-lobed placenta (vasa praevia type 1) or the presence of aberrant fetal vessels running between one or more accessory lobes of the placenta (vasa praevia type 2). Velamentous insertion of the cord (VCI) is a well-defined pathological entity with a frequency around 1% of pregnancies (55, 56). Approximately 90% of women with vasa praevia have VCI and 3–4% of women with a VCI have vasa praevia. VCI of one of the umbilical cords is eight times more common in twins than in singletons. Monochorionicity doubles the risk for VCI. The incidence of VCI, vasa praevia, or marginal cord insertion is higher in assisted reproductive technology than in spontaneously conceived singletons, but is similar in both types of twins (73, 74).

Vasa praevia is more common in women in whom the placenta was low lying in the mid pregnancy, but appears to migrate with advancing gestation.

In vasa praevia, vessels are vulnerable to compression changes since they are not supported by Wharton's jelly, and when the cervix is dilated and the rupture of the membranes occurs these unprotected vessels are at risk of rupture and fatal fetal haemorrhage. The classic presentation of undiagnosed vasa praevia in labour is the presence of painless vaginal bleeding usually after the rupture of the membranes associated with acute fetal distress evidenced by CTG changes or fetal demise. The absence of a normal insertion of the umbilical cord in the placenta, VCI, can be reliably detected by the use of colour Doppler ultrasound (**Figure 9.10**). Thus women with VCI, multiple pregnancies, bi-lobated placenta, and placenta praevia should be screened for vasa praevia (59, 60).

Placental examination at delivery

The utility of histopathological examination of the placenta and umbilical cord after delivery is directly relevant to many different aspects of perinatology from the epidemiology of specific obstetric complications to malpractice litigation.

The macroscopic examination of the placenta starts in the delivery room with identification of placental and membranes completeness and the number of vessels in the umbilical cord. This examination is performed by the midwife and/or birth attendant to alert the clinicians to possible retention of placental tissue *in utero* and undetected fetal anomalies associated with the SUA. A complete macroscopic report should also include placental weight as the evaluation of placenta-to-birth weight ratio or fetal-to-placental weight ratio (FPR) provides indirect information on placental development and function during pregnancy. An abnormal FPR has been shown to be a good predictor for short- and long-term adverse outcome during childhood and adulthood such as cardiovascular diseases

(51, 75). In cases of multiple gestation pregnancy, labelling of placentas and umbilical cords, using different sizes or forms of clips, is essential for further investigations. The identification of structure of intertwin membranes in twins, site of insertion and number of vessels in each umbilical cord, and evaluation of vascular anastomoses in monochorionic twins can also be clinically useful (54).

The microscopic examination is performed in the laboratory by a specialist fetoplacental pathologist. The Amsterdam Placental Workshop Group has recently proposed a classification of placental lesions (76). This classification covers clinically significant microscopic placental lesions, which cannot be diagnosed antenatally.

REFERENCES

1. Martin A, Holloway K. Something there us that doesn't love a wall: histories of the placental barrier. *Stud Hist Philos Biol Biomed Sci* 2014;**47**:300–10.
2. O'Leary MA, Bloch JI, Flynn JJ, et al. The placental mammal ancestor and the post-K-Pg radiation of placentals. *Science* 2013;**339**:662–67.
3. Carter AM. IFPA Senior Award Lecture: Mammalian fetal membranes. *Placenta* 2016;**48** Suppl 1:S21–30.
4. Jaffe R, Jauniaux E, Hustin J. Maternal circulation in the first-trimester human placenta – myth or reality? *Am J Obstet Gynecol* 1997;**176**:695–705.
5. Burton GJ, Jauniaux E. What is the placenta? *Am J Obstet Gynecol* 2015;**213**:S6.e1–4.
6. Romano-Keeler J, Weitkamp JH. Maternal influences on fetal microbial colonization and immune development. *Pediatr Res* 2015;**77**, 189–95.
7. Reus AD, El-Harbachi H, Rousian M, et al. Early first-trimester trophoblast volume in pregnancies that result in live birth or miscarriage. *Ultrasound Obstet Gynecol* 2103;**42**:577–84.
8. Jauniaux E, Poston L, Burton GJ. Placental-related diseases of pregnancy: Involvement of oxidative stress and implications in human evolution. *Hum Reprod Update* 2006;**12**:747–55.
9. James JL, Carter AM, Chamley LW. Human placentation from nidation to 5 weeks of gestation. Part I: What do we know about formative placental development following implantation? *Placenta* 2012;**33**:327–34.
10. Pijnenborg R, Vercruysse L, Brosens I. Deep placentation. *Best Pract Research Clin Obstet Gynaecol* 2011;**25**:273–85.
11. Knöfler M. Critical growth factors and signalling pathways controlling human trophoblast invasion. *Int J Dev Biol* 2010;**54**:269–80.
12. Plaisier M. Decidualisation and angiogenesis. *Best Pract Research Clin Obstet Gynaecol* 2011;**25**:259–71.
13. Filant J, Spencer TE. Uterine glands: biological roles in conceptus implantation, uterine receptivity and decidualization. *Int J Dev Biol* 2014;**58**:107–16.
14. Burton G, Jauniaux E, Charnock-Jones DS. Human early placental development: potential roles of the endometrial glands. *Placenta* 2007;Suppl A:S64–69.
15. Al-Lamki RS, Skepper JN, Burton GJ. Are human placental bed giant cells merely aggregates of small mononuclear trophoblast cells? An ultrastructural and immunocytochemical study. *Hum Reprod* 1999;**14**:496–504.
16. Ramsey EM, Donner MW. *Placental Vasculature and Circulation: Anatomy, Physiology, Radiology, Clinical Aspects, Atlas and Textbook*. Stuttgart: Georg Thieme; 1980.
17. Burton GJ, Woods AW, Jauniaux E, Kingdom JC. Rheological and physiological consequences of conversion of the maternal spiral

arteries for uteroplacental blood flow during human pregnancy. *Placenta* 2009;**30**:473–82.

18. Jauniaux E, Jurkovic D, Campbell S. In vivo investigations of anatomy and physiology of early human placental circulations. *Ultrasound Obstet Gynecol* 1991;**1**:435–45.

19. Jauniaux E, Jurkovic D, Campbell S, Hustin J. Doppler ultrasound study of the developing placental circulations: correlation with anatomic findings. *Am J Obstet Gynecol* 1992;**166**:585–87.

20. Boyd JD, Hamilton WJ. *The Human Placenta*. Cambridge: Heffer and Sons; 1970.

21. Jauniaux E, Jurkovic D, Henriet Y, Rodesch F, Hustin J. Development of the secondary human yolk sac: correlation of sonographic and anatomic features. *Hum Reprod* 1991;**6**:1160–66.

22. Hustin J, Schaaps JP. Echographic and anatomic studies of the maternotrophoblastic border during the first trimester of pregnancy. *Am J Obstet Gynecol* 1987;**157**:162–68.

23. Burton GJ, Jauniaux E, Watson AL. Maternal arterial connections to the placental intervillous space during the first trimester of human pregnancy: the Boyd collection revisited. *Am J Obstet Gynecol* 1999;**181**:718–24.

24. Burton GJ, Watson AL, Hempstock J, Skepper JN, Jauniaux E. Uterine glands provide histiotrophic nutrition for the human fetus during the first trimester of pregnancy. *J Clin Endocrinol Metab* 2002;**87**:2954–59.

25. Jauniaux E, Watson A, Burton G. Evaluation of respiratory gases and acid-base gradients in human fetal fluids and uteroplacental tissue between 7 and 16 weeks. *Am J Obstet Gynecol* 2001;**184**:998–1003.

26. Jauniaux E, Gulbis B, Burton GJ. The human first trimester gestational sac limits rather than facilitates oxygen transfer to the foetus: a review. *Placenta* 2003;**24** Suppl A:S86–93.

27. Burton GJ. Oxygen, the Janus gas; its effects on human placental development and function. *J Anat* 2009;**215**:27–35.

28. Burton GJ, Fowden AL. The placenta: a multifaceted, transient organ. *Philos Trans R Soc Lond B Biol Sci* 2015;**370**:20140066.

29. Gulbis B, Jauniaux E, Cotton F, Stordeur P. Protein and enzyme pattern in the fluid cavities of the first trimester human gestational sac: relevance to the absorptive role of the secondary yolk sac. *Molec Hum Reprod* 1998;**4**:857–62.

30. Jauniaux E, Cindrova-Davies T, Johns J, et al. Distribution and transfer pathways of antioxidant molecules inside the first trimester human gestational sac. *JCEM* 2004;**89**;1452–59.

31. Jauniaux E, Gulbis B, Jurkovic D, Gavriil P, Campbell S. The origin of alpha-fetoprotein in first trimester anembryonic pregnancies. *Am J Obstet Gynecol* 1995;**173**:1749–53.

32. Hay WW. Placental transport of nutrients to the fetus. *Horm Res* 1994;**42**:215–22.

33. Stulc J. Placental transfer of inorganic ions and water. *Physiol Rev* 1997;**77**:805–36.

34. Illsley NP. Glucose transporters in the human placenta. *Placenta* 2000;**21**:14–22.

35. Regnault TR, de Vrijer B, Battaglia FC. Transport and metabolism of amino acids in placenta. *Endocrine* 2002;**19**:23–41.

36. Costa MA. The endocrine function of human placenta: an overview. *Reprod Biomed Online* 2016;**32**:14–43.

37. Fournier T, Guibourdenche J, Evain-Brion D. hCGs: different sources of production, different glycoforms and functions. *Placenta* 2015;**36**:S60–65

38. Pineda-Torres M, Flores-Espinosa P, Espejel-Nunez A, et al. Evidence of an immunosuppressive effect of progesterone upon in vitro secretion of proinflammatory and prodegradative factors in a model of choriodecidual infection. *BJOG* 2015;**122**:1798–807.

39. Mendelson CR, Jiang B, Shelton JM, Richardson JA, Hinshelwood MM. Transcriptional regulation of aromatase in placenta and ovary. *J Steroid Biochem Mol Biol* 2005;**95**:25–33.

40. Cocquebert M, Berndt S, Segond N, et al. Comparative expression of hCG beta-genes in human trophoblast from early and late first-trimester placentas. *Am J Physiol Endocrinol Metab* 2012;**303**:E950–58.

41. Burton GJ, Jauniaux E. Oxidative stress. *Best Pract Res Clin Obstet Gynaecol* 2011;**25**:287–99.

42. Hustin J, Jauniaux E, Schaaps JP. Histological study of the materno-embryonic interface in spontaneous abortion. *Placenta* 1990;**11**:477–86.

43. Jauniaux E, Zaidi J, Jurkovic D, Campbell S, Hustin J. Comparison of colour Doppler features and pathologic findings in complicated early pregnancy. *Hum Reprod* 1994;**9**:243–47.

44. Jauniaux E, Watson AL, Hempstock J, Bao Y-P, Skepper JN, Burton GJ. Onset of maternal arterial blood flow and placental oxidative stress; a possible factor in human early pregnancy failure. *Am J Pathol* 2000;**157**:2111–22.

45. Hempstock J, Jauniaux E, Greenwold N, Burton GJ. The contribution of placental oxidative stress to early pregnancy failure. *Hum Pathol* 2003;**34**:1265–75.

46. Tranquilli AL, Landi B. The definition of severe and early-onset pre-eclampsia. Statements from the International Society for the Study of Hypertension in Pregnancy. *Pregnancy Hypertens* 2013;**3**:44–47.

47. Brosens I, Pijnenborg R, Vercruysse L, Romero R. The 'Great Obstetrical Syndromes' are associated with disorders of deep placentation. *Am J Obstet Gynecol* 2011;**204**:193–201.

48. Hung TH, Skepper JN, Burton GJ. In vitro ischemia-reperfusion injury in term human placenta as a model for oxidative stress in pathological pregnancies. *Am J Pathol* 2001;**159**:1031–43.

49. Redman CW, Staff AC. Preeclampsia, biomarkers, syncytiotrophoblast stress, and placental capacity. *Am J Obstet Gynecol* 2015;**213**:S9–11.

50. Suri G, Muttukrishna S, Jauniaux E. 2D-ultrasound and endocrinologic evaluation of placentation in early pregnancy and its relationship to fetal birthweight in normal pregnancies and preeclampsia. *Placenta* 2013;**34**:745–50.

51. Burton GJ, Jauniaux E. Pathophysiology of placental-derived fetal growth restriction. *Am J Obstet Gynecol* 2018;**218**:S745–S761.

52. Yung HW, Atkinson D, Campion-Smith T, Olovsson M, Charnock-Jones DS, Burton GJ. Differential activation of placental unfolded protein response pathways implies heterogeneity in causation of early- and late-onset pre-eclampsia. *J Pathol* 2014;**234**:262–76.

53. Jauniaux E, Alfirevic Z, Bhide AG, Burton GJ, Collins SL, Silver R. Royal College of Obstetricians and Gynaecologists. Vasa Praevia: Diagnosis and Management: Green-top Guideline No. 27b. *BJOG* 2019;**126**:e49–e61.

54. Hubinont C, Lewi L, Bernard P, Marbaix E, Debiève F, Jauniaux E. Anomalies of the placenta and umbilical cord in twin gestations. *Am J Obstet Gynecol* 2015;**213**:S91–102.

55. Jauniaux E, Collins S, Burton GJ. Placenta accreta spectrum: pathophysiology and evidence-based anatomy for prenatal ultrasound imaging. *Am J Obstet Gynecol* 2018;**218**:75–87.

56. Jauniaux E, Burton GJ. Pathophysiology of Placenta Accreta Spectrum Disorders: A Review of Current Findings. *Clin Obstet Gynecol* 2018;**61**:743–54.

57. Jauniaux E, Chantraine F, Silver RM, Langhoff-Roos J. FIGO Placenta Accreta Diagnosis and Management Expert Consensus Panel. FIGO consensus guidelines on placenta accreta spectrum disorders: Epidemiology. *Int J Gynaecol Obstet* 2018;**140**:265–73.

58. Jauniaux E, Ayres-de-Campos D, Langhoff-Roos J, Fox KA, Collins S. FIGO Placenta Accreta Diagnosis and Management Expert Consensus Panel. FIGO classification for the clinical diagnosis of placenta accreta spectrum disorders. *Int J Gynaecol Obstet* 2019;**146**:20–24.

59. Jauniaux E, Alfirevic Z, Bhide AG, Burton GJ, Collins SL, Silver R. Royal College of Obstetricians and Gynaecologists. Vasa Praevia: Diagnosis and Management: Green-top Guideline No. 27b. *BJOG* 2019;**126**:e49–e61.

60. Melcer Y, Maymon R, Jauniaux E. Vasa previa: prenatal diagnosis and management. *Curr Opin Obstet Gynecol* 2018;**30**:385–91.

61. Jauniaux E, Ramsay B, Campbell S. Ultrasonographic investigation of placental morphology and size during the second trimester of pregnancy. *Am J Obstet Gynecol* 1994;**170**:130–37.

62. Veerbeek JH, Nikkels PG, Torrance HL, et al. Placental pathology in early intrauterine growth restriction associated with maternal hypertension. *Placenta* 2014;**35**:696–701

63. Deans A, Jauniaux E. Prenatal diagnosis and outcome of subamniotic hematomas. *Ultrasound Obstet Gynecol* 1998;**11**:367–77.

64. Johns J, Hyett J, Jauniaux E. Obstetric outcome after threatened miscarriage with and without a hematoma on ultrasound. *Obstet Gynecol* 2003;**102**:483–87.

65. Johns J, Jauniaux E. Threatened miscarriage as a predictor of obstetric outcome. *Obstet Gynecol* 2006;**107**:845–50.

66. Jauniaux E, Memtsa M, Johns J, Ross JA, Jurkovic D. New insights in the pathophysiology of complete hydatidiform mole. *Placenta* 2018;**62**:28–33.

67. Jauniaux E. Ultrasound diagnosis and follow-up of gestational trophoblastic disease. *Ultrasound Obstet Gynecol* 1998;**11**:367–77.

68. Jauniaux E. Partial moles: from postnatal to prenatal diagnosis. *Placenta* 1999;**20**:379–88.

69. Johns J, Greenwold N, Buckley S, Jauniaux E. A prospective study of ultrasound screening for molar pregnancies in missed miscarriages. *Ultrasound Obstet Gynecol* 2005;**25**:493–97.

70. Jauniaux E, Ogle R. Colour Doppler imaging in the diagnosis and management of chorioangiomas. *Ultrasound Obstet Gynecol* 2000;**15**:463–67.

71. Iacovella C, Chandrasekaran N, Khalil A, Bhide A, Papageorghiou A, Thilaganathan B. Fetal and placental vascular tumors: persistent fetal hyperdynamic status predisposes to poorer long-term neurodevelopmental outcome. *Ultrasound Obstet Gynecol* 2014;**43**:658–61.

72. Heifetz SA. Single umbilical artery. A statistical analysis of 237 autopsy cases and review of the literature. *Perspect Pediatr Pathol* 1984;**8**:345–78.

73. Gavriil P, Jauniaux E, Leroy F. Pathologic examination of placentas from singleton and twin pregnancies obtained after in vitro fertilization and embryo transfer. *Pediatr Path* 1993;**13**:453–62.

74. Jauniaux E, Ben-Ami I, Maymon R. Do assisted-reproduction twin pregnancies require additional antenatal care? *Reprod Biomed Online* 2013;**26**:107–19.

75. Risnes KR, Romundstad PR, Nilsen TI, Eskild A, Vatten LJ. Placental weight relative to birth weight and long-term cardiovascular mortality: findings from a cohort of 31.0307 men and women. *Am J Epidemiol* 2009;**170**:622–31.

76. Redline RW. Classification of placental lesions. *Am J Obstet Gynecol* 2015;**213**:S21–28.

10

Fetal growth

Jane E. Hirst and Aris T. Papageorghiou

Introduction

Human growth and development from conception to birth is a complex, highly regulated, and orchestrated process. Suboptimal fetal growth places the baby at increased risk of stillbirth and fetal distress in labour, while excessive growth can predispose to birth complications.

Low birth weight (LBW) has been defined by the World Health Organization (WHO) as a weight at birth of 2500 g or less, regardless of gestational age or sex. The selection of 2500 g was based on epidemiological observations that babies were approximately 20 times more likely to die when born below this weight (1). However, this method of denoting small babies does not take into account the fact that LBW can occur because of infants being born preterm, or because of intrauterine growth restriction (IUGR), or both (2). It is essential to differentiate these conditions if evidence-based strategies are to be appropriately targeted. This threshold also fails to recognize that there are physiological differences between the sexes, with girls being lighter than boys at every gestational age; however, boys experience worse survival and perinatal outcomes in most populations. Finally, LBW is also a non-specific marker of several potential adverse exposures. Therefore the value of LBW to monitor and compare the state of perinatal health between countries or over time has been queried (2).

In order to improve the definition and detection of babies with suboptimal growth, an expert committee from the WHO defined small for gestational age (SGA) as a birth weight less than the tenth percentile when compared to a reference for gestational age and sex (3). The terms average for gestational age (AGA, 50th centile) and large for gestational age (LGA, 90th centile) are also used. It is important to note that SGA is not the same as IUGR—which is defined as failure to reach growth potential. It is possible for a fetus to be SGA but not IUGR (rather, to be a healthy small baby); in contrast, it is possible to be IUGR while not being SGA. Nevertheless, as growth potential is not possible to accurately define, SGA is the most commonly accepted proxy for IUGR used in the perinatal literature. The definition of SGA requires accurate gestational age estimation.

The burden of low birth weight around the world

The WHO estimated that 15.5% of all births, equating to more than 20 million infants, were born with LBW in 2004 (1). The estimate for the number of babies born with LBW in low- and middle-income countries in 2010 was very similar, 18 million babies (4); however, as the total number of babies born continues to increase, even allowing for the uncertainly in these estimates, the rate of LBW is likely to be falling. In 2010, it was calculated that 59% of LBW babies were born at term (after 37 completed weeks of gestation) and 41% were preterm.

Evidence-based interventions to reduce mortality from preterm birth exist, but if inappropriately administered there is also a potential for harm. It is therefore essential to differentiate babies that are preterm from those that are term but growth restricted before birth. An example of the importance of correctly recognizing preterm birth was inadvertently demonstrated in the ACT trial, a large cluster-randomized controlled trial to assess the efficacy of antenatal corticosteroids to reduce deaths from prematurity in Africa, Latin America, and South Asia. Antenatal corticosteroid administration has been a mainstay of obstetric management of preterm labour for decades, with evidence from a Cochrane meta-analysis to support survival benefit when given to mothers in preterm labour at less than 34 weeks of gestation. In the ACT trial, staff in the intervention sites were trained to identify and administer steroids to women likely to deliver with either a birth weight below the fifth centile or gestational age less than 36 weeks, while in the control arm no additional interventions were introduced. The trial ran for 18 months and during this time 51,523 women delivered in the control sites, and 48,219 in the intervention sites. The result, however, was surprising, with an increased risk of perinatal death in the intervention group (relative risk (RR) 1.12; 95% confidence interval (CI) 1.02–1.22) (5). Correct differentiation of preterm from term but small babies is essential if interventions are to be appropriately given and outcomes improved.

Defining small for gestational age

The importance of gestational age estimation

In order to overcome the problem of the definition of LBW capturing fetuses with suboptimal growth and preterm birth, the definition of SGA is used. This presupposes accurate gestational age estimation, an essential component of pregnancy management. This not only allows appropriate scheduling of a woman's antenatal care but also informs obstetric management decisions—for example, whether administration of prophylactic corticosteroids for fetal lung maturity and transfer to another healthcare setting is appropriate in cases of preterm labour; or, at the other extreme, determines if labour induction should be scheduled in the post-term period

Knowledge of gestational age is also integral in the correct interpretation of clinical or ultrasonographic fetal growth assessment: abnormal fetal growth patterns such as SGA or LGA may be missed or incorrectly diagnosed if gestational age is unknown or incorrect. Accurate dating is not only important in individual pregnancy care, but also at population and health policy level: the lack of accurate gestational age estimation, in particular in those areas of the world at greatest risk of these conditions, means that preterm birth and SGA rates are merely estimates in much of the world—it is thought that preterm birth rates in over half of all births worldwide depend upon modelled data and are of uncertain accuracy (6) while estimates of SGA are based on the proxy of LBW (<2500 g) (7) which of course also include many preterm births.

Traditionally, gestational age is estimated using the first day of the last menstrual period. This assumes that ovulation occurs 14 days after the last menstrual period. Irregular menses, unknown or uncertain dates, oral contraceptive use, or recent pregnancy or breastfeeding may all influence the accuracy of this method, and this inaccuracy is significant in a large proportion of women (8, 9).

Because of this, early ultrasound measures of fetal crown–rump length (CRL) is recommended to assess gestational age in the first trimester before 14 weeks of gestation; various studies have been conducted to derive CRL reference charts for the estimation of gestational age, mostly in single institutions or geographical locations; a review of 29 available studies showed several limitations in study design and approaches to statistical analysis and reporting for most studies (10). The large number of charts relating CRL to gestational age can lead to significant variation. However, when using those with the lowest risk of methodological bias (10–14), very small differences in gestational estimation arise when compared with the remaining charts. Nevertheless, these charts were developed on local populations; international standards for evaluating fetal linear size in the first trimester and for the estimation of gestational age from CRL that can be used across countries and populations are now available. This is in close agreement with the studies with a low risk of methodological bias mentioned previously conducted in populations from developed countries, suggesting that when high methodological standards are met and populations adequately selected, early fetal growth is similar across populations (15).

It is generally the case that such first-trimester gestational age assessment is more accurate than late pregnancy dating; this is because fetal ultrasound measurements are associated with a larger absolute error with advancing gestation (16), and because fetal growth disturbances become more prevalent, meaning that an abnormally small fetus could be misjudged to have lower gestational age while a macrosomic fetus may be ascribed a more advanced gestation. Finally, once the gestational age has been ascribed using the earliest reliable ultrasound scan, this should not be changed as this can lead to potential dating errors.

The effects of different charts

Although the WHO defined SGA as a birth weight less than the 10th percentile when compared to a reference for gestational age and sex (3), which reference should be used was not defined, resulting in a long-running debate around the most appropriate chart (2).

The recognition of pathological growth is dependent on the existence of reliable standards. However, the establishment of normal charts for key biometric variables, such as biparietal diameter, head circumference, abdominal circumference, and femur length, is not straightforward. In a systematic review of 83 fetal growth charts available at the time (2012), Ioannou et al. showed that differences in study design, data analysis, and presentation contributed to significant discrepancies between studies of fetal growth. The resulting different fetal size charts will have an obvious effect on the ability to discriminate appropriate from inappropriately grown fetuses. The study called for international standards of fetal growth in order to be able to unify screening and diagnosis (6).

As an example, using the 1991 United States national reference, it was estimated that 27% of all live births (32.4 million babies) were born SGA in low- and middle-income countries in 2010, with the highest prevalence of term-SGA being born in south Asia (41.5%) (4). If a different reference chart had been chosen, however, this figure could be quite different (17). Without definition of a reference against which centiles are judged, SGA is also a problematic indicator. In practice, this can lead to the confusing scenario of a woman identified as having a SGA baby in a clinic using one reference, then being referred for a second opinion only to be being told that her baby is normal if a different chart is used (18).

Complicating the definition of SGA babies further is the concept that the tenth centile should be individualized, or customized, for each pregnancy. This has led to customized charts that adjust expectations of fetal growth based on maternal characteristics, most commonly maternal ethnicity, height, weight, and parity (19). These charts have been used extensively in the United Kingdom (20) based on observational data suggesting they may better detect babies with growth problems at risk of stillbirth (21). In the United States, customization tends to be limited to adjusting growth expectations based on ethnicity. A multicentre study which followed the growth of 1737 babies in the United States demonstrated small differences in the growth curves of African American and Hispanic babies when compared to non-Hispanic white babies. However, in this study, women from the three groups had very different baseline characteristics and socioeconomic backgrounds (22). It is difficult therefore to determine whether much of the difference in the growth of babies was attributable to ethnicity per se, or to socioeconomic characteristics that are associated with ethnicity. Thus, while customization may be an appealing concept, the construct of size being predetermined based on maternal height and ethnicity has been challenged by recent scientific evidence. A Cochrane review concluded that customized charts demonstrate no evidence of superiority compared to population-based references (23).

Given this confusion around charts and indicators for size at birth, there has been a move towards aiming instead to optimize development in the fetus (24) with the goal of maximizing human capital and outcomes. Achieving this goal requires a comprehensive approach focusing on maintaining adequate (not excessive) preconceptual maternal nutrition, optimizing health, and minimizing exposure to substances that can adversely influence growth (nutritional, pharmacological, environmental, and other) (25).

What is 'normal' fetal growth?

With the advent of ultrasonography, it has become possible to monitor the skeletal growth, soft tissue deposition, and organ development of the baby, as well as functional parameters of placental function such as blood flow in the maternal uterine vessels, umbilical arteries, and fetal circulation. However, in order to identify abnormal growth, there must be an understanding of physiological or optimal fetal growth trajectories. This has proven controversial in obstetric ultrasound practice. A systematic review of the literature identified over 70 published fetal growth charts, most with potential major methodological sources of bias (17).

In 1995, the WHO recommended the use of standards for the measurement of human anthropometry (3). Standards describe growth under near-optimal conditions, and are prescriptive: they demonstrate how growth should be, rather than descriptive as reference charts are, which describe how growth has occurred at a particular time or place.

The concept of growth standards has been widely accepted in paediatrics, following the landmark publication of the findings of the WHO Multicentre Growth Reference Study (MGRS) in 2006 (26). This longitudinal, international study followed the growth and development of children born in cities in six countries with arguably distinct ancestral lineages around the world (Brazil, Oman, Norway, United States, India, and Ghana). The study demonstrated that when mothers were free from complications in pregnancy, lived in non socially deprived settings, did not smoke, and exclusively breastfed the infants for the first 6 months of life, the growth of their children was remarkably similar. In 2006, the WHO Child Growth Standards were released, defining optimal growth trajectories for children everywhere. Definitions of poor growth, including the clinical conditions of stunting and wasting, are thereby near universally accepted. The WHO Child Growth Standards have been adopted in over 130 countries (27). International standards have been shown to be useful both at an individual level screening for problems of growth, as well as at the population and global level to identify and compare nutrition around the world. With advancing socioeconomic progress, the population-level distribution of childhood growth gradually shifts closer to the optimal population (28).

Until recently, lack of knowledge about of the optimal growth of babies *in utero* and preconceived ideas about fetal growth in relation to maternal characteristics have prohibited similar comparisons in the perinatal period.

The INTERGROWTH-21st Project

The INTERGROWTH-21st Project was established to address this fundamental gap in our understanding of early human growth. The Project aimed to determine how fetal growth, preterm postnatal growth, and neurodevelopment in the first 1000 days of life occur under *optimal* conditions, and whether or not this growth is similar enough around the world to justify the use of a single set of international growth standards (29).

The INTERGROWTH-21st Project was based on uniquely detailed methodology (29) and all study protocols and primary findings are available freely online (https://intergrowth21.tghn.org). Briefly, eight diverse urban populations living in demarcated geographical or political areas were selected where environments were free from major known pollutants; altitude was less than 1600 m; most women accessed antenatal and delivery care in institutions; mean birth weight was greater than 3100 g; rates of LBW (<2500 g) were less than 10%; and perinatal mortality was less than 20 per 1000 births. The study sites were Pelotas, Brazil (30); Shunyi County Beijing, China (31); Central Nagpur District, India (32); Turin, Italy (33); Parklands Suburb, Nairobi (34); Muscat, Oman (35); Oxford, United Kingdom (36); and Seattle, United States (37). From 2009 to 2014, mothers from these populations were screened for eligibility to enter the Fetal Growth Longitudinal Study (FGLS), to monitor growth and development from early pregnancy until infancy.

From 9 weeks onwards and every 5 weeks until birth, fetal biometry was measured by ultrasound using a highly standardized, blinded, and scientifically rigorous protocol designed to minimize intra- and interobserver bias (38). At birth, the same rigour was applied to measure the weight, length, and head circumference of all newborns born in the entire population (39). Infants were then followed up to the age of 2 years.

The statistical approaches to determine whether the measurements from the eight study sites could be pooled to produce standards were the same as those used in the WHO MGRS (40). Skeletal (i.e. fat-free) measurements were compared across sites as they are less likely to be skewed by overnutrition. Measurements selected were CRL in the first trimester, fetal head circumference from 14 weeks until birth, and birth head circumference and length. The variability of measurements between sites was compared by examining the crude values from each country; by conducting sensitivity analysis to assess the effect of removing one country at a time on the overall trend; by comparing the standardized site differences, that is, assessing whether the standard deviation of measurements for each country were within 0.5 of the overall standard deviation; and by conducting analysis of variance to determine the amount of variation in growth due to intersite differences

The analysis demonstrated that between 1.9% and 3.5% of the variation observed between linear fetal growth and newborn size at birth was due to intersite differences (41). Therefore, as previously observed with infant and child growth patterns, fetal growth and newborn size at birth are remarkably similar around the world when constraints on growth are minimal. At 12 months of age, height-for-age z-scores in the FGLS children aligned almost exactly with the distribution observed in the MGRS children (42). These findings provide the most robust evidence to date that under relatively optimal conditions, the growth trajectories of human beings are very similar around the world, with ethnicity playing a minor role in the variation of the size of babies that is observed.

The INTERGROWTH-21st Standards challenge how growth problems should be identified and defined. Changing physicians' concepts about 'normal' fetal growth is challenging. Further research is needed on the best approach to implement the standards in clinical practice at scale (43), as well as appropriate and evidence-based guidelines adapted for different contexts for the management of pregnancies where growth problems are suspected. Like in childhood, evidence of faltering growth is rarely diagnostic in itself, and this information must be considered in light of findings of functional parameters, fetal morphology, maternal conditions, and possible toxins or infectious exposures.

The growing problem of larger babies

In addition to the problem of small babies, large babies are also at risk of perinatal and long-term complications (44). In many high-income populations, birth weight was observed to increase during the 1970s to 2000s (45); more recently, however, declines in birth weight have been observed (46–48). This could correlate with increases in iatrogenic preterm deliveries, or possibly improved screening and treatment of gestational diabetes mellitus (GDM). Further investigation is needed in specific settings to see what factors are most likely driving these trends.

Large babies frequently pose a dilemma for obstetric care providers. Large size at birth increases the risks of slow or obstructed labour, which in turn increases the risk of emergency caesarean section and postpartum haemorrhage. In those women who do progress to vaginal birth with a large baby, there is an increased risk of shoulder dystocia and the associated maternal and neonatal birth trauma. It is therefore important to recognize LGA and macrosomia before birth so that there can be appropriate counselling of the parents and planning for the timing and mode of delivery.

The definition of macrosomia most commonly used in perinatal medicine is a birth weight more than 4.0 kg. Other definitions used include 3.8, 4.5, and 5 kg, often based on the distribution of birth weight and perinatal outcomes in different populations around the world. While it has been argued that the risk of adverse outcomes is greatest in the group weighing over 4.5 kg, the risk of shoulder dystocia has been shown to increase steeply from 4 to 4.25 kg (49). In mothers who are stunted (adult height <150 cm), malnourished, or with skeletal problems such as rickets caused by vitamin D deficiency, a baby much smaller than 4 kg may increase the risk of labour dystocia and the need for operative birth.

Aetiologies and risk factors for LGA

Diabetes in pregnancy

Rates of diabetes in pregnancy around the world have now reached epidemic levels. The vast majority of cases of diabetes in pregnancy are GDM, with smaller proportions of women entering pregnancy with known type1 or type 2 diabetes (50). The International Diabetes Federation estimated in 2015 that one in seven pregnant women had GDM (51). Most of these women are unaware of their diagnosis and live in societies with poorly developed health systems to screen or manage diabetes and the associated complications in pregnancy.

During pregnancy, placental hormones create a state of relative insulin resistance in the mother to facilitate the transfer of amino acids and glucose to the fetus. The degree of insulin resistance that develops by the third trimester is similar to that observed in people with type 2 diabetes, requiring the maternal pancreas to increase insulin secretion by almost 250% to maintain, who are either unable to increase their insulin secretion, or who already have borderline levels of peripheral insulin resistance, or both.

The high proportion of women with GDM has been attributed to current unprecedented rates of overweight and obesity in reproductive-aged women (52); women delaying childbearing until the fourth decade; and a relative abundance of calorie-rich and nutrient-poor foods, particularly in deprived social areas and in countries undergoing economic transition (53).

The other important contributor to the rate of GDM relates to changes in the definition of the condition itself. The landmark Hyperglycemia and Adverse Pregnancy Outcomes (HAPO) study demonstrated a linear and increasing association between maternal glycaemia at 28 weeks and birth weight, need for primary caesarean section, cord blood C peptide (a marker of fetal hyperinsulinaemia), and neonatal hypoglycaemia (54). These findings formed the basis for a revised definition of GDM. This was based on an increased relative risk of 1.75 of one or more adverse perinatal outcomes associated with GDM, including LGA (based on birthweight >90th centile on local charts), primary caesarean section, neonatal hypoglycaemia, and cord C peptide (55).

In 2015, the National Institute for Health and Care Excellence (NICE) in the United Kingdom updated its recommendations on the screening and treatment of GDM (50). Women who experienced GDM in a prior pregnancy are offered oral glucose tolerance testing as early as possible in pregnancy, while other women with risk factors are screened for GDM around 26–28 weeks' gestation. While there remains controversy around diagnostic thresholds for GDM, values higher than the current diagnostic criteria should trigger a system to provide dietary advice, advice on blood glucose monitoring, and multidisciplinary care (50). Frequently, the diagnosis of LGA is not made until late in pregnancy in women without GDM. Interpreting results from glucose tolerance tests very late in pregnancy can be challenging and there is little evidence to guide appropriate screening for diabetes in women detected to have a large baby close to term. A sensible compromise would be to exclude overt diabetes in these women, through either a fasting blood glucose or 2-hour oral glucose tolerance test.

The aim of clinical management in women with all forms of diabetes in pregnancy is to normalize blood glucose to decrease the risk of complications associated with hyperglycaemia. In women with GDM there is level 1 evidence that screening and treatment of GDM can reduce birthweight (56) and severe adverse outcomes in the offspring (death, brachial plexus injury, skull fracture) (57). Normalizing glycaemic control in women with diabetes is one of the few interventions that have been shown to decrease birth size, although tight control of blood glucose in pregnancy can increase the chance of maternal hypoglycaemia, poor fetal growth, and low newborn body fat percentage (58), highlighting how difficult this condition can be to optimally control.

Maternal overweight and obesity

Another risk factor for LGA is maternal obesity, with estimates indicating the risk of macrosomia to be approximately doubled when compared to women with a normal body mass index (BMI) (odds ratio 2.1; 95% CI 1.6–2.6) (59). Several approaches have been taken to reduce fetal overgrowth associated with obesity, including intensive lifestyle and pharmacological interventions; however, results have been disappointing.

The UK Pregnancies Better Eating and Activities Trial (UPBEAT) and the Limiting Weight Gain in Overweight and Obese Women during Pregnancy to Improve Health Outcomes (LIMIT) trial, both assessed the effects of lifestyle interventions to improve pregnancy outcomes in obese pregnant women. The UPBEAT trial was conducted in the United Kingdom and involved 1555 obese pregnant women (772 allocated to standard antenatal care and 783 to the intervention). The intervention involved weekly lifestyle and dietary counselling informed by social change theories. There was no difference between the groups in the primary endpoints of a difference in rates of GDM and LGA babies, although some secondary outcomes such as maternal weight gain were improved in the intervention group (60). The LIMIT trial was conducted in Australia and reported similar findings (61).

The effect of metformin to reduce birthweight in obese women without gestational diabetes has also been assessed in two randomized controlled trials from the United Kingdom. The Efficacy of Metformin in Pregnant Obese Women, a Randomised controlled (EMPOWaR) trial assessed the effect of 2.5 g of metformin daily from 16–18 weeks gestation on birth outcomes in 449 women. A second United Kingdom study assessed the effect of 3 g of metformin in 450 obese women. Neither of these studies demonstrated any evidence of effect on birthweight (62).

The effects of maternal obesity on fetal growth may have their origins very early in pregnancy. In animal models there is evidence that exposure to obesity in either parent changes the molecular structure of the oocyte or sperm, and that this can alter the process of epigenetic reprogramming that occurs after conception (63). Current interventions targeting gestational weight gain in obese gravidas may therefore be coming too late, with a life course focus on women's health needed if we are to seriously tackle the problem of intergenerational obesity.

Gestational weight gain

Excessive gestational weight gain is also associated with accelerated fetal growth. Despite decades of research, however, there remains controversy in the value and recommendations for optimal gestational weight gain in pregnancy with most of the evidence which current recommendations are based on being poor (64). The INTERGROWTH-21st Project has published weight gain trajectories in low-risk women with normal BMIs (65). Robust evidence for women in other weight groups is lacking, and it is often women in these weight groups who pose the greatest clinical challenge. The Institute of Medicine 2009 guidelines for gestational weight gain are widely used in clinical practice. These guidelines are an expert synthesis of the best available evidence and try to balance the perinatal risks of inadequate or excessive weight gain with the risks of postpartum weight retention, a significant contributor to obesity in many women. Evidence for the use of the Institute of Medicine guidelines in populations outside the United States is lacking.

Fetal genetic overgrowth syndromes

Detection of very severe LGA, particularly early in pregnancy or in the presence of other abnormalities, should prompt expert review in a fetal medicine unit. Somatic overgrowth syndromes, while relatively rare, can begin in the prenatal period and can be associated with genetic syndromes that are associated with neurodevelopmental delay and increase the risks of neoplasia. Generalized overgrowth syndromes that can be detected *in utero* include Beckwith–Wiedemann syndrome, Simpson–Golabi–Behmel syndrome, Sotos syndrome, Weaver syndrome, Marchall–Smith syndrome, and Perlman syndrome. For an overview of these rare conditions, the reader is referred to the review by Yachelevich, published in 2015 (66).

Detection of LGA

Traditionally, the detection of LGA babies was made clinically, either by palpation, symphysiofundal height measurement, or by maternal suspicion; however, all these methods have been reported to have poor detection rates of less than 50% (67). If a large baby was suspected, commonly ultrasound biometry would be performed to measure the size of the baby and approximate the volume of amniotic fluid. The diagnosis of LGA from ultrasound is usually based on the finding of the estimated fetal weight at greater than the 90th or 97th centile, depending on local practice. As this value is based on regression equations combining two or more measures of fetal biometry, it can be inaccurate at the upper weight limits. The density of babies is not uniform across the size distribution, and typically accuracy of estimated weight reduces in larger babies. A review of the published literature found the post-test probability of ultrasound to predict LGA to range from 15% to 79% (68).

Given these limitations, several groups have attempted to improve the diagnosis of LGA by utilizing three-dimensional volumetric measures of fetal structures, such as the thigh volume, or novel two-dimensional measurements of fetal fat deposits, such as cheek-to-cheek diameter, abdominal wall thickness, and upper arm diameter.

While these procedures show promise in improving diagnostic accuracy, due to technical difficulty, cost, and time they are currently limited largely to research settings.

Evidence for clinical management

The clinical management of LGA babies in pregnancy depends on the individual factors likely to be driving the growth and other comorbid complications. For obstetricians, the most important decisions need to be made around the timing and mode of delivery. These decisions will be different in women with LGA and diabetes compared to those women with LGA who are not known to have diabetes.

LGA in pregnancies complicated by diabetes

Decisions for delivery timing and mode for women with all forms of diabetes in pregnancy are based on concerns of excessive fetal growth, an increased risk of shoulder dystocia with disproportionate fat deposition in the fetus, as well as a fivefold increased risk of stillbirth in women with pre-existing diabetes. The 2015 NICE guideline recommends delivery by 41 weeks for women with well-controlled GDM with dietary modifications (50). Delivery should be sooner in women with pre-existing diabetes (37–38 weeks), or in women with GDM requiring medication with either poor glycaemic control or signs of macrosomia (50).

Non-diabetic pregnancies

In women without diabetes carrying a LGA baby, there has been little evidence to support induction before term to prevent shoulder dystocia. In 2015, however, a multicentre randomized controlled trial published in *The Lancet* and examining whether induction of labour by 39^{+6} weeks in babies estimated to have a birth weight greater than the 90th centile compared to expectant management could actually reduce this risk. The trial recruited 822 women (409 in the induction group and 413 in the expectant management group) and demonstrated a significant reduction in the primary outcome, shoulder dystocia (RR 0.32; 95% CI 0.15–0.71; *P* = 0.004) with planned induction of labour. The women in the induction group did not experience a higher rate of caesarean section and were actually more likely to delivery spontaneously (RR 1.14; 95% CI 1.01–1.29) (69). This trial is the largest and most rigorous to address the management of LGA babies. While none of the babies who experienced the primary outcome of shoulder dystocia in labour suffered permanent brachial plexus injury or death, the lack of harm from the intervention and potential for improved spontaneous vaginal birth rates are important. Based upon this evidence, a policy of detection of LGA in the third trimester and induction of labour before 39 weeks would seem sensible, although international guidelines have not yet endorsed this change in practice. Before clinical practices are changed there must be consideration of local resource constraints for the provision of ultrasound to detect LGA, as well as the capacity of the unit to provide safe induction of labour. As with all evidence from randomized trials, there must also be consideration as to whether this evidence is applicable to individual patients, for example, the small risk of shoulder dystocia may be outweighed by the risk of induction of labour in women with a previous caesarean section hoping to have a vaginal birth.

Longer-term outcomes associated with LGA

Around the world, children are getting heavier and childhood overweight and obesity is recognized to be a significant global problem (70). Being born large is associated with an increased risk of childhood obesity, although establishing the direct causal link is challenging due to multiple potential confounding dietary and socioeconomic factors (71). The observational epidemiological data consistently support a positive association between size at birth and childhood weight. Part of the effort to reduce childhood obesity must include strategies to limit excessive fetal growth in pregnancy where possible (72). As previously discussed, this is not an easy outcome to change, and any advice to expectant mothers must be given in a way that balances the real risks of fetal overgrowth with risks of mothers drastically altering their food intake to prevent these outcomes and causing problems of inadequate fetal growth.

REFERENCES

1. Wardlaw T, Blanc A, Zupan J, et al. *Low Birthweight: Country Regional and Global Estimates.* Geneva: World Health Organization, UNICEF; 2004.
2. Kramer MS. The epidemiology of low birthweight. *Nestle Nutr Inst Workshop Ser* 2013;**74**:1–10.
3. World Health Organization (WHO). *Physical Status: The Use and Interpretation of Anthropometry. Report of a WHO Expert Committee.* WHO Technical Report Series. Geneva: WHO; 1995.
4. Lee AC, Katz J, Blencowe H, et al. National and regional estimates of term and preterm babies born small for gestational age in 138 low-income and middle-income countries in 2010. *Lancet Glob Health* 2013;**1**:e26–36.
5. Althabe F, Belizan JM, McClure EM, et al. A population-based, multifaceted strategy to implement antenatal corticosteroid treatment versus standard care for the reduction of neonatal mortality due to preterm birth in low-income and middle-income countries: the ACT cluster-randomised trial. *Lancet* 2015;**385**:629–39.
6. Blencowe H, Cousens S, Oestergaard MZ, et al. National, regional, and worldwide estimates of preterm birth rates in the year 2010 with time trends since 1990 for selected countries: a systematic analysis and implications. *Lancet* 2012;**379**:2162–72.
7. de Onis M, Blossner M, Villar J. Levels and patterns of intrauterine growth retardation in developing countries. *Eur J Clin Nutr* 1998;**52** Suppl 1:S5–15.
8. Campbell S, Warsof SL, Little D, et al. Routine ultrasound screening for the prediction of gestational age. *Obstet Gynecol* 1985;**65**:613–20.
9. Nguyen TH, Larsen T, Engholm G, et al. Evaluation of ultrasound-estimated date of delivery in 17,450 spontaneous singleton births: do we need to modify Naegele's rule? *Ultrasound Obstet Gynecol* 1999;**14**:23–28.
10. Napolitano R, Dhami J, Ohuma E, et al. Pregnancy dating by fetal crown-rump length: a systematic review of charts. *BJOG* 2014:**121**;556–65.
11. Robinson HP, Fleming JE. A critical evaluation of sonar 'crown-rump length' measurements. *Br J Obstet Gynaecol* 1975;**82**:702–10.
12. McLennan AC, Schluter PJ. Construction of modern Australian first trimester ultrasound dating and growth charts. *J Med Imaging Radiat Oncol* 2008;**52**:471–79.
13. Sahota DS, Leung TY, Leung TN, et al. Fetal crown-rump length and estimation of gestational age in an ethnic Chinese population. *Ultrasound Obstet Gynecol* 2009;**33**:157–60.
14. Verburg BO, Steegers EA, De Ridder M, et al. New charts for ultrasound dating of pregnancy and assessment of fetal growth: longitudinal data from a population-based cohort study. *Ultrasound Obstet Gynecol* 2008;**31**:388–96.
15. Papageorghiou AT, Kennedy SH, Salomon LJ, et al. International standards for early fetal size and pregnancy dating based on ultrasound measurement of crown-rump length in the first trimester. *Ultrasound Obstet Gynecol* 2014;**44**:641–48.
16. Sarris I, Ioannou C, Ohuma EO, et al. Standardisation and quality control of ultrasound measurements taken in the INTERGROWTH-21st Project. *BJOG* 2013;**120** Suppl 2:33–37.
17. Ioannou C, Talbot K, Ohuma E, et al. Systematic review of methodology used in ultrasound studies aimed at creating charts of fetal size. *BJOG* 2012;**119**:1425–39.
18. Westerway SC, Papageorghiou AT, Hirst J, et al. INTERGROWTH-21st- time to standardise fetal measurement in Australia. *AJUM* 2015;**18**:91–128.
19. Gardosi J, Chang A, Kaylan B, et al. Customized antenatal growth charts. *Lancet* 1992;**339**:283–87.
20. Royal College of Obstetricians and Gynaecologists (RCOG). *Small-for-Gestational-Age Fetus, Investigation and Management.* Green-top Guideline No. 31. London: RCOG; 2013.
21. Gardosi J, Madurasinghe V, Williams M, et al. Maternal and fetal risk factors for stillbirth: population based study. *BMJ* 2013;**346**:f108.
22. Buck Louis GM, Grewal J, Albert PS, et al. Racial/ethnic standards for fetal growth: the NICHD Fetal Growth Studies. *Am J Obstet Gynecol* 2015;**213**:449.e1–49.
23. Carberry AE, Gordon A, Bond DM, et al. Customised versus population-based growth charts as a screening tool for detecting small for gestational age infants in low-risk pregnant women. *Cochrane Database Syst Rev* 2011;**12**:CD008549.

24. World Health Organization (WHO). *Promoting Optimal Fetal Development: Report of a Technical Consultation.* Geneva: WHO; 2006.

25. WHO Multicentre Growth Reference Study Group. Assessment of differences in linear growth among populations in the WHO Multicentre Growth Reference Study. *Acta Paediatr Suppl* 2006;**450**:56–65.

26. Borghi E, de Onis M, Garza C, et al. Construction of the World Health Organization child growth standards: selection of methods for attained growth curves. *Stat Med* 2006;**25**:247–65.

27. de Onis M, Onyango A, Borghi E, et al. Worldwide implementation of the WHO Child Growth Standards. *Public Health Nutr* 2012;**15**:1603–10.

28. Stevens GA, Finucane MM, Paciorek CJ, et al. Trends in mild, moderate, and severe stunting and underweight, and progress towards MDG 1 in 141 developing countries: a systematic analysis of population representative data. *Lancet* 2012;**380**:824–34.

29. Villar J, Altman D, Purwar M, et al. The objectives, design and implementation of the INTERGROWTH-21 Project. *BJOG* 2013;**120** Suppl 2:9–26.

30. Silveira MF, Barros FC, Sclowitz IK, et al. Implementation of the INTERGROWTH-21st Project in Brazil. *BJOG* 2013;**120** Suppl 2:81–86.

31. Pan Y, Wu MH, Wang JH, et al. Implementation of the INTERGROWTH-21st Project in China. *BJOG* 2013;**120** Suppl 2:87–93.

32. Purwar M, Kunnawar N, Deshmukh S, et al. Implementation of the INTERGROWTH-21st Project in India. *BJOG* 2013;**120** Suppl 2:94–99.

33. Giuliani F, Bertino E, Oberto M, et al. Implementation of the INTERGROWTH-21st Project in Italy. *BJOG* 2013;**120** Suppl 2:100–104.

34. Carvalho M, Vinayak S, Ochieng R, et al. Implementation of the INTERGROWTH-21st Project in Kenya. *BJOG* 2013;**120** Suppl 2:105–10.

35. Jaffer YA, Al Abri J, Abdawani J, et al. Implementation of the INTERGROWTH-21st Project in Oman. *BJOG* 2013;**120** Suppl 2:111–16.

36. Roseman F, Knight HE, Giuliani F, et al. Implementation of the INTERGROWTH-21st Project in the UK. *BJOG* 2013;**120** Suppl 2:117–22.

37. Dighe MK, Frederick IO, Andersen HF, et al. Implementation of the INTERGROWTH-21st Project in the United States. *BJOG* 2013;**120** Suppl 2:123–28.

38. Papageorghiou AT, Sarris I, Ioannou C, et al. Ultrasound methodology used to construct the fetal growth standards in the INTERGROWTH-21st Project. *BJOG* 2013;**120** Suppl 2:27–32.

39. Cheikh Ismail L, Knight HE, Bhutta Z, et al. Anthropometric protocols for the construction of new international fetal and newborn growth standards: the INTERGROWTH-21st Project. *BJOG* 2013;**120** Suppl 2:42–47.

40. Altman DG, Ohuma EO, International F, et al. Statistical considerations for the development of prescriptive fetal and newborn growth standards in the INTERGROWTH-21st Project. *BJOG* 2013;**120** Suppl 2:71–76.

41. Villar J, Papageorghiou AT, Pang R, et al. The likeness of fetal growth and newborn size across non-isolated populations in the INTERGROWTH-21 Project: the Fetal Growth Longitudinal Study and Newborn Cross-Sectional Study. *Lancet Diabetes Endocrinol* 2014;**2**:781–92.

42. Villar J, Papageorghiou AT, Pang R, et al. Monitoring human growth and development: a continuum from the womb to the classroom. *Am J Obstet Gynecol* 2015;**213**:494–99.

43. Chatfield A, Caglia JM, Dhillon S, et al. Translating research into practice: the introduction of the INTERGROWTH-21st package of clinical standards, tools and guidelines into policies, programmes and services. *BJOG* 2013;**120** Suppl 2:139–42.

44. Weissmann-Brenner A, Simchen MJ, Zilberberg E, et al. Maternal and neonatal outcomes of large for gestational age pregnancies. *Acta Obstet Gynecol Scand* 2012;**91**:844–49.

45. Hadfield RM, Lain SJ, Simpson JM, et al. Are babies getting bigger? An analysis of birthweight trends in New South Wales, 1990–2005. *Med J Aust* 2009;**190**:312–15.

46. Shan X, Chen F, Wang W, et al. Secular trends of low birthweight and macrosomia and related maternal factors in Beijing, China: a longitudinal trend analysis. *BMC Pregnancy Childbirth* 2014;**14**:105.

47. Diouf I, Charles MA, Blondel B, et al. Discordant time trends in maternal body size and offspring birthweight of term deliveries in France between 1972 and 2003: data from the French National Perinatal Surveys. *Paediatr Perinat Epidemiol* 2011;**25**:210–17.

48. Catov JM, Lee M, Roberts JM, et al. Race disparities and decreasing birth weight: are all babies getting smaller? *Am J Epidemiol* 2016;**183**:15–23.

49. Campbell S. Fetal macrosomia: a problem in need of a policy. *Ultrasound Obstet* Gynecol 2014;**43**:3–10.

50. National Institute for Health and Care Excellence (NICE). *Diabetes in Pregnancy: Management from Preconception to the Postnatal Period.* NICE guideline [NG3]. London: NICE; 2015.

51. International Diabetes Federation. IDF Diabetes Atlas. 2015. Available at: http://www.diabetesatlas.org.

52. Heslehurst N, Rankin J, Wilkinson JR, et al. A nationally representative study of maternal obesity in England, UK: trends in incidence and demographic inequalities in 619 323 births, 1989-2007. *Int J Obes (Lond)* 2010;**34**:420–28.

53. Popkin BM, Adair LS, Ng SW. Global nutrition transition and the pandemic of obesity in developing countries. *Nutr Rev* 2012;**70**:3–21.

54. HAPO Study Cooperative Research Group, Metzger BE, Lowe LP, et al. Hyperglycemia and adverse pregnancy outcomes. *N Engl J Med* 2008;**358**:1991–2002.

55. Diagnosis and classification of diabetes mellitus. *Diabetes Care* 2010;**33** Suppl 1:S62–69.

56. Landon MB, Spong CY, Thom E, et al. A multicenter, randomized trial of treatment for mild gestational diabetes. *N Engl J Med* 2009;**361**:1339–48.

57. Crowther CA, Hiller JE, Moss JR, et al. Effect of treatment of gestational diabetes mellitus on pregnancy outcomes. *N Engl J Med* 2005;**352**:2477–86.

58. Au CP, Raynes-Greenow CH, Turner RM, et al. Body composition is normal in term infants born to mothers with well-controlled gestational diabetes mellitus. *Diabetes Care* 2013;**36**:562–64.

59. Jolly MC, Sebire NJ, Harris JP, et al. Risk factors for macrosomia and its clinical consequences: a study of 350,311 pregnancies. *Eur J Obstet Gynecol Reprod Biol* 2003;**111**:9–14.

60. Poston L, Bell R, Croker H, et al. Effect of a behavioural intervention in obese pregnant women (the UPBEAT study): a multicentre, randomised controlled trial. *Lancet Diabetes Endocrinol* 2015;**3**:767–77.

61. Dodd JM, Turnbull D, McPhee AJ, et al. Antenatal lifestyle advice for women who are overweight or obese: LIMIT randomised trial. *BMJ* 2014;**348**:g1285.

62. Chiswick C, Reynolds RM, Denison F, et al. Effect of metformin on maternal and fetal outcomes in obese pregnant women (EMPOWaR): a randomised, double-blind, placebo-controlled trial. *Lancet Diabetes Endocrinol* 2015;**3**:778–86.

63. Lane M, Zander-Fox DL, Robker RL, et al. Peri-conception parental obesity, reproductive health, and transgenerational impacts. *Trends Endocrinol Metab* 2015;**26**:84–90.

64. Ohadike CO, Cheikh-Ismail L, Ohuma EO, et al. Systematic review of the methodological quality of studies aimed at creating gestational weight gain charts. *Adv Nutr* 2016;**7**:313–22.

65. Cheikh Ismail L, Bishop DC, Pang R, et al. Gestational weight gain standards based on women enrolled in the Fetal Growth Longitudinal Study of the INTERGROWTH-21st Project: a prospective longitudinal cohort study. *BMJ* 2016;**352**:i555.

66. Yachelevich N. Generalized overgrowth syndromes with prenatal onset. *Curr Probl Pediatr Adolesc Health Care* 2015;**45**:97–111.

67. Walsh JM, McAuliffe FM. Prediction and prevention of the macrosomic fetus. *Eur J Obstet Gynecol Reprod Biol* 2012;**162**:125–30.

68. Chauhan SP, Grobman WA, Gherman RA, et al. Suspicion and treatment of the macrosomic fetus: a review. *Am J Obstet Gynecol* 2005;**193**:332–46.

69. Boulvain M, Senat MV, Perrotin F, et al. Induction of labour versus expectant management for large-for-date fetuses: a randomised controlled trial. *Lancet* 2015;**385**:2600–705.

70. Lobstein T, Jackson-Leach R, Moodie ML, et al. Child and adolescent obesity: part of a bigger picture. *Lancet* 2015;**385**:2510–20.

71. Gaillard R, Felix JF, Duijts L, et al. Childhood consequences of maternal obesity and excessive weight gain during pregnancy. *Acta Obstet Gynecol Scand* 2014;**93**:1085–89.

72. Hirst JE, Villar J, Papageorghiou AT, et al. Preventing childhood obesity starts during pregnancy. *Lancet* 2015;**386**:1039–40.

11

Prenatal diagnosis

Ana Piñas Carrillo and Amarnath Bhide

Introduction

Prenatal diagnosis has vastly developed over the last 50 years. Until the 1970s, the assessment of the fetus was limited to determining the position using the Leopold manoeuvres and registering the fetal heart beat by ultrasonography. Ultrasound examination was introduced in the 1980s in the United Kingdom as part of routine antenatal care. However, uniformity on the timing and requirements of routine ultrasound scanning has only been standardized relatively recently across the country. Obstetric ultrasound scanning has advanced rapidly since its inception, which has aided earlier and better diagnosis of fetal abnormalities.

Ultrasound is generally accepted to be safe for antenatal use. However, the development of ultrasound has led to equipment capable of higher energy output. Potential risks of thermal or mechanical damage exist with prolonged exposure to ultrasound in general, and the use of pulsed wave Doppler in particular. The advice is to limit the exposure to as low as is reasonably achievable (ALARA). Ultrasound should always be used prudently.

Universal screening and case finding

Screening is the systematic application of a test to identify individuals at sufficient risk of a specific disorder to benefit from further investigations. The concept of universal screening for prenatal diagnosis started in the United Kingdom in the 1980s.

The screening for chromosomal abnormalities started with the introduction of maternal age as a risk factor. Any pregnant woman over 35 years old was offered an invasive test to detect chromosomal defects, in particular trisomy 21 (Down syndrome). This initial approach detected about 50% of trisomy 21 cases with a high false-positive rate (1). In the 1980s, the screening consisted of maternal serum biochemistry and a detailed anomaly scan in the second trimester. The combined first-trimester screening was introduced in the 1990s. It combines maternal age, nuchal translucency (NT), and biochemical markers in maternal serum (beta-human chorionic gonadotropin (hCG) and pregnancy-associated plasma protein A (PAPP-A)). This test increased the detection rate to 90% with a false-positive rate of 5% for trisomy 21 and is the currently recommended method for screening in the United Kingdom and most developed countries (2). It was recently discovered that small fragments of cell-free fetal DNA are present in maternal blood, and can be used to test for chromosomal abnormalities. The introduction of cell-free fetal DNA testing (also known as non-invasive prenatal testing or NIPT) has improved the detection rates of trisomy 21 to 99%. However, it is still not universally available (3).

Parallel to the screening for chromosomal defects, the introduction of a routine anomaly scan in the second trimester (18–21 weeks) was aimed at prenatal identification of major structural abnormalities.

In order to obtain uniformity in the prenatal screening, and to improve the neonatal morbidity and mortality, the National Health Service (NHS) Fetal Anomaly Screening Programme (FASP) (4) guidelines have introduced a series of recommendations:

- Ensure access to a uniform screening programme which conforms to an agreed level of quality.
- Provide appropriate information for women so that they can make an informed choice.
- Offer choices to women about their screening options and pregnancy management.
- Identify serious fetal abnormalities, either incompatible with life or associated with morbidity, allowing women to make reproductive choices.
- Identify abnormalities that may benefit from antenatal intervention.
- Identify abnormalities that require early intervention following delivery.

The lower limit of the gestational age window was selected to acknowledge the ability to examine the fetal anatomy thoroughly and competently from 18 completed weeks (i.e. 18^{+0} weeks) as a few of the abnormalities could be missed at an earlier gestation. The upper limit of 20^{+6} weeks was selected to allow sufficient time for referral to a tertiary centre, subsequent assessment to be undertaken, and, when indicated, termination of pregnancy to be available before the legal limit for pregnancy termination (24 weeks in the United Kingdom). The Standards (Standard 4—Clinical arrangements) also recommend that a woman with a suspected or confirmed fetal anomaly should be seen by an obstetric ultrasound specialist within three working days of the referral being made or by a fetal medicine unit within five working days of the referral being made (4, 5).

There are two approaches with screening—one is to offer ultrasound to all women (universal screening), and the other is targeted screening to those deemed at high risk. The majority of fetal abnormalities are encountered in women without risk factors. Therefore, the policy of universal screening is appropriate.

Earlier studies have shown that the sensitivity and specificity of ultrasound in detecting fetal anomalies in a low-risk population are 40% and 85% respectively (6–8). The Routine Antenatal Diagnostic Imaging with Ultrasound Study (RADIUS) concluded that the sensitivity was only 35% for major fetal anomalies (9).

It is acknowledged that there are some cohorts deemed at high risk for having an affected fetus:

- Women with type 1 diabetes have a higher risk of congenital heart abnormalities (10).
- Women with epilepsy and on antiepileptic medication have a higher risk of neural tube defects (11).
- Fetuses with an increased NT have an increased risk of various structural abnormalities in addition to chromosomal abnormalities (12).
- Women with a previous fetus affected by a structural abnormality (e.g. spina bifida) (13).
- Women found to have a high serum alpha-fetoprotein are known to be associated with a higher risk of neural tube defects and abdominal wall defects.

When ultrasound scanning is performed on an indication basis on these 'high-risk' women, the sensitivity is much higher, in the range of 86–99%. But it could be argued that many of the anomalies occur in low-risk women, so it is reasonable to offer screening universally.

Chromosomal abnormalities

Chromosomal abnormality refers to a missing, extra, or irregular portion of a chromosome or part of a chromosome. They occur due to an error in cell division, either during mitosis or meiosis, and they can be classified into numerical or structural anomalies. Rarely, they can be inherited from a parent.

The presence of a chromosomal abnormality is a major cause of perinatal mortality and childhood disability. The incidence of the majority of chromosomal defects increases with advancing maternal age and this incidence decreases as pregnancy advances due to the increased risk of miscarriage of fetuses with chromosomal defects. The rate of fetal death between 12 weeks and term in euploid fetuses is 1–2%; however, this rate increases to 30% in trisomy 21 (14) and is as high as 80% in trisomies 18 and 13 (1).

Screening for chromosomal abnormalities

The most common chromosomal defects are trisomy 21 (Down syndrome), accounting for 50% of the chromosomal abnormalities; 25% are trisomy 13 (Patau syndrome) or trisomy 18 (Edward syndrome); 10% are monosomy X (Turner syndrome); 5% are triploidies; and 10% are other aneuploidies.

First-trimester screening

The first-trimester ultrasound scan was initially introduced with the only purpose of measuring the crown–rump length (CRL) and dating the pregnancy accordingly.

After the initial screening tests based on maternal age alone and maternal serum biochemistry on the second trimester (15, 16), the screening programmes moved towards the first trimester for the purpose of screening for chromosomal abnormalities. This started with the introduction of the NT as the main method of screening combined with the biochemical markers (17, 18). The NT is the measurement of the ultrasound echo-free space (translucency) between the skin and the soft tissue overlying the cervical spine. It needs to be performed between 11 weeks and 13 weeks and 6 days (or a CRL between 45 and 84 mm), on a sagittal section of the fetal head and with appropriate magnification of the image (**Figure 11.1**).

While early studies used fixed cut-off values for NT, it is now understood that NT is a dynamic measurement that increases as gestational age advances. The 95th centile is therefore dependent on the gestational age (and, therefore, CRL). NT is increased (>95th centile) in approximately 70% of fetuses with trisomy 21. An increased NT can also be associated with other chromosomal abnormalities (trisomy 13, trisomy 18, Turner syndrome, and triploidy among others), genetic conditions, and fetal structural abnormalities (most commonly cardiac defects) (19, 20). It is also known that the higher the value is, the higher the risk of fetal death.

The NT is combined with the maternal serum biochemical markers (free beta-hCG and PAPP-A) to improve the detection rate. Typically, in trisomy 21 the maternal serum free beta-hCG is increased to about twice as high and the PAPP-A is halved compared to euploid pregnancies (2, 21). In the case of trisomies 18 and 13, both beta-hCG and PAPP-A are decreased (22).

Other sonographic markers described in the first trimester are the nasal bone (23), ductus venosus flow (24), and tricuspid regurgitation (25). The combination of maternal age, NT thickness, biochemical markers, and these three additional markers shows detection rates as high as 96% for trisomy 21 with a false-positive rate of 3% (26).

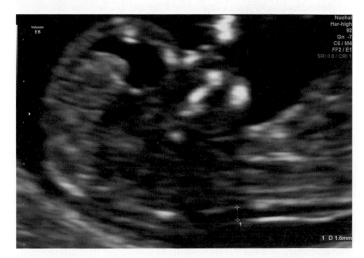

Figure 11.1 Mid-sagittal ultrasound view of the fetal head with measurement of the nuchal translucency at 12 weeks.

A detailed first-trimester scan performed by an experienced operator can detect a number of major structural abnormalities.

Trisomy 18 can be suspected in the first trimester in the presence of a strawberry-shaped head, heart defects, diaphragmatic hernia, oesophageal atresia, exomphalos, single umbilical artery, megacystis, radial aplasia, overlapping fingers, and talipes. Common ultrasound features of trisomy 13 that can be detected in the first trimester are holoprosencephaly, facial abnormalities, cardiac abnormalities, echogenic kidneys, exomphalos, and postaxial polydactyly.

Second-trimester screening

Routine second-trimester ultrasound scanning was introduced in the United Kingdom in the 1980s. However, uniform criteria on how to perform and what to look for in this scan were only introduced recently by the NHS FASP.

During the first trimester, the most frequent marker of chromosomal abnormality is the increased NT. In the second trimester, each chromosomal defect can have its own specific structural abnormalities:

- *Strawberry-shaped head*: this feature is characteristic of trisomy 18, and is present in up to 80% of cases. The frontal skull is narrow with a flat occiput.
- *Holoprosencephaly*: the incidence at birth is 1:10,000. It includes a heterogeneous group of cerebral malformations as a result of a failed or incomplete cleavage of the forebrain. Around 30% of them are associated with chromosomal defects, in particular trisomy 18 and trisomy13, the latter sometimes associated with microcephaly. The holoprosencephaly can be associated with facial clefts or other defects and the incidence of chromosomal defects is higher if it is associated with extrafacial abnormalities.
- *Choroid plexus cysts* (CPCs): the presence of CPCs together with other structural abnormalities raises the suspicion of trisomy 18. However, isolated CPCs can be found in 2% of the fetuses in the second trimester and is mostly benign. They typically disappear by 28 weeks.
- *Agenesis of the corpus callosum*: the incidence is 1:1000 births and it is related to chromosomal defects, especially trisomy 18 and trisomy 13. It can be suspected by the absence of cavum septum pellucidum (CSP) in the biparietal diameter view or by the presence of abnormalities in the lateral ventricles.
- *Ventriculomegaly*: this is defined by the increase in the transverse diameter of the atrium of the lateral ventricle by more than 10 mm. It can be secondary to infection, haemorrhage, or obstruction or associated with genetic conditions or chromosomal defects in around 10% of cases. The most frequent are trisomies 21, 13, and 18 and triploidy. The incidence of chromosomal defects is higher with mild to moderate, rather than severe ventriculomegaly.
- *Dandy–Walker malformation*: there is a spectrum of defects of the cerebellar vermis, cystic dilatation of the fourth ventricle, and enlargement of the cisterna magna. The incidence of chromosomal defects in the presence of Dandy–Walker malformation is as high as 40%, more frequent in trisomy 18, trisomy 13, and triploidy.
- *Facial cleft*: the term facial cleft includes cleft lip and palate that may present together. The incidence of chromosomal defects is around 10%, most frequently trisomy 13 and trisomy 18.

- *Micrognathia*: this entity is common in numerous genetic syndromes. Among the chromosomal defects, trisomy 18 and triploidy are the most likely ones.
- *Nasal bone hypoplasia*: the presence of a small nasal bone on the sagittal view of the face is defined as a hypoplasic nasal bone and is seen in 60% of the fetuses with trisomy 21. Only 1–2% of normal fetuses present with this feature and it is considered the most sensitive and specific isolated second-trimester marker of trisomy 21 (27).
- *Nuchal oedema*: this is the equivalent of the increased NT thickness in the second trimester. It is defined as an increase in the subcutaneous tissue greater than 5 mm measured on a suboccipitobregmatic view of the head. It is present in about 30% of fetuses with trisomy 21. It can also be associated with infection and other genetic conditions.
- *Cystic hygroma*: this is a congenital malformation of the lymphatic system. On the ultrasound scan, it is possible to identify a bilateral swelling of the posterolateral aspect of the fetal neck. It is typically septated and often there is a thick midline septum corresponding to the nuchal ligament. It is strongly associated with chromosomal defects, mostly Turner syndrome but also trisomy 21 and trisomy 18. About 20% of the fetuses have a normal karyotype. There is also an association with generalized hydrops that carries a worse prognosis.
- *Cardiac abnormalities*: the presence of cardiac defects is seen in 90% of the fetuses with trisomy 13 and trisomy 18, 50% with trisomy 21, and 40% with Turner syndrome. Some studies have reported a 25% incidence of chromosomal defects in the presence of a cardiac abnormality. The presence of intracardiac hyperechogenic foci is considered one of the soft markers of chromosomal defects on the second-trimester scan and may be seen in up to 25% of fetuses with trisomy 21 (27).
- *Congenital diaphragmatic hernia*: the incidence is around 1:4000 live births. It can be an isolated finding but in 30–50% of the cases there is an underlying chromosomal defect, most frequently trisomy 18 and tetrasomy 12p (Pallister–Killian syndrome).
- *Oesophageal atresia*: oesophageal atresia is a relatively common gastrointestinal tract defect with an incidence of 1:4000 births. It is associated with aneuploidy in 5% of the cases, most frequently trisomy 13 and trisomy 18. It can also be part of the VACTERL syndrome (vertebral abnormalities, anal atresia, cardiac defect, tracheo-oesophageal fistula, renal and radial limb abnormalities) or CHARGE (choanal atresia, renal abnormalities, tracheo-oesophageal fistula, micrognathia, cleft lip/palate, and exomphalos). The diagnosis is suspected if there is failure to visualize the stomach bubble or a very small stomach is seen on serial ultrasound scans. At later stages in pregnancy, it can be associated with polyhydramnios. Most cases are associated with a tracheo-oesophageal fistula, and antenatal identification is possible in less than half of all cases.
- *Duodenal atresia*: the incidence is 1:10,000 births. Up to 50% of the cases are associated with other abnormalities: cardiac malformations (10–20%), trisomy 21 (30%), skeletal dysplasias, and intrauterine growth restriction. The classical sign is the 'double bubble' as a result of the enlarged stomach and proximal duodenum.
- *Exomphalos*: the reported incidence varies between 1:4000 and 1:7000 livebirths. In 40% of the cases there is an underlying

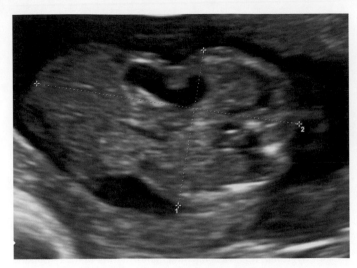

Figure 11.2 Exomphalos containing bowel and stomach.

chromosomal defect, usually trisomy 13 or 18, most commonly if there is only small exomphalos containing bowel rather than a large exomphalos containing liver as well as small bowel. Even in the absence of aneuploidy, additional structural abnormalities are encountered in 80% of the cases, cardiac defects in 30% of these. Other associations are Beckwith–Wiedemann syndrome, cloacal exstrophy, pentalogy of Cantrell, and Meckel–Gruber syndrome (**Figure 11.2**).

- *Hyperechogenic bowel*: this is found in 1–2% of all fetuses in the second trimester. In 50% of the cases there is spontaneous resolution. It can be associated with cystic fibrosis, chromosomal abnormalities (in particular, trisomies 21, 18, or 13 and triploidy), intra-amniotic bleeding, congenital infection, growth restriction, and bowel obstruction.
- *Renal/urinary tract anomalies*: although mild renal pelvic dilatation is relatively common, the presence of a mild hydronephrosis is also common in fetuses with trisomy 21 (10–25%). A diagnosis of moderate to severe hydronephrosis, polycystic kidneys, or renal agenesis is more common in trisomies 18 and 13. Megacystis (>7 mm longitudinal diameter in the first trimester) raises the possibility of trisomy 18.
- *Skeletal dysplasias*: there is a wide variety of skeletal dysplasias and the suspicion of any abnormality of the bones should trigger further investigations and detailed ultrasound examination to exclude other structural abnormalities. A short femur is present in 40% of the fetuses with trisomy 21; also characteristic are clinodactyly and the sandal gap sign. The presence of polydactyly, overlapping fingers, and rocker-bottom feet are classical signs of trisomy 18.
- *Growth restriction*: this is a common finding in many chromosomal defects and genetic syndromes, but not trisomy 21. Trisomy 18 and triploidy are classically associated with severe growth restriction from very early stages of pregnancy. In addition, in triploidy there is a marked disproportion of the head size compared to a marked reduction in the growth of the abdomen and femur.

In addition to a detailed second-trimester ultrasound scan, risk assessment for chromosomal abnormalities can be performed using maternal serum biochemistry (quadruple test). It combines maternal age with maternal serum levels of alpha-fetoprotein, free beta-hCG, unconjugated oestriol, and inhibin A and has a detection rate of 70–75% with a 5% false-positive rate (15, 16). Due to the low detection rate compared to the combined first-trimester screening, the use of this test is mainly limited to women who missed the first-trimester risk assessment using the combined test.

Diagnostic procedures

Screening tests such as combined screening, serum biochemistry, as well as tests of free fetal DNA are not diagnostic. All have false positives and false negatives, and a confirmatory diagnostic procedure is required. The choice of diagnostic procedures depends on the gestational age, risk versus benefit, and the availability of expertise.

Indications for diagnostic procedures (28) include:

- increased risk of Down syndrome on screening tests (see 'Screening for chromosomal abnormalities').
- identification of structural abnormalities known to be associated with chromosomal imbalance
- parental (usually maternal) carrier status of chromosomal rearrangement
- increased NT even in the apparent absence of other structural abnormalities
- parental carrier status or affection of single gene disorders or chromosomal microdeletions
- genetic disorders for which molecular genetic diagnosis is available.

Advances in technology have resulted in changes in the indications and choices of diagnostic procedures. The advantage of these techniques is that they can be performed on uncultured amniocytes or trophoblasts. Most centres have discontinued conventional karyotyping using light microscopy. The type of tests performed on the sample depends on the indication for sampling:

- Increased risk for commonly seen trisomies—this risk assessment can be on maternal age, or on some form of tests (ultrasound, maternal serum biochemistry, or both) in addition to maternal age. It can also be following a high-risk result for cell-free DNA analysis on maternal plasma. In these cases, most centres will test only for commonly seen trisomies (21, 18, and 13). Sometimes, monosomy X (Turner syndrome) is also checked for. Usually quantitative fluorescent polymerase chain reaction is the technique utilized to check chromosomal copy number.
- Identification of structural abnormalities, suspicion of rare chromosomal abnormalities (other than trisomy 13/18/21), or imbalance of genetic material including (micro-) deletions or translocations—this is usually looked for using chromosomal microarray analysis.
- Single gene disorder or methylation defects—specific genes must be tested to identify a mutation for prenatal identification of single gene disorders.

With all diagnostic procedures there is a small chance of a laboratory failure. The usual reason for failure to obtain a result by the laboratory is because more than one cell line is identified, raising the suspicion of maternal contamination or mosaicism, which may or may not be confined to the placenta. The risk of confined placental mosaicism is particularly relevant to the chorionic villus sampling (CVS) procedure.

The following diagnostic tests are available:

Chorionic villus sampling

CVS can be performed transabdominally, or by a transcervical approach. CVS is usually performed after 11 (11^{+0}) weeks of gestation. The transabdominal route is perhaps the most commonly used method for CVS. This is performed under direct ultrasound guidance. The single-needle technique uses a single 20–21-gauge needle or a double-needle technique with a 17–18-gauge outer needle and a 19–20-gauge inner sampling needle. The double-needle technique avoids the use of multiple skin punctures in the event of obtaining an inadequate sample with the first pass. The transvaginal technique uses a specially designed transcervical CVS cannula. A biopsy forceps appears to be a safe alternative.

The procedure is associated with a small risk of a miscarriage. Wijnberger and co-workers substantiated a learning curve for CVS and showed that the safety and success of this procedure was strongly related to the number of prior procedures performed by an operator (29).

Amniocentesis

Amniocentesis involves insertion of a thin needle into the amniotic cavity to aspirate amniotic fluid. This contains cells from the fetus, which can be used to obtain genetic information. The current recommendation is not to perform amniocentesis before 15 weeks. CVS provides the advantage of earlier diagnosis, albeit accompanied by a 1–2% chance of encountering confined placental mosaicism. The procedure-related miscarriage rate for both CVS and amniocentesis is widely quoted as 1%, but is thought to be much lower than that (30).

Fetal blood sampling

This procedure involves passing a thin needle into the umbilical cord (usually the placental end) to obtain a sample of the fetal blood. With advances in newer genetic tests, fetal blood sampling is rarely necessary. The procedure is also associated with a small risk of a miscarriage.

A written consent should be obtained before performing a diagnostic test. Women should be informed about the reason for a diagnostic test, what tests will be performed, and how long the results would take.

Consent should have the following:

- The national and local risks of procedure-related pregnancy loss.
- The accuracy and limitations of the particular laboratory test(s) being performed, with information about failure rates and estimation of when reports will be available.
- How the results will be communicated.
- The reasons for seeking medical advice following the test.
- Anti-D should be administered post procedure if the woman is rhesus D negative.

It is recommended that units and operators should keep a record of frequencies of multiple insertions, failures, bloody taps, and post-procedure losses.

Structural abnormalities

Since the introduction of routine ultrasound scanning as part of the antenatal care in the 1980s, there has been a continuous development of both the technology as well as the knowledge and experience of the clinicians.

The prevalence of fetal structural abnormalities is approximately 2% with congenital malformations accounting for 20% of the neonatal deaths.

Cardiac defects are perhaps the most common abnormalities encountered in approximately 5–10 out of every 1000 births. The second most common defects are abnormalities of the central nervous system with an incidence of 5:1000 of neural tube defects.

Detection in the first and second trimester using ultrasound

Currently, there are two ultrasound examinations offered to all pregnant women, each with different aims. The first trimester ultrasound is performed between 11 and 14 weeks of gestational age. The primary objectives are confirmation of viability, dating the pregnancy accurately according to the CRL, and to offer screening for common chromosomal abnormalities. The technological advances in ultrasonography have improved resolution and capabilities to such an extent that it has changed our understanding and ability to visualize early fetal anatomy. In doing so, structural abnormalities are being detected at an earlier stage, allowing for early counselling and intervention when required. This is the case for lethal malformations such as anencephaly, holoprosencephaly, and body-stalk anomaly. Other malformations that can be detected in the first trimester are defects of the anterior abdominal wall (gastroschisis, exomphalos), congenital diaphragmatic hernia, and megacystis.

The second ultrasound scan is performed between 18 and 21 weeks. The purpose of this scan is to identify major fetal structural abnormalities. The NHS FASP has identified 11 structural abnormalities with anticipated detection rates of greater than 50%, that should be routinely screened for (Table 11.1). Although some other conditions can be detected during the anomaly scan, there is insufficient published data on detection rates to establish a standard. If any of these or any other abnormality is suspected, a referral to a

Table 11.1 Screening for fetal structural abnormalities

Abnormality	Expected detection rate (%)
Anencephaly	98
Open spina bifida	90
Cleft lip	75
Diaphragmatic hernia	60
Gastroschisis	98
Exomphalos	80
Serious cardiac abnormalities	50
Bilateral renal agenesis	84
Lethal skeletal dysplasia	60
Edward syndrome (trisomy 18)	95
Patau syndrome (trisomy 13)	95

fetal medicine unit should be made to confirm diagnosis and offer appropriate management. Identification of any malformation at this stage allows the parents to make decisions regarding continuation of pregnancy, and if the pregnancy continues, appropriate management with intervention or supportive care if required (antenatal or in the early postnatal period). Table 11.1 shows the anticipated prenatal detection rates of these 11 structural abnormalities.

The FASP committee has established a series of routine views, measurements, and images that should be obtained and stored during the anomaly scan. It is important to have a systematic approach when examining the fetus. Before starting the fetal biometry, it is advisable to examine the uterus and its contents, the fetal position, and orientation within the uterine cavity, confirming viability, number of fetuses, and chorionicity in multiple pregnancies. In addition, it is essential to assess the amniotic fluid volume and the placental site as well as its structure. Once this has been established, the sonographer should proceed with fetal biometry. The standard measurements that should be obtained are as follows:

1. *Head circumference* (HC). This can be measured in a thalamic plane (as established by the International Society of Ultrasound in Obstetrics & Gynecology Education Committee guidelines) (31) or in a transventricular plane (NHS FASP) (3). The landmarks are the CSP, the thalami, and the posterior lateral ventricles. It can be measured by placing an ellipse directly around the outside if the skull bone or by measuring the biparietal diameter and the occipitofrontal diameter and calculating the HC (**Figure 11.3**).

2. *Abdominal circumference* (AC). This is measured on a transverse plane of the abdomen. The landmarks of the AC plane are the stomach, the umbilical vein at the level of the portal sinus, and one entire rib should be seen (**Figure 11.4**). The AC may be measured placing an ellipse or measuring the anteroposterior abdominal diameter and the transverse abdominal diameter placing the callipers from the skin covering the abdomen.

3. *Femur length* (FL). The landmarks to measure the FL are an angle of insonation of 30 degrees, both ends of the ossified diaphysis, and tissue beyond them needs to be seen (**Figure 11.5**).

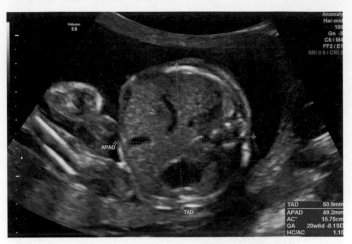

Figure 11.4 Transverse section of the fetal abdomen showing measurement of the transverse abdominal diameter (TAD) and the anteroposterior diameter (APAD) to obtain the abdominal circumference (AC).

These measurements need to be plotted on appropriate charts according to gestational age. If the pregnancy has not been previously dated (according to CRL in the first trimester), this needs to be done according to the HC and documented in the report.

A systematic examination of fetal anatomy needs to include the following:

1. *Skull, brain, and spine.* Shape and ossification of the fetal skull. In the brain, measures of the atrium of the posterior horn of the lateral ventricles, transcerebellar diameter, cisterna magna, and nuchal fold. The anatomy of these structures and the presence of the CSP need to be assessed. The spine is examined in three planes, coronal, sagittal, and transverse, allowing spina bifida, scoliosis, and agenesis of the sacrum among other possible structural defects to be excluded.

2. *Face.* The soft tissues are best assessed on a coronal plane to evidence the nostrils and lips. In the profile view, it is possible to assess the presence of a nasal bone and the shape of the maxilla and chin. Transverse planes are needed to assess the orbits and the alveolar ridge.

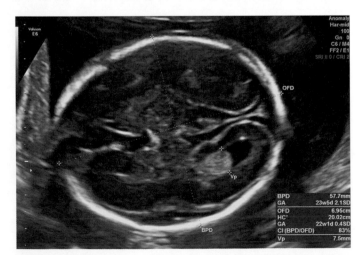

Figure 11.3 Transventricular plane of the fetal head showing measurement of the biparietal diameter (BPD), occipitofrontal diameter (OFD), and posterior ventricular atrium (Vp).

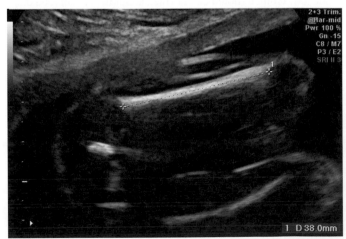

Figure 11.5 Femur length.

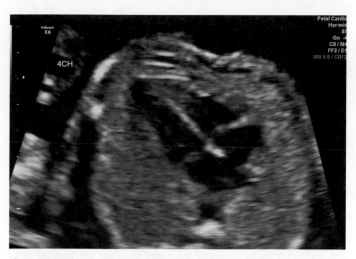

Figure 11.6 Four-chamber view of the heart.

3. *Thorax.* Examination of the lungs (uniform echogenicity), ribs (ossification, shape, number), and the integrity of the diaphragm. The diaphragm can be assessed on a sagittal plane as an echolucent line separating the thorax from the abdomen. The presence of the stomach in the thorax should raise the suspicion of congenital diaphragmatic hernia.

4. *Heart.* Basic routine examination of the heart includes three views: a four-chamber view, the left outflow tract arising from the left ventricle, and the three-vessel view showing the right outflow tract, the aorta, and the superior vena cava. The four-chamber view is obtained on a transverse plane and allows examination of the integrity of the interventricular septum, the morphology and size of both atria and ventricles, the atrioventricular valves moving freely and their insertion, and the foramen ovale moving in the left atrium (**Figure 11.6**).

5. *Abdomen.* Examination of the abdomen in a transverse section allows visualization of the stomach bubble at the level used to measure the AC. Moving caudally, the insertion of the umbilical cord in the abdominal wall must be evidenced to assess its integrity. At the same level, the bowels should have uniform echogenicity and no sign of dilatation in the second trimester.

6. *Urinary tract.* The kidneys are best visualized on a transverse view lower than the plane used for the abdomen. They appear like two rounded structures on both sides of the spine. In this view, it is possible to examine and measure the renal pelvises to exclude hydronephrosis. The fetal bladder is seen on a transverse section of the pelvis. The two arteries in the umbilical cord can be seen with colour Doppler on both sides of the bladder.

7. *Limbs.* All four limbs need to be assessed. In the lower limbs, it is important to confirm the presence of all long bones (femur, fibula, and tibia) and the angle of the leg with the foot to assess the presence of talipes. In the upper limbs, similarly, the presence of all long bones (humerus, radius, and ulna). In addition, the five metacarpals and five metatarsals in the hands and feet respectively and the density, length, and shape of bones need to be assessed.

8. *Genitalia.* Examination of the genitalia is not part of the routine fetal anomaly scan but it is good practice to assess normal anatomy especially if other structural abnormalities have been diagnosed.

Common structural abnormalities

Central nervous system

Neural tube defects arise from abnormal closure of the neural folds in the third and fourth weeks of development. They can involve the meninges, vertebrae, muscles, and skin. Neural tube defects include anencephaly, encephalocoele, and spina bifida. The incidence is about 5:1000 births in the United Kingdom with the majority being spina bifida (95% of cases).

Anencephaly is the absence of the cranial vault. Ossification of the fetal skull is normally complete by 11 weeks' gestation. At the end of the first trimester, the absence of the cranial bones (acrania) may be noted which allows early diagnosis and management. It is a lethal condition and the majority of patients opt for termination of pregnancy.

Encephalocoele is a defect in the cranium, which results in the herniation of a sac containing either fluid or part of the brain. The most common location is in the occipital region. The prognosis depends on the degree of herniation and the integrity of the underlying brain. In view of this, the parents may opt to terminate the pregnancy. Some cases are associated with Meckel–Gruber syndrome. The inheritance is autosomal recessive, and therefore the recurrence risk is one in four. Genetic referral is advised for further counselling.

In spina bifida, the defect is in the neural arch and is most commonly seen in the lumbosacral region. The spinal defect may be identified during the examination of the spine in lateral and transverse views by an interruption on the skin covering the spine and the presence of a myelocoele or a myelomeningocoele. Two additional cranial signs of spina bifida have been described: the 'lemon sign', defined as a deformity in the frontal bones seen between 16 and 24 weeks, and the 'banana sign', referring to the characteristic shape of the cerebellum that can be seen from 15 weeks (32).

Ventriculomegaly occurs in 1% of pregnancies and refers to the enlargement (diameter >10 mm) of the posterior lateral ventricles. The severe form, hydrocephalus, is often associated with other defects such as spina bifida (**Figure 11.7**).

Holoprosencephaly consists of several disorders characterized by the incomplete cleavage of the forebrain. It occurs in 1:10,000 pregnancies and can be associated with facial clefts and trisomy 13.

Face

The commonest facial abnormalities seen on ultrasound are cleft lip and palate. However, the antenatal detection rate is 30–35% at best. The face needs to be examined in sagittal, transverse, and coronal planes by ultrasound. In 75% of cases the abnormality is unilateral with the left side affected more often. It is important to be aware that there is a close relationship between midline facial clefts and abnormalities of the forebrain such as holoprosencephaly. The FASP aims at improving the detection of cleft lips and palates.

Cardiac defects

Congenital cardiac defects are one of the commonest fetal malformations occurring in 5–10:1000 live births. There is a huge regional variation in the prenatal detection rates of cardiac abnormalities by ultrasound ranging from 16.7% to 94% for major abnormalities. However, prenatal diagnosis of cardiac defects can improve significantly the outcome of the pregnancy. This is particularly true in the case of transposition of the great arteries, hypoplastic left heart

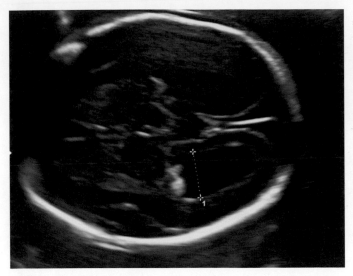

Figure 11.7 Ventriculomegaly, borderline measurement 10.6 mm.

syndrome, and coarctation of the aorta. Basic examination of the fetal heart should include the four-chamber view and ventricular outflow tracts. The detection rate of congenital heart disease is increased from 48% to 78% with the addition of the outflow tracts to the four-chamber view. If an abnormality is suspected, a fetal echocardiogram should be offered.

Thorax

The most common thoracic anomaly is congenital diaphragmatic hernia. The defect on the diaphragm allows the abdominal contents to shift into the thorax and the stomach may be visualized on the same plane as the heart that may be shifted to the right. The incidence is in 1:4000 pregnancies with 85% of cases occurring on the left side. The prognosis is worse if there is herniation of the fetal liver. The most commonly associated chromosomal abnormality is trisomy 18. Complications for the fetus arise from pressure on the heart and lungs causing mediastinal shift, pulmonary hypoplasia, pulmonary hypertension, and rarely hydrops.

Other malformations found in the chest are pleural effusions, cystic lesions of the lung, the most frequent one being congenital cystic adenomatoid malformation (CCAM) and less frequently bronchogenic cysts, lung sequestration, and bronchial atresia. The CCAM occurs in 1:4000 births. The condition may be bilateral involving all lung tissue, which is a lethal condition, or unilateral confined to a single lobe. The lesions are described as macrocystic (cysts >5 mm) or microcystic (cysts <5 mm) or mixed, according to their appearance on ultrasound imaging. The fetus will require assessment in the neonatal period with computed tomography of the thorax to confirm the diagnosis and treatment options.

Abdomen

Abdominal wall defects occur in approximately 1:4000 births. Exomphalos occurs secondary to a failure of the bowel to return to the body cavity from its physiological herniation between the sixth and tenth weeks. Gastroschisis is the herniation of the abdominal contents directly into the abdominal cavity with the defect usually occurring lateral to the umbilicus. It is therefore possible to make a prenatal diagnosis at the end of the first trimester.

It is important to also assess the fetal bladder and chest to exclude bladder exstrophy and ectopia cordis. It is essential to differentiate between the two defects sonographically, as the management and prognosis differ significantly. In gastroschisis, there is a defect in the abdominal wall, most commonly on the right side of a normally inserted umbilical cord, allowing the herniated loops of intestine to float freely within the amniotic cavity. It is usually isolated and not related to chromosomal defects. In exomphalos, there is a herniation of the abdominal contents into the umbilical cord. Bowel, liver, spleen, and stomach can be herniated and covered by a layer of peritoneum and amnion. Exomphalos is associated with other structural abnormalities or aneuploidy in over 50% of cases.

Gastrointestinal tract

Oesophageal and duodenal atresia are difficult to diagnose at a routine second-trimester scan as the signs often do not present until after 26–28 weeks' gestation. At this gestation stage, there may be an abnormally small stomach and the presence of polyhydramnios. The majority of cases of oesophageal atresia are associated with tracheo-oesophageal fistula so the stomach may appear normal on scanning and prenatal diagnosis may be impossible. Duodenal atresia is associated with chromosomal defects in about 40% of the cases.

Gastrointestinal obstruction may result from atresia, stenosis, agenesis, or fistula of any part of the bowel. It is usually detected during the third trimester when the dilatation of the preceding segment is more evident or there is associated polyhydramnios.

Kidneys and urinary tract

The fetal bladder can be seen in over 80% of fetuses at 11 weeks' gestation and in over 90% of fetuses over 13 weeks. Urine production commences between 10 and 11 weeks and by 16 weeks it contributes to the majority of amniotic fluid production. It is reasonable to assume that a normal amount of amniotic fluid after 16 to 18 weeks' gestation is associated with good renal function. The commonest renal tract abnormality is hydronephrosis, occurring in 2–4% of pregnancies. In most of the cases, this disappears before or shortly after birth. In a minority, dilatation will be persistent (about 5%) and may require surgery, depending on the underlying cause of either reflux or obstruction. If the renal dilatation is persistent on renal ultrasound of the neonate then prophylactic antibiotics are commenced to prevent urinary infection.

Bilateral renal agenesis carries a very poor prognosis with complications from pulmonary hypoplasia due to anhydramnios and the onset of renal failure in the neonatal period. Bilateral renal agenesis can be reliably diagnosed by ultrasound after 16 weeks' gestation by the anhydramnios coupled with failure to visualize the fetal bladder. This is not the case in unilateral agenesis, where a fetal bladder and normal amniotic fluid are seen. The prognosis is excellent provided the existing kidney has normal functioning.

Cystic renal disease includes many conditions, the most common being multicystic dysplastic kidney occurring in 1:1000 births.

Limbs and skeleton

This group includes skeletal dysplasias, arthrogryposis syndromes, talipes, limb-reduction defects, and digital abnormalities.

Skeletal dysplasias occur in 1:4000 pregnancies and there are around 150 different entities described in the literature. Limb reduction defects occur in 1:20,000 births. About 50% of them have multiple malformations, chromosomal defects, or syndromes associated.

Talipes equinovarus ('clubfoot') is a common anomaly with an incidence of 1:1000. About 50% are associated with chromosomal defects, syndromes, or neuromuscular disorders.

Role of fetal magnetic resonance imaging

Although ultrasound remains the routine imagining to assess the fetus, over the last 10 years, fetal magnetic resonance imaging (MRI) has developed an important role as a complement to ultrasound. Prenatal MRI complements ultrasound because of a larger field of view, superior soft tissue contrast, easier and more precise volumetric measurement, and greater accuracy in the demonstration of intracranial and spinal abnormalities.

The safety of MRI in pregnancy has been extensively studied and none of the studies have reported any adverse effects. The contraindications for MRI are the same as outside pregnancy: magnetically activated implanted devices such as pacemakers that may need to be deprogrammed, cerebral aneurysm clips, and hip prosthesis, among others.

The main drawbacks of MRI are the artefacts or poor resolution of the images if there are fetal movements especially in the early second trimester. The spread of MRI as a complementary test is helping professionals to become more experienced in the interpretation of fetal MRI images.

The benefits of fetal MRI are proven for intracranial and intrathoracic abnormalities. Fetal MRI is particularly good for the assessment of fetal cerebral cortex and abnormalities of sulcation. However, the development of the brain is very dynamic and it is essential to time adequately the MRI to maximize the information obtained as the brain appearances can change on a weekly basis (33).

Impact of the screening programmes

It is evident that the introduction of universal screening programmes increases the detection rate but whether this improves neonatal morbidity and mortality is controversial and depends on the abnormalities found, the diagnostic expertise, and the availability of termination of pregnancy in the population.

The two important questions to be answered when introducing ultrasound as a screening tool are the effectiveness of ultrasound in detecting the pathologies and the implications of this on the perinatal outcome. A study published in 2005 reported on the detection rates for the specific anomalies. An overall detection rate of about 60% was reported.

Another recent study from the EUROCAT (34) database assessed prenatal screening policies and the impact on detection rates and termination of pregnancy. It looked at neural tube defects as an indicator of assessing the efficacy of ultrasound anomaly screening in an attempt to map the current state of prenatal screening in Europe. The study concluded that in countries with an established national screening programme for prenatal diagnosis of neural tube defects, 91% of all abnormalities were detected prenatally at a median gestation of 17 weeks and resulted in 84% of all affected pregnancies undergoing termination. Countries that did not have a national screening programme for fetal anomalies but did perform routine ultrasound had 17% lower detection rates than those with a national screening programme. The study uncovered large differences in screening policies in Europe. In addition, it pointed out that even with the existence of a national or recommended policy on screening for abnormalities, the service was not always delivered. Responsible factors were lack of resources, lack of uptake, or late booking—the latter two influenced by social and cultural factors.

Although the detection of fetal anomalies is enhanced by ultrasound, any beneficial effect is far from proven. The Helsinki ultrasound trial in 1990 showed that the perinatal mortality was significantly lower in the group screened with ultrasound, and that a 49% reduction in the perinatal mortality was achieved due to early detection of abnormalities and the termination that followed. This contrasted with the findings of the RADIUS trial that showed the perinatal outcome and the frequency of induced abortion was unchanged with or without routine ultrasound screening. Both these studies were published more than 20 years ago. Since then, there have been significant improvements in equipment quality and training as well as knowledge of operators performing the screening. Even in the absence of robust evidence based on randomized controlled trials, routine ultrasound screening is now established as part of antenatal care (35).

Ultrasound is an established practice in the prenatal diagnosis of structural abnormalities in developed countries. As the standard of practice varies widely, many countries such as the United Kingdom are adopting national programmes in an attempt to improve the quality of service for all pregnant women. The management of women diagnosed with a fetus with a structural abnormality requires a multidisciplinary approach. The aim is to provide the required information, support, and time to enable parents to decide how they wish to manage the pregnancy.

REFERENCES

1. Snijders RJM, Holzgreve W, Cuckle H, Nicolaides KH. Maternal age-specific risks for trisomies at 9–14 weeks gestation. *Prental Diagn* 1994;**14**:543–52.
2. Nicolaides KH. Screening for fetal aneuplodies at 11 to 13 weeks. *Prenatal Diagn* 2011;**31**:7–15.
3. Gil MM, Akolekar R, Quezada MS, Bregant B, Nicolaides KH. Analysis of cell-free DNA in maternal blood in screening for aneuploidies: meta-analysis. *Fetal Diagn Ther* 2014;**35**:156–73.
4. National Institute for Health and Clinical Excellence (NICE). Antenatal care for uncomplicated pregnancies. Clinical guideline [CG62], updated 2019. London: NICE; 2008.
5. Royal College of Obstetricians and Gynaecologists (RCOG). *Routine Ultrasound Screening in Pregnancy: Protocol, Standards and Training*. Report of the RCOG Working Party. London: RCOG; 2000.
6. Rosendahl H, Kivinen S, Antenatal detection of congenital malformations by routine ultrasonography. *Obstet Gynaecol* 1989;**73**:947–59.
7. Saari-Kemppainen A, Karajalainen O, Ylostalo P. Ultrasound screening and prenatal mortality: controlled trial of systematic one-stage screening in pregnancy. The Helsinki ultrasound trial. *Lancet* 1990;**336**:387–91.
8. Shirley IM, Bottomley F, Robinson VP. Routine radiographer screening for fetal abnormalities in unselected population. *Br J Radiol* 1992;**65**:564–69.

9. Ewigman BG, Crane JP, Frigoletto FD, et al. Effect of prenatal ultrasound screening on perinatal outcome. RADIUS Study Group. *N Eng J Med* 1993;**329**:821–27.

10. Eidem I, Stene LC, Henriksen T, et al. Congenital anomalies in newborns of women with type 1 diabetes: nationwide population-based study in Norway, 1999–2004. *Acta Obstet Gynecol Scand* 2010;**89**:1403–11.

11. Rosa F. Spina bifida in infants of women treated with carbamazepine during pregnancy. *N Engl J Med* 1991;**324**:674–77.

12. Jouannic JM, Thieulin AC, Bonnet D, et al. Measurement of nuchal translucency for prenatal screening of congenital heart defects: a population-based evaluation. *Prenat Diagn* 2011;**31**:1264–69.

13. Collins JS, Canfield MA, Pearson K, et al. Public health projects for preventing the recurrence of neural tube defects in the United States. *Birth Defects Res A Clin Mol Teratol* 2009;**85**:935–38.

14. Snijders RJM, Sundberg K, Holzgreve W, et al. Maternal age and gestation-specific risk for trisomy 21. *Ultrasound Obstet Gynecol* 1999;**13**:167–70.

15. Wald NJ, Watt HC, Hackshaw AK. Integrated screening for Down's syndrome on the basis of tests performed during the first and second trimesters. *N Engl J Med* 1999;**341**:461–67.

16. Wald NJ, Rodeck C, Hackshaw AK, et al. SURUSS Research group. First and second trimester antenatal screening for Down's syndrome: the results of the Serum, Urine and Ultrasound Screening Study (SURUSS). *Health Technol Assess* 2003;**7**:1–88

17. Snijders RJ, Noble P, Sebire N, et al. Fetal Medicine Foundation First Trimester Screening Group. UK multicentre project on assessment of risk of trisomy 21 by maternal age and fetal nuchal-translucency thickness at 10–14 weeks of gestation. *Lancet* 1998;**352**:343–46.

18. Nicolaides KH, Azar G, Byrne D, et al. Fetal nuchal translucency: ultrasound screening for chromosomal defects in first trimester of pregnancy. *Br Med J* 1992;**304**:867–89.

19. Souka AP, Von Kaisenberg CS, Hyett JA, et al. Increased nuchal translucency with normal karyotype. *Am J Obstet Gynecol* 2005;**192**:1005–1021.

20. Nicolaides KH, Snijders RJM, Gosden RJM, et al. Ultrasonographically detectable markers of fetal chromosomal abnormalities. *Lancet* 1992;**340**:704–707.

21. Wright D, Kagan KO, Molina FS, et al. A mixture model of nuchal translucency thickness in screening for chromosomal defects. *Ultrasound Obstet Gynecol* 2008;**31**:376–83.

22. Spencer K, Souter V, Tul N, et al. A screening program for trisomy 21 at 10–14 weeks using fetal nuchal translucency, maternal serum free ß-human chorionic gonadotropin and pregnancy-associated plasma protein-A. *Ultrasound Obstet Gynecol* 1999;**13**:231–37.

23. Cicero S, Curcio P, Papageorghiou A, et al. Absence of nasal bone in fetuses with trisomy 21 at 11–14 weeks of gestation: an observational study. *Lancet* 2001;**358**:1665–67.

24. Maiz N, Wright D, Ferreira AF, et al. A mixture model of ductus venosus pulsatility index in screening for aneuploidies at 11–13 weeks' gestation. *Fetal Diagn Ther* 2012;**31**:221–29.

25. Kagan KO, Valencia C, Livanos P, et al. Tricuspid regurgitation in screening for trisomies 21, 18 and 13 and Turner syndrome at 11+0 to 13+6 weeks of gestation. *Ultrasound Obstet Gynecol* 2009;**33**:18–22.

26. Nicolaides KH. *Ultrasound Markers for Fetal Chromosomal Defects*. Carnforth: Parthenon Publishing; 1996.

27. Agathokleous M, Chaveeva P, Poon LCY, et al. Meta-analysis of second-trimester markers for trisomy 21. *Ultrasound Obstet Gynecol* 2013;**41**:247–61.

28. Royal College of Obstetricians and Gynaecologists (RCOG). *Amniocentesis and Chorionic Villus Sampling*. Green-top Guideline No. 8. London: RCOG; 2010.

29. Wijnberger LD, van der Schouw YT, Christiaens GC. Learning in medicine: chorionic villus sampling. *Prenat Diagn* 2000;**20**:241–46.

30. Akolekar R, Beta J, Picciarelli G, Ogilvie C, D'Antonio F. Procedure-related risk of miscarriage following amniocentesis and chorionic villus sampling: a systematic review and meta-analysis. *Ultrasound Obstet Gynecol* 2015;**45**:16–26.

31. International Society of Ultrasound in Obstetrics & Gynecology Education Committee. Sonographic examination of the fetal central nervous system: guidelines for performing the 'basic examination' and the 'fetal neurosonogram' *Ultrasound Obstet Gynecol* 2007;**29**:109–16.

32. Pilu G, Nicolaides KH. *Diagnosis of Fetal Abnormalities—The 18–23 Week Scan*. Carnforth: The Parthenon Publishing Group; 1994.

33. Sohn YS, Kim MJ, Kwon JY, Kim YH, Park YW. The usefulness of fetal MRI for prenatal diagnosis *Yonsei Med J* 2007;**48**:671–77.

34. Boyd P, DeVigan C, Khoshnood B, et al. Survey of prenatal screening policies in Europe for structural malformations and chromosome anomalies, and their impact on detection and termination rates for neural tube defects and Down's syndrome. *BJOG* 2008;**115**:689–96.

35. Garne E, Loane M, Dolk H, et al. Prenatal diagnosis of severe structural congenital malformations in Europe. *Ultrasound Obstet Gynecol* 2003;**22**:555–58.

12

Cardiac disease in pregnancy

Philip Steer

Changes in cardiovascular physiology in pregnancy and implications for women with heart disease

The most striking cardiovascular change in early pregnancy is a marked decrease in peripheral resistance, which falls by up to 30% of its prepregnancy value (1). This is most likely due to the changes in maternal hormone levels (particularly progesterone, relaxin, prostacyclin, and prolactin) brought about by the developing conceptus, stimulated in part by its secretion of human chorionic gonadotropin (similar in structure to luteinizing hormone), although exactly how these hormones act to do this remains uncertain (2). It is probably mediated in part by the increases in nitric oxide production in the endothelium (3), and by increased resistance to the effects of angiotensin II and norepinephrine (noradrenaline). As pregnancy progresses, the placental circulation is established, and its blood flow of up to 700 mL per minute by the third trimester (about 10% of cardiac output) acts as a low resistance shunt which contributes to the loss of peripheral resistance (4). These changes would produce a marked decrease in blood pressure if their effect was not counteracted by the increase in circulating blood volume of up to 50% (there is a large increase in plasma volume and a somewhat smaller increase in the circulating red cell mass, resulting in a decrease in haemoglobin concentration—the 'physiological anaemia of pregnancy'). This increase occurs because the decrease in blood pressure stimulates the production of renin in the kidney leading to the formation of angiotensinogen and angiotensin I, which is then converted into angiotensin II by a converting enzyme (2). This would normally produce vasoconstriction, but this action is blocked by the hormone changes described earlier. However, its effects on the adrenal cortex and kidney are not blocked, resulting in a three- to fourfold increase in aldosterone levels, causing cumulative sodium and water retention which expands the circulating volume and restores cardiac preload. The overall net change is an up to 50% increase in resting cardiac output, which peaks between 26 and 36 weeks of pregnancy, and which represents a considerable challenge to anyone with impaired cardiac function.

Clinically, these changes are manifested by a small (about 10 mmHg) decrease in blood pressure as pregnancy progresses, reaching a nadir between 26 and 34 weeks of gestation, and then rising slowly thereafter back to the prepregnancy level by about 40 weeks (5). Resting heart rate increases by about 15–20 beats per minute (bpm) by the early third trimester; a resting heart rate of 90–100 bpm is common but rates higher than this should be investigated. Both cardiac output and blood pressure can decrease in pregnant women who are allowed to lie on their back in late pregnancy, because the weight of the uterus compresses the inferior vena cava and obstructs venous return. This can cause the woman to feel faint and may if prolonged lead to a reduction in placental perfusion and fetal hypoxia; the supine position should therefore be avoided in late pregnancy and labour, especially if the mother has an epidural anaesthetic (which also encourages venous pooling in the legs).

The stress and pain of labour also places an increased demand on the heart (6), which can largely be avoided by the use of regional anaesthetic for pain relief. Because rapid onset of sympathetic blockade can decrease blood pressure acutely, it is usual to administer such a blockade very slowly with careful monitoring.

Prepregnancy counselling

The major cardiac causes of maternal mortality and morbidity

Congenital cardiovascular malformation is the single commonest group of congenital abnormalities seen in newborn children, occurring about 0.8–1% (7). Before the introduction of open heart surgery in the 1960s (requiring the development of heart–lung bypass technology, and the use of hypothermia), about two-thirds of affected babies died in the first year of life (8). Accordingly, the majority of women with cardiac disease becoming pregnant before the 1960s had acquired disorders, mostly secondary to rheumatic fever. Mitral stenosis (caused by autoimmune damage to the valve associated with the immune response to rheumatic fever caused by streptococcal infections) was the commonest lesion, and in 1957 the maternal mortality due to acquired heart disease was approximately 5 per 100,000 maternities. However the widespread use of penicillin greatly reduced the incidence of rheumatic fever, and by 1990 the maternal mortality rate due to acquired disease had fallen to only 0.38 per 100,000 maternities. In contrast, by the 1990s two-thirds of women with congenital heart disease were surviving into their 20s and were therefore eligible to become parents themselves

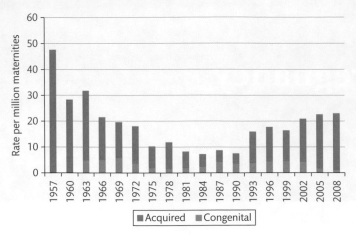

Figure 12.1 Cardiac deaths 1957–2008.
Source data from Cantwell R, Clutton-Brock T, Cooper G, Dawson A, Drife J, Garrod D et al. Saving Mothers' Lives: Reviewing maternal deaths to make motherhood safer: 2006-2008. The Eighth Report of the Confidential Enquiries into Maternal Deaths in the United Kingdom. *BJOG* 2011; 118 Suppl 1:1–203.

(8); and they now accounted for half of maternal deaths due to cardiac disease (also 0.38 per 100,000 maternities). However, since that time, in the United Kingdom, the rate of death due to acquired heart disease has increased again—it has almost trebled, to 2.18 per 100,000 maternities in 2008, while those due to congenital heart disease had fallen to 0.13 per 100,000 maternities (**Figure 12.1**) (9). The United Kingdom Confidential Enquiries into Maternal Deaths and Morbidity report for the triennium 2009–2011 confirmed the fact that cardiac disease now represents the single most common cause of maternal death related to pregnancy (10) (**Figure 12.2**). What lies behind this worrying increase?

Currently, one-third of maternal deaths from cardiac disease are the result of myocardial infarction/ischaemic heart disease. This is in part due to the growing number of women having babies later in life. **Figure 12.3** illustrates the changing age distribution of maternal age in the United Kingdom from 1938 through 2013. The most striking feature is a more than halving of births to women under the age of 25 since the early 1970s, paralleled by a more than fourfold increase in

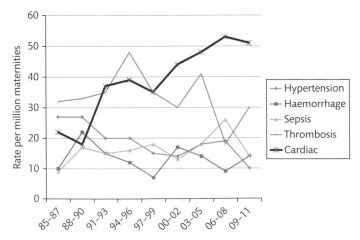

Figure 12.2 Number of deaths by cause by year.
Source data from MBRRACE-UK. Saving lives, Improving Mother's Care. https://www.npeu.ox.ac.uk/downloads/files/mbrrace-uk/reports/Saving%20Lives%20Improving%20Mothers%20Care%20report%202014%20Full.pdf.

births to women aged 35 and over. This is a trend seen in most developed countries, and has resulted in a major increase in age-related complications such as hypertension, diabetes, and obesity (11), all of which contribute to the aetiology of ischaemic heart disease.

A further third of deaths are associated with cardiomyopathy. This comprises a variety of conditions, the commonest being hypertrophic cardiomyopathy and the specific pregnancy-related condition of peripartum cardiomyopathy, as well as less common conditions such as restrictive cardiomyopathy, arrhythmogenic right ventricular cardiomyopathy, and left ventricular non-compaction. The overall prevalence of dilated cardiomyopathy is difficult to define because many affected individuals are apparently healthy; about a third of cases are familial (12). The common feature in all cases is left ventricular dilatation and systolic dysfunction in the absence of any obvious cause such as hypertension. The aetiology of peripartum cardiomyopathy remains conjectural, but may include genetic susceptibility, viral myocarditis, immunologically mediated damage, and the antiangiogenic 16 kDa fragment of the hormone prolactin (13).

Rheumatic heart disease, congenital heart disease, and pulmonary hypertension are currently each responsible for about 5–10% of deaths.

Implications for the baby

Fetal growth is very dependent upon efficient placental perfusion and gas and nutrient exchange. This in turn is determined partly by maternal cardiac output (affecting the maternal blood supply to the placenta), the structure and function of the placenta itself (including the microvasculature), and the efficiency of the fetal circulation. In women with heart disease, even when apparently normal cardiac output is maintained, there is a tendency for babies to be smaller than average (**Figure 12.4**). The reasons for this are not clear, but might in some cases be associated with reduced maternal stature, impaired nutrition, or genetic effects. Easier to understand is a greater reduction in mean centile birthweight when there is reduced cardiac output. Beta-blockers are commonly used in women with cardiac disease who have a tendency to arrhythmia (myocardial excitability is increased by the hormonal changes of pregnancy) and these are known to cause (usually mild) fetal growth restriction (14). However, the most serious forms of growth restriction are associated with maternal cyanosis, due not only to the lower oxygen tension in the blood, but also to the compensatory maternal high haemoglobin concentrations, which increase blood viscosity and impair placental blood flow. In such cases, moderate to severe fetal growth restriction almost always occurs, commonly requiring early delivery even if the mother's condition remained stable.

The priorities in prepregnancy counselling

The number one priority in prepregnancy counselling is to make sure that the mother and her family are fully and correctly informed of the risks facing both the mother and the baby in any future pregnancy. At one time it was traditional to separate cardiac conditions into three categories: mild, moderate, or severe. Mild lesions are those where the maternal risk of mortality is less than 1%, and this will include such common conditions as mitral valve prolapse or a well-functioning bicuspid aortic valve. However, it must be remembered that even a risk of death of 1 in 1000 is still more than 10 times higher than the background risk for a healthy woman in a developed

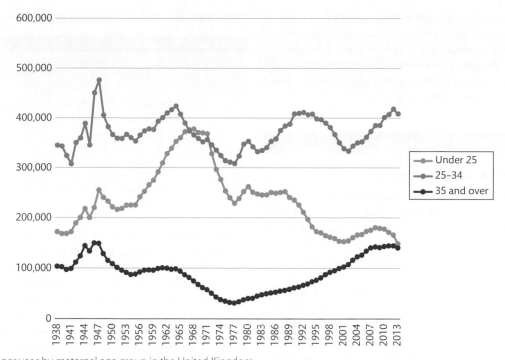

Figure 12.3 Births per year by maternal age group in the United Kingdom.

Source data from http://www.ons.gov.uk/peoplepopulationandcommunity/birthsdeathsandmarriages/livebirths/bulletins/livebirthsinenglandandwalesbycharacteristicsofmother1/2014-10-16.

country, so one must be careful to explain that 'low risk' does not mean 'no risk'. A moderate-risk lesion is one where the risk of maternal mortality or morbidity is between 1% and 10%, and includes significant mitral or aortic stenosis, women with a systemic right ventricle, cyanotic lesions without pulmonary hypertension, or a Fontan type circulation (a single systemic ventricle where the blood returning from the body travels to the lungs via direct blood vessel connections without a pumping chamber). Some women faced with up to a one in ten chance of dying in pregnancy will choose to remain childless. It must also be appreciated that some of these conditions confer a particularly high risk of growth restriction, particularly, for example, in women with a Fontan circulation, where in one series the mean birthweight was just over 2 kg (15).

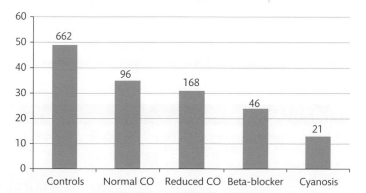

Figure 12.4 Centile birthweight by cardiac lesion group. CO, cardiac output.

Source data from Gelson E, Curry R, Gatzoulis MA, Swan L, Lupton M, Steer P, Johnson M. The effect of maternal heart disease on fetal growth. *Obstet Gynecol* 2011, Apr;117(4):886–91.

It has been traditional in the past for women with a risk of mortality exceeding 10% (such as women with Eisenmenger syndrome, truncus arteriosus syndrome, pulmonary hypertension, or Marfan syndrome with an aortic root dilated to more than 4 cm) to be advised against pregnancy. However, the principle of patient autonomy has now superseded the traditional paternalistic model of healthcare, and shared decision-making has become the new standard of practice (16). The perception of risk is subjective and varies from one person to another. Sometimes women, their partners, and family will not consider having children to be a major priority and instead value longevity for the woman. On the other hand, some women feel that their lives are incomplete without having children, and will be prepared to take even high risks to achieve motherhood. In this regard, it is vital that women understand that there may also be a risk to their baby, both of the recurrence of their heart disease if it is congenital, and fetal growth restriction and/or preterm birth.

It is the clinician's responsibility to ensure that all decisions are taken in full knowledge of the facts. Sometimes these facts are unwelcome, for example, one might have to tell a woman who has not previously thought much about it, that her life expectancy is reduced. Even if she survives her pregnancy, she might face the prospect of needing major surgical intervention or even dying while her children are young. While it might seem harsh to have to confront her with these unwelcome facts, a 2015 United Kingdom Supreme Court judgment in the case of Nadine Montgomery ruled that women should be given full information and stated that 'the onus should not be upon the patient (to ask), who may not know that there is anything to ask about' (17, 18). Counselling should be done jointly by an obstetrician and a cardiologist, and risks should be discussed in a sensitive manner, aiming to inform but not frighten unnecessarily. It is also important to say that risk assessment can never be precise. A 10% risk of dying is a population statistic; for the one woman in ten who dies the outcome is 100% mortality. In terms of whether the decision is contraception or a pregnancy, only women themselves can decide because only they have the full insight into their own priorities. Preconception counselling should not be aimed at discouraging women from becoming pregnant; rather, it should empower them to make informed choices.

General aspects of antenatal care

Maternal monitoring and investigation

Women who are known to have pre-existing heart disease should be advised to seek medical care as soon as pregnancy is confirmed, so that they can have a plan of care established by the multidisciplinary team. This team should include a cardiologist (preferably with experience of dealing with pregnant women) and an obstetrician (preferably with experience of dealing with women with heart disease). Joint consultation is the ideal because although each specialist may acquire considerable knowledge of the other specialty, they will not have the breadth of experience, or the regular updating of their knowledge, that is required to give the best advice and care. The team should regularly also include an anaesthetist, and when appropriate, a specialist nurse, a midwife, an intensivist, and a neonatologist. Geneticists, ultrasonographers, radiologists, haematologists, and other specialists will need to be involved when appropriate.

A detailed plan of care should be established and fully documented in the woman's notes, and shared with all relevant professionals including the family doctor. Women should carry their notes at all times so that key information is available in case of emergencies.

The women should be seen frequently by the obstetrician, usually every 2–4 weeks in the first half of pregnancy (depending on the severity of their lesion) and then weekly thereafter. Continuity of care is very important as it enables the detection of subtle signs of deterioration, such as increases in shortness of breath and palpitations. At each consultation, exercise tolerance should be assessed (watching the woman walk down the corridor to the consulting room can be informative) and enquiries should be made about any new symptoms such as palpitations or shortness of breath. There should be a careful clinical examination at each consultation, assessing the pulse rate and rhythm, and the heart should be auscultated to detect any change in murmurs. Auscultation of the lung bases is also important to detect early signs of pulmonary oedema.

There should also be regular review by the multidisciplinary team, at a minimum for delivery planning once the baby has reached viability, and more frequently in high-risk cases. Echocardiography is a key investigation, and should be undertaken in all cases at the beginning of pregnancy, with further scans according to the nature and severity of the lesion. For example, it is usual in women with Marfan syndrome (a genetic deficiency in fibrillin structure leading to a loss of elasticity, most critically in the aortic root) to undertake measurement of the aortic root diameter at least every 8 weeks.

Women are increasingly being assessed and monitored using scoring systems such as that first described by the New York Heart Association in 1928 (**Table 12.1**).

This relatively simple system was updated in 2001 by incorporating the results of modern investigative techniques such as echocardiography to derive the CARPREG ('CARdiac disease in PREGnancy')

Table 12.1 New York Heart Association scoring system

NYHA class	Symptoms
I	Cardiac disease, but no symptoms and no limitation in ordinary physical activity, e.g. no shortness of breath when walking, climbing stairs etc.
II	Mild symptoms (mild shortness of breath and/or angina) and slight limitation during ordinary activity
III	Marked limitation in activity due to symptoms, even during less-than-ordinary activity, e.g. walking short distances (20–100 m). Comfortable only at rest
IV	Severe limitations. Experiences symptoms even while at rest. Patients are usually bedbound

score, which was derived and then validated in a prospective multicentre study of 599 pregnancies in women with a variety of congenital and acquired heart disease (19). The score varies from 0 to 4, depending on the number of criteria met (**Box 12.1**).

In 2011, the Task Force on the Management of Cardiovascular Diseases in Pregnancy of the European Society of Cardiology modified the World Health Organization classification to devise a new score related more closely to the nature of the cardiac lesion rather than just the overall maternal condition before pregnancy (20)—deterioration during pregnancy can be more rapid with some types of lesions than with others. For example, mitral incompetence is better tolerated during pregnancy than stenosis. This is because with incompetence, the percentage impairment varies little with the cardiac output, whereas with stenosis, the resistance to flow increases exponentially as cardiac output increases. This classification was further refined by Regitz-Zagrosek et al. in 2014 (21).

Fetal screening

Fetal assessment usually starts with an ultrasound scan at 10–14 weeks of gestational age. This is routinely done to assess whether the baby's size is consistent with the presumed gestational age, and to assess the nuchal thickness (thickness of the tissues at the back of the neck). This is done as part of screening for Downs syndrome, but a raised nuchal translucency (4 mm or more) is also associated with an increased risk of congenital cardiac disease. Most women with congenital heart disease will have a risk of recurrence of the condition in their baby. For polygenic conditions such as tetralogy of Fallot, the recurrence risk is about 3–5% (compared with a background risk of congenital cardiac anomaly of 0.8%) (22). The risk is increased if the father of the baby has the same condition because it increases the likelihood of recurrence of the particular combination of genes which produced the

---

Box 12.1 CARPREG score

- Prior episodes of heart failure, transient ischaemic attack, stroke before pregnancy, or arrhythmias
- Baseline functional class greater than class II or cyanosis
- Left heart obstructive lesions
- Low systemic ventricular ejection fraction (<40%)

Source data from Siu SC, Sermer M, Colman JM, Alvarez AN, Mercier LA, Morton BC et al. Prospective multicenter study of pregnancy outcomes in women with heart disease. *Circulation* 2001; 104(5):515–521.

abnormality. Some conditions (such as Marfan syndrome) are autosomal dominant and therefore the recurrence rate is 50% and specialized antenatal diagnosis (such as preimplantation genetic diagnosis or chorionic villus sampling) can be offered. It is important that for each specific condition, the multidisciplinary team obtain the latest information about inheritance risk (a useful source is the Online Mendelian Inheritance in Man website, available at http://www.omim.org/).

In addition to the routine fetal anomaly scan at 20 weeks gestational age, it is also usual to offer women with a congenital heart lesion that may recur in the baby detailed ultrasound screening by a fetal cardiologist. In most places this is done at 22 weeks of gestation, when the baby's heart is big enough to provide a good view, although in units with more resources, it can be done as a two-stage procedure, with an early look at 16 weeks followed up by a more detailed scan at 22 weeks.

Due to the increase in the risk of fetal growth restriction in nearly all cases, it is usual to organize serial fetal biometry scans to assess growth. If these scans suggest that growth is impaired, the next step is the assessment of flow velocity waveforms in the umbilical artery using Doppler techniques, and if they are abnormal, daily monitoring should be carried out using cardiotocography until there is either a maternal or fetal indication for delivery.

Specific lesions of major importance

Ischaemic heart disease

Pregnancy itself raises the risk of acute myocardial infarction three- to fourfold (e.g. the risk is 30 times higher for women over the age of 40 compared with women aged <20 years) (23). If a myocardial infarction occurs during pregnancy, the mortality is up to 1 in 13 (9). Unfortunately, most women suffering this condition will have no history of heart disease and will have been asymptomatic before pregnancy. Management is similar during pregnancy to that outside pregnancy, and the first step is a high index of suspicion for myocardial ischaemia/infarction in any pregnant woman presenting with chest pain. The other important possibility to consider is aortic dissection, another significant cause of maternal mortality during pregnancy.

All women presenting with chest pain in pregnancy should have an electrocardiogram (ECG) and this needs to be interpreted by someone who is used to interpreting it against the background changes seen during pregnancy. Because an initial ECG may be normal, ECGs should be repeated at least every 2 hours until the pain subsides. Serum troponin levels are important to confirm a suspected diagnosis; they need to be taken at least 3–4 hours after the onset of pain to avoid false-negative results. If they are elevated, there should be a low threshold for investigation by angiography. If the diagnosis is not clear, computed tomography (CT) or a magnetic resonance imaging (MRI) scan should be undertaken. Although there was concern at one time regarding the radiation exposure from CT scanning, the modern generation of scanners use substantially reduced amounts of X-rays and their use in demonstrating coronary anatomy has improved. MRI and CT scanning are both useful for detection of previously unsuspected aortic dissection.

Cardiomyopathy

The wide variety of proposed aetiologies for cardiomyopathy has already been alluded to earlier in this chapter. A key distinction is whether the cardiomyopathy was already present/diagnosed before pregnancy, or whether it was detected for the first time during pregnancy. The pregnancy prognosis for pre-existing cardiomyopathy (the most common form of which is idiopathic dilated cardiomyopathy) is very dependent upon the cardiac ejection fraction (24). This is the proportion of the left ventricular volume which is ejected with each heartbeat, and it should normally be 60% or more (as the heart does not collapse completely during each beat, there is always a substantial amount of blood left in the ventricular cavity at the end of each contraction). The majority of women with previously diagnosed cardiomyopathy will have an ejection fraction of approximately 45% or more, and their prognosis is relatively good. An ejection fraction of 30–45% is likely to be associated with decompensation during pregnancy, and an ejection fraction of less than 30% indicates that termination of pregnancy should be considered because the pregnancy may result in a fatal decompensation. Most women with this pre-existing cardiomyopathy will survive pregnancy, but complications such as cardiac failure and arrhythmia will occur in a third or more of women. Management is mainly directed towards minimizing the risk of pulmonary oedema secondary to low cardiac output (diuretics such as furosemide can be life-saving) and prophylaxis against arrhythmia using a beta-adrenergic blocking drug such as bisoprolol. There should be a low threshold for the use of prophylactic anticoagulation with low-molecular-weight heparin because of the risk of thrombus formation in a poorly contractile ventricle, and therapeutic anticoagulation is indicated if atrial fibrillation occurs.

Peripartum cardiomyopathy (cardiomyopathy appearing for the first time in relation to pregnancy or in the puerperium) has a highly variable incidence according to racial origin (25), with particularly high rates in women of black African origin. It is usually diagnosed when a woman presents with rapidly increasing shortness of breath and pulmonary oedema; diagnosis is by echocardiography and the demonstration of a severely reduced ejection fraction. There is currently some optimism that treatment with bromocriptine can prevent or ameliorate peripartum cardiomyopathy (26–28). Management is in other respects supportive (the use of diuretics to combat pulmonary oedema, inotropic agents to improve cardiac contractility). The most important prognostic feature in relation to the outlook for future pregnancies is the rate and completeness of the recovery of cardiac function. If after 12 months cardiac function has returned to entirely normal, then the risk of recurrence of heart failure in a future pregnancy is about 20%, but the mortality is low. However, in the presence of persistently impaired left ventricular function, almost half will have recurrent heart failure in their next pregnancy, and about one in five will die (13). In general therefore, women who do not recover their cardiac function are advised against a further pregnancy.

Mitral stenosis

The majority of mitral stenosis cases are secondary to rheumatic fever. It is common for it to present for the first time during pregnancy, particularly in immigrants who have never had any form of cardiac assessment previously and who are unaware that they have had rheumatic fever (in the developing world, non-specific fevers are common and the diagnosis of rheumatic fever is frequently missed). A simple 'rule of thumb' for severity is that the normal mitral valve area is 8 cm², a value less than 4 cm² is abnormal, a value less than 2 cm² is concerning, and a value less than 1 cm² is likely to require intervention during pregnancy. As explained previously, the obstruction to blood flow increases exponentially with stenosis, and therefore the clinical status of most women with mitral stenosis will deteriorate during pregnancy because of the increased circulating blood volume and cardiac output. The reduction in output from the left side of the heart results in the blood 'backing up' in the lungs, leading to pulmonary oedema. This can occur acutely if the left atrium (which is commonly dilated due to the back pressure from the constricted valve) starts to fibrillate. Symptoms are commonly those of orthopnoea, a dry cough, and paroxysmal nocturnal dyspnoea. Diagnosis is readily made using echocardiography.

Treatment is bed rest (reduces cardiac output), oxygen therapy, beta-blockade, and a diuretic (29). As with cardiomyopathy, treatment anticoagulation with low-molecular-weight heparin should be given if there is atrial fibrillation. In severe cases with a valve area less than 1 cm², a balloon valvotomy or even an open valvotomy may be needed.

Aortic stenosis

Most aortic stenosis is secondary to bicuspid aortic valve disease, a congenital lesion. A common method of assessment is to measure the gradient across the valve using Doppler echocardiography. A normal gradient is less than 5 mmHg, but it can be as high as 25 mmHg with only mild stenosis. The gradient commonly doubles during pregnancy because of the increased blood flow, and therefore a gradient up to about 60 mmHg during pregnancy suggests mild-to-moderate stenosis only. Values above 60 mmHg are likely to be clinically significant, and values above 80 mmHg are commonly associated with symptoms and morbidity (29). The majority of women with aortic stenosis will have a congenital aetiology and therefore should have had preconception counselling. Ideally, in severe cases, there will have been prepregnancy treatment to improve function during pregnancy. One such treatment is the Ross procedure, where the mother's tricuspid valve is used to replace the damaged aortic valve, and a tissue homograft/xenograft (from a human, pig, or cow) is placed in the tricuspid position. The value of this exchange is that the native tissue will survive longer in the high pressure of the left heart than a tissue homograft or xenograft, while the latter will survive longer in the low pressure of the right heart. Unlike with the mitral valve, surgical valvotomy commonly results in severe regurgitation and thus valve replacement is preferable. This requires the use of cardiopulmonary bypass, and in its usual form this has a high fetal mortality (20–30%). This can be reduced by using higher perfusion pressures than would usually be used with non-pregnant patients, and avoiding the use of hypothermia; this makes the technique particularly challenging during pregnancy, as does the need for full anticoagulation during the procedure (30).

Aortopathies

There is a wide range of congenital and acquired aortopathies, many of which have a genetic component. The most common is probably Marfan syndrome, and there are about 10,000 individuals with this syndrome in the United Kingdom, associated with approximately 150 pregnancies per year (31). It is due to a defect (at least a dozen different defects have been identified) in the gene responsible for the production of fibrillin-1. This is associated with an increase in a protein called transforming growth factor beta, which causes problems in connective tissues throughout the body. Those affected tend to be very tall and slim, with a span (width from the tip of the fingers of an outstretched arm to the tips of the fingers on the other side) which exceeds their height. Other signs include eye problems, particularly dislocation of the lens. The expression of the defect is very variable from one individual to another. From the perspective of pregnancy complications, the main problem is excessive dilatation of the aortic root. The interquartile range of the aortic root diameter at the level of the sinuses of Valsalva in healthy women is from 26 to 34 mm (32). Some dilatation occurs in pregnancy due to the circulatory volume expansion; the likelihood of dissection during pregnancy is generally said to be no more than 1% if the aortic root diameter is less than 40 mm, but increases to 10% if the diameter is greater than this (33). Of course there is no sudden jump in the likelihood of dissection between 39 mm and 41 mm; the risk is probably also increased if there is a sudden expansion even within the normal range. There is no specific management other than a recommendation for the woman to take beta-blockers to reduce the cardiac impulse and thus limit the stretch on the aortic root, and careful monitoring of the aortic root diameter with elective delivery if it shows a worrying increase. Elective aortic root replacement is then recommended during the puerperium (34).

Right heart lesions

These comprise a wide variety of conditions including systemic right ventricles (transposition of the great arteries after an atrial switch operation (Mustard or Senning)), or congenitally 'corrected' transposition of the great arteries), functionally univentricular hearts with or without a Fontan-type operation, atrial septal defects, tetralogy of Fallot, and Ebstein's anomaly of the tricuspid valve. Accordingly, the risk of an adverse outcome depends very much on the specific lesion and associated factors such as arrhythmia, impaired cardiac output due to tricuspid regurgitation, heart failure, cyanosis, myocardial dysfunction, and the severity of outflow tract obstruction.

Tetralogy of Fallot is the most common cyanotic congenital heart lesion (it comprises up to 10% of cases of congenital heart disease) and consists of a large ventricular septal defect, right ventricular outflow tract obstruction, right ventricular hypertrophy, and overriding of the aorta. Genetic testing should be offered before pregnancy, as the recurrence risk of DiGeorge syndrome is 50%. In its absence, the risk for recurrence in the fetus is about 2–3%. Repair is usually to relieve the outflow tract obstruction with a transannular patch, resulting in free pulmonary valve regurgitation (35). In pregnancy, the degree of pulmonary regurgitation is the main variable influencing the degree of fetal growth restriction, with which it is commonly associated (36). Tetralogy of Fallot can be part of the DiGeorge syndrome (present in 15% of tetralogy of Fallot patients). Pulmonary valve regurgitation is also the main concern with Ebstein's anomaly.

Women who rely on a systemic right ventricle need to be observed carefully for any signs of decompensation during pregnancy. This will be manifest as a decrease in blood pressure and signs of pulmonary oedema.

Pulmonary hypertension

Although pulmonary hypertension is relatively rare, it is one of the most serious conditions in women who become pregnant, because it limits severely their ability to adapt to the cardiovascular changes of pregnancy. The outcome for the fetus is also commonly poor, with high rates of preterm delivery, fetal growth restriction, and perinatal mortality (37). Until the beginning of the twenty-first century, maternal mortality rates of 50% were sometimes quoted, and pulmonary hypertension was widely regarded as a complete contraindication to pregnancy. However recent series show some improvement in outcomes, with a mortality of perhaps only (!) 20% (37, 38). This improvement has been attributed to new therapies, such as the routine use of sildenafil, and the use of prostanoids such as intravenous prostacyclin. These therapies have a specific vasodilator in action in the lungs, helping to reduce the impedance to blood flow. Specific pregnancy care involves routine full anticoagulation with low-molecular-weight heparin, monitored by the measurement of antifactor Xa levels (target 0.6–1). In the typical case, failing fetal growth and increasing maternal compromise at about 34 weeks of pregnancy mandate delivery, which is then usually by caesarean section under either regional block or general anaesthetic.

Arrhythmias

The most common arrhythmia is extrasystole; these often occur in healthy individuals. They increase in frequency during pregnancy because of the increase in myocardial excitability, and commonly become noticeable to the woman because of the increased stroke volume associated with the pregnancy circulatory expansion. They are readily investigated by the use of 24-hour ECG recording (commonly called the Holter test). As a rule of thumb, up to 10,000 isolated unifocal ventricular extrasystoles per day can be regarded as normal; above this number it is wise to investigate further with an echocardiogram. The largest number the author has seen recorded in a single day in a woman who was subsequently normal on all investigations was 24,000. Runs of ventricular tachycardia of no more than seven consecutive beats occur less frequently but provided they only occur occasionally and are associated with an otherwise normal ECG do not usually justify further investigation unless they are associated with symptoms such as syncope. Other common conduction disturbances including the Wolff–Parkinson–White syndrome are relatively common and generally innocuous during pregnancy. However, there are rare but serious conditions such as the long QT syndrome and Brugada syndrome which are associated with sudden cardiac arrest and may require the insertion of an implanted cardiac defibrillator. Chronic atrial fibrillation can lead to embolism of clot from the poorly contracting atria and therapeutic anticoagulation with low-molecular-weight heparin is therefore indicated. Persistent arrhythmia is increasingly being treated successfully with catheter thermoablation, when the abnormal myocardium where the arrhythmia originates is destroyed (39).

Prosthetic heart valves

Women who need a heart valve replacement before pregnancy face a difficult choice. Replacement of a damaged valve with a homograft/xenograft has the major advantage that anticoagulation is not required because while it is still structurally intact, the valve functions in much the same way as a normal human valve. This makes pregnancy straightforward and relatively low risk. Unfortunately, the tissue has to be denatured before being implanted so that it does not create an immune response, and therefore is not self-repairing. This means that it gradually wears out and after about 12–15 years a tissue valve on the left (high pressure) side of the heart usually needs replacing. This means once again undergoing major open-heart surgery, which even in the best hands carries a 1–2% mortality rate. A metal valve on the other hand will usually last a lifetime. Unfortunately, its mechanical structure makes it prone to act as a focus for the formation of thrombus, with the potential for embolus. On the left side of the circulation, this embolism can be to the brain, causing a disabling stroke. As a result, permanent anticoagulation, usually with warfarin, is required. Unfortunately, warfarin crosses the placenta and in the first trimester, once the placental circulation has formed, it can cause warfarin embryopathy (this has many features but typically comprises epiphyseal stippling, nasal hypoplasia, limb abnormalities, and developmental delay) and miscarriage. It also anticoagulates the fetus, and in the second trimester this can result in intracranial haemorrhage and death of the fetus. If the baby survives, it may have neurological disability (40). The alternative to warfarin is therapeutic low-molecular-weight heparin. Unfortunately, this is less effective as an anticoagulant than warfarin, and results in a 5–10% risk of valve thrombosis, requiring an urgent repeat valve replacement with associated morbidity and mortality, especially during pregnancy.

A 2015 study in the journal *Circulation* reported on the outcomes of pregnancy in 212 women with mechanical valves and 134 women with tissue valves (41). Although mortality was similar (1.4% vs 1.5%), complications were more common with mechanical valves (42% vs 21%), largely due to miscarriage (28.6% vs 9.2%), haemorrhage (23.1% vs 4.9%), and late fetal loss (7.1% vs 0.7%).

Currently, the balance of counselling tends to encourage the use of tissue valves in young women who have expressed an intention to have one or more pregnancies with the aim of completing their pregnancies and then when their tissue valve needs replacement, changing to a metal valve. However, if they already have a metal valve when they become pregnant, the choice of anticoagulant is very difficult as there is no entirely satisfactory solution. Therefore, current practice is to explain to women the pros and cons of each approach and allow them to choose (42).

Endocarditis

Endocarditis in pregnancy is so rare that in 2008 the National Institute for Health and Care Excellence recommended that routine prophylaxis not be given for any obstetric procedure (43, 44). However, some clinicians still prefer to give appropriate broad-spectrum antibiotic prophylaxis to women who have had previous endocarditis, or who have a mechanical valve.

Intrapartum care including anaesthesia

Delivery is a particularly risky time for any woman, and is additionally risky for women with significant heart disease. This is because the stress of labour adds to the strain on her heart, and during the birth there can be major cardiovascular stressors such as postpartum haemorrhage. The general approach to managing intrapartum care is to aim for a birth which is as non-stressful as possible, and consequently it is usual to hope for a spontaneous onset of labour at term (presuming that maternal decompensation has not indicated delivery before this), with a vaginal birth (avoiding the stress and potential haemorrhage/infection from a caesarean section). At one time it was common for women with heart disease to be advised to have a caesarean section because of a common perception that this was less stressful than labour. In fact, the stress of labour can be effectively reduced by the use of regional (epidural) anaesthesia, using slow incremental top-ups of low-dose Marcaine to avoid any sudden changes in blood pressure, and vaginal delivery avoids both the increased haemorrhage and infection risk of caesarean section. Moreover, it is beneficial for the baby (45) because it avoids the respiratory difficulties associated with elective caesarean delivery (46). In cases with more severe cardiac impairment it is common to recommend the avoidance of prolonged bearing down (which is in effect repeated Valsalva manoeuvres, which can compromise venous return) and instead assist the birth of the baby using a vacuum extractor, although there are no prospective studies which show this to be necessary. The delivery is commonly straightforward because the baby tends to be smaller than average.

It is particularly important to avoid acute emergencies, as these will always increase the risk in women with compromised cardiac function. Induction of labour when necessary is therefore preferably carried out using artificial rupture of membranes and a low-dose oxytocin infusion, because the use of prostaglandins is associated with a 3–5% risk of uterine hyperstimulation. If hyperstimulation occurs, the usual tocolytics such as ritodrine or salbutamol are contraindicated because they induce maternal tachycardia. When oxytocin is used as a prophylactic against postpartum haemorrhage, it should be given as a bolus of no more than 2 units given slowly over 10 minutes (47) because acute administration can cause marked hypotension (48). Ergometrine is generally avoided because it causes vasoconstriction and hypertension, and can also cause spasm of the coronary arteries (49).

Careful planning of clinical management during labour is essential, and is commonly undertaken at about 34–36 weeks of pregnancy, when the woman's ability to cope with the stress of pregnancy has become apparent, and preterm birth is no longer likely. Planning should be done by the multidisciplinary team, and the recommendations for care are best entered onto a pro forma of the sort illustrated in **Figure 12.5.**

Care in the puerperium

The mother with heart disease continues to be at risk during the puerperium. The first risk is from the major changes in fluid distribution and the diuresis that occurs secondary to the hormone changes following delivery of the placenta; this can destabilize the cardiovascular system. The second risk is that of thrombosis. The incidence of thrombosis is six times higher during pregnancy and 11 times higher in the puerperium than in the non-pregnant woman. Routine prophylaxis with low-molecular-weight heparin is now recommended for 7 days following caesarean section in all women, and will be additionally be recommended after a vaginal delivery to

any woman with cardiac disease who has impaired cardiac output or whose mobility is in any way restricted.

Long-term outcome

In general, the long-term prognosis for women with heart disease is not adversely affected by pregnancy. There is some evidence of minor long-term deterioration in cardiac function in women with a systemic right ventricle, Marfan syndrome, pulmonary hypertension, and peripartum cardiomyopathy.

Contraception

Contraception is most commonly used to space pregnancies, rather than to avoid them permanently. Because of this, many methods of contraception are used which have a significant failure rate (50). For example, one of the most popular forms of contraception is the male condom, and even with 'perfect use' this is associated with 2 unintended pregnancies for every 100 women-years of use. A more typical failure rate is 15%. For more effective contraception, women most commonly use the combined oral contraceptive pill, which has a 'perfect use' failure rate of 0.3 per 100 women-years, and a typical failure rate of 8%. However, even this high efficacy may not be adequate in women for whom an unintended pregnancy could be fatal (those in the high-risk groups). Moreover, both the oestrogen and progestogen component of the combined oral contraceptive confer a 3.5 times increased relative risk of thrombosis in users compared with non-users (51). The 'low-dose progestogen-only pills' such as Micronor are considered medically safe in all forms of heart disease, but their failure rate is similar to that of the combined pill and they should not therefore be recommended for high-risk women when avoidance of pregnancy is a high priority. They also suffer from the disadvantage that the pregnancy rate after a single missed pill is substantially higher than with the combined oral contraceptive.

As a result of these considerations, the three most widely used reversible forms of contraception in women with heart disease are the oral contraceptive progestogen-only pill Cerazette/Cerelle, containing desogestrel (75 mg), the progestogen implant (Nexplanon), and the progestogen intrauterine contraceptive device (LNG-IUS (Mirena)). Cerazette/Cerelle has a failure rate similar to that of the combined oral contraceptive pill, its major disadvantage being an increased incidence of progestogenic side effects such as irregular bleeding when compared with the low-dose progestogen-only pills. The progestogen implant has the lowest failure rate of any form of contraception, 1 in 2000 women-years, and once inserted remains effective for at least 3 years. The major reason for discontinuation is irregular bleeding, which occurs in about 20%. The progestogen intrauterine contraceptive device has a failure rate of 1 in 500 women-years but has the advantage of commonly producing amenorrhoea (useful in women prone to anaemia) and being effective for at least 5 years. The major disadvantage is a small (0.1%) risk of syncope during insertion, and therefore in women with cardiac disease it should only be inserted in an environment fully equipped for resuscitation, and preferably with an anaesthetist in attendance. The copper T intrauterine device is not recommended for routine use because of

If admitted to LW Please Inform	Cons Obstetrician on Call ☐ Y ☐ N Obstetric SpR on Call **Senior / junior** Cons Anaesthetist on Call ☐ Y ☐ N Anaesthetic SpR on Call **Senior / junior** Maple Midwifery Team ☐ Y ☐ N	If advice is needed, please contact one of the following via switchboard at: (Obstetricians) (Cardiologists)
Mode of Delivery	Elective LSCS / Trial of Vaginal Delivery	
Elective LSCS (see anaesthetic sheet for anaesthetic details)	Prophylactic Compression Suture Syntocinon 2 units over 10–20 mins Syntocinon-low dose infusion (8–12 munits/min – see over for details) Anaesthetic technique......................... Maternal Monitoring......................	*Inform consultant on call if admitted in labour before scheduled date* **Epid/Spin/CSE/GA** ECG/SaO₂/Non-invasive BP/arterial line BP/CVP
Vaginal Delivery 1st stage Mx (see anaesthetic sheet for anaesthetic details)	TED stockings in labour/HDU chart Prophylactic Antibiotics: If operative delivery / in all situations...... Search DATIX under "bacterial endocarditis" for details of antibiotics **Epidural for analgesia......................** Maternal Monitoring............................ Continuous EFM is recommended for all women with cardiac disease	Medications to be continued: .... ☐ As soon as in established labour/ ☐ If and when requested ECG SaO₂ Non-invasive BP arterial line BP CVP
Vaginal Delivery 2nd stage Mx	☐ Normal second stage **OR** ☐ Short second stage................. **OR** ☐ Elective assisted delivery only	assist if not delivered in................... minutes
Vaginal Delivery 3rd stage Mx	1. Normal active Mx (oxytocin 5IU I/M and CCT, or 2IU I/V over ten mins) <u>OR</u> 2. Syntocinon infusion 8–12 mU/min (For details, see overleaf)	**DO NOT GIVE Ergometrine** Continue .... hours
Post Delivery	Simpson Unit Yes No For .... hours LMW heparin Yes No Dose...................Duration...................... List medications to be given... and continued for......................days/weeks Recommended post-natal stay ......days Cardiac review **Y/N** weeks............	

Figure 12.5 Example of a clinical management plan for delivery.

its failure rate of 1 in 120 women-years, but it can be useful for post-coital contraception because inserting it within 7 days of unprotected intercourse prevents implantation in the great majority of cases.

Sterilization can also be considered if the woman is sure she does not want children, or if she considers her family is complete. Male sterilization can be inappropriate if the woman's life expectancy is substantially reduced because he may wish to have a pregnancy with a future partner. The commonest form of female sterilization, clipping the fallopian tubes at laparoscopy, is contraindicated because the generation of a carbon dioxide pneumoperitoneum can compromise cardiac function in susceptible women. However, there is a more recent form of sterilization in which coils are inserted into the base of the fallopian tubes via a hysteroscope (Essure). This can be performed under sedation as an outpatient provided resuscitation facilities are immediately available in case of syncope. Occasionally, salpingectomy at caesarean section is appropriate. Clearly, all forms of reversible contraception require detailed counselling before they are undertaken.

Examples of Clinical Situations	Consider the following
Spontaneous Labour & Recent thromboprophylaxis use e.g. LMWH/Warfarin	Inform Anaesthetist asap
An epidural can be given more than 12 hours after prophylactic dose or more than 24 hours after therapeutic dose, or earlier at the discretion of the anaesthetist.	D/W Consultant anaesthetist on call For additional advice, contact Drs X, Y, Z via switchboard, or obstetricians listed overleaf
Need for Syntocinon Augmentation in Labour	- Use of double strength syntocinon but halve rate to reduce total volume of fluids given ***(this decision needs to be taken at consultant level)***
Syntocinon as prophylaxis against PPH;	Low dose infusion (12mU/min) use either: 5 IU in 50 ml at 7ml per hour *or* 10 IU in 500 ml at 36 ml per hour *Continue for 4 hours (longer if concerns)*
Postpartum Haemorrhage	- Inform Anaesthetic and Obstetric Consultant on call - For uterotonic, misoprostol 600mcg rectally is preferred but monitor for hyper-pyrexia. **Avoid hemabate or high dose syntocinon** - Consider use of compression suture - Consider use of intrauterine balloon (antibiotic cover is recommended) - Strict input /output charts to be maintained - Consider central access or arterial monitoring
Preterm Labour	Atosiban (Tractocile) is the first line Mx **Do not use Ritodrine or Salbutamol**
Pacemaker	**Do not use unipolar diathermy** **Beware** pacemaker in unusual places (e.g. abdominal wall) when performing CS If patient has a defibrillator and needs a CS programme therapies off for the case or in emergency situation use a magnet.
Induction of labour	Prostaglandins are best avoided as they cause hyperstimulation in about 2% of women and the tocolytics usually used to control tachysystole (beta sympathomimetics) are relatively contraindicated. The rapidity required for emergency caesareans for 'fetal distress' poses an increased risk. Accordingly, ARM and syntocinon are preferred in most cases.

Please inform the Consultant Obstetrician on call if there is departure from planned management or if unexpected clinical situations develop in women with cardiac disease

Figure 12.5 Continued

REFERENCES

1. Clapp JF, Seaward BL, Sleamaker RH, Hiser J. Maternal physiologic adaptations to early human pregnancy. *Am J Obstet Gynecol* 1988;**159**:1456–60.
2. Johnson MR, von Klemperer K. Cardiovascular changes in normal pregnancy. In: Steer PJ, Gatzoulis MA (eds), *Heart Disease and Pregnancy*, 2nd edn, pp. 19–28. Cambridge: Cambridge University Press; 2016.
3. Moncada S, Palmer RM, Higgs EA. Nitric oxide: physiology, pathophysiology and pharmacology. *Pharmacol Rev* 1991;**43**:109–42.
4. Wang Y, Zhao S. Placental blood circulation. In: *Vascular Biology of the Placenta*, pp. 3–12. San Rafael, CA: Morgan and Claypool Life Sciences; 2010.
5. Steer PJ, Little MP, Kold-Jensen T, Chapple J, Elliott P. Maternal blood pressure in pregnancy, birth weight, and perinatal mortality in first births: prospective study. *BMJ* 2004;**329**:1312.
6. Robson SC, Dunlop W, Boys RJ, Hunter S. Cardiac output during labour. *Br Med J (Clin Res Ed)* 1987;**295**:1169–72.
7. Stout K. Pregnancy in women with congenital heart disease: the importance of evaluation and counselling. *Heart* 2005;**91**:713–14.
8. Somerville J. Near misses and disasters in the treatment of grown-up congenital heart patients. *J Roy Soc Med* 1997;**90**:124–27.
9. Cantwell R, Clutton-Brock T, Cooper G, et al. Saving Mothers' Lives: Reviewing maternal deaths to make motherhood safer: 2006–2008. The Eighth Report of the Confidential Enquiries into Maternal Deaths in the United Kingdom. *BJOG* 2011;**118** Suppl 1:1–203.
10. MBRRACE-UK. Saving Lives, Improving Mother's Care. 2014. Available at: https://www.npeu.ox.ac.uk/downloads/files/mbrrace-uk/reports/Saving%20Lives%20Improving%20Mothers%20Care%20report%202014%20Full.pdf.
11. Scott-Pillai R, Spence D, Cardwell C, Hunter A, Holmes V. The impact of body mass index on maternal and neonatal outcomes: a retrospective study in a UK obstetric population, 2004–2011. *BJOG* 2013;**120**:932–39.
12. Stergiopoulos K, Shiang E, Bench T. Pregnancy in patients with pre-existing cardiomyopathies. *J Am Coll Cardiol* 2011;**58**:337–50.
13. Elkayam U. Clinical characteristics of peripartum cardiomyopathy in the United States: diagnosis, prognosis, and management. *J Am Coll Cardiol* 2011;**58**:659–70.
14. Ersboll AS, Hedegaard M, Sondergaard L, Ersboll M, Johansen M. Treatment with oral beta-blockers during pregnancy complicated by maternal heart disease increases the risk of fetal growth restriction. *BJOG* 2014;**121**:618–26.
15. Cauldwell M, Von Klemperer K, Uebing A, et al. A cohort study of women with a Fontan circulation undergoing preconception counselling. *Heart* 2016;**102**:534–40.
16. Cauldwell M, Steer PJ, Johnson M, Gatzoulis M. Counselling women with congenital cardiac disease. *BMJ* 2016;**352**:i910.
17. Montgomery (Appellant) *v* Lanarkshire Health Board (Respondent) (Scotland) [2015] (UKSC 11). Available at: https://www.supremecourt.uk/decided-cases/docs/UKSC_2013_0136_Judgment.pdf.
18. Bolton H. The Montgomery ruling extends patient autonomy. *BJOG* 2015;**122**:1273.
19. Siu SC, Sermer M, Colman JM, et al. Prospective multicenter study of pregnancy outcomes in women with heart disease. *Circulation* 2001;**104**:515–21.
20. Regitz-Zagrosek V, Lundqvist CB, Borghi C, et al. ESC Guidelines on the management of cardiovascular diseases during pregnancy: the Task Force on the Management of Cardiovascular Diseases during Pregnancy of the European Society of Cardiology (ESC). *Eur Heart J* 2011;**32**:3147–97.
21. Regitz-Zagrosek V, Gohlke-Barwolf C, Iung B, Pieper PG. Management of cardiovascular diseases during pregnancy. *Curr Probl Cardiol* 2014;**39**:85–151.
22. Burn J, Brennan P, Little J, et al. Recurrence risks in offspring of adults with major heart defects: results from first cohort of British collaborative study. *Lancet* 1998;**351**:311–16.
23. Roos-Hesselink JW, van Hagen IM. Ischemic heart disease. In: Steer PJ, Gatzoulis MA (eds), *Heart Disease and Pregnancy*, 2nd edn, pp. 174–79. Cambridge: Cambridge University Press; 2016.
24. Grewal J, Siu SC, Ross HJ, et al. Pregnancy outcomes in women with dilated cardiomyopathy. *J Am Coll Cardiol* 2009;**55**:45–52.
25. Nelson-Piercy C, Head C. Peripartum and other cardiomyopathies in pregnancy. In: Steer PJ, Gatzoulis MA (eds), *Heart Disease and Pregnancy*, 2nd edn, pp. 160–73. Cambridge: Cambridge University Press; 2016.
26. Elkayam U, Goland S. Bromocriptine for the treatment of peripartum cardiomyopathy. *Circulation* 2010;**121**:1463–64.
27. Desplantie O, Tremblay-Gravel M, Avram R, Marquis-Gravel G, Ducharme A, Jolicoeur EM. The medical treatment of new-onset peripartum cardiomyopathy: a systematic review of prospective studies. *Can J Cardiol* 2015;**31**:1421–26.
28. Bouabdallaoui N, Mouquet F, Lebreton G, Demondion P, Le Jemtel TH, Ennezat PV. Current knowledge and recent development on management of peripartum cardiomyopathy. *Eur Heart J Acute Cardiovasc Care* 2017;**6**:359–66.
29. Thorne SA. Management of mitral and aortic stenosis in pregnancy. In: Steer PJ, Gatzoulis MA (eds), *Heart Disease and Pregnancy*, 2nd edn, pp. 125–30. Cambridge: Cambridge University Press; 2016.
30. Yates MT, Soppa G, Smelt J, et al. Perioperative management and outcomes of aortic surgery during pregnancy. *J Thorac Cardiovasc Surg* 2015;**149**:607–10.
31. Swan L. Management of aortopathies, including Marfan syndrome, in pregnancy. In: Steer PJ, Gatzoulis MA (eds), *Heart Disease and Pregnancy*, 2nd edn, pp. 115–24. Cambridge: Cambridge University Press; 2016.
32. Vriz O, Aboyans V, D'Andrea A, et al. Normal values of aortic root dimensions in healthy adults. *Am J Cardiol* 2014;**114**:921–27.
33. Curry RA, Gelson E, Swan L, et al. Marfan syndrome and pregnancy: maternal and neonatal outcomes. *BJOG* 2014;**121**:610–17.
34. Mayet J, Steer P, Somerville J. Marfan syndrome, aortic dilatation, and pregnancy. *Obstet Gynecol* 1998;**92** 4 II Suppl:713.
35. Jensen AS, Sondergaard L, Uebing A. Management of right heart lesions in pregnancy. In: Steer PJ, Gatzoulis MA (eds), *Heart Disease and Pregnancy*, 2nd edn, pp. 131–43. Cambridge: Cambridge University Press; 2016.
36. Gelson E, Gatzoulis M, Steer PJ, Lupton M, Johnson M. Tetralogy of Fallot: maternal and neonatal outcomes. *BJOG* 2008;**115**:398–402.
37. Curry RA, Fletcher C, Gelson E, et al. Pulmonary hypertension and pregnancy – a review of 12 pregnancies in nine women. *BJOG* 2012;**119**:752–61.
38. Kiely DG, Elliot CA, Sabroe I, Condliffe R. Pulmonary hypertension: diagnosis and management. *BMJ* 2013;**346**:f2028.
39. Enriquez AD, Economy KE, Tedrow UB. Contemporary management of arrhythmias during pregnancy. *Circ Arrhythm Electrophysiol* 2014;**7**:961–67.
40. Basude S, Hein C, Curtis SL, Clark A, Trinder J. Low-molecular-weight heparin or warfarin for anticoagulation in pregnant women with mechanical heart valves: what are the risks? A retrospective observational study. *BJOG* 2012;**119**:1008–13.

41. van Hagen IM, Roos-Hesselink JW, Ruys TP, et al. Pregnancy in women with a mechanical heart valve: data of the European Society of Cardiology Registry of Pregnancy and Cardiac Disease (ROPAC). *Circulation* 2015;**132**:132–42.

42. Suri V, Keepanasseril A, Aggarwal N, et al. Mechanical valve prosthesis and anticoagulation regimens in pregnancy: a tertiary centre experience. *Eur J Obstet Gynecol Reprod Biol* 2011;**159**:320–23.

43. National Institute for Health and Care Excellence (NICE). *Prophylaxis Against Infective Endocarditis: Antimicrobial Prophylaxis Against Infective Endocarditis in Adults and Children Undergoing Interventional Procedures.* Clinical guideline [CG64], updated 2016. London: NICE; 2008. Available at: https://www.nice.org.uk/guidance/cg64/chapter/Recommendations.

44. Stokes T, Richey R, Wray D. Prophylaxis against infective endocarditis: summary of NICE guidance. *Heart* 2008;**94**:930–31.

45. Ruys TP, Roos-Hesselink JW, Pijuan-Domenech A, et al. Is a planned caesarean section in women with cardiac disease beneficial? *Heart* 2015;**101**:530–36.

46. Steer PJ, Modi N. Elective caesarean sections – risks to the infant. *Lancet* 2009;**374**:675–76.

47. Sartain JB, Barry JJ, Howat PW, McCormack DI, Bryant M. Intravenous oxytocin bolus of 2 units is superior to 5 units during elective Caesarean section. *Br J Anaesth* 2008;**101**:822–26.

48. Thomas JS, Koh SH, Cooper GM. Haemodynamic effects of oxytocin given as i.v. bolus or infusion on women undergoing Caesarean section. *Br J Anaesth* 2007;**98**:116–19.

49. Tsui BC, Stewart B, Fitzmaurice A, Williams R. Cardiac arrest and myocardial infarction induced by postpartum intravenous ergonovine administration. *Anesthesiology* 2001;**94**:363–64.

50. World Health Organization. Medical Eligibility Criteria for Contraceptive Use, 5th edn. 2015. Available at: http://wwwwhoint/reproductivehealth/publications/family_planning/Ex-Summ-MEC-5/en/ (accessed 15 November 2015).

51. de Bastos M, Stegeman BH, Rosendaal FR, et al. Combined oral contraceptives: venous thrombosis. *Cochrane Database Syst Rev* 2014;**3**:CD010813.

13

Diabetes in pregnancy

Michael Permezel and Alexis Shub

Introduction

The importance of diabetes in pregnancy arises through two unre lated phenomena: an increased predisposition to impaired glucose tolerance in late pregnancy and an adverse impact of the increased glucose on important obstetric outcomes.

There are marked differences in clinical outcomes and management between pregnancies in which a clinically significant impairment of glucose tolerance was first noticed during pregnancy ('gestational diabetes mellitus' (GDM)) and those where type 1 or type 2 diabetes mellitus had been known prior to pregnancy ('prepregnancy diabetes'). These will be discussed separately in the following sections.

Gestational diabetes mellitus

Background

The incidence of GDM will vary according to the definition used (see 'Definition') and the population being studied but would usually be within the range 5–20%. The higher levels mostly are in centres using the International Association of Diabetes and Pregnancy Study Groups (IADPSG) criteria with an ethnically predisposed population.

What impairs glucose tolerance in pregnancy?

The hormonal environment in pregnancy impairs glucose tolerance. In a predisposed patient, the insulin secretion will not be able to keep up with insulin demand and the plasma glucose concentration will rise—hence the condition of GDM.

The principal hormone responsible is probably human placental lactogen which is structurally analogous to human growth hormone and carries the same property of impairing glucose tolerance. The increased levels of progesterone and corticosteroid may also contribute to hyperglycaemia in pregnancy. Given that all these hormones do not reach high levels until the latter half of pregnancy, GDM is most often a third-trimester condition and diagnosed by a glucose tolerance test at 24 28 weeks' gestation.

Why is there a clinical impact of raised plasma glucose in pregnancy?

Medical colleagues have sometimes thought it strange that obstetricians are concerned about lower levels of plasma glucose than would raise concern in the non-pregnant population. This comes about for two reasons. Firstly, the fetus appears particularly sensitive to increased plasma glucose levels in terms of the impact on fetal growth. The clinical consequences of excessive fetal size will be discussed in a later section. The second issue is that, like non-pregnant diabetes mellitus, the increased plasma glucose may lead to inadequate placental blood flow. This may create a critical mismatch of poor maternal placental perfusion but increased fetal demands on the placenta for oxygenation.

Definition

Historically, GDM has been defined as the diagnosis of clinically significant impaired glucose tolerance in pregnancy in a woman not previously known to be diabetic. This has recently been complicated by recognizing that some diabetes mellitus will present for the first time in pregnancy and lack of clarity as to where the lower threshold for diagnosis should best be placed.

Upper threshold for diagnosis

Where the impairment of glucose tolerance is severe such that the criteria for diagnosing diabetes mellitus outside pregnancy would be met, the condition is better termed 'diabetes mellitus in pregnancy' (rather than GDM). This would apply to a fasting level of at least 7.0 mmol/L or a 2-hour level of at least 11.1 mmol/L on a 75 g glucose tolerance test.

Lower threshold for diagnosis

It has proved difficult to set a lower threshold for diagnosis, given a remarkably linear relationship of glucose tolerance with such outcomes as birthweight, caesarean section rate, neonatal hypoglycaemia, and cord blood C-peptide levels (1). This is discussed in the following section.

Screening for GDM

Early pregnancy diagnosis

As alluded to previously, impaired glucose tolerance in the first half of pregnancy is unlikely to be the consequence of pregnancy but rather a pre-existing tendency to diabetes mellitus. There is remarkably little research that explores the consequences of minor impairments of glucose tolerance in early pregnancy. Most centres will undertake testing in early pregnancy only where there are significant predisposing factors (**Box 13.1**) and then treat if GDM criteria are met. Interestingly, the New Zealand health system has chosen to screen all women using glycated haemoglobin (HbA1c) in early pregnancy and treat if the HbA1c level is 6.5% or greater. This may reflect a high incidence of impaired glucose tolerance in the Polynesian population in that country.

Late second-trimester diagnosis

The IADPSG recommend the performance of a 75 g fasting glucose tolerance test on all women not previously diagnosed with diabetes at 24–28 weeks' gestation. Their criteria for diagnosis (Table 13.1) have been endorsed by the World Health Organization and numerous national organizations (2).

The introduction of the IADPSG criteria created significant controversy—largely in relation to the subsequent increase in incidence of GDM in most populations. The thresholds were set at the plasma glucose levels associated with a 1.75-fold increase in the risk of complications based on the Hyperglycemia and Adverse Pregnancy Outcome (HAPO) study (1). It is true that this threshold is somewhat arbitrary but more logical than having fasting and 2-hour thresholds at different levels of clinical risk as was the case with previous definitions.

Given that there is a linear correlation of glucose tolerance with measurable clinical outcomes, the benefits of treating GDM will be less with levels closer to the threshold values. At least one study (3) investigated as to whether there is any benefit to treating mild GDM. Although using different diagnostic criteria to those subsequently

suggested by the IADPSG, the study found that treating mild GDM resulted in reduced rates of macrosomia, shoulder dystocia, caesarean birth, and pre-eclampsia. A benefit in treating mild GDM therefore appears likely but the magnitude of that benefit and the cost-effectiveness of treating marginal GDM is uncertain. The issue is likely to be long debated as an effective randomized controlled trial of sufficient magnitude would not be feasible if it is recognized that even a small clinical benefit is likely to be of significance to most women (4). Additionally, such a study would not be the best use of limited research resources when so little is known about other aspects of GDM such as the impact of minor impairments of glucose tolerance through the second trimester of pregnancy.

Clinical consequences of GDM

The clinical consequences of GDM are listed in Box 13.2. Many are a direct impact of increased fetal and placental size which in turn correlates with blood glucose control as well as maternal body weight and pregnancy weight gain. Shoulder dystocia is particularly noteworthy as it occurs at a lower fetal weight than in the absence of diabetes—presumably due to the disproportionately large shoulders.

Most controversial is the increase in perinatal mortality. While an important feature in the early report of O'Sullivan et al. (5), some subsequent observational studies have not shown an increase in perinatal death. This may be explained by the current management of GDM: effecting birth in most centres at or prior to 40 weeks' gestation appears to result in an overall perinatal mortality no worse than the non-GDM population. This is at least in part attributable to avoiding perinatal deaths after 40 weeks that are relatively common in all pregnancies and avoided in the GDM group if birth is recommended before 40 weeks (6)

Antenatal management of GDM

Crowther et al. (7) in the Australian Carbohydrate Intolerance Study in Pregnant Women (ACHOIS) study established that treatment of GDM improved a composite perinatal outcome. Given that the rationale for therapy is in part due to that study, the therapeutic regimen used underpins the treatment protocols of many units today. In broad terms, antenatal management comprises maternal and fetal surveillance, diet and exercise, and insulin or an oral hypoglycaemic drug. Further important care includes the timing and mode of birth, intrapartum care, postnatal and neonatal care, and long-term follow-up.

Table 13.1 IADPSG threshold values for diagnosis of gestational diabetes mellitus or overt diabetes in pregnancy

	Glucose concentration (mmol/L)	Glucose concentration (mg/dL)
Gestational diabetes mellitus diagnosis[a]		
Fasting plasma glucose	5.1	92
1-hour plasma glucose	10.0	180
2-hour plasma glucose	8.5	153
Overt diabetes in pregnancy diagnosis[b]		
Fasting plasma glucose	7.0	126
Random plasma glucose	11.1	200

[a] One or more of these values from a 75 g oral glucose tolerance test must be equalled or exceeded for the diagnosis of GDM.

[b] One or more of these values must be equalled or exceeded for the diagnosis of overt diabetes in pregnancy. Also diagnosed if the HbA1c level is at least 6.5% (Diabetes Control and Complications Trial/United Kingdom Prospective Diabetes Study standardized).

Source data from IADPSG Consensus Panel, 2010.

Maternal and fetal surveillance

GDM is commonly managed in a multidisciplinary setting that incorporates expertise in both diabetes and maternity care. Home monitoring of blood glucose should be instigated that initially includes measurements of fasting blood glucose and 2-hour postprandial levels. The target levels for capillary blood glucose in the ACHOIS study were 5.5 mmol/L and 7.0 mmol/L respectively. If all glucose measurements were in the target range over a 2-week period, home monitoring could be reduced to once per day—varying the time of sampling between fasting and the three postprandial measurements.

All pregnant women should receive specific instructions with respect to reporting unsatisfactory fetal movements. There is no general consensus as to whether routine ultrasonography is indicated in a pregnancy complicated by GDM. The threshold for ultrasonography should be low whenever there is a clinical suspicion of poor fetal growth or maternal obesity makes clinical estimation of fetal growth less reliable. Ultrasound estimation of fetal weight is notoriously inaccurate in the macrosomic fetus but should be performed at approximately 35 weeks' gestation where there is a clinical suspicion of macrosomia.

Diet and exercise

Advice regarding diet and exercise is key to the control of blood sugar levels in GDM, with less than 20% of women requiring insulin or metformin. Dietary advice should focus on the replacement of rapidly absorbed sucrose (high glycaemic index foods) with foods that produce a slower rise in blood glucose (low glycaemic index foods) particularly fruit and vegetables. Total calories should be adjusted to achieve the desired weight gain in pregnancy. The Institute of Medicine recommendations are listed in **Table 13.2** but in the presence of morbid obesity (body mass index $\geq$40 kg/m²), no weight gain or even weight loss may be recommended. Regular exercise also is important in the control of blood sugar but should be limited to mild to moderate levels of exertion only. A common recommendation is a 30-minute walk during the day or after the evening meal.

Medications to control hyperglycaemia

When diet and exercise are unable to maintain satisfactory glucose levels, medical therapy should be initiated. There are many thresholds used but the ACHOIS study recommended that insulin be initiated if there were more than two capillary blood glucose measurements above target (fasting 5.5 mmol/L; 2-hour postprandial 7.0 mmol/L) in a week of testing. In the study by Landon et al. (3), insulin was prescribed if the majority of fasting values or postprandial values

Table 13.2 Institute of Medicine recommendations for total and average rate of weight gain during pregnancy

Pre-pregnancy body mass index (kg/m²)	Total weight gain range (kg)
Underweight (<18.5)	12.5–18
Healthy weight (18.5–24.9)	11.5–16
Overweight (25.0–29.9)	7–11.5
Obese ($\geq$30.0)	5–9

Source data from Institute of Medicine recommendations.

between study visits were elevated (fasting glucose level $\geq$5.3 mmol/L or 2-hour $\geq$6.7 mmol/L).

Considerable research has now investigated the relative benefits of metformin and insulin as first-line treatments when diet and exercise prove insufficient to control glucose levels. In the most important study (8), there was no apparent superiority of insulin over metformin and the latter appeared to be associated with a notable reduction in gestational hypertension. Although some centres continue to prefer insulin as first-line treatment, the United Kingdom National Institute for Health and Care Excellence (NICE) (9) now recommends metformin as first-line treatment. Metformin is unlikely to be adequate where there is more severe impairment of glucose tolerance (e.g. fasting blood glucose $\geq$7.0 mmol/L) and insulin should be the first-line treatment in this circumstance.

Where insulin is used, a once-daily long-acting insulin (e.g. Protaphane) will often be adequate initially but as insulin requirements rise, better control may be achieved by supplementing the long-acting insulin with boluses of short-acting (soluble) insulin before meals.

Timing and mode of birth in GDM

Perinatal morbidity and mortality increase with advancing gestation beyond 38 weeks in all pregnancies and to a marginally greater degree in the presence of GDM (6). The gestation at which induction of labour becomes recommended varies widely. Most units will recommend birth for GDM pregnancies between 38 and 40 weeks' gestation; earlier in that range in the presence of macrosomia, poor glucose control, or high doses of insulin and closer to 40 weeks if these are not present. The NICE guideline (9) allows pregnancies in GDM to progress up to 40 weeks and 6 days. The added mortality and morbidity of that extra week will be low but probably not justifiable given the low tolerance that most women have for even small risks to their offspring (4).

The mode of birth is not commonly affected by GDM. If there are no contraindications to vaginal birth, induction of labour is appropriate if the predetermined 'maximum gestation' is reached before the onset of spontaneous labour. As for prepregnancy diabetes, with extremes of fetal macrosomia (e.g. birthweight anticipated $\geq$4500 g), consideration may be given to recommending caesarean section in place of induction.

Intrapartum care

This will mostly not differ greatly from intrapartum care of all women. Where the woman has been on significant doses of insulin, a plan for glucose surveillance and insulin according to tests should be made antenatally. Continuous electronic fetal surveillance is not mandated by most units in the presence of GDM but should be used in the presence of macrosomia as further hypoxia may be anticipated at the time of birth if manipulations prove necessary for the management of shoulder dystocia.

The woman should birth in a position where shoulder dystocia can be effectively managed should it occur and in the presence of an obstetrician with experience in management of shoulder dystocia.

Postnatal and neonatal care

Insulin is rarely required postpartum in the woman with GDM. Removal of the diabetogenic hormones following delivery of the placenta, leads to the return of normal glucose tolerance in the early puerperium. The neonate is at risk of hypoglycaemia and should have glucose levels monitored until satisfactory. Neonatal respiratory distress is also more common and neonatal respiratory observations are indicated.

Long-term follow-up

Women who have had GDM are at increased risk of future type 2 diabetes mellitus. A glucose tolerance test is performed at approximately 6 weeks postpartum to determine whether this is already present. Tests should then be performed at least every 2 years for the early detection of type 2 diabetes. Life-table studies indicated that the prevalence post GDM is approximately 17% at 10 years and 25% at 15 years (10).

Prepregnancy diabetes mellitus

Background

Before the advent of insulin, women with type 1 diabetes had almost no chance of having a live baby. However, with contemporary high-quality, intensive, multidisciplinary care, outcomes are usually very good. The complications of diabetes are thought to arise from underlying micro- and macrovascular disease and the effects of glucose on the fetus as discussed in the following sections. Type 1 diabetes is present in approximately 0.2% of pregnant women, and the numbers are largely stable. In contrast, type 2 diabetes was once uncommon in pregnancy but is now also as high as 0.2%. This is likely to continue to increase as increased numbers of overweight and obese women enter the reproductive years. Prepregnancy diabetes provides the model of how pregnancy and maternal disease impact each other, and how good preconception, antenatal, and intrapartum care can make an enormous difference for these women and their babies.

Clinical consequences of type 1 and type 2 diabetes in pregnancy

Impact of pregnancy on diabetes

The same hormonal changes referred to in the earlier sections on GDM also further impair glucose tolerance in prepregnancy diabetes. Other factors also may conspire to impair control of blood glucose including changes in dietary intake (e.g. a pregnancy affected by vomiting in early pregnancy) and changes in physical activity. Poor glucose control during pregnancy may accelerate diabetic medical complications including nephropathy or retinopathy. For a small number of women, there may be a permanent deterioration in renal function or eyesight.

Impact of diabetes on pregnancy

Women with prepregnancy diabetes are at increased risk of obstetric complications including miscarriage, preterm birth, pre-eclampsia, shoulder dystocia, caesarean section, instrumental birth, and perineal trauma. The neonate is at increased risk of congenital anomalies, macrosomia (**Figure 13.1**), growth restriction, birth trauma, neonatal respiratory distress, and hypoglycaemia. Higher rates of perinatal mortality may relate to congenital anomalies, fetal growth restriction, and birth trauma but approximately half of stillbirths in diabetic pregnancies are unexplained.

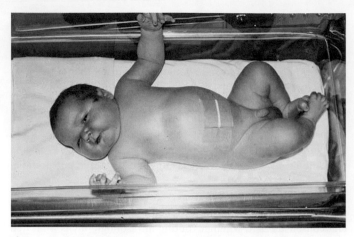

Figure 13.1 The 6700 g infant of a diabetic mother delivered by caesarean section after a failed attempt at forceps delivery.

Management of type 1 or 2 diabetes at the prepregnancy visit

Prepregnancy management for women with underlying diabetes provides a very important chance to change the outcome for the women and her baby. At a preconception visit, all the usual aspects of prepregnancy care (see Chapter 6) should be discussed, but in addition, special attention should be paid to a number of specific issues.

Assessment

Diabetes assessment

The therapeutic regimen for the diabetes should be assessed along with the glucose control being achieved. The incidences of both miscarriage and congenital abnormalities are directly related to diabetic control in the periconceptual period. The HbA1c level is an accepted marker of glucose control and women should aim for an HbA1c level less than 6.5%. Where the HbA1c level is greater than 10%, the woman should be advised to delay pregnancy until improved control is achieved (11).

The prepregnancy visit is also an opportunity to assess and stabilize complications of diabetes including nephropathy and retinopathy. Renal function should be evaluated with a serum creatinine and urinary albumin:creatinine ratio. Retinopathy should be assessed by an ophthalmologist.

Assessment of comorbidities

Type 1 diabetes may be associated with other autoimmune disorders including thyroid disease and coeliac disease.

Common comorbidities in type 2 diabetes include obesity and hypertension. Weight loss prior to pregnancy may enable some women to return to normal glucose tolerance. Bariatric surgery may be appropriate for some markedly obese diabetic women, but pregnancy should be delayed until the weight loss has stabilized after surgery. Smoking is of particular concern in women with diabetes, and a planned pregnancy may provide motivation to quit.

Treatment

Optimizing control of blood glucose

Oral hypoglycaemic agents will be changed to insulin in some centres, but in others, women will continue on metformin throughout pregnancy. Other oral hypoglycaemic agents are usually not recommended in pregnancy.

For those with relatively poor control, obtaining good blood glucose control may take a number of months. For some women, this will involve changing the insulin regimen to a more intensive method with insulin administered three or four times daily. For women with type 1 diabetes, an insulin pump may provide better control, but this has not been shown to unequivocally improve obstetric outcomes.

Folic acid—5 mg daily

Women with diabetes are at increased risk of having a baby with a neural tube defect, (anencephaly or spina bifida), and should take 5 mg of folate from 1 month prior to conception until 3 months of gestation to reduce this risk. This is in contrast to the usual 0.5 mg of folate recommended for other women.

Other medications

Many women with diabetes will be on angiotensin-converting enzyme (ACE) inhibitors, statins, diuretics, or oral hypoglycaemic agents. These should be changed to safer alternatives, in the preconception period if possible, or as soon as pregnancy is confirmed. Statins can usually be ceased. ACE inhibitors should be ceased. If an antihypertensive is required, control should be achieved with those documented to be safe in pregnancy such as methyldopa or labetalol.

Advice regarding a pregnancy with diabetes

The woman and her family should be informed of what to expect during pregnancy and possible outcomes. They should be made aware of the increased numbers of antenatal visits and the need for strict adherence to glucose control. They should also be informed of the increased rates of congenital abnormality, miscarriage, pre-eclampsia, preterm birth, and obstetric intervention and that these risks will relate to the degree of diabetic control.

Most women can be reassured that they are likely to successfully navigate pregnancy without long-term harm to their own health or that of their child. For the small number of women with significant renal impairment from diabetic nephropathy, pregnancy may cause a permanent deterioration in renal function—even to the extent of requiring renal dialysis. Decisions around whether or not to counsel against pregnancy should be undertaken with a multidisciplinary team.

First antenatal visit

Antenatal care should start as early in pregnancy as possible, especially if preconception care has not taken place. All of the aspects discussed earlier in prepregnancy care should be addressed again at the first antenatal visit.

Accurate dating is very important because of the risks of preterm delivery and the need for timed delivery. An ultrasound scan should be performed in the first trimester for accurate estimation of gestational age, and an agreed due date calculated and documented.

Congenital anomalies, especially cardiac abnormalities and neural tube defects, are increased, and the risk is proportional to the degree of maternal glycaemic control in the periconceptual period. Ultrasound assessment of fetal anatomy should be performed by an experienced sonographer at 20–22 weeks' gestation. An additional ultrasound assessment for structural abnormalities may also be performed at 12–16 weeks' gestation in those women who would consider termination of pregnancy in the presence of a serious congenital anomaly.

Women with diabetes, especially those with underlying hypertension or obesity, are at an increased risk of pre-eclampsia. This risk can be reduced by commencing 150 mg daily of aspirin and 1200 mg of calcium supplementation before 16 weeks of pregnancy.

Subsequent antenatal care

Care should be with a multidisciplinary team where possible, including an obstetrician, endocrinologist, diabetes educator, dietician, neonatologist, and midwife. Antenatal visits occur at increased frequency to enable increased maternal and fetal surveillance and careful management of the diabetes in the presence of changing glucose tolerance as the pregnancy advances and hormonal milieu changes.

Fetal surveillance

All women should pay attention to fetal movements and present for review early if there are any concerns that fetal movements have decreased. As women with diabetes are at increased risk of fetal loss, additional fetal surveillance is indicated in the third trimester. A common surveillance regimen includes ultrasound for fetal growth, amniotic fluid, and umbilical artery Doppler at 28, 32, and 36 weeks' gestation. These 4-weekly fetal growth assessments may be supplement with weekly cardiotocography and ultrasound for amniotic fluid and fetal Dopplers from 34 weeks.

Diabetes management

Women with type 1 diabetes will have increased difficulty with blood sugar control in early pregnancy if there is significant nausea or vomiting. Extra care must be taken to avoid hypoglycaemia or ketoacidosis in these situations. In this circumstance, glucose targets may need to be revised and multiple admissions to hospital may prove necessary.

For the reasons specified earlier, insulin requirements will increase during pregnancy. Home blood glucose monitoring should be performed multiple times each day, but the preferred regimen varies in different units. A suggested testing plan is a morning fasting level, and either 1 or 2 hours after each meal. Some women may require more frequent testing, including overnight. A period of continuous glucose monitoring can be helpful if glucose control has been very difficult. Blood glucose targets vary but, as a guide, women should aim for fasting levels of 5.3 mmol/L, and either 1 hour of 7.8 mmol/L or 2 hours of 6.4 mmol/L. Regular HbA1c assessment during the pregnancy will help women and clinicians assess control of blood glucose.

Exercise should be encouraged in most women with diabetes as it improves glucose control, weight management, and feelings of well-being. Daily walking is generally recommended. Women with type 1 diabetes undertaking more strenuous exercise should monitor blood glucose more often while exercising to exclude hypoglycaemia.

Dietary management is very similar to women with gestational diabetes, but many women will benefit from additional individualized advice from a dietitian with experience in diabetes and pregnancy.

Assessment of retinopathy should be performed in early pregnancy and repeated later in pregnancy. Treatment of diabetic eye disease can be undertaken safely in pregnancy.

As women with diabetes are at increased risk of pre-eclampsia, frequent antenatal visits with measurement of blood pressure and urinalysis contribute to earlier detection of pre-eclampsia. Women with underlying hypertension and proteinuria are at particularly high risk of developing pre-eclampsia but diagnosis is more difficult. Aspirin commenced in early pregnancy with a view to preventing pre-eclampsia is commonly ceased at 36 weeks' gestation.

Pregnancy in women with diabetes can be very stressful because of the increased focus on risks and the increased workload for the woman in terms of visits and careful control of diabetes. Support and education for the woman and her family may help manage these extra stressors.

Timing and mode of birth

As the gestation advances toward and beyond the due date, the fetus of the woman with diabetes is at increased risk of fetal death *in utero* and birth trauma. To minimize these risks, birth is usually recommended at 37–38 weeks' gestation in an otherwise uncomplicated diabetic pregnancy.

For many women with pregnancy diabetes, a vaginal delivery can be recommended, subject to the same contraindications as for other women. However, macrosomia is a common complication of diabetes and shoulder dystocia is more likely than with an infant of the infant of a non-diabetic woman with the same birth weight. If the fetus is estimated to weigh more than 4500 g at the time of planned delivery, a caesarean section is usually recommended.

If an elective caesarean section is planned, antenatal corticosteroids may be recommended in the days prior birth to reduce the rate of respiratory distress syndrome in the newborn. Corticosteroids in women with diabetes will result in an increase in blood sugar levels, and this will often require a short-term increase in insulin.

The overall primary caesarean section rate is increased in women with prepregnancy diabetes due to macrosomia and increased rates of fetal compromise in labour. For the woman with a prior caesarean section, vaginal birth rates are low because of the need for timed delivery and a reluctance to induce labour in a diabetic woman with a uterine scar.

Intrapartum care

Delivery should take place in a hospital equipped to manage intrapartum and neonatal complications.

A plan should be made with the woman prior to labour with respect to insulin. Blood glucose levels should be measured every hour during labour. For women with type 2 diabetes, long-acting insulin should be stopped or reduced and short-acting insulin administered as needed according to test results. Women with type 1 diabetes will usually require an insulin and dextrose infusion to maintain stable blood glucose. Women having an elective caesarean section should be first on the elective list in the morning to better manage fasting, and there should be a staff member present at the time of delivery responsible for neonatal resuscitation.

Continuous electronic fetal monitoring should be used during labour because the fetus is at increased risk of intrapartum hypoxia. An experienced obstetrician should be present for delivery, and preparations made in anticipation of shoulder dystocia.

Postpartum care

In the first 24 hours after birth, insulin demand is usually low. Insulin requirements then usually return rapidly to prepregnancy levels. As lactation is established, further modification of the insulin regimen will be required. Tight control of diabetes may be difficult in the postpartum period as the woman adjusts to the needs of the baby and the changes in her own sleeping and food patterns.

Breastfeeding should be encouraged in women with diabetes, both to manage neonatal hypoglycaemia, and because breastfeeding may have a role in reducing the long-term risks to the baby of obesity and cardiovascular disease. In the past, infants of diabetic mothers were often routinely separated from their mothers and cared for in a neonatal special care or intensive care setting. The common consequence was increased difficulty in establishing breastfeeding.

Many women with diabetes choose to limit family size. All pregnancies in women with diabetes should be planned, so discussion and provision of postpartum contraception is very important. All of the available contraceptive options are acceptable for women with diabetes, limited only by the avoidance of oestrogen-based contraception in women who are breastfeeding, as for all other women.

Neonates

Babies of women with diabetes have increased rates of hypoglycaemia, hyperbilirubinaemia, and respiratory distress syndrome. Less commonly, they may have clinical or imaging/laboratory evidence of cardiomyopathy, polycythaemia, hypocalcaemia, or hypomagnesaemia. The impact of diabetes on the baby is explained by the 'Pederson' hypothesis. High levels of glucose cross the placenta and result in high blood glucose in the fetus. The fetus responds appropriately by increasing insulin and insulin-like growth factor (IGF) secretion. The IGF encourages fetal growth, and the high levels of insulin are maintained in the first days of life, resulting in neonatal hypoglycaemia.

The baby of a woman with diabetes should not be routinely separated from the mother, but will need regular measurements of blood glucose during the first few hours of life and additional observation for signs of clinical hypoglycaemia. Early feeding is recommended. The baby should have careful clinical examination for congenital abnormalities.

REFERENCES

1. HAPO Study Cooperative Research Group, Metzger BE, Lowe LP, et al. Hyperglycemia and adverse pregnancy outcomes. *N Engl J Med* 2008;**358**:1991–2002.
2. International Association of Diabetes and Pregnancy Study Groups Consensus Panel, Metzger BE, Gabbe SG, et al. International association of diabetes and pregnancy study groups recommendations on the diagnosis and classification of hyperglycemia in pregnancy. *Diabetes Care* 2010;**33**:676–82.
3. Landon MB, Spong CY, Thom E, et al. A multicenter, randomized trial of treatment for mild gestational diabetes. *N Engl J Med* 2009;**361**:1339–48.

4. Walker SP, McCarthy EA, Ugoni A, Lee A, Lim S, Permezel M. Cesarean delivery or vaginal birth: a survey of patient and clinician thresholds. *Obstet Gynecol* 2007;**109**:67–72.

5. O'Sullivan JB, Gellis SS, Dandrow RV, Tenney BO. The potential diabetic and her treatment in pregnancy. *Obstet Gynecol* 1966;**27**:683–89.

6. Rosenstein MG, Cheng YW, Snowden JM, Nicholson JM, Doss AE, Caughey AB. The risk of stillbirth and infant death stratified by gestational age in women with gestational diabetes. *Am J Obstet Gynecol* 2012;**206**:309.e1–7.

7. Crowther CA, Hiller JE, Moss JR, et al. Effect of treatment of gestational diabetes mellitus on pregnancy outcomes. *N Engl J Med* 2005;**352**:2477–86.

8. Rowan JA, Hague WM, Gao W, et al. Metformin versus insulin for the treatment of gestational diabetes. *N Engl J Med* 2008;**358**:2003–2015

9. National Institute for Health and Care Excellence (NICE). *Diabetes in Pregnancy: Management from Preconception to the Postnatal Period*. NICE guideline [NG3]. London: NICE; 2015.

10. Lee AJ, Hiscock RJ, Wein P, Walker SP, Permezel M. Gestational diabetes mellitus: clinical predictors and long-term risk of developing type 2 diabetes: a retrospective cohort study using survival analysis. *Diabetes Care* 2007;**30**:878–83.

11. Jensen DM, Korsholm L, Ovesen P, et al. Peri-conceptional A1C and risk of serious adverse pregnancy outcome in 933 women with type 1 diabetes. *Diabetes Care* 2009;**32**:1046–8.

14

Renal disease in pregnancy

David Williams

Physiological changes to the kidney during healthy pregnancy

Renal glomerular function during pregnancy

Renal adaptation to pregnancy is anticipated during the luteal phase of each menstrual cycle. Renal blood flow and glomerular filtration rate (GFR) increase by 10–20% before menstruation (1). If pregnancy is established, the corpus luteum persists and these haemodynamic changes continue (2). By 16 weeks' gestation, GFR is 55% above non-pregnant levels (2). This increment is mediated through an increase in renal blood flow that reaches a maximum of 70–80% above non-pregnant levels by the second trimester and then falls to around 45% above non-pregnant levels at term (3).

The changes to renal physiology in healthy pregnancy can both hide and mimic renal disease. The gestational increase in GFR leads to a fall in serum creatinine (SCr) concentration, so that values considered normal in the non-pregnant state may be abnormal during pregnancy (Table 14.1). Serum creatinine is not, however, linearly correlated with creatinine clearance and is influenced by muscle mass, physical exercise, racial differences, and diet.

The gestational rise in renal blood flow also causes the kidneys to swell so that bipolar renal length increases by approximately 1 cm (Figure 14.1). During the third trimester renal blood flow falls, leading to a decrease in creatinine clearance and an increase in serum creatinine (1). Serum urea levels, however, continue to fall in the third trimester due to reduced maternal hepatic urea synthesis.

The renal pelvis and ureters dilate and appear obstructed to those unaware of these changes. The right renal pelvis dilates by up to 0.5 mm each week from 6 to 32 weeks, reaching a maximum diameter of 2 cm (90th centile) until term (4). The left renal pelvis reaches a maximum diameter of 8 mm (90th centile) at 20 weeks' gestation (4).

Other physiological changes simulate the classic features of nephrotic syndrome. For example, in healthy pregnancy, proteinuria increases as pregnancy progresses. However, a random urinary protein (mg):creatinine (mmol) ratio (PCR) should not normally exceed 0.20 mg/mmol (95th centile), while a PCR greater than 0.27 mg/mmol is a good predictor of significant proteinuria (5). In healthy pregnancy, the serum albumin level falls by 5–10 g/L, serum cholesterol and triglyceride concentrations increase markedly (Table 14.1), and towards term, dependent oedema affects most pregnancies.

Renal tubular function during healthy pregnancy

Increased alveolar ventilation causes respiratory alkalosis to which the kidney responds by increased bicarbonaturia and a compensatory metabolic acidosis. The result is that maternal pH remains stable at 7.4. Reduced tubular glucose reabsorption leads to glycosuria in approximately 10% of pregnant women, even when maternal blood glucose levels are normal. During the first trimester urinary urate excretion increases, but then decreases towards term so that plasma urate rises again to non-pregnancy levels.

A healthy pregnant mother gains a total of 6–8 kg of fluid, of which approximately 1.2 L is intravascular plasma. Plasma osmolality falls by 10 mOsmol/kg by 5–8 weeks' gestation due to a decrease in both the threshold for thirst and for the release of antidiuretic hormone (vasopressin) (6). During pregnancy, vasopressin is degraded by placental vasopressinase, such that the maternal posterior pituitary produces four times as much vasopressin to maintain physiological concentrations at term. Failure of the maternal pituitary to keep up with the increased metabolic clearance of vasopressin leads to a transient polyuric state in the third trimester, which is known as transient diabetes insipidus of pregnancy (7). This condition can be controlled with desmopressin and cured by childbirth.

Renal endocrine function during pregnancy

The kidney also acts as an end1ocrine organ, producing three hormones, namely erythropoietin, active vitamin D, and renin. The production of all three hormones increases during healthy pregnancy but their effects are masked by other changes. In early pregnancy, peripheral vasodilatation exceeds renin–aldosterone-mediated plasma volume expansion, so diastolic blood pressure decreases by 12 weeks. Conversely, plasma volume expansion exceeds the erythropoietin-mediated increase in red cell mass, causing a 'physiological anaemia', which should not normally lead to a haemoglobin concentration of less than 95 g/L (8). Similarly, extra active-vitamin D produced by the placenta circulates at twice non-gravid levels, but concomitant halving of parathyroid hormone levels, hypercalciuria, and increased fetal requirements keep plasma ionized calcium levels unchanged (9).

Table 14.1 Physiological changes to common indices of renal function during healthy pregnancy (mean ± SD)

	Non-pregnant	First trimester	Second trimester	Third trimester
Effective renal plasma flow (mL/min)	480 ± 72	841 ± 144	891 ± 279	771 ± 175
GFR (mL/min) inulin clearance	105 ± 24	162 ± 19	174 ± 24	165 ± 22
GFR (mL/min) 24-hour creatinine clearance	98 ± 8	151 ± 11	154 ± 15	129 ± 10
Serum creatinine (mmol/L)	73 ± 10	60 ± 8	54 ± 10	64 ± 9
Plasma urea (mmol/L)	4.3 ± 0.8	3.5 ± 0.7	3.3 ± 0.8	3.1 ± 0.7
Plasma urate (mmol/L)	246 ± 59	189 ± 48	214 ± 71	269 ± 56
Plasma osmolality (mOsmol/kg)	290 ± 2.2	280 ± 3.4	279 ± 2.9	279 ± 5.0
Fast. cholesterol (mmol/L)	5.0 ± 0.3	5.5 ± 0.4	6.9 ± 0.4	7.8 ± 0.4

Acute kidney injury in pregnancy

Acute kidney injury (AKI) has replaced the term acute renal failure, as kidneys can be injured before function fails. The common causes of AKI are outlined in **Box 14.1**. AKI is rare in early pregnancy. When it does occur, it is usually associated with septic abortion, a complication largely confined to low-resource nations or those without legalized abortion services. Rarely, severe hyperemesis gravidarum can cause dehydration and prerenal AKI. AKI at the time of childbirth is most commonly caused by gestational syndromes such as pre-eclampsia and abruption placentae (**Box 14.1**).

Pregnancy is a prothrombotic state, associated with changes to the vascular endothelium and clotting factors that predispose pregnant women to acute glomerular capillary thrombosis. Whereas non-pregnant patients who suffer an acute prerenal insult (e.g. haemorrhage, dehydration, or septic shock) may develop AKI if inadequately treated, the same prerenal insult in pregnancy is more likely to develop into renal cortical necrosis with permanent renal impairment.

The principles of AKI management are aimed at identification and correction of the precipitating cause (summarized in **Table 14.2**). While definitive management to treat the cause of AKI is carried out, the patient should be supported with optimal fluid resuscitation guided by fluid balance monitoring. If oliguria persists despite euvolaemia, with deteriorating renal function or fluid overload, then fluid restriction followed by renal replacement therapy should be considered. The indications for acute renal replacement therapy (dialysis) in pregnancy include hyperkalaemia (potassium >7.0 mmol/L) refractory to medical treatment, pulmonary oedema refractory to diuretics, acidosis producing circulatory problems, and uraemia. There is no absolute level of uraemia above which dialysis is mandatory for new-onset AKI, but a serum urea over 25–30 mmol/L or SCr greater than 500–700 mmol/L (5.65–7.91 mg/dL), usually indicates a need for dialysis.

Pre-eclampsia and the kidney

Women with pre-existing renal disease are more vulnerable to pre-eclampsia, especially with associated chronic hypertension (10, 11). Pregnant women with moderate to severe renal disease (chronic

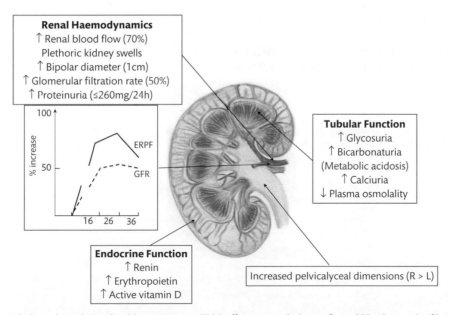

Figure 14.1 Changes to renal physiology during healthy pregnancy. ERPF, effective renal plasma flow; GFR, glomerular filtration rate.
Reproduced from Williams D and Davison JM. Chronic Kidney Disease in Pregnancy. *BMJ* 2008; 336: 211–215 with permission from BMJ Publishing Group Ltd.

Box 14.1 Causes of acute kidney injury in pregnancy

Prerenal

- Volume depletion: hyperemesis gravidarum, peripartum haemorrhage, diabetes insipidus
- Oedematous states: nephrotic syndrome, peripartum cardiomyopathy
- Hypotension: sepsis, peripartum cardiomyopathy, amniotic fluid embolus
- Renal hypoperfusion: drugs (e.g. NSAIDS)
- Renovascular disease: renal artery stenosis, more commonly congenital in young women

Intrinsic renal disease

- Pre-eclampsia: glomerular endotheliosis
- Microangiopathic haemolytic anaemia (MAHA) (e.g. HUS, TTP)
- Acute fatty liver of pregnancy (AFLP)
- Acute-on-chronic kidney disease (e.g. flare of lupus nephritis)
- Vasculitis (e.g. granulomatosis with polyangiitis, formerly Wegener's granulomatosis)

Post-renal disease; obstructive

- Acute obstruction of renal tracts (e.g. calculi, papillary necrosis)
- Congenital urological anomalies (e.g. pelviureteric junction or vesico-ureteric junction obstruction, even if previously 'surgically corrected')

---

kidney disease (CKD) stages 2–5) should be offered low-dose aspirin (50–150 mg/each evening from 12 weeks' gestation) to reduce their risk of pre-eclampsia and perinatal death (12).

Suspected proteinuria on urinary dipstick testing (≥1+ proteinuria) should be assessed with a spot urinary PCR, rather than a 24-hour urine collection (13, 14). New-onset proteinuria (PCR >30 mg/mmol) in conjunction with new-onset hypertension is sufficient to make a diagnosis of pre-eclampsia (14). However, the level of proteinuria is a poor predictor of maternal and neonatal complications and taken in isolation should not be used as an indication for premature delivery. Pregnant women who develop proteinuria (PCR >100–300 mg/mmol; the threshold depends upon other maternal risk factors for thrombosis) should be offered thromboprophylaxis with low-molecular-weight heparin until at least 4 weeks postpartum and fully mobile.

Pre-eclampsia itself is often associated with mild AKI (SCr up to 125 μmol/L; 1.41 mg/dL) and complete postpartum recovery of

renal function is usual. Only if pre-eclampsia is associated with another renal insult such as peripartum haemorrhage, will AKI be severe enough to require transient renal replacement therapy.

Postpartum, only 2–5% of women who had pre-eclampsia are found to have underlying renal disease (15). Women who have had pre-eclampsia should nevertheless be checked for persistent postpartum hypertension and proteinuria. Gestational hypertension usually resolves within 3 months of delivery, but severe pre-eclampsia-induced hypertension and heavy proteinuria can take up to 24 months to disappear (16). Persistent microalbuminuria is suggestive of underlying renal disease and may also herald a predisposition to future cardiovascular disease (17).

The diagnosis of pre-eclampsia is difficult if there is chronic hypertension and pre-existing proteinuria, especially as these two parameters become more marked in late pregnancy. Furthermore, hyperuricaemia and fetal growth restriction are common features of both pre-eclampsia and chronic renal impairment, but new-onset hepatic transaminitis and thrombocytopenia support a diagnosis of pre-eclampsia (18).

Pre-eclampsia and AKI: clinical management of renal impairment and fluid balance

The cure for pre-eclampsia is delivery of the fetus, but the maternal condition can transiently deteriorate postpartum (19). A rise in maternal SCr concentration from around 70 μmol/L (0.79 mg/dL) to greater than 120 μmol/L (1.36 mg/dL) would be an indication for delivery to prevent irreparable renal impairment. Dialysis is very rarely necessary, but is most common in women who double their SCr in the first 24–48 hours after birth (20).

Fluid balance is critical to the successful management of AKI during pregnancy. Too little intravascular fluid provokes prerenal failure, especially damaging to chronically impaired kidneys, while too much fluid risks pulmonary oedema, adult respiratory distress syndrome, and maternal death. Furthermore, transient oliguria (<100 mL/4 hours) is common in the first 24 hours after normal childbirth. If a pre-eclamptic woman is not obviously hypovolaemic and has a serum urea less than 5 mmol/L and SCr not higher than 90 μmol/L, repeated fluid challenges to increase urine output are unnecessary and will only increase the maternal risk of pulmonary oedema.

Table 14.2 Targeted management of acute kidney injury according to precipitating complications commonly associated with pregnancy

AKI with presenting complication	Identify cause of presenting complication	Targeted treatment of presenting complication
Sepsis	Pyelonephritis or abortion or intra-partum sepsis or abscess	Antibiotics/surgical drainage
Intravascular volume depletion	Hyperemesis or ovarian hyper-stimulation syndrome or nephrotic syndrome	Rehydration/antiemetic/steroids. Give thromboprophylaxis
Haemorrhage	Placental abruption or atonic uterus or coagulopathy with amniotic fluid embolus	Resuscitation with blood and clotting factors/surgery
Microangiopathic haemolytic anaemia (MAHA)	Haemolytic uraemic syndrome (HUS) or thrombotic thrombocytopenic purpura (TTP)	HUS: eculizumab (anti-C5 antibody). TTP: plasmapheresis/steroids/low-dose aspirin
Lupus nephritis	Usually known systemic lupus erythematosus (SLE)	Immunosuppression guided by nephrologist
Urinary tract obstruction	Congenital renal tract anomaly/calculi/papillary necrosis from sickle cell disease	Identify and bypass obstruction usually with guidance from a urologist
Nephrotoxic drugs	Often, peripartum non-steroidal anti-inflammatory drugs (NSAIDs)	Stop prescription

Women with intrapartum AKI (approximate SCr >90 μmol/L; 1.0 mg/dL) should have their fluid balance guided by clinicians on a high dependency unit. The rate of fluid replacement should take account of an assessment of current volume status, assessed by jugular venous pressure, lung fields, oxygen saturations, skin turgor, hourly urine output, and estimated insensible loses. Once euvolaemic, the rate of intravenous fluid replacement should equal the previous hour's urine output plus insensible losses—usually 30–50 mL/hour if apyrexial and not bleeding. The amount of intravenous fluid replacement can be reduced once the mother can take oral fluid and her renal impairment starts to improve. Intravenous fluid regimens that stick to a fixed hourly replacement can lead to fluid overload in oliguric woman and to reduced intravascular volume in those having a diuresis. Fluid replacement should include blood to replace blood losses, then isotonic sodium chloride or compound sodium lactate (Hartmann's solution). Dextrose solutions are hypotonic and lead to maternal hyponatraemia (5% dextrose contains only 30 mmol/L NaCl, compared with 150 mmol/L NaCl in 0.9% sodium chloride solution). Low-dose 'renal' dopamine infusions should not be used.

If AKI progresses with oliguria and a rising SCr, despite adequate intravascular volume and blood pressure, then fluid intake should be restricted to avoid fluid overload. Under these circumstances, renal replacement therapy will eventually be necessary. This is a rare eventuality affecting less than 1:10,000 pregnancies. Women who have had a pregnancy affected by AKI are at increased risk of adverse outcome in a future pregnancy, even if they make a full recovery from the initial insult (21).

Thrombotic microangiopathies and pregnancy

Thrombotic microangiopathies (TMAs) are rare, life-threatening causes of AKI during pregnancy. They are characterized by platelet consumption within microvascular thrombi leading to thrombocytopenia, haemolysis, and multiorgan failure (22). TMAs can be triggered by several disease processes, but the final common pathway results in activated, proinflammatory, procoagulant endothelial cells (23). A careful medical history, elucidation of organ involvement, and correct interpretation of blood tests will identify the type of TMA, which is essential for successful management.

During pregnancy, the HELLP (haemolysis, elevated liver enzymes, low platelets) syndrome is the most frequently observed TMA. HELLP syndrome has overlapping features with preeclampsia, thrombotic thrombocytopenic purpura (TTP), and antiphospholipid syndrome. HELLP syndrome usually presents with acute hepatic pain and marked elevation of liver transaminases, suggestive of liver infarction (24). Although delivery is the cure for HELLP syndrome, the postpartum clinical condition can progress for several days before improvement. Hypertension, proteinuria, abnormal clotting, and fetal growth restriction are more evident in women with HELLP syndrome compared with other forms of TMA. In the absence of postpartum resolution, rarer forms of TMA should be considered, namely TTP, which most commonly affects the nervous system and haemolytic uraemic syndrome (HUS), which most commonly causes AKI. Pregnancy predisposes to both TTP and HUS.

Haemolytic uraemic syndrome

HUS is characterized by severe AKI with thrombocytopenia and haemolysis and usually presents in late pregnancy or peripartum.

Women with HUS typically have a much higher serum creatinine (creatinine>150 μmol/L) than is seen in pre-eclampsia/HELLP syndrome with marked thrombocytopenia (<50 × 10⁹/L) and haemolysis (Hb <90 g/L, low haptoglobin, raised lactate dehydrogenase and bilirubin, elevated reticulocytes, and red cell fragments on a blood film) (23). Women with HUS usually have a normal coagulation screen.

HUS can be caused by infection or coexisting diseases such as malignancy, solid-organ transplantation, drugs, and autoimmune disease (23). HUS associated with pregnancy has most in common with a genetic or acquired dysregulation of the alternative complement pathway, complement-mediated HUS also known as atypical-HUS (aHUS) (22, 23). If a pregnant woman presents with features of HUS and has a personal or family history of aHUS, first-line treatment should be with the 'complement blocker' eculizumab, a monoclonal anti-C5 antibody (23). Eculizumab has transformed the management of aHUS and has been successfully used during pregnancy to prevent end-stage renal failure (25).

There is no quick and specific diagnostic test for HUS, therefore pregnant women who present with a first episode of TMA should be investigated for TTP (23, 25). TTP is caused by an acquired (autoimmune) or congenital deficiency of ADAMTS13, a plasma metalloprotease which cleaves von Willebrand factor multimers to prevent microthrombi (22). Deficiency of ADAMTS13 leads to ultra-large von Willebrand factor multimers, which trap platelets within micro-arterioles to cause arteriolar thrombosis, organ ischaemia, and dysfunction. The plasma levels of ADAMTS13 gradually decrease during healthy pregnancy. Women with a congenital or acquired deficiency of ADAMTS13 are therefore predisposed to pathologically low levels by the end of pregnancy. Very low levels of ADAMTS13 (<10% of normal) or anti-ADAMTS13 antibodies support a diagnosis of TTP (22, 25). While results of ADAMTS13 levels are pending, plasma exchange should be started to treat suspected TTP (23). Plasma exchange may also improve the haematological aspects of HUS, but it will not improve AKI secondary to HUS (23). In the presence of a TMA and ADAMTS13 levels greater than 10% of normal, a diagnosis of aHUS is more likely and treatment should be switched from plasma exchange to eculizumab (22, 23, 25). While disease-modifying treatment is taking effect, supportive care with renal replacement therapy is sometimes necessary.

Acute renal cortical necrosis

Prolonged hypotension causing reduced renal artery perfusion leads to irreparable ischaemic destruction of the renal cortex: renal cortical necrosis. During pregnancy, activation of maternal endothelium and hypercoagulability predispose women to renal cortical necrosis. The main cause of reduced renal artery perfusion during early pregnancy is septic abortion and in late pregnancy, massive haemorrhage, sepsis, and amniotic fluid embolus. The reduced incidence of septic abortion has reduced the frequency of AKI developing into irreparable renal cortical necrosis and CKD (26). However, inadequate support of the maternal circulation at the time of massive peripartum haemorrhage, especially when associated with disseminated intravascular coagulation is still a rare cause of renal cortical necrosis in well-resourced nations (27). A large international study has demonstrated that early use of 1 g intravenous tranexamic acid reduces maternal mortality due to postpartum haemorrhage without increasing the risk of renal failure (28).

Acute fatty liver of pregnancy

Acute fatty liver of pregnancy (AFLP) is a rare metabolic disorder of fatty acid oxidation leading to multiorgan failure in the third trimester of pregnancy. AFLP affects 1:10,000 to 1:15,000 maternities and is cured by delivery (29). Women with AFLP present after several days of nausea and vomiting, but despite prolonged fasting, they have an absence of ketonuria (personal observation). Key laboratory findings reveal impaired synthetic liver function with prolonged international normalized ratio, hypoglycaemia, hypoalbuminaemia, moderately elevated transaminases and bilirubin, and AKI with an elevated level of uric acid (29). Eventually women with AFLP develop hepatic encephalopathy and placental failure leading to sudden fetal demise. The subacute onset of AFLP is supported by the observation that babies born to mothers with AFLP are usually well grown. A recessively inherited fetal inborn error of mitochondrial fatty acid oxidation has been found in a minority of pregnancies affected by AFLP (30). Other defects in fatty acid oxidation may explain other cases of AFLP.

AKI associated with AFLP is often aggravated by hypotension secondary to haemorrhage, due to a prolonged international normalized ratio at the time of emergency operative delivery. Women with AFLP should therefore be managed by a multidisciplinary team of hepatologists, nephrologists, intensivists, anaesthetists, and obstetricians in an intensive care setting, ideally in an acute liver unit. Management is supportive, aimed at maintaining adequate fluid balance for renal perfusion, replacing blood, and correcting the coagulopathy. Hypoglycaemia should be corrected with 10% dextrose solution, mindful that this may aggravate hyponatraemia and predispose to cerebral oedema. Temporary dialysis may be necessary, but with good supportive care, recovery of normal renal and liver function is usual. Perinatal survival is improving, but is dependent on the early recognition of the maternal condition, close fetal surveillance, timely delivery, and excellent neonatal care.

Nephrotoxic drugs during pregnancy

Non-steroidal anti-inflammatory drugs (NSAIDs) are frequently given peripartum. NSAIDs reduce renal blood flow and in combination with hypotension and hypertension can lead to AKI (31). Women with reduced intravascular volume, especially with pre-existing renal impairment, are particularly vulnerable and should not be prescribed NSAIDs. Aminoglycosides are also nephrotoxic and should be prescribed with care and attention to drug plasma levels in women with CKD.

Acute renal tract obstruction in pregnancy

Obstruction of the renal tracts during pregnancy may be due to renal calculi, congenital renal tract abnormalities, or gestational overdistension syndrome.

Nephrolithiasis

Gestational dilatation of the renal tracts, urinary stasis, and hypercalciuria all create an ideal environment for renal stone formation. However, renal colic is no more common during pregnancy than the non-gravid state, due to increased excretion of renal stone inhibitors. These include magnesium, citrate, nephrocalcin, and uromodulin. Renal colic affects approximately 1:200 to 1:1000 pregnancies, usually in the second and third trimester, and creates challenging management issues (32).

The passage of a renal calculus down the ureter causes intense intermittent pain. Renal colic is often associated with fever, urinary tract infection (UTI), and haematuria. Renal ultrasound will identify a renal calculus in about half of these women. In those with a normal ultrasound, but suggestive symptoms, magnetic resonance urography will avoid radiation, or if magnetic resonance urography is contraindicated, low-dose computed tomography can be used with minimal radiation exposure to the fetus (33).

Uncomplicated cases are those with a unilateral stone less than 1 cm in diameter, no sign of infection, good pain control, and normal maternal renal function. Under these circumstances, conservative management will result in up to 75% of pregnant women passing their stone spontaneously (32). Conservative management includes generous hydration, antibiotics, and pain relief with opiates, or prior to the third trimester, NSAIDs.

Failure of conservative management, or pregnant women with an obstructed single kidney or bilateral ureteric obstruction, or signs of infection, or a large stone larger than 1 cm require surgical intervention. If infection is suspected, drainage with an ultrasound-guided percutaneous nephrostomy or ureteric stent may be considered. However, both a nephrostomy and stent usually need to remain in place for the rest of pregnancy, require regular changes to avoid infection or encrustation, and only delay the need for definitive treatment. Ureteroscopy is now regularly used to insert a double J stent or accurately deliver local stone crushing lithotripsy. These techniques have been successfully and safely used in all stages of pregnancy (34).

Women who are recurrent stone formers with persistent hypercalciuria despite increased fluid intake can use thiazide diuretics in pregnancy to increase distal tubular reabsorption of calcium. Uric acid and cystine stones rarely form in pregnancy due to gestational bicarbonaturia, which naturally alkalinizes the urine. If problematic, both conditions may be controlled by increasing urine output and further alkalinization of the urine to a pH higher than 6. During pregnancy, D-penicillamine may be necessary for severe cases of stone-forming cystinurics and xanthine oxidase inhibitors for uric acid stones (35). However, data on these two drugs in pregnancy are limited and there are concerns about allopurinol causing major malformations when used in the first trimester (36).

Congenital ureteric obstruction

Women with congenital obstructive uropathies at the renal pelvis or vesicoureteric junction are at increased risk of acute urinary outflow obstruction in the second half of pregnancy, even if the original obstruction had been surgically corrected. Ultrasonography of the renal pelvis at the end of the first trimester provides a useful baseline with which to compare future imaging. A repeat renal ultrasound scan is indicated if there is pain suggestive of obstruction, persistent or recurrent infections, or a rise in serum creatinine. Gestational urinary outflow obstruction may require a temporary nephrostomy or ureteric stent (**Figure 14.2**).

Women with a single kidney and ureteric abnormalities are particularly vulnerable to develop outflow tract obstruction and AKI during pregnancy. An incomplete obstruction can cause renal impairment with an apparently good urine output. High back-pressure compresses and damages the renal medulla, leading to a loss of renal concentrating ability and production of dilute urine that is passed through an incomplete obstruction. Women born with a single

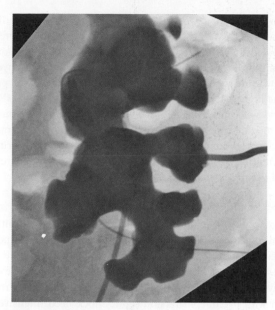

Figure 14.2 A postpartum nephrostogram of an obstructed pelviureteric junction showing a dilated collecting system in a solitary cross-fused left kidney. A 28-year-old primigravida presented with loin pain at 22 weeks' gestation. She had severe hypertension (180/110 mmHg) and a SCr concentration that rose rapidly to 298 µmol/L, despite a urine output of 4 L/24 hours. Pelvicalyceal dilatation (36 mm diameter) was noted and within days of a nephrostomy, her symptoms, hypertension, and SCr had all returned to normal. The pregnancy continued to 37 weeks and the nephrostomy remained *in situ* until 6 weeks postpartum, at which time it was replaced by a ureteral stent. The nephrostomy tube and ureteral stent can be seen on the nephrostogram.

kidney may also have other Mullerian duct anomalies that impact on pregnancy outcome, most notably a unicornuate uterus (37).

Gestational renal overdistension syndrome

During pregnancy, the renal tracts rarely become grossly overdistended. Women with renal tract overdistension present with severe loin pain, most commonly on the right side and radiating to the lower abdomen. The pain is positional, inconstant, and characteristically relieved by lying on the opposite side and tucking the knees up to the chest. Urinalysis will reveal haematuria. A renal ultrasound scan will detect a hydronephrotic kidney and grossly dilated pelvicalyceal system. Occasionally, a urinoma will be evident around the kidney indicating rupture of the renal pelvis.

Women with severe unremitting pain, haematuria, and grossly distended renal tracts on ultrasonography usually have immediate pain relief following decompression of the system with either a ureteric stent or nephrostomy. Gestational overdistension can rarely unmask a previously asymptomatic weakness in a diseased kidney, leading to kidney rupture (38). Under these circumstances, immediate surgery and almost invariably an emergency nephrectomy is needed (38).

Urinary tract infection

Urinary frequency, nocturia, urge incontinence, and strangury are common symptoms of both healthy pregnancy and UTI. If these symptoms coexist with dysuria or offensive-smelling urine, a UTI should be suspected. Microscopy and culture of a freshly voided mid-stream urine (MSU) sample will allow quantification of pyuria

(white blood cells in the urine) and growth of a urinary pathogen. Bacterial UTI is the most common cause of pyuria and is considered significant if microscopy of an un-spun MSU reveals more than ten white blood cells/µL. Urine culture is conventionally recognized as significant if there is growth of greater than 10^5 colony-forming units (CFU)/mL of a single recognized uropathogen, in association with pyuria. Low counts of bacteriuria (10^2–10^4 CFU/mL) may still be significant if symptomatic women have a high fluid intake or are infected with a slow-growing organism. If left untreated, most symptomatic women with 'low-count bacteriuria' will develop 10^5 CFU/mL within days. Haematuria and proteinuria are unreliable indicators of an UTI, but are important signs of renal disease.

The most common uropathogens are Gram-negative bacteria: *Escherichia coli*, *Proteus mirabilis*, *Enterobacter* species, and *Klebsiella pneumoniae*. Pregnant women who are symptomatic of a UTI, which is dipstick positive for nitrite (produced by most uropathogens) and leucocyte esterase (produced by white blood cells) should start empirical antibiotic treatment. As *E. coli* and enterococci are responsible for about 75% of uncomplicated UTIs, empirical treatment with nitrofurantoin 100 mg twice daily for 3 days is a good first-line choice. After 48 hours, the results of urine culture will allow a definitive choice of antibiotic. Women with glucose-6-phosphate dehydrogenase (G6PD) deficiency should avoid nitrofurantoin. Some authorities recommend that nitrofurantoin is avoided in the third trimester due to theoretical concerns it will cause neonatal haemolysis. Despite hundreds of thousands of prescriptions, there are no well-documented cases of nitrofurantoin-induced neonatal haemolysis (39). It is the author's practice to prescribe nitrofurantoin in the third trimester to women at high risk of pyelonephritis and at low risk of G6PD deficiency.

Trimethoprim 200 mg twice daily for 3 days is more likely to be active against *E. coli* and *Enterococcus* than ampicillin or cephalosporins and can be used as a second-line choice for empirical treatment of a suspected UTI. Trimethoprim should be avoided in the first trimester as it is a folic acid antagonist associated with an increased risk of neural tube defect (40). Bacterial multidrug resistance is induced by empirical antibiotic treatment. However, until new technologies accelerate our choice of antibiotic through point of care testing, an empirical choice of antibiotic remains necessary (41).

Asymptomatic bacteriuria

Asymptomatic bacteriuria, growth of a uropathogen in the absence of symptoms, occurs in 2–10% of pregnant women. Onsite tests, including dipstick testing for nitrites and the dipslide with Gram staining, have good specificity to rule out asymptomatic bacteriuria, but lack sensitivity and therefore miss many cases of asymptomatic bacteriuria (42). Currently, culture of a MSU sample remains a useful screen for asymptomatic bacteriuria.

Pregnancy-induced structural and immune changes to the urothelium make it more likely that a lower UTI will ascend to cause acute pyelonephritis (43, 44). Women with underlying renal disease are particularly at risk of UTI and pyelonephritis and should be screened for asymptomatic bacteriuria every 6 weeks (**Box 14.2**). Healthy women with a singleton pregnancy and asymptomatic bacteriuria also have an increased relative risk of pyelonephritis, but the absolute risk is much lower (2.4%) than previously estimated (30%) (43, 44). A previous Cochrane review concluded that antibiotic treatment of asymptomatic bacteriuria reduced the incidence

Box 14.2 Pregnant women at risk of asymptomatic bacteriuria and ascending urinary tract infection and for whom screening with MSU every 4-6 weeks is recommended

- Past history of asymptomatic bacteriuria
- Previous recurrent UTIs
- Pre-existing renal disease, especially scarred kidneys due to reflux nephropathy
- Structural and neuropathic abnormalities of the renal tracts
- History of renal calculi
- Pre-existing diabetes mellitus but not gestational diabetes
- Sickle cell disease and trait
- Low socioeconomic group and less than 12 years of higher education

of pyelonephritis compared to placebo or no treatment (odds ratio 0.24; 95% confidence interval 0.19–0.32) (45). For this reason, antibiotics have been readily prescribed for asymptomatic bacteriuria. However, there are concerns that widespread antibiotic use may lead to bacterial multidrug resistance, and also of a possible increased risk of cerebral palsy in children exposed to antibiotics *in utero*. Hence it seems prudent to reserve the treatment of asymptomatic bacteriuria to women at high risk of renal complications (**Box 14.2**). Asymptomatic bacteriuria has also been thought to be associated with an increased risk of preterm delivery and low birth weight (46), but a contemporary multicentre study has shown no such association between asymptomatic bacteriuria in mid-trimester and preterm birth or growth restriction (44).

Screening for recurrent infections should begin 1 week after completion of initial treatment and then 6-weekly for the rest of pregnancy. Recurrent infections or a first infection in a pregnant woman at high risk of pyelonephritis (**Box 14.2**) should be treated with an antibiotic that reflects antibacterial sensitivities for 7–10 days. Women with renal disease who have had two episodes of asymptomatic bacteriuria or cystitis should be considered for low-dose antibiotic prophylaxis—guided by the sensitivities of the most recent infective organism. Antibiotic prophylaxis will reduce the risk of pyelonephritis for the remainder of pregnancy and until 4–6 weeks postpartum (47). Suitable regimens for long-term antibiotic prophylaxis include nitrofurantoin 50–100 mg every night (nocte), trimethoprim 100–150 mg nocte, amoxicillin 250 mg nocte, or cephalexin 125–250 mg nocte (47). These women should have a renal ultrasound scan to check for structural abnormalities or renal calculi.

Acute pyelonephritis

The same uropathogens that cause asymptomatic and symptomatic infections are responsible for acute pyelonephritis. Therefore, the prevalence of asymptomatic bacteriuria in a pregnant population dictates the incidence of acute pyelonephritis. In the United States, acute pyelonephritis affects approximately 1:200 pregnancies (48). Unless acute pyelonephritis is treated promptly there is an increased risk of AKI, respiratory distress, anaemia, sepsis, and preterm birth (48).

Most women with acute pyelonephritis present with back ache, fever, rigors, and costovertebral angle tenderness, while about half have lower urinary tract symptoms, nausea, and vomiting. Bacteraemia is present in approximately 20% of pregnant women with acute pyelonephritis and a small proportion of these women

will develop septic shock, and increased capillary leak leading to pulmonary oedema (48). It is important however to differentiate the hypotension due to reduced intravascular volume (fever, nausea, and vomiting) from that due to septic shock. Women with pyelonephritis who are at risk of serious complications are those who present with the highest fever, tachycardia, at greater than 20 weeks' gestation, and who have received tocolytic agents and injudicious fluid replacement. Acute pyelonephritis can trigger uterine contractions and preterm labour (49). Antibiotic treatment of pyelonephritis will reduce uterine activity, but those with recurrent infection are at increased risk of preterm labour.

Management of acute pyelonephritis

Women suspected of acute pyelonephritis should be admitted to hospital for at least 24 hours. Laboratory tests should include full blood count, SCr, electrolytes, C-reactive protein, urine, and blood culture. Renal tract ultrasound scanning is recommended to identify any underlying structural abnormality or calculi. Pregnant women with pyelonephritis and septic shock need intensive care. Assessment of hydration will optimize fluid balance, aiming for a urine output greater than 30 mL/hour to minimize renal impairment and reduce the risk of pulmonary oedema. Intravenous antibiotics should be started empirically until sensitivities of blood and urine cultures are known.

Gram-negative bacteria causing pyelonephritis in pregnancy are usually sensitive to intravenous cefuroxime 750 mg–1.5 g every 8 hours, or ceftriaxone 1 g depending on the severity of the maternal condition and until sensitivities are known (48). Women allergic to beta-lactam antibiotics can be given intravenous gentamicin (1.5 mg/kg every 8 hours) for the initial treatment of acute pyelonephritis. A single-dose regimen (7 mg/kg every 24 hours) should be avoided during pregnancy to reduce the small risk of eighth nerve damage to the fetus (50). Serum concentrations of gentamicin should be measured and dose adjustments made according to levels. Intravenous antibiotics should be continued until the patient has been afebrile for 24 hours. Oral antibiotics should then be given for 7–10 days, according to bacterial sensitivities, or if not available, as for symptomatic lower UTI (50).

Following one episode of pyelonephritis, pregnant women should have monthly urine cultures to screen for a recurrence (51). The risk of recurrent pyelonephritis can be reduced with antimicrobial prophylaxis, according to the sensitivities of the initial bacterial infection until 4–6 weeks postpartum (51).

Chronic kidney disease

CKD is often clinically and biochemically silent until renal function has deteriorated significantly. Symptoms are unusual until the GFR declines to less than 25% of normal and more than 50% of renal function can be lost before the SCr concentration rises above 120 μmol/L. However, women who become pregnant with a SCr concentration above 120 μmol/L are at increased risk of an accelerated decline in renal function and poor pregnancy outcome (10, 52, 53). Women with the most severe prepregnancy CKD have the greatest risk of adverse pregnancy outcome and the greatest risk of a pregnancy-related decline in renal function, especially if associated with hypertension (10, 52–55). Clinical management of pregnant women with

CKD aims to prevent pregnancy-induced harm to the mother's renal function and CKD-induced harm to the developing fetus.

CKD is classified into five stages according to the level of renal function, (estimated glomerular filtration rate; eGFR) (Table 14.3) (56). In a prepregnancy Norwegian population, the overall prevalence of women with CKD was 3.3% (54). CKD stage 1 affected 2.4%, CKD 2, 0.8%, and CKD stage 3, 0.1% (54). There were no cases of CKD stages 4 and 5, which in other populations affects between 1:500 and 1:1000 women of childbearing age (20–39 years). Due to reduced fertility and an increased rate of early miscarriage, ongoing pregnancy in women with CKD stage 4 or 5 is rare. Conversely, up to 20% of women who develop early pre-eclampsia (≤30 weeks' gestation), especially those with heavy proteinuria, are found to have previously unrecognized CKD (57).

Women with CKD are less able to make the renal adaptations of healthy pregnancy. Their inability to boost renal hormones leads to normochromic normocytic anaemia (reduced erythropoietin), attenuated plasma volume expansion (reduced renin), and vitamin D deficiency (reduced 1,25 dihydroxycholecalciferol). The gestational rise in GFR is blunted in women with moderate renal impairment and usually absent in those with a SCr concentration greater than 200 µmol/L (2.26 mg/dL) (58, 59).

The impact of pregnancy on maternal chronic kidney disease

Mild renal impairment during pregnancy (CKD stages 1–2)

Most women with CKD who become pregnant have mild renal dysfunction and pregnancy usually succeeds without affecting renal prognosis (Table 14.3). A case-controlled study of 360 women with primary glomerulonephritis and only mild prepregnancy renal dysfunction (SCr <110 µmol/L), minimal proteinuria (<1 g/24 hours), and absent or well-controlled hypertension, showed that pregnancy had little or no adverse effect on long-term (up to 25 years) maternal renal function (60).

Moderate to severe renal impairment (CKD stages 3–5)

Women with the worst prepregnancy renal function are at greatest risk of an accelerated decline in renal function due to pregnancy (Table 14.4). Pre-existing proteinuria and hypertension both add to this risk (52, 54, 58). One retrospective series of women with CKD (87 pregnancies) found that those with initially moderate renal impairment (SCr 124–168 mmol/L) had a 40% risk of a pregnancy-related decline in renal function, which persisted postpartum in about half of those affected (61). Of those women with severe renal impairment (SCr >177 mmol/L; 2.0 mg/dL), 13/20 (65%) had a decline in renal function during the third trimester, which persisted in almost all and deteriorated to end-stage renal failure in 7/20 (35%) (61).

The first prospective study to assess the rate of decline of maternal renal function before and after pregnancy in 49 women with prepregnancy CKD stages 3 to 5 confirmed these earlier observations (52). Specifically, women with a prepregnancy eGFR less than 40 mL/min/1.73 m² and proteinuria greater than 1 g/24 h, but not either factor alone, showed an accelerated decline in renal function after their pregnancy (52). Chronic hypertension, which predisposes women to pre-eclampsia, may explain why those with milder renal dysfunction also have a gestational decline in renal function (52–55). This risk is reduced when hypertension is controlled and prophylaxis with low-dose aspirin started around 12 weeks' gestation (62).

The impact of maternal chronic kidney disease on pregnancy outcome

Maternal hypertension, proteinuria, and recurrent urinary infection often coexist in women with CKD. Each factor is individually and cumulatively detrimental to pregnancy outcome (10, 52–55, 59–61). Furthermore, the risk of adverse pregnancy outcome increases at every stage of CKD (Tables 14.3 and 14.4) (10, 55). Women with CKD stages 1–2 have a low risk of adverse pregnancy outcome in the absence of hypertension (Table 14.5) (54).

Women with severe renal impairment have the greatest difficulty conceiving, the highest rate of miscarriage, and poorest fetal outcome (10, 52–55, 61). There is, however, a spectrum of poor outcomes, including pre-eclampsia, fetal growth restriction, preterm delivery, and fetal death, correlating with the level of renal dysfunction (Tables 14.3 and 14.4).

Optimal antenatal care for women with CKD requires the input of a multidisciplinary obstetric-nephrology team from before conception. With few exceptions, the most important aspects of the

Table 14.3 Definition, description, and prevalence of chronic kidney disease in women of reproductive age

CKD stage K/DOQI guidelines	Description of prepregnancy renal function	Mean eGFR ± SD (mL/min/1.73 m²)	Estimated prevalence of CKD in women aged 20–45 years HUNT 2 (%)	Relative risk of pre-eclampsia or SGA or preterm birth HUNT 2
	Normal renal function			
G1	Kidney damage with normal or increased GFR	≥90 with persistent microalbuminuria	2.5	1.0
G2	Kidney damage with mildly decreased GFR	60–89 with persistent microalbuminuria	0.5	eGFR 75–89: OR 1.13 (0.90–1.45) n = 153 eGFR 60–74: OR 1.65 (0.97–2.83) n = 25
G3a	Mild to moderately decreased GFR	45–59	<0.5	n = 1 OR 2.53 (0.25–25.35)
G3b	Moderately to severely decreased GFR	30–44	0.1	See Table 14.6
4	Severely decreased GFR	15–29	<0.1	See Table 14.6
5	Kidney failure	<15 or dialysis	<0.005	See Table 14.6

HUNT, Nord-Trøndelag Health Study (54); K/DOQI, Kidney Disease Outcomes Quality Initiative; OR, odds ratio; SD, standard deviation; SGA, small for gestational age.

Table 14.4 Prepregnancy renal function (SCr) with estimated rates for pregnancy outcome (>24 weeks) and impact on maternal renal function

SCr μmol/L (mg/dL)	Rate of fetal growth restriction (%)	Rate of preterm delivery (%)	Rate of pre-eclampsia (%)	Perinatal deaths (%)	Loss of >25% renal function		
					Pregnancy (%)	Persists postpartum (%)	ESRF in 1 year (%)
<125 (<1.4)	25	30	22	1	2	–	–
125–180 (1.4–2.0)	45	65	50	5	40	20	2
>180 (>2.0)	75	90	60	10	70	50	35
Dialysis	>90	90	75	50[a]	N/A	N/A	N/A

ESRF, end-stage renal failure.

Estimates are based on literature from 1985 to 2011, with all pregnancies attaining at least 24 weeks' gestation.

[a] If conceived on dialysis, 50% of infants survival; if conceived before introduction of dialysis, there is 75% infant survival (10).

management of CKD in pregnancy relate to the management of associated clinical features rather than the type of renal disease. Regular monitoring of maternal renal function (serum creatinine and urea levels, not eGFR), full blood count, blood pressure, MSU for infection and proteinuria, and when appropriate ultrasound imaging of renal tracts will identify most subclinical pathological changes and allow timely intervention to optimize perinatal and maternal renal outcome (Table 14.6).

Prepregnancy preparation for women with chronic kidney disease

Ideally, all women with CKD should be made aware of the effects that pregnancy may have on their own long-term renal function, and of the risks of adverse pregnancy outcome, before they conceive (Table 14.5). Women with CKD often have amenorrhoea, but may still ovulate and should be considered fertile. Sexually active women with CKD who do not wish to become pregnant should therefore take appropriate contraceptive measures that consider clinical comorbidities.

Folic acid 400 mcg daily should be given as usual before conception until 12 weeks' gestation. Low-dose aspirin (50–150 mg/day) should be started in early pregnancy to reduce the risk of pre-eclampsia and improve perinatal outcome (62). Regular drugs should be reviewed so that fetotoxic drugs (e.g. angiotensin-converting enzyme inhibitors and angiotensin II receptor blockers) can be stopped as soon as pregnancy is confirmed.

Care of pregnant women with chronic kidney disease

CKD includes a wide range of different conditions and monitoring during pregnancy needs to be tailored according to the severity of CKD and associated complications (Table 14.7). In general, all factors should be checked more frequently as pregnancy progresses, or if there are changes to suggest deteriorating kidney function. Specialist care of pregnant women with CKD should begin early in

Table 14.6 Management plan for pregnant women with chronic kidney disease

Maternal renal parameter	Action
Renal function	Check serum creatinine and urea each trimester if asymptomatic, normotensive CKD stages 1 and 2.[a] Check more frequently for CKD stages 3–5 and during the second half of pregnancy
Blood pressure	1. Check BP regularly and according to maternal BP control. 2. Aim to keep BP <140/90 mmHg with antihypertensive treatment
Mid-stream urine	Every 4–6 weeks screen for (1) urinary tract infection (UTI)—treat first UTI with sensitive antibiotic. Consider prophylactic antibiotic after 2 UTIs. (2) Proteinuria—use thromboprophylaxis with low-molecular-weight heparin if >1 g proteinuria/24 hours. (3) Haematuria—if present, perform microscopy for red cell casts, which suggest active renal parenchymal disease. Normal red cell morphology suggests urological pathology—seek urological advice
Ultrasound of renal tracts	Perform baseline renal ultrasound scan at booking (around 12 weeks' gestation) for pelvicalyceal dimensions. Repeat if symptoms suggest obstruction
Full blood count	Check haemoglobin: aim for haemoglobin >100 g/L. If low serum ferritin, give iron supplement. If iron replete normochromic normocytic anaemia, consider erythropoietin

Table 14.5 Odds ratio for pre-eclampsia, small for gestational age, or preterm birth by kidney function and blood pressure

Blood pressure	eGFR >90 mL/min	eGFR 75–89 mL/min	eGFR 60–74 mL/min
<140/90 mmHg	1.0 (ref) (n = 4352)	1.18 (95% CI 0.85–1.63; P = 0.31) (n = 906)	1.65 (95% CI 0.97–2.83; P = 0.066) (n = 25)
>140/90 mmHg	1.82 (95% CI 1.12–2.97; P = 0.015) (n = 304)	2.58 (95% CI 1.40–4.75; P <0.001) (n = 93)	10.09 (95% CI 2.38–42.87; P <0.001)

CI, confidence interval.

Adjusted for maternal age, parity, follow-up time, previous pre-eclampsia, preterm birth or small for gestational age, body mass index, diabetes, smoking, history of cardiovascular disease, and education

Source data from Munkhaugen J et al. *Nephrol Dial Transplant* 2009; 24: 3744–3750.

[a] United Kingdom laboratories have been encouraged to report eGFR using the validated Modification of Diet in Renal Disease formula, whereby serum creatinine is adjusted for age, sex, and race. In pregnancy, this formula significantly underestimates the rate and is not recommended for use in clinical practice.

Table 14.7 Summary points: specific chronic kidney diseases during pregnancy

Renal disease	Complicating factors	Key management issues
Primary glomerulonephritis	Hypertension, impaired renal function, proteinuria, recurrent infection	Control blood pressure <140/90 mmHg; serial assessment of SCr. If protein:creatinine ratio >100 mg/mmol, consider thromboprophylaxis with low-molecular-weight heparin; screen and treat for UTIs
Autosomal dominant polycystic kidney disease	Impaired renal function, hypertension	As for 'Primary glomerulonephritis' and the child has a 50% risk of inheriting the ADPKD
Congenital renal tract obstruction	Risk of renal tract obstruction, even if surgically corrected	Renal ultrasound in early pregnancy. Serial assessment of SCr, blood pressure
Vesicoureteric reflux nephropathy	Recurrent UTIs (28–65%), ureteral obstruction (5%), pre-existing renal impairment, blood pressure	Consider prophylactic antibiotics. Drain obstruction as necessary
Nephrolithiasis	Renal colic, ureteric obstruction	Involve a urologist. Ureteroscopy or magnetic resonance urography can be used to remove or treat stones, while avoiding radiation exposure
Diabetic nephropathy	Renal function, hypertension, and proteinuria	Maintain good control of maternal glucose, blood pressure, and screen for urinary infection
Lupus nephritis	Distinguish from pre-eclampsia	Ask patient if it feels like a lupus flare. Check double-stranded DNA levels. Link with rheumatologist or nephrologist
Dialysis	Mimic physiological changes of pregnancy	Almost daily haemodialysis allows mimicking of gestational physiological change
Renal transplant	Pre-eclampsia, fetal growth restriction, deteriorating graft function	Delay pregnancy until stable graft function and allow immunosuppression to low–normal levels

pregnancy, but much of the monitoring of women with CKD stages 1–2 can be done by primary care physicians.

Optimal management of pregnant women with CKD will often involve the combined expertise of specialists in obstetrics, nephrology, urology, fetal medicine, and neonatology. Impressive improvements in perinatal outcome over recent decades have been driven by advances in these specialties. Maternal renal conditions that have a genetic basis require specialist fetal medicine and genetic advice.

Specific kidney conditions during pregnancy

Primary glomerulonephritis

The histological type of primary glomerulonephritis does not affect pregnancy outcome as much as the clinical parameters of hypertension, level of renal impairment, proteinuria, and recurrent urinary infections (10). Severe vascular lesions on renal biopsy are associated with increased perinatal mortality, which probably reflects maternal clinical parameters (63). On the rare occasion that sudden renal impairment (SCr >120 μmol/L), or an active urinary sediment with red cell casts occurs before 34 weeks' gestation in the absence of pre-eclampsia, a renal biopsy may detect a glomerular lesion that would benefit from targeted therapy. However, in pregnancy the plethoric kidney is more prone to bleed and more awkward to biopsy, so should only be undertaken by an experienced operator (64). New-onset heavy proteinuria (nephrotic range, >5 g/24 hours) could be managed with a trial of steroids and in the absence of a prompt clinical response, a renal biopsy should be considered. After 34 weeks, early delivery becomes an option. Postpartum, pregnancy-induced proteinuria and renal impairment will improve, therapeutic options broaden, and clinical management, including renal biopsy, becomes less difficult.

Immunoglobulin A nephropathy

Immunoglobulin (Ig)-A nephropathy is the commonest primary glomerulonephritis in young people and is consequently highly represented in pregnant women (65). IgA nephropathy presents with macroscopic haematuria, often during an acute gastrointestinal or respiratory tract illness. The diagnosis is made by histological examination of a renal biopsy that shows IgA deposits in the glomerular mesangium (65). The clinical course is variable, but progression towards end-stage renal failure is more common in the presence of hypertension, proteinuria, and severe histological lesions (65). Initial treatment is aimed at controlling hypertension and proteinuria with an angiotensin-converting enzyme inhibitor or angiotensin II receptor blocker, but both agents are fetotoxic and need to be replaced by other antihypertensive agents during pregnancy. Thromboprophylaxis with low-molecular-weight heparin is prudent if there is proteinuria (PCR >100 mg/mmol). Progressive IgA nephropathy has been treated with immunosuppression with limited success.

Pregnancy and renal outcomes for women with IgA nephropathy follow the same general principles stated for all women with CKD. Those with preconception CKD stage 3 or 4, (but not CKD stage 1 or 2), hypertension, nephrotic range proteinuria, and the most severe histological lesions on renal biopsy are more likely to have an accelerated decline in renal function postpartum compared with women who have IgA nephropathy, but don't become pregnant (66). Similarly, these clinical features increase the risk of pre-eclampsia, fetal growth restriction, and preterm labour (67).

Henoch–Schönlein purpura nephritis

Henoch–Schönlein purpura (HSP) is a small vessel vasculitis that predominantly affects children. Renal involvement (HSP nephritis) is present in approximately 50% of cases and shares histological similarities with IgA nephropathy (65). Women who had HSP nephritis as children usually make a good recovery, but are at an increased risk of recurrent proteinuric hypertension during their pregnancies (68). Immunosuppressive treatment appears to be of no proven benefit. Management aims to control hypertension and reduce the risk of pre-eclampsia with low-dose aspirin.

Lupus nephritis

Systemic lupus erythematosus (SLE) is a multisystem autoimmune disorder directed against nuclear antigens, which predominantly affects young women (69). Lupus nephritis affects up to 50% of women with SLE and is often subclinical (70). Active lupus nephritis is characterized by an increase serum creatinine concentration, active urinary sediment (haematuria, red cell casts, and leucocytes), proteinuria, and hypertension (69). Lupus nephritis runs a relapsing and remitting course and during pregnancy is best managed by a multidisciplinary team of obstetricians, nephrologists, and rheumatologists.

Women who have well-controlled SLE before conception are at low risk of an adverse pregnancy outcome (71). Furthermore, it is rare for women with SLE to develop lupus nephritis for the first time during pregnancy (72). The risk of a flare of lupus nephritis during pregnancy is influenced by clinical disease activity at conception and predicted using subclinical markers of immunological activity (72, 73). These include elevated levels of anti-double-stranded (ds) DNA and anti-C1q antibodies and low levels of complement C3 and C4 (73). The risk of pre-eclampsia, fetal growth restriction, and preterm labour is driven by the usual prepregnancy clinical factors that drive an adverse pregnancy outcome with other renal diseases. These include maternal hypertension, the level of renal impairment, proteinuria, elevated maternal body mass index, and specific to lupus nephritis, a longer clinical history of lupus nephritis with renal flares (73). Low-dose aspirin, 75–150 mg nocte from 12 weeks' gestation until childbirth, is recommended to reduce the risk of pre-eclampsia (74).

During the second half of pregnancy, a relapse of lupus nephritis may present with similar clinical signs as pre-eclampsia: specifically, hypertension, proteinuria, elevated serum creatinine, thrombocytopenia, and hyperuricaemia. Indeed, women with lupus nephritis are at increased risk of pre-eclampsia (73). Distinguishing features of lupus nephritis include haematuria with an active urinary sediment (red cell casts) and extrarenal manifestations affecting the skin and joints or other visceral organs. Furthermore, most pregnant women with lupus nephritis will recognize the symptoms associated with a typical lupus flare. Active lupus nephritis is associated with a rising titre of anti-dsDNA antibodies and a failure of the gestational rise in serum complement (C3 and C4) levels from the first to second half of pregnancy (72).

Women with active lupus nephritis are at an increased risk of adverse fetal outcomes, especially if associated with antiphospholipid antibodies (lupus anticoagulant, anticardiolipin IgG antibodies, and anti-beta-2 IgG antibodies) (75). Maternal hypertension and a high SLE disease activity index (SLEDAI) compounds these risks (75).

Management of lupus nephritis in pregnancy

Prednisolone, azathioprine, and hydroxychloroquine have all been safely used during pregnancy and while breastfeeding to keep lupus nephritis in remission (76). Mycophenolate mofetil is widely used outside pregnancy for the control of lupus nephritis, but it is teratogenic. Women who switch from mycophenolate mofetil to azathioprine while their lupus nephritis is quiescent and in anticipation of pregnancy, have good pregnancy outcomes and rarely develop renal flares (77). Rituximab is a monoclonal antibody that depletes B cells and has shown promise to ameliorate lupus nephritis. However, rituximab crosses the placenta to deplete B cells in the fetus and should not be used during pregnancy (76).

A flare of lupus nephritis during pregnancy can be treated with intravenous methylprednisolone 500 mg and an increase of oral prednisolone to around 40 mg daily. During pregnancy, steroid-resistant and progressive lupus nephritis has been successfully treated with tacrolimus and intravenous cyclophosphamide. However, when a severe flare of lupus nephritis occurs during pregnancy, the effects of this life-threatening condition on the mother, as well as the effects of toxic drugs on the fetus, need to be balanced against the likelihood of a successful fetal outcome. Sometimes, difficult decisions regarding continuation of the pregnancy need to be taken. Additional treatment includes antihypertensive medication to control blood pressure (to ≤140/90 mmHg) and thromboprophylaxis with low-dose aspirin and low-molecular-weight heparin, especially in the presence of antiphospholipid antibodies and proteinuria greater than 1 g/24 hours. Lupus nephritis is slightly more likely to flare postpartum, but there is no evidence to support the use of prophylactic steroids in anticipation of a peripartum disease flare.

Autosomal dominant polycystic kidney disease

Women with autosomal dominant polycystic kidney disease (ADPKD) who have normal renal function and blood pressure, usually have a successful, uncomplicated pregnancy (78). However, pre-existing hypertension in ADPKD is a significant risk factor for pre-eclampsia and fetal prematurity (78). Children born to mothers with ADPKD will of course have a 50% risk of inheriting the gene associated with ADPKD. New treatments for slowing the progression of renal cysts and reducing the decline in renal function are emerging, but are not yet recommended in pregnancy (79).

Reflux nephropathy/vesicoureteral reflux

Reflux nephropathy or vesicoureteral reflux (VUR) is a congenital urological abnormality that usually presents in childhood with recurrent urinary tract infections. Retrograde passage of urine is associated with renal scars and is a common cause of CKD in young women. During pregnancy, women with VUR are at risk of ureteric obstruction, even if VUR has been surgically corrected. An ultrasound scan of the renal tracts before pregnancy, or in the first trimester can be a useful comparator, if symptoms of urinary outflow obstruction develop in later pregnancy. Relief of the obstruction may require nephrostomy or ureteric stenting.

Pregnant women with persistent VUR are twice as likely to develop acute pyelonephritis compared with those who have had spontaneous or surgical resolution of VUR (80). These women should therefore be screened for asymptomatic bacteriuria every 4–6 weeks throughout pregnancy. There should be a low threshold for prescribing prophylactic antibiotics to reduce the risk of recurrent UTIs and preserve renal function. Women with persistent VUR, especially those with a history of upper UTI, and who are contemplating pregnancy should consider prepregnancy correction of VUR to reduce maternal and fetal morbidity. As with other forms of CKD, women with VUR and reduced GFR, proteinuria, and hypertension have the greatest risk of adverse pregnancy outcome (80, 81). Almost 50% of neonates born to mothers with VUR will themselves have VUR and should therefore be offered screening with a micturating cystogram (81).

Diabetic nephropathy

Diabetic nephropathy is the most common cause of end-stage renal disease (ESRD) in high-resource nations (82). However, the early stages of diabetic nephropathy are asymptomatic. An initial rise in glomerular capillary pressure leads to renal hyperfiltration, elevated GFR, and microalbuminuria. Pregnancy augments the hyperfiltration of early diabetic nephropathy, which implies that diabetic and gestational hyperfiltration work through separate, but synergistic mechanisms. This explains why women with diabetic nephropathy show a gestational increase in proteinuria, which does not necessarily indicate pre-eclampsia. Women with diabetes can also be reassured that pregnancy does not trigger the onset of diabetic nephropathy and those who have established diabetic nephropathy with well-preserved renal function and normal blood pressure, do not progress more rapidly to ESRD due to pregnancy.

Diabetic nephropathy (urinary albumin:creatinine ratio >300 mg/g) affects approximately 2.5% of pregnant women with both type 1 and type 2 diabetes (83). Microalbuminuria (urinary albumin:creatinine ratio 30–299 mg/g) is also equally prevalent among pregnant women with type 1 and type 2 diabetes at approximately 4% (83). Good control of maternal blood glucose levels and hypertension before conception and during pregnancy improve both perinatal and maternal outcomes (83, 84). Conversely, poor glycaemic control and blood pressure greater than 130/80 mmHg are associated with an increased rate of pre-eclampsia and preterm childbirth (85).

Over time, diabetic nephropathy leads to a gradual reduction in GFR. Women with diabetic nephropathy and moderate to severe renal impairment (SCr >125 µmol/L) have more than a 40% chance of an accelerated decline in renal function, usually associated with pre-eclampsia or an exacerbation of hypertension (86).

Renal replacement therapy and pregnancy

Pregnancy on dialysis

Women with ESRD have reduced fertility, which may be associated with amenorrhoea or anovulatory cycles and they are predisposed to premature menopause. Improved haemodialysis (HD) systems and intensified dialysis regimens have however increased the likelihood of women conceiving while on HD (87). Diagnosis of pregnancy can be difficult, due to irregular menses and a raised beta-human chorionic gonadotropin which is not diagnostic of pregnancy in women with ESRD. Transvaginal ultrasonography is therefore necessary if pregnancy is suspected. Pregnancy outcomes for women on HD have improved markedly over recent years with HD regimens that successfully mimic the physiological increase in GFR of healthy pregnancy. Live birth rates of up to 85% have been found in women on the most intensive HD regimens (88). A dedicated multidisciplinary renal and obstetric team is crucial for a good pregnancy outcome.

Fewer women conceive on peritoneal dialysis (PD) than on HD (89). There are, however, several case reports of successful pregnancies in women on PD. Meeting the increased GFR and physiological demands of healthy pregnancy is challenging on PD. Furthermore, women with large polycystic kidneys or polyhydramnios may be unable to accommodate peritoneal fluid in the third trimester. A switch to HD may therefore be necessary to maintain a pregnancy. When it is necessary to initiate dialysis during pregnancy HD is the preferred modality. Complications of PD include peritonitis that should be treated in the same way as non-pregnant patients with intraperitoneal antibiotics.

Women who conceive with residual renal function but then start dialysis have a better pregnancy outcome compared with women who conceive on an established dialysis regimen (90). For this reason, HD should be considered in women with a serum urea concentration greater than 20 mmol/L (87). Urea crosses the placenta to the fetus and a high fetal urinary urea concentration causes an osmotic diuresis, which is associated with polyhydramnios on less rigorous dialysis regimens. Preterm rupture of membranes and maternal hypertension are other causes for preterm delivery. Frequent dialysis will also reduce the need for large fluid shifts which may compromise uteroplacental blood flow. In those women who have some residual renal function, fluid balance is easier to manage, which increases the likelihood of a successful pregnancy outcome.

Women who increase their HD regimen to between 37 and 56 hours per week are more likely to have a successful pregnancy outcome compared with women on a lower HD intensity regimen (Figure 14.3) (88). Fluid balance and weight gain should recognize an average gestational weight gain of 0.5 kg per week during the second and third trimesters. Maternal blood pressure should be kept below 140/90 mmHg. Rises in blood pressure might initially respond to extra fluid removal, but resistant hypertension in a euvolaemic woman may herald gestational hypertension requiring antihypertensive medication. Women on HD with anuria will clearly not produce proteinuria and therefore the obstetrician will have to use other symptoms and signs of pre-eclampsia to make the diagnosis.

Increased dialysis will lead to hypokalaemia and a higher concentration of potassium in the dialysate or potassium supplements may be necessary. Furthermore, a gestational reduction in serum sodium concentration necessitates a concomitant reduction in dialysate sodium concentration to around 135 mmol/L and the gestational reduction in serum bicarbonate concentration (18–22 mmol/L) should be matched with a low-bicarbonate dialysate. Increased dialysis frequency will also allow a greater protein intake, which is variably recommended to be between 1.2 and 1.8 g/kg/day.

Anaemia and haemorrhage are common in the dialysis population. Haemoglobin and iron status need to be monitored monthly; iron supplements and erythropoietin should be given to maintain Hb between 100 and 110 g/L. The dose of erythropoietin needs to be increased by 50–100% during pregnancy. It does not cross the placenta and consequently there have been no reports of teratogenicity or polycythemia in the infant. The dialysis circuit should be heparinized as usual. Folic acid supplementation (2–5 mg/day) is recommended throughout pregnancy and low-dose aspirin (50–150 mg/day) taken from shortly after conception may reduce the risk of pre-eclampsia. The requirement for calcium and vitamin D supplements is also likely to change as pregnancy progresses and plasma levels of calcium, phosphate, and vitamin D need to be monitored and doses of phosphate binders and vitamin D analogues adjusted accordingly.

If preterm labour has not eventuated, planned induction of labour at 37 weeks' gestation is recommended (87). Caesarean section is reserved for clinical indications. Breastfeeding on dialysis is possible if maternal euvolaemia is maintained and drugs toxic to the neonate are avoided.

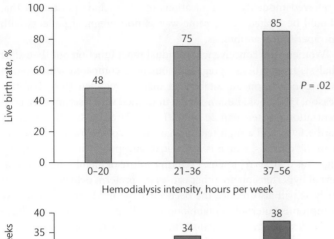

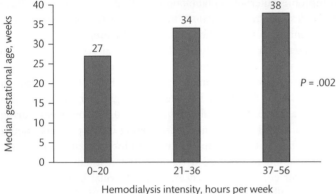

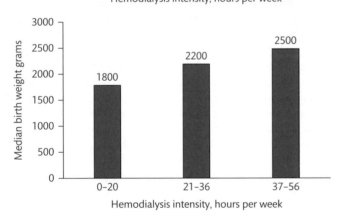

0–20, n = 46; 21–36, n = 16; 37–56, n = 13.
In written with established ESRD.

Figure 14.3 Improved pregnancy outcomes with greater haemodialysis intensity.

Reproduced from Hladunewich M, Schatell D. Intensive dialysis and pregnancy. *Hemodialysis International* 2016; 20: 339–348 with permission from John Wiley and Sons.

Renal transplantation and pregnancy

A successful pregnancy outcome is much more likely and much easier to manage if a woman with ESRD receives a renal transplantation. Fertility usually returns within 6 months of a transplantation, by which time renal function and immunosuppressive therapy have usually stabilized. Over 1500 pregnancies from women with renal transplants have been reported (91, 92). Among these pregnancies, approximately 75–80% result in a live birth (92). As for all CKD, pregnancy outcome depends on clinical parameters, specifically

level of renal function at conception, maternal hypertension, recurrent UTIs, and proteinuria. Pregnancy appears to have no long-term influence on maternal survival or graft function (92).

Immunosuppression for renal transplants during pregnancy

Despite physiological immune tolerance during pregnancy, continued therapeutic immunosuppression is necessary to maintain graft survival. Prednisolone is safe in pregnancy as only one-tenth of the maternal concentration is found in cord blood. Azathioprine passes easily across the placenta, but it is not converted to its active metabolite, 6-mercaptopurine, by the immature fetal liver. Azathioprine has had an excellent safety record during pregnancy.

During pregnancy, the gestational rise in plasma volume leads to a fall in plasma concentration of calcineurin inhibitors (e.g. tacrolimus and ciclosporin). If trough drug levels are to be kept within the prepregnancy therapeutic range, the dose of tacrolimus or ciclosporin needs to be increased as pregnancy progresses (93). To avoid toxic side effects during pregnancy (e.g. hypertension), the dose of calcineurin inhibitor should be adjusted to keep levels at the lower end of the therapeutic range. Postpartum, the plasma volume returns to non-pregnancy levels within a few days and calcineurin inhibitor doses should be promptly reduced to prepregnancy levels.

Women taking mycophenolate mofetil should be switched to azathioprine. Women taking sirolimus should be switched to tacrolimus, despite several reports of good pregnancy outcomes with sirolimus. In anticipation of pregnancy, it is prudent to switch from drugs with an unknown or harmful safety profile to those known to be safe.

High-dose steroids remain a first-line therapy for an acute rejection episode during pregnancy. In steroid-resistant rejection, difficult decisions may need to be taken about escalating the immunosuppression to prevent graft rejection and unknown harm to the fetus. There are many case reports of good pregnancy outcomes using multiple immunosuppressant therapies (94).

Pregnant women on immunosuppression should receive prophylactic antibiotics for all surgical interventions, including childbirth. Furthermore, immunosuppressed women should be screened regularly for asymptomatic bacteriuria, and treated when pathogenic bacteria is isolated. Just one UTI during pregnancy in a transplant patient is an indication for low-dose antibiotic prophylaxis for the duration of the pregnancy.

The pelvic transplant kidney does not obstruct childbirth. A spontaneous vaginal delivery should therefore be the aim if obstetric circumstances allow. Caesarean section is, however, often necessary. The dose of corticosteroids should be temporarily increased in the perioperative period.

Postpartum care

Breastfeeding should be encouraged in women with renal transplants and a thriving infant. Small amounts of ciclosporin and tacrolimus are detectable in breast milk, but none is evident in the breastfed infant. Azathioprine is not detectable in breast milk. In general, mothers taking immunosuppressive drugs and who are keen to breastfeed should continue to do so as long as the neonate is thriving.

REFERENCES

1. Chapman AB, Zamudio S, Woodmansee W, et al. Systemic and renal hemodynamic changes in the luteal phase of the menstrual cycle mimic early pregnancy. *Am J Physiol (Renal Physiol)* 1997;**273**:F777–82.

2. Chapman AB, Abraham WT, Zamudio S, et al. Temporal relationships between hormonal and hemodynamic changes in early human pregnancy. *Kidney Int* 1998;**54**:2056–63.

3. Sturgiss SN, Dunlop W, Davison JM. Renal haemodynamics and tubular function in human pregnancy. *Baillieres Clin Obstet Gynaecol* 1994;**8:2**:209–34.

4. Faundes A, Bricola-Filho M, Pinto e Silva LC. Dilatation of the urinary tract during pregnancy: proposal of a curve of maximal caliceal diameter by gestational age. *Am J Obstet Gynecol* 1998;**178**:1082–86.

5. Baba Y, Yamada T, Obata-Yasuoka M, et al. Urinary protein to creatinine ratio in pregnant women after dipstick testing: prospective observational study. *BMC Pregnancy Childbirth* 2015;**15**:331.

6. Davison JM, Shiells EA, Philips PR, Lindheimer MD. Serial evaluation of vasopressin release and thirst in human pregnancy. Role of human chorionic gonadotrophin in the osmoregulatory changes of gestation. *J Clin Invest* 1988;**81**:798–806.

7. Williams DJ, Metcalfe KA, Skingle L, Stock AI, Beedham T, Monson JP. Pathophysiology of transient cranial diabetes insipidus during pregnancy. *Clin Endocrinol* 1993;**38**:595–600.

8. Steer PJ. Maternal haemoglobin concentration and birth weight. *Am J Clin Nutr* 2000;**71** Suppl:1285S–87S.

9. Prentice A. Calcium in pregnancy and lactation. *Annu Rev Nutr* 2000;**20**:249–72.

10. Williams D, Davison JM. Chronic kidney disease in pregnancy. *BMJ* 2008;**336**:211–15.

11. Davidson NL, Wolski P, Callaway LK, et al. Chronic kidney disease in pregnancy: maternal and fetal outcomes and progression of kidney disease. *Obstet Med* 2015;**8**:92–98.

12. Coomarasamy A, Honest H, Papaioannou S, Gee H, Khan KS. Aspirin for prevention of preeclampsia in women with historical risk factors: a systematic review. *Obstet Gynecol* 2003;**101**:1319–32.

13. Verdonk K, Niemeijer IC, Hop WC, et al. Variation of urinary protein to creatinine ratio during the day in women with suspected pre-eclampsia. *BJOG* 2014;**121**:1660–65.

14. Visintin C, Mugglestone MA, Almerie MQ, et al. Management of hypertensive disorders during pregnancy: summary of NICE guidance. *BMJ* 2010;**341**:c2207.

15. Lopes van Balen VA, Spaan JJ, Cornelis T, Spaanderman MEA. Prevalence of chronic kidney disease after preeclampsia. *J Nephrol* 2017;**30**:403–409.

16. Berks D, Steegers EA, Molas M, Visser W. Resolution of hypertension and proteinuria after preeclampsia. *Obstet Gynecol* 2009;**114**:1307–14.

17. Bellamy L, Casas JP, Hingorani AD, Williams DJ. Pre-eclampsia and risk of cardiovascular disease and cancer in later life: systematic review and meta-analysis. *BMJ* 2007;**335**:974.

18. Hypertension in pregnancy. Report of the American College of Obstetrics and Gynecologists' task force on hypertension in pregnancy. *Obstet Gynecol* 2013;**122**:1122–31.

19. Drakely AJ, Le Roux PA, Anthony J, Penny J. Acute renal failure complicating severe pre-eclampsia requiring admission to an obstetric intensive care unit. *Am J Obstet Gynecol* 2002;**186**:253–56.

20. Hildebrand AM, Liu K, Shariff SZ, et al. Characteristics and outcomes of AKI treated with dialysis during pregnancy and the postpartum period. *J Am Soc Nephrol* 2016;**26**:3085–91.

21. Tangren JS, Powe CE, Ankers E, et al. Pregnancy outcomes after clinical recovery from AKI. *J Am Soc Nephrol* 2017;**28**:1566–74.

22. Scully M, Cataland S, Coppo P, et al. Consensus on the standardization of terminology in thrombotic thrombocytopenic purpura and related thrombotic microangiopathies. *J Thromb Haemost* 2017;**15**:312–22.

23. Fakhouri F, Zuber J, Fremeaux-Bacchi V, Loirat C. Haemolytic uraemic syndrome. *Lancet* 2017;**390**:681–96.

24. Pauzner R, Dulitzky M, Carp H, et al. Hepatic infarctions during pregnancy are associated with the antiphospholipid syndrome and in addition with complete or incomplete HELLP syndrome. *J Thromb Haemost* 2003;**8**:1758–63.

25. Thomas MR, Robinson S, Scully MA. How we manage thrombotic microangiopathies in pregnancy. *Br J Haematol* 2016;**173**:821–30.

26. Prakash J, Singh VP. Changing picture of renal cortical necrosis in acute kidney injury in developing country. *World J Nephrol* 2015;**4**:480–86.

27. Frimat M, Decambron M, Lebas C, et al. Renal cortical necrosis in postpartum haemorrhage: a case series. *Am J Kidney Dis* 2016;**68**:50–57.

28. Woman Trial Collaborators. Effect of early tranexamic acid administration on mortality, hysterectomy, and other morbidities in women with post-partum haemorrhage (WOMAN): an international, randomised, double blind, placebo-controlled trial. *Lancet* 2017;**389**:2105–16.

29. Knight M, Nelson-Piercy C, Kurinczuk JJ, et al. A prospective national study of acute fatty liver of pregnancy in the UK. *Gut* 2008;**57**:951–56.

30. Yang Z, Zhao Y, Bennett MJ, Strauss AW, Ibdah JA. Fetal genotypes and pregnancy outcomes in 35 families with mitochondrial trifunctional protein mutations. *Am J Obstet Gynaecol* 2002;**187**:715–20.

31. Carmelina G, Garovic VD, Gullo A, et al. Kidney injury during pregnancy: associated comorbid conditions and outcomes. *Arch Gynecol Obstet* 2012;**286**:567–73.

32. Semins MJ, Matlaga BR. Kidney stones during pregnancy. *Nat Rev Urol* 2014;**11**:163–68.

33. Masselli G, Weston M, Spencer J. The role of imaging in the diagnosis and management of renal stone disease in pregnancy. *Clin Radiol* 2015;1462–71.

34. Zhang S, Liu G, Duo Y, et al. Application of ureteroscope in emergency treatment with persistent renal colic patients during pregnancy. *PLOS One* 2016;**11**;e0146597.

35. Gregory MC, Mansell MA. Pregnancy and cystinuria. *Lancet* 1983;**2**:1158–60.

36. Hoeltzenbein M, Stieler K, Panse M, Wacker E, Schaefer C. Allopurinol use during pregnancy: outcome of 31 prospectively ascertained cases and a phenotype possibly indicative for teratogenicity. *PLOS One* 2013;**8**:e66637.

37. Khati NJ, Frazier AA, Brindle KA. The unicornuate uterus and its variants. *J Ultrasound Med* 2012;**31**:319–31.

38. Wolff JM, Jung PK, Adam G, Jakse G. Non-traumatic rupture of the urinary tract during pregnancy. *Br J Urol* 1995;**76**:645–48.

39. Gait JE. Hemolytic reactions to nitrofurantoin in patients with glucose-6-phosphate dehydrogenase deficiency: theory and practice. *DICP* 1990;**24**:1210–13.

40. Hernandez-Diaz S, Werler MM, Walker AM, Mitchell AA. Neural tube defects in relation to use of folic acid antagonists during pregnancy. *Am J Epidemiol* 2001;**15**:961–68.

41. Davenport M, Mach KE, Dairiki Shortliffe LM, et al. New and developing diagnostic technologies for urinary tract infections. *Nat Rev Urol* 2017;**14**:296–310.

42. Rogozinska E, Formina S, Zamora J, et al. Accuracy of onsite tests to detect asymptomatic bacteriuria in pregnancy: a systematic review and meta-analysis. *Obstet Gynecol* 2016;**128**;495–503.

43. Kincaid Smith P, Bullen M. Bacteriuria in pregnancy. *Lancet* 1965;**191**:359–99.

44. Kazemier BM, Koningstein FN, Schneeberger C, et al. Maternal and neonatal consequences of treated and untreated asymptomatic bacteriuria in pregnancy: a prospective cohort study with an embedded randomised controlled trial. *Lancet Infect Dis* 2015;**15**:1324–33.

45. Smaill F. Antibiotics for asymptomatic bacteriuria in pregnancy. *Cochrane Database Syst Rev* 2001;**2**;CD000490.

46. Romero R, Oyarzun E, Mazor M, et al. Meta-analysis of the relationship between asymptomatic bacteriuria and preterm delivery/low birth weight. *Obstet Gynecol* 1989;**73**:576–82.

47. Dwyer PL, O'Reilly M. Recurrent urinary tract infection in the female. *Curr Opin Obstet Gynaecol* 2002;**14**:537–43.

48. Wing DA, Fassett MJ, Getahun D. Acute pyelonephritis in pregnancy: an 18-year retrospective analysis. *Am J Obstet Gynecol* 2014;**210**:219.e1–6.

49. Farkash E, Weintraub AY, Sergienko R, et al. Acute antepartum pyelonephritis in pregnancy: a critical analysis of risk factors and outcomes. *Eur J Obstet Gynecol Reprod Biol* 2012;**162**:24–27.

50. Duff P. Antibiotic selection in obstetrics: making cost-effective choices. *Clin Obstet Gynaecol* 2002;**45**:59–72.

51. Wing DA. Pyelonephritis in pregnancy. Treatment options for optimal outcomes. *Drugs* 2001;**61**:2087–96.

52. Imbasciati E, Gregorinin G, Cabiddu G, et al. Pregnancy in CKD stages 3 to 5: fetal and maternal outcomes. *Am J Kidney Dis* 2007;**49**:753–62.

53. Bramham K, Briley AL, Seed PT, et al. Pregnancy outcome in women with chronic kidney disease: a prospective cohort study. *Reprod Sci* 2011;**18**:623–30.

54. Munkhaugen J, Lydersen S, Romundstad PR, et al. Kidney function and future risk for adverse pregnancy outcomes: a population-based study from HUNT II, Norway. *Nephrol Dial Transplant* 2009;**24**:3744–50.

55. Piccoli GB, Attini R, Vasario E, et al. Pregnancy and chronic kidney disease: a challenge in all CKD stages. *Clin J Am Soc Nephrol* 2010;**5**:844–55.

56. Kidney Disease: Improving Global Outcomes (KDIGO) CKD Work Group. KDIGO clinical practice guideline for the evaluation and management of chronic kidney disease. *Kidney Int Suppl* 2013;**3**:1–150.

57. Murakami S, Saitoh M, Kubo T, Koyama T, Kobayashi M. Renal disease in women with severe preeclampsia or gestational proteinuria. *Obstet Gynecol* 2000;**96**:945–49.

58. Jungers P, Chauveau D, Choukroun G, et al. Pregnancy in women with impaired renal function. *Clin Nephrol* 1997;**47**:281–88.

59. Cunningham FG, Cox SM, Harstad TW, Mason RA, Pritchard JA. Chronic renal disease and pregnancy outcome. *Am J Obstet Gynecol* 1990;**163**:453–59.

60. Jungers P, Houillier P, Forget D, et al. Influence of pregnancy on the course of primary chronic glomerulonephritis. *Lancet* 1995;**346**:1122–24.

61. Jones DC, Hayslett JP. Outcome of pregnancy in women with moderate or severe renal insufficiency. *N Eng J Med* 1996;**335**:226–32.

62. Visintin C, Mugglestone MA, Almerie MQ, et al. Management of hypertensive disorders during pregnancy: summary of NICE guidance. *BMJ* 2010;**341**:c20207.

63. Packham DK, North RA, Fairley KF, et al. Primary glomerulonephritis and pregnancy. *QJM* 1989;**266**:537–53.

64. Lupton M, Williams DJ. The ethics of research on pregnant women: is maternal consent sufficient? *BJOG* 2004;**111**:1307–12.

65. Wyatt RJ, Julian BA. IgA nephropathy. *N Engl J Med* 2013;**368**:2402–14.

66. Su X, Lv J, Liu Y, et al. Pregnancy and kidney outcomes in patients with IgA nephropathy: a cohort study. *Am J Kidney Dis* 2017;**70**:262–69.

67. Liu Y, Ma X, Zheng J, Liu X, Yan T. A systematic review and meta-analysis of kidney and pregnancy outcomes in IgA nephropathy. *Am J Nephrol* 2016;**44**:187–93.

68. Ronkainen J, Nuutinen M, Koskimies O. The adult kidney 24 years after childhood Henoch-Schönlein purpura: a retrospective cohort study. *Lancet* 2002;**360**:666–70.

69. Lech M, Anders H-J. The pathogenesis of lupus nephritis. *J Am Soc Nephrol* 2013;**24**:1357–66.

70. Wakasugi D, Gono T, Kawaguchi Y, et al. Frequency of class III and IV nephritis in systemic lupus erythematosus without clinical renal involvement: an analysis of predictive measures. *J Rheumatol* 2012;**39**:79–85.

71. Buyon JP, Kim MY, Guerra MM, et al. Predictors of pregnancy outcome in a prospective, multi-ethnic cohort of lupus patients. *Ann Intern Med* 2015;**163**:153–63.

72. Buyon JP, Kim MY, Guerra MM, et al. Kidney outcomes and risk factors for nephritis (flare/de novo) in a multi-ethnic cohort of pregnant patients with lupus nephritis. *Clin J Am Soc Nephrol* 2017;**12**:940–46.

73. Moroni G, Doria A, Giglio E, et al. Maternal outcome in pregnant women with lupus nephritis. A prospective multicentre study. *J Autoimmun* 2016;**74**:194–200.

74. Bertsias GK, Tektonidou M, Amoura Z, et al. Joint European League Against Rheumatism and European Renal Association-European Dialysis and Transplant Association (EULAR/ERA-EDTA) recommendations for the management of adult and paediatric lupus nephritis. *Ann Rheum Dis* 2012;**71**:1771–82.

75. Moroni G, Doria A, Giglio E, et al. Fetal outcomes and recommendations of pregnancies in lupus nephritis in the 21st century. A prospective multicentre study. *J Autoimmunity* 2016;**74**:6–12.

76. Flint J, Panchal S, Hurrell A, et al. BSR and BHPR guideline on prescribing drugs in pregnancy and breastfeeding – Part 1: standard and biologic disease modifying anti-rheumatic drugs and corticosteroids. *Rheumatology (Oxford)* 2016;**55**:1693–97.

77. Fischer-Betz R, Specker C, Brinks R, et al. Low risk of renal flares and negative outcomes in women with lupus nephritis conceiving after switching from mycophenolate mofetil to azathioprine. *Rheumatology* 2013;**52**:1070–76.

78. Chapman AB, Johnson AM, Gabow PA. Pregnancy outcome and its relationship to progression of renal failure in autosomal dominant polycystic kidney disease. *J Am Soc Nephrol* 1994;**5**:1178–85.

79. Torres VE, Chapman AB, Devuyst O, et al. Multicenter, open-label, extension trial to evaluate the long-term efficacy and safety of early versus delayed treatment with tolvaptan in autosomal dominant polycystic kidney disease: the TEMPO 4:4 trial. *Nephrol Dial Transplant* 2018;**33**:477–89.

80. Jungers P, Houillier P, Chauveau D, et al. Pregnancy in women with reflux nephropathy. *Kidney Int* 1996;**50**:593–99.

81. North RA, Taylor RS, Gunn TR. Pregnancy outcome in women with reflux nephropathy and the inheritance of vesico-ureteric reflux. *Aust N Z J Obstet Gynaecol* 2000;**40**:280–85.

82. Collins AJ, Foley RN, Herzog C, et al. US Renal Data System 2010 Annual Data Report. *Am J Kidney Dis* 2011;**57** 1 Suppl 1:A8. e1–526.

83. Damm JA, Asbjornsdottir B, Callesen NF, et al. Diabetic nephropathy and microalbuminuria in pregnant women with type 1 and type 2 diabetes. *Diabetes Care* 2013:**36**:3489–94.

84. Nielsen LR, Muller C, Damm P, et al. Reduced prevalence of early preterm delivery in women with type 1 diabetes and microalbuminuria—possible effect of early antihypertensive treatment during pregnancy. *Diabet Med* 2006;**23**:426–31.

85. Klemetti MM, Laivouri H, Tikkanen M, et al. Obstetric and perinatal outcome in type 1 diabetes with diabetic nephropathy during 1988-2011. *Diabetologia* 2015;**58**:678–86.

86. Purdy LP, Hantsch CE, Molitch ME, et al. Effect of pregnancy on renal function in patients with moderate to severe diabetic renal insufficiency. *Diabetes Care* 1996;**19**:1067–74.

87. Hladunewich M, Schatell D. Intensive dialysis and pregnancy. *Hemodial Int* 2016;**20**:339–48.

88. Hladunewich M, Hou S, Odutayo A, et al. Intensive hemodialysis associates with improved pregnancy outcomes: a Canadian and United States cohort comparison. *J Am Soc Nephrol* 2014;**25**:1103–109.

89. Cabiddu C, Castellino S, Gernone G, et al. Best practices on pregnancy on dialysis: the Italian study group on kidney and pregnancy. *J Nephrol* 2015;**28**:279–88.

90. Jesudason S, Grace BS, McDonald SP. Pregnancy outcomes according to dialysis commencing before or after conception in women with ESRD. *Clin J Am Soc Nephrol* 2014;**9**:143–49.

91. Coscia LA, Constantinescu S, Moritz MJ, et al. Report from the national transplantation pregnancy registry (NTPR): outcomes of pregnancy after transplantation. *Clin Transpl* 2010;**7**:65–85.

92. Richman K, Gohh R. Pregnancy after renal transplantation: a review of registry and single-centre practices and outcomes. *Nephrol Dial Transplant* 2012;**27**:3428–34.

93. Kim H, Jeong JC, Yang J, et al. The optimal therapy of calcineurin inhibitors for pregnancy in kidney transplantation. *Clin Transplant* 2015;**29**:142–48.

94. Kutzler HL, Ye X, Rochon C, martin ST. Administration of antithymocyte globulin (rabbit) to treat a severe mixed rejection episode in a pregnant renal transplant recipient. *Pharmacotherapy* 2016:**36**:e18–22.

15

Haematological disorders in pregnancy

Amanda Ali and Hassan Shehata

Antiphospholipid syndrome in obstetrics

Definition

Antiphospholipid syndrome (APS) is an autoimmune condition characterized by recurrent arterial or venous thromboembolic episodes and adverse pregnancy outcomes such as recurrent miscarriage, stillbirth, and severe pre-eclampsia/toxaemia (PET); in association with persistent antiphospholipid antibodies.

The antibodies associated with this condition are lupus anticoagulant, anticardiolipin, and anti-beta-2 glycoprotein-1. APS and antiphospholipid antibodies can occur in isolation as primary APS or secondary, in association with other diseases such as systemic lupus erythematosus.

Background

Antiphospholipid antibodies can be found in up to 1–5% of healthy women, this rises to 15% in women with recurrent miscarriages and up to 20% in women having a stroke before the age of 50 (1). Recent studies reported a lower prevalence in women with recurrent miscarriage, when current diagnostic criteria for positive antiphospholipid antibodies were followed (2).

Thrombosis may occur in 30% of patients with antiphospholipid antibodies, and 30% of women with severe early PET may have positive antibodies (3).

The prevalence of APS in the general population is 0.5% (4); the female-to-male ratio is 3.5:1 in primary disease, and 7:1 in secondary disease related to systemic lupus erythematosus, with a mortality rate of 5% (5). Approximately 30–40% of patients with systemic lupus erythematosus have antiphospholipid antibodies.

Pathogenesis

The hallmarks of APS are thrombosis and inflammation in the venous and arterial beds and placental circulation leading to placental insufficiency. Placental thrombosis is not exclusive to patients with APS, and may be seen in patients with PET. Conversely; inflammation rather than thrombosis may be found in some patients with APS and obstetric complications (6, 7).

Endothelial cells, neutrophils, monocytes, platelets, cytokines, and complement all contribute to thrombosis and fetal loss.

Antiphospholipid antibodies binding to negative phospholipids and protein-binding phospholipids may trigger endothelial activation, which in turn plays a role in abnormal placentation (8). Activated endothelial cells upregulate tissue factor production, which initiates a coagulation cascade and plays a key role in thrombosis and inflammation and the hypercoagulability state seen in APS (9). There is also trophoblast dysfunction and impaired transplacental exchange which leads to early miscarriage, PET, fetal growth restriction, and fetal death (10).

Effect of pregnancy on APS

The prothrombotic state in pregnancy increases the risk of new-onset, and recurrent venous (deep vein thrombosis and pulmonary embolism) and arterial (stroke and transient ischaemic attacks) thrombosis, which classically recur in the same region as previous thrombotic events (3).

There is also a risk of worsening of pre-existing thrombocytopenia.

Effect of APS on pregnancy

There is an increased risk of maternal and fetal complications (5, 11, 12), this risk is particularly raised in patients with lupus antibodies (13).

Maternal

- PET, which is usually of early onset and severe
- Eclampsia
- Haemolysis, elevated liver enzymes, and low platelets (HELLP) complete or partial syndrome
- Placental abruption
- Catastrophic APS—some studies have shown a 0.9% occurrence of this rare life threatening cause of multiorgan failure in pregnancy (5).

Fetal

- Recurrent miscarriages
- Intrauterine fetal growth restriction
- Preterm labour
- Intrauterine fetal death.

Classification criteria and diagnosis

The presence of antiphospholipid antibodies alone does not constitute APS. The international classification criteria—*Sapporo criteria*—were introduced in 1998 and revised in 2008 (14). To fulfil

Table 15.1 Revised classification criteria for antiphospholipid syndrome

Clinical criteria	Laboratory criteria
Vascular thrombosis • One or more clinical episodes of arterial, venous, or small vessel thrombosis, in any tissue or organ • Thrombosis must be confirmed by objective validated criteria (i.e. unequivocal findings of appropriate imaging studies or histopathology). For histopathological confirmation, thrombosis should be present without significant evidence of inflammation in the vessel wall	• Lupus anticoagulant present in plasma, on two or more occasions at least 12 weeks apart, detected according to the guidelines of the International Society on Thrombosis and Haemostasis (Scientific Subcommittee on Lupus anticoagulant/phospholipid-dependent antibodies) • Anticardiolipin antibody of IgG, IgM isotype, or both, in serum or plasma, present in medium or high titres (i.e. >40 GPL or MPL, or greater than the 99th percentile), on two or more occasions, at least 12 weeks apart, measured by a standardized enzyme-linked immunosorbent assay • Anti-β_2 glycoprotein-I antibody of IgG, IgM isotype, or both, in serum or plasma (in titres greater than the 99th percentile), present on two or more occasions, at least 12 weeks apart, measured by a standardized enzyme-linked immunosorbent assay, according to recommended procedures
Pregnancy morbidity[a] • (a) One or more unexplained deaths of a morphologically normal fetus at or beyond the 10th week of gestation, with normal fetal morphology documented by ultrasound or by direct examination of the fetus; OR • (b) one or more premature births of a morphologically normal neonate before the 34th week of gestation because of (1) eclampsia or severe pre–eclampsia defined according to standard definitions or (2) recognized features of placental failure; OR • (c) three or more unexplained consecutive spontaneous abortions before the 10th week of gestation, with no maternal anatomic or hormonal abnormalities and paternal and maternal chromosomal causes excluded	

IgG, immunoglobulin G; IgM, immunoglobulin M.

[a] In studies of populations of women who have more than one type of pregnancy morbidity, investigators are strongly encouraged to stratify groups of women according to a, b, c as listed.

Reproduced from Miyakis S, Lockshin MD, Atsumi T, et al. International consensus statement on an update of the classification criteria for definite antiphospholipid syndrome (APS). *J Thromb Haemost.* 2006;4:295–306 with permission from John Wiley and Sons.

the criteria, there must be at least one clinical feature—thrombosis or pregnancy morbidity—in addition to at least one laboratory abnormality including lupus anticoagulant, anticardiolipin, and anti-beta-2 glycoprotein-1 antibodies detected in medium or high titre on two occasions at least 12 weeks apart. Classification details are shown in Table 15.1.

Early recognition of APS helps prevent thrombosis and adverse obstetric outcomes. Situations (12, 15, 16) where patients should be tested for antiphospholipid antibodies are summarized in Box 15.1.

Management

Preconceptual care

Prepregnancy counselling is recommended to discuss the risk of potential complications and formulate a management plan (17):

• Women with a history of recurrent miscarriage, intrauterine fetal death, early-onset PET, severe fetal growth restriction,

Box 15.1 Situations in which antiphospholipid antibodies should be tested

• Systemic autoimmune diseases carriers.
• Women who have a history of:
  – recurrent miscarriages
  – fetal loss after 10 weeks' gestation
  – severe early intrauterine fetal growth restriction
  – stillbirth
  – early onset severe pre-eclampsia or eclampsia (<34 weeks of gestational age)

or thrombosis should be screened for lupus anticoagulant or anticardiolipin antibodies.
• A detailed obstetric history and history of previous thrombotic events should be obtained. In patients with APS, previous obstetric outcome is the best predictor of pregnancy outcome.
• Women on long-term warfarin should be counselled about the teratogenic effects and a plan made to convert to low-molecular-weight heparin either before or shortly after conception.
• Low-dose aspirin (75–150 mg) is recommended preconceptually because of its antithrombotic effect (18) and its role in reducing the risk of PET (19).

Antenatal care

A multidisciplinary team should be involved in the management of pregnant patients with APS.

Women with antiphospholipid antibodies, with no history of adverse obstetric outcome and no history of thrombosis

There is no robust data to guide treatment of these patients; however, some studies have shown an increase rate of pregnancy loss in this group (20). The consensus is to commence low-dose aspirin for the duration of pregnancy.

Women with APS, but no history of thrombosis

Meta-analysis of trials comparing the use of a combination of aspirin and low-molecular-weight heparin (LMWH) versus aspirin alone in this group of patients has shown a reduction of pregnancy loss (21, 22) and increased life birth rates (23). These studies, however, have several limitations including sample size, poor study design,

Table 15.2 Recommended treatment of APS in pregnancy

Antiphospholipid syndrome with poor obstetric outcomes	Antiphospholipid syndrome with thrombosis
Recurrent early (pre-embryonic or embryonic) miscarriage: low dose aspirin alone or plus: low-molecular-weight heparin: usual thromboprophylactic doses (e.g. enoxaparin 40 mg/d sc. or dalteparin 5000 U/d sc. or tinzaparin 4500 U/day sc.)	Low-dose aspirin plus: Low-molecular-weight heparin: full anticoagulation doses (e.g. enoxaparin 1 mg/kg sc. or dalteparin 100 U/kg, sc. every 12 h or enoxaparin 1.5 mg/kg/day sc. or dalteparin 200 U/kg/day sc.)
	In all cases associate supplementary:
	calcium 1000 mg/day
	vitamin D 800 IU/day
Fetal death (>10 weeks' gestation) or prior early delivery (<34 weeks' gestation) due to severe pre-eclampsia or placental insufficiency: low-dose aspirin plus: low-molecular-weight heparin: usual thromboprophylactic doses (e.g. enoxaparin 40 mg/day sc. or dalteparin 5000 U/day sc or tinzaparin 4500 U/day sc.)	

sc., subcutaneous.

Reproduced from Ruiz-Irastorza G, Crowther M, Branch W et al. Antiphospholipid syndrome. *Lancet* 2010; 376: 1498–1509 with permission from Elsevier.

and inconsistent selection criteria. Due to a lack of robust evidence to support aspirin alone or combination therapy, an individualized assessment by the obstetrician and haematologist and a discussion with the woman is recommended to formulate a management plan. Table 15.2 summarizes a suggested treatment protocol.

Women with APS, plus a history of thromboembolism

This group of women are at a significant risk of further thrombosis during pregnancy and during the puerperium. It is imperative that these women are started on a therapeutic dose of LMWH (e.g. dalteparin 100 IU/kg twice daily) as early as possible.

Some women may already be on long-term anticoagulation with warfarin; it is important to switch to LMWH preconceptually or prior to 6 weeks' gestation to avoid the teratogenic side effects of warfarin. A therapeutic dose of LMWH is needed in this high-risk group of women due to the magnified risk of thrombosis in pregnancy.

An increased risk of thromboembolism continues up to 12 weeks postnatally (24); however, the absolute risk beyond 6 weeks is small. Therefore, thromboprophylaxis beyond 6 weeks is usually only needed for very high-risk women, such as those on long-term anticoagulation outside of pregnancy.

Surveillance during pregnancy

These women should be seen in an obstetric medicine or high-risk pregnancy clinic throughout pregnancy, with regular visits every 4–6 weeks initially and more frequent visits towards the end of pregnancy or if complications arise:

- Regular blood pressure monitoring and urine analysis to detect the development of PET.
- Uterine artery Doppler assessment is recommended at around 20 weeks and repeated at 24 weeks of gestation if abnormal, to predict PET and placental insufficiency (25).
- Regular ultrasounds for fetal growth, umbilical artery Doppler, and amniotic fluid index is recommended to detect fetal growth restriction and placental insufficiency (26).

Postpartum care

- Women who were on long-term warfarin prior to pregnancy may be recommended on it 5–7 days postnatally provided that there are no ongoing obstetric risk factors.
- Oestrogen-containing contraceptives are contraindicated due to the significant risk of thrombosis (27).
- Both heparin and warfarin are safe to use while breastfeeding (28).

Disseminated intravascular coagulation in obstetrics

Definition

Disseminated intravascular coagulation (DIC) is a serious life-threatening condition in which endothelial damage leads to activation of the haemostatic system, microvascular thrombosis, and activation of the coagulation system leading to increased production and degradation of coagulation factors (29). This leads to uncontrolled bleeding, microthrombi, and thrombi in small and large vessels (30), which if untreated leads to complete consumption of coagulation factors and ultimately death.

DIC is not a disease in itself; it is usually secondary to an underlying disorder that leads to activation of the coagulation system.

Causes of DIC in obstetrics

The incidence of DIC in pregnancy is influenced by patient demographics and variations in obstetric practice; studies have reported figures ranging from 0.03% (31) to 0.35% (32).

The main causes of DIC in obstetric patients are as follows:

- Obstetric haemorrhage:
  - Antepartum haemorrhage—particularly placental abruption
  - Intrapartum and postpartum haemorrhage
- Hypertensive disorders:
  - PET
  - Eclampsia
  - Haemolysis, elevated liver enzymes, and low platelets (HELLP) syndrome
  - Acute fatty liver of pregnancy
- Sepsis
- Amniotic fluid embolism
- Retained dead fetus

Diagnosis

There is no single specific test to diagnose DIC and the majority of diagnosis lies in clinical assessment. An important message is that due to the dynamic process of DIC; tests need to be repeated during the clinical incident to reflect the progression and response to treatment. A downward trend is diagnostic of DIC.

- Thrombocytopenia—low platelet count is the commonest feature seen, although levels may be normal in the early stages of DIC.
- Prolonged prothrombin time, thrombin time, and activated partial thromboplastin time.
- Reduced fibrinogen—fibrinogen levels are usually higher in pregnancy, so a fibrinogen level of less than 2 g/L is diagnostic.
- Increased fibrinogen degradation products.
- Point-of-care testing—novel methods such as thromboelastography and thromboelastometry can be used to provide rapid results in the acute setting (33).

Management

There are four elements to managing patients with DIC (1) treatment of the underlying cause; (2) multidisciplinary care and early specialist involvement; (3) correction of coagulopathy with blood and blood products; and (4) serial clinical and laboratory assessment.

Obstetric haemorrhage, hypertensive disorders, and sepsis should be managed in line with current Royal College of Obstetricians and Gynaecologists (RCOG) guidance and local agreed protocols, in conjunction with anaesthetic, haematology, and microbiology teams.

Treatment of coagulopathy:

- Blood (red cell) transfusion—each unit increases the haemoglobin count by 1 g/dL and the haematocrit by 3%.
- Fresh frozen plasma—contains all the coagulation factors, a ratio of fresh frozen plasma:red cell transfusion of 1:1 reduces coagulopathy in obstetric haemorrhage (34, 35).
- Cryoprecipitate—especially recommended if fibrinogen level is less than 1.5 g/L—two pools of cryoprecipitate will raise the fibrinogen level by 1 g/L if there is no continued bleeding.
- Fibrinogen concentrate.
- Platelet transfusion—may be given in obstetric haemorrhage if platelet count is less than 80×10^9/L.
- Recombinant factor VIIa—is expensive but effective in controlling massive obstetric haemorrhage (36). It should be reserved to cases that are refractory to treatment with conventional methods (37).
- Repeated measurement of haemoglobin, platelet count, and coagulation profile including fibrinogen is essential to guide management and assess response to treatment.

Due to the pathophysiology of DIC, there is also an additional increased risk of thrombosis.

Patients must have measures to reduce the risk of thromboembolism such as compression stockings initially and thromboprophylaxis once the coagulopathy is corrected and there are no further ongoing risks of haemorrhage.

Inherited bleeding disorders in pregnancy

Women with inherited bleeding disorders face multiple challenges in pregnancy and delivery. A multidisciplinary approach to management reduces maternal and fetal morbidity and mortality.

The commonest inherited bleeding disorder is von Willebrand disease (vWD), followed by haemophilia A and haemophilia B.

Rarer types of bleeding disorders include fibrinogen, factor II, V, VIII, VII, X, XI, XIII deficiencies, and multiple deficiencies of vitamin K-dependent factors.

Physiological changes in pregnancy

Multiple haemostatic changes occur in normal pregnancy to prepare for the challenges of delivery. These changes also occur in women with bleeding disorders and may act to normalize their existing haemostatic abnormality. There is a large variation in this response however, even in women with the same condition. The various changes are summarized in Table 15.3.

Von Willebrand disease

This is the commonest inherited bleeding disorder, occurring in about 1% of the general population (38, 39). The mode of inheritance is usually autosomal dominant, and it is due to either a quantitative or qualitative defect in von Willebrand factor (vWF) which acts as a carrier for factor VIII. There are three types of vWD: type 1, which is due to partial deficiency of vWF, is autosomal dominant, usually mild, and accounts for 70–80% of cases. Type 2, is due to a functional defect in the vWF protein, has four subtypes based on pathogenesis, and is also autosomal dominant. Type 3, due to a complete absence of vWF, is autosomal recessive and typically severe.

Diagnosis

There is no single simple test to diagnose vWD; the diagnosis is made using a combination of specific investigations.

vWF and FVIII levels may be reduced and the activated partial thromboplastin time may be prolonged. Specific tests to measure vWF activity using ristocetin cofactor may be used in addition to a quantitative immunoassay assessment of vWf (vWf:Ag).

Due to the physiological increase in vWF levels in pregnancy, most women have uncomplicated pregnancies and usually do not have complications such as antepartum haemorrhage (40, 41). This rise is not as established in the first trimester, so these women do have an increased risk of bleeding with miscarriage and ectopic pregnancies. Due to the dramatic decrease in vWF levels postnatally,

Table 15.3 Haemostatic changes during normal pregnancy

Clotting factors	Changes
Fibrinogen	Increase
FVII	Increase
FVIII	Increase
FX	Increase
FXII	Increase
vWF	Increase
FII	No significant change
FV	No significant change
FIX	No significant change
FXI	Inconsistent
FXIII	Decrease

F, factor; vWF, von Willebrand factor.

these women are at a significant risk of primary and secondary post-partum haemorrhage.

Haemophilia A and B

Haemophilia A is caused by a deficient or defective coagulation factor VIII and haemophilia B is caused by a deficient or defective coagulation factor IX. They are X-linked recessive conditions, therefore males are affected and females are obligate carriers. Haemophilia can cause significant complications such as bruising, muscle and joint bleeding, spontaneous bleeding, bleeding after surgery, and intracranial bleeding. Carriers of haemophilia usually have a clotting factor level of 50% of normal and are therefore also at risk of bleeding complications.

Some studies have shown an increased risk of miscarriage and bleeding in pregnancy in haemophilia carriers (42–44), but at present the evidence is not robust enough to support antenatal prophylaxis to prevent early pregnancy loss. Replacement may be indicated, however, in some women with significant bleeding.

Preconceptual counselling

Preconceptual counselling is important in patients who are either affected or are carriers of a bleeding disorder to allow appropriate counselling and discuss the option of prenatal diagnosis, and make an appropriate plan for pregnancy and delivery, and perform a trial of desmopressin if indicated.

It is also an opportunity to discuss and arrange hepatitis immunization for women who are more likely to need blood transfusions during pregnancy.

Prenatal diagnosis

Prenatal diagnosis is a vital part of the management of patients with bleeding disorders, specifically in patients who are haemophilia carriers, as they have a 50% chance of having an affected male fetus and a 50% chance of a carrier female. Invasive diagnostic tests such as chorionic villous sampling and amniocentesis are available, but they are associated with a risk of miscarriage of approximately 1%. The uptake of prenatal diagnosis and termination for patients with haemophilia remains generally low (45)—possibly due to the effect that improvement in management has made to the quality of life of most affected individuals.

Preimplantation genetic diagnosis using *in vitro* fertilization to selectively transfer unaffected embryos is another option. **Table 15.4** summarizes the options for prenatal diagnosis.

Antenatal care

Patients with inherited bleeding disorders should be cared for in an obstetric medicine clinic, or by obstetricians who have experience in managing high-risk pregnancies with close liaison with a haematologist:

- Clotting factors levels should be checked at booking if there are no recent prepregnancy readings, and they should ideally be repeated at 28 and 34 weeks' gestation, specifically in women with low levels prior to pregnancy.
- Desmopressin, fibrinogen concentrate, recombinant factor VIII, platelets, and plasma have all been used to manage bleeding disorders. These are all specialised treatments and should only be used by experienced clinicians and in conjunction with a

Table 15.4 Prenatal diagnosis options for haemophilia carriers

Prenatal testing	Timing (weeks gestation)	Risk of miscarriage (%)	Comments
Non-invasive determination of fetal gender			
ffDNA	≥6–8	–	Currently only available in certain centres
USS	11–14	–	First-trimester USS fetal sexing available at certain centres
	≥15	–	
Prenatal diagnosis of haemophilia			
ffDNA	≥6–8	–	Under research, case report
CVS	11–14	1–2	Known causative mutation
Amniocentesis	≥15	1	Known causative mutation
Cordocentesis	18–20	1–2	Causative mutation unknown

CVS, chorionic villus sampling; ffDNA, free fetal DNA in maternal blood; USS, ultrasound

haematologist. Recombinant products are preferable to reduce the risk of viral transmission. Treatment options are summarized in **Table 15.5**.

- A clear plan for delivery must be made and documented in the patient's notes; this plan should also include provisions for unexpected early delivery. There is no evidence to suggest a caesarean section for all women; a careful assessment must be made antenatally to highlight any additional risk factors that may affect the mode of delivery

Intrapartum care

- Intravenous access, full blood count, coagulation screen, and a sample for group and antibody screen should be taken upon arrival to the delivery suite.
- Clotting factor levels are generally not available in an emergency, so clinicians should be guided by third-trimester levels.
- Knowledge of fetal sex is useful, but since it is not always available, it is recommended to follow the same plan for all patients as there is a 50% chance of a male fetus.
- Fetal scalp electrode and fetal blood sampling should not be performed—a caesarean section should be carried out if there is a suspicion of fetal distress (46).
- Delivery by vacuum, mid-cavity, or rotational forceps should be avoided due to the high risk of cephalohaematoma and intracranial bleeding (47).
- Delivery by outlet forceps may be considered as it is safer than a caesarean section in advanced labour. This should be conducted by a senior practitioner to minimise the risk of potential complications.
- The majority of haemophilia A carriers do not need prophylactic cover during labour unless their levels are persistently low at term (48–50). Conversely, the majority of haemophilia B carriers will have persistently low levels and require treatment in labour to maintain factor levels greater than 50 IU/dL.

Table 15.5 Therapeutic options for women with inherited bleeding disorders in pregnancy.

Bleeding disorder	Preferred therapeutic option	Other options
vWD	Desmopressin or vWF-containing concentrates	Platelet (type 2B)
		rFVIII or FVIII concentrate (type 2N)
Carriers of haemophilia A	Desmopressin or rFVIII	FVIII concentrate
Carriers of haemophilia B	rFIX	FIX concentrate
Fibrinogen abnormalities	Fibrinogen concentrate	SD plasma
Prothrombin II deficiency	PCC	SD plasma
FV deficiency	SD plasma	SD plasma
FV and FVIII deficiency	SD plasma rVIII	FVIII concentrate
FVII deficiency	rVIIa	FVII concentrate
FX deficiency	PCC	SD plasma
FXI deficiency	FXI concentrates or tranexamic acid	SD plasma rVIIa
FXIII deficiency	FXIII concentrates	SD plasma
VKCFD	Vitamin K	SD plasma PCC

F, factor; PCC, prothrombin complex concentrates; r, recombinant; SD plasma, fresh frozen plasma virally inactivated using a solvent detergent technique; VKCFD, hereditary combined deficiency of the vitamin K-dependent clotting factors; vWD, von Willebrand disease.

- Treatment is usually not required in patients with type1 vWD, type 2 patients usually require vWF concentrate and desmopressin especially if a caesarean section is required. Treatment is usually indicated for all types of delivery in patients with type 3 vWD.
- Intramuscular injections should be avoided in patients with untreated coagulopathy due to the risk of haematoma.
- Spinal or epidural anaesthetic use is controversial in women with bleeding disorders. It is contraindicated in patients with a significant coagulopathy but studies have shown that it may be used safely in patients with normal or corrected factor levels (51). An assessment and decision should be made antenatally and a plan documented in the patient's records.

Postnatal care

There is a significant increased risk of primary and secondary postpartum haemorrhage in these patients. This risk is usually proportional to the factor levels. The key factor in the management of these patients is prevention; active management of the third stage of labour, careful haemostasis during caesarean section, operative vaginal delivery, and perineal repair are all measures that reduce the incidence of bleeding following delivery (14, 15). Management of postpartum haemorrhage may be challenging and input from the haematologists and anaesthetists is required.

Prophylactic cover using desmopressin is required for patients with vWF, factor VIII, or factor IX levels less than 50 IU/dL and this level should be maintained for a minimum of 3 days following vaginal delivery and 5 days following caesarean section (52, 53). There is an ongoing risk of bleeding (54) and women should be counselled and given follow-up advice prior to discharge from hospital (55).

Neonatal care

- Cord blood samples should be taken and tested for coagulation profile and clotting factor levels.
- A cranial ultrasound scan should be performed if there has been a traumatic delivery or if there are signs of intracranial bleeding (56).
- Intramuscular injections should be avoided and any surgical procedures delayed until the coagulation status is known.
- It is important to be aware that clotting factor levels correlate with gestational age and some do not reach adult levels until 6 months after birth.
- Haemophilia A is the only bleeding disorder that can be reliably diagnosed at birth.

Management of haematological malignancy in pregnancy

Introduction

Haematological malignancies are rare in pregnancy, with an incidence that ranges from 1:1000 to 1:10,000. This is a diverse group which presents several diagnostic and therapeutic dilemmas to the clinician, as both the maternal and fetal well-being need to be addressed. Management is complex and requires multidisciplinary input. The mother needs to be informed about the disease progression, the requirement for immediate treatment, and the effect of delay in treatment to enable her to make an informed decision about continuation of pregnancy.

Diagnosis

Symptoms and signs of haematological malignancy are similar to non-pregnant women. Bone marrow aspiration (57) and lymph node biopsy under local or general anaesthetic may safely be performed in pregnancy (58). Magnetic resonance imaging without contrast can also safely be used and carries no radiation risk to the fetus.

Chemotherapy in pregnancy

All chemotherapeutic agents can cross the placenta (59) and can cause a spectrum of effects ranging from teratogenesis, carcinogenesis, and organ toxicity to abnormal neurodevelopment. This risk is reduced when single-agent chemotherapy is used (60, 61).

The effect on the fetus is determined by the gestation at exposure to treatment and the stage of fetal development:

- Pre-embryonic stage (from conception to 17 days post conception): exposure has little or no effect.
- Embryonic stage (3–4 weeks post conception): exposure may result in permanent damage to an end organ.
- Fetal stage (from 8 weeks post conception): exposure may result in damage to the cerebral cortex, gastrointestinal tract, and renal glomeruli.
- Second and third trimester: exposure carries an increased risk of fetal growth restriction, intrauterine fetal death, preterm labour, and low birth weight (62). There is no associated increased risk, however, of neurodevelopmental delay or childhood malignancy (63, 64).

Radiotherapy in pregnancy

Radiotherapy in pregnancy can cause a number of significant adverse effects on the fetus. It can cause organ malformation, reduced intelligence quotient, developmental delay, severe intellectual disability, and an increased risk of childhood cancer (65). Treatment with radiotherapy should therefore be reserved for cases where it is essential, and to limit the total amount the fetus is exposed to less than 0.1 Gy.

Hodgkin's lymphoma in pregnancy

Lymphoma is the fourth commonest malignancy in pregnancy; Hodgkin's is the commonest lymphoma in pregnancy, with an estimated prevalence of 1:1000 to 1:6000 (66).

The standard treatment regimen is a combination of doxorubicin, bleomycin, vinblastine, and dacarbazine (ABVD).

In early disease diagnosed in the first trimester, treatment may be delayed to the second trimester to avoid the teratogenic side effects of drugs. In advanced disease in the first trimester, termination of pregnancy is recommended followed by ABVD. In early disease limited to the supradiaphragmatic area in the first trimester, radiotherapy with abdominal shielding and a fetal dose of less than 0.1 Gy may be an alternative option. The prognosis of pregnant women with Hodgkin's lymphoma is similar to non-pregnant women (67).

Non-Hodgkin's lymphoma in pregnancy

Non-Hodgkin's lymphoma is less common in pregnancy; it consists of two types; indolent lymphomas and aggressive lymphomas.

- *Indolent lymphoma (follicular)*: this progresses slowly and is incurable; expectant management is recommended unless the patient is symptomatic, in which single-agent chemotherapy may be used; preferably in the second or third trimester.
- *Aggressive lymphoma (diffuse large B-cell lymphoma, mantle cell lymphoma, mature T and natural killer cell lymphoma)*: these require treatment due to their aggressive nature. Counselling about termination of pregnancy is recommended if diagnosed in the first trimester. Treatment may be given safely in the second and third trimesters, and early delivery may be considered if the patient is diagnosed from 32 weeks of gestation onwards.

Acute leukaemia

Acute leukaemia occurs in 1:100,000 pregnant women (68). The majority, two-thirds of cases, are myeloid, and one-third are lymphoid leukaemias. This is an aggressive malignancy and treatment should not be delayed or modified due to pregnancy (69).

- *Acute myeloid leukaemia*: the standard treatment is using a combination of cytarabine and an anthracycline. Treatment should not be delayed due to pregnancy as this will minimise the chance of remission. Women should be counselled about termination if diagnosed in the first trimester followed by chemotherapy (70). If diagnosed in the second or third trimester, standard chemotherapy should be given with increased fetal surveillance due to the risk of limb anomalies and cardiac arrhythmias (71).
- *Acute lymphocytic leukaemia*: this is a very aggressive type of leukaemia and any delay in treatment will affect survival. All treatment protocols contain methotrexate which is highly teratogenic.

Therefore, if acute lymphocytic leukaemia is diagnosed before 20 weeks, women should be counselled and offered termination of pregnancy. If it is diagnosed after 20 weeks' gestation, treatment could be given with the omission of methotrexate until the third trimester, elective early delivery from 32 weeks, and continuing treatment postnatally.

Myeloproliferative neoplasms

These encompass essential thrombocythaemia, polycythaemia vera, primary myelofibrosis, chronic myelogenous leukaemia (CML), and the rarer types; myeloproliferative neoplasm unclassified, mast cell disorders, chronic neutrophilic leukaemia and hypereosinophilic syndrome.

- *Chronic myelogenous leukaemia*: the incidence is 0.6–2 per 100,000 per year, chronic myelogenous leukaemia accounts for 15% of leukaemia in adults, 10% of which occurs in women of reproductive age (72). Standard treatment is with imatinib mesylate which may be teratogenic; women should be counselled and offered termination depending on the gestation at diagnosis. In women who present in the chronic phase of chronic myelogenous leukaemia, treatment may be delayed until after delivery.
- *Philadelphia-negative myeloproliferative neoplasms*: these are essential thrombocythaemia, polycythaemia vera, and primary myelofibrosis, and collectively they occur in about 6–9 per 100,000. Essential thrombocythaemia has a peak incidence in women of reproductive age, and 15% of patients diagnosed with polycythaemia are less than 40 years of age. There is a high risk of thrombosis with this condition in pregnancy, which may also lead to microthrombi at the placental bed, placental insufficiency, PET, stillbirth, preterm labour and low birth weight.

Treatment options include aspirin, heparin, venesection, and cytoreductive agents such as interferon-alpha.

Thalassaemia in pregnancy

Introduction

Thalassaemia is a heterogonous group of autosomal recessive haemolytic anaemias with a decreased synthesis of one or more globin chains. There are two main types classified according to the chain involved: alpha thalassaemia and beta thalassaemia. It is the commonest monogenetic disease worldwide, with an estimated prevalence of 16% in southern Europe, 10% in Thailand, and 3–8% in India, Pakistan, Bangladesh, and China (73, 74).

Alpha thalassaemia

The alpha chains are produced by four alpha-globin genes, two (one each of *HBA1* and *HBA2*) on each copy of chromosome 16. Alpha thalassaemia is caused by a decrease in the synthesis of these alpha chains; the severity of the condition depends on how many genes are affected (75).

The heterozygous form, alpha thalassaemia minor, may be asymptomatic, or the patient may have mild anaemia.

If three genes are mutated, the result will be a condition called haemoglobin H disease. Patients will have chronic anaemia and may require repeated blood transfusions.

The homozygous form, alpha thalassaemia major (Bart's Hb), where there is complete absence of the gene, is incompatible with life and results in a stillborn infant with severe hydrops fetalis.

Beta thalassaemia

There are two beta genes (*HBB*), one on each copy of chromosome 11. Beta thalassaemia is caused by a decrease in synthesis of these beta chains, and again, the severity depends on how many genes are affected (76).

The heterozygous form, beta thalassaemia minor, is asymptomatic or the patient may have mild anaemia.

The homozygous form, beta thalassaemia major, is complicated by marked hypochromic microcytic anaemia from a few months after birth and the patient is blood transfusion dependent.

Beta thalassaemia intermedia, is a milder form, where a mutation causes moderate impairment of beta chain production. Here the patient's condition fluctuates between minor and major beta thalassaemia, also known as 'non-transfusion-dependent thalassaemia'.

Diagnosis

- *Full blood count*: patients present with a hypochromic microcytic anaemia with a mean corpuscular haemoglobin cut-off of 27 pg for thalassaemia carriers and 25 pg in the homozygous forms (77, 78).
- *Iron studies*: can be used to differentiate from iron deficiency anaemia—which also leads to a hypochromic microcytic anaemia.
- *Haemoglobin electrophoresis*: presence of haemoglobin H inclusion bodies is diagnostic of alpha thalassaemia. Haemoglobin A2 and haemoglobin F levels are elevated in beta thalassaemia carriers.
- *Partner screening*: this is important to enable genetic analysis and counselling about the risk of an affected child.

Diagnosis in the fetus

Once the couple's carrier status is confirmed, they should be informed that the risk of an affected child with thalassaemia major is one in four. The severity of disease in the fetus will depend on the type of thalassaemia in the parents:

- Non-invasive prenatal tests for beta thalassaemia (79):
  - Free fetal DNA
  - Preimplantation genetic diagnosis
- Invasive tests:
  - Chorionic villous sampling
  - Amniocentesis
- Ultrasound surveillance for alpha thalassaemia (Bart's):
  - Fetuses affected with alpha thalassaemia will have major abnormalities detected early on ultrasound; increased cardiothoracic ratio, thickened placenta, abnormal middle cerebral artery Doppler and finally, hydrops fetalis in the second or third trimester (80).

Effect of thalassaemia on pregnancy

Maternal

- Pregnancy-induced hypertension and PET
- Gestational diabetes

- Anaemia
- Polyhydramnios
- Placental abruption
- Urinary tract infection
- Multiple pregnancy—there is a higher rate of multiple pregnancy, possibly due to the high rate of assisted reproduction (81)
- Cardiac failure
- Caesarean section
- Mirror syndrome—fluid retention and symptoms similar to PET; this occurs in women carrying a fetus with alpha thalassaemia and hydrops fetalis.

Fetal

- Miscarriage
- Intrauterine fetal growth restriction
- Preterm labour
- Stillbirth
- Increased neural tube defects (81).

Preconceptual care

Patients with thalassaemia may have cardiac, endocrine, and haematological comorbidities, it is therefore prudent to adopt a multidisciplinary approach in their care to optimize maternal and perinatal outcome:

- Echocardiogram: multiple transfusions may lead to iron load and cardiac failure in these patients, an echocardiogram must be performed to assess ventricular function.
- Liver function test.
- Optimise diabetes control and ascertain adequate thyroid replacement.
- Iron toxicity may lead to multiple endocrine disorders such as diabetes and hypothyroidism.
- Screen for viral infections: there is a high risk of hepatitis B and C and HIV due to repeated blood transfusions.
- Review medications: discontinue iron chelation therapy, and prescribe a pregnancy safe antihypertensive if indicated.
- Folic acid, calcium, and vitamin D supplementation.
- Partner screening: this will enable adequate genetic counselling.

Antenatal care

Patients should be seen by obstetricians with experience in high-risk pregnancy, in conjunction with a fetal medicine specialist and multidisciplinary input from the relevant specialties. Management includes the following:

- Screening and treatment of anaemia: there is a high incidence of anaemia, use of oral iron should be individualised and women may need a blood transfusion for the first time in pregnancy.
- Glucose tolerance test.
- Blood pressure and urinalysis during each visit.
- Mid-stream urine sample during each visit.
- Serial ultrasounds for fetal growth and umbilical artery Doppler assessment.
- Vaginal delivery is recommended. A caesarean section should only be performed for obstetric reasons.

Postnatal care

- Postnatal thromboprophylaxis—high risk of thrombosis in alpha thalassaemia trait and beta thalassaemia intermedia and major.
- Breastfeeding is recommended.
- Resume iron chelation therapy if indicated.

Thrombocytopenia in pregnancy

Definition

Thrombocytopenia is defined as a low platelet count of less than 150×10^9/L (83–85), but only counts of less than 100×10^9/L are clinically significant.

It is classified as mild—platelet count $100–150 \times 10^9$/L; moderate—platelet count $50–100 \times 10^9$/L; and severe—platelet count less than 50×10^9/L. Platelet counts of less than 20×10^9/L are associated with significant maternal and perinatal morbidity (86).

Incidence

Thrombocytopenia is the second commonest haematological disorder in pregnancy after anaemia. It affects 6–10% of all pregnancies, and while some studies show a 10% decrease in platelet counts in the third trimester in normal pregnancy, the absolute count remains well within normal levels (87, 88). Approximately 8% of pregnant women will have a platelet count between 100 and 150×10^9/L (2).

Causes

The main causes of thrombocytopenia are (1) gestational; (2) autoimmune—immune thrombocytopenic purpura, systemic lupus erythematosus, or APS; (3) hypertensive disorders, PET, and HELLP syndrome; (4) thrombotic thrombocytopenic purpura (TTP), haemolytic uraemic syndrome (HUS); (5) human immunodeficiency virus (HIV); and (6) bone marrow suppression.

Gestational thrombocytopenia

This is the commonest type of thrombocytopenia and accounts for 75% of cases of thrombocytopenia diagnosed in pregnancy (1). It usually occurs in the third trimester and is thought to be due to the increased platelet consumption and plasma volume expansion in pregnancy. It is a diagnosis of exclusion and the following criteria should be met for diagnosis:

- There is mild to moderate thrombocytopenia.
- The platelet count seldom falls below 70×10^9/L.
- Patients are asymptomatic.
- It usually occurs in the third trimester and platelet levels are normal in the first trimester.
- Platelet levels normalise rapidly following delivery.

Gestational thrombocytopenia is distinguished from immune thrombocytopenic purpura based on the gestation at onset, the absence of symptoms, and normal platelet levels prior to pregnancy (89).

There are usually no adverse effects to the mother or fetus, and no intervention other than reassurance is required.

Immune thrombocytopenic purpura

This is caused by autoantibodies against platelet surface glycoproteins, which leads to platelet destruction by the reticuloendothelial system. The exact cause is unknown; the majority of cases are idiopathic but some cases could be secondary to chronic infections such as HIV or connective tissue disorders. The antibody is immunoglobulin G (IgG), and can therefore cross the placenta and cause fetal thrombocytopenia. Management of this condition in pregnancy is divided into a maternal care plan and a fetal care plan. Patients should be managed by obstetricians experienced in high-risk pregnancy with haematologist involvement (90).

Maternal care plan

- Platelet level should be checked every 4 weeks in the first and second trimester and more frequently in the third trimester to initiate treatment if required.
- Treatment should be initiated in the first trimester only if the platelet levels fall below 20×10^9/L.
- Vaginal delivery is safe, and a caesarean section should only be performed for usual obstetric indications.
- A general guide is to maintain platelet levels above 20×10^9/L for vaginal delivery, above 50×10^9/L for caesarean section, and above 80×10^9/L for regional anaesthesia.
- Levels below 80×10^9 in the third trimester generally require treatment to provide the patient the option of regional anaesthesia for delivery.
- Corticosteroids are the first-line treatment; different protocols exist but generally the dose is 1 mg/kg/day which will increase platelet levels in about 1–2 weeks. After 2 weeks of treatment, the dose can be reduced by 10–20% per week to the minimum dose effective at keeping platelet levels between 50 and 80×10^9/L.
- Intravenous immunoglobulins (IVIGs) may be given as second line, and are reserved for women with platelet levels below 10×10^9/L or women who do not respond to steroid therapy. They increase platelet count rapidly—within 6–72 hours—but the level is not sustained and falls rapidly within days returning to pretreatment levels within 4 weeks.
- Platelet transfusions are a last resort as they will increase antibody titres and they do not cause a sustained increase in platelet levels. They should be used as directed by a haematologist.
- Splenectomy can be performed if there is severe immune thrombocytopenic purpura and medical treatment has failed. If indicated, it should be performed in the first or second trimester, and women should subsequently be offered immunization against *Haemophilus influenzae*, pneumococcus, and meningococcus and given penicillin prophylaxis.

Fetal care plan

- Cord blood samples should be taken to measure platelet count.
- Bleeding complications are not as common as previously stated, and platelet levels rarely fall below 50×10^9/L in neonates.
- The platelet level reaches its nadir between 2 and 5 days of life, so it is important to monitor neonates closely during this period.
- Treatment with IVIG is recommended if platelet levels are below 20×10^9/L and a cranial ultrasound scan should be performed to rule out bleeding.

Thrombotic thrombocytopenic purpura and haemolytic uraemic syndrome

The hallmarks of TTP and HUS are a microangiopathic haemolytic anaemia and thrombocytopenia. The incidence of both conditions is increased in pregnancy, and may be difficult to differentiate from each other and from other hypertensive disorders in pregnancy such as PET and HELLP syndrome.

Management

The absence of hypertension is the main differentiating factor between TTP/HUS and PET or HELLP syndrome. Making this distinction is imperative, as the ultimate treatment of hypertensive disorders of pregnancy is delivery; while in TTP and HUS delivery does not alter the course of the disease (91).

Treatment:

- Corticosteroids.
- Plasmapheresis and plasma exchange.
- Dialysis in patients with acute kidney injury.
- Neurological support for patients with seizures and further imaging to rule out other causes of seizures.
- The use of platelet transfusion is controversial; there have been some reports of deterioration and microthrombi formation with their use (92). However, a review did not demonstrate any evidence of complications from platelet transfusion (93). Current recommendations are that platelet transfusion should be reserved for the prevention or management of life-threatening haemorrhage.

Thrombophilia and early pregnancy loss

Definition

Thrombophilia is an abnormality of blood coagulation that increases the risk of thrombosis (e.g. deep vein thrombosis and pulmonary embolism) (94). There are two types of thrombophilias: inherited and acquired. Thrombophilias are thought to cause pregnancy loss due to thrombosis in the uteroplacental circulation leading to placental insufficiency and inflammation (95).

Inherited thrombophilia

This group includes factor V Leiden, prothrombin G20210A gene mutation, protein S and protein C deficiency, and antithrombin III deficiency.

The correlation between inherited thrombophilia and pregnancy loss is debatable, with some previous studies showing an association of as high as 50–60% (96, 97)—although the majority of first-trimester miscarriage is due to a chromosomal abnormality (98).

Acquired thrombophilia

- APS: this is the most recognised acquired thrombophilia; it is characterised by obstetric complications (e.g. recurrent miscarriages, fetal growth restriction, and early-onset PET) and/or thromboembolic events, in association with antiphospholipid antibodies (99, 100). In one study, APS, the only thrombophilia that has been shown to have a direct adverse effect on miscarriages, was found in 15% of women with recurrent miscarriages (7); however, when revised diagnostic criteria are applied, this figure is much lower and recent evidence suggests figures of around 2% (2).

- Acquired activated protein C resistance (APCR): acquired APCR is associated with lupus anticoagulant and elevated coagulation factor VIII. It is a well-documented risk factor for recurrent miscarriages (101), and studies have shown a higher association with acquired rather than inherited protein C resistance (102). There is also an increased incidence of thromboembolism with acquired APCR (103).

Recurrent miscarriages

The European Society for Human Reproduction and Embryology defines recurrent miscarriage as three or more consecutive pregnancy losses before 20 weeks gestation (104). About 15% of pregnancies will end in a miscarriage, and the incidence of recurrent miscarriage is 1% in the general population. A careful history and examination is important to highlight other causes of recurrent miscarriage, however, in over 50% of cases the cause is unexplained (105). Different protocols have been proposed in the management of couples with recurrent miscarriage, many of them with unproven efficacy (106, 107). An evidence-based approach is recommended to avoid prescribing unnecessary medications in pregnancy.

Thrombophilia and recurrent miscarriages

There is much debate about the association between inherited thrombophilia and recurrent miscarriage. A positive result, even after a recent miscarriage, has not been shown to have an effect on future pregnancy outcome (108). The benefit of screening is questionable given that the prevalence of inherited thrombophilia in women of reproductive age is 20% (109), which is similar to the background risk of miscarriage. Nonetheless, most centres routinely offer screening for thrombophilia following recurrent miscarriage and offer anticoagulation if the result is positive (110). Conversely, there is a proven association between APS and recurrent miscarriage.

Treatment of inherited thrombophilia and recurrent miscarriages

A variety of treatment protocols have been used in patients with inherited thrombophilia and recurrent miscarriages, mostly adapted from treatment protocols for patients with APS.

Various studies have shown different efficacies with aspirin monotherapy versus combination therapy with aspirin and heparin (111–113). Many of the studies supporting the use of anticoagulation have significant flaws and limitations, and results from larger studies have shown no difference in outcomes (114), and in fact, higher live births in patients managed expectantly (115).

Treatment of APS and recurrent miscarriage

APS is an established, curable cause of recurrent miscarriages (116). Without treatment, some studies have shown a poor pregnancy outcome with a miscarriage rate as high as 90% (117).

Several treatment protocols have been suggested: aspirin alone, aspirin and LMWH, and aspirin and unfractionated heparin. Similar outcomes were found when comparing aspirin alone and aspirin in combination with LMWH (118, 119). Some studies have questioned the benefit of heparin use, but until more robust research data are available, current guidelines advocate the addition of heparin if the patient had previously miscarried with aspirin monotherapy (12, 120, 121).

A Cochrane review of treatment of APS patients with corticosteroids has not shown improved efficacy compared to placebo in improving live birth rates (122). The incidence of gestational diabetes and hypertension was significantly higher in patients treated with corticosteroids (123); hence, steroids are not used for APS in miscarriages.

The role of IVIG in APS and recurrent miscarriage has been reviewed in a number of studies (124). There was no substantial evidence to support the use of IVIG and recent consensus is to limit its use to research trials.

Anaemia in pregnancy

Definition

Anaemia is defined by a low haemoglobin level of less than 110 g/L which is two standard deviations below the mean for a matched healthy population (125). Due to the physiological haemodilution of pregnancy, haemoglobin levels vary each trimester, with levels of less than 105 g/L in the second and third trimesters and less than 100g/L postpartum used to diagnose anaemia (1, 126).

Haemoglobin measurement identifies the presence of anaemia but not the cause of anaemia. There are many causes, with iron deficiency being the commonest cause, leading to approximately 50% of cases of anaemia (3, 127). This percentage varies among different populations in different geographical areas (1). Other causes of anaemia include deficiency of macronutrients such as folate and vitamin B_{12}; acute and chronic infections such as malaria, tuberculosis, and HIV; malignancies; and inherited or acquired haemoglobin synthesis disorders, and red blood cell production or function such as haemoglobinopathies (1, 3).

Background

Anaemia in pregnancy is a global problem, in 2011 the World Health Organisation estimated the prevalence of anaemia in pregnant women to be 38%, and 29% in all women of reproductive age. This translates to 32 million pregnant women and 496 million women of reproductive age affected globally. This prevalence varies depending on geographical area, the highest being in Africa, where 55% of pregnant women are affected compared to North America which has the lowest prevalence of 6.1% (128).

Causes

Iron deficiency is the commonest cause of anaemia in pregnancy. The second commonest cause is folate deficiency; anaemia related to folate deficiency varies considerably with nutritional variation and socioeconomic status (129). The common causes of anaemia are summarized in Table 15.6.

Effect of pregnancy on anaemia

Many women enter pregnancy with depleted iron stores, the increased demands and increased mobilisation of iron from circulating red blood cells leads to further depletion and has a direct effect on maternal and perinatal mortality and morbidity. Conditions such as multiparity, multiple pregnancy, teenage pregnancy, and smoking, in addition to intrapartum and postpartum

Table 15.6 Causes of anaemia in pregnancy

Nutritional deficiencies	Iron
	Folic acid
	Vitamin B_{12}
	Vitamin C, vitamin A
	Protein
Haemolysis and abnormal haemoglobin synthesis	Malaria
	Glucose-6-phosphate dehydrogenase deficiency
	Thalassaemias
	Sickle cell disease
Blood loss and defective iron absorption and metabolism	Helminthiasis, especially hookworm infestation
	Amoebiasis and giardiasis
	Schistosomiasis
	Abnormal iron metabolism
	Bleeding haemorrhoids
	Antepartum haemorrhage
	Trauma
	High parity
Chronic conditions	Malignancies
	Tuberculosis
	Chronic renal including disease including urinary tract infection
	Sexual transmitted infections including bacterial vaginosis
	Human immune deficiency virus infection
	Chronic rheumatic and rheumatoid disease

Source data from Goonewardene M, Shehata M, Hamad A. Anaemia in pregnancy. *Best Pract Res Clin Obstet Gynaecol* 2012;26:3–24.

blood loss all contribute to increase incidence and worsening of pre-existing anaemia.

Effect of anaemia on pregnancy

Adequate iron and folate are needed for normal tissue enzyme function. Initially the fetus compensates by upregulating placental iron transport proteins (130), but further depleted stores increase the risk of developing anaemia in the first 3 months of life. Some of the reported obstetric outcomes in relation to anaemia are as follows:

Maternal

- Lower immunity and increased susceptibility to infections
- Tiredness
- Lethargy
- Poor concentration and work performance
- Postpartum depression
- Spinal and peripheral nerve involvement with vitamin B_{12} deficiency.

Fetal

- Impaired psychomotor and/or mental development

- Low birth weight
- Preterm birth
- Placental abruption
- Postpartum haemorrhage
- Neural tube defects with vitamin B_{12} and folate deficiency.

Diagnosis

Clinical symptoms and signs of anaemia in pregnancy are non-specific and can sometimes be difficult to differentiate from normal symptoms of pregnancy, unless the anaemia is severe. Fatigue is the most common presenting symptom. Women may also complain of weakness, palpitations, dyspnoea, dizziness, and irritability.

Laboratory tests include the following:

- *Full blood count, blood film, and red cell indices*: in iron deficiency anaemia, this will show low Hb less than 11 g/dL, mean cell volume less than 80 fL, mean cell haemoglobin less than 30 mg/dL, and mean cell haemoglobin concentration less than 30%; a blood film may show microcytic hypochromic red cells and characteristic 'pencil cells' (131).
  - A raised mean cell volume greater than 100 fL is indicative of folate deficiency, but can also be raised with liver disease and alcohol consumption.
- *Serum ferritin*: ferritin is a glycoprotein which reflects iron stores. It is the first laboratory test to become abnormal as iron stores decrease and it is not affected by recent iron ingestion. It is an acute phase reactant, so levels may rise in the presence of infection or inflammation. Ferritin levels increase initially in pregnancy, followed by a progressive decrease in the third trimester due to haemodilution and iron mobilization. Nevertheless, a ferritin concentration of less than 15 µg/L indicates iron depletion (132).
- *Serum iron and total iron binding capacity (TIBC)*: serum iron and TIBC are unreliable in predicting availability of iron to tissues due to fluctuation of levels with infection, diurnal variation, and ingestion of iron. Levels decline in normal pregnancy but serum iron of less than 12 µg/L and TIBC of less than 15% indicate iron deficiency.
- *Soluble transferrin receptor*: the transferrin receptor is a transmembrane protein that transports iron into the cell (133). It is a sensitive measure of tissue iron supply and is not an acute phase reactant. Initially there is little change in concentration, but in established iron deficiency the soluble transferrin receptor concentration will increase in direct proportion to the total transferrin receptor concentration. However, this is an expensive test which limits its use in pregnancy.
- *Reticulocyte haemoglobin content and reticulocytes*: reticulocyte haemoglobin concentration and reticulocyte count is reduced in iron deficiency anaemia. Erythropoietic activity in anaemia can be assessed early by measuring reticulocyte cellular characteristics. This is not widely available and there are limited data in pregnancy.
- *Serum and red cell folate*: folate deficiency results in macrocytosis (mean cell volume >100 fL) and the development of megaloblastic change in the bone marrow. A serum folate of less than 2.0 µg/L, and red cell folate concentration of less than 160 µg/L is diagnostic of folate deficiency.
- *Vitamin B_{12} (cobalamin) level*: vitamin B_{12} deficiency also leads to macrocytosis and megloblastic change in the bone marrow.

Cobalamin level vary in pregnancy with the lowest being in the third trimester, a level of less than 100 pg/mL is diagnostic of vitamin B_{12} deficiency.
  - An adjunct to diagnosis of B_{12} deficiency is a reduction in holotranscobalamin level, and an increase in methylmalonic level and lactate dehydrogenase level. The latter is due to destruction of red blood cells in the bone marrow.
- *Bone marrow biopsy*: a bone marrow sample is considered the gold standard for assessment of iron stores; however, this test is very invasive and should only be used in complicated cases where the underlying cause cannot be identified by simpler methods.
- *Haemoglobin electrophoresis*: can be used to measure amounts of normal HbA and HbA2, and measure abnormal haemoglobin levels such as HbS, HbF, and HbC which can be elevated in conditions such as sickle cell disease (SCD).

Prevention

The type of nutritional deficiency anaemia varies with geographic location.

Dietary advice is important in all types of nutritional anaemias especially in vegan and vegetarian women—a balanced diet, rich in iron, protein, and folic acid-fortified breads and cereals is advised. In countries with a high prevalence of anaemia, a daily supplement of 60 mg of elemental iron and 400 mg of folic acid should be given to all pregnant women throughout pregnancy and continued for 3–6 months postpartum to ensure adequate iron stores (134, 135). This can be associated with considerable gastrointestinal side effects and lead to poor compliance, so a weekly dose may be appropriate in areas with less prevalence of anaemia.

Treatment

All pregnant women should be screened for anaemia at booking and again at 28 weeks' gestation (136).

Iron deficiency anaemia

Oral iron

A trial of iron therapy can be used as a diagnostic and therapeutic measure. Oral iron should demonstrate a rise in haemoglobin within 2 to 3 weeks. A rise confirms the diagnosis, if there is no rise in haemoglobin—further tests must be carried out.

Oral iron is a cheap and effective way to restore iron stores. There are only marginal differences between the different ferrous salts. Ferrous salts available include ferrous fumarate, ferrous sulphate, and ferrous gluconate.

The recommended dose of elemental iron for treatment of iron deficiency is 100–200 mg daily.

Haemoglobin concentration should rise by 20 g/L in 3–4 weeks, although compliance and intolerance to oral iron may limit efficacy. Repeat testing should be performed 2–3 weeks following initiation of treatment to assess response. Once haemoglobin levels normalize, treatment should be continued for 3 months and carried on for 6 weeks postnatally to replace stores.

Parenteral iron

Parenteral iron should be reserved for women with poor compliance, malabsorption, or non-tolerance to oral iron (137).

Several authors have reported faster increase in haemoglobin levels, quicker replenishment of iron stores, and less need for blood transfusions with parenteral iron therapy (138–140).

Different preparations are available, iron III carboxymaltose (Ferrinject) and iron III isomaltoside (Monofer) are examples of fast-acting intravenous iron preparations.

Intramuscular preparations

The only intramuscular preparation available in the United Kingdom is low-molecular-weight iron dextran. Significant pain at the injection site and the risk of permanent skin discolouration limit its use in clinical practice (141).

Blood transfusion

Blood transfusion should be given in obstetric haemorrhage as indicated, in line with local guidelines. Efforts should be made to reduce unnecessary blood transfusions by appropriate assessment of women in the postpartum period and balancing the risks of transfusion against potential benefit (142).

Folic acid

A prophylactic dose of 400 mcg daily is recommended for all women at least 3 months preconceptually. A therapeutic dose of 5 mg is recommended in women with haemolytic anaemias such as SCD, or on medications affecting folate metabolism such as antiepileptic drugs (143).

Vitamin B$_{12}$

Vitamin B$_{12}$ levels must be measured prior to giving folate supplements as this may mask B$_{12}$ deficiency.

Women with a balanced diet rarely need vitamin B$_{12}$ supplementation, but vegans or patients with pernicious anaemia benefit from treatment. Treatment is usually in the form of hydroxocobalamin intramuscular injections.

Sickle cell disease in obstetrics

Definition

Sickle Cell Disease (SCD) is an autosomal recessive disorder caused by valine replacing glutamic acid at position six on the haemoglobin (Hb) beta chain. This abnormal haemoglobin leads to the formation of fragile rigid sickle-shaped red cells in low-oxygen conditions. There are various types of abnormal haemoglobin: homozygous HbSS or heterozygous forms, HbSC or HbS-beta thalassaemia, which arise when HbS is co-inherited with HbC or beta-thalassaemia. Other less common heterozygous forms are HbD, HbE, and HbO-Arab. HbS combined with normal Hb leads to a carrier (trait) state, and these patients are generally asymptomatic. The different types have varying severity of symptoms, with HbSS patients having more severe disease (144).

Background

SCD is the commonest inherited disorder worldwide, with over 300,000 affected children born each year (145, 146), with two-thirds of these births occurring in Africa (147). In the United Kingdom,

there are over 300 affected children born and 100–200 pregnant women affected each year (148).

Pathophysiology

The polymerisation of abnormal haemoglobin in low-oxygen conditions leads to formation of fragile rigid red blood cells that are prone to increased breakdown causing haemolytic anaemia, which in turn leads to a decrease in red cell lifespan. Vaso-occlusion of small blood vessels is the main event that leads to the clinical features of this condition. Vaso-occlusion in the bone causes acute bony pain and is associated with chronic multiorgan complications.

Clinical features

SCD is a multiorgan disorder with lifelong complications. Most patients will have a chronic anaemia with a haemoglobin level of 6–9 g/dL, although patients with the milder HbSC type may have higher or normal haemoglobin levels. Recurrent acute, severe episodes of bone pain are the predominant clinical feature; it affects the fingers and toes in children and the trunk and long bones in adults. These painful episodes or 'crisis' occur with variable severity and can be precipitated by dehydration, stress, and infection. Other features are an increased risk of stroke, renal disease, pulmonary hypertension, retinal disease, avascular necrosis, and leg ulcers.

Pregnancy may unmask any of these conditions and they may be diagnosed for the first time in pregnancy. Previously, SCD was associated with early mortality, but with improved medical care the average life expectancy has improved and most children born in the United Kingdom will reach childbearing age (149, 150).

Effect of pregnancy on sickle cell disease

There is a large variation in reported maternal mortality, varying from 0.07% in the studies from the United States (151) to over 9.2% in Nigeria (152). A national cohort study—the UK Obstetric Surveillance System(UKOSS)—comparing sickle cell anaemia (HbSS) with HbSC disease, showed a high rate of maternal and fetal complications in mothers with SCD, even in women with HbSC, who were previously considered to be at lower risk of complications during pregnancy (153).

Pregnancy can increase the frequency and severity of painful episodes leading to multiple hospital admissions even in patients with mild disease outside of pregnancy (154–156). There is also an increase in infections, pulmonary complications (157–159), and thromboembolic events (160).

Effect of sickle cell disease on pregnancy

Maternal

- Painful crisis
- Antepartum haemorrhage
- PET
- Pulmonary thrombosis
- Thromboembolism
- Bone marrow embolism
- Sepsis.

Fetal

- Miscarriage
- Intrauterine growth restriction
- Stillbirth
- Placental abruption
- Preterm labour
- Four- to sixfold increase in perinatal mortality.

Diagnosis

Most patients have an established diagnosis prior to pregnancy and are regularly reviewed in a haematology or specialist clinic.

High-pressure liquid chromatography (HPLC) is the most commonly used diagnostic test. Alternative tests are isoelectric focusing, cellulose acetate electrophoresis at alkaline pH, or capillary electrophoresis. All pregnant women in England have antenatal screening for SCD at their booking visit.

Management

Preconceptual care

- Partner screening should be offered ideally prior to pregnancy, this enables clinicians to offer the couple appropriate counselling about the risk of having an affected child.
- The risk of pulmonary hypertension is increased in patients with SCD (161); an echocardiogram should be offered prior to any planned pregnancy if it has not been performed in the preceding year.
- Patients with SCD commonly have elevated blood pressure and proteinuria which may progress to end-stage renal disease. Measurement of blood pressure, urinalysis, and assessment of renal function is important to identify patients with nephropathy.
- Women who are on prophylactic antibiotics (penicillin or erythromycin if allergic to penicillin) to reduce the risk of infection particularly from encapsulated bacteria, are encouraged to continue them throughout pregnancy (162).
- Other medication such as hydroxycarbamide given to reduce the incidence of acute chest syndrome is teratogenic and should be stopped 3 months before conception (163). Women on angiotensin-converting enzyme inhibitors and angiotensin receptor blockers should be switched to a suitable alternative antihypertensive that is safe in pregnancy.
- High dose—5 mg folic acid per day is recommended due to associated folate deficiency (164).
- Pneumococcal vaccine is recommended every 5 years and the influenza vaccine is recommended annually.
- Some patients with SCD are at a high risk of developing proliferative retinopathy. An assessment by an ophthalmologist should be offered preconceptually in such patients.
- Iron overload is common in women who require multiple transfusions. A cardiac and hepatic magnetic resonance imaging scan should be offered preconceptually, and iron chelation therapy offered prior to pregnancy if indicated.

Antenatal care

Antenatal care should be provided by a multidisciplinary team: an obstetrician with special interest in high-risk pregnancy, a specialist midwife and a haematologist. It is important to have clear clinical pathways and referral channels to a specialist centre if complications arise during pregnancy.

Ideally patients with SCD should be booked early to enable clinicians to make an appropriate plan for the pregnancy and arrange referrals as necessary. They should receive general advice about maintaining adequate nutrition, warmth, and hydration during pregnancy.

- If the patient has not been seen preconceptually, partner screening should be carried out as soon as possible and appropriate genetic counselling offered regarding the risk of having an affected child.
- Generally, patients should be seen every 4 weeks up to 28 weeks, then every 2 weeks thereafter—more frequent visits may be needed if there are any maternal or fetal complications.
- Medications that are teratogenic in pregnancy should be discontinued preconceptually.
- Blood pressure and urine should be checked each visit.
- Folic acid 5 mg daily and antibiotic prophylaxis should be taken throughout pregnancy.
- Aspirin 75 mg should be given daily to reduce the risk of PET (165).
- There is an increased risk of venous thromboembolism in patients with SCD (166). Thromboprophylaxis should be offered if the patient is admitted to hospital or if there are additional risk factors
- In addition to routine antenatal ultrasound scans, a uterine artery Doppler assessment should be offered at 24 weeks (167). Due to the increased incidence of fetal growth restriction, regular growth scans every 4 weeks from 24 weeks should be offered.
- There is conflicting evidence of benefit from prophylactic transfusion (168–170), although some centres offer it routinely. Women who are on a long-term transfusion protocol for secondary stroke prevention should follow the same protocol throughout pregnancy.
- Women with SCD will usually have a chronic anaemia due to haemolysis; however, an acute anaemia with a haemoglobin level of less than 6 g/dL or a decrease by more than 2 g/dL from baseline is an indication for blood transfusion.
- Red cell alloimmunization is common due to repeated transfusions and can occur in up to 29% (171, 172) of patients. Red cell phenotyping should be performed at booking, and only C-, E-, and Kell-matched blood given if a transfusion is needed.
- Delivery is recommended by 38–40 weeks due to the increased risk of perinatal mortality in late gestation. Vaginal delivery is recommended, and caesarean section should only be performed for obstetric indications.

Intrapartum care

The stress of labour may potentiate crises in patients with SCD, so patients should be delivered in units that are able to manage high-risk pregnancy complications.

- Hydration—oral hydration is usually sufficient, but intravenous hydration may be needed in women who are unable to tolerate oral fluids. Patients should have strict fluid balance monitoring and early warning scoring charts should be used.
- Oxygenation—oxygen saturation should be monitored throughout labour and supplemental oxygen given if the saturation falls below 94%.

- Progress in labour—prolonged labour should be avoided and an early recourse to caesarean section should be made if progress is not adequate.
- Antibiotics—prophylactic antibiotics are not indicated unless there is evidence of infection.
- Continuous fetal monitoring—continuous monitoring during labour is recommended due to the increased risk of fetal growth restriction, placental abruption, and fetal distress (172, 173).
- Analgesia/anaesthesia—patients may receive analgesia and regional anaesthesia as per normal, with the exception of pethidine as it may provoke seizures in women with SCD.
- Thromboprophylaxis—routine thromboprophylaxis should be offered in line with RCOG guidance (174).

Postnatal care

There is an increased incidence of acute sickle pain, occurring in 7–25% of patients in the postpartum period (175, 176). Adequate analgesia in the form of opioids should be offered and fluid balance and oxygenation should be monitored carefully.

- Thromboprophylaxis—should be given for the duration of hospital admission, for 7–10 days following vaginal delivery and 6 weeks following caesarean section.
- Breastfeeding—there are no restrictions on breastfeeding and women should be encouraged to breastfeed.
- Contraception—progesterone preparations such as the progesterone-only pill, injectable (Depo-Provera), Mirena coil, and the implant (Implanon) are the first-line recommended contraceptives. Progestogens have been shown to reduce the frequency and severity of painful crisis (177). Second-line contraceptives include the combined oral contraceptive pill, copper intrauterine device, vaginal ring, and combined contraceptive patch. Oestrogen-containing contraceptives are associated with an increased risk of thrombosis—a careful risk assessment must be made prior to prescribing them to women with SCD.

Management of acute sickle crisis in pregnancy

There is an increased incidence of painful crisis in pregnancy, with some studies showing an occurrence in about 27–50% of women (13, 178, 179):

- Mild sickle pain: patients with mild pain can be managed as an outpatient with rest, fluids, and analgesia (paracetamol and weak opioids)
- Moderate to severe pain: these patients should be assessed promptly in hospital for signs of infection or acute chest syndrome. The mainstay of management is rapid analgesia and hydration:
  - Analgesia—strong oral or parenteral opioids should be given rapidly with frequent reassessment of pain score and further analgesia given until the patient is pain free (180).
  - Hydration—oral fluids should be given at 60 mL/kg/24 hours, or intravenous fluids if oral fluids are not tolerated.
  - Monitoring—fluid balance, oxygenation, and sedation score should be monitored using an early warning scoring chart. Patients should be managed jointly by the obstetric, haematology, and anaesthetic teams.

- Investigations—urinalysis, full blood count, and renal function, and blood cultures and chest X-ray if there is a suspicion of infection.
- Thromboprophylaxis—should be given for the duration of hospital admission.
- Antibiotics—should be prescribed if there is a risk or evidence of infection.
- Acute chest syndrome (ACS): this is seen in 7–20% (181–183) of pregnant patients with SCD and is associated with high morbidity and mortality.
  - It is characterized by new infiltrates on chest X-ray in conjunction with respiratory signs and symptoms. One of the earliest signs is hypoxia, therefore women who develop hypoxia should have a clinical assessment, arterial blood gas measurement, and a chest X-ray to rule out acute chest syndrome.
  - The senior and multidisciplinary team should be involved in the management if acute chest syndrome is suspected, and the patient should be nursed in a high dependency unit. Treatment is with respiratory support, antibiotics, and blood transfusions. An emergency exchange transfusion should be performed if there is severe hypoxia. Pulmonary embolism may have a similar presentation and should be considered as an alternative diagnosis, specifically if the chest X-ray is normal.
- Other acute complications: acute neurological complications such as haemorrhagic or ischaemic stroke are increased in patients with SCD (183). Urgent brain imaging and assessment should be performed in women presenting with symptoms, with urgent involvement of the haematology and neurology teams. Emergency exchange transfusion is imperative and can reduce long-term neurological disability.

REFERENCES

1. Ruiz-Irastorza G, Crowther M, Branch W, et al. Antiphospholipid syndrome. *Lancet* 2010;**376**:1498–509.
2. Bowman ZS, Wünsche V, Porter TF, Silver RM, Branch DW. Prevalence of antiphospholipid antibodies and risk of subsequent adverse obstetric outcomes in women with prior pregnancy loss. *J Reprod Immunol.* 2015 Feb;**107**:59–63. doi: 10.1016/j.jri.2014.09.052. Epub 2014 Oct 13
3. Cervera R, Font J, Khamashta MA, et al. Antiphospholipid syndrome: clinical and immunologic manifestations and patterns of disease expression in a cohort of 1000 patients. *Arthritis Rheum* 2002;**46**:1019–27.
4. Cohen D, Berger SP, Steup-Beekman GM, et al. Diagnosis and management of the antiphospholipid syndrome. *BMJ* 2010;**340**:1125–32.
5. Cervera R, Khamashta MA, Shoenfeld Y, et al. Morbidity and mortality in the antiphospholipid syndrome during a 5-year period: a multicentre prospective study of 1000 patients. *Ann Rheum Dis* 2009;**68**:1428–32.
6. Alijotas-Reig J, Vilardell-Tarres M. Is obstetric antiphospholipid syndrome a primary nonthrombotic, proinflammatory, complement-mediated disorder related to antiphospholipid antibodies? *Obstet Gynecol Surv* 2010;**65**:39–45.
7. Alijotas-Reig J. The complement system as a main actor in the pathogenesis of obstetric antiphospholipid syndrome. *Med Clin (Barc)* 2010;**134**:30–34.
8. Stone S, Khamashta MA, Poston L. Placentation, antiphospholipid syndrome and pregnancy outcome. *Lupus* 2001;**10**:67–74.

9. Girardi G, Mackman N. Tissue factor in antiphospholipid antibody-induced pregnancy loss: a pro-inflammatory molecule. *Lupus* 2008;**17**:931–36.

10. Cohen D, Berger SP, Steup-Beekman GM, et al. Diagnosis and management of the antiphospholipid syndrome. *BMJ* 2010;**340**:1125–32.

11. Bick RL. Antiphospholipid syndrome in pregnancy. *Hematol Oncol Clin North Am* 2008;**22**:107–20.

12. Clark EA, Silver RM, Branch DW. Do antiphospholipid antibodies cause preeclampsia and HELLP syndrome? *Curr Rheumatol Rep* 2007;**9**:219–25.

13. Ruffatti A, Bagatella P, Pengo V. Laboratory classification categories and pregnancy outcome in patients with primary antiphospholipid syndrome prescribed antithrombotic therapy. *Thromb Res* 2009;**123**:482–87.

14. Miyakis S, Lockshin MD, Atsumi T, et al. International consensus statement on an update of the classification criteria for definite antiphospholipid syndrome (APS). *J Thromb Haemost* 2006;**4**:295–306.

15. Silver RM, Heuser CC. Stillbirth workup and delivery management. *Clin Obstet Gynecol* 2010;**53**:681 90.

16. Silver RM, Heuser CC. Stillbirth workup and delivery management. *Clin Obstet Gynecol* 2010;**53**:681–90.

17. Ruiz-Irastorza G, Khamashta MA. Lupus and pregnancy: ten questions and some answers. *Lupus* 2008;**17**:416–20.

18. Bates SM, Greer IA, Middeldorp S, et al. VTE, thrombophilia, antithrombotic therapy, and pregnancy: Antithrombotic Therapy and Prevention of Thrombosis, 9th ed: American College of Chest Physicians Evidence-Based Clinical Practice Guidelines. *Chest* 2012;**141** Suppl 2:e691S–736S.

19. Farquharson RG, Quenby S, Greaves M. Antiphospholipid syndrome in pregnancy: a randomized, controlled trial of treatment. *Obstet Gynecol* 2002;**100**:408–13.

20. Lynch A, Marlar R, Murphy J, et al. Antiphospholipid antibodies in predicting adverse pregnancy outcome. A prospective study. *Ann Intern Med* 1994;**120**:470–75.

21. Laskin CA, Spitzer KA, Clark CA, et al. Low molecular weight heparin and aspirin for recurrent pregnancy loss: results from the randomized, controlled HepASA Trial. *J Rheumatol* 2009;**36**:279–87.

22. Ziakas PD, Pavlou M, Voulgarelis M. Heparin treatment in antiphospholipid syndrome with recurrent pregnancy loss: a systematic review and meta-analysis. *Obstet Gynecol* **2010**;**115**:1256–62.

23. Mak A, Cheung MW, Cheak AA, et al. Combination of heparin and aspirin is superior to aspirin alone in enhancing live births in patients with recurrent pregnancy loss and positive anti-phospholipid antibodies: a meta-analysis of randomized controlled trials and meta-regression. *Rheumatology (Oxford)* 2010;**49**:281–88.

24. Kamel H, Navi BB, Sriram N, et al. Risk of a thrombotic event after the 6-week postpartum period. *N Engl J Med* 2014;**370**:1307–15.

25. Cnossen JS, Morris RK, ter Riet G, et al. Use of uterine artery Doppler ultrasonography to predict pre-eclampsia and intra-uterine growth restriction: a systematic review and bivariable meta-analysis. *Can Med Assoc J* 2008;**178**:701–11.

26. Le Thi Huong D, Wechsler B, Vauthier-Brouzes D, et al. The second trimester Doppler ultrasound examination is the best predictor of late pregnancy outcome in systemic lupus erythematosus and/or the antiphospholipid syndrome. *Rheumatology (Oxford)* 2006;**45**:332 38.

27. Faculty of Sexual and Reproductive Health Care. UK Medical Eligibility Criteria for Contraceptive Use (UK MEC). 2009. Available at: http://www.fsrh.org/admin/uploads/UKMEC2009.pdf.

28. Østensen M, Khamashta M, Lockshin M, et al. Anti-inflammatory and immunosuppressive drugs and reproduction. *Arthritis Res Ther* 2006;**8**:209.

29. Levi M, Ten Cate H. Disseminated intravascular coagulation. *N Engl J Med* 1999;**341**:586–92.

30. Levi M, van der Poll T. Disseminated intravascular coagulation: a review for the internist. *Intern Emerg Med* 2013;**8**:23–32.

31. Rattray DD, O'Connell CM, Baskett TF. Acute disseminated intravascular coagulation in obstetrics: a tertiary centre population review (1980 to 2009). *J Obstet Gynaecol Can* 2012;**34**:341–47.

32. Erez O, Novack L, Beer-Weisel R, et al. DIC score in pregnant women—a population based modification of the International Society on Thrombosis and Hemostasis score. *PLoS One* 2014;**9**:e93240.

33. Mallaiah S, Barclay P, Harrod I, Chevannes C, Bhalla A. Introduction of an algorithm for ROTEM-guided fibrinogen concentrate administration in major obstetric haemorrhage. *Anaesthesia* 2015;**70**:166–75.

34. Mercier FJ, Bonnet MP. Use of clotting factors and other prohemostatic drugs for obstetric hemorrhage. *Curr Opin Anaesthesiol* 2010;**23**:310–16.

35. Cotton B, Au B, Nunez T, et al. Predefined massive transfusion protocols are associated with a reduction in organ failure and post injury complication. *J Trauma* 2009;**66**:41–48.

36. Franchini M, Franchi M, Bergamini V, et al. The use of recombinant activated FVII in postpartum haemorrhage. *Clin Obstet Gynecol* 2010;**53**:219–27.

37. Franchini M, Lippi G, Franchini M. The use of recombinant activated factor VII in obstetric and gynaecological haemorrhage. *BJOG* 2007;**114**:8–15.

38. Rodeghiero F, Castaman G, Dini E. Epidemiological investigation of the prevalence of von Willebrand's disease. *Blood* 1987;**69**:454–59.

39. Werner EJ, Broxson EH, Tucker EL, et al. Prevalence of von Willebrand disease in children: a multiethnic study. *J Pediatr* 1993;**123**:893–98.

40. Kadir RA, Lee CA, Sabin CA, et al. Pregnancy in women with von Willebrand's disease or factor XI deficiency. *Br J Obstet Gynaecol* 1998;**105**:314–21.

41. James AH, Jamison MG. Bleeding events and other complications during pregnancy and childbirth in women with von Willebrand disease. *J Thromb Haemost* 2007;**5**:1165–69.

42. Kadir RA, Economides DL, Braithwaite J, et al. The obstetric experience of carriers of haemophilia. *Br J Obstet Gynaecol* 1997;**104**:803 10.

43. Chi C, Lee CA, Shiltagh N, et al. Pregnancy in carriers of haemophilia. *Haemophilia* 2008;**14**:56–64.

44. Guy GP, Baxi LV, Hurlet-Jensen A, et al. An unusual complication in a gravida with factor IX deficiency: case report with review of the literature. *Obstet Gynecol* 1992;**80**:502–505.

45. Varekamp I, Suurmeijer TP, Brocker-Vriends AH, et al. Carrier testing and prenatal diagnosis for hemophilia: experiences and attitudes of 549 potential and obligate carriers. *Am J Med Genet* 1990;**37**:147–54.

46. Pachydakis A, Belgaumkar P, Sharmah A. Persistent scalp bleeding due to fetal coagulopathy following fetal blood sampling. *Int J Gynaecol Obstet* 2006;**92**:69–70.

47. Ljung R, Lindgren AC, Petrini P, et al. Normal vaginal delivery is to be recommended for haemophilia carrier gravidae. *Acta Paediatr* 1994;**83**:609–11.

48. Kadir RA, Economides DL, Braithwaite J, et al. The obstetric experience of carriers of haemophilia. *Br J Obstet Gynaecol* 1997;**104**:803–10.

49. Greer IA, Lowe GD, Walker JJ, et al. Haemorrhagic problems in obstetrics and gynaecology in patients with congenital coagulopathies. *Br J Obstet Gynaecol* 1991;**98**:909–18.

50. Chi C, Lee CA, Shiltagh N, et al. Pregnancy in carriers of haemophilia. *Haemophilia* 2008;**14**:56–64.

51. Chi C, Lee CA, England A, et al. Obstetric analgesia and anaesthesia in women with inherited bleeding disorders. *Thromb Haemost* 2009;**101**:1104–11.

52. Conti M, Mari D, Conti E, et al. Pregnancy in women with different types of von Willebrand disease. *Obstet Gynecol* 1986;**68**:282–85.

53. Roque H, Funai E, Lockwood CJ. von Willebrand disease and pregnancy. *J Matern Fetal Med* 2000;**9**:257–66.

54. Hoveyda F, MacKenzie IZ. Secondary postpartum haemorrhage: incidence, morbidity and current management. *BJOG* 2001;**108**:927–30.

55. Chi C, Bapir M, Lee CA, Kadir RA. Puerperal loss (lochia) in women with or without inherited bleeding disorders. *Am J Obstet Gynecol* 2010;**203**:56.e1–56.

56. Lee CA, Chi C, Pavord SR, et al. The obstetric and gynaecological management of women with inherited bleeding disorders: review with guidelines produced by a taskforce of UK Haemophilia Centre Doctors' Organization. *Haemophilia* 2006;**12**:301–36.

57. Weisz B, Meirow D, Schiff E, et al. Impact and treatment of cancer during pregnancy. *Exper Rev Anticancer Ther* 2004;**4**:889–902.

58. Cohen-Kerem R, Railton C, Oren D, et al. Pregnancy outcome following non obstetric surgical intervention. *Am J Surgery* 2005;**190**:467–73.

59. Pacifici GM, Nottoli R. Placental transfer of drugs administered to the mother. *Clin Pharmacokinet* 1995;**28**:235–69.

60. Doll DC, Ringenberg QS, Yarbro JW. Management of cancer during pregnancy. *Arch Intern Med* 1998;**148**:2058–64.

61. Randall T. National registry seeks scarce data on pregnancy outcomes during chemotherapy. *JAMA* 1993;**269**:323.

62. Cardonick E, Iacobucci A. Use of chemotherapy during human pregnancy. *Lancet Oncol* 2004;**5**:283–91.

63. Aviles A, Neri N. Hematological malignancies and pregnancy: a final report of 84 children who received chemotherapy in utero. *Clin Lymphoma* 2001;**2**:173–77.

64. Nulman I, Laslo D, Fried S, et al. Neurodevelopment of children exposed in utero to treatment of maternal malignancy. *Br J Cancer* 2001;**85**:1611–18.

65. Kal HB, Struikmans H. Radiotherapy during pregnancy: fact and fiction. *Lancet Oncol* 2005;**6**:328–33.

66. Pavlidis NA. Coexistence of pregnancy and malignancy. *Oncologist* 2002;**7**:279–87.

67. Lishner M, Zemlickis D, Degendorfer P, et al. Maternal and foetal outcome following Hodgkin's disease in pregnancy. *Br J Cancer* 1992;**65**:114–17.

68. Hass JF. Pregnancy in association with a newly diagnosed cancer: a population based epidemiological assessment. *Int J Cancer* 1984;**34**:229–35.

69. Rizack T, Mega A, Legare R, et al. Management of haematological malignancies during pregnancy. *Am J Hematol* 2009;**84**:830–41.

70. Yang D, Hladnik L. Treatment of acute promyelocytic leukemia during pregnancy. *Pharmacotherapy* 2009;**29**:709–24.

71. Terada Y, Shindo T, Endoh A, et al. Fetal arrhythmia during treatment of pregnancy-associated acute promyelocytic leukemia with all-trans retinoic acid and favourable outcome. *Leukemia* 1997;**11**:454–55.

72. Cortes J. Natural history and staging of chronic myelogenous leukaemia. *Haematol Oncol Clin North Am* 2004;**18**:569–84.

73. Leung TN, Lau TK, Chung TKH. Thalassaemia screening in pregnancy. *Curr Opin Obstet Gynecol* 2005;**17**:129–34.

74. Kham SK, Quah TC, Loong AM, et al. A molecular epidemiologic study of thalassaemia using newborns' cord blood in a multiracial Asian population in Singapore: results and recommendations for a population screening program. *J Pediatr Hematol Oncol* 2004;**26**:817–19.

75. Old JM. Screening and genetic diagnosis of haemoglobin disorders. *Blood Rev* 2003;**17**:43–53.

76. Cao A, Galanello R. Beta-thalassaemia. *Genet Med* 2010;**12**:61–76.

77. Ryan K, Bain BJ, Worthington D, et al. Significant haemoglobinopathies: guidelines for screening and diagnosis. *Br J Haematol* 2010;**149**:35–49.

78. Lafferty JD, Crowther MA, Ali MA, et al. The evaluation of various mathematical RBC indices and their efficacy in discriminating between thalassemic and non-thalassemic microcytosis. *Am J Clin Pathol* 1996;**106**:201–205.

79. Lo YM, Chiu RW. Noninvasive approaches to prenatal diagnosis of hemoglobinopathies using fetal DNA in maternal plasma. *Hematol Oncol Clin North Am* 2010;**24**:1179–86.

80. Tongsong T, Wanapirak C, Sirichotiyakul S, et al. Fetal sonographic cardiothoracic ratio at midpregnancy as a predictor of Hb Bart disease. *J Ultrasound Med* 1999;**18**:807–11.

81. Ansari S, Kivan A, Tabaroki A. Pregnancy in patients treated for beta thalassaemia major in two centers (Ali Asghar Children's Hospital and Thalassaemia Clinic): outcome for mothers and newborn infants. *Pediatr Hematol Oncol* 2006;**23**:33–37.

82. Ibba RM, Zoppi MA, Floris M, et al. Neural tube defects in the offspring of thalassaemia carriers. *Fetal Diagn Ther* 2003;**18**:5–7.

83. Shehata N, Burrows R, Kelton JG. Gestational thrombocytopenia. *Clin Obstet Gynecol* 1999;**42**:127–34.

84. Burrows RF, Kelton JG. Thrombocytopenia at delivery: a prospective survey of 6715 deliveries. *Am J Obstet Gynecol* 1990;**42**:327–34.

85. Levy JA, Murphy LD. Thrombocytopenia in pregnancy. *J Am Board Fam Pract* 2002;**15**:290–97.

86. Sullivan CA, Martin JN Jr. Management of the obstetric patient with thrombocytopenia. *Clin Obstet Gynecol* 1995;**38**:521–34.

87. McCrae KR. Thrombocytopenia in pregnancy: differential diagnosis, pathogenesis and management. *Blood Rev* 2003;**17**:7–14.

88. James TR, Reid HL, Mullings AM. Are published standards for haematological indices in pregnancy applicable across populations: an evaluation in healthy pregnant Jamaican women. *BMC Pregnancy Childbirth* 2008;**8**:8.

89. Strong J. Bleeding disorders in pregnancy. *Curr Obstet Gynecol* 2003;**13**:1–6.

90. McCrae KR. Thrombocytopenia in pregnancy. *Haematology* 2010;**4**:397–402.

91. Egbor M, Johnson A, Harris F, Makanjoula D, Shehata H. Pregnancy-associated atypical haemolytic uraemic syndrome in the postpartum period: a case report and review of the literature. *Obstet Med* 2011;**4**:83–85.

92. Harkness DR, Byrnes JJ, Lian EC, Williams WD, Hensley GT. Hazard of platelet transfusion in thrombotic thrombocytopenic purpura. *JAMA* 1981;**246**:1931–33.

93. Swisher KK, Terrell DR, Vesely SK, Kremer Hovinga JA, Lämmle B, George JN. Clinical outcomes after platelet transfusions in patients with thrombotic thrombocytopenic purpura. *Transfusion* 2009;**49**:873–87.

94. Kaandorp S, Di Nisio M, Goddijn M, et al. Aspirin or anticoagulants for treating recurrent miscarriage in women without antiphospholipid syndrome. *Cochrane Database Syst Rev* 2009;**1**:CD004734.

95. Rey E, Kahn SR, David M, Shrier I. Thrombophilic disorders and fetal loss: a meta analysis. *Lancet* 2003;**361**:901–908.

96. Bick RL. Recurrent miscarriage syndrome and infertility caused by blood coagulation protein or platelet defects. *Hematol Oncol Clin North Am* 2000;**14**:1117–31.

97. Meinardi JR, Middeldorp S, de Kam P, et al. Increased risk for fetal loss in carriers of the factor V Leiden mutation. *Ann Intern Med* 1999;**130**:737–39.

98. Balasch J, Reverter JC, Fabregues F, et al. First trimester repeated abortion is not associated with activated protein C resistance. *Hum Reprod* 1997;**12**:1094–97.

99. Urbanus RT, Derksen RH, de Groot PG. Current insight into diagnostics and pathophysiology of the antiphospholipid syndrome. *Blood Rev* 2008;**22**:93–105.

100. Lassere M, Empson M. Treatment of antiphospholipid syndrome in pregnancy: a systematic review of randomized therapeutic trials. *Thromb Res* 2004;**114**:419–26.

101. Dawood F, Farquharson R, Quenby S, et al. Acquired activated protein C resistance maybe a risk factor for recurrent fetal loss. *Fertil Steril* 2003;**80**:649–50.

102. Rai R, Shelbak A, Cohen H, et al. Factor V Leiden and acquired activated protein C resistance among 1000 women with recurrent miscarriage. *Hum Reprod* 2001;**16**:961–65.

103. Lindqvist PG, Svensson PJ, Marsaal K, et al. Activated protein C resistance (FV: Q506) and pregnancy. *Thromb Haemost* 1999;**81**:532–37.

104. Jauniaux E, Farquharson RG, Christianson OB, et al. Evidence-based guidelines for the investigation and medical treatment of recurrent miscarriage. *Hum Reprod* 2006;**21**:2216–22.

105. Jaslow CR, Carney JL, Kutteh WH. Diagnostic factors identified in 1020 women with two verses three or more recurrent pregnancy losses. *Fertil Steril* 2010;**2009**:1234–43.

106. Clark P, Walker ID, Langhorne P, et al. SPIN: the Scottish Pregnancy Intervention Study: a multi-centre randomized control trial of low molecular weight heparin and low dose aspirin in women with recurrent miscarriage. *Blood* 2010;**115**:4162–67.

107. Kaandorp SP, Goddijn M, Van Der Post JA, et al. Aspirin plus heparin or aspirin alone in women with recurrent miscarriage. *N Engl J Med* 2010;**362**:1586–96.

108. Coppens M, Folkeringa N, Teune MJ, et al. Outcome of subsequent pregnancy after a first loss in women with the factor V Leiden or prothrombin 20210A. *Thromb Haemost* 2007;**5**:1444–48.

109. American College of Obstetrics and Gynaecologists. ACOG practice bulletin. Management of recurrent pregnancy loss. *Int J Gynaecol Obstet* 2002;**78**:179–90.

110. Norrie G, Farquharson RG, Greaves M. Screening and treatment for heritable thrombophilia in pregnancy failure: inconsistencies among UK early pregnancy units. *Br J Haematol* 2008;**144**:241–44.

111. Carp H, Dolitzky M, Inbal A. Thromboprophylaxis improves the live birth rate in women with consecutive recurrent miscarriages and hereditary thrombophilia. *J Thromb Haemost* 2003;**1**:433–38.

112. Gris JC, Mares P. The long and winding road towards LMWH for pregnancy loss. *J Thromb Haemost* 2005;**3**:224–26.

113. Folkeringa N, Leendert J, Brouwer P, et al. Reduction of high fetal loss rate by anticoagulant treatment during pregnancy in antithrombin, protein C or protein S deficient women. *Br J Haematol* 2007;**136**: 656–61.

114. Lindqvist PG, Merlo J. The natural course of women with recurrent fetal loss. *J Thromb Haemost* 2006;**4**:896–97.

115. Lindqvist PG, Svensson PJ, Marsaal K, et al. Activated protein C resistance (FV: Q506) and pregnancy. *Thromb Haemost* 1999;**81**:532–37.

116. Rai R, Regan L. Recurrent miscarriage. *Lancet* 2006;**368**:601–11.

117. Rai RS, Clifford K, Cohen H, et al. High prospective fetal loss rate in untreated pregnancies of women with recurrent miscarriage and antiphospholipid antibodies. *Hum Reprod* 1995;**10**:348–49.

118. Laskin CA, Spitzer KA, Clark CA, et al. Low molecular weight heparin and aspirin for recurrent pregnancy loss: results from the randomized, controlled HepASA Trial. *J Rheumatol* 2009;**36**:279–87.

119. Farquharson RG, Quenby S, Greaves M. Antiphospholipid syndrome in pregnancy: a randomized, controlled trial of treatment. *Obstet Gynecol* 2002;**100**:408–13.

120. Brenner B. Antithrombotic prophylaxis for women with thrombophilia and pregnancy complications. *Thromb Haemost* 2003;**1**:2070–72.

121. Dawood F, Mountford R, Farquharson R, et al. Genetic polymorphisms on the factor V gene in women with recurrent miscarriage and acquired APCR. *Hum Reprod* 2007;**22**:2546–53.

122. Flint Porter T, La Coursiere Y, Scott JR. Immunotherapy for recurrent miscarriage. *Cochrane Database Syst Rev* 2006;**2**:CD000112.

123. Laskin CA, Bombardier C, Hannah ME, et al. Prednisone and aspirin in women with autoantibodies and unexplained recurrent fetal loss. *N Engl J Med* 1997;**368**:148–53.

124. Triolo G, Ferrante A, Ciccia F, et al. Randomized study of subcutaneous low molecular weight heparin plus aspirin versus intravenous immunoglobulin in the treatment of recurrent fetal loss associated with antiphospholipid antibodies. *Arthritis Rheum* 2003;**48**:728–31.

125. de Benoist B, Mclean E, Egli I, Cogswell M (eds). *Worldwide Prevalence of Anaemia 1993– 2005: WHO Global Database on Anaemia*. Geneva: World Health Organization; 2008.

126. World Health Organization. *Haemoglobin concentrations for the diagnosis of anaemia and assessment of severity*. Vitamin and Mineral Nutrition Information System. Geneva: World Health Organization; 2011.

127. World Health Organization. *Iron Deficiency Anaemia: Assessment Prevention and Contro. A Guide for Programme Managers*. Geneva: World Health Organization; 2001.

128. Stevens GA, Finucane MM, De-Regil LM, et al. Global, regional, and national trends in haemoglobin concentration and prevalence of total and severe anaemia in children and pregnant and non-pregnant women for 1995–2011: a systematic analysis of population-representative data. *Lancet Glob Health* 2013;**1**:E16–E25.

129. Aslinia F, Mazza JJ, Yale SH. Megaloblastic anemia and other causes of macrocytosis. *Clin Med Res* 2006;**4**:236–41.

130. Gambling L, Danzeisen R, Gair S, et al. Effect of iron deficiency on placental transfer of iron and expression of iron transport proteins in vivo and in vitro. *Biochem J* 2001;**356**:883–89.

131. Pavord S, Myers B, Robinson S, et al, UK guidelines on the management of iron deficiency in pregnancy. *Br J Haematol* 2012;**156**:588–600.

132. Shehata HA, Ali MM, Evans-Jones JC, Upton GJ, Manyonda IT. Red cell distribution width (RDW) changes in pregnancy. *Int J Gynaecol Obstet* 1998;**62**:43–46.

133. Punnonen K, Irjala K, Rajamaki A. Serum transferrin receptor and its ratio to serum ferritin in the diagnosis of iron deficiency. *Blood* 1997;**89**:1052–57.

134. United Nations Children's Fund, United Nations University, World Health Organization. *Iron Deficiency Anaemia: Assessment, Prevention, and Control. A Guide for Programme Managers*. Geneva: World Health Organization; 2001. Available at: http://www.who.int/nutrition/publications/en/ida_assessment_prevention_control.pdf.

135. World Health Organization. *Guideline: Daily Iron and Folic Acid Supplementation in Pregnant Women*. Geneva: World Health Organization; 2012.

136. National Institute for Health and Care Excellence (NICE). Antenatal Care for Uncomplicated Pregnancies. Clinical guideline [CG62], updated 2019. London: NICE; 2008. Available at: https://www.nice.org.uk/guidance/CG62.

137. Royal College of Obstetricians and Gynaecologists (RCOG). *Blood Transfusions in Obstetrics*. Green-top Guideline No. 47. London: RCOG; 2007.

138. Al RA, Unlubilgin E, Kandemir O, Yalvac S, Cakir L, Haberal A. Intravenous versus oral iron for treatment of anemia in pregnancy: a randomized trial. *Obstet Gynecol* 2005;**106**:1335–40.

139. Bayoumeu F, Subiran-Buisset C, Baka N-E, Legagneur H, Monnier-Barbarino P, Laxenaire MC. Iron therapy in iron deficiency anaemia in pregnancy: Intravenous route versus oral route. *Eur J Obstet Gynecol Reprod Biol* 2005;**123**:S15–19.

140. Van Wyk DB, Martens MG. Intravenous ferric carboxymaltose compared with oral iron in the treatment of postpartum anaemia: a randomized controlled trial. *Obstet Gynecol* 2007;**110**:267–78.

141. Solomons NW, Schumann K. Intramuscular administration of iron dextran is inappropriate for treatment of moderate pregnancy anaemia, both in intervention research on underprivileged women and in routine prenatal care provided by public health services. *Am J Clin Nutr* 2004;**79**:1–3.

142. Department of Health. *Better Blood Transfusion – Safe and Appropriate Use of Blood*. HSC 2007/001. London: Department of Health.

143. Scholl TO, Johnson WG. Folic acid: influence on the outcome of pregnancy. *Am J Clin Nutr* 2000;**71** Suppl:1295S–303S

144. Weatherall D, Akinyanju O, Fucharoen S, Olivieri N, Musgrove P. Inherited disorders of haemoglobin. In: Jamison DT, Breman JG, Measham AR, et al. (eds), *Disease Control Priorities in Developing Countries*, 2nd edn, pp. 663–80. Washington, DC: The World Bank; 2006.

145. Angastiniotis M, Modell B, Englezos P, et al. Prevention and control of haemoglobinopathies. *Bull World Health Organ* 1995;**73**:375–86.

146. Serjeant GR. Sickle cell disease. *Lancet* 1997;**350**:725–30.

147. Diallo D, Tchernia G. Sickle cell disease in Africa. *Curr Opin Hematol* 2002;**9**:111–16.

148. Streetley A, Latinovic R, Hall K, et al. Implementation of universal newborn bloodspot screening for sickle cell disease and other clinically significant haemoglobinopathies in England: screening results for 2005–7. *J Clin Pathol* 2009;**62**:26–30.

149. Telfer P, Coen P, Chakravorty S, et al. Clinical outcomes in children with sickle cell disease living in England: a neonatal cohort in East London. *Haematologica* 2007;**92**:905–12.

150. Wierenga KJ, Hambleton IR, Lewis NA. Survival estimates for patients with homozygous sickle-cell disease in Jamaica: a clinic based population study. *Lancet* 2001;**357**:680–83.

151. Villers MS, Jamison MG, De Castro LM, et al. Morbidity associated with sickle cell disease in pregnancy. *Am J Obstet Gynecol* 2008;**199**:125.e1–125.

152. Dare FO, Makinde OO, Faasuba OB. The obstetric performance of sickle cell disease patients and homozygous haemoglobin C disease patients in Ile-Ife Nigeria. *Int J Gynaecol Obstet* 1992;**37**:163–68.

153. Oteng-Ntim E, Ayensah B, Knight M, Howard J. Pregnancy outcome in patients with sickle cell disease in the UK—a national cohort study comparing sickle cell anaemia (HbSS) with HbSC disease. *Br J Haematol* 2015;**169**:129–37.

154. Al Jama FE, Gasem T, Burshaid S, et al. Pregnancy outcome in patients with homozygous sickle cell disease in a university hospital, Eastern Saudi Arabia. *Arch Gynecol Obstet* 2009;**280**:793–97.

155. Rajab KE, Issa AA, Mohammed AM, et al. Sickle cell disease and pregnancy in Bahrain. *Int J Gynecol Obstet* 2006;**93**:171–75.

156. Ngo C, Kayem G, Habibi A, et al. Pregnancy in sickle cell disease: maternal and fetal outcomes in a population receiving prophylactic partial exchange transfusions. *Eur J Obstet Gynae Reprod Biol* 2010;**152**:138–42.

157. Howard RJ, Tuck SM, Pearson TC. Pregnancy in sickle cell disease in the UK: results of a multicentre survey of the effect of prophylactic blood transfusion on maternal and fetal outcome. *Br J Obstet Gynaecol* 1995;**102**:947–51.

158. Powars DR, Sandhu M, Niland-Weiss J, et al. Pregnancy in sickle cell disease. *Obstet Gynecol* 1986;**67**:217–28.

159. Sun PM, Wilburn W, Raynor BD, et al. Sickle cell disease in pregnancy: twenty years of experience at Grady Memorial Hospital, Atlanta, Georgia. *Am J Obstet Gynecol* 2001;**184**:1127–39.

160. El Shafei AM, Sandhu AK, Dhaliwal JK. Maternal mortality in Bahrain with special reference to sickle cell disease. *Aust NZ J Obstet Gynaecol* 1988;**28**:41–44.

161. Ataga KI, Moore CG, Jones S, et al. Pulmonary hypertension in patients with sickle cell disease: a longitudinal study. *Br J Haem* 2006;**134**:109–15.

162. Sickle Cell Society. Standards for the Clinical Care of Adults with Sickle Cell Disease in the UK. 2008. Available at: https://www.sicklecellsociety.org/resource/standards-clinical-care-adults-sickle-cell-disease-uk/standards-for-the-clinical-care-of-adults-with-sickle-cell-disease-in-the-uk/.

163. Charache S, Terrin ML, Moore RD, et al. Effect of hydroxycarbamide on the frequency of painful crisis in SCD. *N Engl J Med* 1995;**332**:1317–22.

164. Lindenbaum J, Klipstein FA. Folic acid deficiency in sickle cell anaemia. *N Engl J Med* 1963;**269**:875–82.

165. Duley L, Henderson-Smart DJ, Meher S, et al. Antiplatelet agents for preventing pre-eclampsia and its complications. *Cochrane Database Syst Rev* 2007;**2**:CD004659.

166. Villers MS, Jamison MG, De Castro LM, et al. Morbidity associated with sickle cell disease in pregnancy. *Am J Obstet Gynecol* 2008;**199**:125.e1–125.e5.

167. National Institute of Health and Clinical Excellence (NICE). *The Management of Hypertensive Disorders during Pregnancy*. Clinical guidelines [CG107]. London: NICE; 2010. Available at: https://www.nice.org.uk/guidance/cg107.

168. Cunningham FG, Pritchard JA. Prophylactic transfusions of normal red blood cells during pregnancies complicated by sickle cell hemoglobinopathies. *Am J Obstet Gynecol* 1975;**135**:994–1003.

169. Koshy M, Burd L, Wallace D, et al. Prophylactic red cell transfusions in pregnant patients with sickle cell disease. *N Engl J Med* 1988;**319**:1447–52.

170. Mahomed K. Prophylactic versus selective blood transfusion for sickle cell anaemia during pregnancy. *Cochrane Database Syst Rev* 2007;**3**:CD000040.

171. El Shafei AM, Sandhu AK, Dhaliwal JK. Maternal mortality in Bahrain with special reference to sickle cell disease. *Aust NZ J Obstet Gynaecol* 1988;**28**:41–44.

172. Anyaegbunam A, Morel MI, Merkatz IR. Antepartum fetal surveillance tests during sickle cell crisis. *Am J Obstet Gynecol* 1991;**165**:1081–83.

173. Anyaegbunam A, Mikhail M, Axioitis C, et al. Placental histology and placental/fetal weight ratios in pregnant women with sickle

cell disease: relationship to pregnancy outcome. *J Assoc Acad Minor Phys* 1994;**5**:123–25.

174. Royal College of Obstetricians and Gynaecologists (RCOG). *Reducing the Risk of Thrombosis and Embolism during Pregnancy and the Puerperium.* Green-top Guideline No. 37(A). London: RCOG; 2009.

175. Howard RJ, Tuck SM, Pearson TC. Pregnancy in sickle cell disease in the UK: results of a multicentre survey of the effect of prophylactic blood transfusion on maternal and fetal outcome. *Br J Obstet Gynaecol* 1995;**102**:947–51.

176. Camous J, N'da A, Etienne-Julan M, et al. Anesthetic management of pregnant women with sickle cell disease—effect on postnatal sickling complications. *Can J Anesth* 2008;**55**:276–83.

177. Legardy JK, Curtis KM. Progestogen-only contraceptive use among women with sickle cell anaemia, a systematic review. *Contraception* 2006;**73**:195–204.

178. Al Jama FE, Gasem T, Burshaid S, et al. Pregnancy outcome in patients with homozygous sickle cell disease in a university hospital, Eastern Saudi Arabia. *Arch Gynecol Obstet* 2009;**280**:793–97.

179. Howard RJ, Tuck SM, Pearson TC. Pregnancy in sickle cell disease in the UK: results of a multicentre survey of the effect of prophylactic blood transfusion on maternal and fetal outcome. *Br J Obstet Gynaecol* 1995;**102**:947–51.

180. Rees DC, Olujohungbe AD, Parker NE, et al. Guidelines for the management of acute painful crisis in sickle cell disease. *Br J Haematol* 2003;**120**:744–52.

181. Serjeant GR, Loy LL, Crowther M, et al. Outcome of pregnancy in homozygous sickle cell disease. *Obstet Gynaecol* 2004;**103**:1278–85.

182. Howard RJ, Tuck SM, Pearson TC. Pregnancy in sickle cell disease in the UK: results of a multicentre survey of the effect of prophylactic blood transfusion on maternal and fetal outcome. *Br J Obstet Gynaecol* 1995;**102**:947–51.

183. Smith JA, Espeland M, Bellevue R, et al. Pregnancy in sickle cell disease: experience of the cooperative study of sickle cell disease. *Obstet Gynaecol* 1996;**87**:199–204.

184. Ohene-Frempong K, Weiner SJ, Sleeper LA, et al. Cerebrovascular accidents in SCD: rates and risk factors. *Blood* 1998;**91**:288–94.

16

Thrombosis and embolism in pregnancy

Ian A. Greer

Epidemiology, risk factors, and clinical features

Venous thromboembolism (VTE) is a leading cause of direct maternal mortality with a substantial number of deaths associated with inadequate approaches to prevention and management of this condition in pregnancy (1). However, it is not just mortality that is important as there is significant morbidity from gestational VTE, due not only to thrombosis per se, but also haemorrhagic problems with therapeutic anticoagulation, and an impact on management of delivery for women with a recent VTE who are on therapeutic anticoagulation. Long-term sequelae include recurrent VTE and post-thrombotic syndrome, as well as an impact on use of hormonal contraception and hormone-replacement therapy in later life (2). Providing sound prophylaxis or management of VTE in pregnancy can impact outcome, with recent reports suggesting that it is associated with reduced mortality (1) and morbidity (3). In the United Kingdom's most recent report on maternal mortality, VTE was the most common cause of direct maternal death with an incidence of 1.08 (95% confidence interval (CI) 0.71–1.59) per 100,000 maternities (4). The overall reported incidence of gestational VTE varies considerably depending on the population studied, but ranges from 0.5 to 2.2 per 1000 (3, 5, 6). In relative terms, there is a 5- to 10-fold increase in the risk of VTE during pregnancy, increasing to a daily risk of 15–35-fold in the puerperium, compared with non-pregnant women of similar age (5). The risk of VTE appears greatest during the first 3 weeks following delivery when 80% of postpartum events occur (6, 7), then declines, although there may be a small increase in risk persisting for up to 12 weeks after delivery (8).

Clinically, it is important to recognize that there are important considerations for VTE in pregnancy that set it apart from VTE in the non-pregnant. Deep venous thrombosis (DVT) in pregnancy is usually left sided (85% in pregnancy vs 55% in non-pregnant), and proximal (72% iliofemoral in pregnancy vs 9% in the non-pregnant) (9). The latter point is important as there is greater potential for thromboembolism from proximal DVT, and also post-thrombotic problems are more likely. The majority of women with VTE in pregnancy have non-specific symptoms and signs, such as leg swelling or breathlessness. These can also occur with the physiological changes of pregnancy, so making clinical diagnosis unreliable and objective diagnosis is required (9, 10). Non-specific lower abdominal pain can occur with extension of thrombus into the pelvic veins or venous distension through the collateral circulation in the pelvis including around the ovary (10).

The increase in risk of VTE in pregnancy is considered due to venous stasis, procoagulant changes, suppressed fibrinolysis, and endothelial injury in the course of delivery (9). Risk factors often exaggerate one or more of these components, and clinical events tend to occur when multiple risk factors coexist (10). The most commonly encountered risk factors are shown in **Table 16.1** (see **Table 16.2** for levels of risk). Previous VTE with a relative risk of over 20-fold (3, 13) is one of the most important risk factors. There are limited data on how these risks interact, but estimates suggest that the interaction leads to a high level of risk. For example, immobility with strict bedrest for at least 1 week in the antenatal period with a pre-pregnancy body mass index (BMI) of at least 25 kg/m² has been estimated to carry a 62-fold increase in VTE risk (5). These risk factors inform the use of thromboprophylaxis which is used where risk is considered to be significant as set out in various guidelines (5, 11, 14).

While heritable thrombophilia in general is a risk factor, the magnitude of risk varies with the type of heritable or acquired thrombophilia (11, 14). Furthermore, the absolute risk is often modest. For example, in non-familial studies of antithrombin and protein C and protein S deficiencies, the estimated absolute risk is less than 1%, and for heterozygous factor V Leiden and prothrombin G20210A is around 1%. The absolute risk is higher in homozygotes; however, estimates still place the risk at under 5% (5). There are data suggesting that a positive family history of VTE in women with thrombophilia is associated with a two- to fourfold higher risk of VTE (15, 16).

Anticoagulants in pregnancy

The key consideration for anticoagulant treatment in pregnancy is the potential for any effect on the fetus, both in terms of impact on development and also any anticoagulant effect consequent upon placental transfer. Warfarin and other vitamin K antagonists cross the placenta. These agents have a potential teratogenic effect, specifically warfarin embryopathy (midface hypoplasia, short proximal limbs, short phalanges, and scoliosis), which complicates a small number of pregnancies exposed to warfarin in the first trimester.

Table 16.1 Risk factors for gestational venous thromboembolism

Patient factors	Pregnancy factors
Previous VTE****	Twin pregnancy**
Immobility***	Antepartum haemorrhage**
BMI >30 kg/m²***	Postpartum haemorrhage (>1 L)***
Weight >120 kg**	Caesarean section**
Smoking (10–30 cigarettes a day before or during pregnancy)**	Pre-eclampsia**
Weight gain >21 kg (vs 7–21 kg)*	Pre-eclampsia with fetal growth restriction***
Parity >1*	Assisted reproductive techniques**/***
Age >35 years*	Blood transfusion**
Medical conditions,[a] e.g. SLE, heart disease, anaemia, sickle cell disease, active infection, varicose veins	Hyperemesis**
Thrombophilia[b]	Postpartum infection***

Typical estimates risk: odds ratios: **** >20; *** >4; ** >2; * >1.

[a] Wide range of risk according to type and severity of medical condition (14).

[b] See Table 16.2 for levels of risk.

Source data from Jacobsen AF, Skjeldestad FE, Sandset PM. Ante- and postnatal risk factors of venous thrombosis: a hospital-based case-control study. *J Thromb Haemost* 2008; 6(6):905–912, Greer IA. Thrombosis in pregnancy: updates in diagnosis and management. *Hematology Am Soc Hematol Educ Program* 2012;2012:203–7, Bates SM, Greer IA, Middeldorp S, Veenstra DL, Prabulos AM, Vandvik PO. VTE, Thrombophilia, Antithrombotic Therapy, and Pregnancy. *Chest* 2012;141(2)(Suppl):e691S–e736S, Robertson L, Wu O, Langhorne P, et al. Thrombosis Risk and Economic Assessment of Thrombophilia Screening (TREATS) Study. Thrombophilia in pregnancy: a systematic review. *Br J Haematol* 2005;132 :171–96, James AH, Jamison MG, Brancazio LR, Myers ER. Venous thromboembolism during pregnancy and the postpartum period: incidence, risk factors, and mortality. *Am J Obstet Gynecol* 2006;194:1311–15 and Royal College of Obstetricians and Gynaecologists. Green-top Guideline No. 37a. Reducing the risk of thrombosis and embolism during pregnancy and the puerperium (April 2015). https://www.rcog.org.uk/en/guidelines-research-services/guidelines/gtg37a/.

With discontinuation of vitamin K antagonists prior to 6 weeks' gestation, the risk of warfarin embryopathy is avoided (11). There are also associations with pregnancy loss and neurodevelopmental deficits (11), and risks from fetal anticoagulation. While generally warfarin should be avoided in pregnancy, there are some high-risk situations where, because of a high risk of maternal thrombosis that is thought to outweigh the fetal risk, warfarin can be considered. In

Table 16.2 Relative risk of gestational venous thromboembolism in asymptomatic women with heritable thrombophilia

Thrombophilia	Typical relative risk for non-familial studies Odds ratio (95% confidence interval)
Antithrombin deficiency	4.7 (1.3–17.0)
Protein C deficiency	4.8 (2.2–10.6)
Protein S deficiency	3.2 (1.5–6.9)
Factor V Leiden, heterozygous	8.3 (5.4–12.7)
Factor V Leiden, homozygous	34.4 (9.9–120.1)
Prothrombin G20201A, heterozygous	6.8 (2.5–18.8)
Prothrombin G20201A, homozygous	26.4 (1.2–559.3)

Source data from 12. Robertson L, Wu O, Langhorne P, et al. Thrombosis Risk and Economic Assessment of Thrombophilia Screening (TREATS) Study. Thrombophilia in pregnancy: a systematic review. *Br J Haematol* 2005;132(2):171–196.

this situation, it is still best to avoid warfarin in the first trimester where possible. For women on long-term oral anticoagulation it is important to discontinue this (and replace with unfractionated heparin (UFH) or low-molecular-weight heparins (LMWHs)) where possible by 6 weeks' gestation to avoid the risk of embryopathy. However, as warfarin does not cross into breastmilk, it can be used postpartum (11). Outside of pregnancy, oral direct thrombin and factor Xa inhibitors are increasingly being used; however, their effects and risks in pregnancy have not been established (11, 17). Given the established safety of alternative established treatments (UFH and LMWH), these agents should generally be avoided in pregnancy. Fondaparinux appears to cross the placenta in small quantities; however, adverse effects have not been described in the increasing number of reports describing its use in pregnancy, particularly in situations where LMWH cannot be used (17–19). It should be noted that most reports on fondaparinux relate to second- and third-trimester use.

In contrast to warfarin, UFH and LMWH do not cross the placenta and therefore do not pose a direct risk to the fetus (11). LMWH has a better safety profile than UFH (5, 9–11, 20, 21) in terms of bleeding complications, heparin-induced thrombocytopenia, and heparin-associated osteoporosis. A systematic review of 18 studies with 981 pregnant women with acute VTE reported a mean incidence of major antenatal bleeding of 1.41% (95% CI 0.60–2.41%), 1.90% (95% CI 0.80–3.60%) in the first 24 hours after delivery, 1.2% (95% CI 0.30–2.50%) for major postpartum bleeding after 24 hours, and 1.97% (95% CI 0.88–3.49%) for recurrent VTE in pregnancy (21). There is a risk of accumulation of LMWH in women with significant renal dysfunction, as these agents depend on renal excretion and dose adjustment may be required in this situation.

Prophylaxis of venous thromboembolism

There is considerable variability between guidelines on the use of prophylactic anticoagulants for VTE. This is because of an insufficient evidence base to inform the estimated risk of gestational VTE and associated risk reduction with prophylaxis, the burdens of long-term (parenteral) anticoagulant therapy, and patient and physician values and preferences. Guidelines are based on evidence obtained from a small number of trials, observational studies, or extrapolated from the non-pregnant situation. An individual risk–benefit assessment is needed when considering thromboprophylaxis with shared decision-making with the woman regarding her preferences and values. Underlining the need for better evidence, the most recent Cochrane systematic review of thromboprophylaxis in pregnancy and the puerperium concluded that the current available evidence is insufficient to make firm recommendations, based on 2592 women in 16 randomized trials (22). The common risk factors for VTE are set out in **Tables 16.1** and **16.2**. Lack of knowledge of how these interact, but an awareness that they do and that the interactions are not simply arithmetic, has led to a pragmatic approach in guidelines based on magnitude and number of risk factors. There is consistency, however, on a preference for long-term subcutaneous LMWH for prophylaxis. **Table 16.3** summarizes existing guidance for thromboprophylaxis according to the clinical features (11, 14, 23). When prophylaxis with LMWH is used, there is also uncertainty regarding duration, particularly postpartum. Mechanical prophylaxis

Table 16.3 Suggested prophylaxis of venous thromboembolism in pregnancy based on guidelines

Patient group	Suggested[a] period of prophylaxis	Suggested[a] thromboprophylactic agent and management
All pregnant women with previous VTE	Postpartum prophylaxis for 6 weeks	Prophylactic or intermediate-dose LMWH[b] or vitamin K antagonists targeted at INR[c] 2.0
Pregnant women at low risk of recurrent VTE (single previous VTE associated with a transient risk factor not related to pregnancy or use of oestrogen such as with the combined oral contraceptive pill)	NA	Clinical vigilance antepartum rather than antepartum prophylaxis (note that if multiple additional risk factors are present, these may lead to antepartum prophylaxis with prophylactic or intermediate-dose LMWH)
Pregnant women at moderate to high risk of recurrent VTE because of (a) previous single VTE that was unprovoked or pregnancy or oestrogen related; (b) multiple previous unprovoked VTE not receiving long-term anticoagulation	Antepartum from diagnosis of pregnancy	Prophylactic or intermediate-dose LMWH[b]
Pregnant women receiving long-term vitamin K antagonists	Antepartum from diagnosis of pregnancy (switching to LMWH before 6 weeks' gestation if possible to avoid embryopathy risk)	Therapeutic-dose LMWH or 75% of a therapeutic dose of LMWH followed by resumption of vitamin K antagonists postpartum
Pregnant women with (a) no previous VTE and (b) homozygous for factor V Leiden or the prothrombin 20210A mutation and (c) have a positive family history for VTE	Throughout the antepartum period from diagnosis of pregnancy and postpartum prophylaxis for 6 weeks	Antepartum: prophylactic- or intermediate-dose LMWH. Postpartum: prophylactic- or intermediate-dose LMWH or vitamin K antagonists targeted at INR 2.0–3.0
Pregnant women with all other heritable thrombophilias and no prior VTE who have a positive family history for VTE	Postpartum prophylaxis for 6 weeks	Antepartum: clinical vigilance Postpartum: prophylaxis with prophylactic or intermediate-dose LMWH
Pregnant women with no previous VTE and known to be homozygous for factor V Leiden or the prothrombin 20210A mutation and who do not have a positive family history for VTE	Postpartum prophylaxis for 6 weeks	Antepartum: clinical vigilance Postpartum: prophylactic or intermediate-dose LMWH or vitamin K antagonists targeted at INR 2.0–3.0
Pregnant women with all other thrombophilias and no previous VTE and no family history for VTE	NA	Antepartum and postpartum clinical vigilance rather than pharmacological prophylaxis
Women at increased risk of VTE after caesarean section because of the presence of one major or at least two minor risk factors[d]	Postpartum while in hospital following delivery	Prophylactic LMWH or mechanical prophylaxis (elastic stockings or intermittent pneumatic compression) if heparin contraindicated. Elastic stockings may be combined with LMWH for those considered at very high risk for VTE
Women at high-risk because of significant risk factors persisting following delivery	Extended prophylaxis (up to 6 weeks following delivery)	Prophylactic LMWH. Elastic stockings may be combined with LMWH for those considered at very high risk for VTE
Women with multiple risk factors (≥3 antenatal or ≥2 postpartum) or with absolute risk considered >1%	Antepartum prophylaxis and postpartum prophylaxis for 6 weeks	Prophylactic LMWH. Elastic stockings may be combined with LMWH for those considered at very high risk for VTE

[a] 'Suggested' rather than recommended due to lack of direct evidence.
[b] Prophylactic LMWH given subcutaneously once daily: examples—dalteparin 5000 units, enoxaparin 40 mg, tinzaparin 4500 units. (Note that at extremes of body weight, modification of dose may be required). Intermediate-dose LMWH: for example, dalteparin 5000 units or enoxaparin 40 mg subcutaneously twice daily.
[c] INR: international normalized ratio
[d] Major risk factors (OR ≥6): the presence of at least one risk factor suggests a risk of postpartum VTE >3% following caesarean section: immobility, postpartum haemorrhage >1000 mL with surgery, previous VTE, pre-eclampsia with fetal growth restriction, thrombophilia (antithrombin deficiency, factor V Leiden (homozygous or heterozygous), prothrombin G20210A (homozygous or heterozygous)), medical conditions (systemic lupus erythematosus, heart disease, sickle cell disease, blood transfusion, postpartum infection. Minor risk factors (OR ≥6 when combined): the presence of at least two risk factors or one risk factor in the setting of emergency caesarean section suggests a risk of postpartum VTE >3% following caesarean section: BMI >30 kg/m², multiple pregnancy, postpartum haemorrhage >1 L, smoking >10 cigarettes/day, fetal growth restriction, thrombophilia (protein C deficiency, protein S deficiency), pre-eclampsia.

Source data from Bates SM, Greer IA, Middeldorp S, Veenstra DL, Prabulos AM, Vandvik PO. VTE, Thrombophilia, Antithrombotic Therapy, and Pregnancy. *Chest* 2012;141(2) (Suppl):e691S–e736S, Royal College of Obstetricians and Gynaecologists. Green-top Guideline No. 37a. *Reducing the risk of thrombosis and embolism during pregnancy and the puerperium* (April 2015). https://www.rcog.org.uk/en/guidelines-research-services/guidelines/gtg37a/, and Chan WS, Rey E, Kent NE; VTE in Pregnancy Guideline Working Group, Chan WS, Kent NE, Rey E, Corbett T, David M, Douglas MJ, Gibson PS, Magee L, Rodger M, Smith RE. Venous thromboembolism and antithrombotic therapy in pregnancy. *J Obstet Gynaecol Can* 2014;36(6):527–53.

with graduated elastic compression stockings is an alternative treatment where there are contraindications to the use of anticoagulants, or as additional prophylaxis in those women considered at high risk. Women considered at significant risk of VTE should be advised of the features of VTE so that they can seek specific medical assessment should such features arise.

Diagnosis of venous thromboembolism

VTE can occur at any time in pregnancy; however, it is noteworthy that over 50% of events occur prior to 20 weeks' gestation (24, 25). The clinical features were noted earlier, but are not in themselves sufficiently reliable to make a firm diagnosis. As clinical diagnosis is unreliable then given the importance of the condition, objective assessment is required when there is clinical suspicion of an event. Less than 10% of clinically suspected cases of VTE are confirmed on objective testing (10). At present, pretest probability assessment is not validated in pregnancy in contrast to the non-pregnant where the Wells score is often used (26). Chan et al. (27) have demonstrated that the pretest probability of gestational DVT using three variables with their LEFt rule (left leg (L), (E for (o)edema), calf circumference difference of at least 2 cm, and first trimester presentation (Ft)) may be effective in excluding DVT. Supporting this, a post hoc analysis of 157 women with suspected gestational DVT (28) reported that the LEFt rule could accurately identify those in whom the incidence of confirmed DVT was very low. The modified Wells score (MWS) has been assessed for risk stratification in the diagnosis of pulmonary embolism (PE) in pregnancy (29): a score of 6 or higher had 100% sensitivity, 90% specificity, and a positive predictive value of 36% for objectively confirmed PE, while a MWS less than 6 had a negative predictive value of 100%. Although encouraging, these data are not yet sufficient to support the introduction of such assessment into routine practice, and prospective evaluation of pretest probability assessment tools is still required.

Compression duplex ultrasonography is the first-line investigation for suspected gestational DVT (30, 31). Where there is a negative ultrasound examination and a high level of clinical suspicion, the ultrasound examination should be repeated within 3–7 days (32). While awaiting the repeat test anticoagulation is usually discontinued. Serial compression duplex ultrasonography has been reported, in a prospective cohort study of over 200 pregnancies, to have a negative predictive value of 99.5% (95% CI 96.9–100%) (32). Occasionally, when iliac vein thrombosis is suspected and where DVT is not confirmed on ultrasonography, alternative techniques such as magnetic resonance imaging or X-ray venography may be used (30).

Where PE is suspected and where there are clinical features of possible DVT, ultrasound examination of the leg may be useful. Where a DVT is confirmed, then anticoagulation can be started, as treatment is the same for both conditions, so avoiding the need for specific radiation-based thoracic imaging, unless life-threatening PE is present. Clearly a negative ultrasound result cannot exclude PE and where specific investigations for PE are required in pregnancy, ventilation–perfusion (V/Q) lung scans may be preferred to CTPA (26). This is because of their high negative predictive value, low maternal radiation dose, and the relatively low prevalence of comorbid pulmonary problems in pregnancy, which outside pregnancy often lead to non-diagnostic intermediate probability results (26). With a normal chest X-ray, the ventilation component may be omitted so minimizing the radiation dose. Computed tomography pulmonary angiography (CTPA) is often avoided in pregnancy despite its high sensitivity and specificity and ability to identify other pathologies such as aortic dissection, because of the maternal radiation dose (up to 20 mGy), which may be associated with an increased risk of breast cancer (26). However, by employing bismuth breast shields the maternal radiation exposure can be reduced considerably (33). CTPA, V/Q, and low-dose perfusion (Q) lung scans are reported to have similar negative predictive values for PE diagnosis in pregnancy of 99% or more (34, 35). CTPA can be of value where the V/Q scan result shows intermediate probability for PE. There has sometimes

been a reluctance to use radiation-based investigations for PE in pregnancy because of concerns relating to exposure of the fetus to potentially harmful radiation (27). However, the fetal radiation dose from such investigations is minimal. For example, a chest X-ray at any gestation exposes the fetus to a negligible dose of radiation (<0.01 mSv) (36), while CTPA and V/Q scanning carry similar levels of exposure (26) that are well below the threshold associated with a risk of teratogenesis. However, there is an association with a very small increase in the risk of childhood cancer (37). These small risks must be set in the context of a potentially fatal condition for the mother.

While reduced arterial partial pressure of oxygen or oxygen saturation may occur with PE, this is only present in a minority of cases. Further, in the majority of cases of PE the chest X-ray is normal, or shows non-specific features such as regional oligaemia; however, it can be of value in identifying an alternative diagnosis (26). Where the chest X-ray is abnormal, CTPA is usually preferred to V/Q scanning for PE diagnosis (26). An electrocardiogram can also show non-specific features of PE, or identify alternative problems such as myocardial ischaemia (26). Outside pregnancy, D-dimer measurements have high sensitivity, and negative predictive value for VTE, but this is not so in pregnancy (26) as D-dimer increases with advancing gestation to levels higher than the normal non-pregnancy range by term and postpartum in most pregnancies (38). Pregnancy complications such as pre-eclampsia also lead to an increase in D-dimer levels (9, 26). Thus D-dimer testing has limited value in pregnancy.

Management of gestational venous thromboembolism

LMWH is usually the first-choice treatment for gestational VTE based on safety, and efficacy (superior to UFH) on extrapolation from trials in the non-pregnant. This is supported by observational data including cohort studies, and systematic reviews of safety and efficacy in pregnancy (11, 20, 21, 26, 39). However, UFH is still preferred for the initial treatment of massive PE. A specific concern when LMWH is used peripartum is bleeding, but LMWHs have not been associated with an increased risk of severe postpartum haemorrhage (11, 20, 21, 26, 39). The treatment dose of LMWH for VTE in pregnancy is shown in Table 16.4 (26). While it is uncertain whether once- or twice-daily dosing is optimal, there are increasing data from observational and pharmacokinetic studies to suggest that once-daily dosing is satisfactory (39, 40). When LMWH is used, there is no need for either routine platelet count monitoring (for heparin-induced thrombocytopenia), or anti-Xa activity. The latter may be of value in women at extremes of body weight (<50 kg or ≥90 kg) or with other complications such as renal impairment (26). Where UFH is used, platelet monitoring should be performed. It is usual to continue therapeutic doses of LMWH for the remainder of the pregnancy, for at least 6 weeks postpartum, and for at least 3 months of treatment in total. So women should be taught to self-inject LMWH and arrangements made to allow safe disposal of needles and syringes. Women with heparin-induced thrombocytopenia or with allergic reactions to heparin should be managed with an alternative anticoagulant under specialist advice (26). There is insufficient evidence to determine whether the dose of LMWH (or UFH) can be reduced to an intermediate dose after an initial period

Table 16.4 Low-molecular-weight heparin doses for treatment of venous thromboembolism in pregnancy

Maternal weight (kg)	Enoxaparin[a]	Dalteparin[a]
<50	40 mg twice daily or 60 mg once daily	5000 IU twice daily or 10,000 IU once daily
50–69	60 mg twice daily or 90 mg once daily	6000 IU twice daily or 12,000 IU once daily
70–89	80 mg twice daily or 120 mg once daily	8000 IU twice daily or 16,000 IU once daily
90–109	100 mg twice daily or 150 mg once daily	10,000 IU twice daily or 20,000 IU once daily
110–125	120 mg twice daily or 180 mg once daily	12,000 IU twice daily or 24,000 IU daily

[a] Dose based on maternal weight and whether once- or twice-daily treatment is used. Dosing: dalteparin 200 IU/kg daily or 100 IU/kg twice daily; enoxaparin 1.5 mg/kg daily or 1 mg/kg twice daily; tinzaparin 175 units/kg daily. As the LMWH may be provided in prefilled syringes, the dose closest to the patient's weight is used (26). At extremes of body weight such as those women weighing more than 125 kg, expert haematological advice should be sought, but dose capping is generally avoided. For women with significant renal compromise, lower doses are required.

of therapeutic anticoagulation; however, dose reduction is practised in some centres. Reducing to an intermediate dose may be useful in pregnant women at increased risk of bleeding or osteoporosis.

In addition to LMWH, graduated elastic compression stockings are of value in the acute treatment as these reduce the pain and swelling associated with DVT. Previously it was considered that prolonged use of graduated elastic compression stockings might reduce the risk of post-thrombotic syndrome, however, in the non-pregnant situation a recent randomized trial has not shown such benefit (41).

In the situation of massive life-threatening PE with haemodynamic compromise or proximal DVT threatening leg viability, thrombolysis should be considered. This can be systemic or catheter-directed thrombolysis, depending in the situation—the latter may be preferable for severe DVT. Bleeding complications in pregnancy appear similar to the non-pregnant based on accumulating case reports and case series (26, 42). There is a role for a temporary inferior vena cava (IVC) filter when recurrent VTE occurs despite adequate anticoagulation, or when anticoagulation is contraindicated. Case reports and case series have reported favourable outcomes with regard to safety and efficacy with the use of IVC filters in pregnancy (26, 43). However, the long-term safety of IVC filters is uncertain. In non-pregnant patients, filters reduce PE, but increase DVT, with no overall change in the frequency of VTE. The hazards of caval filters include filter migration (>20%), filter fracture (around 5%), and IVC perforation (up to 5%) (26).

Peripartum anticoagulant therapy

It is important to advise the woman taking LMWH for maintenance therapy following VTE that if she considers that she might be in labour that she should not inject any further LMWH. When VTE occurs at term close to delivery, a number of factors need to be taken into account. These include risk of thrombosis, mode of delivery, bleeding risk, and use of neuraxial anaesthesia. A number of options

can be considered. Intravenous UFH may be of value in unstable situations where delivery is imminent as it is more easily manipulated and can be quickly stopped. With planned delivery, either by elective caesarean section or induction of labour, LMWH maintenance therapy should be discontinued 24 hours prior to planned delivery to allow neuraxial anaesthesia and reduce the risk of bleeding. Neuraxial anaesthesia or analgesia should be avoided until at least 24 hours after the last dose of therapeutic LMWH and LMWH should not be given for at least 4 hours after the use of spinal anaesthesia or after the epidural catheter has been removed. The epidural catheter should not be removed within 12 hours of the last LMWH injection (26). There is an increased incidence of wound complications in women receiving peripartum anticoagulation (44), so it is prudent to anticipate this and with caesarean delivery the use of drains and interrupted skin sutures may be of value in preventing or draining wound haematomas (26).

Postpartum issues

As discussed previously, therapeutic anticoagulant treatment for gestational VTE should be continued for the duration of the pregnancy, for at least 6 weeks postpartum, and for at least 3 months total duration. The use of LMWH for more than 12 weeks is associated with a significantly lower risk of developing post-thrombotic syndrome. Before discontinuing treatment the risk of recurrent thrombosis should be assessed. As warfarin does not cross the breast in significant amounts it can be used postpartum for anticoagulation. However, because of bleeding risks, especially at the transition between LMWH and warfarin in the postpartum period (26), it is best to avoid starting warfarin until at least the fifth postpartum day and for longer where there is an increased risk of postpartum haemorrhage. Therefore, women can be offered a choice of LMWH or warfarin for postpartum therapy. In contrast to LMWH, warfarin will require regular monitoring with the INR particularly during the first 10 days of treatment, which may be problematic for a woman with a young baby.

REFERENCES

1. Cantwell R, Clutton-Brock T, Cooper G, et al. Saving Mothers' Lives: Reviewing maternal deaths to make motherhood safer: 2006–08. The Eighth Report of the Confidential Enquiries into Maternal Deaths in the United Kingdom. *BJOG* 2011;**118** Suppl 1:57–64.
2. Wik HS, Jacobsen AF, Sandvik L, Sandset PM. Prevalence and predictors for post-thrombotic syndrome 3 to 16 years after pregnancy-related venous thrombosis: a population-based, cross-sectional, case-control study. *J Thromb Haemost* 2012;**10**:840–47.
3. Kane EV, Calderwood, C, Dobbie R, Morris, CA, Roman E. Greer IA. A population-based study of venous thrombosis in pregnancy over 25 years. *Eur J Obstet, Gynecol Reprod Biol* 2013;**169**:223–29.
4. Knight M, Kenyon S, Brocklehurst P, et al. *Saving Lives, Improving Mothers' Care: Lessons Learned to Inform Future Maternity Care from the UK and Ireland Confidential Enquiries into Maternal Deaths and Morbidity 2009–12.* Oxford: National Perinatal Epidemiology Unit, University of Oxford; 2014.
5. Bates SM, Middeldorp S, Rodger M, James AH, Greer IA. Guidance for the treatment and prevention of obstetric-associated venous thromboembolism. *J Thromb Thrombolysis* 2016;**41**:92–128.

6. Heit JA, Kobbervig CE, James AH, Petterson TM, Bailey KR, Melton LJ 3rd. Trends in the incidence of venous thromboembolism during pregnancy or postpartum: a 30-year population-based study. *Ann Intern Med* 2005;**143**:697–706.

7. Jacobsen AF, Skjeldestad FE, Sandset PM. Ante- and postnatal risk factors of venous thrombosis: a hospital-based case-control study. *J Thromb Haemost* 2008;**6**:905–12.

8. Kamel H, Navi BB, Sriram N, Hovsepian DA, Devereux RB, Elkind MS. Risk of a thrombotic event after the 6-week postpartum period. *N Engl J Med* 2014;**370**:1307–15.

9. Greer IA. Thrombosis in pregnancy: updates in diagnosis and management. *Hematology Am Soc Hematol Educ Program* 2012;**2012**:203–207.

10. Greer IA. Pregnancy complicated by venous thrombosis. *N Eng J Med* 2015;**573**:540–47.

11. Bates SM, Greer IA, Middeldorp S, Veenstra DL, Prabulos AM, Vandvik PO. VTE, thrombophilia, antithrombotic therapy, and pregnancy: Antithrombotic Therapy and Prevention of Thrombosis, 9th ed: American College of Chest Physicians Evidence-Based Clinical Practice Guidelines. *Chest* 2012;**141** Suppl 2:e691S–736S.

12. Robertson L, Wu O, Langhorne P, et al. Thrombosis Risk and Economic Assessment of Thrombophilia Screening (TREATS) Study. Thrombophilia in pregnancy: a systematic review. *Br J Haematol* 2005;**132**:171–96.

13. James AH, Jamison MG, Brancazio LR, Myers ER. Venous thromboembolism during pregnancy and the postpartum period: incidence, risk factors, and mortality. *Am J Obstet Gynecol* 2006;**194**:1311–15.

14. Royal College of Obstetricians and Gynaecologists (RCOG). *Reducing the Risk of Thrombosis and Embolism during Pregnancy and the Puerperium.* Green-top Guideline No. 37a. London: RCOG; 2015. Available at: https://www.rcog.org.uk/en/guidelines-research-services/guidelines/gtg37a/.

15. Bezemer ID, van der Meer FJ, Eikenboom JC, Rosendaal FR, Doggen CJ. The value of family history as a risk indicator for venous thrombosis. *Arch Intern Med* 2008;**169**:610–15.

16. Zoller B, Ohlsson H, Sundquist J, Sundquist K. Familial risk of venous thromboembolism in first-, second- and third-degree relatives: a nation-wide family study in Sweden. *Thromb Haemost* 2013;**109**:361–62.

17. Tang A-W, Greer I. A systematic review on the use of the new anti-coagulants in pregnancy. *Obstet Med* 2013;**6**:64–71.

18. Knol HM, Schultinge L, Erwich JJHM, Meijer K. Fondaparinux as an alternative anticoagulant therapy during pregnancy. *J Thromb Haemost* 2010;**8**:1876–79.

19. Elsaigh E, Thachil J, Nash MJ, et al. The use of fondaparinux in pregnancy. *Br J Haematol* 2015;**168**:762–64.

20. Greer IA, Nelson Piercy C. Low molecular weight heparins for thromboprophylaxis and treatment of venous thromboembolism in pregnancy: a systematic review of safety and efficacy. *Blood* 2005;**106**:401–407.

21. Romualdi E, Dentali F, Rancan E, et al. Anticoagulant therapy for venous thromboembolism during pregnancy: a systematic review and a meta-analysis of the literature. *J Thromb Haemost* 2013;**11**:270–81.

22. Bain E, Wilson A, Tooher R, Gates S, Davies L-J, Middleton P. Prophylaxis for venous thromboembolic disease in pregnancy and the early postnatal period. *Cochrane Database Syst Rev* 2014;**2**:CD001689.

23. Chan WS, Rey E, Kent NE, et al. Venous thromboembolism and antithrombotic therapy in pregnancy. *J Obstet Gynaecol Can* 2014;**36**:527–53.

24. Gherman RB, Goodwin TM, Leung T, et al. Incidence, clinical characteristics, and timing of objectively diagnosed venous thromboembolism during pregnancy. *Obstet Gynecol* 1999;**94**:730–34.

25. James AH, Tapson VF, Goldhaber SZ. Thrombosis during pregnancy and the postpartum period. *Am J Obstet Gynecol* 2005;**193**:216–19.

26. Royal College of Obstetricians and Gynaecologists (RCOG). *Thromboembolic Disease in Pregnancy and the Puerperium: Acute Management.* Green-top Guideline No. 37b. London: RCOG; 2015. Available at: https://www.rcog.org.uk/en/guidelines-research-services/guidelines/gtg37b/.

27. Chan WS, Lee A, Spencer FA, et al. Predicting deep venous thrombosis in pregnancy: out in 'LEFt' field? *Ann Intern Med* 2009;**151**:85–92.

28. Righini M, Jobic C, Boehlen F, et al. Predicting deep venous thrombosis in pregnancy: external validation of the LEFT clinical prediction rule. *Haematologica* 2013;**98**:545–48.

29. O'Connor C, Moriarty J, Walsh J, Murray J, Coulter-Smith S, Boyd W. The application of a clinical risk stratification score may reduce unnecessary investigations for pulmonary embolism in pregnancy. *J Matern Fetal Neonatal Med* 2011;**24**:1461–64.

30. Bates SM, Jaeschke R, Stevens SM, et al. Diagnosis of DVT: Antithrombotic Therapy and Prevention of Thrombosis, 9th ed: American College of Chest Physicians Evidence-Based Clinical Practice Guidelines. *Chest* 2012;**141**:Suppl 2:e351S–418S.

31. Le Gal G, Kercret G, Yahmed KB, et al. Diagnostic value of single complete compression ultrasonography in pregnant and postpartum women with suspected deep vein thrombosis: prospective study. *BMJ* 2012;**344**:e2635.

32. Chan WS, Spencer FA, Lee AY, et al. Safety of withholding anticoagulation in pregnant women with suspected deep vein thrombosis following negative serial compression ultrasound and iliac vein imaging. *CMAJ* 2013;**185**:E194–200.

33. Hurwitz LM, Yoshizumi TT, Goodman PC, et al. Radiation dose savings for adult pulmonary embolus 64-MDCT using bismuth breast shields, lower peak kilovoltage, and automatic tube current modulation. *Am J Roentgenol* 2009;**192**:244–53.

34. Shahir K, Goodman LR, Tali A, Thorsen KM, Hellman RS. Pulmonary embolism in pregnancy: CT pulmonary angiography versus perfusion scanning. *Am J Roentgenol* 2010;**195**:W214–20.

35. Ridge CA, McDermott S, Freyne BJ, Brennan DJ, Collins CD, Skehan SJ. Pulmonary embolism in pregnancy: comparison of pulmonary CT angiography and lung scintigraphy. *Am J Roentgenol* 2009;**193**:1223–27.

36. Nguyen CP, Goodman LH. Fetal risk in diagnostic radiology. *Semin Ultrasound CT MR* 2012;**33**:4–10.

37. Schembri GP, Miller AE, Smart R. Radiation dosimetry and safety issues in the investigation of pulmonary embolism. *Semin Nucl Med* 2010;**40**:442–54.

38. Khalafallah AA, Morse M, Al-Barzan AM, et al. D-Dimer levels at different stages of pregnancy in Australian women: a single centre study using two different immunoturbidimetric assays. *Thromb Res* 2012;**130**:e171–77.

39. Nelson-Piercy C, Powrie R, Borg JY, et al. Tinzaparin use in pregnancy: an international, retrospective study of the safety and efficacy profile. *Eur J Obstet Gynecol Reprod Biol* 2011;**159**:293–99.

40. Patel JP, Green B, Patel RK, Marsh MS, Davies JG, Arya R. Population pharmacokinetics of enoxaparin during the antenatal period. *Circulation* 2013;**128**:1462–69.

41. Kahn SR, Shapiro S, Wells PS, et al. Compression stockings to prevent post-thrombotic syndrome: a randomised placebo-controlled trial. *Lancet* 2014;**383**:880–88.

42. te Raa GD, Ribbert LSM, Snijder RJ, Biesma DH. Treatment options in massive pulmonary embolism during pregnancy: a case-report and review of literature. *Thromb Res* 2009;**124**:1–5.

43. Milford W, Chadha Y, Lust K. Use of a retrievable inferior vena cava filter in term pregnancy: case report and review of literature. *Aust N Z J Obstet Gynaecol* 2009;**49**:331–33.

44. Limmer JS, Grotegut CA, Thames E, Dotters-Katz SK, Brancazio LR, James AH. Postpartum wound bleeding complications in women who received peripartum anticoagulation. *Thromb Res* 2013;**132**:e19–23

17

General and specific infections in pregnancy including immunization

Austin Ugwumadu

General characteristics of innate immunity and fetal host response to infection

The innate immune system is primitive and critical for survival. Therefore, during fetal life it develops first before the adaptive immune system. It is the first line of defence particularly in the immature fetus. The frontline components of this system include genetically encoded pattern recognition receptors, which are expressed on macrophages, monocytes, and other cell types (1). These receptors are programmed by millennia of evolution to recognize structural patterns such as lipopolysaccharide, which form components of microbial cell walls and are very potent activators of innate immune responses and expression of proinflammatory cytokines (1). The resultant cytokines, particularly tumour necrosis factor alpha (TNF-α), produce cerebral (2) or generalized endothelial damage, systemic vasodilatation, tissue hypoperfusion, increased vascular permeability, shock, and myocardial depression (3). These processes may lead to profound circulatory disturbances within vulnerable regions of the developing fetal brain, impair cerebrovascular regulation, and increase the risk of hypoxic–ischaemic injury.

Several biological pathways of intrauterine infection/inflammation leading to fetal and perinatal brain damage have been documented. These pathways clarify the multiple links between maternal and perinatal inflammation, cerebral palsy, and other associated complications. Three newer concepts related to infection/inflammation and perinatal brain damage may be considered to put these pathways in perspective:

1. Inflammatory responses of both the fetus and the mother to ascending or blood-borne intrauterine infections are mediated by each individual's genetically controlled inflammatory process (4).
2. Infection may precede pregnancy or be established very early in pregnancy. Endometrial or decidual infection may remain clinically unrecognized and may even persist from one pregnancy to the next (5).
3. The end results of infection/inflammation include cellulitis, abscess formation, thrombosis, embolization, ischaemia, and infarction, but also cell damage from reactive oxygen species and other damaging molecules, altered immune recognition, and apoptosis. The brain-damaging mechanisms may persist and cause damage after the original harmful processes have been removed or corrected (5, 6).

Within the brain, cytokines may also attenuate the fetal blood–brain barrier (7, 8) and mediate transendothelial migration of leucocytes and inflammatory damage. The brain phagocytes, microglial cells, express interleukin (IL)-1β, IL-6, and TNF-α in response to stimulation by lipopolysaccharide (9). TNF-α, IL-1β, and interferon-gamma exert a direct neurotoxic effect on oligodendrocytes progenitors (10–12), which are destined at maturity to myelinate the axons (white matter) of neural cells, and induce gliosis and release of nitric oxide leading to mitochondrial dysfunction and cellular energy failure (13).

Developmental vulnerability to infection-driven brain damage

Several developmental anatomical, metabolic, and immuno-endocrinological factors, act synergistically to promote fetal tissue injury. Developing neurons are vulnerable to insults during the period of neuronal and glial mitosis, the stage of orderly cellular migration, and during the formation and organization of the microarchitecture. The premyelination stage appears to be the period of maximum susceptibility of the oligodendrocyte. In addition, the germinal matrix zone is another developmental structure with increased vulnerability to injury.

The germinal matrix zone is a transient embryonic tissue of the developing fetal brain located immediately adjacent to the lateral ventricles and spanning across the vascular boundaries of the cerebral circulation. It involutes at about 32 weeks of gestation. Between 23 and 32 weeks, the motor nerve cells and their axons (white matter) in the matrix are perfused by a loose network of fragile and immature blood vessels, which are supported by only a single cell layer of endothelium with no muscularis or muscle coats. This deficiency provides the platform for the high incidence of intraventricular haemorrhage (IVH) in preterm infants when there is fluctuation in the fetal blood pressure.

Collectively, the incompletely developed vascular supply of the cerebral white matter (14), dysregulation of cerebral blood flow related to immaturity (15, 16), and the vulnerability of the oligo-dendroglial precursors to attack by free radicals (17, 18) predispose the preterm brain to pressure-passive circulation and ischaemic injury. The end result is a fatal accumulation of reactive oxygen species and apoptotic death of the oligodendroglia resulting in neuronal loss.

The developmental predisposition, maturity-dependent pathophysiological mechanisms, and oligodendrocyte vulnerability discussed previously may exert their effects on the premature brain to produce a set of clinical disorders including neonatal depression, periventricular leucomalacia (PVL), cerebral palsy, and IVH. The mechanism through which infection drives fetal brain damage in the term and near-term infant is less well defined but is likely to involve the inflammatory cascade acting synergistically with other factors. Respiratory morbidity in the form of bronchopulmonary dysplasia has also been linked with fetal exposure to intrauterine infection.

Periventricular leucomalacia and cerebral palsy

PVL is the main precursor lesion of cerebral palsy and predicts 60–100% of cases in affected preterm infants (19). It consists of two major components, namely focal, which is located deep in the white matter and characterized by a localized but non-selective necrosis of all cellular elements with subsequent cyst formation, and the diffuse component, characterized by a more diffuse but selective injury directed at the oligodendrocyte precursors (20). The inflammatory mediators of infection and hypoxia–ischaemia exert a direct neurotoxic damage on the oligodendroglial precursors through the generation of reactive oxygen species. In fetal rabbits, induction of maternal infection led to cerebral white matter lesions (21, 22) while in humans the incidence of PVL and cerebral palsy in preterm infants is increased with maternal (23, 24), placental (25, 26), or fetal (27, 28) infection. Infants at risk of developing PVL and subsequently cerebral palsy at 3 years of age can be identified by prior antenatal exposure to high concentrations of proinflammatory cytokines (27, 29–31).

Intraventricular haemorrhage

Fetuses with fetal systemic inflammatory response syndrome (FSIRS) or severe hypoxia–ischaemia lose their autoregulatory capacity required to maintain steady cerebral blood flow (15). The resultant dramatic alterations in the cerebral blood flow may rupture the tenuous germinal matrix vasculature with bleeding into the matrix and subsequent extension through the single ependymal cell layer, which separates the matrix zone from the lateral ventricle into the ventricles resulting in IVH (32). Alternatively, the inflammatory adhesion of leucocytes to the fragile vessels of the matrix zone may lead to vascular damage and bleeding into the germinal matrix. Subsequent ventriculomegaly arising from IVH may further compress adjacent periventricular capillaries causing ischaemia and further white matter damage. Infants with chorioamnionitis and raised amniotic fluid IL-6 have a three- to fourfold increase in the risk of IVH compared to their peers without membrane inflammation (33–35).

Chorioamnionitis

The term chorioamnionitis applies to the inflammation of the fetal membranes and the placenta as a result of the entry of microorganisms usually from the maternal lower genital tract into the amniotic sac. The membranes bear the brunt of the inflammatory process rather than the placenta. Maternal polymorphs first infiltrate the lower pole of the amniotic sac followed by their accumulation in the intervillous space immediately beneath the chorionic plate, the so-called intervillositis (36). Inflammatory cells are rarely seen elsewhere in the intervillous space and villitis is very rarely seen except in listeriosis (36) and vertical transmission of blood-borne maternal infections. Later in the process, fetal leucocytes migrate out from fetal vessels in the chorionic plate, and subsequently an angiitis of the umbilical cord vessels occurs with migration of fetal leucocytes into the Wharton's jelly, the so-called funisitis, a marker of more generalized FSIRS (37), probably mediated in part by widespread endothelial injury (**Figure 17.1**) (38).

FSIRS is associated with hypotension, neonatal seizures, need for intubation, meconium aspiration syndrome, multiorgan dysfunction, chorioamnionitis, preterm delivery, a clinical diagnosis of hypoxic ischaemic encephalopathy or neonatal encephalopathy (39–41), IVH (42), white matter damage, periventricular leucomalacia, bronchopulmonary dysplasia, and cerebral palsy in the term and near-term infant (**Figure 17.1**) (43). It is probably the most common antecedent of low Apgar scores and other indicators of neonatal depression (41, 44). Fetal demise from overwhelming sepsis or growth restriction may occur (45), as well as polymicrogyria (a migratory disorder of the cerebral cortex) (46). In a meta-analysis, clinical chorioamnionitis had a relative risk (RR) of 1.9 (95% confidence interval (CI) 1.4–2.5) for development of cerebral palsy in preterm infants and a RR of 4.7 (95% CI 1.3–16.2) in term infants (47). However, the literature is relatively silent on the risk of cerebral palsy associated with intrauterine infection before the peripartum period in term infants and on the contribution of extrauterine infection.

Chorioamnionitis is a strong risk factor for neonatal encephalopathy and cerebral palsy (48). It accounts for 11–22% of cases of cerebral palsy in term and near-term infants, and carries an odds ratio of 9.3 for unexplained cerebral palsy (49). Fetal exposure to chorioamnionitis has two potent noxious elements, namely, hyperthermia and inflammation. Current diagnosis of clinical chorioamnionitis is based on maternal fever of at least 38.0°C, and any two of uterine fundal tenderness, purulent and/or foul-smelling vaginal discharge, fetal tachycardia, maternal tachycardia, raised inflammatory markers including C-reactive protein, and white cell count. However, 10% or less of cases with histological chorioamnionitis had signs of clinical chorioamnionitis. Uterine tenderness is subjective and abolished after epidural analgesia. Purulent or offensive vaginal discharge is subjective and attenuated by antiseptic gels and lubricants used for vaginal examination during labour. Labour is an inflammatory process and is associated with increase in the levels of inflammatory markers. Collectively, the criteria used for the diagnosis of clinical chorioamnionitis are

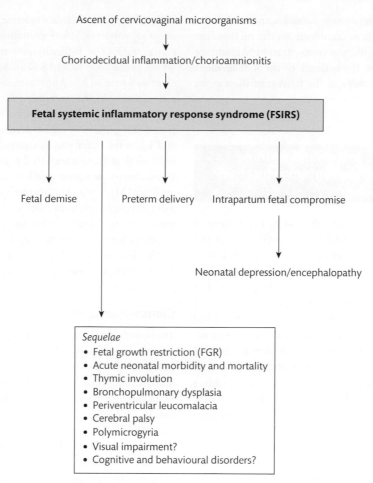

Ascent of cervicovaginal microorganisms

↓

Choriodecidual inflammation/chorioamnionitis

↓

Fetal systemic inflammatory response syndrome (FSIRS)

Fetal demise   Preterm delivery   Intrapartum fetal compromise

Neonatal depression/encephalopathy

Sequelae
- Fetal growth restriction (FGR)
- Acute neonatal morbidity and mortality
- Thymic involution
- Bronchopulmonary dysplasia
- Periventricular leucomalacia
- Cerebral palsy
- Polymicrogyria
- Visual impairment?
- Cognitive and behavioural disorders?

Figure 17.1 Short-, medium-, and long-term complications of chorioamnionitis.

insensitive and reflects the fact that the fetal compartment is sequestrated and not contiguous with the maternal. In the authors' institution, maternal temperature and fetomaternal tachycardia are the most commonly used criteria to make the diagnosis of clinical chorioamnionitis.

Intrapartum maternal fever

Although maternal oral temperature is the best indicator of intrauterine temperature, it still underestimates intrauterine temperature by approximately 0.8°C (50). Furthermore, fetal core temperature is another 0.75°C higher than fetal skin and intrauterine temperature (51). Maternal pyrexia is therefore inevitably associated with elevated fetal temperature and the threshold temperature of 38.0°C, which is widely used as an essential parameter for the definition and diagnosis of intrapartum fever and clinical chorioamnionitis will be associated with fetal brain temperatures of 39.5°C or greater. The impact of this is observed in the risk of encephalopathy to the exposed fetus. For example, the background risk of neonatal encephalopathy of 0.12% among term infants is amplified nearly tenfold to 1.13% with fetal exposure to maternal fever alone (50). In experimental rats, raised brain temperature correlated directly with increased susceptibility to a host of neurotoxic factors (52, 53). In the human newborn, maternal pyrexia was associated with an increased risk of neonatal seizures regardless of whether the pyrexia was of non-infectious origin, for example, epidural analgesia (54). Unsurprisingly, there has recently been a great deal of interest and success with brain cooling for the newborn with significant neonatal encephalopathy.

The risk of neonatal encephalopathy with fetal exposure to acidosis alone, defined as a cord pH less than 7.05, is 1.58%. However, the combination of maternal fever and neonatal acidosis results in over a tenfold increase in the risk of neonatal encephalopathy to 12.5%, and this is independent of neonatal sepsis (50). It has been hypothesized that maternal fever increases fetal oxidative stress depleting cellular energy reserves, and increases fetal susceptibility to hypoxic injury. Prophylactic antioxidants have been shown to provide neuroprotection and reduce fetal injury in lipopolysaccharide-based animal models of chorioamnionitis (55–57).

Clinical management

The clinical management of isolated intrapartum maternal fever is based on administration of antipyretics such as paracetamol, tepid sponge, cooling fan, and intrapartum antibiotic prophylaxis in the form of benzylpenicillin every 4 hours until delivery. These antipyretics at least in theory restore the fetomaternal temperature gradient and allow the fetus to rid itself of its metabolic heat. However, there is scant evidence that they improve the prognosis for the baby. In contrast, many clinicians presume that the outlook for the baby improves when the maternal temperature subsides and antibiotics have been administered. There is no antibiotic on the market that crosses the placental barrier in sufficient concentration to eradicate intrauterine infection. Therefore, the bedrock of the management of chorioamnionitis remains delivery of the fetus regardless of its gestational age.

Intra-amniotic infection, meconium staining of the amniotic fluid, and meconium aspiration syndrome: what is the link?

The fetus ingests and inhales the amniotic fluid as part of its normal behavioural state. Earlier studies of fetal sheep concluded that the egress of lung fluid was towards the amniotic cavity (58, 59), suggesting that the fetus could not aspirate amniotic fluid and therefore meconium. However, recent ultrasound and colour Doppler studies have demonstrated clearly that there is an influx as well as efflux of fluid in the nasopharynx, the nose, and in the trachea (60–62). Fetal gasping has long been accepted as the precursor of meconium aspiration syndrome (MAS) and it has been described in the human fetus 24–72 hours before death in the absence of labour (63), in fetal lambs that died from antenatal infection, hypoxia, and other causes (64), and in primate fetuses before death (65). Therefore, we know that amniotic fluid can be inhaled *in utero*, especially when the fetus is in a pre-agonal state (65–68) and meconium has conclusively been demonstrated in the fetal lung of stillborn fetuses (69).

The amniotic fluid is normally sterile and has antimicrobial activity, which helps it to protect the fetus against ascending microorganisms from the lower genital tract. However, meconium staining of the amniotic fluid (MSAF) facilitates the growth of bacterial species (70) by inhibiting the phagocytic ability of macrophages to ingest bacteria (71–73) and impairing oxidative burst and bacterial killing by polymorphonuclear leucocytes (74). This general rule does not apply to group B *Streptococcus* (GBS), which has the capability to grow and multiply rapidly within normal and clear amniotic fluid (70). If ascending microorganisms invade the amniotic fluid they may gain access into the fetal systemic circulation via the immature intestinal and/or pulmonary epithelium and elicit a fetal host inflammatory response. Fetal ingestion of amniotic fluid contaminated with microorganisms, bacterial products, and inflammatory mediators may elicit enteritis and enhanced colonic motility leading to discharge of meconium. Patients with MSAF in spontaneous term labour have a higher frequency of positive amniotic fluid culture, a higher IL-6 concentration, more common Gram-negative bacterial isolates, and more frequent endotoxin assays, compared to those with clear amniotic fluid (75). The infected meconium discharged from the bowels contains microorganisms, bacterial products, inflammatory cytokines, and complements, and if inhaled into the lungs may induce local inflammatory damage within the lungs. However, a more generalized FSIRS may enhance this local effect and extend it to the pulmonary circulation, which ultimately may lead to persistent pulmonary hypertension (76–80) linking MSAF, intra-amniotic inflammation, funisitis, and MAS (81). The fact that these events leading to meconium aspiration are already established *in utero* and occur before birth explains the limited success of suction and clearing meconium out of the airway at birth to prevent MAS.

Based on the available evidence, Romero et al. proposed that *in utero* aspiration of MSAF containing bacteria, endotoxin, and high concentrations of inflammatory mediators creates the conditions which predispose to MAS (75). MSAF is necessary but not sufficient to cause MAS. Approximately one of every seven pregnancies will have MSAF and only 5% of exposed infants develop MAS. A recent study found that newborns who developed MAS were exposed to significantly higher levels of intra-amniotic inflammation, and when the latter was associated with funisitis had a higher rate of MAS than their unexposed peers (RR 4.3; 95% CI 1.5–12.3). Of 89 newborns for whom amniotic fluid and placental histology were available, MAS was significantly more common in those with both intra-amniotic inflammation and funisitis than in those without intra-amniotic inflammation and funisitis while the rate of MAS did not differ between patients with intra-amniotic inflammation alone (without funisitis) and those without intra-amniotic inflammation and funisitis, suggesting that it is the fetal host response characterized by funisitis, which determines the outcome (81).

Clinical management

The obstetrician's task is to manage the labour complicated by MSAF with the aim of preventing MAS if this has not occurred already. In practice, this involves continuous fetal heart rate (FHR) monitoring and avoiding intrapartum asphyxia of sufficient severity to induce MAS such as very prolonged bradycardia. Some obstetricians advocate routine fetal blood sampling to exclude fetal acidaemia if there was MSAF. This is unwarranted in the presence of a normal FHR pattern. Moreover, as discussed previously, a significant proportion of cases of MAS have normal or near normal acid–base status and have no signs of significant asphyxia and fetal blood sampling will be falsely reassuring under those circumstances. The majority of fetuses with MAS will exhibit a monotonous FHR pattern without fetal cycling activity or long-term variability and these patterns have recently been reviewed (82). Depending on the timing of the original insult, the baseline FHR may be raised or within the normal range and unless the fetus is acidaemic there may be no FHR decelerations associated with maternal contractions. Such babies should be delivered expeditiously to avoid exacerbation of the pre-existing injury. In some parts of the world amnioinfusion is deployed to dilute MSAF and reduce the frequency of variable deceleration but it has no impact on the risk of MAS if the fetus had continuous FHR monitoring. It also is associated with fetal and maternal infectious morbidity and therefore not recommended in the United Kingdom.

Intrapartum fetal monitoring in the presence of infection and MSAF

For the infected fetus, labour is markedly hazardous. The fetus is at risk of overwhelming intrauterine sepsis, or severe injury at lower levels of asphyxial insult, or both. Unfortunately, there are no consistent FHR patterns that predict fetal infection. However, FHR tachycardia is a sensitive marker of intrauterine infection and FSIRS especially when this is associated with MSAF in early labour where the risk of infection is 51-fold (83). The same study showed a weak or no association with maternal tachycardia or maternal fever (83). There is no place for fetal blood sampling in the assessment of the infected fetus or one suspected to be infected. There are no significant differences in the mean arterial pH values of fetuses exposed to intrauterine infection and controls, however, the fetuses exposed to intrauterine infection had significantly lower Apgar scores (84). The risk to the fetus under these circumstances is largely mediated by inflammation rather than acidaemia although the fetus is primed for greater damage by hypoxia. Obstetricians should also avoid complicated and/or traumatic delivery in the inflamed fetus.

Abnormal vaginal flora and selected bacterial infections

Bacterial vaginosis

Bacterial vaginosis (BV) is an ecological disorder of the vagina characterized by varying degrees of depletion or total absence of the normally protective *Lactobacillus* species and an overgrowth of anaerobes (Figure 17.2). Over 60% of BV-positive women are asymptomatic (85) but the condition is associated with significant complications of pregnancy including late miscarriage, preterm delivery, preterm prelabour rupture of membranes, low birth weight, amniotic fluid infection, chorioamnionitis, and postpartum

(a)

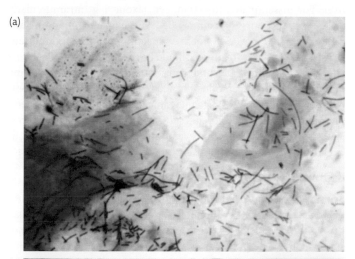

(b)

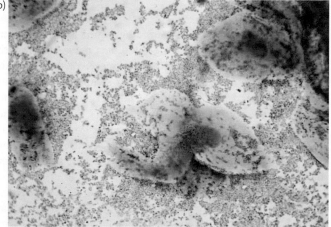

Figure 17.2 Gram stain of normal vaginal smear showing the dominant *Lactobacillus* species (a), and bacterial vaginosis showing a depletion of the protective *Lactobacillus* species and an increase in other bacterial species (b).

Reproduced from Ugwumadu A. Managing bacterial infections in pregnancy and the puerperium. *The Prescriber*; 2010;21(21):53–57 with permission from John Wiley and Sons.

endometritis. The role of screening for and treating BV in the general population of pregnant women at low risk of adverse pregnancy outcome is controversial. However, there is strong and persuasive evidence of benefit for screening and treating high-risk women with a prior history of late miscarriage or preterm delivery for BV (86, 87). When treatment is indicated in pregnancy, the authors prefer oral clindamycin because of its wider spectrum of activity against the range of organisms associated with BV, anti-inflammatory properties, and fewer recurrences after treatment, compared to metronidazole, which is an antianaerobe only. There is consensus that symptomatic women should be treated, however, there is debate whether clindamycin is superior to metronidazole, what gestational age to initiate treatment, the optimal route of antibiotic administration, and the dosage and duration of therapy.

Group B *Streptococcus*

Approximately 20–30% of pregnant women are GBS carriers, with higher rates of colonization in black than in white or Asian women (88). It emerged in the 1970s as the leading cause of neonatal sepsis and trials showed that intravenous (IV) penicillin or ampicillin during labour prevented neonatal disease (89), in contrast to antenatal eradication of genital GBS colonization before labour (90, 91). There are no efficacy data on oral or intramuscular antibiotic prophylaxis during labour.

Prevention of early-onset neonatal GBS disease

Two competing strategies for the prevention of early-onset neonatal GBS disease (EOGBSD) are widely recognized, the cheaper but less effective one is the treatment of women with known risk factors for EOGBSD, namely intrapartum fever (20% of GBS-positive women), preterm labour, prolonged rupture of membranes (≥18 hours), GBS bacteriuria, previously affected infant, and isolation of GBS at any other time; the other is a culture-based screening of all women before labour (35–37 weeks in practice) to identify and offer intrapartum antibiotic prophylaxis to those colonized by GBS. Implementation based on this resulted in a nationwide reduction of 70% in the incidence of EOGBSD (from 1.5–2 cases/1000 live births to 0.5 cases/1000 live births) in the United States (92). However, a subsequent large, retrospective cohort study showed that late antenatal culture-based screening was over 50% more effective in reducing the EOGBSD than the risk-based approach (93), leading to its adoption (94). The improvement may be related to the detection and treatment of the 20% of colonized women who do not display any risk factors. For optimal detection rates (up to 27%), a rectovaginal or vaginal/perianal swab inoculated into a selective medium was recommended in addition to intrapartum treatment of women who have had a previously affected infant, GBS bacteriuria, or whose GBS status was unknown.

Intrapartum antibiotic prophylaxis and risk of resistant organisms

The recommended regimens for intrapartum antibiotic prophylaxis include penicillin G, 5 million units IV initially followed by 2.5 million units every 4 hours until delivery, or ampicillin 2 g IV initially, then 1 g IV every 4 hours until delivery. Patients who are allergic to penicillin but not at risk of anaphylaxis should receive cefazolin 2 g IV initially, then 1 g IV every 4 hours until delivery, or either clindamycin 900 mg IV every 8 hours or erythromycin

500 mg IV every 6 hours until delivery, if they were at risk of anaphylaxis. At present, GBS remains universally sensitive to penicillin and the narrow spectrum of penicillin G drives the mistaken belief that there is less selective pressure for the emergence of resistant organisms. However, recent studies have shown that intrapartum administration of both benzylpenicillin and ampicillin was associated with a 35% increase in vaginal colonization with ampicillin-resistant *Enterobacter* species, 36 hours postpartum (95). One large study found a significant increase in the rate of early-onset *Escherichia coli* sepsis, although this was restricted to low-birthweight neonates (96, 97), and the total Gram-negative bacterial sepsis declined despite the increase in *E. coli* infections.

Some clinicians wrongly presume that clindamycin and erythromycin are automatically effective as prophylaxis for GBS in women who are sensitive to penicillin but the frequency of strains of GBS which are resistant to erythromycin (currently 47%) or clindamycin (15%) is rising. Vancomycin 1 g IV every 12 hours until delivery is recommended if the susceptibility was unknown. Clinicians should request sensitivity studies when taking samples for possible GBS colonization from women who volunteered a history of penicillin allergy. The risk-based approach, associated with a 55% reduction in the incidence of EOGBSD, is adopted in the United Kingdom. It is noteworthy that the baseline incidence of EOGBSD in the United Kingdom is estimated at 0.5–1.15/1000 live births (98) in contrast to the 1.5–2.5/1000 rate in the United States prior to the introduction of mass screening in late pregnancy. The introduction of screening for the prevention of EOGBSD in the United Kingdom may not be appropriate or cost-effective. The current United Kingdom NICE guidelines do not recommend intrapartum antibiotic prophylaxis for women with prolonged rupture of membranes (≥24 hours) or their babies, if there is no evidence of infection such as pyrexia in labour (http://www.nice.org.uk/CG55). This is a significant deviation from current understanding of the risk factor-based approach to the prevention of EOGBSD, particularly as 20% of colonized women do not display any risk factors.

Gonorrhoea

Gonorrhoea is a sexually transmitted infection caused by *Neisseria gonorrhoeae*, a Gram-negative diplococcus bacteria.

Epidemiology

Gonorrhoea is spread by contact with the penis, vagina, mouth, or anus. The incidence of newly diagnosed gonorrhoea in the United Kingdom increased by 6% from 16,629 cases in 2008 to 17,385 cases in 2009 (99–101). Some of the risk factors associated with infection include young age, previous sexually transmitted infections, inconsistent condom use, drug abuse, and new or multiple sexual partners. *N. gonorrhoeae* may infect the genitourinary tract, rectum, pharynx, or eye. Spread of infection to the upper genital tract can cause pelvic inflammatory disease. The perinatal implications include transmission to the neonate causing conjunctivitis and blindness if untreated. Disseminated infections may cause septic arthritis, endocarditis, and meningitis. Pregnant women are at greater risk for disseminated infection than non-pregnant women (101).

Clinical diagnosis

In most cases, gonorrhoea is asymptomatic but some women may complain of dysuria or mucopurulent vaginal discharge. Screening

women at high risk for sexually transmitted infections is essential for infection control. Pregnant women should be screened at the first prenatal visit if they are at risk or if there is a high rate of gonorrhoea in the population (101). Patients who continue to be at high risk should be screened again in the third trimester. Although Gram stain of the endocervical fluid has a high positive predictive value, diagnosis is usually made by culture, nucleic acid hybridization, or nucleic acid amplification tests (NAATs) of samples obtained from the endocervix, vagina, male urethra, or urine. The patient should be evaluated also for other sexually transmitted infections including chlamydia, syphilis, and human immunodeficiency virus (HIV), and have all their sexual contacts traced and offered treatment.

Treatment

Due to spread of resistant strains of bacteria, the recommended regimens for uncomplicated urogenital and anorectal gonorrhoea include single-dose intramuscular ceftriaxone 250 mg or oral cefixime 400 mg with treatment for chlamydia if the latter has not been excluded (102). Alternative regimens include single-dose intramuscular spectinomycin 2 g or cefotaxime 500 mg. Cefpodoxime 400 mg and cefuroxime axetil 1 g have been suggested as oral alternatives. For disseminated infection, ceftriaxone 1 g intramuscularly or IV every 24 hours is recommended; alternative regimens include cefotaxime 1 g IV every 8 hours or spectinomycin 2g intramuscularly every 12 hours. Treatment should be continued for 24–48 hours after clinical improvement and then continued with cefixime 400 mg orally twice daily or cefpodoxime 400 mg orally twice daily to complete 1 week of therapy. Pregnant women should not be treated with fluoroquinolones or tetracyclines. It is good practice to treat empirically for chlamydia infection even if this has not been tested for, as concurrent infection is frequent.

Syphilis

Syphilis is a sexually transmitted infection caused by the spirochete *Treponema pallidum*. Without treatment the disease progresses through different stages over time. Syphilis may cause miscarriage, stillbirth, hydrops, polyhydramnios, or fetal abnormalities.

Epidemiology

In 2001, the World Health Organization estimated that 12 million new cases of syphilis occurred in adults per year across the globe (103). There has been a recent resurgence of syphilis in developed countries after many years of low seroprevalence. For example, a rapid increase of infectious syphilis occurred in the United Kingdom between 1999 and 2008 mostly among men who have sex with men (104). This was attributed to increased IV drug misuse and HIV infection. Risk factors associated with infection include multiple sexual partners, drug abuse, poor socioeconomic status, and young age.

Vertical transmission results in more than 1 million infants born with congenital syphilis annually worldwide (105). Rates of perinatal transmission of infection vary depending on the stage of maternal disease—almost 100% if the fetus is exposed to the chancre during delivery in primary syphilis, 50% during secondary syphilis as a result of transplacental infection, 40% during early latent disease, and about 10% during late latent and tertiary syphilis (106). Vertical transmission is decreased to 1–2% in women who are adequately treated during pregnancy.

Clinical diagnosis

The infection has a long natural history progressing through recognized stages:

1. Primary syphilis—this is characterized by the chancre (a raised, indurated, exudative, and painless ulcer) at the site of entry of the spirochete. There may be non-tender regional lymphadenopathy (bubo). The chancre usually resolves spontaneously within 3–6 weeks even without treatment. The incubation period averages 3 months but may lie between 3 and 90 days depending on the size of the inoculum at infection.

2. Secondary syphilis—this is the stage during which the spirochetes become systemic and begins from about 6 weeks and may last up to 6 months after initial infection. It is seen in about 25% of untreated individuals. Clinical signs include extensive maculopapular rash particularly involving the palms and soles, lymphadenopathy, and genital condyloma lata.

3. Latent syphilis is the diagnosis of asymptomatic infection documented with positive serology but absent manifestation on physical examination. If this occurs within 1 year of inoculation it is called early latent; if the diagnosis occurs after 1 year or cannot be determined, it is defined as late latent syphilis.

4. Tertiary (late) syphilis occurs after the initial stages of syphilis and the onset may vary from 1 year to 30 years after the initial inoculation. It is slowly progressive and may involve the central nervous system, the cardiovascular system, or the skin and subcutaneous tissues. The typical lesion of tertiary syphilis, the gumma, is an area of chronic inflammatory destruction presenting as an indolent lesion with a necrotic centre. Gumma may be single or multiple and are variable in size from microscopic to large tumour-like areas. They have a predilection for the skin, liver, bones, and spleen.

Congenital syphilis occurs via transplacental transmission of *T. pallidum* to the fetus and can occur at any time during pregnancy. Congenital transmission is extremely high during the first 4 years after inoculation. It may result in intrauterine growth restriction, intrauterine fetal demise, neonatal death, preterm birth, and congenital infection and anomalies.

Diagnosis of primary or secondary syphilis can be made with dark-field microscopy and direct visualization of spirochetes or serological testing. Serological tests remain the method of choice for diagnosis. The Venereal Disease Research Laboratory (VDRL) test and rapid plasma reagin (RPR) tests are simple and inexpensive with high sensitivity during early infection (106). Specific treponemal serological tests include fluorescent treponemal antibody absorption (FTA-ABS), the microhaemagglutination test for antibodies to *T. pallidum* (MHA-TP), and the *T. pallidum* particle agglutination assay (TPPA). False-positive results may occur with both non-treponemal and treponemal methods, therefore single-test syphilis diagnosis is inadequate. A false-positive result is associated with febrile illness, immunizations, autoimmune conditions particularly systemic lupus erythematosus, IV drug use, chronic liver disease, and HIV infections. Yet other tests for detecting syphilis include direct fluorescence antibody testing (DFA-TP) and multiplex polymerase chain reaction (PCR). Cerebrospinal fluid analysis via lumbar puncture is essential in anyone with latent syphilis, ophthalmic/neurological signs or symptoms, treatment failure, coexistent HIV infection, and active tertiary syphilis.

Screening for syphilis is recommended at the first prenatal visit, and repeated during the third trimester and at delivery for patients at high risk. If positive for VDRL, further specific tests from a reference laboratory should be arranged along with referral to a specialist in genitourinary medicine. During pregnancy, ultrasonography can be used to determine the extent of fetal disease during the second half of pregnancy. If there are ultrasonographic signs of fetal disease such as hepatosplenomegaly or hydrops fetalis, a multidisciplinary team including genitourinary medicine and perinatology/fetal medicine specialists should be consulted. An abnormal ultrasound scan is an indication for antepartum FHR monitoring prior to instituting antibiotic treatment. Sonographic signs of fetal syphilis combined with an abnormal FHR pattern may indicate a severely affected and possibly moribund fetus (103).

Treatment

Penicillin continues to be the gold standard treatment for syphilis in and outside of pregnancy. Treatment is effective for maternal disease, prevention of vertical transmission to the fetus, and eradication of early fetal disease. Primary syphilis may be treated with a single dose of penicillin G (benzathine 2.4 million units intramuscularly). In all other cases, the disease should be considered latent and of unknown duration and treated with a course of *three* intramuscular injections of penicillin G (benzathine 2.4 million units) spaced a week apart. An alternative treatment regimen is daily intramuscular injections of procaine penicillin (0.6–0.9 million units) for 10–14 days. Neurosyphilis requires aqueous crystalline penicillin G between 12 and 24 million units daily in divided IV doses for 10–14 days.

Treatment of maternal syphilis is complicated in pregnant woman with a penicillin allergy (5–10% of cases). Confirmation of the penicillin allergy with skin testing is recommended, unless there is a documented anaphylactic reaction. In this situation, penicillin desensitization followed by penicillin treatment is the next treatment option of choice. Oral penicillin desensitization is given in small, gradually increasing doses with inpatient monitoring over approximately 4 hours, followed by the administration of the therapeutic dose intramuscularly 30 minutes after completion. Most adverse reactions can be managed supportively without discontinuation of the desensitization protocol. The Jarisch–Herxheimer reaction is a common systemic reaction to the treatment of syphilis occurring in approximately 40–45% of pregnant women, during the first course of penicillin (107). It is thought to result from the release of an endotoxin-like substance when a large number of spirochetes are killed by the antibiotics. The Jarisch–Herxheimer reaction is characterized by headache, pyrexia, malaise, rash, tachycardia, and hypotension usually 1–12 hours after the administration of an initial antibiotic dose and should be managed supportively. It may precipitate FHR abnormalities and/or preterm labour, therefore fetal monitoring is recommended (108). However, the reaction is usually not seen with subsequent antibiotic doses. The therapeutic response to treatment should be followed up with serological testing at 1-, 3-, 6-, 12-, and 24-month intervals.

Treatment of the baby at birth is recommended if maternal treatment was with alternative antibiotics such as macrolides. If delivery occurred within 30 days of treatment completion, the neonate needs empirical treatment (108). The neonatologists should be informed before delivery of the baby so that appropriate examination, management, and follow-up may be arranged for the neonate. If the neonate's serum is negative on screening and there are no signs of congenital syphilis, no further testing is necessary and the mother can be reassured. About 75% of infected babies may not show any symptoms at birth with signs of congenital syphilis manifesting many weeks, months, or years after birth. These can present as skin lesions, snuffles, hepatosplenomegaly, lymphadenopathy, and failure to thrive (108). Women diagnosed with syphilis should be offered testing for other sexually transmitted infections including HIV infection and their sexual contacts traced and offered treatment.

Listeriosis

Listeriosis is a rare infection caused by the bacterium *Listeria monocytogenes*, a Gram-positive, rod-shaped organism, which may contaminate raw food such as soft cheese, cured meat, and prepacked raw items such as smoked fish, sandwiches, or salads. Infection occurs when contaminated food is ingested.

Epidemiology

The incidence of listeriosis in pregnancy is 12 per 100,000 compared with a rate of 0.7 per 100,000 in the general population (109). Infection is mostly seen in neonates, however, listeriosis is 20 times more likely in pregnancy and 300 times more likely with acquired immunodeficiency syndrome (AIDS) (110). Elderly and immunocompromised individuals are at high risk of infection. Neonatal infection is caused mainly by vertical transmission of maternal infection via the placenta or occasionally as an ascending infection to the fetus.

Clinical diagnosis

In immunocompetent individuals, infection is often asymptomatic or presents as acute fever and gastroenteritis with full recovery within 2 days. Maternal symptoms include fever, malaise, headache, sore throat, conjunctivitis, abdominal or back pain, diarrhoea/vomiting, stiff neck, and confusion. Among pregnant women, about 20–30% of cases may result in stillbirth or neonatal death, and miscarriage is common (110). (111). Seventy per cent of pregnancies with listeriosis result in preterm delivery below 35 weeks' gestation and about 66% of infants surviving a pregnancy complicated by listeriosis will have neonatal listeriosis (112). Mortality in the infected neonate is 30–50%.

Pregnant women with listeriosis may show signs of chorioamnionitis such as uterine fundal tenderness, contractions, fever, vaginal discharge, or ruptured membranes. Early-onset neonatal disease (<7 days) is characterized by sepsis, respiratory distress, and hepatosplenomegaly while late-onset infection manifests as fever, meningitis, lethargy, irritability, and feeding problems.

Diagnosis is made by culture of the Gram-positive bacilli from blood, cerebrospinal fluid, amniotic fluid, or the placenta. Maternal vaginal secretions or stool cultures are not diagnostic as they can occur in carriers of listeria not necessarily indicating active infection. Infection must be suspected in any pregnant woman presenting with fever accompanied by gastrointestinal symptoms. Blood culture is recommended.

Treatment

High-dose IV antibiotics administered to the mother has been proposed for listeria chorioamnionitis in the preterm period to avoid preterm birth (113). Infection control precautions with gowning, gloves, and careful hand washing are important to prevent nosocomial spread. Pregnant or immunocompromised individuals should be empirically treated with ampicillin and an aminoglycoside after cultures have been obtained. Treatment regimens include ampicillin (2 g IV every 4 hours) or penicillin G (4 million units IV every 4 hours) (112). Gentamicin or another aminoglycoside should be used in combination with ampicillin or penicillin to treat complicated infections involving nervous system, neonates, endocarditis, and immunocompromised patients. A combination of amoxicillin and erythromycin can also be used. Treatment must be continued for 2 weeks in immunocompetent patients with bacteraemia and 2–4 weeks for complicated infections or in immunocompromised individuals. Prevention of infection centres on food safety including cooking raw food, avoiding unpasteurized products, and preventing cross-contamination of cooking surfaces by thorough washing of hands, cutting boards, or cooking surfaces. Pregnant women should avoid eating delicatessen meats, soft cheese, refrigerated pâtés, meat spreads, and packaged salads containing meat or smoked seafood. Raw vegetables should be thoroughly washed before consumption.

Selected viral infections

Cytomegalovirus

Cytomegalovirus (CMV) is a double-stranded DNA virus of the *Herpesviridae* family, which causes cytomegalic inclusion disease. The disease is characterized by large cells containing prominent intranuclear inclusion bodies.

Epidemiology

CMV is a ubiquitous virus. Most primary CMV infections in adults are asymptomatic although a minority present with flu-like illness (10%). Forty to eighty per cent of adults have been affected by CMV at some time in life, usually in childhood (114). CMV may be cultured from the cervix or urine of 2–28% of pregnant women (115).

Following primary infection, CMV like other herpes viruses remains latent but may cause infection due to reactivation during pregnancy. Although CMV infection is common, serious illness occurs only in fetuses and in immunodeficient or immunosuppressed individuals. Congenital CMV infection is acquired *in utero*, primarily from transplacental transmission. Congenital CMV infections may occur after either primary or recurrent maternal infection. The incidence of congenital CMV is 0.3–0.6% with the risk of transmission distributed across all trimesters. In the majority of cases where CMV is transmitted from the mother to the fetus, no damage is caused to the baby. In 10% of cases, the baby may be born with symptoms at birth (116). Congenital CMV infections may occur after either primary or recurrent maternal infection. Symptomatic congenital CMV infection occurs mainly with primary maternal infection.

Common manifestations of CMV infection acquired *in utero* include mental impairment and hearing loss. Infants with clinically apparent disease at birth have mortality rates as high as 20–30% and 90% may have late complications (115).

Clinical diagnosis

The spectrum of disease in the fetus and neonate is wide. The manifestations in the severely affected neonates include hepatosplenomegaly, jaundice, thrombocytopenia, purpura, microcephaly, deafness, chorioretinitis, optic atrophy, and cerebral calcifications. A characteristic tetrad includes intellectual disability, chorioretinitis, cerebral calcification, and microcephaly or hydrocephaly (117). The diagnosis of primary CMV infection is by the demonstration of seroconversion of CMV-specific immunoglobulin (Ig)-G antibodies from negative to positive (117). A rise of IgG titre is not useful as this can also occur with recurrent infection.

Diagnosis of primary maternal CMV infection in pregnancy should therefore be based on the *de novo* appearance of virus-specific IgG in the serum of the pregnant woman who was previously seronegative or on detection of specific IgM antibody associated with low IgG avidity. IgM specific to CMV is not a reliable marker for diagnosis of primary infection because the CMV IgM, though suggestive of recent infection, can remain positive for many months. IgM can also indicate reactivation of past infection (118). The diagnosis of secondary infection should be based on a significant rise of IgG antibody titre with or without the presence of IgM and high IgG avidity.

Ultrasound scan findings of microcephaly, hepatosplenomegaly, ventriculomegaly, calcifications of the brain, liver, or placenta, intrauterine growth restriction/oligohydramnios, ascites, pericardial or pleural effusion, hypoechogenic bowel, and/or hydrops may raise suspicion of fetal infection. Amniotic fluid culture for CMV or PCR for DNA identification should be offered to pregnant women with documented primary CMV infection or sonographic findings suggestive of CMV infection. A high CMV viral load in the amniotic fluid is associated with a higher risk of an affected fetus (119).

Treatment

At present there is no therapy for the *in utero* treatment of primary infection. There is also no CMV vaccine available at the present time. Routine screening for CMV infection in pregnancy is not recommended. Antenatal management options include counselling followed by either expectant management or termination of pregnancy. Termination of pregnancy should be offered if a significant CMV viral load is confirmed on prenatal testing. Specific treatment strategies such as therapies with adenosine arabinoside, cytosine arabinoside, ganciclovir, and foscarnet have been used for severe clinical infection (119). In view of their toxicity profiles, advice should be sought from perinatal infection specialists prior to using these agents. Research studies are exploring the use of CMV-specific IV immunoglobulins in affected pregnancies.

Rubella

The rubella virus is an RNA virus of the *Togaviridae* family. The infection is also known as German measles.

Epidemiology

Prior to the introduction of the rubella vaccine the infection was seen mainly in children of school age but the incidence in most countries has fallen in recent times with the introduction of the vaccine (120). The number of women of reproductive age who remain susceptible varies widely between countries as rubella vaccine is not universally available. Rubella infection during pregnancy may lead to intrauterine fetal demise, miscarriage, fetal growth restriction, hydrops, or congenital rubella syndrome characterized by sensorineural deafness, cataracts, glaucoma, chorioretinitis, microphthalmia, patent ductus arteriosus, peripheral pulmonary

artery stenosis, atrial or ventricular septal defect, microcephaly, meningoencephalitis, and intellectual disability (121). Other associations include hepatosplenomegaly, thrombocytopenia, bone defects, and purpuric skin lesions resulting in the classic 'blueberry muffin' presentation.

Clinical diagnosis

In most of the developed world, pregnant women are routinely screened for immunity to rubella and advised to avoid contact with rubella if they are non-immune. Evaluation for rubella infection should be done in susceptible pregnant women if clinical features consistent with rubella infection occurred or following exposure to an active case. Rubella causes a febrile illness with transient rash, fever, arthralgia, and postauricular and suboccipital lymphadenopathy. The rash often migrates from the face to the rest of the body. The incubation period is 12–24 days. Complications of rubella infection include encephalitis, myocarditis, pericarditis, hepatitis, and thrombotic thrombocytopenic purpura/haemolytic uraemic syndrome. The risk of fetal anomaly is over 90% with infection before 11 weeks of pregnancy, dropping down to the background risk after 20 weeks (105). Serology is the usual method for the diagnosis of rubella infection. It involves the detection of specific IgM antibodies or a significant rise in specific IgG titres. If recent infection is suspected, rubella IgM and rubella-specific IgG avidity may be used to confirm primary infection. Fetal infection may be confirmed by testing for viral DNA in a chorionic villus sample in the first trimester or by PCR of the amniotic fluid or fetal blood.

Treatment

If fetal infection is confirmed at an early stage, termination of pregnancy should be offered as an option. Management is limited to supportive care since there is no specific treatment available.

Rubella vaccine is available as a single live attenuated vaccine or in combination with the measles and mumps vaccine (MMR). It should be offered to all non-immune and seronegative women of reproductive age outside of pregnancy. Vaccination should be offered to non-immune women post delivery and they should be advised to avoid pregnancy for 3 months after vaccination. There is no contraindication to breastfeeding with the vaccine. Approximately 5% of women may not respond to the vaccine and remain susceptible to rubella (105).

Measles (rubeola)

Measles is an acute, highly infectious illness caused by the rubeola virus and is transmitted via droplet infection. The virus belongs to the *Paramyxoviridae* family, which are enveloped negative single-stranded RNA viruses.

Epidemiology

Although measles is highly contagious, the infection is uncommon in industrialized nations because of a safe and effective vaccine (122). The disease remains one of the leading causes of death among young children globally. In 2015, there were 134,200 measles deaths globally—about 367 deaths every day or 15 deaths every hour (122). Most epidemics occur in the spring and summer of alternate years. The spread of infection occurs by direct contact with droplets from respiratory secretions of infected persons.

Clinical diagnosis

The incubation period following exposure is 10–14 days. Exposure to the virus results in entry via the respiratory mucosa and/or conjunctiva. There may be transient respiratory symptoms, fever, or a rash during this period. There is a prodromal phase of 2–4 days followed by fever, conjunctivitis, coryza, and Koplik's spots (white, irregular lesions on the buccal mucosa opposite the upper premolars) on day 2 of the fever. By day 3 to 4, an erythematous maculopapular rash appears starting initially at the forehead, and behind the earlobes moving to the trunk and feet by the third day. The early lesions become confluent, although peripherally, the lesions remain discrete. It begins to fade by the third day in the order of its appearance.

Most measles-related deaths are caused by complications associated with the disease including disseminated disease and pneumonia. Post-infectious encephalitis can occur in 1 in 800–1600 cases. It has a mortality rate of up to 15% with neurological sequelae in half of the survivors (123). Subacute sclerosing panencephalitis is another rare (1 in 100,000 cases) late-appearing complication occurring most often in children (123). Measles during pregnancy is associated with increased maternal mortality secondary to pneumonia. Hence women with suspected pneumonia should be referred to a tertiary centre (105). Measles infection in pregnancy increases the risk of preterm birth and fetal growth restriction (105). Serum testing for measles-specific IgG and IgM antibodies is utilized for the confirmation of acute infection.

Treatment

Measles usually runs a self-limiting course, resulting in full recovery with supportive therapy such as hydration and antipyretics. Secondary bacterial infections (otitis or pneumonia) should be treated appropriately as soon as a diagnosis is made. Live attenuated measles vaccine is highly effective in controlling epidemic disease as well as the rare neurological sequelae (123). Two doses of the vaccine are recommended to ensure immunity and prevent outbreaks. In non-immune women of childbearing age, two doses of MMR vaccine can be given separated by a 3-month interval. In susceptible exposed women, passive immunization with pooled immunoglobulins may be offered within 72 hours of exposure as postexposure prophylaxis.

Parvovirus

Parvovirus B19 is a DNA virus of the *Parvoviridae* family. It causes erythema infectiosum or 'fifth disease'. Outbreaks usually occur in nurseries or schools with seasonal peaks.

Epidemiology

Parvovirus B19 infection is common among school children and 60% of women are immune to it by the age of 20 years (124). The cellular receptor for B19 parvovirus is the erythrocyte P antigen, thus its main target is erythroid progenitor cells. The infection is spread via respiratory secretions. Mothers, nursery teachers, and health workers who come in contact with school-aged children are at highest risk of contracting the infection. The virus is also transmissible via blood and blood products. There is a 50% risk of transmission from an infected mother to her fetus *in utero* (125).

Clinical diagnosis

Parvovirus B19 infection is characterized by a flu-like illness (fever, malaise, arthropathy, and lymphadenopathy) followed by a malar rash with the characteristic 'slapped cheeks' appearance and a lace-like rash in the extremities. The rash may reappear for several weeks following stimulus, including changes in temperature, sunlight exposure, or emotional stress. While in some cases, the infection may be asymptomatic, in others, the symptoms may persist for several months. Fetal infection may be asymptomatic or result in serious consequences such as miscarriage or fetal loss (10–15%) or hydrops fetalis (3–10%) as a result of haemolytic anaemia and congestive cardiac failure (126). If infection occurs after 20 weeks' gestation, the fetal loss rate is 2% (124). Spontaneous recovery of hydropic fetuses with delivery of normal infants has been reported (127).

Serological testing with enzyme-linked immunosorbent assay (ELISA) to detect IgG and IgM antibodies to B19 parvovirus may be used for diagnosis. Susceptible individuals will have negative status to both antibodies. A positive IgG and negative IgM suggests immunity or infection of more than 120 days prior. Recently infected patients will have positive IgM and negative IgG, and, finally, those who have had an infection more than 7 days but less than 120 days prior will show seropositivity to both G and M immunoglobulins. DNA detection by PCR is the other diagnostic test available. If primary infection during pregnancy is confirmed, serial fetal ultrasound scans should be offered starting from 2 to 4 weeks after infection or seroconversion to detect any hydrops fetalis. Monitoring by scanning should continue every 1–2 weeks until 34 weeks of pregnancy.

Treatment

Maternal treatment is just supportive care since the infection is self-limited. Cordocentesis and intrauterine transfusion are recommended if hydrops occurs, and fetal medicine specialists should be involved in the care. If hydrops has not occurred by 8 weeks after maternal infection, it is unlikely to occur (127). Parvovirus B19 infection is not associated with congenital anomalies in the fetus and there is no indication for therapeutic termination of pregnancy. Currently, routine screening for infection is not justifiable and no prophylaxis or vaccine is available.

Herpes simplex virus

Over 70% of primary genital herpes infections pass asymptomatically. Recurrent episodes tend to be milder in severity and shorter in duration than the primary infection. Transmission of herpes simplex virus (HSV) from mother to child around the time of delivery can cause potentially fatal disease in the newborn; however, routine antenatal screening for the detection of HSV 1 and 2 in the cervix, or antibodies from patients with a history of recurrent HSV, is not recommended. Therefore, if genital herpes infection is suspected, it is essential to determine whether the infection is primary or a recurrence and establish the gestational age of the pregnancy. Women who suffer their first genital HSV infection during pregnancy are at the highest risk of transmitting the virus to their newborn. Efforts to prevent vertical transmission of HSV disease may be summarized as follows:

1. Prevention of acquisition of maternal genital HSV infection.
2. Prevention of transmission of HSV during pregnancy and delivery.
3. Prevention of disease in an exposed newborn postnatally.

At the present time, there is no vaccine licensed to prevent genital herpes, although a number of clinical trials are ongoing. The potential role of intrapartum antiviral therapy and postnatal strategies to prevent neonatal HSV disease is yet to be determined. Oral aciclovir and valaciclovir given prophylactically in late pregnancy have been shown to reduce recurrences of genital herpes, shedding of HSV at delivery, and is the mainstay of prevention of HSV acquisition (128). There is insufficient evidence to determine the effect of antiviral prophylaxis in pregnancy on neonatal HSV disease. Neonatal HSV disease should always be treated with systemic antiviral therapy. Opinion is still divided on the use of caesarean section for the management of recurrent HSV. If the infection is primary, the woman should be referred urgently to the local sexual health clinic. A primary episode of HSV at 34 weeks' gestation or more but before the onset of labour is managed with prophylactic aciclovir until delivery. However, a primary episode in labour is managed by caesarean section provided the membranes have not been ruptured for more than 4 hours. If the interval between initiating prophylactic antiviral therapy and delivery is more than 4 weeks, vaginal delivery is appropriate. With infections prior to 34 weeks, aciclovir should be started from 34 weeks until delivery with the aim of vaginal delivery.

Varicella zoster virus

Varicella zoster virus (VZV) is the cause of chickenpox, a highly contagious infection. Like other viruses in the herpes family the infection is characterized by an acute illness, which is followed by the persistence of the virus within body tissues where they lie dormant for prolonged periods of time and may become reactivated subsequently. The zoster virus persists in the dorsal root ganglia of the spinal cord from where reactivation may give rise to shingles long after the primary infection.

Epidemiology

Over 90% of the antenatal population in the United Kingdom have had chickenpox infection, usually as a mild self-limiting illness in childhood, which confers lifelong immunity. As a result, the incidence of chickenpox in pregnancy in the United Kingdom is low, estimated to be 3 per 1000 (129). In contrast, the infection is usually acquired at older ages in the tropics resulting in higher susceptibility among adults from those populations. Therefore, immigrant women from tropical countries are at a greater risk of chickenpox infection than their counterparts who grew up in the United Kingdom (129, 130).

Clinical diagnosis

The infection is transmitted via respiratory droplets. The symptoms include malaise, fever, pruritic maculopapular rash, vesicles, crusts, and lesions at different stages of healing. If the infection is suspected or diagnosed, the woman should avoid contact with other pregnant women, immunosuppressed patients, and neonates for more than 5 days, or until the lesions crust over. Pregnant women are at greater risk of pulmonary complications particularly if they smoked, had chronic lung disease, took immunosuppressant drugs, had over 100 vesicles, or are in the second half of pregnancy. Other maternal complications include hepatitis, encephalitis, acute cerebella ataxia, thrombocytopenia, purpura, and haemorrhagic gangrene. These women and those with mucosal lesions or new lesions after 6 days should be referred urgently to the hospital. Shingles is usually mild and there is no risk to the fetus or neonate. Viraemia is rare with shingles unless in the immunocompromised host. Since the introduction of antiviral therapy, mortality from VZV pneumonia in pregnant women has become rare (130).

Risk assessment and prevention

Susceptible pregnant women should avoid contact with people with chickenpox and report any potential exposure. If a pregnant woman presents with a history of significant contact with chickenpox (defined as living in the same household, being in the same room for ≥15 minutes, face-to-face conversation for >5 minutes with someone who has chickenpox or shingles in an exposed part of the body, or any contact with a case of chickenpox during the period of 'infectiousness') immunity should be assumed if she gives a definite history of chickenpox (130). However, an urgent VZV IgG assay should be ordered if the history is negative or vague. Immunity (VZV IgG) can also be determined on the booking serum sample. Varicella zoster immunoglobulin (VZIG) should be administered as soon as possible (up to 10 days) if a woman with significant exposure is found to be non-immune. VZIG has no therapeutic benefit once chickenpox has developed and it does not prevent intrauterine infection. The woman should be referred to the fetal medicine unit between 16 and 20 weeks or 6 weeks after the infection for ultrasound scan assessment (130). After birth, the infant should undergo ophthalmic assessment and VZV IgM, and IgG at 7 months (130).

Fetal risks

Chickenpox infection is not associated with an increased risk of first- or second-trimester miscarriage. Fetal varicella syndrome is characterized by segmental skin loss, scarring, limb deformities, microcephaly, intellectual disability, hypotonia, bladder and/or bowel sphinteric dysfunction, cataracts, and chorioretinitis, and the risk of its occurrence is about 1% if maternal infection occurred before 28 weeks. Fetal varicella syndrome is due to the reactivation of VZV *in utero*. Since transplacental transfer of maternal antibodies is limited before 28 weeks' gestation, maternal immunity does not usually protect fetuses less than 28 weeks' gestation (130).

Perinatal chickenpox

Maternal chickenpox infection near the time of delivery or in the immediate postpartum period results in early neonatal chickenpox because of insufficient production and transfer of protective antibodies to the infant. Approximately 50% of infants delivered within 1–4 weeks of maternal infection are infected even in the presence of high antibody titres suggesting that in the short term, these antibodies may be less protective. Severe neonatal chickenpox is likely if delivery occurred within seven days of the onset of maternal rash. VZIG should be administered at birth in this situation and also if maternal chickenpox occurred within 2 days of delivery (130). The infant should be monitored for signs of infection for 14–16 days and treated with IV aciclovir if neonatal chickenpox occurred. Consideration should be given if possible to delaying the delivery for 5–7 days after the onset of maternal illness to allow transfer of maternal antibodies. If a neonate of a non-immune mother comes into contact with chickenpox, VZIG should be administered (130).

Hepatitis B

The hepatitis B virus (HBV) is a partially double-stranded DNA hepatotropic virus. It is estimated that 240 million people worldwide are chronically infected with hepatitis B (131).

Epidemiology

Hepatitis B is a potentially life-threatening liver infection and more than 686,000 people die every year from complications of hepatitis B infection, including cirrhosis and liver cancer (132). The virus is transmitted through contact with infected blood or other body fluids including sexual transmission. Hepatitis B is an important occupational hazard for health workers. In highly endemic areas, hepatitis B is most commonly spread from mother to child at birth (perinatal transmission) or through horizontal transmission (exposure to infected blood), especially from an infected child to an uninfected child during the first 5 years of life.

Clinical diagnosis

The HBV can survive outside the body for at least 7 days. The virus remains infectious during this time if it enters the body of a susceptible individual. The incubation period is approximately 75 days but can vary from 30 to 180 days. The virus may be detected within 30–60 days of infection and may persist and develop into chronic hepatitis B.

Hepatitis B viral infection has a wide spectrum of clinical manifestations ranging from acute hepatitis, through asymptomatic carriage, to liver cirrhosis and hepatocellular carcinoma. While most affected individuals are asymptomatic during the acute infection, some experience acute illness manifesting as fatigue, nausea, vomiting, jaundice, and abdominal pain, which may persist for several weeks. A small subset of patients with acute hepatitis may develop acute liver failure, which can be fatal. The likelihood of chronic infection is inversely related to the age of acquisition of the virus. The majority of infected adults recover and develop long-lasting immunity, defined as loss of hepatitis B surface antigen (HBsAg) and development of antibodies against the surface antigen (anti-HBsAb). In contrast, vertical transmission at birth or infection in early childhood carries a high risk of chronic liver infection, which may progress to liver cirrhosis or hepatocellular carcinoma. Children less than 6 years of age who become infected with the HBV are the most likely to develop chronic infection. The diagnosis of the infection is based on the clinical picture and serological detection of:

- HBsAg—current infection
- HB e antigen (HBeAg)—active viral replication
- anti-HBsAb (antibodies)—indicating immunity either from infection or vaccination.

Treatment

There is no specific treatment for acute hepatitis B. Therefore, care is aimed at maintaining comfort and adequate nutritional balance, including replacement of fluids lost from vomiting and diarrhoea. Chronic hepatitis B infection with high viral load can be treated with antiviral agents such lamivudine. It is now well established that HBV infection and its complications can be prevented by active and passive vaccination. A vaccine against hepatitis B has been available since 1982. The vaccine is 95% effective in preventing infection and the development of chronic disease and liver cancer (131). All pregnant women should be screened for HBV at booking. High-risk women (commercial sex workers and IV drug abusers) should be counselled and vaccinated before pregnancy. Acute HBV infection in pregnancy is per se not associated with an increase in maternal morbidity or mortality and does not increase the risk of fetal congenital abnormalities. An increased risk of preterm labour has been reported. The risk of perinatal transmission is high especially in the third trimester or postpartum period.

The risk of perinatal infection in chronic carriers depends on maternal HBeAg status. Without immunoprophylaxis and depending on maternal viral load, up to 90% of infants born to HBeAg-positive mothers acquire the infection compared to approximately 10% of babies born to HBeAg-negative mothers (133). If chronic HBV infection is diagnosed in pregnancy, complete serological work-up including liver ultrasound, liver function tests, viral load estimation, and if indicated serum levels of alpha-fetoprotein should be determined to assess liver damage. Hepatologists should be involved in the care of the pregnant woman to determine the need for and type of antiviral therapy required during or after delivery. The risk of fetal hepatitis B infection through amniocentesis is low; however, if amniocentesis is required, insertion of the needle through the placenta should be avoided. During labour, invasive procedures such as fetal blood sampling, fetal scalp electrode, or instrumental delivery should be avoided. Neonatal infection may be fatal or result in chronic carrier status with significant lifelong risks of cirrhosis and liver cancer. Babies whose mothers have acute or chronic HBV should receive HBV IgG (immunoglobulins) and vaccination within 24 hours of delivery with the aim of completing the schedule. This is thought to be up to 95% effective at preventing neonatal HBV infection (131).

Hepatitis C

Hepatitis C virus (HCV) infection is a major global health problem. The infection is caused by a single-stranded virus, which is transmitted through infected blood and sexual (rare) route.

Epidemiology

The average time from exposure to the HCV to seroconversion is about 8–9 weeks. Women with risk factors for HCV such as IV drug abusers and HIV-positive women should be counselled and offered screening.

Clinical diagnosis

Acute infection may present with loss of appetite, nausea, vomiting, abdominal pain, and jaundice. However, up to two-thirds of infections are asymptomatic.

The diagnosis is confirmed by detecting anti-HCV antibodies or HCV RNA in blood. HCV may remain quiescent for many years before progression to chronic infection (85%), cirrhosis (20%), or hepatocellular carcinoma (134, 135) (<5%). The risk of vertical transmission of HCV is about 5% but is higher if the woman is co-infected with HIV (136). Risk factors for perinatal transmission include high viral load, co-infection with HIV, and female infant (137).

Treatment

There is no vaccine or treatment for chronic HCV infection during pregnancy. During labour, invasive procedures such as fetal blood sampling, fetal scalp electrode, or instrumental delivery should be avoided. Although the evidence is slim, some treatment programmes advocate elective caesarean section for HCV-positive women with a high viral load who are also co-infected with HIV. A hepatologist should be involved in the care of the woman to ensure long-term hepatological follow-up.

Human immunodeficiency virus

HIV infection is associated with serious morbidity and mortality and is one of the world's most significant public health challenges. HIV is a retrovirus, which means that it has the ability to synthesize DNA from viral RNA through the action of the enzyme reverse transcriptase. The viral DNA is subsequently integrated into the host cell genome with instructions for the production of viral elements required for replication.

Epidemiology

HIV-1 is responsible for majority of HIV infections worldwide while HIV-2 is generally confined to West Africa and has a much lower virulence and transmission (138). HIV is transmitted via sexual intercourse, IV drug abuse, transfusion of blood products, and vertical transmission from mother to child. The three established routes of vertical transmission include *in utero*, during the time of delivery (commonest), and breastfeeding. HIV preferentially targets lymphocytes expressing CD4 molecules, also known as helper cells. Following infection, viral replication and integration results in a gradual loss of the CD4 lymphocyte count causing immune deficiency, indicated by a cell count less than 350 cells/mm³. This predisposes the patient to a variety of opportunistic infections and malignancies, and eventually development of AIDS. The time taken to develop AIDS from seroconversion is variable, ranging from months to more than a decade.

Improved access to antiretroviral therapy (ART) has led to longer life expectancy and healthier lives among HIV-positive individuals. In addition, ART prevents onward transmission of HIV. Progress has also been made in reducing mother-to-child transmission and keeping mothers alive. In 2015, almost eight out of ten pregnant women living with HIV, or 1.1 million women, received ART (139). Factors which have been consistently associated with transmission include maternal viral load, duration of membrane rupture, delivery before 32 weeks, mode of delivery, and breastfeeding. At a viral load of greater than 100,000 copies/mL there is a 40% risk of transmission, falling to 1% at 1000 copies/mL, and less than 1% at undetectable viral load (<40 copies/mL) (138).

Clinical diagnosis

It is recommended that all pregnant women are screened for HIV infection in early pregnancy usually at their booking antenatal visit. Women who decline HIV testing at booking are reoffered screening at 28 weeks of pregnancy while those considered to be at ongoing risk are reoffered screening still, particularly if they presented with symptoms consistent with seroconversion. Women at risk should also be screened for other sexually transmitted infections such as chlamydia, syphilis, hepatitis B, gonorrhoea, and herpes. Screening for sexually transmitted infections should be performed twice during pregnancy, once in the first trimester and again in the third trimester. Recurrent HSV type 2 infection is common in HIV-positive women and all women should have type-specific HSV serology if they have no previous diagnosis of genital herpes and present with genital ulcers (138).

Treatment

Bottle feeding instead of breastfeeding, ART, and appropriate management of delivery have reduced mother-to-child transmission rates from 25–30% to less than 1% (140). Women with HIV in pregnancy should be managed by a multidisciplinary team including an HIV physician, obstetrician, specialist midwife, virologist, health advisor, and neonatologist. Women who test positive for HIV should be encouraged to disclose their HIV status to their partners so they can be tested appropriately and any existing children of unknown HIV status should also be tested for HIV (140).

Women who require HIV treatment for their own health should take highly active antiretroviral therapy (HAART) and continue treatment postpartum. They may also require prophylaxis against *Pneumocystis jirovecii* pneumonia depending on their CD4 count. HAART usually involves combinations of nucleoside reverse transcriptase inhibitors, non-nucleoside reverse transcriptase inhibitors, protease inhibitors, and integrase inhibitors. Those not on HAART for their own health should be initiated on therapy between 20 and 28 weeks and discontinued through delivery. Women already taking HAART and/or *Pneumocystis jirovecii* pneumonia prophylaxis before pregnancy should not discontinue their medication. It is important to start ART earlier than 20–24 weeks when the baseline viral load is high, the CD4 count is low, in the presence of co-infections such as hepatitis B/C or recurrent genital HSV, and if there is history of preterm delivery (138).

Invasive prenatal diagnostic testing should not be performed until the HIV status of the woman has been determined and ideally deferred until the viral load is suppressed although the risks from the procedure should be weighed against the benefits. Maternal viral load should be estimated at 36 weeks of pregnancy and a decision regarding the mode of delivery made. Historically, planned elective caesarean section has been the method of choice for delivery of HIV-positive women; however, effective suppression of the viral load with HAART has led to many women having vaginal deliveries with similar low rates (<1%) of vertical transmission as caesarean section. Delivery by elective caesarean section at 38 weeks of pregnancy is recommended in women taking HAART who have a viral load greater than 50 copies/mL and in women with hepatitis C co-infection. During caesarean section, the risk of transmission may be minimized by keeping a haemostatic operating field, attempting to deliver the fetal head with the membranes intact, and clamping the cord as early as possible (140). A planned vaginal delivery may be offered to women taking HAART who have a plasma viral load of less than 50 copies/mL. In women with such levels of viral load who do decline vaginal birth, caesarean section should be carried out after 39 completed weeks. Although unlikely to confer an increased risk of vertical transmission, intrapartum invasive procedures such as fetal scalp electrode or fetal blood sampling should be avoided in women with undetectable viral load. Membranes should be kept intact for as long as possible during labour. To prevent chorioamnionitis and perinatal transmission, labour should be expedited for all women with rupture of membranes at term.

If a woman presents in labour and is not on treatment, she should be given a stat dose of nevirapine as this rapidly crosses the placenta. While the obstetric management continues, if time permits prior to caesarean section, more potent ART, which crosses the placenta and results in rapid reduction of the viral load should be administered (136). If delivery is indicated before 34 weeks, the risk of prematurity-related complications, availability of neonatal facilities, and the risk of perinatal HIV transmission should be considered in timing of the delivery.

ART to the newborn is an example of pre-exposure prophylaxis and should be decided before the delivery. The main antiretroviral therapies licensed for neonates are oral preparations and therefore it is necessary to treat the mother in order to optimize the prognosis for the preterm neonate. ART should be commenced in the neonate as soon after birth as possible. Infants born to HIV-positive mothers should have an HIV test on day 1, at 6 weeks, and at 12 weeks of age. If breastfeeding has not occurred and all these tests are negative, the infant is classified as HIV negative and a confirmatory blood test should only be offered at 18 months of age. In the postpartum period, women should be advised not to breastfeed, although in resource-poor settings breastfeeding may need to continue in the absence of valid alternatives. HIV-positive mothers should be offered appropriate vaccines and given advice regarding contraception and regular cervical screening (140). A multidisciplinary care plan should be put in place during and after pregnancy for women with HIV as many of them may suffer from consequences of chronic HIV infection, opportunistic infections, stigma, poverty, homelessness, domestic violence, drug abuse, and mental illness.

Selected parasite

Toxoplasma

Toxoplasmosis is an infection caused by the intracellular parasite *Toxoplasma gondii*. The infection is acquired by ingestion of toxoplasma tissue cysts (sporocysts). This may be secondary to eating inadequately washed vegetables or salads contaminated with cat litter, or from inadequate hand washing following gardening, or consumption of undercooked or cured meats containing viable parasitic tissue cysts.

Epidemiology

In developed countries, improvements in hygiene have led to a fall in the incidence of toxoplasma infection. In the United Kingdom, 90% of women of childbearing age are susceptible to toxoplasma infection and the incidence of maternal infection is approximately 2 per 1000 pregnancies (141). Reproductive-age women are at risk of acquiring an infection if they live in a high prevalence area, eat undercooked/raw meat, have contact with contaminated soil, drink contaminated water, and/or own a cat. Fetal transmission risk increases with gestational age at seroconversion (from 1% before 4 weeks, between 4–15% at 13 weeks, to 60% at 36 weeks) (142–145). The risk of congenital abnormality is greatest when infection occurs during the first trimester.

Clinical diagnosis

Primary infection is often asymptomatic (60–70%) but some women suffer from fever, fatigue, and lymphadenopathy. Toxoplasmosis mainly affects the central nervous system and eyes and can cause microcephaly, ventriculomegaly, hydrocephalus, and chorioretinitis. The affected child may experience learning difficulties, convulsions, spasticity, chorioretinitis, and blindness. Other consequences of congenital toxoplasmosis include hepatosplenomegaly, anaemia, rash, pneumonitis, and jaundice.

Diagnosis is mainly serological and based on testing for *Toxoplasma*-specific IgG and IgM antibodies. Diagnosis should be confirmed in relation to maternal history and with a specialist virologist's opinion. An acute infection in pregnancy is most accurately diagnosed when at least two blood samples drawn at least 2 weeks apart show seroconversion from negative to positive. Cases of confirmed primary maternal infection should be referred to a fetal medicine unit. Fetal diagnosis is based on the detection of *T. gondii* DNA in amniotic fluid. Amniocentesis should be considered from 16 weeks of gestation, as a positive result would lead to a change from treatment with spiramycin to a pyrimethamine/sulfadiazine regimen (125).

Treatment

When primary maternal infection is confirmed before 16 weeks of gestation, it is advisable to treat with spiramycin empirically rather than delay starting until after amniocentesis (125). Spiramycin administered to the mother reduces the risk of fetal infection by 60–70% (146, 147). In cases where amniocentesis is not possible, spiramycin should be started and continued throughout pregnancy with the aim of reducing transmission to the fetus. In cases where the amniotic fluid is positive for *Toxoplasma* DNA, transmission to the fetus is assumed. In proven fetal infection with ultrasound abnormalities, the outcome can be poor including fetal demise, neonatal death, neurological impairment (intellectual disability, seizures, need for ventricular shunt placement), and/or chorioretinitis. In cases of confirmed fetal infection, the treatment options include termination of pregnancy or maternal drug therapy with a pyrimethamine/sulfadiazine regimen throughout pregnancy along with ultrasound surveillance for assessment of fetal damage. Prevention of infection is the best strategy. This involves thorough cooking of meats and thorough washing of fruits, vegetables, cutting boards, dishes, utensils, and hands. Pregnant women should wear gloves when gardening and should avoid changing a cat litter box.

Immunization in pregnancy

Ideally, preconceptional administration of vaccines to prevent fetal and maternal disease is a better strategy than immunization during pregnancy. There is no evidence that vaccinating pregnant women with an inactivated virus, bacterial vaccines, or toxoids poses a risk. However, live vaccines pose a theoretical risk to the fetus of transmission of the organism.

When administering a live or live attenuated vaccine to a pregnant woman, the risk of exposure to disease and its adverse effects must be balanced against the efficacy of the vaccine. The obstetric care provider should counsel the pregnant woman about the risks and benefits of vaccine as well as potential exposure to the disease.

Starting at the first prenatal visit, attention should be paid to the immunization history of each pregnant woman. Women who have inadvertently received immunization with a live or live attenuated vaccine during pregnancy should not be advised to terminate the pregnancy because of the teratogenicity. Non-pregnant women immunized with a live or a live attenuated vaccine should be counselled to delay pregnancy for at least 4 weeks. Pregnant women should be offered the influenza vaccine during the influenza season. Neither inactivated nor live attenuated vaccine administered to lactating women affect the safety of breastfeeding for mothers or infants. Breastfeeding is not a contraindication for any vaccine except smallpox vaccine.

Tables **17.1** and **17.2** summarize the vaccines used for active and passive immunization during pregnancy.

Table 17.1 Active immunization during pregnancy

Vaccine	Virus	Maternal risk from disease	Fetal risk from disease	Fetal risk from vaccine	Immunization in pregnancy	Dose schedule	Comment
Measles	Live attenuated	High morbidity, low mortality	High miscarriage rate, may cause malformations	None confirmed	Contraindicated	Single dose SC	Performed postpartum
Mumps	Live attenuated	Low morbidity, low mortality	Possible high miscarriage rate	None confirmed	Contraindicated	Single dose SC	Performed postpartum
Rubella	Live attenuated	Low morbidity, low mortality	High miscarriage rate, congenital rubella syndrome	None confirmed	Contraindicated	Single dose SC	Performed postpartum Theoretic teratogenicity not confirmed
Poliomyelitis	Live attenuated	High morbidity	Anoxic fetal damage reported	None confirmed	Not routinely recommended in USA, except women at increased risk of exposure	Two doses SC at 4–8 weeks interval and third dose 6–12 months from second dose	Indicated for susceptible pregnant women travelling in endemic areas
Yellow fever	Live attenuated	High morbidity, high mortality	Unknown	Unknown	Contraindicated	Single dose SC	
Varicella	Live attenuated	Possible increase in severe pneumonia	Congenital varicella 2% if infected during second trimester	None confirmed	Contraindicated	Two doses needed 4–8 weeks apart	Performed postpartum
Influenza	Inactivated	Increase in morbidity and mortality during epidemic of new antigenic strain	Possible increased miscarriage rate	None confirmed	Any time	Single dose IM	
Rabies	Killed	100% fatality	Determined by maternal disease	Unknown	Indication for prophylaxis considered individually		Public health authorities consulted for indications, dosage and route
Hepatitis B	Purified surface antigen	Possible increased severity in third trimester	Possible increased miscarriage rate and preterm birth	None reported	Pre exposure and post exposure for women at risk of infection	Three-doses series IM at 0, 1, and 6 months	Used with hepatitis B immunoglobulin for some exposure
Hepatitis A	Inactivated	No increased risk during pregnancy		None reported	Pre exposure and post exposure for women at risk of infection	Two doses 6 month apart	
Pneumococcus	Polyvalent polysaccharide	No increased risk	Unknown, but depends on maternal illness	None reported	Recommended in case of asplenia; metabolic, renal, cardiac, pulmonary diseases; smokers; immunosuppressed.	Single dose SC or IM	Consider repeat dose in 6 years in high risk women
Meningococcus	Quadrivalent polysaccharide	High morbidity, high mortality	Unknown, but depends on maternal illness	None reported	Recommended in unusual outbreak situations	Single dose SC	Public health authorities consulted
Typhoid	Killed or live attenuated	High morbidity	Unknown	None confirmed	Recommended for close, continued exposure or travel in endemic areas	Killed: Primary: two injection SC. Booster: single dose SC	Oral vaccine preferred
Anthrax	Preparation from cell-free filtrate of B anthracis	High morbidity, high mortality	Unknown, but depends on maternal illness	None confirmed	Not routinely recommended	Six-dose primary vaccination SC, then annual booster	Teratogenicity of vaccine theoretical
Tetanus/diphtheria	Combined toxoids	Tetanus mortality 30%, diphtheria mortality 10%	Neonatal tetanus mortality 60%	None confirmed	Lack of primary series or no booster within past 10 years		Updating immune status during antepartum care

SC, subcutaneously; IM, intramuscularly.

Reproduced from Sabaratnam Arulkumaran, Lesley Regan, Aris Papageorghiou, Ash Monga, and David Farquharson, (Chapter 8) in *Oxford Desk Reference Obstetrics and Gynaecology*, Oxford University Press, pp. 259–260 with permission from Oxford University Press.

Table 17.2 Passive immunization during pregnancy

Vaccine	Virus	Maternal risk from disease	Fetal/neonatal risk from disease	Fatal risk from vaccine	Immunization in pregnancy	Dose schedule	Comment
Hepatitis B	Hepatitis B immune globulin	Possible increased severity in third trimester	Possible increase in miscarriage and preterm birth, neonatal hepatitis may occur	None reported	Postexposure prophylaxis	Consult Practice Advisory Committee recommendation	Usually given with hepatitis B vaccine
Rabies	Rabies immune globulin	100% fatality	Determined by maternal disease	None reported	Postexposure prophylaxis	Half dose at injury site and half in deltoid	Used in conjunction with rabies killed virus vaccine
Tetanus	Tetanus immune globulin	High morbidity, mortality 60%	Neonatal tetanus with 60% mortality	None reported	Postexposure prophylaxis	Single dose IM	Used in conjunction with tetanus toxoid
Varicella	Varicella zoster immune globulin	Possible increase in severe varicella pneumonia	Can cause congenital varicella with increased mortality in neonatal period	None reported	Considered for healthy pregnant women exposed to varicella to protect against maternal, not congenital infection	Single dose IM within 96 hours of exposure	Indicated in newborn of women who developed varicella within 4 days before delivery or 2 days following delivery, not indicated for prevention of congenital varicella
Hepatitis A	Standard immune globulin	Possible increased severity during third trimester	Possible increase in miscarriage and preterm birth,	None reported	Post exposure prophylaxis, but the vaccine should be used with immune globulin	Single dose IM	Immune globulin should be given as soon as possible and within 2 weeks of exposure

IM, intramuscularly.

Reproduced from Sabaratnam Arulkumaran, Lesley Regan, Aris Papageorghiou, Ash Monga, and David Farquharson, (Chapter 8) in *Oxford Desk Reference Obstetrics and Gynaecology*, Oxford University Press, pp. 259-260 with permission from Oxford University Press.

Conclusion

Subclinical perinatal infections exert direct fetal harm and make the fetus vulnerable to hypoxic damage. Numerically, this group of infections contribute a greater proportion of adverse outcome compared to specific bacterial or viral infection. Unfortunately, current clinical tests are targeted at the mother and are insensitive for the detection of intrauterine infection. Clinicians should consider intrauterine infection in the fetus with FHR tachycardia particularly if there was MSAF. The 'TORCHES' group of infections remain important but with the introduction of screening and vaccines contribute fewer cases of adverse perinatal outcome.

REFERENCES

1. Choi KS, Scorpio DG, Dumler JS. Anaplasma phagocytophilum ligation to toll-like receptor (TLR) 2, but not to TLR4, activates macrophages for nuclear factor-kappa B nuclear translocation. *J Infect Dis* 2004;**189**:1921–25.
2. Brian JE Jr, Faraci FM. Tumor necrosis factor-alpha-induced dilatation of cerebral arterioles. *Stroke* 1998;**29**:509–15.
3. van Deuren M, Dofferhoff AS, van der Meer JW. Cytokines and the response to infection. *J Pathol* 1992;**168**:349–56.
4. Eschenbach DA. Amniotic fluid infection and cerebral palsy. Focus on the fetus. *JAMA* 1997;**278**:247–48.
5. Goldenberg RL, Hauth JC, Andrews WW. Intrauterine infection and preterm delivery. *N Engl J Med* 2000;**342**:1500–507.
6. Yoon BH, Romero R, Kim CJ, et al. High expression of tumor necrosis factor-alpha and interleukin-6 in periventricular leukomalacia. *Am J Obstet Gynecol* 1997;**177**:406–11.
7. Saija A, Princi P, Lanza M, Scalese M, Aramnejad E, De Sarro A. Systemic cytokine administration can affect blood-brain barrier permeability in the rat. *Life Sci* 1995;**56**:775–84.
8. Wright JL, Merchant RE. Blood-brain barrier changes following intracerebral injection of human recombinant tumor necrosis factor-alpha in the rat. *J Neurooncol* 1994;**20**:17–25.
9. Hopkins SJ, Rothwell NJ. Cytokines and the nervous system. I. Expression and recognition. *Trends Neurosci* 1995;**18**:83–88.
10. Robbins DS, Shirazi Y, Drysdale BE, Lieberman A, Shin HS, Shin ML. Production of cytotoxic factor for oligodendrocytes by stimulated astrocytes. *J Immunol* 1987;**139**:2593–97.
11. Kahn MA, De Vellis J. Regulation of an oligodendrocyte progenitor cell line by the interleukin-6 family of cytokines. *Glia* 1994;**12**:87–98.
12. Andrews T, Zhang P, Bhat NR. TNFalpha potentiates IFNgamma-induced cell death in oligodendrocyte progenitors. *J Neurosci Res* 1998;**54**:574–83.
13. Almeida A, Bolanos JP, Medina JM. Nitric oxide mediates glutamate-induced mitochondrial depolarization in rat cortical neurons. *Brain Res* 1999;**239**:580–86.
14. Altman DI, Powers WJ, Perlman JM, Herscovitch P, Volpe SL, Volpe JJ. Cerebral blood flow requirement for brain viability in newborn infants is lower than in adults. *Ann Neurol* 1988;**24**:218–26.
15. Pryds O, Greisen G, Lou H, Friis H. Vasoparalysis associated with brain damage in asphyxiated term infants. *J Pediatr* 1990;**117**:119–25.
16. Boylan GB, Young K, Panerai RB, Rennie JM, Evans DH. Dynamic cerebral autoregulation in sick newborn infants. *Pediatr Res* 2000;**48**:12–17.
17. Oka A, Belliveau MJ, Rosenberg PA, Volpe JJ. Vulnerability of oligodendroglia to glutamate: pharmacology, mechanisms, and prevention. *J Neurosci* 1993;**13**:1441–53.

18. Back SA, Gan X, Li Y, Rosenberg PA, Volpe JJ. Maturation-dependent vulnerability of oligodendrocytes to oxidative stress-induced death caused by glutathione depletion. *J Neurosci* 1988;**18**:6241–53.

19. Paneth N, Rudelli R, Kazam E, Monte W. Prognosis. In: *Brain Damage in the Preterm Infant*, pp. 171–185. London: MacKeith; 1994.

20. Volpe JJ. Neurobiology of periventricular leukomalacia in the premature infant. *Pediatr Res* 2001;**50**:553–62.

21. Yoon BH, Kim CJ, Romero R, et al. Experimentally induced intrauterine infection causes fetal brain white matter lesions in rabbits. *Am J Obstet Gynecol* 1997;**177**:797–802.

22. Debillon T, Gras-Leguen C, Verielle V, et al. Intrauterine infection induces programmed cell death in rabbit periventricular white matter. *Pediatr Res* 2000;**47**:736–42.

23. Perlman JM, Risser R, Broyles RS. Bilateral cystic periventricular leukomalacia in the premature infant: associated risk factors. *Pediatrics* 1996;**97**:822–27.

24. Zupan V, Gonzalez P, Lacaze-Masmonteil T, et al. Periventricular leukomalacia: risk factors revisited. *Dev Med Child Neurol* 1996;**38**:1061–67.

25. Wu YW, Colford JM Jr. Chorioamnionitis as a risk factor for cerebral palsy: a meta-analysis. *JAMA* 2000;**284**:1417–24.

26. De Felice C, Toti P, Laurini RN, et al. Early neonatal brain injury in histologic chorioamnionitis. *J Pediatr* 2001;**138**:101–104.

27. Yoon BH, Romero R, Yang SH, et al. Interleukin-6 concentrations in umbilical cord plasma are elevated in neonates with white matter lesions associated with periventricular leukomalacia. *Am J Obstet Gynecol* 1996;**174**:1433–40.

28. Yoon BH, Jun JK, Romero R, et al. Amniotic fluid inflammatory cytokines (interleukin-6, interleukin-1beta, and tumor necrosis factor-alpha), neonatal brain white matter lesions, and cerebral palsy. *Am J Obstet Gynecol* 1997;**177**:19–26.

29. Yoon BH, Romero R, Jun JK, et al. Amniotic fluid cytokines (interleukin-6, tumor necrosis factor-alpha, interleukin-1 beta, and interleukin-8) and the risk for the development of bronchopulmonary dysplasia. *Am J Obstet Gynecol* 1997;**177**:825–30.

30. Yoon BH, Romero R, Park JS, et al. Fetal exposure to an intra-amniotic inflammation and the development of cerebral palsy at the age of three years. *Am J Obstet Gynecol* 2000;**182**:675–81.

31. Gomez R, Ghezzi F, Romero R, Munoz H, Tolosa JE, Rojas I. Premature labor and intra-amniotic infection. Clinical aspects and role of the cytokines in diagnosis and pathophysiology. *Clin Perinatol* 1995;**22**:281–342.

32. Sarnat HB. Role of human fetal ependyma. *Pediatr Neurol* 1992;**8**:163–78.

33. Morales WJ. The effect of chorioamnionitis on the developmental outcome of preterm infants at one year. *Obstet Gynecol* 1987;**70**:183–86.

34. Salafia CM, Minior VK, Rosenkrantz TS, et al. Maternal, placental, and neonatal associations with early germinal matrix/intraventricular hemorrhage in infants born before 32 weeks' gestation. *Am J Perinatol* 1995;**12**:429–36.

35. Yoon BH, Romero R, Kim CJ, et al. Amniotic fluid interleukin-6: a sensitive test for antenatal diagnosis of acute inflammatory lesions of preterm placenta and prediction of perinatal morbidity. *Am J Obstet Gynecol* 1995;**172**:960–70.

36. Fox H. Infections and inflammatory lesions of the placenta. In: *Pathology of the Placenta*, 2nd edn, pp. 294–343. Philadelphia, PA: W.B. Saunders; 1997.

37. Gomez R, Romero R, Ghezzi F, Yoon BH, Mazor M, Berry SM. The fetal inflammatory response syndrome. *Am J Obstet Gynecol* 1998;**179**:194–202.

38. Garcia-Fernandez N, Montes R, Purroy A, Rocha E. Hemostatic disturbances in patients with systemic inflammatory response syndrome (SIRS) and associated acute renal failure (ARF). *Thromb Res* 2000;**100**:19–25.

39. Grether JK, Nelson KB. Maternal infection and cerebral palsy in infants of normal birth weight. *JAMA* 1997;**278**:207–11.

40. Badawi N, Kurinczuk JJ, Keogh JM, et al. Antepartum risk factors for newborn encephalopathy: the Western Australian case-control study. *BMJ* 1998;**317**:1549–53.

41. Badawi N, Kurinczuk JJ, Keogh JM, et al. Intrapartum risk factors for newborn encephalopathy: the Western Australian case-control study. *BMJ* 1998;**317**:1554–58.

42. Verma U, Tejani N, Klein S, et al. Obstetric antecedents of intraventricular hemorrhage and periventricular leukomalacia in the low-birth-weight neonate. *Am J Obstet Gynecol* 1997;**176**:275–81.

43. Nelson KB, Willoughby RE. Infection, inflammation and the risk of cerebral palsy. *Curr Opin Neurol* 2000;**13**:133–39.

44. Alexander JM, McIntire DM, Leveno KJ. Chorioamnionitis and the prognosis for term infants. *Obstet Gynecol* 1999.**94**;274–78.

45. Williams MC, Brien WF, Nelson RN, Spellacy WN. Histologic chorioamnionitis is associated with fetal growth restriction in term and preterm infants. *Am J Obstet Gynecol* 2000;**183**:1094–99.

46. Toti P, De F, Palmeri ML, Villanova M, Martin JJ, Buonocore G. Inflammatory pathogenesis of cortical polymicrogyria: an autopsy study. *Pediatr Res* 1998;**44**:291–96.

47. Wu YW, Colford JM, Jr. Chorioamnionitis as a risk factor for cerebral palsy: a meta-analysis. *JAMA* 2000;**284**;1417–24.

48. Wu YW, Escobar GJ, Grether JK, et al. Chorioamnionitis and cerebral palsy in term and near term infants. *JAMA* 2003;**290**:2677–84.

49. Banerjee S, Cashman P, Yentis SM, Steer PJ. Maternal temperature monitoring during labor: concordance and variability among monitoring sites. *Obstet Gynecol* 2004;**103**:287–93.

50. Impey LW, Greenwood CE, Black RS, Yeh PS, Sheil O, Doyle P. The relationship between intrapartum maternal fever and neonatal acidosis as risk factors for neonatal encephalopathy. *Am J Obstet Gynecol* 2008;**198**:49.e1–6.

51. Macaulay JH, Bond K, Steer PJ. Epidural analgesia in labor and fetal hyperthermia. *Obstet Gynecol* 1992;**80**:665–69.

52. Dietrich WD, Busto R, Valdes I, Loor Y. Effects of normothermic versus mild hyperthermic forebrain ischemia in rats. *Stroke* 1990;**21**:1318–25.

53. Dietrich WD, Busto R, Halley M, Valdes I. The importance of brain temperature in alterations of the blood-brain barrier following cerebral ischemia. *J Neuropathol Exp Neurol* 1990;**49**:486–97.

54. Lieberman E, Eichenwald E, Mathur G, Richardson D, Heffner L, Cohen A. Intrapartum fever and unexplained seizures in term infants. *Pediatrics* 2000;**106**:983–88.

55. Beloosesky R, Weiner Z, Khativ N, et al. Prophylactic maternal N-acetylcysteine before lipopolysaccharide suppresses fetal inflammatory cytokine responses. *Am J Obstet Gynecol* 2009;**200**:665.e1–5.

56. Paintlia MK, Paintlia AS, Contreras MA, Singh I, Singh AK. Lipopolysaccharide-induced peroxisomal dysfunction exacerbates cerebral white matter injury: attenuation by N-acetyl cysteine. *Exp Neurol* 2008;**210**:560–76.

57. Buhimschi IA, Buhimschi CS, Weiner CP. Protective effect of N-acetylcysteine against fetal death and preterm labor induced by maternal inflammation. *Am J Obstet Gynecol* 2003;**188**:203–208.

58. Fewell JE, Johnson P. Upper airway dynamics during breathing and during apnoea in fetal lambs. *J Physiol* 1983;**339**:495–504.

59. Harding R, Bocking AD, Sigger JN. Upper airway resistances in fetal sheep: the influence of breathing activity. *J Appl Physiol* 1986;**60**:160–65.

60. Kalache KD, Chaoui R, Bollmann R. Doppler assessment of tracheal and nasal fluid flow during fetal breathing movements: preliminary observations. *Ultrasound Obstet Gynecol* 1997;**9**:257–61.

61. Kalache KD, Chaoui R, Marcks B, et al. Differentiation between human fetal breathing patterns by investigation of breathing-related tracheal fluid flow velocity using Doppler sonography. *Prenat Diagn* 2000;**20**:45–50.

62. Kalache KD, Chaoui R, Marks B, et al. Does fetal tracheal fluid flow during fetal breathing movements change before the onset of labour? *BJOG* 2002;**109**:514–19.

63. Boddy K, Dawes GS. Fetal breathing. *Br Med Bull* 1975;**31**:3–7.

64. Patrick JE, Dalton KJ, Dawes GS. Breathing patterns before death in fetal lambs. *Am J Obstet Gynecol* 1976;**125**:73–78.

65. Manning FA, Martin CB Jr, Murata Y, et al. Breathing movements before death in the primate fetus (Macaca mulatta). *Am J Obstet Gynecol* 1979;**135**:71–76.

66. Byrne DL, Gau G. In utero meconium aspiration: an unpreventable cause of neonatal death. *Br J Obstet Gynaecol* 1987;**94**:813–14.

67. Burgess AM, Hutchins GM. Inflammation of the lungs, umbilical cord and placenta associated with meconium passage in utero. Review of 123 autopsied cases. *Pathol Res Pract* 1996;**192**:1121–28.

68. Kearney MS. Chronic intrauterine meconium aspiration causes fetal lung infarcts, lung rupture, and meconium embolism. *Pediatr Dev Pathol* 1999;**2**:544–51.

69. Mortensen E, Kearney MS. Meconium aspiration in the midtrimester fetus: an autopsy study. *Pediatr Dev Pathol* 2009;**12**:438–42.

70. Eidelman AI, Nevet A, Rudensky B, et al. The effect of meconium staining of amniotic fluid on the growth of Escherichia coli and group B streptococcus. *J Perinatol* 2002;**22**:467–71.

71. Florman AL, Teubner D. Enhancement of bacterial growth in amniotic fluid by meconium. *J Pediatr* 1969;**74**:111–14.

72. Larsen B, Galask RP. Host resistance to intraamniotic infection. *Obstet Gynecol Surv* 1975;**30**:675–91.

73. Hoskins IA, Hemming VG, Johnson TR, et al. Effects of alterations of zinc-to-phosphorus ratios and meconium content on group B Streptococcus growth in human amniotic fluid in vitro. *Am J Obstet Gynecol* 1987;**157**:770–73.

74. Clark P, Duff P. Inhibition of neutrophil oxidative burst and phagocytosis by meconium. *Am J Obstet Gynecol* 1995;**173**:1301–305.

75. Romero R, Yoon BH, Chaemsaithong P, et al. Bacteria and endotoxin in meconium-stained amniotic fluid at term: could intra-amniotic infection cause meconium passage? *J Matern Fetal Neonatal Med* 2014;**27**:775–88.

76. Wu JM, Yeh TF, Wang JY, et al. The role of pulmonary inflammation in the development of pulmonary hypertension in newborn with meconium aspiration syndrome (MAS). *Pediatr Pulmonol Suppl* 1999;**18**:205–208.

77. Kallapur SG, Nitsos I, Moss TJ, et al. IL-1 mediates pulmonary and systemic inflammatory responses to chorioamnionitis induced by lipopolysaccharide. *Am J Respir Crit Care Med* 2009;**179**:955–61.

78. Kallapur SG, Kramer BW, Nitsos I, et al. Pulmonary and systemic inflammatory responses to intra-amniotic IL-1 alpha in fetal sheep. *Am J Physiol Lung Cell Mol Physiol* 2011;**301**:L285–95.

79. Ban R, Ogihara T, Mori Y, Oue S, Ogawa S, Tamai H. Meconium aspiration delays normal decline of pulmonary vascular resistance shortly after birth through lung parenchymal injury. *Neonatology* 2011;**99**:272–79.

80. Jobe AH. Effects of chorioamnionitis on the fetal lung. *Clin Perinatol* 2012;**39**:441–57.

81. Lee J, Romero R, Lee KA, et al. Meconium aspiration syndrome: a role for fetal systemic inflammation. *Am J Obstet Gynecol* 2016;**214**:366.e1–9.

82. Ugwumadu A. Understanding cardiotocographic patterns associated with intrapartum fetal hypoxia and neurologic injury. *Best Pract Res Clin Obstet Gynaecol* 2013;**27**:509–36.

83. Blot P, Milliez J, Breart G, et al. Fetal tachycardia and meconium staining: a sign of fetal infection. *Int J Gynaecol Obstet* 1983;**21**:189–94.

84. Maberry MC, Ramin SM, Gilstrap LC 3rd, Leveno KJ, Dax JS. Intrapartum asphyxia in pregnancies complicated by intra-amniotic infection. *Obstet Gynecol* 1990;**76**:351–54.

85. Eschenbach DA, Hillier S, Critchlow C, Stevens C, DeRouen T, Holmes KK. Diagnosis and clinical manifestations of bacterial vaginosis. *Am J Obstet Gynecol* 1988;**158**:819–28.

86. Ugwumadu A, Manyonda I, Reid F, Hay P. Effect of early oral clindamycin on late miscarriage and preterm delivery in asymptomatic women with abnormal vaginal flora and bacterial vaginosis: a randomised controlled trial. *Lancet* 2003;**361**:983–88.

87. Lamont RF, Duncan SL, Mandal D, Bassett P. Intravaginal clindamycin to reduce preterm birth in women with abnormal genital tract flora. *Obstet Gynecol* 2003;**101**:516–22.

88. Regan JA, Klebanoff MA, Nugent RP. The epidemiology of group B streptococcal colonization in pregnancy. Vaginal Infections and Prematurity Study Group. *Obstet Gynecol* 1991;**77**:604–10.

89. Boyer KM, Gotoff SP. Prevention of early-onset neonatal group B streptococcal disease with selective intrapartum chemoprophylaxis. *N Engl J Med* 1986;**314**:1665–69.

90. Gardner SE, Yow MD, Leeds LJ, et al. Failure of penicillin to eradicate group B streptococcal colonisation in the pregnant woman. A couple study. *Am J Obstet Gynecol* 1979;**135**:1062–65.

91. Hall RT, Barnes W, Krishnan L, et al. Antibiotic treatment of parturient women colonized with group B streptococci. *Am J Obstet Gynecol* 1976;**124**:630–34.

92. White K, Rainbow J, Johonson S, et al. Early onset group B streptococcal disease, US 1998–1999. *MMWR* 2000;**49**:793–996.

93. Regan JA, Klebanoff MA, Nugent RP, et al. Colonisation with group B streptococci in pregnancy and adverse outcome. VIP Study Group. *Am J Obstet Gynecol* 1996;**174**:1354–60.

94. Schrag SJ, Zell ER, Lynfield R, et al. A population-based comparison of strategies to prevent early-onset group B streptococcal disease in neonates. *N Engl J Med* 2002;**347**:233–39.

95. Schrag S, Gorwitz R, Fultz-Butts K, Schuchat A. Prevention of perinatal group B streptococcal disease. Revised guidelines from CDC. *MMWR Recomm Rep* 2002;**51**:1–22.

96. Moore MR, Schrag SJ, Schuchat A. Effects of intrapartum antimicrobial prophylaxis for prevention of group-B-streptococcal disease on the incidence and ecology of early-onset neonatal sepsis. *Lancet Infect Dis* 2003;**3**:201–13.

97. Stoll BJ, Hansen NI, Sánchez PJ, et al. Early onset neonatal sepsis: the burden of group B Streptococcal and E. coli disease continues. *Pediatrics* 2011;**127**:817–26.

98. Beardsall K, Thompson MH, Mulla RJ. Neonatal group B streptococcal infection in South Bedfordshire, 1993–1998. *Arch Dis Child Fetal Neonatal Ed* 2000;**82**:F205–7.

99. Health Protection Agency (HPA). *Rise in New Diagnoses of Sexually Transmitted Infections in the United Kingdom in 2009*. London: HPA; 2010.

100. Health Protection Agency (HPA). *All New Episodes Seen at GUM Clinics: 1998–2007. United Kingdom and Country Specific Tables.* London: HPA; 2008.

101. Carey J. Gonorrhoea in maternal medicine and infections. In: Arulkumaran S, Regan L, Papageorghiou A, Monga A, Farquharson D (eds), *Oxford Desk Reference Obstetrics and Gynaecology*, pp. 218–19. Oxford: Oxford University Press; 2011.

102. Brocklehurst P. Antibiotics for gonorrhoea in pregnancy. *Cochrane Database Syst Rev* 2002;**2**:CD000098.

103. Witzeman K. Syphilis in maternal medicine and infections. In: Arulkumaran S, Regan L, Papageorghiou A, Monga A, Farquharson D (eds), *Oxford Desk Reference Obstetrics and Gynaecology*, pp. 306–308. Oxford: Oxford University Press; 2011.

104. Public Health England. Sexually transmitted infections and chlamydia screening in England, 2013. Health Protection Report. 2014. Available at: https://webarchive.nationalarchives.gov.uk/20140714084352/http:/www.hpa.org.uk/hpr/archives/2014/hpr2414_AA_stis.pdf.

105. Khare MM, Khare MD. Infections in pregnancy. In: Greer I, Nelson-Piercy C, Walters B (eds), *Maternal Medicine: Medical Problems in Pregnancy*, pp. 217–35. London: Elsevier Ltd; 2007.

106. Allstaff S, Wilson J. The management of sexually transmitted infections in pregnancy. *TOG* 2012;**14**:25–32.

107. De Santis M, De Luca C, Mappa I, et al. Syphilis infection during pregnancy: fetal risks and clinical management. *Infect Dis Obstet Gynecol* 2012;**2012**:430585.

108. Narayan H. Syphilis in maternal infections. In: *Compendium for the Antenatal Care of High-Risk Pregnancies*, pp. 102–103. Oxford: Oxford University Press; 2015.

109. Hof H. History and epidemiology of listeriosis. *FEMS Immunol Med Microbiol* 2003;**35**:199–202.

110. Janakiraman V. Listeriosis in pregnancy: diagnosis, treatment, and prevention. *Rev Obstet Gynecol* 2008;**1**:179–85.

111. Gilbert GL. Infections in pregnant women. *Med J Aust* 2002;**176**:229–36.

112. Heinrichs G. Listeriosis in maternal medicine and infections. In: Arulkumaran S, Regan L, Papageorghiou A, Monga A, Farquharson D (eds), *Oxford Desk Reference Obstetrics and Gynaecology*, pp. 272–73. Oxford: Oxford University Press; 2011.

113. Temple ME, Nahata MC. Treatment of listeriosis. *Ann Pharmacother* 2000;**34**:656–61.

114. Gaytant MA, Steegers EA, Semmekrot BA, Merkus HM, Galama JM. Congenital cytomegalovirus infection: review of the epidemiology and outcome. *Obstet Gynecol Surv* 2002;**57**:245–56.

115. Gibbs R. Cytomegalovirus in maternal medicine and infections. In: Arulkumaran S, Regan L, Papageorghiou A, Monga A, Farquharson D (eds), *Oxford Desk Reference Obstetrics and Gynaecology*, pp. 197–97. Oxford: Oxford University Press; 2011.

116. Narayan H. Cytomegalovirus in maternal infections. In: *Compendium for the Antenatal Care of High-Risk Pregnancies*, pp. 67–69. Oxford: Oxford University Press; 2015.

117. Society of Obstetricians and Gynaecologists of Canada (SOGC). *Cytomegalovirus Infection in Pregnancy*. Clinical Practice Guideline No. 240. Ottawa: SOGC; 2010.

118. Adler SP. Screening for cytomegalovirus during pregnancy. *Infect Dis Obstet Gynecol* 2011;**2011**:942937.

119. McCarthy FP, Jones C, Rowlands S, Giles M. Primary and secondary cytomegalovirus in pregnancy. *TOG* 2009;**11**:96–100.

120. Alston M. Rubella in maternal medicine and infections. In: Arulkumaran S, Regan L, Papageorghiou A, Monga

A, Farquharson D (eds), *Oxford Desk Reference Obstetrics and Gynaecology*, pp. 302–303. Oxford: Oxford University Press; 2011.

121. Marret H, Golfier F, Di Maio M, Champion F, Attia-Sobol J, Raudrant D. Rubella in pregnancy. Management and prevention. *Presse Med* 1999;**28**:2117–22.

122. World Health Organization. Measles. Fact sheet. November 2016. Available at: http://www.who.int/mediacentre/factsheets/fs286/en/.

123. Stiglich N. Measles: rubeola in maternal medicine and infections. In: Arulkumaran S, Regan L, Papageorghiou A, Monga A, Farquharson D (eds), *Oxford Desk Reference Obstetrics and Gynaecology*, pp. 278–79. Oxford: Oxford University Press; 2011.

124. Narayan H. Parvovirus in Maternal infections. In: *Compendium for the Antenatal Care of High-Risk Pregnancies*, pp. 99–100. Oxford: Oxford University Press; 2015.

125. To M, Kidd M, Maxwell D. Prenatal diagnosis and management of fetal infections. *TOG* 2009;**11**:108–16.

126. Royal College of Obstetricians and Gynaecologists (RCOG) Safety and Quality Committee. *Parvovirus in Pregnancy*. Safety Alert No. 3. London: RCOG; 2012.

127. Miranda-Seijo P. Parvovirus in maternal medicine and infections. In: Arulkumaran S, Regan L, Papageorghiou A, Monga A, Farquharson D (eds), *Oxford Desk Reference Obstetrics and Gynaecology*, p. 280. Oxford: Oxford University Press; 2011.

128. Royal College of Obstetricians and Gynaecologists (RCOG). *Management of Genital Herpes in Pregnancy*. Green-top Guideline No. 30. London: RCOG; 2007.

129. Public Health England. *Varicella: The Green Book, Chapter 34*. London: Public Health England; 2012. Available at: https://www.gov.uk/government/publications/varicella-the-green-book-chapter-34.

130. Royal College of Obstetricians and Gynaecologists (RCOG). *Chickenpox in Pregnancy*. Green-top Guideline No. 13. London: ROCG; 2007.

131. World Health Organization. Hepatitis B. Fact sheet. Updated July 2016. Available at: http://www.who.int/mediacentre/factsheets/fs204/en/.

132. GBD 2013 Mortality and Causes of Death Collaborators. Global, regional, and national age–sex specific all-cause and cause-specific mortality for 240 causes of death, 1990–2013: a systematic analysis for the Global Burden of Disease Study 2013. *Lancet* 2015;**385**:117–71.

133. Forton D, Gess M. Hepatitis B in maternal medicine and infections. In: Arulkumaran S, Regan L, Papageorghiou A, Monga A, Farquharson D (eds), *Oxford Desk Reference Obstetrics and Gynaecology*, pp. 238–41. Oxford: Oxford University Press; 2011.

134. Di Bisceglie AM. Hepatitis C. *Lancet* 1998;**351**:351–55.

135. Center for Disease Control and Prevention. Recommendations for prevention and control of hepatitis c virus (HCV) infection and HCV-related chronic disease. *MMWR Recomm Rep* 1998;**47**:1–39.

136. Pembrey L, Newell ML, Tovo PA. Antenatal hepatitis C virus screening and management of infected women and their children: policies in Europe. *Eur J Pediatr* 1999;**158**:842–46.

137. European Paediatric Hepatitis C Virus Network. A significant sex—but not elective cesarean section—effect on mother-to-child transmission of hepatitis C virus infection. *JID* 2005;**192**:1872–79.

138. Bull L, Khan AW, Barton S. Management of HIV infection in pregnancy. *Obstet Gynaecol Reprod Med* 2015;**25, 10**:273–78.

139. World Health Organization. 10 facts on HIV/AIDS. Updated November 2016. Available at: http://www.who.int/features/factfiles/hiv/en/.

140. Lack N. HIV in pregnancy. In: Bhide A, Divakar H, Arulkumaran S (eds), *Handbook of Obstetrics and Gynaecology for Asia and Oceania*, pp. 216–20. New Delhi: Jaypee Brothers Medical Publishers (P) Ltd; 2016.

141. Joynson DH. Epidemiology of toxoplasmosis in the UK. *Scand J Infect Dis Suppl* 1992;**84**:65–69.

142. Thulliez P. Maternal and fetal infection. In: Joynson DHM, Wreghitt TG (eds), *Toxoplasmosis: A Comprehensive Clinical Guide*, pp. 193–213. Cambridge: Cambridge University Press; 2001.

143. Desmonts G, Couvreur J. Congenital toxoplasmosis. Prospective study of the outcome of pregnancy in 542 women with toxoplasmosis acquired during pregnancy. *Ann Pediatr (Paris)* 1984;**31**:805–809.

144. Antsaklis A, Daskalakis G, Papantoniou N, Mentis A, Michalas S. Prenatal diagnosis of congenital toxoplasmosis. *Prenat Diagn* 2002;**22**:1107–11.

145. Foulon W, Pinon JM, Stray-Pedersen B, et al. Prenatal diagnosis of congenital toxoplasmosis: a multicenter evaluation of different diagnostic parameters. *Am J Obstet Gynecol* 1999;**181**:843–47.

146. Wong SY, Remington JS. Biology of Toxoplasma gondii. *AIDS* 1993;**7**:299–316.

147. McCabe RE. Antitoxoplasma chemotherapy. In: Joynson DHM, Wreghitt TG (eds), *Toxoplasmosis: A Comprehensive Clinical Guide*, pp. 319–59. Cambridge: Cambridge University Press; 2001.

18

Psychiatric disorders in pregnancy and the postpartum

Arianna Di Florio and Ian Jones

Introduction

Psychiatric disorders in pregnancy and the postpartum period are common and have an impact not only on the health of the mother, but also on the well-being of her offspring. A 2015 report has estimated that the cost of perinatal psychiatric disorders in the United Kingdom is approximately 8.1 billion GBP for each year's birth cohort (1), with the majority of costs due to the consequences of maternal illness on the child. Despite their importance, maternal psychiatric disorders are underdiagnosed and undertreated.

In this chapter, we provide a concise introduction to perinatal psychiatric disorders and emphasize the role of prevention, early detection, and collaborative care. We are aware that the term perinatal is not used in exactly the same way in different contexts. We here use it to indicate pregnancy and the first few months after childbirth. Although the perinatal and postpartum specifier in the American Psychiatric Association *Diagnostic and Statistical Manual of Mental Disorders*, fifth edition (DSM-5) (2) and the World Health Organization International Classification of Diseases, tenth edition (ICD-10) (3) respectively cover the first 4 and 6 weeks after delivery, in clinical practice it is common to extend the postpartum period to 6 months after childbirth or even up to 1 year. Indeed, the United Kingdom National Institute for Health and Care Excellence (NICE) 'Antenatal and Postnatal Mental Health: Clinical Management and Service Guidance' defined the postpartum period as up to 1 year after childbirth (4).

We discuss both disorders with first onset in the perinatal period and the course and management of women with pre-existing illness. We discuss the presentation, epidemiology, risk factors, prognosis, and management of a range of common mental disorders, such as depression and anxiety, and less prevalent, but more severe disorders, such as postpartum psychosis, bipolar disorder, and schizophrenia. We then briefly overview other important conditions that can have a significant impact at this time, namely substance misuse, eating disorders, and personality disorders. A final section will consider the impact of perinatal mental illness and its treatment on the fetus and child. In three separate boxes we present information relevant to all disorders, including hormone sensitivity, suicide and violence, and general principles of care.

Common mental disorders

Depression

Major depression is the leading cause of disability worldwide (5) and common during pregnancy and in the postpartum period. The nosological status of depressive episodes associated with reproductive events is controversial (6). The American Psychiatric Association (2) and the World Health Organization (3) in their classification systems currently do not consider them as separate disorders but rather subtypes of major depression.

Epidemiology

The point-prevalence of major depression during pregnancy and postpartum varies widely across studies and countries, ranging from 0% to over 30% (7–10). Although cultural differences may play a role, it is likely that methodological heterogeneity and, in particular, differences in the assessment of depression are likely to contribute to the large variability observed.

Evidence on whether pregnancy is protective and the postpartum period is a high-risk period for depression is also inconsistent. According to a Danish registry-based study, the relative risk of being admitted to hospital for major depression for the first time is halved during pregnancy, but more than doubled in the first 2 months after childbirth compared to 1 year postpartum (11). This research, however, considered only first-onset cases. In a retrospective study on 546 women with recurrent major depression, over 35% of the 1189 pregnancies followed by live births were affected by a postpartum depressive episode, while depression during pregnancy was less frequent (12). A prospective study in the United States, however, has questioned the temporal association between childbirth and depression and estimated that one-third of postpartum depressive episodes begin in pregnancy and an additional 27% prior to conception (13).

Established risk factors for postpartum depression are a history of depression or anxiety, recent stressful life events, poor social support, and domestic violence (reviewed in (14)). A recent systematic review identified similar risk factors for depression during pregnancy (poor social support; adverse life events; domestic violence;

history of mental illness; unplanned or unwanted pregnancy; present/past pregnancy complications, including miscarriage) (15).

Clinical presentation

The symptomatology is similar to that of non-childbearing depression (6, 16). The validity of somatic symptoms of depression (i.e. fatigue, loss of libido, appetite, and weight and sleep changes) in the perinatal period has, however, been debated, because they overlap with the normal physical experience of pregnancy and childbirth (8). It has been described that intrusive violent thoughts and psychosis are more common in women with postpartum-onset than in those with pregnancy-onset depression (17). In a United States national survey, 30% of women who screened positive for postpartum depression endorsed thoughts of self-harm (13). Suicide in pregnancy and postpartum is a rare event, but represent a major, neglected, cause of maternal mortality (**Box 18.1**). The same study found that the majority (65.7%) of women with postpartum depression had comorbid anxiety disorders including generalized anxiety disorder and obsessive–compulsive disorder.

Screening

A study in the United Kingdom has estimated that about 50% of cases of maternal depression go undetected with high costs for the woman, the child, and the entire society (1). Given the high prevalence and the detrimental consequences of untreated perinatal depression, universal screening of perinatal women has been advocated in many countries worldwide, most recently in the United States by the US Preventative Services Task Force (18).

Self-reported measures of depression, specifically designed to identify women who need further clinical assessment in the postpartum period, include the Bromley Postnatal Depression Scale, the Edinburgh Postnatal Depression Scale, and the Postpartum Depression Screening Scale. NICE (4) recommends that healthcare professionals in contact with women in the perinatal period (including midwives, obstetricians, health visitors, and general practitioners) should ask two questions to identify possible depression (Whooley questions), at the woman's first contact with primary care, at her booking visit, and postpartum (first year after childbirth):

- During the past month, have you often been bothered by feeling down, depressed, or hopeless?
- During the past month, have you often been bothered by having little interest or pleasure in doing things?

If there is a positive answer to either question, or a high risk of developing a mental health problem, or clinical concern, the clinician should consider using the Edinburgh Postnatal Depression Scale or the Patient Health Questionnaire as part of a full assessment or referring the woman to her family physician or, if a severe mental health problem is suspected, to a mental health professional. Although formal screening programmes for maternal depression remain controversial, what is not in doubt is that all health professionals who come into contact with women in pregnancy or following childbirth should be aware of her mental health in addition to her physical well-being.

Differential diagnosis

'Organic' disorders, such as thyroid dysfunction, anaemia, or substance abuse, should always be ruled out. Postpartum major depression needs to be distinguished from minor mood disorders, such as postpartum blues, and from postpartum psychosis (discussed in detail in a later section). Postpartum blues is common and characterized by transient emotional liability during the first week after birth that does not impair the care of the baby. It is self-limiting, but assessment should ensure that the woman is not and does not become more severely depressed.

Clinicians need to be aware that postpartum depression can be a manifestation of a bipolar disorder. One study found that over 50% of cases of bipolar postpartum depression were initially misdiagnosed as unipolar disorder by clinicians (19) and a further study found that over 20% of women who screen positive for postpartum depression had bipolar disorder (13). The differential diagnosis between bipolar and unipolar depression is important, as the treatment of bipolar episodes with antidepressants may be associated with the risk of a manic switch, rapid cycling, and treatment resistance (19). The use of tools designed to detect manic symptomatology such as the Mood Disorder Questionnaire, the Hypomania Checklist-32, or the Highs Scale can help the clinician in the identification of hypomanic symptoms (19). Episodes of psychotic depression in the immediate postpartum period should raise the possibility of an underlying bipolar diathesis, even in the absence of manic symptoms (20).

Treatment

The proportion of women taking antidepressants during pregnancy has increased in recent decades but varies widely with studies finding rates of around 3% in Denmark (21) to over 13% in the United States (22).

A longitudinal study in the United States on 201 euthymic pregnant women taking antidepressants found that 68% of those who discontinued the treatment had a relapse during pregnancy compared with 26% of those who maintained it (23). Another study, however, of 778 pregnant women with a history of major depression found that staying on or stopping antidepressant treatment had little influence on

---

Box 18.1 Suicide, violence, and perinatal mental health

According to recent estimates, women with postpartum psychiatric disorders have an over 80-fold increased risk of violent death and are about 290 times more likely to commit suicide in the first year postpartum compared to mothers without mental disorders. Over 40% of women with postpartum mental disorders who die in the first year after giving birth, die of suicide, homicide, or accident (94).

Estimates of perinatal (defined as 1 year preconception, in pregnancy, and 1 year after childbirth) intimate partner violence vary considerably, from less than 1% to over 80% (41), with higher prevalence in women with low socioeconomic status and in those with perinatal mental disorders, including anxiety, depression, and PTSD (95). The majority of the current evidence is based on findings for high-income countries, but it is likely that the cultural context influences the prevalence and risk factors of perinatal psychiatric disorders associated with domestic violence (95).

Untreated postpartum severe disorders are associated with an increased risk of both suicide (94, 96) and infanticide (97). According to the Eighth Report of the Confidential Enquiries into Maternal Deaths in the United Kingdom, a substantial proportion of women who committed suicide following postpartum psychosis were misdiagnosed by clinicians as suffering from anxiety, moderate depression, or adjustment disorder and did not receive adequate treatment (51). Similarly, a retrospective study on 45 filicidal mothers found that two out of three women were initially erroneously diagnosed as having unipolar depression (58).

psychiatric outcome (24). It is likely that differences in the nature of the depressive histories in the two groups of women account for these conflicting findings. The first study was in women treated in a specialist mood disorder service who are likely to have a severe unipolar depression. The latter study, in contrast, was of women recruited in a community maternity setting with consequently less severe mood disorder histories. The different results from these studies emphasize the need to individualize decisions based on the particular woman's history.

If a pregnant woman is taking an antidepressant, NICE (4) recommends to discuss the therapeutic options with her and to choose the treatment approach according to the level of severity of the symptomatology, the previous psychiatric history, the stage of the pregnancy, and her preferences (4).

For new-onset moderate or severe episodes, NICE (4) recommends either a high-intensity psychological intervention or antidepressant medications, according to the woman's preferences and psychiatric history. If there is no or only a limited response to the high-intensity psychological intervention or medication alone, a combination of the two is recommended.

There is little specific evidence for the pharmacological management of postpartum depression and for evaluating the comparative harms and benefit of specific antidepressants (25). Research comparing psychological intervention to pharmacological treatments is also lacking. Decisions must therefore be made on the basis of evidence for the efficacy of approaches accumulated in the non-perinatal context. Women requiring psychological treatment should be seen for treatment quickly, ideally within 1 month of initial assessment (26). There are many psychological approaches that have been shown to be effective in the perinatal period. A Cochrane meta-analysis of ten trials of psychological and psychosocial interventions concluded that peer support and nondirective counselling, cognitive behavioural therapy, psychodynamic psychotherapy, and interpersonal therapy are all effective in postpartum depression (27). In addition, the Scottish Intercollegiate Guidelines Network (SIGN) suggests specific interventions directed to the improvement of the mother–baby relationship are offered, if this is impaired (28).

Similarly to pregnancy, in breastfeeding women the risk–benefit balance of pharmacological therapy is altered, and antidepressant therapy should be considered if the woman expressed a preference for medication, or she declines psychological interventions or they are not available, or her symptoms have not responded to psychological interventions (4), or are severe. As with all drugs taken during breastfeeding, the infant should be monitored regularly for sedation, irritability, and any alteration in sleep, feeding, or growth pattern.

As new data on medication safety in pregnancy and during lactation are emerging regularly, up-to-date advice from specialist services may be useful in individual cases.

Emerging therapies proposed for perinatal depression include oestrogens and progestins (**Box 18.2**), omega-3 fatty acids, such as eicosapentaenoic acid and docosahexaenoic acid, exercise, and integrated yoga. Evidence of effectiveness is, however, based on small studies or is inconsistent (28–31).

Prognosis

Data on prognosis are difficult to interpret, because of the heterogeneous methodologies and definitions used. Episodes of postpartum depression last 3–6 months on average, but about 30% of women remain depressed beyond the first postpartum year (8). Having a

---

Box 18.2 Gonadal steroid sensitivity and mood disorders

The exact pathophysiology of perinatal mood disorders is not known, especially for non-psychotic postpartum depression. It is likely to be complex and multifactorial. Although not all perinatal episodes may be aetiologically linked to the biological changes observed in the perinatal period (6), the onset of mood disorders in relation to the dramatic changes in neuroendocrine function seen in pregnancy and immediately after delivery have generated interest in the role of gonadal steroids in affective dysregulation.

It is increasingly recognized that ovarian sex steroids have important functions in the central nervous system. Oestrogen and progesterone receptors are widespread in the brain, where they modulate neurotransmission and neuroplasticity via both genomic and non-genomic mechanisms and regulate not only maternal behaviour, but also emotion processing, arousal, cognition, and motivation (98–101). Gonadal steroids have been implicated in a number of neuropsychiatric illnesses, including migraine, neurodegenerative disorders, and premenstrual dysphoric disorders (101, 102).

The brain is a steroidogenic organ able to synthetize pregnane neurosteroids, either *de novo* or from peripherally derived sources. Some progesterone metabolites, including allopregnanolone, are potent stereoselective, positive allosteric modulators of the gamma-aminobutyric acid type A (GABA-A) receptor and may be involved in the susceptibility to affective dysregulation (101, 103).

Studies investigating the role of gonadal steroids in perinatal mood disorders have mainly focused on non-psychotic depression. It has been suggested that the hormonal trigger of postpartum depression is characterized by an abnormal response to normal concentrations of gonadal steroids, rather than abnormal basal hormone levels. In a milestone experiment, euthymic women with a history of postpartum depression and a group of matched controls underwent a hormone manipulation protocol that simulated the changes in oestradiol and progesterone observed during pregnancy and immediately after delivery (104). The protocol consisted of three phases: (1) endogenous hormone suppression with a gonadotropin-releasing hormone agonist, (2) an 8-week add-back phase with supraphysiological doses of oestradiol and progesterone, and (3) withdraw of both steroids under double-blind conditions. While controls were not affected by the manipulation protocol, five out of eight women with a history of postpartum depression developed significant mood symptoms. Interestingly, although symptoms were more severe during the hormone withdrawal phase, significant depressive symptoms started to develop during the add-back phase simulating the hormone conditions of pregnancy (104).

Research into the role of gonadal steroids in the pathogenesis of perinatal mood disorders is still in very early stages and its clinical implications are unclear. A Cochrane review on oestrogens and progestins for preventing and treating postpartum depression has suggested that synthetic progestins should be used with significant caution in the postpartum period and that oestrogen therapy may be of modest value and should not be part of routine management (29).

A recent randomised, controlled, phase 3 trial has reported some promising findings for brexanolone, an analog of allopregnanolone, for the treatment of postpartum depression (PMID: 30177236). The place of brexanolone in the treatment of postpartum depression is still considered emerging and further research is warranted (PMID: 31241747, PMID: 31255297, PMID: 31255300).

---

depressive episode in relation to childbirth increases the risk of subsequent depressive episodes, with recurrence rates around 40% for both perinatal and non-perinatal episodes (32).

Anxiety disorders

Perinatal anxiety disorders are often overlooked (4, 8), commonly occurring in association with other psychiatric conditions, especially depression (13, 33, 34). Prevalence rates of anxiety disorders in studies ranges widely from 6% to 39% in pregnancy (35) and from

16% to 50% in the postpartum period (36). There is inconsistent evidence of a specific link between the perinatal period and anxiety disorders, with the exception of obsessive–compulsive disorder (8, 35). According to a meta-analysis, both pregnant and postpartum women have an increased risk of developing obsessive–compulsive disorder (risk ratios 1.45 and 2.38 respectively) (37). While some obsessional thinking is common in pregnancy and following childbirth, some women are much more significantly affected with thoughts concerning contamination or aggression against the child that can lead to compulsive behaviours such as cleaning, avoidance of the child, or excessive checking on the child's well-being. Although causing significant distress to women, these aggressive thoughts are not acted on and only in a small proportion of cases lead to significant distress and functional impairment. Clinical episodes of obsessive–compulsive disorder in the perinatal period are much less common than obsessional symptoms, affecting about 2.5% of women (37). Obsessions need to be distinguished from delusions that may pose a risk to the baby. Delusions are strongly held false beliefs that persist even when there is evidence that the beliefs are not true or logical. Obsessions are intrusive, reoccurring thoughts or urges, or mental images that cause anxiety and distress. However, the distinction between delusions and obsessions is not always clear-cut and can be a diagnostic challenge.

Randomized controlled trials for the treatment of anxiety disorders in the perinatal period are lacking and even non-controlled, naturalistic study evidence is also scarce (8). The treatment of perinatal anxiety disorders largely relies on information on the treatment in the wider population. It is, however, not clear whether and to what extent psychosocial and psychological interventions need to be modified to be effective in the perinatal period (8). Mind–body interventions have been increasingly popular, but strong, rigorous evidence to support their effectiveness for the management of anxiety during pregnancy or postpartum is lacking (38).

Post-traumatic stress disorder

Perinatal post-traumatic stress disorder (PTSD) is not very well studied and recognized, with the majority of studies concerning symptoms occurring after miscarriage, termination, stillbirth (39), or traumatic birth (40). In case of perinatal loss, gestational age is positively associated with the likelihood for PTSD (39). The prevalence of perinatal PTSD is estimated at around 1–8% (8, 41), with a higher prevalence in low-income countries compared to high-income countries and showing a high comorbidity with major depression, anxiety, alcohol or illicit drugs use, and suicidality (8, 42). PTSD is highly prevalent (40% according to a recent study (41)) among low-income pregnant women exposed to intimate partner violence in pregnancy and following childbirth.

Little research has been conducted on the management of perinatal PTDS, especially in women with a preconception history of trauma. However, what is clearer is that a recent Cochrane systematic review found little or no evidence to support psychological debriefing for women who perceive giving birth as psychologically traumatic (43).

Severe mental illness

Although not as common as those conditions considered earlier, severe mental illnesses have a significant impact in the perinatal period. Severe postpartum episodes can be a recurrence of an existing mental illness, such as bipolar disorder or schizophrenia, or in around 50% of cases, the first episode of psychiatric illness. Just as with common mental disorders, the use of diagnostic labels such as postpartum psychosis for severe episodes of illness is controversial and confused. In this section, we discuss the management in the perinatal period of women with pre-existing, recurrent bipolar disorder and schizophrenia and the diagnosis and treatment of severe episodes of affective psychosis with onset in the immediate postpartum. While for many women with a postpartum episode of bipolar disorder it is the first time they have been unwell, schizophrenia at this time is usually the continuation of a pre-existing condition (11, 44).

Postpartum psychosis

The term 'puerperal' or 'postpartum psychosis' is commonly used in clinical practice and research for a heterogeneous group of psychiatric episodes with onset in the immediate postpartum period (in 90% of cases within 2 weeks after delivery) (45). The word 'psychosis' in this context can, however, be confusing (46). In the majority of cases, the symptomatology and prognosis resemble that of an affective disorder rather than that of schizophrenia. Patients usually present with severe manic, depressive, or mixed symptoms. Positive psychotic symptoms such as delusions and hallucinations, confusion, and perplexity are also common. Some women may present with the typical symptoms of the so-called polymorphic/cycloid psychosis (47). In other cases, however, the term 'postpartum psychosis' is used to describe manic or mixed episodes without psychotic symptoms. In the assessment of women with significant psychiatric symptoms with onset in the immediate postpartum, one evaluation is usually not enough, as the picture fluctuates over time, can escalate rapidly, and severity is sometimes difficult to recognize (48, 49).

The debate on the validity and nosology of postpartum psychosis, especially in relation to bipolar disorder, is ongoing. The current classification systems DSM-5 and ICD-10 do not recognize postpartum psychosis as a separate nosological entity. However, some authors have maintained that there are several advantages in adopting a separate diagnosis of puerperal psychosis for both research and clinical practice (50).

Differential diagnosis

The Eighth Report of the Confidential Enquiries into Maternal Deaths in the United Kingdom has underscored that a number of maternal deaths are due to the misattribution of psychotic symptoms to postpartum psychosis rather than to 'organic' disorders (51). Several 'organic' disorders can cause psychosis: infections; pre-eclampsia and eclampsia (52); autoimmune (53), metabolic (54–56) and para-neoplastic disorders; encephalitis and cerebral vascular diseases (57); and syndromes associated with substance abuse and withdrawal.

On the other hand, the tendency to label all psychiatric perinatal episodes as 'postpartum depression' can lead to the wrong management and to an underestimation of the risk of suicide and infanticide, sometimes with dramatic consequences (51, 58).

Epidemiology

Although postpartum psychosis can be considered a rare disorder (50), certainly when compared to postpartum mood disorders more generally, it can have a potentially fatal impact and is therefore important to identify and manage. Studies based on hospital admission have estimated an incidence of 1–2 per 1000 deliveries (11). This estimate, however, does not account for women treated as outpatients and will also include women admitted for other reasons than an episode that could be labelled as postpartum psychosis.

The specific link between childbirth and the triggering of manic/affective psychosis is well established (11, 12, 44, 50, 59, 60). The relative risk of having a first lifetime manic episode in the first month postpartum is over 23 times higher than 1 year after childbirth (11). Even if a woman without a previous psychiatric history is admitted for another psychiatric disorder, a first admission within the first month after childbirth increases by four times the likelihood of developing bipolar disorder within 15 years compared to any first psychiatric admission outside the childbearing period (59).

For the majority of women affected (two in three according to a retrospective study), postpartum psychosis represents the first psychiatric episode (61). In this group without a psychiatric history, postpartum psychosis is very difficult to predict (61). There are, however, risk factors that have been associated with postpartum psychosis. Women with a history of bipolar disorder have a one in five chance of a delivery affected (12); a previous episode of postpartum psychosis confers an even higher risk, around one in two (62). A family history of postpartum psychosis has also been identified as a risk factor (63), although molecular genetic studies have yet to fulfil their promise (64). Although several factors associated with pregnancy and delivery have been explored, the only robust risk factor identified is primiparity (65, 66). The association between primiparity and postpartum psychosis is not a mere reflection of the fact that women with a history of postpartum psychosis tend not to have further pregnancies and it has been hypothesized that it may be due to the biological differences between first and subsequent pregnancies (66). Research, in fact, has failed to demonstrate an association between psychosocial factors and postpartum psychosis (67, 68). A particularly intriguing hypothesis is that postpartum psychosis may be underpinned by immune dysregulation. This hypothesis is based on the observation of a marked increase in the rates of postpartum autoimmune thyroiditis and immune biomarkers alterations in women with postpartum psychosis (69). It has also been hypothesized that there is an aetiological link between postpartum psychosis and eclampsia. Eclampsia and postpartum psychosis in fact share the association with primiparity and are both inversely correlated with tobacco smoking (70).

Treatment

In the majority of cases, postpartum psychosis is the first contact with psychiatric services in women without apparent risk factors (61). A prompt diagnosis and treatment are therefore paramount. Postpartum psychosis is a psychiatric emergency. Admission is necessary in the majority of cases, even when the family is supportive (48). NICE recommends the admission of the mother with the baby to specialized mother and baby units; however, these are not always available. There is accumulating evidence that mother and baby units not only are preferred by the women (71), but also lead to better outcomes and shorter durations of admission (64).

Postpartum psychosis requires pharmacological treatment. However, there are no randomized controlled trials specifically addressing postpartum psychosis. A recent clinical study conducted in the Netherlands followed up for 9 months women with postpartum psychosis to evaluate the efficacy of an empirical treatment algorithm consisting sequentially of (a) benzodiazepines, then (b) benzodiazepines and antipsychotics, then (c) benzodiazepines, antipsychotics, and lithium. With adherence to this stepped regimen, they observed a complete remission of the symptomatology in more than 98% and 80% of women maintained the remission for the entire period of observation. In addition, significantly higher relapse rates were seen in women treated with an antipsychotic only compared to those treated with lithium only (plasma concentrations 0.6–0.8 mmol/L) (72).

Severe psychotic symptoms in pregnancy, catatonia, lack of response to pharmacological treatment, and suicidality are among the most common indications for electroconvulsive therapy (64). Although there are no randomized controlled trials for electroconvulsive therapy in the perinatal period, the evidence of effectiveness is promising (73). The possible side effects (anterograde amnesia (18%) and prolonged seizures (11%) according to a recent study (74)) need to be evaluated against (a) the efficacy in cases resistant to pharmacotherapy; (b) the rapidity of treatment action and its impact on the lives of the mother and the baby; and (c) the lack of side effects of drugs on the mother and, in case of breastfeeding, on the baby.

A referral to social services should not be made routinely and should be supported by a careful risk–benefit evaluation (64) (see 'Schizophrenia').

One study has suggested that women with a history of isolated postpartum psychosis (without bipolar episodes outside the puerperium) may be at lower risk for a recurrence in pregnancy than women who also have experienced non-postpartum episodes of illness. The risk of recurrence after childbirth, however, is elevated in this group and women should consider starting prophylactic pharmacotherapy immediately after delivery (62).

Prognosis

If promptly identified and treated the prognosis is good, with over 95% of patients achieving remission within 1 year (72). The median duration of illness is considerably shorter for women treated with pharmacotherapy (40 days) (72) than for those without (8 months) (75). If misdiagnosed or untreated, postpartum psychosis is one of the major risk factors for suicide after childbirth and in tragic but rare circumstances may also be linked with infanticide (Box 18.3).

In a retrospective study on 116 women with postpartum psychosis, only 58% of women had a further pregnancy (61). Recurrence rates are around 50% for further postpartum episodes and between 50% and 70% for bipolar recurrences outside the puerperium (76, 77).

Postpartum psychosis has a negative impact on the life of the woman, with one study reporting 18% of marriages ending after the severe postpartum episode (61). The stigma affecting all mental disorders is in this case accompanied by that of being a 'bad mother' and by feelings of guilt for the consequences of the illness on the baby (71).

Bipolar disorder

As we have discussed, over 50% of episodes of postpartum psychosis are the first episode of illness, but there is strong evidence of a specific relationship to bipolar disorder.

Clinical presentation and epidemiology

Over 70% of mothers with bipolar disorder have suffered at least one episode of mood disorder in the perinatal period, and over one in four have experienced an episode of postpartum psychosis (12). Although the emphasis for women with bipolar disorder has always been on psychotic/manic episodes, a large retrospective study on 1212 women with bipolar disorder found that non-psychotic depression is the most common mood episode in the perinatal period (12). It does appear, however, that there is a closer relationship between childbirth and episodes of mania and psychosis. Over 90% of manic/psychotic episodes occur within the first 4 weeks after childbirth, while one depressive episode in four has its onset later in the postpartum period, after the first month (12).

The association between childbearing and bipolar disorder is specific for delivery and for manic/psychotic episodes. The risk of manic/psychotic episodes is significantly lower after miscarriage or termination than after delivery whereas depressive episodes are equally common following each of these pregnancy outcomes (60). The high risk of recurrence after delivery does not seem merely related to the discontinuation of medications during pregnancy, as recurrences are three times more frequent postpartum when lithium (a first-line treatment for bipolar disorder) is discontinued due to pregnancy than when the woman stops taking it for other reasons (70% vs 24%) (78).

Treatment

The pharmacological treatment of bipolar disorder during pregnancy often requires difficult decisions and needs to be evaluated in light of the high risk of recurrence and the negative impact that the illness may have on the fetus (4, 48, 64). The discontinuation of lithium during pregnancy, especially if abrupt, doubles the risk of a recurrence (79). A women's psychiatric history can help individualize these decisions. A longitudinal study found that not one of

29 women with a history of postpartum psychosis with no episodes outside the perinatal period had a recurrence during a subsequent pregnancy, while 10 of 41 women with a history of bipolar disorder outside the puerperium had a recurrence during pregnancy, with a risk doubled in those without mood-stabilizing therapy (19% vs 40%) (62).

Similar to postpartum psychosis, there is a lack of randomized controlled trials on the treatment of postpartum bipolar depression. A naturalistic study on 34 women with postpartum bipolar depression initially misdiagnosed as unipolar showed that the discontinuation of antidepressants and the introduction of a mood-stabilizing therapy improved symptoms in 88% of cases (19).

Psychological interventions and psychoeducation should always be considered, even if specific evidence for these approaches in the perinatal period is lacking (64).

Schizophrenia

Schizophrenia is a chronic, highly disabling, and severe mental disorder that affects about 1% of the general population. Symptoms usually start in early adulthood and are commonly grouped in three categories: positive (hallucinations, delusions, thought and movement disorders), negative (blunted expression of emotions, anhedonia, difficulty beginning and sustaining activities, reduced speaking), and cognitive (poor executive functioning and working memory, trouble focusing or paying attention).

Although women with schizophrenia may have lower fertility, with the development of newer antipsychotic medications that impact less on prolactin levels, more women with this disorder are becoming mothers (64). The close relationship of episodes of illness following childbirth observed in bipolar disorder is not found for schizophrenia, a marked distinction between the two disorders (11, 44). Women with schizophrenia may, however, require hospital admission to monitor and facilitate the mother–baby relationship, even in the absence of a severe symptomatic recurrence (81).

There is a paucity of evidence on the management of schizophrenia in the perinatal period. A preliminary study found that a collaboration between services and the women's partner in the care of the baby leads to an improvement in the symptomatology (82). Although women with schizophrenia may successfully parent, many do have difficulties. Indeed, studies have shown that the diagnosis of schizophrenia, together with that of personality disorders and substance abuse or dependence, are associated with an increased risk of involvement of social services (64). The loss of custody of a child represents a severe threat and a traumatic event (71) that can precipitate a crisis and a worsening clinical picture. According to the Eighth Report of the Confidential Enquiries into Maternal Deaths in the United Kingdom, 31% of mothers who committed suicide during pregnancy had been referred to social services (83). The fear of losing custody can also have a negative impact on the patient–doctor relationship and may induce the woman to deny the symptoms in the hope of maintaining the maternal role (71, 84). Although schizophrenia is associated with problems with the maternal role and a 25-fold increased risk of social service supervision compared to psychotic depression, women with schizophrenia are not necessarily unable to fulfil the maternal role (64). Among the factors that should be considered in assessing the potential for successful parenting are (valid also for other psychiatric disorder) (a) psychotic symptoms involving the baby or passivity experiences; (b) the partner's psychiatric history, and (c) the social context, including intimate partner violence and abuse (64).

Other disorders

Personality disorders

Personality disorders are difficult to define and diagnose but can cause significant difficulties in pregnancy and the postpartum period. According to the American Psychiatric Association, they are characterized by 'an enduring pattern of inner experience and behaviour that deviates markedly from the expectations of the culture of the individual who exhibits it' (83). There is a paucity of evidence on the impact of personality disorders in the perinatal period. According to a Scandinavian survey, the prevalence of personality disorders in pregnancy, assessed by self-report, is about 6% (85). Personality disorders often occur in comorbidity with other disorders and are associated with poor prognosis (8, 85).

Eating disorders

Although eating disorders may be associated with fertility problems (86), a clinical study has estimated the prevalence of some form of eating disorders during pregnancy at around 7.5%, compared to 9.2% prior to pregnancy (87). Some women symptomatically improve in pregnancy. A Norwegian survey reported remission rates between 29% and 78%, depending on the specific eating disorder (88). Over half of women with a history of a prepregnancy eating disorder have a continuation or recurrence in the postpartum (8). The continued presence of eating disorder symptoms increases the risk of postpartum depression compared to women whose symptoms remit (8). Apart from binge-eating disorder, the incidence of other eating disorders in pregnancy is rare (8).

Substance abuse and dependence

The United States 2012 National Survey on Drug Use and Health estimated that 9.0% of pregnant women aged 18–25 and 3.4% of those aged 26–44 use illicit drugs (including cannabis, stimulants, cocaine, heroin, hallucinogens, and inhalants) or misuse prescription-type drugs. These estimates are roughly half the rates observed in non-pregnant women in the same age group (89).

There are significant barriers to care for pregnant women with substance use disorders (89). Universal antenatal screening with validated questionnaires has been advocated and should be preferred to urine drug testing, that does not identify women with significant, but sporadic, use and may prevent women to seek prenatal care (89). Perinatal women with substance use disorders require intensive and multidisciplinary care. They often present comorbidity with other medical and psychiatric disorders and environmental stressors that need to be addressed. A harm reduction approach, aimed to extend periods of abstinence while recognizing the likelihood of relapse, should be adopted (89).

Opioid use in pregnancy is an increasing concern, with rates raised from 0.1% in 2000 to 0.6% in 2009 in the United States. Opioid-containing pain medications are ten times more commonly used than heroin during pregnancy (89). Opioid replacement therapy has specific benefits for pregnant women, including the prevention of intoxication and withdrawal and the mitigations of the negative effects on fetal growth and length of gestation. Significant constipation is a common side effect of all opioids, including replacement therapy, and should be enquired about and addressed by clinicians (89).

The impact of perinatal mental illness on the baby

It is difficult to disentangle the effects of maternal mental disorders on the fetus and child from the effects of genetic contribution, medications, poor parenting, and lifestyle, including smoking, poverty, poor nutrition, and substance use.

Depression during pregnancy is associated with an increased risk of premature delivery, while evidence for birth weight is equivocal (90). Maternal perinatal depression has been associated with emotional dysregulation, impaired social skills, internalizing and externalizing disorders, attachment problems, and increased risk of depression during adolescence (90). It has been hypothesized that the mechanisms underpinning the association between depression in the offspring and maternal antenatal and postnatal depression are different (91). There is little or inconsistent evidence for an effect of perinatal depression on cognitive development (90).

There is a paucity of studies investigating the effects of other mental disorders and evidence is often inconsistent. A study conducted on multiparae admitted to mother and baby units found that the risk of psychiatric disorders in adulthood was higher in offspring of puerperal episodes (34%) compared to their siblings from unaffected pregnancies (15%) (92).

The study of the effect of alcohol and illicit substances during pregnancy on the fetus is complicated by the use of multiple substances, comorbidity with other psychiatric disorders, and the association with disadvantaged socioeconomic status. Teratogenic effects include intrauterine death, dysmorphism, growth restrictions, and behavioural changes (93).

Conclusion

Obstetricians will frequently be involved in the care of women with the new onset or recurrence of a psychiatric illness. There are significant barriers to care for women with psychiatric disorders in the perinatal period. Universal screening for the most prevalent disorders, depression and anxiety, but also for eating disorders and substance abuse has been advocated but remains controversial. What is not in doubt, however, is that a woman's mental health is as important as her physical health in pregnancy and all healthcare professionals should be making an assessment of her mental health at each contact. Women with chronic and recurrent psychiatric disorders require monitoring, increased contact, and multidisciplinary, coordinated care, including a specific mental health management plan. Women with psychiatric disorders often present with significant medical comorbidities and environmental stressors that both need to be addressed. Care should be provided in a non-judgemental, compassionate way, and involve, if the woman agrees, her partner and wider family.

REFERENCES

1. Bauer A, Parsonage M, Knapp M, Iemmi V, Adelaja B. *Costs of Perinatal Mental Health Problems*. London: London School of Economics and the Centre for Mental Health; 2014.

2. American Psychiatric Association. *Diagnostic and Statistical Manual of Mental Disorders, Fifth Edition*. Arlington, VA: American Psychiatric Association; 2013.

3. World Health Organization. *ICD-10: The ICD-10 Classification of Mental and Behavioural Disorders: Clinical Descriptions and Diagnostic Guidelines*. Geneva: World Health Organization; 1992.

4. National Institute for Health and Care Excellence (NICE). *Antenatal and Postnatal Mental Health: Clinical Management and Service Guidance*. Clinical guideline [CG192]. London: NICE; 2014. Available at: http://www.nice.org.uk/guidance/cg192 (accessed 19 March 2015).

5. Whiteford HA, Degenhardt L, Rehm J, et al. Global burden of disease attributable to mental and substance use disorders: findings from the Global Burden of Disease Study 2010. *Lancet* 2013;**382**:1575–86.

6. Di Florio A, Meltzer-Brody S. Is postpartum depression a distinct disorder? *Curr Psychiatry Rep* 2015;**17**:76.

7. Halbreich U, Karkun S. Cross-cultural and social diversity of prevalence of postpartum depression and depressive symptoms. *J Affect Disord* 2006;**91**:97–111.

8. Howard LM, Molyneaux E, Dennis CL, Rochat T, Stein A, Milgrom J. Non-psychotic mental disorders in the perinatal period. *Lancet* 2014;**384**:1775–88.

9. Gavin NI, Gaynes BN, Lohr KN, Meltzer-Brody S, Gartlehner G, Swinson T. Perinatal depression: a systematic review of prevalence and incidence. *Obstet Gynecol* 2005;**106**:1071–83.

10. Fisher J, Cabral de Mello M, Patel V, et al. Prevalence and determinants of common perinatal mental disorders in women in low- and lower-middle-income countries: a systematic review. *Bull World Health Organ* 2012;**90**:139H–49H.

11. Munk-Olsen T, Laursen TM, Pedersen CB, Mors O, Mortensen PB. New parents and mental disorders. *JAMA* 2006;**296**:2582–89.

12. Di Florio A, Forty L, Gordon-Smith K, et al. Perinatal episodes across the mood disorder spectrum. *JAMA Psychiatry* 2013;**70**:168–75.

13. Wisner KL, Sit DK, McShea MC, et al. Onset timing, thoughts of self-harm, and diagnoses in postpartum women with screen-positive depression findings. *JAMA Psychiatry* 2013;**70**:490–98.

14. Di Florio A, Jones I. Postpartum depression. *BMJ Best Practice*. Last updated February 2019. Available at: http://bestpractice.bmj.com/best-practice/monograph/512/resources/credits.html.

15. Biaggi A, Conroy S, Pawlby S, Pariante CM. Identifying the women at risk of antenatal anxiety and depression: a systematic review. *J Affect Disord* 2016;**191**:62–77.

16. Cooper C, Jones L, Dunn E, et al. Clinical presentation of postnatal and non-postnatal depressive episodes. *Psychol Med* 2007;**37**:1273–80.

17. Altemus M, Neeb CC, Davis A, Occhiogrosso M, Nguyen T, Bleiberg KL. Phenotypic differences between pregnancy-onset and postpartum-onset major depressive disorder. *J Clin Psychiatry* 2012;**73**:e1485–91.

18. O'Connor E, Rossom RC, Henninger M, Groom HC, Burda BU. Primary care screening for and treatment of depression in pregnant and postpartum women: Evidence report and systematic review for the US preventive services task force. *JAMA* 2016;**315**:388–406.

19. Sharma V, Khan M. Identification of bipolar disorder in women with postpartum depression. *Bipolar Disord* 2010;**12**:335–40.

20. Bergink V, Koorengevel KM. Postpartum depression with psychotic features. *Am J Psychiatry* 2010;**167**:476–77.

21. Munk-Olsen T, Gasse C, Laursen TM. Prevalence of antidepressant use and contacts with psychiatrists and psychologists in pregnant and postpartum women. *Acta Psychiatr Scand* 2012;**125**:318–24.

22. Cooper WO, Willy ME, Pont SJ, Ray WA. Increasing use of antidepressants in pregnancy. *Am J Obstet Gynecol* 2007;**196**:544.e1–5.

23. Cohen LS, Altshuler LL, Harlow BL, et al. Relapse of major depression during pregnancy in women who maintain or discontinue antidepressant treatment. *JAMA* 2006;**295**:499–507.

24. Yonkers KA, Gotman N, Smith MV, et al. Does antidepressant use attenuate the risk of a major depressive episode in pregnancy? *Epidemiology* 2011;**22**:848–54.

25. Molyneaux E, Howard LM, McGeown HR, Karia AM, Trevillion K. Antidepressant treatment for postnatal depression. *Cochrane Database Syst Rev* 2014;**9**:CD002018.

26. Musters C, McDonald E, Jones I. Management of postnatal depression. *BMJ* 2008;**337**:a736.

27. Dennis CL, Dowswell T. Psychosocial and psychological interventions for preventing postpartum depression. *Cochrane Database Syst Rev* 2013;**2**:CD001134.

28. Scottish Intercollegiate Guidelines Network (SIGN). *Management of Perinatal Mood Disorders*. SIGN 127. Edinburgh: SIGN; 2012. Available at: https://www.sign.ac.uk/sign-127-management-of-perinatal-mood-disorders.html (accessed 14 April 2016).

29. Dennis CL, Ross LE, Herxheimer A. Oestrogens and progestins for preventing and treating postpartum depression. *Cochrane Database Syst Rev* 2008;**4**:CD001690.

30. Gong H, Ni C, Shen X, Wu T, Jiang C. Yoga for prenatal depression: a systematic review and meta-analysis. *BMC Psychiatry* 2015;**15**:14.

31. Miller BJ, Murray L, Beckmann MM, Kent T, Macfarlane B. Dietary supplements for preventing postnatal depression. *Cochrane Database Syst Rev* 2013;**10**:CD009104.

32. Cooper PJ, Murray L. Course and recurrence of postnatal depression. Evidence for the specificity of the diagnostic concept. *Br J Psychiatry* 1995;**166**:191–95.

33. Navarro P, García-Esteve L, Ascaso C, Aguado J, Gelabert E, Martín-Santos R. Non-psychotic psychiatric disorders after childbirth: prevalence and comorbidity in a community sample. *J Affect Disord* 2008;**109**:171–76.

34. Matthey S, Barnett B, Howie P, Kavanagh DJ. Diagnosing postpartum depression in mothers and fathers: whatever happened to anxiety? *J Affect Disord* 2003;**74**:139–47.

35. Goodman JH, Chenausky KL, Freeman MP. Anxiety disorders during pregnancy: a systematic review. *J Clin Psychiatry* 2014;**75**:e1153–84.

36. Marchesi C, Ossola P, Amerio A, et al. Clinical management of perinatal anxiety disorders: a systematic review. *J Affect Disord* 2016;**190**:543–50.

37. Russell EJ, Fawcett JM, Mazmanian D. Risk of obsessive-compulsive disorder in pregnant and postpartum women: a meta-analysis. *J Clin Psychiatry* **74**:377–85.

38. Marc I, Toureche N, Ernst E, et al. Mind-body interventions during pregnancy for preventing or treating women's anxiety. *Cochrane Database Syst Rev* 2011;**7**:CD007559.

39. Daugirdaitė V, van den Akker O, Purewal S. Posttraumatic stress and posttraumatic stress disorder after termination of

pregnancy and reproductive loss: a systematic review. *J Pregnancy* 2015;**2015**:646345.

40. James S. Women's experiences of symptoms of posttraumatic stress disorder (PTSD) after traumatic childbirth: a review and critical appraisal. *Arch Womens Ment Health* 2015;**18**:761–71.

41. Kastello JC, Jacobsen KH, Gaffney KF, Kodadek MP, Bullock LC, Sharps PW. Posttraumatic stress disorder among low-income women exposed to perinatal intimate partner violence: posttraumatic stress disorder among women exposed to partner violence. *Arch Womens Ment Health* 2016;**19**:521–28.

42. Smith MV, Poschman K, Cavaleri MA, Howell HB, Yonkers KA. Symptoms of posttraumatic stress disorder in a community sample of low-income pregnant women. *Am J Psychiatry* 2006;**163**:881–84.

43. Bastos MH, Furuta M, Small R, McKenzie-McHarg K, Bick D. Debriefing interventions for the prevention of psychological trauma in women following childbirth. *Cochrane Database Syst Rev* 2015;**4**:CD007194.

44. Munk-Olsen T, Laursen TM, Mendelson T, Pedersen CB, Mors O, Mortensen PB. Risks and predictors of readmission for a mental disorder during the postpartum period. *Arch Gen Psychiatry* 2009;**66**:189–95.

45. Heron J, McGuinness M, Blackmore ER, Craddock N, Jones I. Early postpartum symptoms in puerperal psychosis. *BJOG* 2008;**115**:348–53.

46. Sharma V, Sommerdyk C. Postpartum psychosis: what is in a name? *Aust N Z J Psychiatry* 2014;**48**:1081–82.

47. Pfuhlmann B, Stöber G, Franzek E, Beckmann H. Cycloid psychoses predominate in severe postpartum psychiatric disorders. *J Affect Disord* 1998;**50**:125–34.

48. Di Florio A, Smith S, Jones I. Postpartum psychosis. *Obstet Gynecol* 2013;**15**:145–50.

49. Jones I, Craddock N. Bipolar disorder and childbirth: the importance of recognising risk. *Br J Psychiatry* 2005;**186**:453–54.

50. Di Florio A, Munk-Olsen T, Bergink V. The birth of a psychiatric orphan disorder: postpartum psychosis. *Lancet Psychiatry* 2016;**3**:502.

51. Cantwell R, Clutton-Brock T, Cooper G, et al. Saving Mothers' Lives: Reviewing maternal deaths to make motherhood safer: 2006–2008. The Eighth Report of the Confidential Enquiries into Maternal Deaths in the United Kingdom. *BJOG* 2011;**118** Suppl 1:1–203.

52. Brockington IF. Eclamptic psychosis. In: *Eileithyia's Mischief: the Organic Psychoses of Pregnancy, Parturition and the Puerperium*, pp. 117–77. Bredenbury: Eyry Press; 2006.

53. Bergink V, Kushner SA, Pop V, et al. Prevalence of autoimmune thyroid dysfunction in postpartum psychosis. *Br J Psychiatry* 2011;**198**:264–68.

54. Patil NJ, Yadav SS, Gokhale YA, Padwa N. Primary hypoparathyroidism: psychosis in postpartum period. *J Assoc Physicians India* 2010;**58**:506–508.

55. Fassier T, Guffon N, Acquaviva C, D'Amato T, Durand DV, Domenech P. Misdiagnosed postpartum psychosis revealing a late-onset urea cycle disorder. *Am J Psychiatry* 2011;**168**:576–80.

56. Häberle J, Vilaseca MA, Meli C, et al. First manifestation of citrullinemia type I as differential diagnosis to postpartum psychosis in the puerperal period. *Eur J Obstet Gynecol Reprod Biol* 2010;**149**:228–29.

57. Brockington IF. Cerebral vascular disease as a cause of postpartum psychosis. *Arch Womens Ment Health* 2007;**10**:177–78.

58. Kim JH, Choi SS, Ha K. A closer look at depression in mothers who kill their children: is it unipolar or bipolar depression? *J Clin Psychiatry* 2008;**69**:1625–31.

59. Munk-Olsen T, Laursen TM, Meltzer-Brody S, Mortensen PB, Jones I. Psychiatric disorders with postpartum onset: possible early manifestations of bipolar affective disorders. *Arch Gen Psychiatry* 2012;**69**:428–34.

60. Di Florio A, Jones L, Forty L, Gordon-Smith K, Craddock N, Jones I. Bipolar disorder, miscarriage, and termination. *Bipolar Disord* **17**:102–105.

61. Blackmore ER, Rubinow DR, O'Connor TG, et al. Reproductive outcomes and risk of subsequent illness in women diagnosed with postpartum psychosis. *Bipolar Disord* 2013;**15**:394–404.

62. Bergink V, Bouvy PF, Vervoort JS, Koorengevel KM, Steegers EA, Kushner SA. Prevention of postpartum psychosis and mania in women at high risk. *Am J Psychiatry* 2012;**169**:609–15.

63. Jones I, Craddock N. Familiality of the puerperal trigger in bipolar disorder: results of a family study. *Am J Psychiatry* 2001;**158**:913–17.

64. Jones I, Chandra PS, Dazzan P, Howard LM. Bipolar disorder, affective psychosis, and schizophrenia in pregnancy and the postpartum period. *Lancet* 2014;**384**:1789–99.

65. Munk-Olsen T, Jones I, Laursen TM. Birth order and postpartum psychiatric disorders. *Bipolar Disord* 2014;**16**:300–307.

66. Di Florio A, Jones L, Forty L, et al. Mood disorders and parity—a clue to the aetiology of the postpartum trigger. *J Affect Disord* 2014;**152–54**:334–39.

67. Brockington IF, Martin C, Brown GW, Goldberg D, Margison F. Stress and puerperal psychosis. *Br J Psychiatry* 1990;**157**:331–34.

68. Dowlatshahi D, Paykel ES. Life events and social stress in puerperal psychoses: absence of effect. *Psychol Med* 1990;**20**:655–62.

69. Bergink V, Gibney SM, Drexhage HA. Autoimmunity, inflammation, and psychosis: a search for peripheral markers. *Biol Psychiatry* 2014;**75**:324–31.

70. Di Florio A, Morgan H, Jones L, et al. Smoking and postpartum psychosis. *Bipolar Disord* 2015;**17**:572–73.

71. Dolman C, Jones I, Howard LM. Pre-conception to parenting: a systematic review and meta-synthesis of the qualitative literature on motherhood for women with severe mental illness. *Arch Womens Ment Health* 2013;**16**:173–96.

72. Bergink V, Burgerhout KM, Koorengevel KM, et al. Treatment of psychosis and mania in the postpartum period. *Am J Psychiatry* 2015;**172**:115–23.

73. Focht A, Kellner CH. Electroconvulsive therapy (ECT) in the treatment of postpartum psychosis. *J ECT* 2012;**28**:31–33.

74. Babu GN, Thippeswamy H, Chandra PS. Use of electroconvulsive therapy (ECT) in postpartum psychosis—a naturalistic prospective study. *Arch Womens Ment Health* 2013;**16**:247–51.

75. Protheroe C. Puerperal psychoses: a long term study 1927–1961. *Br J Psychiatry* 1969;**115**:9–30.

76. Chaudron LH, Pies RW. The relationship between postpartum psychosis and bipolar disorder: a review. *J Clin Psychiatry* 2003;**64**:1284–92.

77. Robertson E, Jones I, Haque S, Holder R, Craddock N. Risk of puerperal and non-puerperal recurrence of illness following bipolar affective puerperal (post-partum) psychosis. *Br J Psychiatry* 2005;**186**:258–59.

78. Viguera AC, Nonacs R, Cohen LS, Tondo L, Murray A, Baldessarini RJ. Risk of recurrence of bipolar disorder in pregnant and nonpregnant women after discontinuing lithium maintenance. *Am J Psychiatry* 2000;**157**:179–84.

79. Viguera AC, Whitfield T, Baldessarini RJ, et al. Risk of recurrence in women with bipolar disorder during pregnancy: prospective study of mood stabilizer discontinuation. *Am J Psychiatry* 2007;**164**:1817–24.

80. Benedetti F, Riccaboni R, Locatelli C, Poletti S, Dallaspezia S, Colombo C. Rapid treatment response of suicidal symptoms to lithium, sleep deprivation, and light therapy (chronotherapeutics) in drug-resistant bipolar depression. *J Clin Psychiatry* 2014;**75**:133–40.

81. Jones I, Heron J, Blackmore ER, Craddock N. Incidence of hospitalization for postpartum psychotic and bipolar episodes. *Arch Gen Psychiatry* 2008;**65**:356.

82. Nishizawa O, Sakumoto K, Hiramatsu KI, Kondo T. Effectiveness of comprehensive supports for schizophrenic women during pregnancy and puerperium: preliminary study. *Psychiatry Clin Neurosci* 2007;**61**:665–71.

83. American Psychiatric Association. *Diagnostic and Statistical Manual of Mental Disorders: DSM-IV-TR.* Washington, DC: American Psychiatric Association; 2000.

84. Boots Family Trust. Perinatal Mental Health: Experiences of Women and Health Professionals. 2013. Available at: https://www.tommys.org/sites/default/files/Perinatal_Mental_Health_Experiences%20of%20women.pdf.

85. Börjesson K, Ruppert S, Bågedahl-Strindlund M. A longitudinal study of psychiatric symptoms in primiparous women: relation to personality disorders and sociodemographic factors. *Arch Womens Ment Health* 2005;**8**:232–42.

86. Easter A, Treasure J, Micali N. Fertility and prenatal attitudes towards pregnancy in women with eating disorders: results from the Avon Longitudinal Study of Parents and Children. *BJOG* 2011;**118**:1491–98.

87. Easter A, Bye A, Taborelli E, et al. Recognising the symptoms: how common are eating disorders in pregnancy? *Eur Eat Disord Rev* 2013;**21**:340–44.

88. Bulik CM, Von Holle A, Hamer R, et al. Patterns of remission, continuation and incidence of broadly defined eating disorders during early pregnancy in the Norwegian Mother and Child Cohort Study (MoBa). *Psychol Med* 2007;**37**:1109–18.

89. Gopman S. Prenatal and postpartum care of women with substance use disorders. *Obstet Gynecol Clin North Am* **41**:213–28.

90. Stein A, Pearson RM, Goodman SH, et al. Effects of perinatal mental disorders on the fetus and child. *Lancet* 2014;**384**:1800–19.

91. Pearson RM, Evans J, Kounali D, et al. Maternal depression during pregnancy and the postnatal period: risks and possible mechanisms for offspring depression at age 18 years. *JAMA Psychiatry* 2013;**70**:1312–19.

92. Abbott R, Dunn VJ, Robling SA, Paykel ES. Long-term outcome of offspring after maternal severe puerperal disorder. *Acta Psychiatr Scand* 2004;**110**:365–73.

93. Holbrook BD, Rayburn WF. Teratogenic risks from exposure to illicit drugs. *Obstet Gynecol Clin North Am* 2014;**41**:229–39.

94. Johannsen BM, Larsen JT, Laursen TM, Bergink V, Meltzer-Brody S, Munk-Olsen T. All-cause mortality in women with severe postpartum psychiatric disorders. *Am J Psychiatry* 2016;**173**:635–42.

95. Howard LM, Oram S, Galley H, Trevillion K, Feder G. Domestic violence and perinatal mental disorders: a systematic review and meta-analysis. *PLoS Med* 2013;**10**:e1001452.

96. Khalifeh H, Hunt IM, Appleby L, Howard LM. Suicide in perinatal and non-perinatal women in contact with psychiatric services: 15 year findings from a UK national inquiry. *Lancet Psychiatry* 2016;**3**:233–42.

97. Spinelli MG. Postpartum psychosis: detection of risk and management. *Am J Psychiatry* 2009;**166**:405–408.

98. Arevalo MA, Azcoitia I, Garcia-Segura LM. The neuroprotective actions of oestradiol and oestrogen receptors. *Nat Rev Neurosci* 2015;**16**:17–29.

99. Jensik PJ, Arbogast LA. Differential and interactive effects of ligand-bound progesterone receptor A and B isoforms on tyrosine hydroxylase promoter activity. *J Neuroendocrinol* 2011;**23**:915–25.

100. Zlotnik A, Gruenbaum BF, Mohar B, et al. The effects of estrogen and progesterone on blood glutamate levels: evidence from changes of blood glutamate levels during the menstrual cycle in women. *Biol Reprod* 2011;**84**:581–86.

101. Belelli D, Lambert JJ. Neurosteroids: endogenous regulators of the GABA(A) receptor. *Nat Rev Neurosci* 2005;**6**:565–75.

102. Rubinow DR, Schmidt PJ. Gonadal steroid regulation of mood: the lessons of premenstrual syndrome. *Front Neuroendocrinol* 2006;**27**:210–16.

103. Schiller CE, Schmidt PJ, Rubinow DR. Allopregnanolone as a mediator of affective switching in reproductive mood disorders. *Psychopharmacology (Berlin)* 2014;**231**:3557–67.

104. Bloch M, Schmidt PJ, Danaceau M, Murphy J, Nieman L, Rubinow DR. Effects of gonadal steroids in women with a history of postpartum depression. *Am J Psychiatry* 2000;**157**:924–30.

19

Fetal therapy

Caitriona Monaghan and Basky Thilaganathan

Introduction

Fetal therapy is defined as any prenatal treatment administered to the mother or fetus with the primary indication to improve perinatal or long-term outcomes for the fetus or newborn (1). The practice of fetal therapy is a relatively new concept in the field of obstetrics. It originated over 55 years ago when Liley et al. first performed intraperitoneal transfusion for the treatment of fetal anaemia. Since then, the practice has evolved from open fetal surgery to minimally invasive techniques used to manage an array of complex conditions.

As well as the clinical challenges of working with a small, mobile fetus, the concept of fetal therapy also evokes a number of ethical issues. These include balancing the benefit versus potential harm to the fetus, particularly in the setting of research where techniques have not yet proven to improve outcome. The majority of fetal therapies are associated with maternal consequences and as such it is extremely important to obtain fully informed consent when commencing treatment or performing surgery. Multiple pregnancies discordant for anomaly prove to be extremely challenging to manage as we face risking the health of one fetus to improve the outcome for another. More recently, the concept of fetal pain and ensuring adequate analgesia *in utero* has also been raised.

Fetal therapy now encompasses a wide range of techniques which can be broadly divided into five categories:

1. Transplacental therapy
2. Ultrasound-guided fetal therapy
3. Fetoscopic procedures
4. Open fetal surgery
5. Peripartum fetal therapy.

Transplacental therapy

Transplacental therapy is a non-invasive method of treating a fetal condition via maternal administration of a drug. The ideal transplacental agent is one which crosses the placenta unaltered to reach the fetus, deliver an appropriate dose of the drug to treat the underlying condition, with limited adverse effects on the mother. One of the first documented cases of transplacental therapy in the literature was described in 1975 when Ampola et al. successfully treated methylmalonic acidaemia in a fetus in the third trimester by administering large doses of vitamin B_{12} to the mother (2). Today, one of the most common indications for transplacental therapy is the administration of maternal corticosteroids to promote fetal lung maturity in the setting of threatened preterm labour. Transplacental therapy is also established in the management of fetal arrhythmias, congenital adrenal hyperplasia (CAH) and fetal alloimmune thrombocytopenia (FMAIT).

Fetal arrhythmias

Fetal arrhythmias affect approximately 2% of pregnancies and account for 10–20% of referrals to fetal cardiologists (3). Rhythm disturbances may be classified as irregular, tachy-, or bradyarrhythmia. The most prevalent fetal dysrhythmias are atrial extrasystoles. These are often found incidentally during routine fetal heart auscultation in the third trimester and tend to resolve spontaneously without intervention. Life-threatening rhythm disturbances in the fetus are rare; however, they are potentially treatable. In order to commence appropriate prenatal therapy, accurate diagnosis is essential. Clinical assessment involves fetal echocardiography to examine the fetal heart for any structural or functional defects. Conservative management is indicated in fetuses with intermittent arrhythmias who are haemodynamically stable. The decision between fetal therapy and birth will largely be based on gestational age (as a proxy for fetal lung maturity) and fetal well-being, including the presence of hydrops fetalis, as the latter are less likely to respond to transplacental antiarrhythmic therapy.

Tachyarrhythmias

Sustained fetal tachycardia at greater than 180 beats per minute (bpm) should prompt urgent referral. Structural congenital heart disease is reported in up to 5% of cases, including Ebstein's anomaly, coarctation of the aorta, and cardiac tumours (4). The most common fetal tachyarrhythmias are supraventricular tachycardia (SVT) and atrial flutter. Approximately 90% of fetal SVT is associated with an atrioventricular re-entry tachycardia caused by an accessory pathway between the atrium and ventricle. There is typically a 1:1 ratio of atrial to ventricular contractions and a fetal heart rate of approximately 220–240 bpm. Presently there is no consensus on first-line therapy for fetal SVT. In the absence of fetal hydrops,

Table 19.1 Common antiarrhythmic agents used in the management of fetal arrhythmias

Antiarrhythmic agent	Indication	Dose	Typical response time	Maternal side effects
Digoxin	SVT AF	1 mg once daily divided doses	1–2 weeks	Proarrhythmia, AV block, nausea, vomiting
Flecainide	SVT, VT	100–400 mg twice daily	48 hours	Proarrhythmia, vertigo, nausea, headache, disturbed vision, paraesthesia
Sotalol	SVT, AF, VT	80–160 mg twice daily	72 hours	Proarrhythmia

AF, atrial fibrillation; AV, atrioventricular; SVT, supraventricular tachycardia; VT, ventricular tachycardia.

sotalol, flecainide, and digoxin are the most commonly used drugs. Transplacental transfer of digoxin is significantly impaired in the presence of hydrops fetalis, where flecainide may be more effective than sotalol (5). Combination therapies may be used when first-line treatments have failed; however, this can increase the maternal side effect profile. Table 19.1 illustrates the common antiarrhythmic agents used in the management of fetal tachyarrhythmias.

Atrial flutter is sustained by a re-entrant pathway in the atrial wall resulting in atrial heart rates between 300 and 500 bpm. There is typically a 2:1 ratio of atrial to ventricular contractions resulting in a ventricular rate of 150–250 bpm. Atrial flutter accounts for 30% of cases of fetal tachycardia and tends to present at later gestations than fetal SVT (5). Digoxin and sotalol are typically the antiarrhythmics of choice with sotalol being the preferred agent in the presence of fetal hydrops. Once converted, maintenance therapy should be continued until after delivery. Postnatally, these neonates require careful monitoring as a significant proportion can relapse. Electro- and echocardiograms should be performed. Refractory or relapsing conditions may require interventions such as cardioversion, pacing, or alternative antiarrhythmic agents.

Bradyarrhythmias

A bradyarrhythmia is defined as a sustained fetal heart rate less than 100 bpm. This may be secondary to sinus bradycardia, blocked atrial ectopic beats, or complete heart block (CHB). CHB is caused by complete dissociation between atrial and ventricular contractions. The atrial rate is regular and normal; however, the ventricular rate is typically between 40 and 90 bpm. In 50% of cases there is associated complex congenital heart disease including left atrial isomerism and congenitally corrected transposition. This association with congenital heart disease carries a significant risk of mortality when hydrops fetalis is present. The predominant aetiology in fetuses with structurally normal hearts is the transplacental passage of maternal antibodies (anti-Ro and anti-La) after 16 weeks' gestation, resulting in damage to fetal cardiomyocytes and conduction tissue. CHB carries a significant mortality of 18–40% and satisfactory treatment is not well established (6). Therapy to date has been aimed at targeting the immune-mediated inflammatory process associated with CHB and treatment with maternal steroids, beta sympathomimetic agents, intravenous immunoglobulin (IVIG), and hydroxychloroquine have all been described. Data on the efficacy of maternal steroid therapy is conflicting. Dexamethasone is thought to be associated with a reduction in maternal autoantibody load but is not directly protective of the fetal myocardium. In 2011, a large retrospective multicentre study examined the outcomes of 175 cases of isolated CHB. Fluorinated corticosteroid therapy was used in 38% of affected cases; however, this had no significant effect

on perinatal mortality or the development of late cardiomyopathy (7). Postnatally, neonates with congenital CHB require immediate cardiac assessment and the vast majority will require a pacemaker.

Congenital adrenal hyperplasia

CAH describes a group of inherited disorders in which enzyme deficiencies result in impaired cortisol biosynthesis. The incidence in Great Britain is approximately 1 in 18,000 live births (8). More than 90% of cases of CAH are caused by a deficiency of 21-hydroxylase resulting in an overproduction of adrenal androgens as well as impaired cortisol production. Exposure to excess androgens *in utero* results in the virilization of the external genitalia of affected female fetuses, a hallmark of this condition. Phenotype can vary depending on the severity of enzyme deficiency. Postnatally these infants often require genitoplasty and have long-term physical and psychological complications. Since 1984, prenatal dexamethasone has been proposed as a therapy to prevent virilization of the external genitalia of affected female fetuses following a case series published by David and Forest (9). Dexamethasone is thought to cross the placenta unaltered and suppress the fetal hypothalamic–pituitary axis, resulting in decreased androgen production; however, its exact mode of action is debated. Despite more than 30 years since the first published case series, and the established clinical effectiveness of transplacental therapy, prenatal treatment of CAH remains a controversial issue. Virilization of the external genitalia occurs between 6 and 8 weeks' gestation, therefore prophylactic treatment needs to be initiated before the sixth week and continued until cell free DNA can determine the fetal gender. However, seven out of eight at-risk fetuses will be unaffected by this condition and exposed to unnecessary high-dose glucocorticoids during early fetal development. Several observational studies have suggested that this exposure *in utero* may negatively impact the child's physical and neuropsychological development (10). In order to evaluate the efficacy and safety of prenatal CAH treatment, a prospective long-term follow-up study (PREDEX) is underway in Europe.

Fetal alloimmune thrombocytopenia

FMAIT results from the production of maternal alloantibodies directed against paternally inherited human platelet antigens (HPAs) located on fetal platelet membrane glycoproteins. It is the leading cause of severe thrombocytopenia in the newborn, affecting approximately 1 in 1500 pregnancies (11). Approximately 85% of cases in Caucasians are caused by antibodies to HPA-1a (12). Immunoglobulin G antibodies cross the placenta and bind to fetal platelets. The antibody-coated platelets are removed from the fetal circulation via the reticuloendothelial system resulting in fetal thrombocytopenia. Despite a similar pathophysiology to haemolytic disease of the fetus and newborn, approximately 50% of cases occur in the first pregnancy. Clinical manifestations of this condition can vary in severity, the most severe complication, intracranial haemorrhage (ICH), arises in 7–26% of untreated cases (13). ICH is associated with a perinatal mortality rate of 1–7% and severe neurological sequelae such as cerebral palsy, cortical blindness, and seizures have been described in 16–26% of those who survive (13).

Presently there is no universal antenatal screening for FMAIT, and it is typically diagnosed on clinical manifestations of fetal haemorrhage. Laboratory diagnosis can be used to confirm the presence of platelet antibodies in the maternal circulation and to perform HPA genotyping. As with haemolytic disease, the familial recurrence rate is dependent on the paternal genotype. Families with homozygous dominant fathers have almost 100% recurrence rate. Given that the severity of clinical manifestations may increase with subsequent pregnancies, it is imperative to perform these investigations for accurate prenatal counselling. In heterozygous affected pregnancies, non-invasive fetal genotyping from maternal blood can now be performed to help guide management. The antenatal management of this condition remains contentious, as its evolution over the last 25 years has been largely based on case series. The main aim of treatment is to prevent fetal thrombocytopenia with the use of IVIG therapy, immunosuppression with corticosteroids, or serial intrauterine platelet transfusions.

IVIG has previously been used to treat autoimmune conditions such as idiopathic thrombocytopenic purpura, but its exact mechanism of action remains unclear. Due to a lack of prospective randomized controlled trials, there is conflicting evidence in the literature with regard to its efficacy in the prevention of ICH. Most centres typically give 0.5–1 g/kg intravenously to the mother on a weekly basis from 16 weeks' gestation. IVIG therapy is expensive and can be associated with side effects such as renal dysfunction, transmission of blood-borne diseases, febrile reactions, and severe headaches. As a result of the cost and associated adversities, some centres stratify IVIG treatment regimens according to the presence or absence of ICH in the previously affected child. Corticosteroids can be administered alongside IVIG therapy, with prednisolone being the corticosteroid of choice. In 2011, a Cochrane review of the antenatal interventions for FMAIT found that IVIG in combination with prednisolone was more effective than IVIG alone at raising the fetal platelet count in high-risk pregnancies (14). Serial intrauterine platelet transfusions have previously been used in the prenatal management of FMAIT. They are associated with a significant risk of fetal loss and for this reason remain second-line therapy for the prevention of ICH associated with this condition.

Ultrasound-guided fetal therapy

Some of the first ultrasound images of the fetus were published in *The Lancet* by Donald et al. in 1958 (15). Over the last 60 years, technological advances have included real-time imaging, colour and power Doppler, transvaginal sonography, and three/four-dimensional imaging. Ultrasound-guided techniques including intrauterine blood transfusion (IUT), direct fetal pharmacological therapy, radiofrequency ablation (RFA), interstitial laser therapy (ILT), selective fetal reduction, and shunting procedures constitute an essential part of fetal therapy.

Intrauterine blood transfusion

Rodeck et al. described the technique of intravascular IUT into the umbilical cord under fetoscopic guidance (16). Despite widespread use of anti-D immunoglobulin, IUT under ultrasound guidance remains the definitive treatment for fetal anaemia secondary to red cell alloimmunization. It has also been described in the management of fetal anaemia secondary to non-immune conditions such as parvovirus, twin-to-twin transfusion syndrome (TTTS), fetomaternal haemorrhage, and placental chorioangioma. Invasive techniques such as amniocentesis and fetal blood sampling were previously used to diagnose fetal anaemia *in utero*. These procedures, however, carry an increased risk of miscarriage, preterm labour, and fetal loss. Today, measurement of the peak systolic velocity in the middle cerebral artery is the standard non-invasive screening technique for fetal anaemia (17). When performing IUT, access to the fetal circulation is via the umbilical cord typically at the placental cord insertion site (Figure 19.1 and ● Video 19.1). The umbilical vein is chosen preferentially as it has a wider diameter and is also less likely to spasm than the umbilical artery. Under circumstances where the umbilical vein is inaccessible (e.g. posterior placenta or advanced gestation), the intrahepatic portion of the umbilical vein or a free loop of umbilical cord may be used as an alternative. Intravascular transfusion into a free-floating loop of umbilical cord is associated with an increased risk of displacement, cord tamponade, and higher fetal loss rate (18). Prior to 20 weeks' gestation, the intraperitoneal route remains the method of choice, where the donor red cells are absorbed into the fetal circulation via the lymphatic system. The intracardiac route via the apex of the left ventricle has also been described in the literature (19). This technique, however, is associated with an increased risk of cardiac tamponade and fetal arrhythmias.

The need for serial IUTs is dependent on the gestation of the first procedure and the severity of fetal anaemia. Monitoring via the middle cerebral artery peak systolic velocity may guide the need for a repeat procedure. This would typically be performed 2–3 weeks following the first transfusion. The interval following the second transfusion is more predictable, however, as the red cells in the fetal circulation are almost exclusively adult and therefore fetal erythropoiesis is suppressed. The fall in the haematocrit is 1% per day due to plasma expansion and fetal growth rather than haemolysis. The

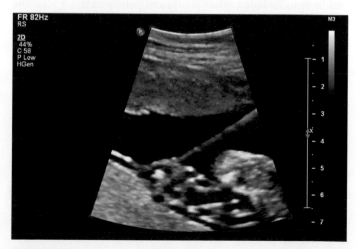

Figure 19.1 Intrauterine transfusion.

interval between the second and third procedure is typically 3–4 weeks. Given the associated risks with this procedure, delivery rather than repeat IUT after 35 weeks is the preferred management strategy. Despite survival rates of greater than 90%, IUT has associated procedure-related complications including fetomaternal haemorrhage, fetal heart rate abnormalities, chorioamnionitis, cord accidents, volume overload, preterm prelabour rupture of membranes (PPROM), and preterm labour. Procedure-related fetal loss rates vary in the literature from 0.9% to 4.9% per procedure and are associated with hydrops, severity of anaemia, early gestational age, transfusion into a free loop of umbilical cord, and the experience of the operator (20). Following delivery, these neonates tend to require more top-up transfusions in the first 6 months of life. Small fetomaternal haemorrhages which occur at the time of IUT, particularly during transplacental puncture, may cause increased sensitization in the current and future pregnancies.

Direct fetal pharmacological therapy

In cases of failed transplacental therapy for the treatment of fetal arrhythmias, direct fetal therapy has been described. This is largely indicated as a measure of last resort in cases of very preterm or hydropic fetuses in which delivery would be inappropriate. Direct therapy may be achieved by intravenous (IV) infusion of an antiarrhythmic drug into the umbilical vein. The technique for performing this procedure would be similar to that for IUT. More rarely, fetal intramuscular (IM) injection may be undertaken under ultrasound guidance. Infusion of digoxin, amiodarone, verapamil, and adenosine via IV or IM routes have all been described in the literature (21, 22).

Radiofrequency ablation

RFA occurs when radiofrequency waves passed through tissue cause an increase in tissue temperature. The application of percutaneous RFA in obstetrics has been reported mostly in the management of twin reversed arterial perfusion (TRAP) sequence and sacrococcygeal teratoma (SCT). TRAP sequence is a rare complication exclusive to monochorionic twin pregnancy in which one twin (acardiac) with varying degree of anomalous cardiac structure is dependent on the circulation of the normal (pump) fetus (23). Placental anastomoses allow blood to flow from the umbilical artery of the healthy pump twin in a reversed direction into the umbilical artery of the acardiac fetus. The clinical consequences for the healthy fetus include cardiac failure and polyhydramnios resulting in preterm delivery. If untreated mortality rates as high as 55% have been reported (24). Previous treatment options have incorporated cord occlusion of the acardiac twin and amniodrainage. Over the last decade, ablative therapies such as RFA have been used to interrupt the vascularization of the acardiac twin.

Fetal SCT is a rare neoplasm, which complicates approximately 1–2 per 20,000 pregnancies (25). Due to improved antenatal detection, the frequency of diagnosis is increasing. Perinatal mortality rates of prenatally diagnosed SCTs range from 25% to 37% (26). Fetuses with solid, rapidly enlarging, highly vascularized teratomas can develop high-output cardiac failure and non-immune hydrops via vascular shunting. Observational studies have determined that SCTs associated with cardiac failure and fetal hydrops have a mortality rate which approaches 100%. If cardiac failure occurs following viability, early delivery, possibly with *ex utero* intrapartum treatment (EXIT)

and postnatal surgery, may be the best management strategy. Prior to viability, therapeutic techniques including open fetal surgical resection and percutaneous coagulation such as RFA to decrease vascular shunting have rarely been described.

RFA is typically carried out under maternal anxiolysis and local anaesthesia. The ablation system is a monopolar device and therefore grounding pads are applied to the maternal skin to complete the circuit. The needle electrode is inserted percutaneously under ultrasound guidance, for example, in TRAP sequence this would typically be adjacent to the umbilical cord insertion of the acardiac twin. Colour Doppler ultrasound can be used during the procedure to demonstrate cessation of flow within the umbilical artery or the vascular supply to the teratoma. An ultrasound scan should be performed 12–24 hours following the procedure to ensure cessation of blood flow. The most common postprocedure complication is PPROM. Cabassa et al. performed a systematic review of twin pregnancies complicated by TRAP sequence managed with RFA. In 78 pregnancies there was an 85% neonatal survival rate with 22% of the treated pregnancies complicated by PPROM and two reports of maternal thermal injury (23). In hydropic SCT fetuses undergoing interstitial laser or RFA, survival was found to be 45% with the major associated complications being PPROM and associated preterm delivery (26). Despite small numbers and in the absence of long-term outcomes, RFA appears to be a relatively safe and effective procedure in the management of twin pregnancies complicated by TRAP sequence and prenatal treatment of fetal SCT.

Interstitial laser therapy

ILT uses an image-guided needle to deliver laser energy into a tumour to heat and destroy the abnormal cells. ILT has been described in the management of fetal SCT and chorioangioma. Chorioangioma are vascular lesions present in approximately 1% of placentae. Giant chorioangiomas (>4 cm in diameter) have a prevalence of 1 in 9000 pregnancies and are associated with a range of fetal complications including anaemia, polyhydramnios, hyperdynamic heart strain, hydrops, growth restriction, and fetal demise in up to 30% of cases (27). Treatment options in early pregnancy include amniodrainage to alleviate polyhydramnios and IUT in the presence of fetal anaemia. These procedures provide symptomatic relief but do not treat the underlying cause. A variety of techniques including ILT have been proposed to ablate the vascular supply to the tumour. The 17–18 G ILT needle is positioned under ultrasound guidance and a 400–600-micron laser fibre is advanced a few millimetres from the tip of the needle into the target tissue (Figure 19.2a). Power is applied until the tissue close to the fibre becomes echogenic and the blood flow ceases (Figure 19.2b) (28). Zanardini et al. published the results of a retrospective analysis of 19 cases of pregnancy complicated by antenatally detected placental chorioangioma. Eighteen of the nineteen cases were associated with a fetal complication. ILT was performed in three cases under ultrasound guidance to devascularize the tumour and prevent the development of fetal hydrops and associated compromise. All three cases were associated with a successful pregnancy outcome (27). The advantages of ILT include the ability to perform this minimally invasive technique under local anaesthetic and that it is technically easier compared to endoscopic laser coagulation (27).

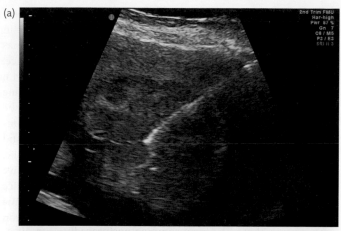

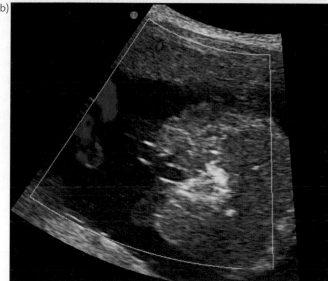

Figure 19.2 (a) Insertion of an 18 G ILT needle under ultrasound guidance into a giant placental chorioangioma. (b) Echogenic tissue adjacent to ILT laser fibre during treatment of the same placental chorioangioma as in (a).

Selective fetal reduction—dichorionic twin pregnancies

While the true incidence of structural anomalies in twin pregnancies is difficult to determine, approximately 2–3% of dizygotic twins are thought to be affected. This is similar to that of singleton pregnancies; however, the risk is increased two- to threefold in monozygotic pairs (29). Dichorionic twin pregnancies lack placental anastomoses and, as such, the passage of substances from one twin into the circulation of the co-twin is unlikely. Selective fetal reduction in dichorionic twin pregnancies that are discordant for anomaly can therefore be performed safely by injection of a drug that will induce asystole in the affected fetus. Injection of potassium chloride into the fetal heart or less frequently the umbilical vein under ultrasound guidance is an established technique. A key principle of this procedure is the importance of meticulous fetal labelling (30). This is particularly relevant in dichorionic pregnancies with concordant gender and minor abnormalities. Following a detailed ultrasound scan the affected fetus is identified. Using aseptic technique and ultrasound guidance, typically a 20–22 G needle is inserted through the maternal

abdomen into the left ventricle and if intracardiac access is not possible, the umbilical vein may be used. A retrospective analysis of 106 feticide procedures concluded that both intracardiac and umbilical routes may be used to achieve feticide effectively without compromising maternal safety (31). Fetal loss rates in the literature vary between 4% and 7% with preterm birth rates of 6% between 25 and 28 weeks' gestation and 22% before 33 weeks' gestation (32).

Fetal shunting procedures

In the early 1980s, several groups introduced the concept of ultrasound-guided fetal shunting procedures for a variety of conditions including fetal hydrocephalus, obstructive uropathy, and hydrothorax. Unfortunately, due to a lack of scientific evidence of therapeutic benefit these techniques have failed to become established fetal therapies.

Hydrocephalus

The improved neurological outcome following postnatal shunting of neonatal hydrocephalus generated significant enthusiasm for attempting prenatal therapy (33). Despite this initial enthusiasm, further studies failed to demonstrate an improvement in neurological outcome. The fetuses that underwent shunting procedures had in fact a poorer prognosis (34). This was thought to be secondary to underlying anomalies including migration disorders which could not be alleviated by shunting. Current clinical practice does not advocate the use of ventriculo-amniotic shunting for the management of fetal hydrocephalus.

Lower urinary tract obstruction

Lower urinary tract obstruction (LUTO) is a group of pathologies most commonly due to urethral atresia or posterior urethral valves which has an incidence of approximately 2.2 per 10,000 births (35). The clinical consequences of LUTO include renal dysplasia and dysfunction leading to oligohydramnios, pulmonary hypoplasia, and positional limb anomalies. Fetal LUTO without intervention is associated with a mortality rate of 45% (35). In those who survive, up to one-third develop end-stage renal impairment requiring dialysis or transplantation. Prenatal intervention was based on the belief that relieving the obstruction would potentially allow for normal lung development and prevent further renal damage. The technique of percutaneous vesicoamniotic shunting (VAS) involves the placement of a double pig-tailed catheter under ultrasound guidance and local anaesthesia, with the distal end of the catheter in the fetal bladder and the proximal end in the amniotic cavity. Amnioinfusion prior to shunt insertion in cases of severe oligohydramnios may facilitate the procedure.

A meta-analysis of prenatal bladder drainage in LUTO demonstrated that despite improvement in survival, neonates who were treated prenatally had significant long-term morbidities (36). Subsequently, the Percutaneous Shunting in Lower Urinary Tract Obstruction (PLUTO) trial was conducted. This multicentre randomized controlled trial to investigate the role of fetal VAS in moderate or severe LUTO has reported short-term outcomes (37). Survival to 28 days and 1 year of life appeared to be higher with VAS than conservative management, but not conclusively so. The prognosis for both groups in terms of renal function was poor and VAS was substantially more expensive and unlikely to be regarded as cost-effective based on the 1-year data (37).

Hydrothorax

Fetal hydrothorax may present as an isolated accumulation of lymphatic fluid in cases of primary fetal hydrothorax or in association with non-immune hydrops secondary to structural anomalies. Primary fetal hydrothorax is a relatively uncommon condition with a prevalence up to 1 in 15,000 pregnancies (38). Although some hydrothoraces will resolve spontaneously, progression predisposes to pulmonary hypoplasia, hydrops, polyhydramnios, and preterm delivery. Approximately 57% of fetuses present with primary fetal hydrothorax complicated by hydrops with anticipated survival of 24% without treatment (39). As a consequence of significant associated morbidity and mortality, intrauterine therapy may be offered depending on gestational age, the size of the pleural collection, and secondary effects including the presence of hydrops. The aim of prenatal therapy is to remove the fluid from the chest in order to relieve intrathoracic pressure and its effects on pulmonary development and cardiovascular function. Therapeutic interventions to date have included thoracocentesis, thoracoamniotic shunting, and more recently pleurodesis. In a systematic review of 278 cases of fetal hydrothorax managed with thoracoamniotic shunting, the reported overall survival was 63%, with a survival of 55% and 85% in hydropic and non-hydropic fetuses, respectively (40). The most common complications associated with the shunting procedure include PPROM, chorioamnionitis, and preterm delivery. Presently, there is no agreed consensus on the management of primary fetal hydrothorax. Most clinicians recommend that intervention should be reserved for hydropic fetuses, but a case may be made for those with large progressive effusions discovered at severe preterm gestations.

Fetoscopic procedures

The term fetoscopy is used to describe the endoscopic visualization of the fetus (41). Today, therapeutic fetoscopy has several indications including laser ablation for TTTS, selective reduction of monochorionic twin pregnancies, and endotracheal occlusion in the prenatal management of congenital diaphragmatic hernia (CDH).

Fetoscopic laser ablation for twin-to twin transfusion syndrome

TTTS arises in approximately 10% of monochorionic twin pregnancies between 16 and 26 weeks' gestation (42). This condition occurs in a previable period, the prognosis is therefore extremely poor and mortality approaches 90% without treatment. Sonographic diagnosis of TTTS is characterized by an amniotic fluid discordance, that is, polyhydramnios and a distended bladder in the volume-overloaded recipient and oligohydramnios and a small or empty bladder in the volume-depleted donor. The pathophysiology of this condition is thought to be secondary to an imbalance in blood flow across placental anastomoses. In 1999, Quintero et al. developed a staging classification system for TTTS after evaluating the prognostic value of sonographic and clinical parameters (43). The limitations of this staging system are associated with the fact that the disease evolution of TTTS is unpredictable. Prior to the introduction of fetoscopic laser coagulation, serial amnioreduction was the mainstay of treatment for TTTS. In 2004, a randomized controlled trial compared the safety and efficacy of endoscopic laser surgery to serial amnioreduction in the treatment of severe TTTS and demonstrated that the perinatal outcomes were significantly better in the laser group (44). The procedure is typically performed with maternal anxiolysis and local anaesthetic. Under ultrasound guidance, a trocar is advanced into the gestational sac of the recipient twin. Endoscopes with diameters of 1–3 mm are available and uterine distension with normal or physiological saline may occasionally be used to improve visualization. Laser photocoagulation of the communicating vessels is performed (**Figure 19.3** and ⊙Video 19.2) and surgery is completed following amniodrainage of the recipient's sac.

Several modifications of the laser technique including selective and sequential selective laser coagulation have been described since the original description of coagulation of all vessels crossing the inter-twin membrane. The Solomon technique involves coagulation of the entire vascular equator from one placental margin to the other, with the aim of reducing the number of residual anastomoses and hence the associated complications of twin anaemia–polycythaemia sequence, or recurrent TTTS. A subsequent trial reported that this method reduces associated postoperative fetal morbidity and recommended that fetoscopic surgeons consider incorporating this technique into their own practice (45). Although fetoscopic laser coagulation is a safe and effective procedure for the management of

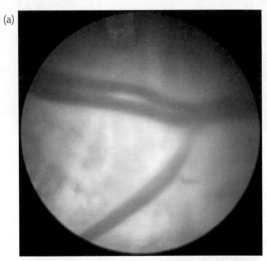

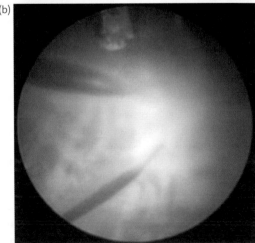

Figure 19.3 Vascular anastomoses during fetoscopic laser treatment of TTTS—(a) before and (b) after photocoagulation.

severe TTTS, it is associated with complications. The survival rates of both fetuses have improved significantly to approach over 70%. Significant complications relating to the procedure include iatrogenic PPROM, twin anaemia–polycythaemia sequence, recurrence of TTTS, and adverse long-term neurological sequelae in 6–18% of survivors (46). The future of fetoscopic laser therapy in the treatment of TTTS will involve evaluating its role in the management of early disease—a randomized controlled trial is currently underway to compare conservative management to laser therapy for the treatment of TTTS stage 1.

Fetoscopic cord occlusion for selective fetal growth restriction or discordant fetal anomaly in monochorionic twin pregnancies

Selective fetal growth restriction affects 12–15% of monochorionic twin pregnancies (47). Isolated selective fetal growth restriction is usually defined as an inter-twin size difference of 25% or greater in the absence of TTTS and is easily differentiated from TTTS due to a lack of polyhydramnios surrounding the appropriately grown fetus. There is also an increased incidence of discordance in fetal anomalies in monochorionic twin pregnancies compared to dichorionic pairs. This is most likely due to the teratogenic effect of embryo cleavage or as a result of shared circulation. Either of these conditions may lead to intrauterine demise of one twin and potential neurological injury to the other. In certain situations, selective feticide of one twin is offered to maximize the chances of survival of the co-twin. As a consequence of shared placental circulation, selective termination is achieved by interrupting the vascular supply of the affected twin. This may be achieved by bipolar cord coagulation, cord ligation, ILT, or RFA.

Fetoscopic cord coagulation requires the insertion of a 3.8 mm operative sleeve into the amniotic sac of the fetus that is to be terminated (48). Sufficient amniotic fluid is required to facilitate insertion of the sleeve and deployment of the device. Complications associated with fetoscopic cord occlusion include membrane rupture, preterm labour, and haemorrhage. Intrauterine demise of the co-twin has been reported in up to 15% of cases (49). Bebbington et al. performed a retrospective review of the outcomes associated with selective termination by bipolar cord coagulation compared to RFA. The overall survival rates of the co-twin associated with bipolar cord coagulation versus RFA were 85.2% and 70.7% respectively (48). The increased overall survival in the bipolar cord coagulation group was attributed to decreased time taken to achieve cessation of blood flow. The optimal therapeutic technique to achieve selective reduction in monochorionic twin pregnancies is yet to be defined.

Fetoscopic endotracheal occlusion for congenital diaphragmatic hernia

CDH is a defect of the diaphragmatic wall which results in protrusion of the abdominal organs into the thoracic cavity. It affects approximately 1 in 4000 live births and is associated with a chromosomal abnormality in 30% of cases (50). Cases of isolated CDH are associated with a 50% mortality rate secondary to pulmonary hypoplasia and hypertension. Over the years, studies have recognized predictors of outcome for CDH including gestational age, additional anomalies, herniation of the liver, and the measurement of the observed to expected fetal lung area to head circumference ratio (51). The concept of intrauterine repair to replace the herniated viscera and subsequently

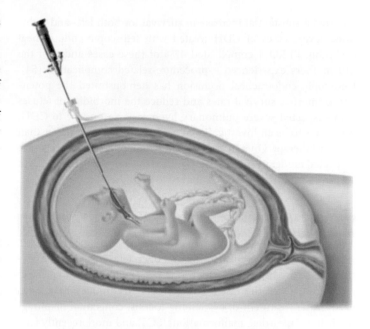

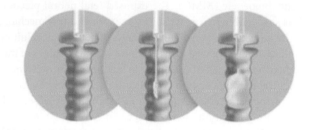

Figure 19.4 Schematic drawing of fetoscopic endoluminal tracheal occlusion using a detachable balloon.
Reproduced from J. Deprest, E. Gratacos, K. H. Nicolaides, Fetoscopic tracheal occlusion (FETO) for severe congenital diaphragmatic hernia: evolution of a technique and preliminary results, *Ultrasound in Obstetrics and Gynaecology*, Vol 24 No 2, August 2004, with permission from John Wiley and Sons.

reverse the effects of pulmonary hypoplasia and pulmonary hypertension were first demonstrated in animal studies. These were abandoned, however, as the procedure was associated with high rates of maternal morbidity and did not confer any significant improvement in neonatal mortality or morbidity (52). Endotracheal occlusion in humans was originally performed via open hysterotomy and subsequently endoscopically by means of tracheal clip application. The removal of these clips required a strict delivery protocol which gave rise to the EXIT procedure. As a consequence of increased rates of preterm delivery and irreversible damage to the trachea, clips were subsequently abandoned in favour of endotracheal balloon occlusion (Figure 19.4). In 1999, a prospective randomized controlled trial of fetal endotracheal occlusion versus standard postnatal care for fetuses with severe isolated left CDH was terminated early after treatment of 24 patients failed to demonstrate a significant benefit in outcome (53). Failure to demonstrate a significant difference in survival to 90 days may be explained by the fact that the fetuses in the interventional group were born at significantly earlier gestations than those in the control group.

Following on from this trial, numerous centres have been involved in the development of endoscopic techniques (fetoscopic endotracheal occlusion) and protocols to tackle the significant complication rate associated with CDH. A case series of 210 procedures reported a substantial increase in survival for both left- and right-sided severe cases of CDH treated with fetoscopic endotracheal occlusion. PPROM complicated 47% of these cases and 7 of the 210 mothers experienced a procedure-related complication (54). Fetoscopic endotracheal occlusion has demonstrated the potential to improve survival rates and reduce the morbidity of fetuses with suspected severe pulmonary hypoplasia secondary to CDH. It remains to be an investigational procedure, however, rather than standard therapy. Ongoing research into its application in cases with suspected moderate hypoplasia as well as the long-term outcomes of survivors remain key issues that need to be addressed.

Open fetal surgery

In 1981, Harrison performed the first open fetal surgical intervention for a case of LUTO, which was not eligible for shunt placement (55). Over the last 30 years, open techniques have been used in the treatment of cystic lung lesions, congenital diaphragmatic hernia, cardiac malformations, SCT, and more recently fetal myelomeningocoele (MMC). The exposed fetal neural placode in MMC is susceptible to further injury *in utero* and this mechanism forms the basis of the 'two-hit' hypothesis of neurological injury in MMC. Individuals affected by MMC have varying degrees of motor and somatosensory deficits resulting in bladder and bowel dysfunction. Central nervous system complications including hydrocephalus requiring ventriculoperitoneal (VP) shunting arise secondary to hind brain herniation also known as an Arnold–Chiari II malformation. Until recently, postnatal surgical treatment of MMC was the only option. The rationale for *in utero* repair is to target the second hit of the hypothesis, that is, to limit the exposure of the neural placode to direct trauma and toxins within the amniotic fluid and to reduce ongoing cerebrospinal fluid leak. One of first reports of open fetal MMC repair came from a Vanderbilt University (Nashville, Tennessee, USA) team in 1999 who conducted a non-randomized observational study over a 9-year period (56). With a study sample size of 29 patients with isolated fetal MMC referred for intrauterine repair, they were able to demonstrate significantly improved hindbrain herniation and decreased need for VP shunting compared with controls. This improvement came at a cost, however, as there were significantly higher levels of preterm delivery in the intervention group (56).

Following on from the work by Bruner et al., the clinical outcomes of early studies varied. The risks associated with open MMC surgery were significant and not only included preterm labour but also placental abruption and hysterotomy scar dehiscence. In order to determine whether the benefits of this surgery outweighed the risks, a multicentre randomized controlled trial comparing safety and efficacy of pre- versus postnatal closure of myelomeningocoele (MOMs trial) was conducted. The primary outcomes were fetal or neonatal death and the need for a VP shunt at less than 12 months of age (57). The need for VP shunting in the prenatal and postnatal surgery groups at 12 months of age were 68% and 98%, respectively (P <0.001). The secondary outcomes demonstrated significant functional and neurological improvement at 30 months of age in the prenatal surgery group (P = 0.007) (57). Significant maternal morbidity related to prenatal surgery included uterine dehiscence, oligohydramnios, placental abruption, spontaneous rupture of membranes, and chorioamniotic separation (57). Following on from the MOMs trial, more recent work has been conducted with the aim of reducing the maternal and fetal morbidity associated with open MMC repair by developing fetoscopic techniques. A meta-analysis comparing open versus fetoscopic repair of fetal MMC concluded that open fetal surgery was associated with lower rates of procedure-related complications compared to endoscopic techniques. The authors advised that these conclusions be interpreted with caution, however, due to the low-quality evidence available (58).

Peripartum fetal therapy

Peripartum fetal therapy techniques such as the EXIT procedure have been developed to overcome difficulties encountered at the time of delivery and the immediate postpartum period.

Ex utero intrapartum treatment procedure

The EXIT procedure was first described as a systematic approach to securing the airway during delivery while managing fetuses with predictable airway obstruction (59). It was primarily indicated in fetuses with neck masses and also to facilitate controlled reversal of tracheal clipping for fetuses with CDH who had undergone *in utero* tracheal occlusion. The aim of the procedure is to establish reliable neonatal airway control while the uteroplacental unit maintains oxygenation during a partial delivery at caesarean section. In order to permit maximal uteroplacental perfusion, the EXIT procedure is performed under deep inhalational general anaesthesia and tocolytic therapy. This facilitates sufficient time to perform complex airway procedures to secure the fetal airway. Current indications for performing the EXIT procedure include reversal of endotracheal occlusion and management of disorders leading to congenital airway obstruction, for example, fetal lung, neck or mediastinal masses, severe micrognathia, or laryngeal atresia. As a consequence of general anaesthesia and tocolytic therapy, the maternal risks associated with the EXIT procedure are commonly increased blood loss secondary to uterine atony and increased operating times. There is also an increased risk of placental abruption which can have consequences for both the mother and the fetus. Fetal risks are dependent on the underlying cause; however, complex cases are associated with increased morbidity and mortality secondary to airway obstruction. In a series of 31 EXIT procedures undertaken predominantly for fetal neck masses and reversal of tracheal occlusion, five fetuses required a tracheostomy and there was one neonatal death due to inability to secure the airway in a case of extensive lymphangioma. The average maternal blood loss was 848 mL and there were two significant maternal complications (60). The EXIT procedure has demonstrated improvement in the outcomes of neonates with upper airway obstruction; however, it can have implications for the mother. In order to adequately coordinate the management of two patients (i.e. the mother and the fetus), a multidisciplinary team approach is essential.

REFERENCES

1. Hui L, Bianchi DW. Prenatal pharmacotherapy for fetal anomalies: a 2011 update. *Prenat Diagn* 2011;**31**:735–43.

2. Ampola MG, Mahoney MJ, Nakamura E, Tanaka K. Prenatal therapy of a patient with vitamin-B12-responsive methylmalonic acidaemia. *N Engl J Med* 1975;**293**:313–17.

3. Wacker-Gussmann A, Strasburger JF, Cuneo BF, Wakai RT. Diagnosis and treatment of fetal arrhythmia. *Am J Perinatol* 2014;**31**:617–28.

4. Api O, Carvalho JS. Fetal dysrhythmias. *Best Pract Res Clin Obstet Gynaecol* 2008;**22**:31–48.

5. Jaeggi ET, Carvalho JS, De Groot E, et al. Comparison of transplacental treatment of fetal supraventricular tachyarrhythmias with digoxin, flecainide, and sotalol: results of a nonrandomized multicenter study. *Circulation* 2011;**124**:1747–54.

6. Srinivasan S, Strasburger J. Overview of fetal arrhythmias. *Curr Opin Pediatr* 2008;**20**:522–31.

7. Eliasson H, Sonesson SE, Sharland G, et al. Isolated atrio-ventricular block in the fetus: a retrospective, multinational, multicenter study of 175 patients. *Circulation* 2011;**124**:1919–26.

8. Khalid JM, Oerton JM, Dezateux C, Hindmarsh PC, Kelnar CJ, Knowles RL. Incidence and clinical features of congenital adrenal hyperplasia in Great Britain. *Arch Dis Child* 2012;**97**:101–106.

9. David M, Forest MG. Prenatal treatment of congenital adrenal hyperplasia resulting from 21-hydroxylase deficiency. *J Pediatr* 1984;**105**:799–803.

10. Lajic S, Nordenström A, Hirvikoski T. Long term outcome of prenatal dexamethasone treatment of 21-hydroxylase deficiency. *Endocr Dev* 2011;**20**:96–105.

11. Bertrand G, Drame M, Martageix C, Kaplan C. Prediction of the fetal status in non invasive management of alloimmune thrombocytopenia. *Blood* 2011;**117**:3209–13.

12. Zdravic D, Yougbare I, Vadasz B, et al. Fetal and neonatal alloimmune thrombocytopenia. *Semin Fetal Neonatal Med* 2016;**21**:19–27.

13. Spencer JA, Burrows RF. Feto-maternal alloimune thrombocytopenia: a literature review and statistical analysis. *Aust N Z J Obstet Gynaecol* 2001;**41**:45–55.

14. Rayment R, Brunskill SJ, Soothill PW, Roberts DJ, Bussel JB, Murphy MF. Antenatal interventions for fetomaternal alloimmune thrombocytopenia. *Cochrane Database Syst Rev* 2011;**5**:CD004226.

15. Donald I, MacVicar J, Brown TG. Investigation of abdominal masses by pulsed ultrasound. *Lancet* 1958;**1**:1188–95.

16. Rodeck CH, Nicolaides KH, Warsof SL, Fysh WJ, Gamsu HR, Kemp JR. The management of severe rhesus isoimmunisaton by fetoscopic intravascular transfusion. *Am J Obstet Gynecol* 1984;**150**:769–74.

17. Pretlove SJ, Fox CE, Khan KS, Kilby MD. Non-invasive methods of detecting fetal anaemia: a systematic review and meta-analysis. *BJOG* 2009;**116**:1558–67.

18. Van Kamp IL, Klumper FJ, Oepkes D, et al. Complications of intra-uterine intravascular transfusion for fetal anaemia due to maternal red-cell alloimmunization. *Am J Obstet Gynecol* 2005;**192**:171–77.

19. Mackie FL, Pretlove SJ, Martin WL, Donovan V, Kilby MD. Fetal intracardiac transfusions in hydropic fetuses with severe anaemia. *Fetal Diagn Ther* 2015;**38**:61–64.

20. Lindenburg IT, van Kamp IL, Oepkes D. Intrauterine blood transfusion: current indications and associated risks. *Fetal Diagn Ther* 2014;**36**:263–71.

21. Hansmann M, Gembruch U, Bald R, Manz M, Redel DA. Fetal tachyarrhythmias: transplacental and direct treatment of the fetus—a report of 60 cases. *Ultrasound Obstet Gynecol* 1991;**1**:162–70.

22. Simpson JM, Sharland GK. Fetal tachycardias: management and outcome of 127 consecutive cases. *Heart* 1998;**79**:576–81.

23. Cabassa P, Fichera A, Prefumo F, et al. The use of radiofrequency in the treatment of twin reversed arterial perfusion sequence: a case series and review of the literature. *Eur J Obstet Gynecol Reprod Biol* 2013;**166**:127–32.

24. Wong AE, Sepulveda W. Acardiac anomaly: current issues in pre-natal assessment and treatment. *Prenat Diagn* 2005;**25**:796–806.

25. Swamy R, Embleton N, Hale J. Sacrococcygeal teratoma over two decades: birth prevalence, prenatal diagnosis and clinical outcomes. *Prenat Diagn* 2008;**28**:1048–51.

26. Van Mieghem T, Al-Ibrahim A, Deprest J, et al. Minimally invasive therapy for fetal sacrococcygeal teratoma: case series and systematic review of the literature. *Ultrasound Obstet Gynecol* 2014;**43**:611–19.

27. Zanardini C, Papageorghiou A, Bhide A, Thilaganathan B. Giant placental chorioangioma: natural history and pregnancy outcome. *Ultrasound Obstet Gynecol* 2010;**35**:332–36.

28. Bebbington M. Selective reduction in multiple gestations. *Best Pract Res Clin Obstet Gynaecol* 2014;**28**:239–47.

29. Rustico MA, Baietti MG, Coviello D, Orlandi E, Nicolini U. Managing twins discordant for fetal anomaly. *Prenat Diagn* 2005;**25**:766–71.

30. Dias T, Ladd S, Mahsud-Dornan S, Bhide A, Papageorghiou AT, Thilaganathan B. Systematic labelling of twin pregnancies on ultrasound. *Ultrasound Obstet Gynecol* 2011;**38**:130–33.

31. Bhide A, Sairam S, Hollis B, Thilaganathan B. Comparison of feticide carried out by cordocentesis versus cardiac puncture. *Ultrasound Obstet Gynecol* 2002;**20**:230–232.

32. Eddleman KA, Stone JL, Lynch L, Berkowitz RL. Selective termination of anomalous fetuses in multifetal pregnancies: Two hundred cases at a single center. *Am J Obstet Gynecol* 2002;**187**:1168–72.

33. Clewell WH, Johnson ML, Meier PR, et al. A surgical approach to the treatment of fetal hydrocephalus. *N Engl J Med* 1982;**306**:1320–25.

34. Manning FA, Harrison MR, Rodeck C. Catheter shunts for fetal hydronephrosis and hydrocephalus. *N Engl J Med* 1986;**315**:336–40.

35. Freedman AL, Johnson MP, Gonzalez R. Fetal therapy for obstructive uropathy: past, present, future? *Pediatr Nephrol* 2000;**14**:167–76.

36. Clark TJ, Martin WL, Divakaran TG, Whittle MJ, Kilby MD, Khan KS. Prenatal bladder drainage in the management of fetal lower urinary tract obstruction: a systematic review and meta-analysis. *Obstet Gynecol* 2003;**102**,:367–82.

37. Morris RK, Malin GL, Quinlan-Jones E, et al. The Percutaneous shunting in Lower Urinary Tract Obstruction (PLUTO) study and randomised controlled trial: evaluation of the effectiveness, cost-effectiveness and acceptability of percutaneous vesicoamniotic shunting for lower urinary tract obstruction. *Health Technol Assess* 2013;**17**:1–232.

38. Longaker MT, Laberge JM, Dansereau J, et al. Primary fetal hydrothorax: natural history and management. *J Pediatr Surg* 1989;**24**:573–76.

39. Aubard Y, Derouineau I, Aubard V, Chalifour V, Preux PM. Primary fetal hydrothorax: a literature review and proposed antenatal clinical strategy. *Fetal Diagn Ther* 1998;**13**:325–33.

40. O'Brien B, Kesby G, Ogle R, Rieger I, Hyett JA. Treatment of primary fetal hydrothorax with OK-432 (Picibanil): outcome in 14 fetuses and a review of the literature. *Fetal Diagn Ther* 2015;**37**:259–66.

41. Mandelbaum B, Evans TN. Life in the amniotic fluid. *Am J Obstet Gynecol* 1969;**104**:365–77.

42. Lewi L, Jani J, Blickstein I, et al. The outcome of monochorionic diamniotic twin gestations in the era of invasive fetal therapy: a prospective cohort study. *Am J Obstet Gynecol* 2008;**199**:514.e1–8.

43. Quintero RA, Morales WJ, Allen MH, Bornick PW, Johnson PK, Kruger M. Staging of twin-twin transfusion syndrome. *J Perinatol* 1999;**8**:550–55.

44. Senat MV, Deprest J, Boulvain M, Paupe A, Winer N, Ville Y. Endoscopic laser surgery versus serial amnioreduction for severe twin-to-twin transfusion syndrome. *N Engl J Med* 2004;**351**:136–14.

45. Slaghekke F, Lopriore E, Lewi L, et al. Fetoscopic laser coagulation of the vascular equator versus selective coagulation for twin-to-twin transfusion syndrome: an open-label randomised controlled trial. *Lancet* 2014;**383**:2144–51.

46. van Klink JM, Koopman HM, van Zwet EW, et al. Improvement in neurodevelopmental outcome in survivors of twin-twin transfusion syndrome treated with laser surgery. *Am J Obstet Gynecol* 2014;**210**:540.e1–7.

47. Lewi L, Van Schoubroeck D, Gratacós E, Witters I, Timmerman D, Deprest J. Monochorionic diamniotic twins: complications and management options. *Curr Opin Obstet Gynecol* 2003;**15**:177–94.

48. Bebbington M. Selective reduction in multiple gestations. *Best Pract Res Clin Obstet Gynaecol* 2014;**28**:239–47.

49. Rossi AC, D'Addario V. Umbilical cord occlusion for selective feticide in complicated monochorionic twins: a systematic review of literature. *Am J Obstet Gynecol* 2009;**200**:123–29.

50. Deprest J, Gratacos E, Nicolaides KH; FETO Task Group. Fetoscopic tracheal occlusion (FETO) for severe congenital diaphragmatic hernia: evolution of a technique and preliminary results. *Ultrasound Obstet Gynecol* 2004;**24**:121–26.

51. Deprest J, Jani J, Gratacos E, et al. Fetal intervention for congenital diaphragmatic hernia: the European experience. *Semin Perinatol* 2005;**29**:94–103.

52. Harrison MR, Adzick NS, Bullard KM, et al. Correction of CDH in utero. VII. A prospective trial. *J Pediatr Surg* 1997;**32**:1637–42.

53. Harrison MR, Keller RL, Hawgood SB, et al. A randomized trial of fetal endoscopic tracheal occlusion for severe fetal congenital diaphragmatic hernia. *N Engl J Med* 2003;**349**: 1916–24.

54. Jani JC, Nicolaides KH, Gratacós E, et al. Severe diaphragmatic hernia treated by fetal endoscopic tracheal occlusion. *Ultrasound Obstet Gynecol* 2009;**34**:304–10.

55. Deprest JA, Flake AW, Gratacos E, et al. The making of fetal surgery. *Prenat Diagn* 2010;**30**:653–67.

56. Bruner JP, Tulipan N, Paschall RL, et al. Fetal surgery for myelomeningocele and the incidence of shunt-dependent hydrocephalus. *JAMA* 1999;**282**:1819–25.

57. Adzick NS, Thom EA, Spong CY, et al. A randomized trial of prenatal versus postnatal repair of myelomeningocele. *N Engl J Med* 2011;**364**:993–1004.

58. Araujo Júnior E, Eggink AJ, van den Dobbelsteen J, Martins WP, Oepkes D. Procedure-related complications of open versus fetoscopic fetal surgery for treatment of spina bifida: systematic review and meta-analysis in the new era of intra-uterine myelomeningocoele repair. *Ultrasound Obstet Gynecol* 2016;**2**:151–60.

59. Mychaliska GB, Bealer JF, Graf JL, Rosen MA, Adzick NS, Harrison MR. Operating on placental support: the ex utero intrapartum treatment procedure. *J Pediatr Surg* 1997;**32**:227–30.

60. Bouchard S, Johnson MP, Flake AW, et al. The EXIT procedure: experience and outcome in 31 cases. *J Pediatr Surg* 2002;**37**:418–26.

20

Multiple pregnancy

Surabhi Nanda and James P. Neilson

Incidence and importance

There has been a sustained rise in the incidence of multiple pregnancy worldwide over the past few decades (1–3). This has largely been due to the rise in use of assisted reproductive techniques including *in vitro* fertilization (IVF), despite the adoption of a single-embryo transfer policy where appropriate in some countries (4). One in eighty births following natural conception in the United Kingdom are multiples and one in four births after IVF (including intracytoplasmic sperm injection) in the United Kingdom result in either twins or triplets. The United Kingdom regulator estimates that about 40% of IVF babies are twins (5, 6). Triplet pregnancies continue to occur at a rate of 0.22 per 1000 livebirths, partly attributable to monozygotic twinning in assisted reproductive technique cycles and partly to spontaneous conception in women of advanced maternal age (7). The Human Fertilization and Embryology Authority (HFEA) reported that the number of women giving birth with multiple pregnancies (twins, triplets, and higher-order multiples) have more than trebled between 1992 and 2006 (from 664 to 2312) (2). This led to the introduction and subsequent implementation of the HFEA multiple pregnancy policy in 2008 with an aim to bring down the United Kingdom IVF multiple birth rate to 10% over a staged period (6, 8–10). The key recommendation to achieve such a reduction was to increase the proportions of elective single-embryo transfer (9). This has led to some reduction in multiple births, with one in four pregnancies being a multiple pregnancy in 2008 to one in six pregnancies in 2013 (9). However, monozygotic twinning may still occur with assisted reproductive techniques and elective single-embryo transfer, especially since the adoption of day 5 blastocyst transfer, to optimize successful pregnancy rates. **Figure 20.1** shows a rise in multiple pregnancy over the years, with advancing maternal age.

Multiple pregnancies are at increased risk for both mother (hypertensive disorders in pregnancy, diabetes in pregnancy, antepartum haemorrhage, obstetric cholestasis, anaemia, cardiovascular complications, postnatal illness, thromboembolic disorders, and maternal mortality) and the fetuses (miscarriage, preterm delivery, congenital malformations, stillbirth, and complications of monochorionic placentation such as twin-to-twin transfusion syndrome (TTTS)) (11). In general, maternal mortality associated with multiple births is 2.5 times that for singleton births. The overall stillbirth rate in multiple pregnancies is higher than in singleton pregnancies, ranging from 12.3 per 1000 twin births and 31.1 per 1000 triplet and higher-order multiple births, compared with 5 per 1000 singleton births. The risk of preterm birth is also considerably higher in multiple pregnancies than in singleton pregnancies, occurring in 50% of twin pregnancies. It has been shown that the rate of cerebral palsy is at least six times higher for twins and 18 times higher for triplets than for singleton babies (12).

Therefore, multiple pregnancies pose an increased workload to fetal medicine units (as well as obstetric services more generally and neonatal units). This includes early chorionicity assessment, recognition and counselling of the increased risks associated with monochorionic placentation, and fetal therapy where appropriate. Besides fetal medicine input, successful maternal and fetal outcomes can be achieved by provision of care for women with twin and triplet pregnancies by a nominated multidisciplinary team consisting of a core team of named specialist obstetricians, specialist midwives, and ultrasonographers, all of whom have experience and knowledge of managing twin and triplet pregnancies. Various national and international guidance on multiple pregnancy corroborate this approach (11). A 2015 Cochrane review, however, has concluded that the value of 'specialized' multiple pregnancy clinics in improving health outcomes for women and their infants has yet to be proven in appropriately powered, randomized controlled trials (13).

Chorionicity and zygosity

Assessment of chorionicity and zygosity is important for prenatal diagnosis, risk stratification of pregnancy, genetic counselling, and planning interventional procedures, particularly in twin pregnancies discordant for structural, chromosomal, or growth abnormalities. With the advent of non-invasive prenatal diagnosis, accurate assessment of chorionicity is important in interpretation of the results.

There are two types of twin pregnancy—dizygotic and monozygotic.

Dizygotic twins occur when two ova are fertilized and have separate amnions, chorions, and placentas (dichorionic diamniotic). The placentas may fuse if the implantation sites are close together. The majority of twin pregnancies are dizygotic. Monozygotic twins

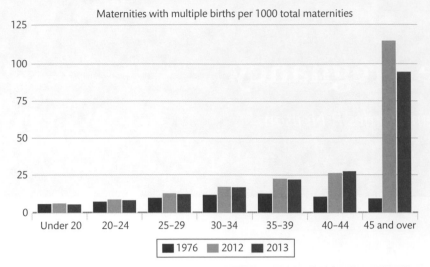

Figure 20.1 Risk in multiple pregnancy over years with advancing maternal age.
Source data from Office for National Statistics.

develop when a single fertilized ovum or zygote divides after conception (**Figure 20.2**).

Early division of the zygote (within 2 days of fertilization) results in separate chorions and amnions (dichorionic diamniotic twins). This occurs in approximately 30% of monozygotic twins. Later division (3–8 days after fertilization) results in a shared chorion and placentation and occurs in approximately 70% of monozygotic twins (monochorionic diamniotic (MCDA) twins). Division of the zygote

between 9 and 12 days after fertilization) results in a shared chorion, amnion, and placentation and is rare, occurring in only 1% of monozygotic twins (monochorionic monoamniotic (MCMA) twins). If twinning occurs more than 12 days after fertilization, then the monozygotic fertilized ovum only partially divides resulting in conjoined twins. This is extremely rare occurring in 1 in 50,000 to 100,000 twin pregnancies. Triplet pregnancies may result from various fertilization and division scenarios involving ovum and sperm. Triplets can

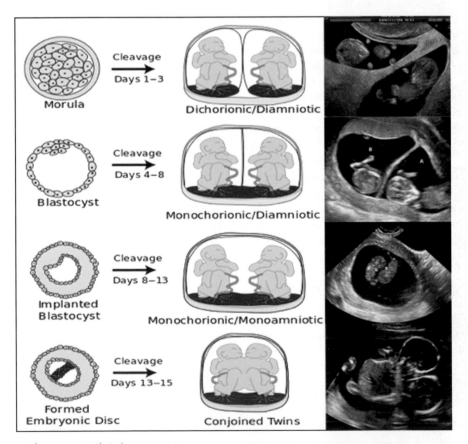

Figure 20.2 Twinning process in monozygotic twin pregnancy.

be trizygotic, dizygotic, or monozygotic. Zygosity in higher-order multiples (quadruplets or more) also varies.

Ultrasound determination of amnionicity and chorionicity is best achieved in the first trimester by examining the inter-twin membrane at its placental attachment and identifying the lambda (λ) or T sign (14). The earliest gestation for determining chorionicity is 5 weeks and for amnionicity 8 weeks. The lambda sign or the 'twin peak' sign is seen in dichorionic twin pregnancy. It appears as a triangular tissue projection extending from the base of the inter-twin membrane, giving the characteristic appearance of the Greek letter lambda (λ) (15). It is produced by extension of chorionic villi into the interchorionic space where the two separate placentas and chorionic attachments meet. Studies suggest a sensitivity and a specificity of 97–100% for accurate determination of dichorionicity using the lambda sign. In MCDA pregnancies, the T sign is evident as there is no triangular chorionic projection and the two amnions meet perpendicularly to the shared placenta. This is a reliable sign in identification of monochorionicity with about 98–100% accuracy. In MCMA pregnancies, there is no inter-twin membrane and the placental cord insertions are close together (16). See (Figure 20.3).

The reliability of using the inter-twin membrane for assessment of chorionicity decreases as the gestation advances. The lambda sign regresses in about 7% of dichorionic twin pregnancies in the late second trimester. If there is no accurate first-trimester detection of

chorionicity, fetal sex determination may be useful in the dizygotic pregnancies. However, one needs to be mindful that a proportion of dichorionic pregnancies (up to one-third) are not discordant for gender. Although measuring inter-twin membrane thickness has been described (the mean measurement is approximately 2.4 mm whereas in monochorionic twins mean thickness is 1.4 mm), it is less reliable, technically more challenging, and affected by inter- and intra-observer variability in the late second and third trimesters (17). Care must be taken in a new diagnosis of monoamniotic twin pregnancy in the second trimester, as this may represent severe TTTS in a MCDA twin pregnancy.

The evaluation of the membranes (amnion and chorion) and placenta(s) after the birth is important in all multiple pregnancies, but it does not always help determine zygosity (dichorionic placenta/like-sex twins).

Diagnosis

Gestational dating

A Cochrane review of 11 trials including 37,505 women showed that early ultrasonography (in the first trimester) improves the early detection of multiple pregnancies (prior to 24 weeks' gestation) and improves gestational dating therefore leading to fewer inductions for post maturity (18). More recently, the Clinical Standards Committee of the International Society of Ultrasound in Obstetrics and Gynecology (ISUOG) have recommended that twin pregnancies should ideally be dated when the crown–rump length (CRL) measurement is between 45 and 84 mm (i.e. 11^{+0} to 13^{+6} weeks of gestation). In pregnancies conceived spontaneously, the larger of the two CRLs should be used to estimate gestational age. Where the twin pregnancy was conceived via IVF, it should be dated using the oocyte retrieval date or the embryonic age from fertilization. If the woman presents after 14 weeks' gestation, the larger head circumference should be used (19). Some studies have recommended using a mean CRL or the smaller CRL for dating. However, a smaller CRL may reflect a fetal growth problem secondary to fetal abnormality. Indeed, the United Kingdom National Institute for Health and Care Excellence (NICE) guidelines on multiple pregnancy also recommend dating by the largest CRL to avoid estimating it from a fetus with early growth pathology, albeit that it is recognized that this may exaggerate this risk causing anxiety (11).

Labelling in twins

It is accepted as a good clinical practice to follow a clear consistent strategy for labelling of twins (3, 19). Various options include labelling according to their site, either left and right, or upper and lower; or mapping in the first trimester according to the insertion of their cords relative to the placental edges and membrane insertion (3). This is particularly important in laterally orientated twins (i.e. left and right twins) where 8.5% change presenting order between the first and last scans, and 20.3% delivered by caesarean versus 5.9% delivered vaginally change birth order (i.e. the twin labelled 'twin 2' delivers first) (20). Correct labelling according to orientation in relation to the mother as lateral maternal left and maternal right or vertical upper and lower, is better than assigning a fetus number as it enables consistency with longitudinal biometric assessment, accuracy when

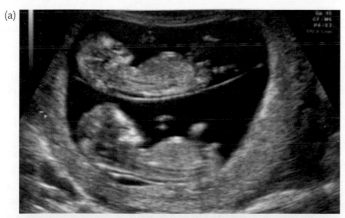

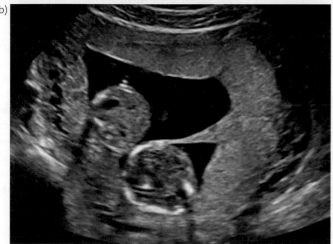

Figure 20.3 (a) T sign in monochorionic twin pregnancy. (b) Lambda or twin peak sign in dichorionic twin pregnancy.

interpreting screening results and undertaking invasive diagnostic tests where necessary, and avoids misconception about birth order ensuring the parents and paediatric team are aware of the possibility of the 'perinatal switch phenomenon' (i.e. possible change in birth order). This is particularly important if one fetus has an abnormality that is not outwardly obvious (e.g. cardiac abnormality). In such a case, it is important to perform an ultrasound scan prior to delivery to ascertain the fetal order and thereby plan any neonatal interventions for the appropriate fetus. It is, however, vital that the nomenclature assigned to twins from early pregnancy is clearly documented at each visit and remains consistent throughout the pregnancy (11).

Prenatal diagnosis

Screening for common trisomies is more complex compared to singletons, and the detection rates vary depending on the chorionicity. It is important that women are appropriately counselled about the implications of detection of a discordant chromosomal abnormality, the risks associated with an invasive or a diagnostic test, and the practicalities and implications of selective fetal reduction, where appropriate.

Zygosity and not chorionicity mediates the risk of chromosomal abnormalities in a multiple pregnancy. In monozygotic twins, the risk of aneuploidy for each fetus is similar to that in singleton pregnancies. Very rarely, heterokaryotic monozygotic twins with chromosomal discordance can be noted due to postzygotic mitotic errors (21). Dizygotic twins are genetically distinct and thus aneuploidy, when present, is usually discordant. Each twin has an independent risk. As a result, the chance of at least one fetus in a dizygotic twin pregnancy being affected by chromosomal defect is broadly twice as high as that for women of the same age with a singleton fetus (22).

First-trimester screening for chromosomal abnormalities

It is recommended that in a twin pregnancy, screening for trisomy 21 should be performed in the first trimester using the combined test, which includes maternal age, measurement of nuchal translucency (NT) and serum beta-human chorionic gonadotrophin (β-hCG), and pregnancy associated plasma protein-A (PAPP-A) levels (3, 11). An alternative is the combination of maternal age and the NT recorded between 11^{+0} and 13^{+6} weeks of gestation (11, 23). In case of a vanished twin, if there is still a measurable fetal pole, β-hCG and PAPP-A measurements are biased and in such cases, NT alone should be used for risk estimation (24). The risk of trisomy 21 in monochorionic twin pregnancy is calculated per pregnancy based on the average risk of both fetuses, whereas in dichorionic twin pregnancy, the risk is calculated per fetus. The detection rate for Down syndrome is thought to be lower in twin compared with singleton pregnancy (11). However, a recent meta-analysis reported similar performance (89% for singletons, 86% for dichorionic twins, and 87% for monochorionic twins, at a false-positive rate of 5%) (25). For triplets or higher-order multiple pregnancies, NT and maternal age is the only available screening method.

Second-trimester screening for chromosomal abnormalities

In twin pregnancies, conventional second-trimester serum screening tests are not as reliable as in singleton pregnancies and do not provide a fetus specific risk. This may not be a problem for monochorionic twins, but for dichorionic twin pregnancies, which are more likely to be discordant for aneuploidy, second-trimester biochemical screening is not an effective or an accurate option. The NICE guidance on multiple pregnancy does, however, recommend offering second-trimester serum screening for twins (11). However, where first-trimester screening is missed or not possible in monochorionic twin pregnancies, the 2017 Royal College of Obstetricians and Gynaecologists (RCOG) guidance does recommend offering the quadruple test (3).

Investigators have suggested calculating a 'pseudo-risk' using the biochemical markers (alpha-fetoprotein, hCG, and oestriol) for twins similar to singletons, albeit with a lower sensitivity of 51–73% for a 5% false-positive rate (26). Some studies have suggested some improvement in performance of screening in the second-trimester twin pregnancy with the quadruple test) (27). As such, the norm is to offer first-trimester combined screening to all pregnancies including twin pregnancies. For triplet or higher-order pregnancy, there are no second-trimester screening options.

Non-invasive prenatal testing in multiple pregnancy

Non-invasive prenatal testing (NIPT) of maternal blood for common fetal trisomies can be offered as early as 10 weeks of pregnancy. It has a better detection rate and lower false-positive rate compared to the conventional combined screening, especially for trisomy 21 and less so for trisomies 18 and 13 (28). NIPT should never replace diagnostic testing in both singletons and twins. In monochorionic twin pregnancies, due to the same genotype (except for a very small incidence of heterokaryotypia), this may be an effective option for screening. For dichorionic twins, with current techniques it is difficult to distinguish individual contribution of the fetuses. The largest series on NIPT in twin pregnancy was a recent prospective study in 438 twin and 10,698 singleton pregnancies undergoing screening for fetal trisomies by cell-free fetal DNA testing at 10^{+0} to 13^{+6} weeks' gestation, showed that in twin pregnancies, the median fetal fraction was lower (8.0% vs 11.0%; P <0.0001) and the failure rate after first sampling was higher (9.4% vs 2.9%; P <0.0001) compared to in singletons. It also showed that the risk of test failure increased with increasing maternal age and body mass index and decreased with fetal CRL. The main contributor to the higher rate of failure in twins was conception by IVF (9.5% singletons and 56.2% twins). In the 417 twin pregnancies with a cell-free fetal DNA result after first or second sampling, the detection rate was 100% for trisomy 21 and 60% for trisomies 18 or 13, at a false-positive rate of 0.25%. However, the overall reported number of trisomy 21 cases in twin pregnancy detected by NIPT are still far less than those in singleton pregnancies. In a recent meta-analysis, the weighted pooled detection rate for trisomy 21 with NIPT in twin pregnancy was 94.4% (29). There is some evidence that newer techniques including single nucleotide polymorphism-based NIPT are more reliable in trisomy 21 detection in cases with vanished twin, previously unrecognized twin, and triploid pregnancies (30).

Invasive prenatal diagnosis

Women with multiple pregnancies are more likely to be offered an invasive test based on the results of combined screening or either equivocal or a high-risk result from NIPT (11). This is because most multiple pregnancies are at a higher risk of aneuploidy due to maternal age, IVF, or multiple gestation. Invasive procedures in multiple pregnancies should be carried out in a tertiary unit with an expertise in such procedures (11). Invasive prenatal diagnosis in multiple pregnancies carries a higher risk of miscarriage compared to singleton pregnancies. Prior to an invasive procedure it is important to be sure of the chorionicity and map the twins carefully (3, 19). It is also vital to discuss the implications of the results if they are positive for a chromosomal abnormality (especially in discordant abnormality). In such cases, selective fetal reduction should be discussed as an option and the complexity of this procedure in monochorionic twins should be highlighted (3).

Chorionic villus sampling

A meta-analysis showed that the overall pregnancy loss rate following chorionic villus sampling (CVS) in twin pregnancy was 3.8%, and following amniocentesis was 3.1% (31). The risk was found to be similar for transabdominal and transcervical approaches, use of a single-needle or double-needle system, and single or double uterine entry. Other studies have reported lower loss rates: 2% following CVS and 1.5–2% following amniocentesis (32). CVS is preferred over amniocentesis in dichorionic twin pregnancies because of the earlier gestation at which it can be performed. This enables earlier counselling and, if needed, selective reduction, and thereby reducing the miscarriage rates with selective reduction (7% risk of loss of the entire pregnancy, and 14% risk of delivery before 32 weeks) (33). In monochorionic twin pregnancies, especially where discordant for anomaly, amniocentesis would be preferred over CVS due to the small risk of heterokaryotypia (3).

Amniocentesis

Traditionally, amniocentesis has been the gold standard invasive procedure for multiple pregnancies, although with the advent of NIPT and increased uptake of first-trimester screening, where the expertise is available CVS (especially for monochorionic twins) is being offered for the reasons mentioned previously. In monochorionicity, if the chorionicity has been confirmed before 14 weeks' gestation and the fetuses appear concordant for growth and anatomy, it is acceptable to sample only one amniotic sac. Otherwise, both amniotic sacs should be sampled because of the possibility of rare discordant chromosomal anomalies in monochorionic pregnancy (3, 19). Techniques include the single-needle (higher risk of fetal contamination, but a slightly lower risk of miscarriage) or a double-needle technique (higher rate of miscarriage due to multiple insertions but minimal fetal contamination) (34). In a meta-analysis of 2026 women with twin pregnancies, compared with women unexposed to the procedure, amniocentesis increased the risk of fetal loss prior to 24 weeks' gestation (odds ratio 2.4; 95% confidence interval 1.2–4.7) with an additional risk of one adverse outcome for every 64 amniocenteses (35). This procedure-related risk of miscarriage can be minimized by delaying amniocentesis until the third trimester, but this is only relevant in those countries in which late termination of pregnancy is permitted. Although there is a small risk of preterm delivery, the risks to the fetus from preterm birth are minimal when invasive testing is performed at or after 32 weeks. In twins, late fetal karyotyping carries an additional advantage of avoiding loss of an unaffected co-twin from earlier selective reduction if twins are discordant for anomaly. Due to the higher risk of

fetal cell contamination and failure to sample each sac with CVS, amniocentesis is the preferred option for prenatal diagnosis in triplets and higher-order multiples.

Fetal risks

Fetal loss/miscarriage

There is a higher risk of fetal loss and miscarriage (pregnancy loss before 24 weeks' gestation) in multiple pregnancy, with risks increasing with the number of fetuses. The higher fetal loss rates are mainly explained by the increased risk of poor implantation, fetal abnormality (aneuploidy and structural), extreme preterm labour, and in monochorionic twins, complications of shared placenta. One study estimates about 12% of all early conceptions start as twins (36). Resorption of one pregnancy in a previously ultrasonographically confirmed twin pregnancy, 'the vanishing twin' phenomenon, occurs in up to 20% of first-trimester twin pregnancies. This has implications in first-trimester screening (24).

Fetal abnormality

The risk of fetal anomaly is greater in twin compared with singleton pregnancy (37). The rate per fetus in dizygotic twins is probably the same as that in singletons, whereas it is two to three times higher in monozygotic twins, being attributed to abnormal cleavage in the latter. In around 1 in 25 dichorionic, 1 in 15 MCDA, and 1 in 6 monoamniotic twin pregnancies, there is a major congenital anomaly that typically affects only one twin (38, 39). Common structural abnormalities in twins include neural tube defects, anterior abdominal wall defects, facial clefts, brain abnormalities, cardiac defects and gastrointestinal anomalies. All multiple pregnancies should have a detailed scan for screening for structural defects, considering that scanning in multiples may take longer than singletons (40). NICE recommends that the ultrasound scans in twin and triplet pregnancies at a slightly later gestational age than in singleton pregnancies. Any discordant anomaly in twins warrants a referral to a tertiary fetal medicine unit (11). Even in monozygotic twins, concordance for a structural anomaly is found in fewer than 20% of cases. One to two per cent of twin pregnancies will have a discordant anomaly, needing specialist assessment and counselling about the options of expectant management and selective reduction.

Selective reduction in twin pregnancy

Selective reduction is an option for multiple pregnancy with discordant anomaly. This is usually offered for a major congenital abnormality or an aneuploidy. The procedure and the timing depend on the chorionicity, the gestation at which a discordant abnormality is picked up as this influences the risk of miscarriage, and/or preterm birth. Such cases should be referred to a tertiary fetal medicine unit with experience in such procedures. In dichorionic twins, a selective feticide is performed by ultrasound-guided intracardiac injection of potassium chloride or lidocaine, preferably in the first trimester, due to lower risk of miscarriage (7% miscarriage, 14% risk of delivery before 32 weeks) (33). A third-trimester feticide is an option only where the law permits, and usually offered when there is a late detection of anomaly, bearing in mind that cardiac and brain abnormalities may continue to evolve till the third trimester, changing the prognosis for the baby (19). In monochorionic twins, selective feticide is performed using cord occlusion, intrafetal laser ablation, or radiofrequency ablation (41). Due to shared placentation, there is still a risk of the healthy twin losing part of its circulating blood volume into the terminated twin following its death. As such, the survival rate of the co-twin is approximately 80% and the risk of premature rupture of the membranes and preterm birth prior to 32 weeks is 20% (41). The risk of adverse neurological sequelae in the surviving co-twin may also be increased compared with that in uncomplicated pregnancy (42, 43).

Complications specific to monochorionic twin pregnancies

Due to their unique shared placentation, monochorionic twin pregnancies are at risk of serious complications. Whereas balanced flow in the shared vascular connections in the monochorionic twin pregnancy is a physiological phenomenon, imbalance in the flow can lead to complications such as TTTS or twin anaemia–polycythaemia sequence (TAPS). There may be discordant growth (one twin growth restricted with a normally grown co-twin) due to unequal sharing of placenta, leading to selective intrauterine growth restriction (sIUGR). When there is early pregnancy disruption in vascular anastomoses, particularly arterial, this results in the 'acardiac twin' or twin reversed arterial perfusion (TRAP) sequence. Monochorionic pregnancies not complicated by TTTS, sIUGR, or TAPS are still at risk of fetal death and neurological abnormality, and parents should be appropriately counselled by the clinicians about the range of complications of such type of twin pregnancy (3).

Twin-to-twin transfusion syndrome

TTTS is the most important cause of death and handicap in monochorionic twin pregnancies (44). It is thought to arise from an inter-twin transfusion imbalance across the vascular anastomoses with hypervolaemia, polyuria, and polyhydramnios in the recipient and hypovolaemia, oliguria, and oligo-anhydramnios in the donor. TTTS occurs in 15% of monochorionic twin pregnancies which overall is about 1 in 2000 pregnancies (**Figure 20.4**). It typically manifests around 16–26 weeks. The presentation of TTTS is variable

and its course can be unpredictable. TTTS may present as a slow-onset disease or be rapidly progressive. If untreated, the condition is associated with an 80% rate of perinatal mortality and a 15–20% risk of brain injury in survivors (45). Diagnosis of TTTS is based on ultrasound criteria of amniotic fluid discordance. Classification and staging of TTTS is currently based on the Quintero system (46) (**Table 20.1**). Although Quintero staging does not always predict accurately outcome or chronological evolution of TTTS, it remains the classification system of choice.

In current practice, most European countries have adopted the gestational age-dependent criteria to define polyhydramnios in the recipient sac: deepest vertical pocket greater than 8 cm prior to 20 weeks and greater than 10 cm after 20 weeks. In contrast, in the United States, the 8 cm cut-off is used more often throughout gestation. The definition of oligohydramnios in the donor's sac is universally accepted to be below 2 cm deepest vertical pocket (46).

Screening for TTTS in monochorionic twin pregnancies should commence from 16 weeks' gestation onwards. Fortnightly assessment of growth, deepest vertical pool of amniotic fluid, and umbilical artery Doppler is recommended. Care should be taken to note a free-floating inter-twin membrane and fetal bladder in both twins. Where there is discrepancy in amniotic fluid or folding of the inter-twin membrane, increased surveillance (usually weekly) should be offered to exclude progression to TTTS (3, 11, 19).

The NICE and RCOG guidance do not support the ultrasound parameters used in first-trimester screening—NT, CRL, and/or ductus venosus blood flow—as predictive for evolution of TTTS (3, 11). A recent meta-analysis of 2009 monochorionic twin pregnancies of which 323 developed TTTS showed that monochorionic twin pregnancies with NT discrepancy greater than 20%, NT greater than 95th centile, CRL discrepancy greater than 10%, or ductus venosus abnormal flow at the first-trimester scan are at significantly increased risk of developing TTTS, with sensitivities of 52.8% and 50% for NT discrepancy and abnormal ductus venosus flow, respectively (47). The ISUOG guidance on ultrasound in twin pregnancy recommends that the management of twin pregnancy with CRL discordance of at least 10% or NT discordance or at least 20% should be discussed with a fetal medicine expert and in these pregnancies

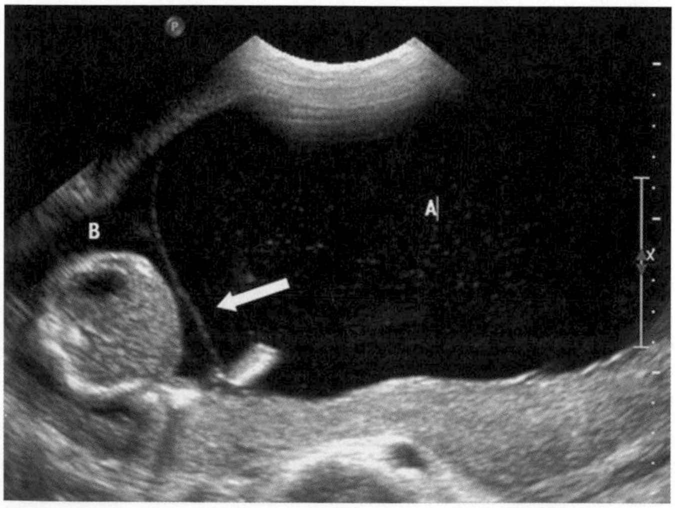

Figure 20.4 Polyhydramnios–oligohydramnios sequence in twin-to-twin transfusion syndrome.

Table 20.1 Quintero staging of TTTS

Stage	Description
I	Discrepancy in amniotic fluid volume with oligohydramnios of a maximum pool depth (MPD) ≤2 cm in one sac and polyhydramnios in other sac (MPD ≥8 cm). The bladder of the donor twin is visible and Doppler studies are normal
II	The bladder of the donor twin is not visible (during length of examination, usually around 1 hour) but Doppler studies are not critically abnormal
III	Doppler studies are critically abnormal in either twin and are characterized as abnormal or reversed end-diastolic velocities in the umbilical artery, reverse flow in the ductus venosus or pulsatile umbilical venous flow in either twin
IV	Ascites, pericardial or pleural effusion, scalp oedema, or overt hydrops present in recipient twin
V	One or both babies are dead

Source data from Quintero RA, Morales WJ, Allen MH, Bornick PW, Johnson PK, Kruger M. Staging of twin-twin transfusion syndrome. *J Perinatol* 1999;19:550–5.

there should be detailed ultrasound assessment and testing for karyotype abnormalities (19).

The gold standard treatment for TTTS diagnosed before 26 weeks is laser ablation, as the evidence suggests that it leads to better outcomes compared with amnioreduction or septostomy (48). Indeed, the Eurofetus randomized trial showed a higher survival after fetoscopic laser (76% of at least one twin) compared with serial amnioreduction (56%) (49). However, the Cochrane review on interventions in twin-to-twin transfusion also suggested that if laser ablation expertise is not available, amnioreduction is an acceptable alternative in pregnancies diagnosed after 26 weeks of gestation. Techniques described in fetoscopic laser for TTTS include the non-selective technique for ablation of all the vessels that cross the inter-twin membrane, the selective technique which identifies specific anastomosis and ablates them, and lastly the 'connecting the dots' or Solomon technique, which involves lasering healthy areas of the placenta between lasered anastomoses in order to create an 'equator' or 'dichorionization' of placenta (50–52). Following laser treatment, the recurrence rate of TTTS is up to 14%, and this risk is reduced by use of the Solomon technique compared with the highly selective technique (53–55).

Fetoscopic laser technique is therefore offered for stage II to stage IV TTTS. At present, there is a variation in offering laser versus expectant management for stage I TTTS. In a systematic review of the management of stage I TTTS pregnancy, overall survival appeared to be similar for those undergoing laser therapy or conservative management (85% and 86%, respectively), but was somewhat lower for those undergoing amnioreduction (77%) (56). Indeed, the management option for stage I TTTS will be debatable till the results of a randomized control trial comparing expectant versus laser management are available (NCT01220011) (57). Another option for the management of severe TTTS is selective termination of pregnancy using bipolar diathermy, laser coagulation, or radiofrequency ablation of one of the umbilical cords. Rarely, parents may opt for termination of the entire pregnancy.

From October 2015, the Twins and Multiple Births Association (TAMBA) have supported a United Kingdom-based registry of complications of monochorionic twins with emphasis on TTTS. This will provide a tool to assist the improvement of clinical skills and practice and also establish a platform to allow long-term follow-up of TTTS survivors at a national level showing the longer-term neurodevelopment outcomes (58).

TTTS has an effect on the cardiovascular status of both babies—possibly more in the recipient. Even early in stage I, up to 55% of fetuses have a degree of myocardial dysfunction (59). Studies have also shown evolution of pulmonary stenosis and functional pulmonary atresia in the recipient twin after laser procedure, suggesting that the cardiovascular status of twins in a pregnancy complicated by TTTS should be evaluated postnatally (60).

In pregnancies complicated by TTTS, cerebral abnormalities have been reported in 5% of those undergoing laser coagulation, 14% following serial amnioreduction, and 21% following expectant management (61). Both donors and recipients are at risk of developing either ischaemic or haemorrhagic lesions. The neurodevelopmental outcome at 6 years of age was similar to that at the age of 2 years and 10 months, with 9% of the children experiencing major neurodevelopmental delay (62). Neurodevelopment outcome was no different in those with TTTS treated by the Solomon technique

versus the standard technique in a subgroup analysis of the survivors recruited in the Solomon randomized trial (63).

Selective fetal growth restriction

sIUGR by definition is applicable to cases in monochorionic pregnancies where the estimated fetal weight (EFW) of the small fetus falls below the tenth percentile and the inter-twin growth discordance is greater than 25%. This condition is present in about 10–15% of all monochorionic twin pregnancies and in a small proportion can coexist with a superimposed TTTS. The pathophysiology behind sIUGR is inadequate placental sharing, possibly in association with very eccentric or velamentous cord insertion, and the presence of vascular anastomoses in the monochorionic placenta (64).

sIUGR is divided into three subtypes depending on whether there is umbilical artery Doppler waveform abnormality. Perinatal outcome differs in these three subtypes. In type I sIUGR, the lowest risk type, there is positive end-diastolic flow in the umbilical artery waveform of the growth-restricted fetus, and if this persists, the outcome can be good with over 90% survival. In type II sIUGR, there is persistent absent or reversed end-diastolic flow in the umbilical artery waveform of the growth-restricted fetus, and there is a risk of fetal death of either twin in up to 29% and neurological sequelae in 15% of cases born before 30 weeks. In type III sIUGR, there is a cyclical pattern present—absent and reversed end-diastolic flow in the umbilical artery waveform of the growth-restricted fetus and a 10–20% risk of sudden death of the growth-restricted fetus, and a high rate of neurological morbidity (up to 20%) in the larger twin (65).

There is limited evidence to guide the management of monochorionic twins affected by sFGR. Options include conservative management followed by early delivery, fetoscopic laser ablation, or cord occlusion of the growth-restricted twin (in order to protect the co-twin) (66). Irrespective of the presence or absence of intervention, such pregnancies are at a high risk of iatrogenic preterm delivery (3).

Twin anaemia polycythaemia sequence

The prenatal diagnosis of TAPS is based on the finding of a discordant middle cerebral artery (MCA) Doppler—MCA peak systolic velocity (PSV) greater than 1.5 multiples of the median (MoM) in the donor, suggesting fetal anaemia, and MCA PSV less than 1.0 MoM in the recipient, suggesting polycythemia. The incidence of TAPS in MCDA twins is up to 5% (spontaneous) and up to 13% (iatrogenic following laser ablation for TTTS) (67). TAPS occurs due to the presence of small arteriovenous anastomoses (<1 mm) which allow slow transfusion of blood from the donor to the recipient, leading to highly discordant haemoglobin concentrations at birth. In pregnancies complicated by TAPS, the risk of neurodevelopmental delay is around 20%. The management options depend on the gestational age at diagnosis, parental choice, severity of the disease, and technical feasibility of intrauterine therapy, and includes conservative management, early delivery, laser ablation, or intrauterine blood transfusion for the anaemic twin, combined intrauterine blood transfusion for the anaemic twin, and partial exchange transfusion to dilute the blood of the polycythaemic twin (68). In cases complicated by TAPS, the ISUOG guidance recommends brain imaging during the third trimester and neurodevelopmental assessment at 2 years of age (19).

Twin reversed arterial perfusion sequence

TRAP sequence is a rare complication of monochorionic twin pregnancy (1% of monochorionic twin pregnancies and 1 in 35,000 pregnancies overall). It is characterized by the presence of a TRAP or acardiac mass perfused by an apparently normal (pump) twin. The perfusion occurs in a retrograde fashion through artery–artery anastomoses, usually through a common cord insertion site. This characteristic vascular arrangement predisposes to a hyperdynamic circulation and progressive high-output cardiac failure in the pump twin. The risk of demise of the pump fetus in TRAP sequence managed conservatively is up to 30% by 18 weeks' gestation. Invasive techniques to treat TRAP sequence that have been described include cord occlusion using bipolar diathermy, intrafetal laser ablation or radiointerstitial thermal ablation. Poor prognostic indicators are (a) if the relative size of the acardiac twin is greater than 50% of the pump twin and (b) if the pump twin is showing signs of cardiovascular compromise. Best outcomes are achieved if intrafetal laser is performed prior to 16 weeks, ideally in the first trimester as reported in a recent meta-analysis (69).

Monochorionic monoamniotic twins

MCMA twin pregnancies constitute approximately 5% of monochorionic twin pregnancies. These pregnancies are associated with a high perinatal loss rate before 16 weeks' gestation, as high as 50%, mostly due to fetal abnormalities and spontaneous miscarriage (70). It is recommended that these pregnancies are managed in centres with the relevant expertise (3, 11). MCMA pregnancies have a slightly lower risk of TTTS than MCDA pregnancies (6%). A recent study reports an incidence of cerebral injury in MCMA twins to be 5%, respectively (71). Most MCMA twins have cord entanglement and are best delivered between 32^{+0} and 34^{+0} weeks, by caesarean section, after corticosteroids (3).

Conjoined twins

Conjoined twins occur in approximately 1 in 100,000 pregnancies (1% of monochorionic twin pregnancies) and are always MCMA twin pregnancies. They occur due to incomplete division of the single blastocyst between 13 and 15 days post conception. Diagnosis is usually made by the first trimester on ultrasound. The classification of conjoined twins depends on the site of the union. The most common form is thoracopagus. There is a high incidence of congenital anomalies, 60–70%, including neural tube defects, orofacial clefts, and cardiac anomalies. Approximately 40% of conjoined twins are stillborn and more than 50% of those born alive die during the neonatal period (72). Although vaginal delivery of conjoined twins has been reported, there is a significant risk of obstructed labour, dystocia, and uterine rupture and caesarean section is almost always offered. Postnatal surgery and rehabilitation depends on the extent of conjoining and the presence of other structural abnormalities. Such pregnancies should be managed in a specialist tertiary fetal medicine unit (3).

Co-twin demise in twin pregnancies

Single twin demise after 14 weeks has been reported to occur between 2.6% and 6.2% of all twin pregnancies (73). Fetal morbid sequelae may include prematurity, death of the surviving fetus, or survival with perinatal morbidity. In addition, maternal morbidity has been reported as increased with higher (than background) rates of pre-eclampsia, coagulopathy, and sepsis (74).

Following single intrauterine death, the following complications are found in monochorionic and dichorionic pregnancies, respectively: death of the co-twin (15% and 3%), preterm delivery (68% and 54%), abnormal postnatal cranial imaging of the surviving co-twin (34% and 16%), and neurodevelopmental impairment of the surviving twin (15–26% and 2%) (19). Management of pregnancies complicated by intrauterine death in a twin may be challenging as controversy exists regarding the optimal time of delivery, the frequency of antenatal surveillance, the appropriate investigations to determine cerebral damage and neurological morbidity, and the effects on maternal well-being (both physical and psychological) of retaining one dead fetus. In addition, co-twin demise in monochorionic twins poses a risk of acute TTTS, and resultant anaemia in the surviving fetus and risk of brain injury. To this effect, it is recommended to follow-up the pregnancy with serial MCA PSV measurements to check for fetal anaemia and offer fetal MRI of the brain 4–6 weeks after the event. Such pregnancies should be managed in a tertiary fetal medicine unit and the child would need neurodevelopmental assessment up to 2 years of age (75). A United Kingdom Obstetric Surveillance System (UKOSS) study is currently being undertaken to address to determine the incidence of single twin demise in monochorionic twin pregnancies and the adverse maternal, fetal, and neonatal outcomes (76).

Maternal risks

Compared to women with singleton pregnancies, mothers with multiple pregnancies are at a higher risk of developing pre-eclampsia, other hypertensive disorders in pregnancy, gestational diabetes, and venous thromboembolism. Other conditions such as obstetric cholestasis and acute fatty liver in pregnancy are more common in mothers with multiples than singletons (77). Some epidemiological studies have reported higher rates of long-term cardiovascular events following multiple pregnancy compared to singletons (78). Due to change in haemodynamics, mothers with multiples are at higher risk of pregnancy-related mortality (79, 80).

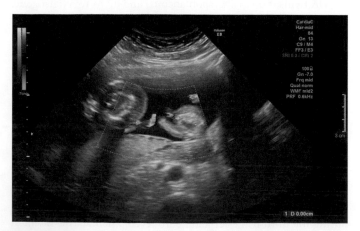

Figure 20.5 Twin reversed arterial perfusion sequence.

NICE guidance recommends blood pressure measurement and testing urine for proteinuria to screen for hypertensive disorders at each antenatal appointment in twin and triplet pregnancies as in routine antenatal care, and for women to take 75 mg of aspirin daily from 12 weeks until delivery if they have one or more of the following risk factors for hypertension: first pregnancy, age 40 years or older, pregnancy interval of more than 10 years, BMI of 35 kg/m² or more at first visit, or family history of pre-eclampsia (11).

Maternal risks should be discussed at the beginning of the pregnancy and appropriate investigations or treatments offered if the risk assessments change over the course of pregnancy.

Preterm labour (prediction, prevention, and treatment)

Multiple pregnancies contribute disproportionately to preterm deliveries. This can be iatrogenic or spontaneous. Overall, 52.2% of twin births deliver before 37 weeks and 10.7% before 32 weeks (81). The neonatal mortality rate of twins is six to seven times that of singleton pregnancies, at 18 per 1000 live births, while neonatal mortality of triplets and higher-order multiple pregnancies reaches 39.6 per 1000 live births. A meta-analysis of observational studies found an increase of preterm birth at less than 37 weeks' gestation in multiple pregnancies conceived through IVF when compared to spontaneous conceptions matched for age and parity (odds ratio: 1.57) (82).

The cause of the high incidence of spontaneous preterm birth in multiple pregnancies is generally attributed to uterine overdistension, precipitating increased myometrial contractility. However, the aetiology is probably more complex. For example, social stress is an important predictor of preterm birth in twin pregnancies (83).

Several factors/tests have been studied as predictors of spontaneous preterm birth in twin and triplet pregnancies, including ultrasonographic cervical length (CL) measurements (one off or serial), fetal fibronectin test, other biomarkers, home uterine activity monitoring, previous history of preterm birth, and a combination of these approaches.

A systematic review of 21 studies comprising 3523 twin pregnancies concluded that transvaginal CL at 20–24 weeks' gestation is a good predictor of spontaneous preterm birth in asymptomatic women with twin pregnancies (84). The NICE guideline recommended that a CL of less than 25 mm at 18–24 weeks' gestation is a good predictor of spontaneous preterm delivery in twin pregnancy and a CL measurement of less than 25 mm at 14–20 weeks' gestation is a good predictor of spontaneous preterm birth in triplet pregnancy (11). A recent study reported serial CL measurements to have a better detection rate (69% vs 28%; $P < 0.001$) and higher positive likelihood ratio (14.54 vs 5.12) for preterm birth at less than 32 weeks' gestation compared with a single measurement of CL (85). However, another recent multicentre, randomized controlled trial of 125 dichorionic or monochorionic/diamniotic twin pregnancies without prior preterm birth at less than 28 weeks showed that routine second-trimester transvaginal ultrasound assessment of CL is not associated with improved outcomes when incorporated into the standard management of otherwise low-risk twin pregnancies (86).

There are emerging data on the association of studies of fetal fibronectin in twin pregnancies and preterm labour. A recent study of 611 women undergoing serial CL measurements including fetal fibronectin showed that in asymptomatic women with twin pregnancies, the CL, fetal fibronectin, and gestational age are all significantly associated with spontaneous preterm birth (87).

Studies have shown that certain biomarkers can be used as predictors of early preterm birth in twins. These include increased concentration of interleukin-8 and matrix metalloproteinase-9 in mid-trimester amniotic fluid (88).

Interventions that have been studied to prevent spontaneous preterm labour, and hence delivery, in twin and triplet pregnancies include bed rest, progesterone (intramuscular or vaginal), cervical cerclage, and tocolytics (oral betamimetics).

A systematic review of five randomized controlled trials evaluating the effectiveness of betamimetics found no evidence to support this intervention to reduce preterm delivery (89). A Cochrane review of 713 women with an uncomplicated twin pregnancy showed that the routine bed rest in hospital for multiple pregnancy did not reduce the risk of preterm birth, or perinatal mortality. In the subgroup analyses for women with an uncomplicated twin pregnancy, with cervical dilation prior to labour with a twin pregnancy and with a triplet pregnancy, no differences were seen in any neonatal outcomes and maternal outcomes (90). A systematic review of six randomized trials of home uterine activity monitoring showed this intervention to be ineffective in predicting spontaneous preterm delivery (91).

Several randomized controlled trials have evaluated the clinical effectiveness of progesterone (intramuscular or vaginal) versus placebo in the prevention of preterm birth in women with twin and triplet pregnancies. None have shown this intervention to be effective (11). A systematic review and meta-analysis of individual patient data from five randomized controlled trials considering the impact of vaginal progesterone in women with asymptomatic short cervix (defined as ≤25 mm on mid-trimester ultrasound) included only 52 twin pregnancies (92). While there was a significant reduction in preterm birth in singleton pregnancy, there was no such effect in twin pregnancies.

A 2014 Cochrane review of five trials, including 128 women, of whom 122 women had twin gestations, and six women had triplet gestations, showed that for multiple gestations, there is no evidence that cerclage is an effective intervention for preventing preterm births and reducing perinatal deaths or neonatal morbidity (93).

More recently, the cervical pessary (Arabin pessary) has been studied in women with a short cervix and while the preliminary results are promising, there are conflicting results from randomized controlled trials showing effectiveness of the Arabin pessary in multiple gestation. A recent randomized controlled trial of 1180 women with twin pregnancy showed no significant differences between the pessary and control groups in rates of spontaneous birth at less than 34 weeks, perinatal death, adverse neonatal outcome, or neonatal therapy. A post hoc subgroup analysis of women with a short cervix (≤25 mm) showed no benefit from the insertion of a cervical pessary (94). However, another well-designed prospective, open-label, multicentre, randomized clinical trial showed that the insertion of a cervical pessary was associated with a significant reduction in the spontaneous preterm birth rate. This trial included 2287 women with twin pregnancy, and showed that the pessary use was associated with a significant reduction in the rate of birthweight less than 2500 g. However, no significant differences were observed in composite neonatal morbidity outcome (95). The results of a third trial on the role of cervical pessary in reduction of preterm birth are awaited (STOPPIT 2) (96).

In the absence of an effective, proven treatment intervention, routine screening to predict preterm delivery is not recommended in twin and triplet pregnancy. There is no evidence to guide management in higher-order pregnancies or for those who have twin and triplet pregnancies and have other risk factors apart from the multiple pregnancy, and therefore this management should be individualized.

Better understanding of the causes, prediction, and prevention of preterm birth in multiple pregnancies should be important research priorities.

Fetal growth and well-being

Fetuses of multiple pregnancies are at increased risk of being small for gestational age and, if there is placental dysfunction, intrauterine growth restricted (IUGR). Both small for gestational age and IUGR fetuses and babies have poorer perinatal outcomes and therefore identifying growth problems is important. Symphysis–fundal height measurement is not effective in identifying growth problems in twin pregnancy, and serial ultrasound scans are required to identify both small babies but also a significant size difference between fetuses (97). There is controversy over using specific twin pregnancy-based charts for plotting ultrasound parameters especially EFW, as there is evidence that there is reduction in the growth velocity in twins compared to singletons (more so in monochorionic twins), especially in the third trimester (98).

From a review of 26 studies assessing ultrasound parameters in multiple pregnancy, NICE concluded that any single fetal biometric parameter is a poor predictor of IUGR or birthweight discordance and an EFW of the tenth centile or less is a moderately useful predictor of IUGR. The guidance proposes that the best cut-off for inter-twin birthweight discordance is an EFW difference of 25% or more, as calculated by the EFW of the larger fetus: EFW of smaller fetus/EFW larger fetus × 100. The guidance recommends that EFW discordance should be calculated using two biometric parameters from 20 weeks' gestation, scans should be undertaken at intervals of less than 28 days, a 25% or greater EFW discordance should be considered significant, and umbilical artery Doppler should not be used to monitor for IUGR or birthweight differences in twin and triplet pregnancies (11). The American College of Obstetricians and Gynecologists considers a difference of 15–25% in the EFW to constitute discordant fetal growth. Based on a consensus of a group of experts in multiple pregnancy, the ISUOG has recently recommended an arbitrary cut-off of 20% for distinguishing pregnancies at increased risk of adverse outcome (19). It must, however, be acknowledged that the discordance cut-off most predictive of adverse outcome is likely to vary with gestational age (99). A United Kingdom-based large cohort study of 2161 twin pregnancies (302 monochorionic and 1859 dichorionic twin pregnancies) showed that both EFW and birthweight discordance are good predictors of adverse outcome (99). The RCOG recommends that growth

discordance should be measured in all monochorionic twin pregnancies at 2-weekly intervals from 16 weeks' gestation onwards and an appropriate referral should be made to the regional fetal medicine unit with expertise in multiple pregnancy if the discordance is 20% or more (3).

Higher-order multiples

Perinatal and maternal risk increases exponentially with increasing fetal number. Every woman/couple with a higher-order multiple pregnancy should have a discussion with a senior obstetrician relating to increased maternal and perinatal risks. This should involve the tactful and sensitive discussion of the option of multiple fetal pregnancy reduction (MFPR). In addition to perinatal mortality rates, parents should be counselled as to the mean gestational age at delivery (33 weeks for triplets, 31 weeks for quadruplets). In addition, 10% of triplets and 25% of quadruplets deliver before 28 weeks' gestation, with severe neurological sequelae rates of 12% and 25% (respectively) in survivors. Higher-order multiple pregnancies should be managed in tertiary perinatal centres with a fetal medicine service (3, 11).

Multifetal pregnancy reduction

To optimize maternal and fetal outcome, MFPR in the first trimester has been recommended. With MFPR, not only are there ethical considerations, but also a significant psychological impact on the parents, including emotional distress, fear, feelings of regret, and guilt. This is often compounded by the fact that the pregnancy is the result of assisted conception and the pregnancy long awaited and much wanted. The consensus views from the RCOG 50th Study Group on multiple pregnancy stated that 'parents of high order multiple pregnancies (≥3) should be counselled and offered MFPR to twins in specialist centres' (3). The procedure is performed between 11 and 14 weeks' gestation as spontaneous reduction may occur before this ('vanishing' fetus) and a detailed scan, including NT measurement to exclude anomalies or features of aneuploidy, may guide selection of fetuses for reduction, aiming to keep the healthiest fetuses.

Recent studies have shown that in dichorionic triamniotic (DCT) and trichorionic triamniotic triplet pregnancies, embryo reduction in the first trimester reduces the risk of preterm birth but increases the risk of miscarriage (100). In the management of dichorionic triamniotic pregnancies, MFPR to dichorionic twins by intrafetal laser is an additional option to the traditional ones of expectant management, embryo reduction by intrafetal injection of potassium chloride to monochorionic twins or embryo reduction by potassium chloride to a singleton (101).

In a recent meta-analysis of five studies, including 331 dichorionic triamniotic triplets, the miscarriage rate was shown to be 8.9% and the severe preterm delivery rate was 33.3% with expectant management; the miscarriage rate was 14.5% with a reduction of the monochorionic pair, 8.8% with a reduction of one fetus of the monochorionic pair, and 23.5% with a reduction of the fetus with a separate placenta. Severe preterm delivery rates were 5.5%, 11.8%, and 17.6%, respectively (102).

Antenatal care for women with a multiple pregnancy

It is recommended that antenatal care to women with a multiple pregnancy should be provided in a dedicated service, whether it be in a clinic staffed by a dedicated multidisciplinary team or delivered by a core team in a specialized model.

Some previous (non-randomized) studies have showed that specialist care might have an impact on some of the important outcomes including fewer women with pre-eclampsia, less preterm birth, fewer low birthweight babies, fewer perinatal deaths, less major neonatal morbidity, and lower infant mortality (103). A Cochrane review of only 162 women with a multiple pregnancy, however, did not show any significant difference in improving maternal and infant health outcomes in women seen in 'specialized' antenatal clinics compared with 'standard' antenatal care (13). A recent retrospective cohort study in 286 women in a single centre showed lower caesarean section rates and fewer late preterm births, in women with antenatal care in a dedicated twins clinic compared to standard care (104).

The United Kingdom NICE guideline recommends that 'clinical care for women with twin and triplet pregnancies should be provided by a nominated multidisciplinary team consisting of a core team of named specialist obstetricians, specialist midwives and ultrasonographers, all of whom have experience and knowledge of managing twin and triplet pregnancies' (11). NICE specifies a schedule of appointments including timing of ultrasound scans depending on whether there are twin or triplets and based on chorionicity and amnionicity (**Table 20.2**). The guidance also covers recommended timing and place of delivery (11).

For higher-order multiple pregnancy, it is recommended that antenatal care should be delivered by fetal medicine specialists and should involve regular serial ultrasound but there is no published literature to guide this care and it would need to be individualized.

Nutritional supplements, diet, and lifestyle advice

A pregnant woman with a multiple pregnancy has a higher metabolic rate compared to a pregnant woman with a singleton pregnancy. However, there are no randomized controlled trials to advise whether specific dietary advice is recommended for women with a multiple pregnancy (105). It needs to be emphasized that women with a multiple pregnancy have a higher incidence of anaemia and it is recommended checking the full blood count at 20–24 weeks' gestation to identify women who may need iron and folic acid supplementation (11). There is no evidence to suggest any advice specific for multiple pregnancy in relation to lifestyle issues, for example, work patterns, sexual activity, and exercise.

Use of corticosteroids

It is well known that antenatal corticosteroids reduce neonatal complications in preterm babies. However, it is better to avoid untargeted routine single or multiple courses of steroids and to advocate targeted steroids when indicated, that is, when preterm labour or birth is imminent, and therefore to shift the focus towards informing all women with twin and triplet pregnancies of the increased risk of preterm birth and the benefits of targeted steroids, and provide information about symptoms and signs to be aware of so that they can present in a timely manner (11).

Planning timing and method of birth

Up to 60% of twins and more triplets and higher-order pregnancies deliver preterm (i.e. before 37 weeks' gestation). For those that are undelivered, appropriate timing of delivery is aimed at optimizing gestation but avoiding stillbirth. For triplets and higher orders, it is rare to get beyond 35 weeks' gestation. Epidemiological studies show that perinatal mortality of twins increases significantly after 37 weeks' gestation. Therefore, for uncomplicated twin pregnancies delivery should be considered from 37 weeks' gestation. A recent systematic review concluded that elective delivery from 36 completed weeks may be the best current strategy to decrease fetal mortality in MCDA twins, and from 37 weeks for uncomplicated dichorionic twins (106).

The United Kingdom NICE guideline recommends delivery of dichorionic twins from 37 completed weeks' gestation, monochorionic twins from 36 completed weeks' gestation, and triplets from 35 weeks' gestation. For monochorionic twin pregnancies

Table 20.2 Schedule for specialist antenatal appointments in multiple pregnancy

Type of multiple pregnancy (uncomplicated)	Minimum contacts with core multidisciplinary team	Timing of appointments plus scans	Additional appointments without scans
MCDA	9[a]	Approximately 11^{+0}–13^{+6} weeks and 16, 18, 20, 22, 24, 28, 32, 34 weeks	–
DCDA	8[a]	Approximately 11^{+0}–13^{+6} weeks and 20, 24, 28, 32, and 36 weeks	16 and 34 weeks
MCTA and DCTA triplets	11[a]	Approximately 11^{+0}–13^{+6} weeks and 16, 18, 20, 22, 24, 26, 28, 30, 32, and 34 weeks	–
DCTA triplets	7[a]	Approximately 11^{+0}–13^{+6} weeks and 20, 24, 28, 32, and 34 weeks	16 weeks

[a] Including two visits with an obstetrician

Source data from National Institute for Health and Clinical Excellence. *Multiple pregnancy: the management of twin and triplet pregnancies in the antenatal period.* (Clinical guideline 129.) 2011. http://www.nice.org.uk/CG129. Last accessed 16 April 2016.

complicated by TTTS, it is reasonable to offer delivery after 34 weeks' gestation. If a monochorionic twin pregnancy is complicated by sIUGR, timing of delivery would be guided by alteration in the pattern of fetal Doppler (ductus venosus) or changes on computerized fetal monitoring (short-term variation or decelerations). If the Doppler pattern remains stable, then delivery can be planned around 34–36 weeks for type I sIUGR and by 32 weeks for types II and III sIUGR (3). It is important to counsel parents that in sIUGR and TTTS (even after apparently successful treatment) there can be acute transfusional events and despite regular monitoring, there may still be adverse perinatal outcomes. For women who decline elective birth, it is recommended to offer weekly appointments with the specialist obstetrician. At each appointment, offer an ultrasound scan, and perform weekly biophysical profile assessments and fortnightly fetal growth scans (3, 11) (**Table 20.2**).

The absolute indications for caesarean section in a multiple pregnancy include monoamniotic twins, conjoined twins and triplets, or higher-order multiples (107). Most clinicians would recommend a caesarean section if the first twin is non-vertex in presentation, due to concerns about locked twins and the associated morbidity and mortality (107, 108).

Care during labour and birth

The Twin Birth Study has clearly shown that *routine* planned elective caesarean section is not advantageous for the fetuses, and this finding applies to both dichorionic and MCDA twins (107). It is, however, important to emphasize that to optimize outcomes, deliveries should be carried out by skilled clinicians, particularly in vaginal breech delivery (if the second twin is non-vertex), and there is access to facilities for emergency caesarean section without delay. The evidence to guide the mode of delivery for preterm twins less than 32 weeks' gestation is not robust and conflicting. There is some evidence to support caesarean section when the fetal weight range is 500–1500 g; however, vaginal delivery is an acceptable practice if the first twin is vertex until more robust data come available (109).

When in labour, there should be one-to-one care with an attending midwife. It is important to ascertain separate fetal heart monitoring, ideally using a cardiotocography machine with twin tracing functions. Indications for delivery by caesarean section when a woman in labour would include usual indications as per NICE intrapartum care guidance for singletons; however, failure to adequately monitor twin 2 or fetal distress would need offering delivery by caesarean section. When in the second stage, the obstetrician and the neonatal team (if there are any concerns about gestation) should be informed. There should be two resuscitaires in the proximity (checked for functioning prior to delivery and switched on and warm). An ultrasound machine should be available, as it would be needed to check the presentation of the second twin after the delivery of the first, and to stabilize fetal lie. Adequate arrangements including oxytocin for the third stage need to be made beforehand as women with multiple pregnancies are at a higher risk of postpartum haemorrhage.

Postnatal care of mother and babies

A survey of experience in pregnancy, labour, and the postnatal period in nearly 26,000 women, of whom 384 delivered twins and 13 delivered triplets, was recently conducted by the National Perinatal Epidemiology Unit, in collaboration with TAMBA and the Multiple Births Foundation (MBF). Results showed that babies delivering as twins or triplets were twice as likely to have an extended neonatal intensive care unit stay compared to singletons and as such, mothers of multiples stayed in hospital for longer. Mothers of multiples were only slightly more likely to report having received practical help with infant feeding. In terms of overall physical health at 3 months or more after the birth, there were no significant differences reported by women who had given birth to a single infant and those who had given birth to twins or triplets. The nationwide survey highlighted the additional needs of postnatal women in particular, mothers of multiples, whose babies are admitted to a neonatal unit following birth. Separation from one or more babies, the need to feed or provide breast milk, and the practical issues associated with discharge home before their infants leave hospital are all aspects of care which can affect women and their babies that need to be taken into account in planning effective care. For parents of multiples there is a need for support with transition to parenthood and early parenting, particularly infant care. The survey recognized the importance of the role of fathers and partners and the need for effective health visitor involvement postnatally for families following multiple birth (110).

Support for women with multiple pregnancy

The risks of multiple pregnancy and the additional elements of antenatal care required to mitigate and identify them can lead to a certain level of anxiety for the woman and her partner/family. It is important to ensure women are given good information, are guided to reputable sources of further information, and have the opportunity to clarify matters that are unclear to them. They should be encouraged to explore socioeconomic issues related to caring for and supporting more than one child. Emotional support becomes paramount when there is a co-twin demise. Various organizations focused on multiple pregnancy including TAMBA, MBF, as well as local support groups including 'twin evenings' in specialist antenatal clinics dedicated to multiple pregnancy can provide much needed support for women with such a high-risk pregnancy.

REFERENCES

1. Royal College of Obstetricians and Gynaecologists. Multiple pregnancy following assisted reproduction. Scientific Impact Paper No. 22. 2011. Available at: https://www.rcog.org.uk/globalassets/documents/guidelines/sip_no_22.pdf (accessed 1 September 2016).
2. Human Fertilisation and Embryology Authority. Fertility treatment 2014 trends and figures. Available at: http://www.hfea.gov.uk/docs/HFEA_Fertility_treatment_Trends_and_figures_2014.pdf (accessed 1 September 2016).
3. Kilby MD, Bricker L, Royal College of Obstetricians and Gynaecologists. Management of monochorionic twin pregnancy. *BJOG* 2017;**124**:e1–45.
4. Braude P (Chair). One child at a time. Reducing multiple births after IVF. Report of the Expert Group on Multiple Births after IVF. 2006. Available at: https://ifqlive.blob.core.windows.net/umbraco-website/1311/one-child-at-a-time-report.pdf.

5. Human Fertilisation and Embryology Authority. Multiple births. Available at: http://www.hfea.gov.uk/docs/Multiple_births_background_and_statistics.pdf.

6. Human Fertilisation and Embryology Authority. Improving outcomes for fertility patients: multiple births. 2011. Available at: https://ifqlive.blob.core.windows.net/umbraco-website/1766/multiple-births-2011.pdf.

7. Martin JAHB, Sutton PD, Ventura SJ, Menacker F, Kirmeyer S. Births: final data for 2004. *Natl Vital Stat Rep* 2006;**55**:26.

8. Human Fertilisation and Embryology Authority. Improving outcomes for fertility patients: multiple births. Available at: https://ifqlive.blob.core.windows.net/umbraco-website/1169/multiple_births_report_2015.pdf.

9. Human Fertilisation and Embryology Authority. Our campaign to reduce multiple births: One at a Time. Available at: https://www.hfea.gov.uk/about-us/our-campaign-to-reduce-multiple-births/.

10. Human Fertilisation and Embryology Authority. Multiple births. What you need to know. Available at: https://ifqlive.blob.core.windows.net/umbraco-website/1315/2017-02-24-multiple-births-leaflet-final.pdf.

11. National Institute for Health and Clinical Excellence (NICE). *Multiple Pregnancy: The Management of Twin and Triplet Pregnancies in the Antenatal Period.* Clinical guideline [CG129]. London: NICE; 2011. Available at: http://www.nice.org.uk/CG129.

12. Centre for Maternal and Child Enquiries (CMACE). *Perinatal Mortality 2009: United Kingdom.* London: CMACE; 2011.

13. Dodd JM, Dowswell T, Crowther CA. Specialised antenatal clinics for women with a multiple pregnancy for improving maternal and infant outcomes. *Cochrane Database Syst Rev* 2015;**11**:CD005300.

14. Hertzberg BS, Kurtz AB, Choi HY, et al. Significance of membrane thickness in the sonographic evaluation of twin gestations. *Am J Roentgenol* 1987;**148**:151–53.

15. Wood SL, St Onge R, Connors G, Elliot PD. Evaluation of the twin peak or lambda sign in determining chorionicity in multiple pregnancy. *Obstet Gynecol* 1996;**88**:6–9.

16. Dias T, Arcangeli T, Bhide A, Napolitano R, Mahsud-Dornan S, Thilaganathan B. First-trimester ultrasound determination of chorionicity in twin pregnancy. *Ultrasound Obstet Gynecol* 2011;**38**:530–32.

17. Senat MV, Quarello E, Levaillant JM, Buonumano A, Boulvain M, Frydman R. Determining chorionicity in twin gestations: three-dimensional (3D) multiplanar sonographic measurement of intra-amniotic membrane thickness. *Ultrasound Obstet Gynecol* 2006;**28**:665–69.

18. Whitworth M, Bricker L, Neilson JP, Dowswell T. Ultrasound for fetal assessment in early pregnancy. *Cochrane Database Syst Rev* 2010;**4**:CD007058.

19. Khalil A, Rodgers M, Baschat A, et al. ISUOG Practice Guidelines: role of ultrasound in twin pregnancy. *Ultrasound Obstet Gynecol* 2016;**47**:247–63.

20. Dias T, Ladd S, Mahsud-Dornan S, Bhide A, Papageorghiou AT, Thilaganathan B. Systematic labeling of twin pregnancies on ultrasound. *Ultrasound Obstet Gynecol* 2011;**38**:130–33.

21. Lewi L, Blickstein I, Van Schoubroeck D, et al. Diagnosis and management of heterokaryotypic monochorionic twins. *Am J Med Genet A* 2006;**140**:272–75.

22. Jenkins TM, Wapner RJ. The challenge of prenatal diagnosis in twin pregnancies. *Curr Opin Obstet Gynecol* 2000;**12**:87–92.

23. Sebire NJ, Snijders RJ, Hughes K, Sepulveda W, Nicolaides KH. Screening for trisomy 21 in twin pregnancies by maternal age and fetal nuchal translucency thickness at 10–14 weeks of gestation. *Br J Obstet Gynaecol* 1996;**103**:999–1003.

24. Sankaran S, Rozette C, Dean J, Kyle P, Spencer K. Screening in the presence of a vanished twin: nuchal translucency or combined screening test? *Prenat Diagn* 2011;**31**:600–601.

25. Prats P, Rodríguez I, Comas C, Puerto B. Systematic review of screening for trisomy 21 in twin pregnancies in first trimester combining nuchal translucency and biochemical markers: a meta-analysis. *Prenat Diagn* 2014;**34**:1077–83.

26. Wald N, Cuckle H, Wu TS, George L. Maternal serum unconjugated oestriol and human chorionic gonadotrophin levels in twin pregnancies: implications for screening for Down's syndrome. *Br J Obstet Gynaecol* 1991;**98**:905–908.

27. Garchet-Beaudron A, Dreux S, Leporrier N, et al. Second-trimester Down syndrome maternal serum marker screening: a prospective study of 11 040 twin pregnancies. *Prenat Diagn* 2008;**28**:1105–109.

28. Taylor-Phillips S, Freeman K, Geppert J, et al. Accuracy of non-invasive prenatal testing using cell-free DNA for detection of Down, Edwards and Patau syndromes: a systematic review and meta-analysis. *BMJ Open* 2016;**6**:e010002.

29. Sarno L, Revello R, Hanson E, Akolekar R, Nicolaides KH. Prospective first-trimester screening for trisomies by cell-free DNA testing of maternal blood in twin pregnancy. *Ultrasound Obstet Gynecol* 2016;**47**:705–11.

30. Curnow KJ, Wilkins-Haug L, Ryan A, et al. Detection of triploid, molar, and vanishing twin pregnancies by a single-nucleotide polymorphism-based noninvasive prenatal test. *Am J Obstet Gynecol* 2015;**212**:79.e1–9.

31. Agarwal K, Alfirevic Z. Pregnancy loss after chorionic villus sampling and genetic amniocentesis in twin pregnancies: a systematic review. *Ultrasound Obstet Gynecol* 2012;**40**:128–34.

32. Gallot D, Vélémir L, Delabaere A, et al. Which invasive diagnostic procedure should we use for twin pregnancies: chorionic villous sampling or amniocentesis? *J Gynecol Obstet Biol Reprod (Paris)* 2009;**38**:S39–44.

33. Evans MI, Goldberg JD, Horenstein J, et al. Selective termination for structural, chromosomal, and mendelian anomalies: international experience. *Am J Obstet Gynecol* 1999;**181**:893–97.

34. Taylor MJ, Fisk NM. Prenatal diagnosis in multiple pregnancy. *Baillieres Best Pract Res Clin Obstet Gynaecol* 2000;**14**:663–75.

35. Millaire M, Bujold E, Morency AM, Gauthier RJ. Mid-trimester genetic amniocentesis in twin pregnancy and the risk of fetal loss. *J Obstet Gynaecol Can* 2006;**28**:512–18.

36. Boklage CE. Survival probability of human conceptions from fertilization to term. *Int J Fertil* 1990;**35**:75, 79–80, 81–94.

37. Hall JG. Twinning. *Lancet* 2003;**362**:735–43.

38. Lewi L, Jani J, Blickstein I, et al. The outcome of monochorionic diamniotic twin gestations in the era of invasive fetal therapy: a prospective cohort study. *Am J Obstet Gynecol* 2008;**199**:514.e1–8.

39. Baxi LV, Walsh CA. Monoamniotic twins in contemporary practice: a single-center study of perinatal outcomes. *J Matern Fetal Neonatal Med* 2010;**23**:506–10.

40. Department of Health. NHS Fetal Anomaly Screening Programme (NHS FASP). Available at: https://www.gov.uk/topic/population-screening-programmes/fetal-anomaly (accessed 1 September 2016).

41. Roman A, Papanna R, Johnson A, et al. Selective reduction in complicated monochorionic pregnancies: radiofrequency ablation vs bipolar cord coagulation. *Ultrasound Obstet Gynecol* 2010;**36**:37–41.

42. van den Bos EM, van Klink JM, Middeldorp JM, Klumper FJ, Oepkes D, Lopriore E. Perinatal outcome after selective feticide in monochorionic twin pregnancies. *Ultrasound Obstet Gynecol* 2013;**41**:653–58.

43. Griffiths PD, Sharrack S, Chan KL, Bamfo J, Williams F, Kilby MD. Fetal brain injury in survivors of twin pregnancies complicated by demise of one twin as assessed by in utero MR imaging. *Prenat Diagn* 2015;**35**:583–91.

44. Ortibus E, Lopriore E, Deprest J, et al. The pregnancy and long-term neurodevelopmental outcome of monochorionic diamniotic twin gestations: a multicenter prospective cohort study from the first trimester onward. *Am J Obstet Gynecol* 2009;**200**:494.e1–8.

45. Lewi L, Gucciardo L, Van Mieghem T, et al. Monochorionic diamniotic twin pregnancies: natural history and risk stratification. *Fetal Diagn Ther* 2010;**27**:121–33.

46. Quintero RA, Morales WJ, Allen MH, Bornick PW, Johnson PK, Kruger M. Staging of twin-twin transfusion syndrome. *J Perinatol* 1999;**19**:550–5.

47. Stagnati V, Zanardini C, Fichera A, et al. Early prediction of twin-to-twin transfusion syndrome: systematic review and meta-analysis. *Ultrasound Obstet Gynecol* 2017;**49**:573–82.

48. Roberts D, Neilson JP, Kilby MD, Gates S. Interventions for the treatment of twin–twin transfusion syndrome. *Cochrane Database Syst Rev* 2014;**1**:CD002073.

49. Senat MV, Deprest J, Boulvain M, Paupe A, Winer N, Ville Y. Endoscopic laser surgery versus serial amnioreduction for severe twin-to-twin transfusion syndrome. *N Engl J Med* 2004;**351**:136–44.

50. Ville Y, Hyett J, Hecher K, Nicolaides K. Preliminary experience with endoscopic laser surgery for severe twin-twin transfusion syndrome. *N Engl J Med* 1995;**332**:224–27.

51. Quintero R, Morales W, Mendoza G, Allen M, Kalter C, Giannina G, Angel J. Selective photocoagulation of placental vessels in twin-twin transfusion syndrome: evolution of a surgical technique. *Obstet Gynecol Surv* 1998;**53**:s97–103.

52. Chalouhi GE, Essaoui M, Stirnemann J, et al. Laser therapy for twin-to-twin transfusion syndrome (TTTS). *Prenat Diagn* 2011;**31**:637–46.

53. Baschat AA, Barber J, Pedersen N, Turan OM, Harman CR. Outcome after fetoscopic selective laser ablation of placental anastomoses vs equatorial laser dichorionization for the treatment of twin-to-twin transfusion syndrome. *Am J Obstet Gynecol* 2013;**209**:234.e1–8.

54. Slaghekke F, Lopriore E, Lewi L, et al. Fetoscopic laser coagulation of the vascular equator versus selective coagulation for twin-to-twin transfusion syndrome: an open-label randomized controlled trial. *Lancet* 2014;**383**:2144–51.

55. Dhillon RK, Hillman SC, Pounds R, Morris RK, Kilby MD. Comparison of Solomon technique against selective laser ablation for twin–twin transfusion syndrome: a systematic review. *Ultrasound Obstet Gynecol* 2015;**46**:526–33.

56. Rossi AC, D'Addario V. Survival outcomes of twin-twin transfusion syndrome stage I: a systematic review of literature. *Am J Perinatol* 2013;**30**:5–10.

57. ClinicalTrials.gov. Randomized Controlled Trial Comparing a Conservative Management and Laser Surgery (TTTS1). NCT01220011. Available at: https://clinicaltrials.gov/ct2/show/NCT 01220011?term=stage+i+twin&rank=1 (accessed 1 September 2016).

58. Twin to Twin Transfusion Syndrome (TTTS) registry. Available at: https://www.medscinet.com/ttts/default.aspx?lang=1 (accessed 1 September 2016).

59. Stirnemann JJ, Mougeot M, Proulx F, et al. Profiling fetal cardiac function in twin-twin transfusion syndrome. *Ultrasound Obstet Gynecol* 2010;**35**:19–27.

60. Ortiz JU, Masoller N, Gómez O, et al. Rate and outcomes of pulmonary stenosis and functional pulmonary atresia in recipient twins with twin-twin transfusion syndrome. *Fetal Diagn Ther* 2017;**41**:191–96.

61. Quarello E, Molho M, Ville Y. Incidence, mechanisms, and patterns of fetal cerebral lesions in twin-to-twin transfusion syndrome. *J Matern Fetal Neonatal Med* 2007;**20**:589–97.

62. Graeve P, Banek C, Stegmann-Woessner G, et al. Neurodevelopmental outcome at 6 years of age after intrauterine laser therapy for twin-twin transfusion syndrome. *Acta Paediatr* 2012;**101**:1200–205.

63. van Klink JM, Slaghekke F, Balestriero MA, et al. Neurodevelopmental outcome at 2 years in twin-twin transfusion syndrome survivors randomized for the Solomon trial. *Am J Obstet Gynecol* 2016;**214**:113.e1–7.

64. Valsky DV, Eixarch E, Martinez JM, Crispi F, Gratacos E. Selective intrauterine growth restriction in monochorionic twins: pathophysiology, diagnostic approach and management dilemmas. *Semin Fetal Neonatal Med* 2010;**15**:342–48.

65. Gratacós E, Lewi L, Muñoz B, et al. A classification system for selective intrauterine growth restriction in monochorionic pregnancies according to umbilical artery Doppler flow in the smaller twin. *Ultrasound Obstet Gynecol* 2007;**30**:28–34.

66. Chalouhi GE, Marangoni MA, Quibel T, et al. Active management of selective intrauterine growth restriction with abnormal Doppler in monochorionic diamniotic twin pregnancies diagnosed in the second trimester of pregnancy. *Prenat Diagn* 2013;**33**:109–15.

67. Slaghekke F, Pasman S, Veujoz M, et al. Middle cerebral artery peak systolic velocity to predict fetal hemoglobin levels in twin anemia-polycythemia sequence. *Ultrasound Obstet Gynecol* 2015;**46**:432–36.

68. Tollenaar LS, Slaghekke F, Middeldorp JM, et al. Twin anemia polycythemia sequence: current views on pathogenesis, diagnostic criteria, perinatal management, and outcome. *Twin Res Hum Genet* 2016;**19**:222–33.

69. Chaveeva P, Poon LC, Sotiriadis A, Kosinski P, Nicolaides KH. Optimal method and timing of intrauterine intervention in twin reversed arterial perfusion sequence: case study and meta-analysis. *Fetal Diagn Ther* 2014;**35**:267–79.

70. Prefumo F, Fichera A, Pagani G, Marella D, Valcamonico A, Frusca T. The natural history of monoamniotic twin pregnancies: a case series and systematic review of the literature. *Prenat Diagn* 2015;**35**:274–80.

71. Hack KE, Derks JB, Schaap AH, et al. Perinatal outcome of monoamniotic twin pregnancies. *Obstet Gynecol* 2009;**113**:353–60.

72. Spitz L, Kiely EM. Conjoined twins. *JAMA* 2003;**289**:1307–10.

73. Pharoah PO, Adi Y. Consequences of in-utero death in a twin pregnancy. *Lancet* 2000;**355**:1597–602.

74. Kilby MD, Govind A, O'Brien PM. Outcome of twin pregnancies complicated by a single intrauterine death: a comparison with viable twin pregnancies. *Obstet Gynecol* 1994;**84**:107–109.

75. Mackie FL, Morris RK, Kilby MD. Fetal brain injury in survivors of twin pregnancies complicated by demise of one twin: a review. *Twin Res Hum Genet* 2016;**19**:262–67.

76. National Perinatal Epidemiology Unit. Single intrauterine fetal death in monochorionic twins. Available at: https://www.npeu.ox.ac.uk/ukoss/current-surveillance/stwin (accessed 1 September 2016).

77. Nelson-Piercy C. *Handbook of Obstetric Medicine*, 5th edn. London: CRC Press; 2015.

78. Sattar N, Greer IA. Pregnancy complications and maternal cardiovascular risk: opportunities for intervention and screening? *BMJ* 2002;**325**:157–60.

79. Cantwell R, Clutton-Brock T, Cooper G, et al. Saving Mothers' Lives: Reviewing maternal deaths to make motherhood safer: 2006–2008. The Eighth Report of the Confidential Enquiries into Maternal Deaths in the United Kingdom. *BJOG* 2011;**118** s1:1–203.

80. Knight M, Tuffnell D, Kenyon S, et al. *Saving Lives, Improving Mothers' Care—Surveillance of Maternal Deaths in the UK 2011–13 and Lessons Learned to Inform Maternity Care from the UK and Ireland Confidential Enquiries into Maternal Deaths and Morbidity 2009–13*. Oxford: National Perinatal Epidemiology Unit, University of Oxford; 2015.

81. Stock S, Norman J. Preterm and term labour in multiple pregnancies. *Semin Fetal Neonatal Med* 2010;**15**:336–41.

82. McDonald S, Murphy K, Beyene J, Ohlsson A. Perinatal outcomes of in vitro fertilization twins: a systematic review and meta-analyses. *Am J Obstet Gynecol* 2005;**193**:141–52.

83. Owen DJ, Wood L, Creed F, Neilson JP. Social stress predicts preterm birth in twin pregnancies. *J Psychosom Obstet Gynaecol* 2017;**38**:63–72.

84. Conde-Agudelo A, Romero R, Hassan SS, Yeo L. Transvaginal sonographic cervical length for the prediction of spontaneous preterm birth in twin pregnancies: a systematic review and metaanalysis. *Am J Obstet Gynecol* 2010,**203**.128.e1–12.

85. Melamed N, Pittini A, Hiersch L, et al. Do serial measurements of cervical length improve the prediction of preterm birth in asymptomatic women with twin gestations? *Am J Obstet Gynecol* 2016;**215**:616.e1–14.

86. Gordon MC, McKenna DS, Stewart TL, et al. Transvaginal cervical length scans to prevent prematurity in twins: a randomized controlled trial. *Am J Obstet Gynecol* 2016;**214**:277.e1–7.

87. Spiegelman J, Booker W, Gupta S, et al. The independent association of a short cervix, positive fetal fibronectin, amniotic fluid sludge, and cervical funneling with spontaneous preterm birth in twin pregnancies. *Am J Perinatol* 2016;**33**:1159–64.

88. Lee SM, Park JS, Norwitz ER, et al. Mid-trimester amniotic fluid pro-inflammatory biomarkers predict the risk of spontaneous preterm delivery in twins: a retrospective cohort study. *J Perinatol* 2015;**35**:542–46.

89. Yamasmit W, Chaithongwongwatthana S, Tolosa JE, Limpongsanurak S, Pereira L, Lumbiganon P. Prophylactic oral betamimetics for reducing preterm birth in women with a twin pregnancy. *Cochrane Database Syst Rev* 2015;**12**:CD004733.

90. Crowther CA, Han S. Hospitalisation and bed rest for multiple pregnancy. *Cochrane Database Syst Rev* 2010;7:CD000110.

91. Colton T, Kayne HL, Zhang Y, Heeren T. A metaanalysis of home uterine activity monitoring. *Am J Obstet Gynecol* 1995;**173**:1499–505.

92. Romero R, Nicolaides K, Conde-Agudelo A, et al. Vaginal progesterone in women with an asymptomatic sonographic short cervix in the midtrimester decreases preterm delivery and neonatal morbidity: a systematic review and metaanalysis of individual patient data. *Am J Obstet Gynecol* 2012;**206**:124.e1–19.

93. Rafael TJ, Berghella V, Alfirevic Z. Cervical stitch (cerclage) for preventing preterm birth in multiple pregnancy. *Cochrane Database Syst Rev* 2014;**9**:CD009166.

94. Nicolaides KH, Syngelaki A, Poon LC, et al. Cervical pessary placement for prevention of preterm birth in unselected twin pregnancies: a randomized controlled trial. *Am J Obstet Gynecol* 2016;**214**:3.e1–9.

95. Goya M, de la Calle M, Pratcorona L, et al. Cervical pessary to prevent preterm birth in women with twin gestation and sonographic short cervix: a multicenter randomized controlled trial (PECEP-Twins). *Am J Obstet Gynecol* 2016;**214**:145–52.

96. STOPPIT-2: An open randomised trial of the Arabin pessary to prevent preterm birth in twin pregnancy, with health economics and acceptability. https://w3.abdn.ac.uk/hsru/STOPPIT2/ (accessed 1 September 2016).

97. Neilson JP, Verkuyl DAA, Bannerman C. Tape measurement of symphysis-fundal height in twin pregnancies. *Br J Obstet Gynaecol* 1988;**95**:1054–59.

98. Stirrup OT, Khalil A, D'Antonio F, Thilaganathan B, Southwest Thames Obstetric Research Collaborative (STORK). Fetal growth reference ranges in twin pregnancy: analysis of the Southwest Thames Obstetric Research Collaborative (STORK) multiple pregnancy cohort. *Ultrasound Obstet Gynecol* 2015;**45**:301–307.

99. D'Antonio F, Khalil A, Dias T, Thilaganathan B, Southwest Thames Obstetric Research Collaborative (STORK). Weight discordance and perinatal mortality in twins: analysis of the Southwest Thames Obstetric Research Collaborative (STORK) multiple pregnancy cohort. *Ultrasound Obstet Gynecol* 2013;**41**:643–48.

100. Chaveeva P, Kosinski P, Puglia D, Poon LC, Nicolaides KH. Trichorionic and dichorionic triplet pregnancies at 10–14 weeks: outcome after embryo reduction compared to expectant management. *Fetal Diagn Ther* 2013;**34**:199–205.

101. Chaveeva P, Kosinski P, Birdir C, Orosz L, Nicolaides KH. Embryo reduction in dichorionic triplets to dichorionic twins by intrafetal laser. *Fetal Diagn Ther* 2014;**35**:83–86.

102. Morlando M, Ferrara L, D'Antonio F, et al. Dichorionic triplet pregnancies: risk of miscarriage and severe preterm delivery with fetal reduction versus expectant management. Outcomes of a cohort study and systematic review. *BJOG* 2015;**122**:1053–60.

103. Bricker L. Optimal antenatal care for twin and triplet pregnancy: the evidence base. *Best Pract Res Clin Obstet Gynaecol* 2014;**28**:305–17.

104. Henry A, Lees N, Bein KJ, et al. Pregnancy outcomes before and after institution of a specialised twins clinic: a retrospective cohort study. *BJOG* 2015;**122**:1053–60.

105. Bricker L, Reed K, Wood L, Neilson JP. Nutritional advice for improving outcomes in multiple pregnancies. *Cochrane Database Syst Rev* 2015;**11**:CD008867.

106. Cheong-See F, Schuit E, Arroyo-Manzano D, et al. Prospective risk of stillbirth and neonatal complications in twin pregnancies: systematic review and meta-analysis. *BMJ* 2016;**354**:i4353.

107. Barrett JFR. Twin delivery: method, timing and conduct. *Best Pract Res Clin Obstet Gynaecol* 2014;**28**:327–38.

108. Hannah ME, Hannah WJ, Hewson SA, Hodnett ED, Saigal S, Willan AR. Planned caesarean section versus planned vaginal birth for breech presentation at term: a randomised multicentre trial. Term Breech Trial Collaborative Group. *Lancet* 2000;**356**:1375–83.

109. Barrett, JF, Hannah ME, Hutton EK, et al. A randomized trial of planned cesarean or vaginal birth for twin pregnancies. *N Engl J Med* 2013;**369**:1295–305.

110. Redshaw M, Henderson J, Kurinczuk JJ. *Maternity Care for Women Having a Multiple Birth*. Oxford: National Perinatal Epidemiology Unit; 2011.

21

Hypertension

Laura A. Magee and Peter von Dadelszen

Introduction

Globally, the hypertensive disorders of pregnancy (HDPs) remain significant causes of maternal and perinatal morbidity and death (1–3), with lifelong health implications for surviving mothers and their infants (4–10). While estimated to cause 30,000 maternal deaths annually (1), unpublished verbal autopsy data from Pakistan suggest that the root cause of an estimated 40% of the 40,000 maternal deaths currently ascribed to postpartum haemorrhage was pre-eclampsia (identified by symptoms), presumably complicated by disseminated intravascular coagulation that, in turn, may have been precipitated by abruption. In addition, it is estimated that 2 million fetuses, neonates, and infants die annually in association with pregnancy complicated by pregnancy hypertension (11).

While approximately 99% of HDP-related deaths occur in less developed countries (12), failures and delays in triage, transport, and treatment commonly precede maternal death in all settings (13). Therefore, an understanding of the diagnosis and management of the HDP is central to the provision of safe and effective maternity care (14, 15).

Diagnosis

In the authors' opinion, the cornerstone of care for women with suspected or confirmed pregnancy hypertension is making an accurate diagnosis of both hypertension and/or proteinuria. To place these diagnostic tests in context a brief review of cardiovascular adaptations to pregnancy is required (16).

The major haemodynamic changes of pregnancy include an increase in sodium and water retention leading to blood volume expansion, an increase in cardiac output, and reductions in both systemic vascular resistance and systemic blood pressure (BP). Beginning in early pregnancy, these changes reach their sustained peak during the second trimester, remaining relatively constant until delivery. While plasma volume expands by approximately 50%, the red cell mass increases by 40%, resulting in the physiological anaemia of pregnancy. Women who are destined to develop pre-eclampsia may not have the mid-trimester fall in BP and have relative haemoconcentration.

Measurement of blood pressure

The definition of hypertension in pregnancy is a challenging task because BP levels in pregnancy are dynamic, have a circadian rhythm, and change by gestational age (16). Therefore, the diagnosis of pregnancy hypertension should be based on outpatient clinic or in-hospital BP measurements. This mirrors recommendations by general hypertension guidelines outside pregnancy, such as those of the Canadian Hypertension Education Program (17).

The accepted definition is a diastolic BP (DBP) of at least 90 mmHg and/or a sustained systolic BP (SBP) of at least 140 mmHg by repeated measurements in the same arm until a steady BP reading is achieved (15, 17, 18), rather than the historical definition of 4 or more hours apart. There is less certainty about a diagnosis of hypertension based on only SBP between 140 and 159 mmHg, as opposed to DBP criteria.

Severe hypertension should be defined, in any setting, as a SBP of at least 160 mmHg or a DBP of at least 110 mmHg based on the average of at least two measurements, repeated either until steady readings are achieved or at least 15 minutes apart, using the same arm (15, 19).

Isolated office ('white coat') hypertension is defined as an outpatient clinic SBP of at least 140 mmHg or a DBP of at least 90 mmHg, but an ambulatory BP monitoring (ABPM) or home BP monitoring (HBPM) SBP less than 135 mmHg and DBP less than 85 mmHg (15). In contrast, a normal office BP with elevated ABPM or HBPM ('masked hypertension') should be defined as an outpatient clinic SBP less than 140 mmHg or a DBP less than 90 mmHg, but an ABPM or HBPM SBP of at least 135 mmHg or DBP of at least 85 mmHg (15).

There are several issues of consideration specific to the measurement of BP during pregnancy. The technique should be standardized, as it should be outside pregnancy. BP can be measured using validated and calibrated auscultatory (mercury or aneroid devices) or automated methods. Factors to consider when selecting a BP measurement device include validation, disease specificity, observer error, and the need for regular recalibration (20).

Validation of BP devices is a process by which the accuracy of a device is assessed, over a range of BP readings, on several occasions and for women with different HDPs. Observer error (e.g. terminal digit preference to numbers ending in '0' and '5') can be eliminated by automated BP measurement devices. Calibration involves comparing readings from an aneroid or automated BP machine with those taken with a mercury manometer. Only some devices have been validated in pre-eclampsia (Dinamap ProCare 400, Microlife 3AS1-2, Microlife 3BTO-A, Nissei DS-400, Omron-MIT, and Omron-MIT Elite) (18, 21–25). Most other automated devices will tend to underestimate both SBP and DBP by 5–15 mmHg—a systematic error that places women at risk.

There are three categories of BP monitoring methods: (a) office BP measurement, (b) ABPM, and (c) HBPM (15, 17). In the past two decades, both ABPM and HBPM have gained popularity in confirming diagnosis and improving BP monitoring, compliance with antihypertensive medication, and achievement of BP targets. Evidence from cross-sectional studies shows that HBPM and ABPM have modest diagnostic agreement and they are similar in identifying patients with 'white coat' effect and 'masked' hypertension. However, HBPM offers some advantages. HBPM is economical, comfortable, engages the patient, and is easy to repeat when disease evolution is suspected, a particularly important issue in pregnancy. Also, pregnant women and practitioners prefer HBPM to ABPM. There is an important cautionary note about HBPM, however; HBPM values have not been validated against adverse pregnancy outcomes, and, to date, no randomized trial has assessed the impact of either HBPM or ABPM on maternal or perinatal outcomes.

However determined, a diagnosis of hypertension in pregnancy in a community setting is consistent with a daytime ABPM or average HBPM of SBP of at least 135 mmHg or DBP of at least 85 mmHg (15).

As stated previously, less developed countries bear a disproportionate burden of maternal morbidity and mortality from the HDP. While regular BP monitoring can cost-effectively reduce this disparity, less developed country health systems face unique challenges which reduce this capacity (26–39). Continued efforts to address these challenges through implementation and evaluation of interventions informed by robust needs assessments is urgently needed to strengthen the capacity of health systems to provide good maternity care and reduce maternal and neonatal outcome disparities in less developed countries.

Measurement of proteinuria

In the authors' opinion, all pregnant women should be assessed for proteinuria, at minimum, at their first antenatal visit, and it should repeated, if not at every antenatal visit, whenever either hypertension is detected or symptoms suggestive of pre-eclampsia are declared (14, 15). Urinary dipstick testing (or sulphosalicylic acid (SSA) or heat coagulation testing if dipsticks are not available) may be used to screen for proteinuria when the suspicion of pre-eclampsia is low, and significant proteinuria should be strongly suspected when urinary dipstick proteinuria is 2+ or greater (14, 15).

Definitive testing for proteinuria (by urinary protein:creatinine ratio or 24-hour urine collection) is encouraged when there is a suspicion of pre-eclampsia, with significant proteinuria defined as at least 0.3g/day in a complete 24-hour urine collection or at least 30 mg/mmol (≥0.3 mg/mg) urinary creatinine in a random urine sample. It should be remembered that 24-hour urine collections are prone to both under- and over-collection approximately half of the time, with even splitting between under- and over-collections (40). Although increasingly used outside pregnancy, currently there is insufficient information to make a recommendation about the accuracy of the urinary albumin:creatinine ratio, although values less than 2 mg/mmol (<18 mg/g) are normal and all values equal or greater than 8 mg/mmol (≥71 mg/g) are elevated (41).

In well-resourced settings with sophisticated fetal monitoring, proteinuria testing does not need to be repeated once the significant proteinuria of pre-eclampsia has been confirmed (19); while in under-resourced settings, proteinuria testing can be repeated to detect 4+ dipstick proteinuria that increases the risk of stillbirth (42, 43).

Classification

During pregnancy, it is important to detect hypertension of any sort, as pregnancy hypertension is associated with increased maternal and perinatal risks. However, not all HDPs carry the same level of risk for women and their babies. Therefore, the classification of the HDPs into pre-existing (chronic) hypertension, gestational hypertension, pre-eclampsia, and 'other' hypertension matters (**Tables 21.1 and 21.2**). Reducing the rates of false-positive and false-negative classification relative to current standard of care should help to better target healthcare spending and lowers overall costs associated with the care of women with pre-eclampsia (44). In the authors' opinion, the term PIH (pregnancy-induced hypertension) should be abandoned, as its meaning in clinical practice is unclear. In some places, PIH means pre-eclampsia, in others it means gestational hypertension without proteinuria, while in others it means both (14, 15).

Although classification of the HDPs is usually straightforward in higher-income countries, this may not be the case in settings where late gestational age at booking is prevalent, and the final diagnosis may only be possible at 6–12 weeks postpartum. Also, as it is critical to identify women who require delivery, the only cure for pre-eclampsia, we endorse the Canadian approach of defining 'severe' pre-eclampsia according to the presence of severe complications that mandate delivery (14, 15).

Healthcare providers should inform pregnant and recently pregnant women about pre-eclampsia, its signs and symptoms, and the importance of timely reporting of symptoms to healthcare providers. Information should be re-emphasized at subsequent visits.

For women with pre-existing hypertension, serum creatinine, fasting blood glucose, serum potassium, and urinalysis should be performed in early pregnancy if not previously documented. Among women with pre-existing hypertension or those with a strong clinical risk marker for pre-eclampsia, additional baseline laboratory testing may be based on other considerations deemed important by healthcare providers.

The presence or absence of pre-eclampsia must be ascertained, given its clear association with more adverse maternal and perinatal outcomes. Tools have been developed that are available in all settings to facilitate identification of women at highest risk of adverse outcomes: the diagnosis of pre-eclampsia and to provide women with a management strategy that has been shown to improve maternal and perinatal outcomes (**Figure 21.1**) (45, 46). Such tools are

Table 21.1 Classification of the hypertensive disorders of pregnancy

	Comments
Pre-existing (chronic) hypertension	
	This is defined as hypertension that was present either prepregnancy or that develops at <20^{+0} weeks gestation
With comorbid conditions(s)	Comorbid conditions (e.g. pre-gestational type 1 or 2 diabetes mellitus or kidney disease) warrant tighter BP control outside of pregnancy because of their association with heightened cardiovascular risk
With evidence of pre-eclampsia	This is also known as 'superimposed pre-eclampsia' and is defined by the development of one or more of the following at ≥20 weeks: • Resistant hypertension, *or* • New or worsening proteinuria, *or* • One/more adverse condition(s),[a] *or* • One/more severe complication(s)[a]
	Severe pre-eclampsia is defined as pre-eclampsia with one or more severe complication(s)
Gestational hypertension	
	This is defined as hypertension that develops for the first time at ≥20^{+0} weeks' gestation
With comorbid conditions(s)	Comorbid conditions (e.g. pregestational type 1 or 2 diabetes mellitus or kidney disease) warrant tighter BP control outside of pregnancy because of their association with heightened cardiovascular risk
With evidence of pre-eclampsia	Evidence of pre-eclampsia may appear weeks after the onset of gestational hypertension
Pre-eclampsia	
	Pre-eclampsia may arise *de novo*. It is defined by gestational hypertension and one or more of the following: • New proteinuria, *or* • One/more adverse condition(s),[a] *or* • One/more severe complication(s)[a]
	Severe pre-eclampsia is defined as pre-eclampsia with one or more severe complication(s)
'Other hypertensive effects'[b]	
Transient hypertensive effect	Elevated BP may be due to environmental stimuli or the pain of labour, for example
White coat hypertensive effect	BP that is elevated in the office (SBP ≥140 mmHg or DBP ≥90 mmHg) but is consistently normal outside of the office (<135/85 mmHg) by ABPM or HBPM
Masked hypertension effect	BP that is consistently normal in the office (SBP <140 mmHg or DBP <90 mmHg) but is elevated outside of the office (≥135/85 mmHg) by ABPM or repeated HBPM

ABPM, ambulatory BP monitoring; BP, blood pressure; DBP, diastolic BP; HBPM, home BP monitoring, SBP, systolic blood pressure after monitoring.

[a] Please see Table 21.2 for definitions of adverse conditions and severe complications of pre-eclampsia.

[b] These may occur in women whose BP is elevated at <20^{+0} or ≥20^{+0} weeks who are suspected at having pre-existing or gestational hypertension/pre-eclampsia, respectively.

Source data from *The FIGO Textbook of Pregnancy Hypertension* (2016) p34.

Table 21.2 Defining adverse conditions and severe pre-eclampsia

Organ system affected	Adverse conditionals (that increase the risk of severe complications)	Severe complications (that warrant delivery)
CNS	Headache/visual symptoms	Eclampsia PRES Cortical blindness or retinal detachment Glasgow coma scale <13 Stroke, TIA, or RIND
Cardiorespiratory	Chest pain/dyspnoea Oxygen saturation <97%	Uncontrolled severe hypertension (over a period of 12 h despite use of three antihypertensive agents) Oxygen saturation <90%, need for ≥50% oxygen for > 1 h, intubation (other than for caesarean section), pulmonary oedema Positive inotopic support Myocardial ischaemia or infarction
Haematological	Elevated WBC count Elevated INR or APTT Low platelet count	Platelet count <50 × 10^9/L Transfusion of any blood product
Renal	Elevated serum creatinine Elevated serum uric acid	Acute kidney injury (creatinine > 150μM with no prior renal disease) New indication for dialysis
Hepatic	Nausea or vomiting RUQ or epigastric pain Elevated serum AST, ALT, LDH, or bilirubin Low plasma albumin	Hepatic dysfunction (INR >2 in absence of DIC or warfarin/coumarin) Hepatic haematoma or rupture
Fetoplacental	Non-reassuring FHR IUGR Oligohydramnios Absent or reversed end-diastolic flow by Doppler velocimetry	Abruption with evidence of maternal or fetal compromise Reverse ductus venosus A wave Stillbirth

ALT, alanine aminotransferase; AST, aspartate aminotransferase; APTT, activated partial thromboplastin time; CNS, central nervous system; DIC, disseminated intravascular coagulation; FHR, fetal heart rate; INR, international normalized ratio; IUGR, intrauterine growth restriction; LDH, lactate dehydrogenase; PRES, posterior reversible leucoencephalopathy syndrome; RIND, reversible neurological deficit <48 hours; RUQ, right upper quadrant; TIA, transient ischaemic attack

Source data from *The FIGO Textbook of Pregnancy Hypertension* (2016) p38.

the miniPIERS (Pre-eclampsia Integrated Estimate of RiSk) outcome prediction model/tool for under-resourced settings and the fullPIERS model for well-resourced settings; both of which are optimized by pulse oximetry and can be accessed online or as mobile health applications (42, 43, 47–51). In resource-constrained settings, the miniPIERS model can provide personalized risk estimation for women with any HDP.

In women with pre-existing hypertension, pre-eclampsia should be defined as resistant hypertension, new or worsening proteinuria, one or more adverse conditions, or one or more severe complications. Similarly, in women with gestational hypertension, pre-eclampsia should be defined as new-onset proteinuria, one or more adverse conditions, or one or more severe complications. The assessment of maternal angiogenic factor balance appears to inform the diagnosis of pre-eclampsia, and other placental complications of pregnancy, where uncertainty exists, especially when 'superimposed pre-eclampsia' is suspected (52–55). In particular, placental growth factor is useful in delineating progression to pre-eclampsia in women with pre-existing hypertension and renal disease (56). However, how to integrate angiogenic balance into the management

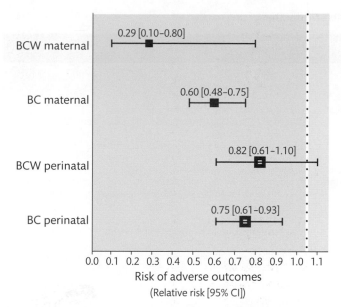

Figure 21.1 Reducing the rate of adverse maternal and perinatal outcomes using standardized care.

of women with suspected or confirmed pre-eclampsia remains to be determined.

Severe pre-eclampsia should be defined as pre-eclampsia complicated by one or more severe complications (**Table 21.2**). Previous paradigms defining 'severe' pre-eclampsia have mixed items that increase the risks of adverse events and those events themselves, and were largely poorly predictive of adverse maternal events when tested in the PIERS dataset (57). The criteria listed here delineate between adverse conditions that should increase surveillance and lower thresholds to deliver a woman and those criteria that mandate delivery irrespective of gestational age.

Women with suspected pre-eclampsia should undergo the maternal laboratory and a schedule of pertinent fetal testing as described in **Table 21.3**. If initial testing is reassuring, maternal and fetal testing should be repeated if there is ongoing concern about pre-eclampsia (e.g. change in maternal and/or fetal condition). For women being managed as outpatients for whom there is either concern about pre-eclampsia or the diagnosis of pre-eclampsia has been confirmed, that testing should occur at least once every week, and once women have been admitted due to either maternal and/or fetal concerns, twice weekly. This twice-weekly paradigm with testing at least as frequently as on admission, the day after admission, on Mondays and Thursdays, the day of delivery, and the day after delivery was associated with an 80% reduction in the incidence of severe adverse events in a single institutional study (45).

Doppler velocimetry-based assessment of the fetal circulation, complemented by maternal fetal movement awareness and fetal heart rate assessment, may be useful to support a placental origin for hypertension, proteinuria, and/or adverse conditions (including intrauterine growth restriction), and for timing of delivery (10, 58–62). However, the biophysical profile is not recommended as part of a schedule of fetal testing in women with a HDP as it appears to falsely reassure practitioners, as it does with intrauterine growth restriction (59–61).

Prediction of pre-eclampsia

Here, we review the risk factors for pre-eclampsia but focus more on the predictors of pre-eclampsia and, to a lesser extent, other placental complications of pregnancy, especially gestational hypertension and intrauterine growth restriction. Early prediction of pre-eclampsia will aid in identifying women at highest risk, allow for preventive interventions such as low-dose aspirin, and guide surveillance to avoid severe complications. Clinically relevant predictors of pre-eclampsia are presented in **Table 21.4**.

The strongest risk factors for pre-eclampsia include previous pre-eclampsia, antiphospholipid antibody syndrome, pre-existing medical conditions, and multiple pregnancy (**Table 21.4**). In the authors' opinion, all women should be screened for clinical risk markers of pre-eclampsia from early pregnancy, recognizing that there is no single predictor of pre-eclampsia among women at either low or increased risk of pre-eclampsia that is ready for introduction into clinical practice. The most promising predictors are the angiogenic factors and uterine artery Doppler velocimetry combined with other biochemical factors using multivariate models (2, 3, 15, 63–66).

However, it should be stated that very little of the informative data have been derived from populations of women who bear the greatest of experiencing complications of pre-eclampsia, namely women in less developed countries (14).

Consultation with an obstetrician or an obstetric internist/physician should be offered to women with a history of previous pre-eclampsia or another strong clinical marker of increased pre-eclampsia risk, particularly multiple pregnancy, antiphospholipid antibody syndrome, significant proteinuria at booking, or a pre-existing condition of hypertension, diabetes mellitus, or renal disease (14, 15).

Prevention of pre-eclampsia

There is a considerable literature devoted to the prevention of pre-eclampsia with the intention of avoiding the associated maternal and perinatal complications. However, preeclampsia, at least in its non-severe form, may serve some adaptive function in terms of improved neonatal outcomes in the neonatal intensive care unit or neurodevelopmental outcome (67, 68).

Therefore, we have based our preventative recommendations on both the prevention of pre-eclampsia and/or the prevention of its associated complications where the literature permits. Preventative interventions may be best started before 16 weeks' when most of the physiological transformation of uterine spiral arteries occurs, or even before pregnancy. Such early intervention has the greatest potential to decrease the early forms of pre-eclampsia that are associated with incomplete transformation of uterine spiral arteries (69).

Pregnant women can be classified as being at 'low' or 'increased' risk of pre-eclampsia most commonly by the presence or absence of one or more of the risk markers (**Table 21.4**). Widespread implementation of the following interventions is recommended to help prevent pre-eclampsia and its complications (15, 19).

Table 21.3 Investigations to diagnose and monitor women with a hypertensive disorder of pregnancy

Investigations for diagnosis	Description in women with pre-eclampsia	Description in women with other conditions
Maternal testing		
Uterine testing		
Urinalysis (routine and microscopy with/without additional tests for proteinuria)	Proteinuria (as discussed under *Proteinuria*) without RBCs or casts	Haemoglobinuria (dipstick 'haematuria' without RBCs): haemolytic anaemia RBCs alone: renal stones, renal cortical necrosis (also associated with back pain and oliguria/anuria) RBCs and/or casts are associated with other glomerular disease and scleroderma renal crisis and (about half of) TTP-HUS Bacteria: UTI or asymptomatic bacteriuria Proteinuria is usually absent in secondary causes of hypertension such as phaeochromocytoma, hyperaldosteronism, thyrotoxicosis, coarctation of the aorta, and withdrawal syndromes
Oxygen saturation		
Pulse oximetry	SpO_2 <97% associated with a heightened risk of severe complications (including non-respiratory)	May be decreased in any cardiorespiratory complication (e.g. pulmonary embolism)
CBC and blood film		
Haemoglobin	↑ due to intravascular volume depletion ↓ if microangiopathic haemolysis (with HELLP)	↑ due to volume depletion from any cause (e.g. vomiting ↓ if microangiopathic haemolysis from other cause ↓ with any chronic anaemia (nutritional or myelodysplasia) ↓ with acute bleeding of any cause
WBC and differential	↔	↑ due to neutrophilia of normal pregnancy ↑ with inflammation/infection ↑ with corticosteroids
Platelet count	↓ associated with adverse maternal outcome	↓ with gestational, immune (ITP), or thrombotic thrombocytopenia (TTP), APS, AFLP, myelodysplasia
Blood film	RBC fragmentation	Microangiopathy due to mechanical causes (e.g. cardiac valvopathy, cavernous haemangioma), DIC or other disorders of endothelial function (e.g. APS, TTP-HUS, vasculitis, malignant hypertension)
Tests of coagulation		
INR and APTT	↑ with DIC which is usually associated with placental abruption ↑ is associated with adverse maternal outcome	May be ↑ in APS, DIC from other causes including sepsis, amniotic fluid embolism, stillbirth, massive haemorrhage, haemangiomas, shock ↑ is prominent in AFLP
Fibrinogen	↔	↓ with all causes of DIC including massive haemorrhage, genetic disorders ↓ more profound with AFLP than with HELLP Usually normal in TTP-HUS (ADAMTS13 vWF cleaving protein may be moderately decreased in HELLP but ADAMTS13 antibody should be absent
Serum chemistry		
Serum creatinine	↑ due to haemoconcentration and/or renal failure ↑ associated with adverse maternal outcome	↑ with other acute or chronic kidney disease. Rental failure prominent in malignant hypertension, TTP-HUS (along with thrombocytopenia), AFLP (along with liver dysfunction)
Serum uric acid	↑ associated with adverse maternal and perinatal outcomes	↑ with dehydration, medication (e.g. HCTZ), genetic causes
Glucose	↔	↓ with AFLP, insulin therapy
AST or ALT	↑ associated with adverse maternal outcome	↑ with AFLP and other 'PET imitators' but to a lesser degree, and usually normal in TTP-HUS
		May be increased in other pregnancy-related conditions (e.g. intrahepatic cholestasis of pregnancy) or conditions not associated with pregnancy (e.g. viral hepatitis or cholecystitis)
LDH	↑ which may be prominent	↑ with AFLP, intravascular haemolysis
	↑ the is associated with adverse maternal outcome	↑ LDH, AST ratio (>22) with TTP-HUS

(continued)

Table 21.3 Continued

Investigations for diagnosis	Description in women with pre-eclampsia	Description in women with other conditions
Bilirubin	↑ unconjugated from haemolysis or conjugated from liver dysfunction	(early) ↑ in AFLP, ↑ with haemolytic anaemia, other liver disease with dysfunction, genetic disease
Albumin	↓ associated with adverse maternal and perinatal outcomes	↓ as negative acute phase reactant with acute severe illness, malnutrition, nephrotic syndrome, crystalloid infusion
Fetal testing		
	Abnormalities are not specific to the cause of poor placentation and/or placental dysfunction	
Uterine artery Doppler velocimetry	Unilateral/bilateral notching, or elevated pulsatility index or resistance index may support a diagnosis of placental insufficiency including pre-eclampsia	

AFLP, acute fatty liver of pregnancy; APS, antiphospholipid syndrome; APTT, activated partial thromboplastin time; CBC, complete blood count; DIC, disseminated intravascular coagulation; HCTZ, hydrochlorothiazide; HUS, haemolytic uraemic syndrome; INR, international normalized ratio; ITP, immune thrombocytopenic purpura; PET, pre-eclampsia; SpO$_2$, oxygen saturation by pulse oximetry; RBC, red blood cell; TTP, thrombotic thrombocytopenic purpura; vWF, von Willebrand factor.
Source data from *The FIGO Textbook of Pregnancy Hypertension* (2016) p42–43.

Prevention of pre-eclampsia in women at low risk

Calcium supplementation (of at least 500 mg/day, orally) is recommended for women with a low dietary intake of calcium (<600 mg/day, corresponding to less than two dairy servings per day) (19, 70–72). While periconceptual and ongoing use of a folate-containing multivitamin, and exercise may be useful, the following are not recommended: dietary salt restriction during pregnancy, calorie restriction during pregnancy for overweight women, low-dose aspirin, vitamins C and E, and thiazide diuretics (14, 15).

There is insufficient evidence to make a recommendation about the following: a heart-healthy diet, workload or stress reduction, supplementation with iron with/without folate, pyridoxine, or foods rich in flavonoids (14, 15).

Prevention of pre-eclampsia in women at increased risk

In women deemed to be at high risk of pre-eclampsia, the following are recommended for its prevention: low-dose aspirin and calcium supplementation (of at least 500 mg/day) for women with low calcium intake (14, 15, 70–72). Low-dose aspirin (75–150 mg/day) should be administered at bedtime, initiated after the diagnosis of pregnancy but before 16 weeks' gestation, and may be continued until delivery. In addition, the following may be useful: L-arginine, metformin in women with polycystic ovarian syndrome and/or overweight women, increased rest at home in the third trimester, and reduction of workload or stress (14, 15).

The following are not recommended: calorie restriction in overweight women during pregnancy, weight maintenance in obese women during pregnancy, antihypertensive therapy specifically to prevent pre-eclampsia, and vitamins C and E (14, 15). Following the results of the Thrombophilia in Pregnancy Prophylaxis Study (TIPPS) trial (73), the chapter authors do not believe that prophylactic doses of low-molecular-weight heparin should be considered in women with previous placental complications (including pre-eclampsia) to prevent the recurrence of 'severe' or early-onset pre-eclampsia, preterm delivery, and/or small-for-gestational age infants. Low-molecular-weight heparin retains a role in the management of women with antiphospholipid syndrome (14, 15).

There is insufficient evidence to make a recommendation about the usefulness of the following: the heart-healthy diet, exercise, selenium, garlic, zinc, pyridoxine, iron (with or without folate), or multivitamins with/without micronutrients (14, 15).

Diet, lifestyle, and place of care

Non-pharmacological management of women with a HDP involves consideration of dietary interventions, lifestyle and place of care. There is scant literature on the role of dietary interventions or lifestyle change (including bed rest and stress reduction) for women with an established HDP; the limited literature has focused on these practices as preventative measures against pre-eclampsia (15, 19). As such, the bulk of this section focuses on place of care, including transport from community to facility. In particular, there is enormous potential benefit of addressing delays in transport to facility in low- and middle-income countries, where more than 99% of HDP-related maternal deaths occur (11). Communities in all settings have a critical role to play in ensuring that women and their families are prepared for birth and HDP-related or any other emergencies that may arise.

Currently, and as stated previously, there is insufficient evidence to make a recommendation about the usefulness of the following: exercise, workload reduction, stress reduction, ongoing salt restriction among women with pre-existing hypertension, new severe dietary salt restriction for women with any HDP, and a heart-healthy diet or calorie restriction for obese women specifically (15, 19).

For women with gestational hypertension (without pre-eclampsia), some bed rest in hospital (compared with unrestricted activity at home) may be useful to decrease severe hypertension and preterm birth (74). However, it should be remembered that for women with pre-eclampsia who are hospitalized, strict bed rest is not recommended (14, 15, 19).

Inpatient care should be provided for women with severe hypertension or 'severe' pre-eclampsia, however defined. A component of care through hospital day units or home care can be considered for women with non-severe pre-eclampsia or non-severe (pre-existing or gestational) hypertension.

In under-resourced settings, transport from community to facility must be considered to be a responsibility of women, their families, their communities, civil society, and their care providers (11).

Fluids, drugs, and transfusion

The management of the HDP encompasses far more than use of antihypertensive therapy. Women with pre-existing or gestational hypertension are at risk of evolving into pre-eclampsia, a multisystem

Table 21.4 Prediction of pre-eclampsia

Maternal				Paternal
Demographics and family history	Past medical or obstetric history	Current pregnancy		
		First trimester	Second or third trimester	
	Previous pre-eclampsia	Multiple pregnancy		
	Antiphospholipid antibody syndrome			
	Pre-existing medical condition(s)			
	• Pre-existing hypertension or booking DBP ≥90 mmHg			
	• Pre-existing renal disease or booking proteinuria			
	• Pre-existing diabetes mellitus			
Afro-Caribbean or South Asian race	Lower maternal birth weight and/or preterm delivery	Short maternal stature ≤164 cm/5′5″	Excessive weight gain in pregnancy	Paternal age ≥45 years
Maternal age ≥35–40 years	Thrombophilias	Overweight/obesity		
Family history of pre-eclampsia (grandmother, mother or sister)	Increased pre-pregnancy triglycerides, total cholesterol and/or non-HDL-cholesterol	Reduced physical activity		Mother had pre-eclampsia
Family history of early-onset cardiovascular disease	Non-smoking	First ongoing pregnancy		Fathered pregnancy complicated by pre-eclampsia with another partner
Rural location (LMICs)	Cocaine and/or methamphetamine use	New partner		
	Previous miscarriage at ≤10 weeks with same partner	Short duration of, or reduced, exposure to sperm of current partner		
	Previous pregnancy complicated by IUGR	Reproductive technologies		
	Maternal uterine anomaly	Inter-pregnancy interval ≥4 years		
	Increased stress	Mental health (depression and/or anxiety)		
		Booking SBP ≥130 mmHg	Elevated BP (gestational hypertension)	
Rural location (LMICs)	(Recurrent miscarriage)	Booking DBP ≥80 mmHg	Gestational proteinuria	
		Vaginal bleeding in early pregnancy		
		Gestational trophoblast disease		
		Anaemia with low vitamin C and E intake (LIMCs)		
		Severe anaemia (Hb <7.0 g/L)		
		Abnormal serum screening analytes	Abnormal serum screening analytes	
		Investigational laboratory markers	Investigational laboratory markers	
		Reduced 25(OH)-vitamin D	Abnormal uterine artery Doppler	
		Female fetus (early onset)	Infection during pregnancy (e.g. UTI, periodontal disease)	
		Male fetus (late onset)		
		Congenital fetal anomalies		

BP, blood pressure; DBP, diastolic blood pressure; Hb, haemoglobin; HDL, high-density lipoprotein; IUGR, intrauterine growth restriction; LMICs, low- and middle-income countries; SBP, systolic blood pressure; UTI, urinary tract infection.
Source data from *The FIGO Textbook of Pregnancy Hypertension* (2016) p77–78.

disorder of endothelial dysfunction (2, 3, 11). As such, attention must be paid to judicious fluid management, antihypertensive therapy of severe and non-severe hypertension with oral or parenteral agents, magnesium sulphate (MgSO₄) for eclampsia prevention and treatment as well as fetal neuroprotection with birth at less than 34^{+0} weeks, antenatal corticosteroids for acceleration of fetal pulmonary maturity, and various therapies for haemolysis, elevated liver enzyme, and low platelet (HELLP) syndrome, including transfusion of blood products and, possibly, corticosteroids (14, 15). The World Health Organization Model List of Essential Medicines includes all of the aforementioned interventions other than fluid therapy for pregnant women (75). It is our responsibility to ensure that we advocate for use of effective interventions whether we practice in well- or under-resourced settings.

Fluids

Plasma volume expansion is not recommended for women with pre-eclampsia, and, indeed, intravenous fluid intake should be minimized to 80 mL/hour in women with pre-eclampsia to avoid pulmonary oedema (14, 15, 76, 77). Fluid should not be routinely administered to treat oliguria (<15 mL/hour for 6 consecutive hours) for the sole purpose of increasing urine output (14, 15). For treatment of persistent oliguria, neither dopamine nor frusemide/furosemide is recommended (14, 15).

Antihypertensive therapy for severe hypertension

Irrespective of its underlying cause or timing in terms of delivery, severe pregnancy hypertension (i.e. SBP ≥160 mmHg and/or DBP ≥110 mmHg) requires a rapid, but considered, response (14, 15, 17, 19). Severe pregnancy hypertension can be confirmed by serial measurements that achieve a steady set of measurements, rather than requiring 15 minutes for confirmation (18). It should be considered as important as the development of pre-eclampsia in terms of maternal and perinatal risks (78).

The goal of BP should be to achieve values of both SBP at less than 160 mmHg and DBP at less than 110 mmHg. However, this can be achieved over hours—generally at a rate of 10% per hour—to avoid a precipitous fall in BP that may result in a non-reassuring fetal status compelling a decision to deliver by caesarean section while the mother remains unstable (14, 15, 17, 19).

Initial antihypertensive therapy in the hospital setting should be with either short-acting nifedipine (capsules), intermediate-acting nifedipine (PA/retard tablets), parenteral hydralazine, or parenteral labetalol (Table 21.5) (14, 15). Alternative antihypertensive medications include oral methyldopa, oral labetalol, oral clonidine, oral captopril (only postpartum), or a nitroglycerine infusion (Table 21.5). Refractory hypertension may be treated with sodium nitroprusside, but most obstetricians will request internal medicine/critical care medicine support for assistance.

Despite urban legends to the contrary, nifedipine and MgSO₄ can be used contemporaneously (79). While it may cause a non-sustained fall in BP, MgSO₄ is not recommended solely as an antihypertensive agent (14, 15).

Despite very careful titration, some women (especially those with contracted intravascular volumes) will be exquisitely sensitive to even small doses of antihypertensives. Therefore, antenatally, at gestational ages and with an estimated fetal weight associated with postnatal viability (according to local standards), continuous fetal heart rate monitoring is advised until BP is stable as a decreasing maternal BP may expose latent uteroplacental insufficiency (14, 15).

As a general rule, the authors' suggest that colleagues initiate continued antihypertensive therapy, or increase the dose or number of agents used in continuous therapy (with one of the agents outlined in the following sections), after every second dose of an antihypertensive used in response to severe pregnancy hypertension.

Antihypertensive therapy for non-severe hypertension

Following the results of the international Control of Hypertension In Pregnancy Study (CHIPS) trial, the evidence suggests that all hypertensive pregnant women should receive antihypertensive drug therapy aiming for a DBP of 85 mmHg (80). The choice of antihypertensive agent for initial treatment should be based on characteristics of the patient, contraindications to a particular drug, and doctor and patient preference (Table 21.6).

Initial therapy in pregnancy can be with one of a variety of antihypertensive agents: methyldopa, labetalol, other beta-blockers (acebutolol, metoprolol, pindolol, and propranolol), and calcium channel blockers (nifedipine). In the authors' opinion, the agent with the best profile is methyldopa, due to better fetal outcomes compared with labetalol (81), reassuring methyldopa data related to initial and long-term neurodevelopmental follow-up (82–88), and the authors' preference to reserve nifedipine for episodes of severe hypertension (89, 90).

It should be remembered that angiotensin-converting enzyme (ACE) inhibitors, angiotensin-II receptor blockers (ARBs), and prazosin should not be used during pregnancy, due to concerns about stillbirth risk. Due to idiosyncratic effects causing reduced fetal growth velocity, atenolol is not recommended prior to delivery. ACE inhibitors (specifically, captopril, enalapril, and quinapril) and prazosin may be used postpartum, even during breastfeeding.

There is no compelling evidence that antihypertensive treatment of hypertension (with labetalol, nifedipine, and probably methyldopa) is associated with adverse effects on child development. However, irrespective of the choice of antihypertensive agent(s), gestational hypertension and pre-eclampsia can be associated with adverse paediatric neurodevelopmental effects, such as inattention and externalizing behaviours (91, 92).

Magnesium sulphate

MgSO₄ is recommended as the first-line treatment of eclampsia and for eclampsia prevention in women with severe pre-eclampsia (93–97). In addition, MgSO₄ may be considered for eclampsia prevention in women with non-severe pre-eclampsia based on both institutional logistics and cost considerations (14, 15). When using the standard regimen of a 4 g intravenous loading dose followed by 1 g/hour, routine monitoring of serum Mg levels is not recommended.

Phenytoin and benzodiazepines should not be used for eclampsia prophylaxis or treatment, unless there is a contraindication to MgSO₄ or it is ineffective. Their use is associated with increased risks for adverse maternal events (93–95).

In addition, for women with any form of pregnancy hypertension, MgSO₄ should be considered for fetal neuroprotection in the setting of imminent preterm birth within the next 24 hours at no longer than 33⁺⁶ weeks (98, 99). The authors suggest that the same dosage regimen be used for simplicity and to avoid dosing errors.

Therapies for HELLP syndrome

Every obstetric centre should be aware of the local delay between ordering and receiving platelet units. For women with a platelet count less than 20×10^9/L, platelet transfusion is recommended, regardless of mode of delivery, and for a platelet count of $20–49 \times 10^9$/L platelet transfusion is recommended prior to caesarean delivery (14, 15). In addition, for women with a platelet count of $20–49 \times 10^9$/L, platelet transfusion should be considered prior to vaginal delivery if there is excessive active bleeding, known platelet dysfunction, a rapidly falling platelet count, or coagulopathy (14, 15).

For a platelet count of at least 50×10^9/L, platelet transfusion should be considered prior to either caesarean or vaginal delivery if there is excessive active bleeding, known platelet dysfunction, a rapidly falling platelet count, or coagulopathy (14, 15).

Table 21.5 Antihypertensives for severe pregnancy hypertension

Agent	Mechanism of action	Dosage	Pharmacoleinetics[a]			Comments
			Onset	Peak	Duration	
Most commonly recommended						
Labetalol	Peripheral[b] alpha-1 and (non-selective) beta-1 and -2 receptor antagonist	Intermittent dosing Start with 20 mg IV over 2 min. Repeat with 40 mg then 80 mg IV (each over 2 min) every 30 min. Continuous infusion 1–2 mg/min (max. dosage 300 mg)	5 min	30 min	4 h	Best avoided in women with asthma or heart failure Neonatology should be informed if the woman is in labour, as parenteral labetalol may cause neonatal bradycardia Parenteral therapy should be followed by ongoing oral therapy to maintain BP
Nifedipine	Calcium channel blocker (vasodilator)	Capsule 5–10 mg to swallow without biting Repeat every 30 min	5–10 min	30 min	6 h	There are three types of nifedipine preparations with which all staff must be familiar capsules, intermediate-release tables (PA, SR, or retard tablet) and slow-release tablets (XL, MR, or LA) Nifedipine may be given at the same time as MgSO$_4$
		PA, SR. or retard tablet 10 mg to swallow	30 min	240 min	6 h	
		Repeat every 30 min (max dosage 30 mg)				
Hydralazine	Direct-acting vasodilator	Intermittent dosing 5 mg IV	5 min	30 min	3–8 h	May increase the risk of maternal hypotension
		Repeat 5–10 mg IV every 30 min (may be given IM but unusual)				
		Continuous infusion				
		0.5–10 mg/h IV (max. dosage 45 mg)				
Labetalol	Peripheral[b] alpha-1 and (non-selective) beta-1 and -2 receptor antagonist	200 mg orally Repeat in 4 h (max. dosage 2400 mg/day in 4 divided doses[c])	20–120 min	1–4 h	8–12 h	Duration is dose dependent
Methyldopa	Centrally acting alpha-2 receptor agonist	750 mg orally Repeat in 6 h (max. dosage 2000 mg/day in 4 divided doses[c])	Not known	4–6 h	24–48 h	Less effective than oral nifedipine
Clonidine[d]	Centrally acting alpha-2 receptor agonist	0.1–0.2 mg orally	30–60 min	2–4 h	6–10 h	Clonidine therapy is not recommended during breastfeeding[e]
		Repeat in 1 h (max. dosage 0.8 mg[c])				
Captopril[d] *only postpartum*	Angiotensin-converting enzyme inhibitor	6.25–12.5 mg orally Repeat in 1 h (max. dosage 75 mg)	30 min	60–90 min	≥8 h	Captopril must NOT be administered before delivery, but it is acceptable for use during breastfeeding.[e] Duration is dose dependent
Nitroglycerine infusion	Direct vasodilators that has its affects veins more than arterioles	5 mcg/min, increased every 5 min (max rate 100 mcg/min)	2–5 min	5 min	5–10 min	Main side effects are headache (due to direct vasodilation) and tachycardia (from reflect sympathetic activation)
						Methaemoglobinaemia has been reported after 24 h of treatment

BP, blood pressure; IM, intramuscular; IV, intravenous; MgSO$_4$, magnesium sulphate.

[a] General reference http://www.drugs.com.

[b] Beta-blockade is three to seven times more than alpha-blockade, especially at lower doses.

[c] Dosing of this drug may continue after the severe hypertension has resolved, as it is used for chronic treatment of non-severe hypertension.

[d] Captopril (25 mg) and clonidine (0.1 mg) are being compared in a postpartum randomized controlled trial (NCT01761916) based on the effectiveness of these medications for severe hypertension treatment outside pregnancy.

[e] http://toxnet.nlm.nih.gov/newtoxnet/lactmed.htm.

Source data from *The FIGO Textbook of Pregnancy Hypertension* (2016) p138–139.

Table 21.6 Antihypertensives for non-severe pregnancy hypertension

Agent	Mechanism of action	Dosage	Comments
Methyldopa	Centrally acting alpha-2 receptor agonist → decreased sympathetic outflow → decreased peripheral vascular resistance	250–500 mg PO BID-QID (max. dosage 2000 mg/day)	There is no evidence to support a loading dose of methyldopa
			Psychological side effects (e.g. drowsiness or depression) may occur but women do not change drugs more frequently than with other medication Within first 6 weeks of therapy, >10% may develop hepatitis or cholestasis that can be detected by laboratory testing; abnormalities should reverse with discontinuation, but liver failure is rare. After 6 months of therapy, 10–20% develop a positive direct Coombs' test, but it does not interfere with typing or cross matching and associated haemolytic anaemia is rare
Labetalol	Peripheral[a] alpha-1 and (non-selective) beta-1 and 2 receptor antagonist → decreased peripheral vascular resistance with no reflex increase in heart rate	100–400 mg PO BID-QID (max. 2400 mg/day)	Some experts recommend a starting dose of 100 mg PO TID because the half-life of labetalol is shorter in pregnancy May be associated with postural hypotension, especially at higher doses
Nifedipine	Calcium channel blocker → vascular smooth muscle relaxation → decrease peripheral vascular resistance	PA, SR, or retard tablets 10–20 mg PO BID-TID (max. 180 mg/day)	Peripheral oedema as a side effect may be more common at doses of 120 mg/day or more
		XL, MR or LA preparation 20–60 mg PO OD–BID (max. 120 mg/day)	

BID, twice a day; PO, per os; QID, four times a day; TID, three times a day.
[a] Beta-blockade is three to seven times more than alpha-blockade, especially at lower doses.
Source data from *The FIGO Textbook of Pregnancy Hypertension* (2016) p 142.

The authors do not recommend corticosteroids for treatment of HELLP syndrome until they have been proven to decrease maternal morbidity through adequately powered randomized controlled trials (14, 15).

The authors recommend against plasma exchange or plasmapheresis for HELLP syndrome, particularly within the first 4 days postpartum (14, 15). These interventions can be important therapies for women with pre-eclampsia mimickers such as haemolytic uraemic syndrome.

Other therapies for treatment of pre-eclampsia

Women with pre-eclampsia before 35^{+0} weeks' gestation should receive antenatal corticosteroids for acceleration of fetal pulmonary maturity (14, 15). In addition, thromboprophylaxis may be considered antenatally among women with pre-eclampsia who have two or more additional thromboembolic risk markers, postnatally among women with pre-eclampsia who have at least one additional thromboembolic risk marker, or postnatally among women any HDP who were on antenatal bed rest for at least 7 days (14, 15).

Timing and mode of delivery for women with a hypertensive disorder of pregnancy

The phrase, 'planned childbirth on the best day in the best way', alludes to the fact that there are a myriad of considerations regarding timing (and mode of) childbirth in women with a HDP, particularly pre-eclampsia (100). Complicating this decision-making can be inaccurate determination of gestational age, and difficulty identifying those women who are at particular risk of an adverse outcome if pregnancy is prolonged. The literature on timing of childbirth has been complicated by the fact that 'severe' pre-eclampsia has been variably defined by international organizations and yet, all list 'severe' pre-eclampsia as an indication for interventionist management, that is, delivery.

Regardless, the last decade has seen the publication of a significant body of work that informs our decisions about timing of delivery in women with a HDP, particularly pre-eclampsia. Delivery is recommended for women with pre-eclampsia or gestational hypertension at term for maternal benefit (101), although expectant care is recommended for women with any HDP at late preterm gestational ages to reduce neonatal respiratory morbidity (associated with labour induction and caesarean delivery) (102). Small trials suggest that expectant care of women with pre-eclampsia from fetal viability to 33^{+6} weeks reduces neonatal morbidity, but the magnitude of maternal risk has not been fully quantified (103). There are no trials to inform management of women with chronic hypertension.

Management should be based on the understanding that giving birth is the manner in which to *initiate* the cure for pre-eclampsia, and women with gestational hypertension or pre-existing hypertension may develop pre-eclampsia antepartum or postpartum (11, 14, 15). General guidance for delivery decisions is summarized in Table 21.7.

Place of delivery

All women with a HDP of any type require, and deserve access to, delivery in a centre that can provide emergency obstetric care, while women with a HDP and serious maternal complications require delivery in a centre capable of providing comprehensive obstetric care.

Timing of delivery

Women with pre-eclampsia

Consultation with an obstetrician is advised in women with pre-eclampsia. (If an obstetrician is not available in under-resourced

Table 21.7 Timing and mode of delivery in women with a HDP

	Gestational age at diagnosis (weeks)				
	20^{+0}–viability	Viability–29^{+6}	30^{+0}–33^{+6}	34^{+0}–36^{+6}	≥37^{+0}
Perinatal prognosis	Survival: 18–50%	Survival: 60–95%	Survival: 98%	Survival: >99%	
	Intact survival: 2–45%	Intact survival: 15–90%	Intact survival: 88–96%	Intact survival: >96%	
Maternal risks (relative to normotensive pregnancy)	Significantly increased	Significantly increased	Significantly increased	Moderately increased	Minimally increased
In utero transfer to tertiary centre	NO as a routine, but centre should be competent with second trimester termination and/or expectant management	YES if stable for transfer	Ideally, but perinatal outcomes unchanged if postpartum transfer	NO, but centre should be competent with expectant management	NO
Expectant management	NO as a routine, but at 22–23 weeks some may attempt to attain perinatal survival	YES rate of adverse maternal outcomes same with expedited delivery; significant perinatal gains		YES acute morbidity and school-age issues are associated with late preterm birth	NO post-HYPITAT
Betamethasone for fetal lungs	NO	YES	YES	YES if non-laboured caesarean	NO
Assessment and surveillance	Minimum standard: on admission, day after admission, every Monday and Thursday until delivery, and on day of delivery; additional testing as indicated by changes in clinical state				
	NOTE: this approach has been associated with >80% reduction in adverse maternal outcomes				
Maternal	Blood: CBC, INR, APTT, fibrinogen, creatinine, electrolytes, uric acid, AST, LDH, bilirubin, albumin, glucose (to R/O AFLP)				
	Urine: dipstick, protein:creatinine ratio; pulse oximetry				
Fetal	Ultrasound: AFI, umbilical artery Doppler, ductus venosus Doppler; NST				
Deciding when to deliver	Women with 'severe pre-eclampsia, as defined in this textbook, should be delivered				Delivery, post-HYPITAT
Route of delivery	Vaginal (misoprostol IOL)	Probable caesarean, unless IUFD	Vaginal; fetal or uterine status may preclude vaginal delivery		

AFI, amniotic fluid index; AFLP, acute fatty liver of pregnancy; APTT, activated partial thromboplastin time; AST, aspartate aminotransferase; CBC, complete blood count; INR, international normalized ratio; IOL, induction of labour; IUFD, intrauterine fetal death; LDH, lactate dehydrogenase; NST, non-stress test; PTB, preterm birth; R/O, role of. Source data from *The FIGO Textbook of Pregnancy Hypertension* (2016) p 170.

settings, consultation with at least a medical practitioner is recommended.)

When using the severity criteria endorsed here, all women with 'severe' pre-eclampsia or eclampsia should be delivered within 24 hours, regardless of gestational age. For women with non-severe pre-eclampsia at less than 24^{+0} weeks' gestation, counselling should include information about delivery within days as an option. In contrast, for women with non-severe pre-eclampsia at 24^{+0}–33^{+6} weeks' gestation, expectant management should be considered, but only in centres capable of caring for very preterm infants. For women with non-severe pre-eclampsia at 34^{+0}–36^{+6} weeks' gestation, expectant management is advised, while for those with pre-eclampsia at 37^{+0} weeks' gestation or greater, initiating delivery within 24 hours is recommended (101, 102).

For women with non-severe pre-eclampsia complicated by HELLP syndrome at 24^{+0}–34^{+6} weeks' gestation, consider delaying delivery long enough to administer antenatal corticosteroids for acceleration of fetal pulmonary maturity as long as there is temporary improvement in maternal laboratory testing (14, 15). All women with HELLP syndrome at 35^{+0} weeks or more of gestation should be considered for delivery within 24 hours.

Women with gestational hypertension (without pre-eclampsia)

For women with gestational hypertension at less than 36^{+6} weeks' gestation, expectant management is advised, while those with gestational hypertension at 37^{+0} weeks or more of gestation, initiating delivery within days should be discussed (101, 102).

Women with pre-existing hypertension

For women with pre-existing hypertension at less than 36^{+6} weeks' gestation, expectant management is advised, even if women require treatment with antihypertensive therapy. On balance from the existing evidence, but in the absence of trial data that are urgently required, for women with uncomplicated pre-existing hypertension who are otherwise well at 37^{+0} weeks or more of gestation, initiating delivery should be considered at some time between 38^{+0} and 39^{+6} weeks' gestation (104).

Mode of delivery

For women with any HDP, vaginal delivery should be considered unless a caesarean delivery is required for the usual obstetric indications (14, 15). If vaginal delivery is planned and the cervix is unfavourable, then cervical ripening should be used to increase the chance of a successful vaginal delivery. At a gestational age remote from term, women with a HDP with evidence of fetal compromise may benefit from delivery by emergent caesarean delivery.

Antihypertensive treatment should be continued throughout labour and delivery to maintain SBP at less than 160 mmHg and DBP at less than 110 mmHg (14, 15). The third stage of labour should be actively managed with oxytocin 5 units intravenously or 10 units intramuscularly, particularly in the presence of either thrombocytopenia or coagulopathy (14, 15). However, ergometrine maleate should not be administered to women with any HDP, particularly pre-eclampsia or gestational hypertension; alternative oxytocics should be considered.

Anaesthesia and fluid management for women with a hypertensive disorder of pregnancy

This section is not designed to be an anaesthetic text but focuses on anaesthetic issues specifically related to parturients with a HDP. As a general rule, early consultation and involvement of anaesthesia will result in the best possible outcome for women with a HDP and their babies (14, 15). Therefore, the duty anaesthetist should be informed when a woman with pre-eclampsia is admitted to the delivery suite. The anaesthetist should assess the woman with pre-eclampsia from the standpoint of possible anaesthetic care and as her status may change, she should be reassessed.

Provision of effective analgesia for labour will not only decrease pain, but will attenuate its effects on BP and cardiac output. In addition, epidural analgesia benefits the fetus by decreasing maternal respiratory alkalosis, compensatory metabolic acidosis, and release of catecholamines. Therefore, early insertion of an epidural catheter (in the absence of contraindications) is recommended. An effective labour epidural can be used should a caesarean delivery be required, avoiding the need for general anaesthesia. To reduce risks associated with neuraxial anaesthesia (epidural, spinal, continuous spinal, and combined spinal epidural), women with pre-eclampsia should have a platelet count on admission to the delivery suite.

In the absence of contraindications, all of the following are acceptable methods of anaesthesia for women undergoing caesarean section: epidural, spinal, continuous spinal, combined spinal epidural, and general anaesthesia (14, 15). The choice of technique will depend on the overall condition of the parturient, the urgency of the situation, and whether there are contraindications to any particular technique. Challenges associated with anaesthesia include maintaining haemodynamic stability during laryngoscopy and intubation with general anaesthesia, or after sympathetic block secondary to neuraxial anaesthesia.

Although neuraxial anaesthesia is preferred to general anaesthesia, due to potential problems with the airway in the woman with pre-eclampsia, neuraxial anaesthesia may not be possible in the presence of a low platelet count or other coagulation abnormality (14, 15). A routine, fixed intravenous fluid bolus should not be administered prior to neuraxial anaesthesia (14, 15). The interaction of non-depolarizing muscle relaxants (as part of general anaesthesia)

and MgSO$_4$ will limit their use in the woman with pre-eclampsia. Adequate analgesia and ongoing monitoring are important components of overall postpartum management.

Arterial line insertion may be used for continuous arterial BP monitoring when BP control is difficult or there is severe bleeding. In addition, an arterial line is useful when repetitive blood sampling is required, for example, in women with HELLP syndrome (14, 15). Central venous pressure monitoring is not routinely recommended and, if a central venous catheter is inserted, it should be used to monitor trends and not absolute values (14, 15). Similarly, pulmonary artery catheterization is not recommended unless there is a specific associated indication and then only in an intensive care setting (14, 15).

Treatment postpartum—immediate and long term

Puerperium

Hypertension may worsen transiently postpartum, especially between days 3 and 6 when BP peaks in all women, whether normotensive or hypertensive. Women with postpartum hypertension should be evaluated for pre-eclampsia (either arising *de novo* or worsening from the antenatal period).

Hypertension and pre-eclampsia may even develop for the first time postpartum. Antihypertensive therapy may be continued postpartum, particularly in women with antenatal pre-eclampsia and those who delivered preterm. Severe postpartum hypertension must be treated with antihypertensive therapy, to keep SBP less than 160 mmHg and DBP less than 110 mmHg. Antihypertensive therapy may be used to treat non-severe postpartum hypertension, to keep BP at less than 140/90 mmHg for all but women with pregestational diabetes mellitus among whom the target should be less than 130/80 mmHg (14, 15, 17). Antihypertensive agents acceptable for use in breastfeeding include nifedipine XL, labetalol, methyldopa, and ACE inhibitors.

Non-steroidal anti-inflammatory drugs should not be given postpartum if hypertension is difficult to control, there is evidence of kidney injury (oliguria and/or elevated creatinine (>90 μmol/L)), or the platelet count is less than 50 × 10^9/L. As stated previously, postpartum thromboprophylaxis should be considered in women with pre-eclampsia who have other risk factors for thromboembolism.

Hypertension, proteinuria, and the biochemical changes of pre-eclampsia begin to resolve by 6 weeks postpartum but may persist for longer, especially when those changes have been extreme. Care in the 6 weeks postpartum includes management of hypertension, ensuring resolution of biochemical changes, and screening for secondary causes of hypertension in women with resistant hypertension, impaired renal function, or abnormal urinalysis.

Long-term treatment

Care providers should be aware of the mental health implications of the HDP, such as anxiety, depression, and post-traumatic stress disorder and refer women for appropriate evaluation and treatment (105).

Women with a history of severe pre-eclampsia (particularly those who presented or delivered at <34^{+0} weeks) should be screened for pre-existing hypertension and underlying renal disease. Referral for internal medicine or renal medicine/nephrology consultation should be considered for women with postpartum hypertension that is difficult to control, or women who had pre-eclampsia and have ongoing proteinuria 3–6 months postpartum, decreased estimated glomerular filtration rate (<60 mL/min), or another indication of renal disease (such as abnormal urinary sediment) (14, 15, 105).

In addition, the HDPs are associated with a number of long-term complications and the postpartum period provides an ideal window of opportunity to address these risks, such as premature cardiovascular disease and chronic kidney disease (14, 15, 105). A woman who delivers preterm with a HDP, and has a baby in the lowest 20% of birth weight for gestational age, acquires a similar risk of premature cardiovascular disease as women who smoke.

Women with a history of a HDP should adopt a heart-healthy lifestyle and should be screened and treated for traditional cardiovascular risk factors according to locally accepted guidelines (14, 15, 105). Therefore, women who are overweight should be encouraged to attain a healthy body mass index to decrease risk in future and for long-term health. Those women with pre-existing hypertension or persistent postpartum hypertension should undergo the following investigations (if not performed previously): urinalysis; serum sodium, potassium, and creatinine; fasting glucose; fasting lipid profile; and standard 12-lead electrocardiography.

Women who are normotensive but who have had a HDP, may benefit from assessment of traditional cardiovascular risk markers, but this remains unclear (14, 15, 105). As a minimum, all women who have had a HDP should pursue a healthy diet and lifestyle.

A comparison of evidence-based guidelines using ADAPTE II

Clinical practice guidelines are developed to assist healthcare providers in decision-making. A systematic review of existing clinical practice guidelines from the United Kingdom, Europe, North America, and Australasia that guide the care of women with HDPs (19) identified the following as consistent recommendations: (a) definitions of hypertension, proteinuria, and chronic and gestational hypertension; (b) pre-eclampsia prevention for women at increased risk—calcium when intake is low and low-dose aspirin, but not vitamins C and E or diuretics; (c) antihypertensive treatment of severe hypertension; (d) $MgSO_4$ for eclampsia and severe pre-eclampsia; (e) antenatal corticosteroids less than 34 weeks when delivery is probable within 7 days; (f) delivery for women with severe pre-eclampsia pre-viability or pre-eclampsia at term; and (g) active management of the third stage of labour with oxytocin. Notable inconsistencies were in (a) definitions of pre-eclampsia and severe pre-eclampsia; (b) target BP for non-severe hypertension; (c) timing of delivery for women with preeclampsia and severe pre-eclampsia; (d) $MgSO_4$ for non-severe pre-eclampsia, and (e) postpartum maternal monitoring.

Acknowledgement

The chapter sections are based on *The FIGO Textbook of Pregnancy Hypertension*, published by the Global Library of Women's Medicine in 2016.

REFERENCES

1. Kassebaum NJ, Bertozzi-Villa A, Coggeshall MS, et al. Global, regional, and national levels and causes of maternal mortality during 1990–2013: a systematic analysis for the Global Burden of Disease Study 2013. *Lancet* 2014;**384**:980–1004.

2. Mol BW, Roberts CT, Thangaratinam S, et al. Pre-eclampsia. *Lancet* 2016;**387**:999–1011.

3. Steegers EA, von Dadelszen P, Duvekot JJ, Pijnenborg R. Pre-eclampsia. *Lancet* 2010;**376**:631–44.

4. Melchiorre K, Sutherland GR, Liberati M, Thilaganathan B. Preeclampsia is associated with persistent postpartum cardiovascular impairment. *Hypertension* 2011;**58**:709–15.

5. Melchiorre K, Sutherland GR, Baltabaeva A, et al. Maternal cardiac dysfunction and remodeling in women with preeclampsia at term. *Hypertension* 2011;**57**:85–93.

6. Melchiorre K, Sutherland GR, Watt-Coote I, et al. Severe myocardial impairment and chamber dysfunction in preterm preeclampsia. *Hypertens Pregnancy* 2012;**31**:454–71.

7. Ray JG, Vermeulen MJ, Schull MJ, Redelmeier DA. Cardiovascular health after maternal placental syndromes (CHAMPS): population-based retrospective cohort study. *Lancet* 2005;**366**:1797–803.

8. Ray JG, Schull MJ, Kingdom JC, Vermeulen MJ. Heart failure and dysrhythmias after maternal placental syndromes: HAD MPS Study. *Heart* 2012;**98**:1136–41.

9. Ray JG, Booth GL, Alter DA, Vermeulen MJ. Prognosis after maternal placental events and revascularization: PAMPER study. *Am J Obstet Gynecol* 2016;**214**:106.

10. Gruslin A, Lemyre B. Pre-eclampsia: fetal assessment and neonatal outcomes. *Best Pract Res Clin Obstet Gynaecol* 2011;**25**:491–507.

11. von Dadelszen P, Magee LA. Preventing deaths due to the hypertensive disorders of pregnancy. *Best Pract Res Clin Obstet Gynaecol* 2016;**36**:83–102.

12. Hutcheon JA, Lisonkova S, Joseph KS. Epidemiology of preeclampsia and the other hypertensive disorders of pregnancy. *Best Pract Res Clin Obstet Gynaecol* 2011;**25**:391–403.

13. Thaddeus S, Maine D. Too far to walk: maternal mortality in context. *Soc Sci Med* 1994;**38**:1091–110.

14. Magee LA, von Dadelszen P, Stones W, Mathai M (eds). *The FIGO Textbook of Pregnancy Hypertension*. London: The Global Library of Women's Medicine; 2016.

15. Magee LA, Pels A, Helewa M, et al. Diagnosis, evaluation, and management of the hypertensive disorders of pregnancy. *Pregnancy Hypertens* 2014;**4**:105–45.

16. Philipp EE, Barnes J, Newton M (eds). *Scientific Foundations of Obstetrics and Gynaecology*, 3rd edn. Oxford: Butterworth-Heinemann Ltd; 1987.

17. Leung AA, Nerenberg K, Daskalopoulou SS, et al. Hypertension Canada's 2016 Canadian Hypertension Education Program guidelines for blood pressure measurement, diagnosis, assessment of risk, prevention, and treatment of hypertension. *Can J Cardiol* 2016;**32**:569–88.

18. Wilton A, de Greef A, Shennan A. Rapid assessment of blood pressure in the obstetric day unit using Microlife MaM technology. *Hypertens Pregnancy* 2007;**26**:31–37.

19. Gillon TE, Pels A, von Dadelszen P, et al. Hypertensive disorders of pregnancy: a systematic review of international clinical practice guidelines. *PLoS One* 2014;**9**:e113715.

20. Shennan AH, Halligan AW. Measuring blood pressure in normal and hypertensive pregnancy. *Bailliers Best Pract Res Clin Obstet Gynaecol* 1999;**13**:1–26.

21. Chung Y, Brochut MC, de Greeff A, Shennan AH. Clinical accuracy of inflationary oscillometry in pregnancy and pre-eclampsia: Omron-MIT Elite. *Pregnancy Hypertens* 2012;**2**:411–15.

22. de Greeff A, Ghosh D, Anthony J, Shennan A. Accuracy assessment of the Dinamap ProCare 400 in pregnancy and pre-eclampsia. *Hypertens Pregnancy* 2010;**29**:198–205.

23. de Greeff A, Shennan AH. Clinical accuracy of a low cost portable blood pressure device in pregnancy and pre-eclampsia: the Nissei DS-400. *Trop Doct* 2015;**45**:168–73.

24. Nathan HL, de Greeff A, Hezelgrave NL, et al. An accurate semiautomated oscillometric blood pressure device for use in pregnancy (including pre-eclampsia) in a low-income and middle-income country population: the Microlife 3AS1-2. *Blood Press Monit* 2015;**20**:52–55.

25. Reinders A, Cuckson AC, Lee JT, Shennan AH. An accurate automated blood pressure device for use in pregnancy and pre-eclampsia: the Microlife 3BTO-A. *BJOG* 2005;**112**:915–20.

26. Akeju DO, Vidler M, Sotunsa JO, et al. Human resource constraints and the prospect of task-sharing among community health workers for the detection of early signs of pre-eclampsia in Ogun State, Nigeria. *Reprod Health* 2016;**13**:111.

27. Akeju DO, Vidler M, Oladapo OT, et al. Community perceptions of pre-eclampsia and eclampsia in Ogun State, Nigeria: a qualitative study. *Reprod Health* 2016;**13** Suppl 1:57.

28. Akeju DO, Oladapo OT, Vidler M, et al. Determinants of health care seeking behaviour during pregnancy in Ogun State, Nigeria. *Reprod Health* 2016;**13** Suppl 1:32.

29. Boene H, Vidler M, Augusto O, et al. Community health worker knowledge and management of pre-eclampsia in southern Mozambique. *Reprod Health* 2016;**13**:105.

30. Boene H, Vidler M, Sacoor C, et al. Community perceptions of pre-eclampsia and eclampsia in southern Mozambique. *Reprod Health* 2016;**13** Suppl 1:33.

31. Firoz T, Vidler M, Makanga PT, et al. Community perspectives on the determinants of maternal health in rural southern Mozambique: a qualitative study. *Reprod Health* 2016;**13**:112.

32. Khowaja AR, Qureshi RN, Sheikh S, et al. Community's perceptions of pre-eclampsia and eclampsia in Sindh Pakistan: a qualitative study. *Reprod Health* 2016;**13** Suppl 1:36.

33. Munguambe K, Boene H, Vidler M, et al. Barriers and facilitators to health care seeking behaviours in pregnancy in rural communities of southern Mozambique. *Reprod Health* 2016;**13** Suppl 1:31.

34. Ramadurg U, Vidler M, Charanthimath U, et al. Community health worker knowledge and management of pre-eclampsia in rural Karnataka State, India. *Reprod Health* 2016;**13**:113.

35. Salam RA, Qureshi RN, Sheikh S, et al. Potential for task-sharing to Lady Health Workers for identification and emergency management of pre-eclampsia at community level in Pakistan. *Reprod Health* 2016;**13**:107.

36. Sheikh S, Qureshi RN, Khowaja AR, et al. Health care provider knowledge and routine management of pre-eclampsia in Pakistan. *Reprod Health* 2016;**13**:104.

37. Sotunsa JO, Vidler M, Akeju DO, et al. Community health workers' knowledge and practice in relation to pre-eclampsia in Ogun State, Nigeria: an essential bridge to maternal survival. *Reprod Health* 2016;**13**:108.

38. Vidler M, Charantimath U, Katageri G, et al. Community perceptions of pre-eclampsia in rural Karnataka State, India: a qualitative study. *Reprod Health* 2016;**13** Suppl 1:35.

39. Vidler M, Ramadurg U, Charantimath U, et al. Utilization of maternal health care services and their determinants in Karnataka State, India. *Reprod Health* 2016;**13** Suppl 1:37.

40. Cote AM, Firoz T, Mattman A, et al. The 24-hour urine collection: gold standard or historical practice? *Am J Obstet Gynecol* 2008;**199**:625–626.

41. De Silva DA, Halstead AC, Cote AM, et al. Random urine albumin:creatinine ratio in high-risk pregnancy—is it clinically useful? *Pregnancy Hypertens* 2013;**3**:112–114.

42. Payne BA, Hutcheon JA, Ansermino JM, et al. A risk prediction model for the assessment and triage of women with hypertensive disorders of pregnancy in low-resourced settings: the miniPIERS (Pre-eclampsia Integrated Estimate of RiSk) multi-country prospective cohort study. *PLoS Med* 2014;**11**:e1001589.

43. Payne BA, Groen H, Ukah UV, et al. Development and internal validation of a multivariable model to predict perinatal death in pregnancy hypertension. *Pregnancy Hypertens* 2015;**5**:315–21.

44. Zakiyah N, Postma MJ, Baker PN, van Asselt AD. Pre-eclampsia diagnosis and treatment options: a review of published economic assessments. *Pharmacoeconomics* 2015;**33**:1069–82.

45. Menzies J, Magee LA, Li J, et al. Instituting surveillance guidelines and adverse outcomes in preeclampsia. *Obstet Gynecol* 2007;**110**:121–27.

46. von Dadelszen P, Sawchuck D, McMaster R, et al. The active implementation of pregnancy hypertension guidelines in British Columbia. *Obstet Gynecol* 2010;**116**:659–66.

47. Dunsmuir DT, Payne BA, Cloete G, et al. Development of mHealth applications for pre-eclampsia triage. *IEEE J Biomed Health Inform* 2014;**18**:1857–64.

48. Lim J, Cloete G, Dunsmuir DT, et al. Usability and feasibility of PIERS on the move: an mHealth app for pre-eclampsia triage. *JMIR Mhealth Uhealth* 2015;**3**:e37.

49. Millman AL, Payne B, Qu Z, et al. Oxygen saturation as a predictor of adverse maternal outcomes in women with preeclampsia. *J Obstet Gynaecol Can* 2011;**33**:705–14.

50. Payne BA, Hutcheon JA, Dunsmuir D, et al. Assessing the incremental value of blood oxygen saturation (SpO(2)) in the miniPIERS (Pre-eclampsia Integrated Estimate of RiSk) risk prediction model. *J Obstet Gynaecol Can* 2015;**37**:16–24.

51. von Dadelszen P, Payne B, Li J, et al. Prediction of adverse maternal outcomes in pre-eclampsia: development and validation of the fullPIERS model. *Lancet* 2011;**377**:219–27.

52. Rana S, Karumanchi SA, Lindheimer MD. Angiogenic factors in diagnosis, management, and research in preeclampsia. *Hypertension* 2014;**63**:198–202.

53. Benton SJ, Hu Y, Xie F, et al. Angiogenic factors as diagnostic tests for preeclampsia: a performance comparison between two commercial immunoassays. *Am J Obstet Gynecol* 2011;**205**:469–468.

54. Benton SJ, Hu Y, Xie F, et al. Can placental growth factor in maternal circulation identify fetuses with placental intrauterine growth restriction? *Am J Obstet Gynecol* 2012;**206**:163–167.

55. Benton SJ, McCowan LM, Heazell AE, et al. Placental growth factor as a marker of fetal growth restriction caused by placental dysfunction. *Placenta* 2016;**42**:1–8.

56. Bramham K, Seed PT, Lightstone L, et al. Diagnostic and predictive biomarkers for pre-eclampsia in patients with established hypertension and chronic kidney disease. *Kidney Int* 2016;**89**:874–85.

57. Menzies J, Magee LA, Macnab YC, et al. Current CHS and NHBPEP criteria for severe preeclampsia do not uniformly

predict adverse maternal or perinatal outcomes. *Hypertens Pregnancy* 2007;**26**:447–62.

58. Grivell RM, Wong L, Bhatia V. Regimens of fetal surveillance for impaired fetal growth. *Cochrane Database Syst Rev* 2012;**6**:CD007113.

59. Kaur S, Picconi JL, Chadha R, et al. Biophysical profile in the treatment of intrauterine growth-restricted fetuses who weigh <1000 g. *Am J Obstet Gynecol* 2008;**199**:264.

60. Payne BA, Kyle PM, Lim K, et al. An assessment of predictive value of the biophysical profile in women with preeclampsia using data from the fullPIERS database. *Pregnancy Hypertens* 2013;**3**:166–71.

61. Shalev E, Zalel Y, Weiner E. A comparison of the nonstress test, oxytocin challenge test, Doppler velocimetry and biophysical profile in predicting umbilical vein pH in growth-retarded fetuses. *Int J Gynaecol Obstet* 1993;**43**:15–19.

62. Winje BA, Wojcieszek AM, Gonzalez-Angulo LY, et al. Interventions to enhance maternal awareness of decreased fetal movement: a systematic review. *BJOG* 2015.

63. Conde-Agudelo A, Villar J, Lindheimer M. World Health Organization systematic review of screening tests for preeclampsia. *Obstet Gynecol* 2004;**104**:1367–91.

64. Rasanen J, Quinn MJ, Laurie A, et al. Maternal serum glycosylated fibronectin as a point-of-care biomarker for assessment of preeclampsia. *Am J Obstet Gynecol* 2015;**212**:82–89.

65. Staff AC, Benton SJ, von Dadelszen P, et al. Redefining preeclampsia using placenta-derived biomarkers. *Hypertension* 2013;**61**:932–42.

66. Widmer M, Cuesta C, Khan KS, et al. Accuracy of angiogenic biomarkers at 20 weeks' gestation in predicting the risk of preeclampsia: a WHO multicentre study. *Pregnancy Hypertens* 2015;**5**:330–38.

67. McCowan LM, Pryor J, Harding JE. Perinatal predictors of neurodevelopmental outcome in small-for-gestational-age children at 18 months of age. *Am J Obstet Gynecol* 2002;**186**:1069–75.

68. von Dadelszen P, Magee LA, Taylor EL, et al. Maternal hypertension and neonatal outcome among small for gestational age infants. *Obstet Gynecol* 2005;**106**:335–39.

69. Ogge G, Chaiworapongsa T, Romero R, et al. Placental lesions associated with maternal underperfusion are more frequent in early-onset than in late-onset preeclampsia. *J Perinat Med* 2011;**39**:641–52.

70. Hofmeyr GJ, Lawrie TA, Atallah AN, et al. Calcium supplementation during pregnancy for preventing hypertensive disorders and related problems. *Cochrane Database Syst Rev* 2014;**6**:CD001059.

71. Hofmeyr GJ, Belizan JM, von Dadelszen P. Low-dose calcium supplementation for preventing pre-eclampsia: a systematic review and commentary. *BJOG* 2014;**121**:951–57.

72. Lassi ZS, Mansoor T, Salam RA, et al. Essential pre-pregnancy and pregnancy interventions for improved maternal, newborn and child health. *Reprod Health* 2014;**11** Suppl 1:S2.

73. Rodger MA, Hague WM, Kingdom J, et al. Antepartum dalteparin versus no antepartum dalteparin for the prevention of pregnancy complications in pregnant women with thrombophilia (TIPPS): a multinational open-label randomised trial. *Lancet* 2014;**384**:1673–83.

74. Josten LE, Savik K, Mullett SE, et al. Bedrest compliance for women with pregnancy problems. *Birth* 1995;**22**:1–12.

75. World Health Organization. *WHO Model List of Essential Medicines, 19th List*. Geneva: WHO; 2015.

76. Thornton C, Hennessy A, von Dadelszen P, et al. An international benchmarking collaboration: measuring outcomes for the hypertensive disorders of pregnancy. *J Obstet Gynaecol Can* 2007;**29**:794–800.

77. Thornton CE, von Dadelszen P, Makris A, et al. Acute pulmonary oedema as a complication of hypertension during pregnancy. *Hypertens Pregnancy* 2011;**30**:169–79.

78. Magee LA, von Dadelszen P, Singer J, et al. The CHIPS Randomized Controlled Trial (Control of Hypertension in Pregnancy Study): is severe hypertension just an elevated blood pressure? *Hypertension* 2016;**68**:1153–59.

79. Magee LA, Miremadi S, Li J, et al. Therapy with both magnesium sulfate and nifedipine does not increase the risk of serious magnesium-related maternal side effects in women with preeclampsia. *Am J Obstet Gynecol* 2005;**193**:153–63.

80. Magee LA, von Dadelszen P, Rey E, et al. Less-tight versus tight control of hypertension in pregnancy. *N Engl J Med* 2015;**372**:407–17.

81. Magee LA, von Dadelszen P, Singer J, et al. Do labetalol and methyldopa have different effects on pregnancy outcome? Analysis of data from the Control of Hypertension In Pregnancy Study (CHIPS) trial. *BJOG* 2016;**123**:1143–51.

82. Cockburn J, Moar VA, Ounsted M, Redman CW. Final report of study on hypertension during pregnancy: the effects of specific treatment on the growth and development of the children. *Lancet* 1982;**1**:647–49.

83. Mutch LM, Moar VA, Ounsted MK, Redman CW. Hypertension during pregnancy, with and without specific hypotensive treatment. II. The growth and development of the infant in the first year of life. *Early Hum Dev* 1977;**1**:59–67.

84. Mutch LM, Moar VA, Ounsted MK, Redman CW. Hypertension during pregnancy, with and without specific hypotensive treatment. I. Perinatal factors and neonatal morbidity. *Early Hum Dev* 1977;**1**:47–57.

85. Ounsted M, Moar V, Redman CW. Infant growth and development following treatment of maternal hypertension. *Lancet* 1980;**1**:705.

86. Ounsted MK, Moar VA, Good FJ, Redman CW. Hypertension during pregnancy with and without specific treatment; the development of the children at the age of four years. *Br J Obstet Gynaecol* 1980;**87**:19–24.

87. Redman CW. Fetal outcome in trial of antihypertensive treatment in pregnancy. *Lancet* 1976;**2**:753–56.

88. Redman CW, Beilin LJ, Bonnar J. Treatment of hypertension in pregnancy with methyldopa: blood pressure control and side effects. *Br J Obstet Gynaecol* 1977;**84**:419–26.

89. Firoz T, Magee LA, MacDonell K, et al. Oral antihypertensive therapy for severe hypertension in pregnancy and postpartum: a systematic review. *BJOG* 2014;**121**:1210–18.

90. Magee LA, Cham C, Waterman EJ, et al. Hydralazine for treatment of severe hypertension in pregnancy: meta-analysis. BMJ 2003;**327**:955–60.

91. Robinson M, Mattes E, Oddy WH, et al. Hypertensive diseases of pregnancy and the development of behavioral problems in childhood and adolescence: the Western Australian Pregnancy Cohort Study. *J Pediatr* 2009;**154**:218–24.

92. Whitehouse AJ, Robinson M, Newnham JP, Pennell CE. Do hypertensive diseases of pregnancy disrupt neurocognitive development in offspring? *Paediatr Perinat Epidemiol* 2012;**26**:101–108.

93. Duley L, Henderson-Smart DJ, Walker GJ, Chou D. Magnesium sulphate versus diazepam for eclampsia. *Cochrane Database Syst Rev* 2010;**12**:CD000127.

94. Duley L, Gulmezoglu AM, Henderson-Smart DJ, Chou D. Magnesium sulphate and other anticonvulsants for women with pre-eclampsia. *Cochrane Database Syst Rev* 2010;**11**:CD000025.

95. Duley L, Henderson-Smart DJ, Chou D. Magnesium sulphate versus phenytoin for eclampsia. *Cochrane Database Syst Rev* 2010;**10**:CD000128.

96. Duley L, Gulmezoglu AM, Chou D. Magnesium sulphate versus lytic cocktail for eclampsia. *Cochrane Database Syst Rev* 2010;**9**:CD002960.

97. Duley L, Matar HE, Almerie MQ, Hall DR. Alternative magnesium sulphate regimens for women with pre-eclampsia and eclampsia. *Cochrane Database Syst Rev* 2010;**8**:CD007388.

98. Bickford CD, Magee LA, Mitton C, et al. Magnesium sulphate for fetal neuroprotection: a cost-effectiveness analysis. *BMC Health Serv Res* 2013;**13**:527.

99. Magee L, Sawchuck D, Synnes A, von Dadelszen P. SOGC Clinical Practice Guideline. Magnesium sulphate for fetal neuroprotection. *J Obstet Gynaecol Can* 2011;**33**:516–29.

100. Tuffnell DJ, Jankowicz D, Lindow SW, et al. Outcomes of severe pre-eclampsia/eclampsia in Yorkshire 1999/2003. *BJOG* 2005;**112**:875–80.

101. Koopmans CM, Bijlenga D, Groen H, et al. Induction of labour versus expectant monitoring for gestational hypertension or mild pre-eclampsia after 36 weeks' gestation (HYPITAT): a multicentre, open-label randomised controlled trial. *Lancet* 2009;**374**:979–88.

102. Broekhuijsen K, van Baaren GJ, van Pampus MG, et al. Immediate delivery versus expectant monitoring for hypertensive disorders of pregnancy between 34 and 37 weeks of gestation (HYPITAT-II): an open-label, randomised controlled trial. *Lancet* 2015;**385**:2492–501.

103. Churchill D, Duley L, Thornton JG, Jones L. Interventionist versus expectant care for severe pre-eclampsia between 24 and 34 weeks' gestation. *Cochrane Database Syst Rev* 2013;**7**:CD003106.

104. Hutcheon JA, Lisonkova S, Magee LA, et al. Optimal timing of delivery in pregnancies with pre-existing hypertension. *BJOG* 2011;**118**:49–54.

105. Firoz T, Melnik T. Postpartum evaluation and long term implications. *Best Pract Res Clin Obstet Gynaecol* 2011;**25**:549–61.

22

Antepartum haemorrhage

Gbemisola Okunoye and Justin C. Konje

Introduction

Antepartum haemorrhage (APH) is defined as bleeding from the genital tract during pregnancy from viability (24 weeks' gestation in the United Kingdom) and before the delivery of the baby (1). In clinical practice, however, most will manage this as such from 20 weeks of gestation. It affects up to 5% of pregnancies and is associated with significant maternal and perinatal morbidity (2, 3). Of the estimated 300,000 maternal deaths in 2015 (4), obstetric haemorrhage (antepartum and postpartum) accounted for one-third of them (6). This highlights the need for a sustained focus on the understanding and popularization of a system-driven, team-based approach in the management of APH. APH also contributes significantly to the global burden of spontaneous and iatrogenic preterm birth (3, 7).

Historical context

Edward Rigby produced one of the earliest recorded essays that began to clarify the understanding, clinical presentation, and management of the distinctive causes of APH (8). In his 1775 published work, Rigby gave the first description of premature separation of the normally sited placenta which he termed 'accidental' haemorrhage in contrast to the 'unavoidable' haemorrhage of placenta praevia. His initial case series of 30 'accidental' haemorrhages and 14 'unavoidable' haemorrhages provided a clear narrative of the impact of APH on maternal and fetal outcome (9). His pioneering essay stimulated further interest and focused work on improving the management and outcome of APH, and two centuries later, the outcome of pregnancies complicated by APH are only marginally better than Rigby's series in many low-resourced countries. This reflection should inform a more decisive commitment to focus on the key drivers for improvement in the quality of care for pregnant women with APH.

Causes of antepartum haemorrhage

The causes of APH are as listed in Box 22.1. The most important are placenta praevia, placental abruption, placenta accreta, and vasa praevia; these, however, account for only about 50% of all cases (7, 9). APH of unknown origin which makes up the remaining is a diagnosis of exclusion and is typically attributed to placental edge (marginal) bleeding.

Initial assessment of patients with antepartum haemorrhage

The initial assessment of pregnant women presenting with APH should follow a streamlined and structured approach aimed at establishing the cause of the bleeding, maternal resuscitation, fetal assessment, and appropriate triaging based on the working or confirmed diagnosis. This assessment should include a focused clinical history and examination, relevant point-of-care testing, and the involvement of a senior obstetrician in the decision-making for a definitive or ongoing management plan.

Clinical history

Clinical history should establish the basic obstetric parameters including the gestational age and any previously known risk factors during the pregnancy (Box 22.2). Focused history should elicit a description of the circumstances of the bleeding, including the time of onset, precipitating factors, the amount of bleeding, previous bleeding episodes, and any associated symptoms of cardiovascular compromise including dizziness and fainting episodes. Importantly, the presence or absence of pain and its characterization should be elicited as well as any changes in fetal movement.

Clinical examination

General examination of the pregnant woman with APH should focus on assessment of pallor (conjunctiva, palm of the hands, oral mucosa, capillary refill), vital signs including blood pressure, pulse rate, oxygen saturation, and respiratory rate. The presence of maternal tachycardia in association with pallor reflects the degree of blood loss and even when the blood pressure remains within the normal range this is indicative of significant blood loss. The presence of hypertension should prompt routine testing for proteinuria in the context of diagnosing pre-eclampsia. Clinical examination of the abdomen should include the fundal height, assessment of tenderness, bruises, contraction, presentation and lie of the fetus, and fetal assessment with cardiotocography. An assessment of ongoing bleeding should be performed by inspecting the vulva and gently

> **Box 22.1** Causes of antepartum haemorrhage
>
> - Placenta praevia
> - Placenta abruption
> - Vasa praevia
> - Local genital causes:
>   – Cervical ectropion
>   – Inflammation/infection-cervicitis, vaginitis
>   – Cervical neoplasia
>   – Polyps
>   – Trauma
> - Bleeding of unknown origin

parting the labia minora. Digital examination of the cervix should be avoided until placenta praevia has been objectively excluded. A gentle speculum examination allows direct visualization of the cervix, to assess ongoing blood loss and exclude local genital causes.

Initial resuscitation, investigations, and triaging

The assessment and resuscitation of patients presenting with APH should ideally occur simultaneously. A large-bore intravenous access (French gauge 14/16) should be inserted and blood drawn for a full blood count including platelets, blood crossmatch, and coagulation profile. Fluid resuscitation should be commenced promptly to restore circulating blood volume particularly in those patients who are bleeding heavily or who are haemodynamically unstable. Up to 2 L of crystalloids can be administered quickly over 1 hour to restore circulating volume and stabilize the patient. A shock index (pulse rate/systolic blood pressure) of greater than 1.2 is a pointer to the severity of the blood loss. The normal shock index range is 0.7–0.9 in pregnant women (10). An ultrasound scan to assess the placenta site forms part of the assessment. Once a working diagnosis has been made, the patient can be triaged into expectant management or a decision to expedite delivery. This decision is usually based on the likely diagnosis, maternal and fetal conditions, and the gestational age. This decision should involve a senior obstetrician.

Placenta praevia

Placenta praevia is the partial or total implantation of the placenta into the lower uterine segment. The word 'praevia' is derived from

> **Box 22.2** Key points in the clinical history of antepartum haemorrhage
>
> - Timing of onset of bleeding in relation to presentation
> - An estimate of the amount of observed blood loss
> - Presence and characterization of pain
> - Previous episodes of bleeding in pregnancy
> - Changes in fetal movements
> - Medication history and history of substance misuse (especially cocaine)
> - Smoking
> - Cervical smear history
> - Symptom of maternal compromise

two Latin words 'prae' (which means before) and 'via' (which means way) (11) and literally implies that placenta praevia is when the placenta lies in the way of childbirth. The diagnosis of placenta praevia is anatomically and physiologically linked to the stage of pregnancy when the lower uterine segment is fully formed, typically in the third trimester. The lower uterine segment is 0.5 cm at around 20 weeks' gestation and stretches to 5 cm by term (12). Indeed, the practice of routine second-trimester ultrasonography will identify a low-lying placenta in approximately 6% of pregnant women between 10 and 20 weeks' gestation; however, the majority of these will resolve by term (13) and only 12% of low-lying placentas identified before 20 weeks will be present at delivery (14); hence, the incidence of placenta praevia from systematic reviews of 58 observational studies ranges from 3.5 to 4.6 per 1000 births (15).

Grading of placenta praevia

Placenta praevia has been traditionally graded as I to IV with the higher grades corresponding to its increasing encroachment of the lower uterine segment down to covering the internal cervical os. In clinical practice, however, placenta praevia is managed as either minor (grades I and II) or major praevia (grades III and IV) in alignment with the anticipated risks of haemorrhage, likelihood of preterm delivery, and determination of mode and timing of delivery Figure 22.1 (16).

Grading scheme

I Placenta extends into the lower uterine segment but does not reach the internal os.

II The lowermost edge of the placenta reaches the internal os but does not cover it.

III The placenta reaches and partially covers the internal os.

IV The placenta completely (symmetrically) covers the internal os.

Risk factors

There are a number of risk factors associated with the development of placenta praevia; the strongest are a previous history of placenta praevia or a previous caesarean section, with increasing risk associated with multiple repeat caesarean sections (13, 16–21). A previous prelabour caesarean section is associated with a higher risk of placenta praevia more than a previous intrapartum caesarean section or vaginal birth (18). Box 22.3 summarizes the risk factors associated with placenta praevia.

Pathophysiology

There is no clear unifying hypothesis for the development of placenta praevia, however, a purported hypothesis suggests that trophoblastic implantation in the upper part of the uterine cavity is inhibited due to the presence of poorly vascularized endometrium resulting from previous pregnancy or uterine surgery leading to implantation in the lower uterine cavity (15). Also, a large placental surface area, as observed in multiple pregnancy, increases the likelihood of the placenta extending into the lower uterine segment. In established placenta praevia, the progressive stretching of the lower uterine segment and changes in cervical morphology as pregnancy advances result in subtle disruption, leading to the observed symptom of bleeding. Physical disruption of the intervillous space

Figure 22.1 Placenta praevia (symmetrical)—illustration of major placenta praevia.

Box 22.3 Risk factors for placenta praevia

- Previous placenta praevia (adjusted odds ratio (OR) 9.7)
- Previous caesarean section (relative risk 2.6; 95% confidence interval (CI) 2.3–3.0 with background risk of 0.5%):
  - One previous caesarean section: OR 2.2 (95% CI 1.4–3.4 with a background risk of 1%)
  - Two previous caesarean sections: OR 4.1 (95% CI 1.9–8.8)
  - Three previous caesarean sections: OR 22.4 (95% CI 6.4–78.3)
- Previous termination of pregnancy
- Multiparity
- Fertility treatment
- Smoking
- Multiple pregnancy
- Advanced maternal age (age >40 years)
- Defective endometrium due to the presence or history of:
  - uterine scar/previous intrauterine surgery
  - endometritis
  - manual removal of placenta
  - curettage
  - submucous fibroids
- Male fetus

can occur with digital examination or intercourse. The bleeding in placenta praevia is maternal in origin, unless there is a coexisting vasa praevia.

Clinical presentation

Placenta praevia classically presents with painless unprovoked or provoked vaginal bleeding, commonly in the second half of pregnancy. This 'classic' presentation occurs in about 80% of cases while the rest will present with bleeding associated with painful contractions, thus mimicking placenta abruption (22) and up 10% of cases of confirmed placenta praevia presenting acutely with bleeding will have coexisting placenta abruption. About a third of patients will present with their first (warning) bleed before 30 weeks' gestation and most patients with placenta praevia will have a bleed by 36 weeks and only 10% of cases of confirmed placenta praevia will remain asymptomatic until delivery (23).

In most cases the bleeding is self-limiting, and usually settles by the time of initial assessment or shortly afterwards. Subsequent bleeding after the 'warning' bleed is more likely to be more significant as the gestation advances with progressive stretching of the lower segment. Uncommonly, previously undiagnosed placenta praevia can present with significant life-threatening haemorrhage, thus supporting the importance of maternity service preparedness for such cases, where prompt resuscitation, and availability of blood transfusion facilities are key lifesaving procedures (24).

Ultrasound diagnosis of placenta praevia

The practice of a routine mid-trimester detailed fetal anomaly scan which includes placenta localization can identify a low-lying placenta in asymptomatic patients. The transvaginal approach is the preferred modality for confirming a low-lying placenta identified on transabdominal ultrasound. Transvaginal ultrasound has been shown to be safe, acceptable with superior views, and will reclassify up to 25% of placentas diagnosed as low lying by abdominal ultrasound (25, 26). Transvaginal ultrasound also enables a more accurate measurement of the lower edge of the placenta from the internal cervical os (27). For those patients identified by transvaginal ultrasound with a low-lying placenta in the first half of pregnancy, a follow-up scan should be performed around 32–34 weeks, and in those with a persistent low-lying placenta, a further scan at 36 weeks is recommended prior to delivery. This is because only about 12% of low-lying placentas identified at 20 weeks will remain low lying at delivery (28) due to the progressive development of the lower segment in the third trimester leading to the process of placenta relative 'migration'. Placenta 'migration' is less likely in previous caesarean section, posterior placenta praevia, and when the placenta extends by up to 2.5 cm over the internal os at 20 weeks (29–31).

There should be no hesitation in undertaking transvaginal ultrasound to determine placenta localization in stable symptomatic patients because the position of the probe is 2–3 cm from the cervix and the angle between the cervix and the vaginal probe is sufficient to prevent the probe from inadvertently slipping into the cervical os (32). **Figure 22.2** shows a low-lying placenta diagnosed by ultrasound scan.

Management

Asymptomatic women

Pregnant women with placenta praevia who are asymptomatic throughout pregnancy can be managed on an outpatient basis until they are admitted for elective delivery at 38–39 weeks' gestation. Patients who remain asymptomatic are at a lower risk of needing emergency delivery (33). While they remain asymptomatic, it is important to ensure that anaemia is corrected aiming for a haemoglobin concentration greater than 10 g/dL by the time of delivery. It is important to advise these patients to avoid penetrative vaginal intercourse and strenuous physical exercises that could potentially stimulate uterine activity and bleeding. Antenatal fetal surveillance should be dictated by the presence of additional risk factors;

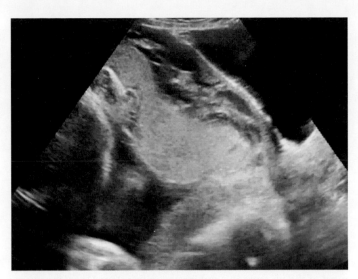

Figure 22.2 Ultrasound scan showing a marginal placenta praevia (not completely covering the os).

however, fetal growth parameters are usually undertaken at the time of ultrasound assessment of placental site. Antenatal care for women with asymptomatic placenta praevia, should be provided in a unit/centre with ready access to inpatient facilities including blood transfusion and emergency caesarean delivery.

Symptomatic stable women

Conservative management

The majority of pregnant women with placenta praevia who present with a first or second episodes of vaginal bleeding will not require immediate delivery as most initial bleeding episodes will subside with the initial resuscitative measures (34). However, these patients should be managed as in-patients initially on the labour ward for ongoing assessment of maternal and fetal well-being. Once the bleeding settles, the decision to embark on conservative management should be based on the need to prolong the pregnancy. This is most appropriate in those cases that are preterm and where the bleeding subsides. The components of conservative management include a course of antenatal corticosteroids for pregnancies between 24 and 34 weeks, blood transfusion to correct a significant drop in haemoglobin, anti-D immunoglobulin in unsensitized rhesus-negative patients, fetal assessment with an ultrasound scan, and cardiotocography. Ongoing management could either be inpatient or outpatient in stable patients after the bleeding episode has settled. The decision on whether to offer outpatient or continued inpatient management should be carefully considered, given that it is difficult to predict accurately the likelihood of rebleeding. However, bleeding episodes are more likely when the placenta completely covers the internal cervical os, in placentas with a thick edge (>1 cm), and when the cervical length is less than 3 cm (35, 36). For patients with the first episode of bleeding that settles spontaneously, outpatient management can be considered after at least a 48-hour bleed-free period, provided the patient is able to attend hospital promptly if she develops further bleeding and she must have someone available with her at home. It is important that the patient fully understands and accepts the risks of outpatient management (37).

Patients with recurrent bleeding episodes and those with additional pregnancy complications are better managed as inpatients until delivery; however, this decision should be individualized taking into consideration maternal and fetal well-being.

The efficacy of cervical cerclage as an intervention for prolonging pregnancy in patients with placenta praevia is unproven and is not recommended in routine clinical practice (38). The cautious use of tocolysis may be considered in selected cases of placenta praevia, particularly those with preterm contractions with minimal or no bleeding to allow the administration of antenatal corticosteroids (39, 40).

Active management-expediting delivery

Prompt resuscitation and expedited delivery is the management strategy for those patients with severe life-threatening bleeding that is refractory to the resuscitation measures, irrespective of the gestational age. Equally, when active bleeding is associated with onset of labour or fetal distress, delivery should be expedited by caesarean section. When patients present with recurrent bleeding after 34 weeks, delivery may be considered if the patient has completed a course of antenatal steroids. Where such bleeding is non-life-threatening, other factors including fetal size and maternal risks must be taken into consideration before making the decision.

Mode and timing of delivery

Asymptomatic women with major placenta praevia and previously symptomatic patients but stable patients should be admitted for elective delivery by caesarean section at 37–38 weeks' gestation. Consideration for vaginal delivery should be limited to those patients where the lower edge of the placenta is greater than 2 cm from the internal os and who have not experienced episodes of vaginal bleeding (41).

Advance planning is an integral part of management prior to delivery, and in cases of major placenta praevia the use of a preoperative care bundle (**Box 22.4**) such as the one proposed for placenta accreta is recommended to ensure a consistent approach in the peripartum period (31).

Consideration should be given to the planning and use of cell salvage where such facilities are available, particularly in those patients who decline donor blood.

At caesarean section, a lower transverse skin incision (Pfannenstiel or Cohen's incision) is usually appropriate. Efforts should be made

---

Box 22.4 Components of the preoperative care bundle

- Senior obstetrician plans and supervises delivery.
- Senior anaesthetist supervises delivery.
- Blood and blood products arranged and confirmed available.
- Multidisciplinary involvement in preoperative planning (midwives, radiologists, haematologists, etc.).
- Discussion and detailed consent to include possible interventions (e.g. hysterectomy, cell salvage, interventional radiology, balloon tamponade, compression suture).
- Availability of a critical care level 2 bed.

Source data from Royal College of Obstetricians and Gynaecologists. *Placenta Praevia, Placenta Praevia Accreta, Vasa Praevia: Diagnosis and Management.* Greentop Guideline No 27. London, RCOG, 2011.

to avoid a uterine incision that traverses the placenta whenever possible, by making the incision above the upper margin of the placenta. This is not always feasible; hence, it might be necessary to incise through the placenta. This must be performed rapidly to deliver the baby and clamp the umbilical cord. Additional surgical procedures may be required to control bleeding in addition to standard oxytocics. Surgical adjuncts include the use of haemostatic sutures on the placenta bed, balloon tamponade, uterine compression sutures (e.g. B-Lynch sutures), and a low threshold for insertion of peritoneal drain.

During the postoperative period, patients who had massive blood loss should be monitored in the critical care unit with close monitoring of ongoing losses from the vagina and intraperitoneal drain, urine output, haematological parameters (complete blood count, platelets, and coagulation studies), and adequate replacement of blood and blood products. Those patients who have undergone very extensive surgery should be offered an extended period of antibiotic prophylaxis for 24–48 hours after surgery. Thromboprophylaxis should be initiated with a pneumatic compression system and subsequently with low-molecular-weight heparin and compression stockings once coagulation and the platelet count returns to normal. These patients are usually stepped down from the critical care unit within 48 hours. Once the patient is fully ambulating, a thorough and detailed debriefing should be carried out by a senior member of the surgical team, ideally in the presence of the patient's partner particularly if the procedure was performed under general anaesthesia. Adequate discharge planning should include follow-up arrangements and a clear instruction on how to access the service in an emergency.

Placenta accreta (morbidly adherent placenta)

Definition

Placenta accreta broadly refers to abnormal placentation of varying degrees of morbid adherence placenta, subclassified into accreta, increta, and percreta based on the degree of penetration of chorionic villi into the uterine wall. It probably results from defective decidualization of the implantation site or implantation in a defective uterine scar (31, 42). In placenta accreta, the chorionic villi are attached to the myometrium instead of the decidua, while in percreta it penetrates into the myometrium and in percreta, the placenta penetrates through the myometrium into the serosal layer and surrounding viscera, commonly the bladder. Accreta is used as an umbrella term for the spectrum of accreta–increta–percreta in this chapter. Increasingly, the term 'morbidly adherent placenta' is being used to encapsulate the various forms of this type of placenta.

Incidence

The incidence of placenta accreta has increased progressively over the past decade in many regions of the world, an increase largely attributable to the increasing caesarean section rates across the world. Rates of up to 1 in 700 deliveries have been reported (43). In a series of histologically confirmed morbidly adherent placenta, placenta accreta accounted for 79% while placenta increta and percreta made up 14% and 7% respectively (44).

Risk factors

The most important risk factor for abnormally adherent placenta praevia is previous caesarean delivery; with risks increasing with the number of prior caesarean sections (Box 22.5). Up to 11% of placenta praevia in a previous caesarean section will be associated with placenta accreta rising to 40% in patients with three previous caesarean sections and placenta praevia (45). A history of prior caesarean section in the absence of placenta praevia is also associated with an increased risk of placenta accreta (46). Box 22.5 summarizes the risk factors for placenta accreta.

Diagnosis

Most cases of placenta accreta are suspected after the routine mid-trimester ultrasound scan or following episodes of bleeding or persistent haematuria in cases of placental extension into the bladder. Transabdominal (Figure 22.3) and transvaginal ultrasound assessment of the placenta in combination with colour Doppler remains the most reliable tool for the diagnosis of abnormally invasive placenta (47–48). Sonographic features of abnormal placenta invasion include the presence of lacunae or venous lakes, loss or disruption of the retroplacental hypoechoic (sonolucent) zone, exophytic mass extending through the serosa, and bulging of the placenta into the posterior wall of the bladder (49). In addition, colour Doppler is highly suggestive of placenta accreta when there is abnormal lacunar flow with prominent vessels over the peripheral subplacental area and hypervascularity of the serosa–bladder interface. The role of magnetic resonance imaging (MRI) in the diagnosis of abnormal placental invasion has been extensively reviewed and found to be comparable to ultrasonography and colour Doppler though with a slightly lower accuracy before 24 weeks' gestation (50–52). MRI is not recommended as the primary diagnostic modality but it has a complementary role where ultrasound findings are inconclusive, in posterior placentas, and to assess the depth or myometrial invasion (53). The MRI features suggestive of placenta accreta include:

- abnormal placenta vascularity
- uterine bulging
- heterogeneous signal intensity on T2-weighted imaging
- heterogeneous signal intensity within the placenta mass
- interruption of the myometrium.

Though not frequently used, three-dimensional ultrasonography has been used in the diagnosis of placenta accreta using

---

Box 22.5 Risk factors for placenta accreta

- Previous caesarean section with placenta praevia
- Previous uterine scarring or surgery:
  - Myomectomy
  - Hysteroscopic resection
  - Adhesiolysis
  - Endometritis
  - Uterine curettage
  - Endometrial ablation
- *In vitro* fertilization
- Caesarean section scar pregnancy
- Maternal age over 35 years

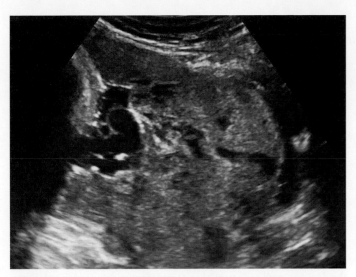

Figure 22.3 Ultrasound diagnosis of placenta accreta—invasive placenta with irregular lacunae.

key diagnostic features such as increased vascularity of the serosa–bladder interphase and irregular tortuous intraplacental vascularization (54).

Timely confirmation of the diagnosis of placenta accreta is crucial to allow sufficient time for advance planning of delivery (Box 22.6). Following the initial ultrasound diagnosis, a further follow-up scan should be performed in the third trimester around 32 weeks in stable patient. An MRI is typically performed at this gestation as well and any additional information gained could be useful in planning the delivery.

Management

The antenatal management of patients with placenta accreta follows the same principles as described for placenta praevia. The distinctive difference, however, is the need for detailed and multidisciplinary advanced planning based on the anticipated complexity of the case. Preoperative planning using the care bundle itemized in **Box 22.4** is recommended in all cases of placenta accreta.

Preterm delivery should be anticipated in patients with placenta accreta and a low threshold for administering antenatal corticosteroids to enhance fetal lung maturity should be adopted in symptomatic patients after 24 weeks of gestation.

Box 22.6 Complications of placenta accreta

- Massive haemorrhage
- Unscheduled hysterectomy
- Preterm delivery (spontaneous and iatrogenic)
- Massive transfusion
- Disseminated intravascular coagulopathy and adult respiratory distress syndrome related to massive transfusion
- Sepsis
- Spontaneous uterine rupture
- Intensive care unit admission
- Maternal mortality

Delivery

The main underlying principle with respect to the timing of delivery is the avoidance of emergency delivery; therefore, elective delivery by caesarean section is recommended at 35–36 weeks of gestation. Earlier delivery at 34 weeks should be considered in patients with recurrent symptoms especially those with placenta percreta that involves adjacent viscera.

The plan for delivery should involve senior clinicians from the relevant specialties including obstetrics, anaesthesia, radiology, and urology and a gynaecological oncologist surgeon and neonatologists. The components of the care bundle could be adapted to the setting based on the skill set and resources available. There should be a comprehensive discussion regarding the intended surgical approach and this should be explained carefully to the patient and documented in her records.

Surgical management

The surgical options for placenta accreta include the following:

- Delivering the baby through an incision away from the site of the placenta, leaving the placenta undisturbed, closing the uterus, and proceeding to a caesarean hysterectomy. This option has been associated with reduced morbidity and blood loss and is ideally recommended in those patients in whom future fertility is not a priority (31).

- Delivering the baby through an incision away from the site of the placenta, leaving the placenta undisturbed, then trimming the umbilical cord and closing the uterus with the placenta *in situ*. The patient is kept for an initial period of monitoring with antibiotics cover and assessment of bleeding. This is followed up by a prolonged period of follow-up with beta-human chorionic gonadotropin and serial ultrasound scans until the placenta mass completely resolves. This is an option in those patients who wish to preserve their uterus. During the follow-up period, this conservative approach is associated with a significant risk of infection and sudden heavy bleeding that would necessitate an emergency caesarean hysterectomy. The role of methotrexate in enhancing the breakdown of placenta trophoblastic tissue is debatable with no clear evidence of benefit and significant drug related morbidity, hence routine use is not advised (55–56).

- Delivering the baby followed by excision of the placenta bed with or without separating the placenta, followed by uterine reconstruction. This option can be associated with significant haemorrhage and adequate blood and blood products must be available. The excisional approach is usually appropriate when there is a clear margin of normal myometrium below the lower edge of the placenta, typically in focal accreta (55). Recently a triple P procedure has been described which is along the same principles as this approach but can retain some chorionic tissue (57)

- In some cases, especially those with bladder involvement, a joint procedure with urologists is advised and the placement of ureteral stents could be of benefit in selected cases to assess the integrity of the urinary tract, particularly during caesarean hysterectomy.

There is a significant risk of haemorrhage when the placenta partially separates and speedily adjunct surgical measures have to be taken to stop bleeding. These measures include internal iliac artery ligation, balloon tamponade, compression sutures (e.g. B-Lynch sutures), and a timely resort to hysterectomy if bleeding persists. The use of a prophylactic catheter placement for balloon occlusion or embolization has become part of the preoperative plan in many centres, though with variable evidence of clear benefit (58). The catheter, if left *in situ*, can be useful in the immediate postpartum period to manage postpartum haemorrhage.

The use of cell saver technology is encouraged where the expertise and facilities are available, especially in those patients who decline donor blood transfusion.

Postoperative care

The management of patients with placenta accreta follows similar principles as previously outlined for major placenta praevia. Access to a critical care bed should be part of the preoperative workup as most patients with prolonged surgery and massive blood transfusion will require postoperative monitoring in the critical care setting in the immediate postoperative period. Careful attention should be paid to assessment of blood loss from pelvic drains, fluid balance, thromboprophylaxis, as well as antibiotic prophylaxis in those patients with placenta tissue *in utero*.

Placenta abruption

Placenta abruption is the premature separation of the placenta prior to the third stage of labour and it is associated with severe maternal and fetal morbidity and increased perinatal mortality of up to 12% (59). Variable incidence rates of placenta abruption have been reported in different populations, with 0.2–1% of pregnancies affected (60).

Risk factors

The major risk factors for the occurrence of placenta abruption include a previous history of abruption, hypertensive disorders, or abdominal trauma, while modifiable risk factors include smoking and cocaine use (Box 22.7). Previous abruption is associated with a recurrence risk of 4.4%. This increases to 19–25% after two or more abruptions (16).

Some of the risk factors associated with abruption have synergistic effects (hypertension and cigarette smoking), hence the importance of antenatal education and intervention to encourage behaviour modifications with regard to substance misuse during pregnancy (61).

Classification

Attempts have been made to classify and grade placental abruption based on the severity in a similar fashion to placenta praevia (Box 22.8); however, this is not consistently used in day-to-day clinical practice where a more practical triaging into mild, moderate, or severe abruption is used based on the overall assessment of maternal and fetal well-being.

Pathophysiology

In a significant number of cases of placenta abruption, an underlying chronic placental disease exists. Abnormalities in the development of the spiral arteries in combination with decidua necrosis and vascular disruption lead to bleeding with or without an obvious trigger (62, 63). The initial bleeding occurs from disruption of maternal vessels in the decidua basalis and the accumulated blood or clot progressively separates the interface between the placenta and the decidua leading to partial or complete separation of the placenta. This process may be self-limiting and contained or continuous especially in the high-pressure arterial bleeding in the central area of the placenta leading to rapid detachment and haemorrhage, with evident maternal and fetal compromise (64). In high-pressure bleeding from maternal vessels in the decidua basalis, some blood will track in between the myometrium towards the uterine serosa leading to the classic appearance of a couvelaire uterus. Abruption resulting from mechanical-related events (abdominal trauma, sudden uterine decompression from ruptured membranes) is thought to be caused by rapid shearing forces applied to the relatively inelastic placenta from sudden stretching or contraction of the uterine wall (62, 63). Placenta abruption resulting from maternal cocaine use may be related to the intense vasoconstriction induced by cocaine with consequent ischaemia and disruption of vessels (65).

The production and release of thrombin accounts for the clinical sequelae observed in placenta abruption. The initial bleeding from the decidua stimulates the production of thromboplastin which then releases thrombin (66). Thrombin is a uterotonic agent and its release in placenta abruption is associated with uterine hypertonia and when in excess in the maternal circulation, it sets the stage for severe bleeding from an overwhelmed haemostatic system and widespread intravascular fibrin deposition (disseminated intravascular coagulopathy) (67).

Box 22.7 Risk factors for placenta abruption

- Hypertensive disorder:
  - Pre-eclampsia
  - Chronic hypertension
- Abdominal trauma
- Placental insufficiency
- Polyhydramnios
- Spontaneous rupture of membranes
- Smoking
- Cocaine use
- Multiparty

Box 22.8 Classification of placenta abruption

0: asymptomatic
Retrospective diagnosis.

1: mild
No or mild bleeding, slightly tender uterus, no maternal or fetal compromise, no coagulopathy.

2: moderate
No or moderate vaginal bleeding, moderate to severe uterine tenderness, maternal haemodynamic compromise, fetal distress, hypofibrinogenaemia.

3: severe
No or heavy vaginal bleeding, tetanic uterus, maternal haemodynamic compromise, coagulopathy, fetal death.

> **Box 22.9** Complications of abruption
>
> - Fetal death
> - Fetal distress
> - Massive obstetric haemorrhage
> - Disseminated intravascular coagulopathy
> - Acute kidney injury
> - Multiorgan failure
> - Caesarean hysterectomy for postpartum haemorrhage

Clinical features

Pregnant women with placental abruption typically present with vaginal bleeding associated with abdominal or lower back pain and uterine contractions. The pain could be constant in nature or intermittent. The presence of known risk factors or triggers should heighten the suspicion of placenta abruption. Clinical examination may reveal pallor, maternal tachycardia, and hypotension in severe blood loss. The abdomen is typically tender with a firm to hard feel. The distinctive feel on abdominal palpation in severe abruption is described as 'woody hard' caused by uterine hypertonus. In severe abruption with more than 50% of the placenta separated, evidence of fetal heart rate abnormalities and coagulopathy may be present. Complications of abruption are listed in **Box 22.9**.

The observed bleeding in these patients does not necessarily reflect the extent of haemorrhage because a significant amount of blood can be trapped in the retroplacental space also termed 'concealed abruption'; therefore, decisions regarding ongoing management should be based on the overall assessment of maternal and fetal status and laboratory investigations.

The diagnosis of placenta abruption is mainly clinical. The investigations performed are aimed at assisting in the triaging and further management.

Assessment and resuscitation

The initial assessment and resuscitation should follow the principles described in the initial assessment of patients with APH. Laboratory investigations in suspected cases include a full blood count, group and crossmatch where it is considered moderate or severe, coagulation profile (prothrombin time, activated partial thromboplastin time, fibrinogen), liver function tests, renal function tests, and Kleihauer–Betke test. A toxicology screen should be performed in suspected cases of substance misuse. Where facilities are available, the use of real-time point-of-care tests of coagulation (e.g. ROTEM), could be particularly helpful in providing an early indication of clotting derangement which allows for timely correction with appropriate blood and blood products.

The role of ultrasonography in the assessment of patients with suspected placenta abruption is limited but this can exclude placenta praevia. However, it has a limited role in those patients who are previously known to have fundal placenta location, as the sensitivity of ultrasound findings for the diagnosis of abruption is relatively low (25–50%) (68).

Transfusion of blood and blood products

The possibility of blood transfusion and transfusion of blood products must always be anticipated in patients with clinical suspicion of abruption. Appropriate preparations must therefore be made. In severe abruption with evidence of maternal haemodynamic compromise, coagulopathy, or fetal death, prompt replacement of blood and blood products must be expeditiously done. This can be achieved in a timely manner by activating the massive blood transfusion protocol. The typical protocol will deliver 6 units of packed red blood cells, 6 units of fresh frozen plasma, two pools of cryoprecipitate (10 units), and six pools of platelets. Fibrinogen at a dose of 2 g should be made available as well. Once the estimated blood loss exceeds 500 mL in placenta abruption, blood transfusion should be initiated while awaiting the results of laboratory investigations. Coagulation studies should be frequently monitored in these patients until there is a trend towards normality.

Delivery

The decision on whether to embark on expediting delivery or to pursue expectant management depends on the presence or absence of significant maternal or fetal compromise. In the presence of fetal compromise or fetal death, delivery should be expedited. This should also be the case when there is evidence of significant coagulopathy and active bleeding.

When vaginal delivery is not imminent and there is evidence of fetal distress, a caesarean delivery should be performed. However, if intrauterine fetal death has already occurred, vaginal delivery is the preferred mode of delivery with transfusion of blood and blood products as required to correct coagulopathy.

In those patients who have been stabilized after the initial resuscitation and are at more than 34 weeks' gestation with regular contractions, expedited vaginal delivery should be the goal unless there are obstetric contraindications to vaginal birth. These patients usually deliver relatively quickly following amniotomy.

Conservative management is only appropriate in stable preterm pregnancies (<34 weeks' gestation) where the initial bleeding episode has subsided and there is no evidence of maternal or fetal compromise. A course of antenatal corticosteroids should be administered given the increased risk of preterm delivery in these patients. The role of tocolysis is debatable and routine use is not recommended. Patients with preterm abruption on expectant management should be monitored very closely until delivery, which should be considered by 37–38 weeks' gestation in those patients who remain stable after initial presentation with preterm mild clinical abruption (69).

Postpartum care

Close monitoring of patients with complications of abruption (**Box 22.8**) should be carried out in a critical care setting after delivery. Monitoring and correction of coagulation status and regular maternal vital signs should be carried out. Patients who have suffered severe abruption particularly those with poor outcome should be properly debriefed about the peripartum events by a senior clinician prior to discharge from the hospital. Additionally, these patients will benefit from a follow-up when a plan of care for any subsequent pregnancies can be discussed. The likelihood of recurrence in a subsequent pregnancy is 3–15% (70) and the need for antenatal awareness should be emphasized.

Vasa praevia

Vasa praevia is the presence of fetal blood vessels running in the membranes in close proximity to the internal os (within 2 cm). It is described as type 1 when it occurs in association with velamentous insertion of the umbilical cord and type 2 when it occurs in association with a bilobed placenta or succenturiate lobe. Vasa praevia is relatively rare and complicates approximately 1 in 2500 births (71) and is associated with significant perinatal mortality especially when diagnosed in acute setting related to ruptured membranes. The significant perinatal mortality results from rapid fetal exsanguination from the disrupted fetal blood vessels.

Placental abnormalities such as placenta praevia, velamentous insertion of the cord, bilobed placenta, succenturiate lobe, multiple pregnancy, and *in vitro* fertilization are known risk factors for vasa praevia (72).

Diagnosis

Although routine screening for vasa praevia is not recommended, a high index of suspicion should be maintained in patients with multiple risk factors linked to vasa praevia. If vasa praevia is suspected in the antenatal period, the diagnosis can be confirmed by transvaginal ultrasound with colour Doppler. This typically shows fetal vessels running in close proximity to the internal cervical os. This should be differentiated from cord presentation, where the vessels are surrounded by Wharton's jelly, and the cord typically floats away when the uterus is gently pushed (73). When vasa praevia is incidentally diagnosed in the second trimester, further assessment by transvaginal ultrasound and colour Doppler should be performed in the third trimester as up to 15% of the cases will resolve by the third trimester (74).

A presumptive diagnosis of vasa praevia is made when brisk bleeding and fetal distress occur immediately after spontaneous or artificial rupture of membranes, particularly in patients with known associations.

Management

When vasa praevia has been diagnosed on a routine ultrasound scan in the antenatal period, fetal surveillance is recommended and antenatal corticosteroids are recommended up to 34 weeks' gestation because of the increased likelihood of preterm delivery. Elective inpatient monitoring from 30 to 34 weeks has been advocated to allow closer fetal surveillance with the added possibility of performing caesarean delivery promptly if labour starts or the membranes rupture (75). Elective delivery by caesarean section is recommended between 35 and 37 weeks once a course of steroid has been completed (31, 76). When there is brisk bleeding and sudden fetal distress or there is a sinusoidal fetal heart rate pattern following ruptured membranes, prompt delivery by caesarean section should be considered with a provisional diagnosis of vasa praevia. There is usually no time to perform a confirmatory test for fetal bleeding (e.g. Apt test or Kleihauer–Betke test) because vasa praevia causes rapid fetal exsanguination and it is imperative to act on the clinical diagnosis to save the fetus in the acute intrapartum scenario.

Local genital causes of antepartum haemorrhage

Once placenta praevia and placenta abruption have been objectively excluded in patients presenting with APH, local genital causes should be explored. The local genital causes include cervical ectropion, cervical polyp, cervicitis, vaginitis, and bleeding from trauma to the vulva and vaginal varicosities (77). Bleeding from cervical ectropion and cervical polyp is usually self-limiting and can present as postcoital bleeding during pregnancy. Reassurance and an explanation is usually all that is required in most cases. Women with cervical polyps should be followed up after the pregnancy to assess the need for polypectomy.

Cervical neoplasia should be suspected when the cervix looks grossly abnormal especially in patients with a poor cervical screening history and these women should be referred urgently for assessment by a gynaecology oncologist. Severe vaginal candidiasis can be associated with vaginal spotting as the yeast plaque sloughs off from the vaginal wall and the symptoms usually resolve with topical antifungal treatment.

Antepartum bleeding of unknown origin

In up to 2% of cases of APH, no cause or source of bleeding will be identified (78). While the patient can be reassured after the initial assessment, the pregnancy should be followed up particularly if the APH is recurrent. These pregnancies are associated with an increased risk of preterm delivery and reduced birth weight babies and fetal death (78, 79). As a minimum, fetal surveillance with growth scans in the third trimester is recommended in cases of recurrent APH of unknown origin.

Conclusion

While significant progress has been made in the understanding and management of pregnancies complicated by APH, sustaining such improvements require a consistent, evidence-based approach in the management of these patients. The implementation of regular team-based obstetric haemorrhage drills is an excellent way of ensuring a system-wide improvement. Such drills should be combined with sentinel event reviews and an audit of the management of major APH. There is also an emerging role for centres of excellence for the multidisciplinary management of placenta accreta.

REFERENCES

1. Giordano R, Cacciatore A, Cignini P, et al. Antepartum haemorrhage. *J Prenat Med* 2010;**4**:12–16.
2. Green J. Placenta abnormalities: placenta praevia and abruptio placentae. In: Creasy RK, Resnik R (eds), *Maternal Fetal Medicine: Principles and Practice*, pp. 141–54. Philadelphia, PA: WB Saunders; 1989.
3. Sinha P, Kuruba N. Ante-partum haemorrhage: an update. *J Obstet Gynaecol* 2008:377–81.
4. Alkema L, Chou D, Hogan D, et al. Global, regional, and national levels and trends in maternal mortality between 1990 and 2015, with scenario-based projections to 2030: a systematic analysis by the UN Maternal Mortality Estimation Inter-Agency Group. *Lancet* 2016;**387**:462–74.
5. Gulland A. Worldwide maternal mortality rate falls by 45% in 13 years. *BMJ* 2014;**348**:g3150.

6. Say L, Chou D, Gemmill A, et al. Global causes of maternal death: a WHO systematic analysis. *Lancet Glob Health* 2014;**2**:e323–33.

7. Bhandari S, Raja EA, Shetty A, Bhattacharya S. Maternal and perinatal consequences of antepartum haemorrhage of unknown origin. *BJOG* 2014;**121**:44–50.

8. Rigby E. *An Essay on the Uterine Haemorrhage, which Precedes the Delivery of the Full Grown Fetus.* London: Johnson; 1775.

9. Dunn MP. Perinatal lessons from the past. *Arch Dis Child Fetal Neonatal Ed* 2000;**82**:F169–70.

10. Le Bas A, Chandraharan E, Addei A, Arulkumaran S. Use of the 'obstetric shock index' as an adjunct in identifying significant blood loss in patients with massive postpartum hemorrhage. *Int J Gynaecol Obstet* 2014;**124**:253–55.

11. Derbala Y, Grochal F, Jeanty P. Vasa praevia. *J Perinat Med* 2007;**1**:2–13.

12. Lavery JP. Placenta previa. *Clin Obstet Gynecol* 1990;**33**:414–21.

13. Oyelese Y, Smulian JC. Placenta previa, placenta accreta, and vasa previa. *Obstet Gynecol* 2006;**107**:927–41.

14. Dashe JS, McIntire DD, Ramus RM, et al. Persistence of placenta previa according to gestational age at ultrasound detection. *Obstet Gynecol* 2002;**99**:692–97.

15. Faiz AS, Ananth CV. Etiology and risk factors for placenta previa: an overview and meta-analysis of observational studies. *J Matern Fetal Neonatal Med* 2003;**13**:175–90.

16. Royal College of Obstetricians and Gynaecologists. *Antepartum Haemorrhage.* Green-top Guideline No. 63. London: RCOG; 2011.

17. Gurol-Urganci I, Cromwell DA, Edozien LC, et al. Risk of placenta previa in second birth after first birth cesarean section: a population-based study and meta-analysis. *BMC Pregnancy Childbirth* 2011;**11**:95.

18. Downes KL, Hinkle SN, Sjaarda LA, et al. Previous prelabor or intrapartum cesarean delivery and risk of placenta previa. *Am J Obstet Gynecol* 2015;**212**:669.e1–6.

19. Rosenberg T, Pariente G, Sergienko R, et al. Critical analysis of risk factors and outcome of placenta previa. *Arch Gynecol Obstet* 2011;**284**:47–51.

20. Macones GA, Sehdev HM, Parry S, et al. The association between maternal cocaine use and placenta previa. *Am J Obstet Gynecol* 1997;**177**:1097–100.

21. Weis MA, Harper LM, Roehl KA, et al. Natural history of placenta previa in twins. *Obstet Gynecol* 2012;**120**:753–58.

22. Silver R, Depp R, Sabbagha RE, et al. Placenta previa: aggressive expectant management. *Am J Obstet Gynecol* 1984;**150**:15–22.

23. Cotton DB, Read JA, Paul RH, Quilligan EJ. The conservative aggressive management of placenta previa. *Am J Obstet Gynecol* 1980;**137**:687–95.

24. McShane PM, Heyl PS, Epstein MF. Maternal and perinatal morbidity resulting from placenta previa. *Obstet Gynecol* 1985;**65**:176–82.

25. Oppenheimer L, Society of Obstetricians and Gynaecologists of Canada. Diagnosis and management of placenta previa. *J Obstet Gynaecol Can* 2007;**29**:261–66.

26. Smith RS, Lauria MR, Comstock CH, et al. Transvaginal ultrasonography for all placentas that appear to be low-lying or over the internal cervical os. *Ultrasound Obstet Gynecol* 1997;**9**:22–24.

27. Leerentveld RA, Gilberts EC, Arnold MJ, Wladimiroff JW. Accuracy and safety of transvaginal sonographic placental localization. *Obstet Gynecol* 1990;**76**:759–62.

28. Dashe JS, McIntire DD, Ramus RM, et al. Persistence of placenta previa according to gestational age at ultrasound detection. *Obstet Gynecol* 2002;**99**:692–97.

29. Oppenheimer L, Holmes P, Simpson N, Dabrowski A. Diagnosis of low-lying placenta: can migration in the third trimester predict outcome? *Ultrasound Obstet Gynecol* 2001;**18**:100–102.

30. Becker RH, Vonk R, Mende BC, et al. The relevance of placental location at 20–23 gestational weeks for prediction of placenta previa at delivery: evaluation of 8650 cases. *Ultrasound Obstet Gynecol* 2001;**17**:496–501.

31. Royal College of Obstetricians and Gynaecologists (RCOG). *Placenta Praevia, Placenta Praevia Accreta, Vasa Praevia: Diagnosis and Management.* Green-top Guideline No. 27. London: RCOG; 2011.

32. Timor-Tritsch IE, Yunis RA. Confirming the safety of transvaginal sonography in patients suspected of placenta previa. *Obstet Gynecol* 1993;**81**:742–44.

33. Love CD, Fernando KJ, Sargent L, Hughes RG. Major placenta praevia should not preclude out-patient management. *Eur J Obstet Gynecol Reprod Biol* 2004;**117**:24–29.

34. Cotton DB, Read JA, Paul RH, Quilligan EJ. The conservative aggressive management of placenta previa. *Am J Obstet Gynecol* 1980;**137**:687–95.

35. Ghi T, Contro E, Martina T, et al. Cervical length and risk of antepartum bleeding in women with complete placenta praevia. *Ultrasound Obstet Gynecol* 2009;**33**:209–12

36. Sekiguchi A, Nakai A, Kawabata I, et al. Type and location of placenta praevia affect preterm delivery risk related to antepartum haemorrhage. *Int J Med Sci* 2013;**10**:1683–88.

37. Mouer JR. Placenta previa: antepartum conservative management, inpatient versus outpatient. *Am J Obstet Gynecol* 1994;**170**:1683–85.

38. Neilson JP. Interventions for suspected placenta praevia. *Cochrane Database Syst Rev* 2003;**2**:CD001998.

39. Besinger RE, Moniak CW, Paskiewicz LS, et al. The effect of tocolytic use in the management of symptomatic placenta previa. *Am J Obstet Gynecol* 1995;**172**:1770–75.

40. Sharma A, Suri V, Gupta I. Tocolytic therapy in conservative management of symptomatic placenta previa. *Int J Gynaecol Obstet* 2004;**84**:109–13.

41. Bhide A, Prefumo F, Moore J, et al. Placental edge to internal os distance in the late third trimester and mode of delivery in placenta praevia. *BJOG* 2003;**110**:860–64.

42. Tantbirojn P, Crum CP, Parast MM. Pathophysiology of placenta accreta: the role of decidua and extravillous trophoblast. *Placenta* 2008;**29**:639–45.

43. Wu S, Kocherginsky M, Hibbard JU. Abnormal placentation: twenty-year analysis. *Am J Obstet Gynecol* 2005;**192**:1458–61.

44. Miller DA, Chollet JA, Goodwin TM. Clinical risk factors for placenta previa-placenta accreta. *Am J Obstet Gynecol* 1997;**177**:210–14.

45. Clark SL, Koonings PP, Phelan JP. Placenta previa/accreta and prior cesarean section. *Obstet Gynecol* 1985;**66**:89–92.

46. National Institutes of Health Consensus Development Conference Panel. National Institutes of Health Consensus Development Conference Statement. NIH Consensus Development Conference: Vaginal Birth After Cesarean: New Insights. March 8–10, 2010. *Obstet Gynecol* 2010;**115**:1279–95.

47. D'Antonio F, Iacovella C, Bhide A. Prenatal identification of invasive placentation using ultrasound: systematic review and meta-analysis. *Ultrasound Obstet Gynecol* 2013;**42**:509–17.

48. Comstock CH. Antenatal diagnosis of placenta accreta: a review. *Ultrasound Obstet Gynecol* 2005;**26**:89–96.

49. Finberg HJ, Williams JW. Placenta accreta: prospective sonographic diagnosis in patients with placenta previa and prior cesarean section. *J Ultrasound Med* 1992;**11**:333–43.

50. Warshak CR, Eskander R, Hull AD, et al. Accuracy of ultrasonography and magnetic resonance imaging in the diagnosis of placenta accreta. *Obstet Gynecol* 2006;**108**:573–81.

51. D'Antonio F, Iacovella C, Palacios-Jaraquemada J, et al. Prenatal identification of invasive placentation using magnetic resonance imaging: systematic review and meta-analysis. *Ultrasound Obstet Gynecol* 2014;**44**:8–16.

52. Horowitz JM, Berggruen S, McCarthy RJ, et al. When timing is everything: are placental MRI examinations performed before 24 weeks' gestational age reliable? *AJR Am J Roentgenol* 2015;**205**:685–92.

53. Maldjian C, Adam R, Pelosi M, et al. MRI appearance of placenta percreta and placenta accreta. *Magn Reson Imaging* 1999;**17**:965–71.

54. Shih JC, Palacios Jaraquemada JM, Su YN, et al. Role of three-dimensional power Doppler in the antenatal diagnosis of placenta accreta: comparison with gray-scale and color Doppler techniques. *Ultrasound Obstet Gynecol* 2009;**33**:193–203.

55. Fox KA, Shamshirsaz AA, Carusi D, et al. Conservative management of morbidly adherent placenta: expert review. *Am J Obstet Gynecol* 2015;**213**:755–60.

56. Sentilhes L, Ambroselli C, Kayem G, et al. Maternal outcome after conservative treatment of placenta accreta. *Obstet Gynecol* 2010;**115**:526–34.

57. Chandraharan E, Rao S, Belli AM, Arulkumaran S. The triple-P procedure as a conservative surgical alternative to peripartum hysterectomy for placenta percreta. *Int J Gynaecol Obstet* 2012;**117**:191–94.

58. Dilauro MD, Dason S, Athreya S. Prophylactic balloon occlusion of internal iliac arteries in women with placenta accreta: literature review and analysis. *Clin Radiol* 2012;**67**:515–20.

59. Tikkanen M, Luukkaala T, Gissler M, et al. Decreasing perinatal mortality in placental abruption. *Acta Obstet Gynecol Scand* 2013;**92**:298–305.

60. Ruiter L, Ravelli AC, de Graaf IM, et al. Incidence and recurrence rate of placental abruption: a longitudinal linked national cohort study in the Netherlands. *Am J Obstet Gynecol* 2015;**213**:573.e1–8.

61. Ananth CV, Savitz DA, Bowes WA Jr, Luther ER. Influence of hypertensive disorders and cigarette smoking on placental abruption and uterine bleeding during pregnancy. *Br J Obstet Gynaecol* 1997;**104**:572–78.

62. Ananth CV, Getahun D, Peltier MR, Smulian JC. Placental abruption in term and preterm gestations: evidence for heterogeneity in clinical pathways. *Obstet Gynecol* 2006;**107**:785–92.

63. Ananth CV, Oyelese Y, Prasad V, et al. Evidence of placental abruption as a chronic process: associations with vaginal bleeding early in pregnancy and placental lesions. *Eur J Obstet Gynecol Reprod Biol* 2006;**128**:15–21.

64. Cheng HT, Wang YC, Lo HC, et al. Trauma during pregnancy: a population-based analysis of maternal outcome. *World J Surg* 2012;**36**:2767–75.

65. Hoskins IA, Friedman DM, Frieden FJ, et al. Relationship between antepartum cocaine abuse, abnormal umbilical artery Doppler velocimetry, and placental abruption. *Obstet Gynecol* 1991;**78**:279–82.

66. Mackenzie AP, Schatz F, Krikun G, et al. Mechanisms of abruption-induced premature rupture of the fetal membranes: Thrombin enhanced decidual matrix metalloproteinase-3 (stromelysin-1) expression. *Am J Obstet Gynecol* 2004;**191**:1996–2001.

67. Elovitz MA, Ascher-Landsberg J, Saunders T, Phillippe M. The mechanisms underlying the stimulatory effects of thrombin on myometrial smooth muscle. *Am J Obstet Gynecol* 2000;**183**: 674–81.

68. Glantz C, Purnell L. Clinical utility of sonography in the diagnosis and treatment of placental abruption. *J Ultrasound Med* 2002;**21**:837–40.

69. Oyelese Y, Ananth CV. Placental abruption. *Obstet Gynecol* 2006; **108**:1005–16.

70. Rasmussen S, Irgens LM, Dalaker K. The effect on the likelihood of further pregnancy of placental abruption and the rate of its recurrence. *Br J Obstet Gynaecol* 1997;**104**:129295.

71. Bronsteen R, Whitten A, Balasubramanian M, et al. Vasa previa: clinical presentations, outcomes, and implications for management. *Obstet Gynecol* 2013;**122**:352–57.

72. Baulies S, Maiz N, Muñoz A, et al. Prenatal ultrasound diagnosis of vasa praevia and analysis of risk factors. *Prenat Diagn* 2007;**27**:595–99.

73. Rebarber A, Dolin C, Fox NS, et al. Natural history of vasa previa across gestation using a screening protocol. *J Ultrasound Med* 2014;**33**:141–47.

74. Society of Maternal-Fetal (SMFM) Publications Committee, Sinkey RG, Odibo AO, Dashe JS. #37: Diagnosis and management of vasa previa. *Am J Obstet Gynecol* 2015;**213**:615–19.

75. Gagnon R, Morin L, Bly S, et al. Guidelines for the management of vasa previa. *J Obstet Gynaecol Can* 2009;**31**:748–53.

76. Robinson BK, Grobman WA. Effectiveness of timing strategies for delivery of individuals with vasa previa. *Obstet Gynecol* 2011; **117**:542–49.

77. Chamberlain G. Antepartum haemorrhage. *BMJ* 1991;**302**: 1526–30.

78. McCormack RA, Doherty DA, Magann EF, et al. Antepartum bleeding of unknown origin in the second half of pregnancy and pregnancy outcomes. *BJOG*.2008;**115**:1451–57.

79. Chan CC, To WW. Antepartum hemorrhage of unknown origin—what is the clinical significance. *Acta Obstet Gynecol Scand* 1999;**78**:186–90.

23

Liver and endocrine diseases in pregnancy

Catherine Williamson

Liver disease

Liver diseases of pregnancy can be divided into disorders specific to pregnancy or diseases incidental to pregnancy. Pregnancy-specific disorders include hyperemesis gravidarum, intrahepatic cholestasis of pregnancy (ICP), acute fatty liver, and pre-eclampsia with hepatic involvement. Many hepatic diseases affect women of reproductive age. Viral hepatitis is very common worldwide. Some non-infectious disorders present in women of reproductive age (e.g. autoimmune hepatitis). While these commonly will have been diagnosed prior to a woman becoming pregnant, some may present *de novo* in pregnancy. It is therefore important to take a thorough history and perform a clinical examination to establish the underlying diagnosis in pregnant women with new symptoms or signs consistent with liver disease. The typical symptoms associated with specific liver disorders are summarized in **Table 23.1**. Not all symptoms are specific to a specific disorder, for example, although pruritus is associated with cholestasis, it may also occur in pregnant women who do not have liver disease. It is also important to know which clinical features are not of concern in pregnancy, and of note, palmar erythema and spider naevi occur in a large number of pregnant women without associated liver disease.

To manage women with gestational liver disease effectively, clinicians should know the normal ranges for liver function tests (LFTs) in pregnancy (**Table 23.2**) (1). The upper end of the normal range for liver transaminases is reduced by approximately 20%, likely secondary to the increase in circulating volume in the second half of pregnancy. There is a similar reduction in the normal range for bilirubin and gamma-glutamyltranspeptidase, but this is not seen for alkaline phosphatase because there is secretion of a placenta-specific isoform in the third trimester.

Disorders specific to pregnancy

Hyperemesis gravidarum

While nausea and vomiting are relatively common in the first trimester, affecting almost 50% of pregnant women, it is much less common to have severe and protracted vomiting (approximately 1%). If women cannot maintain normal fluid and food intake or weight, they should be assessed for dehydration and for coexisting pathology (**Table 23.3**). Blood tests should be taken to ensure they do not have electrolyte disturbance, abnormal LFTs, or biochemical abnormalities of thyroid function tests. Many women with protracted vomiting have hyponatraemia, and this should be corrected slowly with normal saline. It is important to also monitor serum potassium concentrations and to correct hypokalaemia. Abnormal LFTs usually indicate starvation, and they typically return to normal once a woman recommences oral intake. Women with severe hyperemesis gravidarum can have biochemical thyrotoxicosis. This is very rarely seen in conjunction with clinical features of hyperthyroidism, and is usually a marker of severe disease that resolves when the underlying hyperemesis has been successfully treated.

Women with hyperemesis gravidarum can be treated with hydration and antiemetics. There are good safety data for most commonly used antiemetic drugs such as doxylamine with pyridoxine, cyclizine, metoclopramide, promethazine, and prochlorperazine. Women should be reassured that use of these drugs is not associated with an increased risk of congenital malformation. The majority of women respond to a combination of these drugs, ideally with doses spaced throughout the day. If women do not respond to these drugs, either ondansetron or glucocorticoids may be used as second-line treatment. Thromboprophylaxis should be given to women who are admitted to hospital or to those that have risk factors for thrombosis, and thiamine replacement is recommended due to the increased risk of deficiency with acute vomiting. This is important as thiamine deficiency is associated with Wernicke's encephalopathy.

Some investigators have reported increased rates of small-for-gestational age babies and preterm birth in women with hyperemesis gravidarum with low weight gain throughout pregnancy, although this was not seen in all studies. However, it is important to ensure adequate food and fluid intake in pregnancy and antiemetic drugs with good safety data to support their use should not be withheld. This is of particular importance given that women with hyperemesis gravidarum are reported as dying in pregnancy approximately once every 1–3 years in the United Kingdom in the Confidential Enquiries into Maternal Deaths.

Table 23.1 Typical symptoms associated with abnormal liver function tests in pregnancy and likely associated diagnosis

Symptom	Likely diagnosis	Other possible diagnoses
Pruritus	ICP	Pre-eclampsia, AFLP, biliary obstruction, pre-existing hepatobiliary disease (PBC, PSC), DILI
Epigastric pain Nausea and vomiting—second and third trimester Headache Visual disturbance	Pre-eclampsia, HELLP syndrome, AFLP	Gallbladder disease, cholangitis, viral hepatitis
Nausea and vomiting—first trimester	Hyperemesis gravidarum	Viral hepatitis
Jaundice	Viral hepatitis	HELLP syndrome, gallbladder disease, cholangitis, DILI, rarely ICP or pre-eclampsia
Pale stools and dark urine	Biliary obstruction secondary to gallstone disease	ICP, cholangitis, viral hepatitis, other rare causes of biliary obstruction

AFLP, acute fatty liver of pregnancy; DILI, drug-induced liver injury; HELLP, haemolysis, elevated liver enzymes, and low platelets; ICP, intrahepatic cholestasis of pregnancy; PBC, primary biliary cholangitis; PSC, primary sclerosing cholangitis.
Source data from Walker I, Chappell LC, Williamson C. Abnormal liver function tests in pregnancy. *BMJ* 2013;347:f6055.

Table 23.2 Typical reference ranges for liver enzymes, by trimester

Liver enzyme	Non-pregnant	Pregnant	First trimester	Second trimester	Third trimester
Alanine transaminase (ALT) (IU/L)	0–40	–	6–32	6–32	6–32
Aspartate transaminase (AST) (IU/L)	7–40	–	10–28	11–29	11–30
Bilirubin (µmol/L)	0–17	–	4–16	3–13	3–14
Gamma-glutamyltranspeptidase (γGT) (IU/L)	11–50	–	5–37	5–43	3–41
Alkaline phosphatase (ALP) (IU/L)	30–130	–	32–100	43–135	133–418
Albumin (g/L)	35–46	28–37	–	–	–
Bile acids (µmol/L)	0–14	0–14	–	–	–

Source data from Walker I, Chappell LC, Williamson C. Abnormal liver function tests in pregnancy. *BMJ* 2013;347:f6055.

Table 23.3 Coexisting pathology that should be considered in a woman with hyperemesis gravidarum

System	Diagnosis	Investigation/initial assessment	Frequency
Obstetric	Molar pregnancy	Ultrasound scan of the uterus	+
Gastrointestinal	Gastritis/peptic ulceration	*Helicobacter pylori* antibodies	+
	Gastroesophageal reflux and ulcerative esophagitis	Endoscopy or empirical proton pump inhibitor therapy	++
	Pancreatitis	Amylase, blood glucose, calcium	+
	Bowel obstruction	Plain supine abdominal X-ray	+
Endocrine	Addison's disease	U&E, early morning cortisol, short Synacthen test with ACTH	+
	Hyperthyroidism	Surveillance for symptoms and signs of hyperthyroidism, TFTs, thyroid autoantibodies	++
	Diabetic ketoacidosis	Blood glucose, urinary dipstick for ketones, glucose tolerance test	++
CNS	Intracranial tumour	CNS examination, brain imaging	+
	Vestibular disease	CNS examination	+
Respiratory	Asthma	Chest examination, peak expiratory flow rate.	++
Other	Urinary tract infection	Mid-stream urine specimen	+++
	Uraemia	U&E	+

ACTH, adrenocorticotropic hormone; CNS, central nervous system; TFTs, thyroid function tests; U&E, urea and electrolytes.

Pre-eclampsia (including HELLP syndrome)

In a study of the underlying diagnosis in women presenting with abnormal LFTs in pregnancy in Wales (2), 71% of the women studied had pre-eclampsia. While HELLP (haemolysis, elevated liver enzymes, and low platelets) syndrome affected one-third of cases, it was much commoner for women to present with pre-eclampsia and isolated abnormal LFTs, in the absence of low platelets or haemolysis. The presentation and management of pre-eclampsia and HELLP syndrome are discussed elsewhere (see Chapter 21). However, it is important to note that some other disorders are more commonly complicated by pre-eclampsia. These include pre-existing hypertension, raised maternal body mass index, diabetes mellitus, renal disease, and a number of other vascular, endocrine, and metabolic disorders.

Intrahepatic cholestasis of pregnancy

ICP, also called obstetric cholestasis, is the commonest liver-specific disorder of pregnancy. ICP affects 1 in 140 pregnant women in the United Kingdom, but there is considerable geographic variation in the prevalence of the condition with higher rates in South America, particularly Chile, and in women of South Asian and Hispanic origin. Most women with ICP are well when they are not pregnant, and present in pregnancy with generalized pruritus, raised serum bile acid concentrations, and the majority also have abnormal LFTs. The serum bile acid level is the most important biochemical abnormality for diagnosis of ICP because high concentrations in the mother's blood are associated with increased rates of adverse pregnancy outcome (3, 4). The first large, national study that demonstrated an association between serum bile acid concentrations and outcomes in ICP reported no increase in adverse outcomes (spontaneous preterm labour, fetal asphyxia events, and meconium-stained amniotic fluid) when the maternal bile acid concentration was less than 40 µmol/L, but these complications were increased with higher concentrations (3). A UK cohort study and subsequent large individual patient data meta-analysis confirmed these results and also demonstrated a significant increase in stillbirth which increased further as the maternal bile acid concentration increased to above 100 µmol/L confirmed these results and also demonstrated a significant increase in stillbirth which increased further as the maternal bile acid concentration became higher (4). The association between maternal alanine aminotransferase (ALT) concentrations and adverse pregnancy outcome is not as clear cut, and hence it is advisable to monitor maternal serum bile acid concentrations regularly after a diagnosis of ICP has been made, as they typically continue to rise with advancing gestation. Although pruritus in ICP is not preceded by a rash, some women develop skin lesions secondary to scratching (**Figure 23.1**).

If a woman presents with ICP, it is important to perform blood tests to evaluate the severity of the elevation in bile acids to consider the risk of adverse pregnancy outcome, and to measure LFTs to evaluate the extent of maternal hepatic damage. While most women have transient cholestasis that resolves after delivery, a small proportion of women with ICP have another underlying disorder (**Table 23.4**) and it is important to monitor the liver function to ensure they do not deteriorate. The pattern of LFTs is typically characterized by raised liver transaminases (e.g. ALT) in addition to elevated serum bile acids, and both usually continue to rise with advancing gestation. The gamma-glutamyltranspeptidase concentration is raised in approximately one-third of women, and bilirubin is rarely elevated

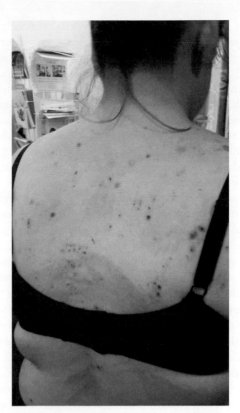

Figure 23.1 Dermatological lesions on the back of a woman with ICP. Excoriations and scarring are secondary to scratching. Figure reproduced with permission of ICP Support.

in ICP. Occasionally, women with ICP have abnormal coagulation tests. This is likely to be secondary to ICP-associated steatorrhoea and vitamin K malabsorption, and treatment with vitamin K should improve this. Tests should be requested to exclude hepatitis C, auto-immune hepatitis, and an abdominal ultrasound scan performed to ensure there is no extrahepatic cause of biliary obstruction. This will demonstrate gallstones in a sizeable proportion of cases because the underlying genetic susceptibility to ICP is caused by some genes that are also associated with an increased risk of gallstones. However, gallstones are very rarely the cause of the cholestasis.

The most commonly used treatment for ICP is ursodeoxycholic acid (UDCA). Several studies have reported improved maternal symptoms and biochemistry with UDCA treatment (5–8). At present it is not established whether UDCA treatment improves adverse pregnancy outcome, although a meta-analysis that considered

Table 23.4 Coexisting pathology that should be considered in a woman with intrahepatic cholestasis of pregnancy

System	Diagnosis
Gestational diseases	Acute fatty liver of pregnancy Pre-eclampsia with abnormal liver function
Disorders not related to pregnancy	Hepatitis C Autoimmune hepatitis Primary biliary cholangitis[a] Primary sclerosing cholangitis Drug-induced liver injury Gallstones ± cholangitis

[a] Also called primary biliary cirrhosis.

all trials of UDCA compared to another drug or placebo reported improved rates of preterm labour, fetal distress, respiratory distress, and prolonged neonatal unit admission in pregnancies treated with UDCA (7). A trial that compared UDCA to placebo treatment in 605 women with ICP, diagnosed in women with serum bile acids of 10 μmol/L or more, in the United Kingdom showed some reduction in pruritus, but no improvement in a composite outcome of all preterm birth, stillbirth or admission to the neonatal unit (8). For women with severe pruritus, aqueous cream with 1–2% menthol may provide symptomatic relief and vitamin K treatment is recommended for women with steatorrhoea.

There is no established form of monitoring that can predict which ICP pregnancies are likely to be complicated by spontaneous preterm labour, fetal distress, or stillbirth. Many hospitals offer regular review in the antenatal day unit, with cardiotocograph checks. While this is reassuring at the time it is performed, it will not give information about the risk of stillbirth after the monitor has been removed. The recent individual patient data meta-analysis (8) showed that the significant increase in stillbirth that occurred in pregnancies where maternal serum bile acids were greater than 100 μmol/L, showed a marked increase in risk between 35–36 weeks' gestation. Therefore early delivery should be considered in this subgroup of women with ICP. It is advisable to check serum bile acids at least weekly from 35 weeks in severe cases as they may rise considerably with advancing gestation. While the increased risk of prolonged admission to the neonatal special care unit has been shown to be associated with higher maternal bile acid concentrations, and there is evidence that bile acid inhibit phospholipase A2, and are likely to cause abnormalities in surfactant (9, 10), it is likely that preterm delivery also contributes to this risk.

For most women, the pruritus and abnormal biochemistry resolve after delivery. It is important to check the serum bile acid concentrations and LFTs to ensure they are returning to normal after delivery. For some women it takes up to 3 months for the tests to return to normal. It is advisable to refer those with ongoing abnormalities to a hepatologist for assessment. Women should be advised that they have a high risk of ICP in subsequent pregnancies, particularly if they have a multiple pregnancy. They should also avoid the combined oral contraceptive pill, although progesterone-only contraception does not cause problems for the majority. They are at increased risk of biliary disease in later life (11).

Acute fatty liver of pregnancy

Acute fatty liver of pregnancy (AFLP) affects 1 in 20,000 pregnancies in the United Kingdom (12). It presents in the third trimester with non-specific symptoms, including nausea, vomiting, polyuria, polydipsia, and feeling generally unwell. Affected women have abnormal LFTs, often with markedly raised liver transaminases, bilirubin, and coexisting elevation of creatinine, leucocytes, abnormal coagulation, and metabolic acidosis. However, the extent of the biochemical abnormalities may vary. It is often useful to consider the 'Swansea criteria' for diagnosis of AFLP (**Table 23.5**). At least six of these clinical features are present in the majority of women with AFLP (12, 13). The condition can deteriorate rapidly, and can result in fulminant hepatic failure. Approximately one woman in the United Kingdom dies from AFLP each year. Most affected women should be cared for in a high dependency or intensive care setting. It is advisable to involve a specialist liver unit early and the input of a multidisciplinary team will be needed, including specialist physicians, obstetricians, midwives,

Table 23.5 Diagnostic criteria for acute fatty liver of pregnancy (AFLP; Swansea criteria); AFLP is the likely diagnosis if six or more features are present

Clinical features	Vomiting Abdominal pain Polydipsia/polyuria Encephalopathy
Blood test abnormalities	Elevated bilirubin Hypoglycaemia Elevated urate Leucocytosis Elevated transaminases Elevated ammonia Renal impairment Coagulopathy
Imaging	Ascites or bright liver on ultrasound
Invasive testing	Microvesicular steatosis on liver biopsy

Source data from Ch'ng CL, Morgan M, Hainsworth I, Kingham JG. Prospective study of liver dysfunction in pregnancy in Southwest Wales. *Gut* 2002;51:876–80.

obstetric anaesthetists, and intensive care specialists. Women with AFLP should be delivered as soon as they have been stabilized as once the placenta has been delivered, the metabolites that cause maternal hepatic impairment will cease to be transported to the mother. Prior to delivery it is important to ensure that coagulopathy and hypoglycaemia have been treated, in addition to correcting any other life-threatening biochemical derangements. AFLP resolves after delivery, although women can deteriorate for a small number of days before they start to improve. Approximately 20% of cases present in the immediate postpartum period, likely related to enhanced release of placental or fetal metabolites that cause hepatic damage at the time of delivery. Providing they do not develop fulminant hepatic failure requiring transplant, most women make a full recovery within a small number of weeks following delivery. A small proportion of cases have children with disorders of beta-fatty acid oxidation (14, 15) and it is therefore advisable to ensure the children of women with AFLP are screened, as they are likely to remain healthy if fed a high-carbohydrate diet. In the United Kingdom, these disorders are detected by neonatal Guthrie spot screening. It is important to ensure that liver function returns fully to normal after pregnancy. The risk of recurrence of AFLP has not been accurately established, with the exception of women who are obligate heterozygotes for fatty acid oxidation disorders, but it is likely to be 10–20%.

Disorders incidental to pregnancy

Women of reproductive age can have a variety of hepatic disorders, and the commoner ones will be discussed in the following sections. The most important issues for the majority of women with pre-existing disease are to ensure they have prepregnancy counselling from a doctor with experience and knowledge of liver disease in pregnancy. This will enable them to embark on pregnancy cognisant of the risks associated with their disease and the drugs used to treat it. Decisions can also be made about where a woman should be managed, whether this should be as part of a multidisciplinary team, at a tertiary referral centre or if she should have shared care.

Viral hepatitis

Hepatitis B infection is the commonest cause of jaundice in pregnancy worldwide. However, acute and chronic maternal disease is managed the same way in pregnancy as in non-pregnant individuals. It is important to give the neonates of affected women immunoglobulin and the hepatitis B vaccine to prevent mother-to-child transmission. Mode of delivery does not influence the rate of vertical transmission. However, this may be increased in women with a high viral load in pregnancy, and in these cases it is advisable to treat with nucleoside analogues (16).

The clinical presentation and treatment of most other forms of viral hepatitis are not affected by pregnancy. An exception is hepatitis E, a virus transmitted by the faecal–oral route, that normally has a mild course in non-pregnant individuals, but can commonly cause fulminant hepatic failure in pregnant women (17, 18). Hepatitis C infection is a blood-borne infection that may present for the first time in pregnancy, typically with symptoms of cholestasis. There is no specific treatment for the infection in pregnancy, but affected women should be referred for treatment postnatally. There is relatively low vertical transmission in the absence of coexisting HIV infection and mode of delivery does not influence this. Breastfeeding should be encouraged as this does not increase the rate of neonatal infection.

Autoimmune hepatitis

Autoimmune hepatitis occurs in women of reproductive age. They have a 25% chance of flare, particularly in the postpartum period, and this is reduced in those that continue immunosuppressive treatment. It is therefore important for hepatologists caring for these women to ensure that they are given appropriate prepregnancy counselling. They should be informed that azathioprine has good safety data to support its use in pregnancy and lactation, and that prednisolone treatment can be used if required (19). Mycophenolate mofetil should not be used in pregnant women as it is associated with high rates of congenital malformations, and if a woman using this drug intends to conceive, her medication should be changed to another drug (e.g. azathioprine, ciclosporin, or tacrolimus). Some women with autoimmune hepatitis have cirrhosis (see later).

Budd–Chiari syndrome

Pregnancy is a prothrombotic state, and a number of new cases of Budd–Chiari syndrome have been diagnosed in pregnancy. However, this is a relatively rare disorder and the majority of cases will have presented before pregnancy. In the rare circumstance when a woman presents *de novo* in pregnancy, the typical symptoms are ascites, jaundice, and right upper quadrant pain. In women with a pre-existing diagnosis of Budd–Chiari syndrome, many have an underlying thrombophilia and it will be important to ensure adequate anticoagulation, usually with low-molecular-weight heparin. A series of 24 pregnancies in 16 patients treated for Budd–Chiari syndrome reported good maternal outcomes but a preterm birth rate exceeding 50% (20).

Primary biliary cholangitis and primary sclerosing cholangitis

Primary biliary cholangitis (PBC), also called primary biliary cirrhosis, is a chronic autoimmune cholestatic disorder that typically affects postmenopausal women. Common symptoms are pruritus and fatigue in conjunction with hepatic impairment, and it may coexist with other autoimmune disorders. Some cases occur at younger ages and the condition can occur in pregnant women. The prognosis of PBC in pregnancy has improved in more recent studies

in which women are treated with UDCA (21). However, despite improved maternal and fetal outcomes most women have a deterioration in liver function postpartum, although this usually resolves after 12 months.

Primary sclerosing cholangitis (PSC) is a chronic inflammatory disorder characterized by fibrosis and stricturing of the intrahepatic and extrahepatic bile ducts, resulting in cholestasis and hepatic damage. Up to 90% of patients have coexisting ulcerative colitis. PSC more commonly affects men, but women are also affected and it usually presents before the age of 40, so it may occur in pregnancy. The most common maternal symptoms are pruritus and abdominal pain (22). UDCA is used less frequently to treat PSC than PBC, and there is no evidence that it improves maternal prognosis during pregnancy. However, given the accumulating data that maternal serum bile acid concentrations of at least 40 µmol/L increase the risk of spontaneous preterm labour, prolonged admission to the neonatal unit, and stillbirth in pregnancies complicated by cholestasis in the absence of PBC or PSC (4), it seems sensible to consider UDCA treatment during pregnancy for women with raised serum bile acids. However, it should be noted that high-dose UDCA treatment is associated with poorer outcomes in PSC outside pregnancy.

Cirrhosis

Many women with chronic cirrhosis have impaired fertility, but some women with treated autoimmune hepatitis, PBC, PSC or long-standing viral hepatitis can become pregnant with cirrhosis. Women with established cirrhosis should be screened for oesophageal varices in the second trimester, and if necessary treatment can be performed with banding or sclerotherapy. Decisions about mode of delivery should be made on a case-by-case basis. The presence of portal hypertension with treated (or minor) varices is not a reason to avoid vaginal delivery.

Bleeding from oesophageal varices

Women with portal hypertension (with or without cirrhosis) are at risk of gastrointestinal haemorrhage. Oesophageal varices may develop in pregnancy in women without liver disease, and in those with portal hypertension this may result in a considerable risk of gastrointestinal bleeding. For women with non-cirrhotic portal hypertension, the risk of bleeding is 10–15%. For those with cirrhosis and untreated oesophageal varices, the risk is very high (70–90%) and is considerably reduced if the varices are treated with banding or sclerotherapy (approximately 10%). In women with life-threatening haemorrhage, vasoconstrictors such as terlipressin can be used, although there are limited safety data for these drugs.

Gallstones

Pregnancy is associated with a tendency to develop cholesterol gallstones. In the majority of women they will be asymptomatic and they may resolve postpartum. Asymptomatic gallstones should not be treated in pregnancy. A small proportion of women may develop acute cholecystitis, and this group should be treated in the same way as they would be managed outside pregnancy with cessation of oral intake, intravenous fluids, antibiotics, and assessment for suitability for surgery. A study that compared outcomes of women with acute cholecystitis treated medically or surgically demonstrated good outcomes for all women treated with surgery, while there was a 38% relapse rate in those that received medical management (23).

Pregnancy following liver transplantation

Fertility typically returns within 6 months of a liver transplant. It is advised to delay conception until 12 months after transplantation as this reduces the risk of transplant rejection. Good outcomes are reported for the majority of women, although there is an increased risk of pregnancy-induced hypertension, pre-eclampsia, and preterm delivery (24). Most immunosuppressive drugs can be used in pregnancy, and there are good safety data for azathioprine, ciclosporin, and tacrolimus. Women treated with mycophenolate should be given prepregnancy advice about the high congenital malformation rate associated with this drug, and their treatment regimen should be changed to include alternative immunosuppressive drugs prior to conception.

Endocrine disease

Endocrine disorders affect many glands and are commonly seen in pregnant women. Most women with endocrine disorders in pregnancy have a condition that is not specific to pregnancy. However, there are a small number of women who develop gestational hyperthyroidism, and hyperemesis has an endocrine component as women with severe disease can develop biochemical thyrotoxicosis (see 'Hyperemesis gravidarum'). Autoimmune endocrine disorders can improve during pregnancy, but typically worsen in the postpartum period. Also, some endocrine tumours can worsen during pregnancy, for example, prolactinomas commonly enlarge and in a subgroup of women with large tumours this can cause visual impairment. Clinicians managing pregnant women with endocrine disease should know about the impact of pregnancy on specific disorders as well as the best strategies for surveillance and safest treatments. It is important to be aware of the normal ranges of specific hormones in pregnancy to enable precise decisions to be made about whether hormones are present in excess or if women have deficiencies. This chapter will consider the commonest endocrine disorders that are seen in pregnancy.

Thyroid disease

The changes over time of specific thyroid hormones are shown in **Figure 23.2**. Human chorionic gonadotropin (hCG) shares some structural similarities to thyroid-stimulating hormone (TSH) and can stimulate the TSH receptor, and this causes a transient increase in tetraiodothyronine (thyroxine) and suppression of TSH in the first trimester. TSH levels will subsequently normalize once hCG levels plateau (**Figure 23.2**).

Also, conditions associated with higher hCG levels (e.g. molar pregnancy, multiple pregnancy, or hyperemesis gravidarum) can result in biochemical derangements suggestive of thyrotoxicosis. Thyroid-binding globulin levels increase in pregnancy, likely secondary to elevated oestrogen levels, and therefore total thyroxine measurement is not helpful, and free thyroxine measurement should be used. The normal ranges of thyroid function tests in each trimester of pregnancy are summarized in **Table 23.6**.

Autoimmune hypothyroidism

Autoimmune hypothyroidism is common, affecting 1% of pregnancies. If well controlled, women should have good pregnancy

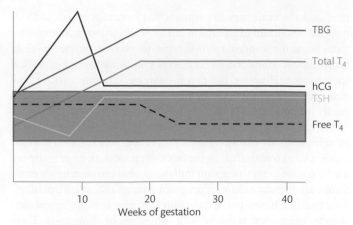

Figure 23.2 Normal ranges for thyroid function tests in pregnancy. hCG, human chorionic gonadotropin; T$_4$, tetraiodothyronine (thyroxine); TBG, thyroid-binding globulin; TSH, thyroid-stimulating hormone.

outcomes. However, overt hypothyroidism is associated with increased risks of adverse pregnancy outcome, including miscarriage, pre-eclampsia, placental abruption, and low birth weight, in addition to having an adverse impact upon the intelligence of the baby (25–27). Therefore it is important to ensure that affected women are adequately treated. However, overtreatment is associated with impaired fetal growth and can cause iatrogenic maternal hyperthyroidism, so overtreatment should be avoided as well (28). While it is clear that overt hypothyroidism causes impaired offspring intelligence, the impact of subclinical hypothyroidism on subsequent intelligence of the fetus is not clearly established. Although some older studies suggested that this could be an issue, there is no clear evidence for this in large, robustly performed studies. Indeed, a well-powered United Kingdom study that evaluated the impact of thyroxine replacement from the end of the first trimester for subclinical hypothyroidism did not show any difference in subsequent intelligence of the offspring at 3 years of age, and nor was there any impact upon birth weight or the rate of preterm birth (29). Therefore it is clearly important to ensure that women with hypothyroidism receive treatment with thyroxine to maintain their thyroid function tests in the normal range for pregnancy, but there is no evidence for treatment of women with normal thyroid function tests (28). There is also no evidence base for taking a TSH concentration of 2.5 mU/L as the threshold above which thyroxine replacement should be commenced in pregnant women with no history of thyroid disease, and recent studies have raised concerns that this practice will be result

Table 23.6 Normal ranges for thyroid function tests in pregnancy

Normal range	FT4 (pmol/L)	TSH (mU/L)
Non-pregnant	11–23	0–4
First trimester	11–22	0–1.6
Second trimester	9–19	0.1–1.2
Third trimester	7–15	0.7–5.5

FT4, free thyroxine; TSH, thyroid-stimulating hormone.
Based on data taken from Parker et al. *BJOG* 1985;92:1234–38; Chan et al. *BJOG* 1988;95:1332–36; Soldin et al. *Ther Drug Monit* 2007;29:553–59.

in unnecessary treatment of up to 15% of pregnant women with no obvious thyroid disease (30).

There is some debate about whether all women need an increase in the dose of thyroxine in early pregnancy. As the thyroid-binding globulin concentration is elevated (**Figure 23.2**), some women will need an increase in thyroxine dose. A study that addressed the need for increased dose of thyroxine in 100 pregnancies in women with autoimmune hypothyroidism found that 50% of women needed more thyroxine, but in the majority of cases this was due to inadequate replacement prior to pregnancy, poor compliance, or recent diagnosis with insufficient time to optimize treatment, rather than a consequence of a gestation-specific need to increased dose (31). Therefore it is advisable to check the thyroid function tests as early as possible in pregnancy (and ideally prepregnancy) and to adjust the thyroxine dose in those that are deficient using normal ranges for pregnancy.

A small number of women present in early pregnancy with overt hypothyroidism and elevated TSH concentration above the normal range for pregnancy. This group of women are often concerned about the potential impact on the intelligence of their children. While there has been no study that specifically focuses on this group of infants, it is likely that the impact will be minimal if thyroxine replacement is optimized in the second and third trimester. Small studies of mild hypothyroxinaemia in the first trimester have shown that there is no impact on subsequent intelligence if the maternal thyroxine concentration returns to normal by the third trimester (32).

There is evidence that pregnant women positive for thyroid autoantibodies are more likely to have a miscarriage and preterm delivery (33). However, the underlying mechanism is not established. It is possible that this may relate to the coexistence of other autoimmune disorders that are associated with these adverse outcomes (e.g. antiphospholipid syndrome). To address the question of whether thyroxine treatment can reduce the risk of adverse pregnancy outcome in euthyroid women with positive thyroid peroxidase antibodies, the TABLET trial randomised 952 euthyroid women to 50 µg thyroxine or placebo from before conception and to be continued throughout pregnancy. This trial did not demonstrate any impact upon live birth rate (34). It is noteworthy that the study of thyroxine replacement for women with subclinical hypothyroidism (29) did not show any change in the rate of miscarriage or preterm labour in the group that received thyroxine replacement.

Hyperthyroidism

Hyperthyroidism affects 1 in 800 pregnancies. The majority of cases have Graves' disease. Rarer causes of hyperthyroidism in pregnancy are toxic nodule, thyroid adenoma, carcinoma, or subacute thyroiditis. Many clinical features of hyperthyroidism also occur in normal pregnancy, for example, palpitations, heat intolerance, and palmar erythema. However, eye signs and pretibial myxoedema are specific to autoimmune thyroid disease and weight loss does not occur in normal pregnancy. The biochemical features of hyperthyroidism are seen in women with hyperemesis gravidarum, but these do not occur in conjunction with clinical signs of thyroid hormone excess.

As most cases of hyperthyroidism occur in women of reproductive age, affected women are likely to need advice about pregnancy and conception. Carbimazole and propylthiouracil are used to treat hyperthyroidism, and both drugs are associated with an increased risk of congenital abnormalities, with the most recent studies suggesting the rate is twice the background rate (35, 36). There are more data to support the association of carbimazole/methimazole with congenital abnormalities, but the 2013 study by Andersen et al. (36) demonstrated that this is a concern for propylthiouracil as well. This is important as guidance from the American Thyroid Association prior to this study recommended that propylthiouracil should be the treatment of choice in pregnant women on the basis of less evidence for an association with congenital malformations, despite the fact that use of propylthiouracil is rarely associated with fulminant hepatic failure in 1:10,000 adults and 1:2000 children (37). A pragmatic approach given the current data is to continue carbimazole in women who are already taking it prior to conception. Either carbimazole or propylthiouracil can be used for newly diagnosed cases in the first trimester of pregnancy, with appropriate advice about the risk of congenital malformations. It should also be explained that untreated thyrotoxicosis is associated with increased risks of fetal loss, growth restriction, preterm labour, and untreated women are at risk of thyroid storm, so treatment should be given. If the diagnosis is made after the first trimester, carbimazole is the most sensible choice. Many women with autoimmune hyperthyroidism find that their disease improves in pregnancy and in some the dose of antithyroid drugs may be reduced or even stopped. However, the requirement for treatment usually returns postpartum.

Women with autoimmune thyroid disease should have TSH receptor antibodies checked as they can cross the placenta and stimulate the fetal thyroid. In women who are taking antithyroid drugs this is unlikely to cause problems until after delivery as carbimazole and propylthiouracil also cross the placenta, but there is a risk of neonatal thyrotoxicosis 2–4 days postpartum. This is because the drugs will clear from the neonatal circulation rapidly, but the maternal antibodies will remain for approximately 3 months. As a consequence, it is important to involve the neonatologists in early fetal assessment. If a woman is not taking antithyroid drugs (e.g. because she has previously had surgery or radioiodine treatment), her pregnancy should be closely monitored for fetal hyperthyroidism or goitre because TSH receptor antibodies can cross the placenta and there will be no antithyroid drugs to prevent fetal disease. Monitoring should include assessment of fetal growth, fetal heart rate, and to ensure there is no goitre.

Carbimazole and propylthiouracil can be given to lactating women. There are no concerns about transfer to the baby with low, maintenance doses of either drug, but if high doses are used, the baby's thyroid function should be monitored.

Adrenal disease

Addison's disease

Adrenal insufficiency can be due to autoimmune destruction of the adrenal gland (Addison's disease), or can be the consequence of prolonged treatment with glucocorticoids causing adrenal suppression, or secondary to ACTH deficiency. Addison's disease is associated with the presence of adrenal antibodies and can have an insidious onset. It should be considered in women with other autoimmune diseases, in particular in those with unexplained lethargy, nausea, vomiting, hypotension or hyponatraemia. Pigmentation of palmar creases, the buccal mucosa, or scars may be seen. If suspected, a short tetracosactrin test should be performed. Glucocorticoid replacement can be given while waiting for the result. Replacement doses of hydrocortisone are usually given, with higher doses in the morning, and this should be decided in collaboration with an endocrinologist. Women with known hypoadrenalism should receive additional glucocorticoids at times of stress, vomiting, and to cover labour. They should also be advised to carry a steroid card and wear a medic-alert bracelet.

Cushing syndrome

Cushing syndrome is caused by glucocorticoid excess. It is caused by tumours of the pituitary or adrenal and by ingestion of excess doses of exogenous glucocorticoids. As adrenal tumours are reported to occur more commonly in pregnancy, likely a consequence of pituitary tumours influencing gonadotrophin secretion, Cushing syndrome will be considered under the heading of adrenal disease. However, the principles relating to complications are the same for both disorders. Cushing syndrome can be difficult to diagnose in pregnancy as many symptoms and signs are also seen in pregnant women, such as weight gain, striae, hypertension, glucose intolerance, and hirsutism. However, the striae in pregnancy are not usually as marked or coloured purple as they are in women with Cushing syndrome. The condition is associated with a number of adverse maternal and fetal outcomes (38–41). Severe hypertension may occur and impaired glucose tolerance or gestational diabetes mellitus affect 25% of cases. There is an increased rate of preterm labour and stillbirth (39). Maternal and fetal outcomes are improved in women who are treated surgically (39). Metyrapone and ketoconazole have also been used in pregnancy with good maternal and fetal outcomes (39, 40).

Phaeochromocytoma

Phaeochromocytoma is rare, affecting 1 in 54,000 pregnancies, but is a cause of severe morbidity and mortality that is important to recognize. The presenting symptoms include sweating, headache, and palpitations and the principal sign is hypertension. The condition may be missed due to these clinical features being attributed to pregnancy. However, the hypertension is often paroxysmal and in women with the classical symptoms and a suggestive history, plasma or urinary catecholamines, and metanephrines should be checked. If phaeochromocytoma remains undiagnosed, the maternal and fetal mortality can be as high as 50%, and this is markedly reduced with active management (41, 42). It is important to involve a multidisciplinary team in the management of women with phaeochromocytoma, particularly to ensure coordinated plans for delivery. The most important treatment is to commence an alpha-adrenoreceptor blocker, and the most commonly used drug is phenoxybenzamine. Once alpha-blockade has been achieved, some women require beta-blockade, but this must not be commenced before alpha-blockade has been achieved. Timing of surgery varies in different studies, with reports of adrenalectomy during the first 24 weeks of pregnancy, usually by a laparoscopic approach. Surgery can also be successfully achieved at the time of delivery or postpartum, providing adequate alpha-blockade has been achieved (43, 44). While there is no contraindication to vaginal delivery in well-controlled women, many cases are delivered by caesarean section. It is important that a team including intensive care physicians, obstetric anaesthetists, endocrinologists, obstetricians, and midwives are involved with peripartum care.

Primary aldosteronism

Primary aldosteronism, also called Conn syndrome, is caused by an aldosterone-producing tumour of the adrenal. The typical presenting features are hypertension and hypokalaemic alkalosis due to autonomous production of aldosterone and secondary renin suppression (45). This condition is rare in pregnancy. The commonest management strategy during pregnancy is to use potassium supplements and antihypertensive drugs with deferral of surgery until after delivery. Potassium-sparing antihypertensive agents (e.g. amiloride) may be used (41).

Pituitary/hypothalamic disease

Prolactinoma and other pituitary tumours

Prolactinomas are the commonest hormone-secreting tumours. They occur in women of reproductive age, and affected women frequently have menstrual irregularity, reduced fertility, and galactorrhoea. Large tumours may present with headache and visual symptoms secondary to compression of the optic chiasm. Prolactinomas respond well to dopamine agonist treatment, and women typically conceive rapidly once they commence treatment. Prolactinomas are subdivided according to size. The commoner subtype is microprolactinomas (measuring <10 mm in diameter) and women with these tumours usually have an uncomplicated course in pregnancy (46). Although most prolactinomas enlarge in pregnancy (47), in the majority of cases this is not associated with symptoms. In contrast, approximately 20–30% of women with macroprolactinomas (≥10 mm diameter) have symptomatic expansion in pregnancy. However, if a woman has previously been treated by radiotherapy or surgery the likelihood of expansion is considerably reduced (48). As there is a significant risk of symptomatic expansion of macroprolactinoma in pregnancy, the guidelines of the Pituitary Society (49) and the Endocrine Society (50) recommend treatment with dopamine agonists in women with symptomatic expansion, and the Endocrine Society guideline supports continuation of therapy in the first trimester in selected high-risk women with macroprolactinoma who have not had prior surgical or radiation therapy. Furthermore, the Pituitary Society guideline recommends close surveillance and that magnetic resonance imaging (MRI) should be performed if there is symptomatic enlargement of a tumour and the Endocrine Society Clinical Practice Guideline recommends formal visual field assessment followed by an MRI scan in pregnant women with prolactinomas who experience severe headaches or visual field changes.

The dopamine agonists bromocriptine and cabergoline have good safety data from large numbers of women who have taken the drugs in pregnancy. Treatment with both drugs in the first trimester is not associated with an increased risk of congenital malformations (46), and offspring intellectual and physical development has been reported as normal in children whose mothers were treated with bromocriptine up to the age of 9 years (51) and in children exposed to cabergoline *in utero* up to 71 months of age (52). In 2008, the British Medicine and Healthcare Products Advisory Authority advised that pregnancy should be excluded prior to administration of cabergoline, due to theoretical concerns about an association between ergot-containing dopamine agonists (bromocriptine and cabergoline) and maternal/fetal cardiac fibrosis. However, there have been no reports of this complication and most clinicians use dopamine agonists in pregnancy if the potential risks of tumour enlargement are perceived to be high. The alternative drug is quinagolide, a non-ergot containing dopamine agonist, but there are fewer safety data about use of this drug in pregnancy, and one study reported 9 congenital malformations in 176 pregnancies where the drug was taken in the first trimester (53). These included three cases of trisomy, unlikely to be related to quinagolide therapy, but more data are required to clarify the risks of quinagolide treatment in pregnancy.

Other pituitary tumours are considerably rarer than prolactinomas. Acromegaly, Cushing's disease and TSHoma can all influence fertility due to gonadotropin-releasing hormone insufficiency, a likely explanation for most affected women having been diagnosed before pregnancy. If a woman has a previous diagnosis of one of these hormone-secreting pituitary tumours that was treated prior to conception, she is likely to have a good pregnancy outcome. Acromegaly and Cushing's disease are associated with hypertension and susceptibility to impaired glucose tolerance and gestational diabetes mellitus, and women should be screened for these disorders. Women with non-functioning pituitary adenomas can present in pregnancy or prior to pregnancy. Although they don't secrete hormones, these tumours may be associated with the same complications that can occur with other pituitary tumours in pregnancy. In particular, they can cause visual symptoms due to optic chiasm compression, likely due to expansion of surrounding pituitary tissue in pregnancy. All pituitary tumours may also be complicated by apoplexy, a rare medical emergency that presents with headache, altered consciousness, visual symptoms, or vomiting (54).

Pituitary insufficiency

Pituitary insufficiency can be caused by infiltrative disorders, lymphocytic hypophysitis, tumours, irradiation, or infection and cause deficiency of one or all pituitary hormones. If pregnant women receive adequate hormonal replacement, they usually have good maternal and fetal outcomes. However, assessment of hormonal concentrations can be challenging due to alterations in normal ranges and binding proteins in pregnant women.

Lymphocytic hypophysitis

Lymphocytic hypophysitis is an inflammatory disorder that occurs more commonly in women than men (8.5:1) and is associated with pregnancy. The commonest presenting symptoms are headache and visual symptoms, and pituitary insufficiency is common. Approximately 30% of cases have panhypopituitarism, and 20% have diabetes insipidus. It is important to distinguish lymphocytic hypophysitis from pituitary tumours as the management is different, and this can usually be achieved with MRI (55). The condition may resolve spontaneously, and also responds to treatment with glucocorticoids or azathioprine.

Diabetes insipidus

Women with pre-existing diabetes insipidus commonly have a deterioration of their symptoms in pregnancy due to placental production of vasopressinase. Most will respond to an increase in dose of desmopressin treatment. The increased requirement for desmopressin will cease rapidly after delivery, so it is important to review the serum sodium concentration and/or plasma and urinary osmolality in women with diabetes insipidus immediately

postpartum as well as at regular intervals during pregnancy. Some women with severe hepatic impairment (e.g. those with AFLP) can develop transient diabetes insipidus, likely a consequence of impaired hepatic degradation of placental vasopressin.

Parathyroid disorders

Primary hyperparathyroidism

Primary hyperparathyroidism occurs in approximately 8 per 100,000 women of reproductive age. In uncomplicated pregnancy, the maternal corrected calcium concentration in serum is usually slightly reduced, and this may explain why women with primary hyperparathyroidism in pregnancy often do not have the typical symptoms of nephrolithiasis or abdominal pain. However, up to 25% present with pre-eclampsia or pregnancy-induced hypertension (56). Maternal hyperparathyroidism is associated with a high perinatal complication rate, including stillbirth and neonatal tetany. A single-centre study of 77 pregnancies in 32 women with hyperparathyroidism reported a 48% fetal loss rate in 62 pregnancies where there was no surgical treatment. In contrast, in the 15 cases where parathyroidectomy was performed in the second trimester, there were good fetal outcomes (57). In this study, the fetal loss rate increased in pregnancies where the maternal serum calcium rate was higher. Given the association with fetal loss, parathyroidectomy is advisable in many cases. Alternatively, the serum calcium can be controlled in some cases with hydration and oral phosphate administration.

Conclusion

Liver and endocrine diseases in pregnancy include pregnancy-specific disorders and diseases incidental to pregnancy. All should be managed by a multidisciplinary team with experts in maternal medicine, high-risk obstetricians, physicians with expertise in managing specific endocrine or liver diseases in pregnancy, and midwives and many will require input from obstetric anaesthetists. Women with pre-existing medical disorders should have prepregnancy counselling with regard to the impact of pregnancy on their disease, and the influence of the disease and drugs used to treat it on a pregnancy. With expert management from appropriate specialists, most women with have good pregnancy outcomes.

Acknowledgement

I would like to thank Leslie McMurtry for help with references and formatting the text, in addition to excellent administrative support.

REFERENCES

1. Walker I, Chappell LC, Williamson C. Abnormal liver function tests in pregnancy. *BMJ* 2013;**347**:f6055.
2. Ch'ng CL, Morgan M, Hainsworth I, Kingham JG. Prospective study of liver dysfunction in pregnancy in Southwest Wales. *Gut* 2002;**51**:876–80.
3. Glantz A, Marschall HU, Mattsson LA. Intrahepatic cholestasis of pregnancy: Relationships between bile acid levels and fetal complication rates. *Hepatology* 2004;**40**:467–74.

4. Ovadia C, Sklavounos A, Geenes V, et al. Adverse perinatal outcomes of intrahepatic cholestasis of pregnancy and association with biochemical markers: results of aggregate and independent patient data meta-analyses. *Lancet* 2019 Feb 14;**393**:899–909. pii: S0140-6736(18)31877-4. doi: 10.1016/S0140-6736(18)31877-4. PMID: 30773280.

5. Chappell LC, Gurung V, Seed PT, et al. Ursodeoxycholic acid versus placebo, and early term delivery versus expectant management, in women with intrahepatic cholestasis of pregnancy: semifactorial randomised clinical trial. *BMJ* 2012;**344**:e3799.

6. Glantz A, Marschall HU, Lammert F, Mattsson LA. Intrahepatic cholestasis of pregnancy: a randomized controlled trial comparing dexamethasone and ursodeoxycholic acid. *Hepatology* 2005;**42**:1399–405.

7. Bacq Y, Sentilhes L, Reyes HB, et al. Efficacy of ursodeoxycholic acid in treating intrahepatic cholestasis of pregnancy: a meta-analysis. *Gastroenterology* 2012;**143**:1492–501.

8. Chappell LC, Bell J, Smith A, Linsell L, Juszczak E, Dixon PH, Chambers J, Hunter R, Dorling J, Williamson C*, Thornton JG*. Ursodeoxycholic acid versus placebo in women with intrahepatic cholestasis of pregnancy (PITCHES): a randomised controlled trial. *Lancet* May 2019; doi: 10.1016/S0140-6736(19)31270-X. PMID: 31378395.

9. Herraez E, Lozano E, Poli E, et al. Role of macrophages in bile acid-induced inflammatory response of fetal lung during maternal cholestasis. *J Mol Med (Berl)* 2014;**92**:359–72.

10. Zhang Y, Li F, Wang Y, et al. Maternal bile acid transporter deficiency promotes neonatal demise. *Nat Commun* 2015;**6**:e8186.

11. Marschall HU, Wikström Shemer E, Ludvigsson JF, Stephansson O. Intrahepatic cholestasis of pregnancy and associated hepatobiliary disease: a population-based cohort study. *Hepatology* 2013;**58**:1385–391.

12. Knight M, Nelson-Piercy C, Kurinczuk JJ, Spark P, Brocklehurst P, UK Obstetric Surveillance System. A prospective national study of acute fatty liver of pregnancy in the UK. *Gut* 2008;**57**:951–56.

13. Ch'ng CL, Kingham JG, Morgan M. Acute fatty liver in pregnancy in the UK. *Gut* 2009;**58**:467–68.

14. Ibdah JA, Bennett MJ, Rinaldo P, et al. A fetal fatty-acid oxidation disorder as a cause of liver disease in pregnant women. *N Engl J Med* 1999;**340**:1723–31.

15. Browning MF, Levy HL, Wilkins-Haug LE, Larson C, Shih VE. Fetal fatty acid oxidation defects and maternal liver disease in pregnancy. *Obstet Gynecol* 2006;**107**:115–20.

16. European Association for the Study of the Liver. EASL clinical practice guidelines: management of chronic hepatitis B virus infection. *J Hepatol* 2012;**57**:167–85.

17. Khuroo MS, Kamili S. Aetiology, clinical course and outcome of sporadic acute viral hepatitis in pregnancy. *J Viral Hepatol* 2003;**10**:61–69.

18. Kumar A, Beniwal M, Kar P, Sharma JB, Murthy NS. Hepatitis E in pregnancy. *Int J Gynecol Obstet* 2004;**85**:240–44.

19. Flint J, Panchal S, Hurrell A, et al. BSR and BHPR guideline on prescribing drugs in pregnancy and breastfeeding—Part I: standard and biologic disease modifying anti-rheumatic drugs and corticosteroids. *Rheumatology* 2016;**299**:1–5.

20. Rautou PE, Angermayr B, Garcia-Pagan JC, et al. Pregnancy in women with known and treated Budd-Chiari syndrome: maternal and fetal outcomes. *J Hepatol* 2009;**51**:47–54.

21. Poupon R, Chretien Y, Chazouilleres O, Poupon RE. Pregnancy in women with ursodeoxycholic acid-treated primary biliary cirrhosis. *J Hepatol* 2005;**42**:418–23.

22. Janczewska I, Olsson R, Hultcrantz R, Broomé U. Pregnancy in patients with primary sclerosing cholangitis. *Liver* 1996;**16**: 326–30.

23. Lu EJ, Curet MJ, El-Sayed YY, Kirkwood K. Medical versus surgical management of biliary tract disease in pregnancy. *Am J Surg* 2004;**188**:755–59.

24. Westbrook RH, Yeoman AD, Agarwal K, et al. Outcomes of pregnancy following liver transplantation: The King's College Hospital experience. *Liver Transpl* 2015;**21**:1153–59.

25. Blazer S. Maternal hypothyroidism may affect fetal growth and neonatal thyroid function. *Obstet Gynecol* 2003;**102**:232–41.

26. Haddow JE, Palomaki GE, Allan WC, et al. Maternal thyroid deficiency during pregnancy and subsequent neuropsychological development of the child. *N Engl J Med* 1999;**341**:549–55.

27. Pop VJ, Kuijpens JL, van Baar AL, et al. Low maternal free thyroxine concentrations during early pregnancy are associated with impaired psychomotor development in infancy. *Clin Endocrinol (Oxf)* 1999;**50**:149–55.

28. Wiles KS, Jarvis S, Nelson-Piercy C. Are we overtreating subclinical hypothyroidism in pregnancy? *BMJ* 2015;**12**:h4726.

29. Lazarus JH, Bestwick JP, Channon S, et al. Antenatal thyroid screening and childhood cognitive function. *N Engl J Med* 2012;**366**:493–501.

30. Maraka S, O'Keeffe DT, Montori VM. Subclinical hypothyroidism during pregnancy—should you expect this when you are expecting? A teachable moment. *JAMA Intern Med* 2015;**175**:1088–89.

31. Kothari A, Girling J. Hypothyroidism in pregnancy: pre-pregnancy thyroid status influences gestational thyroxine requirements. *BJOG* 2008;**115**:1704–708.

32. Pop VJ, Brouwers EP, Vader HL, Vulsma T, van Baar AL, de Vijlder JJ. Maternal hypothyroxinaemia during early pregnancy and subsequent child development: a 3-year follow-up study. *Clin Endocrinol* 2003; **59**:282–88.

33. Thangaratinam S, Tan A, Knox E, Kilby MD, Franklyn J, Coomarasamy A. Association between thyroid autoantibodies and miscarriage and preterm birth: meta-analysis of evidence. *BMJ* 2011;**9**:342:d2616.

34. Dhillon-Smith RK, Middleton LJ, Sunner KK, et al. Levothyroxine in Women with Thyroid Peroxidase Antibodies before Conception. N Engl J Med. 2019 Apr 4;380(14):1316–1325. doi: 10.1056/NEJMoa1812537. PMID: 30907987.

35. Yoshihara A, Noh JY, Yamaguchi T, et al. Treatment of Graves' disease with antithyroid drugs in the first trimester of pregnancy and the prevalence of congenital malformation. *J Clin Endocrinol Metab* 2012;**97**:2396–403.

36. Andersen SL, Olsen J, Wu CS, Laurberg P. Birth defects after early pregnancy use of antithyroid drugs: a Danish nationwide study. *JCEM* 2013;**98**:4373–81.

37. Bahn RS, Burch HS, Cooper DS, et al. The role of propylthiouracil in the management of Graves' disease in adults: report of a meeting jointly sponsored by the American Thyroid Association and the Food and Drug Administration. *Thyroid* 2009;**19**:673–74.

38. Lindsay JR, Jonklaas J, Oldfield EH, Nieman LK. Cushing's syndrome during pregnancy: personal experience and review of the literature. *JCEM* 2005;**90**:3077–83.

39. Vilar L, Conceição Freitas M, LimaII LHC, LyraII R, Kater CE. Cushing's syndrome in pregnancy: an overview. *Arq Bras Endocrinol Metabol* 2007;**51**:1293–302.

40. Lim WH, Torpy DJ, Jeffries WS. The medical management of Cushing's syndrome during pregnancy. *Eur J Obstet Gynecol Reprod Biol* 2013;**168**:1–6.

41. Quartermaine G, Lambert K, Rees K, et al. Women with hormone-secreting adrenal tumours in pregnancy have severe hypertension and increased rates of adverse pregnancy outcome. *BJOG* 2017;DOI: 10.1111/1471-0528.14918. PMID: 28872770.

42. Biggar MA, Lennard TW. Systematic review of phaeochromocytoma in pregnancy. *Br J Surg* 2013;**100**:182–90.

43. Pacak K, Eisenhofer G, Ahlman H, et al. Pheochromocytoma: recommendations for clinical practice from the First International Symposium. *Nat Clin Pract Endocrinol Metab* 2007;**3**:92–102.

44. Lan BY, Taskin HE, Aksoy E, et al. Factors affecting the surgical approach and timing of bilateral adrenalectomy. *Surg Endosc* 2015;**29**:1741–45.

45. Monticone S, Auchus RJ, Rainey WE. Adrenal disorders in pregnancy. *Nat Rev Endocrinol* 2012;**8**:668–78.

46. Molitch ME. Endocrinology in pregnancy: management of the pregnant patient with a prolactinoma. *Eur J Endocrinol* 2015;**172**:R205–13.

47. Lebbe M, Hubinont C, Bernard P, Maiter D. Outcome of 100 pregnancies initiated under treatment with cabergoline in hyperprolactinaemic women. *Clin Endocrinol (Oxf)* 2010;**73**:236–42.

48. Lambert K, Rees K, Seed P, et al. Pituitary tumours in pregnancy: a 3 year prospective UK national cohort study. *Obstet Gynecol.* 2017 Jan; 129(1):185–94. PMID: 27926659. DOI: 10.1097/AOG.0000000000001747.

49. Casanueva FF, Molitch ME, Schlechte JA, et al. Guidelines of the Pituitary Society for the diagnosis and management of prolactinomas. *Clin Endocrinol (Oxf)* 2006;**65**:265–73.

50. Melmed SF, Casanueva F, Hoffman AR, et al. Diagnosis and treatment of hyperprolactinemia: an Endocrine Society clinical practice guideline. *J Clin Endocrinol Metab* 2011;**96**:273–78.

51. Raymond JP, Goldstein E, Konopka P, Leleu MF, Merceron RE, Loria Y. Follow-up of children born of bromocriptine-treated mothers. *Horm Res* 1985;**22**:239–46.

52. Robert E, Musatti L, Piscitelli G, Ferrari CI. Pregnancy outcome after treatment with the ergot derivative, cabergoline. *Reprod Toxicol* 1996;**10**:333–37.

53. Webster J. A comparative review of the tolerability profiles of dopamine agonists in the treatment of hyperprolactinaemia and inhibition of lactation. *Drug Saf* 1996;**14**:228–38.

54. De Heide JLM, van Tol KM, Doorenbos B. Pituitary apoplexy presenting during pregnancy. *Neth J Med* 2004;**62**:393–96.

55. Gutenberg A, Larsen J, Lupic I, Rohdea V, Catureglid P. A radiologic score to distinguish autoimmune hypophysitis from nonsecreting pituitary adenoma preoperatively. *AJNR* 2009;**30**:1766–72.

56. Schnatz PF, Thaxton S. Parathyroidectomy in the third trimester of pregnancy. *Obstet Gynecol Surv* 2005;**60**:672–82.

57. Norman J, Politz D, Politz L. Hyperparathyroidism during pregnancy and the effect of rising calcium on pregnancy loss: a call for earlier intervention. *Clin Endocrinol (Oxf)* 2009;**71**:104–109.

58. Casey BM, Leveno KJ. Thyroid disease in pregnancy. *Obstet Gynecol* 2006;**108**:1283–89.

59. Chan BY, Swaminathan R. Serum thyrotrophin concentration measured by sensitive assays in normal pregnancy. *BJOG* 1988;**95**:1332–36.

60. Parker JH. Amerlex free triiodothyronine and free thyroxine levels in normal pregnancy. *BJOG* 1985;**92**:1234–38.

61. Soldin OP, Soldin D, Sastoque M. Gestation-specific thyroxine and thyroid stimulating hormone levels in the United States and worldwide. *Ther Drug Monit* 2007;**29**:553–59.

24

Neurological disorders in pregnancy

Judith N. Wagner and Tim J. von Oertzen

Pregnancy-related issues of pre-existing conditions

Epilepsy

Epilepsy, with a prevalence of 0.8% and an incidence of 0.05%, is one of the most common chronic neurological conditions in women of childbearing age (1). The classification of epilepsy was revised in 2010 and includes the aetiology of epilepsy as genetic (previously idiopathic), structural/metabolic (previously symptomatic), and of unknown cause (previously cryptogenic) (2). Treatment with antiepileptic drugs (AEDs) should be tailored to the epilepsy syndrome and seizure types, comorbidities, interactions with comedication (e.g. contraception), and individual circumstances. In general, epilepsy responds well to AED treatment in approximately 65–70% of cases with monotherapy (3). Of the remaining 30–35% of people with epilepsy who suffer from drug-refractory epilepsy, approximately 10–15% will become seizure free with add-on AEDs (4). This results in about 20–25% of epilepsies being drug resistant (5). A neurologist or epilepsy specialist should manage the diagnosis and treatment of epilepsy. All women and girls of childbearing age on AEDs should be offered 5 mg of folic acid before the possibility of pregnancy (6).

With respect to pregnancy, most women will develop epilepsy prior to pregnancy given that the prevalence peak is before the age of 25 and after the age of 65. However, a minority of women will develop epilepsy or seizures during pregnancy. In those cases, acute symptomatic seizures due to eclampsia, intracranial venous thrombosis, reversible posterior leucoencephalopathy, or other acute conditions have to be excluded.

AED-associated risk to the fetus

Most women with epilepsy (WwE) are on AEDs. There are several issues to consider: pregnancies in WwE should be planned as AEDs may impact the major congenital malformation (MCM) risk. Several pregnancy in epilepsy registers have been established worldwide addressing this question. Results of the main registers for AEDs in monotherapy are summarized in **Table 24.1**. A dose-dependent effect on MCM rate has been shown for valproate, carbamazepine, lamotrigine, and phenobarbital (7, 8). All studies identified valproate as having a particularly increased MCM rate. In general, it

has been shown that polytherapy carries a higher risk for MCMs (9–11). However, when analysed for particular AEDs, polytherapies including valproate were identified with a higher MCM rate whereas other combinations showed no significantly increased MCM rate (12, 13). MCMs of AEDs include cardiac malformations, neural tube defects, cleft palate and lip, and hypospadias (for review, see Tomson and Battino (14)). Next to MCMs, which result from exposure to AEDs in the first trimester, cognitive effects in children of mothers taking AEDs at any stage during pregnancy were identified. Children exposed to valproate antenatally showed reduced right handedness and verbal abilities at the age of 3 and 6 years compared to those exposed to carbamazepine, lamotrigine, and phenytoin (15, 16). Again, this effect is dose dependent. Additionally, exposure of valproate is linked to an increased risk of autism spectrum disorders in the offspring with a relative risk of 2.6 (17, 18). In view of the increased risk related to valproate, the European Medicines Agency Pharmacovigilance Risk Assessment Committee and the Coordination Group for Mutual Recognition and Decentralised Procedures strengthened warnings on the use of valproate in girls and women (19). A clinical guidance on the use of valproate in this patient group was published jointly by the International League against Epilepsy and European Academy of Neurology (20).

Epilepsy, AEDs, seizures, and pregnancy

Approximately two out of three WwE will remain seizure free during pregnancy, which is more likely in idiopathic generalized epilepsies compared to localization-related epilepsies. Generalized tonic–clonic seizures occur in 15% of women in pregnancy and are associated with a higher risk for preterm birth and low birth weight (21). Worsening of seizure frequency during pregnancy is noted in 15% and is more common with lamotrigine including generalized tonic–clonic seizures (22). This is partly due to increased AED clearance during pregnancy and is doubled for lamotrigine and levetiracetam (23). Seizures in the 9–12 months preceding conception are a risk factor for seizures during pregnancy (23, 24). Regular therapeutic drug monitoring of AEDs including proactive dose adjustment is recommended during pregnancy (22).

Pregnancy-related risks

WwE have a slightly increased risk of spontaneous miscarriage, ante- or postpartum haemorrhage, hypertensive disorder, caesarean

Table 24.1 Rates of major congenital malformations for the most commonly used anti-epileptic drugs in pregnancy registries for women with epilepsy.

Antiepileptic drug	EURAP Internatl register (1)	UK and Ireland pregnancy register§ (2, 3)	North American pregnancy register (4)	Australian Pregnancy register§ (5)
Carbamzepine	1.3-7.7*	2.6	3.0	6.3
Lamotrigine	1.7-3.6*	2.3	2.0	5.2
Levetiracetam		0.7	2.4	0
Phenytoin			2.9	2.9
Sodium-Valproate	4.2-23.0*	6.7	9.3	16.3
Topiramate			4.2	3.2
No AED			1.1	5.2**

* Dose dependent, ** women with epilepsy not on AEDs; § also part of EURAP

1. Tomson T, Battino D, Bonizzoni E, Craig J, Lindhout D, Sabers A, et al. Dose-dependent risk of malformations with antiepileptic drugs: an analysis of data from the EURAP epilepsy and pregnancy registry. Lancet Neurol. 2011;10:609–17.

2. Campbell E, Kennedy F, Russell A, Smithson WH, Parsons L, Morrison PJ, et al. Malformation risks of antiepileptic drug monotherapies in pregnancy: updated results from the UK and Ireland Epilepsy and Pregnancy Registers. J Neurol Neurosurg Psychiatry. 2014;85:1029–34.

3. Mawhinney E, Craig J, Morrow J, Russell A, Smithson WH, Parsons L, et al. Levetiracetam in pregnancy: results from the UK and Ireland epilepsy and pregnancy registers. Neurology. 2013;80:400–5.

4. Hernández-Díaz S, Smith CR, Shen A, Mittendorf R, Hauser WA, Yerby M, et al. Comparative safety of antiepileptic drugs during pregnancy. Neurology. 2012;78:1692–9.

5. Vajda FJE, Graham J, Roten A, Lander CM, O'Brien TJ, Eadie M. Teratogenicity of the newer antiepileptic drugs--the Australian experience. J Clin Neurosci. 2012;19:57–9.

section, and fetal growth restriction with an odds ratio (OR) between 1.3 and 1.5. Risk for induction of labour is slightly higher (OR 1.7) whereas preterm birth (<37 weeks) is lower (OR 1.2). There is no difference relating to the risk for early preterm birth, gestational diabetes, fetal death or stillbirth, perinatal death, or admission to the neonatal intensive care unit in pregnancies of WwE compared to healthy women (25). The risk for pre-eclampsia seems to be increased 1.7-fold (26). Maternal mortality is tenfold higher in woman with epilepsy than without. This effect has been fairly stable over the last two decades (27, 28).

Delivery in WwE

The highest risk for seizures occurs within the peripartum period. During delivery, around 2–3% of WwE experience a seizure (29, 30). This effect might be partly caused by low-dose AED therapy. Hence, it is recommended that WwE bring their AEDs to the delivery suite and careful observation should be performed on AED compliance during this period. Epilepsy in itself is not regarded as an indication for induction in uncomplicated pregnancies (29). Epidurals, gas and air, and a transcutaneous electrical nerve stimulation (TENS) can be used for pain relief during delivery. Pethidine and other opioids should be avoided as they may trigger seizures in some patients. In case of seizure occurrence during delivery, administration of magnesium and 1–2 mg lorazepam is recommended. If the mother is treated with enzymes inducing AEDs, 1 mg of vitamin K should be given to the baby parenterally at birth (6).

Postpartum considerations

In the postpartum period, attention should be given to the therapeutic drug monitoring of AEDs, particularly if AED dosage was increased during pregnancy. The AED dosage should be adjusted, most commonly reduced, as appropriate. Breastfeeding is recommended and WwE should be encouraged to do so. AED concentrations in breast milk depend on various factors including plasma protein binding. Recent studies have shown that the development of babies of WwE is favourable in the breastfeeding group. In case of concern (e.g. sleepiness of the baby), the AED serum concentrations of the baby should be analysed (31). Mothers with epilepsy should be advised of the risk of epilepsy on the care of their baby, particularly in active epilepsy. In case contraception is discussed, detailed information is available in the epilepsy guidelines of the National Institute for Health and Care Excellence in the United Kingdom (6).

Multiple sclerosis

Multiple sclerosis (MS) is an inflammatory demyelinating disorder of the central nervous system. Signs and symptoms are diverse, ranging from focal deficits (e.g. sensorimotor or visual disturbances) to more complex complaints such as fatigue or cognitive deficits. Typically characterized by a relapsing–remitting course, MS may take a secondary progressive evolution in later stages. Primary progressive manifestations occur in only about 10% of patients (32).

With a sex ratio (male:female) of approximately 1:2 and a peak incidence around 30 years of age (33), childbearing issues are an important aspect of patient management. Multiple analyses have confirmed a significant decrease of relapse frequency during pregnancy, particularly in the third trimester, and a notable peak postpartum (34). However, the long-term effect of pregnancy on MS-associated disability appears to be negligible (35, 36) or even beneficial (37). A low annualized relapse rate and the use of disease-modifying treatment during the 24-months prior to conception seem to be protective against postpartum relapses (38).

Disabling MS relapses during pregnancy are treated with a 3–5-day course of high-dose steroids. The majority of prednisone, prednisolone, and methylprednisolone is converted into inactive metabolites by the placenta. In contrast, betamethasone and dexamethasone are only minimally metabolized and should therefore not be administered during pregnancy. Corticosteroid use during the first trimester may be associated with an increased risk of cleft lip and palate (39, 40).

With the emergence of a plethora of new disease-modifying drugs in recent years, the therapeutic management of women with MS planning to get pregnant has become more challenging and generally needs to be based upon individualized counselling. This is complicated by the lack of adequate data on the safety of use during pregnancy and lactation for most of the disease-modifying drugs.

Clinicians tend to advise discontinuation of disease-modifying drugs prior to conception (41). This tendency is well founded for drugs with serious indications of embryo-fetal toxicity—such as mitoxantrone and teriflunomide—but more arguable for other agents. In particular, glatiramer acetate and interferon beta may be continued in patients with highly active disease after thorough counselling (42, 43); available data on currently used disease-modifying drugs are summarized in **Table 24.2**). Alternatively, intermittent application of high-dose corticosteroids or intravenous immunoglobulin may be considered for relapse prevention during pregnancy and postpartum (39, 40). The caveats applying to corticosteroid use during gestation were discussed previously.

As to the outcome of pregnancy in MS patients, some studies describe an increased risk of intrauterine growth restriction and of the need for induction and instrumental delivery (44, 45). These findings could not be reproduced in other evaluations, in which mothers with MS were no more likely to experience significant pregnancy complications or adverse fetal outcomes than healthy females (46–48).

Myasthenia gravis

Myasthenia gravis (MG) is an antibody-mediated autoimmune disease affecting the nicotinic acetylcholine receptors (AChRs) blocking the initiation of muscle contraction. It is more common in women then man (male:female ratio of 2:3) and its peak incidence is in the third decade of life. MG can be exacerbated with certain medications or conditions such as pregnancy (for a list, see http://www.myaware.org). Clinically, patients present with muscular weakness which might affect the ocular muscles only, or appear more generalized. Dysphagia and dyspnoea can occur and in severe cases or myasthenic crisis, ventilation might be required. Typically, there is a fatigability and circadian rhythm with more prominent symptoms in the evening hours. In case of appropriate clinical features, diagnosis is confirmed by neurophysiological studies, and AChR antibodies. In case of negative AChR antibody studies, anti-muscle-specific kinase (MuSK) antibodies might differentiate from seronegative patients. In cases of doubt, intravenous injection of edrophonium chloride (Tensilon) reverses the antibody binding to AChR temporarily and reverses symptoms (49). The safety of this test during pregnancy has not been established (50). Thymoma is associated with MG in approximately 15%. Hence, thymoma should be excluded by computed tomography (CT) or magnetic resonance imaging (MRI) studies particularly in AChR-positive patients (51). As thymectomy should be considered prior to pregnancy or in the postnatal period, scanning during pregnancy must be carefully considered in view of therapeutic relevance.

Pregnancy in woman with MG should be carefully planned. If possible, pregnancy should be avoided within the first 2 years of the disease as disease activity is particularly high during this period. If indicated, thymectomy should be performed prior to conception. Treatment of MG usually includes pyridostigmine as first-line therapy and if progressive, with steroids (e.g. prednisolone). When long-term immunosuppression is required, azathioprine is added to reduce the steroid dose. In severe cases, methotrexate, ciclosporin, mycophenolate mofetil, or rituximab might be indicated. In some severe, unstable cases of MG, pregnancy might be contraindicated. Where appropriate, medication should be optimized well before conception.

The course of MG during pregnancy is highly variable. Whereas 80% of patients experience a stable condition or improvement, 20% will worsen within pregnancy including relapses of asymptomatic patients (52). The course of MG in further pregnancies is also variable. Additionally, exacerbation of newly presenting MG in pregnancy occurs. Deterioration during pregnancy usually occurs in the first trimester or in the last 4 weeks. Up to 20% experience respiratory crisis during pregnancy with the need for ventilation. Woman with MG should be closely monitored during pregnancy. Treatment options are similar to the prepregnancy period with the exception of immunosuppressants other than steroids. There are limited safety data on most drugs used but pyridostigmine, neostigmine, intravenous immunoglobulins, azathioprine, and ciclosporin appear to be safe in pregnancy (53). Prednisone and prednisolone show a 3.4-fold increased risk of cleft palate (54). Women with MG who are stable on prednisolone and azathioprine should continue this medication. Plasmapheresis and immunoadsorption are well tolerated during pregnancy if necessary.

Magnesium sulphate which is a standard treatment for eclampsia should be avoided in pregnant women with MG as magnesium inhibits acetylcholine release. In case magnesium sulphate has to be used, worsening of MG should be expected and intensive care unit treatment including ventilation should be available. Alternatively, other AEDs, narcotics, or sedatives can be used (55). MG mimicking eclampsia can be treated with pyridostigmine or intravenous neostigmine (56).

Caesarean section should be discussed for the delivery mode as muscular fatigue can occur during spontaneous delivery. Caution is again advised for those anaesthetic drugs and antibiotics which worsen myasthenia. A list of drugs with a risk of worsening myasthenia can be found online (e.g. http://www.myaware.org). If spontaneous delivery is decided upon, regular doses of pyridostigmine should be continued.

Caution is advised for postnatal care of the newborn as neonatal myasthenia might occur with a frequency of 1:12. Immunoglobulin G(IgG) autoantibodies cross the placenta and are secreted in the breast milk causing a transient myasthenic condition in the newborn. Pyridostigmine is the treatment of choice for the newborn. Symptoms will disappear within a few weeks.

Migraine and other types of headache

Headache is a common complaint in the neurological patient. Primary and secondary headaches are distinguished, with each category comprising a multitude of different entities (see the International Headache Society classification (57)). The most frequent types of headache in a primary care setting are migraine, tension-type headache, and headache related to systemic disorders (e.g. infectious diseases) (58).

Migraine typically presents with attacks of a unilateral throbbing headache, which is accompanied by nausea and vomiting, phonophobia, and/or photophobia, and aggravated by physical activity. Atypical bilateral presentations exist. In migraine with aura,

Table 24.2 Summary of available data on embryofetal safety of currently used MS therapeutics (disease-modifying drugs, DMDs) during pregnancy and lactation. The wash-out period denotes the time span that should be allowed to pass between last application of the DMD and conception.

	Pregnancy	Wash-out period	Breastfeeding
Alemtuzumab (1–3, 15)	Animal studies: association with fetal death and altered lymphocyte counts Humans: preliminary data only, no positive evidence for embryofetal toxicity so far; potential negative impact on pregnancy by therapy-associated hypothyroidism Recommendation: use during pregnancy only if the potential benefit justifies the potential risk to the fetus	3 - 4 months	Drug detected in animal milk. No data on human milk. Avoid breastfeeding during treatment and up to 4 months after last infusion.
Dimethyl fumarate (2–4)	Animal studies: adverse effects on offspring survival, growth, sexual maturation, and neurobehavioral function Humans: no adequate and well-controlled studies; preliminary data show no increased risk of fetal abnormalities or adverse pregnancy outcomes Recommendation: use during pregnancy only if the potential benefit justifies the potential risk to the fetus.	0 - 1 months	Not known if excreted into human milk. Avoid while breastfeeding.
Fingolimod (2,3,5,6)	Animal data: studies demonstrate teratogenicity and embryolethality Humans: no adequate and well-controlled studies; preliminary data demonstrate rate of spontaneous abortion slightly exceeding that in the general population and abnormal fetal development at the upper limit of that expected in the general population Recommendation: use during pregnancy only if the potential benefit justifies the potential risk to the fetus	2 months	Drug detected in animal milk. No data on human milk. Avoid breastfeeding during treatment.
Glatiramer acetate (2,3,7–9)	Animal data: no adverse effects on embryo-fetal development observed Humans: no adequate and well-controlled studies; available data do not demonstrate negative effects on embryofetal development Recommendation: use during pregnancy may be considered in women with highly active MS	0 - 1 month	Unknown if excreted into human milk; use not recommended while breastfeeding
Interferon Beta (2,8–10)	Animal data: no positive proof of teratogenicity, but data insufficient Humans: no adequate and well-controlled studies; data thus far suggest association with shorter mean birth length, lower mean birth weight, and preterm birth but not with low birth weight (< 2500g), cesarean delivery, congenital anomaly, lower mean gestational age, or spontaneous abortion. Recommendation: use during pregnancy only if the potential benefit justifies the potential risk to the fetus	0 - 1 month	Minimal excretion of IFN-β1a in human milk. Unknown if excretion of IFN-β1b in human milk. Administration not recommended during breastfeeding.
Mitoxantrone (2,11,12)	Animal studies: evidence of premature delivery and fetal growth retardation Humans: no adequate and well-controlled studies; anecdotal evidence of teratogenic effect Recommendation: contraindicated during pregnancy	6 months	Significant concentrations detected in human milk for 28 days after last application. Discontinue breastfeeding before starting treatment.
Natalizumab (1,2,9,13)	Animal studies: may cause fetal harm Humans: no adequate and well-controlled studies; current limited data do not provide evidence for substantial teratogenicity Recommendation: use during pregnancy only if the potential benefit justifies the potential risk to the fetus	1 - 3 months	Has been detected in human milk. The effects of this exposure on infants are unknown. Avoid during breastfeeding.
Teriflunomide (14)	Animal studies: high incidence of fetal malformation and embryofetal death Humans: no adequate data Recommendation: contraindicated during pregnancy	May stay in the blood for up to 2 years after last dose. Accelerated elimination procedure available to achieve plasma level < 0.02 mg/l.	Has been detected in the milk in animal models. Avoid breastfeeding while on teriflunomide.

LITERATURE

1. Bove R, Alwan S, Friedman JM, Hellwig K, Houtchens M, Koren G, u. a. Management of multiple sclerosis during pregnancy and the reproductive years: a systematic review. Obstet Gynecol. Dezember 2014;124(6):1157–68.

2. Coyle PK. Multiple sclerosis and pregnancy prescriptions. Expert Opin Drug Saf. December 2014;13(12):1565–8.

3. Amato MP, Portaccio E. Fertility, pregnancy and childbirth in patients with multiple sclerosis: impact of disease-modifying drugs. CNS Drugs. March 2015;29(3):207–20.

4. Prescribing information Dimethyl fumarate [Internet]. http://www.accessdata.fda.gov/drugsatfda_docs/label/2016/204063s014lbl.pdf (accessed April 24 2016)

5. Prescribing information Fingolimod [Internet]. Verfügbar unter: https://www.accessdata.fda.gov/drugsatfda_docs/label/2012/022527s008lbl.pdf (accessed July 18 2019)

6. Karlsson G, Francis G, Koren G, Heining P, Zhang X, Cohen JA, u. a. Pregnancy outcomes in the clinical development program of fingolimod in multiple sclerosis. Neurology. 25. February 2014;82(8):674–80.

7. Prescribing information Glatiramer acetate [Internet]. Verfügbar unter: http://www.accessdata.fda.gov/drugsatfda_docs/label/2009/020622s057lbl.pdf (accessed April 24 2016)

8. Lu E, Wang BW, Guimond C, Synnes A, Sadovnick AD, Dahlgren L, u. a. Safety of disease-modifying drugs for multiple sclerosis in pregnancy: current challenges and future considerations for effective pharmacovigilance. Expert Rev Neurother. March 2013;13(3):251–260; quiz 261.

9. Lu E, Wang BW, Guimond C, Synnes A, Sadovnick D, Tremlett H. Disease-modifying drugs for multiple sclerosis in pregnancy: a systematic review. Neurology. 11. September 2012;79(11):1130–5.

10. Prescribing information Interferon beta [Internet]. Verfügbar unter: http://www.accessdata.fda.gov/drugsatfda_docs/label/2015/103780s5172lbl.pdf (accessed April 24 2016)

11. Prescribing information Mitoxantrone [Internet]. Verfügbar unter: http://www.accessdata.fda.gov/drugsatfda_docs/label/2009/019297s030s031lbl.pdf (accessed April 24 2016)

12. Hellwig K, Schimrigk S, Chan A, Epplen J, Gold R. A newborn with Pierre Robin sequence after preconceptional mitoxantrone exposure of a female with multiple sclerosis. J Neurol Sci. 15. August 2011;307(1–2):164–5.

13. Prescribing information Natalizumab [Internet]. Verfügbar unter: http://www.accessdata.fda.gov/drugsatfda_docs/label/2015/125104s950lbl.pdf (accessed April 24 2016)

14. Prescribing information Teriflunomide [Internet]. Verfügbar unter: http://www.accessdata.fda.gov/drugsatfda_docs/label/2014/202992s001lbl.pdf (accessed April 24 2016)

15 https://www.accessdata.fda.gov/drugsatfda_docs/label/2017/103948s5158lbl.pdf (accessed July 18 2019)

the aura is visual in greater than 90% of patients. It characteristically occurs within 60 minutes before onset of cephalalgia (note that aura symptoms may be present without subsequent headaches) (57).

Tension-type headaches manifest as episodic or chronic bilateral, mild-to-moderate-intensity headaches of a pressing or tightening quality, which are not exacerbated by routine physical activities. Chronic tension-type headaches often concur with medication-overuse headache (57).

The diagnostic approach to headaches rests on a detailed history and physical examination. If these reveal red flags—such as a new-onset headache, altered characteristics of a pre-existing headache, or concomitant neurological signs—further diagnostic evaluation is warranted. Depending on the suspected pathology, this may include neuroimaging (during gestation preferably by MRI), a spinal tap, and specific laboratory studies. Blood pressure should be taken in gravid women presenting with headache to screen for pre-eclampsia (the incidence of which may be higher in women with a previous history of migraine) (59). Further important causes of secondary headaches that need to be excluded in the pregnant or lactating patient include venous sinus thrombosis, reversible cerebral vasoconstriction syndrome, posterior reversible encephalopathy syndrome, idiopathic intracranial hypertension, pituitary apoplexy, and intracerebral/subarachnoid haemorrhage (60).

Many migraine sufferers will experience an abatement of symptoms during pregnancy (61, 62). In those who do not, non-pharmacological measures—such as maintaining a regular lifestyle, avoiding known triggers, and application of behavioural treatment strategies—may suffice (60). If medication is deemed necessary, care should be taken to select those drugs with the best maternal–fetal safety profile. Regarding the drugs commonly used in acute migraine attacks, there are no controlled safety studies in pregnant women showing no harm. Acetaminophen is frequently used for this indication, alone or in combination with metoclopramide or caffeine. Study data connecting its use with an increased incidence of childhood asthma are so far not entirely conclusive (63). For non-steroidal anti-inflammatory drugs (NSAIDs), first-trimester use has been associated with a potentially increased risk of miscarriage, and third-trimester use with premature ductal closure and an adverse effect on fetal renal function. There is conflicting evidence on the safety of aspirin during the first trimester, when its use may be associated with an increased risk of gastroschisis (64, 65). In the third trimester, analgesic doses of aspirin ought to be avoided due to its effect on the ductus arteriosus and platelet inhibition (66). Current evidence is reassuring as to the fetal safety of triptans with most trials failing to demonstrate associated teratogenicity (67–69). The most solid data are available for sumatriptan. Ergotamine is contraindicated during pregnancy for its potential to cause vasoconstriction and uterine contractions (60, 61). In patients with frequent migraine attacks, prophylactic treatment may be considered. Beta-blockers such as propranolol and metoprolol are first-line agents, although they have been linked to mild fetal growth restriction and respiratory depression (70). According to limited data, calcium channel blockers such as verapamil seem to be safe (71). Acupuncture has been shown to be effective for migraine prophylaxis, although sham acupuncture was not superior to 'true' intervention (72).

There are no adequate data on the use of CGRP-antagonists in pregnancy. Acute treatment of tension-type headaches is based on NSAIDs and aspirin. During pregnancy, the caveats previously discussed apply. Care should be taken to avoid medication overuse.

Disorders with increased incidence during pregnancy

Vascular disease

Ischaemic stroke

The incidence of cerebral ischaemia associated with pregnancy is about 25–34:100,000 deliveries, peaking in the third trimester and puerperium. Its aetiology can be subdivided into thrombotic, embolic (arterio-arterial or cardiac), and haemodynamic. Generally, atherosclerosis is the most common source of cerebral ischaemia. However, rare causes of stroke (e.g. arterial dissection and vasculitis) tend to be more prevalent in a young population. A recent study identified maternal smoking as an independent risk factor for perinatal arterial ischaemic stroke (73). Furthermore, pregnancy predisposes to ischaemia secondary to hypercoagulability (such as cerebral venous thrombosis). Some strokes occur due to conditions exclusively seen in the pregnant (i.e. eclampsia, peripartum cardiomyopathy, and amniotic fluid embolism). Other predisposing conditions include the commonly recognized cerebrovascular risk factors, particularly arterial hypertension (74).

Signs and symptoms of cerebral ischaemia depend on the site of the lesion. Common signs of supratentorial infarction include hemiparesis, aphasia, hemianopsia, and hemineglect. Dizziness, ataxia, diplopia, dysarthria, and central facial palsy may herald brainstem/cerebellar ischaemia. An altered level of consciousness—particularly if associated with other brainstem symptoms or bilateral Babinski signs—should prompt immediate investigations for basilar thrombosis.

Diagnosis of ischaemic cerebral infarction is based on radiographic findings. MRI is the method of choice as it does not involve ionizing radiation, is more sensitive for small infarctions and ischaemia in the posterior fossa, and may contribute to determining the exact onset and aetiology of the stroke (e.g. by showing multiple foci in embolic infarction). The time-of-flight technique permits magnetic resonance angiography without the use of contrast agent. If CT is the only imaging technique available, radiation dose-reduction methods and proper shielding protection ought to be used (75). Ultrasonography provides additional haemodynamic and structural information of the intra- and extracranial vessels.

All patients diagnosed with acute cerebral ischaemia should be monitored on a specialized stroke unit. Further aetiological workup includes a transthoracic echocardiogram, which may be combined with a bubble study to evaluate for a right-to-left shunt (e.g. patent foramen ovale). A transoesophageal echocardiogram may be considered, particularly if conditions requiring specific treatment—such as infective endocarditis or intracardiac thrombi—are suspected. A 24-hour electrocardiogram recording should be performed to exclude relevant cardiac arrhythmias such as atrial fibrillations.

Laboratory tests include a thrombophilia workup. The genetic panels are not influenced by pregnancy. However, the other parameters (e.g. antiphospholipid antibodies) are frequently falsely positive and may have to be postponed until several weeks postpartum (74).

After screening for contraindications, intravenous recombinant tissue plasminogen activator (rtPA; 0.9 mg/kg, maximum dose 90 mg) may be used in patients presenting within a time frame of up to 4.5 hours after onset of symptoms (and in select patients with salvageable tissue as determined by cerebral imaging). In patients with mild

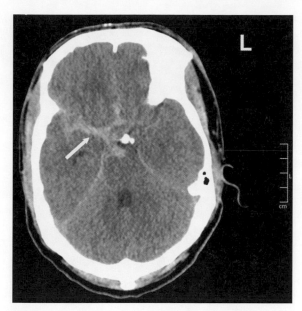

Figure 24.1 Subarachnoid haemorrhage (SAH, arrow) of Hunt and Hess grade III due to rupture of an aneurysm arising from the right middle cerebral artery bifurcation. Courtesy of Dept. of Neuroradiology, Kepler University Hospital, Linz, Austria.

that would require anticoagulation outside of pregnancy—such as mechanical heart valves—the use of unfractionated heparin or low-molecular-weight heparin (LMWH) is recommended (81). LMWH compares more favourably regarding the risk of obstetric bleeding complications, osteoporosis, and heparin-induced thrombocytopenia (82). Doses should be normalized for body weight changes, and anti-Xa activity ought to be monitored (83). LMWH may be discontinued 24 hours or more before a planned delivery (81). Vitamin K antagonists are better avoided due to the risk of embryopathy and fetal bleeding. Data on direct oral anticoagulants regarding their safety during pregnancy are hitherto insufficient; these agents should therefore not be used in the pregnant (84).

In situations in which antiplatelet therapy would be recommended outside of pregnancy, low-dose aspirin (50–150 mg/day) can safely be used after the first trimester (81, 85). There is no clear consensus on the use of aspirin in the first trimester: a meta-analysis found no evidence of an overall increase of congenital malformations, but showed a possible association with an increased risk of gastroschisis (65). Given the paucity of data concerning the risk–benefit ratio of secondary prevention of non-cardioembolic stroke during the first trimester, the American Heart Association/American Stroke Association guidelines consider low-dose aspirin, unfractionated heparin/LMWH, or no treatment acceptable treatment options (81). There are no adequate data on other antiplatelet agents (clopidogrel, dipyridamole) regarding their safety in pregnancy.

Cerebral haemorrhage

Haemorrhagic stroke includes intracerebral parenchymal and subarachnoid haemorrhage (**Figure 24.1**). At 4–6 per 100,000 deliveries, the incidence of haemorrhagic stroke seems to be higher in the pregnant or postpartum population than in age-matched, non-pregnant women (relative risk of 2.5/28.5 during pregnancy/postpartum period) (86).

The major causes of intracranial haemorrhage in pregnancy are ruptured aneurysms, arteriovenous malformations (**Figure 24.2**), and (pre-)eclampsia. Other risk factors include advanced maternal

deficits, risks of thrombolytic treatment have to be weighed against anticipated impairments (76). There are no randomized trials on the use of rtPA in pregnancy and experience is limited to case reports (77), but rtPA is not known to be teratogenic and it is too large a molecule to cross the placenta (78). The decision pro or contra thrombolysis has to be made after individualized appraisal of the case. The indication for endovascular intervention (intra-arterial thrombolysis or mechanical thrombectomy) is subject to interdisciplinary discussion between the stroke specialist and an interventional neuroradiologist (79).

Recurrence rates of cerebral ischaemia during subsequent pregnancies depend on the aetiology of the stroke but generally seem to be low (80). For pregnant women with high-risk conditions

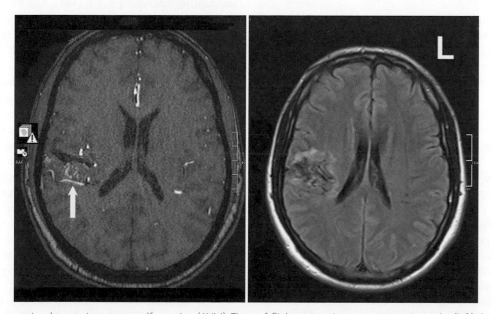

Figure 24.2 Right temporoinsular arteriovenous malformation (AVM). Time-of-flight magnetic resonance angiography (left) shows the AVM, which is fed by temporal branches of the middle cerebral artery and drains via a prominent cortical vein (arrow). Fluid attenuation inversion recovery (FLAIR) imaging (right) shows mild residual oedema and haemosiderin deposits suggesting prior haemorrhage of the AVM. Courtesy of Dept. of Neuroradiology, Kepler University Hospital, Linz, Austria

age, African American race, hypertension, coagulopathy, and tobacco abuse (87, 88).

Signs and symptoms comprise focal neurological deficits corresponding to the site of the lesion, altered state of consciousness, headache (which is typically sudden and severe in subarachnoid haemorrhage), nausea and vomiting, and signs of meningeal irritation such as nuchal rigidity.

Neuroimaging is the most important diagnostic procedure in suspected haemorrhagic stroke. During pregnancy, MRI is preferred over CT. As both methods may yield a small rate of false-negative results, lumbar puncture ought to be considered in patients in whom there is a high suspicion of subarachnoid haemorrhage (89). If further therapeutic planning requires a cerebral angiogram, proper shielding protection of the fetus should be applied (90).

Treatment of intracerebral haemorrhage comprises supportive care (cardiovascular and neurological monitoring, correction of coagulopathies, treatment of intracranial hypertension), symptomatic measures (e.g. treatment of headache, nausea, and epileptic seizures), and possibly elimination of the source of the bleeding. The latter should be subject to careful risk–benefit evaluation in the individual patient (90, 91). The risk of intracranial aneurysm rupture peaks in the third trimester. This situation is associated with a high maternal and fetal mortality, which increases further in the case of a rebleed (no current figures available; in an older study maternal/fetal mortality due to recurrent subarachnoid haemorrhage amounted to 63%/27%, respectively (92)). Thus, symptomatic aneurysms should be controlled by endovascular or surgical means (90).

Data concerning the risk of bleeding from a previously asymptomatic arteriovenous malformation during pregnancy are inconclusive. However, early intervention should be considered once an arteriovenous malformation has ruptured (90, 93).

If the vascular pathology has been treated, the woman may undergo vaginal delivery. Controversy continues whether or not to recommend caesarean section in patients with untreated aneurysms and arteriovenous malformations (94, 95).

Venous sinus thrombosis

Cerebral venous thrombosis (CVT) (**Figure 24.3**) affects the dural sinuses and/or cerebral veins. It represents approximately 0.5–1% of all strokes, affecting 5 people/million/year (96, 97). The incidence of CVT in pregnancy increases to about 8–12:100,000 deliveries, accounting for approximately one-third of pregnancy-associated strokes (98, 99). Peak incidence is in the third trimester and postpartum.

CVT can be subclassified into septic and aseptic thrombosis. The former is caused by local inflammation such as sinusitis, otitis, facial and dental infections, and dental infections. The latter is associated with hypercoagulable states. These include inherited abnormalities of coagulation and acquired conditions, among them pregnancy and puerperium.

Signs and symptoms result from either one of two mechanisms: increased intracranial pressure due to impaired venous drainage and focal brain injury secondary to venous infarctions and/or haemorrhage (100). Headache is the most common presentation, reported by 90% of patients with CVT (101). In approximately 25% of patients it is the only presenting symptom (96). Other signs include visual disturbances, focal neurological deficits (most commonly hemiparesis (102)), and epileptic seizures. Bilateral brain involvement is a

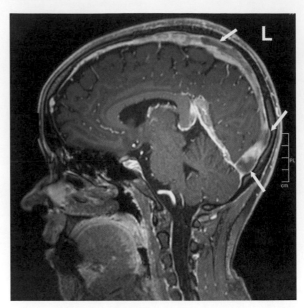

Figure 24.3 Cerebral venous thrombosis (CVT). Contrast-enhanced T1-imaging shows extensive CVT of the superior sagittal sinus (arrows). Courtesy of Dept. of Neuroradiology, Kepler University Hospital, Linz, Austria

distinguishing feature of CVT: reduced consciousness, for example, may be due to bilateral thalamic injury secondary to impairment of the deep venous drainage system (96).

All patients with suspected CVT should be screened for predisposing factors such as hypercoagulable states, infections or inflammatory processes. D-dimer assays have a high negative predictive value (99.6%) (103). However, with a strong clinical suspicion of CVT, a normal level should not preclude further diagnostic evaluation. In pregnant women, D-dimer levels are frequently elevated, particularly in the third trimester. Therefore, the specificity and positive predictive value of elevated D-dimer levels decrease during pregnancy.

MRI with magnetic resonance venography is considered the gold standard in diagnosing CVT (104). The time-of-flight technique permits magnetic resonance venography without the use of contrast agent. Despite the theoretical risks for the fetus, pregnant patients can undergo MRI at any stage of pregnancy if justified after careful risk–benefit considerations (105).

Patients with CVT should be monitored on a stroke unit for early diagnosis and management of complications such as seizures, hydrocephalus, cerebral haemorrhage, and intracranial hypertension. In septic CVT, the infectious focus needs to be eradicated. Once the diagnosis of CVT is made, anticoagulation (unfractionated heparin adjusted to achieve an activated partial thromboplastin time twice the pretreatment value or body-weight adapted LMWH) should be started to prevent thrombus growth. This also applies to patients presenting with secondary intracerebral haemorrhage (106). Preliminary data suggest that LMWH may be more effective than unfractionated heparin (107). In individual cases, endovascular interventions may be considered if there is clinical deterioration due to incomplete sinus recanalization. However, no controlled studies exist to support this approach (96).

Anticoagulation should be continued for 3–6 months in patients with provoked CVT and for 6–12 months in unprovoked CVT. For women with pregnancy-associated CVT, the American Heart

Association/American Stroke Association recommend LMWH treatment throughout the remaining pregnancy and LMWH or vitamin K antagonists for at least 6 weeks postpartum, aiming at a total minimum duration of therapy of 6 months. In patients with recurrent CVT or high-risk thrombophilia, indefinite anticoagulation may be considered (96).

In the largest study available on the prognosis of CVT, the outcome was favourable (modified Rankin Scale 0–2) in 86.6% of patients (101). Pregnancy-related CVT is associated with a low risk of recurrence (101, 108), but prophylaxis with LMWH may be considered during subsequent pregnancies (96).

Reversible cerebral vasoconstriction syndrome and posterior reversible encephalopathy syndrome

Reversible cerebral vasoconstriction syndrome (RCVS) is characterized by hyperacute severe headaches and segmental dynamic vasoconstriction (109). Different trigger factors have been identified, particularly the use of vasoactive drugs and the postpartum state (110). The typical onset of RCVS is at 1–3 weeks postpartum. It may be associated with (pre-)eclampsia (111).

The hallmark symptom of RCVS is a thunderclap headache defined as severe, with throbbing cephalalgia reaching peak intensity within 60 seconds of onset. It is the sole symptom in about 70% of patients and typically shows a waxing and waning course (110). Other variably associated symptoms include nausea, vomiting, photo- and phonophobia, seizures, and focal neurological deficits. The latter are usually transient but may persist if an ischaemic stroke ensues.

Diagnosis of RCVS rests on visualization of the typical 'string-of-beads' appearance of one or more intracranial vessels caused by segmental narrowing and dilatation. The vasoconstriction is dynamic and early angiographies may be normal (112).

Differential diagnoses comprise aneurysmal subarachnoid haemorrhage, primary angiitis of the central nervous system, sinus venous thrombosis, pituitary apoplexy, cervical artery dissection, and other primary and secondary headache syndromes. Brain scans in RCVS patients are usually normal but may show sequelae of vascular dysregulation such as cerebral infarction, and intracerebral, subarachnoid, or subdural haemorrhage. Vasoconstriction may be monitored by transcranial ultrasonography. Lumbar puncture should be performed to exclude aneurysmal subarachnoid haemorrhage (109).

Management of the RCVS patient is based on symptomatic treatment and elimination of precipitating factors. Vasodilating medication (nimodipine/verapamil, magnesium sulphate) have been used to relieve vasoconstriction. However, use of these agents is mostly based on anecdotal data and a positive effect on the evolution of the disease has not been convincingly demonstrated so far (109). The same is true for intra-arterial administration of vasodilators and balloon angioplasty (110).

RCVS is usually self-limiting. However, if associated with the postpartum period, it seems to carry a higher risk of permanent deficits or death: only 50% of patients went on to full recovery in one small study (111).

Posterior reversible encephalopathy syndrome (PRES) is characterized by a heterogeneity of neurological symptoms associated with (sub-)cortical vasogenic oedema. PRES (**Figure 24.4**) has been related to endothelial dysfunction caused by abrupt blood pressure changes or cytokine effects (113). It may be precipitated by a variety

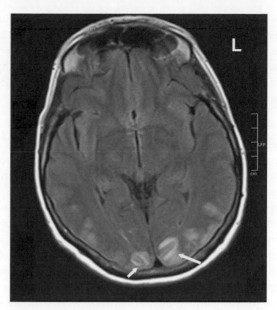

Figure 24.4 Posterior reversible encephalopathy syndrome (PRES). Fluid attenuation inversion recovery (FLAIR) sequences demonstrate confluent temporoparietal signal alterations (arrows) compatible with (sub-)cortical vasogenic oedema. Courtesy of Dept. of Neuroradiology, Kepler University Hospital, Linz, Austria

of factors, such as hypertension, autoimmune disorders, immunosuppression, and (pre-)eclampsia.

PRES is characterized by a (sub-)acute onset of encephalopathic changes, seizures, and visual disturbances. These symptoms are typically accompanied by a dull headache. Focal findings occur in 5–15% of patients (113). PRES is frequently associated with RCVS (109).

Diagnosis is based on the clinical findings and MRI. T2-weighted sequences reveal subcortical—and sometimes cortical—vasogenic oedema, which is usually bilateral, asymmetric, and located in the parieto-occipital regions. However, other cerebral regions may be involved (114).

Management of PRES is symptomatic (e.g. antiepileptic) and by treatment of the causative factor (e.g. hypertension). Its prognosis is usually favourable (113).

Peripheral nervous system disorders

Peripheral nerve compression syndromes

Carpal tunnel syndrome is one of the most frequent peripheral nerve compression syndromes in pregnancy, with a peak incidence in the third trimester. Its occurrence has been associated with increased fluid retention in pregnant women (115). Carpal tunnel syndrome is diagnosed clinically by demonstrating compromised median nerve function. The diagnosis is supported by nerve conduction studies. Patients may benefit from wearing a wrist splint at night. Corticosteroid injections or surgery to release the flexor retinaculum are rarely indicated during pregnancy due to the favourable prognosis of pregnancy-related carpal tunnel syndrome. Symptoms tend to resolve during the weeks and months after delivery, but may recur in subsequent pregnancies (116).

Postpartum compression neuropathies tend to affect the femoral, lateral femoral, cutaneous, and obturator nerves. They are associated with variables related to the fetus (e.g. macrosomia) or to the process of delivery (e.g. prolonged lithotomy position and compression by leg stirrups). The prognosis for recovery is excellent (117). If there is already a history of peripheral nerve compression syndromes or evidence of multiple nerves involved, hereditary neuropathy with liability to pressure palsies should be excluded, a rare genetic neuropathy with a good prognosis (118).

Lumbago and lumbosacral radiculopathies

Lumbago is frequently encountered in pregnant women and is mostly due to local mechanical factors. Disc bulges or prolapses seem to be no more frequent in pregnant than in non-pregnant women (119).

Symptoms of nerve root compression include radiating pain, loss of sensibility, muscular paresis, and bladder/bowel dysfunction. The most commonly affected levels are at L4/L5 and L5/S1.

Physical examination should evaluate for focal neurological deficits. Imaging studies will not be required in the majority of patients but lumbar MRI should be performed in the presence of severe or progressive neurological deficits or when a serious underlying condition is suspected (120).

Conservative management will suffice in most patients. If an analgesic is needed, acetaminophen has one of the best safety profiles in pregnancy (121). Indications for disc surgery during pregnancy are incapacitating pain, severe or progressive neurological deficits, and bladder or bowel dysfunction (122).

Cranial nerve syndromes: Bell's palsy

Bell's palsy denotes idiopathic peripheral paralysis of the facial nerve. Its incidence seems to be increased during pregnancy (although data are not entirely conclusive), particularly in the third trimester and the postpartum period (123).

The diagnosis is based upon the clinical findings. Electrodiagnostic studies can provide prognostic information. MRI or lumbar puncture may be warranted to exclude symptomatic paralysis, particularly in areas endemic for Lyme disease.

Treatment of idiopathic Bell's palsy is steroid based (e.g. prednisone 60–80 mg/day for 1 week). Use during the first trimester of pregnancy may be associated with an increased incidence of cleft palate (123, 124). Careful eye care should be performed in the case of incomplete lid closure.

Restless legs syndrome

Restless legs syndrome (RLS) is characterized by an unpleasant sensation in the legs relieved by movement. Symptoms are worse at rest and in the evening/during the night. Its prevalence during pregnancy is approximately two to three times higher than in non-pregnant females (highest in the third trimester and in multiparous women).

Primary and secondary RLS are distinguished. The latter may be due to iron-deficiency, peripheral neuropathy, or renal disease. Endocrine and metabolic changes have been attributed to pregnancy-related RLS (125).

RLS is a clinical diagnosis based upon the criteria proposed by the International RLS Study Group (126). Secondary RLS should be excluded by appropriate laboratory investigations.

Mild forms of RLS may be treated non-pharmacologically (127). Drugs known to aggravate RLS (e.g. neuroleptics) should be withdrawn. Iron supplementation is to be used in iron-deficient patients.

In refractory RLS, low-dose carbidopa–levodopa or clonazepam have been recommended (128). There is little data on fetal safety for alternative agents (dopamine agonists, opioids, benzodiazepines, anticonvulsants).

Symptoms of RLS disappear or markedly improve within days after delivery in the majority of women (125). However, patients with pregnancy-related RLS are at an increased risk of developing chronic RLS in the future (129).

Pregnancy-specific conditions presenting with neurological symptoms

(Pre-)Eclampsia

Pre-eclampsia is a multisystem disorder characterized by *de novo* hypertension (systolic blood pressure >140 mmHg or diastolic blood pressure >90 mmHg) present after 20 weeks of gestation combined with one or more of the following: proteinuria greater than 300 mg/day, other maternal organ involvement (renal/hepatic/neurological/haematological complications), or uteroplacental dysfunction (130). The progression to eclampsia is defined by new-onset generalized tonic–clonic seizures or coma.

Pre-eclampsia complicates approximately 3–5% of pregnancies. Genetic disposition seems to exist at least in a subset of patients. Further risk factors include pre-eclampsia/hypertension in previous pregnancies, a positive family history for eclampsia, nulliparity, chronic kidney disease, hypertension, diabetes, maternal obesity, and autoimmune disorders (131).

Neurological signs and symptoms of (pre-)eclampsia include headache, visual disturbances due to cortical blindness or retinal detachment, hyperreflexia, seizures, cerebral ischaemia, confusion, and altered levels of consciousness secondary to cerebral oedema. It is a predisposing factor for PRES.

Women with suspected or diagnosed (pre-)eclampsia should be subject to regular monitoring of blood pressure, urine protein, haematological, renal, and hepatic parameters, and fetal assessment. The occurrence of neurological complications may warrant cerebral imaging by MRI or electroencephalographic studies (90).

The definitive treatment for (pre-)eclampsia is delivery, which should be indicated based upon gestational age, the severity of the disease, and maternal and fetal condition. Severe hypertension requires pharmacological intervention. The benefit of treating mild hypertension is less clear (131, 132). Magnesium sulphate is effective for seizure prophylaxis in women at risk for eclampsia (133).

Women who have suffered from pre-eclampsia during their first pregnancy carry a risk of about 15% for recurrence (134). Furthermore, they are at increased risk of developing cardiovascular disease later in life (131). Low-dose aspirin (50–150 mg/day) has some benefit for preventing pre-eclampsia, particularly if initiated at 16 weeks or less of gestation (135). For a discussion of the safety of aspirin in the first trimester, see 'Ischaemic stroke'. The World Health Organization recommends calcium supplementation for women with a low dietary calcium intake (131).

Amniotic fluid embolism

Amniotic fluid embolism is caused by the entry of amniotic fluid into the maternal circulation, causing vaso-occlusion by mechanical and possibly humoral and immunological mechanisms. Although amniotic fluid embolism is rare (2–8:100,000 deliveries), it is one of the leading causes of maternal death resulting directly from childbirth due to its high mortality (136).

Amniotic fluid embolism occurs during delivery and up to 48 hours postpartum (136). Risk factors include maternal age of 35 years or above, multiparity, induction of labour using any method, placenta praevia, instrumental vaginal delivery, and caesarean section (137). Diagnosis is based on clinical criteria (one or more of the following: acute fetal compromise, cardiac arrest, cardiac arrhythmia, coagulopathy, hypotension, maternal haemorrhage, premonitory symptoms such as anxiety, seizures, dyspnoea) (138) and exclusion of any other cause of acute cardiovascular decompensation such as pulmonary embolism and myocardial infarction.

Therapy is interdisciplinary and focuses on stabilizing haemodynamic and cardiorespiratory function and correcting coagulopathies. This will usually require an intensive care setting. Emergency caesarean section ought to be considered (136).

Maternal/fetal mortality in amniotic fluid embolism ranges from 13% to 44% and 7% to 38% respectively (136). Reported rates of neurological morbidity vary widely with 6–61% of survivors suffering from permanent neurological sequelae secondary to hypoxia or cerebrovascular accidents. Although there is little data, amniotic fluid embolism does not seem prone to recurrence (139).

Sheehan syndrome

Sheehan syndrome denotes postpartum hypopituitarism due to pituitary necrosis caused by hypovolaemic shock after severe peripartum haemorrhage. A secondary autoimmune process may also play a role in delayed pituitary dysfunction (140, 141).

The suggested diagnostic criteria for Sheehan syndrome include an obstetric history of significant postpartum vaginal bleeding resulting in severe hypotension/shock, failure of postpartum lactation, failure to resume regular menses after delivery, partial or panhypopituitarism, and empty sella on CT scanning or MRI (142).

Symptoms predominantly result from failure of the *anterior* pituitary endocrine axis (e.g. hypotension, fatigue, and hypopigmentation). With severe insufficiency, coma and death resulting from Addisonian crisis may ensue. Clinically overt involvement of the *posterior* pituitary is rare (140). Sheehan syndrome may manifest itself with considerable postpartum latency (143).

Diagnosis of Sheehan syndrome is made based on the patient's history, basal hormone levels, and pituitary functioning tests. Cerebral imaging may demonstrate an empty sella. Sheehan syndrome should be differentiated from pituitary adenoma infarction, which may require decompressive surgery (140). Treatment is by substitution of deficient hormones, particularly hydrocortisone and levothyroxine.

Chorea gravidarum

Chorea is characterized by brief, involuntary, irregular movements involving multiple parts of the body. Chorea beginning during pregnancy has been termed chorea gravidarum. Important causes include antiphospholipid antibody syndrome, systemic lupus erythematosus, and rheumatic fever. Patients should also be screened for Wilson's and Huntington's diseases, hyperthyroidism, basal ganglia infarction, drug-/toxin-induced chorea, and hyperglycaemia (144). In about half of the cases, chorea gravidarum is idiopathic (145).

Symptoms usually start during the second to fifth month of pregnancy and tend to remit spontaneously within weeks or months or shortly after delivery (146).

If pharmacological treatment is required in severe cases, low-dose haloperidol may be utilized if the potential benefit justifies the potential risk to the fetus (144).

REFERENCES

1. Hauser WA, Annegers JF, Kurland LT. Incidence of epilepsy and unprovoked seizures in Rochester, Minnesota: 1935–1984. *Epilepsia* 1993;**34**:453–68.
2. Berg AT, Berkovic SF, Brodie MJ, et al. Revised terminology and concepts for organization of seizures and epilepsies: report of the ILAE Commission on Classification and Terminology, 2005–2009. *Epilepsia* 2010;**51**:676–85.
3. Kwan P, Brodie MJ. Early identification of refractory epilepsy. *N Engl J Med* 2000;**342**:314–19.
4. Neligan A, Bell GS, Elsayed M, Sander JW, Shorvon SD. Treatment changes in a cohort of people with apparently drug-resistant epilepsy: an extended follow-up. *J Neurol Neurosurg Psychiatry* 2012;**83**:810–13.
5. Kwan P, Arzimanoglou A, Berg AT, et al. Definition of drug resistant epilepsy: consensus proposal by the ad hoc Task Force of the ILAE Commission on Therapeutic Strategies. *Epilepsia* 2010;**51**:1069–77.
6. National Institute for Health and Care Excellence (NICE). *Epilepsies: Diagnosis and Management*. Clinical guideline [CG137], updated 2018 London: NICE; 2012. Available at: https://www.nice.org.uk/guidance/cg137.
7. Tomson T, Battino D, Bonizzoni E, et al. Dose-dependent risk of malformations with antiepileptic drugs: an analysis of data from the EURAP epilepsy and pregnancy registry. *Lancet Neurol* 2011;**10**:609–17.
8. Campbell E, Kennedy F, Russell A, et al. Malformation risks of antiepileptic drug monotherapies in pregnancy: updated results from the UK and Ireland Epilepsy and Pregnancy Registers. *J Neurol Neurosurg Psychiatry* 2014;**85**:1029–34.
9. Samrén EB, van Duijn CM, Christiaens GC, Hofman A, Lindhout D. Antiepileptic drug regimens and major congenital abnormalities in the offspring. *Ann Neurol* 1999;**46**:739–46.
10. Meador K, Reynolds MW, Crean S, Fahrbach K, Probst C. Pregnancy outcomes in women with epilepsy: a systematic review and meta-analysis of published pregnancy registries and cohorts. *Epilepsy Res* 2008;**81**:1–13.
11. Vajda FJE, O'Brien T, Lander C, Graham J, Eadie M. The efficacy of the newer antiepileptic drugs in controlling seizures in pregnancy. *Epilepsia* 2014;**55**:1229–34.
12. Vajda FJE, Hitchcock AA, Graham J, O'Brien TJ, Lander CM, Eadie MJ. The teratogenic risk of antiepileptic drug polytherapy. *Epilepsia* 2010;**51**:805–10.
13. Holmes LB, Mittendorf R, Shen A, Smith CR, Hernandez-Diaz S. Fetal effects of anticonvulsant polytherapies: different risks from different drug combinations. *Arch Neurol* 2011;**68**:1275–81.
14. Tomson T, Battino D. Teratogenic effects of antiepileptic drugs. *Lancet Neurol* 2012;**11**:803–13.
15. Meador KJ, Baker GA, Browning N, et al. Cognitive function at 3 years of age after fetal exposure to antiepileptic drugs. *N Engl J Med* 2009;**360**:1597–605.

16. Meador KJ, Baker GA, Browning N, et al. Fetal antiepileptic drug exposure and cognitive outcomes at age 6 years (NEAD study): a prospective observational study. *Lancet Neurol* 2013;**12**:244–52.

17. Bromley RL, Mawer G, Clayton-Smith J, Baker GA, Liverpool and Manchester Neurodevelopment Group. Autism spectrum disorders following in utero exposure to antiepileptic drugs. *Neurology* 2008;**71**:1923–24.

18. Christensen J, Grønborg TK, Sørensen MJ, et al. Prenatal valproate exposure and risk of autism spectrum disorders and childhood autism. *JAMA* 2013;**309**:1696–703.

19. European Medicines Agency. Procedure under Article 31 of Directive 2001/83/EC resulting from pharmacovigilance data. 2014. Available at: http://www.ema.europa.eu/docs/en_GB/document_library/Referrals_document/Valproate_and_related_substances_31/Recommendation_provided_by_Pharmacovigilance_Risk_Assessment_Committee/WC500177352.pdf (accessed 7 May 2016).

20. Tomson T, Marson A, Boon P, et al. Valproate in the treatment of epilepsy in girls and women of childbearing potential. *Epilepsia* 2015;**56**:1006–19.

21. Rauchenzauner M, Ehrensberger M, Prieschl M, et al. Generalized tonic-clonic seizures and antiepileptic drugs during pregnancy—a matter of importance for the baby? *J Neurol* 2013;**260**:484–88.

22. Battino D, Tomson T, Bonizzoni E, Craig J, et al. Seizure control and treatment changes in pregnancy: observations from the EURAP epilepsy pregnancy registry. *Epilepsia* 2013;**54**:1621–27.

23. Reisinger TL, Newman M, Loring DW, Pennell PB, Meador KJ. Antiepileptic drug clearance and seizure frequency during pregnancy in women with epilepsy. *Epilepsy Behav* 2013;**29**:13–18.

24. Harden CL, Hopp J, Ting TY, et al. Management issues for women with epilepsy-Focus on pregnancy (an evidence-based review): I. Obstetrical complications and change in seizure frequency: Report of the Quality Standards Subcommittee and Therapeutics and Technology Assessment Subcommittee of the American Academy of Neurology and the American Epilepsy Society. *Epilepsia* 2009;**5**:1229–36.

25. Viale L, Allotey J, Cheong-See F, et al. Epilepsy in pregnancy and reproductive outcomes: a systematic review and meta-analysis. *Lancet* 2015;**386**:1845–52.

26. MacDonald SC, Bateman BT, McElrath TF, Hernández-Díaz S. Mortality and morbidity during delivery hospitalization among pregnant women with epilepsy in the united states. *JAMA Neurol* 2015;**72**:981–88.

27. Adab N, Kini U, Vinten J, et al. The longer term outcome of children born to mothers with epilepsy. *J Neurol Neurosurg Psychiatry* 2004;**75**:1575–83.

28. Edey S, Moran N, Nashef L. SUDEP and epilepsy-related mortality in pregnancy. *Epilepsia* 2014;**55**:e72–74.

29. EURAP Study Group. Seizure control and treatment in pregnancy: observations from the EURAP epilepsy pregnancy registry. *Neurology* 2006;**66**:354–60.

30. Thomas SV, Syam U, Devi JS. Predictors of seizures during pregnancy in women with epilepsy. *Epilepsia* 2012;**53**:e85–88.

31. Veiby G, Bjørk M, Engelsen BA, Gilhus NE. Epilepsy and recommendations for breastfeeding. *Seizure* 2015;**28**:57–65.

32. McKay KA, Kwan V, Duggan T, Tremlett H. Risk factors associated with the onset of relapsing-remitting and primary progressive multiple sclerosis: a systematic review. *BioMed Res Int* 2015;**2015**:817238.

33. Confavreux C, Vukusic S. Natural history of multiple sclerosis: a unifying concept. *Brain* 2006;**129**:606–16.

34. Finkelsztejn A, Brooks JBB, Paschoal FM, Fragoso YD. What can we really tell women with multiple sclerosis regarding pregnancy? A systematic review and meta-analysis of the literature. *BJOG* 2011;**118**:790–97.

35. Langer-Gould A, Beaber BE. Effects of pregnancy and breast-feeding on the multiple sclerosis disease course. *Clin Immunol* 2013;**149**:244–50.

36. Ramagopalan S, Yee I, Byrnes J, Guimond C, Ebers G, Sadovnick D. Term pregnancies and the clinical characteristics of multiple sclerosis: a population based study. *J Neurol Neurosurg Psychiatry* 2012;**83**:793–95.

37. Runmarker B, Andersen O. Pregnancy is associated with a lower risk of onset and a better prognosis in multiple sclerosis. *Brain* 1995;**118**:253–61.

38. Hughes SE, Spelman T, Gray OM, et al. Predictors and dynamics of postpartum relapses in women with multiple sclerosis. *Mult Scler* 2014;**20**:739–46.

39. Tsui A, Lee MA. Multiple sclerosis and pregnancy. *Curr Opin Obstet Gynecol* 2011;**23**:435–39.

40. Bove R, Alwan S, Friedman JM, et al. Management of multiple sclerosis during pregnancy and the reproductive years: a systematic review. *Obstet Gynecol* 2014;**124**:1157–68.

41. Coyle PK. Multiple sclerosis and pregnancy prescriptions. *Expert Opin Drug Saf* 2014;**13**:1565–68.

42. Pozzilli C, Pugliatti M, ParadigMS Group. An overview of pregnancy-related issues in patients with multiple sclerosis. *Eur J Neurol* 2015;**22** Suppl 2:34–39.

43. Lu E, Wang BW, Guimond C, et al. Safety of disease-modifying drugs for multiple sclerosis in pregnancy: current challenges and future considerations for effective pharmacovigilance. *Expert Rev Neurother* 2013;**13**:251–60.

44. Kelly VM, Nelson LM, Chakravarty EF. Obstetric outcomes in women with multiple sclerosis and epilepsy. *Neurology* 2009;**73**:1831–36.

45. Dahl J, Myhr K-M, Daltveit AK, Hoff JM, Gilhus NE. Pregnancy, delivery, and birth outcome in women with multiple sclerosis. *Neurology* 2005;**65**:1961–63.

46. Mueller BA, Zhang J, Critchlow CW. Birth outcomes and need for hospitalization after delivery among women with multiple sclerosis. *Am J Obstet Gynecol* 2002;**186**:446–52.

47. Jalkanen A, Alanen A, Airas L, Finnish Multiple Sclerosis and Pregnancy Study Group. Pregnancy outcome in women with multiple sclerosis: results from a prospective nationwide study in Finland. *Mult Scler* 2010;**16**:950–55.

48. van der Kop ML, Pearce MS, Dahlgren L, et al. Neonatal and delivery outcomes in women with multiple sclerosis. *Ann Neurol* 2011;**70**:41–50.

49. Haider B, von Oertzen J. Neurological disorders. *Best Pract Res Clin Obstet Gynaecol* 2013;**27**:867–75.

50. Keesey JC. Clinical evaluation and management of myasthenia gravis. *Muscle Nerve* 2004;**29**:484–505.

51. Choi Decroos E, Hobson-Webb LD, Juel VC, Massey JM, Sanders DB. Do acetylcholine receptor and striated muscle antibodies predict the presence of thymoma in patients with myasthenia gravis? *Muscle Nerve* 2014;**49**:30–34.

52. Batocchi AP, Majolini L, Evoli A, Lino MM, Minisci C, Tonali P. Course and treatment of myasthenia gravis during pregnancy. *Neurology* 1999;**52**:447–52.

53. Sussman J, Farrugia ME, Maddison P, Hill M, Leite MI, Hilton-Jones D. Myasthenia gravis: Association of British Neurologists' management guidelines. *Pract Neurol* 2015;**15**:199–206.

54. Park-Wyllie L, Mazzotta P, Pastuszak A, et al. Birth defects after maternal exposure to corticosteroids: prospective cohort

study and meta-analysis of epidemiological studies. *Teratology* 2000;**62**:385–92.

55. Ferrero S, Esposito F, Biamonti M, Bentivoglio G, Ragni N. Myasthenia gravis during pregnancy. *Expert Rev Neurother* 2008;**8**:979–88.

56. Sikka P, Joshi B, Aggarwal N, Suri V, Bhagat H. Distinguishing myasthenia exacerbation from severe preeclampsia: a diagnostic and therapeutic challenge. *J Clin Diagn Res* 2015;**9**:QD05–QD06.

57. Headache Classification Committee of the International Headache Society (IHS). The International Classification of Headache Disorders, 3rd edition (beta version). *Cephalalgia* 2013;**33**:629–808.

58. Bigal ME, Bordini CA, Speciali JG. Etiology and distribution of headaches in two Brazilian primary care units. *Headache* 2000;**40**:241–47.

59. Facchinetti F, Allais G, Nappi RE, et al. Migraine is a risk factor for hypertensive disorders in pregnancy: a prospective cohort study. *Cephalalgia* 2009;**29**:286–92.

60. Wells RE, Turner DP, Lee M, Bishop L, Strauss L. Managing migraine during pregnancy and lactation. *Curr Neurol Neurosci Rep* 2016;**16**:40.

61. Tepper D. Pregnancy and lactation—migraine management. *Headache* 2015;**55**:607–608.

62. Rasmussen BK. Migraine and tension-type headache in a general population: precipitating factors, female hormones, sleep pattern and relation to lifestyle. *Pain* 1993;**53**:65–72.

63. Cheelo M, Lodge CJ, Dharmage SC, et al. Paracetamol exposure in pregnancy and early childhood and development of childhood asthma: a systematic review and meta-analysis. *Arch Dis Child* 2015;**100**:81–89.

64. Østensen ME, Skomsvoll JF. Anti-inflammatory pharmacotherapy during pregnancy. *Expert Opin Pharmacother* 2004;**5**:571–80.

65. Kozer E, Nikfar S, Costei A, Boskovic R, Nulman I, Koren G. Aspirin consumption during the first trimester of pregnancy and congenital anomalies: a meta-analysis. *Am J Obstet Gynecol* 2002;**187**:1623–30.

66. Becker WJ. Acute migraine treatment in adults. *Headache* 2015;**55**:778–93.

67. Ephross SA, Sinclair SM. Final results from the 16-year sumatriptan, naratriptan, and treximet pregnancy registry. *Headache* 2014;**54**:1158–72.

68. Marchenko A, Etwel F, Olutunfese O, Nickel C, Koren G, Nulman I. Pregnancy outcome following prenatal exposure to triptan medications: a meta-analysis. *Headache* 2015;**55**:490–501.

69. Nezvalová-Henriksen K, Spigset O, Nordeng H. Triptan exposure during pregnancy and the risk of major congenital malformations and adverse pregnancy outcomes: results from the Norwegian Mother and Child Cohort Study. *Headache* 2010;**50**:563–75.

70. Easterling TR. Pharmacological management of hypertension in pregnancy. *Semin Perinatol* 2014;**38**:487–95.

71. Magee LA, Schick B, Donnenfeld AE, et al. The safety of calcium channel blockers in human pregnancy: a prospective, multicenter cohort study. *Am J Obstet Gynecol* 1996;**174**:823–28.

72. Linde K, Allais G, Brinkhaus B, Manheimer E, Vickers A, White AR. Acupuncture for migraine prophylaxis. *Cochrane Database Syst Rev* 2009;**1**:CD001218.

73. Darmency-Stamboul V, Chantegret C, Ferdynus C, et al. Antenatal factors associated with perinatal arterial ischemic stroke. *Stroke* 2012;**43**:2307–12.

74. Grear KE, Bushnell CD. Stroke and pregnancy: clinical presentation, evaluation, treatment, and epidemiology. *Clin Obstet Gynecol* 2013;**56**:350–59.

75. Wang PI, Chong ST, Kielar AZ, et al. Imaging of pregnant and lactating patients: part 1, evidence-based review and recommendations. *AJR Am J Roentgenol* 2012;**198**:778–84.

76. Jauch EC, Saver JL, Adams HP, et al. Guidelines for the early management of patients with acute ischemic stroke: a guideline for healthcare professionals from the American Heart Association/American Stroke Association. *Stroke* 2013;**44**:870–947.

77. Murugappan A, Coplin WM, Al-Sadat AN, et al. Thrombolytic therapy of acute ischemic stroke during pregnancy. *Neurology* 2006;**66**:768–70.

78. Demchuk AM. Yes, intravenous thrombolysis should be administered in pregnancy when other clinical and imaging factors are favorable. *Stroke* 2013;**44**:864–85.

79. Moatti Z, Gupta M, Yadava R, Thamban S. A review of stroke and pregnancy: incidence, management and prevention. *Eur J Obstet Gynecol Reprod Biol* 2014;**181**:20–27.

80. Del Zotto E, Giossi A, Volonghi I, Costa P, Padovani A, Pezzini A. Ischemic Stroke during pregnancy and puerperium. *Stroke Res Treat* 2011;**2011**:606780.

81. Kernan WN, Ovbiagele B, Black HR, et al. Guidelines for the prevention of stroke in patients with stroke and transient ischemic attack: a guideline for healthcare professionals from the American Heart Association/American Stroke Association. *Stroke* 2014;**45**:2160–236.

82. Greer IA, Nelson-Piercy C. Low-molecular-weight heparins for thromboprophylaxis and treatment of venous thromboembolism in pregnancy: a systematic review of safety and efficacy. *Blood* 2005;**106**:401–407.

83. Lebaudy C, Hulot JS, Amoura Z, et al. Changes in enoxaparin pharmacokinetics during pregnancy and implications for antithrombotic therapeutic strategy. *Clin Pharmacol Ther* 2008;**84**:370–77.

84. Burnett AE, Mahan CE, Vazquez SR, Oertel LB, Garcia DA, Ansell J. Guidance for the practical management of the direct oral anticoagulants (DOACs) in VTE treatment. *J Thromb Thrombolysis* 2016;**41**:206–32.

85. Coomarasamy A, Honest H, Papaioannou S, Gee H, Khan KS. Aspirin for prevention of preeclampsia in women with historical risk factors: a systematic review. *Obstet Gynecol* 2003;**101**:1319–32.

86. Kittner SJ, Stern BJ, Feeser BR, et al. Pregnancy and the risk of stroke. *N Engl J Med* 1996;**335**:768–74.

87. Sharshar T, Lamy C, Mas JL. Incidence and causes of strokes associated with pregnancy and puerperium. A study in public hospitals of Ile de France. Stroke in Pregnancy Study Group. *Stroke* 1995;**26**:930–36.

88. Bateman BT, Schumacher HC, Bushnell CD, et al. Intracerebral hemorrhage in pregnancy: frequency, risk factors, and outcome. *Neurology* 2006;**67**:424–29.

89. Connolly ES, Rabinstein AA, Carhuapoma JR, et al. Guidelines for the management of aneurysmal subarachnoid hemorrhage: a guideline for healthcare professionals from the American Heart Association/American Stroke Association. *Stroke* 2012;**43**:1711–37.

90. Razmara A, Bakhadirov K, Batra A, Feske SK. Cerebrovascular complications of pregnancy and the postpartum period. *Curr Cardiol Rep* 2014;**16**:532.

91. Hemphill JC, Greenberg SM, Anderson CS, et al. Guidelines for the Management of Spontaneous Intracerebral Hemorrhage: A Guideline for Healthcare Professionals From the American Heart Association/American Stroke Association. *Stroke* 2015;**46**:2032–60.

92. Dias MS, Sekhar LN. Intracranial hemorrhage from aneurysms and arteriovenous malformations during pregnancy and the puerperium. *Neurosurgery* 1990;**27**:855–65.

93. Gross BA, Du R. Hemorrhage from arteriovenous malformations during pregnancy. *Neurosurgery* 2012;**71**:349–55.

94. Treadwell SD, Thanvi B, Robinson TG. Stroke in pregnancy and the puerperium. *Postgrad Med J* 2008;**84**:238–45.

95. Lee MJ, Hickenbottom S. Cerebrovascular disorders complicating pregnancy. UpToDate. Available at: https://www.uptodate.com/contents/cerebrovascular-disorders-complicating-pregnancy#H10 (accessed 31 December 2015).

96. Saposnik G, Barinagarrementeria F, Brown RD, et al. Diagnosis and management of cerebral venous thrombosis: a statement for healthcare professionals from the American Heart Association/American Stroke Association. *Stroke* 2011;**42**:1158–92.

97. Stam J. Thrombosis of the cerebral veins and sinuses. *N Engl J Med* 2005;**352**:1791–98.

98. Jaigobin C, Silver FL. Stroke and pregnancy. *Stroke* 2000;**31**:2948–51.

99. Liang C-C, Chang S-D, Lai S-L, Hsieh C-C, Chueh H-Y, Lee T-H. Stroke complicating pregnancy and the puerperium. *Eur J Neurol* 2006;**13**:1256–60.

100. Bousser MG, Chiras J, Bories J, Castaigne P. Cerebral venous thrombosis—a review of 38 cases. *Stroke* 1985;**16**:199–213.

101. Ferro JM, Canhão P, Stam J, Bousser M-G, Barinagarrementeria F, ISCVT Investigators. Prognosis of cerebral vein and dural sinus thrombosis: results of the International Study on Cerebral Vein and Dural Sinus Thrombosis (ISCVT). *Stroke* 2004;**35**:664–70.

102. Pfefferkorn T, Crassard I, Linn J, Dichgans M, Boukobza M, Bousser M-G. Clinical features, course and outcome in deep cerebral venous system thrombosis: an analysis of 32 cases. *J Neurol* 2009;**256**:1839–45.

103. Chan W-S, Lee A, Spencer FA, et al. D-dimer testing in pregnant patients: towards determining the next 'level' in the diagnosis of deep vein thrombosis. *J Thromb Haemost* 2010;**8**:1004–11.

104. Linn J, Ertl-Wagner B, Seelos KC, et al. Diagnostic value of multidetector-row CT angiography in the evaluation of thrombosis of the cerebral venous sinuses. *AJNR Am J Neuroradiol* 2007;**28**:946–52.

105. Expert Panel on MR Safety, Kanal E, Barkovich AJ, et al. ACR guidance document on MR safe practices: 2013. *J Magn Reson Imaging* 2013;**37**:501–30.

106. Coutinho J, de Bruijn SF, Deveber G, Stam J. Anticoagulation for cerebral venous sinus thrombosis. *Cochrane Database Syst Rev* 2011;**8**:CD002005.

107. Misra UK, Kalita J, Chandra S, Kumar B, Bansal V. Low molecular weight heparin versus unfractionated heparin in cerebral venous sinus thrombosis: a randomized controlled trial. *Eur J Neurol* 2012;**19**:1030–36.

108. Mehraein S, Ortwein H, Busch M, Weih M, Einhäupl K, Masuhr F. Risk of recurrence of cerebral venous and sinus thrombosis during subsequent pregnancy and puerperium. *J Neurol Neurosurg Psychiatry* 2003;**74**:814–16.

109. Ducros A. Reversible cerebral vasoconstriction syndrome. *Lancet Neurol* 2012;**11**:906–17.

110. Miller TR, Shivashankar R, Mossa-Basha M, Gandhi D. Reversible cerebral vasoconstriction syndrome, part 1: epidemiology, pathogenesis, and clinical course. *AJNR Am J Neuroradiol* 2015;**36**:1392–99.

111. Fugate JE, Ameriso SF, Ortiz G, et al. Variable presentations of postpartum angiopathy. *Stroke* 2012;**43**:670–76.

112. Chen S-P, Fuh J-L, Wang S-J, et al. Magnetic resonance angiography in reversible cerebral vasoconstriction syndromes. *Ann Neurol* 2010;**67**:648–56.

113. Fugate JE, Rabinstein AA. Posterior reversible encephalopathy syndrome: clinical and radiological manifestations, pathophysiology, and outstanding questions. *Lancet Neurol* 2015;**14**:914–25.

114. Fugate JE, Claassen DO, Cloft HJ, Kallmes DF, Kozak OS, Rabinstein AA. Posterior reversible encephalopathy syndrome: associated clinical and radiologic findings. *Mayo Clin Proc* 2010;**85**:427–32.

115. Meems M, Truijens S, Spek V, Visser LH, Pop VJM. Prevalence, course and determinants of carpal tunnel syndrome symptoms during pregnancy: a prospective study. *BJOG* 2015;**122**:1112–18.

116. Wand JS. Carpal tunnel syndrome in pregnancy and lactation. *J Hand Surg* 1990;**15**:93–95.

117. Wong CA, Scavone BM, Dugan S, et al. Incidence of postpartum lumbosacral spine and lower extremity nerve injuries. *Obstet Gynecol* 2003;**101**:279–88.

118. van Paassen BW, van der Kooi AJ, van Spaendonck-Zwarts KY, Verhamme C, Baas F, de Visser M. PMP22 related neuropathies: Charcot-Marie-Tooth disease type 1A and hereditary neuropathy with liability to pressure palsies. *Orphanet J Rare Dis* 2014;**9**:38.

119. Weinreb JC, Wolbarsht LB, Cohen JM, Brown CE, Maravilla KR. Prevalence of lumbosacral intervertebral disk abnormalities on MR images in pregnant and asymptomatic nonpregnant women. *Radiology* 1989;**170**:125–28.

120. Chou R, Qaseem A, Snow V, et al. Diagnosis and treatment of low back pain: a joint clinical practice guideline from the American College of Physicians and the American Pain Society. *Ann Intern Med* 2007;**147**:478–91.

121. Black RA, Hill DA. Over-the-counter medications in pregnancy. *Am Fam Physician* 2003;**67**:2517–24.

122. Garmel SH, Guzelian GA, D'Alton JG, D'Alton ME. Lumbar disk disease in pregnancy. *Obstet Gynecol* 1997;**89**:821–22.

123. Hilsinger RL, Adour KK, Doty HE. Idiopathic facial paralysis, pregnancy, and the menstrual cycle. *Ann Otol Rhinol Laryngol* 1975;**8**:433–42.

124. Vrabec JT, Isaacson B, Van Hook JW. Bell's palsy and pregnancy. *Otolaryngol Head Neck Surg* 2007;**137**:858–61.

125. Srivanitchapoom P, Pandey S, Hallett M. Restless legs syndrome and pregnancy: a review. *Parkinsonism Relat Disord* 2014;**20**:716–22.

126. Allen RP, Picchietti DL, Garcia-Borreguero D, et al. Restless legs syndrome/Willis-Ekbom disease diagnostic criteria: updated International Restless Legs Syndrome Study Group (IRLSSG) consensus criteria—history, rationale, description, and significance. *Sleep Med* 2014;**15**:860–73.

127. Gupta R, Dhyani M, Kendzerska T, et al. Restless legs syndrome and pregnancy: prevalence, possible pathophysiological mechanisms and treatment. *Acta Neurol Scand* 2016;**133**:320–29.

128. Picchietti DL, Hensley JG, Bainbridge JL, et al. Consensus clinical practice guidelines for the diagnosis and treatment of restless legs syndrome/Willis-Ekbom disease during pregnancy and lactation. *Sleep Med Rev* 2015;**22**:64–77.

129. Cesnik E, Casetta I, Turri M, et al. Transient RLS during pregnancy is a risk factor for the chronic idiopathic form. *Neurology* 2010;**75**:2117–20.

130. Tranquilli AL, Dekker G, Magee L, et al. The classification, diagnosis and management of the hypertensive disorders of pregnancy: A revised statement from the ISSHP. *Pregnancy Hypertens* 2014;**4**:97–104.

131. Mol BWJ, Roberts CT, Thangaratinam S, Magee LA, de Groot CJM, Hofmeyr GJ. Pre-eclampsia. *Lancet* 2016;**387**:999–1011.

132. Abalos E, Duley L, Steyn DW. Antihypertensive drug therapy for mild to moderate hypertension during pregnancy. *Cochrane Database Syst Rev* 2014;**2**:CD002252.

133. Altman D, Carroli G, Duley L, et al. Do women with pre-eclampsia, and their babies, benefit from magnesium sulphate? The Magpie Trial: a randomised placebo-controlled trial. *Lancet* 2002;**359**:1877–90.

134. Mostello D, Kallogjeri D, Tungsiripat R, Leet T. Recurrence of preeclampsia: effects of gestational age at delivery of the first pregnancy, body mass index, paternity, and interval between births. *Am J Obstet Gynecol* 2008;**199**:55.e1–7.

135. Roberge S, Nicolaides KH, Demers S, Villa P, Bujold E. Prevention of perinatal death and adverse perinatal outcome using low-dose aspirin: a meta-analysis. *Ultrasound Obstet Gynecol* 2013;**41**:491–99.

136. Rath WH, Hoferr S, Sinicina I. Amniotic fluid embolism: an interdisciplinary challenge: epidemiology, diagnosis and treatment. *Dtsch Ärztebl Int* 2014;**111**:126–32.

137. Fitzpatrick KE, Tuffnell D, Kurinczuk JJ, Knight M. Incidence, risk factors, management and outcomes of amniotic-fluid embolism: a population-based cohort and nested case-control study. *BJOG* 2016;**123**:100–109.

138. Knight M, Tuffnell D, Brocklehurst P, Spark P, Kurinczuk JJ, UK Obstetric Surveillance System. Incidence and risk factors for amniotic-fluid embolism. *Obstet Gynecol* 2010;**115**:910–17.

139. Conde-Agudelo A, Romero R. Amniotic fluid embolism: an evidence-based review. *Am J Obstet Gynecol* 2009;**201**:445. e1–13.

140. Karaca Z, Tanriverdi F, Unluhizarci K, Kelestimur F. Pregnancy and pituitary disorders. *Eur J Endocrinol* 2010;**162**: 453–75.

141. De Bellis A, Kelestimur F, Sinisi AA, et al. Anti-hypothalamus and anti-pituitary antibodies may contribute to perpetuate the hypopituitarism in patients with Sheehan's syndrome. *Eur J Endocrinol* 2008;**158**:147–52.

142. Keleştimur F. Sheehan's syndrome. *Pituitary* 2003;**6**:181–88.

143. Dökmetaş HS, Kilicli F, Korkmaz S, Yonem O. Characteristic features of 20 patients with Sheehan's syndrome. *Gynecol Endocrinol* 2006;**22**:279–83.

144. Kranick SM, Mowry EM, Colcher A, Horn S, Golbe LI. Movement disorders and pregnancy: a review of the literature. *Mov Disord* 2010;**25**:665–71.

145. Kim A, Choi CH, Han CH, Shin JC. Consecutive pregnancy with chorea gravidarum associated with moyamoya disease. *J Perinatol* 2009;**29**:317–19.

146. Cardoso F. Chorea gravidarum. *Arch Neurol* 2002;**59**:868–70.

25

Respiratory diseases in pregnancy

Catherine Nelson-Piercy and Stephen Lapinsky

Normal pulmonary physiological changes

Hormonal changes in pregnancy produce hyperaemia and oedema of the upper airway, resulting in symptoms of rhinitis. Placental growth hormone and oestrogens are likely to be responsible for many of these effects (1). These changes will have implications for endotracheal intubation and other upper airway interventions, increasing the risk of the procedures and necessitating smaller endotracheal tubes. The thoracic cage is altered both by the enlarging uterus and hormonal effects producing ligamentous laxity. The diaphragm is elevated by up to 4 cm, but an increase in the anteroposterior and transverse diameters and widening of the subcostal angle help partially offset the loss of total lung capacity. Diaphragmatic function remains normal and diaphragmatic excursion is not reduced.

Although total lung capacity is only minimally decreased, the changes in the chest wall produce a progressive decrease in functional residual capacity (FRC) by 10–25% by term (2). FRC is made up of the residual volume and the expiratory reserve volume, both of which demonstrate a decrease (2). These changes can be measured as early as 16–24 weeks of gestation and progress to term. Vital capacity remains unchanged, and measurements of airflow and lung compliance are not affected by pregnancy. Measurements of air flow, such as the forced expiratory volume in 1 second (FEV_1) are thus valuable in assessing dyspnoea during pregnancy. Chest wall and total respiratory compliance are reduced in the third trimester due to the chest wall changes and increased abdominal pressure.

The most striking respiratory physiological changes are the functional effects, namely an increase in respiratory drive mediated by progesterone (3). Minute ventilation increases markedly in pregnancy, produced mainly by an increase in tidal volume of approximately 30–35%. These effects begin in the first trimester and minute ventilation reaches 20–40% above baseline by term (**Figure 25.1**). The respiratory rate is unchanged initially and rises only about 10% later in pregnancy. A respiratory alkalosis occurs with partial arterial pressure of carbon dioxide ($PaCO_2$) decreasing to 3.8–4.3 kPa (28–32 mmHg), despite increased carbon dioxide production. Acid–base balance is compensated for by renal excretion of bicarbonate, with plasma bicarbonate falling to 18–21 mEq/L (4). Alveolar-to-arterial oxygen tension differences ($PAO_2 – PaO_2$) are not changed by pregnancy, and mean PaO_2 usually exceeds 13 kPa (100 mmHg) throughout pregnancy (at sea level). An increased alveolar–arterial gradient may develop in the supine position because of airway closure, as FRC diminishes near term. Oxygen consumption increases by 20–33% in pregnancy, due to both maternal and fetal metabolic demands. The combination of a reduction in FRC and an increase in oxygen consumption makes the pregnant patient susceptible to the rapid development of hypoxia in response to apnoea (5).

During labour, pain and anxiety may produce hyperventilation resulting in marked respiratory alkalosis, which may be aggravated by volume depletion and/or vomiting. Alkalosis adversely affects uterine blood flow and therefore fetal oxygenation. In some patients, mild hypoxaemia may result from severe pain and anxiety producing rapid, shallow breathing with alveolar hypoventilation, and atelectasis. Pain relief with narcotics or epidural analgesia blunts this ventilatory response and can correct these gas exchange abnormalities associated with active labour.

Dyspnoea of pregnancy

Many women with an otherwise normal pregnancy may complain of shortness of breath. Dyspnoea may develop in the first or second trimester, and by the third trimester 70% of women complain of some difficulty in breathing (6). The mechanism is not entirely clear and does not seem to correlate purely with uterine size. It appears to be more related to the physiological increase in minute ventilation. This hyperventilation produces an increased respiratory effort and increased motor cortical stimulation of the respiratory centre. The dyspnoea reflects a normal awareness of increased ventilation in some women (7).

The diagnosis of this benign dyspnoea of pregnancy is made in the presence of isolated dyspnoea not usually affecting daily activities, with physiological measurements within the accepted range for pregnancy, the absence of associated symptoms, and the exclusion of other pathologies. Sudden, episodic dyspnoea is more likely to be associated with a pathological condition. Increased exercise-induced dyspnoea may also occur in pregnancy.

Pneumonia

Lower respiratory tract infections are a leading cause of maternal and fetal morbidity and mortality (8). Pneumonia is the commonest reason for antenatal admission to critical care units (9). The reported

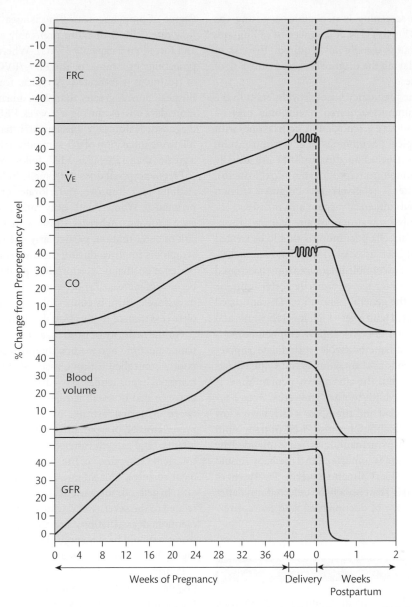

Figure 25.1 Physiological changes occurring during pregnancy and the postpartum period. CO, cardiac output; FRC, functional residual capacity; GFR, glomerular filtration rate; V̇$_E$, minute ventilation.

Reproduced with permission from the American Thoracic Society. Copyright © 2016 American Thoracic Society. Lapinsky SE et al, 1995; *Am J Respir Crit Care Med* 152:427–455.

incidence is probably not higher than that in the general population. Pneumonia in pregnancy is due to the usual bacterial pathogens such as *Streptococcus pneumoniae*, *Haemophilus influenzae*, and *Mycoplasma pneumoniae* but the pregnant woman is at increased risk of complications such as respiratory failure and empyema (10). Due to alterations in cell-mediated immunity in pregnancy, pregnant women are at increased risk of developing severe respiratory disease related to some viral infections, particularly influenza and varicella infection. Critical illness and mortality from influenza in pregnant women is more common than in the general population (11). Varicella infection is more severe in adults than children, likely even more so during pregnancy. Coccidioidomycosis may produce more severe disease than in non-pregnant patients, related to impairment of cell-mediated immunity and to a stimulatory effect of progesterone and 17-β (β)-oestradiols on fungal proliferation (12).

Pneumocystis jirovecii pneumonia may be seen in HIV-positive patients, and has a more aggressive course during pregnancy (13). Pregnancy does not affect the course or incidence of reactivation of tuberculosis. Postpartum pneumonia occurs in the first 6 weeks after delivery and is more common after caesarean section (14).

Pneumonia increases the risk of preterm labour, as well as the incidence of small-for-gestational age infants and intrauterine and neonatal death rates (8). Chronic illness in the mother is a predictor of adverse outcome in both fetus and mother. Although pneumonia is associated with an increased risk of maternal mortality, this may be attributable to the presence of predisposing underlying diseases rather than to the pneumonia itself.

The diagnosis of pneumonia is often delayed because of reluctance on the part of physicians or patients to obtain a chest radiograph. The radiation risk to the fetus of a posteroanterior radiograph performed with abdominal screening is negligible, exposing the fetus to less than 1 mrad (0.01 mGy) (15). A lateral chest radiograph produces greater exposure but is usually not required. The risk to both fetus and mother of delaying the diagnosis exceeds any risk of this very small radiation dose.

Treatment of pneumonia in pregnancy is not very different to the non-pregnant patient. Community-acquired pneumonia may be treated with a β-lactam antibiotic (e.g. amoxicillin, ceftriaxone) with or without coverage for atypical pneumonias (e.g. clarithromycin, azithromycin). Tetracyclines (including doxycycline) are usually avoided in pregnancy as are quinolones (ciprofloxacin, moxifloxacin), although the risk for the latter is relatively low. Pregnant women should receive the inactivated influenza vaccine and if disease occurs, treatment with oseltamivir, zanamivir, or amantadine are acceptable during pregnancy. Varicella pneumonitis should be treated with aciclovir, which has not been associated with fetal anomalies, and decreases mortality (16). Susceptible pregnant women exposed to varicella should be evaluated for use of varicella zoster immune globulin in the same way as the general population. Disseminated coccidioidomycosis is associated with a very high mortality rate, and should be treated with amphotericin (17). *P. jirovecii* pneumonia is treated with trimethoprim–sulfamethoxazole with folate supplementation (5 mg daily) (17). Folic acid antagonists and sulpha drugs carry some risks for the fetus, but the alternative, pentamidine, is associated with higher risks for both mother and fetus. Active tuberculosis is treated with isoniazid and rifampin, which have a low risk of adverse fetal effects. Ethambutol is also used initially until sensitivities are available, and pyrazinamide is recommended by some authorities. Contact tracing is important and the baby should receive immunization with bacillus Calmette–Guérin. Treatment of latent tuberculosis ('prophylaxis') can usually be deferred until after the pregnancy, except in the case of documented skin test conversion and recent exposure.

Asthma

Asthma is the commonest chronic medical illness to complicate pregnancy, affecting up to 7% of women of childbearing age. It is often undiagnosed and when recognized, may be undertreated. Pregnancy provides an opportunity to diagnose asthma, and to optimize the treatment of women already known to have asthma.

Reversible bronchoconstriction is caused by smooth-muscle spasm in the airway walls and inflammation with swelling and excessive production of mucus. The clinical features include cough, breathlessness, wheezy breathing, and chest tightness. Symptoms demonstrate diurnal variation and are commonly worse at night and in the early morning. There may be clear provoking trigger factors, such as pollen, animal dander, dust, exercise, cold, emotion, and upper respiratory tract infections. Signs are often absent but during an acute attack there may be increased respiratory rate, inability to complete sentences, wheeze, use of accessory muscles, and tachycardia.

Diagnosis is based on the recognition of a characteristic pattern of symptoms and signs in the absence of an alternative explanation. Eliciting a careful history is key. A personal or family history of asthma or atopy makes the diagnosis more likely. A hallmark of asthma is variability and reversibility of the bronchoconstriction. The

degree of bronchoconstriction is measured with a peak expiratory flow rate (PEFR) or more preferably spirometry to measure FEV_1 and forced vital capacity (FVC). Where the history suggests a high probability of asthma, or the FEV_1/FVC ratio is less than 0.7, a trial of treatment is indicated. A typical feature is morning 'dipping' in the peak flow. A greater than 20% diurnal variation in PEFR for 3 or more days a week during a 2-week PEFR diary is diagnostic. Other diagnostic features include a greater than 15% improvement in FEV_1 following inhalation of a β-sympathomimetic bronchodilator and/or a greater than 15% fall in FEV_1 following 6 minutes of exercise.

Pregnancy itself does not usually influence the severity of asthma. Asthma may improve, deteriorate, or remain unchanged during pregnancy. Women with only mild disease are unlikely to experience problems, whereas those with severe asthma are at greater risk of deterioration, particularly late in pregnancy. Women whose symptoms improve during the last trimester of pregnancy may experience postnatal deterioration. Acute asthma in labour is unlikely because of increased endogenous steroids at this time. Deterioration in disease control is commonly caused by reduction or even complete cessation of medication due to fears about its safety.

For the majority of women, asthma has no adverse effect on pregnancy outcome, and women should be reassured accordingly. Severe, poorly controlled asthma, associated with chronic or intermittent maternal hypoxaemia, may adversely affect the fetus. Retrospective, uncontrolled or small studies have demonstrated associations between maternal asthma and pregnancy-induced hypertension/pre-eclampsia, preterm births and preterm labour, low-birthweight infants, fetal growth restriction, and neonatal morbidity, including transient tachypnoea of the newborn, neonatal hypoglycaemia, neonatal seizures, and admission to the neonatal intensive care unit (18). In general, adverse effects on pregnancy outcome are small and related to the severity and control of the asthma. Most of the above-mentioned associations are uncommon in clinical practice and women should be reassured that those with well-controlled asthma mostly have normal pregnancies with healthy babies.

Poorly controlled severe asthma presents more of a risk to the pregnancy than the medication used to prevent or treat it. This small risk is minimized with good control. Women should be advised that their asthma is unlikely to adversely affect their pregnancy and maintaining good control of asthma throughout pregnancy is important. Emphasis in the management of asthma is on the prevention, rather than the treatment, of acute attacks. Complete control is defined as the absence of daytime symptoms, night-time awakening due to asthma, need for rescue medication, exacerbations, limitation on activity including exercise, and normal FEV_1 or PEFR greater than 80% predicted. It is important to check the woman's inhaler technique, since failure to do this may result in unnecessary escalation of therapy. Some women require a breath-actuated inhaler.

Management follows a stepwise approach and readers are directed to the British Thoracic Society/Scottish Intercollegiate Guidelines Network guideline on the management of asthma (19). Mild intermittent asthma is managed with inhaled short-acting 'reliever' (β₂-agonist) medication as required (step 1). If usage of a 'reliever' (β₂-agonist) inhaler exceeds three times/week, regular inhaled anti-inflammatory medication with a steroid 'preventer' (e.g. beclomethasone, budesonide) inhaler (400 mcg/day) should be commenced (step 2). The next step up in therapy is either the addition of a long-acting 'reliever' β₂-agonist (LABA;

e.g. salmeterol), or an increase in the dose of inhaled steroid (800 mcg/day) (step 3). Further steps involve a trial of additional therapies such as leukotriene receptor antagonist (see 'Safety profile of medications used to treat asthma'). Alternatively the dose of inhaled steroid can be increased to 2000 mcg/day (step 4). If these measures fail to achieve adequate control then continuous or frequent use of oral steroids becomes necessary. The lowest dose providing adequate control should be used, if necessary with steroid-sparing agents (step 5).

The aim of treatment is to achieve virtual total freedom from symptoms, such that the lifestyle of the individual is not affected. Regrettably, many people with asthma accept chronic symptoms such as wheezing or 'chest tightness' on waking as an inevitable consequence of their disease. This is inappropriate and pregnancy provides an ideal opportunity to educate women with asthma. Women should be advised to stop smoking and encouraged to avoid known trigger factors. They should receive explanation and reassurance regarding the importance and safety of regular medication in pregnancy (19). This is essential to ensure compliance. Home peak-flow monitoring and written personalized self-management plans should be encouraged. Use of a large-volume spacer may improve drug delivery and is recommended with high doses of inhaled steroid. Women should be counselled about indications for an increase in inhaled steroid dosage and if appropriate given an 'emergency' supply of oral steroids.

The treatment of asthma in pregnancy is essentially no different from the treatment of asthma in non-pregnant women. All the drugs in widespread use to treat asthma, including systemic steroids, appear to be safe in pregnancy and during lactation (see 'Safety profile of medications used to treat asthma'). The challenge in the management of pregnant women with asthma is to ensure adequate preconception or early pregnancy counselling so that women do not stop important anti-inflammatory inhaled therapy. Education and reassurance, ideally prior to pregnancy, concerning the safety of asthma medications during pregnancy are integral parts of management.

Safety profile of medications used to treat asthma

β_2-agonists from the systemic circulation cross the placenta rapidly, but very little of a given inhaled dose reaches the lungs, and only a minute fraction of this reaches the systemic circulation. Studies show no difference in perinatal mortality, congenital malformations, birthweight, Apgar scores, or delivery complications when pregnant women with asthma treated with inhaled β_2-agonists are compared with women with asthma not using β_2-agonists and non-asthmatic controls. The LABAs such as salmeterol (Serevent) are also safe in pregnancy (20). Long-acting β-agonists should only be used concurrently with long-acting inhaled corticosteroids. They should not be discontinued or withheld in those who require them for good asthma control.

Use of both inhaled and oral steroids is safe in pregnancy. Only minimal amounts of inhaled corticosteroid preparations are systemically absorbed. There is no evidence for an increased incidence of congenital malformations or adverse fetal effects attributable to the use of inhaled beclomethasone (Becotide) or budesonide (Pulmicort). Fluticasone propionate (Flixotide) is a longer-acting inhaled corticosteroid that may be used for those requiring high doses of inhaled steroids.

Combination inhalers of corticosteroids plus LABA, for example, budesonide/formoterol (Symbicort) and fluticasone/salmeterol (Seretide), are widely available and may aid compliance. They also ensure that the LABA is not taken without an inhaled steroid although to increase the dose of inhaled steroid without exceeding the maximum dose of LABA may necessitate changing the strength of the inhaler rather than asking the patient to take more puffs. The addition of systemic corticosteroids to control exacerbations of asthma is safe, and these must not be withheld if current medications are inadequate. Prednisolone is metabolized by the placenta, and very little (10%) active drug reaches the fetus. Although some workers have found an increased incidence of cleft palate with first-trimester exposure to steroids, this finding is refuted in larger prospective case–control studies and database linkage studies (21). There is no evidence of an increased risk of miscarriage, stillbirth, other congenital malformations, or neonatal death attributable to maternal steroid therapy.

There is a non-significant increase in the relative risk of pre-eclampsia in women with asthma treated with oral but not inhaled steroids. However, it is unclear whether this is an effect of steroids or asthma control and severity. Although suppression of the fetal hypothalamic–pituitary–adrenal axis is a theoretical possibility with maternal systemic steroid therapy, there is little evidence from clinical practice to support this. Long-term, high-dose steroids may increase the risk of preterm rupture of the membranes. There are concerns regarding the potential adverse effects of steroid exposure in utero (such as from repeated high-dose intramuscular betamethasone or dexamethasone to induce fetal lung maturation) and neurodevelopmental problems in the child. It is unlikely that lower doses of prednisolone that do not cross the placenta as well as betamethasone or dexamethasone will have similar adverse effects. Oral steroids will increase the risk of infection, gestational diabetes, and cause deterioration in blood-glucose control in women with established diabetes in pregnancy. Blood glucose should be checked regularly; the hyperglycaemia is amenable to treatment with diet, metformin, and, if required, insulin, and is reversible on cessation or reduction of the steroid dose. The development of hyperglycaemia is not an indication to discontinue or decrease the dose of oral steroids, the requirement for which must be determined by the asthma. Oral steroids for medical disorders in the mother should not be withheld because of pregnancy.

It is important to treat any gastroesophageal reflux as this can exacerbate asthma. No adverse fetal effects have been reported with the use of inhaled chromoglycates (e.g. disodium cromoglycate (Intal) and nedocromil (Tilade)) or inhaled anticholinergic drugs (e.g. ipratropium bromide (Atrovent)).

Methylxanthines are no longer recommended as a first-line treatment of asthma, but have been used extensively in the past. No significant association has been demonstrated between major congenital malformations or adverse perinatal outcome and exposure to methylxanthines. In those few women who are dependent on theophylline, alterations in dose should be guided by drug levels. Both theophylline and aminophylline readily cross the placenta and fetal theophylline levels are similar to those of the mother.

Leukotriene receptor antagonists (e.g. montelukast and zafirlukast) block the effects of cysteinyl leukotrienes in the airways. Studies do not suggest any increased risk of congenital malformations or other adverse outcomes with their use in pregnancy.

If leukotriene antagonists are required to achieve adequate control of asthma then they should not be withheld or discontinued in pregnancy (19).

It is important to consider the possibility of 'aspirin sensitivity' and severe bronchospasm in a minority of women with asthma. Low-dose aspirin is indicated in pregnancy as prophylaxis for women at high risk of pre-eclampsia and in women with antiphospholipid syndrome. Pregnant women with asthma should be asked about a history of aspirin sensitivity before being advised to take low-dose aspirin and before using non-steroidal anti-inflammatory drugs for pain relief postpartum.

Acute severe attacks of asthma are dangerous and should be vigorously managed in hospital. The treatment is no different from the emergency management of acute severe asthma in the non-pregnant patient. Deaths in women with severe asthma are often linked to one or more adverse psychosocial factors including psychiatric illness, drug or alcohol abuse, unemployment, and denial regarding their diagnosis.

The features of acute severe asthma are a PEFR of 33–50% of best/predicted, respiratory rate greater than 25 breaths per minute, heart rate greater than 110 beats per minute and inability to complete sentences in one breath. The management of acute severe asthma should include high-flow oxygen, and β_2-agonists (e.g. salbutamol 5 mg) administered via a nebulizer driven by oxygen. β_2 agonists can be administered by repeated activations of a metered dose inhaler via an appropriate large-volume spacer. Repeated doses or continuous nebulization (salbutamol 5–10 mg/hour) may be indicated for those with a poor response. Nebulized ipratropium bromide (0.5 mg 4–6-hourly) should be added for severe or poorly responding asthma. Corticosteroids (intravenous (hydrocortisone 100 mg) and/or oral (40–50 mg prednisolone) should be given without delay and continued for at least 5 days. Intravenous rehydration is often appropriate. Chest radiography should be performed if there is any clinical suspicion of pneumonia or pneumothorax, or if the woman fails to improve. If the PEFR does not improve to greater than 75% predicted, the woman should be admitted to hospital. If she is discharged, this must be with a course of oral steroids and arrangements for review. Steroids are more likely to be withheld from pregnant than non-pregnant women with asthma presenting via emergency departments. This is inappropriate and leads to an increase in ongoing exacerbation of asthma.

The clinical features of life-threatening asthma are a PEFR less than 33% predicted, oxygen saturation less than 92%, PO_2 less than 8 kPa, and a normal or raised PCO_2 greater than 4.6 kPa. There may be absent breath sounds, cyanosis, feeble respiratory effort, bradycardia, arrhythmia, hypotension, exhaustion, confusion, and coma. Management of life-threatening or acute severe asthma that fails to respond should involve consultation with the critical care team and consideration should be given to intravenous β_2-agonists, intravenous magnesium sulphate 1.2–2 g infusion over 20 minutes, and/or intravenous aminophylline (19). If intubation and ventilation is required then strong consideration should be given to delivery by caesarean section depending on gestational age.

Asthma attacks in labour are exceedingly rare because of endogenous steroid production. Women should not discontinue their inhalers during labour, and there is no evidence to suggest that β_2-agonists given via the inhaled route impair uterine contraction or delay the onset of labour. Women receiving oral steroids (prednisolone >7.5 mg/day for >2 weeks prior to delivery), should receive parenteral hydrocortisone (50–100 mg three or four times/day) to cover the stress of labour, and until oral medication is restarted. Prostaglandin E_2, used to induce labour, to ripen the cervix, and prostaglandin E_1 (misoprostol) for termination of pregnancy or for treatment or prevention of postpartum haemorrhage, are bronchodilators and are safe to use. The use of prostaglandin $F_2\alpha$ to treat life-threatening postpartum haemorrhage may be unavoidable, but it can cause bronchospasm and should be used with caution in women with asthma. All forms of pain relief in labour, including epidural analgesia and Entonox can be used safely by women with asthma, although in the unlikely event of an acute severe asthmatic attack, opiates for pain relief should only be used with extreme caution. Epidural, rather than general, anaesthesia is preferable because of the decreased risk of chest infection and atelectasis. Ergometrine has been reported to cause bronchospasm, in particular in association with general anaesthesia, but this does not seem to be a practical problem when Syntometrine (oxytocin and ergometrine) is used for the prophylaxis of postpartum haemorrhage.

All the drugs previously discussed, including oral steroids, are safe to use in breastfeeding mothers. Prednisolone is secreted in breast milk, but there have been no reported adverse clinical effects in infants breastfed by mothers receiving prednisolone. Concerns regarding neonatal adrenal function are unwarranted with doses less than 30 mg/day.

Sarcoidosis

Sarcoidosis is uncommon in pregnancy, affecting 0.05% of all pregnancies in the United Kingdom. It is a multisystem non-caseating granulomatous disorder of unknown aetiology. Chest symptoms include breathlessness and cough, but the patient is often asymptomatic. The commonest feature is bilateral hilar lymphadenopathy seen on chest radiography or lung computed tomography (CT). There may be extensive pulmonary infiltration progressing to fibrosis. Although there may be no obvious infiltration in the lung fields, the lung parenchyma is usually involved and diagnosis is made by high-resolution CT, bronchoalveolar lavage, and transbronchial biopsy. Lung function may be affected causing an obstructive or restrictive pattern and the transfer factor (diffusing capacity) is reduced. This measurement is not affected by pregnancy and can be used to monitor disease activity. Serum levels of angiotensin-converting enzyme may be altered in normal pregnancy and cannot therefore be used to help diagnosis or monitor disease activity as in the non-pregnant patient.

Extrapulmonary manifestations of sarcoidosis include erythema nodosum (which may also occur as an isolated finding in pregnancy without evidence of an underlying associated cause), anterior uveitis, hypercalcaemia, abnormal liver function tests, arthropathy, fever, and central nervous system involvement.

Sarcoidosis may be unaffected or improved by pregnancy. Those with active disease may have resolution of their X-ray changes during pregnancy and there is a tendency for sarcoidosis to relapse in the puerperium. Any improvement that is seen antenatally may be due to the increased levels of endogenous cortisol present in pregnancy.

Sarcoidosis often resolves spontaneously, but indications for steroid treatment include extrapulmonary, especially central nervous system disease, and functional respiratory impairment. Steroids should be continued or started in pregnancy if clinically indicated. Women receiving maintenance steroids should receive 'stress-dose' steroids in labour and delivery if they are taking more than 7.5 mg daily of prednisolone. Care should be taken with supplemental vitamin D, which may precipitate hypercalcaemia in patients with sarcoidosis.

Cystic fibrosis

Cystic fibrosis (CF) is a common genetic disease occurring in about 1 in 1500 white people and 1 in 17,000 black people. It is an autosomal recessive disorder affecting the CF transmembrane conductance regulator protein, a chloride ion channel. Clinical manifestations affect the lungs (bronchiectasis), pancreas (malabsorption, diabetes), and intestines. Advances in the management of patients with CF have extended life expectancy to a median age of 37 years, well into the childbearing age.

Although fertility may be impaired due to thickened cervical mucous, ovarian dysfunction (22) and malnutrition, about 50% of women with CF are able to conceive naturally (23). Pregnancy in CF patients may be associated with adverse fetal and maternal outcomes, but case series now demonstrate good maternal and neonatal outcome in women with CF, with appropriate management (24, 25). Pregnancy does not appear to negatively impact CF prognosis (26). The rate of hospitalization and outpatient visits increases during pregnancy but the rate of decline in lung function is not higher in women who have been pregnant. FVC less than 50% predicted and the presence of pulmonary hypertension are associated with an increased risk.

Complications during pregnancy include gestational diabetes and increased perinatal mortality, related predominantly to preterm delivery occurring spontaneously or due to maternal complications of CF. A review of 680 pregnant women enrolled in a United States registry demonstrated that survival was better in this group than in 3327 matched control patients with CF (26). Women with CF who became pregnant had less severe disease based on FEV_1 and body weight. However, even after adjustment for severity of illness, pregnancy did not appear to shorten survival. Nevertheless, most studies suggest that risk of pregnancy stratifies according to severity of illness, and prepregnancy counselling is essential to mitigate maternal and fetal risk. Reports from centres with significant experience demonstrate good outcome with normal birth weight and near-term gestation, although women with more severe respiratory disease tend to have lower-weight babies (24, 25).

Management of the pregnant woman with CF requires a multidisciplinary team approach with close attention to nutrition and glucose control (27). Hypoglycaemia may occur postpartum. Exacerbations of lung disease require early aggressive therapy, with consideration of the potential fetal toxicity of antibiotics such as aminoglycosides and quinolones. Genetic testing of the partner and genetic counselling is obviously also essential.

Acute respiratory distress syndrome

Acute respiratory distress syndrome (ARDS) is a condition of widespread inflammation in the lungs, characterized by bilateral infiltrates on chest radiography and impaired gas exchange, not associated with left heart failure. Increased capillary permeability results in a non-cardiogenic pulmonary oedema. ARDS occurs more frequently in pregnant women than in the general population, with an incidence of 1:6000 deliveries (28). The mechanisms of this increased incidence may be related to increased blood volume, decreased colloid osmotic pressure, and upregulation of components of the acute inflammatory response (29). ARDS in pregnancy may result from complications of pregnancy (e.g. amniotic fluid embolism, placental abruption, and chorioamnionitis) or from non-obstetric causes (e.g. pneumonia, sepsis, and gastric acid aspiration).

Management of ARDS is supportive and not different to the non-pregnant patient. Endotracheal intubation in the pregnant patient is associated with an increased risk of failure compared with the non-pregnant patient, and should preferably be performed by someone with experience in obstetric anaesthesia. Mechanical ventilatory support should target tidal volumes of 6 mL/kg (predicted body weight) and plateau pressures less than 30 cmH_2O. The reduced chest wall compliance in pregnancy may require slightly higher airway pressures than in the non-pregnant patient. Non-conventional modes of ventilation have been used successfully in pregnancy as a rescue intervention, including extracorporeal membrane oxygenation (30). Delivery is sometimes, but not always, beneficial to the mother and should be considered on an individualized basis by the multidisciplinary team (31).

Amniotic fluid embolism

Although small amounts of amniotic fluid are likely to enter the circulation during uncomplicated pregnancy, occasionally the catastrophic syndrome of amniotic fluid embolism results. The onset is usually during labour and delivery or following uterine manipulation. Initial manifestations may be acute severe dyspnoea and hypoxaemia, following which seizures, cardiovascular collapse, or cardiac arrest may occur. Surviving patients often go on to develop disseminated intravascular coagulation and ARDS. The maternal mortality rate has been reported as high as 86% but a more recent report suggests a lower mortality of 11–43% (32). The mechanism involves traumatic opening of uterine vessels, with constituents of the amniotic fluid producing the pathological effects. These constituents may include leukotrienes, arachidonic acid metabolites, and fetal squamous cells. An immunological mechanism may play a role. The haemodynamic effects include acute pulmonary hypertension followed by left ventricular dysfunction (33). The diagnosis is usually by exclusion—several biomarkers have been evaluated, with poor sensitivity and specificity. Low levels of C1 esterase inhibitor may be a useful marker and may play a pathological role (34).

Gastric acid aspiration

Contributing factors for gastric acid aspiration include the effect of progesterone lowering the tone of the oesophageal sphincter, the increased intra-abdominal pressure due to the enlarged uterus, and use of the supine position for delivery. The majority of cases of aspiration occur in the delivery suite, and all pregnant women should be considered to have a full stomach. Limited data suggest that a combination of antacids and H_2 antagonist are optimal for increasing gastric pH in this situation (35) Acidic gastric contents produce a chemical pneumonitis and permeability oedema in the lung, that is, ARDS. Bacterial pneumonia may follow in some cases.

Transfusion-related acute lung injury

Transfusion-related acute lung injury (TRALI) may complicate blood component therapy, and is not uncommon in pregnancy (36). The clinical presentation is of a sudden onset of dyspnoea occurring during or within 6 hours of transfusion of plasma-containing blood products. The differential diagnosis includes circulatory overload, which should respond to diuresis. Most patients with TRALI improve within a few days, although the condition may be fatal.

Other causes

Influenza pneumonitis is an important cause of severe ARDS in the pregnant woman, highlighted during the 2009 influenza A (H1N1) epidemic (**Figure 25.2**) (11). Preeclampsia may be complicated by pulmonary oedema, which may be a combination of a hydrostatic mechanism (related to increased afterload) and increased permeability (ARDS). Sepsis, either obstetric or non-obstetric, may be complicated by ARDS. Several series have demonstrated an association between pyelonephritis in pregnancy and ARDS (37). This is likely due to the fact that pyelonephritis is the most common cause of severe sepsis during pregnancy.

Restrictive lung disease

Restrictive lung disease appears reasonably well tolerated in pregnancy as the lungs have relatively more reserve than the heart (38). Many women with restrictive lung disease and markedly reduced FVC due to conditions such as kyphoscoliosis, neuromuscular disease, and parenchymal lung disease have successful pregnancy outcomes. In general, a FVC of greater than 1 L is sufficient but each case must be assessed individually and successful pregnancy with FVC less than 1 L have been reported (39). Whatever the underlying

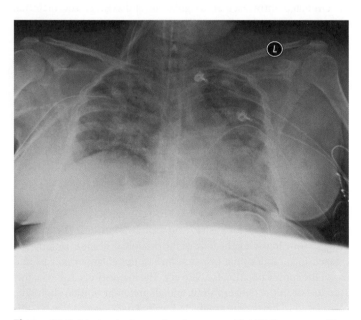

Figure 25.2 Mechanically ventilated woman with H1N1 pneumonitis. Note bilateral airspace disease, bilateral chest tubes for barotrauma, elevated diaphragms, and lead shielding of abdomen.

cause of respiratory insufficiency, significant hypercapnia or hypoxia, and pulmonary hypertension and cor pulmonale are associated with less favourable pregnancy outcomes.

Polycythaemia gives an indirect assessment of the degree of hypoxia and in itself is associated with an increased risk of thrombosis due to hyperviscosity. Women are often delivered preterm due to deterioration in respiratory function in the third trimester, and by caesarean section because of associated abnormalities of the bony pelvis and of abnormal presentations of the fetus.

Management should start with prepregnancy counselling. Multidisciplinary care and delivery planning is essential. Women with nocturnal hypoxia/hypercapnia may require supplemental oxygen and non-invasive ventilation. Liaison with obstetric anaesthetists is important. Regional analgesia/anaesthesia where the block is high may be dangerous in a woman with limited respiratory reserve. In addition, some women have had Harrington rods inserted that may preclude regional anaesthesia. Elective caesarean section may occasionally be indicated for anaesthetic reasons in women in whom regional techniques are not possible and emergency general anaesthesia is deemed too risky because of airway concerns.

Interstitial lung disease

Reduced diffusing capacity may cause difficulty in meeting the increased oxygen consumption requirements of pregnancy. Associated pulmonary hypertension carries significant risks. Interstitial lung disease is encountered most commonly in pregnancy as a manifestation of connective tissue disease (CTD) or sarcoid (discussed earlier). It is the most common pulmonary manifestation of connective tissue disease. It may be seen as a feature of rheumatoid arthritis, scleroderma, systemic lupus erythematosus, polymyositis, and Sjögren syndrome (40). High-resolution lung CT (which may safely be performed in pregnancy) is used to evaluate the extent and subtype of disease (**Figure 25.3**). Management of the acute presentation is usually with high-dose intravenous pulsed methyl prednisolone and management of the chronic disease is immunosuppression with steroids, azathioprine, cyclophosphamide, methotrexate, or biologicals such as rituximab. Immunosuppression, usually with prednisolone or azathioprine, should be continued in pregnancy. Mycophenolate mofetil, methotrexate, and rituximab are usually avoided in pregnancy but cyclophosphamide can be used in the second and third trimester for severe disease (41).

Pneumothorax

Most cases of pneumothorax in pregnancy occur in those with underlying lung pathology such as emphysema, Marfan syndrome, or bronchiectasis. It has also been described in those with pleural endometriosis. Pneumothorax may rarely occur during the second stage of labour secondary to rupture of a bulla during prolonged Valsalva manoeuvres. Chest drains can be inserted in pregnancy and for resistant cases video-assisted thoracoscopic surgery and pleurodesis should not be withheld.

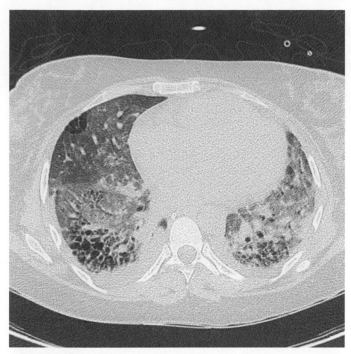

Figure 25.3 CT axial slice of pregnant patient showing fibrotic lung disease secondary to connective tissue disease.

Pulmonary arteriovenous malformations

Pulmonary arteriovenous malformations (PAVMs) are most commonly seen in association with Osler–Weber–Rendu syndrome—hereditary haemorrhagic telangiectasia. This is an autosomal dominant vascular dysplasia characterized by epistaxis, mucocutaneous telangiectasias, and arteriovenous malformations in the brain, lung, liver, gastrointestinal tract, or spine. The risks included bleeding leading to potentially catastrophic haemoptysis, infectious and ischaemic neurological manifestations due to paradoxical emboli, and high-output cardiac failure due to systemic arteriovenous shunting.

Those with PAVMs that bleed in pregnancy should be treated as outside pregnancy with coiling of the PAVMs using interventional radiology. Women should therefore deliver in facilities with interventional radiology support.

Lymphangioleiomyomatosis

Lymphangioleiomyomatosis is a rare lung disease most commonly affecting women of childbearing age, which occurs sporadically or associated with tuberous sclerosis complex. Pathological findings are interstitial proliferation of abnormal smooth muscle, which obstructs lymphatics and causes multiple thin-walled pulmonary cysts. Patients with lymphangioleiomyomatosis present with progressive dyspnoea, recurrent pneumothoraces, chylous collections, or haemoptysis. Extrapulmonary masses may also be found. Elevated serum vascular endothelial growth factor-D levels have been demonstrated in this condition. Lymphangioleiomyomatosis is thought to be accelerated by oestrogen and is believed to progress during pregnancy. However, successful pregnancies have been reported in women with

mild disease. Treatment is usually supportive with oxygen, management of airflow obstruction, and treatment of pneumothorax if it occurs. Recently, genetic findings have suggested a benefit of mechanistic target of rapamycin inhibitors such as sirolimus.

Sleep-disordered breathing

Sleep-disordered breathing includes the spectrum of snoring, upper airway resistance syndrome, and obstructive sleep apnoea and hypopnoea syndrome. It is assessed using the Epworth sleepiness scale and sleep studies measuring transcutaneous PCO_2 and apnoeic/hypopnoeic episodes.

Maternal obesity together with the physiological changes of pregnancy discussed previously predispose to the development of sleep disordered breathing (42). Since nasal obstruction is a risk factor for snoring and sleep-disordered breathing in the general population, it is possible that the nasal hyperaemia and rhinitis of pregnancy increase the risk in pregnancy. Upper airway size at the oropharyngeal junction is also reduced in pregnancy and especially in pre-eclampsia. However, because women in the second half of pregnancy sleep in the lateral position and spend less time in rapid eye movement sleep they are less prone to apnoeic and hypopnoeic events. The risk is also lower because of the respiratory stimulatory effect of progesterone (43).

Continuous positive airway pressure is the treatment of choice of sleep-disordered breathing in the general population and can be safely and effectively used in pregnancy. Women should be advised to limit weight gain. Continuous positive airway pressure has been associated with lower nocturnal blood pressure measurements in patients with preeclampsia (44). Sleep-disordered breathing may improve after delivery.

REFERENCES

1. Ellegard EK. Clinical and pathologic characteristics of pregnancy rhinitis. *Clin Rev Allergy Immunol* 2004;**26**:149–59.
2. Cugell DW, Frank NR, Gaensler EA. Pulmonary function in pregnancy. I. Serial observations in normal women. *Am Rev Tuberc* 1953;**67**:568–97.
3. Contreras G, Gutierrez M, Berioza T, et al. Ventilatory drive and respiratory function in pregnancy. *Am Rev Respir Dis* 1991;**144**:837–41.
4. Lucius H, Gahlenbeck HO, Kleine O, et al. Respiratory functions, buffer system, and electrolyte concentrations of blood during human pregnancy. *Respir Physiol* 1970;**9**:311–17.
5. Archer GW, Marx GF. Arterial oxygen tension during apnoea in parturient women. *Br J Anaesth* 1974;**46**:358–60.
6. Milne JA, Howie AD, Pack AI. Dyspnoea during normal pregnancy. *Br J Obstet Gynaecol* 1978;**85**:260–63.
7. Jensen D, Webb KA, Davies GA, O'Donnell DE. Mechanisms of activity-related breathlessness in healthy human pregnancy. *Eur J Appl Physiol* 2009;**106**:253–65.
8. Goodnight WH, Soper DE. Pneumonia in pregnancy. *Crit Care Med* 2005;**33**:S390–97.
9. Intensive Care National Audit & Research Centre (ICNARC). Female admissions (aged 16–50 years) to adult, general critical care units in England, Wales and Northern Ireland reported as 'currently pregnant' or 'recently pregnant' 2009–2012. ICNARC; 2013.

Available at: https://www.oaa-anaes.ac.uk/assets/_managed/cms/files/Obstetric%20admissions%20to%20critical%20care%202009-2012%20-%20FINAL.pdf.

10. Briggs RG, Mabie WC, Sibai BM. Community acquired pneumonia in pregnancy. *Am J Obstet Gynecol* 1996;**174**:389.

11. ANZIC Influenza Investigators and Australasian Maternity Outcomes Surveillance System. Critical illness due to 2009 A/H1N1 influenza in pregnant and postpartum women: population based cohort study. *BMJ* 2010;**340**:c1279.

12. Catanzaro A. Pulmonary mycosis in pregnant women. *Chest* 1984;**86** Suppl 3:14S–18S.

13. Ahmad H, Mehta NJ, Manikal VM, Lamoste TJ, Chapnick EK, Lutwick LI, Sepkowitz DV. Pneumocystis carinii pneumonia in pregnancy. *Chest* 2001;**120**:666–71.

14. Belfort MA, Clark SL, Saade G, et al. Hospital readmission after delivery: evidence for an increased incidence of nonurogenital infection in the immediate postpartum period. *Am J Obstet Gynecol* 2010;**202**:35.e1–7.

15. Ratnapalan S, Bentur Y, Koren G. 'Doctor, will that x-ray harm my unborn child?' *CMAJ* 2008;**179**:1293–96.

16. Lamont RF, Sobel JD, Carrington D, Mazaki-Tovi S, Kusanovic JP, Vaisbuch E, Romero R. Varicella-zoster virus (chickenpox) infection in pregnancy. *BJOG* 2011;**118**:1155–62.

17. Goodnight WH, Soper DE. Pneumonia in pregnancy. *Crit Care Med* 2005;**33** Suppl 10:S390–97.

18. Schatz M, Dombrowski MP. Asthma in pregnancy. *N Engl J Med* 2009;**360**:1862–69.

19. British Thoracic Society, Scottish Intercollegiate Guidelines Network. British guideline on the management of asthma. Guideline 141. 2014. Available at: https://www.brit-thoracic.org.uk/document-library/clinical-information/asthma/btssign-asthma-guideline-2014/.

20. Lim A, Stewart K, König K, George J. Systematic review of the safety of regular preventive asthma medications during pregnancy. *Ann Pharmacother* 2011;**45**:931–45.

21. Hviid A, Mølgaard-Nielsen D. Corticosteroid use during pregnancy and risk of orofacial clefts. *CMAJ* 2011;**183**:796–804.

22. Schram CA, Stephenson AL, Hannam TG, Tullis E. Cystic fibrosis (CF) and ovarian reserve: a cross-sectional study examining serum anti-mullerian hormone (AMH) in young women. *J Cyst Fibros* 2015;**14**:398–402.

23. Sueblinvong V, Whittaker LA. Fertility and pregnancy: common concerns of the aging cystic fibrosis population. *Clin Chest Med* 2007;**28**:433–43.

24. Gilljam M, Antoniou M, Shin J, Dupuis A, Corey M, Tullis DE. Pregnancy in cystic fibrosis. Fetal and maternal outcome. *Chest* 2000;**118**:85–91.

25. Cheng EY, Goss CH, McKone EF, et al. Aggressive prenatal care results in successful fetal outcomes in CF women. *J Cyst Fibros* 2006;**5**:85–91.

26. Goss CH, Rubenfeld GD, Otto K, Aitken ML. The effect of pregnancy on survival in women with cystic fibrosis. *Chest* 2003;**124**:1460–68

27. Edenborough FP, Borgo G, Knoop C, et al. Guidelines for the management of pregnancy in women with cystic fibrosis. *J Cyst Fibros* 2008;**7** Suppl 1:S2–32.

28. Catanzarite V, Willms D, Wong D, Landers C, Cousins L, Schrimmer D. Acute respiratory distress syndrome in pregnancy and the puerperium: causes, courses, and outcomes. *Obstet Gynecol* 2001;**97**:760–64.

29. Lapinsky SE. Pregnancy joins the hit list. *Crit Care Med* 2012;**40**:1679–80.

30. Nair P, Davies AR, Beca J, et al. Extracorporeal membrane oxygenation for severe ARDS in pregnant and postpartum women during the 2009 H1N1 pandemic. *Intensive Care Med* 2011;**37**:648–54.

31. Lapinsky SE, Rojas-Suarez JA, Crozier TM, et al. Mechanical ventilation in critically-ill pregnant women: a case series. *Int J Obstet Anesth* 2015;**24**:323–28.

32. Knight M, Berg C, Brocklehurst P, et al. Amniotic fluid embolism incidence, risk factors and outcomes: a review and recommendations. *BMC Pregnancy Childbirth* 2012;**12**:7.

33. Martin RW. Amniotic fluid embolism. *Clin Obstet Gynecol* 1996;**39**:101–106.

34. Tamura N, Kimura S, Farhana M, et al. C1 esterase inhibitor activity in amniotic fluid embolism. *Crit Care Med* 2014;**42**:1392–96.

35. Paranjothy S, Griffiths JD, Broughton HK, Gyte GM, Brown HC, Thomas J. Interventions at caesarean section for reducing the risk of aspiration pneumonitis. *Cochrane Database Syst Rev* 2014;**2**:CD004943.

36. Cantwell R, Clutton-Brock T, Cooper G, et al. The Eighth Report on Confidential enquiries into Maternal Deaths in the United Kingdom. *BJOG* 2011;**118** Suppl 1:1–203

37. Towers CV, Kaminskas CM, Garite TJ, Nageotte MP, Dorchester W. Pulmonary injury associated with antepartum pyelonephritis: can patients at risk be identified? *Am J Obstet Gynecol* 1991;**164**:974–78

38. Boggess KA, Easterling TR, Raghu G. Management and outcome of pregnant women with interstitial and restrictive lung disease. *Am J Obstet Gynecol* 1995;**173**:1007–14.

39. Lapinsky SE; Tram C, Mehta S, Maxwell CV. Restrictive lung disease in pregnancy. *Chest* 2014;**145**:394–98.

40. Mathai SC, Danoff SK. Management of interstitial lung disease associated with connective tissue disease. *BMJ* 2016;**352**:h6819.

41. Nelson-Piercy C, Agarwal S, Lams B. Lesson of the month: selective use of cyclophosphamide in pregnancy for severe autoimmune respiratory disease. *Thorax* 2016;**71**:667–68.

42. Bourjeily G. Sleep disorders in pregnancy. *Obstet Med* 2009;**2**:100–106.

43. Bourjeily G, Ankner G, Mohsenin V. Sleep-disordered breathing in pregnancy. *Clin Chest Med* 2011;**32**:175–89.

44. Edwards N, Blyton DM, Kirjavainen T, Kesby GJ, Sullivan CE. Nasal continuous positive airway pressure reduces sleep-induced blood pressure increments in preeclampsia. *Am J Respir Crit Care Med* 2000;**162**:252–57.

SECTION 3

Management of Labour

26

The management of labour

Devendra Kanagalingam

Introduction

Normal labour

Normal labour is defined as painful uterine contractions accompanied by effacement and dilatation of the cervix that finally leads to delivery of the newborn, placenta, and membranes. For management purposes, labour is divided into three stages:

1. The first stage is defined as the duration of observed onset of painful contractions that is associated with cervical changes to full dilatation. The first stage is conventionally divided into a latent phase and an active phase. The latent phase is characterized by progressive cervical effacement and early cervical dilatation. This may be accompanied by mild, irregular uterine contractions and may occur insidiously before the woman presents to the delivery suite. A fully effaced cervix signals the end of the latent phase. There is less agreement on the cervical dilatation at which the latent phase ends and the active phase begins. Traditionally, this was thought to be at 3–4 cm but a limit of 6 cm has been more recently proposed (1). This observation established the rate of cervical dilatation at various points in labour in nulliparae as set out in **Table 26.1**.

    This and earlier observations identify an active phase, characterized by more rapid cervical dilatation that culminates in full dilatation, commencing at 6 cm. Following the more recent observations, many centres in the United States consider the active phase to commence at 6 cm cervical dilatation. Prospective studies are needed to adopt such an approach into routine clinical practice.

2. The second stage is the period from full dilatation of the cervix to delivery of the fetus. In a nullipara, it is considered prolonged if the diagnosed second stage lasts more than 3 hours in a woman who has received regional anaesthesia and 2 hours in the absence of regional anaesthesia. Thresholds of 2 hours and 1 hour are usually applied in multiparous women in the presence and absence of regional anaesthesia, respectively. These thresholds are somewhat arbitrary in that they refer to the diagnosed duration of the second stage. There is a popular view that, with modern methods of fetal surveillance, the second stage can be prolonged beyond these limits without adverse effects.

3. The third stage is the period from delivery of the fetus to complete delivery of the placenta and membranes. Expectant and active management of the third stage are possible. Active management is shown to be beneficial as discussed further in this chapter.

The mechanism of labour

The mechanism of labour involves changes in the position of the fetal presenting part during labour and is described in relation to a vertex presentation. The following discrete steps are described:

1. Engagement.
2. Descent.
3. Flexion.
4. Internal rotation of the fetal head from an occipitotransverse to occipitoanterior position. This is termed internal rotation because it occurs within the pelvis.
5. Extension is the mechanism by which the fetal head is delivered.
6. Restitution—the rotation of the head to be in alignment with the shoulders.
7. External rotation of the fetal head outside the pelvis with rotation of the fetal shoulders within the pelvis. This is termed external rotation as it is visible to birth attendants, the fetal head having been delivered.
8. Expulsion of the rest of the fetus.

The partogram

A partogram is a continuous, pictorial/graphical overview of labour on which clinicians record labour observations. Modern partograms have three distinct sections to record details with regard to maternal condition, fetal condition, and labour progress. Friedman was the first obstetrician to describe the progress of normal labour graphically when he studied 500 primigravid women in labour (2). By plotting the progress of cervical dilatation in centimetres against duration of labour, he described a sigmoid- or 'S'-shaped curve which became known as the cervicograph. Philpott devised a partogram (3) based on Friedman's cervicograph which he used for clinical benefit in Zimbabwe (then Rhodesia). Philpott's partogram had an alert

Table 26.1 Rate of cervical dilatation in spontaneously labouring nulliparae

Cervical dilatation (cm)		Duration (hours)	
From	To	Median	95th centile
3	4	1.8	8.1
4	5	1.3	6.4
5	6	0.8	3.2
6	7	0.6	2.2
7	8	0.5	1.6
8	9	0.5	1.4
9	10	0.5	1.8

line which represented the mean rate of dilatation of the slowest 10% of primigravid women. An action line was plotted parallel and 4 hours to the right of the alert line (**Figure 26.1**a). This partogram was an attempt to utilize midwives efficiently in a hospital where doctors were in short supply. The clinical protocol stipulated that women would be transferred from a peripheral unit to a central unit if progress of cervical dilatation crossed the alert line. If progress was further slowed such that it crossed the action line, an intervention such as amniotomy and/or oxytocin infusion for augmentation of labour would be introduced. More simplified versions of the partogram have been proposed including a version by the World Health Organization (WHO) (**Figure 26.1**b). These simplified versions omit a latent phase on the basis that women in spontaneous labour usually present in the active phase of labour. Other versions may omit action and alert lines (**Figure 26.2**), allowing the obstetrician to draw these when required. Another modification is the active management of labour (AML) partogram used by the National Maternity Hospital in Dublin, Ireland (**Figure 26.3**). The AML partogram similarly dispenses with a latent phase and places emphasis on establishing full effacement of the cervix as the sine qua non of labour rather than the degree of cervical dilatation. There is evidence that these simplified versions are preferred by clinicians.

Research into whether a partogram reduces the caesarean section rate or improves maternal and neonatal outcomes has largely yielded divided results. A large multicentre trial showed a reduction in prolonged labours, caesarean sections in labour, and intrapartum stillbirths when the WHO partogram was utilized in units not previously using a partogram (4). Conversely, a Cochrane review showed no differences in clinical outcomes with or without partogram use (5).

Other modifications in the partogram include using a 2-hour or 3-hour action line as opposed to the original 4-hour action line. Some authors propose an alert line alone without an action line. These modifications also do not appear to alter clinical outcomes. Using an action line with a shorter duration results in more women receiving interventions such as amniotomy or augmentation with oxytocin (5).

Despite the lack of conclusive scientific evidence to support its use, it is widely accepted that the partogram is a useful tool in the management of labour. The pictorial nature of the partogram allows for easy identification of labours which are not progressing normally. The partogram also allows for systematic documentation of labour details as well as maternal and fetal parameters which may minimize omissions.

The management of normal labour

Labour is a physiological process and the management of normal labour should focus on fetal and maternal monitoring and the provision of analgesia when required or requested. Surveillance of the progress of labour allows interventions to be introduced when appropriate.

The first stage

Evidence suggests that the low-risk woman in spontaneous labour can have intermittent auscultation of the fetal heart rate for 1 minute every 15 minutes in the first stage of labour. A landmark randomized controlled trial (6) showed that continuous electronic fetal monitoring in these women did not significantly improve fetal outcomes when compared to intermittent auscultation but resulted in higher intervention rates such as caesarean sections and operative vaginal deliveries. In this study, the incidence of neonatal seizures was higher in the intermittent auscultation group but short-term and long-term neurological and developmental outcomes were similar in both groups.

Friedman proposed that, in the active phase of the first stage of labour, cervical dilatation should progress at the rate of at least 1 cm/hour (2). This represented the lower tenth centile of the rate of cervical dilatation in a cohort of spontaneously labouring nulliparous women. Expectant management is appropriate in labours which are progressing normally. Routine amniotomy is not shown to be beneficial (7). Proponents of amniotomy argue that this allows visualization of the colour of the amniotic fluid which, if clear, is a hallmark of the healthy fetus. There may also be a modest shortening of the duration of labour following amniotomy (8).

The second stage

Women who have reached the second stage of labour and who are being monitored by intermittent auscultation should have the fetal heart rate recorded for 1 minute every 5 minutes soon after a contraction. There is evidence that delayed pushing or allowing a period of passive second stage ('pelvic phase'), that is, not encouraging bearing down efforts immediately, reduces the need for operative vaginal delivery (9). An upright or squatting position during the second stage is also associated with a reduction in need for this intervention. Some birth attendants use a 'hands-on' technique for vaginal delivery where their hands are used to guard the maternal perineum in an attempt to prevent perineal lacerations. Evidence appears to show that both a 'hands-on' or a 'hands-poised' approach give similar outcomes (10) though expert consensus on this matter is quite divided. Performing an episiotomy routinely for delivery is not recommended. A policy of restricted versus liberal use of an episiotomy is shown to reduce the risk of severe perineal injury (11). An episiotomy is more commonly performed when a big baby is suspected, in the presence of malposition of the fetal head and during operative vaginal delivery with the forceps or ventouse. If an episiotomy is performed, a mediolateral episiotomy is less likely to be associated with obstetric anal sphincter injuries than a midline episiotomy (12).

The third stage

Following delivery of the fetus, the uterus contracts. Shortening muscle fibres in the myometrium result in a reduction in the surface area underlying the placenta. This causes detachment of the placenta. Active management of the third stage of labour is a

a. Composite partograph (WHO 1994)

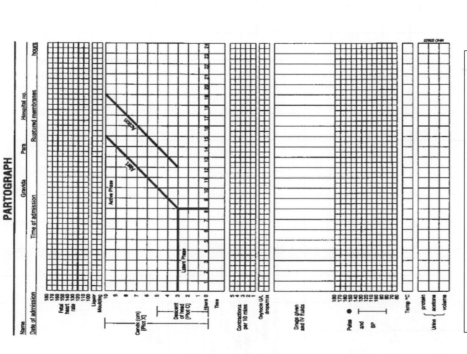

Composite partograph includes graphical
representation of the latent phase of labour.

b. Modified partograph (WHO 2000)

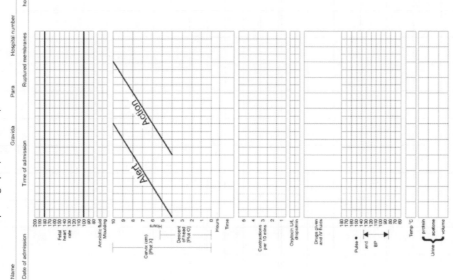

Modified partograph contains no latent
phase and is only plotted once active labour begins.

Figure 26.1 Two versions of the WHO partogram: the composite partogram includes a latent phase with 'Alert' and 'Action' lines as proposed by Philpott. The modified partogram does not include a latent phase.

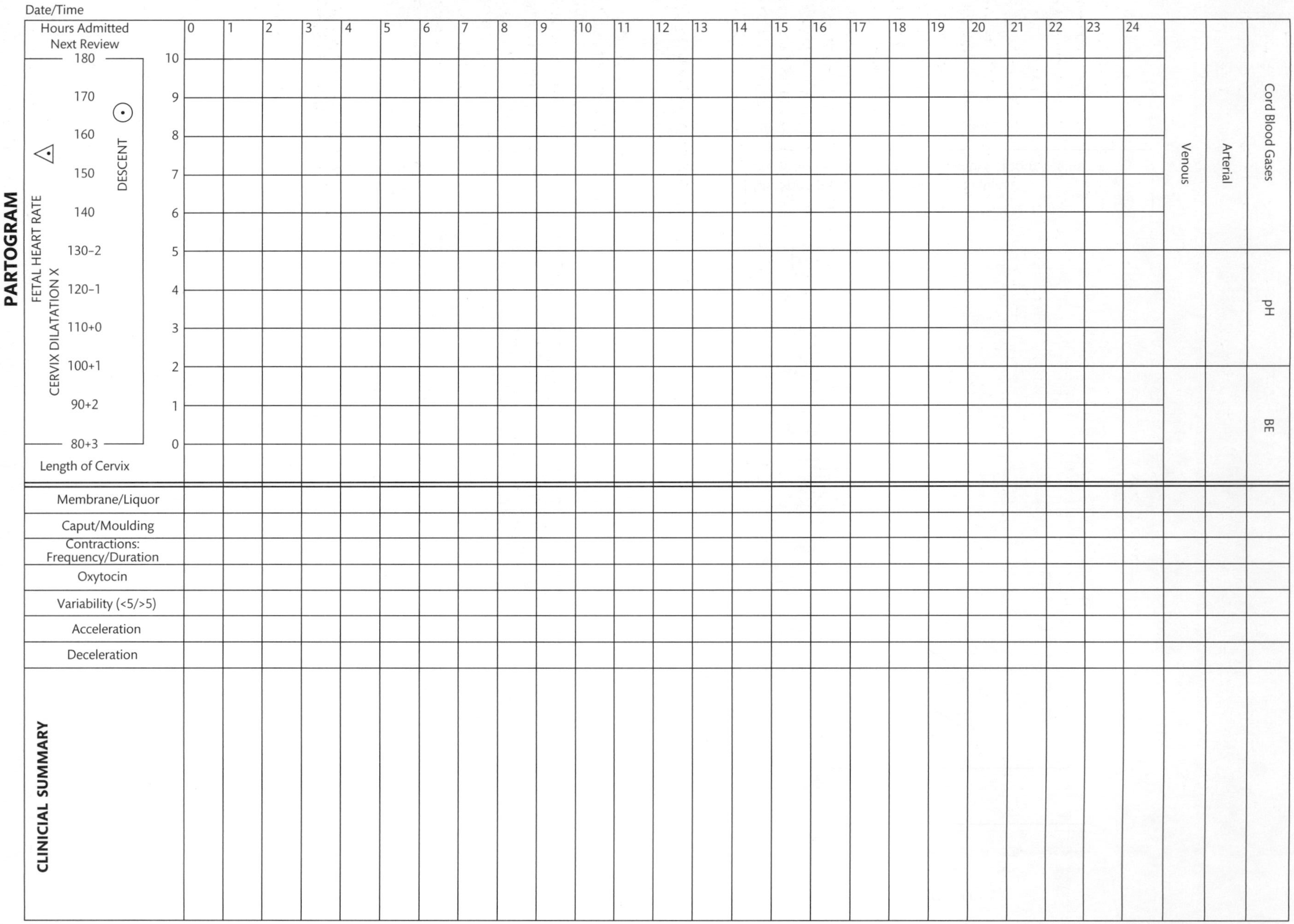

Figure 26.2 The partogram used at the Singapore General Hospital. 'Action' and 'Alert' lines are omitted. Spaces are allocated for clinical documentation.

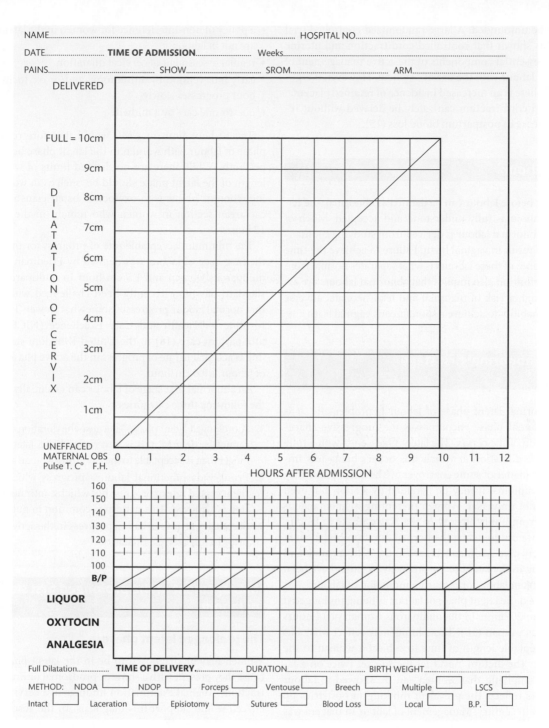

Figure 26.3 The active management of labour partogram used at the National Maternity Hospital in Dublin, Ireland, which does not include a latent phase.

fundamental aspect of modern obstetrics and has been shown to reduce postpartum blood loss. Active management of third stage refers to administration of a uterotonic, controlled cord traction, and uterine massage. The WHO recommends oxytocin as the first-choice prophylactic uterotonic (13) though, in clinical practice, a combination of oxytocin and ergometrine is also commonly used. Both preparations show similar efficacy in reducing postpartum haemorrhage but the combination of oxytocin and ergometrine is associated with a higher incidence of hypertension as well as nausea and retching.

Delayed clamping of the umbilical cord refers to the practice of occluding the umbilical cord between 1 and 3 minutes following delivery and not immediately after. Evidence shows that this practice is beneficial because it reduces neonatal anaemia and reduces the prevalence of iron deficiency in the infant at 4 months (14). This may have potentially positive effects on neonatal development. It has also been shown that delayed cord clamping does not result in adverse effects with the exception of a modest increase in neonatal jaundice. Fears that delayed cord clamping may result in increased postpartum blood loss because controlled cord traction is also delayed have proven to be unfounded. A large randomized controlled trial by the WHO has shown that controlled cord traction and uterine massage are not essential components of the active management of the third stage of labour with the use of oxytocin. However, if ergometrine is used, there is an increased incidence of retained placenta. Hence, controlled cord traction can safely be delayed without resulting in an increase in postpartum blood loss (15).

Abnormal labour

It is essential that before labour can be defined as abnormal, the nature of normal labour is fully understood and accepted. Much of what defines an abnormal labour is derived from studying spontaneous labours that result in vaginal birth. Failure to achieve the time limits and milestones of these labours is what separates normal from abnormal. The definition also implies that abnormal labours are associated with a higher risk of maternal and fetal/neonatal adverse outcomes or an inability to achieve a spontaneous vaginal birth.

Defining the abnormal first stage of labour

Defining an abnormal latent phase of labour is problematic. It is known that the latent phase encompasses the progressive effacement and dilatation of the cervix. The latent phase ends with a fully effaced cervix, the dilatation at which this occurs being less important and also a matter of some controversy. The latent phase may occur without symptoms. It may be heralded by a show but even this symptom is not universal. Women presenting in spontaneous labour are more commonly already in the active phase of labour. This makes any attempt to define the normal duration of the latent phase purely speculative. Women who are in the delivery suite and diagnosed as being in the latent phase are likely to either have been misdiagnosed to be in labour or requiring induction of labour.

Friedman defined the latent phase of labour as being prolonged if it lasted more than 20 hours in the nulliparous woman or 14 hours in the multiparous woman (16). These limits may reflect what was viewed as an acceptable length of time to subject a woman to the stresses of labour. The dictum 'never let the sun set twice on a labouring woman', implying that women can be allowed to labour for up to 48 hours reflects the prevalent thinking in obstetrics up to the mid twentieth century. Management of labour in that era was largely expectant. With improvements in asepsis and anaesthesia, the caesarean section evolved from a potentially lethal procedure reserved for dire situations to save a mother's life to a safe operation that is used for maternal and fetal benefit. Prolonged labours can also be emotionally traumatic for women and increase demands on staff and resources. Adverse maternal and fetal sequelae may also result. It is for these reasons that in present-day obstetrics, labours are not usually allowed to continue for as long as initially suggested by Friedman. O'Driscoll and colleagues at the National Maternity Hospital in Dublin, Ireland proposed the concept of the AML which comprises a package of measures including a limit of 12 hours on the duration of active labour (17). It is noteworthy that the other tenets of AML are:

- a policy of non-interference for women in the latent phase or who are not in labour
- regular assessment of cervical dilatation
- early intervention by amniotomy and/or oxytocin infusion if labour progresses slowly
- one-to-one care by a midwife.

The 12-hour limit in AML would therefore refer to the active phase of labour with women in the latent phase being managed expectantly. While there are no defined limits of what the observed length of the latent phase should be, such as in women undergoing induction of labour with oxytocin, obstetricians may intervene by caesarean section in women who remain in the latent phase for 12 hours.

The minimum acceptable rate of progress for the active phase of the first stage of labour was defined by Friedman as 1 cm/hour in nulliparous women and 1.5 cm/hour in multiparous women. This standard has more recently been challenged with the suggestion that normal labour progresses somewhat slower. The 2014 National Institute for Health and Care Excellence (NICE) guidelines for intrapartum care (18) in the United Kingdom state that the minimum acceptable rate of progress in the active phase of the first stage of labour is 0.5 cm/hour.

An abnormal first stage of labour can essentially be classified into the following three categories:

1. A prolonged latent phase—because the duration of the latent phase cannot be defined, this is best defined as a latent phase that lasts longer than is acceptable to the labouring woman and her caregivers.
2. Primary dysfunctional labour—progress which is slower than the accepted rate of progress but which continues until full dilatation is achieved. This pattern is common in nulliparous women.
3. Secondary arrest—a halt in progress in the active phase of labour prior to full cervical dilatation.

Management of the prolonged first stage of labour

The prolonged latent phase

Women may be diagnosed to be in the latent phase of labour because they present with a show or prodromal or Braxton-Hicks contractions. Vaginal examination findings of a cervix that is not fully effaced would support this diagnosis. In the absence of a medical indication to expedite delivery, these women are best managed expectantly. If left alone, these women often return to the delivery suite in the active phase of labour at a later time.

If an amniotomy is performed inadvertently or intentionally in these women, delivery becomes mandated. The next intervention is an oxytocin infusion to optimize uterine contractions in the hope that labour will progress beyond the latent phase and into the active phase of the first stage. If labour does not progress within the time limits which are acceptable, intervention by caesarean section becomes necessary. Reference was made earlier in this chapter to the 20-hour limit for nulliparous women and 14 hours for multiparous women proposed by Friedman and the fact that shorter durations would be the norm in modern obstetrics.

Primary dysfunctional labour

This pattern of labour exhibits a slow but continued progress in the active phase and is common in nulliparous women. The treatment for primary dysfunctional labour is to ensure efficient uterine contractions. This is achieved by performing an amniotomy, if the membranes are intact, or commencing an oxytocin infusion. The aim is to achieve five uterine contractions every 10 minutes but not more frequent than this. More than five contractions in 10 minutes is termed tachysystole and may induce fetal intolerance as manifested by abnormal fetal heart rate patterns.

Once contractions are optimized, progress of labour is often restored. If this does not happen, there is still a place for expectant management as long as progressive cervical dilatation occurs. The NICE intrapartum care guideline recommendation of at least 0.5 cm/hour (or 2 cm/4 hours) would seem a reasonable target.

Secondary arrest

Causes of an arrest in progress of cervical dilatation in the active phase can be classified as the three Ps. These factors must be present to ensure normal progress of labour:

1. Powers—adequate uterine contractions.
2. Passages—an adequately large pelvic cavity as a conduit for the fetus.
3. Passenger—a fetus which is not excessively large.

The only 'P' over which the obstetrician has any control is the powers. Confirming that efficient uterine activity is present is the first step in managing secondary arrest. An amniotomy (if membranes are intact) or an oxytocin infusion are the available interventions to correct inadequate uterine contractions. There is a case to consider an oxytocin infusion even in women who demonstrate regular uterine contractions as the strength of the contractions is not possible to assess clinically. This is particularly so in nulliparous women who more frequently require augmentation with oxytocin. Augmentation is also safer in nulliparous women whose risk of uterine rupture from this intervention is so low that they are often termed to be immune to it (19).

Once uterine contractions have been optimized, secondary arrest of labour is due to either cephalopelvic disproportion (CPD) or fetal malposition.

Cephalopelvic disproportion

As the name suggests, this cause of secondary arrest is due to a mismatch in fetal size and diameters of the pelvis. Fetal macrosomia can be as a result of maternal diabetes or genetic predisposition (a 'constitutionally large' fetus). A contracted bony maternal pelvis is a rare cause of CPD today but was a common sequelae of rickets two centuries ago. Occasionally, women with an acquired cause of a contracted pelvis such as a history of traumatic fractures of the pelvis may be encountered. As neither an excessively large fetus or an abnormally small pelvis are common in clinical practice, CPD is more likely to be a subtle mismatch between fetus and pelvis with the diagnosis being inferred by demonstrating secondary arrest in the absence of fetal malposition. In addition to poor cervical dilatation there may be signs of increasing caput and moulding.

Fetal malposition

The fetus in the occiput anterior presentation adopts a well-flexed attitude. This results in a vertex presentation where the presenting diameter, the suboccipitobregmatic diameter, is the smallest possible anteroposterior fetal cephalic diameter to negotiate the maternal pelvis. As a result, occipitoanterior positions are optimal for spontaneous vaginal birth unless an unusually large baby or unusually small maternal pelvis is present. The same is not true in malpositions such as an occipitoposterior or occipitotransverse position. In these situations, although there is no cephalopelvic disproportion in the absolute sense, the wider and therefore less optimal fetal diameters must negotiate the maternal pelvis. This can result in secondary arrest of labour. Often, optimizing uterine contractions may correct the malposition and allow the labour to progress. If this spontaneous flexion and rotation to an occiput anterior position does not occur, with persistent malposition and failure to progress with increasing moulding and caput, recourse to caesarean section may need to be considered.

Defining the abnormal second stage of labour

Reference is made in the previous section to the fact that there is no clear consensus on the acceptable duration of the second stage of labour. Traditionally, in the presence of regional anaesthesia, the cut offs are 3 hours and 2 hours in nulliparous women and multiparous women respectively. These limits are reduced by 1 hour if regional anaesthesia is not used in labour. In a 2014 obstetric care consensus statement, the American College of Obstetricians and Gynaecologists (ACOG) and the Society for Maternal-Fetal Medicine made the following statements (20):

1. Nulliparous women can be allowed 3 hours of pushing and multiparous women can be allowed 2 hours of pushing.
2. Longer durations can be allowed on an individual basis if fetal and maternal condition is satisfactory.
3. No absolute maximum length of time for the second stage has been identified.

It is also clear that the practice of delayed pushing, which refers to allowing a period of time after full cervical dilatation during which the woman is not actively encouraged to bear down, will have a bearing on the duration of the second stage. Delayed pushing is shown to increase the likelihood of a spontaneous vaginal delivery (21). Another consideration is that, although a longer second stage may not have harmful fetal or maternal effects, it may not always be possible in practice as maternal exhaustion may set in.

Management of the prolonged second stage of labour

Whatever the limits applied to the second stage, a proportion of fetuses will remain undelivered despite the mother's best efforts. A prolonged second stage can be approached as follows:

1. Ensure uterine contractions are optimal and consider oxytocin augmentation if appropriate—this step is best considered before the agreed limits of the second stage are reached. If delayed pushing is practised, an opportune time to start oxytocin augmentation is when active bearing-down efforts by the mother commence. If ACOG recommendations for a longer period of bearing down are adopted, commencing augmentation after 1 hour of pushing would seem reasonable.

2. Consider operative vaginal delivery by forceps or ventouse, if appropriate. In the presence of malposition, rotational operative vaginal delivery or manual rotation to the occiput anterior position followed by operative vaginal delivery may be possible. Operative vaginal delivery is discussed further in Chapter 33. Manual rotation to the occiput anterior position by an experienced clinician appears to be effective (22) and is a promising intervention, especially in light of the decreasing use of rotational forceps for these deliveries.

3. Caesarean section if operative vaginal delivery is not possible.

In deciding between operative vaginal delivery and caesarean section, careful consideration of the clinical situation including abdominal and vaginal examination findings, the fetal heart rate pattern, and maternal cooperation is essential. The experience of the obstetrician is also a key factor in choosing the appropriate mode of delivery.

REFERENCES

1. Zhang J, Landy HJ, Branch DW, et al. Contemporary patterns of spontaneous labour with normal neonatal outcomes. *Obstet Gynecol* 2010;**116**:1281–87.

2. Friedman EA. The graphic analysis of labor. *Am J Obstet Gynecol* 1954;**68**:1568–75.

3. Philpott RH, Castle WM. Cervicographs in the management of labour in primigravidae—the alert line for detecting abnormal labour. *J Obstet Gynaecol Br Commonw* 1972;**79**:592–98.

4. World Health Organization maternal health and safe motherhood programme. World Health Organization partograph in the management of labour. *Lancet* 1994;**343**:1399–404.

5. Lavender T, Hart A, Smyth RM. Effect of partogram use on outcomes for women in spontaneous labour at term. *Cochrane Database Syst Rev* 2013;**7**:CD005461.

6. MacDonald D, Grant A, Sheridan-Pereira M, et al. The Dublin randomized control trial of intrapartum fetal heart rate monitoring. *Am J Obstet Gynecol* 1985;**152**:524–29.

7. Smyth RM, Alldred SK, Markham C. Amniotomy for shortening spontaneous labour. *Cochrane Database Syst Rev* 2007;**4**:CD006167.

8. Brisson-Carroll G, Fraser W, Bréart G, Krauss I, Thornton J. The effect of routine early amniotomy on spontaneous labor: a meta-analysis. *Obstet Gynecol* 1996;**87**:891–96.

9. Lemos A, Amorim MM, Dornelas de Andrade A, de Souza AI, Cabral Filho JE, Correia JB. Pushing/bearing down methods for the second stage of labour. *Cochrane Database Syst Rev* 2017;**3**:CD009124.

10. Aasheim V, Nilsen ABV, Reinar LM, Lukasse M. Perineal techniques during the second stage of labour for reducing perineal trauma. *Cochrane Database Syst Rev* 2017;**6**:CD006672.

11. Argentine Episiotomy Trial Collaborative Group. Routine vs selective episiotomy: a randomised controlled trial. *Lancet* 1993;**342**:1517–18.

12. Coats PM, Chan KK, Wilkins M, Beard RJ. A comparison between midline and mediolateral episiotomies. *Br J Obstet Gynaecol* 1980;**87**:408–12.

13. World Health Organization (WHO). *WHO Recommendations for the Prevention and Treatment of Postpartum Haemorrhage.* Geneva: WHO; 2012.

14. McDonald SJ, Middleton P, Dowswell T, Morris PS. Effect of timing of umbilical cord clamping of term infants on maternal and neonatal outcomes. *Cochrane Database Syst Rev* 2013;**7**:CD004074.

15. Gülmezoglu AM, Widmer M, Merialdi M, et al. Active management of the third stage of labour without controlled cord traction: a randomized non-inferiority controlled trial. *Reprod Health* 2009;**6**:2.

16. Friedman EA. Primigravid labor; a graphicostatistical analysis. *Obstet Gynecol* 1955;**6**:567–89.

17. O'Driscoll K, Jackson RJA, Gallagher JT. Prevention of prolonged labour. *BMJ* 1969;**ii**:477–80.

18. National Institute for Health and Care Excellence (NICE). *Intrapartum Care: Care of Healthy Women and their Babies during Childbirth.* Clinical Guideline [CG109]. London: NICE; 2014. Available at: http://www.nice.org.uk/guidance/cg190.

19. Walsh CA, Baxi LV. Rupture of the primigravid uterus: a review of the literature. *Obstet Gynecol Surv* 2007;**62**:327–34.

20. American College of Obstetricians and Gynecologists, Society for Maternal-Fetal Medicine. Obstetric care consensus no. 1: safe prevention of the primary cesarean delivery. *Obstet Gynecol* 2014;**123**:693–711.

21. Lemos A, Amorim MM, Dornelas de Andrade A, de Souza AI, Cabral Filho JE, Correia JB. Pushing/bearing down methods for the second stage of labour. *Cochrane Database Syst Rev* 2017;**3**:CD009124.

22. Shaffer BL, Cheng YW, Vargas JE, Caughey AB. Manual rotation to reduce caesarean delivery in persistent occiput posterior or transverse position. *J Matern Fetal Neonatal Med* 2011;**24**:65–72.

27

Fetal monitoring during labour

Vikram Sinai Talaulikar and Sabaratnam Arulkumaran

Methods of intrapartum fetal monitoring

About one out of every ten newborns who later develop cerebral palsy has evidence of isolated intrapartum hypoxia as a cause. Despite its low specificity for hypoxia, cardiotocography (CTG) continues to be the central documentary evidence for all claims for fetal asphyxia (1, 2).

Although it is clear that in some of the cases interventions may have prevented or decreased the severity of cerebral palsy, it has been shown overall that fetal heart rate (FHR) patterns are poor predictors of cerebral palsy (1–4). The low specificity of CTG for fetal hypoxia therefore necessitates secondary or definitive tests to confirm fetal acid–base status in labour such as fetal blood sampling, vibroacoustic stimulation, fetal oximetry, or ST segment analysis of the fetal electrocardiogram (ECG).

Intermittent auscultation

Intrapartum intermittent auscultation of the FHR is probably the commonest and most widely used method of fetal surveillance in labour throughout the world. Its advantages include the ease of monitoring, low cost, and minimal training requirements.

When performing auscultation, a Doppler device is preferable to a Pinard stethoscope. The mother should be asked about fetal movements and a baseline FHR recorded. An attempt should then be made to feel the fetal movements per abdomen and look for any FHR accelerations associated with these movements. When the uterus contracts, the presence or absence of any obvious decelerations immediately after the contractions should be noted and an attempt made to estimate the depth and duration of deceleration, and whether it recurs with the next few contractions with the mother on her left lateral side. FHR accelerations associated with fetal movements and no decelerations should reassure the mother and the healthcare professional of good fetal health. Subsequent observations should be auscultation of FHR soon after contraction every 15 minutes for 1 minute in the first stage of labour and every 5 minutes or after every alternate contraction in the second stage. A change to electronic monitoring should be considered (where available) when recurrent or prolonged decelerations or abnormalities of baseline especially a rising baseline rate are detected on auscultation.

Randomized controlled trials (RCTs) undertaken in the 1970s and 1980s demonstrated no differences in the perinatal mortality, Apgar scores, or neonatal intensive care unit admissions when one-to-one intermittent auscultation (every 15 minutes in the first stage of labour and every 5 minutes in the second stage of labour) was compared to EFM (5–10). However it is important to recognize that the results with intermittent auscultation are poor as compared to EFM when there is no one-to-one care. Thus, in most situations of a busy maternity service when it is not possible to ensure that each healthcare personnel attend a single woman in labour, the success of auscultation may be less than what was observed in RCTs.

As part of the initial assessment (at first contact with the woman in labour, and at each further assessment), the National Institute for Health and Care Excellence (NICE) guideline recommends auscultation of FHR for a minimum of 1 minute immediately after a contraction. The maternal pulse should be palpated to differentiate between maternal heart rate and FHR. Any accelerations and decelerations, if heard, should be documented clearly (11). The biggest drawback of auscultation is that although it may provide the baseline FHR and indicate the presence of accelerations/decelerations, baseline variability is not audible to the unaided ear and quantification/description of the type of decelerations is difficult. It also does not provide objective evidence such as a paper trace for medicolegal purposes.

Electronic fetal monitoring

Since its introduction in the 1960s, the intrapartum and admission use of EFM has increased rapidly in well-resourced countries. Despite its shortcomings, continuous intrapartum CTG remains the predominant method of intrapartum fetal surveillance wherever facilities allow. This is because of medicolegal reasons (it provides a graphical trace record of the FHR throughout labour), also because it is helpful in identifying possible fetal hypoxia during labour and because there is no other better independent monitoring modality yet established for widespread clinical use. When intrapartum CTG was introduced in clinical practice, it was the expectation that this method would reduce the incidence of cerebral palsy and intellectual disability by 50%. However, this dream was not realized. As reviewed in 2002 by Freeman (3), the disappointing outcomes associated with EFM may be because (a) the asphyxial damage may begin before labour, (b) acute asphyxia associated with events such as prolapsed cord or ruptured uterus may not sometimes allow sufficient time for intervention before damage is done, (c) a large proportion of surviving very low birth weight infants contribute to the existing cases of cerebral palsy, (d) a fetal inflammatory response to infection/pyrexia may be responsible and (e) the amount of asphyxia required to cause permanent neurological damage is very near the amount that causes fetal death so the number of patients who develop cerebral palsy caused by intrapartum asphyxia is probably quite small. It is also possible that in some of the studies, the study sample size was not large enough.

Evidence

One large analysis of initial studies concluded that intrapartum fetal death was significantly less common in patients who were observed with electronic FHR monitoring than in those who had auscultation without one-to-one care (12). However, subsequent RCTs comparing EFM with intensive one-to-one auscultation in term patients found no differences with respect to perinatal mortality, Apgar scores, or neonatal intensive care unit admissions (5–10). The effectiveness of continuous CTG in labour was also a subject of a Cochrane systematic review in 2013 which included 13 trials (randomized and quasi-randomized controlled trials with >37,000 women). Compared with intermittent auscultation, continuous CTG showed no significant improvement in overall perinatal death rate (risk ratio (RR) 0.86; 95% confidence interval (CI) 0.59–1.23; $n = 33,513$; 11 trials), but was associated with a halving of neonatal seizures (RR 0.50; 95% CI 0.31–0.80; $n = 32,386$; nine trials). There was no significant difference in cerebral palsy rates (RR 1.75; 95% CI 0.84–3.63; $n = 13,252$; two trials). There was a significant increase in caesarean sections associated with continuous CTG (RR 1.63; 95% CI 1.29–2.07; $n = 18,861$; 11 trials). Women were also more likely to have an instrumental vaginal birth (RR 1.15; 95% CI 1.01–1.33; $n = 18,615$; 10 trials). Data for subgroups of low-risk, high-risk, preterm pregnancies and high-quality trials were consistent with overall results. Access to fetal blood sampling did not appear to influence the difference in neonatal seizures nor any other prespecified outcome. The authors suggested that the real challenge was how best to convey this uncertainty to women to enable them to make an informed choice without compromising the normality of labour (13). Most clinical guidelines that subsequently emerged recommended continuous CTG for women at high risk and intermittent auscultation for those considered at low risk in labour.

Challenges of electronic fetal monitoring

Intrapartum monitoring of FHR presents its own challenges. The report from the Centre for Maternal and Child Enquiries in 2008 and the Chief Medical Officer's report in 2006—'Intrapartum related deaths: 500 missed opportunities' in the United Kingdom have identified problems with interpreting and acting on fetal surveillance in labour (14, 15). It is not uncommon in clinical practice to unexpectedly find normal-size babies born asphyxiated while those delivered operatively for severe fetal distress to be born in good condition. Herein lie the challenges for healthcare professionals trying to interpret the intrapartum FHR patterns and base their management decisions on them. Presently, there appears to be a consensus regarding the reassuring value of a normal reactive CTG pattern (**Figure 27.1**) with accelerations, normal baseline rate, and normal baseline variability without any decelerations. On the other hand, patterns containing absent variability associated with persistent late or variable decelerations (**Figure 27.2**) are considered ominous and those with shallow late decelerations (**Figure 27.3**) and prolonged decelerations where FHR is less than 80 beats per minute (bpm) for longer than 15 minutes (**Figure 27.4**) are considered preterminal and indicate the need for immediate delivery to avoid hypoxic damage. However, the clinician is often challenged with a CTG trace that falls between these two extremes and needs to decide the further action depending on their interpretation of the findings based on overall clinical assessment of the case. Besides, hypoxia may not be the only damaging

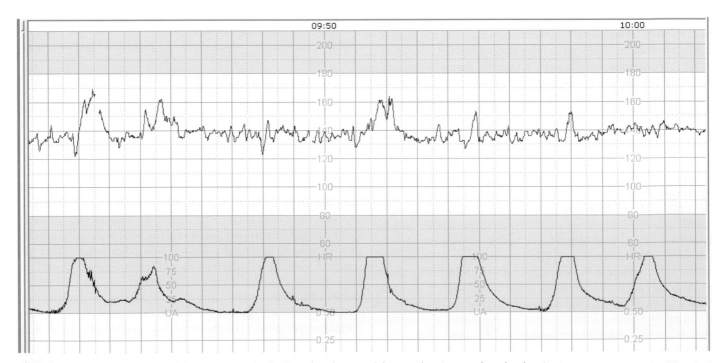

Figure 27.1 A normal reactive CTG with normal baseline rate, baseline variability, accelerations, and no decelerations.

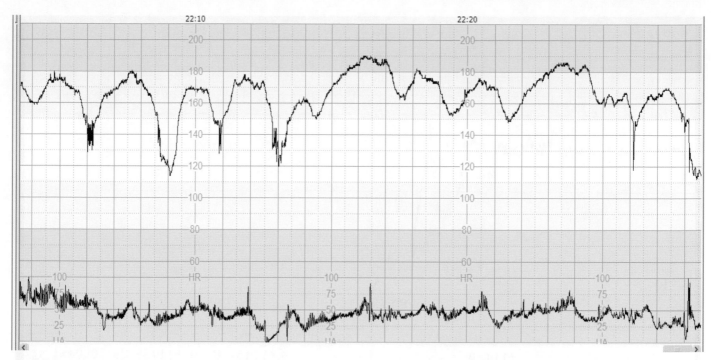

Figure 27.2 An ominous trace with reduced baseline variability, tachycardia, no accelerations, and variable decelerations.

factor during labour. Recent studies suggest a fetal inflammatory response due to infection/pyrexia as a cause of central nervous system damage (16, 17). The patterns of CTG associated with such insults may vary considerably and need to be carefully interpreted based on the overall clinical scenario.

Admission test

The labour admission test (LAT) is a test of fetal well-being that is performed when a woman with a low-risk pregnancy is admitted in labour. Its aim is to assess fetal well-being at the onset of labour and identify those fetuses that may be already hypoxic or may not

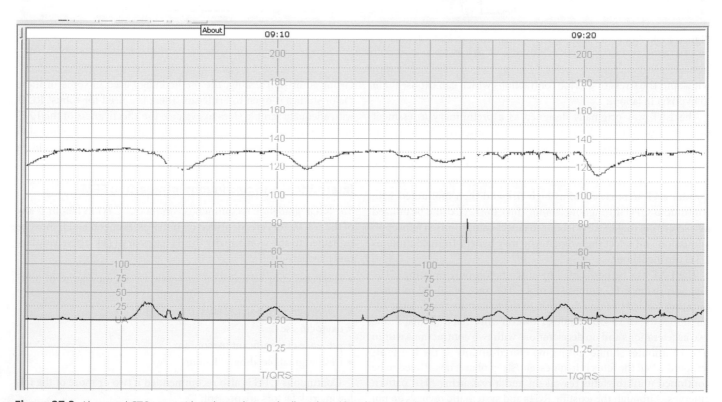

Figure 27.3 Abnormal CTG trace with tachycardia, markedly reduced baseline variability, and shallow late decelerations—a pre-terminal trace.

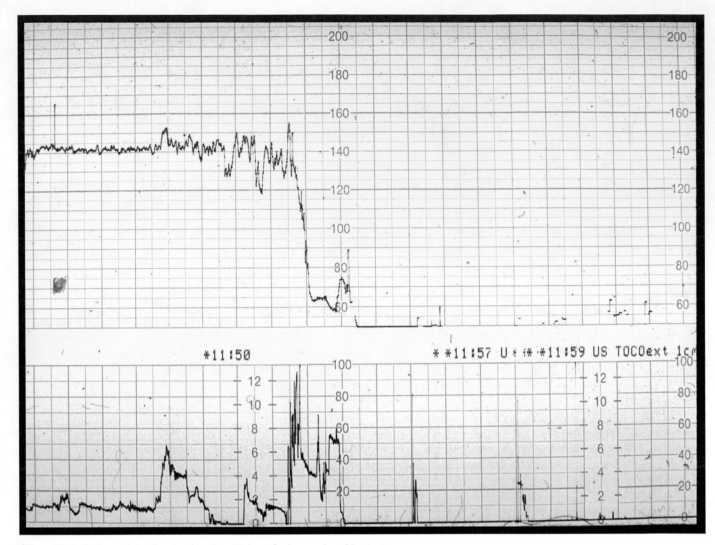

Figure 27.4 Prolonged deceleration less than 80 bpm for longer than 15 minutes.

withstand the stress of uterine contractions which can expose them to hypoxia in labour.

The LAT was originally designed as a preliminary assessment of women with low-risk pregnancies at the onset of labour so that those with non-reassuring FHR patterns could be subjected to additional tests of fetal surveillance or delivered depending on the severity of fetal jeopardy. It often meant that women with an abnormal LAT were classified as high risk and then monitored with continuous CTG throughout labour. Thus, the LAT could be utilized as a screening tool in early labour to detect compromised fetuses on admission and select the women who may benefit from continuous CTG during labour.

The LAT can be performed by auscultation only or using CTG. The admission CTG comprises of a CTG trace of 20–30 minutes' duration carried out on admission to the maternity ward. Most admission tests last 15–30 minutes. However a normal trace that shows two accelerations and no decelerations with two contractions within 5 to 10 minutes should not be monitored unduly. If the test is attempted when the fetus is in quiescent/sleep phase, it will need to be continued until the fetus reawakens and a reassuring FHR pattern emerges. Although the existing RCTs and systematic reviews do not favour admission testing, the methodology used in some of these major studies is open to criticism. There is a need for robust RCTs with adequate sample sizes to evaluate the effectiveness of the LAT. NICE guidelines do not recommend performing CTG on admission for low-risk women in suspected or established labour in any birth setting as part of the initial assessment (11).

Intermittent and continuous intrapartum EFM

The NICE guideline recommends continuous CTG in labour if any of the risk factors are identified on initial assessment, and it must be explained to the woman why this is necessary (11). These risk factors may be:

- suspected chorioamnionitis or sepsis, or a temperature of 38°C or higher
- severe hypertension (≥160/110 mmHg)
- oxytocin use
- presence of significant meconium
- fresh vaginal bleeding in labour.

Continuous CTG is also recommended if two or more of the following risk factors are present:

- Prolonged period since rupture of membranes (≥24 hours).
- Moderate hypertension (150/100 to 159/109 mmHg).
- Confirmed delay in the first or second stage of labour.
- Presence of non-significant meconium.

CTG is also recommended if one of the above-listed factors is present with any of the following:

- Maternal pulse over 120 bpm on two occasions 30 minutes apart.
- A single reading of either raised diastolic blood pressure of 110 mmHg or more, or raised systolic blood pressure of 160 mmHg or more.
- Either raised diastolic blood pressure of 90 mmHg or more, or raised systolic blood pressure of 140 mmHg or more, on two consecutive readings taken 30 minutes apart.
- A reading of 2+ of protein on urinalysis and a single reading of either raised diastolic blood pressure (≥90 mmHg) or raised systolic blood pressure (≥140 mmHg).
- Temperature of 38°C or higher on a single reading, or 37.5°C or higher on two consecutive occasions 1 hour apart.
- Any vaginal blood loss other than a show.
- The presence of significant meconium.
- Pain reported by the woman that differs from the pain normally associated with contractions.
- Confirmed delay in the first or second stage of labour.
- Request by the woman for additional pain relief using regional analgesia.
- Obstetric emergency—including antepartum haemorrhage, cord prolapse, maternal seizure, or collapse.

If continuous CTG is needed, it should be explained to the woman that it will restrict her mobility, particularly if conventional monitoring is used. The woman should be encouraged to be as mobile as possible and to change position as often as she wishes. It should be borne in mind that it is not possible to categorize or interpret every CTG trace; senior obstetric input is important in these cases (11).

CTG is also recommended if intermittent auscultation indicates possible FHR abnormalities. The CTG can be discontinued if the trace is normal after 20 minutes.

Whenever CTG is used as a form of fetal monitoring at the beginning of labour, the woman should be offered an explanation that a normal trace is reassuring and indicates that the baby is coping well with labour, but if the trace is not normal there is less certainty about the condition of the baby and further continuous monitoring will be advised.

Systematic CTG interpretation

A crucial advantage of the CTG is the ability to assess all parameters of FHR including baseline variability. Presence of accelerations, normal baseline heart rate, variability greater than 5–25 bpm, and absence of any decelerations are features of a normal reassuring CTG (Figure 27.1). With a normal baseline CTG, a gradually developing hypoxia will be reflected by no accelerations, repeated decelerations, and gradually rising baseline rate (Figure 27.5). Furthermore, it is known that if a well-grown fetus with clear amniotic fluid and a reactive CTG trace starts to develop an abnormal FHR pattern, it takes some time with these FHR changes before acidosis develops. A study estimated that in situations with abnormal FHR pattern,

for 50% of the babies to become acidotic, it took 115 minutes with repeated late decelerations, 145 minutes with repeated variable decelerations, and 185 minutes with a flat trace (18). Fetuses with a reactive admission CTG will show the following features prior to or becoming hypoxic—all will exhibit decelerations (100%), and almost all will have reduced baseline variability (93%) and baseline tachycardia (93%) (19) (Figure 27.5). A rising baseline associated with reduced variability therefore may be an ominous sign of fetal hypoxia where the fetus tries to increase oxygen delivery to vital organs by increasing cardiac output. On the other hand, if the baseline CTG is non-reactive, the development of further abnormal features with progress of labour are variable and subtle; this is difficult to recognize by intermittent auscultation (20) (Figure 27.6). This is because there might be pre-existing hypoxic damage and the fetus is unable to respond. Such a fetus may not withstand the stress of uterine contractions and runs the risk of death within a few hours of admission (Figure 27.7).

When interpreting a CTG trace, it is important to follow a systematic approach (Box 27.1) (21). The use of vague descriptors such as 'sleepy trace', 'bad CTG', or 'fetal distress' should be avoided. The NICE evidence-based clinical guideline (11) (Tables 27.1 and 27.2) promotes a systematic approach to CTG interpretation, with individual features classified as reassuring, non-reassuring, or abnormal and the overall CTG as normal/non-reassuring and abnormal. Continuous EFM should be systematically assessed at least once an hour in labour and more often if indicated.

Management of non-reassuring or abnormal intrapartum CTG

In general, a 'non-reassuring CTG' can be managed conservatively. An 'abnormal CTG' requires institution of conservative measures and fetal scalp blood sampling (FBS) where appropriate/feasible, otherwise delivery should be expedited. Interventions for non-reassuring or abnormal trace will depend on the suspected underlying cause for the abnormalities in FHR and the clinical situation. These features may be reversed by conservative measures such as changing maternal position, treating hypotension or pyrexia, hydration, reducing or stopping oxytocin, or tocolysis for hyperstimulation.

When the baseline FHR is greater than 180 bpm with no other non-reassuring or abnormal features on the CTG, possible underlying causes (such as infection) should be sought. The woman's temperature and pulse should be checked and if either is raised, fluids and paracetamol should be offered. FBS to measure lactate or pH should be considered if the rate stays higher than 180 bpm despite conservative measures.

Baseline variability will usually be 5–25 bpm. Intermittent periods of reduced baseline variability are normal, especially during periods of quiescence ('sleep'). Mild or minor pseudo-sinusoidal patterns (oscillations of amplitude 5–15 bpm) are also of no significance especially if it is short lasting and the trace preceding or followed by is a reactive trace.

Timely action is crucial in cases of prolonged decelerations or bradycardia (Figure 27.5) for longer than 3 minutes where urgent intervention may be required. Possible causes include abruption, cord prolapse, and scar rupture. In the event of such a catastrophic 'accident', immediate delivery should occur. In the absence of these, the '3-, 6-, 9-, 12-, 15-minute' guidance can be followed. Interventions such as cessation of oxytocin and treatment of maternal hypotension

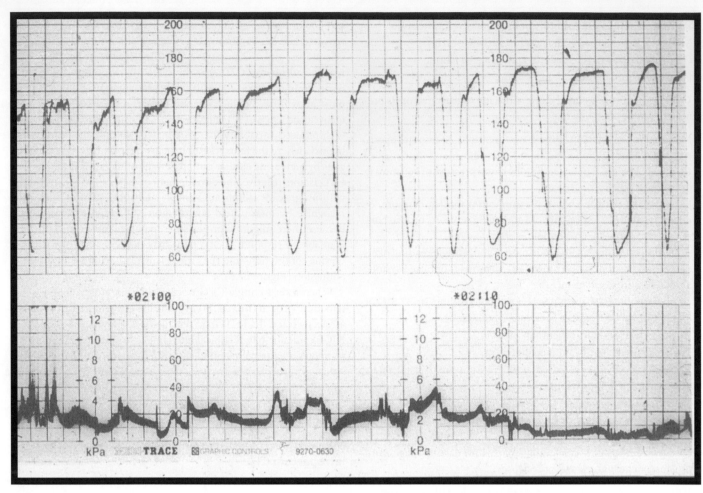

Figure 27.5 Tachycardia (rise from 140 to 170 bpm over 5 hours), absent baseline variability. and variable/late decelerations.

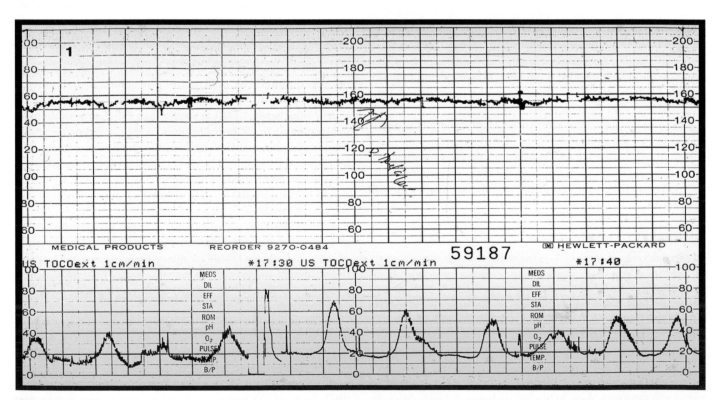

Figure 27.6 CTG trace from the time of admission showing reduced baseline variability, absent accelerations, and shallow late decelerations suggestive of ongoing/pre-existing hypoxia. The clinical history is likely to have thick meconium, reduced fetal movements, intrauterine growth restriction, infection, prolonged pregnancy, or bleeding.

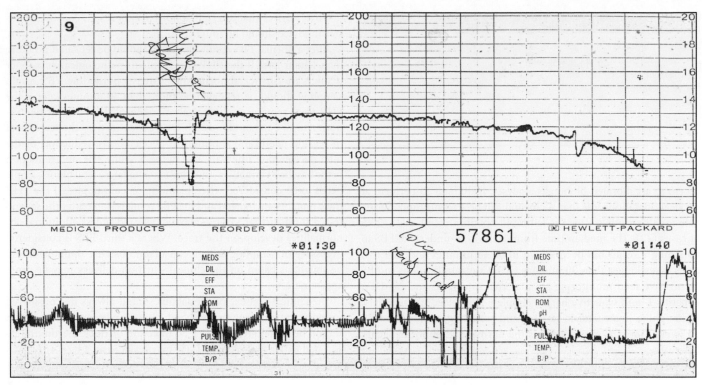

Figure 27.7 The fetal heart rate showing sudden bradycardia and collapse without showing obvious decelerations or rise in the baseline rate.

should commence. If there are no signs of recovery at 6 minutes, preparations should be made to transfer to theatre by 9 minutes. Caesarean section should commence by 12 minutes with the aim of delivery by 15 minutes. If instrumental delivery is possible this should be achieved within 15–20 minutes but a difficult instrumental delivery should be avoided. An experienced neonatal team should attend the delivery if resuscitation is anticipated. Many cases will recover by 9 minutes (especially if they had a normal CTG prior to this event) and caesarean section may not be necessary unless there are additional reasons for concern. If the FHR recovers at any time up to 9 minutes, the decision to expedite the birth should be reassessed, in discussion with the woman. Appropriate debriefing and explanation of events to the mother and partner should follow expedited delivery.

Some of the CTG patterns pose a challenge to the obstetrician regarding their interpretation and management. The following features in isolation are unlikely to be associated with significant acidosis (22): (a) moderate bradycardia (100–109 bpm), (b) moderate uncomplicated tachycardia (161–180) with accelerations present, (c) absence of accelerations, and (d) variable decelerations without complicating features.

Some of the important issues which need to be considered while recording or evaluating a CTG trace include:

- patient identity
- maternal pulse
- quality of the trace
- storage of CTG
- misinterpretation of CTG
- education and training in CTG interpretation
- teamwork and communication of findings
- action with non-reassuring or abnormal CTG
- overall clinical picture and pattern evolution of CTG
- role of infection and inflammation
- documentation of events and risk management.

At all times, it should be ensured that the focus of care remains on the woman rather than the CTG trace and no decisions about a woman's care in labour should be made on the basis of CTG findings alone.

Fetal scalp blood sampling

CTG is an imperfect tool and many of the indicators used to identify early hypoxia are non-specific. Thus, if CTG is used as the sole method of intrapartum fetal surveillance, unnecessary operative deliveries will be performed. FBS for pH analysis and lactate measurement is used to assess fetuses with pathological FHR patterns. FBS is recommended with pathological CTGs to identify those fetuses that require delivery and ideally all maternity units where CTG is used should have ready access, 24 hours a day, to an accurate blood gas analyser. To obtain a fetal scalp capillary sample, the cervix has to be at least 3–4 cm dilated. With the mother in the left lateral position, an amnioscope is introduced into the vagina and kept against the fetal scalp to exclude amniotic fluid entering the sera of sampling and the scalp is cleaned dry. Hyperaemia is induced with ethyl chloride spray and a small sample (approximately 35 μL) is obtained in a capillary tube after making a stab incision. Once FBS has been done, pressure with a swab to the site of the puncture should stop the bleeding. Automated blood gas analysis is performed and management depends on the clinical situation as well as the absolute values of the scalp pH and base excess. In some labours, pH sampling may be required more than once. The test requires technical skill and

Box 27.1 Systematic interpretation of CTG trace

- Determine risk
- Contraction frequency and duration
- Baseline rate
- Accelerations
- Variability
- Decelerations
- Overall impression and care plan

access to a calibrated blood gas analyser, is difficult to perform at cervical dilatations less than 4 cm, and can be stressful/uncomfortable for the mother. There is failure to obtain a result in 11–20% of cases (22). The median time from decision to undertake FBS to obtaining a result has been shown to be 18 minutes and in 9% of cases takes longer than 30 minutes (22). Contraindications to FBS or invasive fetal monitoring are maternal infections such as HIV, hepatitis B and C, active herpes simplex, fetal bleeding disorders, haemophilia (male fetus in carrier), and preterm gestation less than 34 weeks. **Table 27.3** summarizes the normal and abnormal acid–base values.

NICE advises that after an abnormal FBS result, consultant obstetric advice should be sought.

After a normal FBS result, sampling should be repeated no more than 1 hour later if the FHR trace remains pathological, or sooner if there are further abnormalities. After a borderline FBS result, sampling should be repeated no more than 30 minutes later if the FHR trace remains pathological or sooner if there are further abnormalities. Further abnormalities are identified by the features of increasing depth and duration of decelerations, reduction of the inter deceleration intervals, rise in the baseline rate, and reduction in the baseline variability. The time taken to take a fetal blood sample needs to be considered when planning repeat samples. If the FHR trace remains unchanged and the FBS result is stable after the second test, a third/further sample may be deferred unless additional abnormalities develop on the trace. Where a third FBS is considered necessary or sampling fails, a consultant obstetric opinion should be sought as based on the clinical situation delivery may be more appropriate.

The clinical context of the labour should always be considered including parity, progress, stage of labour, and maternal wishes. It should be remembered that fetal infection or thick meconium associated with a pathological CTG may result in an adverse neonatal

Table 27.1 Description of cardiotocograph trace features

Accelerations
- The presence of fetal heart rate accelerations is generally a sign that the unborn baby is healthy
- If a fetal blood sample is indicated and the sample cannot be obtained, but the associated scalp stimulation results in fetal heart rate accelerations, decide whether to continue the labour or expedite the birth in light of the clinical circumstances and in discussion with the woman

Description	Feature		
	Baseline (beats/minute)	Baseline variability (beats/minute)	Decelerations
Normal/reassuring	100–160	5 or more	None or early
Non-reassuring	161–180	Less than 5 for 30–90 minutes	Variable decelerations: • dropping from baseline by 60 beats/minute or less *and* taking 60 seconds or less to recover • present for over 90 minutes • occurring with over 50% of contractions *Or* Variable decelerations: • dropping from baseline by more than 60 beats/minute *or* taking over 60 seconds to recover • present for up to 30 minutes • occurring with over 50% of contractions *Or* Late decelerations: • present for up to 30 minutes • occurring with over 50% of contractions
Abnormal	Above 180 *or* below 100	Less than 5 for over 90 minutes	Non-reassuring variable decelerations (see row above): • still observed 30 minutes after starting conservative measures • occurring with over 50% of contractions *Or* Late decelerations: • present for over 30 minutes • do not improve with conservative measures • occurring with over 50% of contractions *Or* Bradycardia or a single prolonged deceleration lasting 3 minutes or more

National Institute for Health and Care Excellence (NICE). *Intrapartum Care for Healthy Women and Babies.* Clinical guideline [CG190]. London: NICE; 2014.

Table 27.2 Management based on interpretation of cardiotocograph traces

Category	Definition	Interpretation	Management
CTG is normal/reassuring	All 3 features are normal/ reassuring	Normal CTG, no non-reassuring or abnormal features, healthy fetus	• Continue CTG and normal care • If CTG was started because of concerns arising from intermittent auscultation, remove CTG after 20 minutes if there are no non-reassuring or abnormal features and no ongoing risk factors

CTG is non-reassuring and suggests need for conservative measures	1 non-reassuring feature *and* 2 normal/reassuring features	Combination of features that may be associated with increased risk of fetal acidosis; if accelerations are present, acidosis is unlikely	• Think about possible underlying causes
			• If the baseline fetal heart rate is over 160 beats/minute, check the woman's temperature and pulse. If either are raised, offer fluids and paracetamol
			• Start 1 or more conservative measures:
			  – encourage the woman to mobilize or adopt a left-lateral position, and in particular to avoid being supine
			  – offer oral or intravenous fluids
			  – reduce contraction frequency by stopping oxytocin if being used and/or offering tocolysis
			• Inform coordinating midwife and obstetrician

CTG is abnormal and indicates need for conservative measures *and* further testing	1 abnormal feature *or* 2 non-reassuring features	Combination of features that is more likely to be associated with fetal acidosis	• Think about possible underlying causes • If the baseline fetal heart rate is over 180 beats/minute, check the woman's temperature and pulse. If either are raised, offer fluids and paracetamol • Start 1 or more conservative measures (see 'CTG is non-reassuring ...' row for details) • Inform coordinating midwife and obstetrician • Offer to take an FBS (for lactate or pH) after implementing conservative measures, or expedite birth if an FBS cannot be obtained and no accelerations are seen as a result of scalp stimulation • Take action sooner than 30 minutes if late decelerations are accompanied by tachycardia and/or reduced baseline variability • Inform the consultant obstetrician if any FBS result is abnormal • Discuss with the consultant obstetrician if an FBS cannot be obtained or a third FBS is thought to be needed
CTG is abnormal and indicates need for urgent intervention	Bradycardia or a single prolonged deceleration with baseline below 100 beats/minute, persisting for 3 minutes or more[a]	An abnormal feature that is very likely to be associated with current fetal acidosis or imminent rapid development of fetal acidosis	• Start 1 or more conservative measures (see 'CTG is non-reassuring ...' row for details) • Inform coordinating midwife • Urgently seek obstetric help • Make preparations for urgent birth • Expedite birth if persists for 9 minutes • If heart rate recovers before 9 minutes, reassess decision to expedite birth in discussion with the woman

CTG, cardiotocography; FBS, fetal blood sample.

[a] A stable baseline value of 90–99 beats/minute with normal baseline variability (having confirmed that this is not the maternal heart rate) may be a normal variation; obtain a senior obstetric opinion if uncertain.

National Institute for Health and Care Excellence (NICE). *Intrapartum Care for Healthy Women and Babies.* Clinical guideline [CG190]. London: NICE; 2014.

outcome even in the absence of fetal acidosis. A normal FBS result in these circumstances does not give the same reassurance.

If a FBS is indicated and the sample cannot be obtained, but the associated scalp stimulation results in FHR accelerations, the clinician should decide whether to continue the labour or expedite the birth considering the clinical circumstances and in discussion with

Table 27.3 The classification of fetal blood sampling results

Lactate (mmol/L)	pH	Interpretation
≤4.1	≥7.25	Normal
4.2–4.8	7.21–7.24	Borderline
≥4.9	≤7.20	Abnormal

These results should be interpreted taking into account the previous pH measurement, the rate of progress in labour and the clinical features of the woman and baby.

National Institute for Health and Care Excellence (NICE). *Intrapartum Care for Healthy Women and Babies.* Clinical guideline [CG190]. London: NICE; 2014.

the woman (11). This is because induced accelerations by stimulation are almost always associated with non-acidotic scalp pH values. If a FBS is indicated but a sample cannot be obtained and there is no improvement in the CTG trace, advise the woman that the birth should be expedited.

Fetal lactate measurement has been proposed as an alternative to scalp pH as the lactate levels reflect anaerobic respiration and thus tissue hypoxia and metabolic acidosis. The invasive procedure for sampling is similar to FBS but requires a smaller volume of blood (5 μL). Available data indicate that levels greater than 4.8 mmol/L are abnormal and require delivery and levels of 4.2–4.8 mmol/L should be regarded as borderline (22).

The Cochrane review in 2013 by Alfirevic et al. found no reduction in caesarean rates or neonatal seizures with access to scalp sampling in addition to EFM (13). A randomized Swedish study found that scalp pH and lactate were no different in diagnosing fetal acidosis compared with pH and base excess but lactate sampling had lower failure rates (1.2% vs 10.4%) (23).

Meconium-stained liquor

Meconium-stained liquor is defined as dark green or black amniotic fluid that is thick or tenacious, or any meconium-stained amniotic fluid containing lumps of meconium. Although passage of meconium may be a function of fetal maturity, it can also indicate possible fetal compromise. Use of prostaglandin and fetal infection are also associated with the passage of meconium. The incidence of meconium staining of the liquor increases from 36 to 42 weeks' gestation, reaching around 20–30% at full term. Although fetuses do not normally draw amniotic fluid into the airway, they gasp when hypoxic and therefore the coexistence of hypoxia and acidosis may precipitate meconium aspiration.

Since meconium passage may indicate acute or chronic hypoxia, continuous FHR monitoring is recommended in these cases to detect possible fetal compromise. Moderate and thick meconium have been linked to abnormal FHR traces and adverse neonatal outcomes. The commonest abnormal FHR features associated with adverse neonatal outcomes are prolonged decelerations, severe variable decelerations, bradycardia, and tachycardia. In the presence of meconium, the fetal scalp pH result may be a less reliable indicator of poor fetal condition than is fetal oximetry.

As part of ongoing assessment in labour, the presence or absence of significant meconium should be clearly documented. If significant meconium is detected, healthcare professionals trained in FBSs and advanced neonatal life support should be available during labour and delivery. The woman should be transferred to obstetric-led care provided that it is safe to do so and the birth is unlikely to occur before transfer is completed.

Fetal pulse oximetry

The critical fetal oxygen saturation above which the fetus does not demonstrate significant acidosis is 30%. This has led to the development of fetal pulse oximetry techniques to allow assessment of fetal oxygenation as a marker for fetal acidosis. An oximeter probe is passed transcervically and placed against the fetal scalp or side of the face. Deoxygenated and oxygenated haemoglobin absorb light at different wavelengths and by using standard curves the oximeter is able to determine the fetal oxygen saturation. The probe is connected to a standard FHR monitor and displays a continuous signal. Although a normal saturation supports fetal well-being, there is insufficient data available to support its routine clinical use. Several factors such as sensor-to-skin contact, uterine contractions, fetal hair, and caput succedaneum may influence the performance and use of pulse oximetry.

A Cochrane review in 2014 which included published trials comparing fetal pulse oximetry and CTG with CTG alone (or when fetal pulse oximetry values were blinded), suggested that the available data provide limited support for the use of fetal pulse oximetry when used in the presence of a non-reassuring CTG, to reduce caesarean section for non-reassuring fetal status. The addition of fetal pulse oximetry did not reduce overall caesarean section rates (24).

Fetal acoustic stimulation

The ability of a fetus to respond to stimulation with an acceleration in FHR implies a well-oxygenated intact nervous system. Stimulation of the fetal head may be attempted by digital vaginal examination or the scalp laceration during FBS. A reassuring response of acceleration can indicate fetal well-being. The vibroacoustic stimulation test uses an artificial larynx placed closed to the maternal abdominal wall to startle and wake up the fetus. If accelerations are noted in the CTG following the test, a pH of less than 7.2 is unlikely.

A meta-analysis assessed the performance of stimulation tests for the prediction of intrapartum fetal acidaemia. Intrapartum stimulation tests appeared to be useful to rule out fetal acidaemia in the setting of a non-reassuring FHR pattern (25). A Cochrane review found insufficient evidence from randomized trials on which to base recommendations for its use in the presence of a non-reassuring CTG trace (26).

Fetal ECG waveform analysis

A growing number of centres are taking up the use of fetal ECG in combination with continuous EFM as an additional test of fetal well-being. Monitoring requires rupture of the membranes and application of a fetal scalp electrode and a maternal skin reference electrode. The fetal ECG is recorded continuously from a specialized scalp electrode and analysed by computer technology. Fetal hypoxia can act on the fetal myocardium and cause alterations to the ST segment of the fetal ECG. The drawback of the method is that the technology relies considerably on human interpretation of the CTG to indicate the appropriate action when ST-segment changes occur.

Various studies have assessed the effectiveness of fetal ECG with heart rate monitoring (27–30). The results showed a significant reduction in severe metabolic acidosis and neonatal encephalopathy. It was also associated with a significant decrease in obstetric interventions such as FBS and operative vaginal delivery. There was no significant difference in caesarean delivery rate. More recently, an RCT in Finland showed neither a significant improvement in neonatal outcome nor a reduction in caesarean section, although there was a reduction in the need for FBS (31). A Cochrane review found modest support for the use of fetal ST waveform analysis when a decision has been made to undertake continuous electronic FHR monitoring during labour (30).

Medicolegal aspects of intrapartum fetal monitoring

Obstetric litigations are on the rise worldwide and it is a major area of concern for maternity service providers. In United Kingdom, a study found 70% of all legal claims related to fetal brain damage to be based on abnormalities noted on FHR tracings (1). Despite its low specificity for hypoxia, the CTG continues to be the central documentary evidence for all claims for fetal asphyxia (2). Other indicators including a low Apgar score at birth have been shown to be subjective and poor predictors of long-term neurological outcomes.

Umbilical cord arterial blood gas analysis at birth has emerged as an important method, used to support or refute a diagnosis of intrapartum asphyxia. Many maternity units now routinely determine umbilical cord arterial and venous blood acid–base status on deliveries where there has been any concern during labour, for example, operative deliveries, cases where a FBS was done, pathological CTG trace, those with meconium-stained amniotic fluid, bleeding in labour, preterm infants, multiple gestations, vaginal breech deliveries, and the depressed infant at birth. Although it is clear that in some of the cases of newborns who later develop cerebral palsy interventions may have prevented or decreased the severity of cerebral palsy, it has been shown overall that FHR patterns are poor predictors of cerebral palsy (3, 4). The low specificity of CTG for fetal hypoxia therefore necessitates secondary or definitive tests to confirm fetal acid–base status in labour.

Patterns of intrapartum hypoxia and nature of birth injury

'Hypoxaemia' describes the condition where there is a reduction in the placental or cord blood flow causing a reduction in the level of oxygen in the peripheral arterial circulation of the fetus. This can happen in a normal labour with uterine contractions and the majority of fetuses can cope well with such episodes for long periods of time without injury. 'Hypoxia' describes the condition where the blood flow is interrupted for more prolonged periods of time and results in a reduction in the delivery of oxygen to the peripheral tissues of the fetus. If hypoxia continues for prolonged periods, the fetus switches to anaerobic metabolism to create energy and metabolic acidosis starts developing. In early stages, buffering will allow a normal pH to be maintained for some time. In fetuses with compromised reserves such as preterm or growth-restricted fetuses, metabolic acidosis occurs earlier. Fetal infection also reduces the reserve to cope with hypoxia. 'Asphyxia' describes the extreme condition where the oxygen delivery to tissues fails, leading to metabolic acidosis in addition to hypoxia. This leads to critical organ damage which may cause brain injury or fetal death *in utero*.

The nature of asphyxia can determine the type of brain injury and the neurological outcome as described by Myers in 1975 (32):

1. Total asphyxia causes damage to the brainstem and thalamus (athetoid or dyskinetic cerebral palsy).
2. Prolonged hypoxia with acidosis causes brain swelling and cortical necrosis (spastic quadriplegic cerebral palsy).
3. Prolonged hypoxia without acidosis causes white matter damage.
4. Total asphyxia preceded by prolonged hypoxia with mixed acidosis causes damage to the cortex, thalamus, and basal ganglia.

Acute hypoxia (**Figure 27.4**) is characterized by a sudden reduction in placental/cord blood flow and develops over minutes. Causes include acute accidents such as cord accident, abruption, hypertonic contractions, or uterine dehiscence and CTG often shows prolonged deceleration or bradycardia. Management demands rapid delivery or treatment of hyperstimulation to prevent death or long-term damage.

Gradually developing hypoxia (**Figure 27.5**): in gradually developing hypoxia accelerations do not appear, the baseline rate increases, and the variability reduces with progress of time. The decelerations get deeper and wider with increasing hypoxia. One needs to consider the clinical picture of parity, cervical dilatation, rate of progress, and high-risk factors, and either perform FBS or consider delivery.

The natural response for the fetus with hypoxic stress that previously had a reactive CTG would be the appearance of decelerations (variable due to cord compression or late due to placental insufficiency), the disappearance of accelerations (fetal response to conserve energy), a gradual rise in the baseline rate (due to hypoxia and catecholamine surge), deepening and widening of the decelerations

(with increasing hypoxia to the myocardium), and finally progressive reduction of the baseline variability (after a maximum baseline rate has been achieved and with further lack of oxygen there is depression of the autonomic nervous system). Within a reasonable time (60–90 minutes) of no baseline variability in the CTG (i.e. flat baseline variability with tachycardia and repeated late or atypical variable decelerations) (**Figure 27.5**), delivery should be carried out in order to avoid a baby with a low Apgar score and cord blood metabolic acidosis. An alternative would be to perform a FBS for determination of the acid–base balance and then to decide the management based on the FBS results.

Long-standing or chronic hypoxia (**Figure 27.6**) happens due to a reduction in placental blood flow over a long period of time and is associated with underlying conditions such as pre-eclampsia or fetal growth restriction. In the antenatal period the fetus will cope for a significant period of time by redistribution of the blood flow to vital organs, reduction in growth or activity, and buffering against lactic acid. Surveillance with Doppler ultrasound can detect the point where decompensation is likely so that delivery can be recommended. In labour, it may present with a CTG trace with no baseline variability and shallow late decelerations.

Subacute hypoxia (**Figure 27.8**): this may occur due to recurrent cord compression in labour. It may be particularly worsened in situations such as oligohydramnios or prolonged pregnancies. The CTG in this situation is characterized by prolonged decelerations where the FHR spends more time below the baseline rate (>90 seconds) and a shorter duration at the baseline rate (<30 seconds). Hypoxic insults that are slow in onset and persistent over time allow the fetus to make homeostatic adaptations. These protective adaptations begin to fail with the development of acidaemia and at a pH less than 7.0, the entire fetal and cerebral oxygen consumption fall substantially. Acidaemia leads to loss of vascular tone, cardiac cell injury, depressed myocardial function, and hypotension with resultant ischaemic brain injury.

Future of intrapartum fetal monitoring

Computerized CTG and ECG analysis

Computer-assisted analysis of the CTG has been introduced in recent times with the aim to improve the reliability of interpretation and remove the subjective component of assessment. The methodology uses spectral analysis of several components of the CTG. There is preliminary evidence that such computer-assisted analysis improves consistency in interpretation of FHR patterns; however, it is presently insufficient to recommend widespread clinical use.

Intelligent CTG interpretation and neural networks

Funded by the National Institute of Health Research Health Technology assessment, the INFANT study is a multicentre randomized controlled study which aims to compare the effect of a computer-based 'intelligent' system to support decision-making in the management of labour using the CTG by clinicians (midwives and doctors) versus review by clinicians (midwives and doctors) with no computer-based decision support in women who require continuous CTG monitoring of their labour (33). The composite primary outcome being analysed for the study is mortality and

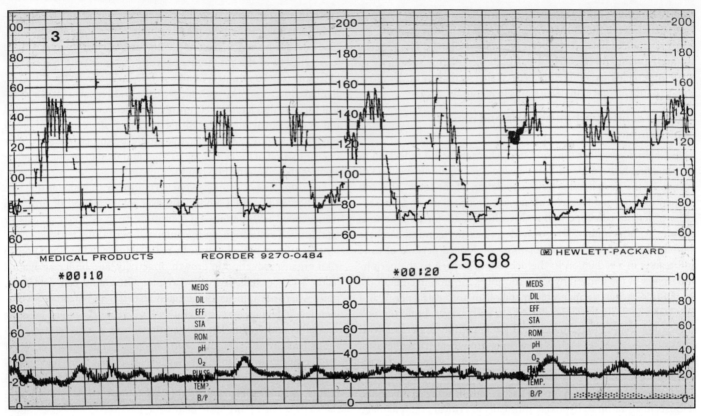

Figure 27.8 Pattern of subacute hypoxia—prolonged decelerations greater than 2 minutes with depth to less than 80 bpm and back to baseline rate for 30 seconds (i.e. suboptimal perfusion).

significant morbidity (neonatal encephalopathy and any admissions to NICU within 48 hours of birth for ≥48 hours). The results have shown no clinical advantage in using computerized CTG.

Artificial neural networks attempt to abstract the complexity and focus on what may hypothetically matter most from an information processing point of view. A study has found neural networks suitable for CTG feature extraction when the problem was reduced to small, well-defined tasks, and numerical algorithms were used to pre-process the raw data before application to the neural networks (34).

Education, training, and assessment

Several Internet-based teaching packages are available which help the users to learn the interpretation of electronic FHR monitoring and include information regarding basic physiology and acid–base balance. 'Electronic Fetal Monitoring' (eFM) is a comprehensive web-based resource developed by the Royal College of Obstetricians and Gynaecologists and the Royal College of Midwives in partnership with e-Learning for Healthcare. eFM provides 17 different subject modules on EFM and several case examples with online assessment learning, written by obstetric and midwifery experts in the field. These knowledge sessions provide learners with information and the case studies encourage learners to practise their skills in a realistic environment with timely feedback. Although most professional organizations have issued standardized nomenclatures for use in interpreting CTGs, there is still a need to optimize and enforce training in intrapartum CTG interpretation (35).

Summary

For last four decades, intrapartum monitoring of fetuses has been commonly performed by either intermittent auscultation or EFM.

EFM has been shown to reduce the incidence of intrapartum deaths and neonatal seizures, but it has not reduced the incidence of cerebral palsy or perinatal mortality and has increased the rates of operative interventions in labour. A large proportion of asphyxial damage begins before labour and intrapartum surveillance and intervention may not benefit these babies. Yet, the aim of fetal monitoring is to correctly identify those fetuses which are becoming hypoxic during labour and to intervene in a timely way to prevent adverse outcomes. The non-specific nature of different CTG patterns as well as the subjective element involved in the interpretation of the traces has made it necessary for additional tests of fetal well-being to be considered before interventions are undertaken during labour. The obstetric population is becoming increasingly complex with rising number of pregnancies with obesity and/or medical conditions. It is important to minimize unnecessary interventions as the vast majority of babies will cope well with normal labour and hypoxia could be avoided. The use of a standardized terminology and systematic approach in the interpretation of CTG as well as documentation is highly recommended. Regular structured training in CTG interpretation should be mandatory for all midwives and doctors. Accurate identification of FHR patterns based on national guidelines, good communication, and evidence-based management are likely to be the key to successful outcomes and avoidance of litigations.

REFERENCES

1. Symonds EM, Senior EO. The anatomy of obstetric litigation. *Curr Opin Obstet Gynecol* 1991;**1**:241–43.

2. Williams B, Arulkumaran S. Cardiotocography and medicolegal issues. *Best Pract Res Clin Obstet Gynaecol* 2004;**18**:457–66.

3. Freeman RK. Problems with intrapartum fetal heart rate monitoring interpretation and patient management. *Obstet Gynecol* 2002;**100**:813–26.

4. Nelson KB, Dambrosia JM, Ting TY, Grether JK. Uncertain value of fetal heart rate monitoring in predicting cerebral palsy. *N Engl J Med* 1996;**334**:613–18.

5. Haverkamp AD, Thompson HE, McFee JG, Cetrulo C. The evaluation of continuous fetal heart rate monitoring in high risk pregnancy. *Am J Obstet Gynecol* 1976;**125**:310–20.

6. Haverkamp AD, Orleans M, Langendoerfer S, McFee J, Murphy J, Thompson HE. A controlled trial of the differential effects of intrapartum fetal monitoring. *Am J Obstet Gynecol* 1979;**134**:399–412.

7. Renou P, Chang A, Anderson I, Wood C. Controlled trial of fetal intensive care. *Am J Obstet Gynecol* 1976;**126**:470–76.

8. Kelso IM, Parsons RJ, Lawrence GE, Arora SS, Edmonds DK, Cooke ID. An assessment of continuous fetal heart rate monitoring in labor: a randomized trial. *Am J Obstet Gynecol* 1978;**131**:526–32.

9. Wood C, Renou P, Oates J, Farrell E, Beischer N, Anderson I. A controlled trial of fetal heart rate monitoring in a low-risk population. *Am J Obstet Gynecol* 1981;**141**:527–34.

10. McDonald D, Grant A, Sheridan-Pereira M, Boylan P, Chalmers I. The Dublin randomized control trial of intrapartum fetal heart rate monitoring. *Am J Obstet Gynecol* 1985;**152**:524–39.

11. National Institute for Health and Care Excellence (NICE). *Intrapartum Care for Healthy Women and Babies*. Clinical guideline [CG190]. London: NICE; 2014. Available at: https://www.nice.org.uk/guidance/cg190.

12. National Institutes of Health. *Antenatal Diagnosis. Report of a Consensus Development Conference*. NIH Publication No. 79-1973. Bethesda, MD: National Institutes of Health; 1979.

13. Alfirevic Z, Devane D, Gyte GM. Continuous cardiotocography (CTG) as a form of electronic fetal monitoring (EFM) for fetal assessment during labour. *Cochrane Database Syst Rev* 2013;5:CD006066.

14. Centre for Maternal and Child Enquiries (CMACE). *Perinatal Mortality 2008: United Kingdom*. London: CMACE; 2010.

15. Department of Health. Intrapartum-related deaths: 500 missed opportunities. In: *On the State of Public Health: Annual Report of the Chief Medical Officer 2006.*, pp. 41–48. London: Department of Health; 2007.

16. Lieberman Richardson DK, Lang J, Frigoletto FD, Heffner LJ, Cohen A. Intrapartum maternal fever and neonatal outcome. *Pediatrics* 2000;**105**:8–13.

17. Impey L, Greenwood C, MacQuillan K, Reynolds M, Sheil O. Fever in labour and neonatal encephalopathy: a prospective cohort study. *Br J Obstet Gynecol* 2001;**108**:594–97.

18. Fleischer A, Schulman H, Jagani N, Mitchell J, Randolph G. The development of fetal acidosis in the presence of an abnormal fetal heart rate tracing. I. The average for gestational age fetus. *Am J Obstet Gynecol* 1982;**144**:55–60.

19. Phelan JP, Ahn MO. Perinatal observations in forty-eight neurologically impaired term infants. *Am J Obstet Gynecol* 1994;**171**:424–31.

20. Gibb D, Arulkumaran S. *Fetal Monitoring in Practice*, 3rd edn. Oxford: Elsevier Ltd. 2008.

21. Bailey RE, Hinshaw K. Intrapartum fetal monitoring. In: *ALSO Provider Manual*, 3rd edn. Leawood, KS: AAFP; 2001.

22. Leslie K, Arulkumaran S. Intrapartum fetal surveillance. *Obstet Gynaecol Reprod Med* 2011;**21**:59–66.

23. Wiberg-Itzel E, Lipponer C, Norman M, et al. Determination of pH or lactate in fetal scalp blood in management of intrapartum fetal distress: randomised controlled multicentre trial. *BMJ* 2008;**336**:1284–87.

24. East CE, Begg L, Colditz PB, Lau R. Fetal pulse oximetry for fetal assessment in labour. *Cochrane Database Syst Rev* 2014;**10**:CD004075.

25. Skupski DW, Rosenberg CR, Eglinton GS. Intrapartum fetal stimulation tests: a meta-analysis. *Obstet Gynecol* 2002;**99**:129–34.

26. East CE, Smyth R, Leader LR, Henshall NE, Colditz PB, Tan KH. Vibroacoustic stimulation for fetal assessment in labour in the presence of a nonreassuring fetal heart rate trace. *Cochrane Database Syst Rev* 2013;1:CD004664.

27. Amer-Wåhlin I, Hellsten C, Norén H, et al. Cardiotocography only versus cardiotocography plus ST analysis of fetal electrocardiogram for intrapartum fetal monitoring: a Swedish randomised controlled trial. *Lancet* 2001;**358**:534–38.

28. Amer-Wåhlin I, Kjellmer I, Maršál K, Olofsson P, Rosén KG. Swedish randomized controlled trial of cardiotocography only versus cardiotocography plus ST analysis of fetal electrocardiogram revisited: analysis of data according to standard versus modified intention-to-treat principle. *Acta Obstet Gynecol Scand* 2011;**90**:990–96.

29. Luzietti R, Erkkola R, Hasbargen U, Mattsson LA, Thoulon JM, Rosén KG. European Community multi-Center Trial 'Fetal ECG Analysis During Labor': ST plus CTG analysis. *J Perinat Med* 1999;**27**:431–40.

30. Neilson JP. Fetal electrocardiogram (ECG) for fetal monitoring during labour. *Cochrane Database Syst Rev* 2012;4:CD000116.

31. Ojala K, Vääräsmäki M, Mäkikallio K, Valkama M, Tekay A. A comparison of intrapartum automated fetal electrocardiography and conventional cardiotocography—a randomised controlled study. *BJOG* 2006;**113**:419–23.

32. Myers RE. Four patterns of perinatal brain damage and their conditions of occurrence in primates. *Adv Neurol* 1975;**10**:223–34.

33. ISRCTN Registry. A multicentre randomised controlled trial of an intelligent system to support decision making in the management of labour using the cardiotocogram (INFANT). ISRCTN98680152. Prof. Peter Brocklehurst, University of Oxford, UK. Available at: http://www.isrctn.com/ISRCTN98680152.

34. Keith RD, Westgate J, Ifeachor EC, Greene KR. Suitability of artificial neural networks for feature extraction from cardiotocogram during labour. *Med Biol Eng Comput* 1994;**32** Suppl 4:S51–57.

35. Ugwumadu A, Steer P, Parer B, et al. Time to optimise and enforce training in interpretation of intrapartum cardiotocograph. *BJOG* 2016;**123**:866–69.

28

Obstetric analgesia and anaesthesia

Sohail Bampoe and Anthony Addei

Introduction

Anaesthetists are involved in the care of over 60% of pregnant women. Effective team working is crucial to maternity care as has been highlighted in a report on safety in maternity services (1). Anaesthesia is not risk free. Preparedness is an integral part of providing safe care. Clear, simple, respectful communication is a key component of teamwork. The anaesthetist must be informed at an early stage of all high-risk patients to allow for timely consultation. A thorough understanding of the basics, including informed consent, a working knowledge of the drugs commonly administered, the availability of emergency airway and resuscitation equipment, as well as personnel trained in cardiopulmonary resuscitation are all critically important resources and skills to have.

Analgesia

Analgesia provides a varying amount of relief for a painful condition. Anaesthesia provides total relief of pain, which is necessary for a surgical operation (2).

Non-pharmacological methods

Many factors can help reduce the need for pharmacological intervention. There is little research proving the effectiveness of these treatments though lots of women say that they found these techniques useful. A calm environment and the presence of a trusted companion throughout labour may reduce the need for pain relief. The use of pools and water baths can also reduce the need for analgesia.

Complementary therapies

Hypnosis, acupuncture, aromatherapy, reflexology, yoga, massage, and homeopathy may all play a role in reducing the need for pharmacological pain relief.

Transcutaneous electrical nerve stimulation

Transcutaneous electrical nerve stimulation (TENS) exerts its analgesic effect by reducing the central transmission of peripheral nociceptive stimuli. It can be effective in early labour, and may postpone the need for pharmacological intervention.

Pharmacological methods

A range of analgesic and anaesthetic options are available in pregnancy. These include non-opioid drugs, opioid drugs, and regional analgesia/anaesthetic techniques.

Non-opioid drugs

Paracetamol

Uses: antenatal period, intra-partum period, and postpartum period.

Mechanism of action: the analgesic actions of paracetamol are poorly understood. It has been shown to inhibit the cyclooxygenase (COX)-3 enzyme in animal studies, but this COX variant has subsequently been shown not to be active in humans. Current theories suggest its analgesic action may be due to the activity of its metabolites. It does, however, exhibit some inhibition of COX enzymes in humans, thereby reducing central prostaglandin production resulting in its antipyretic and limited anti-inflammatory effects.

Dose: 4 g daily in divided doses (or 15 mg/kg if weight is <50 kg). Intravenous or oral administration.

Adverse effects: paracetamol is generally considered safe in pregnancy. Overdose can cause signs of toxicity including abdominal pain, nausea and vomiting, and fulminant hepatic failure.

Ibuprofen

Uses: postpartum analgesia.

Mechanism of action: ibuprofen is a non-specific COX inhibitor. It exerts its anti-inflammatory and antipyretic effects by inhibiting prostaglandin synthesis.

Dose: up to 2.4 g daily in divided doses administered orally.

Adverse effects: ibuprofen should be avoided in pregnancy and its use should be restricted to the management of post-delivery pain. When given antenatally, particularly in the third trimester, it has been associated with premature closure of the patent ductus arteriosus. All non-steroidal inflammatory drugs (NSAIDs) can cause acute kidney injury by reducing renal perfusion. They should be used with caution in patients with asthma. Prolonged use can result in gastric irritation and haemorrhage. Ibuprofen has the best safety profile of all the NSAIDs at low doses.

Diclofenac

Uses: postpartum analgesia.

Mechanism of action: diclofenac is a non-specific COX inhibitor. It has more potent analgesic effects than ibuprofen but a worse safety profile.

Dose: a loading dose of 100 mg via the rectal route (PR) is often given after operative procedures. The daily maximum dose is 75–150 mg in two to three divided doses.

Adverse effects: toxicity is common and increases with duration of therapy; 20% of long-term users will experience side effects. A recent study identified an increased risk of thrombotic vascular events in patients taking NSAIDs (3). This has led to widespread avoidance of diclofenac for longer-term analgesia in the postoperative period beyond a single PR dose. NSAIDs prevent platelet aggregation and should be avoided in patients at risk of significant bleeding, or in patients with disorders of pregnancy that also affect platelet function, for example pre-eclampsia. In 2013, the Medicines Healthcare products Regulation Authority (MHRA) recommended the avoidance of diclofenac in patients with serious cardiovascular disease (4) and in 2015 it became a prescription-only medicine.

Nitrous oxide (Entonox)

Uses: intrapartum analgesia.

Mechanism of action: Entonox is a 50:50 mix of nitrous oxide and oxygen. It is inhaled using a mouthpiece during labour and provides rapid-onset pain relief of short duration during contractions. Its onset time is 30 seconds (one lung–brain circulation time) and its offset time is approximately 60 seconds. Its use in between contractions should be discouraged to prevent unwanted side effects.

Adverse effects: in some patients, nitrous oxide can cause extreme dizziness accompanied by nausea and vomiting. Heavy use of nitrous oxide may cause signs of hypocapnia and hyperventilation including paraesthesia and muscle cramps.

Midazolam is a water-soluble benzodiazepine with anxiolytic, amnestic, and hypnotic properties. When used in combination with opioids, it has a marked synergistic effect that increases the likelihood of life-threatening complications, such as hypoxaemia and apnoea. It is not an analgesic and maternal amnesia can be very distressing for mothers. It is better to supplement inadequate pain relief with other anaesthetic techniques including conversion to a general anaesthetic as appropriate.

Opioid drugs

Pethidine

Uses: intrapartum analgesia.

Dose: 50–150 mg (intramuscular injection).

Mechanism of action: pethidine is a synthetic opioid. It crosses the placenta and can cause significant neonatal depression, with peak effect at 4 hours after maternal dose.

Adverse effects: pethidine has significant anticholinergic effects including dry mouth and mydriasis. It can precipitate seizures in patients with a history of epileptogenic seizures and in those taking monoamine oxidase inhibitors. Its duration of action is up to 150 minutes. In the United Kingdom, it can be prescribed by midwives. Its effects are not reversed by naloxone.

Codeine

Uses: antenatal, intrapartum, postnatal.

Dose: 30–60 mg administered orally every 6 hours. (Co-codamol administered as two tablets of 8/500 mg or 30/500 mg orally every 6 hours.)

Mechanism of action: codeine is a prodrug and is metabolized to morphine. The rate of metabolism can vary between individuals due to variable *CYP* gene expression and therefore caution should be exercised with its use. Codeine is often given as a combination with paracetamol in a preparation called co-codamol. Dihydrocodeine is structurally similar to codeine but is twice as potent and it can also be combined with paracetamol as co-dydramol.

Adverse effects: in 2013, the MHRA issued new guidance recommending the restriction of the use of codeine in breastfeeding mothers due to the risk of neonatal opioid toxicity (4, 5). Subsequently, a significant reduction in its use in the peripartum period has been observed. Signs of opioid toxicity in mothers and neonates may include a reduced conscious level and respiratory depression.

Remifentanil

Uses: intrapartum analgesia. Remifentanil is an effective alternative to epidural analgesia in labour where epidural analgesia may be contraindicated.

Dose: a typical regimen would be a 0.5 mcg/kg intermittent bolus administered using a patient-controlled analgesia pump with a 2-minute lockout period.

Mechanism of action: remifentanil is a potent opioid, which acts at the mu-receptor and is over a hundred times as potent as morphine. Most opioids are metabolized in the liver, but remifentanil is rapidly metabolized by esterase enzymes in the plasma and tissues resulting in a very short duration of action. This property is unique among opioids and prevents the accumulation of remifentanil over time, allowing it to be used for long periods during labour.

Adverse effects: like all potent opioids, remifentanil can cause significant respiratory depression and a reduced conscious level. Oxygen saturations should be monitored continuously when it is used. Significant sedation or respiratory depression can be reversed with naloxone. Remifentanil can also cause hypotension and bradycardia which can be treated with antimuscarinics such as atropine or glycopyrrolate. Remifentanil does cross the placenta, but is most probably rapidly metabolized by the fetus with minimal effect of the neonate.

Morphine

Uses: antenatal, intrapartum*, postnatal.

Dose: 0.1 mg/kg administered intravenously and titrated to effect or 0.3 mg/kg orally every 3–4 hours.

Mechanism of action: morphine exerts its action at the opioid receptors in the brain and spinal cord. Its onset of action is 3–4 minutes with peak effect at 20 minutes. Peak effect occurs at 60 minutes after an oral dose. It crosses the placenta and is contraindicated during labour (*of a live fetus) due to the risk of neonatal respiratory depression. It can be safely administered for pain relief in labour if the mother is not carrying a live fetus.

Adverse effects: morphine causes a decrease in conscious levels and can cause respiratory depression. It can cause significant nausea and vomiting. Morphine can also cause haemodynamic instability with marked hypotension. Its effects can be reversed with naloxone.

Regional analgesia

Regional analgesia is used to provide pain relief in labour. Regional anaesthesia is, on the other hand, used to facilitate operative interventions in theatre. The clinical situation and the urgency of the situation often dictate which method of regional analgesia or anaesthesia is used. Effective epidural/spinal block can allow caesarean section, or the trial of operative vaginal birth in theatre with immediate conversion to a caesarean section if necessary (6).

Epidural analgesia

Anatomy

The epidural space extends from the foramen magnum to the sacrococcygeal membrane. It lies anterior to the ligamentum flavum and posterior to the posterior longitudinal ligament. It contains fat, veins (Batson's plexus), connective tissue, nerve roots, and the dural sac. The innervation for the uterus is derived from T10 to L1 nerve

roots and anaesthesia to this dermatomal level, or higher is necessary for effective analgesia or anaesthesia in labour (**Figure 28.1**).

Indications

Epidural analgesia is indicated primarily for pain relief in labour (7). It also has the advantage of providing pain relief for episiotomy and perineal suturing. Epidural anaesthesia can be used as an adjunct in the management of severe pre-eclampsia due to the vasoactive hypotensive effect of the sympathetic blockade resulting from epidural local anaesthetic administration. Epidural anaesthesia can also be performed *de novo* for operative intervention where spinal block may not be appropriate. A dose of concentrated local anaesthetic can be administered in order to 'top up' a labour epidural for operative delivery. Anaesthesia to the T4 dermatome level bilaterally is necessary to minimize the chances of the parturient experiencing pain during a caesarean section.

Contraindications

- Patient refusal.
- Prophylactic low-molecular-weight heparin within 12 hours.
- Treatment dose low-molecular-weight heparin within 24 hours.
- Platelet count less than 100×10^9/mL with an abnormal clotting screen.
- Platelet count less than 80×10^9/mL.
- Systemic sepsis.
- Local skin infection.

Technique

A soft plastic catheter is introduced into the epidural space using a specially designed needle called a Tuohy needle. An intervertebral space is identified by palpating the spinous processes. Traditionally, the L3/4 interspace is chosen because the spinal cord ends at L1/2. In theory, an epidural may be inserted at any interspace but a spinal

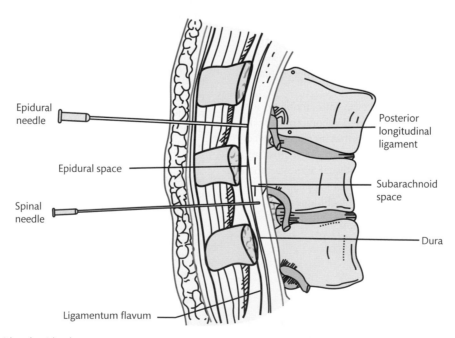

Epidural needle

Epidural space

Spinal needle

Ligamentum flavum

Posterior longitudinal ligament

Subarachnoid space

Dura

Figure 28.1 Subarachnoid and epidural spaces.

needle should only be inserted at a level below where the spinal cord ends to avoid injury to the spinal cord. The L3/4 level can be identified by palpating the iliac crests. An imaginary line between the two crests transects the L3/4 interspace (Tuffier's line). A 'loss of resistance to saline' technique is used to safely advance the needle into the epidural space. The catheter is introduced through the Tuohy needle, which is then removed, leaving the catheter in place (8). Between 3 and 5 cm of catheter is left in the epidural space, through which a local anaesthetic solution can be administered. A low-dose concentration of local anaesthetic is delivered in combination with an opioid which improves the quality and duration of analgesia. A typical regimen uses 0.1% levobupivacaine with 2 mcg/mL fentanyl. The anaesthetic solution can be administered as intermittent boluses, continuous infusion, or patient-controlled boluses (patient-controlled epidural analgesia).

Risks and complications

Epidural analgesia is safe. The third national audit project of the Royal College of Anaesthetists reported an incidence of permanent harm of 0.6 per 100,000.

Other complications include:

- permanent nerve damage (1:100,000)
- temporary nerve damage (1:1000)
- increased likelihood of instrumental delivery (1:10)
- epidural abscess
- epidural haematoma
- postdural puncture headache (1:250).

Spinal anaesthesia

Spinal block is typically used to facilitate operative interventions. A fine-gauge spinal needle is used to puncture the dura in order to deliver an intrathecal dose of local anaesthetic, usually combined with an opioid. Onset of anaesthesia is much more rapid than with epidural anaesthesia and is often accompanied by turbulent haemodynamic changes which can cause significant hypotension and consequent nausea and vomiting. The injected local anaesthetic mixture is typically denser than cerebrospinal fluid (CSF), allowing manipulation of the height of the block by applying Trendelenburg or reverse-Trendelenburg positioning to the patient. The patient may experience residual block for up to 6 hours after injection. A combined spinal and epidural injection allows a 'low-dose' spinal injection to be performed in combination with the placement of an epidural catheter to provide rapid pain relief in labour. It can also be used for operative interventions in theatre instead of a single-shot spinal.

Contraindications are the same as for epidural injection, but in addition may include any clinical scenario where there is already haemodynamic instability such as massive obstetric haemorrhage or maternal sepsis. In these situations, the patient must be resuscitated and stabilized first if time allows. If time is critical and full-volume resuscitation is not possible, then a spinal blockade is relatively contraindicated and general anaesthesia may be necessary.

Complications of neuraxial anaesthesia

Local anaesthetic toxicity

Local anaesthetic drugs are commonly used in obstetrics. These drugs can cause significant neurological and cardiovascular compromise including cardiac arrest if administered in excessive doses or accidentally injected into blood vessels. Local anaesthetics exert their action by reversibly blocking the transmission of action potential in sensory, motor, and sympathetic nerve fibres. Local anaesthetic molecules inhibit the passage of sodium through voltage-sensitive ion channels in the neuronal membrane. In excessive doses, the molecules can bind to ion channels in other excitable tissues resulting in cardiovascular arrhythmias and cardiac arrest. Neurological side effects include an altered mental state, perioral tingling, and seizures. Neurological adverse effects tend to develop before cardiovascular complications become evident. Local anaesthetic toxicity is a medical emergency and should be treated according to nationally agreed protocols using advanced life support algorithms and intravenous lipid solution (9). The Association of Anaesthetists of Great Britain and Ireland (AAGBI) have produced a safety guideline for the management of severe local anaesthetic toxicity (10). This can be found at the AAGBI website (https://www.aagbi.org/).

Postdural puncture headache

Postdural puncture headache is a low-pressure headache that results from a persistent leak of CSF (11). This is usually the consequence of an inadvertent puncture of the dura with the Tuohy needle. The reduction in CSF pressure causes traction on intracranial structures that are pain sensitive. The resultant headache is typically occipitofrontal, and may also involve neck pain. It is intermittent in nature and characteristically improves on lying flat. Many cases will respond to conservative management such as simple analgesics, adequate hydration, and increased caffeine intake. In cases where a severe headache persists, an autologous epidural blood patch may be required. This procedure involves the aseptic withdrawal of a small volume (typically around 20 mL) of the patient's blood which is then injected into the epidural space. The injected blood reduces the headache by exerting a direct positive volume–pressure effect, and also by forming a clot which effectively 'patches' the dural puncture site thereby minimizes further CSF leak.

High block and respiratory arrest

Regional anaesthesia causes a blockade of the spinal transmission of sensory nerve signals. Motor nerve signals are also blocked to a variable extent. The magnitude of this blockade depends on both the density of the block and also the anatomical level of the block, with higher blocks causing loss of function of more anatomical regions. A block from T4–S5 dermatome levels is required for adequate anaesthesia for caesarean section. At the T4 level, a number of intercostal nerves will be anaesthetized resulting in reduced respiratory function. If the block rises to affect the phrenic nerve roots (C3, C4, C5), respiratory arrest can occur necessitating intubation and temporary mechanical ventilation. The cardio-acceleratory fibres originate from T1–T5 and their blockade results in the bradycardia frequently observed with high neuraxial blockade. A 'total spinal' occurs when the block is so high that parts of the brainstem are anaesthetized. This causes a loss of consciousness, apnoea, severe hypotension, and bradycardia. Early recognition is important. The management is supportive and may require sedation, mechanical ventilation, haemodynamic support, and intensive care unit admission until the local anaesthetic wears off.

General anaesthesia

The National Health Service maternity data suggest that between 2% and 4% of deliveries are carried out under general anaesthesia annually. General anaesthesia in obstetrics is indicated for immediate operative deliveries, and in situations where regional anaesthesia for operative intervention is contraindicated or has been performed and found to be inadequate for surgical anaesthesia.

Technique

The risk of hypotension from aortocaval compression should be reduced by placing the parturient in a supine position with a 15-degree left lateral tilt.

- *Induction*—thiopentone is the induction agent most frequently used for induction of anaesthesia in the obstetric population. The use of propofol is slowly gaining popularity in obstetrics. Both drugs rapidly cross the placenta but do not cause excessive neonatal depression when standard doses are used. Ketamine is useful in the presence of hypotension from haemorrhage. It does not cause a reduction in blood pressure because of its sympathomimetic effects. Ketamine may cause delirium and hallucinations in the mother and can be rapidly detected in the fetus.
- *Muscle relaxation*—suxamethonium is the muscle relaxant of choice for obstetric general anaesthesia because its fast onset time (<30 seconds) enables rapid sequence intubation and thereby minimizes the risk of aspiration and delays to obtaining optimal operating conditions.
- *Analgesia*—opioids rapidly cross the placenta to the baby. Once the baby is delivered, the mother is given an adequate dose of opioid to ensure she wakes up reasonably pain free. Drugs such as fentanyl, alfentanil, and morphine are most frequently used for intraoperative analgesia.
- *Maintenance*—anaesthesia is maintained using inhaled volatile agents. Halogenated ethers such as sevoflurane or isoflurane cause relaxation of uterine tone at higher concentrations and may exacerbate postpartum haemorrhage. Often, nitrous oxide is used together with a volatile anaesthetic agent in order to reduce the concentration of volatile agent required to avoid awareness. This facilitates appropriate anaesthesia without excessive uterine atony.

General anaesthesia in the obstetric population presents the anaesthetic team with a number of challenges including the following:

Difficult airway management

A difficult airway is encountered in 1:300 of the obstetric population having general anaesthesia. This is ten times more prevalent than in the non-obstetric population. The main reasons for this occurrence are progesterone-related engorgement of the pharyngeal and laryngeal tissues coupled with the often stressful conditions in which immediate intubation is necessary (12).

Risk of rapid desaturation and hypoxia

A number of physiological factors result in a more rapid desaturation of pregnant women. These include a reduced functional residual capacity coupled with greater tissue oxygen consumption. There is a 20% increase in maternal oxygen consumption at term. Careful preoxygenation before induction of anaesthesia is mandatory regardless of the urgency for delivery. This will ensure that several minutes could elapse during the inevitable apnoea that occurs at induction of general anaesthesia before haemoglobin oxygen saturation begins to fall.

Risk of aspiration of gastric contents

Although rare, aspiration of gastric contents can cause significant and fatal lung injury. The risk of pulmonary aspiration is increased in the obstetric population for a number of reasons. The lower oesophageal sphincter usually has a resting pressure of approximately 20 mmHg above gastric pressure which helps to reduce the likelihood of reflux (known as the gastric barrier pressure). In pregnancy, progesterone causes relaxation of the lower oesophageal sphincter. The gravid uterus causes an increase in intra-abdominal pressure, and therefore an increase in gastric pressure. The combined effect of these phenomena is a reduction in gastric barrier pressure, and an increased risk of reflux of gastric contents.

A number of strategies can be used to reduce the risk of aspiration, and to minimize the damage to the lungs if aspiration does occur:

- *Metoclopramide* is routinely administered for its prokinetic effects to promote gastric emptying.
- *Antacids and H_2 receptor antagonists*, for example, sodium citrate and ranitidine, are given to reduce the acidity of gastric contents.
- *Rapid sequence induction* is used for the induction of anaesthesia to secure and protect the airway as quickly and safely as possible.

Increased risk of awareness

The Fifth National Audit Project of the Royal College of Anaesthetists revealed a 1 in 19,000 risk of awareness under anaesthesia. In the obstetric population, the incidence is reported as high as 1 in 670. This is likely in part, to be due to the urgency with which surgical anaesthesia is often required. However, the true cause of awareness is thought to be multifactorial.

Difficult postoperative pain management

A proportion of parturients who have a general anaesthetic will have had no neuraxial block. The implication of this is primarily that there is a significantly higher likelihood of postoperative pain. Analgesic options include opioids delivered by patient-controlled analgesia and regional anaesthetic techniques such as the rectus sheath block or the transversus abdominis plane block designed to block the nerves supplying the anterior abdominal wall. It is performed at the end of surgery but before the patient wakes up.

Other local anaesthetic techniques

Direct infiltration of local anaesthetic is a useful technique to supplement an incomplete block and reduce the pain of incision or discomfort during manipulations.

Pudendal blocks may be performed via a transvaginal or transperineal route. This block is useful for low assisted vaginal delivery with forceps or vacuum and for the manipulations necessary for assisted breech and delivery of the second twin.

Paracervical blocks may result in the rapid absorption of local anaesthetic from the highly vascular paracervical tissues. Several cases of intrauterine death following fetal bradycardia have occurred after a paracervical block. The technique may, however, be useful in cases where the fetus is dead or non-viable.

Caesarean section using local anaesthetic infiltration until delivery of the baby, followed by intravenous opioid such as morphine while using inhalational nitrous oxide throughout has been described.

Advice on pain relief and resources available

When it comes to giving birth, most women want to know how much it is going to hurt and whether they will be able to cope with the pain. Unfortunately, these questions cannot be answered with certainty. However, there is a huge resource of information available for a parturient, both printed and on the Internet, to help her understand the options available for pain relief and its impact on her, the course of her labour, and her baby.

Options for pain relief should ideally be discussed with parturients before the onset of labour. The broad range of options and their associated risks and benefits should be discussed without bias. Excellent resources can be found on the Obstetric Anaesthetists' Association website (https://www.oaa-anaes.ac.uk) including printable patient information cards in multiple languages.

REFERENCES

1. The King's Fund. *Safe Births: Everybody's Business*. London: The King's Fund; 2008.
2. Addei A, Baskett TF. Analgesia and anaesthesia. In: Baskett TF, Calder AA, Arulkumaran S (eds), *Munro Kerr's Operative Obstetrics*, 12th edn, pp. 236–41. London: Elsevier Health Sciences; 2014.
3. Coxib and traditional NSAID Trialists' (CNT) Collaboration, Bhala N, Emberson J, et al. Vascular and upper gastrointestinal effects of non-steroidal anti-inflammatory drugs: meta-analyses of individual participant data from randomised trials. *Lancet* 2013;**382**:769–79.
4. Medicines and Healthcare products Regulatory Authority. Codeine for analgesia: restricted use in children because of reports of morphine toxicity. *Drug Safety Update* 2013;**6**:A1.
5. Koren G, Cairns J, Chitayat D, Andrea G, Leeder S. Pharmacogenetics of morphine poisoning in a breastfed neonate of a codeine-prescribed mother. *Lancet* 2006;**368**:704.
6. Afolabi BB, Lesi FE. Regional versus general anaesthesia for caesarean section. *Cochrane Database Syst Rev* 2012;**10**:CD00435.
7. Anim-Somuah M, Smyth RM, Jones L. Epidural versus non-epidural or no analgesia in labour. *Cochrane Database Syst Rev* 2011;**12**:CD000331.
8. Odor PM, Bampoe S, Hayward J, Chis Ster I, Evans E. Intrapartum epidural fixation methods: a randomised controlled trial of three different epidural catheter securement devices. *Anaesthesia* 2016;**71**:298–305.
9. Picard J, Ward SC, Zumpe R, Meek T, Barlow J, Harrop-Griffiths W. Guidelines and the adoption of 'lipid rescue' therapy for local anaesthetic toxicity. *Anaesthesia* 2009;**64**:122–25.
10. Association of Anaesthetists of Great Britain & Ireland and Obstetric Anaesthetists' Association. *Guidelines for Obstetric Anaesthesia Services*. London: AAGBI; 2013.
11. Amorim JA, Gomes de Barros MV, Valença MM. Post-dural (post-lumbar) puncture headache: risk factors and clinical features. *Cephalalgia* 2012;**32**:916–23.
12. Djabatey EA, Barclay PM. Difficult and failed intubation in 3430 obstetric general anaesthetics. *Anaesthesia* 2009;**64**:1168–71.

29

Obstetric emergencies

Kiren Ghag, Cathy Winter, and Tim Draycott

Introduction

Obstetric emergencies can be unpredictable and sudden, and may result in significant morbidity and mortality. Successful management requires a rapid coordinated response from multiprofessional maternity teams.

In the recent Confidential Enquiry into Maternal Deaths in the United Kingdom, substandard care was identified in over 50% of cases and one-third of these could have been prevented with better care (1). Recurring problems were identified, including a lack of multiprofessional team working, poor communication, and late recognition of the severely unwell woman.

Multiprofessional training for obstetric emergencies has been demonstrated to reduce intrapartum harm and improve maternal and neonatal outcomes (2, 3). Official organizations have recommended multiprofessional training for many years. Most recently, *Better Births* (4), by the National Maternity Review, recommends multiprofessional training as a standard part of continued professional development: 'Those who work together should train together … Maternity services are multi-professional; teams should learn and train together, breaking down barriers between midwives, obstetricians and other professionals to deliver safe and personalized care for women and their babies.'

This chapter focuses on the immediate management of obstetric emergencies and is largely derived from the authors' work with the PROMPT Maternity Foundation (5) and the contents of the PROMPT (PRactical Obstetric Multi-Professional Training) course manual that is published by Cambridge University Press (6) (https://www.youtube.com/channel/UCh8PZGugxqDKBUcpTrulAfw).

There are a number of key components for the effective management of all emergencies:

- Early recognition of an obstetric emergency or an unwell woman.
- Call for help.
- State the problem clearly.
- Multiprofessional team working.
- Early senior involvement.
- Closed-loop communication: clear, addressed to specific individuals, delivered calmly, acted upon and acknowledged (7).
- A structured approach to managing emergencies, using simple tools that make it easy for teams to provide the correct care.

Additionally, simple tools can help facilitate best practice (3):

- Modified Obstetric Early Warning Score (MOEWS) charts aid identification of the unwell woman. Trends in observations are clear to see and abnormal observations are highlighted in amber or red, necessitating prompt referral.
- Treatment algorithms containing the key investigations and management of emergencies using a structured, step-by-step approach.
- Many maternity units have emergency boxes containing algorithms, medications, and equipment for the immediate management of emergencies such as pre-eclampsia and haemorrhage to enable prompt, effective management. All maternity staff need to be aware of the location of their emergency boxes, so that one of the team members can collect it promptly.
- Clear documentation of timings, actions, and outcomes is essential. The use of a standardized pro forma may improve documentation.
- SBAR (Situation, Background, Assessment, and Recommendation) sheets can be used at handover, to aid the transfer of information.

Obstetric emergencies can be very traumatic for women and their families. During the emergency, it is important to communicate with them and explain what is happening. Interestingly, women want almost the same information as staff, namely the problem, reassurance about their baby and themselves, followed by an explanation of the management required. Furthermore, there are some data suggesting that providing information (careful commentary) during traumatic situations may reduce post-traumatic stress (8).

After the event, full debriefing and support should be offered. Staff members can also be emotionally affected and a formal debrief session may be helpful.

Maternal collapse

Maternal collapse is severe respiratory or circulatory distress that may lead to a sudden change in the level of consciousness or cardiac arrest if untreated. The possible causes of maternal collapse are listed in **Figure 29.1** (6).

Signs of maternal collapse include:

- obstructed or noisy airway
- respiratory rate less than 5 or greater than 35 breaths per minute

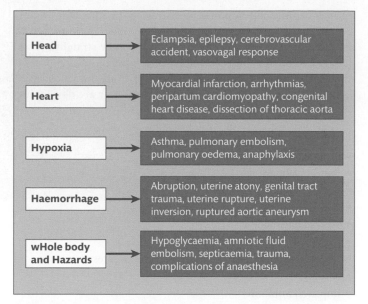

Figure 29.1 Possible causes of maternal collapse.
Reproduced from Winter C, Crofts J, Laxton C, Barnfield S, Draycott T, (eds.) *PROMPT: PRactical Obstetric Multi-Professional Training. Practical locally based training for obstetric emergencies. Course Manual.* 2nd edition. Cambridge: Cambridge University Press; 2012.

Head	How responsive is the patient? Is she alert, responsive to voice, responsive to painful stimuli or unresponsive (AVPU)? Is the patient fitting?
Heart	What is the capillary refill like? What is the pulse rate and rhythm? Is there a murmur?
Chest	Is there good bilateral air entry? What are the breath sounds like? Is the trachea central?
Abdomen	Is there an 'acute' abdomen (rebound and guarding)? Is there tenderness (uterine or non-uterine)? Is the fetus alive? Is there a need for a laparotomy or delivery?
Vagina	Is there bleeding? What is the stage of labour? Is there an inverted uterus?

Figure 29.2 A primary obstetric survey.
Reproduced from Winter C, Crofts J, Laxton C, Barnfield S, Draycott T, (eds.) *PROMPT: PRactical Obstetric Multi-Professional Training. Practical locally based training for obstetric emergencies. Course Manual.* 2nd edition. Cambridge: Cambridge University Press; 2012.

- heart rate less than 40 or greater than 140 beats per minute (bpm)
- blood pressure less than 80 or greater than 180 mmHg
- sudden decrease in level of consciousness
- unresponsive or responding to painful stimuli only
- seizures.

Initial management should follow the same basic principles of management of any critically unwell patient; call for help and assess airway, breathing, and circulation (ABC). If there are no signs of life, commence basic life support, as per United Kingdom Resuscitation Council Guidelines (9). Manually displace the uterus to the left to reduce aortocaval compression from the gravid uterus. Alternatively, this can be achieved with a 30-degree tilt if on a firm surface (e.g. theatre table).

If there are signs of life, place the woman in the recovery position and administer high-flow oxygen. Obtain intravenous access and send blood samples for full blood count, group and save, glucose, urea and electrolytes, liver function tests, and clotting screen. Check vital observations: blood pressure, heart rate, respiratory rate, oxygen saturations, and temperature. Establish continuous monitoring if possible. Perform an electrocardiogram. Commence intravenous fluids, providing there are no obvious contraindications (e.g. eclampsia).

After the initial management, perform a primary obstetric survey, as per **Figure 29.2** (6).

If the diagnosis is not evident, consider key treatment decisions:

- Should the baby be delivered to improve maternal resuscitation?
- Is fluid resuscitation a priority? Are there any contraindications to fluids?
- Is the likely cause severe sepsis and therefore are intravenous antibiotics a priority?
- Is intensive care support required?

Once the woman is stable, perform a secondary obstetric survey to guide further investigations and management, as outlined in **Figure 29.3** (6).

Resuscitation of a pregnant woman

Maternal cardiac arrest is rare, with a very high maternal and fetal mortality rate. Although management follows the same principles of

ACTION	DETAIL
History	Revisit the history of the collapse and the previous history of the woman
	Read the notes and ask the partner or relatives
Examine	Repeat the examination going from top to toe
Investigate	Take arterial blood gases, troponins, blood glucose, lactate, blood cultures, ECG, chest X-ray, and ultrasound of the abdomen, high vaginal swab
Monitor	Continue monitoring of ECG, respirations, pulse, blood pressure and pulse oximetry
	Consider arterial and central venous pressure lines to aid monitoring
Pause and think further	Consider further investigations such as CT/MRI scans and echocardiography
	Ask relevant experts for their opinions

Figure 29.3 A secondary obstetric survey. CT, computed tomography; ECG, electrocardiogram; MRI, magnetic resonance imaging.
Reproduced from Winter C, Crofts J, Laxton C, Barnfield S, Draycott T, (eds.) *PROMPT: PRactical Obstetric Multi-Professional Training. Practical locally based training for obstetric emergencies. Course Manual.* 2nd edition. Cambridge: Cambridge University Press; 2012.

basic and advanced life support, resuscitation of a pregnant woman is more difficult. There are several important factors to consider:

- When a pregnant woman is lying flat, the gravid uterus compresses the aorta and vena cava, decreasing venous return to the heart and resulting in up to 70% decrease in cardiac stroke volume. This will hinder resuscitation efforts, specifically the effectiveness of cardiopulmonary resuscitation (CPR). Aortocaval compression will be relieved by manual displacement of the uterus to the left or a 30-degree tilt on a firm surface.
- The baby should be delivered within 5 minutes of cardiac arrest, to aid maternal resuscitation. This will improve the effectiveness of CPR by removing the oxygen and circulating volume requirement of the fetus and placenta and by relieving aortocaval compression from the gravid uterus. Expediting the birth of the baby should be considered as soon as the woman arrests and the procedure should be commenced by 4 minutes if CPR is not successful. The baby should be born by the quickest means possible; often by caesarean section, although operative vaginal birth can be considered if the woman is fully dilated. CPR should be continued throughout the birth procedure. The neonatal team should also be summoned.
- Intubation is a priority. Aspiration of gastric contents is more likely due to hormonal relaxation of the oesophageal sphincter and delayed gastric emptying. Intubation can be more difficult because of oedema and the physiological changes of pregnancy causing a larger tongue and breasts.
- Ventilation is more difficult due to the increased intra-abdominal pressure from the gravid uterus.

Maternal sepsis

Maternal sepsis is the most common cause of maternal death in the United Kingdom (1). Although *direct* causes such as genital tract sepsis have decreased, there have not been any improvements in *indirect* causes such as pneumonia, urinary tract infection, breast abscess, and meningitis. Between 2009 and 2012, the incidence of maternal deaths from direct and indirect causes of sepsis was 1.56 per 100,000 maternities (1).

During this time period, almost a quarter of women who died had sepsis. Nearly 10% of women died from influenza. The influenza vaccine may have prevented more than half of these cases. Influenza vaccination for pregnant women is a public health priority.

Sepsis is defined as the presence of infection with systemic manifestations. Severe sepsis is defined as sepsis with organ dysfunction or tissue hypoperfusion. Septic shock is defined as sepsis-induced hypotension persisting despite adequate fluid resuscitation (10). Severe sepsis has a mortality rate of 20–40%, which increases to 60% if septic shock develops (11).

Sepsis is often insidious in onset. Pregnant women are usually young and fit, compensating well with infection until sudden cardiovascular decompensation. Presentation is often late, preceded by a short duration of illness and rapidly deteriorating into septic shock, disseminated intravascular coagulation, and multiorgan failure.

Recognition of sepsis

The clinical picture may not always reflect the severity of the underlying infection. The woman may just feel 'not quite right' or may be unusually anxious or distressed. In antenatal women, an abnormal or absent fetal heartbeat may indicate sepsis. Postpartum women may have had a completely straightforward labour and no obvious risk factors. Observing trends in observations on MOEWS charts and performing a full clinical examination will help to identify women who have, or are developing, sepsis.

Risk factors

- Prolonged ruptured membranes
- Preterm labour
- Retained products of conception
- Caesarean birth
- Wound haematoma
- Cervical suture
- Invasive intrauterine procedure (e.g. amniocentesis)
- Obesity
- Impaired immunity
- Diabetes mellitus
- Working with, or having, young children.

Group A *Streptococcus* is the most common organism identified in maternal deaths from genital tract sepsis. Up to 30% of the population are asymptomatic carriers of this organism in their throat or skin. Streptococcal sore throat is one of the commonest bacterial infections of childhood. Spread is common via person-to-person contact and droplet spread. Symptoms can be non-specific and difficult to differentiate from less serious conditions such as gastroenteritis.

Symptoms of genital tract sepsis

- Abdominal pain
- Fever
- Diarrhoea
- Vomiting
- Offensive vaginal discharge
- Sore throat
- Upper respiratory tract infection
- Wound infection.

Signs of genital tract sepsis

- Rash: typically developing over 12–48 hours, initially appearing as blanching, erythematous patches on the chest and axillae, spreading to the trunk and extremities.
- Tachycardia greater than 100 bpm.
- Increased respiratory rate greater than 20 breaths per minute.
- Temperature less than 35°C or greater than 38°C (or a rise or fall in temperature).
- Systolic blood pressure less than 80 mmHg.
- Low oxygen saturations less than 95% on air.
- Poor peripheral perfusion: capillary refill greater than 2 seconds.
- Pallor.
- Clamminess.
- Confusion.
- Mottled skin.
- Low urine output less than 0.5 mL/kg/hour.

Initial management of maternal sepsis

An algorithm for the initial management of maternal sepsis is displayed in **Figure 29.4**.

Activate the emergency buzzer to call for urgent help from the multiprofessional team: senior midwives, obstetricians, and anaesthetists. Critical care consultants may also need to be involved in the woman's care. Assess ABC and administer high-flow oxygen.

Administer high-dose broad-spectrum antibiotics immediately, according to local antibiotic guidelines. Do not wait for laboratory blood results. Ideally send blood cultures prior to giving antibiotics, but do not delay the commencement of antibiotics.

Commence rapid fluid resuscitation. If the woman is hypotensive or has an elevated serum lactate of greater than 4 mmol/L, give at least 30 mL/kg of intravenous crystalloid, for example, a 70 kg woman should be given at least 2 L of Hartmann's solution (10). If the blood pressure or lactate level does not improve, consider transfer to an intensive care unit for vasopressors, to maintain the mean arterial pressure at greater than 65 mmHg. Women with septic shock often require aggressive fluid resuscitation. It is important to closely monitor fluid balance and for signs of fluid overload.

Full clinical examination

Perform a full clinical examination, including vaginal examination, to identify the cause of sepsis.

Send blood samples

- Full blood count: an increased or decreasing white cell count may be indicative of sepsis.

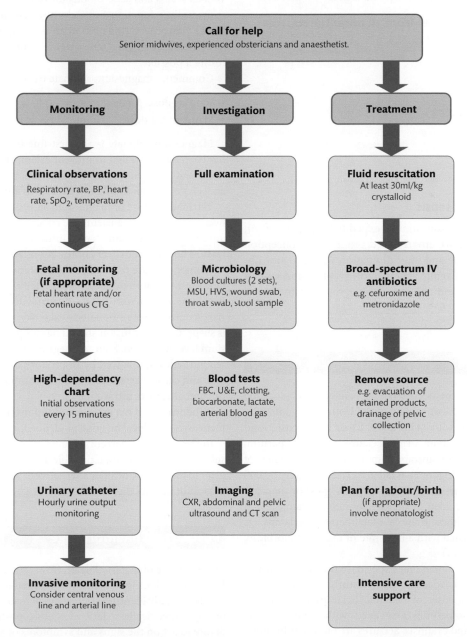

Figure 29.4 Algorithm for the initial management of maternal sepsis.

Reproduced from Winter C, Crofts J, Laxton C, Barnfield S, Draycott T, (eds.) *PROMPT: PRactical Obstetric Multi-Professional Training. Practical locally based training for obstetric emergencies. Course Manual.* 2nd edition. Cambridge: Cambridge University Press; 2012.

- C-reactive protein, urea and electrolytes, and liver function tests.
- Clotting screen (including fibrinogen): disseminated intravascular coagulation can arise as a result of severe sepsis. Clinical signs include undue bleeding or bruising.
- Lactate: a serum lactate concentration greater than 2 mmol/L signifies poor tissue perfusion secondary to severe sepsis or septic shock. A lactate level greater than 4mmol/L indicates a poor prognosis (12). The lactate level is particularly useful for identifying women with tissue hypoperfusion who are at risk of septic shock but are not yet hypotensive or exhibiting obvious signs. An arterial blood gas analyser on the labour ward or in the neonatal intensive care unit will often be able to measure a serum lactate level from a venous or arterial blood sample.
- Arterial blood gas: this will likely show metabolic acidosis due to the production of lactate and will worsen as shock progresses.

Send microbiology samples from all potential sources of sepsis

- Blood cultures
- Urine culture
- Vaginal swabs
- Placental swab (if applicable)
- Throat swab
- Wound swab
- Stool sample
- Sputum sample.

Remove the source of sepsis

If there are signs of chorioamnionitis, expedite birth and inform the neonatal team. Remove any retained products of conception once the woman is stable and after discussion with a senior obstetrician. Consider imaging: chest radiography, abdominal/pelvis ultrasonography, and computed tomography of the chest/abdomen/pelvis.

Eclampsia

Eclampsia is defined as the occurrence of convulsions associated with pre-eclampsia (13). Most women in the United Kingdom who have an eclamptic seizure will not have established hypertension and proteinuria prior to this. About 44% of seizures occur postpartum, 38% antepartum, and 18% intrapartum (14). The incidence of eclampsia in the United Kingdom has fallen to 27.5 cases per 100,000 maternities (15) since the introduction of guidelines for management of pre-eclampsia, guided by the Collaborative Eclampsia and Magpie trials (16, 17). Although the case fatality rate of eclampsia is low, eclampsia is associated with a high rate of maternal morbidity and perinatal mortality (14).

Prior to a seizure, the woman may experience the classical symptoms of pre-eclampsia: headache, visual disturbance, severe epigastric pain, and rapid onset of oedema. Eclampsia presents as generalized seizures, sometimes associated with tongue biting, urinary incontinence, and cyanosis. Seizures are often self-limiting, resolving within 90 seconds. The recurrence rate is up to 30%.

Initial management of eclampsia

An algorithm for the initial management of eclampsia is displayed in **Figure 29.5**.

Activate the emergency bell to call for urgent help from the multiprofessional team: senior midwives, obstetricians, and anaesthetists. State the problem clearly: 'This is an eclamptic seizure'. Request a team member to collect the eclampsia emergency box and to inform the consultant obstetrician and consultant anaesthetist. An example of an eclampsia box and its contents is shown in **Figure 29.6**.

Support ABC. During the seizure, move the woman into the left-lateral position to maintain her airway, administer high-flow oxygen, and remove any obvious hazards in the environment. Once the seizure has resolved, ensure the airway is patent. Obtain intravenous access and send bloods for full blood count, urea and electrolytes, liver function tests, clotting screen, and group and save. Check vital observations: blood pressure, heart rate, respiratory rate, oxygen saturations, and temperature. Commence continuous monitoring if possible.

Commence magnesium sulphate treatment to control seizures:

- Loading dose: 4 g magnesium sulphate over 5 minutes.
- Maintenance dose: 1 g/hour.

Magnesium sulphate is the first-line treatment for eclampsia. It has been demonstrated to prevent eclampsia and is associated with the lowest recurrence rate of seizures (16, 17). Diazepam, phenytoin, and a lytic cocktail should not be used as alternative treatment.

The loading dose of magnesium sulphate should be given slowly over 5 minutes, as transient side effects of flushing and tachycardia are common. The maintenance infusion should be continued for at least 24 hours after delivery or the last seizure (whichever is longest).

Women who are receiving a magnesium sulphate infusion should be closely monitored for signs of toxicity. Toxicity is not common; however, women with renal impairment or oliguria are at greater risk, as magnesium sulphate is excreted by the kidneys. If toxicity is suspected, the infusion should be stopped and the serum magnesium level measured. Signs of magnesium toxicity are a loss of deep tendon reflexes, followed by respiratory depression, respiratory arrest, and cardiac arrest. The antidote for magnesium sulphate is 1 g calcium gluconate intravenously.

If the woman is hypertensive, administer antihypertensive treatment as per the local hospital guideline for severe pre-eclampsia.

In the event of recurrent seizures, give a 2 g bolus of magnesium sulphate over 5 minutes. If possible, take blood for magnesium levels prior to the bolus. Consider alternative causes of the seizures and discuss additional medications for seizure control with an anaesthetist.

Postpartum haemorrhage

The incidence of maternal death from obstetric haemorrhage in the United Kingdom is 0.55 per 100,000 maternities (1). Substandard care is regularly identified in reviews of maternal deaths from haemorrhage: specifically, a lack of routine postpartum monitoring, a failure to act on the signs and symptoms of a deteriorating woman, and a lack of early senior multiprofessional involvement (15).

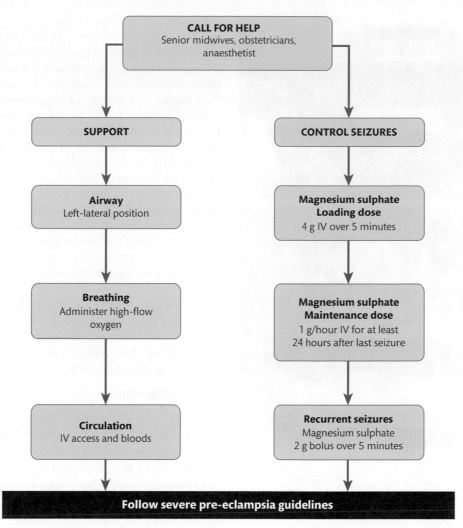

Figure 29.5 Algorithm for the initial management of eclampsia.
Reproduced from Winter C, Crofts J, Laxton C, Barnfield S, Draycott T, (eds.) *PROMPT: PRactical Obstetric Multi-Professional Training. Practical locally based training for obstetric emergencies. Course Manual.* 2nd edition. Cambridge: Cambridge University Press; 2012.

Primary postpartum haemorrhage (PPH) is traditionally defined as blood loss of 500 mL or more within the first 24 hours after birth. Major PPH is categorized as blood loss of greater than 1000 mL, and can be divided into moderate PPH (1000–2000 mL) and severe PPH (>2000 mL) (18).

Primary PPH is usually caused by at least one of what are often classified as the 'the four Ts':

- Tone (e.g. uterine atony)
- Tissue (e.g. retained membranes or placenta)
- Trauma (e.g. tears of the genital tract)
- Thrombin (e.g. coagulopathies).

Secondary PPH is a blood loss of 500 mL or more from 24 hours after birth until 12 weeks postpartum. The most common cause is endometritis, which usually responds to antibiotic treatment and removal of any retained products of conception.

Immediate management of a major PPH

Key tips to enable effective management:

- Prompt recognition.
- Call for help.
- Uterine massage or bimanual compression (the most likely cause of a primary PPH is an atonic uterus).
- Fluid resuscitation.
- Administer uterotonics if appropriate.
- Restore blood volume and oxygen-carrying capacity.
- Replace blood products early.
- Low threshold for transfer to theatre.
- Early recourse to hysterectomy.

PPH is usually overt due to vaginal bleeding. However, bleeding can be concealed (e.g. broad ligament haematoma). The only indication may be a deterioration of postpartum observations or the woman exhibiting signs of shock. It is important to closely monitor the postpartum woman, ideally documenting observations on a MOEWS chart and promptly acting upon any concerning features.

An algorithm for the initial management of a major PPH is displayed in **Figure 29.7**.

(a)

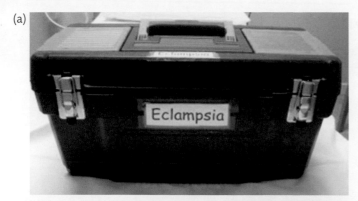

(b)

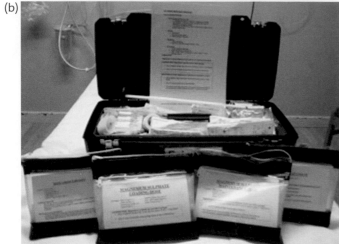

Figure 29.6 An eclampsia emergency box.

Activate the emergency buzzer to call for urgent help from the multiprofessional team: senior midwives, obstetricians, and anaesthetists. State the problem clearly: 'This is a postpartum haemorrhage'. Request the PPH emergency box; an example is shown in **Figure 29.8**. Consider activation of the code red major obstetric haemorrhage protocol.

Each maternity unit should have a major obstetric haemorrhage protocol with agreed criteria for activation. This will usually alert additional team members and initiate the preparation of blood products. The blood transfusion laboratory technicians, porters, and consultant clinical haematologist must be informed and on standby should urgent blood products be required. The theatre team should prepare the operating theatre for possible urgent transfer. The consultant obstetrician and anaesthetist should be informed early in cases of major PPH with ongoing blood loss.

Initial actions

- Lie the woman flat.
- Administer high-flow oxygen.
- Massage the uterus to rub up a contraction and expel any clots.
- Assess ABC.
- Obtain intravenous access with two large-gauge cannulae.
- Send bloods for full blood count, urea and electrolytes, and clotting screen including fibrinogen and crossmatch 4 units of blood.
- Rapid fluid resuscitation with at least 2 L of Hartmann's solution.

Restoration of the blood volume and oxygen-carrying capacity is vital for aiding resuscitation. Up to 3.5 L of fluid can be infused: 2 L of crystalloid as rapidly as possible, followed by up to 1.5 L of colloid if blood is not available. Intravenous fluids should be warmed, as the woman can become cold due to the massive transfusion, further exacerbating the risk of disseminated intravascular coagulation.

Blood products should be replaced early. The woman's clinical picture will determine whether blood products are required, rather than awaiting laboratory blood results. If cell salvage is available, this should be set-up and commenced. If cell salvage is not possible, crossmatched blood is preferable. O rhesus-negative blood or non-crossmatched group-specific blood can be given if crossmatched blood is not available. Additional blood products such as fresh frozen plasma and cryoprecipitate may be indicated at a later stage; obtain advice from the haematologist and consultant anaesthetist.

During the management of the PPH, constantly re-evaluate the condition of the woman, her response to treatment, and the estimated blood loss. Point-of-care testing, such as ROTEM, can be used for a quick assessment of coagulation. Monitor blood pressure, heart rate, respiratory rate, and pulse oximetry continuously if possible. Document observations, including temperature and fluid input and output, on a high-dependency chart. Assign a scribe to document all timings and actions.

Stop the bleeding

- Investigate the cause of the bleeding:
  - Check the uterine tone and height of the fundus.
  - Massage the uterus to expel any clots.
  - Examine for tears of the vagina, cervix, or perineum.
  - Ensure the placenta has delivered and check it is complete.
  - Examine the woman for signs of clotting disorders, such as bleeding from wound or cannula sites.
- Perform bimanual compression if the uterus is atonic: uterine atony is the most common cause of PPH. Bimanual compression, as demonstrated in **Figure 29.9**, encourages contraction of the uterus and is especially useful as a holding measure if travelling in an ambulance or awaiting transfer to the labour ward or theatre.
  - *How to perform bimanual compression*: gently insert one hand into the vagina and form a fist. Apply pressure against the anterior wall of the uterus. With the other hand on the abdomen, press on the uterine fundus and compress the uterus between both hands. Continue bimanual compression until the uterus contracts.
- Administer oxytocic medication: active management of the third stage of labour is recommended for all women (19). First-line medication is 10 mg Syntocinon (oxytocin) or 1 ampoule of Syntometrine (oxytocin plus ergometrine), both administered intramuscularly. If the woman has not received any oxytocics, administer one dose. If the woman has already had an oxytocic, a second dose can be given.
  - The blood pressure must always be checked prior to giving Syntocinon or Syntometrine. Syntocinon boluses should be used with caution in women with severe hypotension, as the blood pressure may drop further (11). Ergometrine can cause hypertension, therefore Syntometrine is contraindicated in women with high blood pressure.

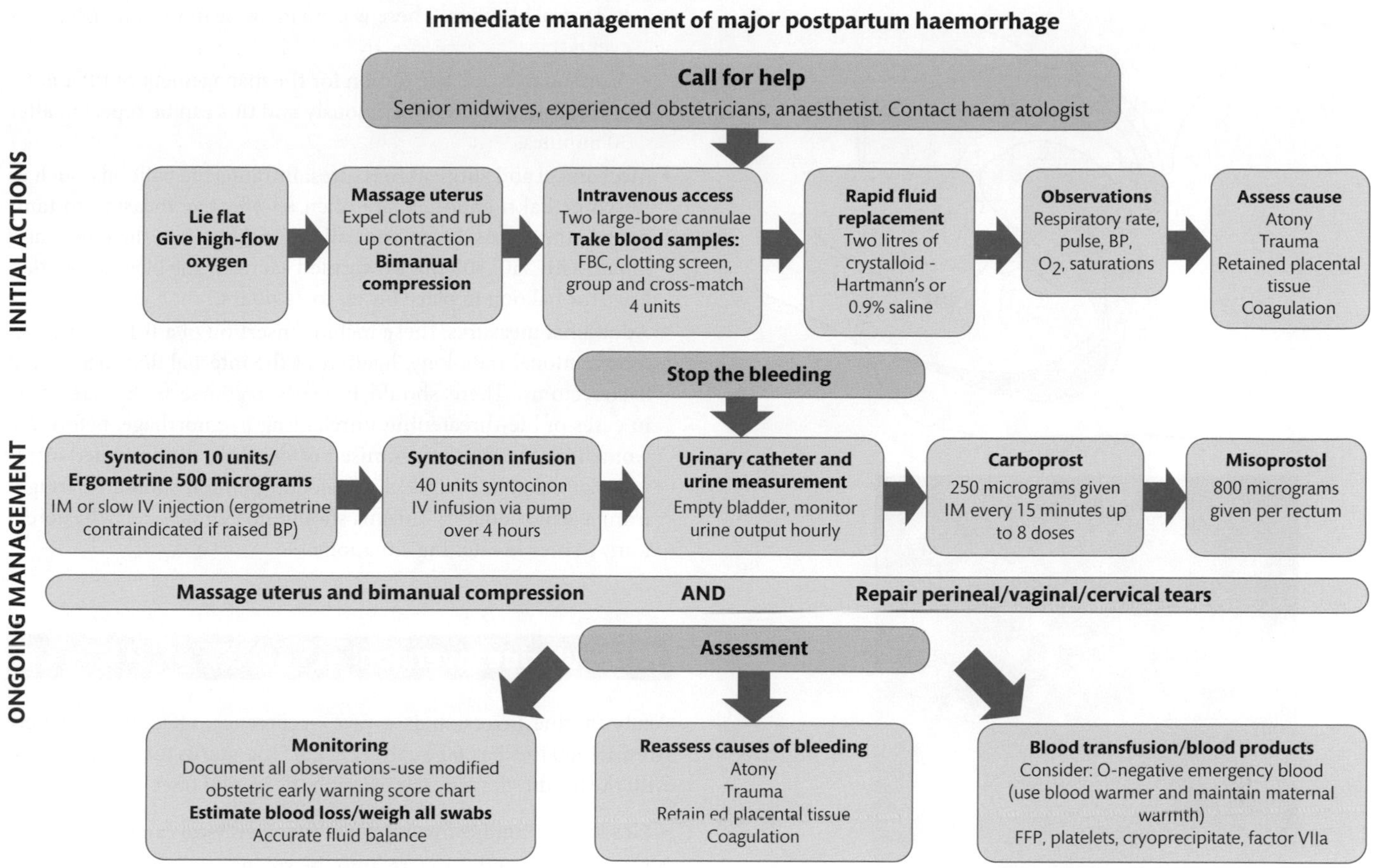

Immediate management of major postpartum haemorrhage

Call for help
Senior midwives, experienced obstetricians, anaesthetist. Contact haematologist

INITIAL ACTIONS

| **Lie flat** Give high-flow oxygen | **Massage uterus** Expel clots and rub up contraction **Bimanual compression** | **Intravenous access** Two large-bore cannulae **Take blood samples:** FBC, clotting screen, group and cross-match 4 units | **Rapid fluid replacement** Two litres of crystalloid - Hartmann's or 0.9% saline | **Observations** Respiratory rate, pulse, BP, O₂, saturations | **Assess cause** Atony Trauma Retained placental tissue Coagulation |

Stop the bleeding

ONGOING MANAGEMENT

| **Syntocinon 10 units/ Ergometrine 500 micrograms** IM or slow IV injection (ergometrine contraindicated if raised BP) | **Syntocinon infusion** 40 units syntocinon IV infusion via pump over 4 hours | **Urinary catheter and urine measurement** Empty bladder, monitor urine output hourly | **Carboprost** 250 micrograms given IM every 15 minutes up to 8 doses | **Misoprostol** 800 micrograms given per rectum |

Massage uterus and bimanual compression   **AND**   **Repair perineal/vaginal/cervical tears**

Assessment

| **Monitoring** Document all observations-use modified obstetric early warning score chart **Estimate blood loss/weigh all swabs** Accurate fluid balance | **Reassess causes of bleeding** Atony Trauma Retained placental tissue Coagulation | **Blood transfusion/blood products** Consider: O-negative emergency blood (use blood warmer and maintain maternal warmth) FFP, platelets, cryoprecipitate, factor VIIa |

Figure 29.7 Algorithm for the initial management of a major postpartum haemorrhage.

Reproduced from Winter C, Crofts J, Laxton C, Barnfield S, Draycott T, (eds.) *PROMPT: PRactical Obstetric Multi-Professional Training. Practical locally based training for obstetric emergencies. Course Manual.* 2nd edition. Cambridge: Cambridge University Press; 2012.

- If the uterus contracts following the oxytocics, consider commencing a Syntocinon infusion (oxytocin 40 units in 500 mL physiological saline infused via a pump at 125 mL/hour over 4 hours) to maintain uterine tone. However, this will not initiate uterine tone, therefore additional measures will be required if the uterus has not contracted.

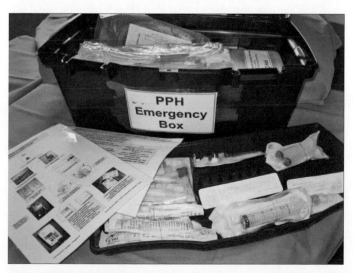

Figure 29.8 A PPH emergency box.

- Catheterize the bladder: a full bladder may inhibit contraction of the uterus. Insert an indwelling Foley catheter to ensure the bladder is empty and enable monitoring of urine output.
- Repair any tears: bleeding from tears is the second most common cause of PPH. If the tear is easily visible in the labour room and analgesia is adequate, repair the tears as soon as possible.
- Transfer to theatre: have a low threshold for transfer to theatre for examination under anaesthesia, particularly in cases of ongoing bleeding, if you suspect retained products of conception or if tears are not easily accessible.
  - The method of anaesthesia (general or regional) should be discussed between the anaesthetist, obstetrician, senior midwife, and the woman (if appropriate).
- Examination under anaesthesia: feel within the uterus to ensure it is empty and systematically inspect the genital tract to identify any tears.
  - Most cases of major haemorrhage will have settled after these measures. If the bleeding is ongoing, consider alternative medications, mechanical and surgical measures.
- Uterotonic medications: if the uterus is still atonic, give carboprost (Haemabate) 250 mcg intramuscularly every 15 minutes up to a maximum of eight doses. Carboprost is a prostaglandin analogue. Side effects include diarrhoea, vomiting, hypertension, headache, and bronchospasm. Carboprost is contraindicated in women with cardiovascular or respiratory disease, including asthma.

(a)

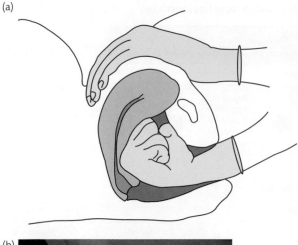

(b)

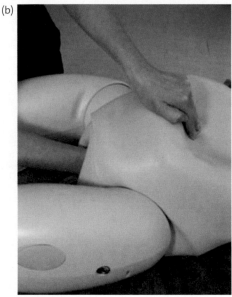

Figure 29.9 Bimanual compression.

- Misoprostol is a less effective, inexpensive prostaglandin ana-logue; 800–1000 mcg per rectum can be administered if other uterotonics are not available or contraindicated.
- Tranexamic acid: tranexamic acid is an antifibrinolytic that is used for prophylaxis and treatment of haemorrhage in many other spe-cialties, including orthopaedics and emergency medicine—1 g of tranexamic acid intravenously is thought to reduce PPH in ob-stetric patients.
  - A systematic review concluded that prophylactic tranexamic acid in conjunction with uterotonics decreased postpartum blood loss after vaginal birth and caesarean section (20). However, these studies were of varying quality and were not large enough to assess the effect on maternal outcomes. Most recently, the World Maternal Antifibrinolytic (WOMAN) trial, an international randomized controlled trial, recruited over 20,000 women with clinically diagnosed PPH to receive tranex-amic acid or placebo. When tranexamic acid was given along-side uterotonics as soon as possible after the onset of primary PPH, the trial demonstrated a significant reduction in maternal deaths from haemorrhage following vaginal and caesarean birth and a reduction in the number of women requiring laparotomy

to control bleeding. There was no increase in vascular occlusive events.
  - A reasonable and safe option for the management of PPH is 1 g of tranexamic acid intravenously and this can be repeated after 30 minutes.
- Mechanical and surgical measures: intrauterine balloons, such as Rusch or Bakri balloons, are often an effective measure to tam-ponade the uterus. Insert the balloon catheter into the uterus and inflate with 250–500 mL of warmed saline. If the bleeding settles, leave the balloon in place for up to 24 hours.
- Additional measures: these include insertion of a B-lynch suture, interventional radiology, ligation of the internal iliac artery, and hysterectomy. There should be early recourse to hysterectomy in cases of life-threatening unrelenting haemorrhage, before the woman is severely compromised or develops disseminated intra-vascular coagulation. Ideally a second opinion should be sought from a senior doctor; but this should not unduly delay hysterec-tomy in life-threatening situations.

Acute uterine inversion

Acute uterine inversion is a rare occurrence, affecting anywhere from 1:1500 to 1:20,000 births (22, 23). The uterus turns 'inside out', with the fundus descending through the genital tract:

- Grade I: the fundus inverts down to the cervical canal.
- Grade 2: the fundus inverts into the vagina.
- Grade 3: the fundus is visible at/outside of the introitus.

Acute uterine inversion most commonly results from early or excessive traction on the umbilical cord. Additional risk factors in-clude fundal pressure, short umbilical cord, adherent placenta, pre-vious caesarean section, manual removal of placenta, abnormalities of the uterus (e.g. unicornuate uterus), connective tissue disorders (e.g. Ehlers–Danlos syndrome), multiparity, previous uterine inver-sion, precipitate labour, and fetal macrosomia.

Diagnosis of acute uterine inversion

The diagnosis may not be obvious as the uterus may not be visible outside of the introitus and vaginal blood loss is often minimal ini-tially. Most commonly, the woman develops presyncopal symp-toms that then progress into signs of neurogenic shock. As the uterus inverts through the cervix, vagal stimulation results in ma-ternal bradycardia and hypotension. The uterus may not be palp-able on abdominal examination. Vaginal examination will often reveal a mass in the vagina, which is the uterus. Atonic PPH ensues in 90% of cases (24, 25), usually once the uterus has been replaced and the placenta has been removed. The woman is likely to develop hypovolaemic shock.

Immediate management of acute uterine inversion

An algorithm for the immediate management of acute uterine inver-sion is displayed in **Figure 29.10**.

Replacement of the uterus is more likely to be successful if at-tempted early. As time progresses, the uterus will become oedema-tous and may develop constriction rings. Uterine relaxation may be useful in these cases but should be used with caution, as they

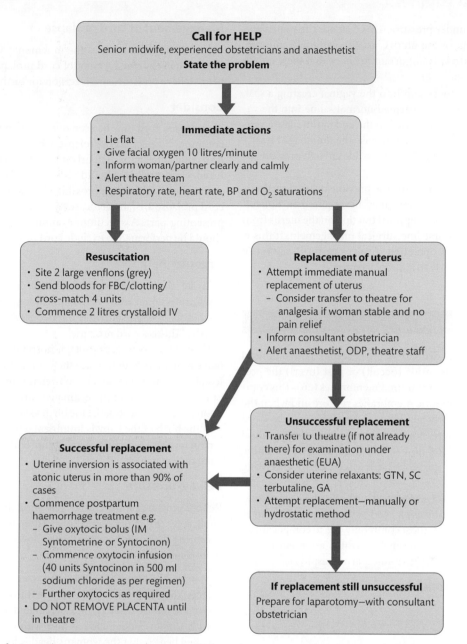

Figure 29.10 Algorithm for immediate management of acute uterine inversion.

Reproduced from Winter C, Crofts J, Laxton C, Barnfield S, Draycott T, (eds.) PROMPT: PRactical Obstetric Multi-Professional Training. Practical locally based training for obstetric emergencies. Course Manual. 2nd edition. Cambridge: Cambridge University Press; 2012.

may conversely exacerbate atonic PPH. Uterine relaxation can be achieved with tocolytics, for example, terbutaline 250 mcg subcutaneously or glyceryl trinitrate spray. General anaesthesia may also relax the uterus.

There should be a low threshold for transfer to theatre. If the woman is bleeding, IS haemodynamically unstable, or has effective analgesia, attempt to manually replace the uterus immediately, wherever the woman is situated. However, if the woman is stable, does not have adequate analgesia, or if initial attempts at manual replacement are unsuccessful, transfer to theatre is advisable. The method of anaesthesia should be chosen according to the woman's clinical status. Once the uterus has been replaced, administer oxytocics to enable uterine contraction and reduce the risk of PPH.

Replacement of the uterus

If the placenta is still *in situ*, do not attempt to remove it until the uterus is replaced. Prophylactic intravenous antibiotics should be administered as per local guidelines.

- Manual replacement: put a hand into the vagina and follow the umbilical cord up to the fundus of the uterus. Gently raise the fundus towards the abdominal cavity with your hand until it reverts into its anatomical position. Leave your hand in position holding the uterus for a few minutes afterwards, to ensure the position is maintained and to encourage uterine contraction.

- Hydrostatic method: hydrostatic pressure is achieved by sealing the introitus with a hand or a silastic ventouse cup and inserting fluid into the vagina under pressure. This distends the vagina and facilitates replacement of the uterus, usually within 10 minutes. Prior to this procedure, it is important to check that there are no large vaginal lacerations.

Place the silastic ventouse cup into the vagina, creating a seal. Rapidly infuse 2 L of slightly warmed normal saline into the vagina, via a blood giving set attached to the end of the silastic ventouse cup. Inflate a pressure jacket or raise the fluid bag at least 1 metre above the level of the vagina to provide enough pressure for insufflation of the vagina.

- Surgical management: it is rare for the previously listed methods to not be successful. Laparotomy may be required in difficult cases. Huntington's operation, upward traction on the uterus from the abdominal cavity, is first-line surgical management. If this is not successful, Haultain's operation involves vertical incision of the cervical ring posteriorly to aid replacement.

Umbilical cord prolapse

Umbilical cord prolapse is defined as the descent of the umbilical cord through the cervix alongside (occult) or past (overt) the presenting part in the presence of ruptured membranes (26). This commonly occurs after the amniotic membranes rupture and when the fetal presenting part is poorly applied to the maternal cervix. Cord prolapse causes cord compression and vasospasm of the umbilical arteries, which reduces blood flow to and from the fetus, resulting in birth asphyxia. Earliest possible birth is crucial to improving outcomes (26).

Cord prolapse occurs in 0.1–0.6% of all births. In breech presentations, the incidence is 1%. The associated perinatal mortality rate is approximately 9% (27). This is most commonly due to complications of prematurity and congenital anomalies, which are predisposing factors for cord prolapse, rather than intrapartum asphyxia.

Risk factors for cord prolapse

Antenatal

- Breech presentation
- Unstable, oblique, or transverse lie
- Polyhydramnios
- Congenital anomalies
- External cephalic version
- Expectant management of premature rupture of membranes
- Previous cord prolapse.

Intrapartum

- Amniotomy (especially with a high presenting part)
- Prematurity
- Breech presentation
- Internal podalic version
- Second twin
- Disimpaction of fetal head during rotational operative vaginal birth
- Fetal scalp electrode application.

Management of cord prolapse

Figure 29.11 demonstrates the mnemonic 'CORD', which outlines the key steps in management of cord prolapse: Consider, Organize help, Relieve pressure, and Decision for birth (26).

Consider

A prolapsed cord may be seen outside of the vagina, but this is uncommon. Suspect cord prolapse when there is an abnormal fetal heart rate pattern, particularly if the membranes have recently ruptured. Cord prolapse should also be considered when there are associated risk factors. Approximately half of the reported cases of cord prolapse are iatrogenic, such as membrane rupture with a high presenting part. A speculum examination or vaginal examination should be performed to exclude cord prolapse in these cases.

Organize help

Activate the emergency bell to call for urgent help from the multiprofessional team: senior midwives, senior obstetricians, anaesthetists, theatre staff, and the neonatal team. State the problem clearly: 'This is a cord prolapse'.

If the emergency occurs outside hospital, call an emergency ambulance immediately to transfer the woman to the nearest consultant-led obstetric unit. Contact the obstetric unit directly to inform them of the emergency and the estimated time of arrival, so that preparations can be made to assist the birth as soon as possible after arrival.

If the birth of the baby is imminent, continue to call a paramedic ambulance in case of neonatal compromise requiring urgent neonatal review in hospital.

Relieve pressure

Relieve pressure on the cord by elevating the presenting part and, if applicable, reducing contractions. These measures are useful while preparing for birth; however, birth should not be delayed by trying to implement them.

- Maternal positioning: advise the woman to adopt a knee–chest face-down position while awaiting transfer to theatre or hospital. For ambulance transfer, the exaggerated Sim's position (left-lateral with a pillow under the left hip) with or without Trendelenburg (tilted bed so that the woman's head is lower than the pelvis) may be more stable and hence safer.
- Digital elevation: manually elevate the presenting part with two fingers to reduce compression of the cord. If the cord has prolapsed outside of the vagina, gently attempt to replace it into the vagina. Handling of the cord must be kept to a minimum, as this may cause vasospasm. Continue manual elevation during transfer to theatre and the administration of anaesthesia, until immediately prior to birth.
- Bladder filling: alternatively, you can fill the bladder to elevate the presenting part. This is often useful when there is a delay, such as awaiting transfer to hospital.
  - Insert a Foley catheter into the bladder and fill with 500–750 mL of sterile physiological 0.9% saline via a blood giving set. Clamp off the giving set once the bladder is filled and leave attached to the catheter, to ensure the volume is maintained. Disconnect the giving set and empty the bladder immediately

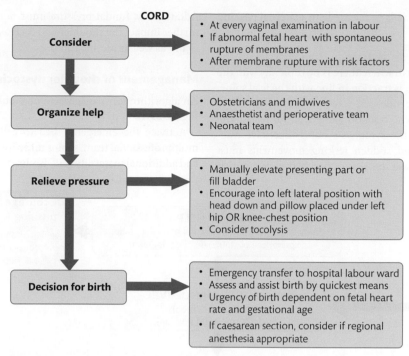

Figure 29.11 'CORD': the key steps for the management of cord prolapse.

Source data from Winter C, Crofts J, Laxton C, Barnfield S, Draycott T, editors. *PROMPT: PRactical Obstetric Multi-Professional Training. Practical locally based training for obstetric emergencies. Course Manual.* 2nd edition. Cambridge: Cambridge University Press; 2012, pp. 169–78.

prior to birth, whether this is by caesarean section or operative vaginal birth.

- Reducing contractions: if an oxytocin infusion is in progress, this should be discontinued. If there are persistent fetal heart rate abnormalities, consider tocolysis with terbutaline 250 mcg subcutaneously. Be prepared for an increased risk of PPH associated with tocolytic administration.

Decision for birth

If the cervix is not fully dilated, perform a caesarean section. The urgency of caesarean section depends on the fetal heart rate pattern and gestational age. If the fetal heart rate pattern is normal, then a category 2 birth may be acceptable. However, you must continually assess the situation and upgrade to category 1 birth if there is any deterioration.

The urgency and timing of birth should be discussed between the anaesthetic, obstetric, and midwifery teams, to ensure the safest method of anaesthesia is chosen. If the anaesthetist is attempting regional anaesthesia, continue to reassess the urgency and timing of birth and avoid prolonged and repeated attempts at regional anaesthesia.

If the cervix is fully dilated and you anticipate that vaginal birth is achievable quickly and safely, consider an operative vaginal birth.

Breech extraction can be considered in certain circumstances, such as after internal podalic version for the second twin.

Shoulder dystocia

Shoulder dystocia is diagnosed when routine axial traction fails to complete the birth of the baby after the birth of the head, and additional manoeuvres are required to release the fetal shoulders.

This is usually due to the anterior fetal shoulder impacting upon the maternal symphysis pubis. The posterior fetal shoulder can impact upon the maternal sacral promontory, but this is less common.

There is a wide variation in the reported incidence of shoulder dystocia (28). Studies involving the largest number of vaginal births report incidences between 0.58% and 0.70% (29–34). Shoulder dystocia is unpredictable, as the majority of cases occur in women without any risk factors, and it is therefore largely unpreventable. Clinicians should be aware of existing risk factors, but should also be alert to the possibility of shoulder dystocia with any birth (35).

Risk factors for shoulder dystocia

- Prelabour:
  - Previous shoulder dystocia
  - Macrosomia greater than 4.5 kg
  - Maternal diabetes mellitus
  - Maternal obesity
- Intrapartum:
  - Prolonged first stage
  - Prolonged second stage
  - Augmentation of labour
  - Operative vaginal birth.

Recognition of shoulder dystocia

- There may be difficulty with the birth of the face and chin.
- When the head is born, it remains tightly applied to the vulva.
- The chin retracts and depresses the perineum—the 'turtle-neck' sign.

- The anterior fetal shoulder fails to release with maternal pushing and routine axial traction.

Routine traction is defined as 'the traction required to release the fetal shoulders in a vaginal birth where there is no difficulty with the shoulders' (36). Axial traction is traction in line with the fetal spine. Traction should be slow and gentle.

In cases of shoulder dystocia, traction alone will not release the fetal shoulder from behind the symphysis pubis. Excessive traction, downward traction, and sudden jerking movements must be avoided, as they all increase the risk of brachial plexus injury.

Additionally, fundal pressure must not be performed, as this will further impact the shoulder and increase the risk of brachial plexus injury as well as uterine rupture.

Management of shoulder dystocia

An algorithm for management of shoulder dystocia is displayed in **Figure 29.12**.

Activate the emergency bell to call for urgent help from the multiprofessional team: senior midwives, experienced obstetricians, and additional maternity staff. Ensure the neonatal team is contacted

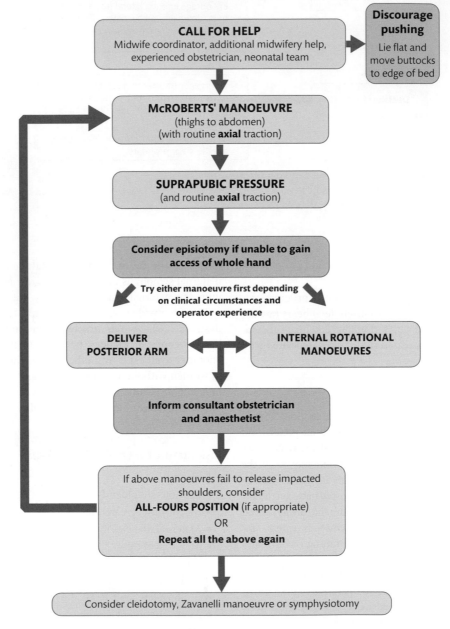

Figure 29.12 Algorithm for management of shoulder dystocia.

Reproduced from Winter C, Crofts J, Laxton C, Barnfield S, Draycott T, (eds.) *PROMPT: PRactical Obstetric Multi-Professional Training. Practical locally based training for obstetric emergencies. Course Manual.* 2nd edition. Cambridge: Cambridge University Press; 2012.

urgently to support neonatal resuscitation if required, and assess the baby for signs of injury after birth. If shoulder dystocia occurs at home, a paramedic ambulance should be immediately requested.

State the problem clearly: 'This is a shoulder dystocia'. Take note of the time of birth of the head and, if possible, assign one team member to document timings and actions. Ask the mother to stop pushing, as this will further impact the shoulder against the symphysis pubis and will not resolve the dystocia.

Manoeuvres

Upon diagnosis of shoulder dystocia, the following manoeuvres should be attempted in a stepwise fashion. After each manoeuvre, apply routine axial traction to assess whether the shoulders have released. If unsuccessful, move on to the next manoeuvre.

These manoeuvres must not be attempted 'prophylactically' in anticipation of shoulder dystocia, as this will make it difficult to assess if there this was definitely a shoulder dystocia and will impact the management of future births and cause maternal anxiety.

McRoberts' manoeuvre

This simple manoeuvre is an effective intervention, with reported success rates as high as 90% (35). It has a low rate of complication and is one of the least invasive manoeuvres. It should therefore be used first, if possible. McRoberts' position increases the relative anteroposterior diameter of the pelvis, by straightening the sacrum relative to the lumbar spine and rotating the maternal pelvis towards the woman's head.

Lay the woman flat and remove any pillows. Bring her to the end of the bed and/or remove the end of the bed to make vaginal access easier. With one assistant on either side, hyperflex the woman's legs so that her thighs are brought close to her abdomen and her knees are up towards her ears. If the woman is in lithotomy, remove her legs from the supports to achieve McRoberts' position.

Apply routine axial traction. If the fetal shoulder is not released, move on to the next manoeuvre.

Suprapubic pressure

Suprapubic pressure aims to rotate the anterior fetal shoulder, releasing it from behind the symphysis pubis into the wider oblique diameter of the pelvis.

Identify the location of the fetal back. Ask an assistant to apply pressure just above the symphysis pubis in a downward, lateral direction from the side of the fetal back. If you are unsure of the location of the fetal back, apply suprapubic pressure from the most likely side of the fetal back, and attempt from the other side if this is unsuccessful.

If the fetal shoulder is not released with routine axial traction, stop suprapubic pressure and move on to the next manoeuvre.

Internal manoeuvres

The two internal vaginal manoeuvres are delivery of the posterior arm and internal rotational manoeuvres. There is no evidence to suggest that one is superior or should be attempted first. Although episiotomy will not relieve the bony obstruction of shoulder dystocia, it can be considered to allow more space to insert the birth attendant's hand to facilitate these manoeuvres.

Both manoeuvres involve gaining access into the vagina. With the woman maintained in McRoberts' position, the most spacious part of the pelvis is the sacral hollow, posteriorly. There is very little room anteriorly or laterally. The whole hand must be inserted into the vagina, as it is otherwise very difficult to perform the manoeuvres. The technique to insert the hand into the sacral hollow is to scrunch up your hand as if putting on a tight bracelet, as demonstrated in **Figure 29.13**.

Delivery of the posterior arm

Delivering the posterior arm will reduce the diameter of the fetal shoulders by the width of the arm. The aim is to grasp the fetal wrist and gently withdraw the baby's hand from the vagina in a straight line. This movement is similar to the action of 'putting your hand up in class'. Once the posterior arm is delivered, routine axial traction will usually achieve birth of the baby.

Babies often lie with their arms flexed, therefore the fetal wrist may be easily felt when you access the vagina. However, if the posterior arm is lying straight against the body, the fetal wrist may be more difficult to reach. The arm will need to be flexed to bring the wrist closer to you. Follow the posterior shoulder and arm with your hand until you reach the elbow. Place your thumb in the antecubital fossa and apply pressure to the back of the elbow with your fingers. This should flex the posterior arm and allow the wrist to be grasped.

If you cannot reach the wrist, move on to the next manoeuvre. Do not pull on the upper arm as this will not bring the wrist closer and may result in a humeral fracture. If the posterior arm is delivered but the shoulder dystocia has not resolved, support the head and posterior arm and gently rotate the baby through 180 degrees. This should resolve the shoulder dystocia, as the posterior shoulder will now become the anterior shoulder and should be below the symphysis pubis.

Internal rotational manoeuvres

Internal rotational manoeuvres aim to move the fetal shoulders into a wider pelvic diameter. As the fetal shoulders rotate within

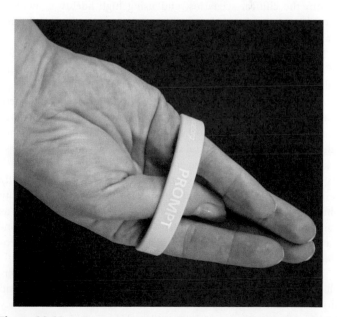

Figure 29.13 A demonstration of the technique for inserting the hand into the sacral hollow.

the pelvis, the fetal shoulder descends through the pelvis due to the bony architecture of the pelvis. Internal rotation can be most easily achieved by applying pressure on the anterior (front) or posterior (back) aspect of the posterior shoulder to guide the shoulders into an oblique or transverse diameter. At the same time, an assistant can apply suprapubic pressure to aid rotation of the shoulders. The direction of suprapubic pressure depends upon the direction you are attempting to rotate the shoulders, that is, ensure you are both attempting to guide the shoulders in the same direction. Birth should then be achieved with routine axial traction.

All-fours position

If these manoeuvres do not work, either try all the manoeuvres again or consider the all-fours position, as the change in position may dislodge the anterior shoulder (37). Some midwives may prefer to try the all-fours position prior to internal rotational manoeuvres.

Last-resort options

These include vaginal replacement of the fetal head (Zavanelli manoeuvre) and maternal symphysiotomy. These procedures are rarely required and are associated with serious maternal morbidity (38–41).

Effective training for obstetric emergencies

Local, multiprofessional training has been associated with improvements in the care administered during an emergency. However, not all training is effective. There are a multitude of training programmes aimed at improving perinatal care: some have demonstrated no improvement in outcomes (42–44) and some have resulted in worse outcomes (45, 46). Current evidence indicates that the most effective training programmes are multiprofessional, training all maternity staff within their own unit annually, integrating teamwork training within the clinical scenarios, and using high-fidelity simulation models and simple tools to facilitate best practice (2, 7). Effective training is very likely to be more than just knowledge transfer.

National enquiries into maternal deaths regularly identify lack of team working and poor communication as key contributors to substandard care (1, 15). Isolated teamwork training does not appear to be effective in intrapartum care (47, 48). In one study, where teamwork and communication skills were integrated throughout the clinical training, the most efficient teams administered magnesium sulphate more quickly during the eclampsia drill (49). These teams were noted to state the emergency earlier, managed the task using structured closed-loop communication, and had significantly fewer exits from the room during the drill. Although high-fidelity simulation models are advantageous for learning techniques such as vaginal breech birth and shoulder dystocia management, the concurrent use of patient actors during drills may improve the perception of safety and communication (50).

Training staff within their own maternity unit enables ownership of their learning, allowing them to address specific issues and drive system changes. Specific unit-based tools such as emergency boxes and algorithms can be introduced during the training and embedded into clinical practice. Local training and subsequent improvements in outcomes may encourage staff to further strive for improvements in care (51).

Training should be sustainable as well as effective. A recent long-term study of shoulder dystocia training in a single maternity unit showed that over 85% of staff were trained annually over 12 years (52). Moreover, the effect of training had improved over time, from a 70% reduction in permanent brachial plexus injury after 4 years of training, to a 100% reduction after 10 years. Sustaining training does require support from hospital management (obstetrics and midwifery) and dedicated staff to run the training. However, this should be associated with improved outcomes and a measurement system is required.

Effective multiprofessional training programmes for obstetric emergencies improve intrapartum care, significantly impacting the lives of women and their families and reducing the burden on health services. All maternity units should implement and sustain a local, evidence-based training programme for all of their staff to attend on an annual basis.

REFERENCES

1. Knight M, Tuffnell D, Kenyon S, et al. (eds). *Saving Lives, Improving Mothers' Care: Surveillance of Maternal Deaths in the UK 2011–13 and Lessons Learned to Inform Maternity Care from the UK and Ireland Confidential Enquiries into Maternal Deaths and Morbidity 2009–13*. Oxford: National Perinatal Epidemiology Unit, University of Oxford; 2015.
2. Bergh A-M, Baloyi S, Pattinson RC. What is the impact of multi-professional emergency obstetric and neonatal care training? *Best Pract Res Clin Obstet Gynaecol* 2015;**29**:1028–43.
3. Draycott TJ, Collins KJ, Crofts, et al. Myths and realities of training in obstetric emergencies. *Best Pract Res Clin Obstet Gynaecol* 2016;**29**:1–10.
4. National Maternity Review. *Better Births: Improving Outcomes of Maternity Services in England: A Five Year Forward View for Maternity Care*. London: NHS England; 2016.
5. PROMPT. Homepage. Available at: http://www.promptmaternity.org.
6. Winter C, Crofts J, Laxton C, Barnfield S, Draycott T (eds). *PROMPT: Practical Obstetric Multi-Professional Training. Practical Locally Based Training for Obstetric Emergencies. Course Manual*, 2nd edn. Cambridge: Cambridge University Press; 2012.
7. Siassakos D, Crofts JF, Winter C, Weiner CP, Draycott TJ. The active components of effective training in obstetric emergencies. *BJOG* 2009;**116**:1028–32.
8. Cornthwaite K, Edwards S, Siassakos D. Reducing risk in maternity by optimising teamwork and leadership: an evidence-based approach to save mothers and babies. *Best Pract Res Clin Obstet Gynaecol* 2013;**27**:571–81.
9. Resuscitation Council (UK). Adult basic life support and automated external defibrillation. Available at: https://www.resus.org.uk/resuscitation-guidelines/adult-basic-life-support-and-automated-external-defibrillation/ (accessed 23 March 2016).
10. Surviving Sepsis Campaign. International guidelines for management of severe sepsis and septic shock: 2012. Available at: http://www.sccm.org/Documents/SSC-Guidelines.pdf (accessed 23 March 2016).

11. Lewis G (ed). *The Confidential Enquiry into Maternal and Child Health (CEMACH). Saving Mothers' Lives: Reviewing Maternal Deaths to Make Motherhood Safer—2003–2005. The Seventh Report on Confidential Enquiries into Maternal Deaths in the United Kingdom*. London: CEMACH; 2007.

12. Weil MH, Afifi AA. Experimental and clinical studies on lactate and pyruvate as indicators of the severity of acute circulatory failure (shock). *Circulation* 1970;**41**:989–1001.

13. National Institute for Health and Care Excellence (NICE). *Hypertension in Pregnancy*. Clinical guideline [CG107]. London: NICE; 2011.

14. Knight M. Eclampsia in the United Kingdom 2005. *BJOG* 2007;**114**:1072–78.

15. Centre for Maternal and Child Enquiries (CMACE). Saving Mothers' Lives: reviewing maternal deaths to make motherhood safer: 2006–08. The Eighth Report on Confidential Enquiries into Maternal Deaths in the United Kingdom. *BJOG* 2011;**118** Suppl 1:1–203.

16. The Eclampsia Trial Collaborative Group. Which anticonvulsant for women with eclampsia? Evidence from the Collaborative Eclampsia Trial. *Lancet* 1995;**345**:1455–63.

17. The Magpie Trial Collaborative Group. Do women with pre-eclampsia, and their babies, benefit from magnesium sulphate? The Magpie Trial: a randomised placebo-controlled trial. *Lancet* 2002;**359**:1877–90.

18. Royal College of Obstetricians and Gynaecologists (RCOG). Green-top Guideline No. 52. *Prevention and Management of Postpartum Haemorrhage*. London: RCOG; 2011.

19. National Institute for Health and Care Excellence (NICE). Clinical guideline [CG190]. *Intrapartum Care*. London: NICE; 2015.

20. Novikova N, Hofmeyr GJ, Cluver C. Tranexamic acid for preventing postpartum haemorrhage. *Cochrane Database Syst Rev* 2015;**6**:CD007872.

21. Shakur H, Elbourne D, Gülmezoglu M, et al. Effect of early tranexamic acid administration on mortality, hysterectomy, and other morbidities in women with post-partum haemorrhage (WOMAN): an international, randomised, double-blind, placebo-controlled trial. *Lancet* 2017;**389**:2105–16.

22. Hussain M, Jabeen T, Liaquat N, Noorani K, Bhutta SZ. Acute puerperal uterine inversion. *J Coll Physicians Surg Pak* 2004;**14**:215–17.

23. Milenkovic M, Kahn J. Inversion of the uterus: a serious complication at childbirth. *Acta Obstet Gynecol Scand* 2005;**84**:95–96.

24. Bhalla R, Wuntakal R, Odejinmi F, Khan RU. Acute inversion of the uterus. *Obstet Gynecol* 2009;**11**:13–18.

25. Watson P, Besch N, Bowes WA. Management of acute and sub-acute puerperal inversion of the uterus. *Obstet Gynecol* 1980;**55**:12–16.

26. Royal College of Obstetricians and Gynaecologists (RCOG). *Umbilical Cord Prolapse*. Green-top Guideline No. 50. London: RCOG; 2014.

27. Murphy DJ, MacKenzie IZ. The mortality and morbidity associated with umbilical cord prolapse. *Br J Obstet Gynaecol* 1995;**102**:826–30.

28. Baskett TF, Allen AC. Perinatal implications of shoulder dystocia. *Obstet Gynecol* 1995;**86**:14–17.

29. Gherman RB, Ouzounian JG, Goodwin TM. Obstetric maneuvers for shoulder dystocia and associated fetal morbidity. *Am J Obstet Gynecol* 1998;**178**:1126–30.

30. McFarland MB, Langer O, Piper JM, Berkus MD. Perinatal outcome and the type and number of maneuvers in shoulder dystocia. *Int J Gynecol Obstet* 1996;**55**:219–24.

31. Ouzounian JG, Gherman RB. Shoulder dystocia: are historic risk factors reliable predictors? *Am J Obstet Gynecol* 2005;**192**:1933–35.

32. Smith RB, Lane C, Pearson JF. Shoulder dystocia—what happens at the next delivery? *Br J Obstet Gynecol* 1994;**101**:713–15.

33. Nesbitt TS, Gilbert WM, Herrchen B. Shoulder dystocia and associated risk factors with macrosomic infants born in California. *Am J Obstet Gynecol* 1998;**1793**:476–80.

34. Bahar AM. Risk factors and fetal outcome in cases of shoulder dystocia compared with normal deliveries of a similar birth-weight. *Br J Obstet Gynecol* 1996;**103**:868–72.

35. Royal College of Obstetricians and Gynaecologists (RCOG). *Shoulder Dystocia*. Green-top Guideline No. 42. London: RCOG; 2013.

36. Metaizeau JP, Gayet C, Plenat F. [Brachial plexus birth injuries. An experimental study (author's transl)]. *Chir Pediatr* 1979;**20**:159–63.

37. Bruner JP, Drummond SB, Meenan AL, Gaskin IM. All-fours maneuver for reducing shoulder dystocia during labor. *J Reprod Med* 1998;**43**:439–43.

38. Sandberg EC. The Zavanelli maneuver—a potentially revolutionary method for the resolution of shoulder dystocia. *Am J Obstet Gynecol* 1985;**152**:479–84.

39. Vaithilingam N, Davies D. Cephalic replacement for shoulder dystocia: three cases. *BJOG* 2005;**112**:674–75.

40. Spellacy WN. The Zavanelli maneuver for fetal shoulder dystocia—3 cases with poor outcomes. *J Reprod Med* 1995;**40**:543–44.

41. Goodwin TM, Banks E, Millar LK, Phelan JP. Catastrophic shoulder dystocia and emergency symphysiotomy. *Am J Obstet Gynecol* 1997;**177**:463–64.

42. Freeth D, Berridge E, Mackintosh N. *Evaluation of Safety Culture and MOSES Training in Four Maternity Units and Two Clinical Simulation Centres*. End of Project Report for the National Patient Safety Agency. London: National Patient Safety Agency; 2008.

43. Markova V, Sorensen JL, Holm C, Norgaard A, Langhoff-Roos J. Evaluation of multi-professional obstetric skills training for postpartum hemorrhage. *Acta Obstet Gynecol Scand* 2012;**91**:346–52.

44. Walsh JM, Kandamany N, Shuibhne NN, Power H, Murphy JF, O'Herlihy C. Neonatal brachial plexus injury: comparison of incidence and antecedents between 2 decades. *Am J Obstet Gynecol* 2011;**204**:1–6.

45. MacKenzie IZ, Shah M, Lean K, Dutton S, Newdick H, Tucker DE. Management of shoulder dystocia: trends in incidence and maternal and neonatal morbidity. *Obstet Gynecol* 2007;**110**:1059–68.

46. Fransen A, van de Ven J, van Tetering A, Schuit E, Mol BW, Oei G. The effect of obstetric team training on perinatal and maternal outcome: a large multicenter randomized controlled trial. *Simul Healthc* 2013;**8**:535.

47. Nielsen PE, Goldman MB, Mann S, et al. Effects of teamwork training on adverse outcomes and process of care in labor and delivery: a randomized controlled trial. *Obstet Gynecol* 2007;**109**:48–55.

48. Riley W, Davis S, Miller K, Hansen H, Sainfort F, Sweet R. Didactic and simulation nontechnical skills team training to improve perinatal patient outcomes in a community hospital. *Jt Comm J Qual Patient Saf* 2011;**37**:357–64.

49. Siassakos D, Bristowe K, Draycott TJ, et al. Clinical efficiency in a simulated emergency and relationship to team behaviours: a multisite cross-sectional study. *BJOG* 2011;**118**:596–607.

50. Crofts JF, Bartlett C, Ellis D, et al. Patient-actor perception of care: a comparison of obstetric emergency training using manikins and patient-actors. *Qual Saf Health Care* 2008;**17**:20–24.

51. The Health Foundation. *Lining Up: How Do Improvement Programmes Work?* London: The Health Foundation; 2014.

52. Crofts JF, Lenguerrand E, Bentham GL, et al. Prevention of brachial plexus injury: 12 years of shoulder dystocia training: an interrupted time-series study. *BJOG* 2016;**123**:111–18.

30

Preterm birth

Angharad Care and Zarko Alfirevic

Definition

Preterm birth (PTB) is usually defined as delivery at any gestation before 37 completed weeks of pregnancy ($<37^{+0}$ weeks, <259 days). The lower limit of PTB and upper limit of late spontaneous miscarriage are blurred as the limit of viability varies with differences in healthcare settings. The World Health Organization recommends using 28 weeks of completed gestation as a cut-off for viability, whereas neonates reaching 23 completed weeks have been successfully resuscitated in the United Kingdom. If the baby is non-viable, spontaneous delivery is termed 'miscarriage'. Despite the difference in semantics, both late spontaneous miscarriage and early spontaneous birth are considered to share the same pathophysiological triggers.

Incidence

Worldwide, an estimated 15 million babies are born before 37 completed weeks of pregnancy. Across 184 countries, the rate of PTB ranges from 5% to 18% and in nearly all countries reporting reliable data, the rates of prematurity are increasing (1).

Being born preterm results in insufficient time *in utero* for complete organ maturation and three-quarters of all perinatal mortality and over half of long-term morbidity is attributable to PTB (2). Many survivors face a lifetime of disability, including cognitive impairment, motor disability, poor respiratory health, behavioural disturbance, and visual and hearing deficiencies. The severity of these risks is inversely proportional to the gestational age at birth (**Figure 30.1**).

Complications of prematurity are the leading cause of death among children under 5 years of age and were responsible for nearly 1 million deaths worldwide in 2015 (3).

The emotional and economic implications of PTB remain a burden to healthcare systems and societies. Parents of neurologically disabled children report social exclusion from parents with normal children, anxiety, relationship breakdown, reduced quality of life, and ending careers to become carers (4). One United Kingdom study (5) estimated the total cost to the public sector for the care of children born prematurely up to 18 years old to be £2.95 billion annually. Based on their decision analytical model, an intervention that could delay PTB by just 1 week would reduce these costs to £1.95 billion.

Classification of preterm birth

As neonatal morbidity and mortality are inversely proportional to the gestational age of birth, PTB is often subclassified into:

- late preterm (34^{+0} to 36^{+6} weeks)
- moderate preterm (32^{+0} to $<34^{+0}$ weeks)
- very preterm (28^{+0} to $<32^{+0}$ weeks)
- extremely preterm ($<28^{+0}$ weeks).

This classification groups neonates based upon their gestation-specific morbidity and mortality risks, and helps us to discuss prognosis in general terms. However, a classification based on gestation tells us little about the phenotype or cause of these births. PTB is the only obstetric pathology defined by a specific time point rather than a common collection of signs and symptoms. There are multiple causes and pathologies under this umbrella term, therefore PTB can also be classified based on phenotype:

- Medically indicated or 'iatrogenic' PTB (30%).
- Spontaneous preterm labour (PTL) with intact membranes (45%).
- Preterm prelabour rupture of the membranes (PPROM) (25%) followed by either (a) medically indicated delivery or (b) spontaneous labour.

Medically indicated or elective PTBs aim to prevent severe maternal or fetal morbidity and mortality from conditions such as pre-eclampsia, intrauterine growth restriction, fetal distress, placental abruption, or maternal medical disease. The rest are due to a spontaneous onset of labour, with regular uterine contractions and progressive dilatation of the cervix, or secondary to spontaneous rupture of the membranes that is not followed by regular uterine contractions and labour (2). Spontaneous PTB (sPTB) is currently viewed as a 'syndrome', rather than a disease entity, encompassing multiple disease mechanisms into a final common pathway of delivery (6).

Risk factors for preterm birth

The triggers of spontaneous labour, both at term and preterm, are still poorly understood—and a precise mechanism is never established in most cases. Therefore, factors associated with PTB have

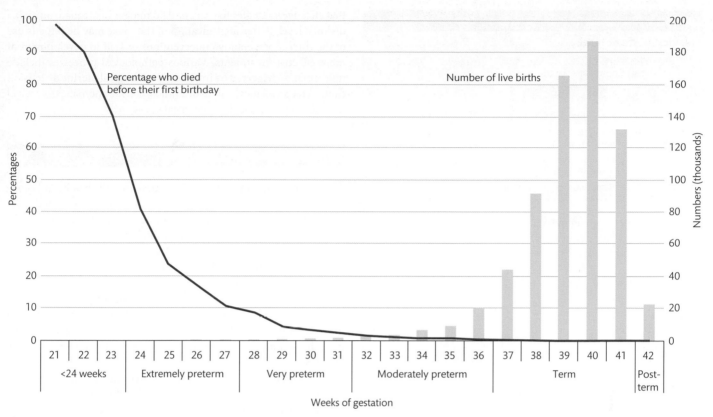

Figure 30.1 Percentage of infant deaths and number of live births per week of gestation in England and Wales.

Source data from Office of National Statistics. Pregnancy and ethnic factors influencing births and infant mortality: 2013–2015 (accessed 25 February 2016). Available at: http://www.ons.gov.uk/peoplepopulationandcommunity/healthandsocialcare/causesofdeath/bulletins/pregnancyandethnicfactorsinfluencingbirthsandinfantmortality/2015-10-14.

been sought to try and identify the most at risk populations. Women with a previous PTB have a recurrence risk of 15–50% depending on the number, gestational age, and characteristics of previous deliveries (2). The risk of a recurrent PTB is inversely related to the gestational age at the first delivery (7). Most risk factors cannot be altered between pregnancies such as genetic influences or uterine abnormalities. Even modifiable risk factors such as social status and body mass index are difficult to change.

Identifying at-risk women in their first pregnancy is particularly challenging. **Box 30.1** lists some of the common risk factors associated with PTB.

Neonatal outcomes following preterm birth

Two United Kingdom cohort studies comparing outcomes of babies born between 22 and 26 weeks in 1995 and 2006 show survival rates of extremely premature infants have been improving (40% to 53%) (8). Overall, more babies are now being admitted for care at earlier gestations, and although healthy survivor numbers are increasing, so are the total number of neonates with moderate or severe disability. The Epicure 2 study showed that in infants born before 26 weeks' gestation in 2006, approximately 44% will survive to 3 years of age and of those 15% will have a severe disability (9). Neonatal clinical networks have now increased centralization of care for babies born at less than 26 weeks' gestation, as survival is greatest in hospitals that are able to provide neonatal intensive care (level 1 service).

Short-term morbidity

Cells in the lung alveoli (type 2 pneumocytes) begin to produce surfactant from 30 weeks of gestational age, decreasing the surface tension within the alveoli. Therefore, babies born below this gestation age are at highest risk of respiratory distress syndrome (RDS). Although rates of RDS have decreased over the last few decades due to the use of antenatal corticosteroids, increased use of surfactant, and improvements in lung ventilation; some preterm neonates treated with oxygen and positive-pressure ventilation will ultimately develop bronchopulmonary dysplasia, a chronic lung injury.

Preterm neonates are particularly susceptible to intraventricular haemorrhage, due to the high levels of vascularization that is occurring during brain development, before 34 weeks. Severe haemorrhage predisposes the child to impairment of cognitive, motor, and visual functions. Periventricular leucomalacia is a white matter brain injury that has long-term sequelae, including cerebral palsy and a low IQ. Even in the late PTB group, between 32 and 36 weeks, there are increased levels of autism, attention deficit hyperactivity disorder, and school difficulties when compared with children born at term (10).

The pathogenesis leading to necrotizing enterocolitis remains unknown. It is a gastrointestinal disorder leading to ischaemic injury and abnormal bacterial colonization. In preterm infants, necrotizing enterocolitis usually presents after the commencement of feeds. It may appear after 2–3 weeks of life once preterm babies have survived the early neonatal period. The mortality for necrotizing enterocolitis

Box 30.1 Risk factors for preterm birth

Medical/obstetric history
- Previous preterm birth
- Anatomical abnormalities of the uterus
- Conceiving through *in vitro* fertilization
- Thrombophilia
- Chronic medical conditions such as diabetes and high blood pressure
- Excisional cervical surgery (e.g. knife cone biopsy, multiple large-loop excision of the transformation zone)
- Other cervical damage—in previous delivery, recurrent second-trimester surgical terminations
- Family history of spontaneous PTB (maternal side only)

Maternal
- Extremely low body mass index (<19 kg/m²)
- Short interpregnancy interval (<6 months)
- Higher social deprivation
- Smoking
- Increasing age
- Domestic violence

Fetal
- Congenital abnormality
- Chromosomal abnormality

Current pregnancy
- Short cervical length (CL) for gestational age
- Positive fetal fibronectin between 22 and 34 weeks
- Certain congenital abnormalities of the fetus
- Vaginal bleeding in pregnancy
- Infections—urinary tract, sexually transmitted, bacterial vaginosis, periodontal disease
- Overdistension of the uterus—multiple pregnancy, polyhydramnios, macrosomia
- Recurrent antepartum haemorrhage
- Pre-eclampsia, uteroplacental insufficiency

can be as high as 50% and operative intervention is necessary in almost 20–40% of cases (11).

Long-term morbidity

Studies examining long-term outcomes for preterm babies show the same inverse relationship with gestational age for both morbidity and mortality. In the United Kingdom, 39% of deaths under the age of 5 years are directly caused by prematurity (12). A risk of ill health during childhood exponentially increases for very preterm and moderately/late preterm (32–36 weeks' gestation) neonates when compared to term counterparts (13). Long-term adverse outcomes include delayed behavioural development at 6 years of age, decreased lung function at 8–9 years of age, increased hospitalization, lower exercise capacity into early adulthood, and increased risk of poor metabolic and cardiovascular health (14–16).

Causes of spontaneous preterm labour

The mechanisms that lead to human term labour, let alone preterm parturition, are not yet fully understood. It is, therefore, unsurprising

that effective strategies to prevent PTB remain inadequate on an individual level. Better identification of the cause may help focus use of the correct preventative interventions or lead to development of more effective treatments. Various pathological processes include inflammation triggered by infection, pathological uterine distension (multifetal pregnancy, polyhydramnios, uterine anomalies), cervical insufficiency, and fetal and maternal stress.

Inflammation and infection

The role of inflammation and infection in PTB has been recognized for many decades. Infection is frequently associated with PTL in both humans and animal models. In pregnant mammals, systemic administration of a microbial load can induce labour (17). In humans, 25–40% of sPTB have evidence of intrauterine infection, particularly in PPROM (18). However, in these cases it can be difficult to elucidate if intrauterine infection preceded ruptured membranes or occurred following the loss of the protective membrane barrier. Ascending infection from the genital tract causing inflammation of the lower uterine segment and triggering cervical shortening and labour has been proposed as one mechanism of sPTB.

The amniotic fluid cavity is a sterile environment, therefore positive cultures of amniotic fluid are considered pathological. The reported rates of positive culture of amniotic fluid detected in women presenting in PTL with intact membranes is 13%, higher than rates of non-labouring preterm patients and term labourers. In women with PPROM, this rises to 32%, and again to 75% by the time these women subsequently labour, demonstrating colonization of microbes both before and during the latent period (19). A third mechanism of infection unrelated to the cervix is haematological spread through the placenta causing microbial invasion of the amniotic cavity (19). This route of infection is supported by the fact that extrauterine infection such as asymptomatic bacteriuria and pyelonephritis (20), periodontal infection (21), and malaria (22) are all associated with an increased risk of PTB.

Changes in cervical ripening during labour have been associated with increased production of inflammatory cytokines such as interleukin (IL)-1, IL-6, IL-8, tumour necrosis factor, and prostaglandins (23). Influx of inflammatory cells into the cervix release matrix metalloproteins, contributing to collagen breakdown, and ultimately a softening or ripening of the cervix.

Uterine stretch

Overdistension of the uterus as a PTB risk has been exemplified clinically by the decrease in the mean age of spontaneous delivery to 35 weeks in twins and 30 weeks in quadruplets. Additionally, women diagnosed with polyhydramnios and unicornuate uterus are also at increased risk of sPTB. *In vitro*, induced mechanical stretch of uterine myometrium causes increases in gap junction proteins such as connexin (Cx)-26 and Cx-43 (24), IL-8, and oxytocin receptor (OTR) expression. This leads to mitogen-activated protein kinase (MAPK) pathway activation (25), and upregulating cyclooxygenase (COX)-2 activity (26) terminating with local prostaglandin release causing increased contractility of the uterine muscle.

Maternal/fetal stress

Stress can be difficult to quantify and disassociate from other risk factors such as smoking, poor nutrition, and low socioeconomic status. Stress in the fetus is thought to arise secondary to abnormal placentation, and may present with growth restriction. This leads to maturation and activation of the fetal hypothalamic–pituitary–adrenal (HPA) axis. The events leading to fetal HPA activation are not fully understood, but it is thought that placental corticotrophin-releasing hormone (CRH) plays a central role. Conversely maternal stress increases biological effectors, including cortisol and adrenaline, which have been postulated to activate placental *CRH* gene expression. CRH is a neuropeptide of predominantly hypothalamic origin; it is also expressed in human placenta and membranes and released in increasing amounts over the course of pregnancy. The exponential rise of CRH has been associated with the length of gestation (27). These findings have led some researchers to suggest that placental CRH may act as a 'placental clock' and regulate the length of gestation (27). Premature senescence of the placenta leading to an earlier trigger for birth or PPROM may be mediated by imbalances in reactive oxygen species causing damage mediated by p38 MAPK pathways (28).

Cervical function

Gradual softening and effacement of the cervix occur in the weeks before labour. Cervical ripening involves a breakdown of collagen, changes in proteoglycan concentration, and an increase in water content that occur in response to increased local prostaglandin release or partial antagonism to progesterone receptors (i.e. action of mifepristone) (29).

The role of the cervix in maintaining pregnancy remains undefined and is probably multifactorial, with two key roles: (a) prevention of ascending infection and (b) physical support to keep the pregnancy *in utero*. Maintenance of a healthy mucus plug and adequate length to the cervix may act to prevent ascending infection that triggers production of local inflammatory cytokines and prostaglandin release.

The quality of strength of the cervix to support the pregnancy *in situ* against gravitational pressure is also required to prevent premature cervical dilatation. Recognized cervical weakness, called cervical insufficiency, causes women to suffer recurrent mid-trimester loss usually with a history of painless dilatation of the cervix. On transvaginal screening of cervical length (CL), funnelling is a feature associated with cervical weakness, and the membranes can be seen prolapsing through the endocervical canal of the cervix. Contributing to the argument for the function of the cervix being related to its length, women who have excisional cervical surgery for cervical intraepithelial neoplasia (CIN) or cervical cancer have an increased risk of sPTB. In the treatment of CIN, the volume/length excised has been shown to correlate with the pregnancy duration (30). However, women with CIN have higher baseline risk for sPTB, suggesting cervical function is not be entirely related to length. (30)

Genomics

Genetics is estimated to play a role in approximately 30% of PTBs (31). In singletons, genetic susceptibility to PTB is based on the evidence of familial aggregation, identification of disease-susceptibility genes, and racial disparity in PTB rate that may be related to differences in risk-predisposing allele frequencies. PTB rates are higher in sisters of women with a history of PTB compared to their sisters-in-law (16% vs 9%). Mothers who were born preterm are more likely to deliver preterm by almost 20% (32). This suggests that PTB is inherited in a matrilineal manner across generations and is unaffected by patterns of PTB in the father's family (33). Several studies have confirmed a twofold increase in risk of sPTB for black American women compared to white American women, even after controlling for socioeconomic factors associated with PTB. The most commonly studied pathways for potential candidate genes are those involved in infection and inflammation. A recent pathway analysis of published studies of different polymorphisms in 274 genes suggested that there may be different gene pathways for women presenting with sPTB and PPROM. An autoimmune or hormonal regulation axis may exist for sPTB, while pathways implicated in the aetiology of PPROM include haematological/coagulation function disorder, collagen metabolism, matrix degradation, and local inflammation (34).

Prediction of spontaneous preterm birth

Obstetric history

There is particular difficulty identifying at-risk women in their first pregnancy; among singletons, a history of sPTB remains the most powerful predictor. Twin pregnancies will be at 40% risk of delivering spontaneously before 37 weeks. A meta-analysis quantifying the risk of recurrence of sPTB based on different subtypes of subsequent pregnancy is summarized in Table 30.1. Women with a previous PTB at less than 37 weeks of gestation are at a significant increased risk for recurrent PTB compared with women who have a previous term birth (odds ratio (OR) 5.43; 95% confidence interval (CI) 4.03–7.31), with an increasing risk of subsequent PTB with decreasing gestational age in the previous pregnancy (7).

Ultrasound measurement of cervical length

Transvaginal ultrasound (TVUS) measurements of CL is consistently one of the strongest predictors of sPTB in women with symptoms of PTL and asymptomatic populations in both singletons and twins (Figure 30.2).

There is an increased likelihood of sPTB as the CL decreases. When using a short CL for risk prediction in an asymptomatic cohort, prediction is improved when screening a predefined high-risk population. For a 10% false-positive rate, the detection rate of spontaneous delivery before 32 weeks was 38% for maternal factors (obstetric history, smoking, etc.), 55% for CL measurement alone, and 69% for combined testing (35). A systematic review of TVUS measurement

Table 30.1 Effect of past obstetric history upon absolute risk of preterm birth

First delivery	Second delivery	Absolute risk of preterm labour
Term singleton	Preterm singleton	4.0% (95% CI 3.9–4.0)
Term twin	Preterm singleton	1.3% (95% CI 0.7–2.0)
Preterm singleton	Preterm singleton	20.2% (95% CI 19.9–20.6)
Preterm twin <30 wks	Preterm singleton	10.0% (95% CI 8.0–12.1)
Term singleton	Preterm twin	25.4% (95% CI 24.3–26.5)

Source data from Kazemier BM, Buijs PE, Mignini L, et al. Impact of obstetric history on the rate of spontaneous preterm birth in singleton and multiple pregnancy: a systematic review. *BJOG* 2014;121(10):1197–208.

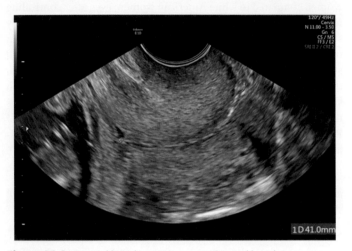

Figure 30.2 Cervical length measurement. Cervical length is defined as the distance between the internal to external os along the endocervical canal.

during the second trimester found that, using ROC curves, the test performs best when a cut off of not more than 20 mm at 24 weeks or less or gestation is used and PTB is defined as less than 35 weeks' gestation. CL can also be plotted on a nomogram of CL in pregnancy (**Figure 30.3**) (36). The advantage of a nomogram is that CL can be plotted serially to ensure CL centiles are being maintained and there is no acute or rapid shortening. One approach is to define a short cervix as less than the third centile, on the nomogram in **Figure 30.3** a CL of 25 mm is below the third centile up to 24 weeks. However, population centiles should be designed specifically for local populations as there is significant variation in the prevalence of women with a short cervix when screening low-risk cohorts for clinical trials.

In women who present with threatened PTL, the resources or skill to perform CL assessment may not be readily available in many units. Therefore, fetal fibronectin (FFN) is frequently the first-line test for prediction of preterm delivery. However, using a CL cut-off of 15 mm or less appears most accurate in predicting spontaneous delivery within 7 days and is associated with a sensitivity and specificity of 74% (95% CI 58–85%) and 89% (95% CI 85–92%), respectively (37). Women with a CL of at least 30 mm or with a CL between 15 and 30 mm with a negative fibronectin result are at low risk (<5%) of spontaneous delivery within 7 days (38).

Fetal fibronectin

Lockwood in 1991 was the first to report an association between FFN and PTB (39). FFN is a glycoprotein that has been described as a biological 'glue' that binds chorion with maternal decidua in the extracellular matrix. After complete fusion of the chorion and decidua at 20 weeks, FFN levels are low (<50 ng/mL) in cervicovaginal secretions

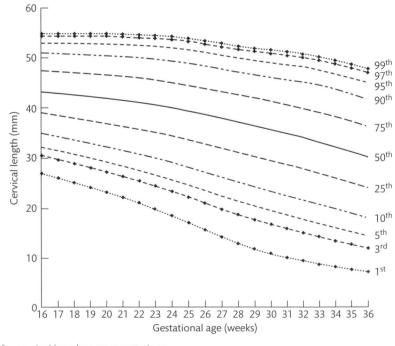

Figure 30.3 Reference ranges for cervical lengths across gestations.

Reproduced from Salomon LJ, Diaz-Garcia C, Bernard JP, Ville Y. Reference range for cervical length throughout pregnancy: non-parametric LMS-based model applied to a large sample. *Ultrasound in Obstetrics & Gynecology: the official journal of the International Society of Ultrasound in Obstetrics and Gynecology.* 2009;33(4):459–64 with permission from John Wiley and Sons.

and are thought to be released through mechanical or inflammatory mediated damage to the membranes before birth. An enzyme-linked immunosorbent assay (ELISA) test against the monoclonal antibody FDC-6 can be used to detect FFN, associated with an increased likelihood of PTB. A concentration of less than 50 ng/mL is considered negative but results may be falsely high if blood is present at the time of taking the test. Although FFN is the best predictor for sPTB at less than 32 weeks even when compared to a short CL (<25 mm) in the asymptomatic population (38), there is not enough evidence to use it as a screening tool as there is currently no preventative treatment with clear benefit. In symptomatic populations, the most advantageous feature of FFN is its high negative predictive value which helps prevent overtreatment with unnecessary antenatal corticosteroids, reduce anxiety, and returns women to normal care pathways. A systematic review demonstrates that the test is most accurate in predicting sPTB within 7–10 days among women with threatened PTB before advanced cervical dilatation, with median likelihood ratios of 5.42 (95% CI 4.36–6.74) (40). Unfortunately the positive predictive value is low (19.7) using a qualitative test (any result >50 ng/mL is considered a positive result), this can be increased to 37.0 or 46.2 using a quantitative test and thresholds of 200 ng/mL or 500 ng/mL respectively. The ability to predict sPTB using TVUS and FFN is improved by concurrent usage (41).

Biomarkers of preterm birth

Biological fluids such as amniotic fluid, blood, cervicovaginal secretions, and saliva are a rich source of protein and metabolites that express the phenotype of gene–environment interactions. Researchers have looked for hundreds of predictive markers but frequently early significant results are not reproducible in validation studies.

In symptomatic women, the phosphorylated insulin-like growth factor binding protein-1 (IGFBP1) test or placental alpha microglobulin 1 (PAMG-1) test are commonly used as alternative predictive bedside tests to FFN, due to comparable negative predictive values (42, 43). These tests are more commonly known as their commercial trade names Actim® Partus and Partosure® respectively. Like FFN detection of these proteins in the cervicovaginal fluid of the posterior fornix indicates a disruption of the choriodecidual interface. Direct comparisons of these tests have been complicated by different study designs and changing or low prevalance of preterm labour between study populations affecting positive and negative predictive values despite stable sensitivities and specificities.

In view of the multiple pathophysiology of PTB, it is unrealistic to expect a single biomarker to be able to predict sPTB in early gestation. The ideal biomarker test or predictive model should try to incorporate the fewest numbers of biomarkers to be measured, be highly sensitive and specific, exist in a biological fluid that is without risk to obtain, and be detectable early enough in pregnancy to allow for preventative measures to be taken.

Prevention of spontaneous preterm birth in singleton pregnancies

Although prediction is key, prevention remains the true goal. Prevention can be classified into primary and secondary preventative strategies. The aim of primary prevention is to lower the incidence of PTB by improving physical and mental well-being and avoiding modifiable behavioural factors associated with PTB. For example, smoking cessation lowers the risk of sPTB by 16% (OR 84%; 95% CI 72–98%) (44). Secondary prevention includes interventions targeted to an at-risk population identified from the general population. At present there are only effective preventative treatments for women identified with a short cervix. As a result, screening clinics have been set up across the United Kingdom to perform TVUS for women at high risk of PTL (45).

17α-hydroxyprogesterone caproate

Progestogens are a class of steroid hormones that bind and activate the progesterone receptor. The role of progestogens in uterine quiescence was first reported in 1954, and they can be classed as natural or synthetic. 17α-hydroxyprogesterone caproate (17-OHPC, often shortened to 17P) is the most investigated synthetic progestogen in the prevention of sPTB. However, the term 'progesterone', a type of natural progestogen, has been erroneously used interchangeably with 'progestogen' for many years. Natural vaginal progesterone and synthetic 17-OHPC (delivered intramuscularly) have very distinct pharmacological and biochemical properties and are not considered to be the same drug (46).

No prior history of PTB, with short or unknown CL

In a low-risk population, with or without a short cervix, no randomized controlled trial (RCT) of 17-OHPC has shown benefit above placebo or a cerclage (short cervix only).

Prior PTB, unknown cervical length

In 463 women with a singleton pregnancy and a history of previous PTB between 20 and 36^{+6} weeks, 17-OHPC 250 mg intramuscularly weekly from 16 weeks was associated with a reduction in incidence of PTB at less than 35 weeks (relative risk (RR) 66%; 95% CI 54–81%), PTB at less than 37 weeks, PTB at less than 32 weeks, as well as intraventricular haemorrhage when compared to placebo (47). Since 2003, 17-OHPC has been recommended routinely for pregnant women in the United States with a singleton gestation (48). In 2011, the US Food and Drug Administration (FDA) approved the use of 17-OHPC during pregnancy to reduce the risk of recurrent PTB in women with a history of prior sPTB. However, the FDA has requested that a second RCT of 17-OHPC versus placebo be conducted before granting full marketing approval under the Food, Drug and Cosmetic Act 505(b).

Prior PTB and short cervical length

In this population, 17-OHPC has only been evaluated in one RCT, which was discontinued after interim analysis ($n = 105$) showed futility in continuing. The PTB rate at less than 37 weeks was 45% in the 17-OHPC arm and 44% in the placebo arm ($P > 0.99$) (49).

Vaginal progesterone

Progesterone is a natural sex steroid produced in pregnancy by the corpus luteum and subsequently the placenta. It plays a key role in maintenance of pregnancy in the first trimester and blocking progesterone receptors (e.g. with RU-486) leads to early pregnancy loss or, if given in the third trimester can result in cervical ripening and sometimes the onset of labour (50).

Short cervix with no prior history of PTB

Fonseca et al. performed an RCT on 250 women of 200 mg nightly vaginal progesterone versus placebo started at 24 weeks in women with a short cervix (CL <15 mm), the majority of whom had no prior history of PTB. There was a significant decrease in sPTB at less than 34 weeks' gestation (19% vs 34%; RR 0.56; 95% CI 0.36–0.86) but no significant effect on neonatal adverse outcome (51). This finding was replicated in a larger trial of 450 women with a CL of 10–20 mm at 19–23[+6] weeks of pregnancy, not only showing a reduction in PTB at less than 33 weeks (9% vs 16%; RR 0.55; 95% CI 0.33–0.92), but also a 43% significant reduction in composite neonatal morbidity and mortality (8% vs 14%; RR 0.57; 95% CI 0.33–0.99) (52).

Prior preterm birth with unknown or normal cervical length

A Cochrane review (53) showed that in women with a previous sPTB, progesterone was associated with a reduction in the risk of perinatal mortality (six studies; 1453 women; RR 0.50; 95% CI 0.33–0.75), PTB less than 34 weeks (five studies; 602 women; average RR 0.31, 95% CI 0.14 to 0.69), and also significant reduction in neonatal morbidity.

Prior PTB and short cervical length

The same Cochrane review has also shown a significant reduction in the risk of PTB at less than 34 weeks in women with a short cervix (<25 mm) and at least one previous PTB (two studies; 438 women; RR 0.64; 95% CI 0.45–0.90) (53). In 2016, OPPTIMUM (54), the largest published clinical trial of vaginal micronized progesterone to date, looked at the effect of progesterone in a heterogeneous group of women all with significant risk factors for sPTB including a previous history of sPTB (77% of participants), a positive FFN test (57%), and/or a short cervix less than 25 mm (36%). Overall, this study showed no association between vaginal progesterone and reduced risk of PTB. However, for women with a singleton pregnancy and a short cervix less than 25 mm, a systematic review and meta-analysis including the results of the OPPTIMUM trial (55) have shown that vaginal progesterone still significantly decreases the risk of PTB at 34 weeks or less or fetal death by 34%. Therefore, clinicians should still offer vaginal progesterone as a treatment for CL of 25 mm or less in singleton pregnancies.

Cervical cerclage

Vaginal cerclage

In 1902, G. Ernest Hermann described the placement of the first three electively placed cervical cerclages through the vaginal route to treat recurrent painless miscarriage resulting in live birth. In 1954 and 1955, MacDonald and Shirodkar respectively described two different methods to place a cerclage for the same indication which became the reference techniques for modern cerclage placement. A MacDonald suture is placed vaginally under a regional or general anaesthetic. Approximately four bites (number of bites can vary) of the cervix are taken to place a purse-string suture as close to the level of the internal cervical os as can be achieved vaginally without suturing the bladder. Several modifications have been made to the original description of the Shirodkar suture which used a portion of fascia lata instead of a suture as a support to the internal os. With a Shirodkar suture the vaginal mucosa is dissected with retraction of the bladder and rectum to expose the cervix at the level of the internal os, achieving a higher placement. The cerclage has to be cut and removed before labour under regional anaesthetic. Evaluation of CL prior to and after cerclage, has shown that CL increases post cerclage, which is also associated with a higher rate of term delivery (56). No benefit of one method of vaginal cervical suture placement over the other has been shown in any RCT or cohort study.

In women with a previous history of PTB, it is unclear whether it is more effective to wait for cervical shortening detected on ultrasound scan or to treat with a history indicated cerclage (HIC). Complications of cervical cerclage include preterm labor, PPROM, chorioamnionitis, cervical trauma, suture displacement and bleeding. The reported rate of chorioamnionitis after HIC is 6.2%, while PPROM ranges from 18% to 38% (57). Therefore, it is important to weigh up individual risks and benefits prior to suture placement.

History-indicated cervical cerclage

Cervical cerclage can be placed because of a prior history of PTB or a previous history of failed elective cervical cerclage (HIC). A history-indicated cerclage is usually placed at 12–13 weeks of pregnancy, once a successful first trimester is completed. The evidence for history-indicated cerclage is much weaker than ultrasound-indicated cerclage and is entirely based on a subgroup analysis of an RCT including just 107 women which showed a decrease in PTB before 33 weeks in women with three or more prior PTB or second-trimester miscarriages (58).

Ultrasound-indicated cerclage–prior preterm birth

In a meta-analysis of five trials of 504 women who were randomized to cerclage placement if they had a previous history of PTB and CL less than 25 mm, before 24 weeks of gestation, PTB less than 37 weeks decreased by 30% and perinatal morbidity and mortality by 36% after cerclage placement (59). However, a Cochrane review of 12 trials involving 3328 women at high risk for PTB showed no statistically significant difference in perinatal deaths despite a similar significant reduction in PTB (average RR 0.80; 95% CI 0.69–0.95; nine trials, 2898 women) (60).

Ultrasound-indicated cerclage–no prior preterm births

In a low-risk singleton population, treatment with a cervical cerclage for a short CL between 16 and 24 weeks has not been shown in any single individual trial (61, 62) to be of benefit in reducing rates of PTB at less than 35 weeks.

Physical exam-indicated cerclage/rescue cerclage

A cerclage placed when (usually) symptomatic women are found to have significant cervical dilatation, detected on vaginal examination, performed either digitally or with a speculum. The evidence remains weak for this practice and there are no long-term safety data to address the effects of keeping a baby to develop in a potentially inflammatory or infected environment. There is only one trial including 23 participants of physical exam-indicated cerclage plus indomethacin versus bed rest alone (63) which drew the conclusion that physical exam-indicated cerclage, indomethacin, antibiotics, and bed rest reduce preterm delivery before 34 weeks' gestation compared with bed rest and antibiotics alone.

Transabdominal cerclage

Vaginal placement of a cervical cerclage has a lower rate of maternal morbidity than placing a cerclage at the level of the internal os through the abdominal route. It is generally reserved for women who have failed a previous vaginal cerclage. A transabdominal cerclage can be sited via (a) open surgery or (b) laparoscopic surgery. Open surgery is performed through a Pfannenstiel incision to the lower abdomen. Currently there are no published RCTs of women receiving abdominal suture but a multicentre randomized trial of high versus low versus abdominal cerclage in women with a previous failed elective stitch shows that transabdominal cerclage is far superior to a repeat vaginal suture (MAVRIC) (64).

Cerclage material

Ongoing clinical trials are looking at the effect of the type of suture used on reduction of PTB rates and particularly infection. Evidence of significant alteration of the vaginal microbiome using a braided suture or tape when compared to a monofilament suggests that monofilament may be better to prevent ascending bacterial infection. The C-STICH trial has been designed to address this question and, at the time of print, is currently recruiting to the study.

Arabin pessary

Pessaries have been used for centuries for the treatment of genital organ prolapse. In 1959, their use was documented in a small case series of women with cervical incompetence or uterus didelphys to take pressure away from the internal cervical os. In the late 1970s, Hans Arabin in West Germany designed a round cone-shaped pessary made of flexible silicone. Its dome-like design resembled the vaginal fornix, with the aim of surrounding the cervix as closely as possible to the internal os. The mechanism of action of the pessary is not completely clear. It has been suggested that after insertion it increases the uterocervical angle, removing direct pressure of the fetal head onto the cervix (65). TVUS images of its use are shown in **Figure 30.4**.

The first randomized trial included 385 women with a CL not greater than 25 mm, and compared Arabin pessary to expectant management. Only 11% of women had previously had a PTB. Spontaneous delivery at less than 34 weeks was significantly less frequent in the pessary group (6%) than the expectant group (27%) (OR 0.18; 95% CI 0.08–0.37) (66). The second trial with the same design was unfortunately underpowered as the rate of short cervix in the screened population was too low (5%) and only recruited 108 women with no significant effect (PTB <34 weeks 9.4% and 5.5%) (67). The largest trial so far randomized 935 women with a short cervix between 20–24 weeks of pregnancy. In this study, all women with a CL less than 15 mm were additionally treated with vaginal progesterone as it was felt unethical to withhold vaginal progesterone from women in view of the previous evidence for its effectiveness. Arabin showed no significant added benefit to being given alongside progesterone (sPTB <34 weeks 12.0% vs 10.8%; OR 1.12; 95% CI 0.75–1.69). There was no benefit in a subgroup of women with mild cervical shortening who were not treated with progesterone (68).

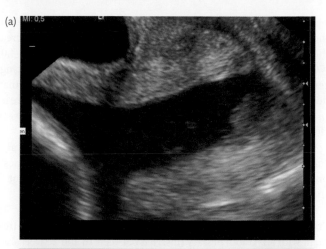

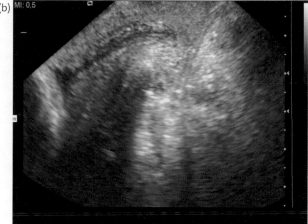

Figure 30.4 Transvaginal sonography of a cervix with U-shaped complete funnelling and sludge in a nulliparous patient at 24 weeks' gestation before (a) and after (b) pessary placement (proximal inner diameter 35 mm, height 21 mm, distal outer diameter 65 mm), showing closer attachment, which suggests normal cervical gland area after placement of pessary. The patient delivered at 37 weeks after pessary removal.

Reproduced from B. Arabin and Z. Alfirevic. Cervical pessaries for prevention of spontaneous preterm birth: past, present and future. *Ultrasound Obstet Gynecol.* 2013 Sep 23; 42(4): 390–399 with permission from John Wiley and Sons.

Prevention of preterm birth in multiple pregnancy

Mechanisms of PTB are likely to overlap with singletons with a higher proportion being related to uterine stretch. However, the same randomized clinical trials into progesterone and cervical cerclage have found considerably different results when compared to singletons. Vaginal progesterone has not shown any decrease in either the rate of PTB at less than 37 weeks nor neonatal morbidity or mortality (53). However, a meta-analysis of individual patient data from twin trials found a 30% non-significant reduction in the rate of preterm birth <33 weeks of gestation (30.4% vs 44.8%; RR 0.70, 95% CI 0.34–1.44), but a statistically significant decrease in the risk of composite neonatal morbidity and mortality (RR 0.52; 95% CI 0.29–0.93) (69).

In asymptomatic twin pregnancies with a CL less than 25 mm, there was initially a suggestion that a cerclage may actually increase the risk of PTB at less than 35 weeks (RR 2.15; 95% CI 1.15–4.01) (70). A more recent Cochrane meta-analysis shows that placing a cerclage is not associated with a significant difference in perinatal death or neonatal morbidity (71). However, overall numbers are low (n = 128) and this area deserves further study before definitive conclusions can be drawn from the data.

Cerclage may still be of use in twin pregnancies where cervical insufficiency is considered to be the cause for recurrent mid-trimester pregnancy loss; however, it should not be used as a treatment for short cervix alone.

Evidence for the use of the Arabin pessary remains unclear. The ProTwin study randomized 813 women with twin pregnancy to treatment with an Arabin pessary (inserted between 16 and 20 weeks' gestation) or to standard treatment (72). Although the pessary did not reduce PTB or the primary neonatal composite outcome overall, both were significantly reduced in the prespecified subgroup of women with a CL less than the 25th centile (n = 143) with a RR of PTB before 32 weeks of 0.49 (95% CI 0.24–0.97) and RR of composite neonatal outcome of 0.42 (95% CI 0.19–0.91). Another study (73) randomized 1180 women at a later stage in pregnancy (20–24^{+6}) to Arabin pessary or no intervention, again there was no significant difference in the rate of sPTB at less than 34 weeks (13.6% vs 12.9%; RR 1.1; 95% CI 0.8–1.4) and a post hoc subgroup analysis of 214 women with a CL less than or equal to 25 mm showed no benefit of insertion of the pessary. The distinct difference between these two trials was the mean gestation at which the Arabin was sited; there is a suggestion that intervention at later gestations may be too late to prevent sPTB. Currently a United Kingdom-led trial, STOPPIT 2, is ongoing to assess the benefit of Arabin pessary in a twin pregnancy population with a short cervix.

Bed rest

Bed rest is not advised to prevent PTB. A Cochrane database meta-analysis concluded that the practice of prescribing antepartum bed rest to prevent PTB should be discontinued until evidence is produced that it is definitely effective. Strict bed rest in pregnancy include adverse side effects such as muscle atrophy, bone loss, maternal weight loss, increased rates of thromboembolism, psychosocial problems including depression, anxiety, and financial burden. However, there is evidence to show that prolonged standing of longer than 3 hours/day, long work hours, and shift work all increase the risk of PTB (OR 1.16–1.29) (74).

Management of acute preterm labour

Confirmation of diagnosis

PTL can present very subtly, particularly in women with cervical insufficiency as painless dilatation can occur without the strong contractions normally associated with labour. In very early gestations, the fetus may pass through only a partially dilated cervix. Therefore PTL must be ruled out in any pregnant woman presenting with abdominal or pelvic symptoms such as pain, increased pelvic pressure, vaginal bleeding, or abnormal vaginal discharge before 37 weeks.

Timely identification of high-risk cases will allow for administration of steroids, tocolytics, and transfer to an appropriate neonatal unit. However, between 70% and 80% of women with symptoms of threatened PTL will continue their pregnancy and deliver at term. As 90% of symptomatic women with threatened PTL will not deliver within 7 days, an accurate diagnosis of PTL should be made before commencing interventions.

When managing a case of threatened PTL, the history of the presenting symptoms should be taken, the gestational age of the pregnancy recorded, and risk factors for PTB evaluated (**Box 30.1**). Other obstetric and non-obstetric causes should also be considered and investigated accordingly.

A physical examination should include vital signs and temperature, an assessment of general well-being, observation of any superficial trauma (particularly to the abdomen), uterine palpation making an assessment of size, tone, tenderness, and the presence of a fetal heart rate should be confirmed.

A speculum examination can be performed to evaluate cervical change, diagnose preterm rupture of the membranes, make an assessment of any bleeding, and take vaginal swabs if there are concerns regarding infection. Unless the cervix is open and the presenting part or bulging membranes can be clearly seen, it is very difficult to make a diagnosis of PTL without further assessment. A sample of urine should be dipstick tested for leucocytes and nitrites, and if positive cultured for antibiotic sensitivities. A positive urine dipstick should not prevent a full assessment for PTL.

If the membranes are intact, the gold standard assessment for prediction of the likelihood of sPTB is measurement of CL with TVUS. TVUS CL greater than 30 mm has a negative predictive value of PTL of 80–100% for PTB at less than 37 weeks and greater than 95% for delivery within 7 days (38). However CL scanning is operator dependent and swab biomarker tests such as FFN, phIGFBP-1 and PAMG-1 are frequently used in the assessment setting for their high negative predictive value.

Symptomatic women with a short CL of less than 15 mm have a risk of 50–57% of delivering within 7 days (41, 75). However, the specificity of TVUS remains poor for women with a CL less than 30 mm and the performance of the test can be improved by the additional use of FFN (41).

Decision on level of intervention

An open discussion with prospective parents regarding potential outcomes and the likelihood of severe handicap is a vital part of management of extreme threatened PTL. Proactive management including tocolysis to allow transfer to a facility with level 1 neonatal care, the use of antenatal steroids, and prompt neonatal resuscitation will increase the likelihood of survival. Ultrasound estimation of fetal weight may help guide management as mortality rates for infants weighing between 400 and 500 g is 83% (75).

Corticosteroids

A single course of antenatal corticosteroids is defined as either betamethasone 12 mg intramuscularly every 24 hours for two doses or dexamethasone 6 mg every 12 hours for four doses. In 1972, the first landmark RCT of antenatal corticosteroids in women at risk of PTB performed was associated with a reduction in neonatal mortality (from 15% to 3.2%) and reduction in RDS (from 25.8% to 9%) (76). Over the following decades further RCTs were performed to replicate these results amid fears that steroid exposure may negatively affect the immune system or alter neurodevelopment. It wasn't until 1990 when Patricia Crowley published the Cochrane review of the 12 RCTs of antenatal corticosteroids showing reductions in neonatal mortality and RDS that it began to be adopted into clinical practice. The most recent Cochrane update still shows significant risk reduction in neonatal death (RR 0.69; CI 0.58–0.81), RDS (RR 0.66; CI 0.59–0.73), cerebroventricular haemorrhage (RR 0.54; CI 0.43–0.69), necrotizing enterocolitis (RR 0.46; CI 0.29–0.74), intensive care admissions, and infections within the first 48 hours of life (77).

Multiple courses of corticosteroids

A Cochrane systematic review of RCTs of women receiving a repeated dose of corticosteroids for risk of PTB at least 7 days after their initial dose (4730 women, 5650 babies) showed a reduced risk of infants having RDS and a reduction in a composite of serious infant outcomes. However, treatment with repeat doses was also associated with a reduction in mean birth weight (mean difference −75.79 g; 95% CI −117.63 to −33.96 g) (78). With no definitive evidence for multiple courses, Cochrane data supports the continued use of only a single course of antenatal corticosteroids to accelerate fetal lung maturation in women at risk of preterm birth (77).

Tocolysis

Tocolytics are medicines given to women in suspected or diagnosed PTL to supress uterine contractions with the aim of delaying birth to improve neonatal outcomes. Comprehensive network meta-analyses have shown tocolytic drugs are effective in delaying delivery by 48 hours and 7 days (79). Despite the general acceptance that neonatal outcomes improve with advancing gestational age at delivery, giving tocolysis has not been shown to significantly improve neonatal outcomes. Tocolytics do, however, allow time for administration of corticosteroids and transfer to a unit with appropriate neonatal care.

It is important to stress that delaying PTB may not always be advantageous to the neonate and there can be detrimental effects of keeping a baby *in utero* in the short term. An overtly septic or inflammatory uterus triggering labour can negatively impact neurodevelopment if the fetus is forced to remain in a 'hostile' environment.

There is considerable variation in clinical practice with respect to the medicinal class, doses, and subgroup of women who receive tocolysis. Additionally, there are very little data for the use of tocolysis before 25 weeks and uncertainty remains over which should be the drug of choice.

Beta-sympathomimetics

Ritodrine and salbutamol were introduced as tocolytics into clinical practice in the 1970s, but are associated with potentially life-threatening side effects. These include pulmonary oedema, myocardial ischaemia, and hyperglycaemia. Since drugs with a better side effect profile are now available, the use of beta-sympathomimetics is now redundant in most high-resource settings.

Oxytocin receptor antagonists

Term labour and PTL are associated with an upregulation of oxytocin receptors in the myometrium. Atosiban is both an oxytocin receptor and a vasopressin receptor antagonist. Unlike other tocolytics it is administered with a bolus injection followed by an intravenous infusion and as a result it is the most expensive tocolytic available. It has a favourable side effect profile with nausea the only statistically significant side effect reported when compared to placebo (OR 2.28; 95% CI 1.26–4.13) (80). Unlike calcium channel blockers, it can be given to hypotensive patients. However, the most recent and largest randomized trial to directly compare atosiban (*n* = 256) and nifedipine (*n* = 249) found similar rates of adverse perinatal outcomes in babies born to women with threatened PTB (81).

Calcium channel blockers

Calcium has a well-recognized role in muscle contractions; reducing calcium influx into cells reduces muscle contractility. Nifedipine is the most widely used drug in this group although it is not currently licensed for this use. The recommended protocol consists of 20 mg orally stat, followed by slow-release 20 mg orally per 6 hours for the following 48 hours. Contraindications include allergy to nifedipine, hypotension, and hepatic dysfunction, and caution should be taken if the woman is using other antihypertensive medications or magnesium. Hypotension is a side effect; however, it is minimal in normotensive patients. Other commonly reported side effects are tachycardia, palpitations, flushing, headaches, dizziness, and nausea. A recent network meta-analysis directly and indirectly comparing all tocolytics using their performance against a common comparator showed that calcium channel blockers were found to be the most clinical and cost-effective treatment overall and have been recommended for use in the most recent National Institute for Health and Care Excellence PTB guideline (82).

Non-steroidal anti-inflammatory drugs/ prostaglandin inhibitors

Indomethacin is the most widely studied non-steroidal anti-inflammatory tocolytic, a non-selective COX inhibitor. It acts by preventing prostaglandin production by inhibiting COX, the enzyme which converts arachidonic acid into prostaglandin. There is concern that COX inhibitors cross the placenta and may interfere with fetal COX production resulting in kidney and cardiac abnormalities such as premature closure of the ductus arteriosus. Its use in clinical practice is typically limited to below 32 weeks' gestation due to fetal concerns. In a recent network meta-analysis of tocolytic agents (79), prostaglandin inhibitors were shown to be more efficacious in delaying delivery by 48 hours when compared with placebo and had a 96% probability of being ranked in the top three most efficacious tocolytics, whereas a Cochrane review (1509 women) showed no clear benefit for COX inhibitors over placebo or any other tocolytic agent. Limitations are recognized due to small numbers and the low quality of studies and there are insufficient data on short- and long-term benefits for COX inhibitors. A larger clinical trial of indomethacin against placebo is expected to finish in June 2018, and may provide a clearer role for indomethacin.

Other tocolytics

Nitric oxide donors, progesterone, and magnesium have all been tested for their possible tocolytic properties.

Nitroglycerine is the only nitric oxide donor to be tested in clinical trials and acts by causing relaxation of the uterine muscle. In a Cochrane meta-analysis including 466 women, nitroglycerine did not prevent prematurity-related outcomes compared with placebo or no treatment (83).

Progesterone is normally used as a prophylactic agent to prevent the onset of PTB; however, it has been used increasingly for acute tocolytic properties. In a randomized, double-blind controlled trial, there was no difference in neonatal morbidity when 200 mg vaginal progesterone was compared with placebo for tocolysis (RR 1.2; 95% CI 0.82–1.8) (84).

Magnesium sulphate is the most commonly used tocolytic in the United States. Extracellularly, it suppresses calcium influx into myometrial cells. Intracellularly, it competes with calcium inhibiting myosin light chain activity. As with other tocolytics contradictory data exist with regards to effectiveness. A Cochrane review failed to prove any delay in PTB when compared with no therapy or placebo (85), but a network meta-analysis found it to be the second most effective drug in delaying PTB for 48 hours (RR 2.76; 95% CI 1.58–4.94) (79). It has a poor side effect profile causing intense flushing and also has to be administered intravenously. Magnesium sulphate is frequently given in PTL for neonatal neuroprotection and there are no known contraindications to giving other tocolytics concomitantly.

Magnesium sulphate for neuroprotection

Preterm babies are at higher risk of poor neurological outcomes including cerebral palsy. It is biologically plausible that magnesium may provide neuroprotection, it is already used to reduce rates of maternal eclamptic seizures and it has been suggested this is due to magnesium's direct haemodynamic effect (86). Blocking voltage-dependent calcium channels in the vascular wall leads to cerebral vasodilatation. For the fetus, this will result in an increased cerebral blood flow possibly counteracting the effects of hypoxia and ischaemia on these tissues. Another mechanism may be related to the anti-inflammatory properties of magnesium causing less apoptosis of cells of the fetal brain (87).

A Cochrane review in 2010 included five large trials (6145 infants) and found a significant reduction in the risk of cerebral palsy (RR 0.68; 95% CI 0.54–0.87). Current guidance recommends magnesium sulphate in cases of threatened PTL with gestational age of less than 32 weeks (88). However more research is required to determine the optimal doses and duration of treatment required to improve outcome.

Management of preterm prelabour rupture of the membranes

PPROM occurs in 2% of all deliveries and accounts for approximately one-third of PTBs. Following PPROM, 50% will deliver within the next 7 days, 75% within 2 weeks, and 85% within the month. As with PTB, the earlier the gestational age at which PPROM occurs, the more negatively this will affect postnatal survival. The presence of amniotic fluid is essential for fetal lung development. Locatelli et al. found that pregnancies with a median residual amniotic fluid pocket persistently less than 2 cm were at highest risk of poor perinatal and long-term neurological outcome while pregnancies with a pocket greater than 2 cm had significantly better perinatal outcome (73–92% survival) and lower pulmonary hypoplasia rates (89, 90).

PPROM prior to viability

Further management following confirmation of PPROM will be dependent on the gestation at which PPROM occurred. Parents require detailed counselling regarding the poor outcomes. Prior to viability (<23 weeks' gestation) there is no evidence to show benefit of antibiotic or corticosteroid use and the options are conservative management or induction of labour. Patients who opt for conservative management may be managed as an outpatient, until the pregnancy reaches viability, if they are asymptomatic of pain or bleeding. Broad-spectrum antibiotics are likely to be of no benefit if the latency period has been a long one and there remain no signs of maternal infection. Corticosteroids should be considered only once viability is reached. AMIPROM, a pilot RCT of amnioinfusion versus expectant management for early PPROM, was the first study to examine outcomes in pregnancies (n = 56) where PPROM occurred between 16 and 24 weeks of pregnancy. The proportion of healthy survivors (without respiratory or neurological disability) was disappointingly only 7% overall. The perinatal mortality rate was extremely high at 67.9%. At present, there is insufficient evidence to recommend amnioinfusion in the management of PPROM and further definitive studies are required (91).

PPROM between 23 and 34 weeks

If PPROM occurs between 23 and 34 weeks' gestation, conservative management is generally adopted if there is no sign of overt chorioamnionitis. Corticosteroids are given in view of the high rate of delivery within 7 days. A vaginal swab for group B *Streptococcus* culture should be taken. Broad-spectrum antibiotics have been evaluated in 22 randomized trials of over 6000 women, classes, doses, and regimens of use show substantial variations but overall, antibiotics improved latency at 48 hours and 7 days, with less chorioamnionitis and a reduction in neonatal morbidity. However there is variation within antibiotics and the largest trial found that ampicillin–clavulanic acid increased rates of necrotizing enterocolitis, and erythromycin alone prolonged pregnancy and reduced the incidence of death and/or major cerebral abnormality and chronic neonatal lung disease (92). Seven-year follow-up of these infants showed no benefit or risk from antibiotic treatment. Therefore,

10 days of erythromycin is given at a dose of 250 mg orally four times a day when PPROM occurs.

PPROM at greater than 34 weeks

If PPROM occurs at or after 34 weeks' gestation, traditionally induction of labour has been recommended due to the low rate of neonatal morbidity and fears that conservative management may increase the risk of infection or uterine cord compression. The largest randomized trial assigning 1839 women to expectant management ($n = 915$) of PPROM versus immediate delivery ($n = 924$) for women with PPROM without signs of infection between 34 and 36^{+6} weeks showed the incidence of neonatal sepsis was not significantly different between the two groups (2% of neonates assigned to immediate delivery vs 3% assigned to expectant management), which has also been reflected in smaller trials (89, 90). Neonates born to mothers in the immediate delivery group had increased rates of respiratory distress syndrome (8% vs 5%), the use of mechanical ventilation (12% vs 9%), and spent more time on special care (median 4.0 days vs median 2.0 days). On the other hand, the expectant management group had higher rates of antepartum/intrapartum haemorrhage, intrapartum fever, postnatal antibiotic use, and longer maternal hospital stay, but a lower risk of caesarean delivery. Therefore, it is reasonable to offer conservative management provided there are no clinical signs of infection and the woman can be adequately monitored as an outpatient.

Mode of delivery

Birth trauma, hypoxia, and metabolic acidosis increase neonatal morbidity and mortality in the preterm infant. Therefore, there have been concerns regarding the best method to manage the second stage of labour when the fetus may be most at risk. In extremely preterm infants, even a partially dilated cervix may allow the fetus to deliver. Due to a disproportionate growth of the head, entrapment of the aftercoming head may occur. At very early gestations, the lower segment of the uterus is not clearly formed and a classical caesarean section, or high transverse incision, may need to be performed. The implications for the next pregnancy include increasing the risk of placenta accreta, uterine rupture, and a repeat caesarean section for delivery. Although caesarean section will reduce intrapartum stillbirths, it is not clear that it improves overall neonatal survival.

A Cochrane meta-analysis of four trials with ($n = 116$) showed less respiratory distress syndrome, less neonatal seizures, and fewer deaths within the caesarean group (93). In contrast, a longitudinal cohort study of women with delivery between 20 and 26 weeks and a subsequent birth, index caesarean delivery ($n = 386$) and index vaginal delivery ($n = 2086$) showed similar risks of composite morbidity (16.1% vs 15.4%; $P = 0.76$) and subsequent haemorrhage (9.6% vs 11.1%; $P = 0.39$). Women with index caesarean were more likely to experience a future uterine rupture (1.8% vs 0.1%; $P < 0.001$), to deliver earlier (35.9 vs 36.9 weeks; $P < 0.001$), and to have lower birth weight (2736 vs 3014 g; $P < 0.001$) subsequently (94). A secondary analysis of a RCT of magnesium sulphate for neuroprotection showed no difference in the 2-year outcomes of babies delivered vaginally ($n = 91$) or by caesarean section ($n = 67$) between 20 and 26 weeks (95).

In later gestations, vacuum delivery should not be used before 34 weeks to assist delivery as the use of ventouse is associated with particularly high rates of subgaleal haematoma (96). Standard use of obstetric forceps is advised should assisted delivery be required.

Conclusion

PTB remains one of the biggest obstetric problems worldwide. Significant advancement has been made in the treatment and care of preterm newborn infants, but little progress has taken place in understanding and better preventing sPTB. The challenge still remains to identify the cause of PTB at an individual level and target therapy accordingly.

REFERENCES

1. Blencowe H, Cousens S, Chou D, et al. Born too soon: the global epidemiology of 15 million preterm births. *Reprod Health* 2013;**10** Suppl 1:S2.
2. Goldenberg RL, Culhane JF, Iams JD, Romero R. Epidemiology and causes of preterm birth. *Lancet* 2008;**371**:75–84.
3. Liu L, Oza S, Hogan D, Chu Y, Perin J, Zhu J, et al. Global, regional, and national causes of under-5 mortality in 2000-15: an updated systematic analysis with implications for the Sustainable Development Goals. Lancet 2016;388(10063):3027–35.
4. McCormick MC. The contribution of low birth weight to infant mortality and childhood morbidity. *N Engl J Med* 1985;**312**:82–90.
5. Mangham LJ, Petrou S, Doyle LW, Draper ES, Marlow N. The cost of preterm birth throughout childhood in England and Wales. *Pediatrics* 2009;**123**:e312–27.
6. Romero R, Dey SK, Fisher SJ. Preterm labor: one syndrome, many causes. *Science* 2014;**345**(6198):760–65.
7. Kazemier BM, Buijs PE, Mignini L, et al. Impact of obstetric history on the risk of spontaneous preterm birth in singleton and multiple pregnancies: a systematic review. *BJOG* 2014;**121**:1197–208.
8. Costeloe KL, Hennessy EM, Haider S, Stacey F, Marlow N, Draper ES. Short term outcomes after extreme preterm birth in England: comparison of two birth cohorts in 1995 and 2006 (the EPICure studies). *BMJ* 2012;**345**:e7976.
9. Marlow N, Bennett C, Draper ES, Hennessy EM, Morgan AS, Costeloe KL. Perinatal outcomes for extremely preterm babies in relation to place of birth in England: the EPICure 2 study. *Arch Dis Child Fetal Neonatal Ed* 2014;**99**:F181–88.
10. Guy A, Seaton SE, Boyle EM, et al. Infants born late/moderately preterm are at increased risk for a positive autism screen at 2 years of age. *J Pediatr* 2015;**166**:269–75.e3.
11. Yee WH, Soraisham AS, Shah VS, et al. Incidence and timing of presentation of necrotizing enterocolitis in preterm infants. *Pediatrics* 2012;**129**:e298–304.
12. World Health Organization. Country statistics and global health estimates by WHO and UN partners 2015. Available at: http://www.who.int/gho/countries/gbr/pdf (accessed 1 March 2016).
13. Boyle EM, Poulsen G, Field DJ, et al. Effects of gestational age at birth on health outcomes at 3 and 5 years of age: population based cohort study. *BMJ* 2012;**344**:e896.
14. Bartha JL, Fernandez-Deudero A, Bugatto F, et al. Inflammation and cardiovascular risk in women with preterm labor. *J Womens Health (Larchmt)* 2012;**21**:643–48.

15. Lapillonne A, Griffin IJ. Feeding preterm infants today for later metabolic and cardiovascular outcomes. *J Pediatr* 2013;**162** Suppl 3:S7–16.

16. Roggero P, Gianni ML, Garbarino F, Mosca F. Consequences of prematurity on adult morbidities. *Eur J Intern Med* 2013;**24**:624–26.

17. McDuffie RS, Jr., Sherman MP, Gibbs RS. Amniotic fluid tumor necrosis factor-alpha and interleukin-1 in a rabbit model of bacterially induced preterm pregnancy loss. *Am J Obstet Gynecol* 1992;**167**:1583–88.

18. Agrawal V, Hirsch E. Intrauterine infection and preterm labor. *Semin Fetal Neonatal Med* 2012;**17**:12–19.

19. Goncalves LF, Chaiworapongsa T, Romero R. Intrauterine infection and prematurity. *Ment Retard Dev Disabil Res Rev* 2002;**8**:3–13.

20. Wing DA, Fassett MJ, Getahun D. Acute pyelonephritis in pregnancy: an 18-year retrospective analysis. *Am J Obstet Gynecol* 2014;**210**:219.e1–6.

21. Parthiban P, Mahendra J. Toll-like receptors: a key marker for periodontal disease and preterm birth—a contemporary review. *J Clin Diagn Res* 2015;**9**:ZE14–17.

22. McDonald CR, Tran V, Kain KC. Complement activation in placental malaria. *Front Microbiol* 2015;**6**:1460.

23. MacIntyre DA, Sykes L, Teoh TG, Bennett PR. Prevention of preterm labour via the modulation of inflammatory pathways. *J Matern Fetal Neonatal Med* 2012;**25** Suppl 1:17–20.

24. Ou CW, Orsino A, Lye SJ. Expression of connexin-43 and connexin-26 in the rat myometrium during pregnancy and labor is differentially regulated by mechanical and hormonal signals. *Endocrinology* 1997;**138**:5398–407.

25. Sooranna SR, Engineer N, Loudon JA, Terzidou V, Bennett PR, Johnson MR. The mitogen-activated protein kinase dependent expression of prostaglandin H synthase-2 and interleukin-8 messenger ribonucleic acid by myometrial cells: The differential effect of stretch and interleukin-1b. *J Clin Endocrinol Metab* 2005;**90**:3517–27.

26. Chen L, Sooranna SR, Lei K, et al. Cyclic AMP increases COX-2 expression via mitogen-activated kinase in human myometrial cells. *J Cell Mol Med* 2012;**16**:1447–60.

27. McLean M, Smith R. Corticotropin-releasing hormone in human pregnancy and parturition. *Trends Endocrinol Metab* 1999;**10**:174–78.

28. Polettini J, Dutta EH, Behnia F, Saade GR, Torloni MR, Menon R. Aging of intrauterine tissues in spontaneous preterm birth and preterm premature rupture of the membranes: a systematic review of the literature. *Placenta* 2015;**36**:969–73.

29. Bennett P. Preterm labour. In: Edmonds DK (ed), *Dewhurst's Textbook of Obstetrics & Gynaecology*, pp. 177–91. Oxford: Blackwell Publishing; 2007.

30. Kyrgiou M, Athanasiou A, Kalliala IEJ, et al. Obstetric outcomes after conservative treatment for cervical intraepithelial lesions and early invasive disease. *Cochrane Database Syst Rev.* 2017;**11**:CD012847.

31. Clausson B, Lichtenstein P, Cnattingius S. Genetic influence on birthweight and gestational length determined by studies in offspring of twins. *BJOG* 2000;**107**:375–81.

32. Porter TF, Fraser AM, Hunter CY, Ward RH, Varner MW. The risk of preterm birth across generations. *Obstet Gynecol* 1997;**90**:63–67.

33. Boyd HA, Poulsen G, Wohlfahrt J, Murray JC, Feenstra B, Melbye M. Maternal contributions to preterm delivery. *Am J Epidemiol* 2009;**170**:1358–64.

34. Capece A, Vasieva O, Meher S, Alfirevic Z, Alfirevic A. Pathway analysis of genetic factors associated with spontaneous preterm birth and pre-labor preterm rupture of membranes. *PloS One* 2014;**9**:e108578.

35. To MS, Skentou CA, Royston P, Yu CK, Nicolaides KH. Prediction of patient-specific risk of early preterm delivery using maternal history and sonographic measurement of cervical length: a population-based prospective study. *Ultrasound Obstet Gynecol* 2006;**27**:362–67.

36. Salomon LJ, Diaz-Garcia C, Bernard JP, Ville Y. Reference range for cervical length throughout pregnancy: non-parametric LMS-based model applied to a large sample. *Ultrasound Obstet Gynecol* 2009;**33**:459–64.

37. Boots AB, Sanchez-Ramos L, Bowers DM, Kaunitz AM, Zamora J, Schlattmann P. The short-term prediction of preterm birth: a systematic review and diagnostic metaanalysis. *Am J Obstet Gynecol* 2014;**210**:54.e1–10.

38. van Baaren GJ, Vis JY, Wilms FF, et al. Predictive value of cervical length measurement and fibronectin testing in threatened preterm labor. *Obstet Gynecol* 2014;**123**:1185–92.

39. Lockwood CJ, Senyei AE, Dische MR, et al. Fetal fibronectin in cervical and vaginal secretions as a predictor of preterm delivery. *N Engl J Med* 1991;**325**:669–74.

40. DeFranco EA, Lewis DF, Odibo AO. Improving the screening accuracy for preterm labor: is the combination of fetal fibronectin and cervical length in symptomatic patients a useful predictor of preterm birth? A systematic review. *Am J Obstet Gynecol* 2013;**208**:233.e1–6.

41. Gomez R, Romero R, Medina L, et al. Cervicovaginal fibronectin improves the prediction of preterm delivery based on sonographic cervical length in patients with preterm uterine contractions and intact membranes. *Am J Obstet Gynecol* 2005;**192**:350–59.

42. Nikolova T, Uotila J, Nikolova N, Bolotshikh VM, Borisova VY, Di Renzo GC. Prediction of spontaneous preterm delivery in women presenting with premature labor: a comparison of placenta alpha microglobulin-1, phosphorylated insulin-like growth factor binding protein-1, and cervical length. *Am J Obstet Gynecol.* 2018;**219**:610.e1–610.e9.

43. Ting HS, Chin PS, Yeo GS, Kwek K. Comparison of bedside test kits for prediction of preterm delivery: phosphorylated insulin-like growth factor binding protein-1 (pIGFBP-1) test and fetal fibronectin test. *Ann Acad Med Singapore* 2007;**36**:399–402.

44. Vanderhoeven JP, Tolosa JE. Tobacco and preterm birth. In: Berghella V (ed), *Preterm Birth: Prevention and Management*, pp. 102–14. Oxford: Wiley-Blackwell; 2010.

45. Sharp AN, Alfirevic Z. Provision and practice of specialist preterm labour clinics: a UK survey of practice. *BJOG* 2014;**121**:417–21.

46. Romero R, Stanczyk FZ. Progesterone is not the same as 17α-hydroxyprogesterone caproate: implications for obstetrical practice. *Am J Obstet Gynecol* 2013;**208**:421–26.

47. Meis PJ, Klebanoff M, Thom E, et al. Prevention of recurrent preterm delivery by 17 alpha-hydroxyprogesterone caproate. *N Engl J Med* 2003;**348**:2379–85.

48. Society for Maternal Fetal Medicine Publications Committee. Use of progesterone to reduce preterm birth. *Obstet Gynecol* 2008;**112**:963–65.

49. Winer N, Bretelle F, Senat MV, et al. 17 alpha-hydroxyprogesterone caproate does not prolong pregnancy or reduce the rate of preterm birth in women at high risk for preterm delivery and a short cervix: a randomized controlled trial. *Am J Obstet Gynecol* 2015;**212**:485.e1–10.

50. Frydman R, Lelaidier C, Baton-Saint-Mleux C, Fernandez H, Vial M, Bourget P. Labor induction in women at term with mifepristone (RU 486): a double-blind, randomized, placebo-controlled study. *Obstet Gynecol* 1992;**80**:972–75.

51. Fonseca EB, Celik E, Parra M, Singh M, Nicolaides KH. Progesterone and the risk of preterm birth among women with a short cervix. *N Engl J Med* 2007;**357**:462–69.

52. Hassan SS, Romero R, Vidyadhari D, et al. Vaginal progesterone reduces the rate of preterm birth in women with a sonographic short cervix: a multicenter, randomized, double-blind, placebo-controlled trial. *Ultrasound Obstet Gynecol* 2011;**38**:18–31.

53. Dodd JM, Jones L, Flenady V, Cincotta R, Crowther CA. Prenatal administration of progesterone for preventing preterm birth in women considered to be at risk of preterm birth. *Cochrane Database Syst Rev* 2013;**7**:CD004947.

54. Norman JE, Marlow N, Messow CM, et al. Vaginal progesterone prophylaxis for preterm birth (the OPPTIMUM study): a multicentre, randomised, double-blind trial. *Lancet* 2016;**387**:2106–16.

55. Romero R, Nicolaides KH, Conde-Agudelo A, et al. Vaginal progesterone decreases preterm birth ≤ 34 weeks of gestation in women with a singleton pregnancy and a short cervix: an updated meta-analysis including data from the OPPTIMUM study. *Ultrasound Obstet Gynecol* 2016;**48**:308–17.

56. Althuisius SM, Dekker GA, van Geijn HP, Hummel P. The effect of therapeutic McDonald cerclage on cervical length as assessed by transvaginal ultrasonography. *Am J Obstet Gynecol* 1999;**180**:366–69.

57. Drassinower D, Poggi SH, Landy HJ, Gilo N, Benson JE, Ghidini A. Perioperative complications of history-indicated and ultrasound-indicated cervical cerclage. Am J Obstet Gynecol. 2011;205:53.e1–53.e5.

58. MRC/RCOG Working Party on Cervical Cerclage. Final report of the Medical Research Council/Royal College of Obstetricians and Gynaecologists multicentre randomised trial of cervical cerclage. *Br J Obstet Gynaecol* 1993;**100**:516–23.

59. Berghella V, Rafael TJ, Szychowski JM, Rust OA, Owen J. Cerclage for short cervix on ultrasonography in women with singleton gestations and previous preterm birth: a meta-analysis. *Obstet Gynecol* 2011;**117**:663–71.

60. Alfirevic Z, Stampalija T, Roberts D, Jorgensen AL. Cervical stitch (cerclage) for preventing preterm birth in singleton pregnancy. *Cochrane Database Syst Rev* 2012;**4**:CD008991.

61. To MS, Alfirevic Z, Heath VC, Cicero S, Cacho AM, Williamson PR, et al. Cervical cerclage for prevention of preterm delivery in women with short cervix: randomised controlled trial. *Lancet* 2004;**363**:1849–53.

62. Rust OA, Atlas RO, Jones KJ, Benham BN, Balducci J. A randomized trial of cerclage versus no cerclage among patients with ultrasonographically detected second-trimester preterm dilation of the internal os. *Am J Obstet Gynecol* 2000;**183**:830–35.

63. Althuisius SM, Dekker GA, Hummel P, van Geijn HP. Cervical incompetence prevention randomized cerclage trial: emergency cerclage with bed rest versus bed rest alone. *Am J Obstet Gynecol* 2003;**189**:907–10.

64. Carter J, Chandiramani M, Seed P, Shennan AH, The MAVRIC Consortium. MAVRIC: Multicentre Abdominal vs Vaginal Randomised Investigation of Cerclage. BJOG 2015;**122**:1–7.

65. Cannie MM, Dobrescu O, Gucciardo L, et al. Arabin cervical pessary in women at high risk of preterm birth: a magnetic resonance imaging observational follow-up study. *Ultrasound Obstet Gynecol* 2013;**42**:426–33.

66. Goya M, Pratcorona L, Merced C, et al. Cervical pessary in pregnant women with a short cervix (PECEP): an open-label randomised controlled trial. *Lancet* 2012;**379**:1800–806

67. Hui SY, Chor CM, Lau TK, Lao TT, Leung TY. Cerclage pessary for preventing preterm birth in women with a singleton pregnancy and a short cervix at 20 to 24 weeks: a randomized controlled trial. Am J Perinatol 2013;30(4):283–8.

68. Nicolaides KH, Syngelaki A, Poon LC, et al. A randomized trial of a cervical pessary to prevent preterm singleton birth. *N Engl J Med* 2016;**374**:1044–52.

69. Romero R, Nicolaides K, Conde-Agudelo A, et al. Vaginal progesterone in women with an asymptomatic sonographic short cervix in the midtrimester decreases preterm delivery and neonatal morbidity: a systematic review and metaanalysis of individual patient data. *Am J Obstet Gynecol* 2012;**206**:124.e1–19.

70. Berghella V, Odibo AO, To MS, Rust OA, Althuisius SM. Cerclage for short cervix on ultrasonography: meta-analysis of trials using individual patient-level data. *Obstet Gynecol* 2005;**106**:181–89.

71. Rafael TJ, Berghella V, Alfirevic Z. Cervical stitch (cerclage) for preventing preterm birth in multiple pregnancy. *Cochrane Database Syst Rev* 2014;**9**:CD009166.

72. Liem S, Schuit E, Hegeman M, et al. Cervical pessaries for prevention of preterm birth in women with a multiple pregnancy (ProTWIN): a multicentre, open-label randomised controlled trial. *Lancet* 2013;**382**:1341–49.

73. Nicolaides KH, Syngelaki A, Poon LC, et al. Cervical pessary placement for prevention of preterm birth in unselected twin pregnancies: a randomized controlled trial. *Am J Obstet Gynecol* 2016;**214**:3.e1–9.

74. Mozurkewich EL, Luke B, Avni M, Wolf FM. Working conditions and adverse pregnancy outcome: a meta-analysis. *Obstet Gynecol* 2000;**95**:623–35.

75. Bruijn M, Vis JY, Wilms FF, et al. Quantitative fetal fibronectin testing in combination with cervical length measurement in the prediction of spontaneous preterm delivery in symptomatic women. *BJOG* 2016;**123**:1965–71.

76. Liggins GC, Howie RN. A controlled trial of antepartum glucocorticoid treatment for prevention of the respiratory distress syndrome in premature infants. *Pediatrics* 1972;**50**:515–25.

77. Roberts D, Brown J, Medley N, Dalziel SR. Antenatal corticosteroids for accelerating fetal lung maturation for women at risk of preterm birth. Cochrane Database Syst Rev. 2017;3(3):CD004454.

78. Crowther CA, McKinlay CJD, Middleton P, Harding JE. Repeat doses of prenatal corticosteroids for women at risk of preterm birth for improving neonatal health outcomes. *Cochrane Database Syst Rev* 2011;**6**:CD003935.

79. Haas DM, Caldwell DM, Kirkpatrick P, McIntosh JJ, Welton NJ. Tocolytic therapy for preterm delivery: systematic review and network meta-analysis. *BMJ* 2012;**345**:e6226.

80. Gyetvai K, Hannah ME, Hodnett ED, Ohlsson A. Tocolytics for preterm labor: a systematic review. *Obstet Gynecol* 1999;**94**:869–77.

81. van Vliet EO, Nijman TA, Schuit E, et al. Nifedipine versus atosiban for threatened preterm birth (APOSTEL III): a multicentre, randomised controlled trial. *Lancet* 2016;**387**:2117–24.

82. National Institute for Health and Care Excellence (NICE). *Preterm Labour and Birth*. NICE guideline [NG25]. London: NICE; 2015.

83. Duckitt K, Thornton S, O'Donovan OP, Dowswell T. Nitric oxide donors for treating preterm labour. *Cochrane Database Syst Rev* 2014;**5**:CD002860.

84. Martinez de Tejada B, Karolinski A, Ocampo MC, et al. Prevention of preterm delivery with vaginal progesterone in women with preterm labour (4P): randomised double-blind placebo-controlled trial. *BJOG* 2015;**122**:80–91.

85. Vogel JP, Nardin J, Dowswell T, West HM, Oladapo OT. Combinations of tocolytic drugs for inhibiting preterm labour. *Cochrane Database Syst Rev* 2014;**7**:CD006169.

86. Scardo JA, Hogg BB, Newman RB. Favorable hemodynamic effects of magnesium sulfate in preeclampsia. *Am J Obstet Gynecol* 1995;**173**:1249–53.

87. Cahill AG, Stout MJ, Caughey AB. Intrapartum magnesium for prevention of cerebral palsy: continuing controversy? *Curr Opin Obstet Gynecol* 2010;**22**:122–27.

88. Vogel JP, Oladapo OT, Manu A, Gulmezoglu AM, Bahl R. New WHO recommendations to improve the outcomes of preterm birth. *Lancet Glob Health* 2015;**3**:e589–90.

89. Locatelli A, Vergani P, Di Pirro G, Doria V, Biffi A, Ghidini A. Role of amnioinfusion in the management of premature rupture of the membranes at <26 weeks' gestation. *Am J Obstet Gynecol* 2000;**183**:878–82.

90. De Carolis MP, Romagnoli C, De Santis M, Piersigilli F, Vento G, Caruso A. Is there significant improvement in neonatal outcome after treating pPROM mothers with amnio-infusion? *Biol Neonate* 2004;**86**:222–29.

91. Roberts D, Vause S, Martin W, et al. Amnioinfusion in very early preterm prelabor rupture of membranes (AMIPROM): pregnancy, neonatal and maternal outcomes in a randomized controlled pilot study. *Ultrasound Obstet Gynecol* 2014;**43**:490–99.

92. Kenyon S, Taylor DJ, Tarnow-Mordi WO, Group OC. ORACLE--antibiotics for preterm prelabour rupture of the membranes: short-term and long-term outcomes. *Acta Paediatr* 2002;**91**:12–15.

93. Alfirevic Z, Milan SJ, Livio S. Caesarean section versus vaginal delivery for preterm birth in singletons. *Cochrane Database Syst Rev* 2012;**13**:CD000078.

94. Lannon SM, Guthrie KA, Reed SD, Gammill HS. Mode of delivery at periviable gestational ages: impact on subsequent reproductive outcomes. *J Perinat Med* 2013;**41**:691–97.

95. Običan SG, Small A, Smith D, Levin H, Drassinower D, Gyamfi-Bannerman C. Mode of delivery at periviability and early childhood neurodevelopment. *Am J Obstet Gynecol* 2015;**213**:578.e1–4.

96. Åberg K, Norman M, Ekéus C. Preterm birth by vacuum extraction and neonatal outcome: a population-based cohort study. *BMC Pregnancy Childbirth* 2014;**14**:1–9.

31

Prolonged pregnancy

Kate F. Walker and Jim G. Thornton

The duration of normal pregnancy

The average pregnancy lasts 40 weeks, or 280 days when measured from the first day of the mother's last menstrual period (LMP). Although conception typically occurs on day 14 of the menstrual cycle, and the 'true' average duration is therefore 266 days, by convention, pregnancies, even those conceived by assisted conception, where there is no LMP and the date of conception is known precisely, are dated from the hypothetical LMP.

Methods for dating pregnancy

The date of the LMP and early scan measurements are both used. If the LMP is uncertain or unknown, the scan will be more accurate. Many authorities suggest that even if the LMP and the menstrual cycle length are known, ultrasound assessment of the crown–rump length before 14 weeks, or the head circumference before 20 weeks, is more accurate. This may well be correct but is almost impossible to prove in modern practice; labour induction based on the agreed due date makes the agreed due date a self-fulfilling prophecy.

Generally, scan dates which are less than menstrual dates are correct because ovulation and conception late in the menstrual cycle is common. Scan dates which are earlier than the menstrual dates by a month or more are also likely to be correct. The issue of scan dates which appear to be 1 or 2 weeks further on than a certain menstrual date is tricky. Ovulation and conception during the LMP or in the first half of the cycle is rare, so it may often be correct to choose the menstrual date as the agreed date in such scenarios.

Variation in the duration of normal pregnancy

The length of gestation is skewed towards preterm delivery. Term is typically regarded as 37^{+0}–42^{+0} and 80% of uninterfered with pregnancies will deliver between these two dates. However, few pregnancies naturally go beyond 43 weeks, while there is a long tail of natural preterm birth right down to 24 weeks. Prolonged pregnancy is defined as a pregnancy that has progressed beyond 42^{+0} weeks. The terms prolonged pregnancy, postdates, and post-term pregnancy are used interchangeably.

Factors causing variation in the length of pregnancy

There is disputed evidence about the relation between parity and length of gestation (1, 2), and there have been claims that it is longer in pregnancies with a male fetus (3). However, given the problems with estimating normality in modern practice with censored data this is probably of little practical importance. Prolonged pregnancy is increased in first pregnancies and in women with a body mass index of greater than 30 kg/m².

Causes of prolonged pregnancy

There are some well-established, albeit fairly uncommon, causes of prolonged pregnancy. Pregnancies with abnormalities in the fetal hypothalamic–pituitary axis, such as anencephaly (4), and pregnancies complicated by the X-linked disease placental steroid sulphatase deficiency (5) are often prolonged. Also, those few extrauterine pregnancies which succeed in obtaining a vascular supply from somewhere in the pelvis and become an advanced abdominal pregnancy also typically fail to go into spontaneous labour.

Risks of prolonged pregnancy

Perinatal risk index

When expressed as risk per 1000 total births, the perinatal mortality rate raises after about 42 weeks (**Figure 31.1**, red circles). But such graphs mislead because the denominator for later deaths includes babies who are already safely delivered. This makes no sense if we are concerned about stillbirth because a delivered baby cannot be stillborn. The correct denominator should be babies still undelivered at the particular gestational age. As this proportion falls after 37 weeks so the risk of stillbirth per undelivered baby starts to rise. But plotting only stillbirth risk is also misleading because babies may also die after birth from complications of labour or prematurity; delivery at 24 weeks would prevent all stillbirths but would hardly be sensible. The most informative data for the risks of prolonged pregnancy the rates of all deaths per 1000 undelivered babies by gestational age at delivery—the perinatal risk index (**Figure 31.1**, blue circles) (6). These show that the safest gestation to be born naturally is between 38 and 39 weeks.

Macrosomia

Although fetal growth tends to level off after about 36 weeks, it is rarely flat. This means that the rate of babies born with a birth weight

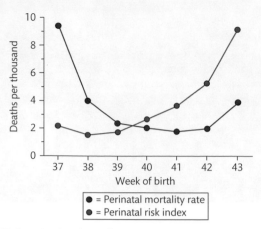

Figure 31.1 Risks of prolonged pregnancy.

over 4000 or 4500 g, that is, macrosomic babies, rises with prolonged pregnancy (7).

Large babies tend to have longer labours, and because the placental reserve tends to fall at later gestational ages they tend to be less able to withstand the stress of labour. This is why there is a measurable increase in caesarean section rates in most settings with each additional week of gestation after 39 weeks. For those postmature babies who deliver vaginally there is also an increased risk of maternal perineal trauma.

Factors associated with increased risks from prolonged pregnancy

If the mother has other complications of pregnancy such as diabetes, hypertension, pre-eclampsia, intrahepatic cholestasis of pregnancy, or fetal growth restriction then the risks associated with prolonged pregnancy are increased. Induction of labour prior to 40 weeks' gestation is commonplace for conditions associated with an increased risk of late antepartum stillbirth.

Fetal growth restriction

Babies weighing less than the tenth centile are at increased risk from prolonged pregnancy than those on or above the tenth centile. In a large, relatively old cohort study of over 400,000 babies comparing term with post-term babies prior to the introduction of a policy of routine induction of labour for prolonged pregnancy, the authors found that of the post-term babies, those less than the tenth centile had an adjusted relative risk of perinatal mortality of 5.68 compared to babies on or above the tenth centile (8).

Diabetes

The association between pregestational diabetes and stillbirth is widely known (9). The perinatal mortality rate for women with pre-existing diabetes (type 1 or 2) is 32 per 1000, compared with 9 per 1000 in the general population. In the United Kingdom, the National Institute for Health and Care Excellence (NICE) recommends that pregnant women with diabetes with a normally grown baby should be offered elective delivery, either by induction of labour or caesarean section if appropriate, from 38 weeks (10).

Past obstetric history

Women who have experienced a stillbirth in their first pregnancy have an increased risk of stillbirth in their second pregnancy (stillbirth rate 16 per 1000 total births) (11).

Advanced maternal age

The overall cumulative risk of antepartum stillbirth throughout gestation (from 20 to 41 completed weeks) for women of all ages is 6.5 per 1000 pregnancies (12). The cumulative risks of stillbirth for women younger than 35 years, 35–39 years, and older than 40 years old were 6.2, 7.9, and 12.8 respectively.

The largest increase in cumulative risk of stillbirth for women over 35 years of age starts at 39 weeks and peaks at 41 weeks. Women over 40 years old have a similar stillbirth risk at 39 weeks as women who are between 25 and 29 years old at 41 weeks, and once they pass 40 weeks' gestation their risk of stillbirth exceeds that of all women less than 40 years old at term (12).

Psychological/social aspects of prolonged pregnancy

Parental preferences

Parental and family views about prolonged pregnancy vary widely. Many people have a strong preference to avoid intervention and are content to allow pregnancy to continue for a long period after the due date. Others place relatively little value on avoiding intervention and become fed up waiting for the birth even in the weeks leading up to the due date. Such opinions are often influenced by the previous experiences of other family members or close friends.

In a prospective questionnaire study of 400 women with uncomplicated pregnancies performed in 1991, completed at 37 weeks and 41 weeks, the authors found that 45% of women at 37 weeks had a preference for conservative management (with serial antenatal monitoring) versus induction of labour if undelivered at 41 completed weeks, falling to 31% of women expressing a preference for conservative management at 41 weeks (13). In a more recent study of 508 women performed in Sweden at 41 weeks, 74% of women preferred to be induced than have serial antenatal monitoring (14). It seems reasonable to conclude therefore that a significant minority of women have a preference for conservative management of prolonged pregnancy.

Treatment/prevention of prolonged pregnancy

Cervical stretch and sweep

Membrane sweeping involves inserting a finger through the cervix and sweeping it round to strip the membranes from the decidua. This causes local release of prostaglandins which sometimes is sufficient to induce labour (15). Randomized trials show that it reduces the chance of not having laboured spontaneously at 48 hours (relative risk (RR) 0.77) and the chance of requiring formal induction of labour (RR 0.60) (16).

Coitus

It is widely believed that penetrative sex with intravaginal ejaculation induces labour. Several plausible mechanisms have been postulated: mechanical pressure on the lower uterine segment, cervical ripening induced by prostaglandin-rich semen, and oxytocin release secondary to orgasm, and observational studies support the idea. The latter suggest that sexual intercourse at term reduces postdates pregnancy (adjusted odds ratio (AOR) 0.28) and the need for postdates induction (AOR 0.28) (17). A rather outdated Cochrane review published in 2001, which included only one trial of 28 women found no differences in delivery within 3 days but was too small to rule out clinically important effects (18).

Induction

Indications for induction

Women with uncomplicated pregnancies are generally given every opportunity to go into spontaneous labour. However, when complications arise either for the mother or the baby whereby delivery is deemed favourable (to either the mother, baby, or both) to continuing the pregnancy then induction of labour is indicated. Examples of indications for induction include prolonged pregnancy, prelabour rupture of membranes (at term and preterm), fetal growth restriction, fetal macrosomia, maternal medical disorders (e.g. pre-existing or gestational diabetes or hypertensive disease), intrauterine fetal death, multiple gestations, advanced maternal age, and even maternal request.

Timing of induction

It is a widely accepted practice in the United Kingdom to offer induction of labour for a pregnancy that continues beyond 41 weeks. This is because the rate of stillbirth increases sixfold from 0.35 per 1000 ongoing pregnancies at 37 weeks to 2.12 per 1000 ongoing pregnancies at 43 weeks (19). The rate of neonatal (up to 28 days) and postneonatal (from 28 days to 1 year of age) mortality falls significantly with advancing gestation up until 41 weeks, when it plateaus and then increases with prolonged pregnancy. As such, the overall risk of pregnancy loss (stillbirth plus death occurring up to the age of 1 year) increases eightfold between 37 weeks and 43 weeks, justifying induction of labour at 41 weeks.

Methods of induction

Traditionally, methods of labour induction have been divided into those which include amniotomy, and therefore irreversibly commit the woman to delivery within a few days, and those which do not, such as vaginal prostaglandins and mechanical methods such as cervical balloons. Many evaluations of the latter describe them as cervical ripening agents for use prior to the definitive labour induction.

Although this is a rather artificial distinction, in that many women labour and deliver after prostaglandins alone, we retain the distinction in what follows.

Prostaglandins

Prostaglandins aid cervical ripening and myometrial contractility and can therefore be used to induce labour. They can be given by a variety of routes: oral, vaginal, intracervical, extra-amniotic, or intravenously. Vaginal preparations of prostaglandins may be in a tablet, gel, or a sustained-release pessary form. Two prostaglandins are in common use: PGE_2 (dinoprostone) and PGE_1 (misoprostol).

PGE_2 is the prostaglandin most commonly used. A systematic review comparing the use of vaginal preparations of PGE_2 with placebo or no treatment for women with an unfavourable cervix, found an increase in successful vaginal delivery rates within 24 hours, an improvement in cervical status within 24 hours, and a reduction in the need for oxytocin augmentation in the treatment group (20). There was no difference in the rate of operative delivery in the two groups.

PGE_1 has also been used for labour induction, although generally 'off label'. This is because until recently no formulations licensed for this indication were available. Instead, drugs licensed for treated gastric ulcer disease, such as Cytotec, were used. Recently, a controlled-release misoprostol formulation has been approved in the European Union and United States. Systematic reviews suggest that misoprostol may have a slightly better efficacy/side effect profile than dinoprostone.

Mechanical methods

Various instruments have been used to mechanically dilate the cervix to allow amniotomy to be performed. Hygroscopic dilators are placed in the cervical canal and work by slowly absorbing water and increasing in size and shape to dilate the cervix mechanically. Foley catheters have also been used.

Hygroscopic dilators Laminaria tents, made from sterile seaweed or synthetic materials (Dilapan), have been compared to prostaglandins for induction of labour and have similar caesarean section rates (RR 1.11; 95% confidence interval (CI) 0.92–1.32) but lower rates of uterine hyperstimulation with fetal heart rate changes (RR 0.13; 95% CI 0.04–0.48).

Balloon catheters Balloon catheters may be used in two ways: (a) inserted through the cervical canal, the balloon is inflated and then traction may or may not be applied, or (b) inserted into the extra-amniotic space and used to instil saline or prostaglandins.

Twenty-three studies comparing balloon catheters with prostaglandins for induction of labour showed similar results to hygroscopic dilators; there were similar rates of caesarean section (RR 1.01; 95% CI 0.90–1.13) and lower rates of uterine hyperstimulation (RR 0.19; 95% CI 0.08–0.43) associated with balloon catheters.

The use of a balloon catheter to infuse saline into the extra-amniotic space when compared to prostaglandins had similar rates of both caesarean section (RR 1.37; 95% CI 0.90–2.08) and uterine hyperstimulation with fetal heart rate changes (RR 0.66; 95% CI 0.30–1.46).

Amniotomy Rupturing the amniotic membrane is performed using an amniotomy hook during a vaginal examination. As mentioned previously, it is more effective as an adjunct in inducing labour when performed following the administration of vaginal prostaglandins. Women with a favourable cervix who have an amniotomy are more likely to require oxytocin augmentation than women who have an amniotomy performed following vaginal prostaglandins. A Drew–Smythe's catheter was used historically to rupture the hind waters in women at high risk of cord prolapse, although concerns about fetal, placental and maternal trauma have rendered it a tool of the past.

Oxytocin

Oxytocin is a hormone secreted by the hypothalamus, then transported to the posterior pituitary from where it is released in a pulsatile manner and acts on oxytocin receptors in the myometrium, causing uterine contractions (21). The frequency and force of contractions is directly proportional to the plasma oxytocin concentration. Oxytocin is given as an intravenous infusion and slowly increased incrementally to achieve three to four contractions in every 10-minute interval. Oxytocin has been used alone, in combination with amniotomy, and following cervical ripening with prostaglandins as an induction agent. One systematic review has compared the effectiveness of oxytocin, when used as a primary agent for induction of labour, in comparison to vaginal prostaglandins. This has shown that when oxytocin is used alone in women with an unfavourable cervix and intact membranes, those women are more likely to have no change to their cervical status after 24 hours, and have a higher risk of needing a caesarean section than women for whom vaginal prostaglandins are used (22). There is insufficient evidence to reach a conclusion whether oxytocin used in combination with amniotomy or vaginal prostaglandins are more likely to result in vaginal delivery within 24 hours (23) but the use of amniotomy and oxytocin in women with a favourable cervix versus vaginal prostaglandins is associated with a significantly increased risk of postpartum haemorrhage (16% vs 2%) and maternal dissatisfaction (RR 53).

Complications of induction

Maternal

Induction of labour is associated with potential complications for the mother and her fetus. Risks to the mother include operative intervention, failure to induce labour, cord prolapse during an amniotomy with a high head, placental abruption with rapid decompression of the uterine cavity at amniotomy, and uterine hyperstimulation. Fortunately, these complications are rare.

Operative intervention It is a commonly held belief that induction of labour results in an increased risk of caesarean delivery. Indeed, examining maternity statistics for England 2010–2011, of those women who laboured spontaneously, 75% achieved a spontaneous vaginal delivery, 12% had an instrumental delivery, and 11% had a caesarean delivery. Of those women who were induced, 59% achieved a spontaneous vaginal delivery, 17% had an instrumental delivery, and 23% had a caesarean delivery. However, it is unscientific to compare these two groups of women, when the reasons for induction of labour (prolonged pregnancy, fetal growth restriction, reduced fetal movements) will all contribute to an increased risk of caesarean delivery.

There is a growing body of evidence that induction of labour at term does not increase emergency caesarean section rates, and does not increase intrapartum deaths.

Cord prolapse Umbilical cord prolapse (UCP) is a rare obstetrical emergency, complicating 1.25–2.1 in 1000 deliveries (24, 25). In one retrospective study of 57 cases over a 10-year period, cord prolapse occurred with amniotomy in 42% of cases (24). However, does amniotomy increase the risk of cord prolapse? A retrospective case–control study of 37 cases of intrapartum UCP and 74 matched control patients with intact membranes found no statistically significant increase in the use of amniotomy in patients who had a cord prolapse (26). A larger retrospective case–control study in which 80 cases of UCP were matched with 800 controls, found that although 63% of the cases of UCP followed amniotomy, in 87% of the control group amniotomy was also performed (27). In 36% of cases of UCP the membranes ruptured spontaneously, while 12% of women in the control group had spontaneous rupture of membranes. They therefore concluded that spontaneous rupture of membranes was associated with a ninefold increase in UCP when compared with amniotomy. A routine policy of amniotomy at 5 cm to accelerate labour at the institution in question, explains the high percentages

of amniotomy seen. In fact, the authors go so far as to advocate early amniotomy to prevent UCP with spontaneous rupture of membranes at a high Bishop score.

Uterine hyperstimulation Uterine hyperstimulation is generally defined as contractions occurring more than five in 10 minutes or contractions lasting more than 2 minutes. It is a complication that arises in 1–5% of cases where pharmacological agents are used to induce labour (15). It may occur with or without fetal heart rate changes. It can also occur in spontaneous labour. During a uterine contraction there is an interruption in the blood flow to the intervillous space where oxygen exchange between the mother and the fetus occurs (28). During the relaxation phase, blood flow is restored. If the interval between contractions reduces or the duration of a contraction increases, then a critical level may be exceeded where fetal hypoxaemia ensues. Simpson et al. found that uterine hyperstimulation was associated with significant fetal oxygen desaturation and non-reassuring fetal heart rate changes (28).

Failed induction of labour There is a lack of consensus in the literature as to what constitutes a failed induction of labour (29). While some authors consider a 'failed induction' to be an induction which doesn't result in a vaginal birth, most consider a failed induction to result either when there is a failure to achieve the active phase of labour following a set period of oxytocin administration, following artificial rupture of the membranes, or an unfavourable cervix despite prostaglandin regimens making artificial rupture of the membranes impossible. NICE defines a failed induction of labour as 'failure to establish labour after one cycle of treatment, consisting of the insertion of two vaginal prostaglandin tablets or gel at 6-hourly intervals or one prostaglandin controlled released pessary over 24 hours' (15).

A recently published randomized controlled trial comparing the efficacy of prostaglandin tablets versus gel found a rate of failed induction (defined as failure of sufficient ripening of the cervix to allow amniotomy following the use of repeated doses of prostaglandin leading to delivery by caesarean section) in primiparous women of 2.78% with gel and 20% with tablets and in multiparous women a rate of 0% with gel and a 16% with tablets (30).

Rouse et al. set out to determine the duration of oxytocin administration following artificial rupture of the membranes, at which if active labour was not achieved, vaginal delivery became unlikely (31). They found that at 6 hours post amniotomy and oxytocin, 14% of nulliparous women remained in the latent phase, of whom 39% went on to deliver vaginally. At 9 hours, 7% remained in the latent phase, of whom 28% went on to deliver vaginally and at 12 hours, 4% remained in the latent phase, of whom 13% then delivered vaginally. Only 4% of nulliparous women had a caesarean section for a failed induction of labour (i.e. lack of cervical dilatation in the latent phase).

Duration There is a paucity of evidence on the duration of active labour in spontaneous versus induced labour. In a retrospective observational study of low-risk women comparing approximately 10,000 women who laboured spontaneously with 1000 women who underwent labour induction for no apparent medical indication, induction was not associated with a prolonged labour. Induction was, however, associated with a longer admission-to-delivery interval and maternal total length of stay was 0.34 days longer with induction compared to spontaneous labour (32).

The findings were similar in a retrospective study of 2681 low-risk multiparous women, where women who were induced had a significantly shorter labour than those who laboured spontaneously (99 vs 161 minutes) (33).

Pain There is evidence that induced labour is more painful than spontaneous labour. United Kingdom data on analgesia in labour reveals that women who have an induced labour are twice as likely to request epidural anaesthesia as women in spontaneous labour (23% vs 11%, NHS Maternity Statistics 2005–2006). A small study ($n = 61$) by Capogna et al. found that the minimum effective analgesic dosage of sufentanil given via an epidural for women with an induced labour was 1.3 times greater than in women with a spontaneous onset of labour ($P = 0.0014$) (34).

Fetal outcomes

Iatrogenic prematurity Most elective caesarean sections are performed at 39 weeks' gestation (35). The timing of this is advised as the risk of neonatal respiratory morbidity falls with advancing gestation until 40 weeks. The risk of respiratory morbidity in infants delivered by elective caesarean at 37 weeks is fourfold higher than infants delivered by mothers intended to have a vaginal delivery at 40 weeks, threefold higher at 38 weeks, and twofold higher at 39 weeks. The risk of developing neonatal respiratory symptoms for babies born by vaginal delivery falls from a probability of 0.07 at 37 weeks to 0.04 at 39 weeks and thereafter plateaus (36). Thus, induction of labour at 39 weeks is the optimal balance between the risk of respiratory morbidity for the neonate and the risk of antepartum stillbirth for the fetus.

Hyperbilirubinaemia There is a reported association between the use of oxytocin in labour and prolonged unconjugated hyperbilirubinaemia in neonates. In a prospective study in Northern India, the use of oxytocin in labour was found to increase the risk of prolonged jaundice in neonates (odds ratio 3.4) (37). In all infants the jaundice disappeared by 8 weeks. However, a randomized controlled trial of the elective use of oxytocin infusion for women using epidural analgesia found no increased risk of neonatal jaundice in the treatment group (38).

Randomized controlled trials of induction

Numerous large, multicentre randomized controlled trials comparing induction of labour with expectant management at term for prelabour rupture of membranes (39), prolonged pregnancies (40), gestational hypertension or mild pre-eclampsia (41), intrauterine growth restriction (42), advanced maternal age (43), and fetal macrosomia (44) found no difference in caesarean section rates between the two groups.

A recent trial of induction of labour at term for women identified as high risk for emergency caesarean section (the higher the risk score, the earlier the induction), found in the treatment group a similar caesarean section rate, a higher uncomplicated vaginal birth rate, and a reduced neonatal intensive care unit admission and adverse outcome rate (45).

Wood et al. published a systematic review of induction of labour versus expectant management in women with intact membranes at term and found that a policy of induction of labour was associated with a 17% reduction in the risk of caesarean section (odds ratio 0.83; 95% CI 0.76–0.92) (46). Two further systematic reviews have confirmed Wood et al.'s findings. Unfortunately, none of the many trials of labour induction around term have followed up either the babies or the mothers longer than the point of discharge from hospital.

Antenatal monitoring

For those women who decline induction of labour for prolonged pregnancy there is no strong evidence supporting an effective monitoring regimen to prevent adverse outcome. Various tests of fetal well-being have been investigated including ultrasound assessment of amniotic fluid, biophysical profile, cardiotocography, formal fetal movement counting, and umbilical artery Doppler velocimetry. NICE recommends that women who decline induction be offered twice-weekly cardiotocography and ultrasound estimation of maximum amniotic pool depth from 42^{+0} weeks onwards (15).

REFERENCES

1. Mittendorf R, Williams MA, Berkey CS, Cotter PF. The length of uncomplicated human gestation. *Obstet Gynecol* 1990;**75**:929–32.
2. Campbell MK, ØStbye T, Irgens LM. Post-term birth: risk factors and outcomes in a 10-year cohort of Norwegian births. *Obstet Gynecol* 1997;**89**:543–48.
3. Divon MY, Ferber A, Nisell H, Westgren M. Male gender predisposes to prolongation of pregnancy. *Am J Obstet Gynecol* 2002;**187**:1081–83.
4. Naeye RL. Causes of perinatal mortality excess in prolonged gestations. *Am J Epidemiol* 1978;**108**:429–33.
5. Rabe T, Hösch R, Runnebaum B. Sulfatase deficiency in the human placenta: clinical findings. *Biol Res Pregnancy Perinatol* 1983;**4**:95–102.
6. Smith GCS. Life-table analysis of the risk of perinatal death at term and post term in singleton pregnancies. *Am J Obstet Gynecol* 2001;**184**:489–96.
7. Stotland NE, Hopkins LM, Caughey AB. Gestational weight gain, macrosomia, and risk of cesarean birth in nondiabetic nulliparas. *Obstet Gynecol* 2004;**104**:671–77.
8. Campbell MK, Ostbye T, Irgens LM. Post-term birth: risk factors and outcomes in a 10-year cohort of Norwegian births. *Obstet Gynecol* 1997;**89**:543–48.
9. Mathiesen ER, Ringholm L, Damm P. Stillbirth in diabetic pregnancies. *Best Pract Res Clin Obstet Gynaecol* 2011;**25**:105–11.
10. National Institute for Health and Clinical Excellence (NICE). *Diabetes in Pregnancy: Management of Diabetes and its Complications from Pre-Conception to the Postnatal Period.* Clinical guideline [CG63]. London: NICE; 2008.
11. Smith G. The relationship between cause and timing of previous stillbirth and the risk of stillbirth in second pregnancies. *Am J Obstet Gynecol* 2012;**206**:S64.
12. Reddy UM, Ko CW, Willinger M. Maternal age and the risk of stillbirth throughout pregnancy in the United States. *Am J Obstet Gynecol* 2006;**195**:764–70.
13. Roberts LJ, Young KR. The management of prolonged pregnancy-an analysis of women's attitudes before and after term. *Br J Obstet Gynaecol* 1991;**98**:1102–106.
14. Heimstad R, Romundstad PR, Hyett J, Mattsson LA, Salvesen KA. Women's experiences and attitudes towards expectant

management and induction of labor for post-term pregnancy. *Acta Obstet Gynecol Scand* 2007;**86**:950–56.

15. National Institute for Health and Clinical Excellence (NICE). *Induction of Labour*. Clinical guideline [CG70]. London: NICE; 2008.

16. Boulvain M, Stan C, Irion O. Membrane sweeping for induction of labour. *Cochrane Database Syst Rev* 2005;**1**:CD000451.

17. Tan PC, Andi A, Azmi N, Noraihan MN. Effect of coitus at term on length of gestation, induction of labor, and mode of delivery. *Obstet Gynecol* 2006;**108**:134–40.

18. Kavanagh J, Kelly AJ, Thomas J. Sexual intercourse for cervical ripening and induction of labour. *Cochrane Database Syst Rev* 2001;**2**:CD003093.

19. Hilder L, Costeloe K, Thilaganathan B. Prolonged pregnancy: evaluating gestation-specific risks of fetal and infant mortality. *Br J Obstet Gynaec* 1998;**105**:169–73.

20. Kelly AJ, Malik S, Smith L, Kavanagh J, Thomas J. Vaginal prostaglandin (PGE2 and PGF2a) for induction of labour at term. *Cochrane Database Syst Rev* 2009;**4**:CD003101.

21. Verrals S. *Anatomy and Physiology Applied to Obstetrics*, 3rd edn. Edinburgh: Churchill Livingstone; 1993.

22. Alfirevic Z, Kelly AJ, Dowswell T. Intravenous oxytocin alone for cervical ripening and induction of labour. *Cochrane Database Syst Rev* 2009;**4**:CD003246.

23. Howarth GR, Botha DJ. Amniotomy plus intravenous oxytocin for induction of labour. *Cochrane Database Syst Rev* 2001;**3**:CD003250.

24. Alouini S, Mesnard L, Megier P, Lemaire B, Coly S, Desroches A. Management of umbilical cord prolapse and neonatal outcomes. *J Gynecol Obstet Biol Reprod (Paris)* 2010;**39**:471–77.

25. Dufour P, Vinatier D, Bennani S, et al. [Cord prolapse. Review of the literature. A series of 50 cases]. *Rev Fr Gynecol Obstet* 1996;**25**:841–45.

26. Roberts WE, Martin RW, Roach HH, Perry KG, Martin JN, Morrison JC. Are obstetric interventions such as cervical ripening, induction of labor, amnioinfusion, or amniotomy associated with umbilical cord prolapse? *Am J Obstet Gynecol* 1997;**176**:1181–83.

27. Dilbaz B, Ozturkoglu E, Dilbaz S, Ozturk N, Sivaslioglu AA, Haberal A. Risk factors and perinatal outcomes associated with umbilical cord prolapse. *Arch Gynecol Obstet* 2006;**274**:104–107.

28. Simpson KR, James DC. Effects of oxytocin-induced uterine hyperstimulation during labor on fetal oxygen status and fetal heart rate patterns. *Am J Obstet Gynecol* 2008;**199**:34.e1–5.

29. Talaulikar VS, Arulkumaran S. Failed Induction of labor: strategies to improve the success rates. *Obstet Gynecol Surv* 2011;**66**:717–28.

30. Taher SE, Inder JW, Soltan SA, Eliahoo J, Edmonds DK, Bennett PR. Prostaglandin E2 vaginal gel or tablets for the induction of labour at term: a randomised controlled trial. *BJOG* 2011;**118**:719–25.

31. Rouse DJ, Owen J, Hauth JC. Criteria for failed labor induction: prospective evaluation of a standardized protocol. *Obstet Gynecol* 2000;**96**:671–77.

32. Glantz JC. Elective induction vs. spontaneous Labor. *J Reprod Med* 2005;**50**:235–40.

33. Hoffman MK, Vahratian A, Sciscione AC, Troendle JF, Zhang J. Comparison of labor progression between induced and noninduced multiparous women. *Obstet Gynecol* 2006;**107**:1029–34.

34. Capogna G, Parpaglioni R, Lyons G, Columb M, Celleno D. Minimum analgesic dose of epidural sufentanil for first-stage labor analgesia: a comparison between spontaneous and prostaglandin-induced labors in nulliparous women. *Anesthesiology* 2001;**94**:740–44.

35. National Institute for Health and Care Excellence (NICE). *Caesarean Section*. Clinical guideline [CG132], updated 2019. London: NICE; 2011.

36. Heinzmann A, Brugger M, Engels C, et al. Risk factors of neonatal respiratory distress following vaginal delivery and caesarean section in the German population. *Acta Paediatr* 2009;**98**:25–30.

37. Gundur NM, Kumar P, Sundaram V, Thapa BR, Narang A. Natural history and predictive risk factors of prolonged unconjugated jaundice in the newborn. *Pediatr Int* 2010;**52**:769–72.

38. Shennan AH, Smith R, Browne D, Edmonds DK, Morgan B. The elective use of oxytocin infusion during labour in nulliparous women using epidural analgesia: a randomised double-blind placebo-controlled trial. *Int J Obstet Anesth* 1995;**4**:78–81.

39. Hannah ME. Induction of labor compared with expectant management for prelabor rupture of the membranes at term. *N Engl J Med* 1996;**334**:1005–10.

40. Gülmezoglu AM, Crowther CA, Middleton P. Induction of labour for improving birth outcomes for women at or beyond term. *Cochrane Database Syst Rev* 2006;**4**:CD004945.

41. Koopmans CM, Bijlenga D, Groen H, et al. Induction of labour versus expectant monitoring for gestational hypertension or mild pre-eclampsia after 36 weeks' gestation (HYPITAT): a multicentre, open-label randomised controlled trial. *Lancet* 2009;**374**:979–88.

42. Boers KE, Vijgen SMC, Bijlenga D, et al. Induction versus expectant monitoring for intrauterine growth restriction at term: randomised equivalence trial (DIGITAT). *BMJ* 2010;**341**:c7087.

43. Walker KF, Bugg GJ, Macpherson M, et al. Randomized trial of labor induction in women 35 years of age or older. *N Engl J Med* 2016;**374**:813–22.

44. Boulvain M, Senat MV, Perrotin F, et al. Induction of labour versus expectant management for large-for-date fetuses: a randomised controlled trial. *Lancet* 2015;**385**:2600–605.

45. Nicholson JM, Parry S, Caughey AB, Rosen S, Keen A, Macones GA. The impact of the active management of risk in pregnancy at term on birth outcomes: a randomized clinical trial. *Am J Obstet Gynecol* 2008;**198**:511.e1–15.

46. Wood S, Cooper S, Ross S. Does induction of labour increase the risk of caesarean section? A systematic review and meta-analysis of trials in women with intact membranes. *BJOG* 2014;**121**:674–85.

32

Malpresentation, malposition, and cephalopelvic disproportion

Deirdre J. Murphy

Introduction

An understanding of fetal malpresentation, malposition, and cephalopelvic disproportion (CPD) is required by every obstetrician and midwife in order to provide safe and effective care in labour. Deviations from normal of the fetal lie, presentation, or position may be apparent in the late antenatal period but in many cases the diagnosis only becomes apparent during the course of labour. A diagnosis of CPD may be suspected in advance of labour but can only be confirmed reliably as labour progresses. Recognition of the aetiological factors that contribute to these abnormalities provides an opportunity for risk assessment which may facilitate preventative strategies. Timely diagnosis is essential for appropriate intervention and overall management. Fetal malpresentation, malposition, and CPD are associated with increased maternal and fetal morbidity—this applies in well-resourced healthcare settings and to an even greater degree in low-resource settings.

Definitions

Fetal lie

The fetus lies within the uterus and is defined in terms of its relationship to maternal anatomical parts. The lie refers to the longitudinal axis of the fetus in relation to the longitudinal axis of the mother. With a longitudinal lie, either the fetal head or breech will be presenting. With a transverse lie, the longitudinal axis of the fetus is perpendicular to the longitudinal axis of the mother. The fetal shoulder or back present or there may be an arm, cord, or placenta presenting. An oblique lie is oriented diagonally and will usually revert to a longitudinal or transverse lie as labour ensues.

Fetal presentation

The presentation refers to the part of the fetus that enters the pelvis first. A cephalic presentation is where the fetal head enters the pelvis first and when the chin is flexed onto the chest it is referred to as a vertex presentation, with the occiput as the leading point descending within the pelvis. The attitude refers to the degree of flexion of the fetal head in relation to its spine, and in normal labour a vertex presentation will be well flexed. Asynclitism refers to an oblique tilt of the vertex with the anterior or posterior parietal bone preceding the sagittal suture. In normal labour there will be minimal asynclitism.

Fetal position

The fetal position is defined as the relationship between the denominator of the presenting part and the maternal pubic symphysis, which is anterior. The denominator is the part of the fetus that defines this relationship and is a fixed bony part. The fetal position changes during the course of labour and the final position at the pelvic outlet determines the relative ease of delivery. The denominator for a vertex presentation is the occiput and in normal labour the optimal position at the pelvic outlet will be occipitoanterior (OA).

Mechanism of normal labour

The mechanism of normal labour refers to a series of changes in position and attitude that the fetus undergoes during its passage through the birth canal. This process is essential so that the optimal diameters of the fetal skull are present at each stage of descent. An understanding of the physiological and anatomical principles involved in labour is best summarized using the '3 Ps' which are the powers, the passages, and the passenger. The 'powers' refers to forces: firstly, the contractions of the uterine muscle that result in propulsion of the fetus through the birth canal, and secondly, the maternal effort of pushing in the second stage of labour. The 'passages' refers to the birth canal itself, which is made up of the bony pelvis, the muscles of the pelvic floor, and the soft tissues of the perineum. The 'passenger' refers to the fetus in terms of its size, presentation, and position. When the 3 Ps are favourable, normal labour is likely to result in a spontaneous vaginal birth with minimal morbidity.

Engagement

The fetal head normally enters the pelvis in a transverse position (more commonly to the left) taking advantage of the widest pelvic diameter. Engagement is said to have occurred when the widest part of the presenting part has passed successfully through the inlet. This occurs in the majority of nulliparous women prior to labour, usually by 37 weeks' gestation, and often later for multiparous women. The number of fifths of the fetal head palpable abdominally is used to describe whether engagement has taken place. If more than two-fifths of the fetal head is palpable abdominally, the head is not engaged.

Descent

Descent of the fetal head is needed before flexion, internal rotation, and extension can occur. During the first stage and passive phase of the second stage of labour, descent of the fetus occurs as a result of uterine contractions. In the active phase of the second stage of labour, further descent of the fetus is assisted by voluntary efforts of the mother using her abdominal muscles and the Valsalva manoeuvre ('active pushing').

Flexion and internal rotation

The fetal head is not always completely flexed when it enters the pelvis. As the head descends into the narrower mid pelvis, flexion occurs. This passive movement occurs, in part, due to the surrounding structures and reduces the presenting diameter of the fetal head. If the head is well flexed, the occiput will be the leading point and on reaching the sloping gutter of the levator ani muscles, it will be encouraged to rotate anteriorly so that the sagittal suture now lies in the anteroposterior (AP) diameter of the pelvic outlet (i.e. the widest diameter).

Extension

Following completion of internal rotation, the occiput is beneath the symphysis pubis and the anterior fontanelle (bregma) is near the lower border of the sacrum. The well-flexed head now extends and the occiput escapes from underneath the symphysis pubis and distends the vulva. This is known as 'crowning' of the head. The head extends further and the anterior fontanelle, face, and chin appear in succession over the posterior vaginal opening and perineal body.

Restitution and external rotation

When the head is delivering, the occiput is directly anterior. As soon as it crosses the perineum, the head aligns itself with the shoulders, which have entered the pelvis in an oblique position. This slight rotation of the occiput through one-eighth of the circle is called 'restitution'. In order to be delivered, the shoulders have to rotate into the direct AP plane (widest diameter at the outlet). When this occurs, the occiput rotates through a further one-eighth of a circle to the transverse position. This is called external rotation.

Delivery of the shoulders and fetal body

When restitution and external rotation have occurred, the shoulders will be in the AP position at the pelvic outlet. The anterior shoulder is under the symphysis pubis and delivers first, and the posterior shoulder delivers subsequently. Normally the rest of the fetal body is delivered easily.

Contributors to abnormal labour

When any of the 3 Ps are unfavourable, labour is likely to be abnormal, resulting in the need for intervention, and an increased risk of morbidity or mortality. Malpresentation, malposition, and CPD are important contributors to abnormal labour and are associated with the following factors:

- Powers:
  - Inefficient uterine activity
  - Inefficient pushing
- Passages:
  - Uterine abnormality—septum, bicornuate uterus, and fibroids
  - Pelvic abnormality—android/anthropoid/platypelloid shape, fractures, and rickets
  - Pelvic floor relaxation—epidural analgesia
  - Placenta praevia
- Passenger:
  - Prematurity
  - Small-for-gestational age/growth-restricted fetus
  - Large-for-gestational age/macrosomic fetus
  - Fetal congenital abnormality
  - Multifetal pregnancy
  - Polyhydramnios.

Malpresentation

Malpresentation refers to any presentation of the fetus other than vertex and includes face, brow and breech, shoulder or back presentation with a transverse lie, and compound presentations with more than one part presenting. The most commonly encountered malpresentation is breech which is discussed in detail in Chapter 33. A firm application of the fetal presenting part on to the cervix is necessary for good progress in labour. A face presentation applies poorly to the cervix and the progress in labour may be slow, although vaginal birth is still possible. Brow presentation is associated with the mentovertical diameter presenting, which is simply too large to fit through the bony pelvis unless flexion occurs to a vertex presentation or hyperextension to a face presentation (**Figure 32.1**). Brow presentation therefore often manifests as poor progress in the first stage of labour, typically in a multiparous woman. Malpresentations relating to an abnormal or unstable lie are often diagnosed and managed prior to the onset of labour. Shoulder presentation cannot deliver vaginally and poor progress will occur if labour proceeds, together with an increased risk of arm or cord prolapse and uterine rupture.

Aetiology

Malpresentations are more common in women of high parity, presumably due to laxity of the uterine muscle and abdomen. They are more common with polyhydramnios and extremes of fetal size, and with multifetal pregnancy (1, 2). They may occur as a result of a uterine malformation such as a bicornuate uterus or uterine septum or in the context of an abnormally located placenta. They may occur as a result of a fetal congenital abnormality such as anencephaly.

Diagnosis

The lie and presentation of the fetus should be determined in the first instance by clinical assessment using the standard approach of inspection, palpation, and auscultation. A transverse or oblique lie and breech presentation should be readily detectable or suspected

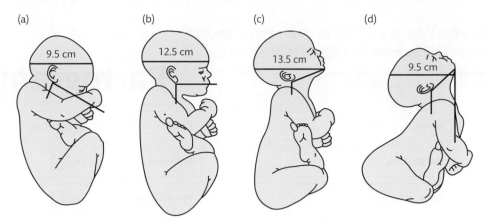

Figure 32.1 Fetal skull dimensions. (a) Flexed vertex presentation—suboccipitobregmatic diameter 9.5 cm. (b) Deflexed occipitoposterior position—occipitofrontal diameter 11.5 cm. (c) Brow presentation—mentovertical diameter 13.5–14.0 cm. (d) Face presentation—submentobregmatic diameter 9.5 cm.
Reproduced from KP Hanretty, *Obstetrics Illustrated*, 7e., Churchill Livingstone 2009, with permission from Elsevier.

clinically. The findings can be confirmed by ultrasonography which has a higher sensitivity and specificity than clinical assessment alone (3) (Table 32.1). A clinical diagnosis of face or brow presentation is usually only suspected for the first time in labour. With a brow presentation, the fetal head may palpate as unengaged abdominally and the orbital ridges and bridge of the nose will be felt on digital vaginal examination with a prominent anterior fontanelle. Abdominal examination of a face presentation may be unremarkable but on digital vaginal examination the orbits, nose, and mouth will be felt with no palpable sutures. It may take a minute or two to differentiate a face presentation from a breech presentation.

Table 32.1 Use of ultrasonography for fetal assessment in labour

Indication	Evidence summary
Confirm presentation	
Singleton preterm	Accepted practice
Multiple pregnancy (especially twin 2)	Accepted practice
Clinical uncertainty	Observational data
Estimate fetal weight/gestational age	
Unbooked patient	Mainly observational data
Threshold of viability/preterm	Accepted practice
Suspected small fetus	Accurate for low birth weight
Suspected large fetus	Inaccurate for macrosomia
Fetal head in the first and second stage of labour	
Engagement and station	Limited data with different techniques used
Descent	Limited data with different techniques used
Position	Observational and RCT data
Cord abnormalities	
Nuchal cord	Limited data
Vasa praevia	Case reports
Placenta	
Placental location	Accepted practice

The partogram may give important diagnostic clues. In nulliparous labour there may be primary arrest or slow progress despite good contractions. In multiparous labour, a secondary arrest or arrest in the second stage of labour warrants early assessment by an experienced obstetrician due to the increased risk of uterine rupture (Figure 32.2). In any of these circumstances, the possibility of a breech, face, or brow presentation should be considered. Ultrasonography may also be helpful in confirming the findings.

Prevention

External cephalic version is the accepted approach to preventing breech presentation in labour. The options for preventing face, brow, shoulder, or compound presentations are less clear and encompass watchful waiting and timely rupture of membranes (4). With a transverse or oblique lie it is usually best to wait until full term or until the lie and presentation have stabilized prior to considering delivery. More than half will convert to a longitudinal lie and cephalic presentation with expectancy (5). Some obstetricians will offer a stabilizing induction of labour with preparations in place in case of cord prolapse or procedural failure requiring immediate caesarean section. Delayed decision-making with a transverse or oblique lie in labour can result in an arm, cord, or compound presentation that might have been prevented by a more timely decision for a caesarean section (Figure 32.3).

In terms of preventing a face or brow presentation, it is best to avoid rupturing the membranes with a high fetal head as the process of flexion takes place during descent of the presenting part within the pelvis. Mobilization, upright positions, and use of a birthing ball may encourage descent in these circumstances. Similarly, for a second twin it is best to wait for the fetal head to descend well into the pelvis prior to rupturing the membranes if a brow, face, or a compound presentation is to be avoided. An oxytocin infusion may facilitate this process.

Management

Face presentation

The incidence of face presentation is approximately 1 in 500 to 1 in 600 births. The presenting diameter is the submentobregmatic

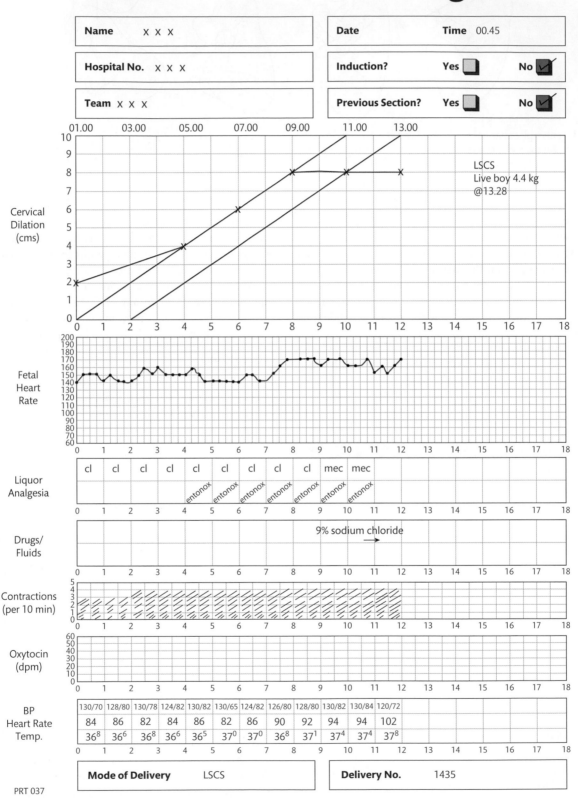

Figure 32.2 Partogram demonstrating secondary arrest in labour.

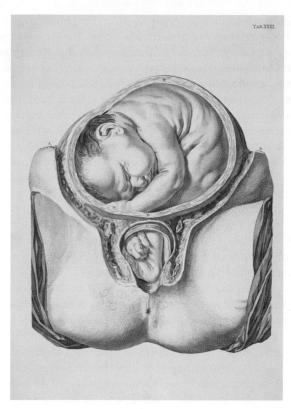

Figure 32.3 Compound presentation (transverse lie).
RCOG Library.

which measures 9.5 cm, similar to a vertex presentation, and as such the labour may not differ greatly from vertex labour (6). Expectancy is the usual approach aiming for a spontaneous vaginal delivery. The mother should be warned that the baby's face may be swollen or bruised at the time of birth but should revert to normal over the following days. The fetal head needs to rotate to a mentoanterior position for vaginal delivery to be achieved. Forceps delivery can be used in a mentoanterior position applying the same safety criteria as for vertex deliveries (**Figure 32.4**). Fetal blood sampling, fetal scalp electrodes, and vacuum extraction are contraindicated. If the position remains mentoposterior, delivery should be by caesarean

section as it is not possible for the fetal head to extend further into the sacrum to allow delivery of the chin (7).

Brow presentation

The incidence of brow presentation is approximately 1 in 700 to 1 in 1000 births. The presenting diameter is the mentovertical which measures 13.5–14.0 cm in term fetuses and usually exceeds the capacity of the pelvis. In most cases this will result in arrested progress in the first stage of labour and delivery by caesarean section. If diagnosed in early labour, expectancy may result in flexion to a vertex presentation or complete extension to a face presentation, both of which may result in vaginal delivery. However, arrested progress in multiparous women and in women with a previous caesarean section requires particular caution as continuing with labour in the context of obstruction could result in uterine rupture. Some authors report success with manual rotation from brow to vertex presentation at full dilatation with a high rate of vaginal delivery (8). This should only be performed by experienced obstetricians under regional anaesthesia and with immediate access to an operating theatre.

Back or shoulder presentation

It is not possible for a term baby in a back or shoulder presentation to deliver vaginally and an early decision should be made to perform a caesarean section if labour starts. Caesarean section for a transverse lie is challenging, particularly with the fetal back down, and requires manipulation of the fetus in order to grasp a leg, aiming to deliver as a breech. This may result in extension of the uterine incision with maternal haemorrhage and/or trauma to the fetus (9). It is one of the potential indications for a classical caesarean incision.

Some authors report success with external version using tocolysis in the intrapartum management of the transverse lie (10). The success rate of conversion to a cephalic presentation is high (75%) but the caesarean section rate in labour is higher than that of vertex presentation from the outset. Nonetheless, caesarean section may be avoided in half the cases where external version is attempted. Internal podalic version in labour is associated with an increased risk of uterine rupture and should be avoided (11). Very preterm fetuses at the limits of viability may present with the back or shoulder deep in the pelvis at full dilatation and gentle manipulation to a

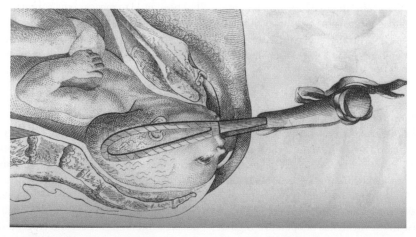

Figure 32.4 Face presentation—mentoanterior forceps delivery.
RCOG Library.

cephalic presentation may result in spontaneous vaginal delivery rather than a technically challenging and potentially traumatic caesarean section.

Compound presentation

Compound presentation occurs more commonly with preterm labour, vaginal delivery of a second twin, or with an abnormal lie (**Figure 32.3**). There may be a fetal head or breech presenting together with an arm or leg, or the cord may present alongside the presenting part. At full cervical dilatation, it may be possible to manipulate the fetus or await descent of the fetal head/breech, and vaginal delivery can be achieved. In term pregnancies, a fetal hand may be palpated alongside the fetal head in the first stage of labour. In the first instance this can be managed expectantly and in many cases the hand will retract as labour progresses and the larger head descends. In some cases, the arm may prolapse through the cervix in which case an urgent caesarean section needs to be performed. These deliveries require advanced obstetric skill in terms of both decision-making and operative delivery.

Malposition

The malpositions associated with a vertex presentation include occipitoposterior (OP) or occipitotransverse (OT) and arrested progress may result from a persistent OP position or deep transverse arrest. The chin (mento) is the denominator for a face presentation and a mentoanterior position is suitable for spontaneous vaginal delivery. Persistent mentotransverse or mentoposterior positions are likely to result in obstructed labour and delivery by caesarean section. For breech presentation, the fetus can deliver vaginally in the optimal sacroanterior position but is considered a malposition if orientated in a sacroposterior position, as the fetal head will be orientated in an OP position following delivery of the body.

If the fetus has engaged in an OP position, internal rotation can occur from an OP to an OA position. This long internal rotation may explain the increased duration of labour associated with OP position. Alternatively, an OP position may persist, resulting in a 'face to pubes' spontaneous delivery. However, the persistent OP position may be associated with deflexion of the fetal head and a resulting increase in the diameter presenting to the pelvic outlet (**Figure 32.1**). This may lead to obstructed labour and the need for instrumental delivery or caesarean section. A deep transverse arrest may occur as a result of a head that has engaged in the transverse position and fails to rotate to OA or a head that engages in an OP position and only partially rotates to OT.

Aetiology

The aetiologies of vertex malposition (OP and OT) are represented by each of the 3 Ps. The fetal head may fail to rotate due to inefficient uterine activity in the first or second stage of labour or insufficient maternal expulsive efforts in the active second stage. This may be precipitated or aggravated by supine positioning of the mother and/or use of epidural analgesia. A Cochrane systematic review reports an average 14-minute increase in the duration of the second stage of labour and 1.4-fold increase in the incidence of operative vaginal delivery (OVD) with use of epidural analgesia in labour (odds ratio (OR) 1.42; 95% confidence interval (CI) 1.28–1.57) (12).

The shape and dimensions of the maternal pelvis have an important contributory role in fetal malposition. The gynaecoid pelvis with a round shape, well-curved sacrum, and subpubic arch of approximately 90 degrees is the preferred shape for labour and an android-, anthropoid-, or platypelloid-shaped pelvis may lead to failure of engagement, descent, or rotation (**Figure 32.5**). Epidural analgesia is thought to relax the pelvic floor musculature and reduce the maternal urge to push which may lead to incomplete flexion and rotation of the presenting part. The extremes of fetal size may contribute to fetal malposition; a very large fetus with relative disproportion may rotate with difficulty and a small fetus may engage with a deflexed attitude or with marked asynclitism that limits spontaneous rotation.

Diagnosis

Vaginal examination during the course of labour allows a systematic assessment of the fontanelles and sutures of the fetal head. The anterior fontanelle is larger, softer, and has four radiating sutures in comparison to the posterior fontanelle which is smaller, firmer, and has three radiating sutures. It should be possible to diagnose OT and OP positions and to define the orientation in terms of direct, right, or left. Examination is more difficult in the context of marked caput, moulding, a high presenting part, maternal obesity, or poor analgesia. Asynclitism results in an oblique orientation of the presenting part and is often associated with malposition. This can complicate assessment, as the sagittal suture will be deviated from the midline to the right or the left for OA–OP positions and deviated superiorly or inferiorly for left OT–right OT positions (13).

The partogram may provide important clues to suggest a malposition. As with malpresentation, there may be primary arrest or slow progress despite good contractions in nulliparous labour. A secondary arrest or arrest in the second stage of labour should raise suspicion of a malposition in both nulliparous and multiparous women (**Figure 32.2**).

The role of ultrasonography in labour has developed in recent years and it is particularly useful when there is clinical uncertainty about the fetal head position (14) (**Table 32.1**). A multicentre randomized controlled trial (RCT) reported a 20% error rate in the clinical diagnosis of the fetal head position immediately prior to instrumental delivery that was reduced to 1.6% with the use of ultrasonography (15) (**Figure 32.6**). Three-dimensional ultrasonography has been used to measure the subpubic arch demonstrating an association between a narrow arch and a higher risk of persistent posterior occiput position at birth (16). The ultimate confirmation of the fetal head position is at the time of birth and this should be documented at emergency caesarean section to help explain the need for operative delivery.

Prevention

Although it is logical to promote maternal positions that widen the pelvic diameters and increase gravitational forces, there is little evidence that manoeuvres such as 'all fours' used prophylactically reduce the incidence of OP or OT positions at delivery (17). However, a systematic review that assessed the benefits and risks of the use of different positions during the second stage of labour reported a reduced duration of the second stage: a weighted mean reduction in duration of 16.9 minutes (95% CI 14.3–19.5 minutes) and a reduction in assisted births (relative risk (RR) 0.84; 95% CI 0.73–0.98) (18).

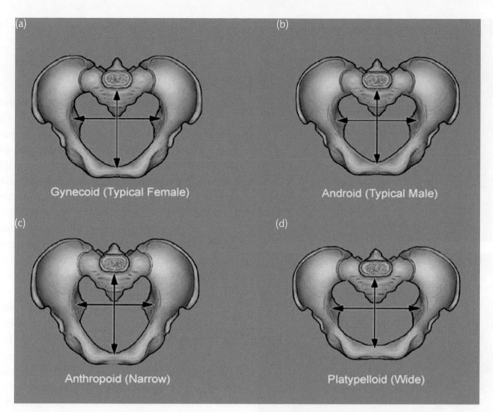

Figure 32.5 Pelvic shapes. (a) Gynaecoid pelvis—'round female shape' favourable for vaginal delivery (50% women). Inlet transverse diameter greater than AP, shallow cavity, short ischial spines, and wide subpubic arch. (b) Anthropoid pelvis—'long oval shape' vaginal delivery possible, favours OP (25% white/40% black women), AP greater than transverse, long narrow canal and sacrum, and wide subpubic arch. (c) Android pelvis—'male heart shape' unfavourable for vaginal delivery (20% women). Narrow inlet, prominent ischial spines, and narrow transverse outlet and subpubic arch. (d) Platypelloid pelvis—'kidney shape' 'unfavourable for vaginal delivery (5% women). Pelvic inlet transverse diameter much greater than AP, sacral promontory pushed forward.

Avoiding epidural analgesia will eliminate the epidural-associated risks of malrotation; however, for women who choose regional analgesia, a passive phase of at least 1 hour should be encouraged to facilitate descent and rotation of the fetal head (19–22). Judicious use of oxytocin should be considered where contractions dissipate; however, an RCT evaluating routine use of oxytocin during the second stage of labour in nulliparous women using epidural analgesia demonstrated a reduction in the operative delivery rate but only when the occiput was anterior (23).

Manual rotation has been explored as a strategy to correct fetal malpositions and is recommended in the guideline of the Society of Obstetricians and Gynaecologists of Canada (24). A large, retrospective cohort study reported a reduction in caesarean delivery associated with the use of manual rotation (9% vs 41%; P <0.001) with no difference in either birth trauma or neonatal acidaemia for neonates who had experienced an attempt at manual rotation versus those who had not (25). Given these data, manual rotation of the fetal occiput for malposition in the second stage of labour warrants further evaluation as a potential preventative strategy.

Management

Fetal malposition in the first stage of labour may result in prolonged labour, a greater need for oxytocin augmentation, and regional analgesia. If progress arrests in the first stage of labour despite standard interventions, the only option is delivery by caesarean section. Fetal malposition in the second stage of labour may be overcome by watchful waiting, use of oxytocin, and prolonged maternal pushing. Some babies will deliver successfully in the OP position 'face to pubes' but only very small babies can deliver vaginally in an OT position. Failure to progress in the second stage of labour with a malposition will require obstetric intervention.

Operative vaginal delivery versus caesarean section

Malposition in the mid pelvis presents the obstetrician with a choice between a potentially difficult OVD and caesarean section at full dilatation, each with inherent risks. The obstetrician must balance the risks of neonatal and maternal morbidity, early and late morbidity, and the potential consequences for future pregnancies. Although there is a published protocol for a Cochrane systematic review comparing OVD with caesarean section for difficult deliveries in the second stage of labour, as yet there have been no RCTs addressing this important question. In current practice, the decision relies on observational data, national guidelines, experience, judgement, and clinical skill (21, 22, 24, 26).

In a United Kingdom-based prospective cohort study of women transferred to theatre for second-stage arrest, two-thirds of whom had a malposition, it was possible to achieve delivery by vacuum or forceps in half the cases (27). The success rate was significantly higher among experienced operators. Caesarean section was associated with an increased risk of major haemorrhage (adjusted odds ratio (aOR) 2.8; 95% CI 1.1–7.6) and prolonged hospital stay (aOR 3.5; 95% CI 1.6–7.6). High rates of obstetric anal sphincter injury

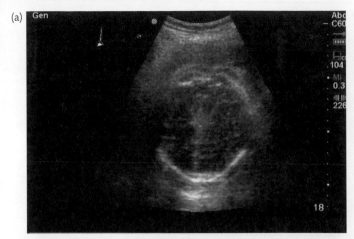

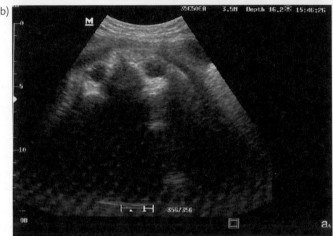

Figure 32.6 Fetal orbits and nose indicating an occipitoposterior position. This image has been taken on a portable ultrasound machine on the labour ward during labour.

(8%) were reported following OVD and there was a threefold increased risk of urinary incontinence at 3 years compared to second-stage caesarean section (28). The comparable morbidity at caesarean section related to extension of the uterine incision into the cervix, vagina, or broad ligaments (24%) and a far higher repeat caesarean section rate in subsequent pregnancies (79% vs 31%) (29).

There is inconsistency in the reported early neonatal morbidity when comparing OVD with caesarean section in the second stage of labour. In the prospective cohort study described earlier, delivery by caesarean section was associated with an increased risk of admission to the special care baby unit (aOR 2.6; 95% CI 1.2–6.0); however, neonatal trauma was significantly less common (aOR 0.4; 95% CI 0.2–0.7) (27). Reassuringly, a 5-year follow-up of the cohort reported low overall rates of neurodevelopmental morbidity with comparable outcomes for each mode of delivery (30). These findings suggest that neonatal complications can be minimized with careful selection of cases for attempted OVD.

Fetal malposition is highlighted in many studies as a risk factor for failed OVD and as such, precautions should be taken to provide immediate access to emergency caesarean section should it be required. The additional time taken to transfer a woman to an operating theatre needs to be balanced with the consequences of a failed attempt at OVD in a delivery room (31). This issue is addressed in

clinical practice guidelines and has been described traditionally as a 'trial of instrumental delivery' (21).

Manual rotation versus rotational vacuum versus rotational forceps

Malposition in the second stage of labour requires both rotation and traction if vaginal delivery is to be achieved. These processes occur simultaneously with rotational vacuum delivery and are consecutive with rotational forceps and manual rotation followed by direct traction forceps. Some operators will choose to deliver an OP position with direct traction forceps 'face to pubes'; however, given the wider presenting diameter, this is a more traumatic delivery with a higher incidence of OASI and should only be contemplated when the vertex is very low in the pelvis. The choice between forceps or vacuum delivery will depend on the operator's competence and preference for the clinical circumstances (32) (**Box 32.1**). As with any OVD, safety criteria have to be met and clear stopping rules should be observed (21, 22).

Successive systematic reviews of RCTs comparing vacuum and forceps report that use of the vacuum extractor is associated with significantly less maternal trauma (OR 0.41; 95% CI 0.33–0.50) (33). However, vacuum failure rates of between 20% and 30% have been reported in two RCTs comparing different vacuum devices, and failure of vacuum delivery was three to four times more likely with a fetal malposition (34, 35). Two United Kingdom-based observational studies compared rotational vacuum, manual rotation with traction forceps, and Kielland's rotational forceps, and reported similar maternal and neonatal morbidity rates but a higher failure rate with attempted rotational vacuum delivery (36, 37). A further

---

Box 32.1 Mid-pelvic rotational delivery

Having judged that attempting OVD is suitable, the following factors influence the selection of a particular method.

- Select manual rotation and traction forceps if:
  - good analgesia
  - rotational movement is possible
  - descent of fetal head with maternal effort
  - birth canal is roomy
  - absence of signs of true CPD.
- Select Kielland's forceps if:
  - dense regional block
  - descent of fetal head with maternal effort
  - birth canal is roomy
  - absence of signs of true CPD.
- Select vacuum (with metal cup or Kiwi OmniCup) if:
  - no dense regional block
  - good maternal effort
  - descent of fetal head with maternal effort
  - no significant caput/moulding
  - no signs of true CPD.
- A method should only be used if the operator is adequately trained.
- The operator should use the instrument he or she prefers.
- Mother's preferences should be taken account of where appropriate.
- Vacuum contraindicated at gestational age <34 weeks and face presentation.
- Fetal status in itself should not determine the choice of instrument.
- There is no evidence that any one instrument leads to quicker delivery.

study compared rotational vacuum, rotational forceps, and second-stage caesarean section applying a propensity score analysis and reported similar outcomes irrespective of mode of delivery (38). The use of Kielland's rotational forceps has decreased in popularity reflecting concerns about morbidity but perhaps more realistically as a result of the need for greater obstetric skill. Greater attention is now being paid to manual rotation which is a skill that encompasses both assessment and intervention (24). An updated Cochrane review places a greater emphasis on choosing an appropriate instrument based on differing risks and benefits (39).

Cephalopelvic disproportion

CPD refers to anatomical disproportion between the fetal head and maternal pelvis. It may be due to a large head, a small pelvis, or a combination of the two relative to each other. True or absolute CPD is where disproportion cannot be overcome and safe vaginal delivery is not possible. Relative CPD is where the degree of disproportion results in slow or arrested progress due to a 'tight fit' that may be overcome by persistent maternal effort or by OVD. Relative CPD may occur as a result of a malposition and can be corrected by rotation of the fetal head. Differentiating between arrested progress due to a malpresentation, malposition, or CPD can be challenging and requires clinical experience and expertise.

Aetiology

Women of short stature (<1.60 m) with a large baby in their first pregnancy are potential candidates to develop this problem. The pelvis may be unusually small because of previous fractures, metabolic bone disease, or nutritional factors such as rickets. Rarely, a fetal anomaly will contribute to CPD. Obstructive hydrocephalus may cause macrocephaly (abnormally large fetal head), and fetal thyroid and neck tumours may cause extension at the fetal neck. Relative CPD is more common and occurs with malpositions of the fetal head. The OP position is associated with deflexion of the fetal head and presents a larger skull diameter to the maternal pelvis (**Figure 32.1**). Fetal macrosomia (e.g. with diabetes in pregnancy) may result in relative or absolute CPD, as indeed may any fetus that is large in proportion to the mother's pelvis.

Diagnosis

CPD should be suspected, particularly in a nulliparous woman, when the head fails to engage at term and the fetus palpates as large. The diagnosis of absolute CPD in labour is clinical. The fetal head will remain palpable abdominally, the vertex on vaginal examination will be above the ischial spines, and there will be marked caput and moulding. Labour is likely to arrest in the first stage, but when full dilatation is reached, these findings preclude any attempt at OVD and delivery will be by caesarean section. The difficulty arises with the correct diagnosis of relative CPD which should be considered with the following features:

- Fetal head is slow to engage.
- Fetus palpates large relative to the maternal size.
- Progress is slow or arrests despite efficient uterine contractions.
- Vaginal examination shows early moulding and caput formation.
- Head is poorly applied to the cervix.

- Progressive oedema of the cervix.
- Haematuria.

As with malpresentation and malposition, the partogram may give clues to the presence of CPD. There may be primary arrest or slow progress despite good contractions in nulliparous labour, and secondary arrest or arrest in the second stage of labour should raise suspicion of potential CPD in both nulliparous and multiparous women (**Figure 32.2**).

Prevention

X-ray pelvimetry has been used in the past to determine the various dimensions of the pelvic inlet, mid pelvis, and outlet, primarily to inform the delivery method for breech presentation or birth after caesarean section. This practice was largely discontinued due to the poor predictive value of pelvimetry for successful vaginal delivery (40). Magnetic resonance imaging and three-dimensional ultrasonography have been evaluated in observational studies but have not been implemented at a population-based level to determine which women are likely to encounter obstructed labour as a result of CPD. Prevention is currently based on case selection with an individualized approach to offering caesarean section, for example, to women who have diabetes in pregnancy complicated by fetal macrosomia. A recent multicentre RCT reported that induction of labour from 38 weeks' gestation compared to expectant management for women with large-for-gestational age fetuses (abdominal circumference >95th percentile) resulted in less traumatic injuries without an increase in delivery by caesarean section (41). It now seems appropriate to offer selected women with large fetuses an induction of labour at term in the interests of avoiding additional fetal weight gain and the potential for CPD.

Management

The principles for managing suspected CPD are similar to that of malposition. In the first stage of labour when progress arrests due to suspected CPD, the only delivery option is caesarean section. Use of an oxytocin infusion may be indicated in nulliparous women with inefficient uterine activity but extreme caution is required in the multiparous woman with secondary arrest or in women with a previous caesarean section, as attempts to overcome the obstruction of CPD with powerful uterine activity could result in uterine rupture, with all its consequences. In the second stage of labour, the operator must decide between attempted OVD and caesarean section, and if OVD is attempted the decision must be made on where to conduct the delivery and which instrument to use (32).

Failed OVD

In an ideal world, there would be no failed vacuum or forceps deliveries, only successfully completed OVDs and appropriately conducted second-stage caesarean sections. In the real world, the diagnosis of CPD is often unconfirmed until there has been an attempt to apply traction with a correctly positioned instrument during a contraction with maternal pushing. Some obstetricians choose not to do this and have abandoned mid-pelvic OVD entirely in favour of caesarean section (26, 42). Other obstetricians will attempt to apply their skills in appropriate circumstances with careful attention to a back-up plan should the attempt be unsuccessful (27, 37, 38).

The Royal College of Obstetricians and Gynaecologists (RCOG) guidelines emphasize that there should be progressive descent with each pull of a correctly applied instrument and that the total number of pulls should be limited (21, 43). With forceps delivery, it will be clear on the first or second pull whether or not CPD is relative or absolute and the delivery can be completed safely or abandoned accordingly. With vacuum extraction, the impression of descent can be more difficult to appreciate but certainly the procedure should be discontinued if the head has not reached the perineum by the third pull. Various studies have shown that a failed attempt at OVD in a setting where immediate recourse to caesarean section is available does not increase the maternal or neonatal morbidity and attempted mid-pelvic OVD will be successful in approximately half the selected cases (27, 38, 44). Nonetheless, every obstetrician should have a clear understanding of appropriate stopping rules and in the event of an abandoned attempt at OVD, the fetal head should be disimpacted to facilitate safe delivery by caesarean section.

Sequential instrument use

Vacuum extraction has become the instrument of choice in many settings and among the majority of obstetricians in training. This has important implications for the management of mid-pelvic arrest with a suspicion of relative CPD. In the prospective cohort study of women with complex deliveries transferred to theatre for arrested progress in the second stage of labour, attempted forceps was more likely to result in completed vaginal delivery than attempted vacuum (63% vs 48%; P <0.01) (27). The difficulty with attempted vacuum delivery is that it may be possible to bring the fetal head low onto the pelvic floor but not to complete the delivery. The decision then has to be made whether or not to complete the delivery by lift-out forceps or by caesarean section.

The use of sequential instruments (vacuum and forceps) has been associated with scalp trauma, intracranial haemorrhage, and neonatal death, and also with an increased risk of maternal morbidity (45–47). These risks need to be weighed up with the significant morbidity associated with performing a caesarean section with the fetal head visible at the perineum (21). In the event that the delivery is completed vaginally, the possibility of shoulder dystocia and postpartum haemorrhage should be considered. In the event that it is completed by caesarean section, strategies to deal with an impacted fetal head and extension of the uterine incision should be anticipated. If speed is of the essence, particularly in the presence of suspected fetal hypoxia, then there is a higher chance of completed OVD with forceps as a single instrument than vacuum, thereby avoiding both the risks of sequential use of instruments and unnecessary delay (31, 45).

Risk management issues

Malpresentation, malposition, and CPD often result in prolonged labour and operative delivery and as such, feature disproportionately in obstetric litigation. Specific risk events include failed OVD, sequential use of instruments, and complicated second-stage caesarean section. Adverse outcomes include perinatal death, cerebral palsy, brachial plexus injury, and pelvic floor morbidity. Causation may relate to a delay in delivery, the conduct of the delivery, or a combination of both. Although morbidity is an inherent risk of abnormal labour, the decision-making processes and conduct of the delivery must stand up to scrutiny at a later date. Good practices at both an individual and organizational level are central to safe delivery, and regular audit should be undertaken to ensure that best practice is maintained (21).

The following issues need to be addressed:

1. *Communication*: good communication is essential before, during, and after operative delivery. An open and positive approach is important in building rapport with the woman and her partner. Professionalism should be maintained at all times, particularly in the context of complications. The obstetrician should review the woman during the postnatal period and offer to schedule a debrief visit at a later date to discuss delivery-related events if required. Inexperienced staff should be supported by senior obstetricians throughout this process and where appropriate should be included in difficult consultations.

2. *Consent*: informed consent should be obtained from the woman after explicit counselling regarding the indication, benefits and risks, and nature of any procedures. Where possible, the birth plan/preferences of the mother should be taken into account and discussed. Verbal consent should be documented as a minimum but written consent is recommended for a 'trial of instruments' in theatre or for caesarean section.

3. *Documentation*: it is essential that the indication for operative delivery, clinical assessment, conduct of the delivery, outcome for mother and baby, and consent process is documented clearly in the medical records. Particular attention should be paid to accuracy and consistency of recorded timings and to legibility of names and signatures. Paired cord blood samples should be processed and recorded in all cases. The use of a structured pro forma, such as the document recommended by the RCOG, reduces the likelihood of incomplete documentation but is not a substitute for documenting the decision-making process (21). The findings at caesarean section and after a failed attempt at OVD should be clearly recorded to inform the decision-making process for future births.

4. *Outcome recognition*: complications will occur and most prospective parents recognize this. However, failure to recognize that a complication has occurred results in anger, upset, complaints, and in some cases litigation. It is essential that obstetricians who perform complex operative deliveries have the skills to recognize and manage pelvic floor injuries and surgical complications. Neonates should be assessed by personnel with the expertise to recognize and manage brachial plexus injury, fractures, intra- and extracerebral haemorrhage, and the consequences of hypoxia.

5. *Incident reporting*: where adverse events occur, these should be reported through the local incident reporting procedures. Every unit should have a risk management structure in place to ensure that adverse events are dealt with in an appropriate and timely manner.

Global perspective

Women who lack access to skilled antenatal and intrapartum care are particularly vulnerable to the adverse consequences of malpresentation, malposition, and CPD. In low-resource settings, where infrastructure and transport are limited, women may present in advanced obstructed labour. This may be exacerbated by nutritional compromise, comorbidities such as malaria, and inability to pay for healthcare. It may result in fetal death, maternal death, or delivery with significant morbidity such as a rectovaginal or vesicovaginal fistula. In the emergency care setting, every attempt should be made to complete a safe delivery for the mother and baby with attention to the cultural and personal importance of preserving future fertility.

Conversely, in high-resource settings there are women who experience intense disappointment following a first birth experience who are willing to take conventionally unacceptable risks in a subsequent birth; for example, homebirth involving attempted vaginal birth after caesarean section with fetal macrosomia. Every effort should be made to regain the trust of these women so that they access expert obstetric care if complications arise during the course of their pregnancy or labour that predispose them to an adverse delivery outcome (48).

Conclusion

The management of malpresentation, malposition, and CPD require obstetric skill that spans the antenatal, intrapartum, and postnatal periods. Imaging by ultrasonography provides useful information but should only be used in conjunction with careful clinical assessment. The dynamic process of labour, particularly in the context of secondary arrest and arrest in the second stage of labour, requires sound diagnostic skills and expertise in both OVD and complex caesarean section. Contingency planning is essential and in many cases this will be an indication for reassessment in an operating theatre. Recourse to OVD, sequential use of instruments, or caesarean section should be individualized to the specific clinical circumstances, the skill of the obstetrician, and wherever possible the preferences of the mother.

REFERENCES

1. Bashiri A, Burstein E, Bar-David J, Levy A, Mazor M. Face and brow presentation: independent risk factors. *J Matern Fetal Neonatal Med* 2008;**21**:357–60.
2. Arsene E, Langlois C, Garabedian C, Cloqueur E, Deruelle P, Subtil D. Prenatal factors related to face presentation: a case-control study. *Arch Gynecol Obstet* 2016;**294**:279–84.
3. Nassar N, Roberts CL, Cameron CA, Olive EC. Diagnostic accuracy of clinical examination for detection of non-cephalic presentation in late pregnancy: cross sectional analytic study. *BMJ* 2006;**333**:578–80.
4. Stitely ML, Gherman RB. Labor with abnormal presentation and position. *Obstet Gynecol Clin North Am* 2005;**32**:165–79.
5. Phelan JP, Boucher M, Mueller E, McCart D, Horenstein J, Clark SL. The nonlaboring transverse lie. A management dilemma. *J Reprod Med* 1986;**31**:184–86.
6. Duff P. Diagnosis and management of face presentation. *Obstet Gynecol* 1981;**57**:105–12.
7. Schwartz Z, Dgani R, Lancet M, Kessler I. Face presentation. *Aust N Z J Obstet Gynaecol* 1986;**26**:172–76.
8. Verspyck E, Bisson V, Gromez A, Resch B, Diguet A, Marpeau L. Prophylactic attempt at manual rotation in brow presentation at full dilatation. *Acta Obstet Gynecol Scand* 2012;**91**:1342–45.
9. Kolas T, Oian P, Skjeldestad FE. Risks for peroperative excessive blood loss in cesarean delivery. *Acta Obstet Gynecol Scand* 2010;**89**:658–63.
10. Phelan JP, Stine LE, Edwards NB, Clark SL, Horenstein J. The role of external version in the intrapartum management of the transverse lie presentation. *Am J Obstet Gynecol* 1985;**151**:724–26.
11. Skelly HR, Duthie AM, Philpott RH. Rupture of the uterus: the preventable factors. *S Afr Med J* 1976;**50**:505–509.
12. AnimSomuah M, Smyth RM, Jones L. Epidural versus non-epidural or no analgesia in labour. *Cochrane Database Syst Rev* 2011;**12**:CD000331.
13. Malvasi A, Barbera A, Di Vagno G, Gomovsky A, Berghella V, Ghi T, Di Renzo GC, Tinelli A. Asynclitism: a literature review of an often forgotten clinical condition. *J Matern Fetal Neonatal Med* 2015;**28**:1890–94.
14. Ramphul M, Murphy DJ. Role of ultrasound on the labor ward. *Expert Rev Obstet Gynecol* 2012;**7**:615–25.
15. Ramphul M, Ooi PV, Burke G, Kennelly MM, Said SA, Montgomery AA, Murphy DJ. Instrumental delivery and ultrasound: a multicentre randomised controlled trial of ultrasound assessment of the fetal head position versus standard care as an approach to prevent morbidity at instrumental delivery. *BJOG* 2014;**121**:1029–38.
16. Ghi T, Youssef A, Martelli F, *et al.* A narrow subpubic arch angle is associated with a higher risk of persistent posterior occiput position at birth. *Ultrasound Obstet Gynecol* 2016;**48**:511–15.
17. Hunter S, Hofmeyr GJ, Kulier R. Hands and knees posture in late pregnancy or labour for fetal malposition (lateral or posterior). *Cochrane Database Syst Rev* 2007;**4**:CD001063.
18. Gupta JK, Hofmeyr GJ. Position for women during second stage of labour. *Cochrane Database Syst Rev* 2003;**3**:CD002006.
19. Roberts CL, Torvaldsen S, Cameron CA, Olive E. Delayed versus early pushing in women with epidural analgesia: a systematic review and meta-analysis. *Br J Obstet Gynaecol* 2004;**111**:1333–40.
20. National Institute for Health and Care Excellence (NICE). *Intrapartum Care: Care of Healthy Women and their Babies during Childbirth*. Clinical guideline [CG190]. London: NICE; 2014.
21. Royal College of Obstetricians and Gynaecologists (RCOG). *Operative Vaginal Delivery*. Green-top Guideline No. 26. London: RCOG; 2011.
22. American College of Obstetricians and Gynecologists. Operative vaginal delivery use of forceps and vacuum extractors for operative vaginal delivery. *ACOG Practice Bull* 2000;**17**:1–6.
23. Saunders NJ, Spiby H, Gilbert L, et al. Oxytocin infusion during second stage of labour in primiparous women using epidural analgesia: a randomized double blind placebo controlled trial. *BMJ* 1989;**299**:1423–26.
24. Cargill YM, MacKinnon CJ, Arsenault MY, et al. Guidelines for operative vaginal birth. Clinical Practice Obstetrics Committee. *J Obstet Gynaecol Can* 2004;**26**:747–61.
25. Shaffer BL, Cheng YW, Vargas JE, Caughey AB. Manual rotation to reduce caesarean delivery in persistent occiput posterior or transverse position. *J Matern Fetal Neonatal Med* 2011;**24**:65–72.
26. Tempest N, Navaratnam K, Hapangama DK. Does advanced operative obstetrics still have a place in contemporary practice? *Curr Opin Obstet Gynecol* 2015;**27**:115–20.
27. Murphy DJ, Liebling RE, Verity L, Swingler R, Patel R. Cohort study of the early maternal and neonatal morbidity associated with operative delivery in the second stage of labour. *Lancet* 2001;**358**:1203–207.
28. Bahl R, Strachan B, Murphy DJ. Pelvic floor morbidity at three years after instrumental delivery and caesarean section in the

second stage of labor and the impact of a subsequent delivery. *Am J Obstet Gynecol* 2005;**192**:789–94.

29. Bahl R, Strachan B, Murphy DJ. Outcome of subsequent pregnancy three years after previous operative delivery in the second stage of labour—cohort study. *BMJ* 2004;**328**:311–14.

30. Bahl R, Patel RR, Swingler R, Ellis N, Murphy DJ. Neuro developmental outcome at 5 years after operative delivery in the second stage of labor: a cohort study. *Am J Obstet Gynecol* 2007;**197**:147.e1–6.

31. Murphy DJ, Koh DM. Cohort study of the decision to delivery interval and neonatal outcome for 'emergency' operative vaginal delivery. *Am J Obstet Gynecol* 2007;**196**:145.e1–7.

32. Bahl R, Murphy DJ, Strachan B. Decision making in operative vaginal delivery: when to intervene, where to deliver and which instrument to use? Qualitative analysis of expert practice. *Eur J Obstet Gynecol Reprod Biol* 2013;**170**:333–40.

33. Johanson RB, Menon BK. Vacuum extraction versus forceps for assisted vaginal delivery. *Cochrane Database Syst Rev* 2000;**2**:CD000224.

34. Attilakos G, Sibanda T, Winter C, Johnson N, Draycott T. A randomised controlled trial of a new handheld vacuum extraction device. *BJOG* 2005;**112**:1510–15.

35. Groom KM, Jones BA, Miller N, Paterson-Brown S. A prospective randomised controlled trial of the Kiwi Omnicup versus conventional ventouse cups for vacuum-assisted vaginal delivery. *BJOG* 2006;**113**:183–89.

36. Tempest N, Hart A, Walkinshaw S, Hapangama DK. A re-evaluation of the role of rotational forceps: retrospective comparison of maternal and perinatal outcomes following different methods of birth for malposition in the second stage of labour. *BJOG* 2013;**120**:1277–84.

37. Bahl R, Van de Venne M, Macleod M, Strachan B, Murphy DJ. Maternal and neonatal morbidity in relation to the instrument used for midcavity rotational operative vaginal delivery: a prospective cohort study. *BJOG* 2013;**120**:1526–32.

38. Aiken AR, Aiken CE, Alberry MS, Brocklesby JC, Scott JG. Management of fetal malposition in the second stage of labor: a propensity score analysis. *Am J Obstet Gynecol* 2015;**212**:355.e1–7.

39. O'Mahony F, Hofmeyr GJ, Menon V. Choice of instruments for assisted vaginal delivery. *Cochrane Database Syst Rev* 2010;**11**:CD005455.

40. Maharaj D. Assessing cephalopelvic disproportion: back to basics. *Obstet Gynecol Surv* 2010;**65**:387–95.

41. Boulvain M, Senat M-V, Perrotin F, et al. Induction of labour versus expectant management for large-for-dates fetuses: a randomized controlled trial. *Lancet* 2015;**385**:2600–605.

42. Bofill JA, Rust OA, Perry KG, Roberts WE, Martin RW, Morrison JC. Operative vaginal delivery: a survey of fellows of ACOG. *Obstet Gynecol* 1996;**88**:1007–10.

43. Murphy DJ, Liebling RE, Patel R, Verity L, Swingler R. Cohort study of operative delivery in the second stage of labour and standard of obstetric care. *Br J Obstet Gynaecol* 2003;**110**:610–15.

44. Alexander JM, Leveno KJ, Hauth JC, et al. Failed operative vaginal delivery. *Obstet Gynecol* 2009;**114**:1017–22.

45. Murphy DJ, Macleod M, Bahl R, Strachan B. A cohort study of maternal and neonatal morbidity in relation to use of sequential instruments at operative vaginal delivery. *Eur J Obstet Gynaecol Reprod Biol* 2011;**156**:41–45.

46. Towner D, Castro MA, Eby-Wilkens E, Gilbert WM. Effect of mode of delivery in nulliparaous women on neonatal intracranial injury. *N Engl J Med* 1999;**341**:1709–14.

47. Ramphul M, Kennelly MM, Burke G, Murphy DJ. Risk factors and morbidity associated with suboptimal instrument placement at instrumental delivery: observational study nested within the Instrumental Delivery & Ultrasound randomized controlled trial ISRCTN 72230496. *BJOG* 2015;**122**:558–63.

48. Dexter SC, Windsor S, Watkinson SJ. Meeting the challenge of maternal choice in mode of delivery with vaginal birth after caesarean section: a medical, legal and ethical commentary. *BJOG* 2014;**121**:133–39.

33

Obstetric procedures

Yvonne Kwan Yue Cheng and Tak Yeung Leung

Introduction

Human childbirth is a natural process but it is not always smooth and successful. To assist in difficult childbirth which may be dangerous to the fetuses and/or mothers, several important obstetric surgical procedures and instruments were invented, modified and refined over centuries, and have become the standard practice in modern obstetrics. In this chapter, the indications, the procedures, and the complications of these commonly practised obstetric surgeries, including caesarean section (CS), instrumental vaginal delivery, episiotomy, repair of perineal tear, routine controlled cord traction for the delivery of the placenta in the third stage of labour, and manual removal of retained placenta, as well as external cephalic version (ECV) will be discussed.

Caesarean section

A brief history of caesarean section

While the exact origin of the name 'caesarean' remains unclear, it is often wrongly attributed to the birth of Julius Caesar, who was mistakenly thought to have been born after his dying mother's abdomen was cut open. Operative abdominal birth was mentioned in legends of various ancient civilizations before Caesar's era, such as the birth of Jilian, the founder of the State of Chu in China 3000 years ago, and that of Bindusara, the second emperor of the Maurya Empire in India in the third century BCE, but perhaps the first well-recorded case of CS with maternal survival was performed in the sixteenth century, by a pig gilder called Jakob Nufer on his wife who suffered from prolonged labour. The maternal mortality of CS remained very high (85% in the nineteenth century in Great Britain) until the introduction of the lower segment uterine incision technique and other surgical improvements since the beginning of the twentieth century.

Indications for a caesarean section

CS is indicated when vaginal delivery is not likely to be successful, or poses substantial risk to the mother or to the fetus. If the fetus (the passenger) is relatively too big to pass through the birth canal (the passage), or when the uterine contraction (power) is insufficient or uncoordinated, vaginal delivery would become unsuccessful, such as in the following conditions:

- Contracted maternal pelvis or cephalopelvic disproportion
- Macrosomia (risk of shoulder dystocia)
- Abnormal fetal lie causing malpresentation (e.g. transverse lie)
- Fibroids in the lower segment causing non-engagement of fetal head
- Poor progress of labour (may be due to obstruction or poor contractions)
- Failed induction of labour
- Failed instrumental delivery
- Congenital malformations with high risk of obstructed labour (e.g. hydrocephalus).

Conditions where vaginal delivery may increase the maternal risks include:

- placenta praevia (causes significant antepartum haemorrhage as well as non-engagement of the fetal head)
- maternal complications (e.g. eclampsia)
- maternal cardiac diseases.

Conditions where vaginal delivery may increase the fetal risks include:

- a severely growth-restricted fetus who cannot sustain the stress of labour
- placental abruption, cord prolapse, intrauterine infection, and other causes of fetal distress which require immediate delivery (some of these conditions also impose maternal risk)
- previous classical CS or previous myomectomy (in particular with an incision entering into the uterine cavity) of which the scars are at risk of rupture during labour, and hence fetal distress (the mother is also at risk of haemorrhage in such a situation)
- vasa praevia where vaginal delivery is associated with a high risk of fetal haemorrhage due to the rupture of the placental vessel
- active genital herpes infection or maternal HIV, in which case avoiding vaginal delivery by planned elective CS may reduce the transmission of the disease to the fetus during labour.

The incidences of CS vary significantly from country to country, with a wide range of below 10% to higher than 50% (1). The very high CS rates in many countries are not because of medical indications but social reasons, such as maternal anxiety towards labour pain and concerns about fetal risk during labour. Although CS is a very safe surgical procedure, it may impose risks on the mothers in their subsequent pregnancy, as well as long-term negative implications for health resources. An unnecessary CS without a medical indication should be avoided.

Types of caesarean incision

Lower segment incision

This is the most common type of caesarean incision performed nowadays (**Figure 33.1**). This involves a transverse incision (Kerr incision) of the lower segment of the uterus, which is developed from the expansion of the isthmic region of the uterus. The risk of rupture of scar at this non-contractile portion of the uterus in the subsequent pregnancy is significantly lower than that of a classical incision (0.2–0.5% vs 4.0–9.0%). Furthermore, it is associated with less blood loss and easier uterine closure because of the thinner muscle wall at the lower segment.

Classical incision

Historically, CS was performed with a vertical incision at the anterior fundus of the uterus. Due to the significantly increased risk of scar rupture and higher complication rate, the classical incision (**Figure 33.1**) has been replaced by lower segment incision, and is nowadays restricted to conditions where access to the lower segment is deemed not possible or with considerable risks, or when the lower segment is not well developed. As the lower segment only begins to form at around 28 weeks' gestation, CS prior to this gestation time may necessitate a classical incision. The indications for classical CS are listed in **Box 33.1**.

Lower vertical (de Lee) incision

This is a vertical incision at the non-contractile lower segment, but it may extend to the upper part of the uterus (**Figure 33.1**). It is seldom

> **Box 33.1** Common indications of classical caesarean section in modern obstetrics
>
> - Preterm caesarean delivery where lower segment is not well formed (especially before 28 weeks).
> - Lower segment fibroid or cervical fibroid.
> - Placenta praevia with large vessels at lower segment.
> - Placenta accreta involving the lower segment.
> - Fetal malformation where the lower segment would not allow sufficient room for infant to be delivered (e.g. conjoined twins).
> - Fetal transverse lie (in particular with fetal back down) may need a classical incision.
> - Perimortem CS (swift delivery is required).

performed but may be required when the transverse incision of the lower segment does not allow enough room for delivery of the fetus (e.g. transverse lie). The combination of a lower vertical and lower segment incisions form an inverted T incision.

J incision

This is a curve-upward extension from one end of a lower segment incision during a difficult delivery, so as to avoid tearing of the uterus laterally to the board ligament (**Figure 33.1**).

Procedure and operative technique

Preoperative preparation

Women are kept fasting before the operation. The risks of the operation must be discussed thoroughly with consent signed. Antacids are given routinely as premedication to reduce the risk of aspiration pneumonitis. Although the chance of transfusion is not high in uncomplicated CSs, a preoperative haemoglobin level should be checked and the type and screen should be saved. Where there is a high risk of bleeding, for example, placenta praevia, blood products must be readily available. A pneumatic cuff or pressure stockings are worn to reduce the risk of deep vein thrombosis. Preoperative ultrasonography may be helpful in certain circumstances, such as mapping the placenta in cases of placenta praevia or accreta. Women are kept in the left lateral tilt position on the operating table to prevent aortocaval compression which could lead to maternal hypotension and uteroplacental insufficiency. A Foley catheter is inserted following anaesthesia to empty the bladder. Prophylactic antibiotics, preferably cephalosporins, are given on induction to prevent wound infection.

Anaesthesia

Regional anaesthesia (either spinal, epidural, or combined spinal–epidural anaesthesia) is the most common and a safer method of anaesthesia compared to general anaesthesia. It allows earlier mobilization and is preferred by most women as they remain awake and can experience the birth of their child. Epidural anaesthesia can also be used for postoperative pain relief. Volume preloading and administration of ephedrine or phenylephrine can reduce the risk of hypotension associated with regional anaesthesia. With general anaesthesia, there are risks of maternal aspiration pneumonitis and difficulty in intubation because of the oedema related to pregnancy (or pregnancy-related complications such as pre-eclampsia). In addition, the anaesthetic agents may cause depression of the infant immediately after birth. Therefore, general anaesthesia is only limited

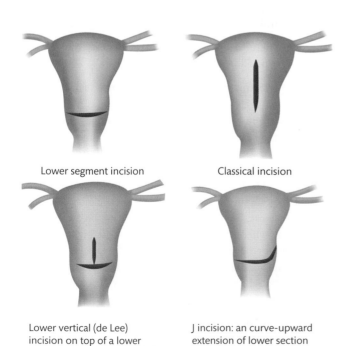

Lower segment incision

Classical incision

Lower vertical (de Lee) incision on top of a lower segment incision (inverted T)

J incision: an curve-upward extension of lower section wound

Figure 33.1 Different types of uterine incisions used in caesarean sections.

to certain cases where regional anaesthesia is contraindicated, or an extremely difficult CS is anticipated.

Abdominal incision

Aseptic reagents (e.g. povidone iodine or chlorhexidine gluconate) are used for skin preparation. The choice of skin incision depends on the gestation, the presence of previous scar, and the need of classical CS. CS is mostly performed through a transverse incision, either through a Pfannenstiel incision or Joel-Cohen incision. The Joel-Cohen incision is made by blunt dissection by fingers in deeper layers of the abdominal wound, which may be more difficult where scar tissues are present in cases of repeat CSs. Transverse incisions are preferable because they reduce wound pain, wound breakdown, incisional hernia, and have a better cosmetic result.

Where classical CS is planned, a subumbilical midline vertical incision should be made to facilitate a longitudinal incision of the uterus. Very occasionally, a paramedian incision is made which allows extension above the umbilicus when necessary.

Uterine incision and wound repair

Lower segment wound

Dissection of the bladder with the bladder flap pushed inferiorly is necessary to allow exposure of the lower segment of the uterus. The uterine incision should not be made too low to avoid injuring the cervix. This is especially true following prolonged labour, CS at the second stage, or after failed instrumental delivery, where the cervix may be drawn upwards. Occasionally, extension of a lower segment incision may be necessary to allow more room for delivery of the infant, either through a J incision or inverted T incision (**Figure 33.1**). With these types of complicated incisions, the risk of scar rupture in future pregnancies may increase. After the delivery of the fetus and the placenta (see later), the lower segment incision is usually closed in two layers.

Classical wound

A vertical incision is made on the anterior uterine wall at the upper part of the uterus (**Figure 33.1**), and hence dissection of the bladder is not necessary. However, this upper part of the uterus has a thick myometrial wall which would lead to more blood loss when compared to a lower segment incision. The classical uterine incision is closed in three layers.

Delivery of the fetus

Cephalic presentation

The posterior aspect of the fetal head is cupped and elevated from the uterine cavity. Fundal pressure can be applied to aid delivery of the fetal head out through the uterine wound. Disimpaction of the fetal head may be necessary if it is engaged into the maternal pelvis, especially in cases of prolonged labour, second-stage CS, or caesarean delivery following failed instrumental delivery. An inferior or lateral uterine tear of the lower segment may result if this step is not performed smoothly. An inferior tear could extend to the cervix or vagina making repair difficult, and a lateral tear could lead to heavy bleeding from the uterine vessels or haematoma formation in the broad ligament. It is crucial that repair is performed properly with haemostasis well secured. In cases where the fetal head is high and has failed to be delivered by fundal pressure, the use of forceps can aid the delivery of the fetal head. Following the delivery of the head, the shoulders and rest of the body can be delivered smoothly.

Breech presentation

In the event of an extended breech, the fetal buttocks are firstly elevated and delivered from the uterine wound. Alternatively, the baby's buttocks can be lifted out from the uterine wound by hooking them bilaterally by the operator. If the baby is in footling breech, the fetal feet are grasped and delivered from the uterine wound. The rest of the baby is delivered by breech extraction, where the arms are delivered by the Lovset manoeuvre, and the fetal head by the Mariceau–Smellie–Viet manoeuvre, in a similar manner as in vaginal breech delivery (as described in the last section of this chapter).

Transverse or other abnormal fetal lie

Ultrasonography prior to the operation may be performed to locate the fetal spine and feet. During the delivery, the fetal lie should first be converted into longitudinal, usually by grasping the fetal feet followed by traction which will then bring the buttocks to the lower segment. The fetus can then be delivered as in breech presentation. Failure to convert into longitudinal lie may occur when the upper limb(s) is/are wrongly grasped and pulled, or when the amniotic membrane is ruptured prematurely, resulting in reduction of amniotic fluid and shrinking of the uterine cavity, which in turn restrict further turning of the fetus. If this happens, extension of the uterine wound or an additional vertical incision may be needed to deliver the transversely lying fetus. Any delay in delivery at this stage may cause fetal hypoxia and birth asphyxia.

Delivery of the placenta

Syntocinon 5 IU is routinely administered intravenously after delivery of the baby to encourage uterine contraction and to reduce blood loss. The placenta may be expelled spontaneously. If not, the placenta can be delivered by applying fundal pressure or controlled cord traction. Only if these measures fail, the placenta can be removed manually by separating it from the uterus by the operator's hand; however, this is associated with an increased risk of blood loss and endometritis. The uterine cavity should always be checked and emptied with complete removal of the placenta.

Closure of the abdominal wall

Closure of the peritoneum is not necessary. The rectus sheath is closed with continuous absorbable sutures. Routine closure of the subcutaneous layer is not necessary, unless the woman has more than 2 cm subcutaneous fat. Skin can be closed by subcuticular continuous sutures. Interrupted mattress sutures are preferred in obese patients.

Postoperative care

Adequate analgesia should be given following CS. Women should be encouraged to have adequate hydration, early mobilization, and graduated stockings to reduce the risk of venous thromboembolism. High-risk women should be given low-molecular-weight heparin. Haemoglobin should be checked if there is significant blood loss. Discussion with the woman about future childbearing and mode of delivery should be provided.

Risks and complications of caesarean section

Short term

Maternal

- Haemorrhage mainly from the uterine wound, occasionally from the wound of the abdominal wall. Small risk of hysterectomy in cases of massive haemorrhage.
- Uterine injury (e.g. uterine tear).
- Wound infection.
- Endometritis.
- Visceral injury, most commonly the bladder.
- Urinary tract infection (after urinary bladder catheterization).
- Venous thromboembolism.
- Complications related to regional or general anaesthesia.

Fetal injury

- Fetal skin lacerations due to an untended cut made during the incision of the uterine wall.
- Fetal musculoskeletal or cranial injury during obstructed delivery through the uterine wound.
- Fetal birth asphyxia due to delayed/obstructed delivery through the uterine wound.

Long-term implications in future pregnancies

- Risk of scar rupture in future pregnancy:
  - Lower transverse scar: 0.2–0.5% (2).
  - Classical scar: 4–9% (3).
- Risk of placenta praevia and placenta accreta in subsequent pregnancy.
- Risk of ectopic scar pregnancy.

Vaginal birth after caesarean section

Vaginal birth after caesarean section (VBAC) can be offered to women with history of a single uncomplicated lower segment CS, and where there are no contraindications for vaginal birth in the current pregnancy. The benefits of a VBAC are the avoidance of the associated anaesthetic and surgical risks involved in a CS, faster recovery, and shorter hospital stay. More importantly, it reduces the risk of placenta praevia or placenta accreta in future pregnancies, as this complication is associated with repeated CSs.

The successful rate of a VBAC is approximately 75% (4). A previous vaginal delivery increases the success rate. With a history of successful VBAC, the success rate increases up to 90%. Contraindications of VBAC include the following:

Absolute contraindications:

- Classical caesarean scar (high risk of scar rupture).
- History of uterine rupture.
- Presence of contraindications for vaginal birth (e.g. placenta praevia).

Relative contraindications:

- Complicated uterine scars.
- Two or more previous lower segment CSs.
- History of myomectomy (especially in the myomectomy incision has entered the uterine cavity).

Complications of VBAC:

- Risk of emergency CS during VBAC.
- Scar rupture (0.2–0.5% following one uncomplicated lower segment CS).
- Fetal asphyxia, perinatal death, and maternal haemorrhage in the event of scar rupture.

Management of labour in women undergoing VBAC (5):

- Delivery should be in a hospital setting where immediate caesarean delivery and advanced neonatal resuscitation facilities are readily available.
- There is a two- to threefold increase in risk of uterine rupture if labour is induced or augmented. If induction of labour is necessary, a mechanical method of induction (e.g. amniotomy, balloon catheter) may be preferred to reduce the risk of scar rupture associated with the use of oxytocin or prostaglandins.
- Continuous cardiotocography (CTG) should be provided.
- Progress of labour should be monitored for evidence of obstructed labour where emergency CS would be necessary.
- Symptoms and signs of scar rupture should be closely monitored. These include:
  - abnormal CTG
  - severe abdominal pain persistent in between contractions
  - scar pain and tenderness
  - vaginal bleeding
  - haematuria
  - evidence of shock of the mother
  - loss of presenting part, change in abdominal contour, fetal parts are easily felt per abdomen.

Instrumental vaginal delivery

A brief history of instrumental vaginal delivery

Instrumental vaginal delivery is performed using either forceps or a vacuum extractor, where traction force is applied on the fetal head to aid delivery in the second stage of labour. The obstetric forceps were probably first invented at the end of the sixteenth century or during the early seventeenth century by the famous Chamberlen family of obstetricians, who took care of the royal family of England at that time. Designed for difficult childbirth, the prototype was kept secret by the Chamberlen family for more than 100 years. Since the mid eighteenth century, a variety of improvements in the design of forceps started to appear which made forceps delivery a popular solution for difficult childbirth. Subsequently, in 1849, Professor James Young Simpson designed the first vacuum extractor for childbirth with a simple design of a metal syringe attached to a soft rubber cup. However, the idea of using vacuum extraction to assist vaginal birth was not popular until the 1950s when Professor Malmstrom developed the ventouse with a metal cup connected to a vacuum pump machine. Vacuum extractors have now become a more favourable choice than forceps in many countries.

Design of forceps

Obstetric forceps consist of two branches, and the basic structure of each branch includes the following (**Figure 33.2**):

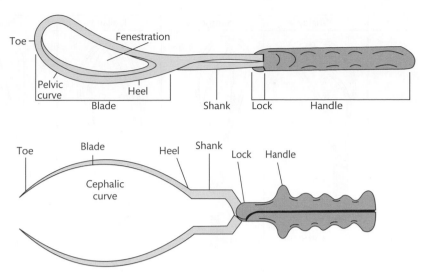

Figure 33.2 Figure showing the basic structure of forceps using Simpson's forceps as an example.

- The blade: this curved portion is to grasp the fetal head, with one blade on each side of the head. It characteristically has two curves, the cephalic and the pelvic curves, shaped to conform to the moulded and elongated fetal head and the birth canal respectively.
- The handle: allows pulling by the operators. In Kielland's forceps, it also allow rotation of malposition and sliding to correct asynclitism.
- The shank: connects the blades and the handles. The axis of the blade is slightly tilted upwards from that of the shank in most of the forceps. However, the axis of the blade and the shanks are on the straight line in Kielland's forceps to facilitate rotation. The shank is shorter in outlet forceps (Wrigely's forceps) but longer in Kielland's forceps. The shank of Piper's forceps is long and bent downwards to facilitate delivery of the aftercoming head in vaginal breech delivery.

The lock is for keeping the two shanks together. Most forceps have a fixed lock design usually located at the junction of the shank and the handle. In rotational forceps (Kielland's), it is a sliding lock design located along the shank.

There are different shapes of forceps which are designed for different purposes. Four characteristic forceps are shown in **Figure 33.3** for comparison.

Design of vacuum extractor

The vacuum extractor consists of a vacuum cup which is designed in various sizes and diameters. The cup is attached or can be connected to a handle which allows the operator to apply traction force. The cup consists of a vacuum port which can be linked to the vacuum pump through a rubber tubing. There are several types as shown in the **Figure 33.4** and described as follows:

- Bird cup (metal cup): this is a metal cup that is most commonly used. It is designed in various sizes of between 4 and 6 cm in diameter, and can be differentiated into an anterior or posterior cup. The posterior cup is specifically designed for use in the occipital posterior or lateral position or when the fetal head is deflexed.
- Silicon cup: the use of this type of soft silastic cup carries a higher incidence of failure than rigid vacuum cups because it is more

likely to result in spontaneous detachment. However, they are less likely to be associated with scalp trauma. They are more suited for occipitoanterior (OA) positions.

- Kiwi OmniCup: this is a single-use, disposable, rigid plastic cup with an integral manual vacuum system incorporated into the hand-held device.

Indications of instrumental vaginal delivery

The incidence of instrumental vaginal delivery is approximately 5–10%, but varies widely between different countries. Instrumental vaginal delivery is indicated in the second stage of labour when vaginal birth is deemed possible but:

- the process has to be hastened because of fetal distress or maternal distress, or
- maternal pushing force needs augmentation because of maternal exhaustion, or
- prolonged second stage of labour
- maternal pushing force is not desirable because of maternal diseases such as cardiac diseases or neuromuscular diseases.

A prolonged second stage may be due to inadequate maternal pushing force or obstructed labour. The latter must be differentiated from the former by careful clinical examination, as it is an absolute contraindication of instrumental delivery. Wrong application of instrumental delivery in obstructed labour not only results in failure but also significant perinatal complications (e.g. birth asphyxia and cranial injury) and maternal complications (e.g. postpartum haemorrhage, perineal injury, and crash CS). Continuous support during labour, use of upright or lateral positions, and avoidance of epidural analgesia can reduce the need for operative vaginal delivery (6).

Classification of instrumental vaginal delivery

Depending on the station and position of the fetal head, instrumental delivery is classified into outlet, low-pelvic, and mid-pelvic levels as shown in **Table 33.1**. More difficulty is anticipated during the procedure when the level moves up. High-pelvic instrumental

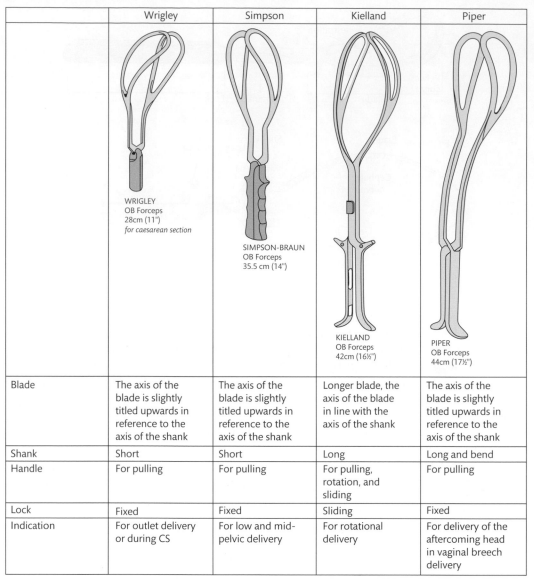

	Wrigley	Simpson	Kielland	Piper
Blade	The axis of the blade is slightly titled upwards in reference to the axis of the shank	The axis of the blade is slightly titled upwards in reference to the axis of the shank	Longer blade, the axis of the blade in line with the axis of the shank	The axis of the blade is slightly titled upwards in reference to the axis of the shank
Shank	Short	Short	Long	Long and bend
Handle	For pulling	For pulling	For pulling, rotation, and sliding	For pulling
Lock	Fixed	Fixed	Sliding	Fixed
Indication	For outlet delivery or during CS	For low and mid-pelvic delivery	For rotational delivery	For delivery of the aftercoming head in vaginal breech delivery

Figure 33.3 Comparison of different types of forceps.

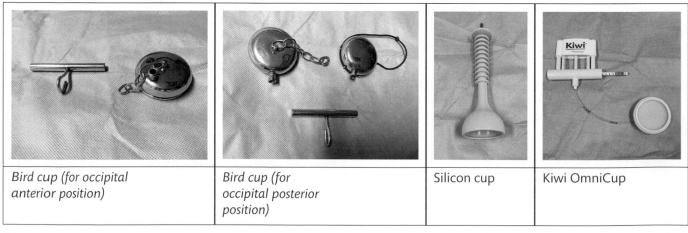

Bird cup (for occipital anterior position)	Bird cup (for occipital posterior position)	Silicon cup	Kiwi OmniCup

Figure 33.4 The Bird cups, both anterior and posterior, silicon cup, and Kiwi OmniCup.

Table 33.1 Classification of instrumental vaginal delivery according to the station and position of the fetal head

Level	Definition
Outlet	Fetal scalp is visible without separating the labia
	Fetal skull has reached the pelvic floor
	Sagittal suture is in the anteroposterior diameter or right or left occiput anterior or posterior position (rotation does not exceed 45 degrees)
	Fetal head is at or on the perineum
Low	Leading point of fetal skull (not caput) is at station +2 or more (lower) and not on the pelvic floor
	Two subdivisions:
	• Rotation of 45º or less from the occipitoanterior position
	• Rotation of more than 45º including the occipitoposterior position
Mid	Fetal head is no more than one-fifth palpable per abdomen
	Leading point of fetal skull is above station +2 but not above the ischial spines (i.e. below station 0)
	Two subdivisions:
	• Rotation of 45º or less from the occipitoanterior position
	• Rotation of more than 45º including the occipitoposterior position
(High)	NOT included in the classification as operative vaginal delivery is not recommended in this situation where the head is two-fifths or more
	palpable abdominally and the presenting part is above the level of the ischial spines

Source data from American College of Obstetricians and Gynecologists. Operative vaginal delivery. *ACOG Practice Bulletin* No. 17. 2000.

delivery is nowadays regarded as a dangerous procedure and has been abandoned.

Prerequisites for instrumental vaginal delivery

The following prerequisites should be fulfilled to ensure a safe and successful instrumental vaginal delivery (8):

- The cervix must be fully dilated and membranes are ruptured.
- The fetal head should be well engaged and not more than one-fifth palpable per abdomen.
- The fetal head position and station must be known.
- The maternal pelvis is assessed to be adequate with no evidence of cephalopelvic disproportion (interspinous distance, subpubic arch, caput, and moulding in addition to station and position of the fetal head).
- The urinary bladder is emptied.
- There is adequate anaesthesia (forceps delivery should be performed under either regional anaesthesia or pudendal block while perineal local anaesthesia is acceptable for vacuum extraction).
- Procedure should be performed by a trained operator.

If vaginal delivery is not possible because of obstructed labour or cephalopelvic disproportion, a CS should be performed.

Choice of instrumental vaginal delivery

The preferences for forceps delivery and vacuum extractions vary between different countries. In the majority of indications, both instruments are applicable. However, forceps should be used instead of vacuum extraction in some less common situations such as gestation less than 34 weeks and face presentation where vacuum pressure may be dangerous to the fetus. In case of vaginal breech delivery, only forceps can be applied for the aftercoming head, and Piper's forceps are the most suitable instrument for this purpose.

In case the fetal head is not in the OA position, ordinary forceps are not applicable. In such situations, rotational forceps (using Kielland's forceps) delivery is more appropriate but it may increase maternal and perinatal morbidity. Hence, vacuum extraction may be a preferred choice to forceps in the non-OA position. This is because when the cup is properly applied over the vertex, it can then facilitate gradual autorotation of the fetal head to direct the OA position around the axis of the cup (over the vertex) as it descends the pelvic floor.

Procedure of forceps delivery

Application of forceps (use direct OA position as an example):

- Bladder is emptied.
- Adequate analgesia given either with pudendal block or regional anaesthesia.
- Check the forceps such that they can be paired and locked correctly.
- Apply lubrication onto the forceps blades.
- Using a pencil-grip to hold the shank of the forceps, the left blade is inserted into the maternal left side, followed by the right blade to the maternal right side.
- If the blades are applied correctly, they should be over the corresponding zygomatic regions of the fetus and the blades should lock easily.
- Check if both shanks are perpendicular to the maternal perineum and at the same length. If not, the forceps are not applied symmetrically and cannot be locked.
- After locking the forceps, check that the sagittal suture is cutting the shank perpendicularly, the space between the heel of the blade and the head allows only one finger (not one on one side and two on the other), and the occiput is 3–4 cm above the shank before traction is applied along the axis of the birth canal, that is, first downward and then upward (**Figure 33.5**).
- An episiotomy may be made when the fetal head crowns.
- Once the head is delivered, the forceps can be removed, and the rest of the body is delivered in the usual manner.

Risks and complications of forceps delivery

- Injury to the baby:
  - Laceration of the face and scalp, especially when the blades are applied incorrectly.
  - Facial nerve palsy.
  - Ocular trauma and retinal haemorrhage.
  - Skull fracture and/or intracranial haemorrhage: occasional but may result in brain injury.
- Injury to the mother:
  - Tears to the perineum and anal sphincters, extension to higher vagina or cervix, and pelvic floor injury.
  - Postpartum haemorrhage secondary to lower genital tract injury.

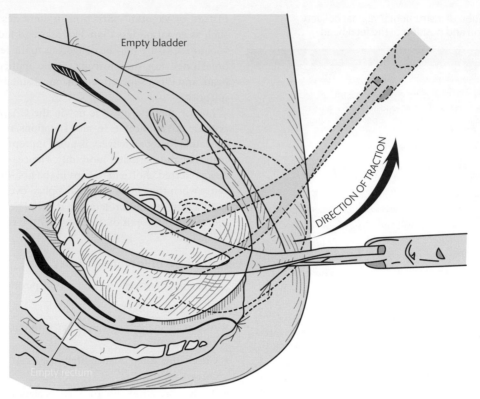

Figure 33.5 The direction of traction in forceps delivery.

Procedure of vacuum extraction

Application of vacuum cup:

- Bladder is emptied.
- Adequate local analgesia is given.
- Apply lubrication onto the vacuum cup.
- The cup is applied to the vertex in the midline over the sagittal suture, with the centre of the cup 3 cm in front of the posterior fontanelle, or 6 cm behind the anterior fontanelle. This is called the flexion point. Therefore, if a 6 cm cup is used, the rim of the cup is touching the posterior fontanelle, or 3 cm behind the anterior fontanelle. Correct placement of the cup at the flexion point (**Figure 33.6**) is crucial to promote flexion of the fetal head during delivery.
- After ensuring that maternal tissue is not trapped in the cup, the vacuum pressure is gradually built up to 60 cmHg in 2 minutes.
- Check again for any maternal tissues trapped between the fetal scalp and the cup.
- Once adequate vacuum pressure is achieved, a pulling force is applied coinciding with uterine contractions and maternal bearing-down effort along the axis of the birth canal (i.e. firstly downwards and then upwards).
- An episiotomy may be made when the fetal head crowns.
- Once the head is delivered, the vacuum cup can be removed, and the rest of the body is delivered in the usual manner.

Risks and complications of vacuum extraction

- Injury to the baby:
  - Subaponeurotic (subgaleal) haemorrhage: an uncommon but potentially life-threatening complication of vacuum extraction.

Bleeding to the subaponeurotic space can be massive, but the diagnosis can be easily missed because of its insidious onset, and the masking effect of the coexisting caput or chignon created by the vacuum cup. It presents as a fluctuant boggy mass developing over the scalp, and in case of delayed diagnosis, the neonate presents with hypovolaemic shock.

- Cephalohaematoma: unlike subaponeurotic haemorrhage, cephalohaematoma is subperiosteal bleeding which is bounded by sutures, and hence is usually self-limiting.
- Intracranial haemorrhage and skull fracture: occasionally happens in difficult vacuum extraction but can result in severe brain injury.

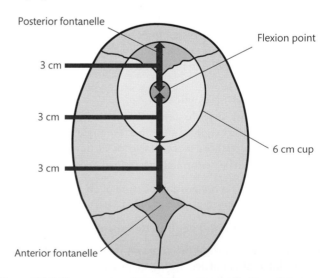

Figure 33.6 The correct position of the cup at the flexion point.

- Injury to the mother:
  - Perineal and pelvic floor injury (less common than forceps delivery).
  - Cervical or vaginal tears if the tissues are accidentally trapped by the vacuum pressure into the cup.
  - Postpartum haemorrhage secondary to lower genital tract injury.

Episiotomy

A brief history of episiotomy

Episiotomy, also known as perineotomy, is a surgical incision of the perineum and the posterior vaginal wall to enlarge the vulval outlet for the baby to pass through. It was introduced to obstetric practice over 200 years ago, yet its value as a prophylactic procedure against perineal or pelvic floor injury during childbirth remains controversial (10).

Indications of episiotomy

Although episiotomy was designed to reduce the risk of an uncontrolled perineal tear, it is not without side effects such as postpartum wound pain, sexual dysfunction, and even major perineal tear and incontinence. Current studies have suggested that a restricted approach would be more beneficial when compared to a routine policy. Episiotomy may be considered when:

- tight perineum: as judged by the birth attendant that the risk of perineal tear is higher without an episiotomy
- instrumental delivery: in which the risk of perineal injury is often high
- shoulder dystocia: episiotomy itself does not relieve shoulder dystocia but may allow more room for the insertion of the operator's hand for internal rotation or delivery of the posterior arm.

Types of episiotomy

Among various types of episiotomy, mediolateral and median are the two most commonly used types.

- Mediolateral: oblique incision downwards and outwards from the midpoint of the fourchette to either the right or left. Ideally it is 45 degrees from the vertical line. However, when the fetal head is stretching the perineal skin, an incision line that deviates from vertical by 60 degrees would be more appropriate.
- Median: midline vertical incision commences from the centre of the fourchette and extends downwards towards but not reaching the anus.

When compared to a median incision, a mediolateral incision has the advantages of avoiding bisecting the perineal body, which is essential for the integrity of the pelvic floor, and reducing the risk of anal tear (12). The potential advantages of a median incision are less blood loss, quicker healing, less postpartum wound pain and dyspareunia, and it is easier to repair, but it may be torn further and result in anal sphincter injury. The latest evidence favours a mediolateral incision if an episiotomy is indicated (13).

Procedure of mediolateral episiotomy

- Timing: the incision should not be made too early when the fetal head has not distended the perineum, or too late when the fetal head is starting to tear the perineum.
- It should begin in the midline at the fourchette.
- It must be made in one single cut.
- Direction: between 45 degrees from the vertical line (when the fetal head is not stretching the perineum) and 60 degrees (when the fetal head is stretching the perineum) (14).
- Length: it is about 2.5–3 cm. A too-small cut will not increase the vulval outlet sufficiently to facilitate delivery, but may itself form a weak point in the perineal tissues from which a tear could extend. On the other hand, a too-large cut may damage the ipsilateral Bartholin's gland.

Risks and complications of episiotomy

Episiotomy is associated with wound pain, bleeding, and infection. Extension of a perineal or vaginal tear, as well as anal sphincter injury may occur. In rare circumstances, an anovaginal fistula may occur if the episiotomy is not repaired properly.

Repair of episiotomy

The aim of episiotomy repair is to achieve haemostasis and tissue reapproximation.

Repair can be done in the labour room provided lighting and exposure is adequate. Local anaesthesia can be given for pain control. Prior to repair, a thorough examination should be performed to look for additional cervical or vaginal tears, and whether the anal sphincters are involved. A digital rectal examination would be useful to assess the rectum and anal sphincters.

Absorbable sutures are used such as Vicryl and Polysorb. Repair begins at approximately 1 cm above the apex of the vaginal wound. The vagina is repaired with continuous sutures around 1 cm apart until the hymenal ring is reached. The suture is then brought forward to the perineal body where the muscular layer of the perineal body is closed with the continuous suture until the posterior apex of the perineal body is reached. Subsequently, the perineal skin is approximated by continuous subcuticular sutures running anteriorly to the introitus and finally, the knot is tied inside the hymenal ring.

Repair of perineal tear

Classification of perineal tear

The severity of perineal tear is classified according to the depth of the perineal tissues involved as well as whether the anal sphincters are damaged, as shown in **Table 33.2** (15).

Complications of perineal tear include severe postpartum haemorrhage, wound breakdown and infection, anovaginal fistula, anal incontinence, and dyspareunia. Repair of first- and second-degree tears is similar to episiotomy repair, but repair of third- and fourth-degree tears, which are also called obstetric anal sphincter injuries (OASIS), require special precaution and skill.

Table 33.2 Definition of different degrees of perineal tears according to the severity

Classification	Definition
First degree	Injury to perineal skin and/or vaginal mucosa
Second degree	Injury to perineum involving perineal muscles but not involving the anal sphincter
Third degree	Injury to the perineum involving the anal sphincter complex:
Grade 3a	Less than 50% of external anal sphincter torn
Grade 3b	More than 50% of external anal sphincter torn
Grade 3c	Both external anal sphincter and internal anal sphincter are torn
Fourth degree	Injury to perineum involving the anal sphincter complex and anorectal mucosa

Repair of third- and fourth-degree perineal tear (OASIS)

Prior to repair of an episiotomy and/or perineal tear, all women should have a systematic examination of the perineum, including a digital rectal examination, to assess the extent and severity of the tear. Failure to identify a major perineal tear (third- or fourth-degree tears) would result in inadequate repair leading to the risk of anal incontinence and other wound complications. Adequate exposure and complete relaxation of the woman are essential for repair of major perineal tears. Hence the procedure should be performed in the operating theatre with good lighting and under either spinal or general anaesthesia.

The anorectal mucosa, internal anal sphincter, and external anal sphincter should be repaired separately to improve the likelihood of subsequent anal continence (16). The anorectal mucosa should be repaired with continuous or interrupted polyglactin sutures, which causes less irritation and discomfort than polydioxanone (PDS) sutures. The internal anal sphincter is to be repaired with interrupted or mattress sutures using either polyglactin or PDS sutures. A third-degree tear where the whole external anal sphincter is torn can be repaired by an overlapping or end-to-end technique using either polyglactin or PDS sutures, whereas if the external anal sphincter is only partially torn, the end-to-end technique is preferred (17). In all three layers of repair, figure-of-eight sutures should be avoided because they may cause tissue ischaemia (18).

Postoperatively, women should be given broad-spectrum antibiotics to reduce the risk of wound infection and dehiscence. Laxatives such as lactulose are prescribed to soften the stool which may allow better healing of the wound. Women should be advised to practise pelvic floor exercises in the postnatal period.

Follow-up after repair

Women should be followed up in 2–3 months after the repair to assess wound healing and to look for complications, especially anal incontinence. About 60–80% of women will become asymptomatic by 12 months after repair. Women who have persistent symptoms should be assessed carefully and endoanal ultrasonography and/or manometry may be necessary to assess for anal sphincter defects. The option of elective caesarean delivery should be discussed in future pregnancies.

Routine management of the third stage of labour and controlled cord traction

This is the period from the delivery of the fetus to the delivery of the placenta, and normally should not last more than 30 minutes. Routine administration of prophylactic oxytocic agents (Syntocinon or ergometrine) is the most effective way to prevent postpartum haemorrhage, and should be given immediately after the birth of the baby (19). Controlled cord traction to deliver the placenta only has a minor contribution to the reduction of postpartum blood loss.

Indication and procedure of controlled cord traction

If the placenta is not delivered spontaneously, controlled cord traction can be performed to shorten the third stage of labour.

One hand of the operator is placed on the abdomen to feel for uterine contractions. When a contraction is felt, the other hand exerts steady traction to the cord such that the placenta could separate from the uterus and is delivered. At the same time, the 'abdominal' hand must exert a counter (upward) pressure at the lower part of the uterus. It is crucial that the traction is applied during a contraction to prevent uterine inversion. The placenta should be examined to be complete after it is delivered. If the placenta fails to be delivered, or part of the placenta is left *in utero*, manual removal of the placenta has to be performed under anaesthesia.

Manual removal of the placenta

Indication

Retained placenta after vaginal delivery, where the placenta failed to separate spontaneously or by controlled cord traction in the third stage of labour. Under such circumstances, manual removal of the placenta will be necessary.

Procedure

The procedure is performed under regional or general anaesthesia in the operating theatre. Prophylactic antibiotics should be given. The operator inserts his/her hand through the dilated cervix into the uterine cavity, identifies the placenta by following the cord, and separates the placenta by shearing movements of the hand between the placenta and the uterus while steadying the uterus abdominally by the other hand. Once the whole placenta is detached from the uterine wall it is removed. The chorionic and the amniotic surfaces of the placenta are checked for completeness. The cavity is checked for any retained tissue at the end of the procedure. The uterus should be massaged to secure a contraction and contraction and retraction is sustained by a Syntocinon infusion to reduce blood loss.

Risks and complications

Possible complications include postpartum haemorrhage, intrauterine infection, and perforation of the uterus.

External cephalic version

A brief history of ECV

ECV has been described in the medical literature since the writings of Hippocrates (around the fourth century BCE) to convert a breech presenting pregnancy to a cephalic presenting one. It did not gain popularity until the beginning of the nineteenth century. However, in the early twentieth century, ECV was often performed in preterm gestation under general anaesthesia and it was associated with high perinatal mortality. That meant that the procedure of ECV was almost abandoned. Since the 1980s, ECV has been revived, due to the assistance of ultrasound surveillance and effective uterine relaxation by tocolytic agents. Both these adjuncts have made ECV a very safe procedure with a high success rate in current obstetric practice.

Indications of ECV

Breech presentation is the most common indication for ECV. ECV may be considered in cases of unstable lie and transverse or oblique lie, provided there is no contracted pelvis or other contraindication to have ECV and vaginal birth has been ruled out. In the cases of abnormal lies, induction of labour immediately after a successful ECV may help to minimize the chance of reverting to abnormal lie.

Contraindications for ECV

Absolute contraindications are few and include conditions where CS is required even if the fetus is in cephalic presentation (such as placenta praevia and contracted pelvis), or there are known structural uterine anomalies (congenital or lower segment fibroids) causing malpresentation or abnormal lie, or the fetal well-being is already compromised (evidenced by an abnormal CTG trace). The umbilical cord tightly wound around the fetal neck, ruptured membranes, or a recent history of antepartum haemorrhage (within 7 days) are also contraindications for ECV.

ECV may be relatively contraindicated if the estimated chance of successful ECV or successful vaginal delivery is low, or if the procedure might be more complicated, such as oligohydramnios, a small-for gestational-age fetus with abnormal Doppler parameters, major fetal anomalies, a scarred uterus, or pre-eclampsia is present (20).

Procedure of ECV

Preoperative preparation

Pre-ECV assessment is an important safeguard of the procedure. First of all, any doubts in gestational age need to be resolved before ECV, as the procedure should not be done prior to 36–37 weeks of gestation, when there is still a good chance of spontaneous cephalic version. Furthermore, if the procedure is complicated, it may result in an iatrogenic preterm delivery. Rhesus-negative mothers must have prophylactic rhesus antibodies immediately after ECV to prevent rhesus isoimmunization. Crossmatching blood and an intravenous line access should be prepared in case emergency CS is required after a complicated ECV. Performing ECV in the labour ward or in a site close to labour ward is preferred. Beta-sympathomimetic tocolytics are contraindicated in maternal cardiac or thyroid disorders which should be ruled out. Ultrasonography and CTG should be performed to rule out any contraindications for ECV. Furthermore, ultrasonography will help to assess the position of the fetal spine and that of the placenta, both of which are important factors for planning the direction of the version.

The turning procedure

The operator firstly has to decide the direction of turning, which will depend on the placenta site and the position of the fetal back. It is important to avoid going against the placenta. If a clockwise direction is decided, the operator should stand on the maternal left side so that he/she will push the fetal breech to the contralateral side (and vice versa). ECV should only be attempted when the uterus is relaxed. Short-acting tocolytics (such as terbutaline and hexoprenaline) are useful to relax the uterus. They may cause palpitation and occasionally induce significant hypotension. Prophylactic fluid loading through an intravenous line may be considered.

If the fetal breech is engaged in the maternal pelvis, a gentle force is needed to elevate it from the pelvis. The breech is then pushed (using the operator's thumbs) to the iliac fossa on the other side. Once it is successful, the breech is maintained in this location by one of the operator's hand. The operator then uses the other hand to pull the fetal head to the cornual region close to himself/herself. Once the fetus is in oblique lie and both the fetal poles are under the control of the operator's hands, the operator can further rotate the fetus to transverse lie by simultaneous forces on both fetal poles. Once the fetal lie becomes transverse, cephalic version can usually be completed in majority of the cases. Forceful or jerky movements should always be avoided. The procedure usually takes about a few seconds to 10 seconds, and seldom more than 20 seconds. If an attempt is failed, the operator may try again but not more than three times.

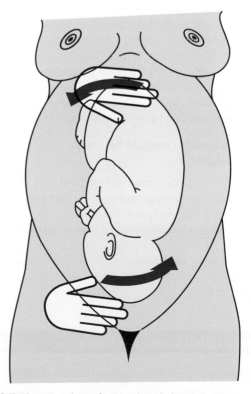

Figure 33.7 The procedure of external cephalic version.

Anaesthesia

In general, ECV is performed without any anaesthesia, which would block a woman's pain sensation and hence unfasten the safeguard against forceful movements of an inexperienced operator. However, recent studies have shown that spinal anaesthesia may relax the maternal abdomen, reduce the force of version, and improve the success rate in experienced hands (21, 22).

Postoperative assessment

After an ECV, the fetal heart rate should be counted immediately with real-time ultrasound to rule out any bradycardia. Transient decelerations are common (3–5%) and should not last for more than 2 minutes. It is often a physiological reaction towards pressure exerted on it (in particular on its head) (23). However, when there is persistent bradycardia, an emergency CS should be considered to minimize fetal risk.

If there is no immediate fetal heart rate disturbance, the fetus should be monitored with CTG for another 30–60 minutes before the patient can be discharged home safely. Any symptoms of rupture of membranes, antepartum haemorrhage, or abdominal pain should be further investigated and managed accordingly.

After a successful ECV, the patient should be followed up a week later to rule out any reversion to breech presentation. If not, then the patient can be managed as other spontaneous cephalic presenting cases, understanding that the risk of intrapartum CS after successful ECV is still higher than that of spontaneous cephalic presenting pregnant women.

Risks and complications of ECV

Major complications of ECV are uncommon (24). Transient fetal bradycardia (<3 minutes) may occur in 5% of cases after ECV. It is most likely a physiological response of the fetuses towards pressure or stress. Prolonged bradycardia or pathological decelerations indicate fetal distress which may be related to placenta abruption or umbilical cord entanglement, haemorrhage, or cord prolapse. Fetal injuries such as fractures of long bones or neurological damage are rarely reported. There is a potential risk of uterine rupture in cases with previous CS scar, but CS scar is not an absolute contraindication for ECV provided that adequate precautions have been taken.

Chance of successful vaginal delivery after successful ECV

Case-controlled studies comparing post-ECV cephalic presenting pregnancies and those with spontaneous cephalic presentation have shown that the former group still has a higher risk of intrapartum CS, due to a higher incidence of fetal distress and failure to progress of labour (25). This may indicate that in women carrying breech presenting pregnancies, their fetuses may have less reserve to sustain stress during labour, or the maternal pelvic size may be less optimal for normal childbirth.

Assisted vaginal breech delivery

A brief history of assisted vaginal breech delivery

As breech presentation is the most common type of malpresentation (3–4% of all pregnancies), vaginal breech delivery was a common practice before the era of safe CS delivery. Planned CS breech delivery had then taken over, after the Term Breech Trial was published in 2000 (26) which showed reduction in the perinatal and maternal safety of planned CS compared with vaginal breech delivery. Although there is criticism on the methodology and results of the Term Breech Trial, more than 90% of breech presenting pregnancies are now delivered by CS in developed countries. Balancing the risk and benefits of different routes of breech delivery, the United Kingdom Royal College of Obstetricians and Gynaecologists in its 2006 guideline has maintained the role and practice of vaginal breech delivery in certain circumstances instead of recommending CS for all breech presenting pregnancies (27). Hence, careful selection of suitable cases, acquisition of the skill to perform vaginal breech delivery, and proper counselling of patients remain the most important safeguarding factors in modern obstetrics.

Contraindications of assisted vaginal breech delivery

The Royal College of Obstetricians and Gynaecologists stated the following to be unfavourable factors for vaginal breech deliveries (27):

- Any other contraindications to vaginal birth (e.g. placenta praevia, compromised fetal condition).
- Clinically inadequate pelvis (radiological pelvimetry is not necessary).
- Footling or kneeling breech presentation (because of higher risk of cord prolapse).
- A large baby (usually defined as >3800 g).
- A growth-restricted baby (usually defined as <2000 g).
- Hyperextended fetal neck in labour (may increase the risk of cervical spinal cord injury; can be diagnosed with ultrasonography or radiography where ultrasonography is not available).
- A lack of presence of a clinician trained in vaginal breech delivery.
- A previous CS.

Procedure of assisted vaginal breech delivery

General labour management

Labour induction for breech presentation may be considered if individual circumstances are favourable, but labour augmentation is not recommended. Continuous electronic fetal heart rate monitoring is essential during labour. In case of a non-reassuring pattern, fetal blood sampling from the buttocks is not advised. CS should be considered if there is a delay in the descent of the breech at any stage in the first or the second stage of labour, or if there is any suspicion of fetal distress. Adequate analgesia for labour pain relief should be offered, preferably with regional anaesthesia. Episiotomy should be performed at the time of perineal distension by the fetal buttocks (27).

Delivery of the fetal legs and trunk

The mother should be encouraged to push to deliver the buttocks and the legs spontaneously. The operator should avoid unnecessary intervention, but may help to flex the knee joint by slightly pressing at the popliteal fossa, and then delivering the flexed thigh by splinting the medial side of the thigh and sweeping it laterally. The operator may also guide the rotation of the buttocks to a sacral anterior position after both legs have been delivered.

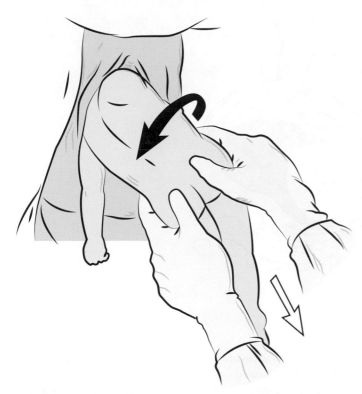

Figure 33.8 Delivery of the shoulders in assisted vaginal breech delivery.

Once the buttocks are delivered, the mother is encouraged to push to deliver the fetal abdomen and the trunk gradually, with or without conjunctional use of gentle downward and rotational force of the operator. The operator should hold the fetal bony pelvis steadily, instead of holding its abdomen, which may result in rupture of the internal organs (e.g. liver) if great force is applied accidentally. Pulling on the legs to promote descent should also be avoided as it may cause hip dislocation or other fetal injury. The umbilical cord may be exposed from the vagina during this stage, and precautions must be taken to avoid any cord compression.

Delivery of the fetal arms

When the scapulas are visible outside the vulva, the next step is to deliver the arms, which are often extended, and the forearms may be even positioned behind the fetal neck (nuchal arm). Continuous downward traction would not help to deliver the arms but further extend it. Hence, at this stage the fetal trunk should be rotated (with operator's hands still on the fetal pelvis) so that one of the shoulders is positioned anteriorly (at 12 o'clock) (**Figure 33.8**). Successful rotation would lead to the sliding of the anterior shoulder and humerus to the vulval level. The operator can then follow the anterior humerus to the elbow, and then with the operator's fingers at the elbow, sweep the fetal arm down in front of the fetal chest. Similar manipulation can be applied on the contralateral side to deliver the other shoulder and arm. Any traction on the humerus should be avoided as it would cause humeral fracture.

If very rarely the rotation cannot facilitate the delivery of the anterior arm, the posterior arm can be approached and delivered first. At this stage, the fetal feet are grasped and drawn upward over the inner thigh of the mother, toward the side that the fetal ventral surface is facing. By doing so, leverage is exerted upon the posterior shoulder, which may slide out over the vulval margin. The operator may then follow the posterior humerus to its elbow and sweep the arm out.

Delivery of the fetal head

The appearance of the fetal hairline outside the vulva indicates that the fetal head is now ready for delivery. Unlike vaginal cephalic delivery in which the fetal cranium has undergone moulding throughout labour as a gradual process, the vaginal delivery of the aftercoming head is potentially more difficult as the base of the skull (not moulded) would come out prior to the cranium. Hence, reducing the presenting diameter of the head by keeping it in a flexed position during the decent of the fetal head is crucial for a smooth delivery. This can be facilitated by the following two common methods:

Mauriceau–Smellie–Veit manoeuvre

In this manoeuvre, the fetal chest and abdomen is first placed on the operator's left palm and forearm, with the fetal legs straddled over the operator's forearm. The operator's left index and middle fingers are inserted into the vagina to identify the fetal maxillas, one on each side. The operator's right index finger and fourth finger are then put over both fetal shoulders, one on each side, to exert a downward traction. The fetal head flexion is facilitated by the simultaneous exertion of force on the maxillas by the left index and middle fingers, and on the occiput by the right middle finger (**Figure 33.9**). Care should be taken to avoid blindly pressing the left fingers on the fetal eyeballs (just above the maxillas), or inserting the fingers into the fetal mouth and to pull the lower jaw. Suprapubic pressure by an assistant may help to facilitate the fetal head flexion. The fetal body is then elevated towards the maternal abdomen, so that the fetal head gradually rotates out of the perineum starting from the fetal mouth, nose, brow, and eventually the occiput.

Forceps to aftercoming head

Grasping the fetal head with a pair of forceps properly can ensure the head flexion during the descent process. Piper's forceps are designed specifically for such a purpose (**Figure 33.3**). In contrast to cephalic forceps delivery, Piper's forceps should be inserted from below the level of the fetal body (**Figure 33.10**), and it is more easily done when the operator kneels down. Secondly, the Piper's forceps should be held horizontally with their shanks parallel to the perineum at the beginning of insertion. With the fetal head in the OA position, the blades are slid into the vagina, one after the other, in a similar manner as in cephalic forceps delivery. After successful locking of the forceps, the fetal head is pulled out by the blades while the shanks and handles are swung upwards to deliver the fetal head in the flexed position.

Burns–Marshall method

The fetal feet are grasped and with gentle traction they are swept over the maternal abdomen, and sometimes the delivery of the fetal head may follow in simple cases. However, unlike the Mauriceau–Smellie–Veit manoeuvre or forceps delivery, the Burns–Marshall

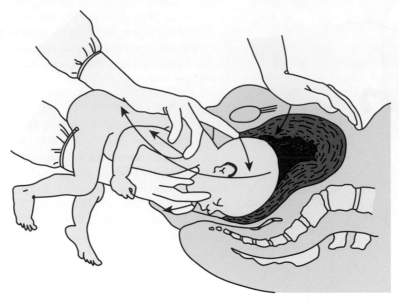

Figure 33.9 The Mauriceau–Smellie–Veit manoeuvre.

method does not promote fetal head flexion, and hence may not help to relieve the aftercoming head. There is also concern about the risks of the Burns–Marshall method if used incorrectly, leading to over-extension of the baby's neck.

Risks and complications of assisted vaginal breech delivery

One of the major risks of vaginal breech delivery is fetal hyp-oxic injury, as the umbilical cord is vulnerable to compression or vasoconstriction once it is outside the cervix during the delivery process. Delayed delivery caused by nuchal arm or head entrap-ment increases the risk of hypoxia. Birth trauma such as frac-tures, nerve injury, and visceral injury can be caused by forceful traction or poor manipulation by inexperienced hands. A recent meta-analysis shows that although planned vaginal delivery is associated with a two to five times higher perinatal complica-tion rate than planned caesarean delivery, its absolute mortality (0.3%), neurological morbidity (0.7%), and birth trauma rate (0.7%) remain at a low level that keep it a viable option in selected cases (28).

Conclusion

The obstetric procedures described in this chapter are effective measures to manage or prevent difficult or complicated childbirth. However, they are not without risk. Hence careful clinical assess-ment of patients, appropriate medical indication of the procedures, and proper training of the skills required are all essential to ensure safe application of these procedures.

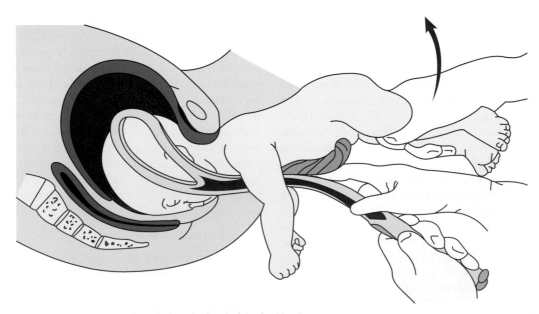

Figure 33.10 Application of Piper's forceps from below the level of the fetal body.

REFERENCES

1. Lumbiganon P, Laopaiboon M, Gülmezoglu AM, et al. Method of delivery and pregnancy outcomes in Asia: the WHO global survey on maternal and perinatal health 2007–08. *Lancet* 2010;**375**:490–99.

2. Crowther CA, Dodd JM, Hiller JE, Haslam RR, Robinson JS, Birth After Caesarean Study Group. Planned vaginal birth or elective repeat caesarean: patient preference restricted cohort with nested randomised trial. *PLoS Med* 2012;**9**: e1001192.

3. Greene RA, Fitzpatrick C, Turner MJ. What are the maternal implications of a classical caesarean section? *J Obstet Gynaecol* 1998;**18**:345–57.

4. Guise JM, Berlin M, McDonagh M, Osterweil P, Chan B, Helfand M. Safety of vaginal birth after cesarean: a systematic review. *Obstet Gynecol* 2004;**103**:420–29.

5. Royal College of Obstetricians and Gynaecologists (RCOG). *Birth after Previous Caesarean Birth*. Green-top Guideline No. 45. London: RCOG; 2015.

6. Anim-Somuah M, Smyth R, Howell C. Epidural versus nonepidural or no analgesia in labour. *Cochrane Database Syst Rev* 2005;**4**:CD000331.

7. American College of Obstetricians and Gynecologists. Operative vaginal delivery. *ACOG Practice Bull* 2000;**17**:1–6.

8. Royal College of Obstetricians and Gynaecologists (RCOG). *Operative Vaginal Delivery*. Green-top Guideline No. 26. London: RCOG; 2011.

9. Chung MY, Wan OY, Cheung RY, Chung TK, Chan SS. Prevalence of levator ani muscle injury and health-related quality of life in primiparous Chinese women after instrumental delivery. *Ultrasound Obstet Gynecol* 2015;**45**:728–33.

10. Gurol-Urganci I, Cromwell DA, Edozien LC, et al. Third- and fourth-degree perineal tears among primiparous women in England between 2000 and 2012: time trends and risk factors. *BJOG* 2013;**120**:1516–25.

11. de Vogel J, van der Leeuw-van Beek A, Gietelink D, et al. The effect of a mediolateral episiotomy during operative vaginal delivery on the risk of developing obstetrical anal sphincter injuries. *Am J Obstet Gynecol* 2012;**206**:404.e1–5.

12. De Leeuw JW, Vierhout ME, Struijk PC, Hop WC, Wallenburg HC. Anal sphincter damage after vaginal delivery: functional outcome and risk factors for fecal incontinence. *Acta Obstet Gynecol Scand* 2001;**80**:830–34.

13. Stedenfeldt M, Pirhonen J, Blix E, Wilsgaard T, Vonen B, Øian P. Episiotomy characteristics and risks for obstetric anal sphincter injuries: a case-control study. *BJOG* 2012;**119**:724–30.

14. National Institute for Health and Care Excellence (NICE). *Intrapartum Care: Care of Healthy Women and their Babies during Childbirth*. Clinical guideline [CG55]. London: NICE; 2007.

15. Sultan AH. Obstetric perineal injury and anal incontinence. *Clin Risk* 1999;**5**:193–96.

16. Royal College of Obstetricians and Gynaecologists (RCOG). *The Management of Third- and Fourth-Degree Perineal Tears*. Green-top Guideline No. 29. London: RCOG; 2015.

17. Mahony R, Behan M, Daly L, Kirwan C, O'Herlihy C, O'Connell PR. Internal anal sphincter defect influences continence outcome following obstetric anal sphincter injury. *Am J Obstet Gynecol* 2007;**196**:217.e1–5.

18. Fernando RJ, Sultan AH, Kettle C, Thakar R. Methods of repair for obstetric anal sphincter injury. *Cochrane Database Syst Rev* 2013;**12**:CD002866.

19. Aflaifel N, Weeks A. Push, pull, squeeze, clamp: 100 years of changes in the management of the third stage of labour as described by ten teachers. *BMJ* 2012;**345**:e8270.

20. Royal College of Obstetricians and Gynaecologists (RCOG). *External Cephalic Version (ECV) and Reducing the Incidence of Breech Presentation*. Green-top Guideline No. 20a. London: RCOG; 2006.

21. Suen SS, Khaw KS, Law LW, et al. The force applied to successfully turn a foetus during reattempts of external cephalic version is substantially reduced when performed under spinal analgesia. *J Matern Fetal Neonatal Med* 2012;**25**:719–22.

22. Khaw KS, Lee SW, Ngan Kee WD, et al. Randomized trial of anaesthetic interventions in external cephalic version for breech presentation. *Br J Anaesth* 2015;**114**:944 50.

23. Lau TK, Lo KW, Leung TY, Fok WY, Rogers MS. Outcome of labour after successful external cephalic version at term complicated by isolated transient fetal bradycardia. *BJOG* 2000;**107**:401–405.

24. Leung KT, Suen SS, Sahota DS, Lau TK, Leung TY. External cephalic version does not increase the risk of intrauterine death: a 17-year experience and literature review. *J Matern Fetal Neonatal Med* 2012; **25**:1774–78.

25. Chan LY, Tang JL, Tsoi KF, Fok WY, Chan LW, Lau TK. Intrapartum cesarean delivery after successful external cephalic version: a meta-analysis. *Obstet Gynecol* 2004;**104**:155–60.

26. Hannah ME, Hannah WJ, Hewson SA, et al. Planned caesarean section versus planned vaginal birth for breech presentation at term: a randomized multicentre trial. *Lancet* 2000;**356**:1375–83.

27. Royal College of Obstetricians and Gynaecologists (RCOG). *The Management of Breech Presentation*. Green-top Guideline No. 20b. London: RCOG; 2006.

28. Berhan Y, Haileamlak A. The risks of planned vaginal breech delivery versus planned caesarean section for term breech birth: a meta-analysis including observational studies *BJOG* 2016;**123**:49–57.

34

Stillbirth

David A. Ellwood and Vicki Flenady

Epidemiology of stillbirth

Definitions

Stillbirth is defined by the World Health Organization as 'death prior to the complete expulsion or extraction from its mother of a product of conception...the fetus does not breathe or show any other evidence of life, such as beating of the heart, pulsation of the umbilical cord, or definite movement of voluntary muscles'. While the term fetal death is most accurate, the word stillbirth is preferred by parents and the community (1, 2). The International Classification of Diseases 10th revision (ICD-10) definitions are as follows:

- Late fetal death: 1000 g or more or 28 weeks or more or 35 cm or more.
- Early fetal death: 500 g or more or 22 weeks or more or 25 cm or more.
- Miscarriage is a pregnancy loss before 22 completed weeks of gestational age (birthweight is given priority over gestational age).

For international comparisons, the World Health Organization recommends reporting of late gestation stillbirths (>28 weeks). The stillbirth rate is commonly expressed as the number of stillbirths per 1000 births. Many high-income countries (HICs) use a lower gestational age and birthweight threshold. For example, the United States, Canada, and Australia use 20 weeks' gestation or 400 g. Different practices for inclusion of medical terminations of pregnancy also result in variations in reported stillbirth rates (3).

Rates and trends in stillbirth rates

Around 2.6 million late gestation stillbirths occur globally each year. The majority (98%) occur in low- and middle-income countries (LMIC) (**Figure 34.1**) (4) with around half during labour or intrapartum (**Figure 34.2**). Applying the lower gestational cut-off definition used across many HICs, the number of stillbirths could be up to 50% higher. A wide variation in stillbirth rates is evident, ranging from 28.7 (sub-Saharan Africa) to 3.4 per 1000 births (developed regions). Reduction in global stillbirth rates has been slow, estimated at 1.4% per year from 2000 to 2015, which is around half that seen for maternal and newborn deaths (5).

While absolute stillbirth rates in HICs are relatively low, variation in rates suggests that further reduction is possible. In the United

States and Australia (using similar definitions of 20 weeks' gestation or 400 g), stillbirth rates are 6.1 and 7.8/1000 births respectively and make up around 70% of total perinatal mortality, with the majority occurring in the antepartum period (3). Overall, around 1 in 140 women who reach 20 weeks' gestation will have a stillborn baby. Using the number of ongoing pregnancies as the denominator, there is a U-shaped risk of stillbirth which is higher in the 20–24 weeks period, falls and then increases from 1 in 2000 at 37 weeks to 1 in 500 at 42 weeks (6).

Risk factors

Two recently reported systematic reviews on risk factors for stillbirth (5, 7) are summarized here with the major factors presented in **Table 34.1**.

Maternal sociodemographic factors

Advanced maternal age (>35 years), overweight (body mass index (BMI) 25–30 kg/m²), and obesity (BMI >30 kg/m²) and smoking are the three largest potentially modifiable contributors to stillbirth across HICs. These risk factors also make an important contribution to stillbirth globally (5). Women of 35 years or older have a 70% increased risk in stillbirth accounting for around 7% of stillbirths globally (7). Women over the age of 40 years have a doubling of the risk of stillbirth. Maternal overweight and obesity has become a global health problem, which also carries an increased risk of stillbirth (20% and 60% respectively). Women with a very high BMI (>40 kg/m²) have a more than twofold increase in the risk (7). The contribution to stillbirth of maternal overweight and obesity globally is estimated at 10% (5) and may be twice that in some disadvantaged groups with higher rates of overweight and obesity (7). Maternal obesity also increases the risk of diabetes and hypertension, which further places women at increased risk of stillbirth. Data from HICs show that while the overall contribution of pre-existing diabetes to stillbirths is small at the population level, it is one of the maternal medical conditions most strongly associated with stillbirth. Despite modern obstetric care, pre-existing diabetes is associated with a threefold increase in stillbirth (7). Chronic/pre-existing hypertension remains an important contributor to adverse pregnancy outcome with almost three times the risk in HICs (7).

The risk of stillbirth for women having their first child is around 40% higher than women who have had a previous birth. In HICs,

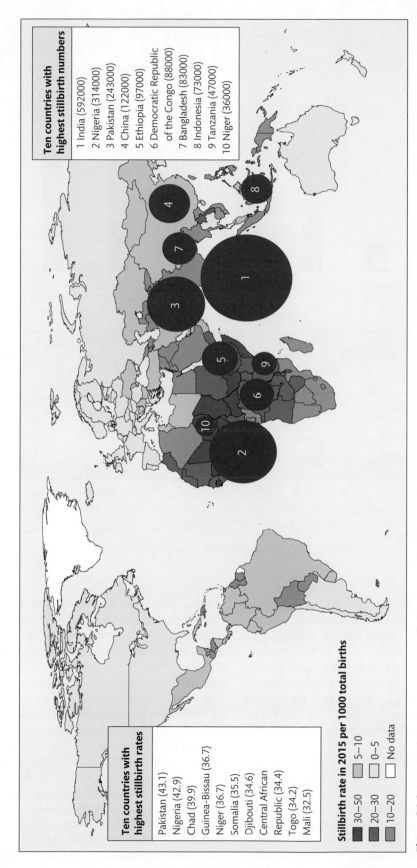

Ten countries with highest stillbirth numbers

1 India (592000)
2 Nigeria (314000)
3 Pakistan (243000)
4 China (122000)
5 Ethiopia (97000)
6 Democratic Republic
of the Congo (88000)
7 Bangladesh (83000)
8 Indonesia (73000)
9 Tanzania (47000)
10 Niger (36000)

Ten countries with highest stillbirth rates

Pakistan (43.1)
Nigeria (42.9)
Chad (39.9)
Guinea-Bissau (36.7)
Niger (36.7)
Somalia (35.5)
Djibouti (34.6)
Central African
Republic (34.4)
Togo (34.2)
Mali (32.5)

Stillbirth rate in 2015 per 1000 total births

- 30–50
- 20–30
- 10–20
- 5–10
- 0–5
- No data

Figure 34.1 Variation between countries in stillbirth rates in 2015 showing the ten countries with the highest rates, and those with the largest numbers.

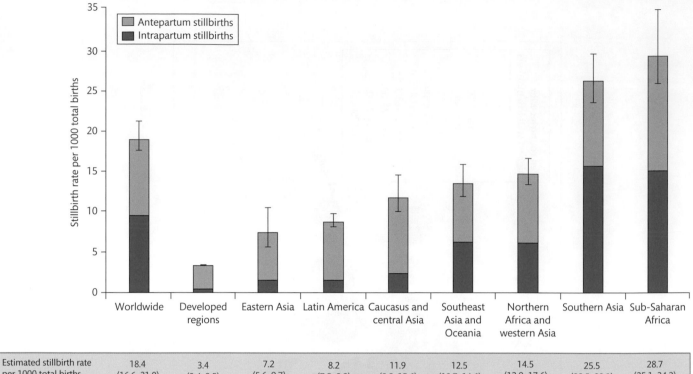

Figure 34.2 Regional variation in estimated stillbirth rates, showing uncertainty ranges, and the proportion of intrapartum stillbirths for 2015. *Based on urban and rural birth cohorts with national stillbirth rates so the values might underestimate rural stillbirth rates, which are expected to be higher than urban rates. Facility and home stillbirth rates are differential, the direction of increased stillbirth rates is unpredictable because the values might be lower at home if high-risk cases are in facilities, or higher at home if very low access to care.

Reproduced from Lawn JE, Blencowe H, Waiswa P, et al. Stillbirths: rates, risk factors and potential for progress towards 2030. *Lancet* 2016; 387: 587–603 with permission from Elsevier.

primiparity is an important contributor accounting for around 15% of stillbirths. Combining risk factors is also important and the stillbirth risk in older primiparous women (i.e. ≥35 years) may be two- to fourfold higher than their counterparts. In HICs particularly, with more women delaying childbearing, the higher rates of primiparous women of advanced age combined with increasing rates of overweight and obesity, sets a real challenge for stillbirth prevention. While rare in many settings, multiparity of five or more births carries increased risk of stillbirth and other adverse pregnancy outcomes (7).

Smoking has a tremendous global impact on health and smoking in pregnancy is causally related to placental pathology and increased risk of stillbirth (around 40%). Heavy smoking (ten or more cigarettes per day) carries a doubling of the risk. Women who are disadvantaged (lower socioeconomic status, poor education, by race/ethnic background, lack of access to quality culturally appropriate care), even in HIC settings, have approximately double or more the risk of stillbirth (7). Higher smoking rates,

and poor antenatal care (which itself is associated with a three-fold increase risk) and maternal medical conditions are important contributors in disadvantaged populations (3). Other factors contributing to this excess includes alcohol consumption (binge drinking) in the first trimester, illicit drugs use in pregnancy, indoor pollution, young maternal age, domestic violence, and possibly short interpregnancy interval. Consanguinity is a risk factor for stillbirth in some regions and cultures. While the adverse effects of alcohol consumption on the developing fetus are well accepted, there is a paucity of high-quality data to assess its true impact. Studies in HICs show a small (around 10%) increase in stillbirth for low intake (one to three drinks per week). One large study in the United States showed the association was stronger for stillbirth at less than 28 weeks' gestation (80% increase). However, the risk was isolated to women with more than five drinks per week. Based on a prevalence of 50% and a 40% increased risk, alcohol intake in pregnancy could account for up to 17% of stillbirth in HIC settings.

Table 34.1 Risk factors for stillbirth

Factor	High-income countries[a]		Globally[b]	
	aOR (95% CI)[c]	PAR (%)[d]	aOR range	PAR (%)[d]
Demographic and fertility				
Maternal age (years)[e]				
35–39	1.5 (1.2–1.7)	–	–	–
40–44	1.8 (1.4–2.3)	–	–	–
≥45	2.9 (1.9–4.4)	–	–	–
>35	1.7 (1.6–1.7)	12	1.7 (1.6–1.7)[a]	6.7
Low education	1.7 (1.4–2.0)	4.9	–	–
Low socioeconomic status	1.2 (1.0–1.4)	9.0	–	–
No antenatal care	3.3 (3.1–3.6)	0.7	–	–
Assisted reproductive technology (singleton pregnancy)	2.7 (1.6–4.7)	3.1	–	–
Primiparity	1.4 (1.4–1.3)	15		
Previous stillbirth	3.4 (2.6–4.4)[f]	1[f]		
Non-communicable disease and obesity				
BMI (kg/m²)[g]				
25–30	1.2 (1.1–1.4)	–	1.2 (1.1–1.4)[a]	–
>30	1.6 (1.4–2.0)	–	1.6 (1.4–2.0)[a]	–
>25		8–18		10
Pre-existing diabetes	2.9 (2.1–4.1)	2–3	2.9 (2.1–4.1)[a]	7.6
Pre-existing hypertension	2.6 (2.1–3.1)	5–10	2.6 (2.1–3.1)[a]	10.4
Pre-eclampsia	1.6 (1.1–2.2)	3.1	1.6 (1.1–2.2)[a]	2.6
Eclampsia	2.2 (1.5–3.2)	0.1	2.2 (1.5–3.2)[a]	2.1
Fetal factors				
SGA (<10th centile)	3.9 (3.0–5.1)	23.3	–	–
Post-term pregnancy (≥42 weeks)	1.3 (1.1–1.7)	0.3	3.3 (1.0–11.1)	14.0
Rhesus disease	2.6 (2.0–3.2)[b]	0.6[b]	2.6 (2.0–3.2)	0.7
Infection				
Malaria	–	–	2.3 (0.8–6.7)	8
Syphilis	–	–	10.9 (6.6–17.9)	7.7
HIV	–	–	1.2 (1.2–2.2)	0.3
Lifestyle factors				
Smoking	1.4 (1.4–1.3)	4–7	1.5 (1.4–1.6)	1.6
Illicit drug use	1.9 (1.2–3.0)	2.1	–	–

[c] Adjusted odds ratio (aOR) (95% confidence interval); [d] PAR, population attributable risk (indicates the proportion of cases that would not occur *in a population* if the factor were eliminated); [e] reference <35 years of age; [g] reference BMI <25 kg/m².

Source data from [a] Flenady V, Koopmans L, Middleton P, et al. Major risk factors for stillbirth in high-income countries: a systematic review and meta-analysis. *Lancet* 2011; 377(9774): 1331–40; and [b] Lawn JE, Blencowe H, Waiswa P, et al. Stillbirths: rates, risk factors and potential for progress towards 2030. *Lancet* 2016; 387: 587–603; [f] sourced from Lamont K, Scott NW, Jones GT, Bhattacharya S. Risk of recurrent stillbirth: systematic review and meta-analysis. *BMJ* 2015; 350: h3080. PAR calculated by chapter authors using a prevalence of 0.05% (V Flenady and D Ellwood).

Pregnancy complications

Previous adverse pregnancy outcome is an indicator of subsequent stillbirth risk. Women who have a previous stillbirth have around three times the risk of stillbirth in a subsequent pregnancy (adjusted for other factors) (8). Previous preterm birth of a small-for-gestational age (SGA) baby also increases the risk of stillbirth in a subsequent pregnancy by three to five times (7). Previous caesarean section may be associated with an increased risk of stillbirth which

is thought to be due to abnormal placentation, however further research is needed (7).

Suboptimal fetal growth is strongly linked with stillbirth. In an analysis of studies across HICs, SGA (less than the tenth centile for gestational age), was independently associated with a fourfold increased risk of stillbirth contributing to 23% of stillbirths (7). This finding points to the important contribution of placental pathologies/insufficiencies in stillbirth in HIC settings. Post-term pregnancy

(≥42 weeks' gestation) is a risk factor for adverse pregnancy outcome estimated to contribute to 14% of stillbirths globally (5). With induction of labour policies before 42 weeks in many developed regions, the contribution to stillbirth of post-term pregnancy in these settings is usually quite small (7).

Multiple pregnancy carries up to a sixfold increase in the odds of stillbirth when controlled for other factors (7). The currently available data suggest that women conceiving using assisted reproductive technology are likely to be at increased risk of neonatal deaths through SGA and preterm birth. While the association between assisted reproductive technologies and stillbirth is unclear, *in vitro* fertilization is definitely associated with an increased risk for singleton pregnancies (7). Male sex is associated with a small increase in the odds of stillbirth which may be through X-linked conditions, increased risk of preterm birth, and poor fetal growth (5).

Causes of stillbirth

Accurate and consistently classified data on the global causes of stillbirth are limited, particularly in LMIC. This is partly due to the difficulty in assigning causation due to the multifactorial circumstances of many stillbirths, underinvestigation, and the use of various, disparate classification systems for assigning cause of death (3). Globally, less than 10% of stillbirths are attributed to congenital abnormality (5) indicating that there is a high degree of potential preventability for cases due to other causes. Even for stillbirth with major abnormalities the potential for primary prevention exists (e.g. folic acid supplementation for neural tube defects). Causes of stillbirth vary with rates, with high-burden settings often reporting much higher proportions of intrapartum-related stillbirths.

Low- and middle-income countries

While data are sparse and vary widely by region across LMIC, the main reported causes of stillbirth include placental abruption accounting for up to one-quarter of stillbirths, pre-eclampsia and eclampsia, infection with malaria and syphilis which is a major problem in some regions, maternal conditions such as pre-existing diabetes and hypertension, and intrapartum complications accounting for up to 40% in some regions (9).

High-income countries

While a global picture of causes of stillbirth across HICs is difficult due to factors previously mentioned, recent population-based data show the most consistently reported categories of causes (3): placental pathology ranging from 13% to 39% (including largely placental abruption and insufficiency), fetomaternal haemorrhage around 2%, infection 5–15%, congenital anomalies 9–27%, maternal hypertensive disorders 3–9%, maternal diabetes 1–3%, cord complications 9%, and intrapartum complications around 3%. Complications of multiple gestation are not well reported but appear to account for around 6% of stillbirths (of which twin–twin transfusion syndrome contributes about 1–3%). Fetal growth restriction (FGR) or SGA, while not strictly a cause of stillbirth, is captured in most stillbirth classification systems with reported proportions ranging widely (3–38%) depending on whether conditions leading to poor fetal growth are classified preferentially. In systems where the scenarios of preterm labour and preterm prelabour rupture of membranes (often in combination with chorioamnionitis) are captured, from 3% to 15% of stillbirths are attributed to these scenarios and

up to 40% of stillbirths at less than 28 weeks' gestation. Unexplained stillbirth ranges from 11% to 31% with adequacy of investigation and the system used being important influencing factors (3). Using a system which takes into account the quality of investigations for stillbirth, one study reported a low proportion of unexplained with thorough investigation (11%), classifying a further 19% as unknown due to insufficient investigation (6).

Quality of care and stillbirth

The stillbirth rate is a key indicator of the health of women in general and the quality of healthcare during pregnancy and childbirth. While the stillbirth rate itself is a valuable indicator (particularly in LMIC settings), to ensure policy and practice change a systematic approach to perinatal outcome audit with feedback to clinicians is needed (10). Perinatal outcome audit has been defined as 'the process of capturing information on the number and causes of all stillbirths and neonatal deaths, or near-misses where applicable, with an aim towards identifying specific cases for systematic, critical analysis of the quality of perinatal care received in a no-blame, interdisciplinary setting in order to improve the care provided to all mothers and babies' (10). Perinatal mortality audits have consistently shown that suboptimal antenatal and obstetric care are frequently associated with stillbirths and neonatal deaths, ranging from 10% to 60% of cases. The main reported factors relate to delayed recognition of emerging clinical disorders, and inadequate or delayed response (most notably around maternal concern of decreased fetal movements (DFMs) and FGR). Other factors include failure to update and use best practice protocols, poor communication between staff, inadequate antenatal care, poor diabetes management, and maternal smoking. In the South African audit programme (Perinatal Problem Identification Programme), almost half of the deaths due to intrapartum asphyxia were found to be probably preventable with better fetal monitoring, use of the partogram, and optimal care in the second stage of labour (11). Although intrapartum stillbirths now make up a small proportion of late gestation stillbirths in HICs, concerns have been raised regarding the contribution of suboptimal care in these cases. In LMIC, high fertility rates coupled with low coverage of care and access to family planning are major contributors to stillbirth and neonatal death. Perinatal mortality audit, when combined with an approach to ensure practice change, can reduce avoidable stillbirth and neonatal deaths and is an essential part of good obstetric practice (10).

Managing the obstetric aspects of stillbirth

The acute presentation, including the diagnosis of stillbirth

Stillbirth presents in many ways but in each case the obstetric management must be compassionate and the multiprofessional team involved should be cognisant of the extreme impact of the diagnosis and the emotional well-being of the woman and her family. A common presentation in the third trimester will be associated with reduced or absent fetal movements, and then an inability to detect the fetal heart using a hand-held Doppler or cardiotocography (CTG) machine. It is important that confirmation of the diagnosis is made with ultrasonography as soon as possible, and that there is senior obstetric and midwifery input at the time. It is essential to avoid any uncertainty. The statement 'I don't think there is a fetal heart present' leaves open the possibility that this could be wrong and can compound the grief reaction when it is finally confirmed. Another common scenario is when an ultrasound examination is being performed, either as part of routine screening or if there is a reduced fundal height, and in this case the sonographer may be the first person to make the diagnosis. Once again, senior input from maternity caregivers is essential, as this is an emotional emergency and how it is handled can impact the grief reaction for many months afterwards. There is no place for delaying the formal diagnosis by ultrasonography until a later, more convenient time.

One particularly difficult situation is when it is discovered that one of twins or triplets has died. For di- or trichorionic pregnancies this will not normally lead to a decision to intervene by delivering the remaining twin or triplets. In the situation of monochorionic twins, especially at more advanced gestations, consideration may need to be given to immediate delivery of the surviving twin to avoid neurological sequelae, although this will depend on the gestational age and the length of time since fetal death occurred.

Delivery care: induction of labour and other obstetric aspects including complications

In many respects, the birth of a stillborn baby is not especially different from that of a live-born baby. Methods of induction of labour are generally going to be the same, although with very early gestations (up to about 30 weeks) other drug combinations such as mifepristone and misoprostol may be used. Local protocols should be consulted but generally a combination of prostaglandins and then artificial rupture of membranes/Syntocinon is used in the third trimester, sometimes with the addition of a cervical catheter to ripen the cervix if very unfavourable.

It is relatively common for women (and their families) to request 'an immediate caesarean section' after fetal death been diagnosed, especially if this is late in the third trimester. This request should be managed respectfully, but it should also be considered to be a natural part of the immediate grief reaction. The desire to deliver the baby by the quickest method possible may be driven by the need to see and hold the baby and protect it from any further harm. While there is no rigorous evidence to support either approach, the experience of many involved in stillbirth care is that careful and expert counselling will lead to a decision to deliver the baby using the method that was originally planned, had the baby survived. It is clearly difficult to raise the issue of the next pregnancy at such a difficult time for parents but avoiding an unnecessary caesarean section may improve outcomes next time, and make management of that pregnancy much easier.

Obstetric complications associated with stillbirth are many, and these need to be explained to the woman before commencing induction of labour. It can be quite unpredictable how long the induction process may take, especially if the pregnancy is still in the second trimester. Stillbirth is more commonly encountered with both FGR and macrosomia, as well as with both oligo- and polyhydramnios, so unstable lie and malpresentations are more common. After the birth it is not unusual to have a retained placenta, and postpartum haemorrhage is also more common as the fetal death may be associated with abnormalities of placentation including abruption. Management of the third stage should be active and the team should be ready to deal with any third-stage complication.

Investigation after stillbirth including postmortem and placental histopathology

In most developed countries there exist protocols for investigation after stillbirth, although there are a number of studies being conducted worldwide into the efficacy and cost-effectiveness of a range of investigations. The purpose of investigations is to try to identify, as far as is possible, a cause of the stillbirth, which should then facilitate discussions about recurrence risks. Investigations are expensive, and all may not be available in every context in which stillbirth occurs. Generally investigations can be discussed under four headings:

Fetal and placental examination (including postmortem (autopsy) and imaging)

The autopsy should be considered the 'gold standard' of the investigations, but there are many considerations around autopsy consent, and availability of expert perinatal pathologists to both perform the autopsy and interpret the results. Many parents will not consent to autopsy as they consider it is highly invasive and in some cases may be against their spiritual or cultural beliefs. This requires careful discussion and senior counselling intervention as the lack of an autopsy will often impede the final diagnosis and classification of the cause, as well as an understanding of any contributory factors. If autopsy is not agreed to, or not available, there are a number of alternatives, which range from external examination by a paediatrician or geneticist to try to identify dysmorphic features, imaging such as radiography or other more complex tests such as computed tomography or magnetic resonance imaging. In some cases, women may consent to a limited autopsy if it is thought that a particular organ system might be involved. It has been recommended that the target autopsy rate should be at least 50% of all stillbirths, but there is some argument for the selective use of this expensive investigation, especially if there is likely to be a low yield or if the cause of the fetal death is obvious. Even if there is no fetal examination performed, placental histopathology should also be done as there is a strong association between various placental pathologies and stillbirth (**Figure 34.3**). The placenta should always be sent to the pathology laboratory fresh, and not placed in formalin.

Microbiological studies

Infection is a relatively common cause of stillbirth but interpretation of microbiological results can be difficult as bacteria will often be present as contaminants, especially if fetal death has been present for some time. Swabs should be taken from the lower genital tract, the fetal membranes and placenta, and also from the fetal skin and internal organs. Generally, to attribute fetal death to bacterial infection it is important to see that the same bacteria is found in multiple sites, that it is considered to be pathogenic, and that there is evidence of some maternal and/or fetal response to the bacteria by eliciting signs of inflammation with histopathology. In some cases not all of these features are present and the conclusion must be drawn that 'infection may have been the cause but it cannot be confirmed'.

Maternal blood tests

In general, the yield from maternal blood tests is quite low. These investigations are aimed at diagnosing a range of maternal medical conditions, such as diabetes, cholestasis, or thyroid disease, and in modern antenatal care it is unusual for these conditions to have been

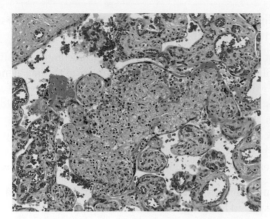

Figure 34.3 Placental histopathology slide showing evidence of chronic villitis, which is strongly associated with fetal growth restriction and stillbirth.

Courtesy of Professor Jane Dahlstrom.

missed prior to the stillbirth. 'TORCH' titres and thrombophilia screens are often part of stillbirth investigation protocols but interpretation of results needs some expertise as they can be misleading. For example, factor V Leiden heterozygosity is found in about 5% of the population and if seen without any evidence of placental infarction it is unlikely to be of significance.

Chromosomal and genetic studies

In the past, a fetal karyotype was always recommended, and this would be done by either taking a skin sample, or else some knee cartilage. Unfortunately, the growth of cells obtained from these sites is often overrun by bacterial growth. More modern molecular techniques are being introduced into practice and there is now some evidence to support the use of microarray technology in stillbirth samples as a range of unusual genetic deletions and duplications have been described in association with third-trimester stillbirth. Recent research with whole genome sequencing is also showing promise as a tool that might reveal previously hidden causes of unexplained stillbirth.

These investigations take time to complete, especially autopsy finalization, and women should be told that there may be a wait of 6–12 weeks to provide results, especially if there is a shortage of expert perinatal pathologists. For this reason, the follow-up from a physical and emotional perspective should be staged, with early appointments scheduled for specific reasons. There must be a clear understanding of when the final results will be available and it is important to avoid giving women and their family results piece by piece. Putting the whole story together requires all the results to be available, for these to be considered in the context of the history, and for an expert in interpretation to be available for the scheduled appointment. This is a highly specialized field and needs to be seen as a tertiary service.

Care in the next pregnancy: recurrence risk, monitoring, timing, and mode of birth

For many women there is a subsequent pregnancy after stillbirth, so care in the next pregnancy is very important although there is little evidence to support the various practices used by clinicians. Surveys of obstetricians show a very high proportion would offer much more intensive fetal monitoring with both ultrasonography and CTG, and many would offer early delivery for women whose previous pregnancy ended in late gestation stillbirth (12).

When managing the next pregnancy, an understanding of the cause of the previous stillbirth is essential to guide clinical decision-making. Early booking, or even pre-pregnancy counselling is helpful in making a comprehensive plan for antenatal care and birth. This plan is inevitably a compromise of both medical and emotional indications for various actions. For some women, normalizing the next pregnancy is important as this helps to reduce their anxiety around recurrence. For others, very intensive monitoring may be welcomed and getting the balance right is essential, as both under- and over-monitoring may fuel anxiety.

The timing and mode of birth are significant variables that both need to be included in the birth plan. Timing will often be influenced by the gestational age at which fetal death occurred previously, although if there is believed to be no or little risk of recurrence it makes no sense to cause iatrogenic prematurity without a good medical indication. Similarly, the view that caesarean section is indicated just because the previous pregnancy resulted in stillbirth is somewhat contentious. The view of these authors is that a request for planned elective caesarean section really should be considered in the same way that this request is considered in any other pregnancy. The option of planned, early induction of labour with close fetal monitoring is a reasonable alternative for the woman who wants to be in control of the timing and circumstances of birth, without the need for planned caesarean section.

Reducing the risk: stillbirth prevention strategies

Stillbirth prevention strategies vary between HICs and LMIC as the causes are very different. In LMIC, the strategies must focus on the provision of basic antenatal and intrapartum care. In many developing countries, lack of access to any form of birth attendant increases the risk of stillbirth, and the inability to intervene in an obstructed labour by either assisted vaginal delivery or caesarean section means that a large proportion of late stillbirths are from intrapartum causes. Infection is also a major contributor with maternal diseases such as malaria and syphilis adding to the burden.

The recent series on stillbirth in *The Lancet* has emphasized the fact that even in HICs there is significant variation in stillbirth rates between countries with similar populations and health systems suggesting that there is a lot that can be done to improve rates through prevention strategies. Even within HICs there are major differences as a result of socioeconomic disadvantage, which is particularly seen in Indigenous populations across the world such as those in Australia and Canada.

The role of risk factors identification and early delivery in stillbirth prevention

The knowledge of healthcare providers in HICs of the importance of risk factors has been surveyed revealing some interesting results, in which some less important risk factors are overemphasized, while the significance of others is underestimated (3). Maternal age, overweight and obesity, and smoking are three significant modifiable risk factors, which collectively contribute to about 30% of stillbirths. However, knowledge of the importance of risk factors does not easily translate into clinical practice. Smoking cessation advice can improve outcomes but as smoking rates fall, this is becoming less important from a population perspective. Average maternal age continues to increase in most HIC, as do rates of overweight and obesity and the most frequently used intervention is early delivery. The problem is when to intervene, and how to target interventions to those at highest risk, without over-intervening to the point that morbidity is increased rather than mortality decreased. In relation to maternal age and BMI, it appears that the increased stillbirth risk is continuous as both risk factors increase, so there is no particular cut-off that can be used to determine when to intervene. One potential approach would be to develop a risk-scoring tool that takes into account the importance of a range of factors, and provides a firm evidence for any early intervention.

The use of ultrasonography in the prediction of stillbirth risk

FGR and placental dysfunction with a range of placental pathologies are frequently found in association with stillbirth. Clinical detection of reduced fetal growth is generally not accurate enough to detect all those late gestation fetuses that are vulnerable. This is in part because of the inherent inaccuracy in fundal height measurements caused by variation in the measurement, but also because some of those at greatest risk may be those that show late slowing of growth. The early randomized trials of routine third-trimester ultrasound scanning, with or without umbilical artery Doppler, did not show improved perinatal outcomes although stillbirth prevention was not the primary outcome of most studies. Ultrasonography is used more frequently in those with risk factors such as maternal obesity but many late gestation stillbirths occur in women without risk factors. There is a resurgence of interest recently in the use of ultrasound biometry to improve the detection of FGR, as well as other modalities such as fetal Doppler making use of the cerebroplacental ratio. The ratio of middle cerebral artery Doppler pulsatility index to that recorded in the umbilical artery is a marker of cerebral redistribution of blood flow. The concept that placental dysfunction may occur in apparently normally grown fetuses, but which show redistribution of blood flow to the fetal brain, is now of significant interest as a stillbirth prevention strategy and requires confirmation by large clinical trials (3). The use of biomarkers in addition to fetal Doppler may be a way to improve the accuracy of this as a screening test.

Predicting stillbirth risk in early pregnancy

In many respects, the ideal strategy is to predict stillbirth risk in early pregnancy and then introduce a treatment that reduces the risk. At present, the only candidate for this is low-dose aspirin but other strategies may be developed in the future. First-trimester uterine artery Doppler, coupled with biomarkers such as pregnancy-associated plasma protein A (PAPP-A), can predict an increased risk of FGR, and indirectly the risk of stillbirth, but this needs further evidence before it can be recommended as an effective prevention strategy. As further research is done there may be other biomarkers identified that can be used for the same purpose.

Monitoring fetal movements, and organizational responses to decreased fetal movements

It has been known for decades that DFM is a predictor of stillbirth, yet evidence from large randomized trials shows that routine fetal

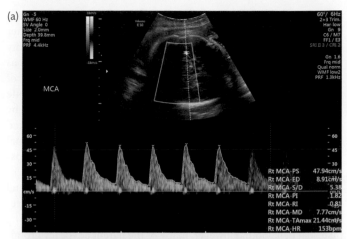

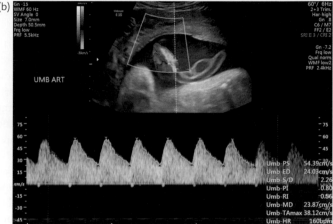

Figure 34.4 Colour Doppler imaging of the fetal circulation enables waveforms from both the (a) cerebral (middle cerebral artery) and (b) umbilical circulations, and enables the calculation of a CU ratio which can show evidence of redistribution of blood flow in the vulnerable fetus.

movement counting does not appear to reduce stillbirth risk. This may be the result of poor response to maternal presentation with DFM, coupled with a lack of appreciation of stillbirth risk factors. A nationwide approach in Norway to raising awareness of DFM has shown promise as a population-based prevention strategy but this is yet to be confirmed in other countries. DFM is a common presentation in the third trimester, and often there is reassurance from a normal CTG, without further investigation or an objective assessment of risk factors for stillbirth. International guidelines promoted by the International Stillbirth Alliance emphasize the importance of a timely institutional response to DFM, accurate and objective CTG interpretation, and ultrasound scanning looking for evidence of FGR if the woman has risk factors for stillbirth. Clinicians need to have a heightened sense of concern for women who represent with DFM several times over a short period. Novel approaches to managing this difficult aspect of stillbirth prevention include the use of mobile phone apps to remind women about fetal movements and/or to count fetal movements, as well as educational programmes for maternity staff to remind them of the importance of following guidelines.

Other interventions (including maternal sleep position)

A potentially important finding was reported in 2011, following a case–control study in Auckland, New Zealand, which showed an association between maternal back sleeping and late gestation still-birth (13). Since then, this observation has been replicated by other similar studies in Sydney, Australia, and West Africa. The possibility that this is part of the causation of stillbirth is an attractive idea as there is some biological plausibility based on the theoretical risk of reduction in uterine blood flow caused by the gravid uterus. Despite considerable interest, the association has not yet been confirmed by studies that prove conclusively the risk of stillbirth can be reduced by not back-sleeping. Part of the problem is the issue of maternal recall of sleeping position after such a traumatic event as the loss of a baby. If maternal sleeping position is part of the mechanism of late gestation stillbirth, possibly coupled with some degree of fetal vulnerability based on placental dysfunction, the intervention to re-duce risk is likely to be an educational campaign aimed at changing maternal behaviour. However, many of the parent advocacy groups involved with stillbirth have already started to promote this idea so it may already be very difficult to study this intervention.

Much of the recent research has focused on late gestation stillbirth as the category where there appears to be the most potential for pre-vention. However, earlier gestation stillbirth (20–28 weeks) is now becoming a more prominent feature of perinatal mortality reports and it is important not to forget that this is an equally tragic outcome of pregnancy. More research needs to be done to try to understand the likely cause of these earlier fetal deaths, as any approach to pre-vention needs to be targeted based on evidence.

Stillbirth prevention strategies must target the most common causes if they are going to have a significant impact. Investigating stillbirths thoroughly, and performing rigorous perinatal mortality audit to classify cases by antecedent cause (including any contribu-tory factors in care), is an essential part of any prevention strategy. Only in this way will interventions be accurately targeted to prevent-able causes of stillbirth.

Quality, respectful care after stillbirth

Stillbirth has a profound impact on the mother, father, and families and also healthcare providers and societies worldwide with substan-tial psychosocial and economic burden (14). Extreme shock and distress is commonly experienced by parents and families at diag-nosis of a fetal death. The majority of grieving mothers have signifi-cant grief-related depressive symptoms which often last for many years (14). Fathers also experience overwhelming and long-lasting grief and may find it difficult to express themselves (15). The life-changing effects of stillbirth on the family extend to siblings, grand-parents, and the wider family (Figure 34.5).

The needs of parents

A recent survey of bereaved parents conducted by the International Stillbirth Alliance (ISA), sought the most important things parents wanted to know when their baby was stillborn. The findings are summarized in Box 34.1. Overwhelmingly, parents wanted to know why their baby died, a question that included both cause of death, reasons for its occurrence, and whether it could have been prevented. These questions were associated with questions about their pregnancy and labour and a pervading sense of guilt among mothers, who asked whether they had done something wrong and if their baby had suffered. Other questions were about the baby's

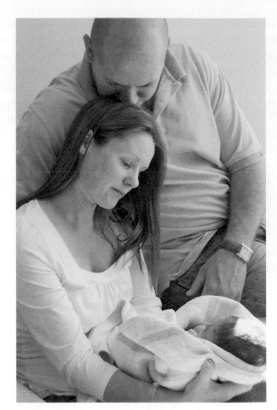

Figure 34.5 Ned and Heidi with Sophie, who was stillborn.

appearance and current location and information about the imme-diate care of the mother. Missed opportunities to answer the parents' questions might be avoided by simple measures that recognize the parents' need to know about their child (Box 34.1). A recent review showed that fathers want to be involved in decision-making and often focus on practical tasks (15).

Parents face many difficult decisions in the context of over-whelming grief and frequently have a diminished capacity to absorb and retain information. Fathers want to protect and support their partner and may feel frustrated and helpless if they cannot do this (15). Maternity staff who provide calm, supportive, and objective information, balancing guidance with parental autonomy, can as-sist parents to make informed decisions and minimize regret. Staff should ensure their own values and opinions do not influence grieving parents. Critical information should be repeated, and verbal information should be reinforced with parent-centred printed ma-terials. Parents need to be given privacy, time, and honesty. The more time dedicated to discussions with parents and the more informa-tion made available, the easier it is for parents to discuss dilemmas and find answers to questions. In the ISA surveys, parents often re-ported less than optimal care after the stillbirth, particularly to do with information sharing and decision support (3) (Figure 34.6).

Acknowledgment and understanding

The grief women experience after stillbirth may be aggravated by social stigma, blame, and marginalization (2). Negative perceptions and misunderstanding of stillbirth are commonplace and are major barriers to appropriate support for parents and families who have a stillborn child. Parents often report feelings that their stillborn child is less valued in the community than the death of an older child. In

Box 34.1 What do parents want to know after their baby is stillborn? Summary of qualitative survey data (n = 3503)

Why and how
- Why did it happen?
- How did it happen?

About the baby
- Where is my baby? What is happening to my baby?
- Did my baby suffer?
- Details about the baby—weight, eye colour, gender, and length.
- How can we create memories of our baby (including holding and caring for the baby and taking the baby home)?
- What are we 'allowed' to do (e.g. baby care, funerals, birth certificates, and taking the baby home)?

About care in pregnancy and labour
- Did I do something wrong?
- Why didn't they listen to me (voiced by women who felt that concerns raised in pregnancy were ignored or dismissed)?
- Why not sooner? This related to a range of care decisions made in their pregnancy.

About their own care
- How do I cope?
- How do I tell other children?

About the future
- Can we have another baby? How soon?
- What are the chances of stillbirth happening again?
- How long will it take to get over this?

Source data from Flenady V, Wojcieszek AM, Middleton P, Ellwood D, Erwich J, Coory M, et al. Stillbirths: recall to action in high-income countries. *The Lancet* 2016;13(387):691–702.

poorer regions of the world in particular, parents also consistently report that their baby was perceived as a taboo object and linked to sins of the mother (2). Even in HICs, negative perceptions are commonplace. Fatalistic attitudes that stillbirth is inevitable ('nature's way') are not only inaccurate and unhelpful to parents but hold back efforts in prevention as many stillbirths are due to conditions that are potentially preventable.

Privacy but not abandonment

Parents should be given privacy during the hospital stay, and generally away from sounds of crying babies, and all staff should be aware of their loss. Parents often report feeling abandoned after a stillbirth and, while privacy is important, this should not impede the provision of optimal care.

Parenting and creating memories

Spending time and parenting the baby is often associated with positive memories and can aid the grieving process by creating a bond and sense of identity of the child. Activities such as seeing and holding a stillborn baby should be carefully and compassionately offered and parents supported in their choice (16). 'Cuddle cots' (or similar) (**Figure 34.7**) provide a cooled environment enabling parents to spend more time with their baby and are being increasingly used. Memory-making activities should be suggested and parents supported in their decision about these options. These activities may include bathing and dressing the baby, talking to the

baby and using the baby's name, engaging in religious or naming ceremonies, introducing the baby to extended family, and capturing interactions in photographs and movies. Having items of memorabilia may reduce negative outcomes and should be offered such as photos, hand/footprints, and special clothing or blankets (17).

Healthcare professional support

While high-quality evidence on specific interventions to improve outcomes for parents after stillbirth is lacking (18), a recent systematic review including non-randomized studies highlighted the importance of actions and attitudes of staff (15). Caring for bereaved parents requires understanding of the current evidence on perinatal loss, the impact of losing a baby, and the diversity of parents' experiences (19). A parent-centred approach that addresses sociocultural context and respects the unique needs of each bereaved parent underpins compassionate communication, and information provision and supported decision-making is vital (19). Continuity of care following diagnosis of stillbirth is important to parents. A coordinated multiprofessional approach to care with staff well known to the parents is critically important from the time of diagnosis and birth through to follow-up visits and ideally, for those wishing to have another baby, into subsequent pregnancies. Stillbirth has a significant impact on obstetricians and midwives, professionally and personally, and many feel inadequate in providing care at this time with training and support often lacking (15, 20). Perinatal bereavement care requires organizational responses including staff development to address training gaps and debriefing and clinical supervision to prevent burnout of staff in highly emotionally demanding roles.

Follow-up after leaving the hospital

With little evidence to guide the type and frequency of follow-up, it is important that parents are aware of support services available to them and that a time is made for a follow-up visit to the hospital. Upon discharge, parents should be provided with the contact number of a staff member known to them to respond to questions that may arise before the follow-up visit, and to also suggest to them to make a list of questions in preparation for their follow-up visit. Many parents find it very distressing to return to the unit where their baby was stillborn and, where possible, these appointments should take place in another setting. If practicable, the option of home visits should be offered to parents. Six to eight weeks is the usual timing of the follow-up appointment with the aim to have all results of investigations available. If important results will not be available at that time (e.g. autopsy), parents need to be made aware and an alternate or additional appointment time made. Once again, compassionate, respectful care is critical to the parents at this time. Referring to the baby by name is important to many parents where a name was given. A coordinated, thoughtful, and multiprofessional approach to care is needed. In addition to discussion on the reasons for the death, counselling about future pregnancy planning should include attention to optimal maternal health including smoking cessation support and weight management if relevant (21). In addition, the visit should include discussion of parent's grief and coping and recommendations or referral for ongoing support if necessary.

Social and tangible support

Adequate social support from family and local social networks can improve outcomes for parents. Family and friends and the wider

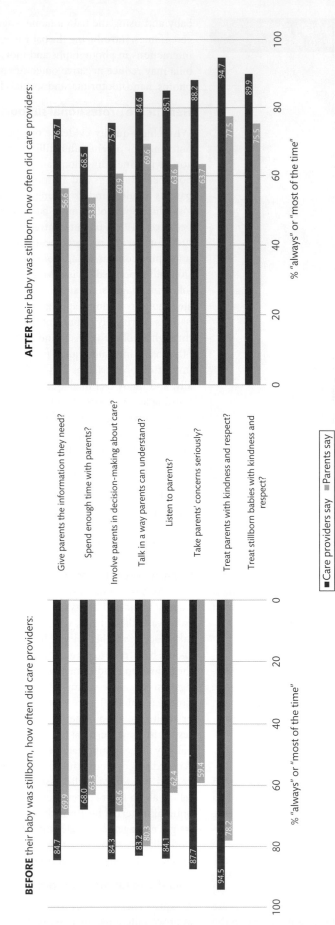

Figure 34.6 Quality antenatal and bereavement care: survey data from parents (*n* = 3503) and care providers (*n* = 2020). Data from parents refers to the care parents, themselves, received in the pregnancy in which their baby was stillborn. Data from care providers refers to the care provided to all parents, in general, at each care provider's facility.

Reproduced from Flenady V, Wojcieszek AM, Middleton P, Ellwood D, Erwich J, Coory M, et al. Stillbirths: recall to action in high-income countries. *The Lancet* 2016; 13(387): 691–702 with permission from Elsevier.

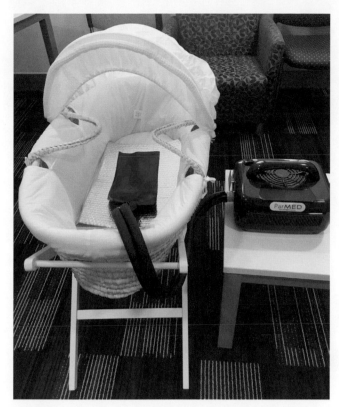

Figure 34.7 A 'cuddle-cot' which is designed to cool a stillborn baby to enable parents to spend longer time with their baby after birth.

community need to understand the enormity of the loss of stillbirth to parents and the need for their child to be acknowledged as part of the family. Effective leave arrangements and tangible support, such as government assistance with funeral costs, and paid leave from work commitments is important for parents (14).

Mental health interventions

Grief is a normal response and most parents and families do not require specialized services including professional counselling. High-risk groups who may have complicated grief such as parents who have previously lost children, and women undergoing termination of pregnancy for fetal anomalies, may benefit from referral to specialists services. Prescribing sedatives for women is common in some settings, despite the addictive nature of these medications and the limited evidence for benefit. Pharmacological management of grief should only be considered in the presence of an established psychological disorder for which medication is indicated.

Acknowledgements

We thank Heidi and Ned Mules for the photo of themselves with their daughter Sophie and for their comments on the chapter. We would like to acknowledge Ms Aleena Wojcieszek, Dr Dell Horey, and Associate Professor Fran Boyle for their contributions to the data presented in this chapter on the findings of the International Stillbirth Alliance survey data on parent and care providers experiences reported in *The Lancet* 'Ending Preventable Stillbirths' series 2016 (3). We also thank Sarah Henry for assistance with compiling the chapter, and Professor Jane Dahlstrom for providing Figure 34.3 on placental histopathology.

REFERENCES

1. de Bernis L, Kinney M, Stones W, et al. Stillbirths: ending preventable deaths by 2030. *Lancet* 2016;**387**:703–16.
2. Froen JF, Cacciatore J, McClure EM, et al. Stillbirths: why they matter. *Lancet* 2011;**377**:1353–66.
3. Flenady V, Wojcieszek AM, Middleton P, et al. Stillbirths: recall to action in high-income countries. *Lancet* 2016;**13**:691–702.
4. Blencowe H, Lawn J. National, regional, and worldwide estimates of stillbirth rates in 2015 with trends since 2000: a systematic analysis. *Lancet Glob Health* 2016;**4**:e98–108.
5. Lawn JE, Blencowe H, Waiswa P, et al. Stillbirths: rates, risk factors and potential for progress towards 2030. *Lancet* 2016;**387**:587–603.
6. Flenady V, Middleton P, Smith GC, et al. Stillbirths: the way forward in high-income countries. *Lancet* 2011;**377**:1703–17.
7. Flenady V, Koopmans L, Middleton P, et al. Major risk factors for stillbirth in high-income countries: a systematic review and meta-analysis. *Lancet* 2011;**377**:1331–40.
8. Lamont K, Scott NW, Jones GT, Bhattacharya S. Risk of recurrent stillbirth: systematic review and meta-analysis. *BMJ* 2015;**350**:h3080.
9. Flenady V. Epidemiology of fetal and neonatal death. In: Khong TY, Malcomson RDG (eds), *Keeling's Fetal and Neonatal Pathology*, 5th edn, pp. 141–64. Heidelberg: Springer International Publishing; 2015.
10. Kerber K. Counting every stillbirth and neonatal death through mortality audit to improve quality of care for every pregnant woman and her baby. *BMC Pregnancy Childbirth* 2015;**15** Suppl 2:S9.
11. Pattinson RC, Rhoda N. Saving babies 2012–2013: ninth report on perinatal care in South Africa. 2014. Available at: https://www.ppip.co.za/wp-content/uploads/Saving-Babies-2012-2013.pdf.
12. Wojcieszek AM, Boyle FM, Belizán JM, et al. Care in subsequent pregnancies following stillbirth: an international survey of parents. *BJOG* 2018;**125**:193–201.
13. McCowan LME, Thompson JMD, Cronin R, Ekeroma A, Lawton B, Mitchell EA. *Supine Sleep Position in Late Pregnancy is Associated with Increased Risk of Late Stillbirth*. Presented at The International Conference on Stillbirth, SIDS and Baby Survival 2014 Amsterdam, 18–21 September, 2014.
14. Heazell AEP, Siassakos D, Blencowe H, et al. Stillbirths: economic and psychosocial consequences. *Lancet* 2016;**387**:604–16.
15. Ellis A, Chebsey C, Storey C, et al. Systematic review to understand and improve care after stillbirth: a review of parents' and healthcare professionals' experiences. *BMC Pregnancy Childbirth* 2016;**16**:16.
16. National Institute for Health and Care Excellence. NICE set to change its advice on holding stillborn babies. *Paediatr Nurs* 2010;**22**:5.
17. Cacciatore J. Psychological effects of stillbirth. *Semin Fetal Neonatal Med* 2013;**18**:76–82.

18. Koopmans L, Wilson T, Cacciatore J, Flenady V. Support for mothers, fathers and families after perinatal death. *Cochrane Database Syst Rev* 2013;**6**:CD000452.

19. Flenady V, Boyle F, Koopmans L, Wilson T, Stones W, Cacciatore J. Meeting the needs of parents after a stillbirth or neonatal death. *BJOG* 2014;**141** Suppl 4:137–40.

20. Nuzum D, Meaney S, O'Donoghue K. The impact of stillbirth on consultant obstetrician gynaecologists: a qualitative study. *BJOG* 2014;**121**:1020–28.

21. Royal College of Obstetricians and Gynaecologists (RCOG). *Late Intrauterine Fetal Death and Stillbirth*. Green-top Guideline No. 55. London: RCOG; 2010.

35

Postpartum care and problems in the puerperium

Stephen J. Robson

Introduction

Across many cultures of the world, the 40 days after childbirth are recognized as a special time of recovery and recuperation for new mothers. During this period, traditionally referred to as the puerperium, women will undergo a series of major transitions. These transitions are not only anatomical and physiological but include changes in self-image, in relationships, and in a woman's place in her family and society. In many modern healthcare settings, women are discharged from care within a few days of birth and may have little contact with their maternity carers for many weeks. Yet the puerperium is a time not only of change, but of great vulnerability for women and their new babies. Women may be vulnerable to a diverse set of problems that have the potential to be very serious. For this reason, a clear understanding of both normal and abnormal recovery in the postnatal period is important for all providers of maternity care.

Recovery from birth

Vagina, perineum, and pelvic floor

For 2 or 3 days after birth the vagina remains capacious and smooth walled, but after this the characteristic rugae reappear and the vaginal capacity reduces quickly. During this time there are histological signs of oestrogen withdrawal, with thinning of the squamous lining and absent glycogen storage granules and basal layer activity (1). This state persists for 1 or 2 months, whereupon there are progressive changes in the vaginal skin bringing structure and function closer to the physiological premenopausal state. A complete return to normal epithelial cyclicity and function does not occur until ovulation commences.

Approximately 85% of vaginal births are complicated by perineal trauma, the majority of which will require suturing to repair (2). In normal circumstances, lacerations, episiotomy, or a combination of the two will heal over 2–3 weeks with healing complete by 4–6 weeks. However, the repair process will be complicated by infection and partial or complete dehiscence in up to 5% of cases.

Careful assessment and management of these complications is required since there is a potential for longer-term sequelae such as painful intercourse and incontinence. Complications of perineal injuries have been associated with postnatal depression and longer-term psychological problems. It is important to provide women with information and support regarding perineal care and hygiene, and regular inspection of the region should be undertaken during the early postpartum period.

Vaginal birth may also cause injury to the endopelvic fascia that supports and holds the vagina in position, and there may be injury to the levator plate. Trauma to the levator muscles, such as partial avulsion from the pelvic sidewall, is a recognized cause of pelvic floor dysfunction characterized by prolapse and incontinence (**Figure 35.1**). The incidence of such injuries is between 10% and 20% following spontaneous vaginal birth and lift-out ventouse delivery, but may be as high as 30% or more following forceps delivery (3). Although there may be no specific additional treatment when these injuries are present, and indeed they can be difficult to diagnose without recourse to imaging, recognition may help women understand changes in pelvic floor function and allow contact with physiotherapists and others skilled in longer-term maintenance of continence.

It has been reported that one or both pudendal nerves are injured during vaginal birth in up to one-third of women (4). Traction injury to the pudendal nerve is associated with incontinence of flatus and sometimes faeces, urinary incontinence and voiding dysfunction, and perineal pain that can lead to sexual difficulties. Fortunately for the majority of women these injuries heal spontaneously although a small proportion of women can have unpleasant symptoms that last for many years.

Caesarean recovery

In many parts of the world, one-quarter or more of births are caesarean and differences in recovery pattern from vaginal birth should be taken into account. Following an uncomplicated caesarean section there is no reason that women should not have a normal oral intake, and early mobilization should be encouraged. Prolonged immobility and dehydration are independent risk factors for thromboembolic complications and should be avoided. Other factors that

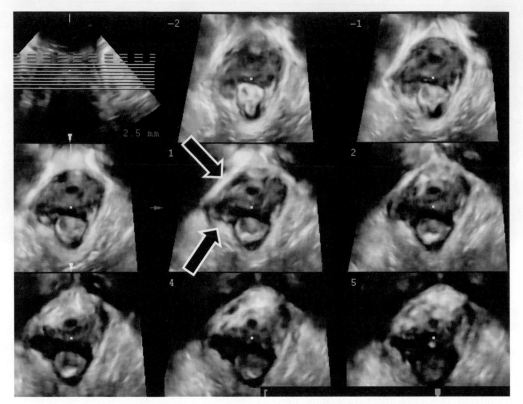

Figure 35.1 Ultrasound image of the pelvic floor in a woman following forceps vaginal delivery, showing avulsion of the levator plate from the right pubic ramus.
Courtesy of Professor HP Deitz.

influence the risk of thrombosis include increasing maternal age, obesity, and inherited thrombophilia: women with these risk factors should be considered for formal anticoagulation in addition to mechanical measures such as compression stockings (5). Recovery in the first few days after birth tends to be slower than that following an uncomplicated vaginal birth, and this can have adverse effects on a woman's ability to manage and care for the newborn and her older children. The majority of women will develop minor health problems that will require treatment whether delivered by caesarean section or vaginally, but women who have had a caesarean section are less likely to have problems than those with a forceps or ventouse delivery (6).

Restrictions on heavy lifting are commonly recommended following caesarean delivery but there is little objective evidence on which to base such advice. It would make sense to reduce activity that might predispose to wound dehiscence or subsequent hernia, but fortunately such complications are rare. An issue of practical concern for many women is driving: advice regarding driving is commonly based on guidelines of insurance companies. When objectively measured, there does not seem to be any difference in women's ability to handle driving irrespective of the mode of birth, and driving seems to be safe from very early in the postnatal period (7). It seems likely that a greater issue is fatigue and its negative effect on driving capacity, with women in the postnatal period subject to sleep deprivation that is likely to have a much greater effect on driving than mode of birth (8).

Uterine involution

When the uterus becomes empty following birth, contraction of the myometrium and continuing uterine tone reduce blood loss. The arterioles and venous channels of the placental bed thread their course through interlacing bundles of uterine muscle, so myometrial contraction acts to compress them. To enhance the mechanical effect of uterine contraction, there are corresponding changes in blood coagulability with a reduction in clotting time and rapid increases in the concentration of clotting factors VIII and V, with a decrease in fibrinogen and a surge in platelet concentration (1). The uterus reduces in size rapidly, following both vaginal birth (**Figure 35.2**) and caesarean section (**Figure 35.3**) reaching prepregnancy dimensions by about 1 month following birth in healthy women. Although it is difficult to obtain tissue for analysis, it seems likely that there is minimal loss of total myometrial cells, but a marked reduction in length and a reduction in the elastin and collagen content of the uterus. The uterine tone is maintained during the early postnatal period although Doppler studies show a steady increase in vascular resistance (1).

Large areas of decidua are shed soon after birth, but new endometrium grows from the deeper portions of the endometrial glands that remain in the basal layer, and a relatively complete surface has usually grown within 2 or 3 weeks of delivery (9). The placental site is slower to heal, and the large arcuate arteries that supplied the placenta become hyalinized and endometrial growth encroaches from the peripheral margins of the placental site to cover it. This process

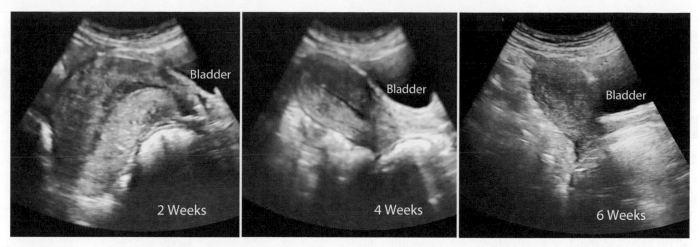

Figure 35.2 Sequential ultrasound images at 2, 4, and 6 weeks postpartum in a primigravid woman, showing involution progressing most rapidly in the first month.

is slow compared to the rest of the uterine surface and can take up to 6 weeks for a full endometrial coverage. The cervix returns to a relatively normal morphology within 2 weeks, although it will have a different shape and characteristics to that of a nulligravid woman.

These physiological changes are characterized by two well-known clinical correlates—'afterpains' and lochia. So-called afterpains are sensations of uterine contraction similar to, but milder than, uterine contractions. They are typically experienced by multiparous women at the time of breastfeeding, presumably a response to oxytocin release, and may herald transient passage of heavier blood loss or clots. Afterpains typically decrease in intensity and level of pain over the first 2 or 3 postnatal days and are rare thereafter. 'Lochia' is the vaginal discharge that occurs following birth. It is usually light but frank blood for the first few hours after birth, changing to a brown light fluid discharge until the third postpartum day. This has classically been termed 'lochia rubra' and contains blood from the placental site, any remaining placental tissue or membranes, some necrotic decidua, and cervical discharge. Beyond the fourth or fifth day the lochia changes to a creamy straw-colour (the 'lochia serosa')

containing serous fluid, leucocytes, and mucus. For another week or two there is a light and clear discharge (the 'lochia alba') that contains sloughed decidual cells and cervical mucus. At this stage, there is commonly contamination with bacteria which gives the lochia a characteristic smell.

Initiation of lactation

The physiological changes necessary for lactation begin in mid pregnancy, and the transition to lactation is completed postnatally. In the prepregnant state the breast has a series of ducts growing inward from the nipple and traversing the fat pad of the breast, ending in terminal duct lobular units. Under the influence of pregnancy-related hormones including prolactin, human placental lactogen, oestrogens, and progesterone, the terminal ductal units grow and expand and from about mid pregnancy some secretory activity begins (10). The initiation of secretory activity in the terminal lobules is termed stage one lactogenesis, but there is a period of quiescence until birth that is likely mediated by the effect of progesterone. With the fall in progesterone after birth, milk secretion begins and

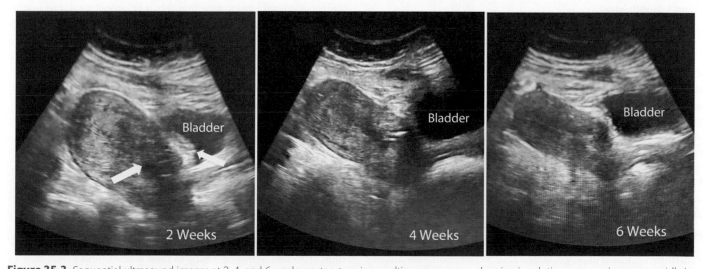

Figure 35.3 Sequential ultrasound images at 2, 4, and 6 weeks postpartum in a multiparous woman, showing involution progressing most rapidly in the first month. The area of haematoma and oedema at the site of the uterine incision is arrowed.

continues in response to prolactin. This transition is referred to as stage two lactogenesis, and with the rapid increase in milk production the alveoli express receptors for oxytocin. Triggering of these receptors leads to contraction of the alveolar myocytes, squeezing milk into the ducts of the breast.

Physiological transition

Cardiovascular

During pregnancy, a woman's cardiac output increases by up to 40% with the maximum increase attained by the beginning of the third trimester. This is brought about by an increase in stroke volume and heart rate, and there is an accompanying increase in left ventricular wall thickness and end-diastolic chamber size. Accompanying this change is an increase in the maternal blood volume and relative dilutional anaemia as the plasma volume expands by almost 50% while the red cell volume increases by only about 20%. During labour, the cardiac output increases to levels approximately 50% greater than those prior to labour as a result of higher heart rate and stroke volume. By late pregnancy, the uterine blood flow increases to almost 700 mL/minute, accounting for about 12% of total cardiac output (11). With delivery, the uterus empties and contracts, increasing resistance and markedly reducing its blood flow and thus diverting the additional blood volume into the general circulation. Maternal cardiac output remains elevated for about 24 hours after birth, then falls steadily over 1–2 weeks (12). Blood pressure tends to fall for about 2 days after delivery then return to levels found at the end of pregnancy. Pregnancy-related changes in stroke volume, heart rate, and thus cardiac output return to prepregnancy levels by about 6 weeks (13). The increased plasma volume falls rapidly with studies suggesting a reduction of between 10% and 20% within a day of birth, partly as a result of diuresis, and partly from either bleeding or accumulation of peripheral oedema. The red cell mass falls quite quickly after birth, perhaps to non-pregnant levels within 1 or 2 days (1). The fall in plasma volume takes longer, leading to a physiological haemodilution. Accompanying these changes is a transient fall in haemoglobin concentration, reaching a nadir about 4 days after birth but thereafter increasing steadily to reach prepregnancy levels about 1 month later.

Thrombosis and coagulation

Delivery of the placenta has the potential to be associated with blood loss greater than the normal physiological bleeding, and as well as the mechanical effect of the contracting uterus occluding the vessels of the placental bed there are changes in haemostasis. Levels of tissue plasminogen activator, released from the placenta, fall abruptly after delivery allowing increased fibrinolysis across the placental bed and release of fibrin degradation products. Although there is consumption of platelets and fibrin, with up to 10% of the body's supplies of both used at the placental site, the fall is very transient and there is a marked rise within a day or two of delivery contributing to an increased risk of thrombosis at this time (1).

Other physiological transitions

With the withdrawal of progesterone after birth, the tidal volume and respiratory rate fall rapidly, however the reduction in diaphragmatic excursion caused by the uterus is relieved allowing normalization of the residual volume and functional residual capacity. The airways also have a reversal of the oedema and vascularity associated with pregnancy. These changes are complete within 2 or 3 weeks. During pregnancy, renal function has been different with an increased glomerular filtration rate, but there is a marked diuresis during the first postpartum week. Changes in the physiological dilatation of the renal pelves and ureters gradually return to normal by 6 weeks. The mechanical effects on the gastrointestinal system are rapidly reversed after birth, with gastric emptying and reflux returning to normal quickly. Other changes that are associated with pregnancy, such as gallbladder emptying and bowel transit time, tend to improve gradually over the puerperium.

Ovarian function

Where breastfeeding is initiated and lactation continues, the normal pulsatile release of gonadotropin-releasing hormone is interrupted and although low levels of follicle-stimulating hormone are secreted and there is some follicular development, the absence of luteinizing hormone leads to inadequate oestradiol secretion and ovulation does not occur (14). This physiological state can persist for long periods, and until lactation ceases women will have few periods or may remain amenorrhoeic. Where breastfeeding is not established, ovulation may occur within a month or two of birth. Only a small proportion of lactating women, perhaps less than 5%, will ovulate during the first 6 months following birth (9). It is likely that increased levels of prolactin play a role in lactational amenorrhoea, but this is transient as prolactin levels may return to normal within 2 months of birth in lactating women.

Emotional transition

Sleep

Adequate sleep is fundamental to good health, and both pregnancy and the puerperium are times when women are especially vulnerable to sleep disturbance. Babies waking and requiring settling, and nocturnal feeding contribute to disturbed sleep and poor sleep quality for many women. Even though short night-time sleep duration is almost universal among new mothers it is important not to underestimate the negative effects these sleep deficits can have on health and well-being (15). Sleep disturbance can impair functioning and predispose to maternal mood and mental health problems so while the overall outlook is good, it is important to provide education to reduce the risk that the normal phase of sleep disturbance does not turn into a chronic problem.

Mood

The arrival of a new baby can be a stressful life event, especially when the expectations set for new mothers regarding their 'role' and 'feelings' do not align with their actual experiences. The transition to motherhood is made more challenging by sleep deprivation and the time-consuming activity required to care for a newborn. Many women who previously participated in the workforce identify a sense of social and professional isolation, and some may view the disruptions attendant in having a baby in their home from a perspective of 'failure' as a parent (16). Additional financial stresses can make these feelings more acute, and contribute to a sense of guilt and shame. Changes in the nature of relationships with intimate partner will also affect a woman's mood and sense of well-being.

All of these changes are a normal part of the transition to parenthood, and in most cases will be resolved as women and their partners adjust to their new circumstances. However, in a proportion of cases more serious disorders of mood will arise, and the mental health of the mother has the potential to affect not only her own well-being but also the health of the baby, other siblings, and her partner. The duration and severity of postpartum mood disorders may be modified by early recognition and adequate treatment (17). The use of a validated instrument such as the Edinburgh Postnatal Depression Scale (EPDS) to screen for perinatal depression and anxiety is of value but should be used as part of a broader assessment of a woman's emotional and psychological well-being. Where there is a suspicion that mental health problems are established or could be developing, a proactive approach must be taken. This will include a full psychosocial assessment and support using a collaborative multidisciplinary team with access to psychiatrists, psychologists, nursing staff, social work resources, and others.

Relationships and sexuality

Having a baby is one of the most challenging events in an intimate relationship, and a newborn can also affect important interactions with other family and friends. Mothers are usually sleep deprived and there is reduced time available for other domestic tasks, for tending friendships and socializing, and simply taking time to rest and recover. In many settings women who have a new baby and who previously participated in the workforce may find there are financial stresses. All couples welcoming a first baby will be affected by the dramatic change from a time of relative freedom to one of attention to a baby's needs that can seem almost oppressive (16). Attention taken away from a partner to attend the baby's needs and conflict over parenting styles and roles can place stress on the most committed relationship.

One of the major adjustments women and couples face is a potential for changes in sexual intimacy. Postpartum sexuality encompasses a range of issues but perhaps most importantly is about a woman's self-perception as a 'sexual being'. Unfortunately, in many settings the paradigm in which postpartum sexuality is viewed, particularly by well-meaning maternity carers, is that of dysfunction rather than function (18). A broad approach to sexuality in the postpartum period should take into account issues such as body image, changes in lifestyle, fears and concerns about discomforts with sexual activity, and the partner's perceptions of, and interest in, sexuality. Studies suggest that difficulties in postnatal sexual adjustment are relatively common but under-reported (19).

Although there is a wide range of normal, many studies report that women's desire for sexual intimacy tends to reduce during pregnancy, and this trend continues after birth (20). Reduced sexual desire is associated with less sexual activity and satisfaction, but enjoyment of sexual activity usually returns in the months after birth. For example, studies suggest that few women find intercourse enjoyable shortly after birth but by about 12 weeks the majority report that sex is 'mostly enjoyable' (21). Fatigue is commonly reported as one of the main factors contributing to a loss of sexual interest, and is clearly related to a reduction in coital frequency. However, perineal pain following vaginal birth and transient atrophy of the vaginal

skin with reduced lubrication can make intercourse unpleasant for many women. One of the important ways of helping women navigate these difficulties in the transition to parenthood is by being proactive, since there are high levels of under-reporting. Fortunately women can be reassured that these changes are usually transient. Persistent reduction in sexual desire and frequency of sexual activity has been associated with perinatal mood disorders so careful inquiry is warranted.

Complications of the puerperium

Infection

The risk of infection is ever present for women after childbirth and some infections have the potential for severe disease and even death. Events during labour and delivery, such as vaginal examinations, prolonged rupture of the membranes, perineal injuries, instrumental delivery, and manual removal of the placenta, all have the potential for associated infectious complications. The presence of devitalized tissues, blood clot, or haematoma anywhere in the genital tract can foster development of infection. For these reasons a high level of suspicion and low threshold for treatment are important in the safe management of puerperal infection.

Vaginal and perineal injuries

Perineal injury, especially if there has been some delay in repair, may become infected. This is particularly so where there has been a third- or fourth-degree injury or where an associated haematoma is present or has been evacuated (**Figure 35.4**). The perineum can be heavily soiled after birth so attention to cleansing and aseptic technique during suturing are important preventive measures. Where anal sphincter or rectal mucosal injuries have been treated, a case can be made for use of antibiotics at the time of repair and in the immediate postpartum period although evidence to guide practice can be difficult to obtain (22). Advice regarding perineal care should be provided, for example, twice-daily showers and avoidance of traumatic drying of the skin. Although perineal infection is relatively uncommon, such infections are important as they are commonly associated with breakdown of the suture line, a particularly unpleasant complication for women (23). Careful surveillance for healing, and early treatment of suspected infection are important principles of care. Perineal infections are usually polymicrobial with facultative and anaerobic species so broad-spectrum antibiotics including metronidazole will usually be required.

Caesarean wound infection and necrotizing fasciitis

As caesarean section rates increase, infection of abdominal incisions has become a more common complication. Some degree of infection of the caesarean section incision occurs in about 10% of cases, and is more common after emergency caesarean section (24). The majority of wound infections are diagnosed after discharge from hospital and are, fortunately, relatively mild. Obesity is a major risk factor for caesarean wound infection and is becoming more common in the obstetric population (25). The use of perioperative antibiotics at the time of caesarean section, and swabbing the vagina with antiseptic solution prior to delivery have been shown to reduce the risk of infection in the incision (26). Despite the best technique and management, caesarean wound infection still occurs and management must

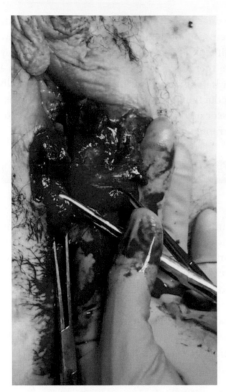

Figure 35.4 Third-degree perineal tear, with complete division of the internal and external anal sphincters. Careful, precise repair of such injuries and close postpartum surveillance and management are the keys to a good long-term outcome from such injuries.

be prompt and careful. Where cellulitis is the primary manifestation, use of intravenous antibiotics is appropriate. However, if there is evidence of purulent discharge or a deeper collection then drainage and debridement, if necessary, should be undertaken without delay (27).

Necrotizing fasciitis following caesarean section is a rare but potentially devastating complication. It occurs when there is a rapidly spreading gangrenous infection of the deep tissues of the abdominal wall, typically polymicrobial in character with *Clostridium* and group A *Streptococcus* (GAS). The presentation may be delayed up to a week or more following birth, with patients reporting increasingly severe pain and debility. Oedema and discolouration of the skin may be seen, and imaging may show gas collections in the abdominal wall. A diagnosis of necrotizing fasciitis following caesarean section is an emergency situation, as the condition is life-threatening and demands urgent action. A combination of high-dose antibiotic therapy and aggressive surgical debridement is necessary, undertaken with a multidisciplinary approach (27).

Mastitis and breast abscess

Mastitis is a relatively common complication of birth, affecting up to one-third of all woman at some point during lactation with the majority of cases occurring within the puerperium (28). Fortunately, the severe complication of mastitis—breast abscess—is rare and affects less than 0.5% of breastfeeding women (29). Some women are prone to mastitis and have repeated episodes, although for most women mastitis is a single event during lactation.

Mastitis typically occurs in women with predisposing factors such as nipple trauma and difficulties in feeding, and possibly reduced frequency of feeds. Maternal fatigue and primiparity may

increase the risk, as does a history of past episodes of mastitis. The commonest pathogen isolated is *Staphylococcus aureus*, followed by various species of streptococci (28).

The pathophysiological mechanism underlying acute mastitis is milk stasis. Milk stasis appears to have an inflammatory effect on the breast tissues, and is associated with maternal fever and breast engorgement. This may be due to the presence of inflammatory mediators in human milk, and a range of proteins not found elsewhere in the body (28). The risk of milk stasis can be reduced by early exclusive breastfeeding, not restricting access to the breast for babies, and support and encouragement of comfortable and functional mother–baby positioning for feeds and correct attachment to the nipple to minimize traumatic injury.

Mastitis can occur very suddenly following a brief prodrome of fever, rigors, and feelings of an influenza-like illness with generalized pain and malaise. Because the infection spreads from the ductal system into the connective tissue, the affected breast becomes painful and may develop an angry erythema that spreads out from the affected area. There is seldom time for breast milk culture and microscopy, and broad-spectrum antibiotics and adequate analgesia should be instituted rapidly. Broad-spectrum antibiotics with anti-staphylococcal sensitivity such as oral cephalosporins are usually indicated. Women will need analgesics with antipyretic properties, such as paracetamol, and possibly non-steroidal anti-inflammatory medication.

It is important that milk stasis is minimized in the affected breast so the baby should continue to feed from the affected side, ideally as the first side to promote effective suckling. Alternatively, a breast pump may be used to empty the breast and this can also be useful after a feed to ensure that the affected breast has been completely emptied. Time spent with the mother to assess and, if necessary, adjust feeding technique or timing is very useful and may help reduce the risk of further episodes. Once antibiotic therapy has been instituted, it should be continued for at least 10 days to reduce the risk of relapse. The support of maternity staff and the woman's family are very important during treatment of mastitis as it is very unpleasant for the women and can be extremely debilitating and stressful.

Incomplete treatment of mastitis may lead to development of a breast abscess. In this case, the woman fails to improve with standard management and the breast may become fluctuant with the woman experiencing spiking fevers. Imaging may be required to demonstrate the presence of an abscess, and where therapy with high-dose intravenous antibiotics does not lead to an improvement in the clinical picture, rarely incision and drainage will be necessary.

Urinary tract infection

Urinary infection is a common cause of fever in the early postpartum period and although women may report urinary frequency and dysuria these symptoms are not invariable and symptoms may be subtle. A high index of suspicion should be maintained where there is a history of catheterization during labour or afterwards, and where there has been perineal or vaginal trauma and swelling. Accurate diagnosis can be difficult due to contamination with lochia, and the presence of white cells in the urine commonly results from bladder trauma during birth.

The commonest organism is *Escherichia coli*, but other pathogens include Gram-negative species such as *Klebsiella* and *Enterobacter*, as well as streptococci (30). Where the woman is febrile and has flank pain, treatment with intravenous antibiotics should be commenced promptly. Due to the high prevalence of resistant bacteria, a broad-spectrum cephalosporin would usually be the treatment of choice. In a clinical setting suspicious for more severe infection, an aminoglycoside should be added to the regimen. Failure to respond to treatment within 2 or 3 days should prompt investigation for underlying complicating factors such as voiding dysfunction, obstruction, or other pathologies such as a renal abnormality or calculus.

Endometritis and retained products of conception

Postpartum endometritis complicates as many as 5% of vaginal births, and a higher proportion of caesarean deliveries (30). The typical presentation is with lower abdominal pain accompanied by malodourous vaginal lochia. Predisposing factors include a history of prior bacterial vaginosis, a prolonged labour, intrapartum fever, and conditions such as diabetes and anaemia. Examination will typically reveal fever and tachycardia with a tender uterus, but absence of fever does not exclude the presence of endometritis. The presence of an elevated white cell count and raised inflammatory markers, such as C-reactive protein, are non-specific but lend support to the clinical diagnosis. Similarly, the results of microscopy and culture of vaginal swabs can be helpful but do not necessarily reflect conditions within the endometrial cavity. Imaging is useful to exclude retained products of conception or pelvic abscess.

Infection is typically polymicrobial with anaerobes and genital mycoplasmas, and occasionally *Chlamydia* species when the onset of clinical infection is delayed (30). Obtaining accurate cultures from the endometrium can be difficult, and is often delayed by several days—pathogens are uncommonly identified in blood cultures or urine specimens. Where the clinical presentation suggests moderate severity with a picture of acute sepsis, purulent discharge, and pain, treatment should begin promptly and consist of fluid resuscitation and pain relief, as well as broad-spectrum antibiotics. Most women will improve quickly, and where there is no improvement over 2–3 days, investigations should aim to exclude pelvic thrombophlebitis or abscess, unsuspected infection elsewhere, or resistant strains (30).

Group A *Streptococcus*

Systemic infection with GAS—puerperal sepsis—is the feared infection for the postnatal women, and there is some evidence that the incidence of GAS is increasing. Although infection can occur antenatally, it is more common and potentially devastating after birth. GAS colonization is common, with as many as one-quarter of the population identified as asymptomatic carriers. The typical presentation is with high fever, rigors, and rapidly progressing malaise. In some cases, women will report a prodromal period with a sore throat or non-specific influenza-like illness. There may be symptoms or signs of endometritis, with vaginal discharge or bleeding and a tender lower abdomen and uterus.

Although many cases have no identifiable risk factors, retained products of conception, prolonged labour, and instrumental delivery may be present. Woman at social disadvantage and those with known immunosuppression or chronic disease may be at higher risk, but overtly healthy women can be affected. A high index of suspicion must be maintained and women who present with high fever and malaise in the postnatal period should have blood cultures, a urine specimen, and swabs taken with a specific request for M-typing

of any GAS isolated from the specimens. Treatment should be aggressive and multidisciplinary with involvement of clinical microbiologists and intensive care teams. High-dose broad-spectrum antibiotics including penicillin and fluid resuscitation with full supportive care are commonly required.

Secondary postpartum haemorrhage

Bloody-stained loss is common in the postnatal period, but secondary haemorrhage is said to occur where there is increasingly heavy frank blood loss beginning more than 24 hours after birth. Unlike primary postpartum haemorrhage (PPH), which is often defined in volume terms (such as 500 mL or more, or 1 L in other definitions), there is no agreed volume in definitions of secondary haemorrhage. Because of the lack of standardization it is difficult to provide a precise incidence rate for secondary PPH with studies estimating that between 0.5% and 1.5% of women will be affected (31). Although much less common than primary PPH, secondary PPH is still a source of morbidity and even maternal death.

The factors predisposing to secondary PPH are those that interfere with the normal involution of the uterus, such as retained placental tissue and membranes, secondary infection, and the presence of leiomyomata (fibroids). Secondary infection may be associated with prolonged prelabour rupture of the membranes, prolonged labour, emergency caesarean section, and manual removal of the placenta (31). Less commonly, secondary PPH occurs with undiagnosed placenta accreta, lower genital tract injuries (especially if there has been haematoma formation), complications of a caesarean section incision such as dehiscence, unrecognized vascular abnormalities such as arteriovenous malformations, and where a coagulopathy develops subsequently to the birth.

The management of secondary PPH should follow a standard approach, with early recognition and action the cornerstone of a good outcome. Although such bleeding is usually light, rarely it can be heavy and potentially catastrophic (32). Resuscitation should be prompt and aggressive as required, with a low threshold to use blood or blood products if early therapy with plasma expanders is unsuccessful. Fortunately, most women will be haemodynamically stable and time can be taken to establish a diagnosis and to tailor treatment to the clinical situation. Examination may reveal potentially helpful signs such as fever, abdominal tenderness, larger-than-expected uterine size, offensive discharge, or local perineal bleeding or haematoma.

Investigations should include a check of haemoglobin concentration and platelet count, with coagulation studies if there is watery loss and absent clotting, as well as grouping of blood in case transfusion is required. Vaginal swabs should be taken to establish whether infection is present, and to guide antibiotic therapy if required. Ultrasound examination is the cornerstone for diagnosis of retained tissues, although in the very early postpartum period interpretation of the findings require experience and judgement (31). Use of colour Doppler, if available, may help distinguish between retained placental tissue (which may retain a blood supply) and necrotic clot or decidua (33). While false-positive results from early postpartum ultrasound scanning may lead to unnecessary surgical intervention, imaging revealing an empty uterus can spare a woman anaesthesia and exploration of the uterus where it is not required.

The therapy for secondary PPH will depend upon the suspected cause. Uterotonic agents such as misoprostol (which can be administered orally or rectally) or prostaglandins (given intramuscularly) may be used to assist with uterine contraction. Although oxytocin is usually readily available, its effectiveness decreases the greater the time since birth. Since infection and resulting endometritis are likely to contribute in many episodes of secondary PPH, antibiotic treatment is commonly instituted (34). Typical bacteria isolated in the setting of secondary PPH include *E. coli, Clostridium perfringens, Bacteroides*, and streptococci (31). When there is either a clinical suspicion or direct ultrasound evidence for retained tissue or clot, and surgical evacuation is planned, antibiotic treatment may be commenced prior to the procedure. Where there is some clinical urgency, use of antibiotics at the time—usually with induction of anaesthesia—should be considered. Although protocols for antibiotic use will vary between institutions, the use of broad-spectrum antibiotics likely to cover the typical range of infective organisms may include penicillins, metronidazole, and gentamicin (31).

There is no single recommended method of uterine evacuation and manual exploration and evacuation, use of a wide-bore suction catheter, and sharp curettage have all been described (35). There is a greater chance of uterine perforation and injury when curettage is performed in the early postnatal period so care and precision are important, particularly in a setting of caesarean section. Fortunately, retained placental tissue is less likely following caesarean section. When infected retained tissues are evacuated surgically, there is an increased risk of uterine synechiae and Asherman syndrome although these are difficult to avoid and the risks must be balanced against continued bleeding and possible escalation of infection (36).

Voiding dysfunction

Voiding difficulty and associated urinary retention is a relatively common occurrence in the puerperium. Although definitions vary, estimates of the incidence of overt voiding dysfunction suggest about 5% of women are affected with a further 10% affected by less obvious dysfunction (37). The pathogenesis of voiding dysfunction is usually multifactorial, resulting from a combination of mechanical, neurological, and physiological processes. Progesterone has an inhibitory effect on smooth muscle tone and this may contribute to reduced detrusor muscle tone.

Voiding dysfunction has a range of clinical presentations, with a complete inability to pass urine in the most severe group. However, there is a spectrum of effect with some women remaining asymptomatic yet having a large postvoid residual bladder volume (38). A high index of clinical suspicion should be maintained in women with recognized risk factors: epidural and regional anaesthesia, primiparity, instrumental delivery, a large baby, and a long duration of labour (38). Women with sequelae of a traumatic vaginal birth, such as prominent vulval oedema, bruising, and tears in the anterior vulva and vagina near the urethra, require special care. Typical presentations include a frequent need for urination with small volumes passed, hesitancy or a need to strain with voiding, a slow or intermittent urinary stream, or urinary urgency. Some women with voiding dysfunction will report a lack of sensation to void.

Proactive surveillance and management are important to avoid short- and longer-term voiding problems. Vulval oedema and trauma should be managed with application of cold packs and selective use of anti-inflammatory medication, and effective, regular analgesia to reduce hesitancy due to pain. Women should be encouraged to ambulate to the toilet and be afforded privacy. Any woman who has not voided within 6 hours of birth should have her residual volumes measured, ideally by catheterization since the results of ultrasound bladder scanners may be affected by the postpartum uterus. Where the woman remains unable to void and has residual bladder volumes of more than 150 mL, an indwelling catheter should be left in place for 24–48 hours then another trial of void undertaken (38). If the voiding dysfunction persists, a catheter should be left in place for 1 week with antibiotic prophylaxis to reduce the risk of cystitis.

With prompt diagnosis and systematic management, most women with voiding dysfunction in the early postnatal period will recover completely and have no enduring difficulties. Although the long-term prognosis is excellent in virtually all cases, persistent voiding dysfunction can necessitate intermittent self-catheterization for weeks which is highly disruptive and predisposes to repeated urinary infections.

Constipation and haemorrhoids

Constipation is a commonly reported problem in the puerperium, affecting up to 20% of women. Although there is wide variation in the normal patterns of bowel function, bowel movements that occur less than three times a week with hard stool that is difficult to pass would generally be diagnosed as constipation. When constipation is diagnosed, careful assessment and management are required. Factors that can exacerbate constipation include opioid pain relief and iron supplements. Physical inactivity and depression are associated with constipation and conditions that make it painful to defecate, such as haemorrhoids and anal fissures, can lead to faecal impaction and sometimes overflow incontinence.

Management should be based on ensuring the woman has an adequate intake of fibre and fluid, and that defecation should not be delayed if there is an urge. Where these measures do not provide adequate relief, stepwise use of bulk-forming laxatives is usually the next step. Agents such as psyllium, ispaghula, and wheat dextrin are safe and effective, but may take a couple of days to work and need to be introduced gradually. Women should be warned about symptoms such as bloating and abdominal discomfort, and need to have a good fluid intake at the same time. If these measures are not successful then osmotic laxatives should be added in addition, either in the form of oral solutions or sometimes by the rectal route. It is uncommon for women still to have problems following these measures, but where success has still not been attained, further and more specialized assistance and advice may be required.

Haemorrhoids are common in pregnancy, and often undergo an acute exacerbation following birth. They result when the supporting tissues of the anal cushions fail, allowing prolapse of the cushions and venous engorgement. There is commonly associated venous thrombosis and a marked inflammatory response, making them very painful to endure (39). Haemorrhoids present as an uncomfortable lump or lumps at the anus, and can cause bleeding during or after defecation. There may be irritation or pruritus associated with faecal soiling, but acute pain is usually associated with either a large acute thrombosis, or with an associated anal fissure.

In general, the management of haemorrhoids in the postnatal period is conservative with the use of Sitz baths up to three times a day, and a pillow or ring cushion to sit on at other times. Women may need to use analgesic and anti-inflammatory creams or ointments before defecation. An important aspect of managing haemorrhoids is to attend to constipation. Women should be reassured that haemorrhoids will settle within a week or two of birth. Where there are continuing problems, the opinion of a general or colorectal surgeon should be sought.

Urinary incontinence

The prevalence of urinary incontinence for women in the post-natal period is surprisingly high, with pooled data from population studies suggesting that one woman in three will report episodes of involuntary urine loss (40). Of note, incontinence is twice as common in women who have had vaginal deliveries when compared to those whose birth was by caesarean section. Reporting urinary incontinence can be embarrassing for many women, so direct questioning may be necessary. In all cases urinary infection should be excluded and other pathology, such as pudendal nerve injury, should be sought. Women who describe incontinence should be managed sensitively in conjunction with an experienced physiotherapist. Therapeutic strategies include coaching in pelvic floor exercises, attention to general fitness, and optimization of weight, and in some cases bladder retraining.

Faecal incontinence

Faecal incontinence following birth is less common than urinary incontinence, but still affects up to 5% of women in the postnatal period, and this figure might be low due to under-reporting (41). The commonest cause is injury to the anal sphincter which complicates up to 3% of all vaginal births. Accurate diagnosis of anal sphincter injuries is important as it allows correct surgical repair and appropriate postnatal management. However, it is likely that many injuries are not recognized at the time of birth and even women who have undergone satisfactory repair are likely to report impairment of bowel control in the postnatal period (42). When there is a sensation of urgency and associated faecal incontinence it is likely that damage to the external anal sphincter has occurred. Injury to the internal sphincter typically presents as passive leakage of flatus or faeces.

There are other causes of these symptoms, including faecal loading of the bowel with overflow. This can be associated with use of narcotic pain relief medications, or where there is significant pain that inhibits normal defecation. When a sphincter injury has occurred, it is important to have frequent contact with the women in the postnatal period, and to provide advice and assessment and ongoing management. Assessment should include careful regular examination of the perineum, anus, and vagina to check that healing is progressing satisfactorily and to assess for asymmetry with voluntary contraction, to assess for reflex contraction with coughing, and to assess sphincter tone. At that same time, haemorrhoids or anal fissure can be excluded, or diagnosed if present and treated appropriately.

Women should be offered advice on diet and the importance of adequate fibre and fluid intake, and also coaching in pelvic floor exercises. One of the most important aspects of care is to offer emotional support, as caring for the newborn is stressful in itself without the added burden of uncertainly and lack of confidence that comes with faecal incontinence. Where women do not respond to conservative measures, referral for further assessment and possibly secondary repair should not be delayed.

Common breastfeeding difficulties

Breastfeeding is an important measure in promoting the health and well-being of children and for this reason should be supported and encouraged. However, almost one-third of women will report difficulties in breastfeeding and these usually fall into two broad categories—pain and a perception of low milk supply (43). Breast and nipple pain are an important symptom and the first condition to exclude is mastitis (discussed previously). Where mastitis is not present, poor attachment of the baby to the nipple is the commonest cause of pain. This can occur when the nipple is inverted and difficult for the baby to grasp, or where there is restricted jaw or tongue movement for the baby. In some cases the frenulum under the baby's tongue may be snipped with sterile scissors and this does not seem to cause undue distress for the baby and may improve attachment.

Where there is trauma to the nipple it is common for the area to be colonized with staphylococci, so use of a topical antibiotic may be of value. Use of purified lanolin has also been shown to be effective in assisting the nipples to heal (43). Where these measures do not provide relief, there has been a presumption that *Candida* infection of the nipples may be a factor and there is certainly some evidence that topical antifungals to both the nipples and the baby's mouth may help (44). Another possible cause is vasospasm, related to Raynaud's phenomenon. This presents with blanching or other colour changes to the nipple, and acute onset of pain radiating into the breast. It commonly occurs in women with a prior history of Raynaud's. The main precipitant is cold so avoidance of cold by covering the nipple immediately after feeds is important. In refractory cases use of the peripheral vasodilator nifedipine has been recommended, although at present there are few trials to confirm this (43).

Low milk supply is commonly reported but is a very difficult problem to define in practical terms. Continuing adequate supply depends upon regular removal of milk from the breasts, a normal hormonal milieu, and adequate breast tissue. Breast hypoplasia is relatively uncommon, and some women will have had breast reduction surgery, but the majority of women will have adequate breast tissue. In many cases the perception of low milk supply results from misinterpretation of feeding patterns or a concern that the breasts are 'soft'. If the baby is gaining weight satisfactorily, the milk supply is likely to be normal and sometimes reassurance is all that is required. A factor that has been demonstrated to contribute to continued successful breastfeeding is skin-to-skin contact after birth, and this should be encouraged (45). Where reduced milk supply is suspected, the use of manual compression of the breast while expressing milk may increase production, along with attention to effective attachment, increasing frequency of feeds, expressing after feeds, and ensuring that the baby is offered both sides (43). Although 'galactogogues' such as domperidone or metoclopramide are commonly prescribed, there is little evidence that they are effective at this time.

Fistula

Obstetric fistula is a major public health problem in developing countries with an incidence rate of up to 1 in 500 births, of which 80% result from obstructed labour (46). A combination of socio-cultural problems promote the occurrence of fistula, including malnourishment leading to skeletal maturation, and marriage at an early age with childbearing before growth of the pelvic bones is complete. In regions where these risk factors are common, there is often a lack of access to obstetric care and facilities for emergency birth by caesarean section (47). In the majority of cases the baby dies, doubling the tragedy for the woman.

Almost half of all women who develop obstetric fistulae are primigravid, and there is often a delay of years between the labour and the seeking of medical attention (48). Findings can be complex and include vesico-, urethro-, and ureterovaginal fistula often with loss of bladder tissue due to pressure necrosis. Rectovaginal fistula formation is also common and is associated with pelvic inflammatory disease and secondary infertility. With these terrible injuries comes chronic skin excoriation due to maceration by urine or faeces. Unsurprisingly, women with fistulae commonly find themselves cast out and abandoned by their families, driving them into social isolation, divorce, poverty, malnutrition, and severe mental health problems sometimes culminating in suicide (47).

Debriefing after adverse outcomes of birth

The desire to talk about birth experiences is very common and for most women this will be accomplished by talking with family, friends, and other social groupings such as mothers' groups (49). Where there have been adverse or unanticipated outcomes of birth, it is important the maternity carers become part of these conversations. For many women, the perception of their birth experience may be different to that of those providing care, and events that seem trivial to staff may have a profound negative impact on women. It is quite possible to have a severe emotional trauma following what, to the maternity carer, may seem like a perfectly acceptable birth outcome. Studies suggest that more than 20% of women report their birth experience as 'traumatic' (50).

While the individual experience of birth is subjective, it is influenced by a number of variables including perceptions of 'medical interference', feelings about personal performance and safety of both mother and baby, cultural expectations, and how well the birth met the woman's expectations (50). An important contributor to the birth experience is the nature and quality of interactions with carers, and this is influenced by verbal and non-verbal behaviours and how the woman judges these in relation to her needs. Feelings of being 'unsupported' or 'abandoned' can leave women feeling that their birth experience was negative or traumatic.

Where there are concerns about a woman's experience of birth, it is ideal to begin a conversation before the woman leaves the place of maternity care. This may simply take the form of inviting women to attend for further discussions or more in-depth counselling (49). The use of open questions, careful reflective listening, acknowledgement of the woman's concerns, and willingness to answer questions are important. Apologies for what has happened are not admissions of wrongdoing and may help the woman deal with the issues. Planning for further follow-up and future pregnancies is an important part of care, and communication with staff involved in the birth is encouraged. To achieve these ends, adequate time must be set aside, and the meeting location should be quiet and appropriate for the discussion. Other family members or advocates may attend to lend support, and staff members involved may also be invited. Timely recognition and the provision of information and support can go a long way to addressing a woman's concerns about her birth outcome.

Contraception choices after birth

The opportunity to space pregnancies is important for many women and their families, and assistance with contraception choices is an important part of care in the puerperium (51). For women who are not breastfeeding, the range of contraceptives is essentially the same as for other women and should be made on an individualized basis. However, for women who are breastfeeding, this can affect and potentially restrict choice and it is important to provide balanced information (52). Progestin-only pill contraceptives have been widely studied and no difference has been demonstrated in breastfeeding outcomes or child health between women using progestin-only pills and those using non-hormonal contraception. Similar conclusions have been reached about the use of depot medroxyprogesterone acetate, even with very early injection before discharge from hospital. Studies of the etonogestrel contraceptive implant in lactating women have also been reassuring. The levonorgestrel-containing intrauterine device is effective and safe during lactation; however, there are reports of a higher incidence of uterine perforation with placement in the postnatal period and possibly longer (53). The literature regarding the use of oestrogen-containing combined oral contraceptives is of limited value, and although there is little direct evidence of an effect on the well-being of the baby, the availability of a range of other safe and effective options renders their use largely irrelevant (52). There are thus a number of safe and effective choices for postnatal contraception available to women, allowing the selection to be tailored to the needs and expectations of the individual woman.

Social support after birth

It is normal for women to find the transition to parenthood challenging and stressful, whether they are welcoming a first child or adding a new sibling to the family. The availability of social support from immediate family members and friends is an important factor in helping women cope, and reduced access to, or dissatisfaction with, social support is strongly associated with adverse outcomes of pregnancy including postnatal depression (54). Barriers to mobilization of support include concerns that asking for help reflects negatively on a woman's capacity as a mother, or that women are in socially isolated situations with minimal support systems available. Women at particular risk are adolescent women and migrant women. Adolescent mothers are at particular risk of intimate partner violence, substance abuse, and postpartum depression (55). These risks are likely due to lack of social supports, high-stress living environments, pre-existing mental health problems, and lack of parenting knowledge. Most of these issues can be addressed by identification of young women at risk during pregnancy and multidisciplinary care and planning for birth and beyond.

With increasing rates of global migration, most large maternity services will be providing care for a diverse group of migrant women. For comprehensive care to be effective, it is important that staff are familiar with, and respectful of, differences in language, culture, socioeconomic status, and traditions related to birth (56).

Women from different cultural and linguistic backgrounds will be familiar with, or may experience pressure from family and friends to conform to, different traditions of care, diet, mobilization, and other postnatal practices. While these should be respectfully addressed, it is important that safe and evidence-based care is available and the reasons for such managements are presented to women in an easily understood and useful way.

REFERENCES

1. Hytten F. The physiology of the puerperium. In: Chamberlain G, Steer PJ (eds), *Turnbull's Obstetrics*, 3rd edn, pp. 635–46. London, Churchill Livingston; 2002

2. Webb S, Sherburn M, Ismail KM. Managing perineal trauma after childbirth. *BMJ* 2014;**349**.

3. Deitz HP, Pardey J, Murray H. Pelvic floor and anal sphincter trauma should be key performance indicators of maternity services. *Int Urogynecol J* 2015;**26**:29–32.

4. O'Brien C, Fitzpatrick M. Managing perineal trauma after childbirth. *BMJ* 2014;**349**:g6829.

5. Jackson N, Paterson-Brown S. Physical sequelae of caesarean section. *Best Pract Res Clin Obstet Gynaecol* 2001;**15**:49–61.

6. Glazener CM, Abdalla M, Stroud P, et al. Postnatal maternal morbidity: extent, causes, prevention and treatment. *Br J Obstet Gynaecol* 1995;**102**:282–87.

7. Harpham M, Shand AW, Lainchbury A, Nassar S, Leung S. Maternal car driving capacity after birth: a feasibility study randomising postnatal women after caesarean section and vaginal birth to early or late driving in a driving simulator. *BJOG* 2015;**122** Suppl 1:345–406.

8. Malish S, Arastu F, O'Brien LM. A preliminary study of new parents, sleep disruption, and driving: a population at risk? *Matern Child Health J* 2016;**20**:290–97.

9. Edmonds DK. Puerperium and lactation. In: Edmonds DK (ed), *Dewhurst's Textbook of Obstetrics and Gynaecology*, pp. 365–76. London: Wiley and Sons, 2012.

10. Neville MC, Morton J. Physiology and endocrine changes underlying human lactogenesis II. *J Nutr* 2001;**131**:3005S–3008S.

11. Thaler I, Manor D, Itskovitz J, et al. Changes in uterine blood flow during human pregnancy. *Am J Obstet Gynecol* 1990;**162**:121–25.

12. Robson SC, Boys RJ, Hunter S, Dunlop W. Maternal hemodynamics after normal delivery and delivery complicated by postpartum haemorrhage. *Obstet Gynecol* 1989;**74**:234–39.

13. Ueland K, Novy MJ, Peterson EN, Metcalfe J. Maternal cardiovascular dynamics. *Am J Obstet Gynecol* 1969;**104**:856–64.

14. McNeilly AS, Tay CC, Glasier A. Physiological mechanisms underlying lactational amenorrhoea. *Ann N Y Acad Sci* 1994;**709**:145–55.

15. Sivertsen B, Hysing M, Dorheim SK, Eberhard-Gran M. Trajectories of maternal sleep problems before and after childbirth: a longitudinal population-based study. *BMC Pregnancy Childbirth* 2015;**15**:129.

16. Ryan B. When career women have children: psychological issues and assistance. *O&G Magazine* 2015;**17**:32–35.

17. Beck CT. Predictors of postpartum depression—an update. *Nursing Res* 2001;**50**:275–85.

18. O'Malley D, Higgins A, Smith V. Postpartum sexual health: a principle-based concept analysis. *J Adv Nurse* 2015;**71**:2247–57.

19. Barrett G, Pendry E, Peacock J, Victor CR, Thakar R. Women's sexual health after childbirth. *Br J Obstet Gynaecol* 2000;**107**:186–95.

20. De Judicibus MA, McCabe MP. Psychological factors and the sexuality or pregnant and postpartum women. *J Sex Res* 2002;**39**:94–103.

21. Lumley J. Sexual feelings in pregnancy and after childbirth. *Aust NZ J Obstet Gynaecol* 1998;**18**:114–17.

22. Robson S, Higgs P. Third- and fourth-degree injuries. *O&G Magazine* 2011;**13**:20–22.

23. Uygur D, Yesildaglar N, Kis S, Sipahi T. Early repair of episiotomy dehiscence. *Aust NZ J Obstet Gynaecol* 2004;**44**:244–46.

24. Johnson A, Young D, Renly J. Caesarean section surgical site infection surveillance. *J Hosp Infect* 2006;**64**:30–35.

25. Lim CC, Mahmood T. Obesity in pregnancy. *Best Pract Res Clin Obstet Gynaecol* 2015;**29**:309–19.

26. McKibben RA, Pitts SI, Suarez-Cuervo C, Perl T, Bass EB. Practices to reduce surgical site infections among women undergoing cesarean section: a review. *Infect Control Hosp Epidemiol* 2015;**36**:915–21.

27. Fitzwater JL, Tita AT. Prevention and management of cesarean wound infection. *Obstet Gynecol Clin North Am* 2014;**41**:671–89.

28. Michie C, Lockie F, Lynn W. the challenge of mastitis. *Arch Dis Child* 2003;**88**:818–21.

29. Osterman KL, Rahm V. Lactation mastitis: bacterial cultivation of breastmilk, symptoms, treatment, and outcome. *J Hum Lact* 2000;**16**:297–302.

30. Gravett MG. Intra-amniotic and postpartum infections. *Global Libr Women Med* 2008. DOI: 10.3843/GLOWM.10176.

31. Groom KM, Jacobson TZ. The management of secondary postpartum hemorrhage. In: Arulkumaran S, Karoshi M, Keith LG, Lalonde AB, Lynch CB (eds), *A Comprehensive Textbook of Postpartum Haemorrhage: An Essential Clinical Reference for Effective Management*, 2nd edn, pp. 466–73. London: Sapiens Publishing; 2012.

32. Neill A, Thornton S. Secondary postpartum haemorrhage. *J Obstet Gynaecol* 2002;**22**:119–22.

33. Zuckerman J, Levine D, McNicholas MM, et al. Imaging of pelvic postpartum complications. *Am J Roentgenol* 1997;**168**:663–68.

34. King PA, Duthie SJ, Dong ZG, Ma HK. Secondary post-partum haemorrhage. *Aust NZ J Obstet Gynaecol* 1989;**29**:394–98.

35. Hoveyda F, MacKenzie I. Secondary postpartum haemorrhage: incidence, morbidity and current management. *BJOG* 2001;**108**:927–30.

36. Schenker JG, Margalioth EJ. Intrauterine adhesions: an updated appraisal. *Fertil Steril* 1982;**37**:593–610.

37. Yip SK, Brieger G, Hin LY, Chung T. Urinary retention in the postpartum period. The relationship between obstetric factors and the post-partum post-void residual bladder volume. *Acta Obstet Gynecol Scand* 1997;**76**:667–72.

38. Lim JL. Post-partum voiding dysfunction and urinary retention. *Aust NZ J Obstet Gynaecol* 2010;**50**:502–505.

39. Lohsiriwat V. Hemorrhoids: from basic pathophysiology to clinical management. *World J Gastroenterol* 2012;**18**:2009–17.

40. Thom DH, Rortveit G. Prevalence of postpartum urinary incontinence: a systematic review. *Acta Obstet Gynecol Scand* 2010;**89**:1511–22.

41. Mackenzie R, Clubb A. Faecal incontinence following childbirth. *Nurs Times* 2007;**103**:40–41.

42. Sultan AH, Kamm MA, Hudson CN, Thomas JM, Bartram CI. Anal-sphincter disruption during vaginal delivery. *N Engl J Med* 1993;**329**:1905–11.

43. Amir LH. Managing common breastfeeding problems in the community. *BMJ* 2014;**348**:g2954.

44. Amir LH, Donath SM, Garland SM, et al. Does Candida and/or Staphylococcus play a role in nipple and breast pain in lactation? A cohort study in Melbourne, Australia. *BMJ Open* 2013;**3**:e002351.

45. Moore ER, Anderson GC, Bergman N, Dowswell T. Early skin-to-skin contact for mothers and their healthy newborn infants. *Cochrane Database Syst Rev* 2012;**5**:CD003519.

46. Hilton P, Ward A. Epidemiological and surgical aspects of urogenital fistula: a review of 25 years' experience in south east Nigeria. *Int Urogynecol J* 1998;**9**:189–94.

47. Wall LL. Obstetric vesicovaginal fistula as an international public health problem. *Lancet* 2006;**368**:1201–209.

48. Wall LL, Karshina J, Kirschner C, Arrowsmith SD. The obstetric vesicovaginal fistula. Characteristics of 899 patients from Jos, Nigeria. *Am J Obstet Gynecol* 2004;**190**:1011–19.

49. Miller M. After the fact. *O&G Magazine* 2011;**13**:32–33.

50. Simpson M, Catling C. Understanding psychological traumatic birth experiences: a literature review. *Women Birth* 2016;**29**:203–207.

51. Gipson JD, Koenig MA, Hindin M. The effects of unintended pregnancy on infant, child, and parental health: a review of the literature. *Stud Fam Plann* 2008;**39**:18–38.

52. Bhardwaj NR, Espey E. Lactation and contraception. *Curr Opin Obstet Gynecol* 2015;**27**:496–503.

53. Heinemann K, Reed S, Moehner S, Minh TD. Risk of uterine perforation with levonorgestrel-releasing and copper intrauterine devices in the European Active Surveillance Study on Intrauterine Devices. *Contraception* 2015;**91**:274–79.

54. Negron R, Martin A, Almog M, Balbierz A, Howell EA. Social support during the postpartum period: mothers' views on needs, expectations, and mobilization of support. *Matern Child Health J* 2013;**17**:616–23.

55. Thompson G, Madigan S, Wentzel K, et al. Demographic characteristics and needs of the Canadian urban adolescent mother and her child. *Paediatr Child Health* 2015;**20**:72–76.

56. Higginbottom G, Vallianatos H, Forgeron J, et al. Food choices and practices during pregnancy of immigrant women with high-risk pregnancies in Canada: a pilot study. *BMC Pregnancy Childbirth* 2014;**14**:370.

36

Induction of labour

Andrew Weeks and Julia P. Polk

Historical background

'Since antiquity various methods, many bizarre and some frankly dangerous, have been used in an attempt to bring on labour.'

Donald I (1955). *Practical Obstetric Problems* (1).

Informal methods for the induction of labour have been described for centuries. The use of 'caster oil, hot bath and emema' has been a common home technique and is thought to date back to Egyptian times. However, it was only in the eighteenth century that induction methods formally entered the medical literature (2). The first technique was amniotomy, described in 1756 by a London obstetrician, Thomas Denman and, as its popularity spread around Europe, it became known as the 'English Method'. But in the absence of a uterotonic, amniotomy had little effect except in multiparous women. The understanding that the ease of induction as well as success rates related to the softness and dilatation of the cervix (not enumerated by Bishop in a formal score until 1964) led to attempts to prepare the cervix prior to amniotomy. This was commonly done forcibly using fingers or rubber bougies. In a detailed review of methods in 1861, Robert Barnes describes the wide variety of options for labour induction:

> Some of these agents act directly upon the spinal marrow…such are ergot of rye, borax, cinnamon, and other drugs. Some evoke the energies of the diastolic system, by stimulating various peripheral nerves – such are rectal injections, the vaginal douche, the colpeurynter [an inflatable bag to distend the cervix], the carbonic-acid-gas douche, probably the irritation of breasts by sinapisms [a mustard plaster] and the air-pump, the cervical plug, whether in the form of sponge-tent or the caoutchouc [rubber] dilator, the separation of the membranes, the placing a flexible bougie in the uterus, the intrauterine injection, the evacuation of the liquor amnii, and galvanism [electrical muscle stimulation]. (3)

He goes on to describe the technique of pushing a rubberized 'fiddle-shaped' bag through the cervix and then filling it with water so that it swelled both on either side of the cervix (3). This was to be repopularized 150 years later with the introduction of the cervical ripening balloon. A variant of this was the de Ribes' bag, named after a Parisian accoucher, which was a reusable, rubber-covered, silk inflatable bag which was inserted through the cervix using special forceps and filled with water to a maximum of 500 mL (**Figure 36.1**).

The changes in medical advice about labour induction (**Table 36.1**) over the next 100 years were traced by Nabi et al. (2014) through the teaching in the 19 editions of the classic textbook *Ten Teachers* (4). Early in the twentieth century, methods were highly invasive, even brutal. As such, their use was restricted to cases of intrauterine fetal demise (IUFD) or severe maternal disease. In a mortality review of eight United Kingdom hospitals from 1925 to 1930, induction of labour was the direct cause of 5% of deaths in an overall maternal mortality rate of 424:100,000 (5). All cases were described as avoidable and were secondary to haemorrhage, sepsis, and anaesthetic complications.

Medical options with oxytocin and then prostaglandins started to become available in the twentieth century. The uterotonic effect of pituitary extract was described in 1909 by Sir Henry Dale, and first introduced into clinical practice by William Blair-Bell, an obstetrician from Liverpool who later founded the Royal College of Obstetrics and Gynaecology. But the major change came in the 1960s with the development of purified prostaglandins by Karim and colleagues in Makerere University, Uganda (6). Initially derived from semen, here was an agent that not only caused uterine contractions, but also simultaneously resulted in cervical ripening. Prostaglandin E_2 is unstable and needs to be kept cold and given intravenously or vaginally. The arrival of the stable prostaglandin E_1 tablets (misoprostol) in the 1980s for gastric protection, allowed the same effect to be achieved by the oral, sublingual, or vaginal route.

Induction rates have fluctuated widely with time and local culture. Despite the difficulties with induction, it became a very common practice in the medicalized days of the 1950s with up to 50% of all women undergoing induction in some hospitals. Rates fell after that, but have recently risen again. In the United Kingdom at the start of the twenty-first century, around 15% of all women were induced, but the rate has been steadily rising since then. Clinicians had been deterred by the association between labour induction and adverse outcomes. However, the recent finding that 'induction without medical indication' did not result in an increase in caesarean section or operative delivery and may even reduce adverse events has led to a steady rise in induction rates. In England today, the average induction rate is 30% with rates of over 40% in some hospitals.

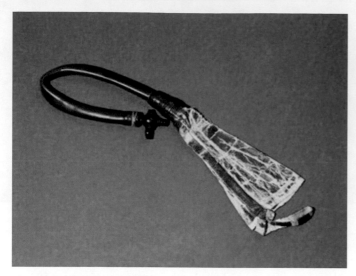

Figure 36.1 De Ribes' bag.

Definitions

Labour is defined by the presence of regular uterine contractions and the resultant cervical change. Induction of labour refers to the use of medications or mechanical methods to stimulate contractions in a patient who is not in labour with the goal of causing labour and vaginal delivery. The initial step is usually cervical ripening, a process which increases the readiness of the cervix to undergo induction. The readiness of the cervix to respond to induction methods is generally calculated by the Bishop score (Table 36.2). This is a widely used calculation, which takes into account the consistency, effacement, position, and dilation of the cervix along with the fetal station. There are modifiers that can be applied to the Bishop score, the most common of which uses the substitution of effacement for cervical length in centimetres. This is what is typically referred to as the 'modified Bishop score'. Additional modifiers are listed in Table 36.2. A Bishop score of 8 or greater is generally considered favourable for induction although various different cut-offs have been reported (between 5 and 8). A favourable Bishop score is also considered the point at which the likelihood of successful vaginal delivery is similar

Table 36.1 Methods of labour induction advised in the *Ten Teachers* textbook between 1917 and 2011

	1917	1922	1925	1931	1935	1938	1942	1948	1955	1961	1966	1972	1980	1985	1990	1995	2000	2006	2011
Medical																			
				Castor oil + quinine															
				Pituitary extract		Oxytocin (IM)					Oxytocin (IV drip)			Oxytocin (IV infusion pump)						
											Buccal oxytocin								
													Prostaglandin E2 (gel/tablet/pessary)						
													F2α	F2α					
															Gemeprost				Misoprostol
						Stillboestrol													
Surgical																			
	Bougies																		
			Oesophageal/stomach tube																
	De Ribes' bag																		
	Amniotomy																		
	Forced dilatation of the cervix (Manual/instrumental)																		
	Vaginal caesarean section																		
													Hypertonic intra-amniotic injection						
																		Membrane sweeping

IM, intramuscular; IV, intravenous.

Bougie: a cylinder of celluloid or gum-elastic. Two or three are inserted through the cervix into the uterus under anaesthetic with vaginal packing to prevent expulsion. Vaginal caesarean section: under anaesthetic, the anterior vaginal wall and the anterior portion of the cervix are incised in the midline and the bladder pushed up. The membranes are ruptured and the baby is delivered through the resulting space.

Reproduced from Nabi HA, Aflaifel NB, Weeks AD. A hundred years of induction of labour methods. *Eur J Obstet Gynecol Reprod Biol* 2014 Aug;179:236–9. doi: 10.1016/j.ejogrb.2014.03.045 with permission from Elsevier.

Table 36.2 Modified Bishop score

Bishop score	Factor				
	Dilatation (cm)	Cervical length (cm)	Station	Cervical consistency	Cervical position
0	<1	<4	−3	Firm	Posterior
1	1–2	2–4	−2	Average	Mid/anterior
2	2–4	1–2	−1/0	Soft	–
3	>4	>1	+1/2	–	–

Additional versions of the modified Bishop score add 1 additional point for every previous vaginal delivery or the presence of pre-eclampsia and 1 point is subtracted for nulliparity, postdate pregnancy, or the presence of PPROM.

to that when in spontaneous labour. Although initially developed only for multiparous women, this relationship is most profound in nulliparous women (7).

If a patient presents in spontaneous labour but requires the use of medication to increase the frequency or strength of contractions, this is referred to as augmentation of labour. This is generally used if there is inadequate cervical change.

Indications

Prevention of maternal disease

Although induction of labour is generally either indicated on behalf of the mother or on behalf of the fetus, in many cases the two overlap and induction is mutually beneficial. Specific clinical situations require individualized treatment plans. However, for the purpose of this chapter, we will provide general guidance which the clinician and woman can modify according to individual clinical scenarios and preferences. More details are provided in the chapters on the individual diseases.

Maternal disease can either be pregestational or gestational; however, the same physiological processes generally mediate the risk to continuation of the pregnancy. Hypertension and diabetes fall along a continuum of maternal vascular disease that has the potential to compromise placentation and thus puts a pregnancy at risk of placental insufficiency as gestational age increases. There are slightly different points at which outcomes are seen to worsen when pregnancies go undelivered depending upon the specific pathology and its severity. Pregnancies affected by either uncomplicated diabetes or hypertension are usually delivered in the early-term period, between 37^{+0} weeks and 40^{+0} weeks (7, 8).

Additional maternal disease, such as coagulopathies, cardiac pathology, or pulmonary pathology, poses a threat to mother or fetus if labour is left to start spontaneously in an uncontrolled setting. For example, if a patient has an active pulmonary embolus and is on anticoagulation therapy, an unplanned delivery may put the patient at risk of haemorrhage if timely discontinuation or change in anticoagulation therapy does not occur. Therefore, there is a whole subset of maternal pathologies that benefit from a controlled induction of labour at a gestation age prior to 40^{+0} weeks or even prior to 39^{+0} weeks when the likelihood of spontaneous labour increases significantly.

International cancer databases have provided a wealth of data on the many pregnancies that have been complicated by cancer. Each type of cancer has a specific gestational age at which delivery is indicated depending on its stage and progression, allowing the mother to return rapidly to her appropriate therapy regimen. Delivery is usually indicated when the risk to the mother becomes greater than the risk for the preterm neonate (9).

In the event of an IUFD, it is beneficial to induce delivery to protect the mother against infection or coagulopathy. As long as it is established that the mother's health is stable, and she has intact membranes, it is appropriate to offer the mother expectant management or induction of labour. Without intervention, 85% of women with an IUFD will deliver within 3 weeks. In the absence of abruption, pre-eclampsia, infection, or bleeding, the risk of an acquired coagulopathy is initially low. Although after 4 weeks only 10% of women will have developed coagulopathy, regular monitoring of coagulation is still prudent. After that point the risk for bleeding and infection begin to rise and it is prudent to induce labour (10).

Prevention of fetal complications

From a fetal perspective, induction of labour is usually carried out in order to prevent IUFD. The risk of this may be related to a specific maternal disease process (e.g. hypertension or diabetes), fetal diseases (e.g. IUGR or macrosomia), or to background risk factors such as maternal age, body mass index (BMI), or advanced gestation. Specific maternal disease processes are covered elsewhere in this textbook.

Maternal obesity is an emerging problem throughout the world. As the medical community learns about the many facets of health affected by obesity it has become obvious that pregnancy complicated by obesity is at increased risk of IUFD. The trend for this phenomenon begins at 40^{+0} weeks, approximately 1–2 weeks prior to that of the remainder of the population. This trend is more profound as maternal BMI increases (11).

Much like increasing BMI, increasing *maternal age* also has a correlation with increase in IUFD rates. It is generally accepted that over the age of 35 a woman is considered at risk of complications such as increased rates of aneuploidies. The rate of IUFD becomes statistically increased over the age of 40 with an odds ratio of 3.04 at 39 weeks in comparison to women aged 25–29 years (12). Many countries acknowledge that it is advisable to recommend induction of labour by 40^{+0} weeks, and this is supported by a randomized trial which found no adverse effects on common outcomes of routine induction of women over the age of 35 at 39 weeks' gestation (13, 14). Whether this translates to fewer perinatal deaths remains unclear.

Oligohydramnios or insufficient amniotic fluid is defined by a single deepest pocket (without umbilical cord or fetal parts) measuring 2 cm or less or an amniotic fluid index of 5 cm or less (7). This condition is associated with uteroplacental insufficiency and resulting low fetal renal blood flow. In the initial evaluation of oligohydramnios, rupture of membranes must be ruled out regardless of gestational age. Induction of labour is usually carried out if isolated oligohydramnios is detected at or beyond 36^{+0} weeks. In oligohydramnios of the preterm fetus, expectant management may be undertaken if fetal testing is feasible along with an investigation for additional aetiologies of oligohydramnios such as fetal anomalies (7). There is some emerging data that expectant management of isolated oligohydramnios at term does not change outcomes and may be a safe alternative to mandated induction (15).

Preterm prelabour rupture of membranes (PPROM) is defined as rupture of membranes prior to 37^{+0} weeks in the absence of labour. In order to reduce the risk of sepsis, induction of labour is commonly conducted once the pregnancy reaches 34 weeks, although randomized trials suggest that expectant management with close monitoring is also a safe option (16). Prior to 34 weeks' gestation, expectant management is appropriate with fetal testing and monitoring for signs of infection (17).

Intrauterine fetal growth restriction is defined as a composite estimated fetal weight less than 10% for gestational age (although different sources may use different cut-offs or terminology). The general timing for delivery for these fetuses is debated, but it is generally acceptable to deliver after 34^{+0} weeks in the setting of growth restriction and abnormal fetal testing such as absent or reverse end-diastolic flow of the umbilical artery Doppler. Otherwise, in the setting of normal fetal testing, delivery is generally recommended after 37^{+0} weeks, prior to 40^{+0} weeks (18). According to current National Institute for Health and Care Excellence (NICE) guidelines, in the setting of severe growth restriction with concern for fetal compromise, induction of labour is not indicated. In these settings, if delivery is indicated it is recommended to proceed with caesarean section (8).

Induction of labour is also sometimes recommended for *fetal macrosomia*, defined as 4000 g or 4500 g depending upon your source. Fetal macrosomia leads to significantly higher rates of IUFD, overall neonatal mortality, birth injury, neonatal asphyxia, failed induction of labour, meconium aspiration, and maternal birth injury (19). In a randomized controlled trial (RCT) conducted in France, Switzerland, and Belgium, 822 women with ultrasound-estimated fetal weight greater than the 95% centile were randomized to delivery between 37 and 38^{+6} weeks or expectant management. Induced babies were 287 g lighter and were significantly more likely to be born vaginally. Furthermore, the risk of the composite outcome (significant shoulder dystocia, delay in delivery of the shoulder by >60 seconds, or fracture) was significantly reduced (by 68% from 6% to 2%). There was no difference in rate of caesarean section (20). This is the largest study of its kind; there are two additional RCTs which investigate induction versus expectant management, however they both utilize 4000 g, they both had much smaller numbers, and they both induced at or close to 40 weeks which is likely why the data was less supportive of labour induction. This suggests that if a fetus has an estimated fetal weight of greater than 95% after 37^{+0} weeks, then induction of labour prior to 39 weeks is beneficial for the fetus without adverse consequences for the mother.

In the general population, a marked increase in IUFD occurs in *'postdates pregnancies'*. The lowest perinatal death rate is at 38 weeks (1.9:1000) with the cumulative probability of death increasing to 5:1000 and 9:1000 at 42 and 43 weeks respectively (21). Additionally, there is an increase in multiple perinatal morbidities such as neonatal convulsions, meconium aspiration, Apgar score less than 4, and admission to neonatal intensive care units. The NICE guideline recommends induction of labour between 41^{+0} and 42^{+0} weeks. If a woman declines induction after 42^{+0} weeks, twice-weekly fetal monitoring with cardiotocography and ultrasonography is recommended to reduce the risk of IUFD (8).

As discussed earlier, there are cases of maternal pathology that necessitate a timed delivery; the same can be said for fetal pathology. If there is a *fetal anomaly* or condition which requires immediate specialist postnatal care, it is often appropriate to perform an induction prior to spontaneous labour. This ensures that the neonate can be born at a time when there are adequate staff and facilities to provide optimal care. The timing of induction is best decided by the providers and should take into account the risks of prematurity, prolonged pregnancy, and timed delivery.

In a pregnancy affected by *isoimmunization* (discussed elsewhere in this textbook), delivery depends upon the severity of fetal haemolysis. If the fetus is stable and has not required intervention, induction of labour is appropriate at 37^{+0} weeks or when fetal lung maturity is documented. In cases where the fetus has undergone multiple transfusions, induction is typically recommended around 32^{+0} weeks (22, 23).

An indication of *'bad obstetric history'* has been given as an indication for induction for many years. It largely refers to a previous stillbirth, but may also include a history of recurrent miscarriage, abruption, prolonged infertility, or adverse fetal outcome in a previous pregnancy. The rationale is that elective induction (often before the gestation of the previous event) will reduce the recurrence risk. While there is little hard evidence behind this, clinicians and women will be reassured by the data on social induction (discussed later in this chapter) that it does not increase the need for operative birth.

Elective/maternal request/maternal discomfort

Induction following maternal request alone and in the absence of medical indication accounts for 6–14% of all inductions of labour in the Western world. This is a controversial topic and the guidelines surrounding this entity are nebulous and differ by nation. According to the 2008 NICE guideline, induction of labour purely due to maternal request should be avoided. However, it states that there may be extenuating social circumstances such as a woman's partner is being deployed for duties during the time of the estimated date of delivery when induction of labour may be considered at or after 40 weeks' gestation (8). The American Congress of Obstetrics and Gynecology (ACOG) supports elective induction of labour without clear medical benefit to mother or fetus, only after fetal lung maturity has been demonstrated or a minimum of 39 weeks of gestation (24).

When compared to expectant management, elective induction of labour at 41^{+0} weeks is associated with a decreased rate of caesarean delivery, and meconium-stained amniotic fluid (25). There is a recent RCT of nulliparous women ages 35 and older who were induced between 39^{+0} days and 39^{+6} days compared to expectant management which showed that no increased rate of caesarean section or maternal and neonatal adverse outcomes (14). Furthermore, a very large retrospective cohort study in Scotland from 1981 to 2007 showed that elective induction between 37^{+0} weeks and 41^{+0} weeks reduced perinatal mortality without increasing the rate of caesarean delivery (26). This was confirmed by a recent randomised trial of induction versus expectant management for 6,106 low risk women, in which induced women had lower rates of CS and improved perinatal adverse outcomes (27). The evidence is sufficient to support elective induction although the ethical caveat is that the alternative of 'expectant management' may carry a variable definition depending upon where one is practising. When feasible or requested, elective induction does not appear to carry added risk to the patient and in most cases appears to have benefit (24, 26, 27).

If avoiding IUFD or poor perinatal outcomes, labour induction is cost-effective when compared to expectant management (26). This cost trade-off is clear after 41 weeks in developed nations, which further supports the use of this gestational age cut-off. Globally, cost-effectiveness is dependent upon resources, distances to healthcare facilities, coverage of prenatal care, and many other factors that when considered together may support the use of elective induction at gestational ages prior to 41^{+0} weeks. For instance, elective induction especially in multiparous patients may be beneficial to avoid unattended births if there are great difficulties for patients to be transported to a health facility.

Contraindications

There are a few circumstances in which induction of labour is contraindicated. Absolute contraindications to labour induction are the same entities which preclude a vaginal delivery. These contraindications include placenta praevia, vasa praevia, or suspected placenta accreta, percreta, or increta; active genital herpes; transverse or oblique fetal presentation; prior classical caesarean section or transfundal uterine surgery; umbilical cord prolapse; and maternal pelvic deformities. Relative contraindications are cervical carcinoma, due to the risk of local disease spread and funic (cord) presentation. Breech presentation is covered elsewhere in this textbook, but generally contraindicates induction. Induction with a previous caesarean section is covered in the 'Special circumstances' section later in this chapter.

Clinical considerations

Prior to embarking upon an induction, one must be sure of the gestational age and presentation. Additionally, the indication for induction must be agreed with the woman and clearly documented. Fetal health should be confirmed by external electronic fetal heart monitoring before starting the induction. If there is evidence that the fetus would not tolerate an induction this is best known prior to administering any medications or performing any procedures to begin the induction. The modified Bishop score, as discussed previously, should also be calculated to decide on the need for pre-induction cervical ripening.

An induction of labour should ideally be carried out in settings with electronic fetal monitoring, facilities for accurately measuring infusion rates, and access to emergency caesarean section.

Outpatient induction is an option for some women, but it should be limited to the use of methods with low rates of hyperstimulation (e.g. mechanical methods, nitric oxide donors, or controlled release prostaglandins). RCTs suggest no difference in clinical outcome between inpatient and outpatient inductions except that outpatient inductions are associated with higher maternal satisfaction rates (28). One recent Australian study of inpatient versus outpatient use of a Foley catheter (see 'Transcervical balloon catheters') showed that the outpatient group was 24% less likely to require oxytocin to achieve vaginal delivery (29).

Ideally, an induction should be started in the morning as they are associated with higher maternal satisfaction and lower operative vaginal delivery rates. If intermittent fetal monitoring is used, it should be conducted before and after every drug administration and once contractions start. Once in labour, most women have continuous monitoring. However, it is safe to forego continuous monitoring in uncomplicated pregnancies without a fetal indication for induction and where oxytocin is not needed for augmentation (8). Induced labours are more painful than spontaneous labours. However, women (and staff) can be reassured that administering epidural analgesia prior to painful contractions or in early labour has no adverse effects on clinical outcomes and increases maternal satisfaction.

A risk of all inductions of labour is hyperstimulation, also known as tachysystole. Hyperstimulation is defined as more than five contractions in 10 minutes averaged over 30 minutes (30). Not all fetuses exposed to hyperstimulation will have fetal heart rate abnormalities, but data from the Parkland Hospital (Dallas, Texas, United States) state that six contractions in 10 minutes is when the rate of fetal heart tone decelerations rapidly increased (30). When using pharmacological methods of induction, uterine hyperstimulation occurs in about 5% of women. One-third of these women will also have fetal heart rate abnormalities (a combination known as 'hyperstimulation syndrome'). Hyperstimulation can be rapidly reversed by stopping an oxytocin infusion, or removing an intravaginal induction system. For those in whom the induction agent cannot be removed or stopped, beta-2-adrenergic therapy (e.g. terbutaline 250 mcg given subcutaneously or intramuscularly) is very effective and without maternal or fetal complications (31).

Mechanical methods

Membrane sweeping

Membrane sweeping is the most basic of mechanical methods of labour induction. It is performed by inserting a finger through the cervical os and sweeping it around between the chorion and the uterine wall to release prostaglandins. Membrane sweeps, if performed more than once after 38 weeks' gestation, are shown to reduce the need for formal induction of labour by 40–50% and to increase the rate of spontaneous labour. The success of membrane sweeping is highest in multiparous women. In the United Kingdom, it is recommended that all women are offered regular membrane sweeps in the 2 weeks after their due date (8). If the cervix will not admit a finger it may not be possible to do a formal membrane sweep. In such cases, massaging around the cervix in the vaginal fornices may achieve a similar effect. A small amount of bleeding and cramping is common following the procedure.

Amniotomy

Amniotomy, or artificial rupture of membranes (ARM), is rarely used alone for induction. If used in isolation, it is most effective in multiparous women with ripe cervixes (7). For these women, when used in combination with oxytocin prior to the start of spontaneous labour, ARM is as effective as vaginal dinoprostone (see later) in achieving vaginal delivery. Dinoprostone is generally given in preference as around half of those induced can progress to delivery without the need for an uncomfortable and intrusive intravenous infusion (8).

Amniotomy may be achieved using a variety of toothed instruments, but a plastic amniotomy hook is most commonly used to tear the membranes. If the fetal head is not engaged in the pelvis, a gradual release of liquor is required and this can be achieved by puncturing the membranes with a needle.

Amniotomy may be a useful adjunct in spontaneous labours to allow visualization of liquor and placement of a fetal scalp electrode in those at risk. However, when performed early in labour or prior to labour, ARM can put a patient at risk of prolonged rupture of membranes and infection (7).

Induction of labour when the head is high in the pelvis increases the risk of cord prolapse and malpresentation. Medical methods (e.g. dinoprostone) should therefore always be used initially. When ARM is necessary, this should be performed along with fundal pressure (a 'controlled ARM'). With polyhydramnios, it is useful to keep the examining hand in the vagina until the liquor has drained and the head descended in case of cord prolapse. The woman should sit upright after the ARM to encourage fetal head descent. If the fetal head is very high, some practitioners prefer to conduct the ARM in theatre so that caesarean delivery can rapidly be carried out in the event of a cord prolapse.

Transcervical balloon catheters

Many versions of transcervical balloon catheters have been in use over the past few centuries. The most common version is a Foley catheter with a large reservoir tip which can hold up to 30–50 mL (typical Foley catheters hold approximately 10 mL). Transcervical catheters are inserted through the cervix manually or using an instrument such as 'sponge holders'. When the position of the balloon is confirmed by inflation of the balloon and pulling back against the cervix, it is inflated to its desired capacity. The distal end of the catheter which hangs outside of the vagina is often taped to the inner thigh to apply tension against the cervix. However, this is probably not necessary as the method was highly effective in the PROBAAT (Dutch for 'approved') and INFORM randomized trials in which a single 30 mL balloon was used with no tension on the catheter (32, 33).

Some models of transcervical balloon have two separate balloons, one sits inside the internal cervical os and one in the vagina; the idea is to apply tension between the two balloons against the cervix. Studies comparing this balloon (commonly known by its trade name 'Cook Balloon' or the 'Cervical Ripening Balloon') to the traditional Foley catheter balloon in women with a previous caesarean section have shown the Foley carries a minimally shorter time to delivery but no difference in time from insertion to active labour, time from balloon expulsion to delivery, caesarean section, instrumental delivery, pain score, need for analgesia, or maternal satisfaction (34). A more recent study, however, has found that that there may be a beneficial effect on both speed and vaginal birth rate, but only in nulliparous women (35). It must be noted that the double-balloon catheter is significantly more costly than the traditional Foley. Some studies have investigated an extra-amniotic saline infusion which runs while the transcervical balloon is in place. The typical rate is approximately 50 mL/hour. This has been shown to decrease the time from balloon insertion to expulsion as well as the time to delivery when used with both single- and double-balloon catheters (36).

Transcervical catheters do not increase the risk of infection according to a meta-analysis (37). They are commonly maintained for up to 12 hours, but this time period was increased up to 4 days in the PROBAAT series of trials without any sign of excessive infective morbidity (32, 33). When the catheter falls out, ARM is performed and oxytocin commenced. Transcervical balloon catheters when compared head-to-head with vaginal misoprostol have longer induction to delivery times but lower rates of hyperstimulation and operative vaginal delivery with no difference in caesarean delivery rates (32).

When comparing mechanical methods to prostaglandins, a Cochrane review from 2012 found that mechanical methods resulted in a similar caesarean section rate, but with a lower risk of hyperstimulation than prostaglandins. No overall increased time to delivery was seen, but there were a larger proportion of multiparous women undelivered at 24 hours when compared to dinoprostone (38).

Laminaria

Laminaria tents are another form of mechanical cervical dilators. They are made from sterile seaweed or synthetic hydrophilic materials, and are introduced into the cervical canal. As these devices absorb water, they increase in diameter and so stretch the cervix. Laminaria appear to be as effective at labour induction as vaginal prostaglandins, but with a markedly reduced incidence of uterine hyperstimulation (38). This may make them safer for women who have had a previous caesarean section. They are commonly used in the outpatient setting for cervical ripening prior to dilation and evacuation of a miscarriage or pregnancy termination above 12 weeks' gestation.

Pharmacological methods

Dinoprostone

There are two major synthetic prostaglandins utilized for cervical ripening and labour induction, dinoprostone (PGE_2) and misoprostol (PGE_1). Dinoprostone is most commonly used for cervical ripening in women with an unfavourable cervix where it is shown to improve the Bishop score, and reduce the need for oxytocin augmentation and caesarean section compared to placebo. However, the relative risk of hyperstimulation is greater compared to placebo (39). Dinoprostone can be administered as a gel, a slow-release drug-eluting tampon (Cervidil or Propess), or tablet. Tablets and gels are seen to be equally effective when given in the vagina. Intracervical dinoprostone results in a slower induction, likely because of the highly absorptive properties of the vaginal mucosa. Dinoprostone has been utilized orally but has a high rate of gastrointestinal side effects.

Misoprostol

Misoprostol, originally intended to treat gastric ulcers (currently its only indicated use from the Food and Drug Administration in the United States), may be used for both cervical ripening and labour induction when used at low doses. It is both cheaper and more heat stable at room temperatures than dinoprostone, making it an attractive option for both low- and high-resource settings. Misoprostol may be used orally, buccally or sublingually, vaginally, or rectally. Some countries have a 25 mcg oral tablet or vaginal pessary available. However, the most commonly available tablets are 200 mcg which require tablets to be cut into very small and typically inaccurate doses. A more accurate dosing regimen is achieved when a 200 mcg tablet is dissolved in 200 mL of water and divided accordingly. This solution is stable at room temperature for approximately 24 hours and should be stirred prior to each use.

Vaginal misoprostol is most typically used for cervical ripening and when given as 25 mcg every 4 hours leads to equivalent outcomes to vaginal dinoprostone. Oral misoprostol solution when dosed as 20 mcg every 2 hours is as effective as vaginal dinoprostone for cervical ripening and has a lower caesarean section rate. Titrated oral misoprostol solution has also been used during induced labour for augmentation (in lieu of oxytocin). Women are given 5–20 mcg orally every 1–2 hours with the goal of maintaining a minimum of three contractions every 10 minutes. This regimen is commonly used following induction with oral misoprostol solution, and appears to be as effective and safe as oxytocin (40).

Oxytocin

Synthetic oxytocin, often referred to as 'pitocin', is identical to the endogenous form produced in the hypothalamus and secreted by the posterior pituitary. Oxytocin is given intravenously, it cannot be given orally; it becomes inactive after breakdown in the gastrointestinal tract. Typically, oxytocin is used for labour induction or augmentation although a few studies document its use for cervical ripening at low continuous dosing. A Cochrane systematic review found that oxytocin used alone for cervical ripening reduced the rate of vaginal births within 24 hours compared to vaginal dinoprostone (21% vs 70%) and led to a 9% higher use of epidural for pain relief (41). The exception to this correlation is the use of only oxytocin in the setting of term, prelabour, spontaneous rupture of membranes where it is seen to be equally effective as prostaglandins followed by oxytocin (42).

Oxytocin binds to receptors in the myometrium which are found after 20 weeks' gestation and increasing over the course of pregnancy as well as during the course of spontaneous labour (7). Theoretically, therefore, oxytocin should be most effective when used to augment existing labour. Its most common uses are for labour augmentation following induction or with ARM following cervical priming. The only alternative for this indication is oral misoprostol, as explained previously. When oxytocin is used in combination with ARM, it is as effective at achieving vaginal delivery as using dinoprostone but with less maternal satisfaction (41). There are no differences in hyperstimulation rates when comparing oxytocin and prostaglandin use (41).

Mifepristone

Mifepristone is a progesterone antagonist that sensitizes the uterus to prostaglandins. When used alone, it results in labour in only 50% of women after 48 hours. When given 24–48 hours before induction in women with IUFD, it reduces the induction to the delivery interval. There have been reports of neonatal antiglucocorticoid effects, as well as fetal renal and hepatic dysfunction when used with live fetuses, and its use is therefore restricted to women with IUFD.

It is also used as the first of two medications given for medical termination of pregnancy which typically includes misoprostol as the second medication in different amounts and delivery methods depending upon the gestation age (43, 44).

Others

There are some additional pharmacological induction methods which have been used over time but not become the mainstay of therapy. For example, vaginal nitric oxide donors (e.g. isosorbide mononitrate or glyceryl trinitrate) are much slower than vaginal dinoprostone but carry lower rates of hyperstimulation. These methods commonly cause mild maternal side effects (headache in 90%), but maternal satisfaction is higher than for dinoprostone. Their gentle uterine effects may make them suitable for outpatient cervical ripening (45).

Oral corticosteroids, intracervical hyaluronidase injection, and oestrogens have all shown some effect, but there is not enough RCT evidence to comment on their safety and efficacy.

Combination methods

Each method previously outlined has its strengths but due to the multitude of options available, various combinations of methods have been investigated over time. Balloon catheters have been used with prostaglandins in multiple different configurations. The overall conclusion from a meta-analysis is that this combination leads to a lower rate of hyperstimulation than when prostaglandins are used alone (38). Many studies also show a shorter time to vaginal delivery, but heterogeneity in the results prevent its recommendation for routine use (38).

Complementary and alternative methods

Many non-traditional medications and methods for labour induction exist. For example, herbal medicines, acupuncture, enemas, castor oil, and homeopathic remedies have all been used. There are Cochrane reviews of all these interventions, but all find insufficient scientific research to recommend their use. Sexual intercourse has been subjected to two randomized trials but neither has shown any benefit in clinical outcome. There is some evidence to support the use of nipple stimulation as a method of induction, but not enough data to support its regular use.

Comparison of methods

The outcomes for the various methods of induction are similar, and this has led to diverse practice worldwide. The choice of one over the other is usually based on side effects, location of induction (inpatient versus outpatient), local experience with the technique, availability of monitoring facilities, patient and provider preference, and cost. It is important therefore to look at the data which compares each method so as to enable a rational choice of induction method for each occasion.

A network meta-analysis (a systematic review method for multiple simultaneous comparisons) attempted to compare the use of the Foley catheter, misoprostol (vaginal and oral), and dinoprostone (vaginal and cervical) in a single review for women with intact membranes (46). In 96 randomized trials, they found that vaginal misoprostol was the most effective cervical ripening method to achieve vaginal delivery within 24 hours, but had the highest incidence of uterine hyperstimulation with fetal heart rate changes. The use of a Foley catheter to induce labour was associated with the lowest rate of uterine hyperstimulation accompanied by fetal heart rate changes. The caesarean section rate was lowest using oral misoprostol for the induction of labour. Sensitivity analysis showed that the results were unaltered with the exclusion of high-dosage regimens. The authors concluded that no method of labour induction demonstrated overall superiority and that decisions regarding the choice of induction method should depend upon the relative importance of the outcomes.

Alfirevic et al. also conducted a much more extensive network meta-analysis of 280 randomized trials, but examined only prostaglandin induction methods (47). They found that low-dose (<50 mcg) titrated oral misoprostol solution had the lowest probability of caesarean section, whereas vaginal misoprostol (≥50 mcg) had the highest probability of achieving a vaginal delivery within 24 hours.

In a discussion of cost, misoprostol is the cheapest medication. Foley catheters follow behind closely but can become more expensive if the bespoke double-balloon version is desired. Dinoprostone is most expensive but has different prices based on the different formulations. The immediate-acting gel is less expensive than the extended-release preparation (slow-eluting tampon). A new vaginal insert version of misoprostol which is 200 mcg and meant to be a corollary to the slow-eluting dinoprostone tampon was shown to significantly reduce time to delivery in comparison to the dinoprostone version but with increased rates of hyperstimulation and fetal heart rate abnormalities (48). It is only available in some countries and is near in price to the dinoprostone slow-eluting tampon.

Induction in special situations

Previous caesarean section

Induction of labour in the setting of a previous uterine scar is not contraindicated but comes with increased risks. The main risk is uterine scar rupture, which brings with it high rates of morbidity and mortality for both mother and fetus. The risk of uterine rupture is approximately 0.5% for women in spontaneous labour or when induced using mechanical methods (49–51). This risk increases to approximately 0.77% if induced with oxytocin alone or around 1% with prostaglandins (32). This risk is not increased in women who have also had a previous vaginal delivery, regardless of the method of induction. Using an intrauterine pressure catheter does not decrease the risk of rupture. According to the 2013 Cochrane review on induction with a previous caesarean section, there is insufficient evidence to recommend one agent over another for induction in this situation (52). Successful vaginal delivery in women undergoing a trial of labour after caesarean section is reduced from approximately 70% in those in spontaneous labour to 50% in women undergoing induction (49–51). In conclusion, induction of labour with a prior caesarean section is not contraindicated, but carries markedly increased risks and so requires careful prior discussion with the woman.

Intrauterine fetal death

IUFD rates vary throughout the world from around 5–6:1000 births in high-income countries to 30–40:1000 births in low-income countries (53). The causes are myriad and addressed in other chapters of this textbook. As discussed previously, the NICE guideline states that in the event of an IUFD when the mother is stable, it is suitable to offer expectant management versus immediate induction of labour. Since most women will deliver within 3 weeks of the fetal demise, this is a reasonable time period for expectant management as long as the mother continues to be stable.

The delivery method depends upon the gestational age, maternal preference, and maternal history of prior uterine scar. Throughout most of the second trimester a *dilation and evacuation* procedure may be offered. Many patients may be opposed to this option due to the damage to the fetus which is not only psychologically difficult but which also precludes a full autopsy. As with a termination of pregnancy, cervical preparation is important if the cervix is closed. The two most common methods are laminaria placed 12–24 hours prior to the procedure and misoprostol 400 mcg given sublingually or vaginally 3 hours prior to the procedure. The risks for infection, bleeding, and uterine perforation along with the level of difficulty of this procedure all increase with the gestational age. At higher gestational ages some practitioners will choose to use ultrasound guidance either during the procedure or after the procedure to confirm its completion. Tissue floating may also be employed, which is a process that involves examining the products of conception to ensure that the contents and quantity are consistent with the gestational age.

Induction of labour after IUFD using prostaglandins may be used at any stage of pregnancy. High-dose intravenous oxytocin can also work in the second and third trimesters but is less effective (54). *Vaginal misoprostol* is considered the best method of induction, and there is evidence that premedication with mifepristone 200 mcg decreases the time to delivery (55). Doses of vaginal misoprostol are higher than those at term. An expert group recommends doses of 200 mcg 6-hourly at 13–17 weeks, 100 mcg 6-hourly at 18–26 weeks, and 25 mcg 6-hourly above 26 weeks (56).

Induction of labour with an IUFD in a patient with a prior uterine scar is a controversial topic. According to the ACOG and the Royal College of Obstetricians and Gynaecologists, vaginal misoprostol use does not increase the risk of uterine rupture up to 28 weeks' gestation. Beyond that, a halving of the misoprostol dose is suggested (54, 56). Caesarean delivery for an IUFD should be avoided as it causes significant risks to the mother such as infection, bleeding, and organ injury, and carries future pregnancy implications.

Multiple pregnancy

Delivery of multifetal pregnancies depends on the type of twin pregnancy, the gestational age, fetal presentation, and general health of the twin pregnancy (58), and is covered in more detail in Chapter 20. In a diamniotic pregnancy without complications, vaginal delivery is a safe option if the presenting twin is cephalic and the gestational age is at least 32 weeks (58). Timing of delivery of the pregnancy is stratified by twin type. In uncomplicated dichorionic diamniotic pregnancies, induction is commonly arranged for 37–38 weeks if delivery has not spontaneously occurred, with monochorionic diamniotic pregnancies a week earlier (58). With higher orders of multiples, vaginal birth and induction of labour are safe options in the presence of an appropriately skilled provider and with an uncomplicated cephalic-presenting first fetus (59).

Methods of induction are the same as for singleton pregnancies. Prior low-transverse caesarean delivery is not on its own a contraindication to vaginal birth or induction in a multifetal gestation (60).

Failed induction

Induction of labour is performed with the goal of achieving a vaginal delivery. There is currently no consensus on the definition of a failed induction, but generally if a patient cannot be put into labour in the time period defined by the clinician as reasonable, this is considered a failed induction. In around 15% of women it is not possible to perform ARM even after cervical ripening with two doses of a prostaglandin (8). Management options at this point depend upon the urgency and indication for delivery. If a patient is of low risk and there is no medical urgency for delivery, medication can be resumed after a 24–48-hour hiatus. If the clinical scenario is more urgent, alternative induction methods or a caesarean section may be indicated (8).

Induction in settings with few resources

Induction indications in low-resource settings are similar to those in high-resource settings. However, due to the lack of technology in prenatal care, there are typically fewer inductions for fetal indications. Without readily available ultrasonography, for example, fewer cases of IUGR are diagnosed. Additionally, with limited resources for monitoring of the fetus or oxytocin infusion rates, induction is more hazardous for mother and baby. As a result, the threshold for induction is raised. When the level of acuity is high and the resources are limited each induction is a risk for everyone involved. In these settings the stillbirth rate may be doubled and the need for neonatal resuscitation is increased. The reasons for such a high rate of stillbirth are multifactorial and probably due to the lack of prenatal diagnostics, limited resources with very limited patient access, and low levels of health literacy.

The World Health Organization has published guidelines on induction of labour in low-resource settings (61). The evidence is similar to that provided previously, and they suggest a choice of oral misoprostol, Foley catheter plus oxytocin, or dinoprostone plus oxytocin depending on the local situations. The Foley catheter has the benefit of low cost and low rates of hyperstimulation, but requires a skilled practitioner for insertion and usually requires an oxytocin infusion. Oral misoprostol is a highly effective method of induction and has probably the best outcomes of any method irrespective of setting. Misoprostol solution or tablets can be given as 25 mcg 2-hourly. It is not commonly available in tablet form and so usually needs to be made up in solution (a detailed explanation is available at http://www.misoprostol.org). It has the added advantages of being low cost, requiring no infusion apparatus, and can be continued at low dose (typically 5–20 mcg/hour) throughout labour in place of oxytocin (62). A recent randomized trial in hypertensive women in an Indian government hospital found that oral misoprostol was more clinically effective and more cost-effective than the Foley catheter (32). Both methods were followed by an oxytocin infusion under gravity control and the fetus was monitored using intermittent auscultation.

REFERENCES

1. Donald I. *Practical Obstetric Problems*. London: Lloyd-Luke Ltd; 1955.
2. Baskett TF, Calder AA, Arulkumaran S. *Munro Kerr's Operative Obstetrics*, 11th edn. Edinburgh: Saunders; 2007.
3. Barnes R. *Obstetric Operations, Including the Treatment of Hemorrhage. Review of Methods*. New York: Appleton and Co; 1861.
4. Nabi HA, Aflaifel NB, Weeks AD. A hundred years of induction of labour methods. *Eur J Obstet Gynecol Reprod Biol* 2014;**179**:236–39.
5. Browne FJ. Antenatal care and maternal mortality. *Lancet* 1932;**2**:1–3.
6. Karim SMM, Hillier K, Trussell RR, Patel RC, Tamusange S. Induction of labour with prostaglandin E2. *J Obstet Gynaecol Br Commonw* 1970;**77**:200–204.
7. Wing DA, Farinelli CK. Abnormal labor and induction of labor. In: Gabbe SG (ed), *Obstetrics: Normal and Problem Pregnancies*, 6th edn, pp. 287–310. Philadelphia, PA: Saunders; 2012.
8. National Institute for Health and Care Excellence (NICE). *Inducing Labour*. Clinical guideline [CG70]. London: NICE; 2008.
9. Van Calseteren K, Hyens L, De Smet F, et al. Cancer during pregnancy: analysis of 215 patients emphasizing the obstetrical and the neonatal outcomes. *J Clin Oncol* 2009;**28**:683–89.
10. Parasnis H, Raje B, Hinduja IN. Relevance of plasma fibrinogen estimation in obstetric complications. *J Postgrad Med* 1992;**38**:183–85.
11. Yao R, Ananth CV, Park BY, Pereira L, Plante LA, Perinatal Research Consortium. Obesity and the risk of stillbirth: a population-based cohort study. *Am J Obstet Gynecol* 2014;**210**:457.e1–9.
12. Bahtiyar MO, Funai EF, Rosenberg V, et al. Stillbirth at term in women of advanced maternal age in the United States: when could the antenatal testing be initiated? *Am J Perinatol* 2008;**25**:301–304.
13. Walker KF, Bugg GJ, Macpherson M, et al. Randomized trial of labor induction in women 35 years of age or older. *N Engl J Med* 2016;**374**:813–22.
14. Walker KF, Malin G, Wilson P, Thornton JG. Induction of labour versus expectant management at term by subgroups of maternal age: an individual patient data meta-analysis. *Eur J Obstet Gynecol Reprod Biol* 2016;**197**:1–5.
15. Bond DM, Gordon A, Hyett J, de Vries B, Carberry AE, Morris J. Planned early delivery versus expectant management of the term suspected compromised baby for improving outcomes. *Cochrane Database Syst Rev* 2015;**11**:CD009433.
16. Van der Ham DP, Vijgen SM, Nijhuis JG, et al. Induction of labor versus expectant management in women with preterm prelabor rupture of membranes between 34 and 37 weeks: a randomized controlled trial. *PLoS Med* 2012;**9**:e1001208.
17. Ehsanipoor R. Premature rupture of membranes. ACOG Practice Bulletin Number 160, January 2016. *Obstet Gynecol* 2016;**127**:e39–51.
18. Galan H, Grobman W. Fetal growth restriction. ACOG Practice Bulletin Number 134, May 2013, reaffirmed 2015. *Obstet Gynecol* 2013;**121**:1122–33.
19. Zhang X, Decker A, Platt RW, Kramer MS. How big is too big? The perinatal consequences of fetal macrosomia. *Am J Obstet Gynecol* 2008;**198**:517.e1–6.
20. Boulvain M, Senat MV, Perrotin F, et al. Induction of labour versus expectant management for large-for-date fetuses: a randomised controlled trial. *Lancet* 2015;**385**:2600–605.

21. Smith GC. Life-table analysis of the risk of perinatal death at term and post term in singleton pregnancies. *Am J Obstet Gynecol* 2001;**184**:489–96.

22. Bowman JM. Maternal alloimmunization and fetal hemolytic disease. In: Reece EA, Hobbins JC (eds), *Medicine of the Fetus and Mother*, 2nd edn, pp. 1241–69. Philadelphia, PA: Lippincott-Raven Publishers; 1999.

23. McKenna DS, Nagaraja HN, O'Shaughnessy R. Management of pregnancies complicated by anti-Kell isoimmunization. *Obstet Gynecol* 1999;**93**:667–73.

24. Ramirez M, Ramin S. Induction of labor. ACOG Practice Bulletin 107, August 2009. *Obstet Gynecol* 2009;**114**:386–97.

25. Vogel JP, Gulmezoglu AM, Hofmeyr GJ, Temmerman M. Global perspectives on elective induction of labor. *Clin Obstet Gynecol* 2014;**57**:331–42.

26. Stock SJ, Ferguson E, Duffy A, Ford I, Chalmers J, Norman JE. Outcomes of elective induction of labour compared with expectant management: population based study. *BMJ* 2012;**344**:e2838.

27. Grobman WA, Rice MM, Reddy UM, Tita ATN, Silver RM, Mallett G, et al. Labor Induction versus Expectant Management in Low-Risk Nulliparous Women *N Engl J Med*. 2018 Aug 9;**379**(6): 513–23.

28. Biem SR, Turnell RW, Olantunbosun A. Randomized controlled trial of outpatient versus inpatient labour induction with vaginal controlled release prostaglandin-E2: effectiveness and satisfaction. *J Obstet Gynaecol Can* 2003;**25**:23–31.

29. Wilkinson C, Adelson P, Turnbull D. A comparison of inpatient with outpatient balloon catheter cervical ripening: a pilot randomized controlled trial. *BMC Pregnancy Childbirth* 2015;**15**:126.

30. Cunningham FG, Leveno KJ, Bloom SL, et al. *Williams Obstetrics*, 24th edn. New York: McGraw Hill Education.

31. Egarter CH, Husslein PW, Rayburn WF. Uterine hyperstimulation after low-dose prostaglandin E2 therapy: tocolytic treatment in 181 cases. *Am J Obstet Gynecol* 1990;**163**:794–96.

32. Mundle S, Bracken H, Khedikar V, Mulik J, Faragher B, Easterling T, et al. Foley catheterisation versus oral misoprostol for induction of labour in hypertensive women in India (INFORM): a multicentre, open-label, randomised controlled trial. *Lancet*. 2017 Aug 12;**390**(10095):669–80.

33. Ten Eikelder ML, Oude Rengerink K, Jozwiak M, et al. Induction of labour at term with oral misoprostol versus a Foley catheter (PROBAAT-II): a multicentre randomised controlled non-inferiority trial. *Lancet* 2016;**387**:1619–28.

34. Rab MT, Mohammed AB, Zahran KA, et al. Transcervical Foley's catheter versus Cook balloon for cervical ripening in stillbirth with a scarred uterus: a randomized controlled trial. *J Matern Fetal Neonatal Med* 2015;**28**:1181–85.

35. Hoppe KK, Schiff MA, Peterson SE, Gravett MG. 30 mL single-versus 80 mL double-balloon catheter for pre-induction cervical ripening: a randomized controlled trial. *J Matern Fetal Neonatal Med* 2016;**29**:1919–25.

36. Mei-Dan E, Walfisch A, Suarez-Easton S, et al. Comparison of two mechanical devices for cervical ripening: a prospective quasi-randomized trial. *J Matern Fetal Neonatal Med* 2012;**25**:723–27.

37. McMaster K, Sanchez-Ramos L, Kaunitz AM. Evaluation of a transcervical Foley catheter as a source of infection: a systematic review and meta-analysis. *Obstet Gynecol* 2015;**126**:539–51.

38. Jozwiak M, Bloemenkamp KWM, Kelly AJ, Mol BWJ, Irion O, Boulvain M. Mechanical methods for induction of labour. *Cochrane Database Syst Rev* 2012;**3**:CD001233.

39. Thomas J, Fairclough A, Kavanagh J, Kelly AJ. Vaginal prostaglandin (PGE2 and PGF2a) for induction of labour at term. *Cochrane Database Syst Rev* 2014;**6**:CD003101.

40. Weeks AD, Navaratnam K, Alfirevic Z. Simplifying oral misoprostol protocols for the induction of labour. *BJOG* 2017 Oct;**124**(11):1642–45.

41. Alfirevic Z, Kelly AJ, Dowswell T. Intravenous oxytocin alone for cervical ripening and induction of labour. *Cochrane Database Syst Rev* 2009;**4**:CD003246.

42. Hannah ME, Ohlsson A, Farine D, et al. Induction of labor compared with expectant management for prelabor rupture of membranes. *N Engl J Med* 1996;**334**:1005–10.

43. Creinin M, Grossman DA. Medical management of first trimester abortion. ACOG Practice Bulletin Number 143, March 2014. *Obstet Gynecol* 2014;**123**:676–92.

44. Steinauer J, Jackson A, Grossman D. Second trimester abortion. ACOG Practice Bulletin Number 135, June 2013, Reaffirmed 2015. *Obstet Gynecol* 2013;**121**:1394–406.

45. Osman I, MacKenzie F, Norrie J, Murray HM, Greer IA, Norman JE. The 'PRIM' study: a randomized comparison of prostaglandin E2 gel with the nitric oxide donor isosorbide mononitrate for cervical ripening before the induction of labor at term. *Am J Obstet Gynecol* 2006;**194**:1012–21.

46. Chen W, Xue J, Peprah MK, et al. A systematic review and network meta-analysis comparing the use of Foley catheters, misoprostol, and dinoprostone for cervical ripening in the induction of labour. *BJOG* 2016;**123**:346–54.

47. Alfirevic Z, Keeney E, Dowswell T, et al. Labour induction with prostaglandins: a systematic review and network meta-analysis. *BMJ* 2015;**350**:h217.

48. Wing DA, Brown R, Plante LA, Miller H, Rugarn O, Powers BL. Misoprostol vaginal insert and time to vaginal delivery: a randomized controlled trial. *Obstet Gynecol* 2013;**122**:201–209.

49. Lydon-Rochelle M, Holt VL, Easterling TR, Martin DP. Risk of uterine rupture during labor among women with a prior cesarean delivery. *N Engl J Med* 2001;**345**:3–8.

50. Smith GC. Factors predisposing to perinatal death related to uterine rupture during attempted vaginal birth after cesarean section: retrospective cohort study. *BMJ* 2004;**329**:75.

51. Royal College of Obstetricians and Gynaecologists (RCOG). *Birth after Previous Caesarean Section*. Green-top Guideline No. 45. London: RCOG; 2015.

52. Dodd, JM, Crowther CA, Grivell RM, Deussen AR. Elective repeat caesarean section versus induction of labour for women with a previous caesarean birth. *Cochrane Database Syst Rev* 2014;**12**:CD004906.

53. Cousens S, Blencowe H, Stanton C, et al. National, regional, and worldwide estimates of stillbirth rates in 2009 with trends since 1995: a systematic analysis. *Lancet* 2011;**377**:1319–30.

54. Fretts R. Management of stillbirth. ACOG Practice Bulletin Number 102, 2009, Reaffirmed 2014. *Obstet Gynecol* 2009;**113**:748–61.

55. Royal College of Obstetricians and Gynaecologists (RCOG). *Late Intrauterine Fetal Death and Stillbirth*. Green-top Guideline No. 55. London: RCOG; 2010.

56. Gómez Ponce de León R, Wing D, Fiala C. Misoprostol for intrauterine fetal death. *Int J Gynecol Obstet* 2007;**99** Suppl 2:S190–93.

57. McMaster K, Sanchez-Ramos L, Kaunitz AM. Evaluation of a transcervical Foley catheter as a source of infection: a systematic review and meta-analysis. *Obstet Gynecol* 2015;**126**:539–51.

58. Hayes EJ, SMFM. Multifetal gestations: twin, triplet, and higher-order multifetal pregnancies. ACOG Practice Bulletin Number 144, May 2014. *Obstet Gynecol* 2014;**123**:1118–32.

59. Grobman WA, Peaceman AM, Haney EI, Silver RK, MacGregor SN. Neonatal outcomes in triplet gestations after a trial of labor. *Am J Obstet Gynecol* 1998;**179**:942–45.

60. Sansregret A, Bujold E, Gauthier RJ. Twin delivery after a previous caesarean: a twelve-year experience. *J Obstet Gynaecol Can* 2003;**25**:294–98.

61. World Health Organization (WHO). *WHO Recommendations for Induction of Labour*. Geneva: WHO; 2011.

62. Kundodyiwa T, Alfirevic Z, Weeks A. Low dose oral misoprostol for induction of labor: a systematic review. *Obstet Gynecol* 2009;**113**:374–83.

Neonatal Care and Neonatal Problems

37

Neonatal care and neonatal problems

Vimal Vasu and Neena Modi

Introduction

Neonatal medicine has advanced considerably in the last four decades. In the United Kingdom, neonatal mortality (Table 37.1) has fallen from 6.3 per 1000 live births in 1982 to 2.7 per 1000 live births in 2014, a reduction of approximately 60% (1). However significant global challenges remain. In 2015, neonatal deaths accounted for 45% of all deaths in children under 5 years, of which 80% were related to preterm birth, infection, or perinatal asphyxia (2). Neonatal medicine continues to evolve rapidly; by the time this textbook is published, many currently accepted wisdoms may have altered. This is of course the nature of medicine, as with hypothesis testing, never seeking absolute truth, but only ever decreasing uncertainty. This chapter will help practitioners anticipate problems, understand the basic principles of newborn care, recognize common newborn problems, and understand the importance of improving newborn services. In doing so, there is emphasis on the importance of (a) having a clear understanding of basic principles that will stand the practitioner in good stead whatever the circumstances, (b) continually questioning accepted wisdoms, and (c) implementing best practice and evaluating outcomes.

Anticipating problems

There are a number of pointers that indicate increased risk to the fetus and newborn. A careful history is key, including maternal obstetric, medical, and family history, medications, antenatal screening tests and sonography, pattern of fetal growth, intrapartum progress, and mode of delivery. Early communication with the neonatal team, well in advance of delivery, is good practice and can help ensure a robust postnatal plan of management is formulated for the newborn. In many cases, the obstetrician is faced with the complex task of balancing maternal benefit and fetal risk. A common example is the timing of delivery in pre-eclampsia where maternal risks must be balanced against the risks to the neonate of preterm delivery. Current evidence helps inform such debate with data from the recent HYPITAT-II trial (3) indicating a more than threefold increase in neonatal respiratory distress syndrome in moderately preterm infants between 34 and 37 weeks' gestation, born to mothers with non-severe hypertensive disorders of pregnancy, randomized to immediate delivery as opposed to expectant management (relative risk (RR) 3.3; 95% confidence interval (CI) 1.4–8.2; $P = 0.005$). The key principles of management, whatever the obstetric condition or concern, are multidisciplinary discussion, shared decision-making, and careful documentation of the rationale for decisions, especially in situations where evidence to guide practice is uncertain.

Preterm birth

The global problem

One in ten babies are born preterm (4) (Table 37.2) with the preterm birth rate continuing to rise globally, especially in low-income countries (5). Currently over 60% of preterm births are in the low-resource, low-income countries of southern Asia and sub-Saharan Africa (5). Though mortality has fallen, there is growing recognition of the increased risk of lifelong morbidity in survivors. In addition to well-recognized respiratory and neurodevelopmental morbidity, a growing research literature points to the adverse impact of preterm birth on cardiometabolic health, longevity, and reproductive outcomes. The prevention and management of preterm birth is thus an important population health issue.

Managing preterm birth from the neonatal perspective

The unexpected birth of a preterm infant is not uncommon, indicating the importance of ensuring that every birth facility has expertise in the basic principles of care. When preterm birth is anticipated, every attempt should be made to transfer the mother to a facility that is able to provide appropriate care for both the mother and her newborn infant. There is growing evidence that care in a high-volume facility improves survival for preterm infants at less than 33 weeks' gestation, an effect that is magnified for extremely preterm infants (<28 weeks' gestation) (6). This, along with the increased risks of postnatal transfer for the preterm infant (7), means that *in utero* transfer of mother and fetus is recommended wherever possible.

Parents must be counselled about problems in the event of preterm birth. Though this advice will vary depending on the gestation of the fetus and other factors (e.g. multiple pregnancy, fetal sex, growth restriction, and congenital anomalies), counselling should ideally be a joint discussion with both neonatal and obstetric personnel. Where possible, information should be provided on more than one occasion verbally, and in writing. It is important that the

Table 37.1 Definition of perinatal, neonatal, postneonatal, and infant mortality

Mortality indicator	Definition
Stillbirth	A baby born after 24 or more weeks completed gestation and who did not, at any time, breathe or show signs of life
Perinatal mortality	Stillbirths and deaths less than 7 days of age per 1000 total births
Neonatal mortality	Deaths under 28 days of age per 1000 live births
Post neonatal mortality	Deaths between 28 days of age and 1 year of age per 1000 live births
Infant mortality	Deaths under 1 year per 1000 live births

information is provided in a clear, consistent, and empathetic way and that decision-making, especially at the limits of gestational viability, genuinely reflects parental views. An opportunity should be provided for the family to visit the neonatal unit.

Preterm health outcomes

Several large population data sets exist such as the EPICURE (8), EXPRESS (9), and EPIPAGE (10) studies and such data can be helpful in providing information about health outcomes to families. Local data on preterm outcomes may also be available but should be used with caution because of the small numbers of extremely preterm infants in any given hospital. In the United Kingdom, the EPICURE 2 cohort provides short- and long-term population-based health outcomes for preterm infants between 22 and 26 weeks' gestation born in 2006 (8). In this cohort comprising preterm infants less than 26 weeks' gestation, 68% developed bronchopulmonary dysplasia (defined as the need for supplemental oxygen at 36 weeks postmenstrual age), 13% had evidence of serious abnormality on cranial sonography, and 16% required laser therapy for treatment of retinopathy of prematurity. Rates of severe impairment at 2–3 years of age were 26% for children born at 22–23 weeks' gestation, 15% at 24 weeks, 14% at 25 weeks, and 10% at 26 weeks. Though population data cannot necessarily be applied to an individual pregnancy, they are nonetheless useful when used in conjunction with a sensitive discussion about pregnancy management options and foreseeable problems for the newborn infant.

Antenatal interventions of benefit to the preterm infant

Antenatal steroids

In the 1960s and 1970s, studies in fetal lambs by Liggins and Howe demonstrated the importance of cortisol in fetal lung maturation

(11). This paved the way for human randomized controlled trials in high-income countries that unequivocally demonstrated the benefit of antenatal corticosteroid administration in reducing neonatal morbidity and mortality (a reduction in respiratory distress syndrome of 34% and a reduction in mortality by 31%) (12). Over the years, further beneficial effects were established including a reduction in necrotizing enterocolitis, periventricular haemorrhage, and infection. However, it was only by the late 1990s that antenatal corticosteroids were established as a standard of care (13).

Based on this evidence, the use of antenatal steroids in threatened preterm delivery has been recommended worldwide. However, recent research raises doubts about its generalizability to low-income countries. A cluster-randomized trial of antenatal steroids versus standard practice in six low-income countries identified no reduction, and a possible increase in neonatal mortality in the treatment arm (RR 1.12; 1.02–1.22; $P = 0.013$) and an excess of maternal infection (odds ratio (OR) 1.45; 1.33–1.58; $P <0.0001$) (14). The long-term effect of antenatal steroid exposure, particularly in relation to multiple doses, also remains an ongoing area of uncertainty (15). The story of antenatal corticosteroids illustrates first the difficulties of translating research into practice; second, the importance of testing interventions in the settings in which they will be used; and third, the difficulties in evaluating the long-term impacts of perinatal interventions.

Cervical length and fetal fibronectin

Antenatal strategies that might enable better prediction of imminent preterm birth are increasing, especially in women who have a history of previous preterm birth. Measurement of cervical length using transvaginal ultrasound with a cut-off value of less than 25 mm in pregnancies between 16^{+0} and 34^{+0} weeks enables consideration of prophylactic interventions (16). Both cervical length and fetal fibronectin measurement are currently considered effective methods for assessing the risk of preterm birth in women with signs of preterm labour, particularly when used in combination (17). Such strategies are important as they enable practitioners to better deploy treatment and management strategies, for example, whether or not to administer antenatal corticosteroids and whether or not to initiate an *in utero* transfer.

Magnesium sulphate

Meta-analysis data indicate that maternal magnesium sulphate administration is neuroprotective to the newborn preterm infant and reduces the risk of cerebral palsy by approximately 30% (18). However evidence of longer-term benefit in respect of childhood educational attainment and motor and cognitive performance remains weak (19).

Intrauterine growth restriction

Fetuses that show growth faltering are at increased risk of perinatal death and neonatal morbidity but optimal criteria for identification are unclear. Clinical assessment has poor sensitivity and the use of ultrasound scanning is now widespread with fetal parameters plotted onto population, intrauterine growth, or customized references. The use of different reference systems leads to confusion for clinical staff and patients. Customization involves adjusting fetal weight for maternal height, weight, parity, and ethnic group on the assumption that a small baby born to a small mother is less likely

Table 37.2 Definitions of extremely, very, moderate and late preterm birth

Preterm birth <37 weeks' gestation	Extremely preterm birth	<28 completed weeks' gestation
	Very preterm birth	$28–31^{+6}$ completed weeks' gestation
	Moderate preterm birth	$32–33^{+6}$ completed weeks' gestation
	Late preterm birth	$34–36^{+6}$ completed weeks' gestation

to be abnormally small than a similar size baby born to a bigger woman. However, a small mother may be small because her own growth was constrained and not because she is constitutionally small. If so, she may be pathologically constraining the growth of her own fetus, hence adjusting for her size would 'normalize' the abnormally small baby, and risks identifying small babies at risk of perinatal death less well than an unadjusted reference. Adding to the confusion is the unhelpful conflation of the term 'small for gestational age' with 'intrauterine growth restriction'. The former is a statistical definition that will apply to 10% of a normal population; the latter also refers to babies who remain above the tenth centile but whose growth is faltering. The widely used Hadlock fetal growth curves were constructed 25 years ago with data from less than 400 'predominantly middle-class white patients' (20) and their effectiveness in identifying at-risk infants in populations around the world is uncertain. The World Health Organization postnatal growth charts developed from longitudinal measurements in infancy show healthy babies across diverse countries that include India, Brazil, and the United States, to have a similar pattern of growth (21). This suggests that all human fetuses, if not constrained by maternal factors, might also exhibit a similar growth pattern. Charts based upon measurements from women around the world have been developed but until maternal health and maternal size are optimal, and until the fetal growth pattern resulting in optimal lifelong health has been identified, these should be considered as a reference, rather than a standard (22). For the moment, a reasonable approach to selecting a reference would be to base this on the sensitivity and specificity for detecting cases of perinatal mortality and morbidity in specific populations.

Caesarean section

Birth by caesarean section is increasing in many parts of the world. Factors suggested as underpinning this trend include maternal choice, social expectation, rise in maternal obesity, a rise in age at first pregnancy (with accompanying comorbidities), and an increased number of mothers with a previous history of caesarean section. Other factors, set against the increased safety of caesarean section as a procedure, include medicolegal concerns, defensive medicine, and the financial incentives of private practice. There are clearly situations where caesarean section is life-saving for either the mother or the fetus, or both, yet paradoxically the procedure is insufficiently available in many parts of the world where both maternal and neonatal morbidity are highest (23).

The short-term neonatal morbidities associated with birth by caesarean section (Box 37.1) are well recognized. To some extent these can be mitigated by the administration of antenatal steroids for elective caesarean section before 38^{+6} weeks' gestation (24). It is perhaps less well known that birth by caesarean section is associated with lower breastfeeding initiation (25). Further, the practising obstetrician needs to also be aware of the emerging evidence relating to possible longer-term health implications of birth by caesarean section (26). Epidemiological studies point to an association between birth by caesarean section and increased body mass index z-score in childhood (0.20 units; 0.07–0.33 increase) (27), diabetes (OR 1.23; 95% CI 1.15–1.32) (28), and childhood asthma (OR 1.20; 95% CI 1.14–1.26) (29). Mechanistic studies are rare and causality has not been established. However, plausible determinant pathways include alterations in the infant microbiome that drive increased intestinal energy harvesting, and epigenetic effects induced by exposure to the inflammatory and endocrine milieu of labour on metabolic and/or immune development.

Multiple births

There has been a fourfold increase between 1992 and 2006 in artificial reproductive technology (ART) such as *in vitro* fertilization (IVF) and intracytoplasmic sperm injection treatment in the United Kingdom (30). This is attributed, at least in part to increased availability, access, and affordability of ART to patients. In addition, the range of ART available has increased to include preimplantation genetic diagnosis and oocyte cryopreservation. Babies born by ART have a significant impact upon neonatal services because of the increased risk of preterm birth, which in turn is associated with a fivefold higher neonatal mortality when compared to singleton pregnancies (11.5 vs 2.4:1000 live births) (31). ART has a major impact upon the numbers of preterm births, and is a growing strain upon neonatal services, especially in countries that have poor regulatory oversight of such practices. In addition, though causality has not been established, there is concern regarding the association between ART and congenital anomalies, epilepsy, genomic imprinting disorders, and an observed fourfold increase in cerebral palsy (32). In the United Kingdom, the Human Fertilisation and Embryology Authority (HFEA) has provided guidance to clinicians and prospective families and requires centres to have clear strategies to reduce multiple births by defining criteria for the use of single embryo transfer. From 2008 to 2010 there has been an increase in the proportion of single embryo transfer IVF pregnancies from 4.8% to 14.7% and a parallel reduction in the proportion of multiple pregnancies from IVF (from 26.7% to 22.0%) (33). HFEA regulation and codes of practice remain an important strategy to ensure that multiple birth-related preterm morbidity and potential adverse health outcomes for the child are mitigated. There is also an increasing call for the health outcomes of children born by newer types of ART to be monitored through the establishment of formal registries.

Congenital anomalies

Congenital anomalies account for approximately 27% of all neonatal deaths in England and Wales (34) and approximately 4.4% of neonatal deaths globally (276,000 neonatal deaths were attributed to congenital anomalies in 2013) (35). Congenital anomaly registers (e.g. National Congenital Anomaly and Rare Disease Registration Service (NCARDRS), British Isles Network of Congenital anomalies register (BINOCAR), European Surveillance of Congenital Anomalies (EUROCAT)) are important means of detecting the prevalence of congenital anomalies, monitoring trends over time and the impact of interventions. United Kingdom data indicate a decline in congenital anomalies between 2007 and 2011 from 264.7

Box 37.1 Short-term newborn health effects related to birth by caesarean section

- Increased rate of neonatal unit admission
- Increased respiratory morbidity
- Impaired thermal adaptation
- Impaired metabolic adaptation (e.g. hypoglycaemia)
- Reduced initiation of breastfeeding

to 249.5 per 10,000 total births (36). Congenital anomalies are important, as though rare individually, as a group they are relatively common. They are also associated with significant long-term disabilities and have considerable impacts upon the affected individual and the family. Maternal risk factors include low socioeconomic status, consanguinity, maternal age, antenatal infections (e.g. syphilis, rubella), diabetes, tobacco, alcohol, illicit drug use, iodine deficiency, and folic acid deficiency. However, antenatal detection rates are anomaly specific (36, 37) as illustrated in **Table 37.3**. Hence, all newborn infants should receive a thorough physical examination following birth. This is particularly so for the detection of serious forms of congenital heart disease where lack of detection (either antenatally or postnatally) can be life-threatening and associated with increased morbidity. Though antenatal detection rates of congenital heart disease are improving (38), the combination of antenatal screening for congenital heart disease and postnatal clinical examination still misses approximately 50% of cases (39). Therefore, to improve detection of these conditions, many countries now recommend universal oxygen saturation screening for all newborns as a moderately sensitive (75%), highly specific (99.9%), cost-effective method in parallel with antenatal sonography and clinical examination (40). This involves applying a pulse oximeter probe to all newborn infants (usually between 4 and 24 hours after birth). A positive test is defined as an oxygen saturation of less than 95% in either pre- or postductal oxygen saturation or a greater than 2% difference between pre- and postductal oxygen saturations. Newborns with a positive test can then undergo further evaluation to establish the cause of their hypoxia. The test has extended utility in that in addition to the detection of asymptomatic congenital heart disease, newborn infants with other pathologies that might require neonatal intervention (e.g. sepsis, meconium aspiration syndrome) may also be identified.

When congenital anomalies are detected in the antenatal period, the clinical team is able to discuss management options with the parents in advance of birth. It is good practice to involve neonatologists (and other relevant specialities, e.g. geneticists) in counselling. This enables decisions to be made about continuation of pregnancy versus termination, helps the family to come to terms with the diagnosis and be provided with relevant information about the condition, and to plan the timing and location of the delivery (e.g. in a centre with surgical neonatal expertise).

Basic principles of newborn care

Healthy babies need only simple measures to promote the natural process of transition from fetal to postnatal life. Following birth, all babies should undergo a rapid assessment of their well-being and need for resuscitation. Other basic principles encompass thermoregulation, cleanliness, breastfeeding, and ability to recognize the sick and at-risk newborn baby.

Cord clamping

The optimal timing of cord clamping (early vs late) continues to fuel considerable debate. Precise definitions of what constitutes early and delayed cord clamping are also uncertain in both routine clinical practice and in the literature. Recent systematic review data indicate no differences in maternal outcomes (maternal death, maternal morbidity, or postpartum haemorrhage). Potential benefits for term-born infants include increased haemoglobin in the first 24–48 hours (mean difference 1.49 g/dL; 95% CI 1.21–1.78 g/dL) and a lower incidence of iron deficiency anaemia (RR 2.65 for the delayed cord clamping groups). No significant differences have been identified between the groups with respect to neonatal mortality (RR 0.37; 95% CI 0.04–3.41) or neonatal unit admission. There is, however, an increased requirement for phototherapy in the late cord clamping groups (RR 1.62; 95% CI 1.41–1.96) (41). This latter consequence is of particular relevance in settings where the incidence of neonatal jaundice is high, and phototherapy may not be readily available. In preterm infants, systematic review data indicate a reduction in anaemia (RR 0.61; 95% CI 0.46–0.81), periventricular haemorrhage (RR 0.59; 95% CI 0.41–0.85) and necrotizing enterocolitis (RR 0.62; 95% CI 0.43–0.90) (42). Other short-term benefits include improved urine output, reduction in hypotension, and improved cardiac function (43). There are limited data on the long-term effects of differing cord clamping regimens but follow-up data from a Swedish randomized controlled trial show delayed cord clamping to be beneficial to fine motor and social skills at 4 years of age (44). Given the available evidence, and to date, the absence of harm, it is reasonable to wait for least a minute before clamping the cord if the baby appears vigorous after delivery. For babies that are in need of newborn resuscitation, the results of considerable ongoing research effort will provide greater insight into the possible benefits of resuscitation prior to cord clamping.

Birth into a clean environment

Newborn infection is one of a triad of problems (with birth asphyxia and prematurity) that are the principal contributors to global neonatal mortality (45). Newborn infection has a high case fatality rate and is thought to account for approximately one-third of neonatal deaths (46). Neonatal sepsis usually presents with non-specific clinical signs (**Table 37.4**) (47) and can

Table 37.3 Antenatal detection rates for selected congenital anomalies

Anomaly	Antenatal detection rate (%)
Anencephaly	96.9
Neural tube defects	95
Cardiac anomalies	35–49.2
Cleft lip ± palate	65–74.5
Congenital diaphragmatic hernia	64–73
Bilateral renal agenesis	89.3
Lethal skeletal dysplasia	94.4
Gastroschisis	91.7–100
Exomphalos	90–92.3
Chromosomal Edward syndrome Patau syndrome	56 76.6 82.7

Source data from Springett A, Budd J, Draper ES, Kurinczuk JJ, Medina J, Rankin J, Rounding C, Tucker D, Wellesley D, Wreyford B, Morris JK. *Congenital Anomaly Statistics 2012: England and Wales.* London: British Isles Network of Congenital Anomaly Registers; 2014 and Kurinczuk JJ, Hollowell J, Boyd PA, Oakley L, Brocklehurst P, Gray R. *The Inequalities in Infant Mortality Project Briefing Paper 4: The Contribution of Congenital Anomalies to Infant Mortality.* National Perinatal Epidemiology Unit, University of Oxford (June 2010).

Table 37.4 Potential indicators of neonatal sepsis

Potential indicators of neonatal sepsis	Comments
Altered behaviour/reduced responsiveness	Healthy term newborn babies should wake for feeds
Feeding difficulties	Lack of interest in breast- or bottle-feeding especially when combined with other signs listed may be a cause for concern
Abnormal heart rate	Tachycardia: heart rate >160 beats per minute Bradycardia: heart rate >60 beats per minute (this may be normal in a sleeping term baby)
Signs of respiratory distress	Tachypnoea, grunting, intercostal recession, subcostal recession, nasal flaring, head bobbing, cyanosis
Seizures	This should prompt investigations and treatment for neonatal central nervous system infection
Temperature instability	Hypothermia: <36°C Hyperthermia: >38°C
Signs of shock	Capillary refill time >3 seconds, poor urine output, metabolic acidosis
Glucose instability	Healthy term infants have a physiological drop in blood glucose following birth and should not have routine measurement of their blood glucose. However, if a newborn is noted to be hypoglycaemic, this may be a sign of sepsis
Jaundice within 24 hours of birth	Jaundice within the first 24 hours of life should always be considered pathological
Evidence of local infection (e.g. skin/eye)	Purulent conjunctivitis/eyelid swelling in the first 24 hours should prompt consideration of a diagnosis of *Neisseria gonorrhoeae* conjunctivitis

Source data from National Institute of Health and Care Excellence (NICE). *Neonatal Infection (Early Onset): Antibiotics for Prevention and Treatment.* Clinical guideline [CG149]. https://www.nice.org.uk/guidance/CG149 (accessed 15 July 2016).

be difficult to treat, especially in low-resource settings where antimicrobials may not be readily available and where antimicrobial resistance is a growing and serious problem. Careful attention should be paid to simple and inexpensive preventive measures, chief among which are scrupulous hand and umbilical cord hygiene. Practitioners should wash their hands or use alcohol hand gels, and utilize the World Health Organization (WHO) 'My five moments of hand hygiene' tool (48). The umbilical cord should be cut with a sterile instrument and then either clamped with a clean device or tied with clean material and allowed to dry and separate naturally by exposure to air. The cord should be kept clean with sterile water until separation occurs. In parts of the world with high rates of newborn infection, current WHO guidance is to recommend 'dry' cord care, though use of topical antiseptics (e.g. chlorhexidine) may also be considered (49). Recent systematic review evidence supports the practice of 'dry' cord care in the hospital setting but also suggests topical antiseptic application of 4% chlorhexidine may be of benefit in home births in low-resource settings (50, 51). Implementation of these simple but highly effective practices requires strong leadership, regular audit of compliance by all healthcare professionals, and access to clean water, soap, and towels.

Resuscitation

All healthcare professional attending a birth should have basic training in newborn resuscitation. This advice extends to obstetric, midwifery, and anaesthetic staff as the need for newborn resuscitation is often unpredictable. Attendance at a recognized neonatal resuscitation training course along with regular multidisciplinary 'skill drills' to ensure ongoing competence is recommended best practice.

Resuscitation equipment should be checked at regular intervals. At birth, the baby should be assessed in accordance with country specific and local guidelines, an example of which is provided in **Figure 37.1** (52). The use of 100% oxygen in neonatal resuscitation of term babies was long considered best practice until research showing this resulted in a 30% increase in neonatal mortality in comparison with resuscitation with air (53). These clinical trials changed neonatal resuscitation guidelines around the world. Room air is now considered the optimal starting gas for the resuscitation of the term baby. Where required, oxygen use should be carefully titrated and ideally utilized with parallel monitoring of oxygen saturation levels to detect both hyperoxia and hypoxia. Though initially considered controversial, this has been accepted into standard practice.

Meconium-stained liquor

The aspiration of meconium into the lungs takes place before delivery and is usually associated with advanced gestational age. The passage of meconium in the preterm infant has historically been associated with maternal and/or congenital infection with *Listeria monocytogenes* but this is not borne out by retrospective case–control studies (54). There are good quality randomized clinical trial data demonstrating no evidence of benefit to the newborn from oropharyngeal suction of the airway prior to delivery of the shoulders (55) and routine intubation of the vigorous infant born through meconium (56), hence these practices are no longer recommended. If a baby born through meconium is not breathing and/or has a low heart rate, then inspection of the oropharynx under direct vision using a laryngoscope, with suctioning of any particulate matter obstructing the airway is recommended, following which resuscitation should proceed along usual lines as outlined in **Figure 37.1**. It is recommended that either a large-bore suction catheter or a meconium aspirator device is used if the newborn airway is thought obstructed with potentially thick particulate matter such as meconium, blood, amniotic fluid, or vernix. The newborn should then be observed (usually for 12–24 hours) according to a locally agreed policy to monitor for clinical signs of meconium aspiration syndrome, which usually presents with respiratory distress.

Thermoregulation

Newborn babies are born with wet skin and have a high surface area-to-weight ratio. They are susceptible to heat loss through the well-described mechanisms of evaporation, conduction, convection, and radiation and so can become hypothermic quickly if attention is not paid to thermoregulation. Every gram of water lost through evaporation results in 0.6 kcal of heat loss (57). Evaporative heat loss is magnified in preterm infants by virtue of their skin immaturity through transepidermal water loss and so these infants require even more attention to their early thermal environment. Hypothermia is associated with increased morbidity and mortality and so measures to actively prevent this are key components of good perinatal care (58). Thermoregulation requirements should be considered by obstetric

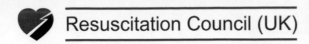

Resuscitation Council (UK) GUIDELINES 2015

Newborn Life Support

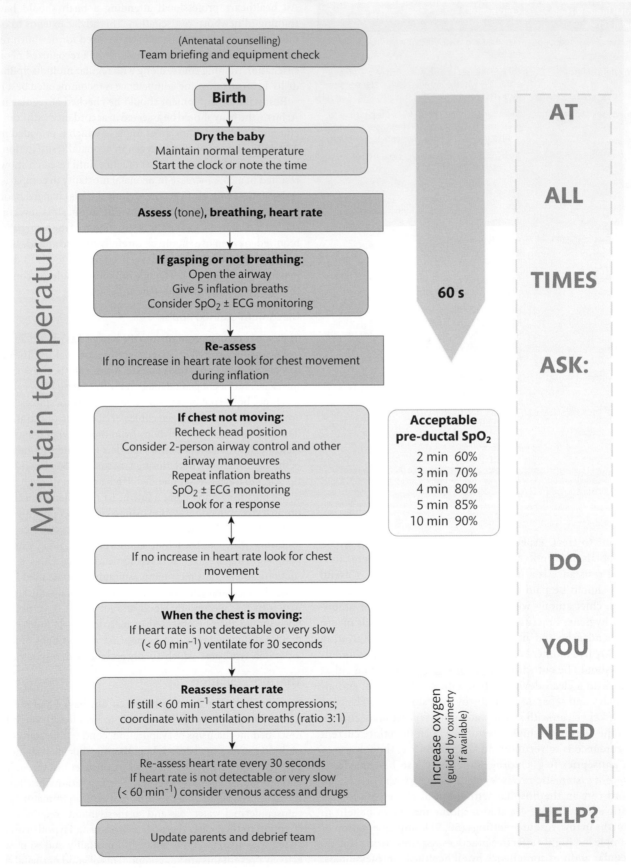

(Antenatal counselling)
Team briefing and equipment check

Birth

Dry the baby
Maintain normal temperature
Start the clock or note the time

Assess (tone)**, breathing, heart rate**

If gasping or not breathing:
Open the airway
Give 5 inflation breaths
Consider SpO_2 ± ECG monitoring

Re-assess
If no increase in heart rate look for chest movement
during inflation

If chest not moving:
Recheck head position
Consider 2-person airway control and other
airway manoeuvres
Repeat inflation breaths
SpO_2 ± ECG monitoring
Look for a response

If no increase in heart rate look for chest
movement

When the chest is moving:
If heart rate is not detectable or very slow
(< 60 min^{-1}) ventilate for 30 seconds

Reassess heart rate
If still < 60 min^{-1} start chest compressions;
coordinate with ventilation breaths (ratio 3:1)

Re-assess heart rate every 30 seconds
If heart rate is not detectable or very slow
(< 60 min^{-1}) consider venous access and drugs

Update parents and debrief team

Maintain temperature

60 s

**Acceptable
pre-ductal SpO_2**

2 min   60%
3 min   70%
4 min   80%
5 min   85%
10 min   90%

Increase oxygen
(guided by oximetry
if available)

AT

ALL

TIMES

ASK:

DO

YOU

NEED

HELP?

Figure 37.1 UK Resuscitation Council Newborn Life Support Guidance.
Reproduced with the kind permission of the Resuscitation Council (UK)
https://www.resus.org.uk/resuscitation-guidelines/.

teams prior to delivery in the same way as the need for neonatal team attendance at high-risk deliveries. The delivery environment (including theatre) should be warm (26°C is recommended), with windows closed and draughts prevented (59). Following birth, a healthy baby should be dried, placed prone on the bare chest of the mother for direct skin-to-skin contact (60) and covered with a warm towel. A hat should be placed on the baby's head as the head is a major source of heat loss in newborn infants. Assessment of well-being by the birth attendant can take place during skin-to-skin contact. If resuscitation is anticipated or required, the first step should be to dry the baby with a warm towel. Once dried, the baby should be wrapped in a fresh warm towel and a hat placed on the head. Preterm infants may also benefit from early skin-to-skin contact especially in low-income settings (61). Systematic review evidence supports the practice of delivery of preterm infants into a plastic bag without drying as a strategy to reduce hypothermia (21–46% reduction in hypothermia defined as a temperature <36.5°C). No effect on neonatal mortality has been observed though none of the included trials were powered to assess this outcome (62).

Breastfeeding

Globally, breastfeeding is the single most important public health intervention. Beneficial effects include, but are not limited to, a reduction in newborn infection and improved neurodevelopment (63). With appropriate consideration for maternal autonomy and choice, antenatal visits should be used as an opportunity to actively encourage later breastfeeding. This is especially important in the case of preterm birth as feeding with maternal milk is associated with better neurodevelopmental outcome (64) and a reduced incidence of necrotizing enterocolitis (65). Suckling at the breast should take place at the earliest opportunity in healthy infants, and consistent advice provided by perinatal healthcare professionals both before and after birth. Where breastfeeding is not initially possible, such as in the case of extremely or very preterm infants, early expression of colostrum and breast milk is recommended. This is provided immediately to the baby by the nasogastric, or orogastric route, or increasingly in small initial volumes as 'mouth washes'. Colostrum contains high concentrations of a wide range of bioactive molecules, prebiotic complex oligosaccharides, and probiotic species. Early administration offers protection against infection and promotes establishment of the newborn intestinal microbiome. In extremely preterm babies, milk feeds are usually initiated at small volumes (12–24 mL/kg/day) and incremented daily as tolerated.

Common newborn problems

Recognizing the range of normal variation, the pattern of postnatal adaptation, and signs that identify the sick newborn baby are important clinical skills. The majority of clinical signs are non-specific; for example, each of the signs listed in Table 37.4 may indicate infection hence examination must always be accompanied by a careful clinical history, supplemented as necessary by appropriate laboratory investigations and imaging (e.g. chest radiography).

Respiratory distress

Respiratory distress is important to recognize as it can be a sign of several different newborn pathologies including systemic infection, pneumonia, surfactant deficiency lung disease (respiratory distress syndrome), meconium aspiration syndrome, pulmonary air leak, congenital diaphragmatic hernia, and congenital heart disease. Signs of respiratory distress include tachypnoea (defined as a respiratory rate of >60 breaths per minute), intercostal recession, subcostal recession, grunting, nasal flaring, and head bobbing. Babies that display any of these clinical signs need an urgent medical assessment including measurement of oxygen saturation and continued regular observation of heart rate, respiratory status, and temperature. Treatment with intravenous antibiotics is usually indicated pending identification of the underlying cause.

Jaundice

Approximately 50–80% of healthy newborn infants will develop visible jaundice. In the majority of infants, jaundice is physiological, occurring due to an increased red cell mass, increased red cell turnover, and hepatic immaturity. Physiological jaundice tends to appear at around 2–3 days, peaks by 5 days, and resolves by 7–10 days of life. Jaundice should be considered pathological until proven otherwise if it is apparent early (within 24 hours of birth), is severe, rises rapidly (>18 μmol/L/hour), or is prolonged (beyond 14 days in term infants and beyond 21 days in preterm infants). Serum or plasma bilirubin levels should be measured or checked using a non-invasive transcutaneous bilirubinometer (not recommended in the first 24 hours, in preterm infants <35 weeks' gestation, and for monitoring bilirubin in babies already receiving phototherapy). The interpretation of serum bilirubin is based upon age-specific nomograms such as that illustrated in **Figure 37.2** (66). Plotting measurements on a gestation-specific neonatal jaundice chart is of help in identifying babies with severe jaundice, monitoring response to treatment, and ensuring consistency in practice (66, 67).

Early and rapidly rising jaundice may be indicative of haemolysis or sepsis and requires urgent neonatal evaluation and treatment with phototherapy. Relevant investigations include a full blood count, blood group (maternal and baby), direct Coombs' test, conjugated/unconjugated bilirubin, and blood culture. Intravenous antibiotics are often initiated pending negative tests for neonatal sepsis. The baby will also require serial measurements of serum bilirubin every 4–6 hours to monitor evolution or resolution of jaundice.

A high level of bilirubin can result in an acute bilirubin encephalopathy and the development of kernicterus. This is characterized by lethargy, high pitched cry, seizures, opisthotonus, and death, resulting in the classic tetrad of choreoathetoid cerebral palsy; high tone, sensorineural hearing loss; oculomotor dysfunction; and dental dysplasia in survivors. Known risk factors for this devastating condition include male sex, gestational age less than 38 weeks, visible jaundice within the first 24 hours, and exclusive breastfeeding at the time of discharge (68). Phototherapy (blue light in the 425–475 nm wavelength) is effective is clearing bilirubin through the production of bilirubin photoproducts (water-soluble photoisomers that can be excreted from the body) and is an effective strategy for preventing the need for exchange transfusion (a procedure associated with significant morbidity) in babies with significant jaundice.

Obstructive jaundice is suggested by a raised conjugated jaundice fraction (>20 mmol/L or >20–25% of total serum bilirubin value), pale stools, and dark urine; there may also be evidence of liver dysfunction (e.g. elevated alkaline phosphatase and/or alanine transaminase). The possibility of obstructive jaundice requires immediate assessment and investigation with referral to a specialist paediatric

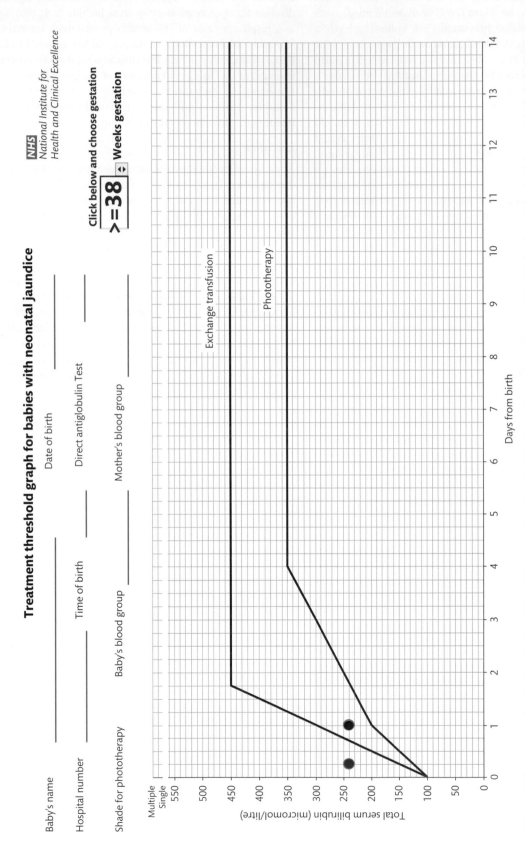

Figure 37.2 Treatment threshold graph for babies with neonatal jaundice. The blue line indicates the total serum bilirubin level at which phototherapy is indicated. The red line indicates the total serum bilirubin at which a double-volume exchange transfusion might be considered. For example, a 38 weeks' gestation newborn infant with a total serum bilirubin of 240 μmol/L at 24 hours of age (indicated by the black circle on the graph above) would require treatment with phototherapy. A similar total serum bilirubin value at 6 hours of age (indicated by the red circle) may require an urgent double-volume exchange transfusion.

Source data from National Institute for Health and Care Excellence (NICE). Neonatal Jaundice. Clinical guideline [CG98]. London: NICE; 2010. https://www.nice.org.uk/guidance/cg98.

liver unit if confirmed (69). There are several potential underlying diagnoses including neonatal sepsis, metabolic conditions, neonatal hepatitis, choledochal cysts, and biliary atresia. Biliary atresia occurs in two forms, syndromic (10–20% of cases) and acquired (80–90% of cases). Though variable in severity, the condition classically presents with conjugated jaundice, pale stools, dark urine, failure to thrive, and hepatomegaly (70). Immediate referral to a specialist liver unit is warranted if biliary atresia is suspected as early surgical treatment (<30 days of age) with a Kasai portoenterostomy to restore bile flow and reduce jaundice is associated with better outcomes (71).

Infection

The possibility of neonatal infection should be considered in the light of a number of perinatal risk factors. These include prolonged rupture of fetal membranes, maternal sepsis, clinical chorioamnionitis, preterm labour, and colonization with group B *Streptococcus*. Though these risk factors indicate an increased risk of neonatal infection, it important to distinguish between the unwell newborn who, irrespective of the presence of risk factors, requires urgent evaluation and intravenous antibiotics, and babies that are well despite the presence of risk factors. This latter group is particularly challenging and the judgement to start antibiotics along with the duration of therapy remain difficult clinical decisions. The majority of infants who receive antibiotics for 'suspected' neonatal infection (based upon risk factors) ultimately do not turn out to have an infection. However, the potential implications of missing a diagnosis of neonatal infection are grave and this perhaps explains the current liberal use of antimicrobials for this purpose. Though several national guidelines are available, for example, the National Institute for Health and Care Excellence (47) which provides pragmatic recommendations on which babies should receive intravenous antibiotics, the clinical conundrum faced by perinatal clinicians around the world is predicated upon carefully balancing the risk of not treating a baby with antibiotics and missing a case of neonatal infection versus unwarranted treatment and investigation. This is a growing problem given widespread antimicrobial resistance (72).

The management of newborn infants with suspected infection involves a careful review of the perinatal history along with serial clinical assessments of the newborn. Blood markers of infection such as white blood cell count, C-reactive protein, and procalcitonin are increasingly used in clinical practice; however, their utility remains questionable, as these acute phase reactants in the main lack adequate sensitivity and specificity. Laboratory investigations should be interpreted in parallel with clinical judgement and caution should be exercised in using them in isolation (73). Of note, clinical signs indicative of possible sepsis usually precede alterations in acute phase reactants. It is important for practitioners to be aware of the local epidemiology of neonatal infections and intravenous antibiotic sensitivities so that appropriate antibiotic regimens can be used. As a general principle, it is recommended that initial antimicrobial therapy be broad spectrum but should be narrow spectrum once the pathogen has been identified. Strict antibiotic discipline is an important means of reducing antimicrobial resistance; this includes facility-based guidelines to ensure that use is consistent and limited to a small range of antibiotics, reserving the use of other antibiotics to specific situations under senior supervision, and stopping antibiotics promptly (usually at 36–48 hours) after initiation for suspected sepsis if the baby is well, and blood cultures are negative. The need for a lumbar puncture to obtain cerebrospinal fluid to diagnose neonatal meningitis should be based upon clinical evaluation first and foremost. The practice of performing routine lumbar punctures in newborns as part of a sepsis workup is not recommended (74).

Poor feeding

The assessment of a baby with poor feeding requires knowledge and experience. Poor feeding can be a sign of an unwell newborn even though specificity is low. Several tools exist to provide mothers and healthcare professionals with indications that infant feeding is progressing well. As a general rule, healthy term babies will take more than eight feeds in a 24-hour period, suckle for between 5–40 minutes, be calm during feeding and contented afterwards, and will have one or two wet nappies and pass meconium within the first 24 hours (75). A common misconception is that the healthy full-term baby who appears to want to suckle frequently in the first 2–3 days before maternal lactation is established is 'hungry' and 'not getting enough'. Healthy term babies require only such colostrum as is available, and will initially suckle at varying frequencies. After a mother's milk has 'come in', a more regular pattern is usually established over the subsequent days. It is important that all healthcare professionals contributing to the care of mothers and babies understand normal postnatal lactation physiology and infant behaviour and are able to provide consistent advice and reassurance if appropriate. Failure to do so may undermine the confidence of a first-time mother and lead her to opt for formula feeding. Every effort should be made to actively promote breastfeeding and this is an important performance metric for perinatal teams.

In the case of a baby who is believed to be feeding poorly, a careful history from the mother and the midwifery or birth attendant staff, observing a feed, and examination of the baby are all essential. A sick baby will not feed well, and feeding may also reflect problems such as an unrecognized cleft palate, genetic syndromes (e.g. unrecognized aneuploidies), infection, and other acute conditions.

Healthy term babies will normally lose 1–2% of their birth weight in the first few postnatal days and regain this by around 7–10 days. Weight loss of greater that 10–15% may be indicative of poor feeding and result in hypernatraemic dehydration. Observation of changing stool colour can also be used as a way of assessing adequacy of feeding. Regular stooling and more than three wet nappies within a 24-hour period are reassuring signs. A healthy, well-fed term baby will pass meconium within the first 24–48 postnatal hours. After this, the stool of a breastfed baby will change to becoming 'transitional' in nature, and then to the characteristic fragrant, soft yellow, seedy appearance.

Bilious vomiting

Bilious vomiting in both term and preterm infants is of concern to the neonatologist as this may indicate a number of underlying medical and surgical pathologies resulting in functional (ileus) or anatomical obstruction (**Table 37.5**). Any baby with bilious vomiting should undergo an urgent medical review to establish the history (antenatal scans and presence of polyhydramnios, family history, passage of meconium, feeding history) and assess well-being. Clinical examination should focus upon whether the abdomen is distended, the anus is patent, and signs of systemic illness. General principles of management include placing the infant nil by mouth, passage of a large-bore nasogastric tube on free drainage, and admission to the neonatal unit. Nasogastric losses in excess of 20 mL/kg/day should be replaced millilitre for millilitre from a 500 mL bag of

Table 37.5 Potential causes of bilious vomiting in newborn infants

Potential causes of bilious vomiting	Comments
Neonatal infection	Associated with a functional gut ileus. Review history for risk factors Serial review of newborn for evolving clinical signs of infection
High gastrointestinal obstruction (duodenal atresia, jejunal atresia, ileal atresia)	Treat newborn with nil by mouth, large-bore nasogastric tube on free drainage, and intravenous antibiotics. Obtain abdominal X-ray. Review antenatal history for known associations (polyhydramnios, requires paediatric surgical referral)
Malrotation and midgut volvulus	Treat newborn with nil by mouth, large-bore nasogastric tube on free drainage, and intravenous antibiotics. Obtain abdominal X ray. Monitor acid–base balance Requires urgent paediatric surgical referral (time critical because of potential for extensive bowel necrosis)
Necrotizing enterocolitis (consider especially in preterm infants)	More likely in preterm infants. Term infants with necrotizing enterocolitis should raise the suspicion of congenital heart disease (76) Treat newborn with nil by mouth, large-bore nasogastric tube on free drainage and intravenous antibiotics. Obtain abdominal X-ray Monitor cardiorespiratory status and acid–base balance If worsening clinical status and/or non-response to medical therapy, requires urgent paediatric surgical referral (time critical because of potential for extensive bowel necrosis)
Meconium ileus	Associated with delayed passage of meconium May be a presentation of cystic fibrosis Treat newborn with nil by mouth, large-bore nasogastric tube on free drainage, and intravenous antibiotics. Obtain abdominal X ray Requires paediatric surgical referral

Source data from National Institute of Clinical Excellence Guideline CG149 https://www.nice.org.uk/guidance/CG149 (accessed 15/07/2016)

Box 37.2 Potential causes of neonatal encephalopathy

- Hypoxic ischaemic encephalopathy (perinatal asphyxia encephalopathy)
- Perinatal stroke
- Perinatal/congenital central nervous system infection (e.g. herpes encephalitis)
- Structural/developmental brain anomalies (e.g. cortical dysplasia)
- Neurometabolic conditions (e.g. Zellweger syndrome, neonatal adrenoleucodystrophy, and non-ketotic hyperglycinaemia)
- Genetic syndromes (e.g. Walker–Warburg syndrome)
- Mitochondrial disorders
- Neuromuscular disorder (e.g. congenital myotonic dystrophy and nemaline rod myopathy)
- Antenatal maternal trauma

presentation of these different causes may share features in common such as fetal distress (e.g. abnormal cardiotocography (CTG) trace, meconium-stained liquor, abnormal cord pH) and need for resuscitation at birth, emphasizing the importance of obtaining a careful history (Table 37.6), examining the newborn and placenta, and carrying out other investigations to help establish the cause. The term hypoxic–ischaemic encephalopathy or birth asphyxia should be reserved for specific cases of neonatal encephalopathy where there is good evidence that the infant has sustained an asphyxial insult likely to have led to impaired cerebral perfusion.

Infants with neonatal encephalopathy may require a multitude of investigations including tests to exclude central nervous system infection, and identify possible underlying genetic, metabolic, structural, or developmental brain anomalies. The placenta and membranes should be sent for histopathological and microbiological analysis. It is important for parents and healthcare professionals that all cases of neonatal encephalopathy have careful documentation of the history, investigations including venous and arterial cord blood gases,

0.9% saline containing 10 mmol of potassium chloride. Imaging (abdominal radiography) and relevant blood tests are first-line investigations followed by gastrointestinal contrast series in discussion with the neonatal surgical team.

Neonatal encephalopathy

This is a clinical syndrome manifest in the early postnatal period comprising disturbed neurological function in term/near-term newborn babies. The features are altered consciousness, and abnormalities of tone; there may be seizures, and apnoeic episodes (77). The initial description of neonatal encephalopathy by Sarnat classified babies into three stages (Sarnat 1, 2, or 3). Sarnat stage 1 is characterized by a duration of less than 24 hours, hyperalertness, uninhibited Moro reflex, and a normal electroencephalogram. Sarnat stage 2 infants are obtunded, hypotonic, with distal limb flexion and clinical seizures. Sarnat stage 3 infants are stuperose, flaccid with absent Moro and suck reflexes, and an abnormal electroencephalogram. Stage 1 generally has a good prognosis with normal development; approximately 25% of stage 2 Sarnat cases develop later neurological problems; stage 3 infants have a very high rates death and cerebral palsy (78). There are many possible causes of neonatal encephalopathy (Box 37.2). The

Table 37.6 Neonatal encephalopathy: important information for the neonatologist

Neonatal encephalopathy	Comments
Antenatal serology	May indicate congenital infection
Maternal medical history, e.g. thrombophilia and medications during pregnancy	Maternal thrombophilia can be associated with neonatal stroke
First-trimester screening results	May indicate aneuploidy
Antenatal scan or liquor volume abnormalities	Polyhydramnios may indicate neurological/neuromuscular problem in newborn
Decreased fetal movements/ abnormal fetal movements	May indicate antenatal origin/may indicate fetal seizure activity
Antenatal maternal trauma	May suggest a sentinel causative event
CTG trace	Provides evidence of fetal distress
Cord blood gas result	Provides evidence of fetal distress
Consanguinity	May be indicative of a rare autosomal recessive disorder in newborn
Family history	May suggest inherited condition
Delivery	Mode of delivery, shoulder dystocia, instrumentation, prolonged second stage

and sequential clinical findings on daily newborn examination. The baby must receive long-term neurodevelopmental surveillance. Multidisciplinary discussion of cases of neonatal encephalopathy can help identify the cause, and promote shared learning.

Therapeutic hypothermia is now a standard of care in most high-income countries for babies older than 36 weeks' gestation who have evidence of moderate to severe perinatal hypoxic–ischaemic encephalopathy. This involves either whole body or head cooling within 6 hours of birth to 33–34°C for 72 hours. The intervention reduces cerebral palsy by approximately 33% at 18 months of age (79). Reassuringly, follow-up data into middle childhood demonstrate persistence of a beneficial effect with respect to higher IQ, reduced cerebral palsy, and less requirement for special educational resources (80). As is common with any emerging evidence-based intervention, many uncertainties remain; examples include whether benefit extends to preterm infants, other causes of neonatal encephalopathy (e.g. perinatal stroke), lesser degrees of compromise, and hypoxic–ischaemic encephalopathy in the presence of sepsis as is particularly common in many low- to middle-income countries (81).

Improving services

The organization of maternal and newborn services

Improvements in obstetric and neonatal services involve collaboration. In a network-based organization of perinatal services, groups of maternity and neonatal units of differing size, services, and complexity collaborate in coordinating the delivery of care. A limited number of centres will provide facilities for the care of the high-risk obstetric patient and critical care for newborn babies (such as mechanical ventilation, therapeutic hypothermia, and surgery). Other neonatal units within a network will provide care of lesser intensity. Babies are transferred between neonatal units according to the intensity of their care needs and the distance from their homes. This structure is cost-effective and efficient, with good evidence that concentrating complex in high-volume neonatal centres results in better outcomes (6). A network structure enables the majority of babies to be looked after within a defined geographical area which in turn reduces the distance between the family home and the place of care for the newborn. This enables the family to visit more easily and the mother to more easily provide her own milk for her baby. A network structure also paves the way for forging strong clinical relationships, developing a network-wide education and governance programme, and the development of clinical practice guidelines for both obstetricians and neonatologists and in team working.

Evaluating and improving practice

Improving the care of newborn infants requires a culture of openness, transparency, a willingness to learn, and robust methods for measuring healthcare processes and health outcomes. Collaboration extends from information sharing between obstetric and neonatal teams through forums such as fetal medicine, clinical governance, 'mortality and morbidity' meetings, and multidisciplinary educational programmes. Systematic capture of clinical information on births and admissions can provide an important opportunity to examine trends, benchmark against other centres, and assess performance against local or national standards. Reliable inferences require consistency in data recording, case definitions, and methods of analysis. The dissemination of league tables of health outcomes is unhelpful if differences in case mix (patient demographic and comorbidities) are not taken into account. Electronic patient records offer an opportunity to streamline surveillance, benchmarking, and audit but ultimately remain dependent on accurate, complete data recording by clinical teams. The United Kingdom benefits from a National Neonatal Audit Programme (82) involving all United Kingdom neonatal units, with central analysis of process and clinical outcome measures utilizing data from a National Neonatal Research Database populated through regular extractions of predefined data from the neonatal Electronic Patient Record (83).

Reducing uncertainties

Testing treatments rigorously and reducing uncertainties in care are a cardinal responsibility of all clinicians. Evidence-based medicine has been embraced as the best approach for ensuring that patients receive treatments and care that are efficacious (they work) and effective (they work in real life). There are any number of examples of the harms that can ensue from the use of non-evidenced-based treatments. Notable examples in newborn care of once standard but now discarded approaches are the routine separation of mother and baby (adverse impact on breastfeeding and bonding), use of 100% oxygen in resuscitation (increased mortality compared with resuscitation in room air), and placing babies prone when sleeping (increases risk of sudden infant death). High-quality care is based on high-quality evidence from high-quality clinical research. It might therefore be considered reasonable that these would form a closely integrated partnership. However, this is not yet the case and much needs to be done to speed the delivery of clinical research, improve the quality of clinical data, and inform professionals and the public about research methods. Not all clinical research involves randomized trials and not all randomized trials involve new treatments. Comparative effectiveness research involves evaluating treatments that are already in standard use, such as, for example, different antibiotic regimens, or different method of feeding newborn babies. Considerable effort is underway to integrate such studies more closely into clinical practice through use of data from existing registries, proportionate research ethics review, short, simple information leaflets, and explanation of the possibility of inclusion benefit through participation (84). Clinicians need to be comfortable with discussing uncertainties with patients and explaining concepts such as 'clinical trial' and 'randomization'. An excellent resource for practitioners and patients alike is 'Testing Treatments', an e-book available in multiple languages (http://www.testingtreatments.org).

Advocacy

Advocacy over the centuries has changed the status of the newborn baby. Child sacrifice was practised in ancient times, and infanticide, especially of female infants, remains a problem in several parts of the world to this day, even though the protection of the newborn baby is now enshrined in law. Other powerful global movements such as the Millennium Development Goals and the WHO 'Every Newborn Action Plan' to end preventable deaths (https://www.everynewborn.org/) have led to an increased focus upon newborn care. The science of epigenetics now provides a plausible mechanistic basis for the many epidemiological associations between early life exposures and later health and disease. Translation of this growing understanding into healthcare and societal policies that lead to incremental improvements in maternal and newborn well-being will require continued and sustained advocacy.

REFERENCES

1. Office for National Statistics. Deaths registered in England and Wales: 2014. 2015. Available at: https://www.ons.gov.uk/peoplepopulationandcommunity/birthsdeathsandmarriages/deaths/bulletins/deathsregistrationsummarytables/2015-07-15.

2. World Health Organization. Newborns: reducing mortality. 2018. Available at: http://www.who.int/mediacentre/factsheets/fs333/en/.

3. Broekhuijsen K, van Baaren GJ, van Pampus MG, et al. Immediate delivery versus expectant monitoring for hypertensive disorders of pregnancy between 34 and 37 weeks of gestation (HYPITAT-II): an open-label, randomised controlled trial. *Lancet* 2015;**385**:2492–501.

4. Boyle EM, Johnson S, Manktelow B, et al. Neonatal outcomes and delivery of care for infants born late preterm or moderately preterm: a prospective population-based study. *Arch Dis Child Fetal Neonatal Ed* 2015;**100**:F479–85.

5. March of Dimes, PMNCH, Save the children, WHO. *Born Too Soon: The Global Action Report on Preterm Birth* (Howson CP, Kinney MV, Lawn JE, eds). Geneva: World Health Organization; 2012.

6. Watson SI, Arulampalam W, Petrou S, et al. The effects of designation and volume of neonatal care on mortality and morbidity outcomes of very preterm infants in England: retrospective population-based cohort study. *BMJ Open* 2014;**4**:e004856.

7. Shlossman PA, Manley JS, Sciscione AC, Colmorgen GH. An analysis of neonatal morbidity and mortality in maternal (in utero) and neonatal transports at 24–34 weeks' gestation. *Am J Perinatol* 1997;**14**:449–56.

8. Costeloe KL, Hennessy EM, Haider S, Stacey F, Marlow N, Draper ES. Short term outcomes after extreme preterm birth in England: comparison of two birth cohorts in 1995 and 2006 (the EPICure studies). *BMJ* 2012;**345**:e7976.

9. EXPRESS Group, Fellman V, Hellström-Westas L, et al. One-year survival of extremely preterm infants after active perinatal care in Sweden. *JAMA* 2009;**301**:2225–33

10. Larroque B, Bréart G, Kaminski M, et al. Survival of very preterm infants: Epipage, a population based cohort study. *Arch Dis Child Fetal Neonatal Ed* 2004;**89**:F139–44.

11. Liggins GC, Howie RN. A controlled trial of antepartum glucocorticoid treatment for prevention of the respiratory distress syndrome in premature infants. *Pediatrics* 1972;**50**:515–25.

12. Roberts D, Dalziel SR. Antenatal corticosteroids for accelerating fetal lung maturation for women at risk of preterm birth. *Cochrane Database Syst Rev* 2006;**3**:CD004454.

13. Reynolds AE, Tansey EM (eds). Prenatal corticosteroids for reducing morbidity and mortality after preterm birth: the transcript of a witness seminar held by the Wellcome Trust Centre for the history of medicine at UCL, London on 15th June 2004. Available at: https://archive.org/details/prenatalcorticos00tans.

14. Althabe F, Belizán JM, McClure EM, et al. A population-based, multifaceted strategy to implement antenatal corticosteroid treatment versus standard care for the reduction of neonatal mortality due to preterm birth in low-income and middle-income countries: the ACT cluster-randomised trial. *Lancet* 2015;**385**:629–39.

15. Wapner RJ, Sorokin Y, Mele L, et al. Long-term outcomes after repeat doses of antenatal corticosteroids. *N Engl J Med* 2007;**357**:1190–98

16. National Institute for Health and Care Excellence (NICE). *Preterm Labour and Birth*. NICE Guideline [NG25]. London: NICE; 2015. Available at: https://www.nice.org.uk/guidance/ng25.

17. Van Baaren GJ, Vis JY, Wilms FF, et al. Predictive value of cervical length measurement and fibronectin testing in threatened preterm labor. *Obstet Gynecol* 2014;**123**:1185–92.

18. Doyle LW, Crowther CA, Middleton P, Marret S, Rouse D. Magnesium sulphate for women at risk of preterm birth for neuroprotection of the fetus. *Cochrane Database Syst Rev* 2009;**1**:CD004661.

19. Chollat C, Enser M, Houivet E, et al. School-age outcomes following a randomized controlled trial of magnesium sulfate for neuroprotection of preterm infants. *J Pediatr* 2014;**165**:398–400.

20. Hadlock FP, Harrist RB, Martinez-Poyer J. In utero analysis of fetal growth: a sonographic weight standard. *Radiology* 1991;**181**:129–33.

21. de Onis M, Garza C, Onyango AW, Martorell R (eds). WHO Child Growth Standards. *Acta Paediatr Suppl* 2006;**450**:100–101.

22. Papageorghiou AT, Ohuma EO, Altman DG, et al. International standards for fetal growth based on serial ultrasound measurements: the Fetal Growth Longitudinal Study of the INTERGROWTH-21st Project. *Lancet* 2014;**384**:869–79.

23. Hofmeyr GJ, Haws RA, Bergström S, et al. Obstetric care in low-resource settings: what, who, and how to overcome challenges to scale up? *Int J Gynaecol Obstet* 2009;**107** Suppl 1:S21–44, S44–45.

24. Stutchfield P, Whitaker R, Russell I, Antenatal Steroids for Term Elective Caesarean Section (ASTECS) Research Team. Antenatal betamethasone and incidence of neonatal respiratory distress after elective caesarean section: pragmatic randomised trial. *BMJ* 2005;**331**:662.

25. Prior E, Santhakumaran S, Gale C, Philipps LH, Modi N, Hyde MJ. Breastfeeding after cesarean delivery: a systematic review and meta-analysis of world literature. *Am J Clin Nutr* 2012;**95**:1113–35.

26. Hyde MJ, Modi N. The long-term effects of birth by caesarean section: the case for a randomised controlled trial. *Early Hum Dev* 2012;**88**:943–49.

27. Huh SY, Rifas-Shiman SL, Zera CA, et al. Delivery by caesarean section and risk of obesity in preschool age children: a prospective cohort study. *Arch Dis Child* 2012;**97**:610–16.

28. Cardwell CR, Stene LC, Joner G, et al. Caesarean section is associated with an increased risk of childhood-onset type 1 diabetes mellitus: a meta-analysis of observational studies. *Diabetologia* 2008;**51**:726–35.

29. Thavagnanam S, Fleming J, Bromley A, et al. A meta-analysis of the association between Caesarean section and childhood asthma. *Clin Exp Allergy* 2008;**38**:629–33.

30. Human Embryology and Fertilisation Authority. Treatments. Available at: https://www.hfea.gov.uk/treatments/.

31. Office for National Statistics. Childhood mortality in England and Wales: 2014. Stillbirths, infant and childhood deaths occurring annually in England and Wales, and associated risk factors. Available at: http://www.ons.gov.uk/peoplepopulationandcommunity/birthsdeathsandmarriages/deaths/bulletins/childhoodinfantandperinatalmortalityinenglandandwales/2014.

32. Topp M, Huusom LD, Langhoff-Roos J, et al. Multiple birth and cerebral palsy in Europe: a multicenter study. *Acta Obstet Gynecol Scand* 2004;**83**:548–53.

33. Human Embryology and Fertilisation Authority. Decisions to make about your embryos. Available at: http://www.hfea.gov.uk/treatments/explore-all-treatments/decisions-to-make-about-your-embryos/.

34. Office for National Statistics. Childhood, infant and perinatal mortality in England and Wales 2013. 2015. Available at: http://www.ons.gov.uk/peoplepopulationandcommunity/birthsdeathsandmarriages/deaths/bulletins/childhoodinfantandperinatalmortalityinenglandandwales/2015-03-10 (accessed 24 June 2016).

35. Liu L, Oza S, Hogan D, et al. Global, regional, and national causes of child mortality in 2000–13, with projections to inform post-2015 priorities: an updated systematic analysis. *Lancet* 2015;**385**:430–40.

36. Springett A, Budd J, Draper ES, et al. *Congenital Anomaly Statistics 2012: England and Wales*. London: British Isles Network of Congenital Anomaly Registers; 2014.

37. Kurinczuk JJ, Hollowell J, Boyd PA, Oakley L, Brocklehurst P, Gray R. *The Inequalities in Infant Mortality Project Briefing Paper 4: The Contribution of Congenital Anomalies to Infant Mortality*. Oxford: National Perinatal Epidemiology Unit, University of Oxford; 2010.

38. NHS England. New congenital heart disease review. 2014. Available at: https://www.england.nhs.uk/wp-content/uploads/2014/09/chd-5-230914.pdf (accessed 15 July 2016).

39. Wren C, Richmond S, Donaldson L. Presentation of congenital heart disease in infancy: implications for routine examination. *Arch Dis Child Fetal Neonatal Ed* 1999;**80**:F49–53.

40. Thangaratinam S, Brown K, Zamora J, Khan KS, Ewer AK. Pulse oximetry screening for critical congenital heart defects in asymptomatic newborn babies: a systematic review and meta-analysis. *Lancet* 2012;**379**:2459–64.

41. McDonald SJ, Middleton P, Dowswell T, Morris PS. Effect of timing of umbilical cord clamping of term infants on maternal and neonatal outcomes. *Cochrane Database Syst Rev* 2013;7:CD004074.

42. Rabe H, Diaz-Rossello JL, Duley L, Dowswell T. Effect of timing of umbilical cord clamping and other strategies to influence placental transfusion at preterm birth on maternal and infant outcomes. *Cochrane Database Syst Rev* 2012;8:CD003248.

43. Raju TN. Timing of umbilical cord clamping after birth for optimizing placental transfusion. *Curr Opin Paediatr* 2013:180–87.

44. Andersson O, Lindquist B, Lindgren M, Stjernqvist K, Domellöf M, Hellström-Westas L. Effect of delayed cord clamping on neurodevelopment at 4 years of age. *JAMA Pediatrics* 2015;**169**:631–38.

45. Allegranzi B, Bagheri Nejad S, Combescure C, et al. Burden of endemic health-care-associated infection in developing countries: systematic review and meta-analysis. *Lancet* 2011;**377**:228–41.

46. Qazi SA, Stoll BJ. Neonatal sepsis: a major global public health challenge. *Pediatr Infect Dis J* 2009;**28** Suppl 1:S1–2.

47. National Institute for Health and Care Excellence (NICE). *Neonatal Infection (Early Onset): Antibiotics for Prevention and Treatment*. Clinical guideline [CG149]. London: NICE; 2012. Available at: https://www.nice.org.uk/guidance/CG14.

48. World Health Organization (WHO). *WHO Guidelines on Hand Hygiene in Health Care*. Geneva: WHO; 2009. Available at: http://apps.who.int/iris/bitstream/10665/44102/1/9789241597906_eng.pdf.

49. Capurro H. *Topical Umbilical Cord Care at Birth: RHL Commentary*. The WHO Reproductive Health Library. Geneva: World Health Organization; 2004.

50. Karumbi J, Mulaku M, Aluvaala J, English M, Opiyo N. Topical umbilical cord care for prevention of infection and neonatal mortality. *Pediatr Infect Dis J* 2013;**32**:78–83.

51. Goldenberg RL, McClure EM, Saleem S. A review of studies with chlorhexidine applied directly to the umbilical cord. *Am J Perinatol* 2013;**30**:699–701.

52. Resuscitation Council UK. Resuscitation guidelines. 2015. Available at: https://www.resus.org.uk/resuscitation-guidelines/.

53. Saugstad OD, Ramji S, Soll RF, et al. Resuscitation of newborn infants with 21% or 100% oxygen: an updated systematic review and meta-analysis. *Neonatology* 2008;**94**:176–82.

54. Tybulewicz AT, Clegg SK, Fonfé GJ, Stenson BJ. Preterm meconium staining of the amniotic fluid: associated findings and risk of adverse clinical outcome. *Arch Dis Child Fetal Neonatal Ed* 2004;**89**:F328–30.

55. Vain NE, Szyld EG, Prudent LM, Wiswell TE, Aguilar AM, Vivas NI. Oropharyngeal and nasopharyngeal suctioning of meconium-stained neonates before delivery of their shoulders: multicentre, randomised controlled trial. *Lancet* 2004;**364**:597–602

56. Wiswell TE, Gannon CM, Jacob J, et al. Delivery room management of the apparently vigorous meconium-stained neonate: results of the multicenter, international collaborative trial. *Pediatrics* 2000;**105**:1–7.

57. Soll RF. Heat loss prevention in neonates. *J Perinatol* 2008;**28** Suppl 1:S57–59.

58. World Health Organization (WHO), Department of Reproductive Health and Research. *Thermal Protection of the Newborn: A Practical Guide*. Geneva: WHO; 1997.

59. Kent AL, Williams J. Increasing ambient operating theatre temperature and wrapping in polyethylene improves admission temperature in premature infants. *J Paediatr Child Health* 2008;**44**:325–31.

60. Moore ER, Anderson GC, Bergman N, Dowswell T. Early skin-to-skin contact for mothers and their healthy newborn infants. *Cochrane Database Syst Rev* 2012;5:CD003519.

61. Leadford AE, Warren JB, Manasyan A, et al. Plastic bags for prevention of hypothermia in preterm and low birth weight infants. *Pediatrics* 2013;**132**:e128–34.

62. Oatley HK, Blencowe H, Lawn JE. The effect of coverings, including plastic bags and wraps, on mortality and morbidity in preterm and full-term neonates. *J Perinatol* 2016;**36** Suppl 1:S83–89.

63. Horta BL, Victora CG. *Long-Term Effects of Breast Feeding: A Systematic Review*. Geneva: World Health Organization; 2013.

64. Rozé JC, Darmaun D, Boquien CY, et al. The apparent breast-feeding paradox in very preterm infants: relationship between breast feeding, early weight gain and neurodevelopment based on results from two cohorts, EPIPAGE and LIFT. *BMJ Open* 2012;2:e000834.

65. Boyd C, Quigley M, Brocklehurst P. Donor breast milk versus infant formula for preterm infants: systematic review and meta-analysis. *Arch Dis Chld Fetal Neonatal Ed* 2006;**92**:F169–75.

66. National Institute for Health and Care Excellence (NICE). *Neonatal Jaundice*. Clinical guideline [CG98], updated 2016. London: NICE; 2010. Available at: https://www.nice.org.uk/guidance/cg98.

67. American Academy of Pediatrics, Subcommittee on Hyperbilirubinemia. Management of hyperbilirubinemia in the newborn infant 35 or more weeks of gestation [published correction appears in *Pediatrics* 2004;114:1138]. *Pediatrics* 2004;**114**:297–316.

68. National Institute for Health and Care Excellence (NICE). Factors that influence hyperbilirubinaemia and kernicterus. In: Neonatal

Jaundice. Clinical guideline [CG98], updated 2016. Available at: http://www.ncbi.nlm.nih.gov/books/NBK65114/.

69. British Society of Paediatric Gastroenterology and Nutrition. Guidelines. Available at: https://bspghan.org.uk/guidelines.

70. Kelly DA, Davenport M. Current management of biliary atresia. *Arch Dis Child* 2007;**92**:1132–35.

71. Nio M, Ohi R, Miyano T, et al. Five- and 10-year survival rates after surgery for biliary atresia: a report from the Japanese Biliary Atresia Registry. *J Pediatr Surg* 2003;**38**:997–1000.

72. The Review on Antimicrobial Resistance. Final report. Available at: http://amr-review.org/Publications (accessed 15 July 2016).

73. Wright KJ, Smith-Collins A, Davis J. G414(P) C-reactive protein without sepsis after birth: development of infant CRP nomograms. *Arch Dis Child* 2016;**101**:A243.

74. Srinivasan L, Harris MC, Shah SS. Lumbar puncture in the neonate: challenges in decision making and interpretation. *Semin Perinatol* 2012;**36**:445–53.

75. UNICEF. Breastfeeding assessment tools. Available at: http://www.unicef.org.uk/BabyFriendly/Resources/Guidance-for-Health-Professionals/Forms-and-checklists/Breastfeeding-assessment-form/.

76. McElhinney DB, Hedrick HL, Bush DM, et al. Necrotizing enterocolitis in neonates with congenital heart disease: risk factors and outcomes. *Pediatrics* 2000;**106**:1080–87.

77. American College of Obstetricians and Gynecologists. Executive summary: neonatal encephalopathy and neurologic outcome. *Obstet Gynecol* 2014;**123**:896–901.

78. Sarnat HB, Sarnat MS. Neonatal encephalopathy following fetal distress. A clinical and electroencephalographic study. *Arch Neurol* 1976;**33**:696–705.

79. Azzopardi DV, Strohm B, Edwards AD, et al. Moderate hypothermia to treat perinatal asphyxial encephalopathy. *N Engl J Med* 2009;**361**:1349–58.

80. Azzopardi D, Strohm B, Marlow N, et al. Effects of hypothermia for perinatal asphyxia on childhood outcomes. *N Engl J Med* 2014;**371**:140–49.

81. Pauliah SS, Shankaran S, Wade A, Cady EB, Thayyil S. Therapeutic hypothermia for neonatal encephalopathy in low- and middle-income countries: a systematic review and meta-analysis. *PLoS One* 2013;**8**:e58834.

82. Royal College of Paediatrics and Child Health, National Neonatal Audit Programme. Available at: http://www.rcpch.ac.uk/nnap.

83. Spencer A, Modi N. National neonatal data to support specialist care and improve infant outcomes. *Arch Dis Child Fetal Neonatal Ed* 2013;**98**:F175–80.

84. Gale C, Hyde M, Modi N, WHEAT trial development group. Research ethics committee decision-making in relation to an efficient neonatal trial. *Arch Dis Child* 2017;**102**:F291–98.

SECTION 5

Gynaecological Problems and Early Pregnancy Loss

38

Miscarriage and recurrent miscarriage

Vikram Sinai Talaulikar and Mushi Matjila

Miscarriage

Definition

Miscarriage is defined as the spontaneous loss of pregnancy before the age of fetal viability. The World Health Organization (WHO) defines miscarriage as expulsion or extraction of a fetus or an embryo weighing 500 g or less from the mother's womb before 20 weeks of pregnancy. The criterion for viability of pregnancy varies from 24 weeks' gestation in the United Kingdom to 28 weeks' gestation in most developing countries. Spontaneous loss of pregnancy up to 12 weeks' gestation is referred to as an early miscarriage while that between 12 to 24 weeks is termed as a late miscarriage.

Epidemiology

Early miscarriage is one of the commonest complications of pregnancy affecting up to 20% of clinical pregnancies (confirmed by ultrasound scan) and early pregnancy loss is responsible for about 50,000 inpatient admissions in the United Kingdom per annum (1). The chance of a subsequent successful pregnancy following one early miscarriage is over 95% and in women with three consecutive miscarriages is over 70% (2).

Aetiology

The most common cause of miscarriage is abnormal development of the embryo or fetus (3). This may be caused by a defect in the number of chromosomes (aneuploidy) or a structural defect in one or many of the chromosomes. Such abnormalities increase with advancing maternal age. Maternal factors which increase the risk of miscarriage include antiphospholipid syndrome (APS), systemic medical disorders (such as uncontrolled diabetes, thyroid disorders, and connective tissue disease), or acute infections during pregnancy. Uterine causes of miscarriage include abnormalities such as cervical insufficiency, submucous fibroids, bicornuate uterus, septate uterus, or other Mullerian abnormalities.

The presence of parental chromosomal translocations and intra-uterine adhesions due to previous uterine instrumentation or endometritis are other less common causes of miscarriage.

Pathology

Histological changes associated with miscarriage include haemorrhage into the decidua basalis and necrotic changes in the adjacent tissues. Placental villi appear thick and oedematous. Changes associated with maceration may be noted in fetal tissue.

In cases of pregnancy of unknown location (where there is no sign of an intrauterine pregnancy, ectopic pregnancy, or retained products of conception in the presence of a positive pregnancy test or serum human chorionic gonadotropin (hCG) concentration >5 IU/L), if uterine curettage is performed as part of management, it is vital to establish histological evidence of chorionic villi in the tissue obtained to exclude the possibility of an ectopic pregnancy.

The Arias-Stella reaction is a benign change in the endometrium associated with the presence of chorionic tissue and may provide the initial histological 'clue' of an ectopic pregnancy. It is a glandular change as a physiological response to the presence of chorionic tissue. The morphological features of the Arias-Stella reaction include nuclear enlargement up to three times normal size and nuclear hyperchromasia, often accompanied by abundant vacuolated cytoplasm (4). The cells typically are stratified and the nuclei hobnail-shaped, bulging into the gland lumen. These large nuclei may contain prominent cytoplasmic invaginations. The degree and extent of the Arias-Stella reaction are highly variable in normal and abnormal intrauterine gestation, in ectopic pregnancy, and in gestational trophoblastic disease. This change occurs as early as 4 days after implantation, although it generally is seen after about 14 days (4).

Assessment of women with a possible early pregnancy loss

Women suspected to have an early pregnancy loss should be cared for in a dedicated outpatient early pregnancy assessment service. Early pregnancy assessment units (EPAUs) offer the advantages of an efficient and high-quality clinical service for women with possible early pregnancy loss, along with significant cost benefits. A systematic approach to management of early pregnancy loss can avoid hospital admissions in 40% of cases and reduce the length of hospital stay in a further 20% (2, 5). Early pregnancy loss is associated with considerable emotional distress and appropriate support and counselling should be offered to all women (1).

Diagnosis

Transvaginal pelvic ultrasound examination is the mainstay in the diagnosis of early miscarriage. Diagnosis is based on a combination of the clinical presentation correlated with ultrasound scan findings.

If a transvaginal ultrasound scan is unacceptable to the woman, a transabdominal ultrasound scan should be offered and limitations of this method of scanning explained. Women should be informed that the diagnosis of miscarriage using one ultrasound scan cannot be guaranteed to be 100% accurate and there is a small chance that the diagnosis may be incorrect, particularly at very early gestational ages (1).

Threatened miscarriage

A transvaginal ultrasound scan shows a viable pregnancy in a woman presenting with cramping pelvic pain and/or vaginal bleeding or spotting. On speculum examination, the cervix appears closed. Some of these women will progress to inevitable miscarriage regardless of the treatment offered. The best predictor of a pregnancy that will continue to viability is the presence of fetal cardiac activity (6). Intrauterine haemorrhages are commonly observed features on ultrasound examinations, especially among patients with clinically evident bleeding in early pregnancy, and the incidence has been reported to be 4–22% (7). Subchorionic haematomas usually appear as hypoechoic or anechoic crescent-shaped areas on ultrasonography (**Figure 38.1**). A meta-analysis suggested that the presence of subchorionic haematomas increases the risk of early or late pregnancy loss by twofold (8).

Complete miscarriage

The woman presents with vaginal bleeding and passage of tissue vaginally (products of conception) along with abdominal pain. The bleeding and pain appear to be settling down. On ultrasound examination, the uterine cavity is empty with a thin endometrium and a vaginal examination confirms the cervix to be closed.

Incomplete miscarriage

The woman presents with active vaginal bleeding, passage of products of conception, and abdominal pain. On ultrasound examination, the uterus has evidence of retained products of conception within the uterine cavity (**Figure 38.2**). Ultrasound features of retained products of conception include a heterogeneous appearance and the presence of irregular tissues with or without a gestational

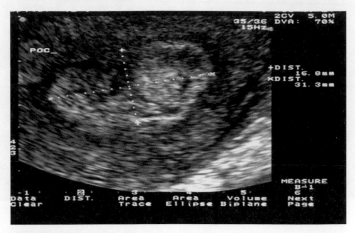

Figure 38.2 Retained products of conception (marked in yellow) within uterine cavity on transvaginal ultrasound.

sac (>15 mm diameter). The midline echo is usually disrupted or distorted.

Missed miscarriage or early pregnancy loss

This term is used when the fetus/embryo has died but is retained in the uterus for a variable period of time without symptoms of miscarriage. The woman presents with receding symptoms of pregnancy with or without vaginal bleeding or brown-coloured discharge. Transvaginal pelvic ultrasound examination confirms an intrauterine pregnancy; however, one of the following observations are made (1):

- Fetal pole with crown–rump length = 7 mm or more but no fetal heart activity (a second opinion should be sought on the viability of the pregnancy and/or a second scan performed a minimum of 7 days after the first before making a diagnosis).
- Fetal pole with crown–rump length less than 7 mm and no fetal heart activity and no change on repeat ultrasound examination performed a week later.
- Mean gestational sac diameter = 25 mm or more but no fetal pole evident (a second opinion should be sought on the viability of the pregnancy and/or a second scan performed a minimum of 7 days after the first before making a diagnosis).
- Mean gestational sac diameter less than 25 mm with no fetal pole evident and no change in scan findings after a week.

A blighted ovum is a term used for an empty gestational sac with absent embryonic pole. A possible complication of unrecognized early pregnancy loss for a prolonged time is consumptive coagulopathy leading to disseminated intravascular coagulation.

Human chorionic gonadotropin

The hCG glycoprotein is produced by the trophoblast of the implanting embryo. Circulating serum hCG concentrations are highly variable and can fluctuate widely during pregnancy. As pregnancy progresses up to 8 weeks' gestation there is a consistent doubling time over 1.94 days (2). Thereafter the doubling time lengthens and the hormone levels stabilize at about 20,000 IU/L by 10–14 weeks' gestation (9). A slower rise or declining hCG concentrations during early pregnancy may indicate an ectopic or a non-viable intrauterine pregnancy (2).

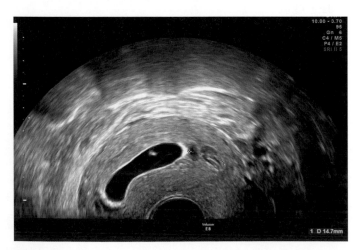

Figure 38.1 Subchorionic haematoma (marked in yellow) next to intrauterine gestational sac on transvaginal ultrasound.

Progesterone

Serum progesterone can be a useful additional test when pregnancy of unknown location is diagnosed as its low level can predict those pregnancies that are most likely to resolve spontaneously (2).

Management

Management of possible early pregnancy loss should ideally be performed in a dedicated EPAU or acute gynaecology unit with suitably trained personnel, modern, high-quality ultrasound machines, and rapid access to serum hCG measurement. Women should be provided with appropriate psychological support and counselling. They should be provided with information about the likely impact of their treatment on future fertility and where to access support services including leaflets, web addresses, and helpline numbers for support organizations (1).

Initial management should focus on haemodynamic stabilization as well as adequate analgesia. Further management should be based on the presenting symptoms, scan findings, and serum hCG measurements. Patient choice should be encouraged at all stages and women should be helped to make informed decisions regarding their own care.

The National Institute for Health and Care Excellence guidelines in the United Kingdom recommend that expectant management for 7–14 days should be offered as the first-line management strategy for women with a confirmed diagnosis of miscarriage (1). If the resolution of bleeding and pain indicate that the miscarriage has completed during 7–14 days of expectant management, the woman should be advised to take a urine pregnancy test after 3 weeks, and to return for individualized care if it is positive. Management options other than expectant management should be explored if (a) the woman is at increased risk of haemorrhage, (b) she has previous adverse and/or traumatic experience associated with pregnancy, (c) she is at increased risk from the effects of haemorrhage, or (d) there is evidence of infection. A repeat ultrasound scan should be offered if, after the period of expectant management, the bleeding and pain have not started (suggesting that the process of miscarriage has not begun) or are persisting and/or increasing (suggesting incomplete miscarriage).

Where clinically appropriate, women undergoing a miscarriage should be offered a choice of manual vacuum aspiration under local anaesthetic in an outpatient/clinic setting, or surgical management in a theatre under general anaesthetic.

Threatened miscarriage

This is best managed by a pelvic ultrasound examination to determine whether a fetus is present and, if so, whether cardiac activity is observed.

Over 90% of women with a live fetus will go on to deliver a baby at term and management of such women consists of reassurance and provision of emotional support (6). Hospitalization, bed rest, or administration of progestogens have not been proven to be of benefit in avoiding pregnancy loss. If the bleeding worsens or persists beyond 14 days after initial presentation, further assessment with pelvic scans should take place. If the bleeding stops, the woman should start or continue routine antenatal care.

Complete miscarriage

In cases of complete miscarriage, women should be informed of the diagnosis sensitively and provided with appropriate counselling and support. They should be offered an easy access to the EPAU in their next pregnancy.

Incomplete miscarriage

Women presenting with incomplete miscarriage should be offered the options of expectant, medical, and surgical management. In the presence of significant active bleeding, hypovolaemia should be initially corrected with crystalloids and later with compatible crossmatched blood. Prophylactic broad-spectrum antibiotics should be administered and once the patient's condition is stabilized, the remaining products of conception should be surgically evacuated from the uterus. In some patients, there may be spontaneous passage of products, thus avoiding the need for surgical evacuation. Medical and expectant management should only be offered when a woman's condition is stable and in units where access to a 24-hour telephone advice line and emergency admission facilities are available.

Expectant management

If retained products of conception measure less than 15 mm and the woman is clinically stable with minimal vaginal bleeding, she may be discharged from EPAU and offered open access to the unit if required (2). If retained products of conception measure greater than 15 mm and the patient is clinically stable with minimal vaginal bleeding she may be reassured that there is a high likelihood (79–96%) that the miscarriage will complete within the next 4 weeks (2, 10–12). The woman may be allowed home with open access to EPAU and reviewed in 2 weeks' time. If the vaginal bleeding subsides subsequently and there are no signs of infection, the woman may be discharged from care (2).

Medical management

Misoprostol is the drug of choice for medical management. The success rate of medical management of incomplete miscarriage varies between 80% and 100% (13). Medical management is more likely to induce complete miscarriage than expectant management. Risks associated with expectant or medical management include retained products of conception, infection (2%), and haemorrhage requiring blood transfusion (0.1%) (2).

Surgical management (evacuation of retained products of conception)

Surgical management has a high success rate (97–100%) but there should be awareness of the possibility of incomplete evacuation of the uterus if symptoms do not settle postoperatively. Associated risks relate to anaesthesia, infection (2%), haemorrhage requiring blood transfusion (0.1%), cervical trauma (1%), intrauterine adhesions causing partial or complete Asherman syndrome, and uterine perforation (0.1–0.2%) (1, 2, 14). Asherman syndrome is characterized by intrauterine adhesions/fibrosis which can lead to partial or complete dysfunction of the endometrium with impairment of fertility, recurrent miscarriage (RM), and/or abnormal menstrual pattern (amenorrhoea or hypomenorrhoea). A pregnant or early pregnant uterus seems to be more susceptible to developing uterine adhesions after curettage especially if complicated by associated infection (15). Risks of incomplete evacuation or of uterine perforation may be lessened by use of transabdominal ultrasound during surgical evacuation, to guide the operator to complete the procedure safely, but this strategy is yet to be subjected to a rigorous clinical trial.

A recent systematic review assessed the effectiveness, safety, and acceptability of any medical treatment for incomplete miscarriage (before 24 weeks) (16). It included 24 randomized controlled studies (5577 women). Three trials involving 335 women compared misoprostol treatment (all vaginally administered) with expectant care. There was no difference in complete miscarriage (average risk ratio (RR) 1.23; 95% confidence interval (CI) 0.72–2.10; two studies, 150 women, random effects; very low-quality evidence), or in the need for surgical evacuation (average RR 0.62; 95% CI 0.17–2.26; 2 studies, 308 women, random effects; low-quality evidence). There were few data on 'deaths or serious complications'. For unplanned surgical intervention, there was no difference between misoprostol and expectant care (average RR 0.62; 95% CI 0.17–2.26; two studies, 308 women, random effects; low-quality evidence). Sixteen trials involving 4044 women addressed the comparison of misoprostol (seven studies used oral administration, six studies used vaginal, two studies sublingual, one study combined vaginal plus oral) with surgical evacuation. There was a slightly lower incidence of complete miscarriage with misoprostol (average RR 0.96; 95% CI 0.94–0.98; 15 studies, 3862 women, random effects; very low-quality evidence) but with the success rate high for both methods. Overall, there were fewer surgical evacuations with misoprostol (average RR 0.05; 95% CI 0.02–0.11; 13 studies, 3070 women, random effects; very low-quality evidence) but more unplanned procedures (average RR 5.03; 95% CI 2.71–9.35; 11 studies, 2690 women, random effects; low-quality evidence). The evidence from the review evidence suggests that medical treatment, with misoprostol, and expectant care are both acceptable alternatives to routine surgical evacuation given the availability of health service resources to support all three approaches (16).

Missed miscarriage

Women with missed miscarriage should also be offered the options of expectant, medical, and surgical management.

Expectant management

The success rates of expectant management vary between 25% and 85% (17). Women should be made aware of the risk of incomplete miscarriage and the need for emergency surgical uterine evacuation in case of acute bleeding, and that there is a lower risk of infection than with surgical management. Women who chose this option should be provided with easy access to the EPAU and they should be followed up within 4 weeks.

Medical management

Medical evacuation can be achieved with the use of prostaglandin analogues (gemeprost or misoprostol) with or without antiprogesterone priming (mifepristone). Misoprostol is recommended as a single dose of 800 mcg (1). Efficacy rates vary between 13% and 96%, and are influenced by several factors including type of miscarriage, gestational sac size, total dose, duration, and route of administration of prostaglandins (2). Vaginal administration is more effective with less side effects. The side effects of the medication are nausea, vomiting, diarrhoea, and mild pyrexia. The medication should be used with caution in women with history of

cerebrovascular or cardiovascular disease. The complications include infection (2%) and haemorrhage requiring blood transfusion (0.1%). Women should be advised to take a urine pregnancy test 3 weeks after medical management unless they experience worsening symptoms, in which case they should be advised to return to the healthcare professional responsible for providing their medical management to consider alternative options.

Surgical management

Women undergoing surgical evacuation for missed miscarriage should have a test for full blood count and blood group and rhesus antibody testing. They should be offered screening for infections including *Chlamydia trachomatis* and bacterial vaginosis. Tissue obtained at the time of evacuation of retained products of conception should be examined histologically to confirm pregnancy and to exclude gestational trophoblastic disease.

A recent systematic review was conducted to compare the safety and effectiveness of expectant management versus surgical treatment for early pregnancy loss (18). It included seven randomized controlled trials with 1521 participants. The expectant-care group was more likely to have an incomplete miscarriage by 2 weeks (RR 3.98; 95% CI 2.94–5.38) or by 6–8 weeks (RR 2.56; 95% CI 1.15–5.69). The need for unplanned surgical treatment was greater for the expectant-care group (RR 7.35; 95% CI 5.04–10.72). The mean percentage needing surgical management in the expectant-care group was 28%, while 4% of the surgical-treatment group needed additional surgery. The expectant-care group had more days of bleeding (mean difference 1.59; 95% CI 0.74–2.45). Further, more of the expectant-care group needed transfusion (RR 6.45; 95% CI 1.21–34.42). Diagnosis of infection was similar for the two groups (RR 0.63; 95% CI 0.36–1.12), as were results for various psychological outcomes. The authors concluded that expectant management led to a higher risk of incomplete miscarriage, need for unplanned (or additional) surgical emptying of the uterus, bleeding, and need for transfusion. Risk of infection and psychological outcomes were similar for both groups. Costs were lower for expectant management. There was lack of clear superiority of either approach (18).

Sepsis associated with miscarriage

This requires urgent hospitalization and prompt institution of parenteral broad-spectrum antibiotic therapy. Once infection is controlled, careful evacuation of the uterus should be performed preferably under ultrasound guidance.

Anti-D rhesus prophylaxis should be offered at a dose of 250 IU (50 mcg) to all rhesus-negative women who have a surgical procedure to manage a miscarriage (1). Anti-D rhesus prophylaxis should not be offered to women who receive solely medical management for a miscarriage or have threatened or complete miscarriage (1).

Recurrent miscarriage

Definition

The definition of RM has been subject of much debate as evidenced by differences in definitions from the European Society of Human Reproduction (ESHRE), the American Society of Reproductive Medicine (ASRM), and the Royal College of Obstetricians and

Gynaecologists (RCOG). More recently, the term recurrent pregnancy loss (RPL) has been adopted. The ASRM defines RPL 'as a disease distinct from infertility, defined by two or more failed pregnancies' (19). The International Committee for Monitoring Assisted Reproductive Technology and the WHO revised glossary of ART terminology define recurrent spontaneous loss/miscarriage as the spontaneous loss of two or more clinical pregnancies (20). Previously ESHRE's Special Interest Group in Early Pregnancy defined recurrent abortion as three consecutive first- trimester clinical losses or two consecutive miscarriages, however a more recent revision states that "A diagnosis of RPL could be considered after the loss of two or more pregnancies" (21, 22, 23). RM is defined by the RCOG as the loss of three or more consecutive pregnancies (24). These differences in definition are important as a much greater number of women have two consecutive early pregnancy losses, followed by a successful pregnancy, than have three consecutive losses. While it is much easier to recruit women with two consecutive losses into research studies on RM, the background (non-treatment related) successful pregnancy rate will be much higher in these studies than in those that recruit only according to the more strict 'three consecutive losses' definition. This must be kept in mind when interpreting research data.

Epidemiology

Unlike sporadic miscarriage with a prevalence of 12–15% in the reproductive population, RM is a much rarer phenomenon occurring in 1–3% of couples attempting conception. Distinct from sporadic miscarriage, the repetitive nature of RM introduces a heavy psychosocial burden to the couple and a unique challenge to clinicians involved. However, this prevalence is much higher than the statistical permutation of consecutive sporadic miscarriage, suggesting a unique pathophysiological entity. Patients with RM have poor reproductive performance across gestation, with higher prevalence of adverse pregnancy outcomes such as preterm delivery, intrauterine growth restriction, and pre-eclampsia in the latter part of pregnancy.

Various medical conditions have been associated with RM although the strengths of these associations are variable. The two strongest associations with RM are embryonic karyotype abnormalities and APS. Other described associations, albeit of weaker strength, include endocrine disturbances, autoimmune disorders, hereditary thrombophilia, and structural uterine abnormalities.

Age (25) and the number of miscarriages are the two most important patient-associated risk factors for RM. However other patient-related risk factors such as obesity (26) and exposure to toxins such as smoking, alcohol, and caffeine are increasingly being recognized as contributory to RM.

The immediate and long-term sequelae associated with RPL are often underestimated and include anxiety, depression, post-traumatic stress disorder, and relationship breakdown (27, 28).

Associated factors

In about 50% of patients investigated for RM, an underlying medical condition will be found. Commonly investigated conditions include genetic, endocrine, autoimmune, thrombotic, and uterine structural abnormalities. However, apart from embryonic karyotype abnormalities, APS, and uterine structural abnormalities, the strength of association between endocrine, autoimmune, and hereditary thrombophilia and RM is comparatively weak.

Genetic

Similar to sporadic miscarriage, the commonest cause of RM, particularly recurrent early miscarriage, is embryonic karyotype abnormalities (29, 30). Commonly identified karyotype aberrations in RM include trisomies 21, 16, and 18 as well as triploidy and monosomy X (31). Detection of an embryonic karyotype abnormality in RM not only unravels underlying aetiology but has prognostic value, as patients with aneuploidy have better livebirth outcomes in subsequent pregnancies (29, 31, 32). More recent and cost-effective approaches to investigating RM recommend initial karyotyping of products of conception and only proceeding to exclude conventional associations (e.g. endocrine, thrombophilia, and APS), in euploid karyotypic losses (33, 34). A practice of routine embryonic karyotype analysis reduces the prevalence of truly unexplained RM from 50% to 24.5% (29).

Investigating for parental karyotype abnormalities to exclude balanced and/or Robertsonian translocations has not been shown to be cost-effective (35). ASRM recommends screening for parental karyotype abnormalities (36), RCOG recommends reactive screening based on a finding of an unbalanced structural embryonic karyotype abnormality (24), while ESHRE recommends selective screening based on maternal age at second miscarriage, number of miscarriages and family history of RM (in parents and siblings) (22). However ESHRE's recent guideline revision states that "Parental karyotyping is not routinely recommended in couples with RPL. It could be carried out after individual assessment of risk" (23).

Endocrine factors

Endocrine factors with reported associations with RM include luteal phase insufficiency, poorly controlled or occult diabetes, polycystic ovary syndrome (PCOS), thyroid dysfunction, and hyperprolactinaemia.

Luteal phase insufficiency

Progressive oestrogen production in the follicular phase is a key mediator of increased luteinizing hormone production and the ultimate surge required for ovulation. The hallmark of the luteal phase is progesterone production and establishment of the corpus luteum. The corpus luteum continues oestrogen and progesterone production and the latter is responsible for decidualization of the endometrium in preparation for implantation (37). Progesterone-driven decidualization involves adaptations in the endometrial glandular epithelium and stroma, resulting in, among others, mucin and glycogen production as well as secretion of prolactin, growth factors, and extracellular matrix proteins (collagen, laminin, and fibronectin), which are all involved in enhancing implantation (38).

Although luteal phase defect or insufficiency remains a controversial entity with a lack of consensus definition and diagnostic criteria, poor follicular growth, oligo-ovulation, inadequate corpus luteal function, and altered endometrial response to oestrogen are thought to play a role in luteal phase defect (39–41). Luteal phase defect has long been associated with RPL and supplementation with progesterone (progestogens), the key endocrine mediator of the luteal phase, has long been the focus of many studies in RM (42, 43). Due to inconsistencies in the definition of RM (two or three losses), population demographics (age and number of previous miscarriage are confounders for future reproductive performance), interventions (different progestogen formulations, dosages and routes of administration), and primary outcome measures (mostly used miscarriage rate rather than live-birth rate), it is unsurprising that these studies have yielded conflicting results (44).

Until recently, the majority of trials examining the effect of progesterone supplementation dated back to the 1950–1960s with considerable methodological limitations (42, 43). The first meta-analysis to examine this subject was by Daya in 1989, which included three studies (45). Different progesterone formulations and routes of administration were used and none of the included studies were sufficiently powered to detect a clinically significant difference in outcome, but pooling resulted in an odds ratio (OR) for pregnancies reaching at least 20 weeks' gestation of 3.09 (95% CI 1.28–7.42). In 2013, a subgroup analysis of patients with RM (three or more consecutive miscarriages) in a Cochrane review that investigated progestogen for preventing miscarriage, showed a statistically significant reduction in miscarriage in favour of those randomized to the progestogens group (Peto OR 0.39; 95% CI 0.21–0.72) (46). This subgroup analysis was based on four trials, three of which were from the 1950s and 1960s. The authors highlighted interpretation of results with caution as numbers were small and the trials were of poor methodological quality. In a systematic review examining the effect of dydrogesterone (Duphaston) on RM by Carp (47), only 3 out of 13 studies were eligible for analysis due to study quality and methodological inadequacies in the others. Of the eligible studies, one was randomized, one quasi-randomized and the other was an open-label study. The conclusion of this systematic review with 409 women for analysis was that administration of dydrogesterone was associated with a 29% odds of miscarrying (OR 0.29; CI 0.13–0.64) (47).

Recently, the results of the Progesterone in Recurrent Miscarriages (PROMISE) trial, the first multicentre, double-blind, placebo-controlled, randomized trial to investigate whether 400 mg of micronized vaginal progesterone in the first trimester of pregnancy would improve pregnancy outcomes in women with unexplained RM, have been published (48). With live-birth rate as the primary outcome and 836 women enrolled, the PROMISE trial reported no significant differences in live-births or maternal and neonatal outcomes in women who were treated with placebo or progesterone in the first half of pregnancy. A recently published randomized controlled trial involving 700 women with unexplained RM (350 in the placebo group and 350 administered 400 mg vaginal progesterone twice daily) started periconceptionally (in the luteal phase prior to pregnancy confirmation), reported significant reduction in miscarriage rate (12.4 vs 23.3% in the placebo group; $P = 0.001$) and improvement in pregnancy continuation and live-birth rate in the progesterone group (87.6 vs 76.7% and 91.6 vs 77.4%, respectively; $P < 0.05$) (49).

Poorly controlled or occult diabetes

Periconception glycaemic control determines maternal and fetal outcomes in pregnancies with pre-existing type 1 or 2 diabetes (50, 51). When periconception glycaemic control is optimized, diabetes-related pregnancy complications such as fetal anomalies, including miscarriage, are comparable to those from the non-diabetic population (52). Although the association between poorly controlled diabetes and adverse pregnancy outcomes is well established, that of RM, hyperinsulinaemia, and impaired glucose tolerance remains poorly defined. In a randomized study, Zolghadri et al. reported improved pregnancy outcomes with metformin, in impaired glucose tolerance patients with RM (53). The ASRM

recommends testing for glycosylated haemoglobin as part of a workup for RM (36). Although also previously recommended by ESHRE (22), its revised guideline strongly recommends against fasting insulin and fasting glucose to improve next pregnancy prognosis in women with RPL (23).

Polycystic ovary syndrome

The association between PCOS and RM remains controversial. The reported prevalence of PCOS from various studies is highly variable and ranges from 4% to 82% (54, 55). The reason for this wide range in reported prevalence is related to the previous lack of consensus in the diagnostic criteria for PCOS and definition of RM and the type of loss (primary or secondary RM) investigated (56). In addition, various studies only focused on particular aspects of the syndrome with some studies investigating the relationship between polycystic ovary morphology alone without the clinical components of the diagnostic criteria (55, 57, 58), while others examined the role of biochemical hyperandrogenism and luteinizing hormone hypersecretion in relation to RM (59).

Postulated mechanisms of pregnancy loss in PCOS include luteinizing hormone hypersecretion resulting in premature oocyte maturation and deleterious effect on the endometrium (60), hyperandrogenaemia contributing to poor oocyte quality and impaired fertilization as well as hyperinsulinaemia leading to increased plasminogen activator inhibitor-1 (PAI-I), and suppression of implantation-enhancing endometrial proteins (PP-12 and PP-14) (61). PCOS is not infrequently accompanied by obesity, itself an independent risk factor for miscarriage. Obesity is associated with hyperinsulinaemia and hyperandrogenism.

Using the widely accepted Rotterdam criteria for the diagnosis of PCOS (62), Cocksedge and colleagues concluded that the prevalence of PCOS in patients with RM was approximately 10% and comparable to that seen in the general population (63). However, this study only included PCOS patients with biochemical hyperandrogenism and excluded those with clinical hyperandrogenism. Another study utilizing the Rotterdam criteria to define PCOS including clinical hyperandrogenism reported a prevalence of 22% (64).

The RCOG does not mention exclusion of PCOS as part of the investigation for RM and ASRM classifies exclusion of PCOS as controversial due to lack of scientific evidence (36). ESHRE strongly recommends against assessment of PCOS in women with RPL (23).

Hyperprolactinaemia

The association between hyperprolactinaemia and RM is based on a single randomized study by Hirahara (65). Out of 352 women with RM (two or more miscarriages), 24 women with hyperprolactinaemia, and 24 with occult hyperprolactinaemia (basal prolactin level, <10 ng/mL, and prolactin level 30 minutes after thyrotropin-releasing hormone administration, <86 ng/mL) were randomized to 2.5–5 mg daily of bromocriptine. Bromocriptine treatment resulted in higher rate of live-births (85.7% vs 52.4% in the non-bromocriptine group; $P < 0.05$). Hyperprolactinaemia is thought to suppress the hypothalamic–pituitary–ovarian system leading to insufficient folliculogenesis and oocyte maturation (65). The study was not placebo controlled and the sample size was small to draw firm conclusions about the findings. The ASRM recommends testing for prolactin in the investigation of patients with RPL, while the RCOG remains silent on the matter. A recent conditional recommendation by ESHRE is that prolactin testing is not recommended in women with RPL in the absence of clinical symptoms of hyperprolactinemia (oligo/amenorrhoea) (23).

Thyroid dysfunction

There is a recognized association between extremes of thyroid dysfunction, in particular hypothyroidism and adverse pregnancy outcomes, in-cluding miscarriage, preterm delivery, and pre- eclampsia. Adequate thyroid reserve is fundamental to sustain the metabolic demands of pregnancy. There is an ongoing debate as to what constitutes adequate thyroid function in pregnancy but there is a realization that thyroid-stimulating hormone concentrations greater than 2.5 mIU/L are associated with poor pregnancy outcomes. The association between RM, subclinical hypothyroidism, and thyroid autoimmunity remains contentious. A meta-analysis including seven studies showed association between thyroid autoantibody positivity and RM (OR 2.26; 95% CI 1.46–3.50) (66). The prevalence of antithyroid peroxidase (TPO-ab) and antithyroglobulin antibodies (TG-ab) has been reported to be 19.5% and 22.5% respectively in women with RM in comparison to 5% and 8% in controls (67). The most commonly associated autoantibodies seen in RM patients with positive antithyroid antibodies are antinuclear antibodies (67). Various mechanisms have been postulated to explain the association between thyroid autoimmunity and RM including binding of autoantibodies to placental or trophoblast antigens, thyroid-stimulating hormone receptor antibodies blocking luteinizing hormone receptors on the corpus luteum, and an association with infertility and delayed age at conception. ESHRE and ASRM recommend thyroid function testing as part of RM workup (22, 36). Additionally, ESHRE strongly recommends testing for thyroid peroxidase (TPO) antibodies in women with RPL (24).

Obesity

Increased body mass index (BMI) is a recognized risk factor for sporadic miscarriage in both spontaneous and assisted conceptions (68, 69). The role of BMI in RM still needs further elucidation but is likely mediated, among others, by hyperinsulinaemia, hyperandrogenism, and leptin. In a nested retrospective case–control study, Lashen et al. found that obese women (BMI >30 kg/m^2) had a higher spontaneous early and recurrent early miscarriage rate in comparison to normal weight, age-matched controls (26). Furthermore, Metwally and colleagues reported a significantly higher risk of miscarriage in subsequent pregnancies of obese and underweight patients with RM (70). Recently, we reported a very high prevalence of obesity in our RM population (64). Obesity does not seem to increase the frequency of aneuploidy embryos in RM (71), but poor oocyte quality and/or endometrial molecular and endocrinological disturbances may be implicated (72). With increasing global burden of obesity, RM may become a less rare phenomenon, and simple strategies such as prepregnancy weight reduction will likely have an impact in obviating pregnancy loss.

Antiphospholipid syndrome

According to the international consensus criteria for APS, APS is present when one clinical and one laboratory criteria are met (73). The clinical criteria consist of vascular thrombosis or pregnancy morbidity (one or more unexplained deaths of a morphologically normal fetus after the tenth week of gestation; one or more premature births of a morphologically normal neonate before 34 weeks' gestation as a result of eclampsia, pre-eclampsia, or recognized features of placental insufficiency; and three or more consecutive spontaneous miscarriages before the tenth week of gestation with maternal anatomical, hormonal, and chromosomal abnormalities excluded). The laboratory criteria consist of positive plasma lupus anticoagulant (LAC), anticardiolipin antibodies (ACA) (>40 GPL or MPL units or >99th centile), and/or anti-beta-2 glycoprotein-1 antibodies (>99th centile) on two or more occasions at least 12 weeks apart.

Antiphospholipid antibodies are directed against anionic phospholipid-binding plasma proteins. Although previously thought to be implicated in pregnancy loss through a thrombotic mechanism, there is recent evidence that antiphospholipid antibodies inhibit trophoblast function and differentiation, suppress expression of key adhesion molecules (alpha-1 integrins, E and VE cadherins) (74), and/or activate complement pathways at the maternal–fetal interface resulting in a local inflammatory response (75). The risk of RPL at less than 13 weeks' gestation in the presence of immunoglobulin G ACA has been reported as 3.16 (95% CI 1.48–8.59) and for anti-beta-2 glycoprotein-1 antibodies 2.12 (95% CI 0.69–6.53) (76). The risk of RPL at less than 24 weeks' gestation with positive ACA antibodies is 5.39 (95% CI 3.72–7.82) and with positive LAC 7.79 (95% CI 2.30–26.45). Among medical conditions associated with RM, APS has the strongest association with RM and is the only one for which treatment has been shown to improve chances of livebirth.

Heparin decreases antiphospholipid antibody binding to trophoblasts, increases cleavage of beta-2 glycoprotein-1, decreases complement activation and trophoblast apoptosis, and enhances trophoblast invasiveness and expression of essential growth (77). There is now abundant evidence that heparin, in combination with aspirin, improves chances of livebirth in APS-related RPL (78–81). However, the combination of heparin and aspirin, or aspirin alone, does not improve pregnancy outcomes in non-APS-related losses, such as in women with unexplained RM (82–84). Most societal guidelines, including those from ESHRE, ASRM, and RCOG, recommend testing for APS in patients with RM (22, 24, 36).

Hereditary thrombophilia

Unlike acquired thrombophilia (APS), the strength of association between RM and hereditary thrombophilias such as factor V Leiden (FVL) mutation, prothrombin gene mutation (G20210A), methylene tetrahydrofolate reductase (MTHFR) gene mutation (C677T), and deficiencies in natural anticoagulants (protein C, protein S and antithrombin III), is rather weak and controversial. While some studies have reported association between FVL, prothrombin gene mutation (PGM), and RPL (85, 86), others have found no association between hereditary thrombophilic defects and RPL (87–89).

The two most common hereditary thrombophilias are PGM and FVL. The first meta-analysis to examine the association between hereditary thrombophilias and fetal loss (not exclusively RPL) was by Rey et al. (90). In this meta-analysis, FVL (OR 2.01; 95% CI 1.13–3.58), activated protein C resistance (3.48; 95% CI 1.58–7.69), and PGM (2.56; 95% CI 1.04–6.29) were associated with early recurrent fetal loss (<13 weeks); however, there was significant heterogeneity between the studies. Although based on one study, an association between FVL and RPL was reported to be even stronger for late RPL (OR 7.83; 95% CI 2.83–21.67) and when other associated conditions with RPL were excluded. Protein S deficiency (14.72; 95% CI 0.99–218.01) was also associated with RPL but not protein C deficiency, antithrombin deficiency, or MTHFR mutation (90). Subsequently, Kovalevsky et al. conducted a meta-analysis that included 16 studies for FVL ($n = 2042$) and 7 studies for PGM ($n = 837$) and reported that carriers of FVL and PGM mutations had double the risk of RPL when compared to non-carriers OR 2.0 (95% CI 1.5–2.7; $P < 0.001$) and 2.0 (95% CI 1.0–4.0; $P = 0.03$), respectively (91).

Unlike with acquired thrombophilia (APS), heparin with or without aspirin does not improve pregnancy outcomes in patients with hereditary thrombophilia (92). The results of the ALIFE2 study, a randomized trial whose objective is to evaluate the efficacy of low-molecular-weight heparin in women with inherited thrombophilia and RM, with livebirth as the primary outcome, are eagerly awaited (93). Currently, recommendations for testing for heritable thrombophilias in patients with RM are diverse. The statement from ESHRE is that larger epidemiological studies are needed to justify testing couples with RM for inherited thrombophilia in routine clinical practice (4). ASRM states that screening for inherited thrombophilia (FVL, PGM, protein C, protein S, and antithrombin deficiencies) may be clinically justified if there is a personal history of venous thromboembolism in the setting of a non-recurrent risk factor (such as surgery) or a first-degree relative with a known or suspected high-risk thrombophilia. However routine testing of women with RPL for inherited thrombophilias is not currently recommended (36). The recommendation from RCOG is that FVL, PGM, and protein S deficiency should be tested for in women with recurrent second-trimester losses (24). ESHRE's conditional suggestion is not to screen for hereditary thrombophilia unless in the context of research, or in women with additional risk factors for thrombophilia (23).

Uterine anomalies

Both congenital and acquired structural uterine abnormalities have been reported to be associated with RM (94–96). In 875 patients with RM (at least two consecutive miscarriages with the same partner) who had imaging, Jaslow and colleagues identified 19.3% with either congenital or structural uterine abnormalities (95).

Congenital

Although congenital uterine anomalies are rare, with an occurrence of 1–6% in the general population, a higher prevalence has been reported in association with RM (94, 96). Of the congenital abnormalities, septate and subseptate uteri were most commonly identified in patients with RM (95, 97). Saravelos and colleagues showed that women with septate or bicornuate uterus suffered from significantly increased second-trimester miscarriages when compared with controls (13.2% and 13.8% vs 1.0%; $P < 0.001$ and $P < 0.05$, respectively) (98).

Arcuate uteri are very common in an unselected population and there is little evidence to suggest an association with RM (94, 97). In a large comparative study, Salim and colleagues showed no significant difference in the prevalence of uterine congenital abnormalities between women with and without RM; however, with both subseptate and arcuate uteri, the length of the remaining uterus was significantly shorter ($P < 0.01$) and the distortion ratio (a fraction of the size of fundal distortion to total uterine length) was significantly higher in patients with RM (97). There is a lack of randomized data

to assess the effect of metroplasty versus conservative management in women with septate uteri and RM (99).

It remains unclear whether didelphic or unicornuate uteri are associated with RM (95). Part of the challenge has been the type of modalities utilized to diagnose uterine anomalies. The most accurate diagnostic procedures are combined hysteroscopy and laparoscopy, sonohysterography (SHG) and three-dimensional ultrasound (3D US). Two-dimensional ultrasound (2D US) and hysterosalpingography (HSG) are inadequate for diagnostic purposes (100). ESHRE's statement on the value of anatomical investigations is that all women with RPL should have an assessment of the uterine anatomy and that the preferred technique to evaluate the uterus is transvaginal 3D ultrasound (3D US), which has a high sensitivity and specificity for distinguishing between septate and bicorporeal uterus with normal cervix. Furthermore that sonohysterography (SHG) is more accurate than hysterosalpingography (HSG) in diagnosing uterine malformations and can be utilised to evaluate uterine morphology when 3D ultrasound is not available, or when tubal patency has to be investigated (23). Lastly, that the MRI is not recommended as first line option for the assessment of uterine malformations in women with RPL, but can be used where 3D ultrasound is not available (23). The ASRM advises HSG and SHG for screening and 3D US or magnetic resonance imaging for further characterization (36). The RCOG recommends that all women with recurrent first-trimester miscarriage and with one or more second-trimester miscarriages should have a pelvic ultrasound scan to assess uterine anatomy and that suspected uterine anomalies may require further investigations to confirm the diagnosis, using hysteroscopy, laparoscopy, or 3D US (24).

Although commonly described, cervical incompetence is in practice a comparatively rare association with RM, with a prevalence of between 4% and 8% (64, 101). Furthermore, there is very little consensus on diagnostic criteria for an incompetent cervix (102). The diagnosis is essentially a clinical one, based on a history of recurrent second-trimester losses and painless cervical dilatation associated with spontaneous rupture of membranes. The RCOG recommends that women with a history of second-trimester miscarriage and suspected cervical weakness who have not undergone a history-indicated cerclage may be offered serial cervical sonographic surveillance (24). Not uncommonly, sonographic cervical shortening is interpreted as cervical weakening warranting reinforcement in the form of cerclage. However, cervical shortening remains the final common pathway in many drivers of miscarriage, irrespective of aetiology.

Acquired

The most common acquired uterine defects associated with RM are uterine fibroids (95). Submucosal and intramural fibroids that result in cavity distortion have been implicated in RM. In a retrospective and prospective data analysis of a tertiary referral RM clinic, Saravelo and colleagues reported the prevalence of fibroids to be 8.2% (103). The same study found that women with intracavitary distortion and undergoing myomectomy significantly reduced their mid-trimester miscarriage rates in subsequent pregnancies from 21.7% to 0% ($P < 0.01$), translating to an increase in live birth rates from 23.3% to 52.0% ($P < 0.05$). The main weakness of this study, as with the many that have reported improvement in live-birth with surgical intervention, is the lack of controlled data. More recently, a systemic review by Russo and co-workers reported a prevalence of submucosal and cavity-distorting myomas to be 4.08% and 5.91% in women with two and three or more pregnancy losses respectively (104). In this review, none of the included studies had proper controls, making it difficult to draw firm conclusions about the association between uterine myomas and recurrent pregnancy loss. In its 2011 guideline, the RCOG makes no mention of uterine myomas as having a potential association with RM (24). The ASRM states that 'the clinical management of pregnancy loss patients with Asherman syndrome or intrauterine synechiae, uterine fibroids, and uterine polyps is controversial, and there is no conclusive evidence that surgical treatment reduces the risk of pregnancy loss. Because randomized trials in this area are lacking and difficult to conduct, the general consensus is that surgical correction of significant uterine cavity defects should be considered' (36). Fibroid size, location, and numbers would be considerations but most RM centres will contemplate surgical management in the presence of cavity-distorting myomas and/or intramural or submucosal fibroids beyond 5 cm in diameter (105, 106).

Current concepts and perspectives

Some of the hypothesis attempting to explain RM suggest that RM may occur in otherwise healthy women with recurrent aneuploid embryos or in women with an underlying medical predilection (endocrine, thrombophilia) driving the recurrent loss of euploid embryos (107). The former RM group is thought to be secondary to a sporadic event, with good prognosis whereas the latter group requires medical intervention aimed at optimization of the pregnancy microenvironment. Many intervention trials have focused on the latter group. Furthermore, RM should be comprehended in the broader perspective, as there is a strong association between RM and unfavourable perinatal outcomes such as intrauterine growth restriction, preterm delivery, and pre-eclampsia (108). Additionally, long-term maternal adverse outcomes such as myocardial infarction, cerebral infarction, and renovascular disease have been associated with RM (107).

Summary

RM remains a challenge to patients and clinicians alike. Recognition of the psychosocial impact should prompt involvement of mental health specialists, counsellors, and social workers in the management of patients with RM. Inconsistencies in definition (two or three consecutive miscarriages) confound research in RM. Although endocrinological, thrombotic, autoimmune, and uterine structural perturbations have been described in association with RM, APS and embryonic karyotype abnormalities remain the two closest conditions for which a reasonable explanation can be offered to patients along with prognostication for future pregnancies. APS is the only diagnosis associated with RM for which there is robust proven efficacy of treatment in improving pregnancy outcomes (in the form of a combination of heparin and aspirin). A diagnosis of RM has additional implications, not only for previable pregnancy loss, but for an association with adverse obstetric and future maternal health outcomes. A global consensus on the definition of RM, along with phenotypic characterization of this heterogeneous condition would improve interpretation of available data and future research. Worsening global trends in diseases of lifestyle such as obesity and non-communicable conditions will likely impact the worldwide prevalence of RM. A thorough understanding of the underlying molecular pathophysiological mechanism in specific phenotypic categories of RM is the fundamental requisite for the advancement of this field.

REFERENCES

1. National Institute for Health and Care Excellence (NICE). *Ectopic Pregnancy and Miscarriage: Diagnosis and Initial Management.* Clinical guideline [CG154]. London: NICE; 2012. Available at: https://www.nice.org.uk/guidance/cg154.
2. Regan L. Miscarriage: early. In: Arulkumaran S, Regan L, Papageorghiou A, Monga A, Farquharson DIM (eds), *Obstetrics and Gynaecology* (Oxford Desk Reference Series), pp. 559–59. Oxford: Oxford University Press; 2011.
3. Regan L, Rai R. Epidemiology and the medical causes of miscarriage. *Baillieres Best Pract Res Clin Obstet Gynaecol* 2000;**14**:839–54.
4. Arias-Stella J. Atypical endometrial changes produced by chorionic tissue. *Hum Pathol* 1972;**3**:450–53.
5. Bigrigg MA, Read MD. Management of women referred to early pregnancy assessment unit: care and cost effectiveness. *BMJ* 1991;**302**:577–79.
6. Everett CB, Preece E. Women with bleeding in the first 20 weeks of pregnancy: value of general practice ultrasound in detecting fetal heart movement. *Br J Gen Pract* 1996;**46**:7–9.
7. Pearlstone M, Baxi L. Subchorionic hematoma: a review. *Obstet Gynecol Surv* 1993;**48**:65–68.
8. Tuuli MG, Norman SM, Odibo AO, Macones GA, Cahill AG. Perinatal outcomes in women with subchorionic hematoma. *Obstet Gynecol* 2011;**117**:1205–12.
9. Konrad G. First-trimester bleeding with falling HCG: don't assume miscarriage *Can Fam Physician* 2007;**53**:831–32.
10. Nielsen S, Hahlin M. Expectant management of first-trimester spontaneous abortion. *Lancet* 1995;**345**:84–86.
11. Shelley JM, Healy D, Grover S. A randomised trial of surgical, medical and expectant management of first trimester spontaneous miscarriage. *Aust N Z J Obstet Gynaecol* 2005,**45**.122–27.
12. Sairam S, Khare M, Michailidis G, Thilaganathan B. The role of ultrasound in the expectant management of early pregnancy loss. *Ultrasound Obstet Gynecol* 2001;**17**:506–509.
13. Neilson JP, Hickey M, Vazquez J. Medical treatment for early fetal death (less than 24 weeks). *Cochrane Database Syst Rev* 2006;**3**:CD002253.
14. Trinder J, Brocklehurst P, Porter R, Read M, Vyas S, Smith L. Management of miscarriage: expectant, medical, or surgical? Results of randomised controlled trial (miscarriage treatment (MIST) trial). *BMJ* 2006;**332**:1235–40.
15. Conforti A, Alviggi C, Mollo A, De Placido G, Magos A. The management of Asherman syndrome: a review of literature. *Reprod Biol Endocrinol* 2013;**11**:118.
16. Kim C, Barnard S, Neilson JP, Hickey M, Vazquez JC, Dou L. Medical treatments for incomplete miscarriage. *Cochrane Database Syst Rev* 2017;**1**:CD007223.
17. Bagratee JS, Khullar V, Regan L, Moodley J, Kagoro H. A randomized controlled trial comparing medical and expectant management of first trimester miscarriage. *Hum Reprod* 2004;**19**:266–71.
18. Nanda K, Lopez LM, Grimes DA, Peloggia A, Nanda G. Expectant care versus surgical treatment for miscarriage. *Cochrane Database Syst Rev* 2012;**3**:CD003518.
19. Practice Committee of the American Society for Reproductive Medicine. Definitions of infertility and recurrent pregnancy loss: a committee opinion. *Fertil Steril* 2013;**99**:63.

20. Zegers-Hochschild F, Adamson GD, de Mouzon J, et al. International Committee for Monitoring Assisted Reproductive Technology (ICMART) and the World Health Organization (WHO) revised glossary of ART terminology, 2009. *Fertil Steril* 2009;**92**:1520–24.

21. Kolte AM, Bernardi LA, Christiansen OB, et al. Terminology for pregnancy loss prior to viability: a consensus statement from the ESHRE early pregnancy special interest group. *Hum Reprod* 2015;**30**:495–98.

22. Jauniaux E, Farquharson RG, Christiansen OB, Exalto N. Evidence-based guidelines for the investigation and medical treatment of recurrent miscarriage. *Hum Reprod* 2006;**21**:2216–22.

23. ESHRE guideline: recurrent pregnancy loss Human Reproduction Open, pp. 1–12, 2018. doi:10.1093/hropen/hoy004.

24. Royal College of Obstetricians and Gynaecologists (RCOG). *The Investigation and Treatment of Couples with Recurrent First-Trimester and Second-Trimester Miscarriage.* Green-top Guideline No. 17. London: RCOG; 2011.

25. Grande M, Borrell A, Garcia-Posada R, et al. The effect of maternal age on chromosomal anomaly rate and spectrum in recurrent miscarriage. *Hum Reprod* 2012;**27**:3109–17.

26. Lashen H, Fear K, Sturdee DW. Obesity is associated with increased risk of first trimester and recurrent miscarriage: matched case–control study. *Hum Reprod* 2004;**19**:1644–46.

27. Kolte AM, Olsen LR, Mikkelsen EM, Christiansen OB, Nielsen HS. Depression and emotional stress is highly prevalent among women with recurrent pregnancy loss. *Hum Reprod* 2015;**30**:777–82.

28. Gold KJ, Sen A, Hayward RA. Marriage and cohabitation outcomes after pregnancy loss. *Pediatrics* 2010:**125**:e1202–207.

29. Sugiura-Ogasawara M, Ozaki Y, Katano K, Suzumori N, Kitaori T, Mizutani E. Abnormal embryonic karyotype is the most frequent cause of recurrent miscarriage. *Hum Reprod* 2012;**27**:2297–303.

30. Ogasawara M, Aoki K, Okada S, Suzumori K. Embryonic karyotype of abortuses in relation to the number of previous miscarriages. *Fertil Steril* 2000;**73**:300–304.

31. Carp H, Toder V, Aviram A, Daniely M, Mashiach S, Barkai G. Karyotype of the abortus in recurrent miscarriage. *Fertil Steril* 2001:**75**:678–82.

32. Stephenson MD, Awartani KA, Robinson WP. Cytogenetic analysis of miscarriages from couples with recurrent miscarriage: a case–control study. *Hum Reprod* 2002;**17**:446–51.

33. Foyouzi N, Cedars MI, Huddleston HG. Cost-effectiveness of cytogenetic evaluation of products of conception in the patient with a second pregnancy loss. *Fertil Steril* 2012;**98**:151–55.e3.

34. Kutteh WH. Novel strategies for the management of recurrent pregnancy loss. *Semin Reprod Med* 2015:**33**:161–68.

35. Barber JC, Cockwell AE, Grant E, Williams S, Dunn R, Ogilvie CM. Is karyotyping couples experiencing recurrent miscarriage worth the cost? *BJOG* 2010;**117**:885–88.

36. The Practice Committee of the American Society for Reproductive Medicine. Evaluation and treatment of recurrent pregnancy loss: a committee opinion. *Fertil Steril* 2012;**98**:1103–11.

37. Lawn, AM, Wilson EW, Finn CA. The ultrastructure of human decidual and predecidual cells. *J Reprod Fertil* 1971;**26**:85–90.

38. Loke Y, King A. *Human Implantation: Cell Biology and Immunology.* Cambridge: Cambridge University Press; 1995.

39. Rosenfeld DL, Chudow S, Bronson RA. Diagnosis of luteal phase inadequacy. *Obstet Gynecol* 1980;**56**:193–96.

40. Wallach E, Jones GS. The luteal phase defect. *Fertil Steril* 1976;**27**:351–56.

41. Ke RW. Endocrine basis for recurrent pregnancy loss. *Obstet Gynecol Clin North Am* 2014;**41**:103–12.

42. LeVine L. Habitual abortion. a controlled study of progestational therapy. *West J Surg Obstet Gynecol* 1964;**72**:30.

43. Swyer G, Daley D. Progesterone implantation in habitual abortion. *Br Med J* 1953;**1**:1073.

44. Walch KT, Huber JC. Progesterone for recurrent miscarriage: truth and deceptions. *Best Pract Res Clin Obstet Gynaecol* 2008;**22**:375–89.

45. Daya S. Efficacy of progesterone support for pregnancy in women with recurrent miscarriage. A meta-analysis of controlled trials. *BJOG* 1989;**96**:275–80.

46. Haas DM, Ramsey PS. Progestogen for preventing miscarriage. *Cochrane Database Syst Rev* 2013;**10**:CD003511.

47. Carp H. A systematic review of dydrogesterone for the treatment of recurrent miscarriage. *Gynecol Endocrinol* 2015;**31**:422–30.

48. Coomarasamy A, Williams H, Truchanowicz E, et al. A randomized trial of progesterone in women with recurrent miscarriages. *N Engl J Med* 2015;**373**:2141–48.

49. Ismail AM, Abbas AM, Ali MK, Amin AF. Peri-conceptional progesterone treatment in women with unexplained recurrent miscarriage: a randomized double-blind placebo-controlled trial. *J Matern Fetal Neonatal Med* 2018;**31**:388–94.

50. Ray JG, O'Brien TE, Chan WS. Preconception care and the risk of congenital anomalies in the offspring of women with diabetes mellitus: a meta-analysis. *QJM* 2001;**94**:435–44.

51. Vääräsmäki MS, Hartikainen A, Anttila M, Pramila S, Koivisto M. Factors predicting peri- and neonatal outcome in diabetic pregnancy. *Early Hum Dev* 2000;**59**:61–70.

52. Jovanovic L, Knopp RH, Kim H, et al. Elevated pregnancy losses at high and low extremes of maternal glucose in early normal and diabetic pregnancy. *Diabetes Care* 2005;**28**:1113.

53. Zolghadri J, Tavana Z, Kazerooni T, Soveid M, Taghieh M. Relationship between abnormal glucose tolerance test and history of previous recurrent miscarriages, and beneficial effect of metformin in these patients: a prospective clinical study. *Fertil Steril* 2008;**90**:727–30.

54. Sagle M, Bishop K, Ridley N, et al. Recurrent early miscarriage and polycystic ovaries. *BMJ* 1988;**297**:1027–28.

55. Rai R, Backos M, Rushworth F, Regan L. Polycystic ovaries and recurrent miscarriage—a reappraisal. *Hum Reprod* 2000;**15**:612–15.

56. Cocksedge KA, Li TC, Saravelos SH, Metwally M. A reappraisal of the role of polycystic ovary syndrome in recurrent miscarriage. *Reprod Biomed Online* 2008;**17**:151–60.

57. Liddell HS, Sowden K, Farquhar CM. Recurrent miscarriage: screening for polycystic ovaries and subsequent pregnancy outcome. *Aust N Z J Obstet Gynaecol* 1997;**37**:402–406.

58. Tulppala M, Stenman UH, Cacciatore B, Ylikorkala O. Polycystic ovaries and levels of gonadotrophins and androgens in recurrent miscarriage: prospective study in 50 women. *BJOG* 1993;**100**:348–52.

59. Cocksedge KA, Saravelos SH, Wang Q, Tuckerman E, Laird SM, Li TC. Does free androgen index predict subsequent pregnancy outcome in women with recurrent miscarriage? *Hum Reprod* 2008;**23**:797–802.

60. Regan L, Owen EJ, Jacobs HS. Hypersecretion of luteinising hormone, infertility, and miscarriage. *Lancet* 1990;**336**:1141–44.

61. Okon MA, Laird SM, Tuckerman EM, Li TC. Serum androgen levels in women who have recurrent miscarriages and their correlation with markers of endometrial function. *Fertil Steril* 1998;**69**:682–90.

62. Rotterdam ESHRE/ASRM-Sponsored PCOS Consensus Workshop Group. Revised 2003 consensus on diagnostic criteria and long-term health risks related to polycystic ovary syndrome. *Fertil Steril* 2004;**81**:19–25.

63. Cocksedge KA, Saravelos SH, Metwally M, Li TC. How common is polycystic ovary syndrome in recurrent miscarriage? *Reprod Biomed Online* 2009;**19**:572–76.

64. Matjila MJ, Hoffman A, van der Spuy ZM. Medical conditions associated with recurrent miscarriage—is BMI the tip of the iceberg? *Eur J Obstet Gynecol Reprod Biol* 2017;**214**:91–96.

65. Hirahara F, Andoh N, Sawai K, Hirabuki T, Uemura T, Minaguchi H. Hyperprolactinemic recurrent miscarriage and results of randomized bromocriptine treatment trials. *Fertil Steril* 1998;**70**:246–52.

66. van den Boogaard E, Vissenberg R, Land JA, et al. Significance of (sub)clinical thyroid dysfunction and thyroid autoimmunity before conception and in early pregnancy: a systematic review. *Hum Reprod Update* 2011;**17**:605–19.

67. Ticconi C, Giuliani E, Veglia M, Pietropolli A, Piccione E, Di Simone N. Thyroid autoimmunity and recurrent miscarriage. *Am J Reprod Immunol* 2011;**66**:452–59.

68. Boots CE, Stephenson MD. Does obesity increase the rate of miscarriage in spontanous conception: a systematic review. *Fertil Steril* 2011;**96** Suppl 3:S284.

69. Metwally M, Ong KJ, Ledger WL, Li TC. Does high body mass index increase the risk of miscarriage after spontaneous and assisted conception? A meta-analysis of the evidence. *Fertil Steril* 2008;**90**:714–26.

70. Metwally M, Saravelos SH, Ledger WL, Li TC. Body mass index and risk of miscarriage in women with recurrent miscarriage. *Fertil Steril* 2010;**94**:290–95.

71. Boots CE, Bernardi LA, Stephenson MD. Frequency of euploid miscarriage is increased in obese women with recurrent early pregnancy loss. *Fertil Steril* 2014;**102**:455–59.

72. Metwally M, Tuckerman EM, Laird SM, Ledger WL, Li TC. Impact of high body mass index on endometrial morphology and function in the peri-implantation period in women with recurrent miscarriage. *Reprod Biomed Online* 2007;**14**:328–34.

73. Miyakis S, Lockshin MD, Atsumi T, et al. International consensus statement on an update of the classification criteria for definite antiphospholipid syndrome (APS). *J Thromb Haemost* 2006;**4**:295–306.

74. Lim W. Complement and the antiphospholipid syndrome. *Curr Opin Hematol* 2011;**18**:361–65.

75. Galli M, Luciani D, Bertolini G, Barbui T. Anti-β2-glycoprotein I, antiprothrombin antibodies, and the risk of thrombosis in the antiphospholipid syndrome. *Blood* 2003;**102**:2717–23.

76. Bates SM. Consultative hematology: the pregnant patient pregnancy loss. *Hematology Am Soc Hematol Educ Program* 2010;**2010**:166–72.

77. Girardi G. Heparin treatment in pregnancy loss: potential therapeutic benefits beyond anticoagulation. *J Reprod Immunol* 2005;**66**:45–51.

78. Backos M, Rai R, Baxter N, Chilcott IT, Cohen H, Regan L. Pregnancy complications in women with recurrent miscarriage associated with antiphospholipid antibodies treated with low dose aspirin and heparin. *BJOG* 1999;**106**:102–107.

79. Kutteh WH. Antiphospholipid antibody-associated recurrent pregnancy loss: treatment with heparin and low-dose aspirin is superior to low-dose aspirin alone. *Am J Obstet Gynecol* 1996;**174**:1584–89.

80. Mak A, Cheung MW, Cheak AA, Ho RC. Combination of heparin and aspirin is superior to aspirin alone in enhancing live births in patients with recurrent pregnancy loss and positive antiphospholipid antibodies: a meta-analysis of randomized controlled trials and meta-regression. *Rheumatology* 2010;**49**:281–88.

81. Rai R, Cohen H, Dave M, Regan L. Randomised controlled trial of aspirin and aspirin plus heparin in pregnant women with recurrent miscarriage associated with phospholipid antibodies (or antiphospholipid antibodies). *BMJ* 1997;**314**:253.

82. Clark P, Walker ID, Langhorne P, et al. SPIN (Scottish Pregnancy Intervention) study: a multicenter, randomized controlled trial of low-molecular-weight heparin and low-dose aspirin in women with recurrent miscarriage. *Blood* 2010;**115**:4162.

83. Kaandorp SP, Goddijn M, van der Post JA, et al. Aspirin plus heparin or aspirin alone in women with recurrent miscarriage. *N Engl J Med* 2010;**362**:1586–96.

84. de Jong PG, Kaandorp S, Di Nisio M, Goddijn M, Middeldorp S. Aspirin and/or heparin for women with unexplained recurrent miscarriage with or without inherited thrombophilia. *Cochrane Database Syst Rev* 2014;**7**:CD004734.

85. Foka ZJ, Lambropoulos AF, Saravelos H, et al. Factor V Leiden and prothrombin G20210A mutations, but not methylenetetrahydrofolate reductase C677T, are associated with recurrent miscarriages. *Hum Reprod* 2000;**15**:458–62.

86. Sarig G, Younis JS, Hoffman R, Lanir N, Blumenfeld Z, Brenner B. Thrombophilia is common in women with idiopathic pregnancy loss and is associated with late pregnancy wastage. *Fertil Steril* 2002;**77**:342–47.

87. Carp H, Dolitzky M, Tur-Kaspa I, Inbal A. Hereditary thrombophilias are not associated with a decreased live birth rate in women with recurrent miscarriage. *Fertil Steril* 2002;**78**:58–62.

88. Carp H, Salomon O, Seidman D, Dardik R, Rosenberg N, Inbal A. Prevalence of genetic markers for thrombophilia in recurrent pregnancy loss. *Hum Reprod* 2002;**17**:1633–37.

89. Jivraj S, Rai R, Underwood J, Regan L. Genetic thrombophilic mutations among couples with recurrent miscarriage. *Hum Reprod* 2006;**21**:1161–65.

90. Rey E, Kahn SR, David M, Shrier I. Thrombophilic disorders and fetal loss: a meta-analysis. *Lancet* 2003;**361**:901–908.

91. Kovalevsky G, Gracia CR, Berlin JA, Sammel MD, Barnhart KT. Evaluation of the association between hereditary thrombophilias and recurrent pregnancy loss: a meta-analysis. *Arch Intern Med* 2004;**164**:558–63.

92. Rodger MA, Hague WM, Kingdom J, et al. Antepartum dalteparin versus no antepartum dalteparin for the prevention of pregnancy complications in pregnant women with thrombophilia (TIPPS): a multinational open-label randomised trial. *Lancet* 2014;**384**:1673–83.

93. de Jong PG, Quenby S, Bloemenkamp KW, et al. ALIFE2 study: low-molecular-weight heparin for women with recurrent miscarriage and inherited thrombophilia-study protocol for a randomized controlled trial. *Trials* 2015;**16**:208.

94. Chan YY, Jayaprakasan K, Zamora J, et al. The prevalence of congenital uterine anomalies in unselected and high-risk populations: a systematic review. *Hum Reprod Update* 2011;**17**:761–71.

95. Jaslow CR, Kutteh WH. Effect of prior birth and miscarriage frequency on the prevalence of acquired and congenital uterine anomalies in women with recurrent miscarriage: a cross-sectional study. *Fertil Steril* 2013;**99**:1916–22.e1.

96. Sugiura-Ogasawara M, Ozaki Y, Kitaori T, Kumagai K, Suzuki S. Midline uterine defect size is correlated with miscarriage of euploid embryos in recurrent cases. *Fertil Steril* 2010;**93**:1983–88.

97. Salim R, Regan L, Woelfer B, Backos M, Jurkovic D. A comparative study of the morphology of congenital uterine anomalies in women with and without a history of recurrent first trimester miscarriage. *Hum Reprod* 2003;**18**:162–66.

98. Saravelos SH, Cocksedge KA, Li TC. The pattern of pregnancy loss in women with congenital uterine anomalies and recurrent miscarriage. *Reprod Biomed Online* 2010;**20**:416–22.

99. Kowalik CR, Goddijn M, Emanuel MH, et al. Metroplasty versus expectant management for women with recurrent miscarriage and a septate uterus. *Cochrane Database Syst Rev* 2011;**6**:CD008576.

100. Saravelos SH, Cocksedge KA, Li TC. Prevalence and diagnosis of congenital uterine anomalies in women with reproductive failure: a critical appraisal. *Hum Reprod Update* 2008;**14**:415–29.

101. Drakeley AJ, Quenby S, Farquharson RG. Mid-trimester loss—appraisal of a screening protocol. *Hum Reprod* 1998;**13**:1975–80.

102. Rai R, Regan L Recurrent miscarriage. *Lancet* 2006;**368**:601–11.

103. Saravelos SH, Yan J, Rehmani H, Li TC. The prevalence and impact of fibroids and their treatment on the outcome of pregnancy in women with recurrent miscarriage. *Hum Reprod* 2011;**26**:3274–79.

104. Russo M, Suen M, Bedaiwy M, Chen I. Prevalence of uterine myomas among women with 2 or more recurrent pregnancy losses: a systematic review. *J Minim Invasive Gynecol* 2016;**23**:702–706.

105. Bailey AP, Jaslow CR, Kutteh WH. Minimally invasive surgical options for congenital and acquired uterine factors associated with recurrent pregnancy loss. *Womens Health* 2015;**11**:161–67.

106. Mukhopadhaya N, Pokuah Asante G, Manyonda IT. Uterine fibroids: impact on fertility and pregnancy loss. *Obstet Gynaecol Reprod Med* 2007;**17**:311–17.

107. Christiansen OB. Recurrent miscarriage is a useful and valid clinical concept. *Acta Obstet Gynecol Scand* 2014;**93**:852–57.

108. Field K, Murphy DJ. Perinatal outcomes in a subsequent pregnancy among women who have experienced recurrent miscarriage: a retrospective cohort study. *Hum Reprod* 2015;**30**:1239–45.

39

Ectopic pregnancy

Mayank Madhra and Andrew W. Horne

Introduction

An ectopic pregnancy (EP) occurs when a fertilized oocyte implants outside the main cavity of the uterus. This places the woman at risk of physical harm, psychological morbidity, and death (1, 2). Remembering to consider an EP as a possibility in all female patients of reproductive age should trigger appropriate investigations and treatment and so limit this potential harm.

EP occurs in 1 in 80 pregnancies (1). The vast majority (around 98%) of EPs result from implantation of the fertilized oocyte in the lumen of the fallopian tube. Other sites of implantation include the ovary, abdominal organs, cervical canal, and interstitial portion of the Fallopian tube. The former two fulfil the definition of implantation outside the normal uterine cavity, as do caesarean section scar EPs. These refer to implantation within a notch of exposed myometrium that communicates with the endometrial cavity. These notches are found after caesarean section and are at a level corresponding to the lower uterine segment in the non-gravid uterus. The aetiology of EP is uncertain, although tubal implantation is probably due to retention of the embryo in the fallopian tube due to impaired embryo-tubal transport and alterations in the tubal microenvironment (3).

EP is the leading cause of maternal death in the first trimester in both resource-rich and resource-poor settings. In the short term, EP causes morbidity from intraperitoneal bleeding and further morbidity arises from the measures necessary to address this, such as emergency surgery, blood transfusion, and postoperative pain. Longer term, women who have suffered from an EP are at risk of a repeat EP, subfertility, and chronic pelvic pain. In the majority of women, an EP is the loss of a wanted pregnancy, and this can also result in psychological morbidity.

Clinical presentation

There is a wide spectrum of clinical presentation in women with EP, ranging from asymptomatic and subacute to collapse with circulatory arrest. Symptoms of EP also overlap with other common conditions, again emphasizing the importance of pregnancy testing in women of reproductive age.

History

Abdominal pain, vaginal bleeding, or a combination of both, in early pregnancy are common presentations in women with EP. There is considerable overlap of symptoms in women with viable pregnancies and miscarriage. The cause of vaginal bleeding may also be from the lower genital tract, as a result of trauma, infection, a cervical polyp, or rarely malignancy. Abdominal pain may result from the presence or torsion of ovarian cysts. Pain may also be entirely non-gynaecological such as constipation, gastroenteritis, irritable bowel syndrome, cystitis, renal colic, or appendicitis.

EPs can result in intraperitoneal bleeding, often associated with rupture of the fallopian tube. The rate of bleeding may be modest; however, changes resultant from the implantation mean that the bleeding is unlikely to stop spontaneously, resulting in a haemoperitoneum. The symptoms associated with this are related to the size of the haemoperitoneum, hypovolaemia, and referred pain. The woman may report abdominal distention with pain, dizziness, and pain at the shoulder tip. The shoulder tip pain is referred pain caused by the extravascular blood in the peritoneum irritating the diaphragm and the phrenic nerve.

There are many established risk factors for EP. Many are related to fallopian tube dysfunction and include smoking, pelvic inflammatory disease, past or present infection with *Chlamydia trachomatis*, endometriosis, previous pelvic surgery (such as appendicectomy, caesarean section, or surgical female sterilization), and previous history of EP (1, 4, 5). A woman with a positive pregnancy test after sterilization has a higher risk of having an EP compared to a non-sterilized woman. However, after sterilization the overall pregnancy rate is much lower, meaning there are fewer EPs overall among sterilized women. Similarly, women who find themselves pregnant despite intrauterine contraception have a higher chance of having an EP compared to those without; however, again the overall pregnancy rate is much lower (6).

An important risk factor for EP is a history of previous EP, with around a 15% recurrence rate after one previous EP. The reasons for this are a combination of ongoing risk factors for cumulative tubal dysfunction, and the mode of treatment for the previous EP (7).

Assisted reproductive technology, particularly *in vitro* fertilization with embryo transfer (IVF-ET), is associated with a higher risk of EP (see Chapter 52). The reasons for this may relate to the underlying reasons necessitating IVF-ET as this technique bypasses the fallopian tube, and also to the techniques involved (8).

When assessing a woman with a possible EP, it is important to enquire about the woman's fertility intent in a sensitive manner. Ascertaining this from the outset will guide any discussion and consent process, particularly with treatments for EP that can affect future fertility.

Examination

The diverse presentation of women eventually diagnosed with EP means a safe and rational approach to each is required. In the 'unwell' patient, key factors of the history will be taken alongside the examination while resuscitation begins.

For the unwell woman with haemodynamic compromise and a positive pregnancy test, the approach should take the form of an 'arrest call'. Airway, breathing, and circulation (ABC) should be assessed and help rapidly summoned to assist with resuscitation. In the case of a women presenting *in extremis*, the diagnosis can be assumed to be ruptured EP with significant haemoperitoneum. The patient requires urgent intravascular volume resuscitation and immediate transfer to theatre for laparoscopy or laparotomy.

The majority of patients present in good condition allowing time for a more detailed assessment. The ABC approach should still be used. Women at an early stage of blood loss from a bleeding EP may have a higher than normal respiratory rate. As blood loss continues, the measures taken by the cardiovascular system to compensate for this can be detect by straightforward observation of blood pressure (BP), heart rate, and respiratory rate. The loss of intravascular volume caused by bleeding in the case of EP first results in an increase in arterial vascular tone to maintain blood pressure. This change can be detected by performing erect and supine blood pressure measurements (10). The normal response in BP when changing position from sitting to standing is for a rise in the systolic BP resultant from the increased vascular tone. This rise in BP is lost when the arteries are maximally constricted in the supine position and is an early sign of intravascular depletion. This is usually associated with a mild increase in respiratory rate. Ongoing blood loss will then be additionally compensated for by an increase in heart rate to maintain cardiac output. Young and normally healthy women will use both these mechanisms to maintain BP and mask significant circulating blood loss. A tachycardia in an otherwise fit and well young woman is a cause for concern.

If the blood loss is ongoing, these mechanisms can no longer maintain BP and the woman becomes hypotensive. The respiratory rate will be high. This matches the description of the 'unwell woman' described previously and demands immediate action. At this stage she will have lost around 40% of her circulating blood volume into her peritoneal cavity. Urgent attention is warranted as this is a life-threatening amount of blood loss. The likelihood is that the EP has concealed the loss of at least 2 L of blood, and at this stage consumption of clotting factors is likely to result in coagulation dysfunction, further compounding the rate of blood loss. The concealed nature of the blood loss can mean appropriate measures are delayed, and care providers are falsely reassured. Formal assessment of the ABC will guide the extent of physiological compromise and balance the urgency and nature of the response.

The 'end-of-the-bed' look at the woman can be revealing about the amount of pain being experienced and if there is pallor. A normal radial pulse and capillary refill under 2 seconds at the fingertips is a reassuring finding. The abdomen may be distended and previous surgical scars noted on inspection. Palpation may reveal guarding or rebound tenderness.

A speculum should be used to examine the lower genital tract and the cervix, particularly so with concurrent symptoms of vaginal bleeding. A cervix open and distended with products of conception is indicative of an inevitable miscarriage (see Chapter 38) and can cause abdominal pain, vaginal bleeding, and hypotension with bradycardia rather than tachycardia (vagal shock). Removing the tissue distending the cervix will stop the stimulation of the vagal nerve causing the cardiovascular depression, quickly relieve the pain, and reverse the bradycardia.

Bimanual examination (see Chapter 1) gives an opportunity to assess for 'cervical excitation'. This is analogous to testing for rebound tenderness during abdominal examination. Gentle rocking of the cervix from side to side causes the pelvic peritoneum to be alternately stretched and relaxed. Movement of inflamed or tethered peritoneum will be experienced as pain and in this context is suggestive of an EP. This finding is typically absent in a normal intrauterine pregnancy. The size of the uterus and the presence of adnexal masses or tenderness can be assessed.

A urinary pregnancy test is usually performed at some point. These are sensitive and accurate with a positive result generated at a corresponding serum concentration of human chorionic gonadotropin (hCG) of 25 IU/L. A false-negative result is occasionally obtained by testing a dilute sample of urine, or reading the result before allowing enough time for the test result to develop. A false-positive result can be produced by cross reaction with other metabolites or toxins, occasionally seen with sepsis (11). For these reasons, and mostly for the interpretation of the following investigations, a serum quantitative hCG should be taken alongside urine hCG testing and other blood tests detailed in the following sections.

Diagnosis and managing uncertainty

Haemodynamically unstable women with a positive pregnancy test can be assumed to have a bleeding EP. They require urgent intervention and circulating volume replacement. There is no alternative.

The diagnosis in haemodynamically stable women in early pregnancy is commonly made by ultrasonography, supported by quantitative serum hCG concentration. The three most common eventual outcomes are of a viable intrauterine pregnancy, non-viable intrauterine pregnancy (commonly referred to miscarriage), and EP. Knowledge of how the diagnosis is made for each is essential in understanding EP.

A transabdominal ultrasound scan is sometimes performed first. The woman requires a full bladder in order to obtain high-quality images. The full bladder facilitates the transmission of ultrasound waves between the body tissues and the transducer (probe) on the skin. The uterus, ovaries, and bladder can be assessed as well as more distant areas as needed such as kidneys and appendix.

A transvaginal ultrasound (TVUS) scan is used to image the uterus, ovaries, and pelvis with higher resolution. This requires the woman's consent, and privacy for her to empty her bladder and to undress. The transvaginal probe is covered in ultrasound gel, a probe cover, and lubricating gel. The probe is inserted into the vagina and the tip gently placed at the posterior fornix of the vagina—better resolution is obtained because the uterus and ovaries are closer to the transducer at the probe tip.

As an embryo implants and begins to grow in size it will at some point cause changes which are detectable by ultrasound. These changes occur long before any changes which would be detected by findings on clinical examination. Deviation from the progression of ultrasound findings in a normally developing intrauterine pregnancy would strongly suggest an alternative pregnancy outcome.

Figure 39.1a shows a normal-sized uterus with a thin endometrium as expected in the non-pregnant female. **Figure 39.1**b shows a thickened endometrium in keeping with secretory phase endometrium or very early stages of pregnancy. The embryo if present is

too small to be seen by modern ultrasound machines. **Figure 39.2a** shows a small sac in the endometrial cavity, which is located towards one side of the cavity. This is known as an eccentrically placed sac and is suggestive of an intrauterine pregnancy. This stage falls short of confirmation that the pregnancy is developing in the uterine cavity. The reason for this is because the sac appears empty, that is, without any other structures visible within it. An empty sac placed centrally in the uterine cavity is a 'pseudosac' and is likely to be a small collection of blood pooling in the uterine cavity.

Pseudosacs are associated with EPs, and if misinterpreted can falsely reassure a woman with an EP that the pregnancy is intrauterine. **Figure 39.2b** shows an intrauterine sac with a yolk sac. The presence of the yolk sac means that the whole intrauterine sac can now be referred to as a gestation sac. This finding means that the pregnancy is intrauterine. The stage of development is in keeping with normally developing pregnancy. A follow-up scan is required

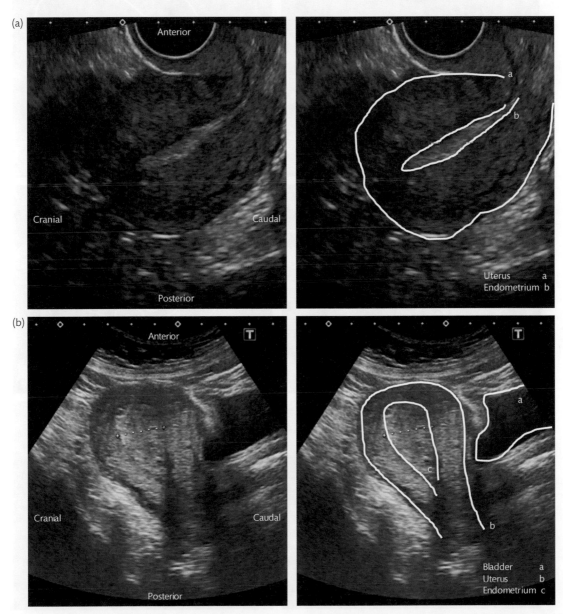

Figure 39.1 Ultrasonography shows (a) a normal-sized uterus with a thin endometrium as expected in the non-pregnant female, and (b) a thickened endometrium in keeping with secretory phase endometrium or very early stages of pregnancy.

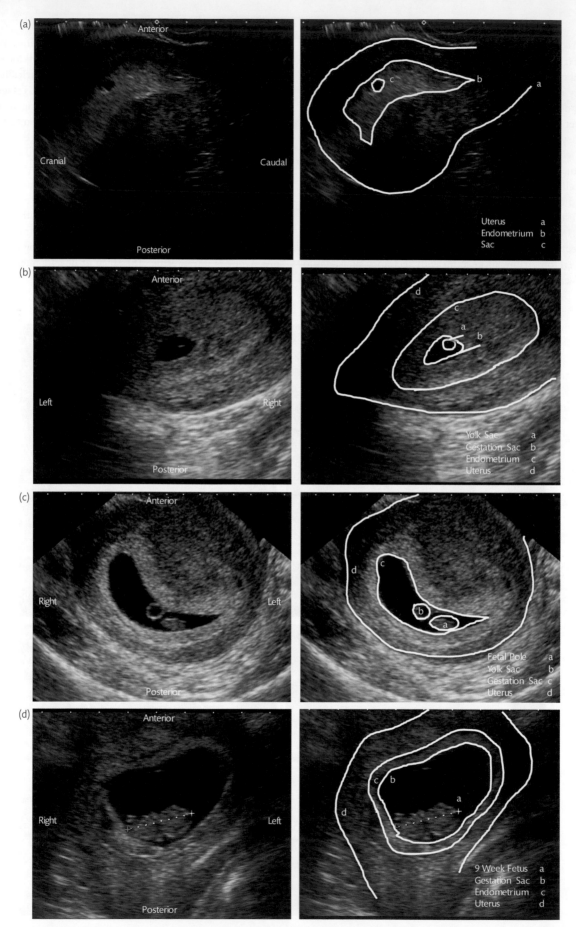

Figure 39.2 Ultrasonography shows (a) a small sac in the endometrial cavity, which is located towards one side of the cavity, and (b) an intrauterine sac with yolk sac. The presence of the yolk sac means that the whole intrauterine sac can now be referred to as a gestation sac; (c) a follow-up scan. Panel (d) shows a developing fetus of 9 weeks' gestation within the uterus with fetal heart motion and fetal movements seen clearly during the scan.

as shown in **Figure 39.2c** to confirm or refute viability. An additional structure, the fetal pole, is now seen in the gestation sac. Using a TVUS scan under ideal conditions, fetal heart motion can be seen when the fetal pole measures 2–3 mm in length, and this would confirm viability. The absence of fetal heart motion with a small fetal pole may suggest miscarriage; however, it may be in keeping with very early stages of a normal pregnancy also. A repeat scan at least 7 days apart should reveal further development in the size of the gestation sac and fetal pole with fetal heart motion now visible confirming a viable pregnancy. The absence of development, the absence of fetal heart motion with a fetal pole greater than 7 mm (in the United Kingdom), or an empty uterus with a thin endometrium suggest a non-viable pregnancy (1). Guidelines for making the diagnosis of miscarriage are designed to minimize the risk of inadvertently reporting an early-stage viable pregnancy as non-viable (1). The absence of a previously seen gestation sac in association with a history of vaginal bleeding strongly suggests that a miscarriage has occurred between scans and the fetal tissue has been passed through the cervix. **Figure 39.2d** shows a developing fetus of 9 weeks' gestation within the uterus with fetal heart motion and fetal movements seen clearly during the scan.

As described previously, there is a point during the normal growth of a viable intrauterine pregnancy in which the developing structures can be detected by ultrasound. This will vary between women and pregnancies. In women with technical obstacles to ultrasound such as a retroverted uterus, fibroids, or obesity, the healthy pregnancy will only be detected at a more advanced stage when larger structures are present. This will also be the case for women in whom only a transabdominal ultrasound scan is acceptable. Correlation of inconclusive scan findings with the serum hCG concentration have led to the development of the concept of the 'discriminatory zone' (12). This is the serum hCG concentration above which a normally developing and normally sited pregnancy should always be visible on ultrasound imaging. The use of TVUS scanning and improvement in the ultrasound technology mean that under optimal conditions this is between serum hCG concentration of 1000 and 1500 IU/L (13). This means that inconclusive scan findings in **Figures 39.1 and 39.2** with a corresponding serum hCG concentration below the discriminatory zone can be in keeping with a healthy pregnancy. The same findings with a serum hCG concentration well above the discriminatory zone would raise concerns about miscarriage or EP. Once the pregnancy is confidently located by ultrasound, the serum hCG concentration adds very little to the information already obtained by ultrasound.

Figure 39.2d demonstrates ultrasound findings with an intrauterine pregnancy with or without fetal viability. A repeat scan after 1–2 weeks is sometimes required to allow development to demonstrate viability, or to demonstrate the lack of development associated with miscarriage.

The presence of an EP can be strongly suggested by scan findings of an empty uterus and *either* identification of an adnexal gestation sac, *or* a heterogeneous adnexal mass as demonstrated in Figures 39.3a and 39.3b. TVUS scanning can have a positive predictive value of 97% and a negative predictive value of 99% in diagnosis of EP in experienced centres (14). The presence of a small or trace amount of free fluid in the pelvis is common in early pregnancy scanning. A large amount of free fluid in the context of a suspected EP can be assumed to be blood, and will usually warrant

surgical management. **Figure 39.3c** shows free fluid with floating small bowel taking the irregular shape of the pelvis and pouch of Douglas.

Of stable women presenting with symptoms in early pregnancy, typically 70% will have an intrauterine pregnancy identified at the initial scan. Approximately half of those will have viability confirmed during the same scan, with the other half requiring further investigation or follow-up to reach a final diagnosis. About 10% of women will have a miscarriage diagnosed on the first scan, and around 2% depending on the local population will have an EP (15). The remainder will fall between the criteria described previously where the pregnancy sac cannot be identified either within or outside the uterus. This includes women with serum hCG concentrations above and below the discriminatory zone. The women are given the working diagnosis 'pregnancy of unknown location' (PUL) (16). This is an intermediate diagnosis for which further or repeat investigation is required to reach a final diagnosis or pregnancy outcome. This could be a viable intrauterine pregnancy, non-viable intrauterine pregnancy, or an EP. Around 20% of women initially classed as PUL will have an EP.

Management of women with uncertain early pregnancy diagnosis

Serial serum hCG measurement at an interval of 48 hours is useful in the management of women with a PUL. Most women are suitable for outpatient management because they are haemodynamically stable and therefore return home between visits for measurement of serum hCG concentrations. Clear advice has to be impressed upon each woman about follow-up, emergency contact numbers out of hours, and about which symptoms should alert her to seek medical help sooner than planned. Worsening of existing symptoms or experiencing symptoms suggestive of intraperitoneal bleeding warrants an urgent review.

A viable intrauterine pregnancy would be expected to be associated with at least a 66% increase from initial serum hCG concentration over 48 hours. The approximate doubling of hCG with healthy pregnancy is a predictable feature in the first trimester. An EP can be associated with a rise of less than 66% or a largely static serum hCG concentration. A 50% drop in serum hCG concentration over 48 hours is strongly suggestive of miscarriage, and associated vaginal bleeding with the passing of the sac through the cervix would further support this.

A stable woman with a serum hCG concentration below the discriminatory zone and PUL on TVUS scanning can safely have serial hCG monitoring. A second serum hCG concentration can suggest a diagnosis based on the hCG trend and if the subsequent serum concentration is above the discriminatory zone, a further TVUS scan may be helpful. Serum hCG concentrations for normal intrauterine pregnancies at equivalent gestation have a wide range. The individual trend in serum hCG concentrations is more useful in establishing a diagnosis and the absolute serum concentration is useful in interpretation of scan findings and subsequent decisions on management options. A normally developing intrauterine pregnancy will approximately double the serum hCG concentration every 48 hours. A rise of more than 66% from the baseline is acceptable. This can roughly predict when a normal intrauterine pregnancy should be

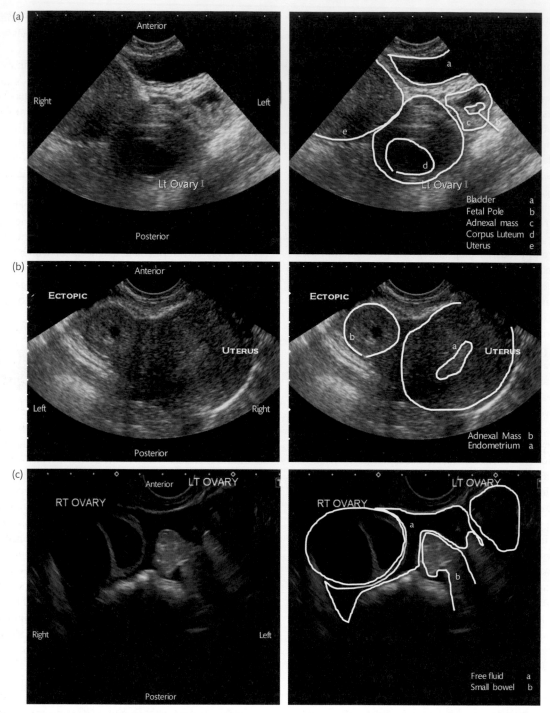

Figure 39.3 Ultrasound scan findings of (a, b) an empty uterus and either identification of an adnexal gestation sac, or a heterogeneous adnexal mass; panel (c) shows free fluid with floating small bowel taking the irregular shape of the pelvis and pouch of Douglas.

above the discriminatory zone and hence located on an ultrasound scan. This would be able to confirm the location of the pregnancy, and some cases confirm the presence of fetal heart motion. Some women may require a further scan to assess viability of the pregnancy, usually after at least 1 week. Once the pregnancy is located by ultrasound, serum hCG concentrations are of little value in determining viability or predicting pregnancy outcome.

A sharp fall in serum hCG concentrations from initial baseline within 48 hours with bleeding symptoms can allow a confident clinical diagnosis of miscarriage and further scans can be avoided. As the

location of the pregnancy had never been confirmed, there is a small remaining possibility of an EP. This small risk is usually mitigated by ensuring follow-up of the women clinically and with serum hCG concentration. In addition, women are advised to re-attend if pain or bleeding worsens, if there are symptoms of intraperitoneal bleeding as described previously, or in those without ongoing contraception if their periods do not resume.

Serial hCG monitoring with PUL can result in the situation where there are several hCG results at 48-hour intervals, all below the discriminatory zone, neither clearly resolving nor doubling. These are known as 'persistent PULs' and either represent an underlying EP or a miscarriage, with the static pattern of the hCG not being consistent with a viable pregnancy. A developing adnexal mass may become apparent in women with a PUL, which would strongly suggest an EP whether the corresponding serum hCG concentration is above or below the discriminatory zone. In those without an adnexal mass visible on ultrasound, taking a conservative approach with close monitoring should see the serum hCG concentration return to normal. Each woman with a PUL should be aware of the possibility of an EP and receive clear advice about action to take if symptoms worsen. Intraperitoneal bleeding is possible even at very low serum hCG concentrations so women and healthcare staff should remain vigilant for complications until the pregnancy has resolved and this has been confirmed by serum hCG concentrations (e.g. decrease to <15 IU/L).

On occasion, when there is uncertainty about the diagnosis despite the measures described previously, an endometrial biopsy can be helpful. This is absolutely contraindicated if there is any possibility of a *viable* intrauterine pregnancy. The presence of trophoblasts in the biopsy sample confirms an intrauterine pregnancy. The absence of trophoblasts or the presence of changes in the endometrium related to hCG exposure without trophoblast presence (Arias-Stella reaction), suggests the presence of an extrauterine pregnancy. Diagnostic laparoscopy is also on occasion required to confirm the diagnosis.

The time course of each particular pregnancy until the diagnosis can be established with certainty can mean multiple visits, blood tests, and scans for the woman. This will incur costs for the healthcare provider and for the woman with losses from employment, travel costs, and cancelling holidays at short notice, adding to what can be already a difficult time (17).

Management of ectopic pregnancy

Removal of the fallopian tube (salpingectomy) containing the pregnancy and causing intraperitoneal bleeding has been the treatment for EP for over 125 years. Commonly performed by laparoscopic means in modern practice, the use of laparotomy (open abdominal incision) is now reserved for the gravely unwell woman. Surgical, medical, and expectant management represent the three main categories of treatment. The final choice will involve considering the woman's wishes, future fertility intent, and safety.

Surgical management

The aims of surgical management are to stop any active bleeding and remove the pregnancy tissue in a manner that takes into consideration the woman's future fertility wishes. It is the most appropriate option for cases of unsuccessful medical or expectant management or in cases where intraperitoneal bleeding is suspected.

For the haemodynamically unstable woman, urgent care from members of the on-call team is required. As previously discussed, an 'ABC' approach is needed with large-bore intravenous access, volume resuscitation, crossmatch of blood, urinary catheter, and assembly of the theatre team in preparation for emergency surgery. These measures can take place simultaneously, so a team-based approach will result in faster stabilization and treatment for the woman. For a tubal EP in this scenario, a salpingectomy is usually

performed. A salpingectomy is removal of the fallopian tube. This will remove the pregnancy tissue, stop bleeding, and allow effective resuscitation of the woman.

The haemodynamically stable woman who requires surgical management for EP will require the same preoperative measures which can be undertaken in a more considered manner. Surgical management is indicated if there is a strong suspicion of EP on ultrasound, when the adnexal mass is considered large (>35 mm in diameter), fetal heart motion is seen in the adnexal mass, there is ultrasound evidence of intraperitoneal bleeding, there is moderate to severe abdominal pain, or if the woman prefers surgical management (1).

Laparoscopy is the preferred alternative to open surgery (laparotomy) as it is associated with a shorter recovery time, less pain, and a faster return to normal activities (18). This involves a general anaesthetic for the woman and insertion of a 5–10 mm laparoscope into the peritoneal cavity, usually through an incision in the umbilicus around the same size. The peritoneal cavity is filled with carbon dioxide gas to lift the anterior abdominal wall away from the abdominal viscera either before or after insertion of the laparoscope, and direct visualization of the pelvis can be made (Figure 39.4a). Once the diagnosis is confirmed, a uterine manipulator is placed to assist optimal positioning of the uterus for any surgery. Other 5–10 mm incisions are made in the abdominal wall to allow surgical instruments to reach the pelvis and perform the necessary surgery (Figure 39.4b), before the instruments are removed, gas released, and skin incisions closed. Less than 1% of cases of EP surgery performed by laparoscopy are converted to laparotomy. Laparoscopy carries a 1 in 500 risk of a serious complication (19). Resort to laparotomy is required when it is felt to be the best approach to repair inadvertent damage to the bowel and blood vessels, and to control bleeding. Half of visceral injuries are related to the entry of the primary port or insufflation, and around 15% of bowel injuries become apparent after the completion of the initial operation with delay and regression of recovery.

The direct visualization of the pelvis is performed first in women with EP. This will allow the surgeon to estimate the amount of blood in the peritoneal cavity and to confirm the diagnosis made by ultrasound imaging.

The surgeon then has the choice of performing a salpingectomy or removing only the pregnancy tissue from the affected tube and leaving the tube *in situ* (salpingotomy). This will depend on the amount of bleeding, the appearance of the other fallopian tube, and the discussion with the woman prior to surgery regarding her wishes. A salpingectomy is indicated if the woman has no future desire for fertility, because of fewer surgical complications and less follow-up requirements. If the other fallopian tube and the rest of the pelvis appear healthy, the reproductive outcomes are similar with salpingectomy or salpingotomy (20).

A salpingotomy is required if the woman wishes to conceive naturally in the future and the contralateral tube appears to be unhealthy, damaged, or absent. This could result from previous infection, surgery, endometriosis, or previous EP. There are equivalent reproductive outcomes after salpingectomy or salpingotomy. It can be difficult to know if all the pregnancy tissue has been removed when performing a salpingotomy, so follow-up serum hCG concentration monitoring is essential until the final resolution. There is an estimated 4–8% risk of residual trophoblast cells in the treated fallopian tube, which can multiply and cause further bleeding. A decrease

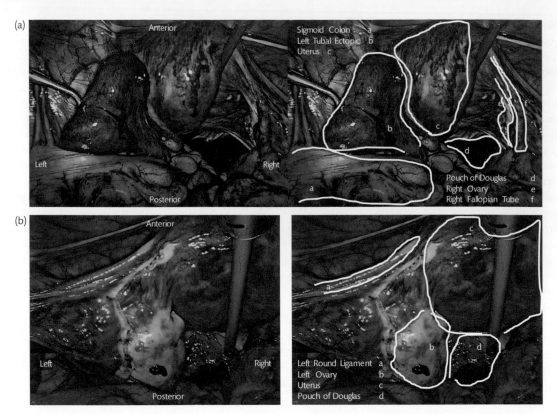

Figure 39.4 (a) The peritoneal cavity is filled with carbon dioxide gas to lift the anterior abdominal wall away from the abdominal viscera either before or after insertion of the camera, and direct visualization of the pelvis can be made. (b) Other 5–10 mm incisions are made in the abdominal wall to allow surgical instruments to reach the pelvis and perform the necessary surgery.

then a subsequent increase in the serum hCG concentration would alert healthcare staff to this possibility. This would require either a second operation to perform a salpingectomy or medical treatment. The risk of recurrent EP following a salpingotomy is 8% with an approximately even distribution between ipsilateral and contralateral tube as the future implantation site (20).

In women who are undergoing IVF-ET, there are further considerations for the surgeon to take into account. It is known that the presence of hydrosalpinges (abnormal fallopian tubes distended with fluid) increases the risk of embryo implantation failure and miscarriage, and that removal of the affected hydrosalpinges, or blocking the fluid from entering the uterine cavity with sterilization clips, reverses this (21). At laparoscopy for EP, a salpingectomy may be used to treat the EP, with contralateral tubal occlusion or contralateral salpingectomy (22). This would mean the chance of spontaneous conception in the future would be almost zero and that IVF would be needed for future pregnancies. The benefits in improved IVF success rate and reduced chance of future EP have to be carefully balanced and discussed with the woman and her fertility team in advance of surgery. If there is doubt or the findings at laparoscopy are unexpected, a conservative approach should be taken.

Surgery for EP is considered a potentially sensitizing event in the United Kingdom in rhesus-negative blood group women without prior sensitization, so 250 IU of anti-D immunoglobulin via intramuscular injection is recommended.

Medical management

This is an option for selected haemodynamically stable women with a suspicion of EP on ultrasonography or a persistent PUL. It can be

a reasonable option when the woman and the gynaecologist wish to avoid laparoscopy. There is no role for medical management in women with severe abdominal pain or suspicion of intraperitoneal bleeding. In either case, expedient surgery is more appropriate.

Methotrexate is widely used for medical management of EP. It is usually given in a single intramuscular injection with a dose of 50 mg/m² body surface area. Methotrexate is a systemic treatment that works by inhibiting dihydrofolate reductase (23). This interrupts the supply of substrate for synthesis of purine DNA base pairs. The downstream effect is to disrupt the cell cycle by preventing duplication of DNA. The effect of methotrexate is concentrated on cells dividing rapidly such as trophoblasts. Systemic methotrexate would disrupt trophoblast cells sited in an EP or in an intrauterine pregnancy equally, so the presence of an intrauterine pregnancy is a contraindication for medical management. The teratogenic nature of methotrexate means a 12-week washout period is recommended before a further attempt to conceive. The common side effects of methotrexate are related to the effect of rapidly dividing cell disruption in the skin, bone marrow, and gastrointestinal tract, namely photosensitivity, leucopenia, stomatitis, and diarrhoea. Women treated with methotrexate maintain their oocyte reserve when it is used as a single dose in this manner, emphasizing the effect on actively dividing rather than quiescent cells (24).

Patient selection for medical management is important. Methotrexate has been successfully used in women with a baseline serum hCG concentration less than 5000 IU/L. Above this level, the frequent resort to surgery, or multiple doses of methotrexate, result in it being considered ineffective and not cost-effective (25). Mirroring criteria for surgical management, women best suited for methotrexate have an adnexal mass less than 35 mm in diameter, without the presence of fetal heart motion in the mass, and at most a small amount of free fluid on ultrasonography. In this context, a small amount of free fluid is considered within normal limits, whereas a moderate or large amount of free fluid would suggest intraperitoneal bleeding. It may be useful in avoiding surgery in women at high risk of surgical complications, such as those with multiple previous abdominal surgeries, provided other requirements are met.

When used as part of the management of persistent PUL, the aim of medical management is to accelerate or promote the complete resolution of the trophoblast. Until this happens and is confirmed by serum hCG concentration, the risk of intraperitoneal bleeding remains. In persistent PUL, the true diagnosis lies between EP and miscarriage. Around 20% of cases of persistent PUL are subsequently discovered to be EPs. Small EP masses can remain undetected by laparoscopy with both fallopian tubes appearing healthy without distention. It is justifiable to treat persistent PUL with methotrexate, and specific management can otherwise be offered should the underlying diagnosis become apparent with subsequent investigations.

Due to the side effect profile of methotrexate, a baseline full blood count, liver function tests, and renal function should be measured alongside serum hCG. Abnormalities in these parameters are likely to be worsened by methotrexate and an alternative to methotrexate should be considered.

Women treated medically are typically managed as an outpatient. Clear advice about symptoms that suggest intraperitoneal bleeding and how to access care swiftly are essential. To facilitate this safely, the woman should have 24-hour access to emergency gynaecology care including resort to urgent surgical management and be able to attend hospital promptly if her symptoms worsen.

After the initial injection, close monitoring is required until the serum hCG concentration is negative. This can take several weeks and women should be prepared to have regular measurement of serum hCG concentrations as part of medical management. Initial response to methotrexate is determined by checking serum hCG concentrations at 4 days and 7 days after the injection. A result showing a greater than 15% decrease in serum hCG concentration when comparing these serum concentrations is indicative of a good initial response. Serum HCG concentrations are checked weekly thereafter to ensure a continuing decrease until complete resolution is achieved. Some units consider medical management a potentially sensitizing event and will offer anti-D immunoglobulin at the same dose for surgical management to unsensitized rhesus negative women.

Between 80% and 90% of women with an EP treated with methotrexate will have successful treatment, meaning surgery or further methotrexate have been avoided. Around 10% of appropriately selected women will required either a second dose of methotrexate or surgical management, both indicating a suboptimal response to medical management. This may become apparent with a worsening of symptoms with clinical or ultrasound suspicion of intraperitoneal bleeding mandating surgical treatment. Alternatively, the woman may no longer wish to continue with medical management. Serum concentrations of hCG after methotrexate which have risen on day 7 give an early indication to move to surgical management. During the serum hCG follow-up phase, the concentrations may plateau or begin to rise again before any symptoms are reported from the woman, indicating failing medical management and giving an opportunity to consider surgical management prior to any clinical deterioration. The risk of intraperitoneal bleeding remains for the woman until the resolution of serum hCG is complete. The risk of recurrent EP after successful medical management is 12%, similar to that after surgery (26).

Expectant management

Careful selection of woman can identify those in whom the EP will resolve spontaneously, avoiding the risks associated with surgical and medical management.

The general characteristics in favour of successful expectant management are a low initial serum hCG concentration, usually less than 1000 IU/L with a downward trend (27). Otherwise the criteria are similar to those required for outpatient medical management.

Serum hCG concentration is monitored at a minimum of weekly intervals until negative, taking an average of less than 3 weeks (14, 28–30). As with methotrexate treatment follow-up, a plateau or rise in serum hCG concentration during monitoring can trigger alternative forms of management to be offered to the woman. Easy access to gynaecology care is essential.

Management of non-tubal ectopic pregnancy

About 2–5% of EPs are located outside the fallopian tubes (8). Surgical access to the location of the implanted pregnancy and the risk of bleeding from the underlying structure determines which mode of treatment is preferred (31, 32).

EPs which have implanted on the surface of the ovary, in the abdomen, or on the omentum are usually managed surgically. The surgeon is able to see the implantation site to assess and take steps to limit any bleeding resulting from removal of the EP tissue. Serum hCG monitoring is required, as with salpingotomy, to detect residual trophoblasts and initiate methotrexate treatment as needed.

EPs can rarely implant in the interstitial portion of the fallopian tube as it passes through the myometrium. This has a characteristic appearance on ultrasonography (33). These can be managed either by surgically removing the pregnancy and surrounding myometrium with the fallopian tube, or with methotrexate. The decision will depend on the gestation and size of the EP mass at diagnosis.

Cervical EPs were traditionally managed by performing a hysterectomy as the diagnosis was previously only made after the onset of unrelenting vaginal bleeding. Caesarean section scar EPs appear to be increasing in prevalence and are located at the expected site of a previous lower segment caesarean section or at a notch visible on ultrasonography at that level. Both of these can be diagnosed by ultrasonography, and as the EP site can be accessed through the vagina, both medical and surgical management for these conditions have been developed (34, 35). The gestation sac can be injected directly with methotrexate, removed by suction evacuation (36), then tamponade performed with a balloon catheter (32, 37). The use of systemic methotrexate works best in those with low initial serum hCG concentrations; however, it is widely used in most cases with patient admission to the ward for close observation and access to operating theatres. The potential for vaginal bleeding with a cervical EP and vaginal and intraperitoneal bleeding with a caesarean EP rupturing the cervico-isthmic junction is present until complete resolution has occurred. Medical management is generally preferred as long as rapid access to surgical management is available in the event of bleeding.

Management of heterotopic pregnancy

A heterotopic pregnancy is the presence of an EP in parallel with a viable intrauterine pregnancy. The natural incidence is around 1 in 30,000 pregnancies. There is a higher rate seen in association with the use of assisted reproductive technology, in particular IVF-ET and more so when more than one embryo is transferred in a single cycle (8). The aim of management is to avoid harm to the mother and preserve the viability of the intrauterine pregnancy where possible.

A heterotopic pregnancy can present as haemodynamic instability and symptoms of intraperitoneal bleeding in a pregnant woman. She may have previously been assumed clinically or with ultrasonography to have only an intrauterine pregnancy. In such a situation, the safest approach will be to treat as if she has a bleeding EP by beginning resuscitation and arranging urgent surgical management. A more common mode of presentation is at the follow-up scan following IVF-ET where intra- and extrauterine gestation sacs can sometimes be seen. The value of the serum hCG concentration lies only in determining if it is above or below the discriminatory zone, as more subtle trends such as a suboptimal rise in hCG from the EP will be masked by the intrauterine pregnancy's production of hCG.

Medical management is contraindicated in the presence of a viable intrauterine pregnancy, and the experience of expectant management is limited to a small number of case reports, meaning the mainstay of treatment is surgical (38). Avoiding maternal blood loss and thereby maintaining an adequate blood supply to the uterus will give the best chance of ongoing viability to the intrauterine pregnancy.

Surgical management can be undertaken with precautions taken to safeguard the intrauterine pregnancy. Laparoscopy is performed without the use of a uterine manipulator and lower intra-abdominal pressures of gas are used. This avoids undue gas pressure on the fundus of the uterus, the muscle of which is further relaxed with general anaesthesia. There is minimal use of electrical energy (diathermy) or its use is avoided altogether by using laparoscopic suturing or 'ultrasonic' instruments. Postoperative analgesia is limited to those safe in pregnancy and non-steroidal anti-inflammatory drugs are avoided. Anti-D immunoglobulin should be given as with rhesus-negative women with EP. A follow-up ultrasound scan to assess viability is essential as despite best practice around 30–40% of intrauterine pregnancies associated with heterotopic pregnancies are found to be non-viable after treatment for the EP (39).

Follow-up care and future pregnancy outcome

There is undoubtedly a psychological and emotional impact associated with EP, both with implications for the current pregnancy and for future pregnancies.

The woman and her partner should be offered testing and treatment for *Chlamydia* infection. Successful treatment may limit further tubal damage, although this may be less relevant in women undergoing IVF-ET where *Chlamydia* screening and clearance is part of the workup for IVF. Similarly, women treated for EP who do not wish to conceive immediately may opt to start or switch their contraception, which will reduce the risk of recurrence.

For women with EP as their first pregnancy, their risk of repeat EP is around 10% regardless of the mode of treatment (7). An early ultrasound scan in the subsequent pregnancy around 6 weeks' gestation can help identified an EP prior to the development of symptoms, or provide reassurance about the intrauterine location of the current pregnancy. Sadly, women with a previous EP have a higher rate of miscarriage in subsequent pregnancies. This is thought to be because of overlapping and persistent risk factors for EP, miscarriage, and subfertility. If the pregnancy progresses beyond the first trimester, the reproductive outcomes are similar to women without a history of EP (7).

Conclusion

EP is the leading cause of maternal death in the first trimester of pregnancy. This can be avoided because this condition can be diagnosed and treated easily. This depends on the healthcare provider and the woman considering the diagnosis and being aware of the overlap of EP symptoms with those of healthy pregnancy and other unrelated medical conditions.

Once the diagnosis is made, laparoscopy is appropriate in the vast majority of cases, and surgery can be avoided entirely in selected women. Careful counselling of women and close monitoring as an outpatient are effective and safe where there is recourse to emergency surgery as the need arises or the woman wishes.

Future research is being directed at identification of a serum marker to diagnose EP at the initial presentation to aid earlier diagnosis (40–42). The combination of methotrexate with gefitinib (an epidermal growth factor receptor inhibitor) is currently being tested in a clinical trial to improve the resolution time and efficacy of medical treatment (43, 44).

REFERENCES

1. National Institute for Health and Care Excellence. *Ectopic pregnancy and miscarriage: diagnosis and initial management.* London: NICE; 2012 [updated Apr 2019] Clinical Guideline NG126. www.nice.org.uk/guidance/ng126.
2. Cantwell R, Clutton-Brock T, Cooper G, et al. Saving Mothers' Lives: Reviewing maternal deaths to make motherhood safer: 2006–2008. The Eighth Report of the Confidential Enquiries into Maternal Deaths in the United Kingdom. *BJOG* 2011;**118** Suppl 1:1–203.
3. Horne AW, Brown JK, Nio-Kobayashi J, et al. The association between smoking and ectopic pregnancy: why nicotine is BAD for your fallopian tube. *PLoS One* 2014;**9**:e89400.
4. Goksedef BP, Kef S, Akca A, Bayik RN, Cetin A. Risk factors for rupture in tubal ectopic pregnancy: definition of the clinical findings. *Eur J Obstet Gynecol Reprod Biol* 2011;**154**:96–99.
5. Menon S, Sammel MD, Vichnin M, Barnhart KT. Risk factors for ectopic pregnancy: a comparison between adults and adolescent women. *J Pediatr Adolesc Gynecol* 2007;**20**:181–85.
6. Heinemann K, Reed S, Moehner S, Minh TD. Comparative contraceptive effectiveness of levonorgestrel-releasing and copper intrauterine devices: the European Active Surveillance Study for Intrauterine Devices. *Contraception* 2015;**91**:280–83.

7. Bhattacharya S, McLernon DJ, Lee AJ, Bhattacharya S. Reproductive outcomes following ectopic pregnancy: register-based retrospective cohort study. *PLoS Med* 2012;**9**:e1001243.

8. Refaat B, Dalton E, Ledger WL. Ectopic pregnancy secondary to in vitro fertilisation-embryo transfer: pathogenic mechanisms and management strategies. *Reprod Biol Endocrinol* 2015;**13**:30.

9. Human Fertilisation and Embryology Authority (HFEA). *A Long Term Analysis of the HFEA Register Data 1991–2006.* London: HFEA; 2007.

10. Yadav K, Akanksha, Jaryal AK, Coshic P, Chatterjee K, Deepak KK. Effect of hypovolemia on efficacy of reflex maintenance of blood pressure on orthostatic challenge. *High Blood Press Cardiovasc Prev* 2016;**23**:25–30.

11. Taylor N. Transient false-positive urine human chorionic gonadotropin in septic shock. *Am J Emerg Med* 2015;**33**:864.e1–2.

12. Mehta TS LD, Beckwith B. Treatment of ectopic pregnancy: is a human chorionic gonadotrophin level of 2,000mIU/mL a reasonable threshold? *Radiology* 1997;**205**:569–73.

13. Kirk E, Bottomley C, Bourne T. Diagnosing ectopic pregnancy and current concepts in the management of pregnancy of unknown location. *Hum Reprod Update* 2014;**20**:250–61.

14. Mavrelos D, Nicks H, Jamil A, Hoo W, Jauniaux E, Jurkovic D. Efficacy and safety of a clinical protocol for expectant management of selected women diagnosed with a tubal ectopic pregnancy. *Ultrasound Obstet Gynecol* 2013;**42**:102–107.

15. Kirk E, Papageorghiou AT, Condous G, Tan L, Bora S, Bourne T. The diagnostic effectiveness of an initial transvaginal scan in detecting ectopic pregnancy. *Hum Reprod* 2007;**22**:2824–28,

16. Barnhart K, van Mello NM, Bourne T, et al. Pregnancy of unknown location: a consensus statement of nomenclature, definitions, and outcome. *Fertil Steril* 2011;**95**:857–66.

17. Unger HW, Starrs L, Scott L, Critchley HO, Duncan WC, Horne AW. The financial costs to patients of diagnosing and excluding ectopic pregnancy. *J Fam Plann Reprod Health Care* 2013;**39**:197–200.

18. Hajenius PJ, Mol F, Mol BW, Bossuyt P, Ankum WM, van der Veen F. Interventions for tubal ectopic pregnancy. *Cochrane Database Syst Rev* 2007;**1**:CD000324.

19. Royal College of Obstetricians and Gynaecologists (RCOG). *Laparoscopic Management of Tubal Ectopic Pregnancy.* Consent Advice No. 8. London: RCOG; 2010.

20. Mol F, van Mello NM, Strandell A, et al. Salpingotomy versus salpingectomy in women with tubal pregnancy (ESEP study): an open-label, multicentre, randomised controlled trial. *Lancet* 2014;**383**:1483–89.

21. Johnson N, van Voorst S, Sowter MC, Strandell A, Mol BW. Surgical treatment for tubal disease in women due to undergo in vitro fertilisation. *Cochrane Database Syst Rev* 2010;**1**:CD002125.

22. Tsiami A, Chaimani A, Mavridis D, Siskou M, Assimakopoulos E, Sotiriadis A. Surgical treatment for hydrosalpinx prior to IVF-ET: a network meta-analysis. *Ultrasound Obstet Gynecol* 2016;**48**:434–45.

23. Electronic Medicines Compendium. Summary of medicinal product characteristics: methotrexate. 2015. Available at: https://www.medicines.org.uk/emc.

24. Boots CE, Hill MJ, Feinberg EC, Lathi RB, Fowler SA, Jungheim ES. Methotrexate does not affect ovarian reserve or subsequent assisted reproductive technology outcomes. *J Assist Reprod Genet* 2016;**33**:647–56.

25. Sowter MC, Farquhar CM, Gudex G. An economic evaluation of single dose systemic methotrexate and laparoscopic surgery for the treatment of unruptured ectopic pregnancy. *BJOG* 2001;**108**:204–12.

26. Fernandez H, Capmas P, Lucot JP, Resch B, Panel P, Bouyer J. Fertility after ectopic pregnancy: the DEMETER randomized trial. *Hum Reprod* 2013;**28**:1247–53.

27. Elson CJ, Salim, R, Potdar N, Chetty M, Ross JA, Kirk EJ on behalf of the Royal College of Obstetricians and Gynaecologists. Diagnosis and management of ectopic pregnancy. *BJOG.* 2016;**123**:e15–e55.

28. van Mello NM, Mol F, Verhoeve HR, et al. Methotrexate or expectant management in women with an ectopic pregnancy or pregnancy of unknown location and low serum hCG concentrations? A randomized comparison. *Hum Reprod* 2013;**28**:60–67.

29. Helmy S, Sawyer E, Ofili-Yebovi D, Yazbek J, Ben Nagi J, Jurkovic D. Fertility outcomes following expectant management of tubal ectopic pregnancy. *Ultrasound Obstet Gynecol* 2007;**30**:988–93.

30. Mavrelos D, Memtsa M, Helmy S, Derdelis G, Jauniaux E, Jurkovic D. beta-hCG resolution times during expectant management of tubal ectopic pregnancies. *BMC Womens Health* 2015;**15**:43.

31. Chetty M, Elson J. Treating non-tubal ectopic pregnancy. *Best Pract Res Clin Obstet Gynaecol* 2009;**23**:529–38.

32. Hunt S, Talmor A, B V. Management of non-tubal ectopic pregnancies at a large tertiary hospital. *Reprod Biomed Online* 2016;**33**:79–84.

33. Chuckus A, Tirada N, Restrepo R, Reddy N. Uncommon implantation sites of ectopic pregnancy: thinking beyond the complex adnexal mass. *Radiographics* 2014;**35**:946–59.

34. Wang CJ, Tsai F, Chen C, Chao A. Hysteroscopic management of heterotopic cesarean scar pregnancy. *Fertil Steril* 2010;**94**:1529. e15–18.

35. Litwicka K, Greco E. Caesarean scar pregnancy: a review of management options. *Curr Opin Obstet Gynecol* 2013;**25**:456–61.

36. Jurkovic D, Knez J, Appiah A, Farahani L, Mavrelos D, Ross JA. Surgical treatment of Cesarean scar ectopic pregnancy: efficacy and safety of ultrasound-guided suction curettage. *Ultrasound Obstet Gynecol* 2016;**47**:511–17.

37. Fuchs N, Manoucheri E, Verbaan M, Einarsson J. Laparoscopic management of extrauterine pregnancy in caesarean section scar: description of a surgical technique and review of the literature. *BJOG* 2015;**122**:137–40.

38. Eom JM, Choi JS, Ko JH, et al. Surgical and obstetric outcomes of laparoscopic management for women with heterotopic pregnancy. *J Obstet Gynaecol Res* 2013;**39**:1580–86.

39. Clayton HB, Schieve LA, Peterson HB, Jamieson DJ, Reynolds MA, Wright VC. A comparison of heterotopic and intrauterine-only pregnancy outcomes after assisted reproductive technologies in the United States from 1999 to 2002. *Fertil Steril* 2007;**87**:303–309.

40. Tong S, Skubisz MM, Horne AW. Molecular diagnostics and therapeutics for ectopic pregnancy. *Mol Hum Reprod* 2015;**21**:126–35.

41. Refaat B. Role of activins in embryo implantation and diagnosis of ectopic pregnancy: a review. *Reprod Biol Endocrinol* 2014;**12**:116.

42. Lekovich J, Witkin SS, Doulaveris G, et al. Elevated serum interleukin-1beta levels and interleukin-1beta-to-interleukin-1 receptor antagonist ratio 1 week after embryo transfer are associated with ectopic pregnancy. *Fertil Steril* 2015;**104**:1190–94.

43. Skubisz MM, Horne AW, Johns TG, et al. Combination gefitinib and methotrexate compared with methotrexate alone to treat ectopic pregnancy. *Obstet Gynecol* 2013;**122**:745–51.

44. Horne AW, Skubisz MM, Doust A, et al. Phase II single arm open label multicentre clinical trial to evaluate the efficacy and side effects of a combination of gefitinib and methotrexate to treat tubal ectopic pregnancies (GEM II): study protocol. *BMJ Open* 2013;**3**:e002902.

40

The menstrual cycle

Lucy H.R. Whitaker, Karolina Skorupskaite, Jacqueline A. Maybin, and Hilary O.D. Critchley

Introduction

The female human reproductive system comprises the hypothalamic–pituitary–ovarian (HPO) axis and the reproductive tract (fallopian tubes, uterus, cervix, and vagina).

The principal functions of this system are to produce an ovum, enable its fertilization and implantation, and allow growth and safe expulsion of the fetus into the external world. The menstrual cycle is critical for facilitation of the initial steps of this *raison d'etre* of the female reproductive system.

Why women menstruate

Menstruation is not a ubiquitous process. All female placental mammals have a uterine lining that is receptive at fertile time points, but menstruation is predominantly limited to primates, several species of bat, and the elephant shrew. In species where there is no outward menstruation, oestrus cycles are followed by 'covert menstruation' in which the endometrium is completely reabsorbed. The benefits of one system over another are not fully understood. Initially menstruation was thought to be an evolutionary defence against sperm-carried pathogens (1) or that the energy expenditure of maintaining the endometrium outweighed shedding and rebuilding (2). However, the current hypothesis is that decidualization is a prerequisite for menstruation. Decidualization is the process of conversion of endometrial stromal cells into specialized decidual cells that have the capacity to nourish an embryo. Decidualization occurs in menstruating women prior to fertilization; in contrast, non-menstruating mammals decidualize only at the point of implantation. Decidualization is thought to confer evolutionary benefits though facilitating placental invasion of healthy embryos, enabling an element of embryo selection by the uterus in menstruating species (3).

Why menstrual problems are a modern problem

Menstruation has traditionally been viewed as a negative process. Aristotle considered it a sign of female inferiority (4) and Pliny the Elder said of menstruating women 'hardly can there be found a thing more monstrous than is that flux and course of theirs' (5). Behavioural dogma are enshrined in elements of Judaism, Christianity, Islam, and Hinduism and only in 2005 was the practice of banishing a woman to the cow shed during her menses banned in Nepal (6). However, the impact of menstruation and menstrual disorders has in some respects increased rather than decreased despite emancipation, decreasing taboos, and improved access to sanitary ware. This is in part because of the increased frequency of menstruation, secondary to earlier menarche, decreased parity (in part as a result of access to contraception), and decreased lactational amenorrhoea. Our ancestors menstruated approximately 40 times (7), but in modern industrialized nations a women can expect to have approximately 450 periods in her lifetime (8). While decreased family size has significant obstetric benefits, the disadvantage is that menstrual disorders have become a relatively modern phenomenon for women and their clinicians. Assessment and evidence-based treatment of these common clinical complaints are underpinned by an understanding of menstrual physiology.

Menstrual physiology

Menstrual cycle physiology may be considered at different levels: hypothalamic, pituitary, ovarian, and endometrial (**Figure 40.1**). Peptide and steroid hormones provide cross-talk and feedback between these levels to regulate menstruation. The predominant hormones of the menstrual cycle are gonadotropin-releasing hormone (GnRH), follicle stimulating hormone (FSH), luteinizing hormone (LH), oestrogen (predominantly oestradiol), and progesterone (**Table 40.1**). Function of this endocrine system is affected by the stage of reproductive life.

Hypothalamic–pituitary regulation of ovarian function

The classical model of the menstrual cycle starts with the hypothalamus and GnRH (**Figure 40.2**). GnRH is produced and released from neurons in the arcuate nucleus of the medial-basal hypothalamus and the preoptic area of the ventral hypothalamus. It is released by axonal transport into the capillaries of the hypophyseal portal system for delivery to the anterior pituitary gland, where GnRH stimulates the synthesis and secretion of LH and FSH from the gonadotrophs.

GnRH is secreted in a pulsatile manner, which is an absolute prerequisite for normal adult reproductive function, including pubertal maturation and fertility (9, 10). The frequency and amplitude of GnRH secretion vary depending on the stage of reproductive life and across the menstrual cycle. In the normal cycling woman,

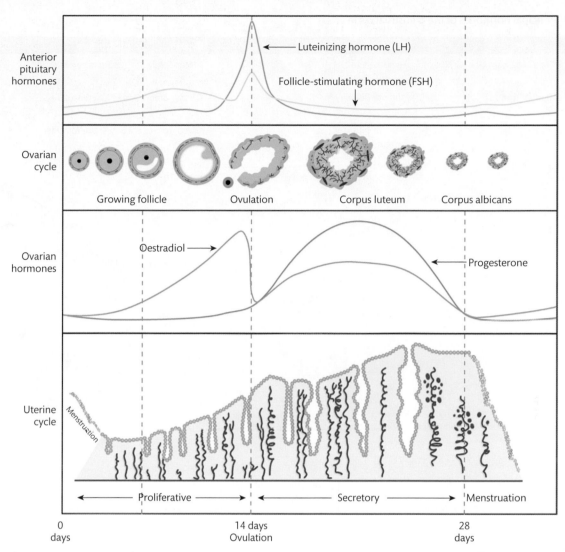

Figure 40.1 Schematic representation of pituitary and ovarian hormones across the menstrual cycle and the response of the ovary and endometrium.

GnRH pulses are of low amplitude, but increase in their frequency during the follicular phase, to a frequency of every 60 minutes during late follicular phase. High GnRH pulse frequency favours LH release, which is also secreted in pulses reflecting those of GnRH and is predominant over FSH in the late follicular phase necessary for ovulation. On the other hand, luteal phase is characterized by high amplitude and low frequency (approximately every 216 minutes) of pulsatile GnRH secretion. Low GnRH pulsatility stimulates FSH secretion, which is released in a more constitutive manner and is dominant over LH in the luteal and early follicular phase necessary for follicular development. Conversely, continuous GnRH exposure (such as with administration of GnRH analogues) results in desensitization of the gonadotrophs and suppression of LH and FSH secretion. Measurement of GnRH in peripheral circulation is difficult due to its short half-life (<3 minutes) and in portal blood is unsound ethically and practically in humans. LH pulses in the peripheral circulation therefore remain a widely used and well-validated surrogate of hypophyseal GnRH secretion.

Upon binding of GnRH to its cognate GnRH receptor (G-protein coupled receptor) on the gonadotrophs it activates phospholipase C and recruits secondary intracellular messengers, inositol triphosphate (IP_3) and diacylglycerol (DAG), which in turn mediate intracellular calcium release. This amplifies the downstream signalling cascade, resulting in transcription and translation of LH and FSH.

LH stimulates androgen production, the hormonal precursor for oestradiol, by binding to theca cells in the ovary; FSH promotes follicular growth, activates aromatase, and induces expression of LH receptors on the granulosa cell in preparation to respond to the preovulatory LH surge. The granulosa cells also produce inhibin B.

During the menstrual cycle GnRH and gonadotropin activity is highly regulated by ovarian feedback loops. In the follicular phase, oestrogen exerts negative feedback at the level of hypothalamus to suppress LH and FSH secretion. Inhibin B more selectively suppresses FSH secretion. However, in the late follicular phase, by yet unclear mechanisms, negative oestrogen feedback switches to positive oestrogen feedback, culminating in the preovulatory LH surge (and to a lesser extent a rise in FSH) necessary for ovulation. Following ovulation, progesterone from the corpus luteum mediates negative feedback to slow down GnRH pulse frequency and subsequently LH secretion. During the luteal phase, inhibin A also suppresses FSH levels. With demise of the corpus luteum in the absence

Table 40.1 Principal hormones of the menstrual cycle

	Source(s)	Type	Structure
Gonadotropin-releasing hormone (GnRH)	Hypothalamus (preoptic area)	Decapeptide	10 amino acids
Follicle-stimulating hormone (FSH)	Anterior pituitary (gonadotrophs)	Glycoprotein	204 amino acids
Luteinizing hormone (LH)	Anterior pituitary (gonadotrophs)	Glycoprotein	204 amino acids
Oestrogen (oestradiol)	Ovary (granulosa cells) Liver, adrenals, breasts, and adipose tissue	Sex steroid	18-carbon molecule
Progesterone	Ovary (theca cells, corpus luteum) Adrenal glands	Sex-steroid	21-carbon molecule

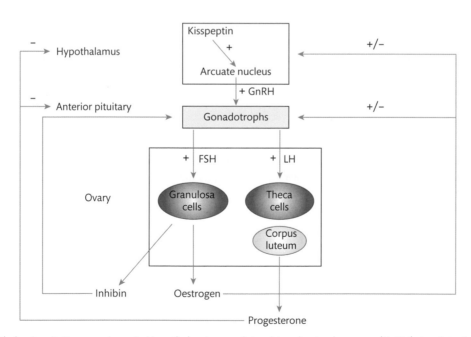

Figure 40.2 The hypothalamic–pituitary–ovarian axis. Hypothalamic gonadotrophin-releasing hormone (GnRH) signals to the anterior pituitary which in turn results in follicle-stimulating hormone (FSH) and luteinizing hormone (LH) secretion. These stimulate the ovary to produce oestradiol and progesterone to regulate the endometrial function. GnRH and gonadotropin signalling is tightly regulated by negative and positive gonadal-steroid loops and is further regulated by other hypothalamic neuropeptides (such as kisspeptin).

of pregnancy, gonadal steroid secretion declines, resulting in menstruation and stimulation of FSH secretion in response to a loss of negative sex-steroid feedback.

Prepubertal development of the HPO axis and menarche

The ovarian germ cells (oogonia) appear at around day 25, and then migrate to the developing gonad at around day 30 of gestation. They undergo meiosis and differentiate into primary oocytes, having arrested during the first meiotic division before entering prophase I.

Pulsatile GnRH secretion is observed during fetal life from around the 16th week of gestation with sustained gonadotropin and sex-steroid secretion. With advancing gestation, LH and FSH secretion is suppressed due to the negative sex-steroid feedback from the developing ovary. Withdrawal of placental steroids following delivery results in rebound GnRH and gonadotropin activity and persists into the early neonatal period. To distinguish this phenomenon from the true puberty, this phase is referred to as 'mini-puberty', where despite the secretion of gonadotropins and sex steroids, ovulation is not present. After the postnatal rise, pulsatile GnRH and gonadotropin secretion become quiescent throughout childhood, with some irregular and low-amplitude pulses, suppressing any activity of the now developed and responsive gonads.

With the onset of puberty there is a nocturnal increase in GnRH secretion and enhanced responsiveness of the pituitary. Slow GnRH pulsatility initially stimulates FSH secretion, resulting in ovarian follicular development and a multicystic appearance of the ovaries, and with the acceleration of GnRH pulsatility LH is secreted. This precedes any external manifestations of puberty by several years. The factors triggering this process are not yet fully elucidated but appear to be centrally regulated either by an activation of stimulatory signals or a suppression of inhibitory signals. Kisspeptin, a hypothalamic neuropeptide, is now recognized as key regulator of pulsatile GnRH secretion (**Figure 40.2**) (11). Its obligate role in human puberty was demonstrated by hypogonadotropic pubertal delay seen in patients with an inactivating mutation in kisspeptin (12) and its receptor (13, 14), and precocious puberty in those with activating mutations in the kisspeptin receptor (15).

The irregular nocturnal pattern of LH secretion gradually increases until regular LH pulses are established, occurring every 90 minutes irrespective of time of day. This results in the production of gonadal steroids and contribution to the development of external sexual characteristics (thelarche—onset of breast development). As circulating concentrations of oestrogens rise, positive feedback develops to induce a preovulatory LH surge with resultant ovulation and the first experience of menstruation (menarche). Of note, adrenarche (axillary and pubic hair growth) reflects the maturation of the hypothalamic–pituitary–adrenal axis. Many of the initial cycles may be anovulatory, which can contribute to the heavy and irregular menstrual bleeding that can affect some girls in adolescence. After 4–5 years the number of anovulatory cycles reduces from 90% to 20% with the consequent experience of more regular menstrual bleeds.

Menopause

Menopause marks the end of the female natural reproductive life and is a retrospective diagnosis based on the absence of periods for 1 year. It occurs when the supply of primordial follicles available for recruitment is exhausted. This process of follicle loss commences while the fetus and her developing gonads are still *in utero* (16–18). At the time of menopause there is a corresponding decline in circulating oestrogen levels and gonadotropin levels (FSH and LH) are elevated. In the perimenopausal transition, fluctuation in oestradiol levels may occur, giving rise to menstruation. While the majority of such cycles are anovulatory, spontaneous ovulation and occasionally pregnancy may occur.

Ovarian function

Ovarian function within the menstrual cycle can be broadly divided into the follicular phase, ovulation, luteal phase, and finally the luteal–follicular transition.

Follicular phase

Throughout ovarian life the oocytes reside within follicles. At any time point in the reproductive years there are follicles at different developmental stages within the ovary.

Initially, they are found in primordial follicles, consisting of a primary oocyte surrounded by a single flattened layer of granulosa cells. At the beginning of each menstrual cycle, a cohort of primordial follicles is activated to initiate growth, regulated by both stimulatory and inhibitory molecular signals. The follicles transition into primary follicles, with the granulosa cells becoming cuboidal in shape, before developing into larger preantral follicles. At this stage, the zona pellucida develops between the oocyte and granulosa cells and surrounding stromal cells differentiate to form the theca. Subsequently, the follicles enlarge, developing a fluid-filled cavity termed the antrum. Preantral and early antral follicles produce anti-Mullerian hormone, which appears to have an inhibitory effect on the growth of nearby primordial follicles, thus preventing their activation. This prevents the ovarian reserve being exhausted too quickly. Anti-Mullerian hormone is also therefore an indirect measure of ovarian reserve as it reflects how many growing follicles there are within the ovary—the higher the serum concentration of anti-Mullerian hormone, the greater the remaining number of follicles (19).

As the follicles grow they acquire FSH and LH receptors and become increasingly gonadotropin dependent, with antral follicles completely dependent on FSH for granulosa cell proliferation and LH for theca cell sex steroidogenesis. The largest follicle in the cohort is termed the dominant follicle, with all other growing follicles undergoing atresia. The dominant follicle produces oestradiol, resulting in a rapid rise in serum oestradiol concentration and consequent reduction in FSH and LH levels by negative feedback at the hypothalamus. This dominant follicle matures into a preovulatory follicle and expresses LH receptors on both granulosa and theca cells. There is a short period of positive feedback in the late follicular phase whereby increasing oestradiol levels result in a surge of LH. The preovulatory follicle responds to this surge by undergoing ovulation.

Ovulation

Following the LH surge and just prior to ovulation, the oocyte responds to its hormonal environment and re-enters meiosis, arresting at metaphase II resulting in a secondary oocyte and a polar body. The granulosa cells decrease oestradiol secretion as a result of decreased sensitivity to FSH. Progesterone production is initiated as a result of LH-driven increased cholesterol side-chain cleavage

(P450scc) levels. This enzyme is critical to steroidogenesis, particularly the conversion of cholesterol to pregnenolone. The rise in LH and FSH causes an increase in antral blood flow. This increased vascularity and local secretion of prostaglandins causes an increase in size of the follicle and it distends the surface of the ovary. Proteolytic enzymes are synthesized in the theca and activated by prostaglandins, causing degradation of the distended follicular wall followed by rupture of the follicle capsule. The oocyte, surrounded by the zona pellucida and attached granulosa cells, is ejected from the ruptured follicle. This occurs on approximately day 14 of the menstrual cycle. Under the influence of oestrogens prior to ovulation, increased tubal motility and elevated activity of the densely ciliated fimbriae allows approximation of the aperture of the distal fallopian tube to the ovary. This promotes passage of the expelled oocyte into the tube to be met by the ascending spermatozoa. If fertilization occurs, meiosis is completed.

Luteal phase

Following ovulation, the walls of the ovarian follicle collapse. Under the influence of LH both the theca and the granulosa cells proliferate and the latter develop into luteal cells. There is an influx of lipid droplets and lutein, which gives the corpus luteum its characteristic yellow appearance. Overall, the corpus luteum enlarges to around 15 mm. The oestrogen and progesterone secreted by the luteal cells negatively feed back to the anterior pituitary and levels of FSH and LH decrease. The corpus luteum is reliant on LH for progesterone production and luteolysis occurs in the absence of pregnancy as the mature corpus luteum becomes less sensitive to the remaining LH. This process remains incompletely understood, particularly with regard to the initiating trigger. In addition to reduced gonadotropins, luteolysis is likely a product of decreased LH sensitivity, altered progesterone receptor isoform ratios, and oestrogen receptor (ERα) levels [20, 21]. Demise of the corpus luteum begins at around day 24 and the corpus luteum is replaced by whitish scar tissue, the corpus albicans. Over subsequent cycles it is replaced by connective tissue, then absorbed.

Luteal–follicular transition

As the corpus luteum degenerates, circulating concentrations of oestradiol and progesterone rapidly decrease. As a result, FSH and LH plasma concentrations rise and a fresh group of follicles are recruited. The withdrawal of progesterone initiates menses.

Maintenance of the corpus luteum in pregnancy

In the event of conception, the developing embryo secretes human chorionic gonadotropin (hCG) from the syncytial trophoblast. This is detectable in maternal serum from around 8 days following conception. hCG rescues the corpus luteum, preventing menstruation and supporting early embryonic growth. Between 7 and 12 weeks' gestation, oestrogen and progesterone production shifts to the placenta and once the second trimester is entered, the corpus luteum slowly involutes and hCG levels decline.

If the corpus luteum is removed prior to 7 weeks' gestation then miscarriage almost inevitably occurs as a result of progesterone and oestrogen withdrawal. A similar effect can be induced by the use of progesterone antagonists such as mifepristone which underpins its use in the medical management of unwanted pregnancy.

Endometrial response to ovarian function

The endometrium consists of two functionally separate layers overlying the myometrium: functional and basal layers. The functional layer is shed during menses and the basal layer is preserved throughout. Both layers comprise glandular epithelial and stromal cells and the functional layer is covered by a surface epithelial layer. The constituent cells may express receptors for progesterone, oestrogen, and androgens as well as receptors for the glucocorticoid hormone, cortisol [22, 23]. The expression of the receptors varies depending on the stage of cycle. Occasional lymphoid follicles may be observed as well as a variety of leucocytes. The endometrium has a complex blood supply arising from the radial branches of the uterine artery and the ovarian vessels. There are both short, straight arteries which supply the basal layer and longer, spiral vessels supplying the whole of the endometrium. The spiral vessels connect with the venous system though capillary networks and direct arteriovenous communications.

The endometrial aspect of the menstrual cycle is divided into proliferative, secretory, and menstrual phases, broadly corresponding to the follicular, luteal, and luteal–follicular transition phases of the ovarian cycle. The classical histological description of the cycling endometrium dates from the 1950s [24] but for research purposes dating may be more robustly determined utilizing histological features combined with the date of the reported last menstrual period and measurement of serum oestradiol and progesterone. More recently, advances in molecular phenotyping have added a greater depth of understanding to the molecular and cellular events that underpin menstrual cycle stage and function [25].

Proliferative phase

Following menstruation, the exposed basal layer of the endometrium proliferates rapidly under the influence of rising oestradiol levels. Concurrently, the glandular cells within the endometrium expand: in the early proliferative phase the glandular cells are initially cuboidal and the glands themselves are small but by the late proliferative phase the glands are tortuous and the individual epithelial cells appear columnar. Proliferation is brisk and mitotic figures are observed (**Figure 40.3**). The stroma is compact throughout the proliferative phase and angiogenesis commences with elongation of the spiral arteries.

Secretory phase

Following ovulation, secretion of progesterone from the corpus luteum inhibits proliferation. The morphological changes associated with progesterone exposure develop between ovulation and approximately 48 hours after progesterone withdrawal (due to demise of the corpus luteum). The endometrial glands become more tortuous and acquire increased secretion of glycoproteins, evident as subnuclear vacuolation (a feature of the early secretory phase). Glandular nuclei move to the centre of cells and mitosis is suppressed. The endometrial spiral arterioles undergo remodelling to become increasingly coiled.

The spiral arterioles have a pivotal role at this time because if implantation is successful, the interaction with invading trophoblasts will play a crucial role in the onward pregnancy outcome.

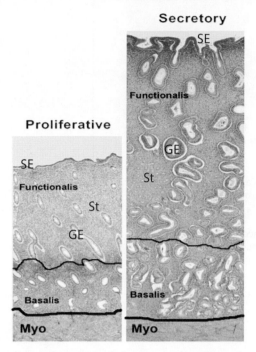

Figure 40.3 Endometrial morphology across the menstrual cycle. Proliferative and secretory endometrium. Surface epithelium (SE), glandular epithelium (GE), and stromal compartment (St) are marked. Note the increased tortuosity of glands in secretory phase and marked thickening of the functional layer.

Adapted from FM Horne and DL Blithe Progesterone receptor modulators and the endometrium: changes and consequences, *Hum Reprod Update* 2007;13:567–580.

Menstruation

In the absence of pregnancy the corpus luteum regresses, resulting in a rapid decrease in circulating progesterone and oestradiol. It is progesterone withdrawal that initiates menstruation (**Figure 40.4**). A local inflammatory response within the endometrium is characterized by cytokine release and infiltration of leucocytes with resultant oedema, activation of matrix metalloproteinases (MMPs), and lysis of the extracellular matrix. This culminates in the shedding of the upper two-thirds of the endometrium (the functional layer). The lower third of the endometrium (basal layer) remains *in situ* but has an exposed, raw mucosal surface that requires efficient repair.

Inflammatory mediators generated within the endometrium upon withdrawal of progesterone include prostaglandins, cyclooxygenase-2, MMPs, and interleukin-8 (**Figure 40.4**). Leucocyte traffic is initially neutrophil dominated although macrophage numbers also increase. Neutrophils contain high levels of MMPs and can activate tissue MMPs and play a critical role in the induction of endometrial shedding. Tight regulation of local endometrial events at the time and appropriate apoptosis is important to secure satisfactory onward endometrial repair. Macrophages are involved in both cytokine production and local remodelling of the endometrium and removal of debris and thus participate in both the breakdown and repair of the endometrium. Tight regulation of localized 'physiological' inflammation is critical to prevent excessive bleeding at menses (4, 26).

An intact endometrial coagulation system is also necessary for the efficient cessation of menstruation. Endometrial blood vessel injury initiates immediate activation and aggregation of platelets to form a 'plug'. Subsequently, fibrin is formed via the intrinsic and extrinsic coagulation cascade. Each pathway culminates in the conversion of factor X to Xa, which drives production of thrombin, ultimately leading to the formation of a stable fibrin clot to seal previously bleeding vessels (**Figure 40.5**) (4). Disorders that interfere with this systemic haemostasis have an impact on menstrual blood loss (see 'Overview of menstrual pathology') (**Figure 40.5**).

Conversely, fibrinolysis is the process of conversion of plasminogen to active plasmin, promoting the degradation of fibrin deposits. Tissue plasminogen activator (tPA) and urokinase plasminogen activator (uPA) drive the production of plasmin. In contrast, plasminogen activator inhibitor (PAI) inhibits fibrinolytic activity. The human endometrium contains tPA and uPA, as well as PAI and the uPA receptor (27, 28). Tight regulation to balance coagulation and fibrinolysis is necessary for normal menstruation.

The pivotal role of the coagulation system in menstruation is evidenced by the association between perturbation of this system and heavy menstrual bleeding (HMB). There is evidence that an overactive fibrinolytic system interferes with haemostasis and contributes to HMB. Women with HMB had raised levels of tPA activity on the second day of bleeding compared to those with normal loss (27). The efficacy of tranexamic acid as a treatment for HMB provides further evidence for overactivation of the fibrinolytic system in the endometrium of these women. The antifibrinolytic, tranexamic acid, reduces tPA and PAI levels in women with HMB and results in a 58% reduction in blood loss (29). Furthermore, up to 13% of women with a complaint of HMB will have von Willebrand disease (30).

During menstruation, the shed surface of the endometrium leads to bleeding from damaged vasculature. Factors influencing blood flow include length and radius of a blood vessel and the viscosity of blood. Of these, vessel radius is the dominant contributory factor (31). Therefore, the endometrium has evolved specialized spiral arterioles that have the ability to undergo intense vasoconstriction during the late secretory and menstrual phases to limit menstrual blood loss. Experiments examining the endometrial vasculature in the non-human primate (rhesus macaque) suggest that this vasoconstriction is so intense that the luminal portion of the endometrium becomes hypoxic during menses (32). There is mounting evidence that this hypoxia may trigger a cellular protective response to increase local repair factors and drive blood vessel and tissue regeneration (33, 34).

The clinical relevance of menstruation

Despite our increasing understanding of menstrual physiology, the mechanisms by which the denuded surface of the endometrium repairs without scarring or loss of function repeatedly throughout a woman's reproductive life remain unknown. The unique physiological inflammatory response, hypoxic insult, and tissue repair and regeneration are only superficially understood. Investigation of the control, regulation, and coordination of menstruation will lead to improved understanding of endometrial physiology and ultimately improve the clinical management of women with menstrual disorders. Furthermore, knowledge of the processes involved in efficient repair may be applied to other tissue sites where persistent inflammation and scarring lead to severe pathology.

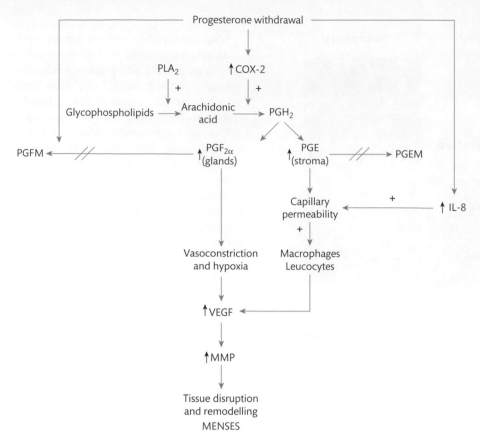

Figure 40.4 Impact of progesterone withdrawal on endometrial inflammation. Progesterone withdrawal in the late secretory phase drives local prostaglandin production. In addition, the withdrawal of progesterone inhibits breakdown of active prostaglandins resulting in a cascade of inflammation at menses. An increase in prostaglandins results in leucocyte influx, vasoconstriction of spiral arterioles, and resultant hypoxia. The process culminates in shedding of the functional layer of endometrium. COX-2, cyclooxygenase-2; IL-8, interleukin-8; MMP, matrix metalloproteinase; PGE, prostaglandin E; PGEM, prostaglandin E metabolites; PGF₂, prostaglandin F2 alpha; PGFM, prostaglandin F2 alpha metabolites; PGH₂, prostaglandin H2; PLA₂, phospholipase A2; VGEF, vascular endothelial growth factor.

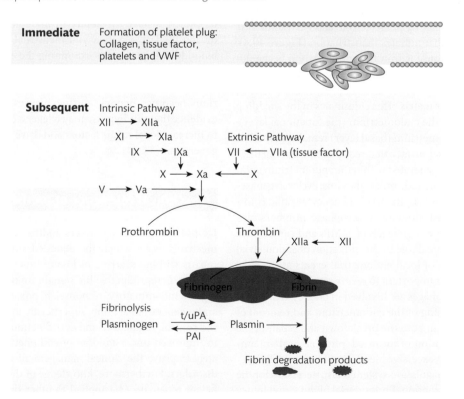

Figure 40.5 Intrinsic and extrinsic coagulation pathways lead to production of fibrin clot and haemostasis. Activation of fibrinolysis is necessary to break down the fibrin clot. Perturbation of these pathways may lead to AUB-C.

Reproduced from JA Maybin and HO Critchley, Menstrual physiology: implications for endometrial pathology and beyond, *Hum Reprod Update* 2015;21:748–761 (https://creativecommons.org/licenses/).

How can we study menstrual physiology?

Human studies

Endometrial tissue

Women frequently undergo hysterectomy for benign conditions. These include abnormal uterine bleeding (AUB), symptomatic fibroids, and uterine prolapse. With informed consent, patients may (anonymously) donate tissue sample surplus to routine histology for laboratory-based studies (molecular and cellular). Such uterine/endometrial tissue may be critically examined for detailed morphological assessment, protein localization with immunohistochemistry, and RNA extracted for gene expression studies (including gene array and more sophisticated sequencing). Furthermore, endometrium may be obtained using tissue samplers allowing serial collection of tissue from the same individual at different time points thereby allowing assessment of the effects of *in vivo* treatments without necessitating removal of the uterus.

Endometrial cells

Both epithelial and stromal cells may be extracted from endometrial tissue samples and cultured *in vitro*. This allows the opportunity for *in vitro* treatment to explore mechanism. Cells may be cultured separately or in co-culture which permits study of paracrine interactions between cell types and simulation of the *in vivo* environment.

Non-invasive imaging—ultrasonography, computed tomography, and magnetic resonance imaging

Imaging methods are well established in gynaecology. High-resolution transvaginal ultrasound scanning can facilitate assessment of follicle development and release as well as the study of endometrial thickness in response to circulating steroid hormones, and myometrial defects such as uterine fibroids and adenomyosis, that can cause menstrual disorders. Computed tomography is less used for the study of menstrual physiology but high-resolution magnetic resonance imaging permits non-invasive and non-ionizing assessment of the reproductive tract and the opportunity to study longitudinal changes over time. Developing modalities of magnetic resonance imaging such as diffusion, dynamic contrast, and functional protocols assessing water content and blood flow respectively are increasing our understanding of dynamic changes in the uterus/endometrium.

Animal models

There are many ethical and practical limitations to the studies that may be conducted on humans. To obtain incisive data on menstrual physiology for onward translation to clinical management, an animal model of menstruation is necessary.

Non-human primate (rhesus macaque)

Old world primates naturally menstruate but the major contribution of this non-human primate model has been due to the ability to exclude hormonal fluctuations that naturally occur between animals/women. Removal of the ovaries and sequential administration of oestradiol and progesterone mimics the human proliferative and secretory phases. Removal of progesterone initiates menstruation in a predictable fashion (35). This is attractive for experimental data

collection. This uniformity of hormone exposure allows a decreased number of animals to generate equally precise experimental data, a significant advantage over human studies.

Murine model of simulated menses

A species that does not naturally menstruate is not an immediately obvious model for studies on the mechanism of menstruation. However, simulating menstruation in the mouse by removal of ovaries, sequential hormone administration, and administration of oil to the uterus to encourage decidualization, results in a process analogous to menstrual bleeding. Various refinements of this model now exist, including pseudopregnancy to decidualize the uterus (36–38). The mouse has major advantages as an experimental model: a rapid breeding time to limit costs, ready availability of laboratory reagents, and the ability to easily perform genetic modifications to enable definitive experimental outcomes. These models have confirmed and increased our knowledge of menstruation and endometrial function.

Overview of menstrual pathology

Pathological disturbances of the menstrual cycle are predominantly reflected in altered bleeding patterns now considered under the umbrella term of abnormal uterine bleeding (AUB). In addition, onset of menarche can be both premature and delayed as can the final cessation of menses (discussed in Chapter 46).

Abnormal uterine bleeding

Chronic AUB is defined as 'bleeding from the uterine corpus that is abnormal in volume, regularity and/or timing that has been present for the majority of the last 6 months' (39, 40).

Normal bleeding patterns are those considered within the 5–95th percentiles (Table 40.2) (39, 40). For the parameter of volume, greater than 80 mL is considered abnormal. However, in clinical practice, objective measurement of loss is redundant, rather a more patient-centred approach is used to define HMB: 'excessive menstrual blood loss which interferes with a woman's physical, social, emotional and/or material quality of life' (41).

Classification of abnormal uterine bleeding

A structured classification of the causes of AUB has been developed by the Fédération International de Gynécologie et d'Obstétrique (FIGO), summarized by the acronym PALM COEIN (Table 40.3) (40).

PALM represents the structural and COEIN the non-structural causes of AUB. It is recommended that the term dysfunctional uterine bleeding (DUB) is discarded. 'DUB' is usually encompassed by AUB-C, -O, or –E.

As well as standardizing nomenclature and definitions of normality, it is hoped that the AUB 'PALM-COEIN' classification system will provide a structured approach to clinical assessment and diagnosis. By the discarding of Latin and Greek derivatives there may be demedicalization of menstrual dysfunction to empower women and decrease the taboos surrounding menstruation, thus reducing the barriers to effective care. Furthermore, by standardizing patient groups with respect to causation it will facilitate research and meta-analyses.

Table 40.2 Suggested normal limits for menstrual parameters

Clinical parameter	Descriptive term	Normal limits (5–95th percentiles)
Frequency of menses (days)	Frequent Normal Infrequent	<24 24–38 >38
Regularity of menses, cycle to cycle (variation in days over 12 months)	Absent Regular Irregular	No bleeding Variation ± 2–20 days Variation >20 days
Duration of flow (days)	Prolonged Normal Shortened	>8.0 4.5–8.0 <4.5
Volume of monthly blood loss (mL)	Heavy Normal Light	>80 5–80 <5

Adapted from Fraser IS, Critchley HO, Broder M, Munro MG. The FIGO recommendations on terminologies and definitions for normal and abnormal uterine bleeding. *Semin Reprod Med.* 2011;29(5):383–390.

Table 40.3 FIGO classification of causes of abnormal uterine bleeding: 'PALM COEIN'

Structural	
Polyp (AUB-P)	Both endometrial and endocervical polyps may contribute to AUB
Adenomyosis (AUB-A)	Both focal and diffuse
Leiomyoma (AUB-L)	Predominantly submucosal and intramural fibroids
Malignancy (AUB-M)	This includes endometrial hyperplasia as well frank endometrial, cervical malignancy, and uterine sarcoma
Non-structural	
Coagulopathy (AUB-C)	von Willebrand disease, disorders of clotting factors, idiopathic thrombocytopenic purpura, platelet storage and release disorders Anticoagulant and antiplatelet medication
Ovulatory disorders (AUB-O)	Extremes of reproductive age Disorders affecting HPO axis: polycystic ovary syndrome, thyroid disease, hyperprolactinaemia, obesity, anorexia, weight loss, mental stress, and extreme exercise Drugs affecting dopamine
Endometrial (AUB-E)	Abnormalities at the endometrial level of molecular and cellular mechanisms regulating the blood lost at menstruation
Iatrogenic (AUB-I)	Oestrogen or progestogen therapy Drugs acting on ovarian steroid release such as GnRH analogues, and aromatase inhibitors SPRMs and SERMs IUS/IUCD-associated endometritis
Not otherwise classified (AUB-N)	Chronic endometritis (non-IUS/IUCD related) AV malformations and pseudoaneurysms Myometrial hypertrophy

AV, arteriovenous; IUS/IUCD, intrauterine system/intrauterine contraceptive device; SERMs, selective oestrogen receptor modulators; SPRMs, selective progesterone receptor modulators.
Adapted from Munro MG, Critchley HO, Fraser IS. The FIGO classification of causes of abnormal uterine bleeding: Malcolm G. Munro, Hilary O.D. Critchley, Ian S. Fraser, for the FIGO Working Group on Menstrual Disorders. *Int J Gynaecol Obstet.* 2011;113(1):3–13.

The most frequent presentation of AUB is HMB. This is a common condition, affecting 20–30% of women of reproductive age and in the United Kingdom is estimated to be the fourth most common reason women are referred to gynaecological services (42). In those with unpredictable bleeding, there may be an ovulatory, iatrogenic, or 'not otherwise classified' cause or a structural abnormality such as a polyp or underlying malignancy; typically those with AUB-A, -L, -C, and –E have predictable HMB.

General principles of management

Specific abnormalities of the menstrual cycle and their management are covered in more detail in Chapter 41. The approach to a woman presenting with perturbation of the menstrual cycle should be patient centred and encompass her contraceptive and reproductive needs and well as reflecting comorbidities and secondary health promotion, particularly with respect to bone mineral density, smoking cessation, cervical screening, and breast examination/enquiry.

Assessment

An accurate history can often identify those with a likely AUB-C, -O, or I as an underlying cause. In particular, a potential coagulopathy may be identified by structured questioning in up to 90% of cases (43, 44). Contributors to AUB-C and -O often then require specific function tests such as to von Willebrand factor and thyroid function tests respectively if pathology is suspected. Imaging, selected histopathology, and direct visualization through hysteroscopy will allow diagnosis of a structural cause ('PALM') or AUB-N. Hysteroscopy in particular may have greater utility than ultrasound scanning in distinguishing between those with AUB-P and submucosal fibroids and offers opportunity for concurrent resection (45). The United Kingdom National Institute for Health and Care Excellence recommends endometrial sampling (outpatient or hysteroscopic) in those with persistent intermenstrual bleeding or age 45 years and older with treatment failure (41), but the Royal College of Obstetricians and Gynaecologists advises sampling those with treatment failure aged 40 years and older (46). With the rise in incidence of endometrial cancer, sampling should be considered on a case-by-case basis in younger women with risk factors for malignancy such as polycystic ovary syndrome, obesity, and type 2 diabetes. AUB-E remains a diagnosis of exclusion as tests of endometrial dysfunction remain the preserve of research studies and there is a current lack of effective biomarkers.

Other investigations aside from imaging and selected endometrial sampling include assessment for anaemia. Tests such as measurement of thyroid function, gonadotropin and prolactin levels, coagulopathy studies, and testing for evidence of chlamydial infection (in those women with intermenstrual bleeding) should be restricted to women who present with relevant symptomatology.

Treatment strategies

For those women with AUB without an infective or a malignant cause, a conservative approach may be adopted with iron replacement for correction of anaemia if required. For those wishing for active treatment, this should be tailored depending on current and future fertility desires and comorbidities. Mefenamic acid and tranexamic acid are the only non-hormonal medical treatments currently available. For women who are not actively seeking pregnancy, the levonorgestrel-releasing intrauterine system (LNG-IUS) remains the first line of treatment (41). However a significant proportion will discontinue treatment either through lack of efficacy or undesirable side effects (47). Alternative hormonal treatments include the combined oral contraceptive pill, progestin-only pill, cyclical progestins, and GnRH analogues (41). For women with AUB and fibroids, myomectomy, uterine artery embolization, and medical management with selective progesterone receptor modulators offer preservation of future fertility potential.

For those women for whom fertility is no longer required, surgical management may be offered and has higher overall patient satisfaction (48). This may be in the form of endometrial ablation (destruction of the endometrium) or hysterectomy. Hysterectomy remains the only definitive treatment for HMB but has higher risks compared to ablation. Therefore, the largest meta-analysis to date concludes that less high-risk surgical procedures should be offered as a first line if surgical intervention is considered (49).

Summary

As a greater understanding of the menstrual cycle biology is garnered, therapies that directly target pathways underpinning the regulation of normal and HMB (e.g. inflammation, angiogenesis, and coagulation) are likely to emerge. Such future targeted therapies have the potential to offer a more personalized approach to management with minimization of undesirable side effects.

Acknowledgements

The authors are most grateful to Mrs Sheila Milne for her assistance with manuscript preparation and Mr Ronnie Grant for his help with the preparation of illustrations. They also wish to thank Dr Cheryl Dunlop for her helpful comments on sections of the manuscript pertaining to ovarian function.

REFERENCES

1. Finn CA. Why do women menstruate? Historical and evolutionary review. *Eur J Obstet Gynecol Reprod Biol* 1996;**70**:3–8.
2. Strassmann BI. The evolution of endometrial cycles and menstruation. *Q Rev Biol* 1996;**71**:181–220.
3. Finn CA. Menstruation: a nonadaptive consequence of uterine evolution. *Q Rev Biol* 1998;**73**:163–73.
4. Maybin JA, Critchley HO. Menstrual physiology: implications for endometrial pathology and beyond. *Hum Reprod Update* 2015;**21**:748–61.
5. Crawford P. Attitudes to menstruation in seventeenth-century England. *Past Present* 1981;**91**:47–73.
6. Sharma S. Women hail menstruating ruling. *BBC News* 15 September 2005. Available at: http://news.bbc.co.uk/1/hi/world/south_asia/4250506.stm.
7. Short RV. The evolution of human reproduction. *Proc R Soc Lond B Biol Sci* 1976;**195**:3–24.
8. Chavez-MacGregor M, van Gils CH, van der Schouw YT, Monninkhof E, van Noord PA, Peeters PH. Lifetime cumulative number of menstrual cycles and serum sex hormone levels in postmenopausal women. *Breast Cancer Res Treat* 2008;**108**:101–12.
9. Fraser HM, Baird DT. Clinical applications of LHRH analogues. *Baillieres Clin Endocrinol Metab* 1987;**1**:43–70.
10. Maggi R, Cariboni AM, Marelli MM, et al. GnRH and GnRH receptors in the pathophysiology of the human female reproductive system. *Hum Reprod Update* 2016;**22**:358–81.
11. Skorupskaite K, George JT, Anderson RA. The kisspeptin-GnRH pathway in human reproductive health and disease. *Hum Reprod Update* 2014;**20**:485–500.
12. Topaloglu AK, Tello JA, Kotan LD, et al. Inactivating KISS1 mutation and hypogonadotropic hypogonadism. *N Engl J Med* 2012;**366**:629–35.
13. de Roux N, Genin E, Carel JC, Matsuda F, Chaussain JL, Milgrom E. Hypogonadotropic hypogonadism due to loss of function of the KiSS1-derived peptide receptor GPR54. *Proc Natl Acad Sci U S A* 2003;**100**:10972–76.
14. Seminara SB, Messager S, Chatzidaki EE, et al. The GPR54 gene as a regulator of puberty. *N Engl J Med* 2003;**349**:1614–27.
15. Teles MG, Bianco SD, Brito VN, et al. A GPR54-activating mutation in a patient with central precocious puberty. *N Engl J Med* 2008;**358**:709–15.
16. Block E. Quantitative morphological investigations of the follicular system in women; methods of quantitative determinations. *Acta Anat (Basel)* 1951;**12**:267–85.
17. Block E. Quantitative morphological investigations of the follicular system in women; variations at different ages. *Acta Anat (Basel)* 1952;**14**:108–23.
18. Block E. A quantitative morphological investigation of the follicular system in newborn female infants. *Acta Anat (Basel)* 1953;**17**:201–206.
19. Ledger WL. Clinical utility of measurement of anti-mullerian hormone in reproductive endocrinology. *J Clin Endocrinol Metab* 2010;**95**:5144–54.
20. Stouffer RL, Bishop CV, Bogan RL, Xu F, Hennebold JD. Endocrine and local control of the primate corpus luteum. *Reprod Biol* 2013;**13**:259–71.
21. Niswender GD, Juengel JL, Silva PJ, Rollyson MK, McIntush EW. Mechanisms controlling the function and life span of the corpus luteum. *Physiol Rev* 2000;**80**:1–29.
22. McDonald SE, Henderson TA, Gomez-Sanchez CE, Critchley HO, Mason JI. 11Beta-hydroxysteroid dehydrogenases in human endometrium. *Mol Cell Endocrinol* 2006;**248**:72–78.
23. Critchley HO, Saunders PT. Hormone receptor dynamics in a receptive human endometrium. *Reprod Sci* 2009;**16**:191–99.
24. Noyes RW, Hertig AT, Rock J. Dating the endometrial biopsy. *Fertil Steril* 1950;**1**:3–25
25. Talbi S, Hamilton AE, Vo KC, et al. Molecular phenotyping of human endometrium distinguishes menstrual cycle phases and underlying biological processes in normo-ovulatory women. *Endocrinology* 2006;**147**:1097–121.
26. Jabbour HN, Kelly RW, Fraser HM, Critchley HO. Endocrine regulation of menstruation. *Endocr Rev* 2006;**27**:17–46.
27. Gleeson N, Devitt M, Sheppard BL, Bonnar J. Endometrial fibrinolytic enzymes in women with normal menstruation and dysfunctional uterine bleeding. *Br J Obstet Gynaecol* 1993;**100**:768–71.
28. Nordengren J, Pilka R, Noskova V, et al. Differential localization and expression of urokinase plasminogen activator (uPA), its receptor (uPAR), and its inhibitor (PAI-1) mRNA and protein in endometrial tissue during the menstrual cycle. *Mol Hum Reprod* 2004;**10**:655–63.
29. Gleeson NC, Buggy F, Sheppard BL, Bonnar J. The effect of tranexamic acid on measured menstrual loss and endometrial fibrinolytic

enzymes in dysfunctional uterine bleeding. *Acta Obstet Gynecol Scand* 1994;**73**:274–77.

30. Shankar M, Lee CA, Sabin CA, Economides DL, Kadir RA. von Willebrand disease in women with menorrhagia: a systematic review. *BJOG* 2004;**111**:734–40.

31. Maybin JA, Critchley HO, Jabbour HN. Inflammatory pathways in endometrial disorders. *Mol Cell Endocrinol* 2011;**335**:42–51.

32. Markee JE. Menstruation in intraocular transplants in the rhesus monkey. *Contrib Embryol* 1940;**28**:219–308.

33. Maybin JA, Battersby S, Hirani N, Nikitenko LL, Critchley HO, Jabbour HN. The expression and regulation of adrenomedullin in the human endometrium: a candidate for endometrial repair. *Endocrinology* 2011;**152**:2845–56.

34. Maybin JA, Hirani N, Brown P, Jabbour HN, Critchley HO. The regulation of vascular endothelial growth factor by hypoxia and prostaglandin F2α during human endometrial repair. *J Clin Endocrinol Metab* 2011;**96**:2475–83.

35. Brenner RM, Slayden OD. Molecular and functional aspects of menstruation in the macaque. *Rev Endocr Metab Disord* 2012;**13**:309–18.

36. Finn CA, Pope M. Vascular and cellular changes in the decidualized endometrium of the ovariectomized mouse following cessation of hormone treatment: a possible model for menstruation. *J Endocrinol* 1984;**100**:295–300.

37. Brasted M, White CA, Kennedy TG, Salamonsen LA. Mimicking the events of menstruation in the murine uterus. *Biol Reprod* 2003;**69**:1273–80.

38. Cousins FL, Murray A, Esnal A, Gibson DA, Critchley HO, Saunders PT. Evidence from a mouse model that epithelial cell migration and mesenchymal-epithelial transition contribute to rapid restoration of uterine tissue integrity during menstruation. *PLoS One* 2014;**9**:e86378.

39. Fraser IS, Critchley HO, Broder M, Munro MG. The FIGO recommendations on terminologies and definitions for normal and abnormal uterine bleeding. *Semin Reprod Med* 2011;**29**:383–90.

40. Munro MG, Critchley HO, Fraser IS. The FIGO classification of causes of abnormal uterine bleeding: Malcolm G. Munro, Hilary O.D. Critchley, Ian S. Fraser, for the FIGO Working Group on Menstrual Disorders. *Int J Gynaecol Obstet* 2011;**113**:3–13.

41. National Institute for Health and Care Excellence (NICE). *Heavy Menstrual Bleeding.* Clinical guideline [CG44]. London: NICE; 2007. Available at: https://www.nice.org.uk/guidance/CG44.

42. Royal College of Obstetricians and Gynaecologists (RCOG). *National Heavy Menstrual Bleeding Audit—First Annual Report.* London: RCOG; 2011. Available at: https://www.rcog.org.uk/globalassets/documents/guidelines/research--audit/nationalhmbaudit_1stannualreport_may2011.pdf.

43. Kadir RA, Economides DL, Sabin CA, Owens D, Lee CA. Frequency of inherited bleeding disorders in women with menorrhagia. *Lancet* 1998;**351**:485–89.

44. Kouides PA, Conard J, Peyvandi F, Lukes A, Kadir R. Hemostasis and menstruation: appropriate investigation for underlying disorders of hemostasis in women with excessive menstrual bleeding. *Fertil Steril* 2005;**84**:1345–51.

45. Mahmud A, Smith P, Clark J. The role of hysteroscopy in diagnosis of menstrual disorders. *Best Pract Res Clin Obstet Gynaecol* 2015;**29**:898–907.

46. Royal College of Obstetricians and Gynaecologists (RCOG). *Standards for Gynaecology—Report of a Working Party.* London: RCOG; 2008. Available at: https://www.rcog.org.uk/globalassets/documents/guidelines/wprgynstandards2008.pdf.

47. Gupta JK, Daniels JP, Middleton LJ, et al. A randomised controlled trial of the clinical effectiveness and cost-effectiveness of the levonorgestrel-releasing intrauterine system in primary care against standard treatment for menorrhagia: the ECLIPSE trial. *Health Technol Assess* 2015;**19**:i–xxv, 1–118.

48. Royal College of Obstetricians and Gynaecologists (RCOG). *National Heavy Menstrual Bleeding Audit—Final Report.* London: RCOG; 2014. Available at: https://www.rcog.org.uk/globalassets/documents/guidelines/research--audit/national_hmb_audit_final_report_july_2014.pdf.

49. Marjoribanks J, Lethaby A, Farquhar C. Surgery versus medical therapy for heavy menstrual bleeding. *Cochrane Database Syst Rev* 2016;**1**:CD003855.

41

Menstrual disorders, amenorrhea, and dysmenorrhoea

Ian S. Fraser and Marina Berbic

Abnormal uterine \bleeding

Introduction to abnormal uterine bleeding

Menstruation is a unique physiological event, occurring approximately once each month for the major part of a woman's reproductive phase of life. The 'reproductive phase' begins at the menarche, the first menstrual period that a young woman will experience, and continues through to the menopause, the last natural menstruation that a woman experiences. The average age of menarche is around 12 years, and the average age of menopause is around 52 years. This means that a woman in modern Western society, experiencing 28-day menstrual cycles, could total as many as 500 menstrual periods in her reproductive lifetime. In fact, this is unlikely to occur because many factors will influence a woman's menstrual cycle at different stages of her life, of which pregnancy and breastfeeding are the most obvious.

An understanding of normal menstruation and the normal menstrual cycle and the various factors which can influence them is critical to determining whether a woman is experiencing abnormal uterine bleeding (AUB) at any one point in time. The patterns of normal menstrual bleeding vary greatly from menarche to menopause, with considerable irregularity and intermittent long cycles being common within the first 2–5 years after menarche and the last 2–5 years before menopause. The menopause is defined as the last natural menstrual period that a woman experiences, a point which can only be determined 1 year later, when no further menstruation has occurred. It needs to be emphasized that there is great variability in normality of menstrual cycles between women, and in some individual women from one phase of their lifetime to another (1). Variability tends to be greater at the extremes of reproductive life.

FIGO recommendations on menstrual terminologies and definitions

Fifteen years ago, understanding of the clinical field of AUB was confused and poorly defined (2). As a consequence, an international meeting of experts was held in Washington DC, United States, 2005 to review all aspects of the definitions, descriptions, terminologies, and causes of AUB. These experts took part in a Delphi process before the conference and then a re-vote (anonymously) on the issues after 3 days of small group and open discussions (3). The agreements by the group were close to unanimous. These included an agreement to abandon a wide range of older, obsolete, and poorly defined menstrual terminologies (**Box 41.1**), and to replace these with simple English terms which can be easily translated into other languages, and which can be understood by women and men in the community (**Box 41.2**).

The three main terms recommended for exclusion from further international use were 'menorrhagia', 'metrorrhagia' (terms of Greek and Latin origin used in the English language without clear definition) and 'dysfunctional uterine bleeding' (a term from the 1930s which was never clearly defined and was an admission of ignorance, which can now be replaced by a much more precise description of three defined underlying causes). These three abandoned terms have all been used in the past to describe both the symptoms and underlying causes of AUB, a very confusing situation! The list of archaic and abandoned terms is included in **Box 41.1**.

Responsibility for the veracity and the educational promotion of this major exercise in revising definitions, terminologies, and causes of abnormal bleeding was accepted by the International Federation of Gynecology and Obstetrics (Fédération Internationale de Gynécologic et d'Obstétrique (FIGO)) (3, 4), and this flexible system has been reviewed and revised on a triennial basis by FIGO since its introduction (known as the FIGO AUB System 1 (description of symptoms)).

The components of normal and abnormal menstrual cycles and menstruation can be clearly defined by a group of four criteria (**Box 41.3**): these criteria all relate to the varied symptoms of normal and AUB (**Box 41.2**):

1. *Regularity* of successive episodes of menstruation (this includes 'variability').
2. *Frequency* of successive episodes of menstruation.
3. *Duration* of each bleeding episode.
4. *Volume* of bleeding, as perceived by the woman on different days of her menstruation.

The limits of each of these parameters in 'normal' menstrual cycles have been clearly defined, based on 5th and 95th percentiles

Box 41.1 Menstrual terminologies which are now obsolete and should no longer be used

They have never been well defined and were used in a very confused manner:

- Menorrhagia (including combination terminology, such as essential menorrhagia, idiopathic menorrhagia, primary menorrhagia, functional menorrhagia, ovulatory menorrhagia, and anovulatory menorrhagia)
- Hypermenorrhoea
- Uterine haemorrhage
- Metropathia haemorrhagica
- Metrorrhagia
- Hypomenorrhoea
- Menometrorrhagia
- Polymenorrhoea
- Polymenorrhagia
- Epimenorrhoea
- Epimenorrhagia
- Functional uterine bleeding
- Dysfunctional uterine bleeding

from population studies (**Box 41.3**). These 'normal limits' have thus allowed the definition of specific abnormalities of uterine bleeding. The Washington experts determined that the overarching term to describe any abnormality of the symptoms of uterine bleeding should be AUB.

Patterns of abnormal uterine bleeding

The most troublesome and frequent patterns of AUB are:

- heavy menstrual bleeding (HMB)
- irregular menstrual bleeding
- prolonged menstrual bleeding
- intermenstrual bleeding
- infrequent or absent menstrual bleeding.

These bleeding patterns are also the commonest departures from the normal limits defined in **Box 41.3**. Sometimes these patterns combine together to provide a more problematic symptom complex. For example, heavy and prolonged episodes of bleeding are often seen in the same woman. Complaints of HMB with or without prolonged bleeding are about ten times more common than complaints of prolonged bleeding on its own.

Box 41.2 Modern descriptive terminologies around menstruation

- Abnormal uterine bleeding (AUB): the overarching symptom.
- Heavy menstrual bleeding (HMB) (replaces 'menorrhagia' and 'hypermenorrhoea').
- Irregular menstrual bleeding (replaces 'metrorrhagia').
- Prolonged menstrual bleeding.
- Infrequent menstrual bleeding (replaces 'oligomenorrhoea').
- Amenorrhoea (absent menstrual bleeding; retained).
- Inter-menstrual bleeding (bleeding in between periods; retained).
- Dysfunctional uterine bleeding is replaced by better defined underlying causes: AUB-C, AUB-O, and AUB-E.

Box 41.3 Parameters of normal menstruation and the menstrual cycle

- *Regularity* of successive episodes of menstruation; variation of less than 7 to 9 days difference between the shortest and longest cycles.
- *Frequency* of successive episodes of menstruation (24–38 days).
- *Duration* of each bleeding episode (up to 8 days in a single period).
- *Volume* of each bleeding episode (as perceived by the woman on different days of menstruation); less than 80 mL.
- *Variability* of any of these parameters can be disturbing for many women.
- Any repeated departure outside these limits is known as *abnormal uterine bleeding*.

Heavy menstrual bleeding

This is one of the commonest and most troublesome complaints of AUB. It is a particularly difficult symptom to evaluate because the volume of menstrual bleeding is impossible to assess accurately without awkward laboratory research assays. In addition, women do not generally discuss details of their menstrual periods with each other, and therefore do not have any good framework of reference to assess their own experiences. On the other hand, this avoidance of discussing menstruation may now be changing with the intense modern focus on social media by young people. Many young women are now sharing information about themselves with their friends in a way that was almost unheard of a decade ago. In some countries, this is leading to a new social movement among educated young women for a 'bleed-free' existence (through the use of tailored hormonal contraceptive regimens to cause pharmacological amenorrhoea) until they are ready to try for a pregnancy.

There are two definitions of HMB

See **Box 41.4**.

The research definition of HMB In the research situation, HMB is defined as a monthly blood loss of greater than 80 mL. This limit has been determined by population studies using objective laboratory measurements of menstrual losses of carefully collected sanitary pads and tampons in general female communities in Sweden and the United Kingdom (5, 6). The laboratory alkaline haematin technique measures the amount of haemoglobin in each sample. The 80 mL upper limit was set by study of circulating iron and haemoglobin parameters indicating that haemoglobin and serum iron were significantly lower in these women. This research technique is not suitable for use in the clinic.

The routine clinical definition of HMB In the clinical situation, HMB should be defined as 'excessive menstrual blood loss, which

Box 41.4 Definitions of heavy menstrual bleeding

- *Research definition of heavy menstrual bleeding*: in most menstrual cycles the measured menstrual blood loss should exceed 80 mL.
- *Clinical definition of heavy menstrual bleeding*: 'Excessive menstrual blood loss, which interferes with the woman's physical, emotional, social and material quality of life, and which can occur alone or in combination with other symptoms.'
- Any intervention should improve quality of life.

interferes with the woman's physical, emotional, social and material quality of life, and which can occur alone or in combination with other symptoms'. Any interventions should therefore aim to improve quality of life measures (7). The woman with HMB presents with a complaint that reflects her perception of the abnormality of her menstrual flow, and as such, her clinical problem requires management. This is a valuable clinical definition, which provides a sound basis for therapy.

Some important clinical messages about HMB

* *Composition of the menstrual flow*: the total menstrual flow is composed of around 50% of venous (and some arteriolar) blood and 50% of an endometrial transudate, hence it is 'very dilute blood'. The research measurement limits of 80 mL of 'whole blood' are based on measurement of haemoglobin lost (in order to assess how much risk the woman faces from her blood loss), so the woman is probably losing and 'seeing' double the volume of fluid that the doctor has in mind.

* *Lack of awareness that periods are abnormally heavy*: many women with HMB are unaware that their menstrual periods are abnormally heavy, and do not complain until they have a really excessive episode of loss.

* *Complaint of HMB when periods are actually normal*: by contrast, there are also many women who complain of heavy bleeding when their measured loss would be within the normal range. This indicates that they probably have experienced a change in their menstrual period, which needs assessment.

* *Women with HMB and menstrual pain are more likely to complain*: those women who have pelvic pain (or other perimenstrual symptoms) accompanying their heavy bleeding are more likely to complain of their HMB, suggesting that they have significantly greater difficulty coping with a combination of symptoms, rather than with the HMB on its own.

* *Cultural differences*: women from different cultures may view their menstrual experiences in different ways. In many countries, women regard a heavy red bleed as a 'good thing', reflecting a thorough 'clean out' of body impurities, when in reality, this red bleed is more likely to signify a heavier period, which may be increasing a woman's risk of developing iron deficiency, especially if she comes from a background of inadequate dietary iron intake. This same woman may find the brownish menstrual loss at the end of her period to be unhealthy looking and unpleasant (especially if it is prolonged in any way), when it is actually a reflection of very light bleeding with healthy partial metabolism of haemoglobin before it reaches the vagina.

* *Hazards of HMB*: the hazards of HMB are mainly twofold. Firstly, a regular monthly loss of greater than 80 mL of 'whole blood' significantly increases that woman's risk of developing iron deficiency (a reduction in circulating levels of serum ferritin—the best reflection of body iron stores) (**Box 41.5**) and a reduction of serum transferrin saturation—the best reflection of circulating 'available' iron, which is in a form immediately accessible by cells in need). Iron deficiency is probably a much greater problem for quality of life than widely recognized, because of the additional troublesome symptoms which it brings. Secondly, other quality of life measures are disturbed by the overlapping symptoms both from HMB and iron deficiency, and by the social problem of 'containment' of the excessive flow.

> **Box 41.5** Definitions and assessment of iron deficiency
>
> * Haemoglobin (to assess anaemia in a non-pregnant woman; should be <120 g/L).
> * Full blood count and film (to assess microcytic and hypochromic changes; and to include a platelet count).
> * Serum ferritin (ferritin is the best measure of iron stores, and should be >30 ng/mL; a measure of <15 ng/mL is severe iron deficiency).
> * Serum transferrin saturation (this is the best measure of available iron in the circulation (<20% indicates deficiency).

* *Variability in menstrual flow*: many women experience considerable variability in their menstrual flow. This variability is more common in the later reproductive years. Women may only experience very heavy bleeds every second or third month, and the worst 'heaviness' may only affect 1 or 2 days in those menstrual periods. Some women are unable to predict in advance which days of their periods may become very heavy, and hence have to stay close to home or use additional sanitary protection throughout their period, based on occasional very heavy 'risk'.

* *Clinical presentations of HMB*: presentation to a doctor may be as an 'acute and severe' or as a chronic problem. FIGO has defined these as follows:
  * *Chronic AUB* is bleeding from the uterine body that is abnormal in duration, volume, regularity, and/or frequency and has been present at least for the majority of the past 6 months.
  * *Acute and severe AUB* is an episode of bleeding that is of sufficient quantity to require immediate intervention to prevent further blood loss. Such acute bleeding will often be found to have occurred on a previously noted chronic basis.

  These presentations will generally require different approaches to investigation and management.

* Other patterns of AUB:
  * *Prolonged menstrual bleeding* is bleeding of greater than 8 days' duration. This is much less common than HMB, and may occur on its own or in combination with HMB. It is also frequently associated with iron deficiency.
  * *Irregular menstrual bleeding* is said to occur when there is a variability of more than 9 days in cycle length between the shortest and the longest cycle that a woman experiences within a year.

Intermenstrual bleeding

This symptom has normal and abnormal components. It is usually a symptom of light bleeding occurring between two otherwise fairly normal menstrual periods, and can occur at any time in between these two periods. It can be 'normal' when a small amount of clinically detectable bleeding appears at around the time of ovulation. This can be found with careful observation in 9% of regularly cycling women, and is thought to be due to the natural drop in circulating oestradiol levels at around mid cycle. On the other hand, significant intermenstrual bleeding can be a reflection of pathology within the reproductive tract, and should be investigated to exclude endometrial or endocervical polyps, early malignancy, and endocervical or endometrial infection (especially with chlamydia).

Infrequent or absent menstrual bleeding

(See later sections on amenorrhoea.)

- *Triggers for 'complaint'*: overall, women are more likely to present to their doctor with a complaint of AUB (typically HMB) if more than one symptom occurs at the same time, especially when pain accompanies HMB.
- *Menstrual mythology*: mistaken beliefs about menstruation are still rife in most communities around the world. These myths mostly began in primitive societies, and have generally been associated with 'fear' of this mysterious process, especially by men. Hence, in primitive cultures, menstruating women have often been placed in seclusion in isolated 'menstrual huts' to protect the men and the tribe from the 'damaging power' of the menstrual blood. So, these menstruating women were not allowed to cook, have sexual intimacy, or take part in communal activities. Negative views of menstruation are still prevalent in many societies, but others have come to believe, erroneously, that a heavy red monthly bleed is healthy for the woman because it results in a more effective 'clean out' of body impurities. However, this does mean that this menstrual blood is unhealthy because of all the impurities that it contains, and therefore must be disposed of safely away from others. Much has been written about the wide range of menstrual beliefs and their continuing influence in modern societies (8).
- *Impact of HMB on women and on society*: several studies have demonstrated the impact that HMB has on different aspects of an individual woman's life and lifestyle. There are clear adverse impacts on a woman's sex life, physical activities, productivity at work, sleep patterns, productivity at home, ability to travel, social life, diet, and relationship with spouse and children.

These impacts on the woman inevitably have a major influence on those around her and on her roles and 'productivity' within the society. Such a common group of symptoms lasting several days each month greatly influences the overall productivity of women in that society. These adverse influences all contribute to the decreased quality of life for the woman with HMB, which the United Kingdom National Institute for Health and Care Excellence guidelines on HMB (7) have expressly highlighted. This decreased quality of life should be a primary target in management of HMB.

Causes of abnormal uterine bleeding (the FIGO PALM-COEIN classification of underlying causes of abnormal uterine bleeding in women in the reproductive years)

The FIGO system of classification of underlying causes of AUB is simply based on dividing the major causes into two groups: the 'structural' causes, where pathology can be imaged by pelvic ultrasound, magnetic resonance imaging (MRI), or direct visualization, and the 'non-structural' causes, which cannot be 'imaged'. These causes are illustrated by the mnemonic PALM-COEIN (**Box 41.6**).

'Structural' lesions (PALM):

- *AUB-P: endometrial or endocervical polyps*, which typically cause intermenstrual bleeding and sometimes HMB.
- *AUB-A: adenomyosis*, which commonly coexists with other causes and may sometimes cause HMB and pelvic pain.
- *AUB-L: leiomyomas*, a very common cause of the heaviest daily bleeding during a period.

> **Box 41.6** The PALM-COEIN system: underlying causes of abnormal uterine bleeding in women in the reproductive years
>
> **Structural causes**
> - AUB-P: endometrial or endocervical polyps
> - AUB-A: adenomyosis
> - AUB-L: leiomyoma
> - AUB-M: malignancy or endometrial hyperplasia
>
> **Non-structural causes**
> - AUB-C: coagulopathy
> - AUB-O: ovulatory disturbances
> - AUB-E: primary endometrial disturbances
> - AUB-I: iatrogenic
> - AUB-N: not otherwise classified

- *AUB-M: endometrial hyperplasia or malignancy* can cause erratic light or heavy bleeding.

Non-structural molecular causes (COEIN):

- *AUB-C: coagulopathies* can be genetically linked causes of very heavy bleeding, but von Willebrand disease can be a common cause of moderate HMB.
- *AUB-O: ovulatory disturbances* are a common cause of disturbed bleeding (light or heavy), particularly in adolescence and in the perimenopausal period.
- *AUB-E: primary endometrial causes* are mainly local disturbances of molecular pathways or a reflection of low-grade, chronic infection (such as chlamydia). Most of the research studies of 'HMB' have been done on women with AUB-E.
- *AUB-I: iatrogenic causes of AUB* include a wide range of drugs causing irregular, light, heavy, or prolonged bleeding. Ceasing the drug therapy will usually correct the AUB rapidly. This section includes intrauterine contraceptive devices.
- *AUB-N: not otherwise classified* is a group of rarities or unusual causes which have not yet been defined or do not easily fit into the other categories. This includes rarities such as arteriovenous malformations in the uterus.

Flexibility of the PALM-COEIN classification allows for the development of subclassifications where needed. This is particularly the case with AUB-L where fibroids in different parts of the uterus and with differing relationships to the endometrium may have very different effects on symptoms and management. This system also allows for more than one cause to be recognized and graded in the same patient. The system also allows for modification of each component with new research, and has an inbuilt requirement for review every 3 years.

Not all genital tract bleeding is uterine

The previous discussion has related specifically to 'uterine' bleeding since this is the commonest and potentially the most complicated aspect of genital tract bleeding. However, it is not uncommon to encounter abnormalities of bleeding arising from the vulva, vagina, or cervix, and these should generally be excluded during history taking and pelvic examination. The possibility of a pelvic malignancy should not be overlooked. Abnormal bleeding from an undiagnosed early pregnancy should also be excluded as a potential cause of symptoms mimicking AUB.

Box 41.7 Potential investigations for abnormal uterine bleeding

- Full blood count, including haemoglobin, film.
- Iron studies (ferritin; transferrin saturation).
- Pap smear.
- High vaginal swab/chlamydia and gonorrhoea polymerase chain reaction.
- Pelvic/transvaginal ultrasound (becoming routine).
- Magnetic resonance imaging (rarely needed).
- Hysteroscopy with or without excision.
- Diagnostic laparoscopy with or without excision.

Box 41.8 A simple screening questionnaire to determine the likelihood that a woman with a complaint of heavy menstrual bleeding will have an underlying coagulopathy

A positive screen comprises any of the following
- HMB from the time of menarche onwards.
- One of the following:
  - Postpartum haemorrhage
  - Excessive bleeding during surgery
  - Bleeding with dental work.
- Two or more of the following symptoms:
  - Significant bruising one or two times per month
  - Epistaxis one or two times per month
  - Frequent bleeding from the gums
  - Family history of bleeding symptoms.
- Patients with a positive screen should be assessed further by a haematologist.

Source data from Kouides PA, Conard J, Peyvandi F, Kadir R. Hemostasis and menstruation: appropriate investigation for underlying disorders of haemostasis in women with excessive menstrual bleeding. *Fertil Steril* 2005;84:1345–49.

Investigations

For most of these patients, there is little need for extensive investigation. The key to good management is usually a 'good clinical history' defining the characteristics of the menstrual pattern and relevant lifestyle features (such as cigarette smoking or risk factors for cervical infection), and a clinical examination, including bimanual pelvic and speculum examinations. Specific investigations should include the following (**Box 41.7**):

1. Full blood count, primarily to assess anaemia and platelet count.
2. Blood film, to assess the possible presence of hypochromia and microcytosis of the red blood cells, and reticulocytes.
3. Iron studies, including serum ferritin and serum transferrin saturation (see **Box 41.5** to assess iron deficiency). We believe that iron deficiency is underdiagnosed in most countries.
4. The pelvic examination should allow collection of a Pap smear, if not up to date with routine collection. Pelvic examination allows assessment of palpable or visible lesions on the vulva, vagina, or ectocervix, and provides information on the presence of tenderness.
5. Transvaginal ultrasound scan has become a technique of central importance in the assessment of AUB. Pelvic scanning has become a complex technology and ideally needs to be carried out by an expert. A good-quality scan carried out with modern equipment and assessed by an expert in pelvic scanning can yield surprising details of the presence and structure of pelvic lesions, and may render other types of scanning or endoscopy unnecessary. Basic ultrasound scanning can be supplemented by the instillation of saline into the uterine cavity (sonohysterography) to outline the endometrial surface and encroaching lesions with much greater clarity. Colour Doppler scanning can provide evidence of the vascularity of endometrial polyps, fibroids, or other structures, and may highlight a rare arteriovenous malformation.

   Basic transvaginal scanning has a relatively high level of error in assessing endometrial polyps and should be supplemented by sonohysterography when polyps may be present, unless a clear feeder vessel is seen in the polyp on colour Doppler.
6. MRI provides very clear images of most pelvic structures and may provide clearer assessments of structural lesions such as fibroids or endometriosis/adenomyosis than ultrasound. However, it is costly and can be difficult to access, and is unnecessary in straightforward cases of menstrual dysfunction.
7. Diagnostic hysteroscopy is an important tool for visualizing lesions encroaching into the uterine cavity, and allows excision or biopsy for assessment of the pathology of the visible lesion. Hysteroscopy can be carried out without local or general anaesthesia in an outpatient clinic situation if the premises and equipment are suitable.
8. Other possible investigations include an initial screening for coagulopathy, if the clinical picture contains suggestive features. A simple, specific, three-question questionnaire will usually give a strong indication whether definitive coagulopathy laboratory investigations are indicated (**Box 41.8**).
9. A small number of centres have extended the availability of these tests so that they can be offered to new patients as a 'one-stop shop', where all necessary investigations can be completed at the first visit and a clear management strategy expeditiously initiated.

Management of abnormal uterine bleeding

Aims of therapy

The acute and severe (or 'acute on chronic') presentations of HMB symptoms and the commoner chronic and less severe HMB symptoms require quite different approaches for initial management.

Management of acute and severe presentations of HMB

Women presenting with acute and severe genital tract blood loss need an urgent history and pelvic examination, aligned with urgent measures to limit further blood loss and stabilize the cardiovascular system (**Boxes 41.9 and 41.10**) and consideration of the principles of 'patient blood management' (see 'Management of chronic presentations of HMB').

Management of chronic presentations of HMB

In most Western societies, 'chronic' presentations are much commoner than 'acute and severe'. An ideal approach to management requires the sequence of menstrual and medical case history, pelvic and speculum examination, and relevant investigations.

Medical therapies for chronic presentations of HMB have been well studied over the past two decades:

Box 41.9 Principles for urgent management of acute and severe heavy menstrual bleeding

1 Insert intravenous line.
2 Take blood for full blood count, biochemistry, and crossmatching.
3 Assess and stabilize cardiovascular status.
4 Assess continuing rate and extent of vaginal blood loss.
5 Complete menstrual, 'HMB', and medical history.
6 Consider transvaginal ultrasound scan.
7 Assessment of patient blood management principles.
8 Plan the best approach to minimizing active blood loss.
9 Consider iron infusion.

1. The most effective medical therapy for HMB is the *levonorgestrel-releasing intrauterine system* (LNG-IUS; marketed as Mirena by the Bayer Healthcare, Berlin). This system reduces menstrual blood loss by around 90%, and is designed to last for up to 5 years. Other LNG-IUS systems are beginning to come onto the market but these have not yet been adequately studied for HMB treatment. It is recommended by all modern guidelines that the LNG-IUS should be offered as first choice unless the woman has contraindications or has other personal preferences.

   There is good evidence that the LNG-IUS can have a strong beneficial effect on reducing menstrual blood loss no matter what is the underlying cause of the HMB. It has highly beneficial effects on HMB in AUB-A, AUB-C, AUB-O, AUB-E, and AUB-M (endometrial hyperplasia; but is not recommended when there is any suspicion of endometrial cancer). It also works well for most cases of AUB-L, provided that the fibroids are not submucous. It appears to be effective in preventing recurrences of endometrial polyps, but when a polyp is present (AUB-P) the usual recommendation is surgical removal.

   The commonest side effect of the LNG-IUS is erratic and 'nuisance-value' light bleeding, sometimes prolonged. This tends to reduce with time, but does sometimes lead to a need for

Box 41.10 Specific active therapies to stop acute and severe HMB

1 Consider uterine balloon tamponade.
2 Consider antifibrinolytic therapy (tranexamic acid)—intravenous or oral.
3 Start hormonal therapies to reduce bleeding and control future bleeding episodes:
   a Many anecdotal regimens.
   b Intravenous conjugated equine oestrogens in countries where this is still available.
   c Oral medroxyprogesterone acetate in moderate dose (10–20 mg three times a day for 7–10 days).
   d Oral norethisterone acetate in moderate dose (5–10 mg three times a day for 7–10 days).
   e Consider intramuscular medroxyprogesterone acetate.
   f Suitable 30 mcg combined oral contraceptive.
   g Plan future hormonal control with LNG-IUS or a suitable oral contraceptive.
4 May need to consider surgery for non-responsive, continuing blood loss.

removal. Amenorrhoea is very common, is reversible following removal of the device unless the woman is perimenopausal, and is usually recognized as a beneficial end-point of the therapy

2. Second-line medical therapies include the following:
   a. *Combined oral contraceptives*:
      i. All modern combined hormonal contraceptives containing ethinyl oestradiol (including vaginal ring and transdermal systems) are effective in reducing menstrual blood loss by an average of 30–50%.
      ii. Oral contraceptives based on oestradiol-17-beta as the oestrogen component seem to be more effective in reducing menstrual blood loss (by 70–80%).
   b. *Tranexamic acid* is a lysine analogue, which has major antifibrinolytic properties by inhibiting the action of plasmin. Hence, it counteracts the breakdown of fibrin by the plasmin system within the endometrium, a tissue which has a very active fibrinolytic system in women with HMB. This drug does not increase the risk of venous thrombosis in large vessels. It works by inhibiting tissue plasminogen activator solely within the tissues. It is highly effective in reducing menstrual blood loss, by around 50%. The drug needs to be taken each month as soon as menstrual bleeding starts, in an oral dosage of 1.0 g three times daily for 3–4 days. Tranexamic acid has a fairly low bioactivity and therefore needs to be taken in this apparently 'high dosage' to maintain its antifibrinolytic effect. This dosage has a low incidence of side effects, mainly mild gastrointestinal symptoms which settle with time. This is a valuable non-steroidal therapy, which only needs to be taken during the heaviest days of menstruation itself. The extensive Scandinavian experience suggests that it can be safely taken on a monthly basis for many years.
   c. *Non-steroidal anti-inflammatory drugs* (NSAIDs) are widely used to treat HMB, although they are generally less effective in reducing the actual blood loss (by around 30%) than other therapies. However, they are often effective in reducing menstrual pain, which is a common accompaniment of HMB. The drugs which have been most thoroughly studied are mefenamic acid, naproxen, and flurbiprofen. These are taken during the time of heavy bleeding, generally in a dosage of 500 mg three times daily. They should not be taken on an empty stomach because they may occasionally cause epithelial erosion within the gastrointestinal tract. Food inhibits this.

3. A new therapy for HMB associated with uterine fibroids is the oral *progesterone receptor modulator*, ulipristal acetate (Esmya). This novel therapy is beginning to establish its place for long-term management of uterine fibroids, and shows great promise in reducing fibroid size and greatly reducing menstrual blood loss (**Box 41.11**).

4. *Third-line medical therapies* (oral danazol and gonadotrophin-releasing hormone (GnRH) analogues) are no longer recommended for treatment of HMB (mainly because of side effects), except in special extenuating circumstances.

5. *Iron therapy* is a critical part of the medical management of HMB, and should be initiated at the same time as the chosen therapy aimed at stopping the heavy bleeding.

Box 41.11 Use of ulipristal acetate for uterine fibroids

- Confirm diagnosis of leiomyomas (uterine fibroids).
- Establish subclassification of fibroid positioning within the uterus.
- Use of ulipristal acetate contraindicated with genital bleeding of unknown origin.
- Each course lasts 3 months (5 mg daily for 84 days; 7-day break before further courses).
- Produces significant reduction in menstrual blood loss.
- Produces significant reduction in individual fibroid size.

Box 41.12 Surgical procedures still used for management of some heavy menstrual bleeding cases of abnormal uterine bleeding

- Surgical procedures for benign gynaecology have greatly reduced (by around 50%) in most countries in the past two decades.
- Surgery is generally now restricted to the structural lesions (PALM).
- Hysterectomy is now usually carried out laparoscopically, unless the structural lesion is extensive.
- Uterine artery embolization is used in some centres for treatment of individual fibroids.
- Endometrial resection can be very effective for AUB-E and AUB-C.
- Modern laparoscopic surgery requires advanced endoscopic training.

Recent research has demonstrated that it takes the average woman with HMB 1 year to recharge her iron stores to normal levels after starting use of a LNG-IUS or having a hysterectomy, unless her iron deficiency is deliberately and adequately treated. Iron therapy can either be with standard oral formulations or, increasingly, with a loading dose of a modern rapid impact intravenous preparation with a low incidence of side effects, such as ferric carboxymaltose.

Patient blood management is a recent concept focusing management strategies for bleeding symptoms around the best health needs of the patient. It can be defined as: 'The timely application of evidence-based medical and surgical concepts designed to maintain haemoglobin concentration, optimize haemostasis, and minimize blood loss in an effort to improve patient outcome' (9, 10). This concept developed along with increasing awareness of the serious hazards and questionable efficacy of allogeneic blood transfusion. Allogeneic blood transfusions are risky, costly, in limited supply and are linked to worsening of patient outcomes. In addition, blood transfusion is a demanding and expensive service to maintain.

Patient blood management has become a multimodal approach to minimize perioperative use of blood products, based on the triad of detection and treatment of preoperative iron deficiency and anaemia, reduction of perioperative blood loss, and harnessing and optimizing patient-specific factors such as inflammation-related hepcidin release.

It is now becoming recognized that menstruating women are at particular risk of the symptoms and complications of iron deficiency and that those with HMB have a condition akin to major surgical blood loss once a month (when they menstruate).

The concepts of patient blood management are reshaping transfusion medicine and the way that blood components are used. Emphasis is increasingly being placed on maximizing iron stores and circulating 'available iron' prior to planned surgery, to minimizing blood loss during surgery, to minimizing transfusion of blood products, and to maintaining iron stores and haemoglobin levels following surgery. There are now many effective oral and intravenous iron preparations that can initiate reasonably rapid restoration of iron stores and support steady replacement of haemoglobin and red blood cells. If the preoperative schedule allows for 3 months before elective surgery in 'at-risk' patients, we tend to use oral iron polymaltose (100 mg twice daily, elemental iron), or if less than 4 weeks is available before urgent surgery, an intravenous total loading dose of ferric carboxymaltose (1000 mg). These preparations are well tolerated in the great majority of patients.

Surgical and procedural approaches to management of AUB

Surgery is still required on a fairly frequent basis for managing the more difficult or persistent cases of HMB (Box 41.12). Structural causes of HMB, such as polyps, adenomyosis, uterine leiomyomas, and endometrial malignancy may all require surgery for management. Surgery may sometimes involve hysteroscopic or laparoscopic resection of the whole lesion (e.g. endometrial polyps, solitary submucous myomas, or multiple myomas). Hysterectomy may still be necessary sometimes, especially if multiple fibroids, adenomyosis, or endometriosis are present. Demographic data from several European countries have demonstrated that the numbers of hysterectomies for benign gynaecological diseases have been reduced by more than 50% in the past 20 years—since the LNG-IUS system has been introduced.

Alternative procedures of lesser degree than hysterectomy, which may effectively treat HMB, include endometrial ablation and uterine artery embolization for leiomyomas or adenomyosis. Endometrial ablation was designed to resect or coagulate the full depth of the endometrium and a small rim of underlying myometrium in those women who chose not to attempt future pregnancy. Overall, endometrial ablation has a similar degree of effectiveness as the LNG-IUS, but the potential disadvantages of being irreversible and not being 'contraceptive'. Newer technologies have allowed modern ablation to be carried out using 'high-tech' programmed devices as an office procedure.

Uterine artery embolization requires precise insertion of a uterine artery catheter under radiological guidance, with the tip being placed close to or in the largest feeder vessel of the targeted leiomyoma. Biodegradable microparticles of polyvinyl alcohol are injected to block the feeder vessels. The technique requires skilled interventional radiology and provides an effectiveness of greater than 90% in greatly reducing fibroid size, blood supply, and HMB symptoms. Side effects include ischaemic pain immediately postoperatively and a small risk of ischaemic damage to surrounding tissues, including ovary. This technique does not necessarily prevent the development of new fibroids in future.

Prognosis

The prognosis for patients with AUB or, more specifically HMB, is closely related to the nature and severity of the underlying cause of the bleeding (PALM-COEIN), and the effectiveness of any targeted therapy. Thus, the prognosis is specifically patient focused. If the underlying cause is not adequately treated, most patients will tend to have worsening symptoms and signs over a period of years, until the menopause.

Summary

This section has focused primarily on HMB since this is the commonest and the most hazardous of the menstrual bleeding symptoms, and is often accompanied by pelvic pain. The main hazard associated with HMB is the development of iron deficiency and iron deficiency anaemia. Many doctors are unaware that iron deficiency without anaemia is so common in menstruating women and that it is just as important in causing symptoms as when anaemia is also present. Hence, iron deficiency needs to be actively treated at the same time as giving therapy to reduce or stop the bleeding.

Amenorrhoea (absence of menstruation) and dysmenorrhoea (menstrually related pelvic pain)

Introduction to amenorrhoea and dysmenorrhoea

Amenorrhoea and dysmenorrhoea are two common symptom groupings presenting at opposite ends of the menstrual cycle symptom spectrum. Amenorrhoea is generally understood to be the complete absence of menstrual bleeding at a time when it would be expected. Hence, the common perimenstrual symptoms which frequently accompany AUB rarely occur in these women. Dysmenorrhoea means pelvic pain accompanying menstruation. Both of these symptoms are common in women within the reproductive ages between menarche and menopause, but the two cannot, by definition, occur in the same patient at the same time! Management of both requires a sound knowledge of the anatomy, physiology, and potential pathophysiology of the reproductive tract.

Amenorrhoea

Amenorrhoea is a very specific type of menstrual disturbance where menstruation does not occur at the specific times when it is expected. The term literally means absence or cessation of bleeding, and the duration of this absence needs to be specified. Amenorrhoea can be divided into two separate categories:

- *Primary amenorrhoea*: failure of natural menstruation to spontaneously begin at the normal age of puberty. If absent at age 15, it should be investigated. However, this symptom needs to be looked at in two ways:
  - The young woman who has had normal onset of other pubertal symptoms and signs, such as breast and pubic hair development, at normal age, but has not menstruated by age 15. She needs to be investigated for '*menstrual delay*'.
  - The young woman who has not yet developed the expected symptoms and signs of puberty. She needs to be investigated for '*delay of onset of normal puberty*', and this investigation should usually begin earlier than age 15.
- *Secondary amenorrhoea*: this is the absence of menstruation for at least 6 months in a woman, who has previously menstruated.

Three other terms are relevant here:

- *Infrequent menstruation*: this category used to be called 'oligomenorrhoea', but that term has now been abandoned. This

term is usually applied to women with long gaps between periods. The upper limit of the normal regular cycle is taken at 38 days. Above this is mild (>38 days), moderate (>50 days), or severely (>90 days) infrequent bleeding. This symptom merges into secondary amenorrhoea, and should be investigated in a similar manner.

- *Physiological amenorrhoea*: this covers those situations where absence of menstruation is expected: prepuberty, postmenopause, pregnancy, and breastfeeding (lactation).
- *Pharmacological amenorrhoea*: occurs when menstruation ceases as a consequence of the administration of specific drugs or of a specific surgical procedure (**Box 41.13**).

Causes of primary amenorrhoea

Primary amenorrhoea typically results from constitutional delay, genetic factors, or from an outflow tract obstruction, such as in the case of imperforate hymen, transverse vaginal septum, or cervical blockage (**Box 41.14**). Constitutional delay is characterized by delayed skeletal growth and is one of the common causes for delayed puberty and menstruation. Chronic illnesses such as diabetes, renal insufficiency, and thyroid disease can further lead to menstrual dysfunction, as can malignancy and its therapies.

History and examination for primary amenorrhoea

A detailed history and examination for the presence, timing, or absence of secondary sexual characteristics is essential. Information regarding past and current medical illness, such as thyroid disease, renal disease, diabetes, malignancy, and therapies should be ascertained. Social history, life stressors, excessive exercise, weight change, potential for anorexia or bulimia, and detailed family history should be explored.

Examination of women with primary amenorrhoea involves recording growth, body mass index (BMI), and pubertal stage. The Tanner system of staging breast and pubic hair development is commonly utilized to compare development of secondary sexual characteristics against normal. In addition to these checks it may be appropriate to perform a pelvic exam (usually only in those who have been sexually active).

Investigations for primary amenorrhoea

After a thorough history and examination, the patients can be grouped into two categories—those with delayed puberty (in whom

---

Box 41.13 Pharmacological amenorrhoea

Drugs
- Combined oral contraceptive pills taken continuously
- Levonorgestrel intrauterine systems
- Progestogen subdermal implants and injectables
- Some antidepressants/antipsychotics
- Some antihypertensives
- Many chemotherapeutic agents

Surgical interventions
- Endometrial destructive techniques such as ablation or resection
- Hysterectomy

Box 41.14 Well-recognized causes of amenorrhoea

- Hypothalamic dysfunction:
  - Excessive exercise
  - Excessive weight loss, anorexia nervosa
  - Rare hypothalamic diseases
- Pituitary dysfunction:
  - Hyperprolactinaemia
  - Pituitary adenoma
  - Medications:
    - Oral contraceptive pill
    - Antidepressants
    - Antihypertensives
- Ovarian dysfunction:
  - Polycystic ovary syndrome
  - Menopause/menopause transition
  - Premature ovarian insufficiency:
    - Autoimmune
    - Endocrine
    - Chemotherapy, radiotherapy
    - Infection
    - Genetic
- Outflow tract (uterus, cervix, and vagina) dysfunction:
  - Mullerian agenesis
  - Intrauterine scarring
  - Intrauterine infections
  - Transverse vaginal septum
  - Cervical stenosis
- Physiological:
  - Prepubertal
  - Pregnancy
  - Lactation
  - Postmenopausal
- Other:
  - Thyroid disease
  - Chronic systemic illness

secondary sexual development has not yet occurred or is minimal) and those with normal puberty (**Figure 41.1** and **Box 41.15**).

Delayed puberty—investigations and differential diagnosis

In patients in whom secondary sexual characteristics have not developed or are minimal, the key investigation is to measure serum follicle-stimulating hormone (FSH). However, we usually choose to measure other relevant hormones at the same time at the initial visit. These include serum luteinizing hormone (LH), oestradiol, prolactin, thyroid-stimulating hormone (TSH), free triiodothyronine (FT_3), and free thyroxine (FT_4).

If FSH is low then the differential diagnosis includes constitutional delay in 'switching on' of hypothalamic mechanisms resulting in the initiation of pulsatile GnRH secretion and any hypothalamic cause, including anorexia, bulimia, and a range of chronic and systemic illnesses, often called hypogonadotropic hypogonadism. A number of genetic mutations have been identified in patients with congenital GnRH deficiency including mutations in genes such as *KAL1, FGFR1*, and *GNRHR* (11) and patients in whom these defects are present may among other things present with amenorrhoea. Kallmann syndrome is a rare but well-recognized condition, which is due to failure of the GnRH-secreting neurons to migrate from their early embryonic origins in the frontal cortex to the adult site in the hypothalamus. This condition is also linked with congenital anosmia and failure of the neurons for sense of smell to develop within the frontal cortex.

If, however, serum FSH and LH levels are high (hypergonadotropic hypogonadism), and oestradiol levels are very low, indicating premature ovarian insufficiency (POI), it is appropriate to investigate further and perform genetic testing. Differential diagnoses include Turner syndrome (45XO), fragile X syndrome (defective gene on X chromosome), XY female, and primary ovarian failure. Turner syndrome is characterized by a 45XO karyotype, and is a condition

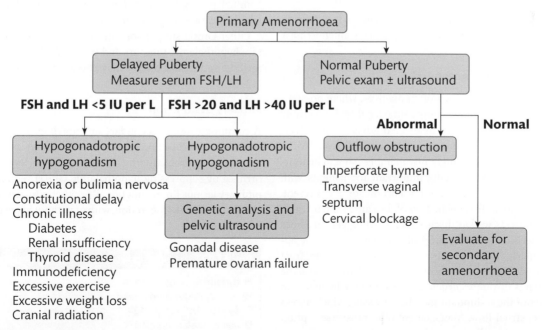

Figure 41.1 Evaluation of primary amenorrhoea.

Source data from Master-Hunter T, Heiman DL. Amenorrhea: evaluation and treatment. *Am Fam Physician* 2006;15:1374–82 and Slap GB. Menstrual disorders in adolescence. *Best Pract Res Clin Obstet Gynaecol* 2003;17:75–92.

> **Box 41.15** The two key questions needed in assessing primary amenorrhoea
>
> 1 Does she have *no signs* of normal puberty? (She has 'delayed puberty'.)
> 2 Does she have *normal pubertal changes* in body shape and normal breast and pubic hair development? (She has 'delayed onset of menstruation'.)

> **Box 41.16** Principles of management of primary amenorrhoea
>
> - Counselling
> - Medical management
> - Surgical management
> - Actively treating infertility factors
> - Prevention of associated side effects

caused by the absence of one complete or partial copy of the X chromosome in some or all of the cells.

Primary ovarian failure commonly results from radiation or chemotherapy exposure in childhood. It may also result from exposure to previous infection (e.g. mumps).

Girls of 15 years or more with normal pubertal changes in body habitus, breasts and public hair but no periods—investigations and differential diagnosis

It is wise to objectively assess pubertal changes in breasts and pubic hair using the Tanner Sexual Maturity Rating scales against a background of body shape and general maturity to ensure that puberty has been normal. Also check whether she has been treated with 'hormones' such as the contraceptive pill.

It is then useful to perform a pelvic ultrasound scan (transvaginal or abdominal, depending on previous sexual activity), which will aid in identifying outflow tract obstruction, or Mullerian agenesis. Outflow tract obstruction can occur at the level of the hymen or within the vagina or cervix. On vaginal examination, obstruction by an imperforate hymen is characterized by a bulging, blue introital membrane through which menstrual effluent can be visualized. Obstruction within the vagina, by a transverse vaginal septum, can occur at any level. Ultrasound scanning may also reveal Mullerian agenesis, characterized by the congenital absence of the uterus, upper (occasionally upper and lower) vagina and cervix, and portions of the fallopian tubes. The ovaries usually appear normal and are normally sited. Ovulation appears to continue in a fairly regular manner.

In the presence of normal ultrasound findings, further investigation should proceed as outlined in the 'Secondary amenorrhoea' section.

Management of primary amenorrhoea

Treatment of primary amenorrhoea often involves, where possible, correcting underlying pathology, improving fertility (or actively treating infertility) and preventing associated adverse side effects that may result from long-term low oestrogen levels (Box 41.16).

In the first instance, patients and family members should be thoroughly counselled. This is especially important for patients with Mullerian agenesis and/or in whom a Y chromosome is present. These patients require careful explanation of the causes and possible management options, as well as discussion regarding gender issues and their future fertility outlook. Surgical management may be appropriate, particularly where there is a need to correct vaginal tract outflow obstruction. Management of outflow tract obstruction at the level of the hymen is through a cruciate incision in the hymen with limited trimming of the redundant membrane tissue, which allows release of the menstrual flow. Management of a transverse septum often requires more complex surgical intervention with some vaginal reconstructive surgery.

Generally for patients with hypo-oestrogenism, hormone replacement therapy or the combined oral contraceptive pill (COCP) is suggested to reduce future cardiovascular or osteoporosis risks. For patients considering pregnancy, referral for assisted reproductive technologies and consultation with an experienced infertility specialist is appropriate. For patients with hypothalamic or pituitary dysfunction, exogenous gonadotrophins or pulsatile GnRH can be administered in a precise manner, and can be combined with other modern *in vitro* fertility technologies. For others, discussion around oocyte donation or surrogacy may be appropriate fertility considerations.

Secondary amenorrhoea

Pregnancy and lactation (planned or unplanned) are the commonest causes of secondary amenorrhoea. However, non-physiological causes of secondary amenorrhoea can be grouped according to the following subgroups in terms of an anatomically based approach (Box 41.17).

Hypothalamic dysfunction

Hypothalamic dysfunction is characterized by suppressed pulsatile GnRH secretion, absence of FSH and LH secretion, absence of ovarian follicle development, and very low serum oestradiol. This dysfunction can be attributed to excessive exercise or major weight reduction, eating disorders, and 'stress'. There is great variability in the degree of weight loss, eating disorders, excessive exercise, and physical and emotional stressors required to induce amenorrhoea. Familial polycystic ovary tendency may contribute. Pathways by which these act are poorly understood.

Other GnRH suppressors include systemic chronic illnesses and rare hypothalamic tumours and infiltrative lesions. Type 1 diabetes mellitus and coeliac disease may also interfere with GnRH secretion (12, 13).

Pituitary dysfunction

A common cause of secondary amenorrhoea is excessive pituitary secretion of prolactin, often from a benign prolactin-secreting adenoma—a 'prolactinoma'. Raised prolactin levels induce amenorrhoea by suppressing hypothalamic GnRH secretion. Other rare pituitary lesions ('non-functional' or other pituitary adenomas), can also suppress GnRH secretion, with or without hyperprolactinaemia.

> **Box 41.17** Anatomical causes of secondary amenorrhoea
>
> H: hypothalamic dysfunction, 35%
> P: pituitary dysfunction, 17%
> O: ovarian dysfunction, 40%
> U: uterine dysfunction, 7%
> Other, 1%

Ovarian dysfunction

Polycystic ovary syndrome (PCOS) accounts for approximately 20% of cases of secondary amenorrhoea. The pathophysiology of PCOS is complex and variable; however, it is usually associated with ovulatory dysfunction, androgen excess, and with increased ovarian antral follicles on ultrasound. Classical signs of hyperandrogenism include oily skin, hirsutism, and acne, and women with PCOS are commonly overweight and have insulin resistance and metabolic syndrome. Women with PCOS typically present with infrequent and irregular periods or secondary amenorrhoea (AUB-O). PCOS is addressed in much more detail in Chapter 42).

Some PCOS patients may develop endometrial hyperplasia (and rarely low-grade endometrial adenocarcinoma at an early age) due to anovulation with excessive ovarian follicular secretion of oestradiol and absence of progesterone secretion. Endometrial hyperplasia may be accompanied by irregular and sometimes very heavy uterine bleeding (AUB-M).

Premature ovarian failure (often nowadays called POI), is characterized by excessive premature depletion of follicles and oocytes prior to the age of 40 years. This can occur at any age, including before puberty. Lack of ovarian endocrine function leads to very low circulating levels of oestradiol and endometrial atrophy. POI may result from a range of rare and poorly known causes of follicular destruction (e.g. the range of blepharophimosis–ptosis–epicanthus inversus syndromes, and carriers of the fragile X premutation) are often combined with POI and amenorrhoea).

Small numbers of women with POI will have moderate numbers of histologically normal follicles and oocytes still present in the ovaries, albeit unresponsive to FSH. Rarely, one or more of these follicles and oocytes may become spontaneously sensitive to FSH and LH and even ovulate.

Genetic and hereditary ovarian causes are likely to present as primary amenorrhoea; however, secondary amenorrhea can occur on a background of autoimmune diseases affecting ovaries (such as in Addison's disease, diabetes mellitus, rheumatoid arthritis, Sjögren syndrome, and systemic lupus erythematosus) or as a result of ovarian toxicity induced by radiation or chemotherapy exposure. Other ovarian causes of amenorrhoea are rare and include rare ovarian tumours, such as fibrothecomas.

Uterine dysfunction

The most common, but still rare, cause of amenorrhoea attributable to uterine dysfunction is the development of intrauterine adhesions following major damage to the endometrium. This is usually referred to as Asherman syndrome (or intrauterine synechiae). These adhesions prevent normal endometrial proliferation, decidualization, and shedding. This scarring is typically secondary to curettage carried out to remove retained placental products postpartum or postabortion in the presence of low-grade endometrial infection and secondary postpartum haemorrhage. This is one of only two situations when amenorrhoea occurs in the presence of regular ovulation, the other being absence of the uterus (either Mullerian agenesis or hysterectomy).

Other causes

A range of other uncommon causes can be implicated in amenorrhoea. Both hyper- and hypothyroidism can cause amenorrhoea, which may be primary or secondary. Appropriate investigation will often pick up thyroid dysfunction and for these patients referral and management by a specialist endocrinologist is indicated. Treatment of underlying thyroid dysfunction will lead to restoration of a normal menstrual cycle.

Evaluation of secondary amenorrhoea

Evaluation of secondary amenorrhoea begins with exclusion of pregnancy, which can occur 'out of the blue' even following a prolonged period of amenorrhoea. This is easily done with urinary and/or serum beta-human chorionic gonadotropin measurement. Detailed history and examination should follow a negative test.

Detailed history to assess secondary amenorrhoea

A thorough history will usually form the basis of the underlying diagnosis. Duration of amenorrhoea and potential recent exacerbating factors (changes in weight, diet, exercise, stressors) are important. Detailed medical, surgical, gynaecological, and family histories are critical. Information should be sought regarding specific signs and symptoms, such as hirsutism, acne and infrequent bleeding (PCOS), neurological symptoms and visual disturbances (hypothalamic–pituitary disease), symptoms of oestrogen deficiency (POI), uterine surgery (Asherman syndrome), or galactorrhoea (hyperprolactinaemia).

Examination for secondary amenorrhoea

Physical examination should include weight and BMI measurements. The patient should be specifically examined for signs of PCOS, oestrogen deficiency, galactorrhoea, thyroid disease, and for signs of other systemic diseases.

Physical examination and investigations for secondary amenorrhoea

Principles of investigations for secondary amenorrhoea are listed in Box 41.18.

Laboratory investigations

Initial laboratory investigations for secondary amenorrhoea are listed in Box 41.19.

Patients in whom prolactin and TSH are normal, and in whom FSH levels are normal or low, are likely to have amenorrhoea attributed to hypothalamic–pituitary dysfunction or PCOS. However, endocrine findings in PCOS can sometimes be complicated and some PCOS patients may have mildly or moderately elevated serum prolactin. In patients with functional hypothalamic amenorrhoea, the 'low' FSH levels are commonly higher than the LH levels, while in PCOS, FSH levels tend to be lower.

Box 41.18 Principles of investigations for secondary amenorrhoea

- Physical examination (weight and BMI); hirsutism, acne, galactorrhoea, thyroid signs
- Laboratory investigations (see Box 41.19)
- Imaging (e.g. transvaginal ultrasound, pituitary MRI)
- Genetic testing
- Hysteroscopy (for Asherman syndrome)

Box 41.19 Laboratory investigations for secondary amenorrhoea

Serum levels of the following:
- Beta-human chorionic gonadotropin
- FSH
- LH
- Prolactin
- TSH, FT_3, and FT_4
- Oestradiol
- Dehydroepiandrosterone sulphate (DHEAS) and 17-hydroxy-progesterone
- Total or free testosterone (if PCOS is suspected)
- Other (HbA1c, fasting blood sugar levels), full blood count, Multi Biochemical Analysis 20 (MBA-20)

Highly elevated FSH levels with low oestrogen levels in conjunction with the presence of hot flushes/symptoms of vaginal atrophy are indicative of POI.

Raised prolactin levels may result on a background of stress or other systemic illness, and therefore initially raised prolactin levels should be repeated. Generally, levels greater than 50 mcg/L (or 500 IU/L) warrant further investigation with imaging. Measuring TSH levels is often all that is needed to elucidate thyroid dysfunction (especially hypothyroidism) and ensure appropriate endocrine referral and treatment.

Greatly raised testosterone levels may be suggestive of PCOS or raise suspicion of a rare androgen-secreting tumour. In the presence of clinical features of hyperandrogenism (hirsutism, acne), serum testosterone levels and transvaginal ultrasound imaging may be diagnostic of PCOS.

Imaging of the pelvic organs and the pituitary gland

Ultrasonography is an extremely useful imagining modality in modern gynaecology and particularly may aid in detection of features suggestive of PCOS (with many follicles) or ovarian failure (with few or no small follicles). It may also be invaluable in assessing the presence, size, and shape of the uterus and the presence of adhesions within the endometrial cavity. For young women who have never been sexually active, it may not be appropriate to attempt a transvaginal scan. An abdominal scan will often reveal all that is necessary, but is less clear and more difficult to interpret.

In patients in whom prolactin levels are raised, imaging of the hypothalamus and pituitary with MRI is indicated to assess the possible presence of a pituitary adenoma. MRI or computed tomography imaging may also be indicated in patients who exhibit neurological signs or symptoms and where there is suspicion of other pituitary or hypothalamic lesions causing local pressure symptoms or tissue damage.

Genetic testing

In cases of POI and where an obvious underlying cause is uncertain, genetic testing for Turner syndrome and fragile X is suggested. In the very near future, genetic testing will become a much more important aspect of management of patients with primary or secondary amenorrhoea, in order to identify uncommon or rare genetic syndromes with significant familial implications.

Hysteroscopy

Hysteroscopy may be indicated in evaluation and active management of intrauterine adhesions, through direct visualization of the endometrial cavity and division of the adhesions themselves, following careful ultrasound assessment.

Management of secondary amenorrhoea

The principles of management of secondary amenorrhoea are listed in **Box 41.20**.

Restoration of menses

For patients with hypothalamic amenorrhoea, restoration of menstruation is often achieved through lifestyle modification and behavioural changes. This may include increased (or decreased) caloric intake, limitation (or increase) of energy expenditure, and nutritional counselling, In addition, appropriate detection, specialist referral, and treatment of underlying systemic diseases is crucial and will aid in restoration of menstruation.

Improving fertility

Various specialized regimens can be used to help induce ovulation, including treatment with the antioestrogenic drugs clomiphene and tamoxifen, and the aromatase inhibitor, letrozole, or more complex fertility regimens utilizing more modern technologies. Therapy for intrauterine adhesions may usually be carried out with hysteroscopic adhesiolysis under direct vision followed by cyclical oestrogen stimulation, aimed to promote regeneration of the endometrial lining.

Prevention of side effects

It is recommended that patients with POI be treated with combined oestrogen–progestogen therapy to prevent bone density loss, through either an oral contraceptive pill or hormone replacement therapy.

Treatment of hyperandrogenism is directed towards treating troublesome signs and symptoms (hirsutism and acne) and preventing long-term sequelae of PCOS (endometrial hyperplasia—or cancer, metabolic dysfunction, or obesity). Antiandrogen therapy can be given using the antiandrogenic steroids spironolactone or cyproterone acetate with the COCP, generally under specialist supervision.

Society concerns, mythology, and changing society perceptions

Amenorrhoea (except in the presence of breastfeeding) has generally been regarded with fear and disfavour in most communities—reflecting influence of 'evil spirits' and effects on fertility. In some

Box 41.20 Principles of management of secondary amenorrhoea

- Restoration of menses
- Treatment of underlying disease
- Improvement of fertility (preservation or treatment)
- Prevention of adverse effects of untreated pathology

cultures, there are beliefs that menstruation is not only necessary for internal 'cleansing', but also for confirming fertility potential.

Emerging evidence supports the safety and efficacy of menstrual suppression with COCP and other hormones and is leading to change in society expectations among women, who often favour a 'bleed-free' existence until pregnancy is desired. For many women, menstrual suppression has substantial advantages in terms of managing a range of benign gynaecological conditions, improving quality of life, reducing menstrual symptoms, and has further benefits in terms of improved contraception compliance.

Dysmenorrhoea: definitions

'Dysmenorrhoea', a term derived from Greek (Dys, difficult; meno, monthly; rhoea, flow), clinically refers to the symptom of menstrually related pelvic pain. It often occurs in association with other symptoms including headache, AUB, nausea, vomiting, and lethargy. Primary and secondary dysmenorrhoea differ in that primary is defined as menstrual pain that occurs in absence of identifiable 'structural' pelvic pathology, while secondary dysmenorrhoea is related to pelvic pathologies which can be 'imaged'.

Primary dysmenorrhoea and secondary dysmenorrhoea are both highly variable symptom complexes, with different types of pain experience for 'primary' or 'secondary' sufferers. Primary dysmenorrhoea is one of the commonest gynaecological complaints among adolescent girls, typically beginning 1–3 years after the onset of menstruation, coinciding with the onset of ovulation, and reaching a peak at around 17–18 years of age. It then has a tendency to spontaneously improve in the 20s and after the first pregnancy.

The secondary type of dysmenorrhoea is usually attributable to a recognizable underlying pelvic 'structural' lesion, which can be 'imaged' and identified in a defined way. Onset of secondary dysmenorrhoea tends to occur in mid to later reproductive years; however, it is now being recognized that the symptoms of pelvic pain with a condition such as endometriosis often have their onset in the adolescent years. Hence, a well-structured history is useful in distinguishing primary and secondary types of menstrual pain, and an important starting point in determining the most appropriate management.

Presentation and symptoms of dysmenorrhoea

Primary and secondary dysmenorrhoea are symptoms or symptom complexes, which may present in different ways in different types of patients (**Box 41.21**). Optimum management therefore depends on symptom characteristics and understanding of likely underlying causes. Young women with 'primary dysmenorrhoea' may experience a spectrum of associated symptoms as well as varying types of pain symptom, ranging from a dull ache and 'tightenings', through obvious contractions to deep colicky-type pain. These pains may range in severity from mild 'cramps' through to some of the most severe pains that a woman can imagine. The pains may radiate to the back, inguinal region, or legs, and can be associated with nausea, vomiting, diarrhoea, fatigue, fever, irritability, myalgia, and headaches.

The pain of primary dysmenorrhoea tends to be 'spasmodic' in nature, and commonly begins just prior to or at the onset of menstruation. The intensity of pain can be very severe and is sometimes associated with the amount of menstrual flow.

Conversely, secondary dysmenorrhoea is associated with a type of pelvic pain often described as 'dragging' or 'congestive' in nature, and

---

Box 41.21 Common characteristics of the symptoms of primary and secondary dysmenorrhoea

Primary
- Intense spasms
- Onset around beginning of menstruation
- Radiating pain (to back/legs)
- Associated symptoms (nausea, headaches)

Secondary
- Dragging-type pain, often prolonged
- May begin several days before menstruation
- Can occur variably throughout menstrual cycle
- Associated symptoms: HMB and deep dyspareunia

---

this may well be a component of more chronic pelvic pain, which tends to be more prolonged or erratic and can occur throughout the menstrual cycle. Chronic pelvic pain is dealt with in more detail in Chapter 44. Typically, this pain begins several days prior to menstruation, peaking with onset of bleeding. Associated symptoms can include HMB and deep dyspareunia associated with uterine tenderness.

Underlying causes, mechanisms, and contributing factors of dysmenorrhoea

Early pathophysiological studies in the 1950s and 1960s investigated the relationship between an intense rise in intrauterine pressure and spasms of pain perception in women with primary dysmenorrhoea.

This lead to the demonstration that a rise in intrauterine pressure on a background of markedly increased myometrial contractile activity caused a reduction in endometrial blood flow, in turn causing uterine ischaemia and release of pain-stimulating metabolites (13). The intrauterine pressures generated by these intense contractions can sometimes exceed 200 mm Hg, substantially higher than is experienced in obstetric labour.

Prostaglandins

Disturbances of endometrial prostaglandin metabolism are also implicated in primary dysmenorrhoea. Endometrial prostaglandins $F_2\alpha$ and E_2 can directly sensitize afferent (sensory) nerve fibres in the uterus leading to generation of pain (14).

Vasopressin and other peptides

Experimental evidence further suggests that raised endometrial and circulatory vasopressin, as well as peptides such as oxytocin, endothelins, and related prostanoid metabolites such as leukotrienes, contribute to increasing myometrial contractility, promote vasoconstriction, and contribute to uterine ischaemia (15).

Imbalance of ovarian hormones

Ovarian hormones can modulate the synthesis and release of prostaglandins and vasopressin and increase myometrial sensitivity. Increased endometrial and circulating oestradiol in the adolescent pelvis appears to stimulate vasopressin release (16).

Figure 41.2 provides a schematic diagram of factors involved in the generation of pain in women with primary dysmenorrhoea. Exacerbating factors can include cigarette smoking, obesity, and local chlamydia infection (17) and there can be a clear familial link (18).

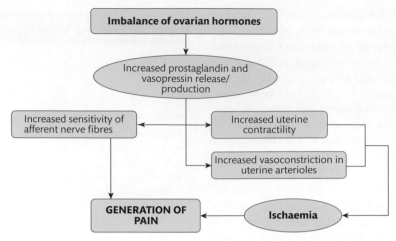

Figure 41.2 Proposed scheme of generation of uterine pain in primary dysmenorrhea.

Secondary dysmenorrhoea

Secondary dysmenorrhoea refers to the painful menstruation that is attributed to certain structurally identifiable, and usually 'inflammatory', pelvic pathologies. These structural lesions can contribute to generation of pain directly by distorting the pelvic anatomy (including nerves) or indirectly via production of inflammatory and other molecules that stimulate the triggering or persistence of pain signals. These lesions are also generally tender to palpation.

Some common causes of secondary dysmenorrhoea are listed and described in **Box 41.22**.

Most ovarian cysts may cause pelvic pain by intermittent torsion, but probably not dysmenorrhoea, except in the case of endometriotic ovarian cysts.

Endometriosis

Endometriosis is a common condition characterized by presence of endometrial-like glands and stroma that develop into lesions at sites outside the uterus, especially on the pelvic peritoneum, in the deeper pelvis, or in the ovaries in the form of local endometriotic cystic lesions, commonly causing intense menstrually related pain. Similar endometriosis pains can also occur at other times of the cycle as erratic, chronic pelvic pain. This disease is a complex and variable condition, which is comprehensively addressed in Chapter 45.

Adenomyosis

Adenomyosis is characterized by the presence of endometrial glands and stroma within the myometrium, and the severity of dysmenorrhoea is often associated with the depth and extent of myometrial 'invasion'. This condition is now recognized to be common in older women in the reproductive age-groups, and it can be well imaged by the latest ultrasound equipment with experienced gynaecological operators, and by modern MRI. It is typically associated with HMB, secondary dysmenorrhoea, and deep dyspareunia; however, many cases of adenomyosis are not associated with obvious symptoms. Many cases of this disease coexist with other benign gynaecological diseases, such as endometriosis, endometrial polyps, leiomyomas, and endometrial hyperplasia, with each or sometimes even none of these diseases contributing to symptoms. These conditions need much more attention with research into their associations and varied symptoms.

Uterine leiomyomas (myomas, fibroids)

Commonly referred to as 'fibroids', uterine leiomyomas (benign, smooth-muscle tumours within the myometrium) can be associated with HMB, and chronic, dragging, and sometimes colicky pain. While many women suffering from myomas can remain asymptomatic, the submucous myomas, which protrude into the uterine cavity are more likely to be associated with dysmenorrhoea and particularly heavy HMB. These tumours are described in detail in Chapter 49.

Chronic pelvic inflammatory disease

Chronic pelvic inflammatory disease usually follows a delayed or inadequately treated acute pelvic infection or, less frequently, spontaneous, induced abortion or normal delivery with retained intrauterine products of conception (Chapter 43). Infection may be caused by specific local bacterial (gonorrhoea), rickettsial (chlamydia) or viral (human papilloma virus, HPV) organisms acting in the sensitized or damaged pelvic tissues. Pelvic inflammatory disease is usually associated with local tenderness, dyspareunia, and chronic, dragging pain, and is often maximal prior to onset of menstruation.

Endometrial polyps

Endometrial and cervical polyps are a common cause of irregular uterine bleeding and sometimes HMB, and dysmenorrhoea is an occasional, accompanying symptom.

Box 41.22 Common causes of secondary dysmenorrhoea

- Structural lesions usually with an inflammatory component:
  - Endometriosis
  - Adenomyosis
  - Leiomyomas
  - Chronic pelvic inflammatory disease
  - Endometrial polyps
- Other causes:
  - Congenital (imperforate hymen, non-communicating uterine horn, transverse vaginal septum)
  - Psychological factors

Ovarian cysts can be associated with ovarian torsion, with intracyst haemorrhage, or with local infection. These pathologies can cause various types of acute or semi-acute pelvic pain, but rarely pain that is labelled as 'dysmenorrhoea'. The only type of ovarian cyst which is frequently associated with 'secondary dysmenorrhoea' is endometriosis.

It should not be forgotten that pain from other organs, such as the bowel or the renal tract, may sometimes mimic dysmenorrhoea.

Mechanisms of pain generation with secondary dysmenorrhoea

Pain associated with endometriosis has been given much more research attention than adenomyosis, leiomyomas, or polyps, and it is clear that the mechanisms of secondary dysmenorrhoea and chronic pelvic pain with endometriosis are complex.

Experimental evidence shows that the endometrium of women with endometriosis is innervated with sensory and sympathetic nerve fibres, which are not usually present in women without the disease. These nerve fibres are also present within the endometriotic lesions and adhesions, along with the expression of multiple inflammatory and neural mediators, contributing to the generation of pain signals. Nociceptors in the sensory nerve fibres, tissue distortion, and ischaemia also contribute to the origin of pain signals.

There are multiple neural pathways through pelvic nerve tracts and neural ganglia leading to the dorsal root ganglia and afferent spinothalamic tracts within the spinal cord. These modulated signals are finally processed in centres within the thalamus and basal brain centres prior to onward referral to the cerebral cortex where they are finally 'perceived'. Other factors, such as psychological factors, influence this interpretation and ultimately perception of pain differs greatly between individuals.

History, examination, and investigations for dysmenorrhoea

History

Initial assessment of dysmenorrhoea begins with a structured history (Box 41.23). This is important in order to characterize pain and to determine the likely origin.

Examination

Examination is not usually indicated when history is suggestive of classical primary dysmenorrhoea and in patients who have not previously been sexually active. However, full examination including

---

Box 41.23 History-taking for dysmenorrhoea

- Nature of pain:
  - Site
  - Onset and duration
  - Character
  - Severity
  - Exacerbating/relieving factors
- General medical history
- Menstrual and sexual history
- Family history (endometriosis, bowel disease, interstitial cystitis, inflammatory conditions and malignancy)
- Effect on quality of life

Box 41.24 Exam characteristics for dysmenorrhoea

- General appearance, abdominal exam
- Pelvic exam—inspection of external genitalia
- Assess for lesions, discharge, point tenderness
- Bimanual exam—cervical motion tenderness, uterine size, mobility, adnexal masses/tenderness, uterosacral nodularity
- Speculum exam
- With or without per rectal exam

---

bimanual and speculum examination may be particularly useful in assessing secondary dysmenorrhoea (Box 41.24).

Investigations

Initial investigations including routine Pap smear and vaginal swabs for infection are an integral part of the pelvic exam. This is often followed by a good-quality transvaginal ultrasound, which may highlight need for further hysteroscopic or laparoscopic intervention (Box 41.25). Hysteroscopy can reveal the appearance of polyps (endometrial and cervical), myomas, adenomyosis, hyperplasia, cancer (although these do not usually present with pelvic pain at an early stage), and infection

Management of primary dysmenorrhoea

A good structured history is often sufficient in identification of primary dysmenorrhoea. These patients should be managed with a trial of suitable analgesics (with strict instructions on how these analgesics should be taken) and this can usually be managed at the level of the general practitioner. Specialist advice may be sought when initial management has failed or in those in whom compliance may be a problem. Optimum medical management depends on precise definition of symptoms and exclusion of structural lesions as possible underlying causes.

Medical management

Mild analgesics

Paracetamol and a wide range of marketed combinations with codeine phosphate, doxylamine, or dextropropoxyphene can be effective in mild dysmenorrhoea.

Prostaglandin inhibitors (NSAIDs)

A range of prostaglandin inhibitors can produce good clinical effect in up to 90% of sufferers. Commonly used NSAIDs include ibuprofen, naproxen sodium, mefenamic acid, and diclofenac sodium. A double dose is usually recommended as the starting dosage to gain initial pain control. Ongoing dosage is usually tailored to response of

---

Box 41.25 Potential investigations for dysmenorrhoea

- Pap smear (at time of speculum examination)
- High vaginal swab/chlamydia and gonorrhoea polymerase chain reaction
- Pelvic/transvaginal ultrasound (becoming routine)
- MRI (rarely needed)
- Hysteroscopy with or without excision
- Diagnostic laparoscopy with or without excision

the primary dysmenorrhoea, but is recommended to be one or two tablets/capsules every 6–8 hours while the pain is severe. Pain relief is not usually needed for more than 2–3 days for primary dysmenorrhoea. Some users experience side effects which are dose related, mainly nausea and gastrointestinal.

Combined oestrogen–progestogen oral contraceptive pills

These agents can be very effective in suppressing moderate to severe primary dysmenorrhoea. Combined oral contraceptives have been shown to reduce prostaglandin and vasopressin receptor activity and thus reduce uterine contractility and sensitivity. Monophasic pills with a strong progestogenic balance tend to be most effective, likely attributed to more effective suppression of endometrial proliferation, development, and prostaglandin production.

Levonorgestrel-releasing intrauterine system

The LNG-IUS is highly effective in suppressing endometrial proliferation and local prostaglandin production. In many patients it induces complete amenorrhoea and markedly reduces any complaint of primary dysmenorrhoea.

Other agents

Other agents, which have been utilized in the past for treatment of primary dysmenorrhoea, include danazol, GnRH agonists, and common antihypertensive agents such as calcium channel blockers and beta-blockers. These agents can induce endometrial atrophy, reduce uterine contractility, and promote relaxation of uterine muscle, reducing the symptoms of dysmenorrhoea. However, these agents are rarely used in modern management and their use is limited by their side effects.

Surgical management

Various surgical methods can be used to aid in diagnosis and management of dysmenorrhoea.

- Diagnostic laparoscopy, lesion biopsy, and endometrial biopsy.
- Presacral neurectomy: is rarely used nowadays, has limited levels of benefit and can have permanent adverse effects on bowel function.
- Laparoscopic laser uterine nerve ablation: has also lost popularity and is now recognized to have limited benefits.
- Hysteroscopic endometrial ablation or hysterectomy: these relatively major surgical procedures are regarded as unnecessarily extensive for primary dysmenorrhoea.
- Cervical dilatation has limited symptomatic benefits, and can cause cervical damage through tearing of the cervical muscular and fibrous structure.

Adjuvant therapy

Numerous other therapies for alleviation of dysmenorrhoea have been tried, and these may include dietary changes, smoking cessation, exercise, heat compresses, acupuncture, and transcutaneous nerve stimulation. Limited benefit occurs in some users.

Management of secondary dysmenorrhoea

Management of secondary dysmenorrhoea usually relies on effective management of underlying pathology. This may require a combination of medical and surgical approaches. Simple analgesics and prostaglandin inhibitors (NSAIDs) generally work less well with the pain symptoms of secondary as opposed to primary dysmenorrhoea, and patients may respond more effectively to a higher NSAID dosage, a combination of agents, or stronger analgesic agents (such as tramadol or oxycodone) to achieve optimum pain control. Nowadays, it is wise to refer to up-to-date pharmacological recommendations on dosage (using a current 'App' such as 'iMIMS').

Management is further challenged by the erratic nature of chronic pelvic pain, which may be exacerbated at menstruation, but may also be present at other times of the cycle. Surgical excision of underlying conditions such as endometriosis, adenomyosis, uterine fibroids, and even endometrial polyps usually requires a highly specialized, skilled, and planned laparoscopic, hysteroscopic, or laparotomy approach.

Society impact

Primary dysmenorrhoea tends to affect women during their early reproductive years (typically during adolescence), while secondary dysmenorrhoea is more commonly seen in the later reproductive years. Both of these two symptoms can have a major impact on quality of life for the woman, and those around her. It may impact self-esteem, time with family, and quality of both social and sexual life. Many women need to take time off from school and from work. In modern Western society, especially among younger, professional women, there is a steadily increasing desire for a 'bleed-free' and 'pain-free' existence, as far as menstruation is concerned. This scenario and these expectations are becoming much more widespread through the impact of modern social media.

The discussed hormonal and other therapies have additional powerful social benefits in that they reduce the amount of monthly bleeding, the associated menstrual pain, other menstrual symptoms, and the associated social impacts for the woman, her quality of life, her family, and her workplace.

Prognosis

Primary dysmenorrhoea tends to spontaneously improve with time as a woman moves into her 20s, and after a first full-term pregnancy, but may continue for many years. Secondary dysmenorrhoea, on the other hand, tends to progress and become worse with time for many women, unless effectively treated. Both types of symptoms can have a severe impact on the quality of life for sufferers.

Summary

This section has presented practical clinical information on two of the commonest symptoms encountered in gynaecology, and has highlighted the important and common underlying causes in a context of the important investigations. These two symptoms can play havoc with the daily lives of women who experience moderate or severe variations.

Understanding of the symptom presentations and the differential diagnoses are critical in determining the most relevant medical or surgical managements for individual women.

Many modern young women (in most cultures) are demonstrating an increasing societal change within health lifestyles in seeking an existence where menstruation is 'switched off' until ovulation is required when seeking a pregnancy. The convenience of pharmacological amenorrhoea is being increasingly recognized as a component of modern business and social lifestyles. This social change is likely to continue and health professionals will need to understand the clinical importance of different causes of amenorrhoea.

Dysmenorrhoea is very common in all societies and can be a major contributor to a significant level of incapacity during menstruation. HMB is often accompanied by menstrual pain, and women with combined HMB and pain are significantly more likely to present with the symptoms to a doctor than women with HMB alone.

These two symptoms are so common and so intrusive into the modern lifestyle that a sound understanding of their impact is essential for the modern doctor. Indeed, these symptoms have an impact, as an important comorbidity, on most medical conditions in women. Further, these are symptoms which rely on a carefully taken case history in order to understand their main impacts on the woman and possible interactions with other medical conditions.

REFERENCES

1. Harlow SD, Lin X, Ho MJ. Analysis of menstrual diary data across the reproductive life span. Applicability of the bipartite model approach and the importance of within woman variance. *J Clin Epidemiol* 2000;**53**:722–33.
2. Fraser IS, Sungurtekin-Inceboz U. Defining disturbances of the menstrual cycle. In: O'Brien PMS, Cameron IT, MacLean AB (eds), *Disorders of the Menstrual Cycle*, pp 141–52. London: RCOG Press, 2000.
3. Fraser IS, Critchley HO, Munro MG, Broder M. Can we achieve international agreement on terminologies and definitions used to describe abnormalities of menstrual bleeding? *Hum Reprod* 2007;**22**:635–43.
4. Munro MG, Critchley HOD, Broder MS, Fraser IS, FIGO Working Group on Menstrual Disorders. FIGO Classification System (PALM-COEIN) for causes of abnormal uterine bleeding in non-gravid women of reproductive age. *Int J Gynecol Obstet* 2011;**113**: 3–13.
5. Hallberg L, Högdahl AM, Nilsson L, Rybo G. Menstrual blood loss—a population study. Variation at different ages and attempts to define normality. *Acta Obstet Gynecol Scand* 1966;**45**:320–51.
6. Cole SK, Billewicz WZ, Thomson AM. Sources of variation in menstrual blood loss. *J Obstet Gynaecol Br Commonw* 1971;**78**:933–39.
7. National Institute for Health and Care Excellence (NICE). *Heavy Menstrual Bleeding: Assessment and Management*. NICE guideline [NG88]. London: NICE; 2007. Available at: https://www.nice.org.uk/guidance/ng88.
8. Tan DA, Haththotuwa R, Fraser IS. Cultural aspects and mythologies surrounding menstruation and abnormal uterine bleeding. *Best Pract Res Clin Obstet Gynaecol* 2017;**40**:121–33.
9. Shander A, Hofmann A, Isbister J, Van Aken H. Patient blood management—the new frontier. *Best Prac Res Clin Anaesthesiol* 2013;**27**:5–10.
10. Clevenger B, Mallett SV, Klein AA, Richards T. Patient blood management to reduce surgical risk. *Br J Surg* 2015;**102**:1325–37.
11. Caronia LM, Martin C, Welt CK. A genetic basis for functional hypothalamic amenorrhea. *N Engl J Med* 2011;**301**:215–25.
12. Codner E, Merino PM, Tena-Sempere M. Female reproducotion and type 1 diabetes: from mechanisms to clinical findings. *Hum Reprod Update* 2012;**18**:568–85.
13. Molteni N, Bardella, MT, Bianchi PA. Obstetric and gynecological problems in women with untreated celiac sprue. *J Clin Gastroenterol* 1990;**12**:37–39.
13. Akerlund M, Anderson KE, Ingemarsson I. Effect of terbutaline on myometrial activity, endometrial blood flow, and lower abdominal pain in women with primary dysmenorrhoea. *Br J Obstet Gynaecol* 1976;**83**:673–78.
14. Lundstrom V, Green K. Endogenous levels of prostaglandin F2alpha and its main metabolites in plasma and endometrium of normal and dysmenorrheic women. *Am J Obstet Gynecol* 1978;**130**:640–46.
15. Stromberg P, Akerlund M, Forsling ML, Granstrom E, Kindahl H. Vasopressin and prostaglandins in premenstrual pain and primary dysmenorrhea. *Acta Obstet Gynecol Scand* 1984;**63**:533–38.
16. Forsling ML, Stromberg P, Akerlund M. Effect of ovarian steroids on vasopressin secretion. *J Endocrinol* 1982;**95**:147–51.
17. Harlow SD, Park M. A longitudinal study of risk factors for the occurrence, duration and severity of menstrual cramps in a cohort of college women. *Br J Obstet Gynaecol* 1996;**103**:1134–42.
18. Sultan C, Jeandel C, Paris F, Trimeche S. Adolescent dysmenorrhea. *Endocr Dev* 2004;**7**:140–47.

42

Polycystic ovary syndrome

Zhongwei Huang and Eu Leong Yong

Introduction

Polycystic ovary syndrome (PCOS) is a common reproductive endocrine disorder that affects up to 15% of women in the reproductive age group using the Rotterdam criteria 2003 (1). The Rotterdam criteria 2003 state that a diagnosis of PCOS is made if two out of the following three criteria of (a) presence of menstrual irregularities, (b) clinical/biochemical evidence of androgen excess, or (c) polycystic ovary morphology on ultrasound assessment are met after excluding other hyperandrogenic conditions such as congenital hyperplasia or androgen secreting tumour (2). Recently, the European Society of Human Reproduction and Embryology (ESHRE) and the American Society of Reproductive Medicine (ASRM)-sponsored Third PCOS Consensus Workshop Group summarized current knowledge on PCOS and identified the knowledge gaps regarding various women's health aspects of PCOS (1). The PCOS Consensus Workshop Group also discussed the challenges in the variations of PCOS phenotypes and defining features of PCOS, which include issues such as ethnic differences in the phenotypes of PCOS (3, 4). Additionally, the diagnosis of PCOS in adolescence, the impact on infertility, and long-term metabolic, cardiovascular, and cancer risks are important aspects of PCOS which require further attention in management of women with this enigmatic condition.

Pathophysiology of polycystic ovary syndrome

Until now, the underlying cause of PCOS remained elusive. However, there are a number of proposed mechanisms which involve hyperandrogenism, hyperinsulinism, and high levels of anti-Mullerian hormone (AMH) associated with anovulation as the pathogenesis of PCOS.

Androgen excess

Hyperandrogenism can be a cause of PCOS but it remains controversial and difficult to prove in humans (5). Clinical studies demonstrated that androgen levels such as total testosterone and androstenedione were consistently elevated in women with PCOS when compared to controls (6, 7). Giving the androgen receptor antagonist flutamide to some women with PCOS restored menstrual regularity and ovulation in these women (8). This study seemed to suggest that androgen receptor-mediated androgen actions could be involved in the pathogenesis of PCOS resulting in the phenotype we recognize in women with PCOS such as irregular periods, polycystic ovarian morphology, or signs of androgen excess. Additionally, an association between short CAG repeat length in the androgen receptor and the subset of anovulatory patients with low serum androgens suggests that the pathogenic mechanism of polycystic ovaries in these patients could be due to the increased intrinsic androgenic activity associated with short androgen receptor alleles (9). Walters reviewed the literature and concluded that rodent, sheep, and primate PCOS models had clearly demonstrated that the reproductive, endocrine, and metabolic characteristics of human PCOS (anovulation, polycystic ovaries, increased anthral follicular count, luteinizing hormone elevation, insulin resistance, dyslipidaemia, obesity) could be consistently induced by androgen excess (5). All in all, the data suggest that androgen excess involving the androgen receptor–androgens pathway is intrinsically linked to PCOS.

Hyperinsulinism

De Leo and colleagues had suggested that insulin resistance and hyperinsulinism could have a central role in the pathogenesis of PCOS (10). Human ovaries had specific receptors for insulin (11, 12) and studies on thecal cells also demonstrated that insulin acted as a co-gonadotropin in steroidogenesis (14) and stimulated proliferation of thecal cells (15) to increase luteinizing hormone-stimulated androgen secretion (16–18) and to increase P450c17 mRNA levels (19) which upregulated luteinizing hormone receptors (20) and ovarian insulin-like growth factor 1 receptors (13). Hyperinsulinaemia therefore increased androgen levels by stimulating ovarian steroidogenesis and inhibiting insulin growth factor binding protein and sex hormone-binding globulin (SHBG) synthesis and secretion (10). Based on the review by De Leo and colleagues, only metformin and the new thiazolidinediones (rosiglitazone and pioglitazone) should be recommended in clinical practice as the balance of opinion seems to favour beneficial effects of insulin-lowering agents on insulin sensitivity, hyperandrogenaemia, menstrual irregularity, and metabolic disorders in a large subset of affected women with PCOS (10). Another study also demonstrated that in women with PCOS, treatment with metformin is effective in the lowering of hyperinsulinaemia, hyperandrogenaemia, and in many women with PCOS, improves the menstrual pattern, but has no effect on hirsutism (21). A recent review by Lautatzis and colleagues also affirmed the efficacy and safety of metformin use throughout pregnancy in women with PCOS as this intervention reduced the rates of early pregnancy loss, preterm labour, and protected against fetal growth restriction. Also, there were no demonstrable teratogenic effects, intrauterine deaths, or developmental delays with the use of metformin in pregnancy (22). Based on the *in vitro* and clinical studies to date, hyperinsulinism can potentially be an aetiological agent for the PCOS phenotype.

Anti-Mullerian hormone

PCOS is a heterogeneous disorder affecting ovarian function primarily, and has features of multiple small follicles growing but which arrest and result in anovulation. Interestingly, AMH is unique and specific to the human ovary and its expression is restricted to the granulosa cells of the ovary in women. AMH begins to be produced at around the 25th week of gestation and continues until menopause (23, 24). AMH is also expressed at all steps of folliculogenesis and is initiated as soon as primordial follicles are recruited to grow into small preantral follicles with its highest expression being observed in preantral and small antral follicles. Thereafter, AMH expression decreases with the selection of follicles for dominance and becomes no longer expressed during the follicle-stimulating hormone-dependent stages of follicular growth (except in the cumulus cells of preovulatory follicles) and in atretic follicles (25, 26). Dumont and colleagues performed a comprehensive review of AMH and its association with PCOS and concluded that in PCOS there were multiple levels of abnormalities in folliculogenesis attributable to the actions by high levels of AMH resulting in an increased number of small growing follicles and inhibition of the terminal follicular growth. This will lead to a lack of selection of the dominant follicle known as 'follicle arrest'. Additionally, a possible follicular apoptosis defect can result in the excess of growing follicles (27).

Henceforth, the most striking reproductive disorder based on the proposed mechanisms results in the clinical presentation of anovulation as irregular (i.e. long intervals between menstrual cycles) or absent periods. This has been demonstrated in a recent study by Zhu and colleagues showing the association between higher AMH levels and longer menstrual cycle length of more than 35 days (28). Due to the anovulatory cycles, women with PCOS may also encounter issues with other endocrine disturbances secondary to the androgen excess and hyperinsulinism. An attempt to look at genetic variants in the AMH signal transduction pathway demonstrated population differences; however, this does not appear to have significant effects on ovarian, endocrine, and metabolic parameters and reproductive outcomes (29).

Clinical manifestations of polycystic ovary syndrome

Prevalence

The prevalence of PCOS is 6–15% of women in the reproductive age group based on the current diagnostic criteria such as the National Institutes of Health criteria (1990) and the Rotterdam criteria (2003) (1, 3). The Androgen Excess and PCOS Society criteria

(2006) defined PCOS as a fulfilling hyperandrogenism (clinical and/or biochemical) and ovarian dysfunction (oligoanovulation and/or polycystic ovaries) after the exclusion of related disorders (30). Henceforth, the most encompassing criteria with the largest group of PCOS phenotypes will be the Rotterdam criteria (2003) (30).

Spectrum of disease

The diagnostic criteria will therefore result in differing permutations of phenotypes observed in women with PCOS (**Table 42.1**). Importantly, although endocrine and metabolic disturbances such as obesity, insulin resistance, and dyslipidaemia are associated with PCOS, the current diagnostic criteria do not take these factors into consideration. Thus, the spectrum of PCOS phenotypes only include women with androgen excess who are disturbed by excessive body and facial hair and/or women with reproductive issues such as irregular menstrual cycles and anovulation trying to conceive or with a desire to have regular menstrual cycles.

Ethnic differences in women with polycystic ovary syndrome

Ethnic differences appeared to exert significant influences on the prevalence of PCOS based on the current diagnostic criteria. This is especially so in the clinical presentation and definition of hirsutism in East Asian women (Chinese, Japanese, Korean, Thai) when compared to Caucasian and Middle Eastern women as it is noted that the modified Ferriman-Gallwey (mFG) score is lower in East Asian women (4). Indeed, the prevalence of PCOS among the Asian populations has been reported to vary from 5.6% in the Southern Chinese population (31), 5.7% in Thai women (32), and 6.3% in Sri Lankan women (33), to 14.3% in Iranian women (34). Even in studies on Caucasian subjects, the prevalence of PCOS ranges from 6% to 15% (3). These differences are likely to be contributed to by ethnic differences. South Asian and Middle Eastern women with PCOS are also known to have a higher prevalence of obesity, diabetes, and metabolic diseases whereas East Asian women are less likely to be afflicted (1). Further work is still required to determine the impact of ethnicity on the reproductive, endocrine, and metabolic disturbances in women with PCOS.

Disease evolution and effects of reproductive ageing

The effect of reproductive ageing in women with PCOS remains poorly understood. However, studies have shown that there is an improvement in the regularity of menstrual cycles with reproductive ageing in women with PCOS (35, 36). Serum testosterone levels decreased in women with PCOS from the third to the fifth decades. Additionally, with age, ovarian size and morphology was also noted to be improved (1). The PCOS phenotype appears to change with ageing, suggesting an amelioration of the phenotype and ovarian dysfunction as indicated by the increase in number of regular menstrual cycles, decrease in serum androgen levels, and decrease in insulin resistance (37). There are still limited data on the long-term fecundity and the precise age of menopause although there are studies reporting that women with PCOS may experience menopause at a later age (38, 39). Long-term, multicentre cohort studies are needed to understand if there is a menopausal phenotype for women with PCOS and the associated long-term health consequences in these women.

Table 42.1 Possible phenotypes of PCOS

Clinical manifestation	Possible phenotypes for PCOS									
Hyperandrogenaemia	1	1	1	1	0	0	1	0	1	0
Hyperandrogenism (hirsutism)	1	1	0	0	1	1	1	1	0	0
Menstrual irregularities	1	1	1	1	1	1	0	0	0	1
Polycystic ovarian morphology on ultrasound	1	0	1	0	1	0	1	1	1	1
Diagnostic criteria										
NIH Criteria 1990	+	+	+	+	+	+				
Rotterdam Criteria 2003	+	+	+	+	+	+	+	+	+	+
Androgen Excess Society/PCOS Society 2006	+	+	+	+	+	+	+	+	+	
1= present 0 = not absent.										

Source data from Azziz R, Carmina E, Dewailly D, Diamanti-Kandarakis E, Escobar-Morreale HF, Futterweit W, Janssen OE, Legro RS, Norman RJ, Taylor AE, Witchel SF; Task Force on the Phenotype of the Polycystic Ovary Syndrome of The Androgen Excess and PCOS Society. The Androgen Excess and PCOS Society criteria for the polycystic ovary syndrome: the complete task force report. *Fertil Steril* 2009;91(2):456–88.

Clinical issues and their management

Women with PCOS tend to have reproductive issues such as oligomenorrhoea and anovulation. Many will need assistance when they are unable to conceive spontaneously. In addition, they are likely to have endocrine problems such as hirsutism and metabolic issues such as obesity, insulin resistance, and dyslipidaemia. The following sections aim to provide an approach to and management of the clinical problems that women with PCOS will face in their life course.

Oligo/amenorrhoea

Up to 79% of women with PCOS will have irregular menstrual cycles (30); many of these women present to the gynaecologist to manage their menstrual periods. Irregular cycles are attributable to anovulation and usually result in a hyperoestrogenic state which may predispose to the risks of developing endometrial hyperplasia and carcinoma (40). Haoula and colleagues observed that women with PCOS have a 2.89-fold (95% confidence interval (CI) 1.52–5.48) increased risk for endometrial cancer (41) and in these women, when intervals between menstruation become longer than 3 months (i.e. fewer than four periods each year), this is associated with endometrial hyperplasia (42). A prospective study of 56 consecutive amenorrhoeic women with PCOS who underwent transvaginal ultrasound to assess the endometrial thickness concluded that the endometrial thickness was positively correlated with endometrial hyperplasia; no cases of endometrial hyperplasia were observed when the endometrial thickness was less than 7 mm (42).

Good clinical practice will involve the regular induction of a withdrawal bleed using cyclical progestogens for at least 12 days (43, 44), or oral contraceptive pills (various formulations with different generations of progesterone preparations), or the intrauterine system with local release of progestogens, commonly known as the Mirena system (Bayer Plc, Newbury, United Kingdom). These interventions are advisable in oligomenorrhoeic women with PCOS (45), but the most effective regimen remains unclear and can be dependent on the patient's preference and risk profile; however, there remains a lack of randomized clinical trials examining this aspect (46).

Another contributing factor to the irregular cycles and potentially other endocrine and metabolic disturbances noted in women with PCOS is the high body mass index (BMI) observed in these women.

A modest but non-significant trend in the prevalence of PCOS with increasing BMI has been reported (47). Obesity and especially abdominal obesity can cause relative hyperandrogenaemia, characterized by reduced levels of SHBG and increased levels of bioavailable androgens delivered to target tissues (48, 49). In adult overweight and obese women with PCOS, menstrual abnormalities and chronic oligoanovulation are more frequent than in normal-weight women (49). In a small study looking at 12 morbidly obese women with PCOS, an average postoperative weight loss of 41 kg in the first year improved hyperandrogenism, insulin resistance, dyslipidaemia, and hypertension and reversed the PCOS diagnosis (50).

A Cochrane review concluded that lifestyle intervention (incorporating diet, exercise, and behavioural modifications) improves body composition, hyperandrogenism (high male hormones and clinical effects), and insulin resistance in women with PCOS. There was no evidence of effect for lifestyle intervention on improving glucose tolerance or lipid profiles and no literature assessing clinical reproductive outcomes, quality of life, and treatment satisfaction (51). Another clinical practice guideline by Legro and colleagues recommended the use of exercise therapy in the management of overweight and obesity in women with PCOS despite there being no large randomized trials of exercise in women with PCOS; exercise therapy, alone or in combination with dietary intervention, improves weight loss and reduces cardiovascular risk factors and diabetes risk in the general population. They also mention that weight loss is likely beneficial for improvement of both reproductive and metabolic dysfunctions but weight loss is likely to be insufficient as a treatment for normal-weight women with PCOS (52).

Subfertility

Women with PCOS are more likely to encounter anovulation—in a large series of women with PCOS, close to half of these women had primary infertility and a quarter of them reported secondary infertility (53). Anovulatory infertility which included PCOS is common and accounts for 25–40% of women with infertility in population-based studies (53, 54). Moreover, PCOS is the most common cause of ovulatory dysfunction, accounting for 70–90% of ovulatory disorders (55) with prolonged periods of anovulation associated with increased infertility (56).

Therefore, in women with PCOS, the first step to regain fertility is to ensure ovulation and this can be performed using various ovulation induction agents such as clomiphene citrate, letrozole, and gonadotropins. Metformin, an insulin sensitizer, has also been tried in women with PCOS not only to correct metabolic disturbances but also to correct hyperandrogenism and for ovulation induction.

Clomiphene citrate has been recommended by the Endocrine Society Clinical Practice Guideline as the first line of therapy for anovulatory infertility for women with PCOS (52). Many multicentre clinical trials had demonstrated the benefits of clomiphene citrate for anovulation (57–59) and that the results are similar to that of gonadotropins (60). Palomba and colleagues (61) also reviewed the literature on metformin usage in PCOS and suggested that in anovulatory infertile therapy-naive PCOS patients, the combined approach of metformin plus clomiphene citrate is not better than clomiphene citrate or metformin monotherapy. Using metformin as a second-line approach, the authors concluded that in women who received gonadotropins as treatment for anovulation, metformin addition reduces the duration of gonadotropins administration and the doses of gonadotropins required and increases the rate of mono-ovulations, reducing the risk of cancelled cycles. Additionally, metformin administration in infertile women with PCOS scheduled for IVF cycles is useful to reduce the risk of ovarian hyperstimulation syndrome (61).

Aromatase inhibitors have been proposed as another oral treatment option to treat anovulatory infertility in women with PCOS. A large National Institutes of Health-sponsored, multicentre, double-blind, randomized, clinical trial which included 750 subjects has been completed with a marked superiority in live birth rate of letrozole over clomiphene for the treatment of anovulatory infertility in women with PCOS together with a comparable safety and tolerance profile between the two drugs (62). Although concerns about the relative teratogenicity of letrozole compared to clomiphene remain, the results of this trial and other publications have been reassuring (63).

Ovarian electrocautery can be considered for selected anovulatory patients with a normal BMI as an alternative to ovulation induction as anovulation associated with PCOS has long been known to be amenable to surgical treatment (64). A long-term cohort study has demonstrated persistence of ovulation as well as normalization of serum androgens and SHBG up to 20 years after laparoscopic ovarian electrocautery in over 60% of subjects, especially if they have a normal BMI (65).

Endocrine issues

Women with PCOS who have marked hyperandrogenism and anovulation are shown to have the highest incidence of metabolic disturbances (66). Insulin resistance is noted to be present in around 65–80% of women with PCOS independent of obesity (67) which is further exacerbated by excess weight (68). Earlier-onset hyperglycaemia and rapid progression to type 2 diabetes mellitus is also reported in women with PCOS (69) and PCOS is classified as a non-modifiable risk factor for type 2 diabetes mellitus (70). Type 2 diabetes mellitus and cardiovascular disease risk are worsened in women with PCOS known to be insulin resistant (71) regardless of their high BMI (72). Lifestyle therapy has been shown to prevent or delay progression to type 2 diabetes, therefore it is important to perform early screening in women with PCOS. An oral glucose

tolerance test is considered to be appropriate for screening women with PCOS for diabetes. However, it would be reasonable to carry out HbA1c measurements where women are unwilling to have oral glucose tolerance tests or where the resources are not readily available (64). Women, particularly of south Asian descent, who are more likely to be insulin resistant, should have an oral glucose tolerance test done regardless of their BMI (73). Rescreening is suggested every 3–5 years, or more frequently if clinical factors such as central adiposity, substantial weight gain, and/or symptoms of diabetes develop in any women with PCOS (52). New compounds such as decanoic acid have been demonstrated to be effective in reversing the endocrine and metabolic abnormalities of the letrozole-induced PCOS rat model, raising the possibility that diets including decanoic acid could be beneficial for the management of both hyperandrogenism and insulin resistance in PCOS (74).

Obesity and the metabolic syndrome

Obesity and especially abdominal obesity can result in relative hyperandrogenaemia, characterized by reduced levels of SHBG and increased levels of bioavailable androgens delivered to target tissues (48, 49). Abdominal obesity is also associated with an increased testosterone production rate and a non-SHBG-bound androgen production rate of dehydroepiandrosterone and androstenedione (75). These mechanisms serve to explain the associations in women with PCOS and obesity. Women with PCOS, as compared with age- and BMI-matched women without the syndrome, appear to have a higher risk of insulin resistance, hyperinsulinaemia, glucose intolerance, dyslipidaemia, and an increased prothrombotic state, thereby resulting in a higher rate of type 2 diabetes mellitus, subclinical atherosclerosis, vascular dysfunction, and cardiovascular disease (76). All women with PCOS should be assessed for cardiovascular disease risk by assessing individual cardiovascular disease risk factors, as stated earlier, at the time of initial diagnosis. The Royal College of Obstetricians and Gynaecologists in the United Kingdom has recommended that in daily clinical practice, hypertension should be treated and lipid-lowering treatment is not recommended routinely and should only be prescribed by a specialist (64). Although statins improve lipid profiles and reduce testosterone levels in women with PCOS, there is no evidence that statins improve resumption of menstrual regularity or spontaneous ovulation, nor is there any improvement of hirsutism or acne based on a Cochrane review (77). The first-line management is to initiate weight-loss strategies with calorie-restricted diets (with no evidence that one type of diet is superior) for adolescents and women with PCOS who are overweight or obese (52). Metformin can be offered as first-line therapy for obesity management and/or management of women with PCOS known to have type 2 diabetes mellitus or impaired glucose tolerance who failed lifestyle modifications. Bariatric surgery may be an option for morbidly obese women with PCOS (BMI of 40 kg/m^2 or more or 35 kg/m^2 or more with a high-risk obesity-related condition) if standard weight loss strategies have failed (64).

Hirsutism and its management

PCOS represents the major cause of hirsutism in women (52) and is present in approximately 65–75% of patients with PCOS (although this figure is lower in Asian populations) (78, 79). Hirsutism may predict the metabolic sequelae of PCOS (80) or failure to conceive with infertility treatment (81), hence treatment of hirsutism is twofold—to correct the hyperandrogenism and metabolic disturbances and for cosmetic purposes. Based on a Cochrane review by van Zuuren and colleagues, treatments for hirsutism may need to incorporate pharmacological therapies, cosmetic procedures, and psychological support (82). For mild hirsutism, there is evidence of limited quality that oral combined contraceptive pills are effective. Flutamide 250 mg twice daily and spironolactone 100 mg daily appeared to be effective and safe, albeit the evidence was low to very low quality. No firm conclusions can be drawn on the use of finasteride 5 mg daily. As the side effects of antiandrogens and finasteride are well known, such drugs must be used with caution in managing women with hirsutism. There was low-quality evidence that metformin was ineffective for hirsutism (82). Therefore, medical treatments can be offered although laser and photoepilation therapies are useful adjuncts and may have to be utilized in conjunction with medical therapies.

Long-term health consequences in women with polycystic ovary syndrome

Ageing and the menopause

The phenotype of women with PCOS appears to ameliorate with ageing as indicated by the increase in frequency in the regularity of menstrual cycles, decrease in serum androgen levels, and decrease in insulin resistance (37). There are studies reporting that women with PCOS may experience menopause at a later age (38, 39) and this may be explained with data showing that women with PCOS have a larger cohort of follicles as compared to age-matched women without PCOS (1). AMH level, a marker of antral follicle number, exhibits a less pronounced longitudinal decrease in ageing women with PCOS, which results in an estimated menopausal age 2 years later than in controls (83). Overall, it appears that ovarian ageing in women with PCOS is delayed compared to control women, but further longitudinal evidence is also needed.

The PCOS menopausal phenotype remained poorly defined and the current diagnostic criteria cannot be used after the menopause. Longitudinal data provide evidence that control women tend to have worsening of some of their metabolic parameters to a range seen in the PCOS subjects over time, whereas women with PCOS have more components of the metabolic syndrome starting at an early age (insulin resistance, abnormal lipid levels, hypertension, obesity) and therefore have a longer exposure to these adverse cardiovascular risk factors (83). Whether the increased cardiovascular risk in reproductive life translates into an increased cardiovascular morbidity and mortality in later life for women with PCOS remains to be unravelled as current data remains conflicting (1, 83). In women who maintain high androgen levels even after menopause, the cardiovascular risk remains increased and can adversely affect these women's risks of cardiovascular disorders later on in life. Further longitudinal data is essential to follow up in women with PCOS to determine their lifetime risks of metabolic and cardiovascular diseases.

Cancer risks in women in PCOS

Women with PCOS share many of the risk factors associated with the development of endometrial cancer including obesity, hyperinsulinism, diabetes, and abnormal uterine bleeding (52). Young women with endometrial cancer are found to be more likely to be nulliparous and infertile, have higher rates of hirsutism, and have a slightly higher chance of oligomenorrhoea (84). Therefore, the Royal College of Obstetricians and Gynaecologists has recommended it is good clinical practice that women with irregular menstrual cycles should receive treatment with progestogens to induce a withdrawal bleed at least every 3–4 months as they are at higher risks of endometrial hyperplasia and cancer later on in life.

Women with PCOS do not have a significant increase in their risk of developing breast cancer compared to those without PCOS (relative risk 0.88; 95% CI 0.44–1.77) based on systematic review (85). A small number of studies have addressed the possibility of an association between PCOS and epithelial ovarian cancer risk and the overall data appear reassuring (86–88). Finally, there does not appear to be an association of PCOS with breast or ovarian cancer. Therefore, no additional surveillance is required beyond that of routine screening for breast and ovarian cancer.

Summary points

- PCOS is diagnosed in women in the reproductive age group based on the Rotterdam criteria when two out of the following three criteria are met—(a) presence of menstrual irregularities, (b) clinical/biochemical evidence of androgen excess, or (c) polycystic ovary morphology on ultrasound assessment.
- The pathophysiology of PCOS remains to be determined but it is likely to involve the androgen, insulin, and AMH pathways.
- Ethnic differences can contribute to the differences in prevalence seen in different populations of women with PCOS such as East Asian, Caucasian, and South Asian populations.
- The spectrum of disease involves various phenotypes based on the current diagnostic criteria and this may have reproductive, metabolic, and endocrine consequences.
- Reproductive issues include irregular menstrual cycles and anovulation. Treatment modalities include lifestyle modifications such as exercise, weight loss, and calorie-restricted diets; and medications such as clomiphene citrate, letrozole, and gonadotropins for ovulation induction. In some cases, especially in women with normal BMI, ovarian electrocautery may be indicated.
- Metabolic disorders such as insulin resistance, obesity, dyslipidaemia, and hypertension must be screened for in all women who are diagnosed with PCOS. Treatment modalities include lifestyle modifications such as exercise, weight loss, and calorie-restricted diets. Medications such as metformin can be useful in obese women with PCOS, although bariatric surgery may be indicated in some women.
- Endocrine issues such as type 2 diabetes mellitus must be treated in women with PCOS.
- Hirsutism can be managed with different medications ranging from oral contraceptive pills to antiandrogens but bearing in mind the side effects of these medications. Physical modalities such as laser and photoepilation therapies may still be necessary.
- Reproductive ageing appears to be increased in women with PCOS and they seem to undergo menopause at a later age.

- Long-term risks of metabolic and endocrine disorders in women with PCOS still need further confirmation with more robust data.
- Women with PCOS are at higher risk of endometrial hyperplasia and cancer but other cancers such as breast and ovarian cancer are not associated with PCOS.

REFERENCES

1. Fauser BCJ, Tarlartzis BC, Rebar RW, et al. Consensus on Women's Health Aspects of polycystic ovarian syndrome (PCOS): the Amsterdam ESHRE/ASRM -Sponsored 3rd PCOS Consensus Workshop Group. *Fertil Steril* 2012;**97**:28–38.

2. The Rotterdam ESHRE/ASRM-Sponsored PCOS Consensus Workshop Group. Revised 2003 consensus on diagnostic criteria and long-term health risks related to polycystic ovary syndrome (PCOS). *Hum Reprod* 2004;**19**:41–47.

3. Zhao Y, Qiao J. Ethnic differences in the phenotypic expression of polycystic ovary syndrome. *Steroids* 2013;**78**:755–60.

4. Huang Z, Yong EL. Ethnic differences: is there an Asian phenotype for polycystic ovarian syndrome? *Best Pract Res Clin Obstet Gynaecol* 2016;**37**:46–55.

5. Walters KA. Androgens in polycystic ovary syndrome: lessons from experimental models. *Curr Opin Endocrinol Diabetes Obes* 2016;**23**:257–63.

6. Keefe CC, Goldman MM, Zhang K, Clarke N, Reitz RE, Welt CK. Simultaneous measurement of thirteen steroid hormones in women with polycystic ovary syndrome and control women using liquid chromatography-tandem mass spectrometry. *PLoS One* 2014;**9**:e93805.

7. Palomba S, Falbo A, Chiossi G, et al. Lipid profile in nonobese pregnant women with polycystic ovary syndrome: a prospective controlled clinical study. *Steroids* 2014;**88**:36–43.

8. Paradisi R, Fabbri R, Battaglia C, Venturoli S. Ovulatory effects of flutamide in the polycystic ovary syndrome. *Gynecol Endocrinol* 2013;**29**:391–95.

9. Mifsud A, Ramirez S, Yong EL. Androgen receptor gene CAG trinucleotide repeats in anovulatory infertility and polycystic ovaries. *J Clin Endocrinol Metab* 2000;**85**:3484–88.

10. De Leo V, la Marca A, Petraglia F. Insulin-lowering agents in the management of polycystic ovary syndrome *Endocr Rev* 2003;**24**:633–67.

11. Poretsky L, Smith D, Seibel M, Pazianos A, Moses AC, Flier JS. Specific insulin binding sites in human ovary. *J Clin Endocrinol Metab* 1984;**59**:809–11.

12. Poretsky L, Cataldo NA, Rosenwaks Z, Giudice LC. The insulin-related ovarian regulatory system in health and disease. *Endocr Rev* 1999;**20**:535–82.

13. Poretsky L, Grigorescu F, Seibel M, Moses AC, Flier JS. Distribution and characterization of insulin and insulin-like growth factor 1 receptors in normal human ovary. *J Clin Endocrinol Metab* 1985;**61**:728–34.

14. Bergh C, Carlsson B, Olsson JH, Selleskog U, Hillensjo T. Regulation of androgen production in cultured human thecal cells by insulin-like growth factor I and insulin. *Fertil Steril* 1993;**59**:323–31.

15. Duleba AJ, Spaczynski RZ, Olive DL. Insulin and insulin-like growth factor I stimulate the proliferation of human ovarian theca interstitial cells. *Fertil Steril* 1998;**69**:335–40.

16. Cara JF, Rosenfield RL. Insulin-like growth factor I and insulin potentiate luteinizing hormone-induced androgen synthesis by rat ovarian thecal-interstitial cells. *Endocrinology* 1988;**123**:733–39.

17. Hernandez ER, Resnick CE, Svoboda ME, Van Wyk JJ, Payne DW, Adashi EY. Somatomedin-C/insulin-like growth factor I as an enhancer of androgen biosynthesis by cultured rat ovarian cells. *Endocrinology* 1988;**122**:1603–12.

18. Wrathall JH, Knight PG. Effects of inhibin-related peptides and oestradiol on androstenedione and progesterone secretion by bovine theca cells in vitro. *J Endocrinol* 1995;**145**:491–500.

19. Kristiansen SB, Endoh A, Casson PR, Buster JE, Hornsby PJ. Induction of steroidogenic enzyme genes by insulin and IGF-I in cultured adult human adrenocortical cells. *Steroids* 1997;**62**:258–65.

20. Adashi EY, Resnick CE, D'Ercole AJ, Svoboda ME, Van Wyk JJ. Insulin-like growth factors as intra-ovarian regulators of granulosa cell growth and function. *Endocr Rev* 1985;**6**:400–20.

21. Krstevska B, Dimitrovski CH, Pemovska G, et al. Metformin improves menstrual patterns, endocrine and metabolic profile in obese hyperinsulinemic women with a polycystic ovary syndrome. *Prilozi* 2006;**27**:57–66.

22. Lautatzis ME, Goulis DG, Vrontakis M. Efficacy and safety of metformin during pregnancy in women with gestational diabetes mellitus or polycystic ovary syndrome: a systematic review. *Metabolism* 2013;**62**:1522–34.

23. Rajpert-De Meyts E, Jorgensen N, Graem N, Muller J, Cate RL, Skakkebaek NE. Expression of anti-Mullerian hormone during normal and pathological gonadal development: association with differentiation of Sertoli and granulosa cells. *J Clin Endocrinol Metab* 1999;**84**:3836–44.

24. Kuiri-Hanninen T, Kallio S, Seuri R, et al. Postnatal developmental changes in the pituitary-ovarian axis in preterm and term infant girls. *J Clin Endocrinol Metab* 2011;**96**:3432–39.

25. Salmon NA, Handyside AH, Joyce IM. Oocyte regulation of anti-Mullerian hormone expression in granulosa cells during ovarian follicle development in mice. *Dev Biol* 2004;**266**:201–208.

26. Durlinger AL, Visser JA, Themmen AP. Regulation of ovarian function: the role of anti-Mullerian hormone. *Reproduction* 2002;**124**:601–609.

27. Dumont A, Robin G, Catteau-Jonard S, Dewailly D. Role of Anti-Müllerian hormone in pathophysiology, diagnosis and treatment of polycystic ovary syndrome: a review. *Reprod Biol Endocrinol* 2015;**13**:137.

28. Zhu R, Lee BH, Huang Z, et al. Anti-müllerian hormone, antral follicle count and ovarian volume predict menstrual cycle length in healthy women. *Clin Endocrinol (Oxf)* 2016;**84**:870–77.

29. Yu ED, Zhu H, Li Y, Chua SE, Indran IR, Li J, Yong EL. Polymorphisms of anti-Müllerian hormone signaling pathway in healthy Singapore women: population differences, endocrine effects and reproductive outcomes. *Gynecol Endocrinol* 2016;**32**:311–14.

30. Azziz R, Carmina E, Dewailly D, et al. The Androgen Excess and PCOS Society criteria for the polycystic ovary syndrome: the complete task force report. *Fertil Steril* 2009;**91**:456–88.

31. Li R, Zhang Q, Yang D, et al. Prevalence of polycystic ovary syndrome in women in China: a large community-based study. *Hum Reprod* 2013;**28**:2562–69.

32. Vutyavanich T, Khaniyao V, Wongtra-Ngan S, Sreshthaputra O, Sreshthaputra R, Piromlertamorn W. Clinical, endocrine and ultrasonographic features of polycystic ovary syndrome in Thai women. *J Obstet Gynaecol Res* 2007;**33**:677–80.

33. Kumarapeli V, Seneviratne Rde A, Wijeyaratne CN, Yapa RM, Dodampahala SH. A simple screening approach for assessing community prevalence and phenotype of polycystic ovary syndrome in a semi-urban population in Sri Lanka. *Am J Epidemiol* 2008;**168**:321–28.

34. Tehrani FR, Simbar M, Tohidi M, Hosseinpanah F, Azizi F. The prevalence of polycystic ovary syndrome in a community sample of Iranian population: Iranian PCOS prevalence study. *Reprod Biol Endocrinol* 2011;**9**:39.

35. Elting MW, Korsen TJ, Rekers-Mombarg LT, Schoemaker J. Women with polycystic ovary syndrome gain regular menstrual cycles when ageing. *Hum Reprod* 2000;**15**:24–28.

36. Elting MW, Kwee J, Korsen TJ, Rekers-Mombarg LT, Schoemaker J. Aging women with polycystic ovary syndrome who achieve regular menstrual cycles have a smaller follicle cohort than those who continue to have irregular cycles. *Fertil Steril* 2003;**79**:1154–60.

37. Brown ZA, Louwers YV, Fong SL, et al. The phenotype of polycystic ovary syndrome ameliorates with aging. *Fertil Steril* 2011;**96**:1259–65.

38. Dahlgren E, Johansson S, Lindstedt G, et al. Women with polycystic ovary syndrome wedge resected in 1956 to 1965: a long-term follow-up focusing on natural history and circulating hormones. *Fertil Steril* 1992;**57**:505–13.

39. Mulders AG, Laven JS, Eijkemans MJ, de Jong FH, Themmen AP, Fauser BC. Changes in anti-Müllerian hormone serum concentrations over time suggest delayed ovarian ageing in normogonadotrophic anovulatory infertility. *Hum Reprod* 2004;**19**:2036–42.

40. Chamlian DL, Taylor HB. Endometrial hyperplasia in young women. *Obstet Gynecol* 1970;**36**:659–66.

41. Haoula Z, Salman M, Atiomo W. Evaluating the association between endometrial cancer and polycystic ovary syndrome. *Hum Reprod* 2012;**27**:1327–31.

42. Cheung AP. Ultrasound and menstrual history in predicting endometrial hyperplasia in polycystic ovary syndrome. *Obstet Gynecol* 2001;**98**:325–31.

43. Sturdee DW, Wade-Evans T, Paterson ME, Thom M, Studd JW. Relations between bleeding pattern, endometrial histology, and oestrogen treatment in menopausal women. *Br Med J* 1978;**1**:1575–77.

44. Judd HL, Mebane-Sims I, Legault C, et al. Effects of hormone replacement therapy on endometrial histology in postmenopausal women. The Postmenopausal Estrogen/Progestin Interventions (PEPI) Trial. *JAMA* 1996;**275**:370–75.

45. Gambrell RD Jr. Prevention of endometrial cancer with progestogens. *Maturitas* 1986;**8**:159–68.

46. Hickey M, Higham JM, Fraser I. Progestogens with or without oestrogen for irregular uterine bleeding associated with anovulation. *Cochrane Database Syst Rev* 2012;**9**:CD001895.

47. Yildiz BO, Knochenhauer ES, Azziz R. Impact of obesity on the risk for polycystic ovary syndrome. *J Clin Endocrinol Metab* 2008;**93**:162–68.

48. Gambineri A, Pelusi C, Vicennati V, Pagotto U, Pasquali R. Obesity and the polycystic ovary syndrome. *Int J Obes Relat Metab Disord* 2002;**26**:883–96.

49. Pasquali R, Gambineri A, Pagotto U. The impact of obesity on reproduction in women with polycystic ovary syndrome. *BJOG* 2006;**113**:1148–59.

50. Escobar-Morreale HF, Botella-Carretero JI, Álvarez-Blasco F, Sancho J, San Millán JL. The polycystic ovary syndrome associated with morbid obesity may resolve after weight loss induced by bariatric surgery. *J Clin Endocrinol Metab* 2005;**90**:6364–69.

51. Moran LJ, Hutchison SK, Norman RJ, Teede HJ. Lifestyle changes in women with polycystic ovary syndrome. *Cochrane Database Syst Rev* 2011;**2**:CD007506.

52. Legro RS, Arslanian SA, Ehrmann DA, et al. Endocrine Society Diagnosis and treatment of polycystic ovary syndrome: an Endocrine Society clinical practice guideline. *J Clin Endocrinol Metab* 2013;**98**:4565–92.

53. Balen AH, Conway GS, Kaltsas G, et al. Polycystic ovary syndrome: the spectrum of the disorder in 1741 patients. *Hum Reprod* 1995;**10**:2107–11.

54. Bhattacharya S, Porter M, Amalraj E, et al. The epidemiology of infertility in the North East of Scotland. *Hum Reprod* 2009;**24**:3096–107.

55. Hull MG Epidemiology of infertility and polycystic ovarian disease: endocrinological and demographic studies. *Gynecol Endocrinol* 1987;**1**:235–45.

56. Imani B, Eijkemans MJ, te Velde ER, Habbema JD, Fauser BC Predictors of patients remaining anovulatory during clomiphene citrate induction of ovulation in normogonadotropic oligoamenorrheic infertility. *J Clin Endocrinol Metab* 1998;**83**:2361–65.

57. Palomba S, Orio F Jr, Falbo A, et al. Prospective parallel randomized, double-blind, double-dummy controlled clinical trial comparing clomiphene citrate and metformin as the first-line treatment for ovulation induction in non-obese anovulatory women with polycystic ovary syndrome. *J Clin Endocrinol Metab* 2005;**90**:4068–74.

58. Moll E, Bossuyt PM, Korevaar JC, Lambalk CB, van der Veen F. Effect of clomifene citrate plus metformin and clomifene citrate plus placebo on induction of ovulation in women with newly diagnosed polycystic ovary syndrome: randomised double blind clinical trial. *BMJ* 2006;**332**:1485.

59. Zain MM, Jamaluddin R, Ibrahim A, Norman RJ. Comparison of clomiphene citrate, metformin, or the combination of both for first-line ovulation induction, achievement of pregnancy, and live birth in Asian women with polycystic ovary syndrome: a randomized controlled trial. *Fertil Steril* 2009;**91**:514–21.

60. Homburg R, Hendriks ML, König TE, et al. Clomifene citrate or low-dose FSH for the first-line treatment of infertile women with anovulation associated with polycystic ovary syndrome: a prospective randomized multinational study. *Hum Reprod* 2012;**27**:468–73.

61. Palomba S, Falbo A, Zullo F, Orio F Jr. Evidence-based and potential benefits of metformin in the polycystic ovary syndrome: a comprehensive review. *Endocr Rev* 2009;**30**:1–50.

62. NIH/NICHD Reproductive Medicine Network Effect of letrozole versus clomiphene on livebirth in women with anovulatory infertility due to polycystic ovary syndrome (PCOS): a randomized double-blind multicenter trial. *Fertil* Steril 2013;**100** Suppl 3:S51.

63. Tulandi T, Martin J, Al-Fadhli R, et al. Congenital malformations among 911 newborns conceived after infertility treatment with letrozole or clomiphene citrate. *Fertil Steril* 2006;**85**:1761–65.

64. Royal College of Obstetricians and Gynaecologists (RCOG). *Long-Term Consequences of Polycystic Ovary Syndrome*. Greentop Guideline No. 33. London: RCOG; 2014.

65. Gjønnaess H. Ovarian electrocautery in the treatment of women with polycystic ovary syndrome (PCOS). Factors affecting the results. *Acta Obstet Gynecol Scand* 1994;**73**:407–12.

66. Moran L, Teede H. Metabolic features of the reproductive phenotypes of polycystic ovary syndrome. *Hum Reprod Update* 2009;**15**:477–88.

67. DeUgarte CM, Bartolucci AA, Azziz R. Prevalence of insulin resistance in the polycystic ovary syndrome using the homeostasis model assessment. *Fertil Steril* 2005;**83**:1454–60.

68. Diamanti-Kandarakis E, Dunaif A. Insulin resistance and the polycystic ovary syndrome revisited: an update on mechanisms and implications. *Endocr Rev* 2012;**33**:981–1030.

69. Norman RJ, Masters L, Milner CR, Wang JX, Davies MJ. Relative risk of conversion from normoglycaemia to impaired glucose tolerance or non-insulin dependent diabetes mellitus in polycystic ovarian syndrome. *Hum Reprod* 2001;**16**:1995–98.

70. Alberti KG, Zimmet P, Shaw J. International Diabetes Federation: a consensus on Type 2 diabetes prevention. *Diabet Med* 2007;**24**:451–63.

71. Meyer C, McGrath BP, Teede HJ. Overweight women with polycystic ovary syndrome have evidence of subclinical cardiovascular disease. *J Clin Endocrinol Metab* 2005;**90**:5711–16.

72. Moran LJ, Misso ML, Wild RA, Norman RJ. Impaired glucose tolerance, type 2 diabetes and metabolic syndrome in polycystic ovary syndrome: a systematic review and meta-analysis. *Hum Reprod Update* 2010;**16**:347–63.

73. Wijeyaratne CN, Seneviratne Rde A, Dahanayake S, et al. Phenotype and metabolic profile of South Asian women with polycystic ovary syndrome (PCOS): results of a large database from a specialist Endocrine Clinic. *Hum Reprod* 2011;**26**:202–13.

74. Lee BH, Indran IR, Tan HM, et al. A dietary medium chain fatty acid, decanoic acid, inhibits recruitment of Nur77 to the HSD3B2 promoter in vitro, and reverses endocrine and metabolic abnormalities in a rat model of polycystic ovary syndrome. *Endocrinology* 2016;**157**:382–94.

75. Pasquali R. Obesity and androgens: facts and perspectives. *Fertil Steril* 2006;**85**:1319–40.

76. Randeva HS, Tan BK, Weickert MO, et al. Cardiometabolic aspects of the polycystic ovary syndrome. *Endocr Rev* 2012;**33**:812–41.

77. Raval AD, Hunter T, Stuckey B, Hart RJ. Statins for women with polycystic ovary syndrome not actively trying to conceive. *Cochrane Database Syst Rev* 2011;**10**:CD008565.

78. Azziz R, Woods KS, Reyna R, Key TJ, Knochenhauer ES, Yildiz BO. The prevalence and features of the polycystic ovary syndrome in an unselected population. *J Clin Endocrinol Metab* 2004;**89**:2745–49.

79. Azziz R, Sanchez LA, Knochenhauer ES, et al. Androgen excess in women: experience with over 1000 consecutive patients. *J Clin Endocrinol Metab* 2004;**89**:453–62.

80. Ozdemir S, Ozdemir M, Görkemli H, Kiyici A, Bodur S. Specific dermatologic features of the polycystic ovary syndrome and its association with biochemical markers of the metabolic syndrome and hyperandrogenism. *Acta Obstet Gynecol Scand* 2010;**89**:199–204.

81. Rausch ME, Legro RS, Barnhart HX, et al. Predictors of pregnancy in women with polycystic ovary syndrome. *J Clin Endocrinol Metab* 2009;**94**:3458–66.

82. van Zuuren EJ, Fedorowicz Z, Carter B, Pandis N. Interventions for hirsutism (excluding laser and photoepilation therapy alone). *Cochrane Database Syst Rev* 2015;**28**;**4**:CD010334.

83. Welt CK, Carmina E. Clinical review: lifecycle of polycystic ovary syndrome (PCOS): from in utero to menopause. *J Clin Endocrinol Metab* 2013;**98**:4629–38.

84. Dahlgren E, Friberg LG, Johansson S, et al. Endometrial carcinoma; ovarian dysfunction—a risk factor in young women. *Eur J Obstet Gynecol Reprod Biol* 1991;**41**:143–50.

85. Chittenden BG, Fullerton G, Maheshwari A, Bhattacharya S. Polycystic ovary syndrome and the risk of gynaecological cancer: a systematic review. *Reprod Biomed Online* 2009;**19**:398–405.

86. Schildkraut JM, Schwingl PJ, Bastos E, Evanoff A, Hughes C. Epithelial ovarian cancer risk among women with polycystic ovary syndrome. *Obstet Gynecol* 1996;**88**:554–59.

87. Olsen CM, Green AC, Nagle CM, et al. Epithelial ovarian cancer: testing the 'androgens hypothesis'. *Endocr Relat Cancer* 2008;**15**:1061–68.

88. Bodmer M, Becker C, Meier C, Jick SS, Meier CR. Use of metformin and the risk of ovarian cancer: a case–control analysis. *Gynecol Oncol* 2011;**123**:200–204.

43

Pelvic inflammatory disease

Gillian Dean and Jonathan Ross

Introduction and definition

Pelvic inflammatory disease (PID) is infection and inflammation of the female upper reproductive tract involving the endometrium, fallopian tubes, ovaries, and pelvic peritoneum. Following breakdown of the physical mucous barrier at the cervix, infection spreads to involve some or all of these structures. The spectrum of disease ranges from asymptomatic or mild disease, through to severe infection with systemic symptoms and the presence of a tubo-ovarian abscess.

Over the last decade, the incidence of pelvic infection in England has fallen by 50% (1) and in the United States it is estimated that from 2004 to 2013 the number of visits to physicians for PID decreased by 39.8% (2). The decrease, at least in part, is thought to be attributable to widespread screening for chlamydia and gonorrhoea which detects uncomplicated infection before it has progressed to PID. Despite this, the cost of PID continues to be a major burden to health economies and is estimated as an average per person lifetime medical cost of $1060–$3180, depending on whether women develop serious sequelae (3).

PID is a polymicrobial infection and the most significant complication of sexually transmitted infections (STIs) in women. Chlamydia and gonorrhoea now account for less than 30% of cases, with many cases having an unidentified microbiological aetiology. Using newer molecular detection methods, new potential pathogens have been identified including *Mycoplasma genitalium, Atopobium, Leptotrichia*, and other bacterial vaginosis (BV) associated bacteria (4).

Diagnosis is based on clinical assessment which is subjective and prone to variation depending on knowledge, training, and experience. The positive predictive value of clinical examination is as low as 65% and no single imaging method is sensitive or specific enough to give a definitive diagnosis. Neither are there any highly accurate laboratory tests nor investigations which reliably confirm or exclude the diagnosis. A low threshold for diagnosis and treatment is required to minimize the adverse effects on the reproductive health of young women. Women presenting with lower abdominal pain with no other identified aetiology, and who have one or more of three minimum criteria (cervical motion tenderness, uterine tenderness, and/or adnexal tenderness), should be treated for PID. The United States Centers for Disease Control and Prevention (CDC) recommends empirical PID treatment in sexually active young women

(≤25 years of age) and other women at risk for STIs (multiple sexual partners or history of STI) if they are experiencing pelvic or lower abdominal pain, when no other cause can be identified, and if these criteria are present on pelvic examination (2). Patients can be treated successfully as an outpatient. Outpatient therapy is as effective as inpatient treatment for patients with clinically mild to moderate PID (5).

PID is associated with major long-term sequelae, including tubal factor infertility, ectopic pregnancy, and chronic pelvic pain, and it remains an important public health problem with far-reaching implications for women's health and high costs for healthcare systems.

Epidemiology

Accurate measures of PID incidence are difficult to obtain due to the asymptomatic and non-specific nature of many cases. To further complicate matters, symptomatic patients present to a variety of services including primary care, gynaecology, and sexual health clinics. This makes precise case-finding challenging and almost certainly leads to widespread under-reporting.

Examination of general practice-based morbidity surveys in England and Wales in 1991–1992, revealed a diagnosis of PID was made in women aged 16–46 at 1.7% of attendances (6). Over the past decade rates have fallen by over 50%. Using data from the Clinical Practice Research Datalink, rates of definite or probable PID in 15–44-year-old women attending general practice decreased in England by 9% per year (from approximately 400:100,000 to 180:100,000) between 2000 and 2011. The reduction was seen in all age groups but was most marked in women aged 15–24 years (**Figure 43.1**) (7).

In the United States there were 1.2 million medical visits for PID in 2000. Here too, the number of annual visits to physicians for PID among women aged 15–44 years has decreased by 39.8% (from 123,000 visits in 2004 to 88,000 visits in 2013) (8). In Canada between 1992 and 2009, PID hospitalizations decreased by 80% and physicians billing for cases of PID decreased by 70% (9). Similar data have been reported from other countries including Sweden, Australia, and Denmark (10).

During this time, all these countries have witnessed an increase in chlamydia diagnoses, partly due to changing sexual behaviour, but also due to increased detection rates through widespread screening.

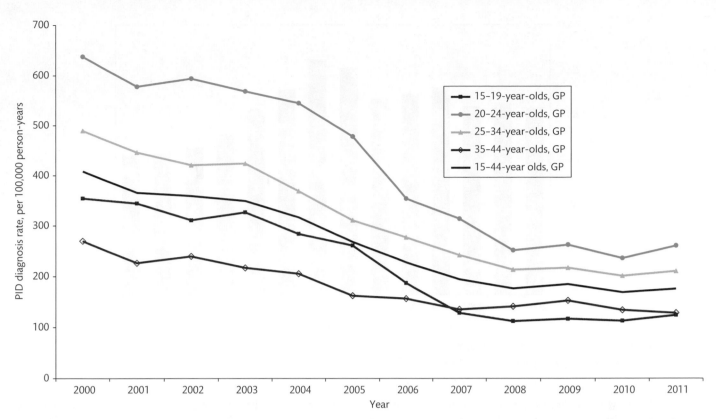

Figure 43.1 PID diagnosis rate by Public Health England centre recorded in general practice (GP) settings from 2000 to 2011. Source data from Public Health England. Rates of pelvic inflammatory disease (PID) in England (2000–2013). *HPR* 2015;9:22.

By decreasing prevalent infection and diagnosing chlamydia at an earlier stage, the risk of progression from simple cervical infection to PID is reduced. Data from randomized controlled trials of chlamydia screening to prevent PID have provided evidence that screening and treatment is a useful intervention, although these studies are not without limitations, and the magnitude of their contribution remains unclear. Certainly the number of cases of PID caused by *Chlamydia trachomatis* seen in many countries has fallen, with chlamydia detected in as few as 10% of cases (11). If chlamydia-associated PID continues to fall, the impact chlamydia screening programmes will have on PID incidence in future may need re-evaluating (**Figure 43.2**).

The estimated medical costs of treating PID range from $700 to $8480 per episode for outpatient and inpatient care respectively (12). Indirect costs relating to sequelae are far higher, and the estimated annual healthcare cost for PID and its complications in the United States is over $2 billion (13).

Risk factors for PID are the same as risks for acquiring STIs. These include unprotected sexual intercourse with multiple sexual partners, young age at onset of sexual activity, previous chlamydia or gonorrhoea infection, low socioeconomic status, lower educational attainment, and a history of PID. Vaginal douching had been previously linked to PID in retrospective studies; however, a prospective study in 2005 showed no causal link. The authors suggested that previous associations had been driven by the symptoms of a genital infection prompting douching, rather than douching causing PID (14).

Aetiology/microbiology

PID has classically been associated with the STIs *Neisseria gonorrhoeae* and *C. trachomatis*. Studies in the 1980s and 1990s detected chlamydia and/or gonorrhoea from over 50% of cases (15–17) and in up to 77% of tubo-ovarian abscesses at laparoscopy (18). More recent literature suggests the proportion of PID cases attributable to *N. gonorrhoeae* or *C. trachomatis* is declining. Price et al. using multiparameter evidence synthesis estimated that in England in 2002, 35% of PID cases in women aged 16–24 years were due to chlamydia, compared to only 20% of women aged 16–44 years (19). In 2011, in patients diagnosed with PID in an emergency department in North America, Burnett et al. found only 4.4% with gonorrhoea, 10% with chlamydia, and 2.6% of individuals with both organisms (11). This left 83% of cases with no identified organism. This would fit with the overall decrease in prevalence of gonorrhoea in some populations, and also the increase in chlamydia screening. Furthermore, as care has shifted to the outpatient setting, invasive tests are less frequently performed with a possible concomitant reduction in rates of organism identification.

Identifying which other organisms are implicated in the pathogenesis of PID is problematic. Firstly it must be considered whether the upper female genital tract is normally sterile. There is some evidence that some microorganisms may be present in healthy, asymptomatic individuals. Even when identified, the role these organisms may play in the disease process is not understood.

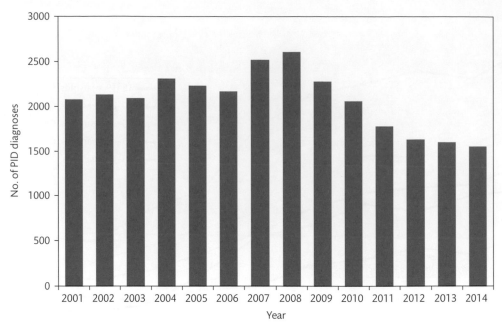

Figure 43.2 PID caused by *C. trachomatis* diagnosed in England 2001–2014.
Source data from https://www.gov.uk/government/statistics/sexually-transmitted-infections-stis-annual-data-tables.

Acute PID is now considered a polymicrobial infection with involvement of a wide variety of microorganisms, many of which are not routinely tested for in clinical practice. This may explain why a large proportion of clinical PID cases have unidentified microbiological aetiology. Included among these are genital tract mycoplasmas (particularly *M. genitalium*) and anaerobic/aerobic bacteria which comprise the endogenous vaginal flora (e.g. black-pigmented Gram-negative anaerobic rods, *Gardnerella vaginalis, Escherichia coli, Haemophilus influenzae*, and aerobic streptococci). Using newer identification techniques, Hebb et al. obtained fallopian tube samples at laparoscopy from Kenyan women with salpingitis, as well as control subjects having tubal ligation (4). Using a broad range 16s rDNA polymerase chain reaction they identified novel, possibly uncultivatable bacteria from fallopian tube specimens in the women with salpingitis. These were sometimes the sole or predominant phylotype. In addition to *N. gonorrhoeae* and *C. trachomatis*, implicated microorganisms included *Leptotrichia* spp., *Atopobium vaginae, Prevotella* spp., *Peptostreptococci* spp., and *Streptococcus pyogenes*.

The exact role of anaerobic bacteria and BV in the pathogenesis of PID remains unclear. Lactobacilli are important in the host defence against STIs, and BV has been shown to increase the risk of incident gonorrhoea and chlamydial infection (20). BV has also been noted to be frequently present in women with PID (up to 70%). But whether BV-associated bacteria *independently* cause PID, whether they facilitate the ascension of *N. gonorrhoeae* or *C. trachomatis* infection, or whether they are simply innocent bystanders following infection with other pathogens are yet to be determined. There are data, however, which suggest anaerobes are capable of causing local tissue damage at the level of the fallopian tube when present (21). The proportion of women with PID who have anaerobes isolated at laparoscopy ranges from 13% to 78% (20). The wide differences are thought to be related to diverse patient populations, different definitions of PID, varying degrees of disease severity, and different microbiological techniques.

Several studies have investigated the role of BV in endometritis or clinically suspected PID. The only prospective study showed no increase in the risk of developing incident PID in women with BV over a 3-year period (22). This study used standard Gram-stained slides and microscopy for the BV diagnosis. However, 1 year later the same authors concluded that women with a heavy growth of BV-associated microorganisms and a new sexual partner appeared to be at particularly high risk of PID (adjusted rate ratio 8.77; 95% confidence interval (CI) 1.11–69.2) (23). Several other studies have also found an association with the presence of anaerobic Gram-negative rods, independent of chlamydia or gonorrhoea infection (24, 25). The differences in these findings have been explained by variable definitions of BV. Although BV as determined by Gram stain is relatively reliable, it does not capture all the microbiological components of the BV ecosystem, in particular anaerobic Gram-negative rods. So when BV was identified by microbial culture, a combination of BV-related microorganisms was shown to significantly increase the risk of acquiring PID (23). There is substantial evidence that anaerobic infection is associated with more severe disease, in particular the formation of tubo-ovarian abscesses (26).

M. genitalium was first identified in the early 1980s in men with non-gonococcal urethritis. The organism was extremely difficult to isolate from clinical specimens, prompting the development of nucleic acid amplification tests (NAATs) which have improved the understanding of pathogenesis and the association with disease processes. *M. genitalium* has been shown to be sexually transmittable in partner studies which demonstrate concurrent infection with concordant strain types (27). Infection with *M. genitalium* is as common as *C. trachomatis* among high-risk women and women with clinical PID, with rates ranging from 2.1% to 16% (28, 29). Studies have increasingly shown an association with cervicitis, PID, and infertility. An independent association was shown in women with histologically confirmed endometritis who were significantly more likely to have *M. genitalium* detected than women without endometritis (16% vs

2%; *P* = 0.02) (30). Similarly, in the PID Evaluation and Clinical Health (PEACH) study women testing positive for *M. genitalium* were more than twice as likely to have histologically confirmed endometritis compared to women without infection (29). More recently, a meta-analysis looking at *M. genitalium* infection and female reproductive tract disease showed this organism is associated with a significantly increased risk of PID, with a pooled odds ratio (OR) of 2.14 (95% CI 1.31–3.49) (31). Women also had an increased risk of cervicitis (OR 1.66; 95% CI 1.35–2.04), preterm birth (OR 1.89; 95% CI 1.25–2.85), and miscarriage (OR 1.82; 95% CI 1.10–3.03). A significant association between *M. genitalium* and PID has implications for current testing algorithms and recommended therapies which specify the use of antibiotics with poor efficacy against this organism.

Pathogenesis

The natural course of *C. trachomatis* infection and ability of individuals to naturally clear infection is incompletely understood. Studies have shown that approximately half of asymptomatic infections are cleared spontaneously at 1 year after initial chlamydia testing. However, most chlamydia natural history studies lack data on when the infection was initially acquired, or whether subsequent detection is persistent or new (32). There is also a lack of consensus regarding the risk of PID following untreated cervical chlamydia infection. However, a recent synthesis of the data from screening trials suggests 14.9% of women will go on to develop symptomatic PID (**Figure 43.3**), and 17.1% of infections if both symptomatic and asymptomatic PID is considered (19). This proportion may be significantly increased by the iatrogenic introduction of organisms into the upper genital tract by procedures involving transcervical instrumentation such as insertion of intrauterine contraceptive devices, hysterosalpingography, hysteroscopy, *in vitro* fertilization, and termination of pregnancy.

The mechanism by which microorganisms ascend spontaneously along the mucosal surfaces from the vagina and cervix to the upper genital tract is unknown. Disruption of the physical mucous barrier, which under normal circumstances would protect the upper genital tract, may be influenced by both microbial and physiological hormonal changes during the menstrual cycle. Both chlamydia and gonorrhoea are known to possess proteolytic enzymes which degrade cervical mucous and associated antimicrobial peptides (33). Physiologically, the cervical mucous barrier will not be as effective during menstruation when the mucous plug is expelled. Similarly, it is likely there is a higher risk of infection at mid cycle, when oestrogen levels are high and progesterone levels relatively low, leading to physiological thinning of the cervical mucous. Endometrial detection of gonorrhoea and chlamydia is more frequent in the proliferative phase of the menstrual cycle. Additionally, at this stage uterine contractions switch from principally 'fundo-cervical' to 'cervico-fundal', favouring transport of sperm, and pathogens, towards the upper genital tract (34).

There is also likely to be an immunological component linked to both virulence of the organism and host factors such as human leucocyte antigen class. While some women clear *C. trachomatis* infection without tissue damage, in others, chlamydia induces a chronic low-grade inflammation. There is almost certainly a role for chlamydia virulence proteins (surface-exposed polymorphic membrane proteins or Pmp) which have been shown to stimulate proinflammatory cytokines and induce different antibody responses with variable effects on the degree of inflammation. In one study, women with a genetic predisposition to a higher expression of PmpA antibody had increased inflammatory markers and decreased pregnancy rates and live births (35).

In gonococcal disease, antibody binding to structural components of the gonococcal surface (lipooligosaccharide and peptidoglycan) activates complement and initiates the prostaglandin cascade in the fallopian tubes. It is important to consider that the diameter of the fallopian tubes varies considerably, but is particularly narrow (<1 mm) at the opening into the uterine cavity. The intense acute inflammatory reaction with the release of oxygen metabolites and proteinases results in cell death and tissue destruction. An influx of polymorphonuclear leucocytes (PMNs) causes purulent secretions and adds to the oedema and vasodilatation within these delicate structures. Ciliated cells are consequently destroyed with irreversible loss of ciliary motility and tubal damage (**Figure 43.4**).

Women with chlamydia-associated salpingitis generally have clinically milder disease. Unlike gonorrhoea, the organism shows little direct cytotoxicity, and although initial infection is also characterized

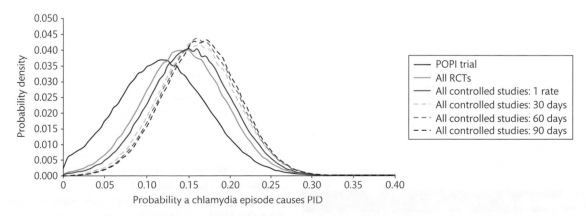

Figure 43.3 The progression risk from *Chlamydia trachomatis* to PID. RCT, randomized controlled trial.

Source data from Price MJ, Ades AE, Soldan K, et al. The natural history of Chlamydia trachomatis infection in women: a multi-parameter evidence synthesis. *Health Technol Assess* 2016;20:1–250.

(a)

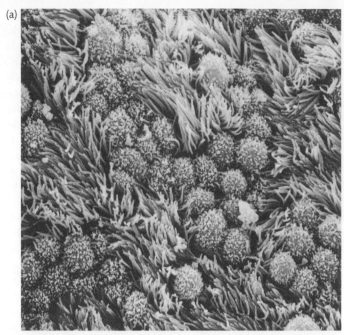

(b)

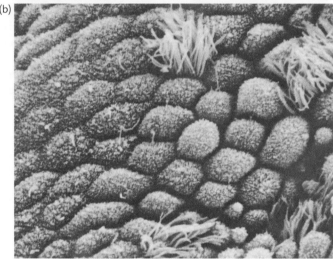

Figure 43.4 Pathological changes in the epithelial surface of the fallopian tube after PID. Scanning electron micrographs show normal human fallopian tube epithelia (a) and the epithelial surface after PID (b). Reproduced with permission from Dorothy L. Patton, University of Washington, Seattle.

by an influx of PMNs and acute inflammation, damage and scarring is thought to be caused by the host inflammatory response. There is evidence that the immunity acquired during initial infection may cause a delayed-type hypersensitivity reaction during reinfection, characterized by the presence of mononuclear cells (cell-mediated immunity). In some studies, more severe inflammatory reactions have been observed following repeat inoculations of chlamydia (36). Regardless of the initiating pathogen, dead epithelial cells are replaced by fibroblasts during the repair process resulting in tubal scarring and functional impairment.

Clinical presentation

Clinical diagnosis of PID is challenging in that no symptoms or signs are pathognomonic of the disease. The proportion of women

with asymptomatic chlamydia has risen in recent years to an estimated 70–95% (19, 37). It is well recognized that asymptomatic infection with chlamydia, mycoplasma, and less commonly gonorrhoea, can lead to pelvic inflammation with a subsequent increased risk of developing long-term complications such as tubal occlusion and infertility. In women undergoing *in vitro* fertilization, the prevalence of serum antibodies to chlamydia, gonorrhoea, and/or mycoplasma were shown to be much higher in individuals with tubal abnormalities (72%) than in infertile women with normal tubes (21%) (38). This is observed in clinical practice where women with tubal factor infertility often do not have a history of classical symptoms and signs of acute PID, but may first be aware of tubal damage during subsequent investigations for infertility, such as a hysterosalpingogram (Figure 43.5). More recently it was shown that women with subclinical PID, proven by endometrial biopsy, were 40% less likely to conceive than women without subclinical PID (39).

When symptoms are present they can range from mild, non-specific disease to severe PID requiring hospitalization. Typically women present in the outpatient setting with mild symptoms, including lower abdominal pain, dyspareunia, vaginal discharge, and abnormal vaginal bleeding. However, even when present, clinical symptoms and signs lack sensitivity and specificity; the positive predictive value of a clinical diagnosis is only 65–90% compared to laparoscopic diagnosis (40) and episodes can go unrecognized if the healthcare provider fails to recognize the implications of these symptoms (2). Clinicians must therefore have a high index of suspicion for making the diagnosis and a low threshold for commencing treatment. A presumptive diagnosis of PID should be made in sexually active young women and other women at risk for STIs if they are experiencing pelvic or lower abdominal pain, if no cause for the illness other than PID can be identified, and if one or more of the following minimum clinical criteria are present on pelvic examination: cervical motion tenderness, uterine tenderness, or adnexal tenderness (2).

Clinical features when present include:

- recent onset of bilateral lower abdominal pain, often described as constant, dull, aching, or cramping
- deep dyspareunia—particularly of recent onset
- abnormal vaginal bleeding—particularly intermenstrual bleeding, postcoital bleeding, or menorrhagia, secondary to associated cervicitis and endometritis
- mucopurulent vaginal discharge—as a result of associated cervicitis
- cervical motion, uterine, and/or adnexal tenderness on bimanual vaginal examination.

The presence of one or more of the following additional criteria will improve the specificity of the minimum criteria:

- Temperature higher than 38.3°C
- Abnormal cervical mucopurulent discharge or cervical friability
- Presence of abundant numbers of white blood cells on saline microscopy of vaginal fluid
- Elevated erythrocyte sedimentation rate; elevated C-reactive protein (41)
- Laboratory documentation of cervical infection with *N. gonorrhoeae*, *C. trachomatis*, or *M. genitalium*.

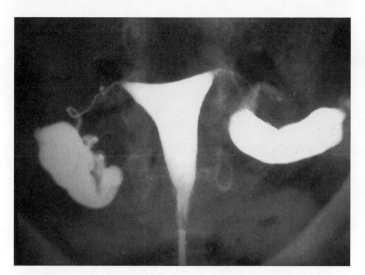

Figure 43.5 Hysterosalpingogram demonstrating left salpingitis isthmica nodosa and right hydrosalpinx.
Reproduced with permission from Mr Peter Greenhouse, Bristol Sexual Health Centre.

The absence of endocervical or vaginal pus cells has a good negative predictive value (95%) for a diagnosis of PID but their presence is non-specific (poor positive predictive value of 17%) (42).

Fever of greater than 38°C can occur, but systemic manifestations are not a prominent feature in patients with mild to moderate PID. Infection and inflammation may spread from the pelvis to the liver capsule via the right paracolic gutter. This is thought to affect 4–14% of women and presents with right upper quadrant pain secondary to perihepatitis (Fitz-Hugh–Curtis syndrome). Subsequent adhesions may form between the liver capsule and the diaphragm, classically described as 'violin string' adhesions (**Figure 43.6**).

The presence and severity of PID symptoms varies by microbiological aetiology. Women with gonococcal PID are more likely to

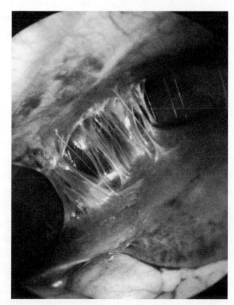

Figure 43.6 Laparoscopic appearance of the Fitz-High–Curtis syndrome showing 'violin string' adhesions between liver capsule and subdiaphragmatic peritoneum with a normal gallbladder.
Reproduced with permission from Mr Peter Greenhouse, Bristol Sexual Health Centre.

have raised systemic inflammatory markers including erythrocyte sedimentation rate and white blood cell count than those with PID caused by chlamydia or mycoplasma. Women with gonococcal PID are also more likely to present with fever, mucopurulent cervicitis, and adnexal tenderness with a higher pelvic pain score (39, 43–46). This may explain why in the PEACH study women with PID associated with *N. gonorrhoeae* presented to care almost 1 week earlier than women with *C. trachomatis* or *M. genitalium* (47). Women with gonococcal PID are also more likely to remember the episode. Miettinen et al. reported that half of the infertile women with positive gonococcal serology recalled a prior episode of PID, compared to only one-quarter of those with positive chlamydia or mycoplasma serology (38). As rates of *N. gonorrhoea* infection have continued to fall in many countries, atypical, milder clinical manifestations have become more common (2, 40, 48).

Diagnosis

The diagnosis of PID remains a challenge due to the wide variation in symptoms and signs which may overlap with other conditions. There is no single symptom, physical finding, or laboratory test that is sensitive or specific enough to definitively diagnose PID. Diagnostic criteria must have a high sensitivity even at the expense of a low specificity to detect as many cases of clinical disease as possible in order to reduce the risk of adverse sequelae (Table 43.1).

Clinical signs

As previously discussed, PID is usually a clinical diagnosis based on pelvic tenderness on bimanual examination indicated by cervical motion tenderness, adnexal tenderness, and uterine tenderness. The positive predictive value of a clinical diagnosis of PID is around 65–90% when compared with laparoscopy. Unsurprisingly, the accuracy of the clinical diagnosis and the experience of the clinician have been shown to be positively correlated (49). Specificity is increased by finding signs of lower genital tract inflammation such as increased friability of the cervix with contact bleeding and a mucopurulent endocervical discharge. Systemic features such as fever and vomiting are rare in mild to moderate disease, but more common in severe infection, particularly with *N. gonorrhoeae*.

Laboratory testing

All patients with suspected PID should have a pregnancy test to rule out possible ectopic pregnancy. Vulvovaginal NAATs for *N. gonorrhoeae* and *C. trachomatis* should be taken, as well as tests for HIV and syphilis. Licensed NAATs for *M. genitalium* are now becoming available and testing should also be performed in women with PID where possible. Microscopy of a saline preparation of vaginal fluid ('wet mount') should be performed looking for increased numbers of white cells (more than one leucocyte per epithelial cell). The absence of endocervical or vaginal pus cells has a good negative predictive value for a diagnosis of PID (94.5%) but their presence is non-specific with a poor positive predictive value (17%) (41). A high peripheral white blood cell count is useful (>10,000 mm³) and raised in approximately 60% of patients (50), but often not immediately available in the primary care or outpatient setting. Although non-specific, elevated inflammatory markers such as C-reactive protein

Table 43.1 Criteria for diagnosis

Minimum diagnostic criteria (one or more of)	Additional diagnostic criteria	Definitive diagnostic criteria
Lower abdominal tenderness	Oral temperature >38.3°C	Endometrial biopsy with histological evidence of endometritis
Adnexal tenderness	Abundant white blood cells on saline microscopy of vaginal secretions/wet mount (white blood cells >epithelial cells)	Transvaginal ultrasound (or other imaging techniques) showing thickened fluid-filled tubes ± free pelvic fluid or tubo-ovarian abscess
Cervical motion tenderness	Abnormal cervical mucopurulent discharge or cervical friability	Laparoscopy demonstrating abnormalities consistent with PID, e.g. fallopian tube erythema ± mucopurulent exudate
	Elevated inflammatory markers (erythrocyte sedimentation rate, C-reactive protein)	
	Laboratory documentation of cervical infection with *N. gonorrhoeae* or *C. trachomatis*	

(>10 mg/L) are also useful and have been found to have good sensitivity (93%) and specificity (83%) in some studies (51).

Imaging

Transvaginal ultrasound (TVUS) scanning is widely available, relatively non-invasive, and useful in ruling out other diagnoses such as a ruptured ovarian cyst or ectopic pregnancy. When the pelvic structures can be visualized, signs such as thickened tubal walls have a high sensitivity and specificity when compared to the gold standards of laparoscopy or endometrial biopsy (85% sensitive, 100% specific) (52). However, fluid must be present in the tubal lumen for this sign to be evaluated. Other features such as free pelvic fluid, tubo-ovarian abscess, pyosalpinx (echogenic fluid in the tube), and the cogwheel sign (protrusion of thickened mucosa into the tubal lumen seen on cross section) increase the specificity of TVUS scanning.

Power Doppler technology detects increased vascularization consistent with hyperaemia and inflammation. Switching to this modality during the examination may increase diagnostic sensitivity. Power Doppler may also allow detection of PID at an earlier stage, before the typical sonographic signs of PID have developed. However, this technique requires a high level of expertise to differentiate significant pathology from 'flash artefacts' generated by iliac and other pelvic vessels adjacent to the adnexae (53).

Magnetic resonance imaging (MRI) is more sensitive (95% vs 81%) and specific (89% vs 78%) than TVUS in women with laparoscopy-proven PID (54), but is more expensive and not typically available for mild to moderate cases. MRI is useful in complex or equivocal cases and may reduce the need for diagnostic laparotomy.

Computed tomography (CT) is not commonly used as it is relatively insensitive, expensive, inaccessible, and leads to unacceptable radiation exposure in women of reproductive age. In hospitalized patients, and where there is diagnostic uncertainty, CT can be useful in confirming alternative diagnoses such as acute appendicitis or urinary tract pathology.

Laparoscopy

Laparoscopy has historically been used as the gold standard diagnostic procedure against which other investigations have been compared; however, as the management of PID has shifted to the outpatient setting, its use has diminished. Finding erythematous, oedematous fallopian tubes, with purulent exudate is highly specific

for a diagnosis of PID, although the sensitivity of this procedure varies depending on the stage of the illness and user experience. Mild or early disease may be confined to the tubal lumen with few macroscopic changes observed within the abdominal cavity. This may explain why one study found laparoscopy had a sensitivity of only 50% in a cohort of women presenting to primary care with pelvic pain, compared to fimbrial histopathological diagnosis (55). Additionally, and also using histopathologically proven PID as the gold standard, others have shown that the overall diagnostic accuracy of laparoscopy was only 78%, and clinicians were only 'poor to fair' at reproducing their previous diagnostic decisions based on laparoscopic images (56).

Indications for laparoscopy include when pelvic or tubo-ovarian abscess is suspected, or where a different diagnosis cannot be excluded. Also, laparoscopy should be considered when there is no clinical improvement after 3 days of adequate antibiotic therapy. As well as confirming (or refuting) the diagnosis, it also offers the chance to perform therapies such as abscess drainage, rinsing and suctioning, lysis of adhesions, or salpingectomy if indicated. However, laparoscopy has the disadvantage of being invasive, requiring a general anaesthetic, and being relatively expensive. Due to these factors and concerns around standardization, it is rarely used for routine diagnosis in mild or moderate disease.

Histology

Endometrial sampling is safe, relatively inexpensive, and less invasive than laparoscopy. Endometrial biopsy showing endometritis on histology has also been used as a gold standard in terms of PID diagnosis. The classic finding of plasma cells in the endometrial stroma gives a sensitivity of 89–92% for predicting laparoscopically confirmed salpingitis (57, 58). In the PEACH study, however, the presence of histological endometritis was not correlated with a greater risk of long-term adverse sequelae (ectopic pregnancy and infertility) when compared with participants without endometritis (5), suggesting not all women with endometritis had tubal inflammation. It is also recognized that 'uncomplicated' endocervical infection can cause endometritis, which would explain the lower specificities reported with this diagnostic test (63–87%). Other drawbacks include the risk of introducing infection, delayed diagnostic reports, and variable histopathological definitions and interpretation. Samples can, however, undergo traditional microbiological analysis or molecular testing for novel organisms. In future, newer methodologies could be used to evaluate the interaction between pathogens and the host response in different individuals.

Differential diagnosis

The differential diagnosis of lower abdominal pain in a young woman includes the following:

- Ectopic pregnancy—pregnancy should always be excluded in women suspected of having PID.
- Acute appendicitis—anorexia is more commonly associated with appendicitis than PID. Nausea and vomiting also occur in most patients with appendicitis but only 50% of those with PID. Cervical movement pain will occur in about a quarter of women with appendicitis (59).
- Endometriosis—the history is usually one of chronic, recurrent pain, typically related to early menstruation, but can occur at any stage of the menstrual cycle. Menorrhagia and dyspareunia are common symptoms of endometriosis. A history of pain radiating to the sacrum or pain on defecation (dyschezia) may be useful discriminators.
- Complications of an ovarian cyst (e.g. torsion or rupture). The pain is often of sudden onset and unilateral.
- Urinary tract infection—usually associated with dysuria, urinary frequency, and haematuria.
- Gastrointestinal origin such as gastroenteritis, irritable bowel syndrome, or diverticulitis—usually associated with a disturbance in bowel habit and cramping abdominal pain.
- Functional pain (Mittelschmerz), or pain with ovulation—a diagnosis of exclusion, usually occurring mid cycle, characterized by unilateral pelvic pain lasting for less than 24 hours.

Treatment

Treatment of PID should produce high rates of clinical and microbiological cure for the principal pathogens described previously, as well as prevent long-term sequelae such as infertility, ectopic pregnancy, and chronic pelvic pain. Treatment is nearly always empirical as therapy must be started as soon as the presumptive diagnosis has been made, and before microbial test results are available. A low index of suspicion is required to minimize potential adverse reproductive health outcomes for young women. Women who delay seeking care are three times more likely to experience infertility and ectopic pregnancy (60). The consequences of other common causes of lower abdominal pain are unlikely to be compromised by early antibiotics in cases where there is diagnostic uncertainty.

The first consideration is whether the woman requires inpatient or outpatient management. The indications for hospitalization include pregnancy, severe illness with high fever and inability to take oral medication, tubo-ovarian abscess, inability to rule out other serious diagnoses, and lack of clinical response to oral therapy. Once started, parenteral treatment should be continued for at least 24 hours after clinical improvement. There is no evidence, however, that treating women with mild to moderate PID in the inpatient setting is more effective than outpatient therapy. In the PEACH study,

both short-term clinical and microbiological cure and long-term reproductive outcomes were similar in both the inpatient and outpatient groups (5). Remarkably, this was despite subjects taking only an average of 70% of the prescribed doses (61).

The choice of treatment should reflect drug availability and cost, antimicrobial susceptibility, local epidemiology of specific infective organisms, and disease severity. Based on an understanding of the polymicrobial aetiology, PID should be treated with antibiotics covering a broad spectrum of pathogens. Antimicrobial agents should be effective against *N. gonorrhoeae* and *C. trachomatis,* even if tests for these organisms are negative, as women may have upper genital tract infection without positive laboratory tests.

There is debate whether to include anaerobic coverage in treatment regimens, which stems from the poor understanding of whether anaerobes are implicated in the pathogenesis of PID. While the prevalence of anaerobes in the upper genital tract of women with PID is variable, it is accepted that when present they can cause local tissue damage. Treatment trials have documented excellent clinical and microbiological cure rates both for regimens that offer adequate anaerobic coverage, and for regimens that do not, although few trials have documented anaerobic microbiological cure data specifically.

While it is recognized that severe disease is usually polymicrobial, and often includes anaerobes, the role of anaerobes in mild to moderate disease is less clear. Many studies have shown that BV-associated organisms are more frequently found in women with PID. In the PEACH study, for example, 53.5% of women had concomitant BV, and women with acute endometritis on endometrial biopsy were commonly infected with BV-associated microorganisms in the upper genital tract (*G. vaginalis* 30.9%, anaerobic Gram-negative rods 31.7%, and anaerobic Gram-positive cocci 22%) (24, 25). The outpatient regimen in the PEACH study, however, had only a single dose of a second-generation cephalosporin (cefoxitin 2 g intramuscularly, plus probenecid 1 g orally) which may not have been sufficient to clear upper genital tract anaerobic infection. Although short- and long-term outcomes were similar in the inpatient and outpatient treatment arms, there were a large proportion of women in both arms with persistent endometritis at 30 days (45.9% outpatient, 37.6% inpatient; $P = 0.09$) (5). If anaerobes can persist and cause ongoing inflammation following treatment with suboptimal antibiotic regimens, including sufficient anaerobic cover would seem to be essential. Following these findings, the PEACH study authors concluded that BV-associated organisms were very commonly present in women with mild to moderate PID and suggested that treatment regimens for all women with PID include antimicrobial agents effective against anaerobes (25). At present, there are no studies illustrating whether short-term treatment of anaerobic organisms influences longer-term outcomes. Consequently, the 2015 CDC guidelines state 'until treatment regimens that do not cover anaerobic microbes have been demonstrated to prevent long-term sequelae (e.g. infertility and ectopic pregnancy) as successfully as the regimens that are effective against these microbes, the use of regimens with anaerobic activity should be considered' (2). This is particularly the case in women where BV or tubo-ovarian abscesses are identified.

Current European and United Kingdom guidelines include agents which cover *N. gonorrhoeae, C. trachomatis*, and anaerobic infection (40, 59) (**Tables 43.2 and 43.3**). As a result of the emergence of quinolone-resistant *N. gonorrhoeae*, regimens that include a quinolone

Table 43.2 Oral treatment regimens for pelvic inflammatory disease

	Drug	Dosage/route/frequency	Duration
First line	Ceftriaxone *plus*	1 g intramuscular	Single dose
	Doxycycline *plus*	100 mg orally BD	14 days
	Metronidazole	400 mg orally BD	14 days
Second line	Ofloxacin[a] *plus*	400 mg orally BD	14 days
	Metronidazole	400 mg orally BD	14 days[b]

BD, twice daily.

[a] Ofloxacin and moxifloxacin should be avoided in patients who are at high risk of gonococcal PID because of increasing quinolone resistance in the United Kingdom (e.g. when the patient's partner has gonorrhoea, in clinically severe disease, following sexual contact abroad). Quinolones should also be avoided as first-line empirical treatment for PID in areas where >5% of PID is caused by quinolone-resistant *N. gonorrhoeae*.

[b] May be discontinued in patients with mild to moderate PID who are unable to tolerate it.

agent are either no longer routinely recommended (2), or only recommended when there is a low probability of *N. gonorrhoeae* being the causative agent. Quinolones should be avoided in patients where the partner has gonorrhoea, in clinically severe disease, or following sexual contact abroad. Quinolones should also be avoided as first-line empirical treatment for PID in areas where more than 5% of PID is caused by quinolone-resistant *N. gonorrhoeae* (40, 59). In 2018 the European Medicines Agency highlighted the potential for disabling and permanent side effects following the use of quinolone antibiotics (62), with the subsequent downgrading of ofloxacin to second-line therapy in UK guidelines (59). For outpatient regimens there are differences in the recommended dosage of intramuscular ceftriaxone between the European and CDC guidelines. The higher dose of intramuscular ceftriaxone is recommended in the European guidelines to reduce the risk of resistance developing in *N. gonorrhoeae*.

The current recommended therapies in most national guidelines specify the use of antibiotics with low efficacy against *M. genitalium*. It has been well documented that clearance of this organism after doxycycline is poor and older fluoroquinolones (ciprofloxacin, ofloxacin) have limited activity against *M. genitalium*. Among women with a positive baseline *M. genitalium* test in the PEACH study, 41% tested positive again at 30 days following intramuscular cefoxitin and oral doxycycline (63). Women with mycoplasma identified in the endometrium were 4.5 times more likely to experience short-term treatment failure. This was defined by histological evidence of endometritis and persistent pelvic pain at 30 days. An extended course of azithromycin (500 mg as a single dose, followed by 250 mg daily for 4 days) has been used successfully for the treatment of mycoplasma infections in the past, but increasing incidence of treatment failure over the last 5 years suggest the rapid emergence of antibiotic resistance (64). Macrolide resistance now appears to be endemic in some areas (65), a phenomenon which will be accelerated by the continuing use of azithromycin 1 g for the treatment of uncomplicated chlamydia infection and non-specific urethritis. Moxifloxacin is currently one of the most active drugs against *M. genitalium* and has been used as a second-line agent in cases with azithromycin treatment failure. In one study, moxifloxacin was effective in 88% of cases failing with azithromycin, although worryingly 12% of patients receiving this antibiotic failed to clear mycoplasma. All of these had pretreatment fluoroquinolone mutations detected. All were able to clear the infection with oral pristinamycin 1 g four times a day for 10 days (65). With respect to EMA guidance, moxifloxacin remains first line therapy for *M. genitalium* associated PID, in the absence of alternative antibiotics (59, 62).

In conclusion, it remains a challenge to provide antibiotic coverage for gonococcal, chlamydial, mycoplasma, and anaerobic infection. Presumptive therapy with moxifloxacin in persistent cases, unresponsive to standard regimens, to cover *M. genitalium* may be warranted. While potentially more effective, combination regimens may

Table 43.3 Parenteral treatment regimens for pelvic inflammatory disease

	Drug	Dosage/frequency	Duration
Option 1	Ceftriaxone *plus*	2 g intravenous (IV) daily	Until 24 hours after clinical improvement
	Doxycycline *plus*	100 mg IV/orally if tolerated BD	To complete 14 days
	Metronidazole	400 mg orally BD	Start when ceftriaxone finishes; to complete 14 days
Option 2	Gentamicin[a]	2 mg/kg loading dose, then 1.5 mg/kg TDS	Until 24 hours after clinical improvement
	Clindamycin	900 mg IV TDS	Until 24 hours after clinical improvement
	Then clindamycin	450 mg orally QDS	To complete 14 days
	or doxycycline *plus* metronidazole	100 mg orally BD 400 mg orally BD	To complete 14 days
Alternative regimen with less evidence:			
Option 3	Ofloxacin[b]	400 mg IV BD	Until 24 hours after clinical improvement
	Metronidazole	500 mg IV TDS	Until 24 hours after clinical improvement
	Then ofloxacin *plus* metronidazole	400 mg orally BD 400 mg orally BD	To complete 14 days

BD, twice daily; QDS, four times a day; TDS, three times a day.

[a] Gentamicin levels need to be monitored if this regimen is used.

[b] Ofloxacin and moxifloxacin should be avoided in patients who are at high risk of gonococcal PID because of increasing quinolone resistance in the United Kingdom (e.g. when the patient's partner has gonorrhoea, in clinically severe disease, following sexual contact abroad). Quinolones should also be avoided as first-line empirical treatment for PID in areas where >5% of PID is caused by quinolone-resistant *N. gonorrhoeae*.

be associated with increased drug cost and more adverse effects, when compared to currently recommended treatments.

Special considerations

Tubo-ovarian abscess

Tubo-ovarian abscess is a serious and potentially life-threatening complication of PID (**Figure 43.7**). Patients are more likely to be systemically unwell, and have higher levels of pelvic pain. The palpation of an adnexal mass, or lack of response to therapy, should prompt imaging studies. Tubo-ovarian abscess is an indication for hospital admission for parenteral antimicrobial therapy, with appropriate anaerobic cover, and to monitor for signs of rupture or sepsis. Conservative management may be effective with studies showing resolution in 70–84% of women, particularly those with smaller abscesses (<9 cm in diameter) (66). Alternatively, in a Norwegian cohort, TVUS-guided aspiration together with antibiotic therapy led to successful treatment and avoidance of surgical intervention in 93.4% (67). Failure of improvement by 72 hours, or clinical deterioration in the interim should be an indication for surgical exploration.

Pregnancy

Pregnant women with suspected PID are at high risk for maternal morbidity and preterm delivery. These women should be hospitalized and treated with intravenous antibiotics. The use of quinolones and doxycycline are contraindicated in pregnancy (and breastfeeding women). Pregnant women should be treated with ceftriaxone, erythromycin, and metronidazole providing there is no documented allergy. It is important to note that doxycycline in very early pregnancy, prior to a pregnancy test becoming positive, is not contraindicated.

HIV

Comprehensive observational and controlled studies have demonstrated that HIV-positive women with PID have similar symptoms when compared with HIV-negative women. There is no evidence

to suggest that HIV-positive women benefit from routine hospitalization or parenteral therapy for uncomplicated PID, although two Kenyan studies have suggested severe disease was more common, particularly in advanced HIV immunosuppression, and time to hospital discharge was longer (68, 69).

Intrauterine device

PID among intrauterine device (IUD) users is most strongly related to the insertion procedure and background risk of STIs. A meta-analysis of 22,908 IUD insertions and 51,399 woman-years of follow-up showed PID was six times higher during the first 20 days after insertion, and an infrequent event thereafter (1.6 cases per 1000 woman-years) (69). If an IUD user is diagnosed with PID, the IUD does not need to be removed immediately. If no improvement occurs after 48–72 hours, then removal should be considered while continuing antibiotics (70). A systematic review of evidence found that treatment outcomes did not generally differ between women with PID who retained the IUD and those who had the IUD removed (70).

Partner notification and other management considerations

Empirical treatment is recommended for all recent male partners. This is stated as the last 60 days (or most recent sexual partner if >60 days ago) in the CDC 2015 guidelines (2). The European and United Kingdom guidelines both recommend tracing contacts within a 6-month period, although recognize this time period is not evidence based (40, 59). Recent partners should receive empirical treatment for chlamydia regardless of symptoms or laboratory results in either individual (59). If adequate screening for gonorrhoea is not available, then empirical treatment for this infection should also be given (40).

To minimize disease transmission, women should be instructed to abstain from sexual intercourse until therapy is completed, symptoms have resolved, and sex partners have been adequately treated. Rest should be advised for those with severe disease, and appropriate analgesia must be provided. Diagnosis and treatment of PID offers an opportunity to provide health promotion information including clear written material (**Box 43.1**).

Follow-up

Clinical symptoms should improve within 3 days of commencing antibiotics. Outpatients should be advised to return for further evaluation if this is not the case. Imaging studies, hospitalization for intravenous therapy, or surgical intervention may be indicated. A routine assessment 2–4 weeks after treatment is recommended to assess the clinical response, adherence to antibiotics, that the individual abstained from sexual contact, and her partners received treatment. It is also an opportunity to check understanding of PID and its sequelae. For those with positive microbiological tests at baseline, repeat testing after 2–4 weeks may be appropriate, particularly in those with persisting symptoms, where poor adherence to antibiotics or partner notification is suspected, or where first-line antibiotic treatment was not used.

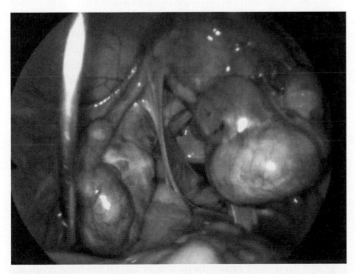

Figure 43.7 Laparoscopic appearances of a right tubo-ovarian abscess/complex.
Reproduced with permission from Mr Peter Greenhouse, Bristol Sexual Health Centre.

Box 43.1 Health promotion messages for patients

- An explanation of what treatment is being given and its possible adverse effects.
- Following treatment, fertility is usually maintained but there remains a risk of future infertility, chronic pelvic pain, or ectopic pregnancy.
- Clinically more severe disease is associated with a greater risk of sequelae.
- Repeat episodes of PID are associated with an exponential increase in the risk of infertility.
- The earlier treatment is given, the lower the risk of future fertility problems.
- Future use of barrier contraception will significantly reduce the risk of PID.
- The need to screen her sexual contacts for infection to prevent her becoming reinfected.

Source data from Ross J, McCarthy G. *UK National Guidelines for the Management of Pelvic Inflammatory Disease 2011*. London, United Kingdom: British Association for Sexual Health & HIV; 2011. (http://www.bashh.org/documents/3572.pdf). (Accessed 8 March 2016).

Sequelae/long-term outcomes

After one episode of PID, a significant proportion of women, up to one in four, will experience long-term complications including infertility, ectopic pregnancy, and chronic pelvic pain (defined as pain lasting >6 months). After repeated episodes, this proportion increases to almost one in two. This was first shown in the seminal paper by Weström et al. who reported on the long-term reproductive outcomes for 1844 women with abnormal laparoscopies. These individuals were followed up for a total of 13,400 woman-years, and compared to 657 women with normal laparoscopy (controls) followed for 3,958 woman-years (71). Of these women, 16% of the patients and 2.7% of controls failed to conceive. A total of 10.8% of patients and 0% of controls had confirmed tubal factor infertility. Each repeated episode of PID doubled the rate of tubal factor infertility. After one episode, the rate was 8%, increasing to 19.5% after two episodes, and 40% after three or more episodes of PID. The ectopic pregnancy rate for first pregnancy was 9.1% among patients and 1.4% in control subjects (P <0.0001).

In this same cohort, the duration of symptoms was shown to be a major determinant of subsequent infertility. Hillis and colleagues demonstrated that, after adjusting for age, organism, year of diagnosis, and history of recent gynaecological events, women who delayed seeking care for PID (≥3 days of symptoms) had a significantly greater infertility rate compared to those who received prompt care (<3 days from symptom onset, 19.7% vs 8.3%) (60). The association was strongest among the 114 women infected with chlamydia, with 17.8% of *C. trachomatis*-positive women who delayed seeking care experiencing impaired fertility compared to 0% who sought care promptly. These data suggest that prompt evaluation and treatment of chlamydia-associated PID can prevent these sequelae.

The PEACH study also reported on long-term outcomes. After 7 years of follow-up, 19% of women were categorized as infertile, 42.7% reported chronic pelvic pain (minimum duration 6 months) (12), and 0.6% had an ectopic pregnancy (74). Recurrent PID was associated with an almost twofold increase in reported infertility (adjusted odds ratio 1.8; 95% CI 1.2–2.8) and more than a fourfold increase in chronic pelvic pain (adjusted odds ratio 4.2; 95% CI

2.8–6.2). Furthermore, women with subsequent STIs of the *lower* genital tract were also 2.3 times more likely to experience chronic pelvic pain compared to those without subsequent STIs (12). More recently, Price et al. have estimated using multiparameter evidence synthesis that 27% (95% credible interval (CrI) 11–46%) of ectopic pregnancies in women aged 16–44 years are due to salpingitis, and 29% (95% CrI 9–56%) of tubal factor infertility is attributable to *C. trachomatis* (19).

The role of different organisms in the development of sequelae is not well understood. As previously discussed, patients with chlamydia or mycoplasma are more likely to delay care which may increase the risk of low-level inflammation and long-term complications. In a further analysis of the PEACH study looking at time to care, Taylor et al. reported that patients waited a mean of 7 days before seeking care for symptoms with time to care being longest among women monoinfected with chlamydia (12.3 ± 9.4 days) and mycoplasma (10.9 ± 8.9 days) and the shortest among women with gonorrhoea (4.6 ± 5 days) or coinfection (5.6 ± 5.1 days; P <0.001). Rates of infertility, recurrent PID, and chronic pelvic pain were frequent overall (17%, 20%, and 36% respectively) and tended to be higher after delayed care (47).

Prevention

In theory, if early infection confined to the cervix can be treated before it ascends to the endometrium and salpinges, then PID should be preventable. Rates of PID have fallen in most countries since chlamydia screening and treatment programmes were initiated and there is considerable evidence to suggest they are leading to decreased rates of PID, ectopic pregnancy, and tubal factor infertility. The first study to show that screening for chlamydia prevented PID was by Scholes et al. in 1996. Women were randomized to screening or usual care and followed up for 12 months. Women assigned to the screening group were found to have a 56% lower incidence of PID than those in the usual care group (relative risk 0.44; 95% CI 0.2–0.9) (75). A Danish study in 2000 compared home sampling (where 93% of women tested) to standard of care (where only 7.6% tested). Forty-three infections were identified in the intervention group, compared to only five in the standard of care. At 1 year, 2.1% of the students in the intervention group were treated for PID versus 4.2% in the control group (Wilcoxon exact value, P = 0.045) (76). Both studies depended on self-reporting or medical records to confirm cases of PID, which may have impacted the results, and some women will have had undiagnosed asymptomatic infection, although these limitations should have been evenly distributed between the groups. However, in the Prevention Of Pelvic Infections (POPI) trial, the incidence of PID was 1.3% (15/1191) in screened women compared with 1.9% (23/1186) in controls who had a stored sample tested for chlamydia at 1 year (relative risk 0.65; 95% CI 0.34–1.22). The authors concluded the risk of PID over 12 months in women screened for chlamydia was non-significantly reduced by 35% (77). In this study, the effect of the intervention may have been reduced by women in the control arm being made aware of the symptoms of PID, and presenting earlier. In fact, in general it has been proposed that if there was better public understanding of the risks and symptoms of PID, women with lower abdominal pain would seek earlier medical attention and avoid the risk of reproductive damage (19).

There is a valuable opportunity to provide health promotion and encourage condom use when women present with PID. There is some evidence that adolescents randomized to watching a short video acknowledging the barriers and benefits of PID self-care at the initial visit, were more likely to attend for follow-up (32% vs 16%). They were also three times more likely to have their partners treated than the control group, thus potentially reducing recurrent disease (78). A further analysis of the PEACH study showed persistent use of condoms during the study reduced the risk of recurrent PID, chronic pelvic pain, and infertility. Consistent condom use at baseline also reduced these risks by 30–60%. The authors concluded that the use of condoms was important in the prevention of PID sequelae (79).

REFERENCES

1. Ross J, Hughes G. Why is the incidence of pelvic inflammatory disease falling? *BMJ* 2014;**348**:g1538.
2. Centers for Disease Control and Prevention. Pelvic inflammatory disease (PID). 2015. Available at: http://www.cdc.gov/std/tg2015/pid.htm. (Accessed 16th July 2019).
3. Yeh JM, Hook EW, Goldie SJ. A refined estimate of the average lifetime cost of pelvic inflammatory disease. *Sex Transm Dis* 2003;**30**:369–78.
4. Hebb JK, Cohen CR, Astete SG, Bukusi EA, Totten PA. Detection of novel organisms associated with salpingitis, by use of 16S rDNA polymerase chain reaction. *J Infect Dis* 2004;**190**:2109–20.
5. Ness RB, Soper DE, Holley RL, et al. Effectiveness of inpatient and outpatient treatment strategies for women with pelvic inflammatory disease: results from the Pelvic Inflammatory Disease Evaluation and Clinical Health (PEACH) Randomized Trial. *Am J Obstet Gynecol* 2002;**186**:929–37.
6. Simms I, Rogers P, Charlett A. The rate of diagnosis and demography of pelvic inflammatory disease in general practice: England and Wales. *Int J STD AIDS* 1999;**10**:448–51.
7. Public Health England. Rates of pelvic inflammatory disease (PID) in England (2000–2013). *HPR* 2015;**9**:22.
8. Centers for Disease Control and Prevention. Pelvic inflammatory disease—initial visits to physicians' offices among women aged 15–44 years, United States, 2004–2013. Sexually Transmitted Disease Surveillance 2014. Available at: http://www.cdc.gov/std/stats14/figures/e.htm. (Accessed 16th July 2019).
9. Rekart, ML, Gilbert, M, Meza, R, et al. Chlamydia public health programs and the epidemiology of pelvic inflammatory disease and ectopic pregnancy. *J Infect Dis* 2013;**207**:30–38.
10. Bender N, Herrmann B, Andersen B, et al. Chlamydia infection, pelvic inflammatory disease, ectopic pregnancy and infertility: cross-national study. *Sex Transm Infect* 2011;**87**:601–608.
11. Burnett AM, Anderson CP, Zwank MD. Laboratory-confirmed gonorrhea and/or chlamydia rates in clinically diagnosed pelvic inflammatory disease and cervicitis. *Am J Emerg Med* 2012;**30**:1114–17.
12. Trent M, Bass D, Ness RB, Haggerty C. Recurrent PID, subsequent STI, and reproductive health outcomes: findings from the PID evaluation and clinical health (PEACH) study. *Sex Transm Dis* 2011;**38**:879–81.
13. Sweet RL. Treatment of acute pelvic inflammatory disease. *Infect Dis Obstet Gynecol* 2011;**2011**:561909.
14. Ness RB, Hillier SL, Kip KE, et al. Douching, pelvic inflammatory disease, and incident gonococcal and chlamydial genital infection in a cohort of high-risk women. *Am J Epidemiol* 2005;**161**:186–95.
15. McCormack W. Pelvic inflammatory disease. *N Engl J Med* 1994;**330**:115–19.
16. Bowie WR, Jones H. Acute pelvic inflammatory disease in outpatients: association with Chlamydia trachomatis and Neisseria gonorrhoeae. *Ann Intern Med* 1981;**95**:685–88.
17. Bevan CD, Johal BJ, Mumtaz G, Ridgway GL, Siddle NC. Clinical, laparoscopic and microbiological findings in acute salpingitis: report on a United Kingdom cohort. *Br J Obstet Gynaecol* 1995;**102**:407–14.
18. Soper DE, Brockwell NJ, Dalton HP, Johnson D. Observations concerning the microbial etiology of acute salpingitis. *Am J Obstet Gynecol* 1994;**170**:1008–14.
19. Price MJ, Ades AE, Soldan K, et al. The natural history of Chlamydia trachomatis infection in women: a multi-parameter evidence synthesis. *Health Technol Assess* 2016;**20**:1–250.
20. Taylor BD, Darville T, Haggerty CL. Does bacterial vaginosis cause pelvic inflammatory disease? *Sex Transm Dis* 2013;**40**:117–22.
21. Walker CK, Workowski KA, Washington AE, Soper D, Sweet R. Anaerobes in pelvic inflammatory disease: implications for the Centers for Disease Control and Prevention's guidelines for treatment of sexually transmitted diseases. *Clin Infect Dis* 1999;**28** Suppl 1:S29–36.
22. Ness RB, Hillier SL, Kip KE, et al. Bacterial vaginosis and risk of pelvic inflammatory disease. *Obstet Gynecol* 2004;**104**:761–69.
23. Ness RB, Kip KE, Hillier SL, et al. A cluster analysis of bacterial vaginosis-associated microflora and pelvic inflammatory disease. *Am J Epidemiol* 2005;**162**:585–90.
24. Hillier SL, Kiviat NB, Hawes SE, et al. Role of bacterial vaginosis-associated microorganisms in endometritis. *Am J Obstet Gynecol* 1996;**175**:435–41.
25. Haggerty CL, Hillier SL, Bass DC, Ness RB. Bacterial vaginosis and anaerobic bacteria are associated with endometritis. *Clin Infect Dis* 2004;**39**:990–95.
26. Lareau SM, Beigi RH. Pelvic inflammatory disease and tubo-ovarian abscess. *Infect Dis Clin North Am* 2008;**22**:693–708.
27. Hjorth SV, Björnelius E, Lidbrink P, et al. Sequence-based typing of Mycoplasma genitalium reveals sexual transmission. *J Clin Microbiol* 2006;**44**:2078–83.
28. Bjartling C, Osser S, Persson K. Mycoplasma genitalium in cervicitis and pelvic inflammatory disease among women at a gynecologic outpatient service. *Am J Obstet Gynecol* 2012;**206**:476.e1–8.
29. Haggerty CL, Taylor BD. Mycoplasma genitalium: an emerging cause of pelvic inflammatory disease. *Infect Dis Obstet Gynecol* 2011;**2011**:959816.
30. Cohen CR, Manhart LE, Bukusi EA, et al. Association between Mycoplasma genitalium and acute endometritis. *Lancet* 2002;**359**:765–66.
31. Lis R, Rowhani-Rahbar A, Manhart LE. Mycoplasma genitalium infection and female reproductive tract disease: a meta-analysis. *Clin Infect Dis* 2015;**61**:418–26.
32. Geisler WM. Duration of untreated, uncomplicated Chlamydia trachomatis genital infection and factors associated with chlamydia resolution: a review of human studies. *J Infect Dis* 2010;**201** Suppl 2;S104–13.
33. Rice PA, Schachter J. Pathogenesis of pelvic inflammatory disease. What are the questions? *JAMA* 1991;**266**:2587–93.
34. Kunz G, Leyendecker G. Uterine peristaltic activity during the menstrual cycle: characterization, regulation, function and dysfunction. *Reprod Biomed Online* 2002; **4** Suppl 3:5–9.
35. Taylor BD, Darville T, Tan C, Bavoil PM, Ness RB, Haggerty CL. The role of chlamydia trachomatis polymorphic membrane proteins

in inflammation and sequelae among women with pelvic inflammatory disease. *Infect Dis Obstet Gynecol* 2011;**2011**:989762.

36. Tuffrey M, Alexander F, Taylor Robinson D. Severity of salpingitis in mice after primary and repeated inoculation with a human strain of Chlamydia trachomatis. *J Exp Pathol (Oxford)* 1990;**71**:403–10.

37. Lanjouw E, Ouburg S, de Vries HJ, Stary, A, Radcliffe K, Unemo M. Background review for the 2015 European guideline on the management of Chlamydia trachomatis infections. *Int J STD AIDS* 2015;Nov 24:0956462415618838.

38. Miettinen A, Heinonen PK, Teisala K, Hakkarainen K, Punnonen R. Serologic evidence for the role of Chlamydia trachomatis, Neisseria gonorrhoeae, and Mycoplasma hominis in the etiology of tubal factor infertility and ectopic pregnancy. *Sex Transm Dis* 1990;**17**:10–14.

39. Wiesenfeld HC, Hillier SL, Meyn LA, Amortegui AJ, Sweet RL. Subclinical PID and infertility. *Obstet Gynecol* 2012;**120**:37–43.

40. Ross J, Judlin P, Jensen J. 2012 European guideline for the management of pelvic inflammatory disease. *Int J STD AIDS* 2014;**25**:1–22.

41. Miettinen AK, Heinonen PK, Laippala P, Paavonen J. Test performance of erythrocyte sedimentation rate and C-reactive protein in assessing the severity of acute pelvic inflammatory disease. *Am J Obstet Gynecol* 1993;**169**:1143–49.

42. Yudin MH, Hillier SL, Wiesenfeld HC, Krohn MA, Amortegui AA, Sweet RL. Vaginal polymorphonuclear leukocytes and bacterial vaginosis as markers for histologic endometritis among women without symptoms of pelvic inflammatory disease. *Am J Obstet Gynecol* 2003;**188**:318–23.

43. Short VL, Totten PA, Ness RB, Astete SG, Sheryl F, Haggerty CL. Clinical presentation of Mycoplasma genitalium infection versus Neisseria gonorrhoeae infection among women with pelvic inflammatory disease. *Clin Infect Dis* 2010;**48**:41–47.

44. Peipert JF, Ness RB, Blume J, et al. Clinical predictors of endometritis in women with symptoms and signs of pelvic inflammatory disease. *Am J Obstet Gynecol* 2001;**184**:856–63.

45. Eschenbach DA, Wölner-Hanssen P, Hawes SE, Pavletic A, Paavonen J, Holmes KK. Acute pelvic inflammatory disease: associations of clinical and laboratory findings with laparoscopic findings. *Obstet Gynecol* 1997;**89**:184–92.

46. Simms I, Warburton F, Weström L. Diagnosis of pelvic inflammatory disease: time for a rethink. *Sex Transm Infect* 2003;**79**:491–94.

47. Taylor BD, Ness RB, Darville T, Haggerty CL. Microbial correlates of delayed care for pelvic inflammatory disease. *Sex Transm Dis* 2011;**38**:434–38.

48. Brunham R, Gottlieb SL, Paavonen J. Pelvic inflammatory disease. *N Engl J Med* 2015;**372**:2039–48.

49. Morris GC, Stewart CMW, Schoeman SA, Wilson JD. A cross-sectional study showing differences in the clinical diagnosis of pelvic inflammatory disease according to the experience of clinicians: implications for training and audit. *Sex Transm Infect* 2014;**90**:445–51.

50. Jaiyeoba O, Soper DE. A practical approach to the diagnosis of pelvic inflammatory disease. *Infect Dis Obstet Gynecol* 2011;**2011**:753037.

51. Hemilä M, Henriksson L, Ylikorkala O. Serum CRP in the diagnosis and treatment of pelvic inflammatory disease. *Arch Gynecol Obstet* 1987;**241**:177–82.

52. Cacciatore B, Leminen A, Ingman-Friberg S, Ylöstalo P, Paavonen J. Transvaginal sonographic findings in ambulatory patients with suspected pelvic inflammatory disease. *Obstet Gynecol* 1992;**80**:912–16.

53. Molander P, Sjöberg J, Paavonen J, Cacciatore B. Transvaginal power Doppler findings in laparoscopically proven acute pelvic inflammatory disease. *Ultrasound Obstet Gynecol* 2001;**17**:233–38.

54. Tukeva TA, Aronen HJ, Karjalainen PT, Molander P, Paavonen T, Paavonen J. MR imaging in pelvic inflammatory disease: comparison with laparoscopy and US. *Radiology* 1999;**210**:209–16.

55. Sellors J, Mahoney J, Goldsmith C, et al. The accuracy of clinical findings and laparoscopy in pelvic inflammatory disease. *Am J Obstet Gynaecol* 1991;**164**:113–20.

56. Molander P, Finne P, Sjöberg J, Sellors J, Paavonen J. Observer agreement with laparoscopic diagnosis of pelvic inflammatory disease using photographs. *Obstet Gynecol* 2003;**101**:875–80.

57. Kivia, NB, Wølner-Hanssen P, Eschenbach DA, et al. Endometrial histopathology in patients with culture-proved upper genital tract infection and laparoscopically diagnosed acute salpingitis. *Am J Surg Pathol* 1990;**14**:167–75.

58. Mitchell C, Prabhu M. Pelvic inflammatory disease: current concepts in pathogenesis, diagnosis and treatment. *Infect Dis Clin North Am* 2013;**27**:793–809.

59. Ross J, Cole M, Evans C et al. *United Kingdom National Guideline for the Management of Pelvic Inflammatory Disease 2019*. London: British Association of Sexual Health and HIV. Available at: https://www.bashhguidelines.org/media/1217/pid-update-2019.pdf (accessed 16th July 2019).

60. Hillis SD, Joesoef R, Marchbanks PA, Wasserheit JN, Cates W, Westrom L. Delayed care of pelvic inflammatory disease as a risk factor for impaired fertility. *Am J Obstet Gynecol* 1993;**168**:1503–509.

61. Dunbar-Jacob J, Sereika SM, Foley SM, Bass DC, Ness RB. Adherence to oral therapies in pelvic inflammatory disease. *J Womens Health* 2004;**13**:285–91.

62. European Medicines Agency. Disabling and potentially permanent side effects lead to suspension or restrictions of quinolone and fluoroquinolone antibiotics. EMA/175398/2019. (https://www.ema.europa.eu/en/medicines/human/referrals/quinolone-fluoroquinolone-containing-medicinal-products). Accessed 16th July 2019.

63. Haggerty CL, Totten PA, Astete SG, et al. Failure of cefoxitin and doxycycline to eradicate endometrial Mycoplasma genitalium and the consequence for clinical cure of pelvic inflammatory disease. *Sex Transm Infect* 2008;**84**:338–42.

64. Jensen JS, Bradshaw CS, Tabrizi SN, Fairley CK, Hamasuna R. Azithromycin treatment failure in Mycoplasma genitalium-positive patients with nongonococcal urethritis is associated with induced macrolide resistance. *Clin Infect Dis* 2008;**47**:1546–53.

65. Bissessor M, Tabrizi SN, Twin J, et al. Macrolide resistance and azithromycin failure in a mycoplasma genitalium-infected cohort and response of azithromycin failures to alternative antibiotic regimens. *Clin Infect Dis* 2015;**60**:1228–36.

66. Reed SD, Landers DV, Sweet RL. Antibiotic treatment of tuboovarian abscess: comparison of broad-spectrum beta-lactam agents versus clindamycin-containing regimens. *Am J Obstet Gynecol* 1991;**164**:1556–61.

67. Gjelland K, Ekerhovd E, Granberg S. Transvaginal ultrasound-guided aspiration for treatment of tubo-ovarian abscess: a study of 302 cases. *Am J Obstet Gynecol* 2005;**193**:1323–30.

68. Cohen CR, Sinei S, Reilly M et al. Effect of human immunodeficiency virus type 1 infection upon acute salpingitis: a laparoscopic study. *J Infect Dis* 1998;**178**:1352–58.

69. Mugo NR, Kiehlbauch JA, Nguti R, et al. Effect of human immunodeficiency virus-1 infection on treatment outcome of acute salpingitis. *Obstet Gynecol* 2006;**107**:807–12.

70. Farley TM, Rosenberg MJ, Rowe PJ, Chen JH, Meirik O. Intrauterine devices and pelvic inflammatory disease. *Lancet* 1992;**3**:280–87.

71. Centers for Disease Control and Prevention. U.S. Selected practice recommendations for contraceptive use, 2013: adapted from

the World Health Organization Selected Practice Recommendations for Contraceptive Use, 2nd edition. June 21, 2013. Available at: http://www.cdc.gov/mmwr/preview/mmwrhtml/rr6205a1.htm. (Accessed 16th July 2019).

72. Tepper NK, Steenland MW, Gaffield ME, Marchbanks PA, Curtis KM. Retention of intrauterine devices in women who acquire pelvic inflammatory disease: a systematic review. *Contraception* 2013;**87**:655–60.

73. Weström L, Joesoef R, Reynolds G, Hagdu A, Thompson SE. Pelvic inflammatory disease and fertility. A cohort study of 1,844 women with laparoscopically verified disease and 657 control women with normal laparoscopic results. *Sex Transm Dis* 1992;**19**:185–92.

74. Ness RB, Trautmann G, Richter HE, et al. Effectiveness of treatment strategies of some women with pelvic inflammatory disease: a randomized trial. *Obstet Gynecol* 2005;**106**:573–80.

75. Scholes D, Stergachis A, Heidrich F, Andrilla H, Holmes KK, Stamm W. Prevention of pelvic inflammatory disease by screening for cervical chlamydial infection. *N Engl J Med.* 1998;**334**:1362–66.

76. Ostergaard L, Andersen B, Møller JK, Olesen F. Home sampling versus conventional swab sampling for screening of Chlamydia trachomatis in women: a cluster-randomized 1-year follow-up study. *Clin Infect Dis* 2000;**31**:951–57.

77. Oakeshott P, Kerry S, Aghaizu A et al. Randomised controlled trial of screening for Chlamydia trachomatis to prevent pelvic inflammatory disease: the POPI (prevention of pelvic infection) trial. *BMJ (Clin Res Ed)* 2010;**340**:c1642.

78. Trent M, Chung S, Burke M, Walker A, Ellen JM. Results of a randomized controlled trial of a brief behavioral intervention for pelvic inflammatory disease in adolescents. *J Pediatr Adolesc Gynecol* 2010;**23**:96–101.

79. Ness RB, Randall H, Richter HE, et al. Condom use and the risk of recurrent pelvic inflammatory disease, chronic pelvic pain, or infertility following an episode of pelvic inflammatory disease. *Am J Public Health* 2004;**94**:1327–29.

44

Chronic pelvic pain

Jacqueline Pui Wah Chung and Tin Chiu Li

Introduction

Chronic pelvic pain (CPP) remains an enigma to the gynaecologists. Up to now, there is no universally agreed definition. According to the latest International Society of Psychosomatic Obstetrics and Gynaecology European Consensus Statement in 2015, CPP is defined as:

> a persistent, severe and distressing pain lasting at least 6 months. It may occur cyclically, intermittently/situationally or chronically. It leads to a major reduction in quality of life. In some patients, physical change/disorders can be regarded as the main cause; while in others, the pain seems to be mainly associated with emotional conflict and psychosocial stress. Both conditions can occur simultaneously. (1)

It is important to remember that it is a symptom, and not in itself a diagnosis (2).

Epidemiology

CPP is a common gynaecological complaint with a similar consultation rate to low back pain, asthma, or migraine. It is estimated that up to 15–20% of women aged 18–50 years have experienced CPP for more than 1 year (3). Nevertheless, the incidence of CPP is likely to be underestimated due to under-reporting.

Causes and differential diagnosis

The pathophysiology of CPP is often multifactorial with significant physical, psychological, and social components. **Box 44.1** shows the differential diagnosis for CPP.

Gynaecological causes

Endometriosis

Endometriosis is the presence of endometrial-like tissue outside the uterus, which induces a chronic inflammatory reaction. The condition is predominantly found in women of reproductive age, from all ethnic and social groups. Up to 30% of women undergoing laparoscopy for CPP are found to have endometriosis (4, 5). The mechanism of endometriosis causing the CPP is still not fully understood but it may be related to the inflammation and adhesion it causes.

Pelvic inflammatory disease

Pelvic inflammatory disease results from ascending infection from the endocervix and vagina into the uterus, tubes, and surrounding structures. The inflammation may cause adhesions leading to CPP, damage to tubal epithelium leading to increased chance of ectopic pregnancy, and infertility. Approximately 85% of cases are acquired via sexual activity, while the remaining 15% of cases are iatrogenic and may occur after invasive procedures such as endometrial biopsies, uterine curettages, or insertion of intrauterine contraceptive devices. Primary pathogens include *Neisseria gonorrhoea* and *Chlamydia trachomatis* and up to 40% of women may have coexisting infections. Secondary pathogens include *Gardnerella vaginalis*, *Mycoplasma*, and other aerobic and anaerobic organisms (6). Patients should also be screened for other sexually transmitted diseases and their sexual partners should also be screened and treated as appropriate. The triad of lower abdominal pain, adnexal tenderness, and tender cervical excitation usually suggests acute pelvic inflammatory disease. Prompt diagnosis and treatment is important as delay in management for a few days may increase morbidity.

Adhesions

Adhesions refer to abnormal attachments between two structures due to the presence of fibrous tissue. Pelvic adhesions are adhesions within the pelvic cavity, which may be produced following previous surgery, pelvic inflammatory disease, endometriosis, previous radiotherapy, peritoneal dialysis, or intra-abdominal abscess. Adhesions do not always cause pain but are more likely to do so if they are dense and vascular, if they involve pain-sensitive structures such as the ovary or parietal peritoneum, or if they restrict mobility. The pain may be more pronounced when certain movement causes stretching of the adhesion tissue, pulling on the tissues attached to it (7, 8).

Adenomyosis

Adenomyosis is defined as the presence of heterotopic endometrial glands and stroma in the myometrium with adjacent smooth muscle hyperplasia. It affects approximately 1% of women and is often found

Gynaecological conditions
- Endometriosis
- Adhesions
- Pelvic inflammatory disease
- Chronic endometritis
- Ovarian cysts
- Ovarian remnant syndrome
- Pelvic congestion syndrome
- Residual ovarian syndrome
- Uterine fibroids
- Vulvodynia
- Vestibulitis
- Adenomyosis
- Cervical stenosis

Urological conditions
- Chronic urinary tract infections
- Interstitial cystitis
- Urolithiasis
- Bladder carcinoma

Gastrointestinal conditions
- Constipation
- Hernias
- Inflammatory bowel disease
- Irritable bowel syndrome

Musculoskeletal conditions
- Nerve entrapment syndrome
- Myofascial pain
- Pelvic floor myalgia
- Surgical scarring

Psychological conditions
- Anxiety
- Depression
- Personality disorders
- Physical/sexual abuse
- Stress

in multiparous women during their late 40s. Apart from pelvic pain, adenomyosis may produce dysmenorrhea, menorrhagia, and dyspareunia. Clinical examination often reveals a tender uterus. Ultrasonography may show characteristic lesions involving the junctional zone and the myometrium that may be focal or diffused. The best diagnostic tool is magnetic resonance imaging (MRI) (9).

Pelvic congestion syndrome

This is a syndrome characterized by the presence of pelvic pain associated with pelvic varicosities and pelvic venous congestion with delayed emptying of the pelvic veins. The pain may be unilateral or bilateral; if it is unilateral it is more often situated in the left iliac fossa than the right as pelvic varicosities are more likely to occur in the left side. The pain is often described as a dull ache or a sensation of heaviness in the pelvic area. It is often exacerbated by menstruation, coitus, or prolonged standing (10).

Ovarian remnant syndrome

Ovarian remnant syndrome refers to the presence of functional ovarian tissue after unilateral or bilateral oophorectomy. It is often associated with severe endometriosis and pelvic adhesions, leading to inadvertent incomplete removal of the ovaries during oophorectomy. The absence of vasomotor symptoms in women not on hormonal replacement therapy (HRT) or the presence of cyclical pain after bilateral oophorectomies should raise suspicion of this condition. Symptoms can occur a few months to several years after surgery (11). Blood test often reveals follicle-stimulating hormone and oestradiol levels in the premenopausal range despite bilateral oophorectomies. Removal of ovarian remnants may lead to resolution of the CPP in 80% of cases as shown in a cohort study (12).

Residual ovarian syndrome or ovarian retention syndrome

Residual ovarian syndrome or ovarian retention syndrome is characterized by the presence of recurrent or intermittent pelvic pain or dyspareunia after hysterectomy with conservation of ovaries. The pain is often due to a combination of development of functional cysts in an ovary involved in adhesion. The pain is often cyclical or intermittent in nature and again can occur a few months to several years after the hysterectomy.

Non-gynaecological causes

Interstitial cystitis and painful bladder syndrome

Different centres and units have different definitions for the term 'interstitial cystitis'. The International Continence Society suggests that 'painful bladder syndrome' may be a better name to describe 'a condition of suprapubic pain related to bladder filling, accompanied by other symptom such as increased day time and night time frequency in the absence of proven urinary tract infection or other obvious pathology'. On the other hand, 'interstitial cystitis' is best used to describe a 'painful bladder syndrome with typical cystoscopic and histological features'. The symptoms often last for more than 6 weeks (13). The exact aetiology of interstitial cystitis or painful bladder syndrome is not known and may be multifactorial.

Irritable bowel syndrome

This is a common gastrointestinal disorder characterized by a chronic, relapsing pattern of lower pelvic pain associating with alteration of bowel function including constipation or diarrhoea. It is defined by the Rome III criteria (available at https://www.theromefoundation.org/assets/pdf/19_RomeIII_apA_885-898.pdf) with recurrent abdominal pain, discomfort for at least 3 days per month in the last 3 months, with a symptom onset at least 6 months prior to diagnosis and associated with two or more of the following: (a) improvement with defecation, (b) onset associated with a change in frequency of stool, or (c) onset associated with a change in form or appearance of stool. The use of a symptom-screening questionnaire may be helpful. The onset is usually during late adolescence to early adulthood and seldom occurs in later life.

Musculoskeletal

It is not uncommon for musculoskeletal conditions to present as CPP. Many musculoskeletal structures of the back and lower limbs share segmental innervation with urogenital structures and may cause referred pain over the lower abdomen and pelvic floor mimicking pelvic pain (14). Direct trauma, operation, overuse, or faulty postures are common causes. Myofascial pain syndrome is a condition where pain is caused by myofascial trigger points in skeletal muscle. Trigger points are hyperirritable, localized painful spots found in any skeletal muscle or its associated fascia and which cause pain after compression or irritation. Pelvic floor tension myalgia is another condition where pelvic pain is associated with tenderness of the pelvic floor muscles including levator ani, coccygeus, or piriformis or their related fascia or insertions. Hypertonus of these muscles may cause pain over the perineum, lower abdominal, and inner thigh regions. Nerve entrapment syndrome may also cause pain when neural tissues are trapped or impinged by nearby musculoskeletal tissues. The ilioinguinal, iliohypogastric, and genitofemoral nerves are commonly entrapped nerves due to their close proximity to the iliopsoas muscle. Postsurgical scarring and inadvertent ligations by sutures may cause entrapment of neural tissue causing pain (15, 16).

Psychosocial factors

Psychosocial factors play an important role in CPP. A patient's personality, psychiatric illness, and coping skills all affect how she perceives the pain and responds to the treatment. Depression may be a cause or a consequence of the CPP. A previous history of sexual or physical abuse and unpleasant life experiences or life stressors is associated with a higher incidence of CPP (17).

Clinical assessment

History taking

History taking and establishing a good patient–doctor relationship are the keys to success in the management of CPP. Building a good rapport with the patient leads to better acceptance, compliance, and therapeutic outcome.

The interview should be carried out in a comfortable, nonintimidating, private room where the patient is relaxed and able to disclose sensitive information to the physician. The patient should feel well respected and believed as many patients worry that their doctors may think that their condition is 'all in their head'. From time to time, patients may find the consultation therapeutic if the doctor is a sympathetic listener, able to validate how they feel, and provides opportunities for them to express their own feelings. Consultations for CPP are usually time-consuming and so sufficient time should be allocated for the interview.

It is helpful to start off with a basic sociodemographic history as it can provide a general overview of the essential background information. Sometimes it is also useful to ask the patient to complete a structured questionnaire which may not only save time, but also elicit sensitive information which the patient may feel uneasy expressing during the consultation. The International Pelvic Pain Society generated a very thorough and useful questionnaire for use and this can be downloaded from their website (http://www.pelvicpain.org.uk).

Details about the pain including the onset, duration, severity, location, radiation, and any exacerbating or relieving factors should be enquired about.

Exactly when the pain started is an important piece of information as it may provide clues to its association with specific events such as a surgical episode, medical illness, trauma, accident, or stressful life experience. CPP that occurs after an adverse life event may point towards a psychological cause. Pain which started shortly after a surgical episode may suggest postoperative adhesions as an underlying cause.

The history should involve a general systematic review of the different organs. The presence of specific associated symptoms and their temporal relationship with the menstrual cycle, coitus, posture, urination, or bowel movements will point towards the likely underlying cause. Cyclical pain, which occurs only at a specific time of the menstrual cycle, is likely to be caused by a gynaecological condition whereas pain associated with a particular posture or physical activity is more likely to be musculoskeletal in origin. Pelvic pain associated with urinary frequency, urgency, or nocturia is typically due to interstitial cystitis. Improvement of pain with defecation and pain associated with a change in bowel movement is indicative of irritable bowel syndrome.

The severity of the pain should be evaluated. Quantifying the severity of the pain may be facilitated by using a pain score of 0–10 or 0–100, a visual analogue scale (marking the pain severity on a 10 cm long line), or a pain questionnaires such as the McGill Pain Questionnaire or more commonly nowadays, the short-form McGill Pain Questionnaire (18, 19), which is less time-consuming and easier to complete. Asking the patient to complete a pain diary also helps to identify potential aggravating factors and assess response to treatments.

The impact of the pain on daily activities should be assessed. The effect on quality of life can be determined by using health-related quality of life questionnaires such as the Short-Form 36 (20). Otherwise, simple questions regarding the effect of pain with reference to work, leisure, sleep, and sexual relationship should be asked. The Society of Obstetricians and Gynaecologists of Canada suggested asking two simple and effective questions: 'On a scale of 0–10, 0 being no pain and 10 being the worst pain imaginable, how is your pain today and how was your pain 2 weeks ago?' (15, 16). Measuring the degree of pain and its effect on daily activities not only help to identify the severity of the problem but are also useful for monitoring the progress after treatment.

Sensitive issues including a previous history of physical or sexual abuse should be elicited. Sexual dysfunction can also lead to CPP. Infrequent sexual intercourse may indicate a need to seek further details of the woman's sexual history. Patients may not be willing to voice out intimate aspects of their relationship during the first visit but they may do so in subsequent visits, after they have developed a certain amount of trust with the doctor. In cases where her partner always accompanies the patient, a separate consultation with the patient alone is required to allow the patient to freely discuss any hidden matters.

Social history is another important aspect. The patient's occupation, lifestyle, and the amount of support she obtains from her partner, family, and friends will influence management options.

A careful drug history especially the patient's response to various analgesics, is necessary to help planning if an additional or alternative analgesic should be offered. Pain improvement after hormonal manipulation is consistent with an underlying gynaecological condition.

At the end of the interview, it is useful to ask about the patient's self-perception of the underlying cause of the pain and her expectations about treatment outcome. Any fears and worries brought up should be addressed. Sometimes, patients need reassurance that there is no cancer or life-threatening condition. Setting a realistic goal together with the patient is an important key in developing a good rapport with the patient.

Physical examination

The examination process should begin as the patient enters the consulting room. The patient's gait, posture, body language, and facial expressions should be observed. An abnormal gait or posture is strongly indicative of an underlying musculoskeletal disorder. In addition, ongoing observation of the patient's response during the interview and examination will enable the examiner to find out about her character and personality.

Physical examination in women with CPP may require a different approach to that used for other gynaecological patients. Pelvic examination may need to be deferred to a later visit depending on the outcome of the initial consultation and the rapport achieved with the patient.

It is good to be open-minded when performing the exam and have the list of differential diagnoses in your mind. Listen to the patient as you perform the examination as she may volunteer valuable clues during the time of examination. General examination should be performed first and the most uncomfortable bimanual examination and speculum examination should be left to the end.

Explain to the patient what will happen and let her know that the examination can be stopped at any time if she feels uncomfortable. Examination should be performed with confidence and in a systematic manner. Documenting your examination findings onto a diagram or chart may be useful and allows better communication and reference between doctors, as well as the patient. Having a checklist will also make the examination easier and ensures completeness of the exam.

The examination should commence with the patient in the standing position. The presence of any scoliosis and the symmetry of the iliac crest should be noted. The inguinal and femoral hernia sites should be palpated while asking the patient to perform the Valsalva manoeuvre. Any local tenderness in the abdominal wall or low back or sacroiliac joint should be carefully looked for. Varicosities or oedema in the lower limb, if present, should be documented. In selected cases, neurological examination of the lower limb should be performed.

When the patient is in the supine position, apart from routine abdominal examination, a single digit palpation should be performed in all four quadrants to illicit any trigger points over the abdominal area. Around 75% of patients with pelvic congestion syndrome have tenderness over the ovarian point during abdominal palpation. The ovarian point lies at the junction of the upper and middle thirds of an imaginary line drawn from the anterior superior iliac spine to the umbilicus (11). Any scars on the abdominal wall should be palpated; if there is significant tenderness, nerve entrapment syndrome may be a possibility. Gently touching the skin in each dermatome can help to identify any hypersensitivity and referred pain. The 'head-raise test' may be used to distinguish pain in the peritoneal cavity or in the abdominal wall: if the pain is reduced when the head is raised, the pain is likely to come from intraperitoneal structures; however, if the pain persists, it is likely to originate from the abdominal wall (15, 16). The pubic symphysis should also be palpated for any tenderness.

The patient should now be placed in the lithotomy position. The patient should be offered a mirror to participate in the examination so to allow better understanding of her anatomy as well as better identification the site of pain. Inspection of the external genitalia is carried out to identify any distorted anatomy, scarring, discoloration, trauma, or lesions. A cotton swab or the 'Q-tip test' is used to identify any trigger points or altered sensation, including the urethral and clitoral region. Care should be taken to identify possible vulval vestibulitis and sometimes further colposcopic examination may be required. Again, any scars from previous episiotomy or perineal repair should be gently palpated to elicit undue tenderness. An intact anal reflex indicates intact pudendal nerve and functional levator ani.

In some cases, vaginal examination may be deferred to a subsequent visit to allow time to establish rapport. It is useful to begin with 'unimanual examination', that is, examination with one finger inserted into the vagina, to verify if there is any evidence of vaginismus. The lateral vaginal walls should be palpated for any tenderness, which may indicate reflex sympathetic hypersensitivity. The levator ani and coccygeus muscles should next be palpated to detect any trigger points or possible pelvic floor pain syndrome. The urethra and bladder base should then be palpated and any tenderness in this region may indicate a urological cause. After palpating the obturator muscles and piriformis muscles, the examination should continue to the cervix, paracervical areas, and vaginal fornixes for any nodularity or tenderness.

Finally, bimanual examination should be performed. The uterus should be examined systemically to ascertain the position, size, contour, consistency, mobility, support, and any tenderness. A fixed retroverted uterus points towards endometriosis, a bulky tender uterus suggests adenomyosis. The adnexal region is also assessed for any tenderness or masses. Speculum examination is performed in the usual way. Sometimes a smaller speculum may be required. Per rectal examination is not routinely performed but may be indicated if there are significant bowel symptoms.

Investigations

The purpose of the investigations is to establish the underlying cause and to rule out the possibility of dual pathology accounting for the symptom. Routine infection screening such as complete blood count, inflammatory markers, urinalysis, or mid-stream urine for culture and sensitivity are performed at the initial stage. Endocervical and vaginal swabs are obtained to rule out *N. gonorrhoea* and *C. trachomatis*. Sexually active women should also be offered screening for other sexually transmitted infections. In case of haematuria, urine for cytology is performed and patient should be referred to an urologist for further investigations.

Ultrasonography

Ultrasonography is a very useful investigation in women with CPP. It can detect many structural pelvic pathology such as uterine fibroids, adenomyosis, ovarian cysts, and hydrosalpinx. However, pelvic ultrasonography may be normal in women with endometriosis or pelvic adhesions. The use of transvaginal ultrasonography to diagnose adenomyosis and pelvic congestion syndrome requires special expertise. The characteristic ultrasound features of adenomyosis are summarized in Box 44.2 (9). It is now recognized that transvaginal ultrasound has a sensitivity between 53% and 89% and a specificity of 50–99% in diagnosing adenomyosis (9). Doppler ultrasound may further help in distinguishing uterine

Box 44.2 Ultrasound features of adenomyosis

- Globularly enlarged uterus
- Asymmetrical myometrial thickening
- Poorly defined, irregular thickened junctional zone
- Linear striations
- Myometrial cysts (anechoic roundish area of 1–7 mm)
- Adenomyoma: ill-defined nodular heterogeneous myometrial mass

Source data from Dueholm M. Transvaginal ultrasound for diagnosis of adenomyosis: a review. *Best Practice & Research Clinical Obstetrics and Gynaecology* Vol. 20, No. 4, pp. 569–582, 2006.
Levy G, Dehaene A, Laurent N, et al. An update on adenomyosis. *Diagn Interv Imaging* 2013;**94**:3–25.

Box 44.3 Indications for laparoscopy in women with chronic pelvic pain

- Past history or history suggestive of:
  - endometriosis with moderate to severe dysmenorrhea, dyspareunia
  - previous pelvic inflammatory disease
  - previous pelvic or abdominal surgery
  - ovarian remnant syndrome.
- Underlying cause of pain remains unexplained despite thorough investigation.
- Persistent pain despite medical treatment.
- Suspicion of adnexal mass or other pelvic pathology.

fibroids from adenomyosis: fibroids often have well-defined rim with few vessels entering the body of the mass while adenomyosis have vessels running perpendicularly into the adenomyoma (9). The use of three-dimensional ultrasound permits a better visualization of the junctional zone in the coronal view and so improves the diagnostic accuracy of adenomyosis compared with two-dimensional ultrasound (21).

Transrectal ultrasonography is particularly useful in assessing lesions in the rectovaginal septum and should be offered to women with symptoms and signs indicative of deep infiltrating endometriosis. Hypoechoic thickening of the torus and uterosacral ligament are often found in deep infiltrating endometriosis (22).

Ultrasound soft markers such as ovarian mobility, probe tenderness, and pouch of Douglas obliteration may help to assess the severity of endometriosis. These soft markers have been used to develop an ultrasound-based endometriosis staging system (UBESS) to help predict the level of complexity of laparoscopic surgery of endometriosis. The presence of soft markers on ultrasound improved the probability of positive findings on diagnostic laparoscopy from 58% to 73% and may help to identify women who may benefit from it (23).

Laparoscopy

Laparoscopy remains the gold standard for diagnosing the underlying cause of CPP. In one series, up to 40% of the indications for laparoscopy performed by gynaecologists were CPP (3). Endometriosis, adhesions, and pelvic inflammatory disease are the most common conditions encountered in women with CPP.

It is helpful to remember that the stage of endometriosis does not correlate with the severity of pain experienced by women. Many women with severe endometriosis may experience little pain; whereas some women with minimal or mild endometriosis may be troubled with severe pain.

Laparoscopy provides an opportunity not only for diagnosis but also treatment at the same setting. Moreover, laparoscopy itself has been shown to have a placebo effect and the reassurance of a negative laparoscopy may improve pain in 30% of the patients, independent of the severity of their disease (24).

However, laparoscopy is not without risks. The procedure is associated with deaths in approximately 3–8 in 100,000 cases and injury to the bowel, bladder, or major blood vessels in 2 in 1000 cases (25). Not everyone presenting with CPP requires a laparoscopy. The decision to proceed with laparoscopy should be made after a careful, individualized assessment, depending partly on how likely there is to be pathology in the pelvis and partly on the response to expectant treatment. **Box 44.3** highlights some of the situations when laparoscopy is suggested. In an earlier series, around 40% of the patients with CPP undergoing laparoscopy had negative findings and some of the positive findings may be coincidental and not necessary be the underlying cause of the CPP (3). A negative laparoscopy, however, may indicate that non-gynaecological causes of the CPP are more likely. A video recording or photographs should be taken during the laparoscopy, as they may be useful during explanation to the patient about her condition and in planning future treatment plans.

Laparoscopic pain mapping

Patient-assisted laparoscopy has been attempted to improve identification of potential sources for CPP. The procedure is performed under conscious sedation and local analgesia by probing and traction of tissue to try and reproduce the patient's symptoms. However, as the procedure may be rather uncomfortable, careful patient selection is crucial. Those with significant cardiopulmonary conditions such as chronic obstructive airway disease, pulmonary hypertension, and heart failure are contraindicated. The procedure is well described elsewhere (26). Gas insufflation pressure is limited to 10 mmHg. The entire pelvis is examined systematically for tenderness on mechanical stimulation and a pain score is given from 0 to 10. Local anaesthetics can be injected at tender sites and the response recorded. A prospective cohort study showed that overall 74% of patients felt that their symptoms had improved after treatment based on findings at pain mapping (27). Further randomized controlled trials (RCTs) with long-term outcome are required to evaluate the role of laparoscopic pain mapping.

Hysteroscopy

Hysteroscopy has a limited role in the diagnosis of CPP. It permits direct visualization of the uterine cavity and may be useful in establishing the diagnosis of adenomyosis. Hysteroscopic findings of irregular endometrium with endometrial defects, hypervascularization, or strawberry pattern or cystic haemorrhagic lesions have been associated with adenomyosis (28). Hysteroscopy also enables visually guided myometrial biopsy for confirmation of the diagnosis.

Pelvic venography

Pelvic venography is the gold standard diagnostic test for pelvic congestion syndrome. It provides assessment of the anatomy of the pelvic veins and allows measurements of venous diameters, venous functions, and grading of the venous plexuses to be made. A scoring system was devised to grade the severity of pelvic venous congestion; a score of 6 is considered diagnostic for pelvic congestion. This scoring system has a diagnostic sensitivity of 91% and specificity of 89% (29). Dihydroergotamine (DHE), a selective venoconstrictor, has been used previously to cause vasoconstriction of the pelvic vein to reduce pelvic congestion syndrome and has been postulated to have diagnostic and therapeutic value in a previous study. In this study, DHE was given intravenously to 12 women with evidence of pelvic congestion. In six women, after administration of DHE, there was a mean reduction of 35% in the diameter of the pelvic veins and the contrast medium was rapidly cleared, showing a visible reduction of pelvic venous congestion. In another six women, DHE was given during an acute attack of pelvic pain. Pain was significantly lower in post-DHE 4 and 8 hours and 2 and 4 days after treatment than after placebo (30). Unfortunately, DHE has now been withdrawn from the market.

Cystoscopy

Cystoscopy should be considered if the CPP is associated with urological symptoms. It is useful in diagnosing interstitial cystitis, bladder stones, granulomatous inflammation, and urological neoplasms. After cystodistension, the bladder is inspected systematically including the trigone and urethral openings. The degree of hyperaemia, trabeculation, and status of the mucosa are carefully examined. Hunner's ulcers are classic features of interstitial cystitis. They are circular areas of reddened bladder mucosa with small vessels radiating toward a central pale scar. These ulcers may rupture during bladder distension causing haemorrhage. Treatment with fulguration with diathermy or laser, resection, or submucosal injection with steroid can be performed during the time of cystoscopy. However, these ulcers represent the most severe form of interstitial cystitis and may only be found in 5–10% of the patients. Other suspicious ulcers should always be biopsied to rule out malignancy. Glomerulations (petechial haemorrhages in bladder lining) after hydrodistension is no longer considered to be pathognomonic for interstitial cystitis and is of limited diagnostic value (31).

Others investigations

Computed tomography and MRI are occasionally required. It should be considered when ultrasonography is equivocal or not diagnostic. MRI can help delineate soft tissue better and may be useful in cases of suspected adenomyosis. The MRI features of adenomyosis are shown in **Box 44.4** (9). However, MRI is expensive and not suitable

---

Box 44.4 MRI features of adenomyosis

- Globular enlarged uterus with smooth contour
- Asymmetrical myometrial thickening
- Thickening of the junctional zone, with a thickness of at least 12 mm
- Largest junctional zone thickness-to-total myometrium ratio greater than 40–50%
- An ill-defined area of low signal intensity in the myometrium on T2-weighted MRI
- Islands of ectopic endometrial tissue identified as punctate foci of high signal intensity on T1-weighted image

Source data from Dueholm M. Transvaginal ultrasound for diagnosis of adenomyosis: a review. *Best Practice & Research Clinical Obstetrics and Gynaecology* Vol. 20, No. 4, pp. 569–582, 2006.
Levy G, Dehaene A, Laurent N, et al. An update on adenomyosis. *Diagn Interv Imaging* 2013;**94**:3–25.

---

in those patients who have metal implants in the body or those who are claustrophobic. Hormonal tests may sometimes be helpful, for example, the finding of low follicle-stimulating hormone level or high oestradiol level typically found in the premenopausal range is consistent with ovarian remnant syndrome in women who have undergone bilateral oophorectomy. Improvement of pain after injection of local anaesthetics to trigger points or scars may be useful in diagnosing myofascial pain syndrome or nerve entrapment conditions.

Management

The treatment of CPP should be patient orientated and individualized for each patient.

Medical treatment

Non-steroidal anti-inflammatory drugs

Non-steroidal anti-inflammatory drugs (NSAIDs) work by inhibiting cyclooxygenase (COX-1 and COX-2) and impeding the production of prostaglandins and thromboxane, which are involved in the pain pathway. NSAIDs have been proven to be effective in randomized control trials for treatment of primary dysmenorrhea (32). NSAIDs are widely used by many physicians as the first-line treatment for CPP.

Oral contraceptive pills

Combined oral contraceptive pills (OCPs) work by inhibiting ovulation by suppressing the release of gonadotrophins. Many studies have shown that they are effective in the treatment of dysmenorrhea. However, there is limited evidence to suggest that it is effective in treating CPP. So far, there is only one RCT which reported on the efficacy of a low-dose OCP for CPP and endometriosis (33). In this study, a 6-month trial of low-dose OCPs was compared with gonadotrophin-releasing hormone (GnRH) agonists in treating women with laparoscopically proven endometriosis. OCPs were shown to be of similar efficacy in relieving dyspareunia and non-menstrual pain as a GnRH agonist but was less effective in reducing dysmenorrhea.

A prospective observational trial showed that continuous low-dose OCPs were more effective than cyclical low-dose OCPs in controlling endometriosis symptoms in patients after surgical treatment for endometriosis but further studies are required to confirm this finding (34). In general, OCP is the first-line hormonal treatment for women with cyclical CPP, given that the OCP has a low-risk profile, is relatively inexpensive, and is widely available.

Danazol

Danazol is a synthetic androgen which inhibits ovarian steroidogenesis and release of pituitary gonadotrophins. A Cochrane review showed that danazol was more effective than placebo in providing pain relief in patients with laparoscopic-confirmed endometriosis and in patients who had not undergone surgery (35). A daily dose of 400–800 mg is effective in treating CPP but it should be given for a minimum of 3 months. However, patients should be warned about the common hyperandrogenic side effects including hirsutism, acne, weight gain, and deepening of the voice (36).

Progestogens

Progestogens such as medroxyprogesterone acetate (MPA) are useful in those with endometriosis. A previous study showed that MPA depot (150 mg every 3 months) had effects comparable to GnRH agonists in a 12-month trial. Although the benefit was not sustained, MPA in an oral dosage of 50 mg daily was found to be effective in reducing pain scores at the end of the therapy (37). Dienogest (2 mg daily) has also been shown to improve the sexual function and quality of life of patients with endometriosis-related pelvic pain (38).

Mirena, the levonorgestrel-releasing intrauterine system (LNG-IUD), is another commonly used option in treating endometriosis. A Cochrane review in 2013 of three RCTs concluded that there was limited but consistent evidence showing that postoperative LNG-IUD use reduces the recurrence of painful periods in women with endometriosis but further well-designed RCTs are needed to confirm these findings (39).

Gonadotrophin-releasing hormone agonists

GnRH agonists such as goserelin, leuprolide, buserelin, and triptorelin create a hormonal milieu similar to a postmenopausal state by downregulating the pituitary–ovarian axis with subsequent hypo-oestrogenism. It can be administrated as a nasal spray, by injection of a short-acting formulation, or by injection of a depot formulation every 1–3 months. Suppression has been found to be more profound and constant with a monthly depot preparation. Again, most evidence available for GnRH agonists is mostly for endometriosis-related pelvic pain and with comparison to danazol, progestogens, or OCPs. Empirical use of a GnRH agonist was evaluated by a RCT in 100 women with noncyclical pelvic pain and clinically suspected endometriosis. After 12 weeks of therapy with depot leuprolide acetate (3.75 mg/month), significant reductions in dysmenorrhea, pelvic pain, and tenderness were noted in the treatment group. Endometriosis was visualized at subsequent laparoscopy in 78% of the leuprolide-treated and 87% of the placebo group. Even those patients with no visualized endometriosis responded favourably to treatment with a GnRH agonist (32, 40).

A Cochrane review also confirmed that GnRH agonists were more effective than no treatment or placebo in pain relief. There was no difference in pain relief between GnRH agonists and danazol or between GnRH agonist and levonorgestrel. However, there were more adverse effects in the GnRH agonist group when compared with danazol (35). Due to the hypo-oestrogenic state caused by GnRH agonists, side effects including hot flushes, vaginal dryness, decreased libido, mood swings, headaches, and osteoporosis are often reported and may ultimately affect compliance of the treatment.

Add-back therapies with steroidal and non-steroidal agents have been used together with a GnRH agonist to suppress the vasomotor symptoms completely and protect against decreasing bone density without affecting its efficacy in controlling pain relief. Add-back therapy is often considered when prolonged use of GnRH agonists is considered beyond 6 months. A number of RCTs have shown the efficacy of add-back regimens with various GnRH agonists for treatment of endometriosis during 6-month courses. A prospective randomized trial showed that long-term use of a GnRH agonist plus immediate add-back HRT is a safe and acceptable approach to the management of intractable cyclical pelvic pain (41). In this study,

women given Zoladex 10.8 mg over 18 months were randomized to receive HRT (tibolone 2.5 mg) either immediately or after 6 months and they were followed up 12 months after treatment. Bone mineral density at 6 months, the end of treatment (18 months), and 12 months later, pain, and quality of life were measured. Women treated with immediate HRT add-back therapy showed less bone mineral density loss at 6 months and less vasomotor symptoms compared with those who had delayed HRT add-back treatment. Long-term follow-up showed that both groups experienced the same bone mineral density loss. Pain and quality of life also showed improvement in both groups and there was evidence of return to baseline levels after ending treatment.

Others

The role of antibiotics is of limited clinical value and they should not be used unless there is good evidence of infection. Antidepressants such as tricyclic antidepressants have been shown to be useful in women with CPP with negative laparoscopy as in the case of other chronic pain syndromes.

Surgery

Adhesions

The role of adhesiolysis in women with CPP associated with adhesions remains controversial. An earlier RCT conducted by Peters et al. suggested adhesiolysis was of benefit (42) while a subsequent RCT by Swank et al. found laparoscopic adhesiolysis was no better than diagnostic laparoscopy (43). In a recently published double-blinded RCT, which was unfortunately was stopped before a statistically powered sample size was reached, Cheong et al. reported that adhesiolysis performed in women with CPP appeared beneficial in terms of improvement of pain and quality of life (7). Overall, current data suggests that women with CPP and adhesions should be offered surgery to remove the adhesions.

Endometriosis

A Cochrane meta-analysis showed that the improvement of pain after laparoscopic treatment of endometriosis was significantly better in those who only underwent diagnostic laparoscopy. Pain relief was significantly higher in patients with moderate and mild endometriosis than those in minimal diseases (44).

Medical treatment of the endometriomas may lead to a temporary reduction in size of the cysts but not complete resolution and thus surgery is the definitive treatment for large symptomatic endometriomas. Laparoscopic ovarian cystectomy with the stripping method has been shown to be more effective than fenestration and ablation alone. Laparoscopic ovarian cystectomy with the stripping method was also shown to be associated with greater improvement in dysmenorrhea, deep dyspareunia, and non-menstrual pain. However, the procedure is associated with a significant risk of damaging the ovarian reserve (45). In women who wish to preserve their fertility, haemostasis with the use of FloSeal, a gelatin haemostatic matrix, rather than haemostasis with the use diathermy should be considered (46).

Pain transmission

The Lee–Frankenhauser sensory nerve plexuses and parasympathetic ganglia in the uterosacral ligaments carry pain from the uterus

(47). It is believed that laparoscopic uterosacral nerve ablation (LUNA) can reduce uterine pain by disrupting the efferent nerve fibres in the uterosacral ligament. Daniels et al. performed an individual patient data meta-analysis of randomized trials to assess the effectiveness of LUNA in treating CPP (48). Raw data were available from 862 women in 5 randomized trials. Pain scores were calibrated to a 10-point scale and were analysed using a multilevel model allowing for repeated measures. They found no significant difference in outcome between those who had and those who had not undergone the LUNA procedure. It seems that current evidence does not support the use of the LUNA procedure in women with CPP. However, the international LUNA IPD Meta-analysis Collaborative Group is collecting further raw individual patient data from randomized trials to reassess its effectiveness (47).

Presacral neurectomy (PSN) disrupts the sympathetic pathways from the uterus. Comparison between LUNA and laparoscopic PSN for primary dysmenorrhea showed no difference in pain relief in the short term. However, long-term laparoscopic PSN was shown to be significantly more effective than LUNA. PSN combined with endometriosis treatment appeared to produce better pain relief than endometriosis treatment alone, although data suggested that this may be specific to laparoscopy and for midline abdominal pain only. In addition, the procedure is not without risks, including haemorrhage from accidental laceration of the middle sacral vein, visceral injury, and disturbance of bladder and bowel function. PSN should not be recommended outside the context of a clinical trial (49).

Hysterectomy and oophorectomy

Hysterectomy with or without oophorectomy is sometimes considered in women who have completed childbearing and who experience debilitating painful symptoms. Hysterectomy without oophorectomy is usually less effective, with higher recurrence and subsequent reoperation rates, than hysterectomy and oophorectomy. However, the implications of oophorectomy need to be fully discussed with the patient and the decision should take into consideration the consequences of surgical menopause. A trial of a GnRH agonist may be considered before a final decision is made. Women who respond to GnRH agonist therapy are more likely to benefit from hysterectomy and oophorectomy.

Others

Pelvic venous congestion

MPA at a dose of 50 mg per day has been shown to produce significant pain relief during 4 months of treatment with 73% of the women reporting at least 50% benefits. The pain reduction was better if MPA treatment was given along with psychotherapy, which also produced longer-lasting benefit (50). In case medical treatment has failed, surgical treatment with ligation, embolization, or sclerotherapy of the pelvic vessels may be considered.

Psychological

Relaxation therapies, behavioural modification, and cognitive behavioural therapies sometimes improve a patient's perception of pain, coping ability, and promote overall wellness, improving a patient's response to pain management. However, a recent systemic analysis failed to confirm the beneficial role of psychological interventions on self-reported pain scores among women with CPP (51).

Alternative treatment options

When medical or surgical treatment fails, women often seek complementary or alternative treatment options, which may include a wide range of treatment methods such as acupuncture, herbal medicine, hypnotherapy, physiotherapy, osteopathy, or chiropractic.

Chinese herbal medication and acupuncture is popular in the Chinese and Asian populations but there is no evidence to confirm that it is effective.

Chinese herbal medication includes the use of an herbal formula containing several different herbs, consumed in the form of herbal soups, powder, or pills. A Cochrane review showed it had comparable benefits to antiprogestogen gestrine as a postoperative adjuvant therapy after surgery for endometriosis but was associated with less adverse effects. The use of herbal medication was also found to produce significantly greater reduction in dysmenorrhea compared with danazol (52).

Acupuncture involves the insertion of fine needles to specific defined (needle) points over the body surface. The exact mechanism of how it may work is still unknown, although it is likely to act by altering the processing of pain in the brain and spinal cord, promoting release of vascular or immune modulatory factors, releasing adenosine, which help reduce sensitivity to painful stimuli and improve microcirculation, leading to reduction in muscle stiffness and tension. There is preliminary evidence that acupuncture is effective in reducing severity of dysmenorrhea when compared to an untreated group (53). Two small trials included in a Cochrane review suggested that acupuncture was superior to standard NSAIDs in the reduction of menstrual symptoms (54).

However, due to a lack of good-quality clinical trials involving these various complementary alternative medicine treatments, it is not possible to make recommendations other than to consider these treatment options as empirical measures.

Multidisciplinary approach

In women with persistent, unexplained CPP refractory to conventional therapy, a multidisciplinary team approach should be adopted. There is good evidence of benefit in integrating psychological interventions into management of chronic pain syndromes. A multidisciplinary team approach has been shown to be more effective than a single treatment modality for CPP (55, 56). The team, which may be formed ad hoc, may involve a gynaecologist, a surgeon, a radiologist, an anaesthetist, a psychologist, a physiotherapist, and a specialist nurse. In this way, it will hasten the treatment process, improve the patient's confidence, compliance, and in some cases, acceptance at the end that there may not be any miraculous cure for the condition.

Conclusion

The management of CPP may be straightforward in many cases but in a significant proportion of cases the underlying cause remains elusive and the pain continues to be debilitating despite conventional treatments. In this situation, a multidisciplinary approach is necessary to help manage this challenging condition. Developing a good doctor–patient relationship is the cornerstone to successful treatment.

REFERENCES

1. Siedentopf F, Weijenborg P, Engman M, et al. ISPOG European Consensus Statement—chronic pelvic pain in women (short version). *J Psychosom Obstet Gynaecol* 2015;**36**:161–70.

2. Royal College of Obstetricians and Gynaecologists (RCOG). *The Initial Management of Chronic Pelvic Pain.* Green-top Guideline No. 41. London: RCOG; 2012.

3. Garry R. Diagnosis of endometriosis and pelvic pain. *Fertil Steril* 2006;**86**:1307–309.

4. Howard FM. The role of laparoscopy as a diagnostic tool in chronic pelvic pain. *Baillieres Best Pract Res Clin Obstet Gynaecol* 2000;**14**:467–94.

5. Howard FM, El-Minawi AM, Sanchez RA. Conscious pain mapping by laparoscopy in women with chronic pelvic pain. *Obstet Gynecol* 2000;**96**:934–39.

6. Paterson N, Jarrell J. Pelvic infections and chronic pelvic pain. In: Vercellini P (ed), *Chronic Pelvic Pain*, pp. 50–64. Chichester: Wiley; 2011.

7. Cheong YC, Reading I, Bailey S, Sadek K, Ledger W, Li TC. Should women with chronic pelvic pain have adhesiolysis? *BMC Womens Health* 2014;**14**:36.

8. Cheong Y, William Stones R. Chronic pelvic pain: aetiology and therapy. *Best Pract Res Clin Obstet Gynaecol* 2006;**20**:695–711.

9. Dueholm M. Transvaginal ultrasound for diagnosis of adenomyosis: a review. *Best Pract Res Clin Obstet Gynaecol* 2006;**20**:569–82.

10. Borghi C, Dell'Atti L. Pelvic congestion syndrome: the current state of the literature. *Arch Gynecol Obstet* 2016;**293**:291–301.

11. Howard FM. The differential diagnosis of chronic pelvic pain. In: Vercellini P (ed), *Chronic Pelvic Pain*, pp. 7–28. Chichester: Wiley; 2011.

12. Abu-Rafeh B, Vilos GA, Misra M. Frequency and laparoscopic management of ovarian remnant syndrome. *J Am Assoc Gynecol Laparosc* 2003;**10**:33–37.

13. Abrams P, Cardozo L, Fall M, et al. The standardisation of terminology of lower urinary tract function: report from the Standardisation Sub-committee of the International Continence Society. *Neurourol Urodyn* 2002;**21**:167–78.

14. Baker PK. Musculoskeletal problems. In: Steege J, Metzger DA, Levy BS (eds), *Chronic Pelvic Pain: An Integrated Approach*, Vol. **24**, pp. 215–40. Philadelphia, PA: Saunders Company; 1998.

15. Jarrell JF, Vilos GA, Allaire C, et al. Consensus guidelines for the management of chronic pelvic pain. *J Obstet Gynaecol Can* 2005;**27**:781–826.

16. Jarrell JF, Vilos GA, Allaire C, et al. Consensus guidelines for the management of chronic pelvic pain. *J Obstet Gynaecol Can* 2005;**27**:869–910.

17. Lampe A, Doering S, Rumpold G, et al. Chronic pain syndromes and their relation to childhood abuse and stressful life events. *J Psychosom Res* 2003;**54**:361–67.

18. Melzack R. The McGill Pain Questionnaire: major properties and scoring methods. *Pain* 1975;**1**:277–99.

19. Melzack R. The short-form McGill Pain Questionnaire. *Pain* 1987;**30**:191–97.

20. Jenkinson C, Layte R, Wright L, Coulter A. *Manual and Interpretation Guide for the UK SF-36.* Oxford: Health Services Research Unit; 1996.

21. Levy G, Dehaene A, Laurent N, et al. An update on adenomyosis. *Diagn Interv Imaging* 2013;**94**:3–25.

22. Guerriero S, Ajossa S, Gerada M, D'Aquila M, Piras B, Melis GB. 'Tenderness-guided' transvaginal ultrasonography: a new method for the detection of deep endometriosis in patients with chronic pelvic pain. *Fertil Steril* 2007;**88**:1293–97.

23. Menakaya U, Reid S, Lu C, Gerges B, Infante F, Condous G. Performance of an Ultrasound Based Endometriosis Staging System (UBESS) for predicting the level of complexity of laparoscopic surgery for endometriosis. *Ultrasound Obstet Gynecol* 2016;**48**:786–95.

24. Baker PN, Symonds EM. The resolution of chronic pelvic pain after normal laparoscopy findings. *Am J Obstet Gynecol* 1992;**166**:835–36.

25. Ahmad G, O'Flynn H, Duffy JM, Phillips K, Watson A. Laparoscopic entry techniques. *Cochrane Database Syst Rev* 2012;**2**:CD006583.

26. Yunker A, Steege J. Practical guide to laparoscopic pain mapping. *J Minim Invasive Gynecol* 2010;**17**:8–11.

27. Swanton A, Iyer L, Reginald PW. Diagnosis, treatment and follow up of women undergoing conscious pain mapping for chronic pelvic pain: a prospective cohort study. *BJOG* 2006;**113**:792–96.

28. Di Spiezio Sardo A, Guida M, Bettocchi S, et al. Role of hysteroscopy in evaluating chronic pelvic pain. *Fertil Steril* 2008;**90**:1191–96.

29. Stones RW, Rae T, Rogers V, Fry R, Beard RW. Pelvic congestion in women: evaluation with transvaginal ultrasound and observation of venous pharmacology. *Br J Radiol* 1990;**63**:710–11.

30. Reginald PW, Beard RW, Kooner JS, et al. Intravenous dihydroergotamine to relieve pelvic congestion with pain in young women. *Lancet* 1987;**2**:351–53.

31. Wittmann D, Clemens JQ. Bladder pain syndrome and other urological causes of chronic pelvic pain. In: Vercellini P (ed), *Chronic Pelvic Pain*, pp. 86–97. Chichester: Wiley; 2011.

32. Gambone JC, Mittman BS, Munro MG, Scialli AR, Winkel CA, Chronic Pelvic Pain/Endometriosis Working Group. Consensus statement for the management of chronic pelvic pain and endometriosis: proceedings of an expert-panel consensus process. *Fertil Steril* 2002;**78**:961–72.

33. Vercellini P, Trespidi L, Colombo A, Vendola N, Marchini M, Crosignani PG. A gonadotropin-releasing hormone agonist versus a low-dose oral contraceptive for pelvic pain associated with endometriosis. *Fertil Steril* 1993;**60**:75–79.

34. Vercellini P, Frontino G, De Giorgi O, Pietropaolo G, Pasin R, Crosignani PG. Continuous use of an oral contraceptive for endometriosis-associated recurrent dysmenorrhea that does not respond to a cyclic pill regimen. *Fertil Steril* 2003;**80**:560–63.

35. Brown J, Pan A, Hart RJ. Gonadotrophin-releasing hormone analogues for pain associated with endometriosis. *Cochrane Database Syst Rev* 2010;**12**:CD008475.

36. Selak V, Farquhar C, Prentice A, Singla A. Danazol for pelvic pain associated with endometriosis. *Cochrane Database Syst Rev* 2007;**4**:CD000068.

37. Stones RW, Mountfield J. Interventions for treating chronic pelvic pain in women. *Cochrane Database Syst Rev* 2000;**4**:CD000387.

38. Caruso S, Iraci M, Cianci S, Casella E, Fava V, Cianci A. Quality of life and sexual function of women affected by endometriosis-associated pelvic pain when treated with dienogest. *J Endocrinol Invest* 2015;**38**:1211–18.

39. Abou-Setta AM, Houston B, Al-Inany HG, Farquhar C. Levonorgestrel-releasing intrauterine device (LNG-IUD) for symptomatic endometriosis following surgery. *Cochrane Database Syst Rev* 2013;**1**:CD005072.

40. Ling FW. Randomized controlled trial of depot leuprolide in patients with CPP and clinically suspected endometriosis. Pelvic Pain Study Group. *Obstet Gynecol.* 1999;**93**:51–58.

41. Al-Azemi M, Jones G, Sirkeci F, Walters S, Houdmont M, Ledger W. Immediate and delayed add-back hormonal replacement

therapy during ultra-long GnRH agonist treatment of chronic cyclical pelvic pain. *BJOG* 2009;**116**:1646–56.

42. Peters AA, Trimbos-Kemper GC, Admiraal C, Trimbos JB, Hermans J. A randomized clinical trial on the benefit of adhesiolysis in patients with intraperitoneal adhesions and chronic pelvic pain. *Br J Obstet Gynaecol* 1992;**99**:59–62.

43. Swank DJ, Swank-Bordewijk SC, Hop WC, et al. Laparoscopic adhesiolysis in patients with chronic abdominal pain: a blinded randomised controlled multi-centre trial. *Lancet* 2003;**361**:1247–51.

44. Jacobson TZ, Duffy JM, Barlow D, Koninckx PR, Garry R. Laparoscopic surgery for pelvic pain associated with endometriosis. *Cochrane Database Syst Rev* 2009;7:CD001300.

45. Jones KD, Sutton CJ. Laparoscopic management of ovarian endometriomas: a critical review of current practice. *Curr Opin Obstet Gynecol* 2000;**12**:309–15.

46. Ebert AD, Hollauer A, Fuhr N, Langolf O, Papadopoulos T. Laparoscopic ovarian cystectomy without bipolar coagulation or sutures using a gelantine-thrombin matrix sealant (FloSeal): first support of a promising technique. *Arch Gynecol Obstet* 2009;**280**:161–65.

47. Xiong T, Daniels J, Middleton L, et al. Meta-analysis using individual patient data from randomised trials to assess the effectiveness of laparoscopic uterosacral nerve ablation in the treatment of CPP: a proposed protocol. *BJOG* 2007;**114**:1580.e1–7.

48. Daniels JP, Middleton L, Xiong T, et al. Individual patient data meta-analysis of randomized evidence to assess the effectiveness of laparoscopic uterosacral nerve ablation in CPP. *Hum Reprod Update* 2010;**16**:568–76.

49. Practice Committee of the American Society for Reproductive Medicine. Treatment of pelvic pain associated with endometriosis: a committee opinion. *Fertil Steril* 2014;**101**:927–35.

50. Farquhar CM, Rogers V, Franks S, Pearce S, Wadsworth J, Beard RW. A randomized controlled trial of medroxyprogesterone acetate and psychotherapy for the treatment of pelvic congestion. *Br J Obstet Gynaecol* 1989;**96**:1153–62.

51. Champaneria R, Daniels JP, Raza A, Pattison HM, Khan KS. Psychological therapies for chronic pelvic pain: systematic review of randomized controlled trials. *Acta Obstet Gynecol Scand* 2012;**91**:281–86

52. Flower A, Liu JP, Lewith G, Little P, Li Q. Chinese herbal medicine for endometriosis. *Cochrane Database Syst Rev* 2012;5:CD006568.

53. Zhu X, Hamilton KD, McNicol ED. Acupuncture for pain in endometriosis. *Cochrane Database Syst Rev* 2011;9:CD007864.

54. Smith CA, Zhu X, He L, Song J. Acupuncture for primary dysmenorrhoea. *Cochrane Database Syst Rev* 2011;1:CD007854.

55. Miller-Matero LR, Saulino C, Clark S, Bugenski M, Eshelman A, Eisenstein D. When treating the pain is not enough: a multidisciplinary approach for chronic pelvic pain. *Arch Womens Ment Health* 2016;**19**:349–54.

56. Twiddy H, Lane N, Chawla R, et al. The development and delivery of a female chronic pelvic pain management programme: a specialised interdisciplinary approach. *Br J Pain* 2015;**9**:233–40.

45

Endometriosis

Arne Vanhie and Thomas D'Hooghe

Introduction

Endometriosis is defined as the presence of endometrial-like tissue outside the uterus, with the most frequent sites of implantation being the pelvic viscera and the peritoneum (1). Although endometriosis is a benign oestrogen-dependent disease, its management is often frustrating due to limited medical treatment options, complex surgical treatment, and high recurrence rates after both surgical and medical treatment (1). While some women with endometriosis experience painful symptoms and/or infertility, others have no symptoms at all (2). In this chapter we will first discuss the prevalence, risk factors, and genetic predisposition for endometriosis, then focus on the pathogenesis and clinical phenotypes of the disease, followed by sections on the diagnosis and staging of the disease, and finally the medical and surgical treatment.

Prevalence and risk factors

Endometriosis is one of the most common benign gynaecological disorders but the exact prevalence is difficult to determine because of the need for a surgical procedure to diagnose the disease (3). Endometriosis is found predominantly in women of reproductive age but has been reported in young adolescents and in postmenopausal women receiving hormonal replacement therapy (3). Estimates of the prevalence of endometriosis among women of reproductive age vary between 2% and 10%, but this prevalence can rise to 30–50% in women with infertility and/or pain (4, 5). The World Endometriosis Research Foundation EndoCost study has shown that the healthcare costs of endometriosis are similar to the costs for diabetes mellitus, Crohn's disease, and rheumatoid arthritis (4). Apart from the economic burden, endometriosis has a significant effect on various aspects of women's lives, including their social and sexual relationships, work, and study (2).

Various factors such as genetic profile, inflammation, menstrual cyclicity, and immunological factors have been suggested to play a role in the pathophysiology of endometriosis (6). From epidemiological studies, nulliparity and short, heavy menstrual cycles are the most consistently reported risk factors (3). An overview of risk factors for endometriosis is presented is **Table 45.1**.

Genetic predisposition

Consistent evidence exists that a family history of endometriosis is more common in women with endometriosis and that the risk of endometriosis is higher in women whose mother or sisters have the disease (3, 7). Twin studies have demonstrated a higher concordance of endometriosis in monozygotic versus dizygotic twins with the proportion of disease variance due to genetic factors estimated at around 52% (9). Studies in rhesus monkeys allowed construction of a detailed multigenerational pedigree with a significantly higher kinship coefficient for affected animals and higher risk for endometriosis in full siblings, underlining the familial aggregation of endometriosis (10).

Meta-analysis of eight genome-wide association studies in patients with endometriosis has shown evidence of a robust association of endometriosis with six risk loci: rs12700667 on 7p15.2, rs7521902 near *WNT4* (wingless-type MMYV integration family member 4), rs10859871 near *VEZT* (vezatin), rs1537377 near *CDKN2B-AS1* (cyclin-dependent kinase inhibitor 2b antisense RNA), rs7739264 near *ID4* (inhibitor of DNA binding 4), and rs13394619 in *GREB1* (growth regulation by oestrogen in breast cancer 1) (11). The 7p15.2 region contains several potential candidate genes such as *NFE2L3* (nuclear factor erythroid derived 2-like 3), *MIR148A* (microRNA 148a), *HOXA10* (homeobox A10), and *HOXA11* (homeobox A11) (11). NFE2L3 protein is a transcription factor suggested to be involved in cell differentiation, inflammation, and carcinogenesis (11). MicroRNA 148a possibly plays a role in the Wnt/β-catenin signalling pathway which has an important role in communication between epithelial and stromal cells in endometrium, fibrogenesis, and sex hormone homeostasis regulation (11). HOXA10 and HOXA11 are members of the homeobox A family of transcription factors that play a role in uterine development (11). *WNT4* encodes a member of the wingless-type MMTV integration site family, which is important for the development of the female reproductive tract and for steroidogenesis (12). *VEZT* encodes an adherens junction transmembrane protein, a putative tumour suppressor gene targeting cell migration and invasion genes, growth genes, cellular adhesion genes, and a functionally validated cell cycle progression gene called *TCF19* (transcription factor 19) (11). CDKN2B-AS1 has been shown to be involved in the regulation of p15, p16-INK4a, and p14ARF

Table 45.1 Risk factors for endometriosis

Risk factor		Description of association	Strength of association
Socioeconomic status		Higher socioeconomic status increases risk	Limited
Family history		Relatives with endometriosis increase risk for endometriosis	Consistent
Constitutional factors			
	Age at menarche	Early age increases risk	Consistent
	Cycle length	Shorter cycle increases risk	Consistent
	Menstrual flow	Longer flow increases risk	Limited
	Dysmenorrhea	Strong predictor	Consistent
	Parity	Higher parity decreases risk	Consistent
	Weight and BMI	Lower BMI increases risk	Limited
	Height	Taller height increases risk	Limited
Lifestyle factors			
	Physical activity	Regular physical activity decreases risk	Limited
	Diet	Possible protective effect of vegetables and fruits. Possible unfavourable effect of red meat, dairy products and unsaturated fats	Limited
	Smoking	No evidence for association	Limited
	Alcohol	Use of alcohol increases risk	Limited
	Caffeine	No evidence for association	Limited
Contraception		Protective effect of combined oral contraceptives	Limited
Environmental factors			
	PCB exposure	Exposure to PCB increases risk	Limited
	Dioxin exposure	Exposure to dioxins increases risk	Limited
Comorbidities			
	GI disease	Possibly increase risk	Limited
	Immunological diseases	Possibly increase risk	Limited
	Cardiovascular diseases	Possibly increase risk	Limited

BMI, body mass index; GI, gastrointestinal; PCB, polychlorinated biphenyl.

Source data from Missmer SA, Cramer DW. *Obstet Gynecol Clin North Am* 2003;30:1–19; Vigano et al. *Best Pract Res Clin Obstet Gynaecol* 2004;18:177–200; Parazzini et al. *Eur J Obstet Gynecol Reprod Biol* 2017;209:3–7.

expression which are all recognized tumour suppressor proteins (12). Rs7739264 is located in an intronic region of lncRNA RP1–167F1.2 (794 bp), of which the biological function remains to be discovered. It is located 52 kb downstream of *ID4*, an ovarian oncogene that is overexpressed in most primary ovarian cancers (11). *GREB1* encodes an early-response gene in the oestrogen receptor-regulated pathway that is involved in hormone-dependent breast cancer (12).

Large genome-wide linkage studies, including more than 1300 families, have identified three linkage regions of endometriosis: on chromosome 10q26, chromosome 20p13, and chromosome 7p13–15 (13). The linkage region on chromosome 10q26 has been studied in more detail and identified a possible role for the *CYP2C19* gene, which is involved in drug and oestrogen metabolism (13). Three candidate genes for the linkage region on chromosome 7p13–15 have been suggested: *INHBA, SFRP4,* and *HOXA10,* which play roles in endometrial development (13). Functional studies and sequencing of the genes in these linkage regions are needed to elucidate their precise role and determine the effects of the variants in underlying pathways (13).

Pathogenesis

The exact pathogenesis and pathophysiology of endometriosis are still not completely elucidated. Theories regarding the pathogenesis of endometriosis can generally be categorized as those proposing that implants originate from uterine endometrium by retrograde menstruation, lymphatic/haematogenous dissemination, or endometrial stem cell implantation and those proposing that implants arise from tissues other than the uterus by coelomic metaplasia or Mullerian remnant abnormalities (14).

The most widely accepted theory on the pathogenesis of endometriosis, proposed by Sampson in the 1920s, is that the disorder originates from retrograde sloughing of endometrial tissue through patent fallopian tubes into the peritoneal cavity (15). This theory is supported by the observation of higher prevalence of endometriosis in patients with obstructed or compromised outflow tracts (14). Furthermore, it has been established that intraperitoneal injection of menstrual blood or iatrogenic obstruction of the outflow tract in a nonhuman primate model results in endometriotic lesions within the peritoneal cavity (16, 17). Nevertheless, it is important to take into account that retrograde menstruation is observed in up to 90% of women and only 2–10% of women have endometriosis, suggesting that additional mechanisms are necessary for the development of endometriotic implants (14).

According to substantial evidence, the endometrium of women with endometriosis is abnormal due to a complex interplay of genetic, environmental, and immunological factors, resulting in the development of endometriotic lesions when retrograde menstruation occurs (15). Indeed, eutopic endometrium from women with endometriosis shares certain alterations with ectopic lesions that are not observed in the endometrium from healthy women (14). Studies comparing gene and protein expression in eutopic endometrium show differences in several pathways resulting in decreased apoptosis and increased cell proliferation in patients with endometriosis (14). Enhanced peritoneal survival of endometrial cells in patients with endometriosis could be an important factor in explaining the higher tendency for implantation in the peritoneal cavity (14). Furthermore, gene expression profiling of the peritoneum has demonstrated cyclic upregulation of several cytokines and proteins (matrix metalloproteinase, intracellular adhesion molecule 1, transforming growth factor-beta, interleukin-1-beta, interleukin-6, RANTES, and vascular cell adhesion molecule-1) in patients with endometriosis (18, 19). The differential expression of these cytokines and growth factors may create a microenvironment that encourages implantation of endometrial cells or protects them from immune-mediated clearance (18, 19).

Normally, refluxed endometrial tissue is cleared from the peritoneum by the immune system and the dysregulation of this clearance mechanism has been implicated in the predisposition to implantation and growth of endometrial cells (15). The eutopic endometrium from women with endometriosis was found to be more resistant to lysis by natural killer cells than the eutopic endometrium from women without disease (20–22). Compromised macrophage function in women with endometriosis may further contribute to decreased clearance of lesions (23). Further support for a fundamentally altered immune system in the predisposition to endometriosis is derived from studies demonstrating a high concordance of autoimmune (systemic lupus erythematosus, rheumatoid arthritis, Sjögren syndrome, and autoimmune thyroid disease) and atopic disease (allergies, asthma, and eczema) in affected women (14).

The alterations in the immune system, endometrium, and peritoneum resulting in decreased immunological clearance of refluxed endometrial tissue, increased cell survival, and higher chances of implantation in the peritoneum are important mechanisms to explain the initial development of endometriotic implants (14). Subsequent survival and growth of these implants is dependent on angiogenesis and an altered hormonal environment (24). Endometriotic implants require neovascularization to guarantee oxygen and essential nutrient supply (24). Correspondingly, a typical clinical feature of endometriotic lesions is their dense vascularization (24). Oestrogens are important for the growth of eutopic and ectopic endometrium. Oestradiol promotes growth of ectopic tissue and is produced by the known steroidogenic organs and locally by the endometriotic implants (12). The ectopic tissue has been consistently shown to express different levels of oestrogen receptor (ER)-α and ERβ than eutopic tissue, with ERβ present in markedly higher levels in ectopic tissue

(12). The pathological overexpression of ERβ in endometriosis diminishes induction of the progesterone receptor in endometriotic cells, resulting in progesterone resistance of the ectopic endometrium (12). Furthermore, inflammation secondary to endometriosis can induce progesterone resistance by altering the progesterone signalling pathway though mechanisms of competition or interference with proinflammatory transcriptional factors (12).

Inflammation is another typical feature of endometriosis, as the presence of ectopic tissue in the peritoneal cavity is associated with overproduction of prostaglandins, cytokines, and chemokines (16). Macrophages infiltrating the ectopic lesions express typical markers of alternative activation, favouring the growth of the lesions and promoting their angiogenesis (12). Macrophages in the peritoneal cavity of affected women are known to accumulate iron, probably as a result of excessive pelvic blood collection (12). Non-protein-bound catalytic iron increases the generation of reactive oxygen species, which in turn favours the progression of endometriosis via peritoneal damage, exposure of submesothelial connective tissue, angiogenesis, and enhanced endometrial cell proliferation (12).

In summary, available evidence suggests that endometriosis originates from retrograde menstruation of endometrial tissue (15) (**Figure 45.1**). Intrinsic alterations in the immune system, endometrium, and peritoneum of patients with endometriosis result in implantation of this endometrial tissue on the peritoneal surface. Local changes in steroid production and angiogenesis support further growth of the lesions. This elicits an inflammatory response accompanied by development of adhesions, fibrosis, scarring, neuronal infiltration, and anatomical distortion, resulting in pain and infertility (15).

Phenotypes and staging of endometriosis

Phenotypes

Endometriosis can present as three different phenotypes: superficial endometriosis, deep endometriosis, and ovarian cystic endometriosis. Superficial or peritoneal endometriosis comprises superficial lesions scattered over the peritoneal, serosal, and ovarian surfaces. Superficial endometriotic lesions or often divided in 'typical' black-brown lesions and 'atypical' or 'subtle' lesions including red implants and clear vesicles (**Figures 45.2 and 45.3**). Ovarian cystic endometriosis refers to an endometrioma or ovarian cyst containing dark-stained blood (chocolate fluid) and lined by a pseudocyst wall covered by ectopic endometrium (**Figures 45.4 and 45.5**). Deep endometriosis, defined as endometriosis infiltrating more than 5 mm beneath the peritoneal surface, is a multifocal pathology that may infiltrate different organs (**Figures 45.6 and 45.7**). The most commonly affected sites are the intestine, vagina, uterosacral ligaments, bladder, and ureter but deep endometriosis is also occasionally observed in remote organs such as lymph nodes, umbilicus, and lungs (25). In women with deep endometriosis, intestinal and urinary tract involvement are estimated to occur in 3.8–37% and in 1–2%, respectively (26, 27).

Deep endometriosis in the bowel is defined as 'bowel endometriosis' only if the muscularis layer is affected (26). Lesions with dense adhesions and/or endometriotic infiltration up to the bowel serosa are not considered bowel endometriosis, because these

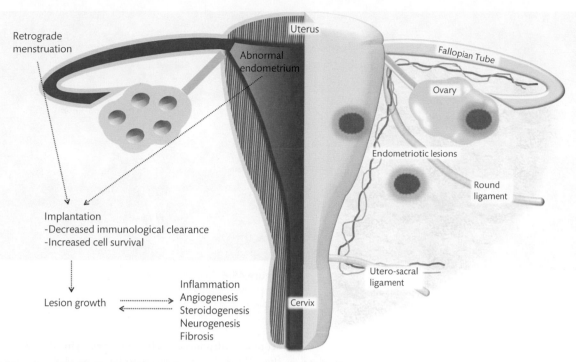

Figure 45.1 Overview of the pathogenesis of endometriosis. Courtesy of Dr Arne Vanhie

lesions are usually less than 5 mm in depth (28). The rectum and rectosigmoid junction together account for 70–93% of all intestinal endometriotic sites (26). In addition to the rectosigmoid junction, the most common intestinal sites are the appendix (2–18%), the distal ileum (2–16%), and the cecum (<2%) (26). Within the urinary system, the bladder is the most commonly affected site (29). A bladder nodule does not represent a risk factor for additional urological lesions. However, different locations of urinary tract endometriosis may coexist, especially bladder and ureters (29). Bladder endometriosis is often described as primary (spontaneously occurring disease) or secondary (iatrogenic lesion,

occurring after pelvic surgery, such as caesarean delivery, hysterectomy, etc.) (29). Ureteral endometriosis is usually confined to the distal third of the ureter but proximal ureteral implants have been described (30). There is a left-sided predominance and bilateral disease has been reported in up to 20–25% of the cases (27). Ureteral endometriosis is often described as intrinsic (lesions infiltrate the muscularis of the ureteral wall) or extrinsic (lesions are responsible for a significant ureteral obstruction but without involvement of the ureteral muscularis) (31). Extrinsic disease is more common than intrinsic disease, but patients with intrinsic disease are more often symptomatic (27).

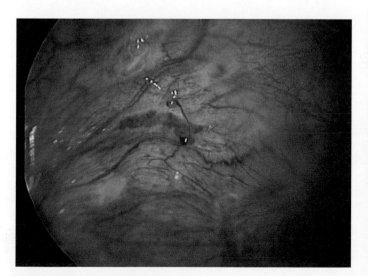

Figure 45.2 Typical black lesion.
Courtesy of Prof Dr Christel Meuleman.

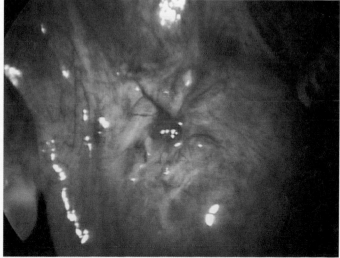

Figure 45.3 Atypical red polypoid lesion.
Courtesy of Prof Dr Christel Meuleman.

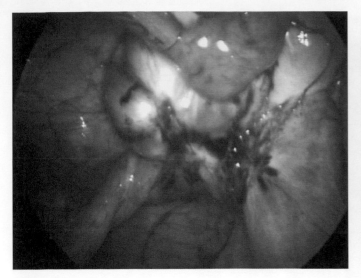

Figure 45.4 Endometrioma.
Courtesy of Prof Dr Christel Meuleman.

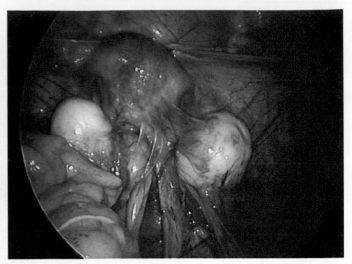

Figure 45.6 Deep endometriotic nodule causing severe distortion of the pelvic anatomy.
Courtesy of Prof Dr Christel Meuleman.

Staging and classification of endometriosis

Endometriosis is a complex disease and there is no 'perfect' staging system available at present. By far the most commonly used and best known staging system is the revised American Society for Reproductive Medicine (rASRM) classification (**Figure 45.8**) (32). This classification system assigns points to the different locations of the disease thus resulting in four stages: minimal, mild, moderate, and severe (32). Major limitations of the rASRM classification are the limited reproducibility and poor correlation with pelvic pain and infertility (33). The Endometriosis Fertility Index (EFI) (**Figure 45.9**) has been shown to predict non-*in vitro* fertilization (IVF) pregnancy rates for patients following surgical staging and treatment of endometriosis, and has been externally validated (34, 35). However, both rASRM and EFI staging systems fail to classify deep endometriosis. In order to supplement the rASRM classification with regard to the description of deep endometriosis, the ENZIAN score was introduced in 2003 and revised in 2011 (36, 37). Although the ENZIAN score appears to be an excellent complement to the rASRM score for morphological description of deep endometriosis and planning of surgery, it is not validated and has rarely been used outside German-speaking European countries.

Diagnosis

The gold standard for the diagnosis of endometriosis remains direct visualization during laparoscopy with histological confirmation of the presence of endometrial glands and/or stroma (2, 38). However, transvaginal ultrasound (TVUS) and magnetic resonance imaging (MRI) can reliably detect deep endometriosis and ovarian endometriomas (39). Barium enema radiography and intravenous pyelography may be necessary to assess ureteric, bladder, and bowel

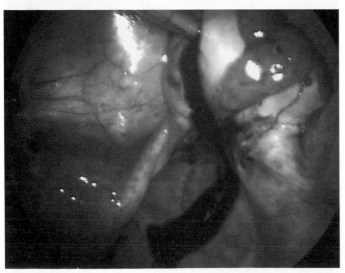

Figure 45.5 Ruptured endometrioma with spilling of 'chocolate fluid'.
Courtesy of Prof Dr Christel Meuleman.

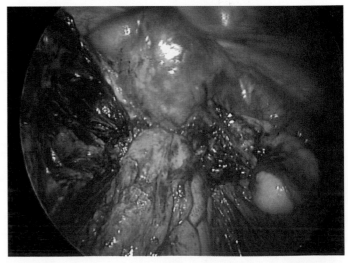

Figure 45.7 Deep endometriotic nodule between the uterus and sigmoid.
Courtesy of Prof Dr Christel Meuleman.

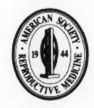

AMERICAN SOCIETY FOR REPRODUCTIVE MEDICINE
REVISED CLASSIFICATION OF ENDOMETRIOSIS

Patient's Name _____   Date _____

Stage I (Minimal) - 1–5
Stage I (Mild) - 6–15   Laparoscopy _____ Laparotomy _____ Photography _____
Stage III (Moderate) - 16–40   Recommended Treatment _____
Stage IV (Severe) - >40

Total _____   Prognosis _____

			<1cm	1.3cm	> 3cm
PERITONEUM	ENDOMETRIOSIS		<1cm	1.3cm	> 3cm
	Superficial		1	2	4
	Deep		2	4	6
OVARY	R	Superficial	1	2	4
		Deep	4	16	20
	L	Superficial	1	2	4
		Deep	4	16	20

	POSTERIOR CULDESAC OBLITERATION	Partial	Complete
		4	40

			< 1/3 Enclosure	1/3–2/3 Enclosure	> 2/3 Enclosure
OVARY	ADHESIONS		< 1/3 Enclosure	1/3–2/3 Enclosure	> 2/3 Enclosure
	R	Filmy	1	2	4
		Dense	4	8	16
	L	Filmy	1	2	4
		Dense	4	8	16
TUBE	R	Filmy	1	2	4
		Dense	4°	8°	16
	L	Filmy	1	2	4
		Dense	4°	8°	16

°If the fimbriated end of the fallopian tube is completely enclosed, change th point assignment to 16.

Denote appearance of superficial implant types as red [(R), red, red-pink, flamelike, vesicular blobs, clear vesicles], white [(W), opacifications, peritoneal defects, yellow-brown], or black [(B) black, hemosiderin deposits, blue]. Denote percent of total described as R___%, W___% and B___%, Total should equal 100%.

Additional Endometriosis: _____   Associated Pathology: _____
_____   _____
_____   _____
_____   _____

To Be Used with Normal   To Be Used with Abnormal
Tubes and Ovaries   Tubes and/or Ovaries

L   R   L   R

Figure 45.8 ASRM Classification of Endometriosis form.

**ENDOMETRIOSIS FERTILITY INDEX (EFI)
SURGERY FORM**

LEAST FUNCTION (LF) SCORE AT <u>CONCLUSION</u> OF SURGERY

Score	Description		Left	Right
4 =	Normal	Fallopian Tube		
3 =	Mild Dysfunction			
2 =	Moderate Dysfunction	Fimbria		
1 =	Severe Dysfunction			
0 =	Absent or Nonfunctional	Ovary		

To calculate the LF score, add together the lowest score for the left side and the lowest score for the right side. If an ovary is absent on one side, the LF score is obtained by doubling the lowest score on the side with the ovary.

Lowest Socre [ ] Left + [ ] Right = [ ] LF Score

ENDOMETRIOSIS FERTILITY INDEX (EFI)

Historical Factors		Points	Surgical Factors		Points
Factor	Description		Factor	Description	
Age			**LF Score**		
	If age is ≤35 years	2		If LF Score = 7 to 8 (high score)	3
	If age is 36 to 39 years	1		If LF Score = 4 to 6 (moderate score)	2
	If age is ≥40 years	0		If LF Score = 1 to 3 (low score)	0
Years Infertile			**AFS Endometriosis Score**		
	If years infertile is ≤3	2		If AFS Endometriosis Lesion Score is <16	1
	If years infertile is >3	0		If AFS Endometriosis Lesion Score is ≥16	0
Prior Pregnancy			**AFS Total Score**		
	If there is a history of a prior pregnancy	1		If AFS total score <71	1
	If there is no history of prior pregnancy	0		If AFS total score ≥71	0
Total Historical Factors			Total Surgical Factors		

EFI = TOTAL HISTORICAL FACTORS + TOTAL SURGICAL FACTORS: [Historical] + [Surgical] = [EFI Score]

Figure 45.9 Endometriosis Fertility Index surgery form.

involvement if there is clinical or anamnestic suspicion of deep endometriosis (40–42). A recent Cochrane review concluded that no imaging modality detects peritoneal endometriosis accurately enough to replace surgical biopsy for diagnosis (39). Furthermore, imaging-based mapping of the extent of endometriosis is indispensable for appropriate planning of surgical management (43, 44).

Clinical signs and symptoms

A history of pelvic pain symptoms will lead to a clinical suspicion for endometriosis. However, endometriosis may be asymptomatic, even in the most advanced stages of the disease. Classic symptoms of endometriosis include infertility, dysmenorrhea, dyspareunia, intestinal complaints (periodic bloating, diarrhoea, constipation), haematuria, dysuria, chronic fatigue, and chronic pelvic pain. The spectrum of complaints depends on the location of the disease and typically increases during menstruation. Bellelis et al. reported dysmenorrhea to be the number one complaint, present in 62% of all women with peritoneal endometriosis (45).

Several studies have tried to analyse the predictive value of certain symptoms in the diagnosis of endometriosis. Overall, the evidence for the use of the 'presence of symptoms' as an indication for the diagnosis of endometriosis is weak with low specificity and sensitivity (2). The European Society of Human Reproduction and Embryology (ESHRE) guideline on management of women with endometriosis states that the following symptoms and patient

characteristics are risk factors for endometriosis: abdominopelvic pain, dysmenorrhea, heavy menstrual bleeding, infertility, dyspareunia, postcoital bleeding, a history of ovarian cyst, irritable bowel syndrome, and pelvic inflammatory disease (2). ESHRE also stated that the presence of multiple factors increases the chance of presence of endometriosis (2). In a prospective study, the presence of dyschezia during menstrual bleeding was a strong predictor for higher stages of endometriosis (ASRM stage III and IV) (46).

Clinical examination can further increase the suspicion of presence of endometriosis and guide the planning of further imaging. However, the clinical examination has a low specificity and sensitivity for the diagnosis of endometriosis, especially peritoneal endometriosis, and clinicians should consider the diagnosis of endometriosis in women suspected of the disease even if the clinical examination is normal (2). There is evidence that the accuracy of the clinical examination is improved when performed during menstruation (47). Although clinical examination might be normal in many women with endometriosis, a routine inspection of the vagina using speculum, bimanual palpation, and rectovaginal palpation is recommended (2, 48, 49). Several studies emphasize the importance of inspection of the posterior fornix and rectovaginal digital examination for the diagnosis of infiltrating nodules of the vagina, uterosacral ligaments or the pouch of Douglas, as well as the detection of infiltration or masses in the rectovaginal septum and ovaries or displacement of the uterus or cervix (47, 48).

Imaging

Transvaginal ultrasound

Both ESHRE and the American College of Obstetricians and Gynecology (ACOG) recommend the use of TVUS in the diagnostic workup of women with suspected endometriosis (2, 50). TVUS is useful in identifying endometriosis, however, the sensitivity and specificity of the examination are dependent on the interest and experience of the sonographer and on the quality of the ultrasound equipment (51, 52).

In the recent Cochrane review by Nisenblat and colleagues, the sensitivity and specificity of TVUS for detecting ovarian endometriosis was 0.93 (95% confidence interval (CI) 0.87–0.99), and 0.96 (95% CI 0.92–0.99) respectively (39). For detection of deep endometriosis, the sensitivity and specificity of TVUS was 0.79 (95% CI 0.69–0.89) and 0.94 (95% CI 0.88–1.00) (39). The authors conclude that the presence of endometriosis (pelvic, ovarian, deeply infiltrating endometriosis) on TVUS could establish the diagnosis with high certainty, whereas the absence of radiological evidence of the disease could not confirm that participants are disease free (39).

The typical ultrasound features of endometriomas were assessed in the large patient cohort of the International Ovarian Tumor Analysis (IOTA) studies (51). Based on these characteristics, the following diagnostic rule for an endometrioma was developed: an ovarian cyst with ground-glass echogenicity of the cyst fluid, one to four locules, and no solid parts (51). This diagnostic rule has a sensitivity of 61.4% (95% CI 57.8–64.9), a specificity of 98.3% (95% CI 97.7–98.7), and a positive predictive value of 90.1% (95% CI 87.1–92.5) (51). It is important to take into account that an endometrioma is only rarely an isolated finding since patients with an endometrioma often have other endometriotic lesions (53). Therefore the diagnosis of an endometrioma should always evoke a detailed investigation for other (peritoneal and deep) endometriotic lesions (2).

The role of TVUS in the diagnosis of deep endometriosis is more complex, given the multitude of possible locations of deep endometriosis. The ESHRE guideline recommends the use of TVUS for identifying or ruling out rectal endometriosis (2). Data on the accuracy of TVUS for diagnosing other bowel endometriosis lesions are more limited but small individual studies displayed similar performance to that demonstrated for rectosigmoid endometriosis (39).

Previously, most of the research on the role of TVUS in deep endometriosis was concentrated on defining the diagnostic sensitivity and specificity of TVUS (54). In recent years, however, the focus has shifted to modified TVUS techniques, which differ from standard TVUS by the introduction of a contrast medium into the vagina or rectum, by preparation of the bowel before the examination or by searching for a landmark linked to the movement of the probe (sliding sign) (39, 54). These new promising techniques have been shown to perform well in a research context, but are also strongly dependent on the operator, with poor repeatability and high interoperator variability when tested in a more routine clinical practice setting (54).

Magnetic resonance imaging

Due to the high costs and limited availability, MRI is not considered as a first-line imaging modality in the diagnosis of endometriosis. However, a growing number of studies suggest that it has a role in the diagnosis of endometriosis because of a greater ability to detect small lesions (55, 56). However, peritoneal endometriotic lesions are only identified by MRI if they are haemorrhagic, greater than 5 mm, or when associated with extensive adhesions distorting the normal anatomy (39).

Since MRI appears to be less accurate for the diagnosis of peritoneal disease, it cannot replace surgery for the diagnosis of endometriosis in general. MRI has a good sensitivity and specificity for the diagnosis of deep endometriosis and endometriomas; however, the added value in addition to TVUS is limited (39). MRI could be useful in the population for whom the risk/benefit ratio of surgery is still unclear (39). The ACOG currently advises MRI, not in routine setting, but only for those with inconclusive ultrasound findings, with high suspicion for rectovaginal or bladder endometriosis (50).

Laparoscopy

Laparoscopic visualization with histological confirmation remains the gold standard for the definite diagnosis of endometriosis (2, 38). A negative diagnostic laparoscopy is highly reliable for the exclusion of endometriosis; however, a positive diagnostic laparoscopy without histological confirmation is inaccurate (57). Data on complication rates of diagnostic laparoscopy for endometriosis are limited. In a systematic review on diagnostic laparoscopy for endometriosis, no direct major complications were reported in any of the included studies, suggesting that laparoscopy is a safe diagnostic intervention, although reporting bias is likely (57).

During laparoscopy, one should systematically evaluate the abdominal cavity, as well as the pelvic cavity for the presence of endometriotic lesions. A good-quality laparoscopy should include systematic checking of (a) the uterus and adnexa; (b) the peritoneum of ovarian fossae, vesicouterine fold, Douglas, and pararectal spaces; (c) the rectum and sigmoid (isolated sigmoid nodules); (d) the appendix and caecum; and (e) the diaphragm. There should also be a speculum examination and palpation of the vagina and cervix under laparoscopic control, to check for 'buried' nodules. A good-quality laparoscopy can only be performed by using at least one secondary port for a suitable grasper to clear the pelvis of obstruction from bowel loops, or fluid suction to ensure the whole pouch of Douglas is inspected (2). When ovarian disease is found, the surgeon should be attentive to deep infiltrating, extensive pelvic, and intestinal diseases. Only 1% of all patients with endometriosis of the ovary have solitary lesions restricted to the ovaries (53). All macroscopic findings may be complicated with signs of retraction, pigmentation, and adhesions to the surrounding peritoneum. A histological confirmation is necessary for the diagnosis of endometriosis, since lesions reported as 'typical' by the surgeon can be microscopically negative in up to 24% of the cases (58).

Women suffering from chronic pelvic pain, dysmenorrhea, and dyspareunia with a high suspicion of endometriosis are often prescribed hormonal medication and analgesics without a prior definitive laparoscopic diagnosis. It is common practice for laparoscopy to be performed if the patient does not react favourably to the prescribed medical or hormonal treatment. In a retrospective study, relief of chronic pelvic pain symptoms, or lack of response, with preoperative hormonal therapy was not an accurate predictor of the presence or absence of histologically confirmed endometriosis at laparoscopy (59). Furthermore, empirical treatment can lead to a delay in diagnosis associated with significant social and psychological disadvantages (59). The ESHRE 2014 guideline recommends to rule out other causes of pelvic pain as far as possible and thoroughly counsel patients with presumed endometriosis before starting empirical treatment (2).

Treatment of endometriosis

Women with endometriosis are confronted with one or both of two major problems: endometriosis-associated pain and infertility. Although endometriosis is a benign gynaecological disorder, its treatment is complex and often frustrating due to the progressive character and high recurrence rates of endometriosis. Management of endometriosis has been based partially on evidence-based practices and partially on unsubstantiated therapies and approaches. Several guidelines have been developed by a number of national and international bodies, yet areas of controversy and uncertainty remain, not at least due to a paucity of firm evidence (38, 50, 60).

Endometriosis should be viewed as a chronic disease that requires a lifelong management with the goal of maximizing the use of medical treatment and avoiding repeated surgical procedures (61). Treatment of endometriosis is very different depending on whether the patient has pain, infertility, or both. It is therefore important to individualize the treatment, with attention to the patient's symptoms and wishes, the impact of the disease, and the effect of treatment on the patient's life.

Treatment of endometriosis should ideally eradicate endometriosis rather than merely relieving its symptoms. However, the currently available medications result in endometriosis suppression rather than cytoreduction and attempt to achieve two main objectives: relief of symptoms (pain) for prolonged periods and prevention of disease progression (61). There is strong evidence that suppression of ovarian function reduces pain associated with endometriosis and currently combined oral contraceptives (COCs), progestogens, antiprogestogens, gonadotropin-releasing hormone (GnRH) agonists, and aromatase inhibitors are in clinical use. There is no evidence that indicates the superiority of one product to the other, but side effects and cost profiles differ (61). Hence, it is recommended that clinicians take patient preferences, side effects, costs, and availability into consideration when choosing hormonal treatment for endometriosis-associated pain (2). In contrast to medical treatment, surgical management has the possibility of eliminating the disease by excision or ablation and restoration of the normal pelvic anatomy can be obtained.

Treatment of endometriosis-associated pain

Medical treatment

Non-steroidal anti-inflammatory drugs

First-line medical treatment of pain due to endometriosis is often a non-steroidal anti-inflammatory drug (NSAID). Good evidence exists to support the use of NSAIDs for primary dysmenorrhea (62), but in a Cochrane meta-analysis there were insufficient data to show that NSAIDs significantly reduce endometriosis-associated pain

(63). It has to be noted that only two studies were available that investigated the role of NSAIDs in the relief of endometriosis-associated pain (63). Nevertheless the ESHRE 2014 guideline recommends that clinicians should consider NSAIDs or other analgesics to reduce endometriosis-associated pain, due to the known benefit of NSAIDs in primary dysmenorrhea (2).

Oestrogens and progestogens

The clinical observation of apparent symptom resolution during pregnancy gave rise to the concept of treating patients with a pseudopregnancy regimen (64). In 1958, Kistner was the first to use combinations of high-dose oestrogens and progestogens, and later progestogens alone (64). Decidualization followed by atrophy of both the eutopic and ectopic endometrial tissue is the generic proposed mechanism of action (38). Additionally, COCs might have a positive effect on endometriosis through reduction of the menstrual blood flow, downregulation of cell proliferation, and enhancement of programmed cell death in the eutopic endometrium (65). Similar to COCs, the chronic administration of progestogens results in decidualization and subsequent atrophy of endometrial tissue (38). Recent research also suggests a possible role of progestogen-induced suppression of matrix metalloproteinases, a class of enzymes important in the growth and implantation of ectopic endometrium, and inhibition of angiogenesis (38).

A Cochrane systematic review from 2007 addressed the use of COCs for pain associated with endometriosis (64). Surprisingly only one study was found, despite the widespread use of COCs in clinical practice (66). In the included study, no significant difference between treatment with a COC and a GnRH agonist was seen (66). Based on this study and on the widespread use of COCs, both the 2013 ESHRE and the ASRM 2014 guideline recommend the consideration of a COC, vaginal contraceptive ring, or transdermal patch in the treatment of endometriosis-associated pain.

The body of evidence supporting the use of progestogens and antiprogestogens in the treatment of endometriosis-associated pain is larger than for COCs. In their systematic review from 2012, Brown and colleagues included 13 articles evaluating progestogens and antiprogestogens (67). Of the two studies comparing progestogens with placebo, only one showed a significant effect. There was no overall evidence of a benefit of progestogens over other medical treatments (COCs, GnRH agonists). The authors concluded that the evidence for progestogens in the treatment of endometriosis pain was limited (67). The 2014 ESHRE guideline considers this evidence as sufficient to recommend the use of some specific progestogens (medroxyprogesterone acetate, dienogest, cyproterone acetate, norethisterone acetate, levonorgestrel-releasing intrauterine system, or danazol) and antiprogestogens (gestrinone) (2). Due to its severe side effects (acne, oedema, vaginal spotting, weight gain, and muscle cramps) the use of danazol is discouraged, and should only be considered if no other medical therapy is available (2).

GnRH agonists

GnRH agonists are synthetic analogues of GnRH that differ from the native hormone with respect to the specific amino acid sequence (68). All are designed either to increase receptor affinity or decrease GnRH degradation (68). Their use therefore leads to persistent activation of GnRH receptors (68). This activation results in an initial release of gonadotropins previously produced and stored in the pituitary (68).

However, the release is rapidly followed by downregulation of GnRH receptor expression and profound suppression of gonadotropin secretion (68). As a result, sex-steroid production in the ovary falls to levels similar to those seen after castration (68). This profound hypo-oestrogenic state inhibits the development, maintenance, and growth of endometriosis, which in turn alters the effect on the immune, nervous, and endocrine systems. The hypo-oestrogenaemia also has direct effects on these systems, further altering their status from that seen in patients with active endometriosis (68). The hypo-oestrogenism induced by GnRH agonists can result in bone loss and severe hypo-oestrogenic symptoms (disturbed sleep pattern, hot flushes, vaginal dryness, etc.). To reduce the negative effects of oestrogen deprivation, hormonal add-back therapy with oestrogens and/or progestogens or tibolone is recommended (2). This is based on the threshold theory, by which lower oestrogen levels are needed to protect the bone and cognitive function and to avoid/minimize menopausal symptoms than to activate endometriotic tissue (69).

GnRH agonists have been studied more extensively for the treatment of endometriosis-associated pain than other medical therapies (68). Multiple randomized trials have pitted GnRH agonists against other known treatments for endometriosis, including COCs, progestogens, and danazol. A Cochrane review compared GnRH agonists at different doses, regimens, and routes of administration, with danazol, intrauterine progestogens, placebo, and analgesics for relieving endometriosis-associated pain symptoms (70). The meta-analysis showed that GnRH agonists were superior to no treatment or placebo for dysmenorrhea and pelvic tenderness with a significant improvement of the Endometriosis Severity Symptom Score. There were no statistically significant differences when GnRH agonists were compared with the levonorgestrel-releasing intrauterine system or oral danazol for dysmenorrhea, dyspareunia, pelvic pain, and pelvic tenderness. Intrauterine progestogens and oral danazol showed a better side effect profile than GnRH agonists without add-back therapy (70). Several studies have demonstrated that add-back therapy reduces the side effects of GnRH agonist treatment without a negative effect on the efficacy of treatment with GnRH agonists (71–74). It can be concluded that GnRH agonists are effective in the relief of endometriosis-associated pain, but evidence is limited regarding dosage or duration of treatment. The severe side effects of monotherapy should be taken into account and therefore the ESHRE guideline recommends that hormonal add-back therapy should be associated from the start of the treatment with GnRH agonists (2). Future studies should compare novel therapies with GnRH agonist with add-back therapy to allow clinically meaningful comparisons.

Aromatase inhibitors

Aromatase inhibitors (AIs) constitute another class of drugs that cause hypo-oestrogenism and are used in the treatment of endometriosis. AIs suppress oestradiol production through reversible (anastrozole, letrozole) or irreversible (exemestane) inhibition of the aromatase P450 enzyme resulting in hypo-oestrogenism (75). The aromatase P450 enzyme plays an important role in the production of oestradiol by converting androstenedione to oestrone (E1) (76). Subsequently, E1 is converted to oestradiol (E2) by the activity of 17-OH-steroid dehydrogenase (76). E2 is mainly produced by the ovary in a cyclic fashion, where it is secreted by the preovulatory follicle. In addition, there is conversion of circulating androstenedione of adrenal origin to E1 in peripheral tissues such as fat, skin, and skeletal muscle (76). There is some evidence that endometriotic tissue, unlike disease-free endometrium, might exhibit a high level of aromatase activity that may result in increased local concentrations of oestradiol that may favour the growth of endometriosis (77). Even though the evidence for increased expression of aromatase P450 in endometriotic tissue is limited and still controversial, AIs have been studied as treatment for pain symptoms in premenopausal women with endometriosis.

A systematic review evaluating the use of AIs to treat endometriosis associated-pain concluded that the existing evidence is of moderate quality and that evidence on the long-term effects are lacking (78). Like GnRH agonists without add-back, AIs have severe side effects such as vaginal dryness, hot flushes, and diminished bone density. Furthermore, in premenopausal women AIs lead to an increase in follicle-stimulating hormone levels and subsequent follicular development and therefore must be used in combination with other agents (progestogens, COCs, or GnRH agonists) to downregulate the ovaries (38). Treatment of endometriosis-associated pain with AIs should be considered experimental and only be prescribed to women after all other options for medical or surgical treatment are exhausted (2, 38).

Surgical treatment

The goal of endometriosis surgery must be to remove all lesions and associated adhesions in order to restore normal anatomy, with attention to preserving fertility. Surgical options for the treatment of endometriosis include surgical excision or ablation and may be performed robotically, laparoscopically, or through laparotomy. Although laparoscopy and laparotomy are equally effective, the laparoscopic approach is now considered routine for the diagnosis and removal of endometriosis as it results in less pain, decreased recovery time, and better cosmetic results (79).

Peritoneal endometriosis

Several randomized controlled trials have evaluated the efficacy of laparoscopic treatment in reducing endometriosis-associated pain compared with diagnostic laparoscopy alone (80). Meta-analysis of these data in a Cochrane review showed that surgical treatment by excision, coagulation, or laser vaporization of endometriotic lesions reduces overall pain associated with endometriosis and is more effective in pain reduction than diagnostic laparoscopy alone (80).

When considering the different types of pain, including pelvic pain, dysmenorrhea, dyspareunia, and dyschezia, there is insufficient evidence to determine which pain type responds best to laparoscopic surgery (80). Two randomized controlled trials compared excision and ablation of endometriosis and found no difference in pain scores up to 1 year after surgery (81, 82). However, the conclusions of these studies should be treated with caution because of the small population of the trial by Wright and colleagues and the suboptimal design of the trial by Healy and colleagues. Consequently, both ASRM and ESHRE recommend surgical treatment of endometriosis when it is identified at laparoscopy since it is effective for reducing endometriosis-associated pain (2, 38). Neither of the guidelines favours excision or ablation, but the ESHRE guidelines states that excision of lesions could be preferred with regard to the possibility of retrieving samples for histology (2, 38).

Endometriomas

Medical therapy for ovarian endometriomas may lead to a temporary reduction in size of the cysts but not complete resolution (38). Surgery is therefore the primary approach for symptomatic or large endometriomas (38). Two surgical approaches can be used for endometriomas: draining and coagulation or cystectomy. A simple draining and coagulation involves opening, aspiration, and irrigation of the cyst followed by destruction/ablation/coagulation of the mucosal lining of the cyst. During cystectomy, the endometrioma is opened and aspirated followed by removal of the cyst wall from the ovarian cortex, with maximal preservation of normal ovarian tissue.

A cystectomy is superior to a simple draining and coagulation, due to a reduction in endometriosis-associated pain and to a carbon dioxide laser evaporation because of a reduction in recurrence of the endometrioma (83, 84). However, with cystectomy there is concern about the risk of ovarian damage and impaired ovarian reserve. A meta-analysis of eight studies on ovarian cystectomy for endometriomas found significantly lower anti-Mullerian hormone levels postoperatively (85). Bilateral cystectomy of ovarian endometriomas is associated with a 2.4% risk of ovarian failure (86). Therefore it is recommended that clinicians counsel women with an endometrioma regarding the risks of reduced ovarian function and ovarian failure after surgical treatment of endometriomas (2).

Deep endometriosis

Deep endometriosis is characterized by involvement of different pelvic and extrapelvic organs with a very diverse and often severe anatomical distortion making surgical excision of deep endometriosis difficult and challenging (43). Similar to surgery for superficial endometriosis and endometriomas the final goal of surgical treatment of deep endometriosis is to achieve complete resection of all deep endometriosis lesions (87). To prevent multiple surgeries, complete excision should be performed in a one-step surgical procedure (87). Taking into account the multifocality of deep endometriosis, this often requires several associated surgical interventions. An overview of the most commonly used surgical interventions for deep endometriosis is presented in **Table 45.2**.

A large number of studies on surgical excision of deep endometriosis have been published but mainly in retrospective designs. A systematic review by Meuleman et al. found that pain and quality of life improvement was reported in most studies (88). In another review on bowel resection for colorectal endometriosis, the authors found excellent pain relief in most studies (89). Hence, surgical treatment is considered to be the treatment of choice for symptomatic deep

Table 45.2 Overview of most commonly used surgical interventions for deep endometriosis

Bowel endometriosis	
Bowel shaving	Superficial excision of bowel serosal and subserosal endometriosis (mechanically, with diathermy, laser, or other energy source) that does not require suturing/closure
Bowel partial thickness discoid excision	Selective excision of the bowel endometriosis lesion (mechanically, with diathermy, laser, or other energy source) without entering the bowel lumen, that requires suturing/closure (i.e. closure of a muscularis defect without a mucosal defect in the bowel wall)

Bowel full thickness discoid excision	Selective excision of the bowel endometriosis lesion (mechanically, with diathermy, laser, or other energy source) with opening of the bowel lumen followed by closure of the bowel
	
	Subtypes:
	
	  Open full thickness disc excision: excision with opening of lumen followed by closure
	
	  Closed full-thickness disc excision: excision with stapler

Bowel resection and re-anastomosis	Resection of a bowel segment affected by endometriosis followed by re-anastomosis by any means
Ureteral endometriosis	

Ureterolysis	Restoration of the normal mobility and anatomical position of the ureter through resection of adhesions and selective dissection of the ureter from a lesion, either mechanically or with diathermy, laser, or any other energy source
	
	Subtypes:
	
	  Without opening of the ureteric wall
	
	  With opening and re-suturing of the ureteric wall.

Ureteral segmental resection	Resection of a ureteral segment affected by endometriosis followed by ipsilateral uretero-ureteral re-anastomosis or ureteral reimplantation into the bladder
Bladder endometriosis	
Bladder shaving	Superficial excision of bladder serosal and subserosal endometriosis (mechanically, with diathermy, laser, or other energy source) that does not require suturing/closure
Bladder partial thickness excision	Selective excision of the bladder endometriosis lesion (mechanically, with diathermy, laser, or other energy source) without opening of the bladder mucosa that requires suturing/closure. (i.e. closure of a muscularis defect without a mucosal defect)
Bladder full thickness excision	Resection of an endometriosis nodule by full thickness partial resection of the bladder wall, including the mucosa and closure of the defect by suture or other device

Source data from Vanhie, A., et al., Consensus on Recording Deep Endometriosis Surgery: the CORDES statement. *Hum Reprod* 2016;31(6):1219–23.

endometriosis, but is complex and associated with significant complication rates (43). The ESHRE guideline on the management of women with endometriosis recommends that treatment of deep endometriosis should be performed by multidisciplinary teams in centres with specific expertise in this area (2).

Several techniques for the excision of deep endometriosis lesions have been described and evaluated, but large, well-designed, prospective randomized controlled trials comparing different techniques are lacking (43). Therefore, the appropriate surgical approach for deep endometriosis remains controversial as little is known about the impact of the different types of surgery on complications, pain, the patients' quality of life, and reintervention and recurrence rates (87). The recently published Consensus On Recording Deep Endometriosis Surgery (CORDES) statement provides a Deep Endometriosis Surgical Sheet (DESS) to record in detail the surgical procedures for deep endometriosis and an international consensus on pre-, intra- and postoperative data that should be recorded in surgical trials on deep endometriosis (43). Future studies on surgical treatment of deep endometriosis should take into account the impact of extensive deep endometriosis surgery on quality of life, sexuality, and bowel and bladder function.

Hysterectomy and interruption of pelvic nerve pathways

Hysterectomy will not necessarily reduce or cure the symptoms of endometriosis. Furthermore, hysterectomy without bilateral salpingo-oophorectomy (BSO) was reported to have a sixfold risk for development of chronic pain recurrence and even an eightfold risk of repeated surgery (90). Therefore, hysterectomy with BSO should be reserved for women with debilitating symptoms who have completed childbearing and in whom other therapies have failed (38). Women should be informed of the limitations of a hysterectomy in the surgical treatment of endometriosis (2).

Laparoscopic uterosacral nerve ablation (LUNA) is a technique designed to disrupt the efferent nerve fibres in the uterosacral ligaments to decrease uterine pain for women with intractable dysmenorrhea (38). Presacral neurectomy (PSN) involves interrupting the sympathetic innervation to the uterus at the level of the superior hypogastric plexus (38). A Cochrane review analysed the effectiveness of surgical interruption of pelvic nerve pathways (91). No benefit of LUNA was found as an adjunct to conservative surgery for endometriosis. Therefore clinicians should not perform LUNA as an additional procedure to conservative surgery to reduce endometriosis-associated pain (2). PSN in addition to conservative surgery did result in a reduction of pain symptoms, but may be specific to midline pain and was associated with an increased risk of complications (bleeding, constipation, urinary urgency, etc.) (91).

Treatment of endometriosis-associated infertility

Medical and surgical treatment

The role of hormonal therapy (i.e. ovarian suppression) in the treatment of endometriosis-associated infertility has been evaluated in a Cochrane review (92). The authors found no significant difference in live birth rate or surrogate markers (conception, pregnancy rate, etc.) for any of the evaluated medical interventions (92). All trials that were included for analysis were in patients with ASRM stages I and II

endometriosis; at present there are no trials in patients with stage III–IV disease. Based on this review, both ASRM and ESHRE guidelines conclude that medical treatment for improving fertility in patients with endometriosis is ineffective and should not be prescribed (2, 60).

There is agreement among international guidelines that laparoscopic surgery is beneficial for infertility associated with endometriosis (2, 60). In a Cochrane review in 2010, the role of laparoscopic surgery for endometriosis-related infertility was addressed (93). The authors conclude that in women with stage I–II endometriosis operative laparoscopy is effective in increasing live birth rate (93). In women with stage III–IV endometriosis there are no controlled studies comparing reproductive outcome after surgery and after expectant management. Observational studies suggest that surgery in patients with stage III–IV disease may increase spontaneous pregnancy rates; however, the significant complication rates of this complex surgery needs to be taken into account (2, 94). Therefore, both the ASRM and ESHRE guidelines recommend surgical treatment for stage I–II endometriosis and in women with stage III–IV endometriosis, operative laparoscopy can be considered to increase spontaneous pregnancy rates (2, 60).

Furness and colleagues assessed the role of pre- and postoperative hormonal therapy in endometriosis (95). No studies were found on the effect on infertility of preoperative hormonal treatment and studies on postoperative therapy showed no increase in pregnancy rates (95). Therefore, preoperative or postoperative adjunctive hormonal therapy to improve the reproductive outcome is not recommended after endometriosis surgery (2). Moreover, pre- and postoperative adjunctive hormonal therapy could unnecessarily delay further fertility therapies (60).

Medically assisted reproduction

Medically assisted reproduction is defined is 'Reproduction brought about through ovulation induction, controlled ovarian stimulation, ovulation triggering, assisted reproductive technology procedures and intrauterine, intracervical and intravaginal insemination with semen of husband/partner or donor' (96). Assisted reproductive technology (ART) is defined as 'all treatments or procedures that include the *in vitro* handling of both human oocytes and sperm or of embryos for the purpose of establishing a pregnancy' (96).

Intrauterine insemination in women with endometriosis

Ovulation induction with intrauterine insemination (IUI) has been used in the treatment of couples with infertility associated with endometriosis, especially of minimal or mild stage. This is supported by limited data from observational studies and small randomized controlled trials (2). The ESHRE guideline states that in women with minimal to mild endometriosis, IUI with controlled ovarian stimulation may be effective in increasing live birth rate when compared with expectant management (2). Several studies on IUI in endometriosis-associated infertility have included women whose endometriosis was treated. One case–control study showed that pregnancy rates following controlled ovarian stimulation plus IUI were not different between women with unexplained infertility and women with surgically treated minimal or mild endometriosis (97). Therefore both the ASRM and ESHRE guidelines recommend controlled ovarian stimulation plus IUI as a viable option for women who have had a surgical diagnosis and treatment of stage I/II endometriosis (60).

Assisted reproductive technology in women with endometriosis

Data on the impact of endometriosis on ART success rates are inconsistent. A review of observational studies reported lower pregnancy rates in patients with endometriosis when compared to patients with tubal factor infertility (98). However, these data were not supported by the observed pregnancy rates in large databases monitoring ART outcomes (2, 60). While endometriosis may or may not affect ART results, IVF likely maximizes cycle fecundity for patients with endometriosis (60). All studies that evaluated the risk of endometriosis recurrence after ovarian stimulation for ART found no increased risk of recurrence (99–102).

A potential role of medical treatment of endometriosis prior to ART has been proposed. GnRH agonists have been studied most extensively for this indication and were reviewed by Sallam and colleagues (103). Although the quality of the studies was poor the results concurred, showing a beneficial effect. The authors concluded that 3–6 months of GnRH agonist treatment before ART increases the odds of clinical pregnancy by more than fourfold (103).

Since surgical treatment of endometriosis is considered to be beneficial for endometriosis-associated infertility, it might also improve ART outcomes. In line with the finding that operative laparoscopy increases (spontaneous) live birth rates in stage I/II endometriosis, Opoien and colleagues showed that complete removal of endometriosis in women with stage I/II disease before ART significantly increased the live birth rate (104). For women who are found to have an (asymptomatic) endometrioma and who are planning to undergo IVF/intracytoplasmic sperm injection, there is insufficient evidence to suggest that removal of the endometrioma will improve IVF success rates (2, 60). However, if the endometrioma is large (>4 cm), surgery should be considered to confirm the diagnosis histologically, to improve access to follicles during oocyte retrieval, and possibly to improve ovarian response (60). However, the patient should be counselled that extensive ovarian surgery could compromise ovarian function and diminish the response to ovarian stimulation (2). In the literature, there is no good evidence for surgical excision of deep endometriosis prior to ART to improve reproductive outcomes. However, the majority of these patients will have pain symptoms, and these symptoms represent a valid indication for endometriosis surgery in addition to or before ART treatment for which surgical treatment is considered the treatment of choice.

Prevention of endometriosis

Primary prevention

Primary prevention is defined as those measures that protect healthy individuals from developing the disease. A typical example is immunization against infectious diseases, but it also includes health promotion and regulation of environmental pollutants.

Given that the exact cause and pathogenesis of endometriosis are unknown, potential interventions for primary prevention are limited. In light of the retrograde menstruation theory, the use of COCs for primary prevention has been suggested (105). COCs suppress ovulation and substantially reduce the amount of monthly uterine blood flow. They are successfully used in the treatment of pain symptoms and progestogens may inhibit expression of matrix

metalloproteinases and angiogenesis. The relationship between COC use and risk of endometriosis was evaluated in a systematic review by Vercellini and colleagues in 2011 (105). The authors conclude that the risk of endometriosis appears reduced during COC use, but that it is not possible to exclude the possibility that the apparent protective effect of COC against endometriosis is the result of postponement of surgical evaluation due to temporary suppression of pain symptoms (105). Based on this meta-analysis, the ESHRE guideline states that the usefulness of oral contraceptives for the primary prevention of endometriosis is uncertain (2).

A second factor that has been investigated is the possible link between the level of physical activity and endometriosis. Physical activity has been hypothesized to be protective against endometriosis because it may increase levels of sex hormone-binding globulin, which would reduce bioavailable oestrogens, and it reduces insulin resistance and hyperinsulinaemia, which has been hypothesized to be related to endometriosis (106). Several case–control studies reported a strong risk reduction of endometriosis associated with physical activity (107–110). Based on prospective collected data from the Nurses' Health Study II, Vitonis and colleagues could not replicate these strong associations. They observed a weak protective effect among fertile participants for total recreational physical activity reported 2 years before diagnosis and a slightly stronger protective effect for aerobic exercise on the rate of laparoscopically confirmed endometriosis (106). Based on these prospective data, the ESHRE guideline states that the usefulness of physical exercise for the primary prevention of endometriosis is uncertain (2).

Secondary prevention

Secondary preventive measures are those interventions used to prevent recurrences, exacerbations, or complications of the disease and its treatment. In the ESHRE guideline, secondary prevention of endometriosis was defined as prevention of the recurrence of pain symptoms (dysmenorrhea, dyspareunia, non-menstrual pelvic pain) or the recurrence of disease (recurrence of endometriosis lesions documented by ultrasound for ovarian endometrioma or by laparoscopy for all endometriosis lesions) in the long term (more than 6 months after surgery) (2).

A frustrating aspect of surgical treatment of endometriosis is the variable recurrence rate, between 10% and 55% within 12 months after excision/removal by an expert in endometriosis surgery, with an extra 10% of recurrence for each additional year after surgery (111). Logically, there has been significant interest in the effect of pre- and postoperative medical therapies for lowering recurrence and complication rates after surgical treatment of endometriosis. A Cochrane review considered both pre-and postoperative treatment in relation to the management of cysts, pain, and infertility. The authors conclude that there is no evidence of a benefit of preoperative medical therapy on the outcome of surgery (95). The ESHRE guideline endorses that preoperative treatment with GnRH analogues to facilitate surgery is common clinical practice, although there are no controlled studies supporting this (2). Based on the same Cochrane review, both the ESHRE and ASRM guidelines recommend the use of long-term (>6 months) postoperative hormonal treatment (COC, levonorgestrel-releasing intrauterine device, progestogens) for the secondary prevention of recurrence of both symptoms and lesions (2, 38). It is important to note that postoperative medical treatment does not improve outcome of surgery and as such there is no clear rationale for short-term (<6 months) adjuvant treatment after surgery (2).

REFERENCES

1. Vanhie A, Tomassetti C, Peeraer K, Meuleman C, D'Hooghe T. Challenges in the development of novel therapeutic strategies for treatment of endometriosis. *Expert Opin Ther Targets* 2016;**20**:593–600.

2. Dunselman GA, Vermeulen N, Becker C, et al. ESHRE guideline: management of women with endometriosis. *Hum Reprod* 2014;**29**:400–12.

3. Viganò P, Parazzini F, Somigliana E, Vercellini P. Endometriosis: epidemiology and aetiological factors. *Best Pract Res Clin Obstet Gynaecol* 2004;**18**:177–200.

4. Simoens S, Dunselman G, Dirksen C, et al. The burden of endometriosis: costs and quality of life of women with endometriosis and treated in referral centres. *Hum Reprod* 2012;**27**:1292–99.

5. Meuleman C, Vandenabeele B, Fieuws S, Spiessens C, Timmerman D, D'Hooghe T. High prevalence of endometriosis in infertile women with normal ovulation and normospermic partners. *Fertil Steril* 2009;**92**:68–74.

6. Giudice LC. Clinical practice. Endometriosis. *N Engl J Med* 2010;**362**:2389–98.

7. Parazzini F, Esposito G, Tozzi L, Noli S, Bianchi S. Epidemiology of endometriosis and its comorbidities. *Eur J Obstet Gynecol Reprod Biol* 2017;**209**:3–7.

8. Missmer SA, Cramer DW. The epidemiology of endometriosis. *Obstet Gynecol Clin North Am* 2003;**30**:1–19, vii.

9. Treloar SA, O'Connor DT, O'Connor VM, Martin NG. Genetic influences on endometriosis in an Australian twin sample. *Fertil Steril* 1999;**71**:701–10.

10. Zondervan KT, Weeks DE, Colman R, et al. Familial aggregation of endometriosis in a large pedigree of rhesus macaques. *Hum Reprod* 2004;**19**:448–55.

11. Rahmioglu N, Nyholt DR, Morris AP, Missmer SA, Montgomery GW, Zondervan KT. Genetic variants underlying risk of endometriosis: insights from meta-analysis of eight genome-wide association and replication datasets. *Hum Reprod Update* 2014;**20**:702–16.

12. Vercellini P, Viganò P, Somigliana E, Fedele L. Endometriosis: pathogenesis and treatment. *Nat Rev Endocrinol* 2014;**10**:261–75.

13. Rahmioglu N, Montgomery GW, Zondervan KT. Genetics of endometriosis. *Womens Health (Lond)* 2015;**11**:577–86.

14. Burney RO, Giudice LC. Pathogenesis and pathophysiology of endometriosis. *Fertil Steril* 2012;**98**:511–19.

15. Giudice LC, Kao LC. Endometriosis. *Lancet* 2004;**364**:1789–99.

16. Tirado-González I, Barrientos G, Tariverdian N, et al. Endometriosis research: animal models for the study of a complex disease. *J Reprod Immunol* 2010;**86**:141–47.

17. D'Hooghe TM, Bambra CS, Raeymaekers BM, De Jonge I, Lauweryns JM, Koninckx PR. Intrapelvic injection of menstrual endometrium causes endometriosis in baboons (Papio cynocephalus and Papio anubis). *Am J Obstet Gynecol* 1995;**173**:125–34.

18. Kyama CM, Overbergh L, Debrock S, et al. Increased peritoneal and endometrial gene expression of biologically relevant cytokines and growth factors during the menstrual phase in women with endometriosis. *Fertil Steril* 2006;**85**:1667–75.

19. Kyama CM, Overbergh L, Mihalyi A, et al. Endometrial and peritoneal expression of aromatase, cytokines, and adhesion factors in women with endometriosis. *Fertil Steril* 2008;**89**:301–10.

20. Oosterlynck DJ, Cornillie FJ, Waer M, Vandeputte M, Koninckx PR. Women with endometriosis show a defect in natural killer activity resulting in a decreased cytotoxicity to autologous endometrium. *Fertil Steril* 1991;**56**:45–51.

21. Somigliana E, Viganò P, Gaffuri B, Guarneri D, Busacca M, Vignali M. Human endometrial stromal cells as a source of soluble intercellular adhesion molecule (ICAM)-1 molecules. *Hum Reprod* 1996;**11**:1190–94.

22. Somigliana E, Viganò P, Gaffuri B, et al. Modulation of NK cell lytic function by endometrial secretory factors: potential role in endometriosis. *Am J Reprod Immunol* 1996;**36**:295–300.

23. Sharpe-Timms KL, Zimmer RL, Ricke EA, Piva M, Horowitz GM. Endometriotic haptoglobin binds to peritoneal macrophages and alters their function in women with endometriosis. *Fertil Steril* 2002;**78**:810–19.

24. Laschke MW, Menger MD. In vitro and in vivo approaches to study angiogenesis in the pathophysiology and therapy of endometriosis. *Hum Reprod Update* 2007;**13**:331–42.

25. Suginami H. A reappraisal of the coelomic metaplasia theory by reviewing endometriosis occurring in unusual sites and instances. *Am J Obstet Gynecol* 1991;**165**:214–18.

26. Meuleman C, Tomassetti C, D'Hoore A, et al. Clinical outcome after CO laser laparoscopic radical excision of endometriosis with colorectal wall invasion combined with laparoscopic segmental bowel resection and reanastomosis. *Hum Reprod* 2011;**26**:2336–43.

27. Kumar S, Tiwari P, Sharma P, et al. Urinary tract endometriosis: review of 19 cases. *Urol Ann* 2012;**4**:6–12.

28. Abrão MS, Petraglia F, Falcone T, Keckstein J, Osuga Y, Chapron C. Deep endometriosis infiltrating the recto-sigmoid: critical factors to consider before management. *Hum Reprod Update* 2015;**21**:329–39.

29. Maccagnano C, Pellucchi F, Rocchini L, et al. Diagnosis and treatment of bladder endometriosis: state of the art. *Urol Int* 2012;**89**:249–58.

30. Ghezzi F, Cromi A, Bergamini V, Bolis P. Management of ureteral endometriosis: areas of controversy. *Curr Opin Obstet Gynecol* 2007;**19**:319–24.

31. Chapron C, Chiodo I, Leconte M, et al. Severe ureteral endometriosis: the intrinsic type is not so rare after complete surgical exeresis of deep endometriotic lesions. *Fertil Steril* 2010;**93**:2115–20.

32. [No authors listed] Revised American Society for Reproductive Medicine classification of endometriosis: 1996. *Fertil Steril* 1997;**67**:817–21.

33. Adamson GD. Endometriosis classification: an update. *Curr Opin Obstet Gynecol* 2011;**23**:213–20.

34. Adamson GD, Pasta DJ. Endometriosis fertility index: the new, validated endometriosis staging system. *Fertil Steril* 2010;**94**:1609–15.

35. Tomassetti C, Geysenbergh B, Meuleman C, Timmerman D, Fieuws S, D'Hooghe T. External validation of the endometriosis fertility index (EFI) staging system for predicting non-ART pregnancy after endometriosis surgery. *Hum Reprod* 2013;**28**:1280–88.

36. Tuttlies F, Keckstein J, Ulrich U, et al. [ENZIAN-score, a classification of deep infiltrating endometriosis.] *Zentralbl Gynakol* 2005;**127**:275–81.

37. Haas D, Shebl O, Shamiyeh A, Oppelt P. The rASRM score and the Enzian classification for endometriosis: their strengths and weaknesses. *Acta Obstet Gynecol Scand* 2013;**92**:3–7.

38. Practice Committee of the American Society for Reproductive Medicine. Treatment of pelvic pain associated with endometriosis: a committee opinion. *Fertil Steril* 2014;**101**:927–35.

39. Nisenblat V, Bossuyt PM, Farquhar C, Johnson N, Hull ML. Imaging modalities for the non-invasive diagnosis of endometriosis. *Cochrane Database Syst Rev* 2016;**2**:CD009591.

40. Faccioli N1, Foti G, Manfredi R, et al. Barium enema evaluation of colonic involvement in endometriosis. *AJR Am J Roentgenol* 2008;**190**:1050–54.

41. Ribeiro HS, Ribeiro PA, Rossini L, Rodrigues FC, Donadio N, Aoki T. Double-contrast barium enema and transrectal endoscopic ultrasonography in the diagnosis of intestinal deeply infiltrating endometriosis. *J Minim Invasive Gynecol* 2008;**15**:315–20.

42. Savelli L, Manuzzi L, Coe M, et al. Comparison of transvaginal sonography and double-contrast barium enema for diagnosing deep infiltrating endometriosis of the posterior compartment. *Ultrasound Obstet Gynecol* 2011;**38**:466–71.

43. Vanhie A, Meuleman C, Tomassetti C, et al. Consensus on recording deep endometriosis surgery: the CORDES statement. *Hum Reprod* 2016;**31**:1219–23.

44. Exacoustos C, Malzoni M, Di Giovanni A, et al. Ultrasound mapping system for the surgical management of deep infiltrating endometriosis. *Fertil Steril* 2014;**102**:143–50.e2.

45. Bellelis P, Dias JA Jr, Podgaec S, Gonzales M, Baracat EC, Abrão MS. Epidemiological and clinical aspects of pelvic endometriosis-a case series. *Rev Assoc Med Bras* 2010;**56**:467–71.

46. Nnoaham KE, Hummelshoj L, Kennedy SH, et al. Developing symptom-based predictive models of endometriosis as a clinical screening tool: results from a multicenter study. *Fertil Steril* 2012;**98**:692–701.e5.

47. Koninckx PR1, Meuleman C, Oosterlynck D, Cornillie FJ. Diagnosis of deep endometriosis by clinical examination during menstruation and plasma CA-125 concentration. *Fertil Steril* 1996;**65**:280–87.

48. Bazot M, Lafont C, Rouzier R, et al. Diagnostic accuracy of physical examination, transvaginal sonography, rectal endoscopic sonography, and magnetic resonance imaging to diagnose deep infiltrating endometriosis. *Fertil Steril* 2009;**92**:1825–33.

49. Chapron C, Dubuisson JB, Pansini V, et al. Routine clinical examination is not sufficient for diagnosing and locating deeply infiltrating endometriosis. *J Am Assoc Gynecol Laparosc* 2002;**9**:115–19.

50. [No authors listed] Practice bulletin no. 114: management of endometriosis. *Obstet Gynecol* 2010;**116**:223–36.

51. Van Holsbeke C, Van Calster B, Guerriero S, et al. Endometriomas: their ultrasound characteristics. *Ultrasound Obstet Gynecol* 2010;**35**:730–40.

52. Hudelist G, English J, Thomas AE, Tinelli A, Singer CF, Keckstein J. Diagnostic accuracy of transvaginal ultrasound for non-invasive diagnosis of bowel endometriosis: systematic review and meta-analysis. *Ultrasound Obstet Gynecol* 2011;**37**:257–63.

53. Redwine DB. Ovarian endometriosis: a marker for more extensive pelvic and intestinal disease. *Fertil Steril* 1999;**72**:310–15.

54. Noventa M, Saccardi C, Litta P, et al. Ultrasound techniques in the diagnosis of deep pelvic endometriosis: algorithm based on a systematic review and meta-analysis. *Fertil Steril* 2015;**104**:366–83.e2.

55. Saba L, Sulcis R, Melis GB, et al. Endometriosis: the role of magnetic resonance imaging. *Acta Radiol* 2015;**56**:355–67.

56. Kinkel K, Frei KA, Balleyguier C, Chapron C. Diagnosis of endometriosis with imaging: a review. *Eur Radiol* 2006;**16**:285–98.

57. Wykes CB, Clark TJ, Khan KS. Accuracy of laparoscopy in the diagnosis of endometriosis: a systematic quantitative review. *BJOG* 2004;**111**:1204–12.

58. Clement PB. The pathology of endometriosis: a survey of the many faces of a common disease emphasizing diagnostic pitfalls and unusual and newly appreciated aspects. *Adv Anat Pathol* 2007;**14**:241–60.

59. Jenkins TR, Liu CY, White J. Does response to hormonal therapy predict presence or absence of endometriosis? *J Minim Invasive Gynecol* 2008;**15**:82–86.

60. Practice Committee of the American Society for Reproductive Medicine. Endometriosis and infertility: a committee opinion. *Fertil Steril* 2012;**98**:591–98.

61. Vercellini P, Crosignani P, Somigliana E, Viganò P, Frattaruolo MP, Fedele L. 'Waiting for Godot': a commonsense approach to the medical treatment of endometriosis. *Hum Reprod* 2011;**26**:3–13.

62. Marjoribanks J, Proctor M, Farquhar C, Derks RS. Nonsteroidal anti-inflammatory drugs for dysmenorrhoea. *Cochrane Database Syst Rev* 2010;**1**:CD001751.

63. Allen C, Hopewell S, Prentice A. Nonsteroidal anti-inflammatory drugs for pain in women with endometriosis. *Cochrane Database Syst Rev* 2009;**2**:CD004753.

64. Davis L, Kennedy SS, Moore J, Prentice A. Oral contraceptives for pain associated with endometriosis. *Cochrane Database Syst Rev* 2007;**3**:CD001019.

65. Meresman GF, Augé L, Barañao RI, Lombardi E, Tesone M, Sueldo C. Oral contraceptives suppress cell proliferation and enhance apoptosis of eutopic endometrial tissue from patients with endometriosis. *Fertil Steril* 2002;**77**:1141–47.

66. Vercellini P, Trespidi L, Colombo A, Vendola N, Marchini M, Crosignani PG. A gonadotropin-releasing hormone agonist versus a low-dose oral contraceptive for pelvic pain associated with endometriosis. *Fertil Steril* 1993;**60**:75–79.

67. Brown J, Kives S, Akhtar M. Progestagens and anti-progestagens for pain associated with endometriosis. *Cochrane Database Syst Rev* 2012;**3**:CD002122.

68. Olive DL. Gonadotropin-releasing hormone agonists for endometriosis. *N Engl J Med* 2008;**359**:1136–42.

69. Barbieri RL. Hormone treatment of endometriosis: the estrogen threshold hypothesis. *Am J Obstet Gynecol* 1992;**166**:740–45.

70. Brown J, Pan A, Hart RJ. Gonadotrophin-releasing hormone analogues for pain associated with endometriosis. *Cochrane Database Syst Rev* 2010;**12**:CD008475.

71. Makarainen L, Ronnberg L, Kauppila A. Medroxyprogesterone acetate supplementation diminishes the hypoestrogenic side effects of gonadotropin-releasing hormone agonist without changing its efficacy in endometriosis. *Fertil Steril* 1996;**65**:29–34.

72. Moghissi KS, Schlaff WD, Olive DL, Skinner MA, Yin H. Goserelin acetate (Zoladex) with or without hormone replacement therapy for the treatment of endometriosis. *Fertil Steril* 1998;**69**:1056–62.

73. Taskin O, Yalcinoglu AI, Kucuk S, Uryan I, Buhur A, Burak F. Effectiveness of tibolone on hypoestrogenic symptoms induced by goserelin treatment in patients with endometriosis. *Fertil Steril* 1997;**67**:40–45.

74. Bergqvist A, Jacobson J, Harris S. A double-blind randomized study of the treatment of endometriosis with nafarelin or nafarelin plus norethisterone. *Gynecol Endocrinol* 1997;**11**:187–94.

75. Ferrero S, Venturini PL, Ragni N, Camerini G, Remorgida V. Pharmacological treatment of endometriosis: experience with aromatase inhibitors. *Drugs* 2009;**69**:943–52.

76. Ferrero S, Remorgida V, Maganza C, et al. Aromatase and endometriosis: estrogens play a role. *Ann N Y Acad Sci* 2014;**1317**:17–23.

77. Bulun SE, Fang Z, Imir G, et al. Aromatase and endometriosis. *Semin Reprod Med* 2004;**22**:45–50.

78. Ferrero S, Gillott DJ, Venturini PL, Remorgida V. Use of aromatase inhibitors to treat endometriosis-related pain symptoms: a systematic review. *Reprod Biol Endocrinol* 2011;**9**:89.

79. Crosignani PG, Vercellini P, Biffignandi F, Costantini W, Cortesi I, Imparato E. Laparoscopy versus laparotomy in

conservative surgical treatment for severe endometriosis. *Fertil Steril* 1996;**66**:706–11.

80. Duffy JM, Arambage K, Correa FJ, et al. Laparoscopic surgery for endometriosis. *Cochrane Database Syst Rev* 2014;**4**:CD011031.

81. Healey M, Ang WC, Cheng C. Surgical treatment of endometriosis: a prospective randomized double-blinded trial comparing excision and ablation. *Fertil Steril* 2010;**94**:2536–40.

82. Wright J, Lotfallah H, Jones K, Lovell D. A randomized trial of excision versus ablation for mild endometriosis. *Fertil Steril* 2005;**83**:1830–36.

83. Carmona F, Martínez-Zamora MA, Rabanal A, Martínez-Román S, Balasch J. Ovarian cystectomy versus laser vaporization in the treatment of ovarian endometriomas: a randomized clinical trial with a five-year follow-up. *Fertil Steril* 2011;**96**:251–54.

84. Hart RJ, Hickey M, Maouris P, Buckett W. Excisional surgery versus ablative surgery for ovarian endometriomata. *Cochrane Database Syst Rev* 2008;**2**:CD004992.

85. Raffi F, Metwally M, Amer S. The impact of excision of ovarian endometrioma on ovarian reserve: a systematic review and meta-analysis. *J Clin Endocrinol Metab* 2012;**97**:3146–54.

86. Busacca M, Riparini J, Somigliana E, et al. Postsurgical ovarian failure after laparoscopic excision of bilateral endometriomas. *Am J Obstet Gynecol* 2006;**195**:421–25.

87. Meuleman C, Tomassetti C, D'Hooghe TM. Clinical outcome after laparoscopic radical excision of endometriosis and laparoscopic segmental bowel resection. *Curr Opin Obstet Gynecol* 2012;**24**:245–52.

88. Meuleman C, Tomassetti C, D'Hoore A, et al. Surgical treatment of deeply infiltrating endometriosis with colorectal involvement. *Hum Reprod Update* 2011;**17**:311–26.

89. De Cicco C, Corona R, Schonman R, Mailova K, Ussia A, Koninckx P. Bowel resection for deep endometriosis: a systematic review. *BJOG* 2011;**118**:285–91.

90. Martin DC. Hysterectomy for treatment of pain associated with endometriosis. *J Minim Invasive Gynecol* 2006;**13**:566–72.

91. Proctor ML, Latthe PM, Farquhar CM, Khan KS, Johnson NP. Surgical interruption of pelvic nerve pathways for primary and secondary dysmenorrhoea. *Cochrane Database Syst Rev* 2005;**4**:CD001896.

92. Hughes E, Brown J, Collins JJ, Farquhar C, Fedorkow DM, Vandekerckhove P. Ovulation suppression for endometriosis. *Cochrane Database Syst Rev* 2007;**3**:CD000155.

93. Jacobson TZ, Duffy JM, Barlow D, Farquhar C, Koninckx PR, Olive D. Laparoscopic surgery for subfertility associated with endometriosis. *Cochrane Database Syst Rev* 2010;**1**:CD001398.

94. Vercellini P, Fedele L, Aimi G, De Giorgi O, Consonni D, Crosignani PG. Reproductive performance, pain recurrence and disease relapse after conservative surgical treatment for endometriosis: the predictive value of the current classification system. *Hum Reprod* 2006;**21**:2679–85.

95. Yap C, Furness S, Farquhar C. Pre and post operative medical therapy for endometriosis surgery. *Cochrane Database Syst Rev* 2004;**3**:CD003678.

96. Zegers-Hochschild F, Adamson GD, de Mouzon J, et al. International Committee for Monitoring Assisted Reproductive Technology (ICMART) and the World Health Organization (WHO) revised glossary of ART terminology, 2009. *Fertil Steril* 2009;**92**:1520–24.

97. Werbrouck E, Spiessens C, Meuleman C, D'Hooghe T. No difference in cycle pregnancy rate and in cumulative live-birth rate between women with surgically treated minimal to mild endometriosis and women with unexplained infertility after controlled ovarian hyperstimulation and intrauterine insemination. *Fertil Steril* 2006;**86**:566–71.

98. Barnhart K, Dunsmoor-Su R, Coutifaris C. Effect of endometriosis on in vitro fertilization. *Fertil Steril* 2002;**77**:1148–55.

99. D'Hooghe TM, Denys B, Spiessens C, Meuleman C, Debrock S. Is the endometriosis recurrence rate increased after ovarian hyperstimulation? *Fertil Steril* 2006;**86**:283–90.

100. Coccia ME, Rizzello F, Gianfranco S. Does controlled ovarian hyperstimulation in women with a history of endometriosis influence recurrence rate? *J Womens Health (Larchmt)* 2010;**19**:2063–69.

101. Benaglia L, Somigliana E, Vercellini P, et al. The impact of IVF procedures on endometriosis recurrence. *Eur J Obstet Gynecol Reprod Biol* 2010;**148**:49–52.

102. Benaglia L, Pasin R, Somigliana E, Vercellini P, Ragni G, Fedele L. Unoperated ovarian endometriomas and responsiveness to hyperstimulation. *Hum Reprod* 2011;**26**:1356–61.

103. Sallam HN, Garcia-Velasco JA, Dias S, Arici A. Long-term pituitary down-regulation before in vitro fertilization (IVF) for women with endometriosis. *Cochrane Database Syst Rev* 2006;**1**:CD004635.

104. Opøien HK, Fedorcsak P, Byholm T, Tanbo T. Complete surgical removal of minimal and mild endometriosis improves outcome of subsequent IVF/ICSI treatment. *Reprod Biomed Online* 2011;**23**:389–95.

105. Vercellini P, Eskenazi B, Consonni D, et al. Oral contraceptives and risk of endometriosis: a systematic review and meta-analysis. *Hum Reprod Update* 2011;**17**:159–70.

106. Vitonis AF, Hankinson SE, Hornstein MD, Missmer SA. Adult physical activity and endometriosis risk. *Epidemiology* 2010;**21**:16–23.

107. Cramer DW, Wilson E, Stillman RJ, et al. The relation of endometriosis to menstrual characteristics, smoking, and exercise. *JAMA* 1986;**255**:1904–908.

108. Signorello LB1, Harlow BL, Cramer DW, Spiegelman D, Hill JA. Epidemiologic determinants of endometriosis: a hospital-based case-control study. *Ann Epidemiol* 1997;**7**:267–74.

109. Dhillon PK, Holt VL. Recreational physical activity and endometrioma risk. *Am J Epidemiol* 2003;**158**:156–64.

110. Heilier JF, Donnez J, Nackers F, et al. Environmental and host-associated risk factors in endometriosis and deep endometriotic nodules: a matched case-control study. *Environ Res* 2007;**103**:121–29.

111. Johnson NP, Hummelshoj L, World Endometriosis Society Montpellier Consortium. Consensus on current management of endometriosis. *Hum Reprod* 2013;**28**:1552–68.

46

Menopause

Jenifer Sassarini and Mary Ann Lumsden

Introduction

Definition

Menopause is part of the normal ageing process and will occur in all women who live long enough. The diagnosis is clinical. Natural menopause is a retrospective diagnosis that can only be made after 12 months of amenorrhoea, that is not associated with some other physiological (e.g. lactation) or pathological cause and, in the United Kingdom, the mean age is 51 years.

STRAW+10

Menopause occurs as a result of oocyte depletion in the ovary. This is associated with an increase in circulating follicle-stimulating hormone (FSH) and a decrease in circulating oestrogen. In 2001, the World Health Organization (WHO) and Stages of Reproductive Ageing Workshop (STRAW) Working Groups defined menopause as the permanent cessation of menstrual periods that occurs naturally or is induced by surgery, chemotherapy, or radiation.

WHO recommended the use of 'perimenopause' and 'menopausal transition' in place of 'climacteric' in 1996 and a model was developed in 2001 to describe the stages of the menopausal transition. The model identifies seven stages of reproductive life and is primarily based on the characteristics of the menstrual cycle and secondarily, on follicular phase FSH concentrations in the circulation. The model was reviewed in 2011, STRAW+10, and has been recommended regardless of women's age, ethnicity, body size, or lifestyle characteristics (**Figure 46.1**).

As women progress through the menopausal transition, the menstrual cycle becomes irregular, and FSH levels are raised in response to decreased ovarian hormone concentrations, normally starting to rise around the age of 38. Menstrual cycles are then missed and ultimately stop, as does ovulation; however, the change in gonadotropins and sex steroids actually starts in the late 30s as the rate of decrease in the ovarian follicle numbers escalates. During the perimenopause, FSH levels can fluctuate considerably in response to spasmodic oestrogen production from the ovary.

Physiology

Figure 46.2 shows a rapid decrease in the number of primordial follicles after the age of 40 years. Fewer follicles result in decreased secretion of inhibin B, with a subsequent increase in FSH that can maintain oestradiol until follicle depletion. Levels of serum FSH begin to increase in women still having regular cycles.

Diagnosis

The recommendation from the National Institute for Health and Care Excellence (NICE) guideline, published in 2015, is to diagnose menopause clinically, on the basis of menstrual history and age. Biochemical measurements are not required in women who are over the age of 45 years. Vasomotor symptoms and irregular periods suggest perimenopause, while menopause may be diagnosed in women who have not had a period in at least 12 months.

NICE recommends measuring FSH levels in women who are between the age of 40 and 45 years, who present with symptoms, including a change in their menstrual cycle, and in women under the age of 40 years, in whom menopause is suspected (2).

Premature ovarian insufficiency

Premature ovarian insufficiency (POI), previously known as premature ovarian failure, is defined as the loss of normal ovarian function before the age of 40 years. Approximately 1% of women in the United Kingdom will experience an early loss of ovarian function secondary to a number of aetiologies. About 1 in 1000 women under the age of 30 years, are affected.

Causes of POI

There are three main identifiable causes of POI—genetic, autoimmune, or iatrogenic:

- Genetic conditions include a strong maternal family history; 45X, 46XX, and 46XY POI; and POI associated with galactosaemia and *FMR1* (fragile X mental retardation 1) gene premutations.
- Women with an autoimmune predisposition may develop autoimmune POI, with or without other autoimmune diseases (diabetes mellitus, Addison's disease, thyroid disease).
- Women with iatrogenic menopause form an increasingly large group. These are women whose treatments for cancer (hormonal, chemotherapy, and/or radiotherapy) have brought about an earlier menopause.

Menarche — n

Final menstrual period (FMP) — 0

Stage		−5	−4	−3b	−3a	−2	−1	+1a	+1b	+1c	+2
Terminology		**Reproductive**				**Menopausal transition**		**Postmenopause**			
		Early	Peak	Late		Early	Late	Early			Late
				Perimenopause							
Duration		variable				variable	1–3 years	2 years (1+1)	3–6 years		Remaining lifespan
PRINCIPAL CRITERIA											
Menstrual cycle		Variable to regular	Regular	Regular	Subtle changes in flow/length	Variable cycle length (persistent 7 or more day difference in length of consecutive cycles)	An interval of amenorrhoea ≥ 60 days				
SUPPORTIVE CRITERIA											
Endocrine FSH AMH Inhibin B				Low Low Low	Variable Low Low	↑ Variable Low Low	↑ ≥ (25IU/l) Low Low	↑ Variable Low Low	Stabilises Low Low		
Antral Follicle Count				Low	Low	Low	Low	Very Low	Very Low		
DESCRIPTIVE CHARACTERISTICS											
Symptoms						Vasomotor symptoms likely	Vasomotor symptoms most likely				Increasing symptoms of urogenital atrophy

Figure 46.1 The STRAW+10 staging system for reproductive ageing in women.

Reproduced from Executive summary of the Stages of Reproductive Aging Workshop + 10: addressing the unfinished agenda of staging reproductive aging. Harlow SD, Gass M, Hall JE, Lobo R, et al. for the STRAW+10 Collaborative Group. *Climacteric* 2012;15:105–114.

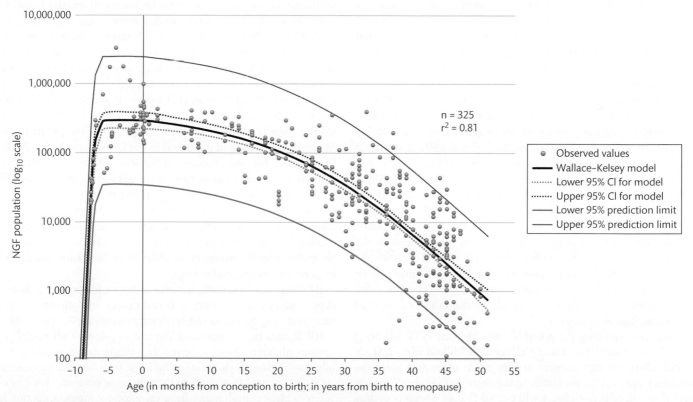

n = 325
$r^2 = 0.81$

- Observed values
— Wallace–Kelsey model
····· Lower 95% CI for model
······ Upper 95% CI for model
— Lower 95% prediction limit
— Upper 95% prediction limit

NGF population ($\log_{10}$ scale)

Age (in months from conception to birth; in years from birth to menopause)

Figure 46.2 The number of non-growing follicles from conception to the menopause.

Reproduced from Wallace WH, Kelsey W. Human ovarian reserve from conception to the menopause. *PLoS One* 2010;5:e8772.

In most women, the cause of an early menopause is unknown.

POI is associated with decreased bone mass and fractures, an increased risk of premature death from cardiovascular disease, as well as dementia and Parkinsonism (3–5). There is also fertility compromise associated not only with the loss of ovarian function but, in those with prepubertal POI, inadequate uterine morphology.

As well as managing clinical and physical issues, these young women need support and holistic care with a number of psychosocial issues, such as infertility, sexuality, and psychological distress.

Diagnosis of POI

The diagnosis should be based on the presence of menstrual disturbance and biochemical confirmation. Take into account previous medical or surgical treatment, and family history when diagnosing premature ovarian insufficiency.

The European Society for Human Reproduction and Embryology (6) recommend diagnosing premature ovarian insufficiency in women aged under 40 years based on:

- oligo/amenorrhoea for at least 4 months, and
- elevated FSH level greater than 25 IU/L on two occasions more than 4 weeks apart.

Anti-Mullerian hormone testing should not routinely be used to diagnose premature ovarian insufficiency, although this test is widely used in reproductive medicine as a means of assessing the woman's 'ovarian reserve' and likely response (or lack of it) to gonadotropin stimulation prior to *in vitro* fertilization.

Management of POI

Treatment should be multidisciplinary, with consideration given to prevention of potential morbidities, reproductive healthcare including fertility and contraception, and the provision of counselling and emotional support. Ideally, these women should be seen in dedicated clinics, with ease of access to a multidisciplinary team.

It is widely accepted that the mainstay of treatment of POI is sex steroid replacement. 17β-oestradiol is preferred to ethinylestradiol or conjugated equine oestrogens for oestrogen replacement (6). Patient preference for route and method of administration of each component of hormonal replacement therapy (HRT) must be considered when prescribing, as should contraceptive needs. About 50% of young women with spontaneous POI experience intermittent and unpredictable ovarian function (7), although there is only a 5–10% chance of spontaneous conception (8). This is vital when considering treatment, as HRT is not a contraceptive, therefore, the combined oral contraceptive pill may be the treatment of choice, rather than HRT. Both provide bone protection, but HRT may provide a beneficial effect on blood pressure compared to the combined oral contraceptive pill (9). Treatment should be continued at least until the average age of menopause.

Concerns regarding the potential risks of using HRT, following the Women's Health Initiative (WHI) and the Million Women Study publications, are not relevant to this group of women since the ovarian failure occurs prematurely and there is no evidence to suggest that risk of breast cancer will exceed that of normally cycling women of similar age.

Symptoms of the menopause

There are a number of symptoms associated with perimenopause, although some women will experience none of these. They include hot flushes and night sweats (vasomotor symptoms), urogenital symptoms, depression, anxiety, irritability and mood swings (psychological effects), joint pains, migraines or headaches, and sleeping problems.

Short-term symptoms

Vasomotor symptoms

The most commonly reported symptoms in the West are hot flushes and night sweats, and a recent study has demonstrated that women may experience symptoms for a median duration of 7.4 years.

Hot flushes are characterized by a feeling of intense warmth, often accompanied by profuse sweating, anxiety, skin reddening, and palpitations, and sometimes followed by chills.

The exact pathophysiology underlying vasomotor symptoms is not known; oestrogens undoubtedly play a role, as flushing occurs at times of relative oestrogen withdrawal, and replacing oestrogen improves symptoms. However, oestrogen levels remain low, and flushing improves with time. Moreover, women who have never been exposed to oestrogen will not flush, unless first treated with oestrogen, which is then withdrawn. This suggests that it is the withdrawal of oestrogen, rather than low circulating levels that are responsible for this symptom, and this would seem to be supported by the symptoms experienced by premenopausal women following surgical removal of the ovaries.

Menopause induced by surgery is associated with about a 90% probability of hot flushes during the first year and symptoms associated with surgical menopause are often more abrupt and severe and can last longer than those associated with a non-surgical menopause.

Hot flushes are the most common indication for the prescription of hormone therapy (HT) since it is effective in over 80% of cases. Concern that the risks of HT outweighed the benefits, following publication of the WHI trials (10), led to a dramatic decrease in the use of HT. Reanalysis of the data as well as analysis of subgroups have led to a global consensus statement, endorsed by the International Menopause Society, and published in 2013, which states that 'MHT [menopausal hormone therapy] is the most effective treatment for vasomotor symptoms associated with menopause at any age, but benefits are more likely to outweigh risks for symptomatic women before the age of 60 years or within 10 years after menopause' (11). The recent publication of the NICE guideline on menopause has recommended that HRT can be offered for the treatment of vasomotor symptoms after discussion of the short-term (less than 5 years) and longer-term benefits and risks (2).

HRT may not be suitable for women with a history of hormone-dependent cancer, for example, breast cancer, and other treatment modalities may be considered; however, none are as effective as HRT.

NICE does not recommend the use of selective serotonin reuptake inhibitors (SSRIs), serotonin noradrenaline reuptake inhibitors (SNRIs), or clonidine as first-line treatment for vasomotor symptoms alone (2), and while there is some evidence that isoflavones or black cohosh may relieve vasomotor symptoms, caution is advised, as interactions with other medicines have been reported. In addition, there are multiple preparations available, these may vary and their safety is uncertain.

Urogenital symptoms

The female urogenital tract arises embryonically from the urogenital sinus, and high-affinity oestrogen and progesterone receptors have been found in the vagina, urethra, trigone of the bladder, and pelvic floor musculature.

A loss of oestrogen results in urogenital ageing. The vaginal walls become pale and thin as a result of reduced collagen, decreased elastin, and thinning of the epithelium. A loss of elasticity, and a reduction in vaginal secretions, leads to a susceptibility to trauma and pain during intercourse, which in turn can lead to pain and irritation after sex.

The vaginal pH becomes less acidic, and increases the likelihood of urinary tract infections. There may also be urinary frequency and urgency, and nocturia, and as such, menopause-related genitourinary changes are not confined to the vulva and vagina. What has long been termed *vulvovaginal atrophy* or *atrophic vaginitis* has now been recognized to be inadequate, and a terminology consensus conference, comprising the International Society for the Study of Women's Sexual Health and the North American Menopause Society, formally endorsed new terminology—genitourinary syndrome of menopause—in 2014.

Genitourinary symptoms attributable to the menopause can affect up to 50% of women; however, these are underdiagnosed and undertreated. They may be chronic and, without treatment, are unlikely to improve over time. By increasing skin collagen content, and increasing acid mucopolysaccharides and hyaluronic acid, oestrogen therapy encourages the growth and development of vaginal epithelial cells which make up the thick layers of the vaginal wall, and condone a moist, supple, and elastic environment.

Vaginal symptoms and sexual dysfunction

Vaginal symptoms become apparent 4–5 years after the menopause and are present in 25–50% of all postmenopausal women. Symptoms may include vaginal dryness (75%), dyspareunia (38%), vaginal itching, burning, and pain (15%). Dyspareunia can adversely affect a postmenopausal woman's sexual quality of life or intensify pre-existing sexual disorders.

Vaginal oestrogens are an effective treatment for menopause-related vulval and vaginal symptoms and a Cochrane review reported equal efficacy across all products tested: creams, pessaries, tablets, and vaginal rings (12). On behalf of the International Menopause Society Writing Group, Sturdee and Panay (13) recommend treatment of established vaginal atrophy to restore physiology and alleviate symptoms. These have subsequently been supported by NICE. Local oestrogen therapy will lower vaginal pH, thicken the epithelium, increase blood flow, and improve vaginal lubrication. Vaginal oestrogens should be offered to women with urogenital atrophy (including those on systemic HRT) and treatment should be continued for as long as required to relieve symptoms (2). Women should be aware that symptoms often come back when treatment is stopped.

A 2009 review of topical oestrogen demonstrated no evidence of endometrial proliferation after 6–24 months of use, therefore progestins and the monitoring of endometrial thickness are not required with topical oestrogens (2, 14). However, any postmenopausal bleeding should be investigated in the usual way.

Use of vaginal oestrogen for women with a history of breast cancer is controversial. Vulval and vaginal symptoms are common in this group of patients particularly those on endocrine therapies such as aromatase inhibitors and antioestrogens. In a case–control study, there was no documented increase in recurrence in those women receiving endocrine therapy and use of local oestrogen compared to non-use (15). However, in another study of breast cancer survivors, there was an initial, albeit unsustained, increase in circulating oestrogen concentrations (16), measured using an ultra-sensitive oestrogen assay. These women should be referred to a specialist clinic, to discuss the risks and benefits of treatment.

Non-hormonal treatment options include lubricants and moisturizers. Lubricants are non-physiological, but may reduce friction-related irritation of vaginal tissues, while moisturizers are hydrophilic, insoluble, cross-linked polymers which reduce vaginal pH. In a trial of vaginal moisturizer compared to low-dose vaginal oestrogen, both preparations were found to be effective, but the moisturizer provided only temporary benefit.

Urinary symptoms

Overactive bladder is a highly prevalent disorder, with higher rates and symptom severity in postmenopausal women. Oestrogen deficiency has been implicated in the aetiology of urinary tract symptoms with up to 70% of women relating the onset of their incontinence to their last menstrual period. Oestrogen has been used for decades to treat this, yet a Cochrane review (17) concluded that there was insufficient evidence to support the use of local oestrogens and that systemic oestrogens may make incontinence worse. The WHI study showed no protective effect of HT against incontinence. In fact, among women who had incontinence at baseline, incontinence episodes were seen to be increased in both studies. However, the mean age in WHI was 63.3 years and women had a greater than average number of comorbidities. In addition, the findings were as a result of secondary analysis and not a primary outcome measure.

The Fourth International Consultation on Incontinence has given oestrogen a grade C recommendation based on a level of evidence of 2 of overactive bladder and concluded that there is no solid evidence to support the use of HT, oral or vaginal, for the treatment of urge urinary incontinence. Grade A recommendations include weight reduction, supervised pelvic floor muscle training, and bladder training and antimuscarinics (18).

Long-term consequences

Osteoporosis

The onset of the menopause, with associated decline in oestrogen, results in a decrease in bone mineral density and a subsequent significant increase in the prevalence of osteoporosis, which continues to increase through the postmenopausal period. The number of hip fractures worldwide due to osteoporosis is expected to rise threefold by 2050, from 1.7 million in 1990 to 6.3 million.

The National Osteoporosis Guideline Group advises that fracture probability should be assessed in postmenopausal women, using a fracture risk assessment tool (FRAX), for cases in which such an assessment would influence management (19).

The optimal management of osteoporosis is aimed at primary prevention for those at risk, while general management includes assessment of the risk of falls and their prevention, maintenance of mobility, and correction of nutritional deficiencies, particularly of calcium, vitamin D, and protein.

Pharmacological interventions include bisphosphonates, denosumab, parathyroid hormone peptides, raloxifene, and strontium ranelate. All have been shown to reduce the risk of vertebral fracture and some have been shown to reduce the risk of non-vertebral fractures (19).

There is evidence from randomized controlled trials (RCTs), including WHI, that HT reduces the risk of spine and hip, as well as other osteoporotic fractures even in women at low risk. It would appear that half of the traditional doses (oestradiol 2 mg, conjugated equine oestrogen 0.625 mg and transdermal 50 mcg patch) may be effective in conserving bone mass although the effect of oestrogen on bone mass is dose dependent.

Regulators do not recommended HT as first-line treatment in the prevention of osteoporosis, because risks outweigh benefits; however, a statement released by the British Menopause Society states that 'whilst this may be true for a population with no increased osteoporosis risk, … the risk-benefit ratio changes favourably when targeting a population with increased osteoporosis risk'. Oestrogen remains the treatment of choice in women with premature ovarian failure, and may be the best option in women under the age of 60, however, 'the initiation of standard dose HT is not recommended solely for fracture prevention in women over 60' (20). All women using oestrogen for symptoms should be made aware that it has a bone protective effect (2).

Cardiovascular disease

Cardiovascular disease is the leading cause of death in women worldwide, but is often unreported in women before the age of 55. Menopausal status has been included in the Framingham risk calculator as an independent risk factor and a premature menopause is associated with a doubling of risk. It has been proposed that hypo-oestrogenism plays a role, but there has been some conflicting data over the years with regard to risk versus benefit of oestrogen replacement.

Before the publication of the WHI results, HT was thought to confer cardiovascular disease risk reduction, particularly in coronary events. The principal results of the WHI trial, the largest randomized controlled primary prevention trial of the most commonly prescribed HT in the United States, demonstrated an increased number of coronary heart disease events and strokes, and concluded that the risks outweighed the benefits.

However, the average age of participants in the WHI was 63 years, 12 years older than the average age of menopause in the United Kingdom; therefore, it is possible that the women in these studies had established subclinical atherosclerosis.

Subgroup analysis of data from the WHI trials examined HT use stratified by age and time since menopause, and demonstrated more favourable results for all-cause mortality and myocardial infarction in women aged 50–59 years, and those close to menopause (21). This 'window of opportunity' has been supported by the Danish Osteoporosis trial (DOPS), which demonstrated a reduction in risk of mortality, heart failure, or myocardial infarction, after 10 years of hormone replacement therapy, started soon after menopause (22).

At present, in women under the age of 60 years, there is no increase in cardiovascular disease risk with HT, but there are insufficient data to support the use of HT for cardiovascular disease prevention. Women should be told that there is a small increased risk of stroke when taking oral (but not transdermal) oestrogen, but it should also be noted that the baseline risk of stroke in women under the age of 60 years is very low.

Dementia

Dementia is not a normal part of ageing; it is a term that is used to describe a set of symptoms that occur when the brain is affected by certain diseases or conditions, with Alzheimer's disease being most common.

Oestrogen facilitates synaptogenesis, induces growth factor production, protects against oxidative stress, and regulates neurotransmission (e.g. serotonin, noradrenaline, and acetylcholine) in brain systems associated with cognition and mood.

Although oestrogens affect brain tissues and brain processes in ways expected to reduce dementia risk and improve the course of cognitive ageing, therapeutic use of oestrogens for dementia is not supported by clinical findings. Many observational studies have implied that oestrogens reduce the rate of Alzheimer's disease; however, better quality evidence now suggests that there is no benefit of hormone treatment for these patients (23).

Isolating the effects of ageing from the effects of the menopause is difficult, but there is currently no evidence to support the use of HT for improvement or prevention of cognitive decline (2).

Management

Hormone therapy

Starting HT

There is now consensus that the minimum effective dose to alleviate symptoms should be used for the shortest duration of time.

The recommended starting doses of oestrogen are:

- 0.3 mg oral conjugated equine oestrogen
- 1 mg oral micronized oestradiol or oestradiol valerate
- 25–50 mcg transdermal oestradiol
- two (0.5 mg) metred doses of oestradiol gel
- 25–50 mcg implanted oestradiol.

Women who have a uterus must be prescribed combined HT (oestrogen and progesterone) because of the risk of endometrial hyperplasia and cancer associated with the effects of unopposed oestrogen on the endometrium. Those women who have had a total hysterectomy may use oestrogen-only preparations.

If the last menstrual period was more than 1 year ago, continuous combined preparations may be used; otherwise sequential (continuous oestrogen with progesterone for 12–14 days per month) preparations should be commenced. After 1 year of therapy, women on sequential preparations may change to continuous combined preparations if they wish to avoid a regular bleed.

Unscheduled vaginal bleeding is common in women with a uterus in the first 3 months of starting HT; however, it should be reported at review appointments.

Risks of HT

Breast

Breast cancer is the most common cancer in women and today there are an estimated 550,000 women in the United Kingdom living with breast cancer.

Female sex and age are the most important risk factors, but family history, particularly in association with *BRCA1* and *BRCA2* gene mutations, are associated with a high risk for developing breast cancer. Personal factors must also be considered: alcohol intake and obesity are considered to be risk factors, while physical activity and breast feeding may be protective. HT has also been implicated as a potential risk factor in randomized and observational studies.

Currently the question of linkage between breast cancer and HT use in women over the age of 50 years is complex. NICE suggests that we explain to women that HRT with oestrogen alone is associated with little or no change in the risk of breast cancer, but HRT with oestrogen and progesterone can be associated with an increase in risk (2). This risk of breast cancer attributable to HT is small, is duration dependent, and decreases after stopping. When counselling women it is also important to emphasize that the baseline risk of breast cancer will vary from women to woman, and other risk factors must be considered (Table 46.1).

Venous thromboembolism

Venous thromboembolism (VTE) is a condition comprising deep vein thrombosis and pulmonary embolism precipitated by conditions such as immobility, compression of the blood vessel, or increased blood viscosity that cause blood flow to slow.

HT is associated with a twofold increased risk of VTE, which appears to be greatest in the first year of use, and in those with increased body mass index (BMI).

Oral HT must undergo first-pass metabolism in the liver, and as such, affects the clotting cascade by increasing resistance to protein C and protein S (anticoagulants), and increasing fibrinogen, and as a result increasing the clotting risk. Transdermal preparations are absorbed directly into the bloodstream through the skin, bypassing this metabolism, and at standard doses are associated with a VTE risk no greater than baseline.

Transdermal preparations should be considered in those women with a BMI greater than 30 kg/m², but those women at high risk of VTE (e.g. inherited thrombophilias) should be referred to a specialist before considering HT.

Prescribed non-hormonal alternatives for flushing

Monoamines have been shown to play an important role in the control of thermoregulation, and animal studies have shown that noradrenaline acts to narrow the thermoregulatory zone. Noradrenergic stimulation of the medial preoptic area of the hypothalamus in primates causes peripheral vasodilation, heat loss, and a drop in core temperature, similar to changes which occur in women during hot flushes.

Clonidine is an alpha-2-adrenergic agonist licensed for use as a non-hormonal alternative for the treatment of flushing. It has been shown, in a meta-analysis of poor to fair quality trials, to reduce hot flush frequency and severity at 4 weeks and at 8 weeks (24); however, adverse effects include dry mouth, insomnia, and drowsiness.

Serotonin is involved in many bodily functions including mood, anxiety, sleep, sexual behaviour, and thermoregulation. Oestrogen withdrawal is associated with decreased blood serotonin levels, and short-term oestrogen therapy has been shown to increase these levels.

A meta-analysis assessed two RCTs comparing paroxetine to placebo and concluded that paroxetine was more effective than placebo in reducing the frequency and severity of hot flushes (24). This same meta-analysis assessed a further two RCTs comparing venlafaxine and placebo. There was an improvement in quality of life in one study, despite no reduction in frequency of flushes, and a decrease in hot flush frequency compared with placebo, in the other. Adverse effects included dry mouth, constipation, decreased appetite, nausea, and sleeplessness. Nausea typically improves in 2–3 days, and can be improved by titrating the dose slowly.

Table 46.1 Absolute risks of breast cancer for different types of HRT compared with no HRT (or placebo), different durations of HRT use, and times since stopping HRT for menopausal women

		Difference in breast cancer incidence per 1000 menopausal women over 7.5 years (95% confidence interval) (baseline population risk in the UK over 7.5 years: 22.48 per 1000[a])			
		Current HRT users	Treatment duration <5 years	Treatment duration 5–10 years	>5 years since stopping treatment
Women on oestrogen alone	RCT estimate[b]	4 fewer (−11 to 8)	No available data	No available data	5 fewer (−11 to 2)
	Observational estimate[c]	6 more (1 to 12)[d]	4 more (1 to 9)	5 more (−1 to 14)	5 fewer (−9 to −1)
Women on oestrogen + progesterone	RCT estimate[b]	5 more (−4 to 36)	No available data	No available data	8 more (1 to 17)
	Observational estimate[c]	17 more (14 to 20)	12 more (6 to 19)	21 more (9 to 37)	9 fewer (−16 to 13)[e]

[a] Office of National Statistics (2010) breast cancer incidence statistics.

[b] For women aged 50–59 years at entry to the RCT.

[c] Observational estimates are based on cohort studies with several thousand women.

[d] Evidence on observational estimate demonstrated very serious heterogeneity without plausible explanation by subgroup analysis.

[e] Evidence on observational estimate demonstrated very serious imprecision in the estimate of effect.

Reproduced from National Institute for Health and Care Excellence (NICE). *Menopause: Diagnosis and Management of Menopause*. NICE guideline [NG23]. London: NICE: 2015. Available at: https://www.nice.org.uk/guidance/ng23.

NICE does not advocate the use of SSRIs/SNRIs or clonidine as first-line therapy for vasomotor symptoms alone (2).

Use of these drugs in women with breast cancer using tamoxifen is common; therefore, consideration must be given to potential interactions. Tamoxifen must be metabolized by the cytochrome P450 enzyme system, predominantly cytochrome P450 isoenzyme 2D6 (CYP2D6), to become active, and CYP2D6 is inhibited to varying degrees by SSRIs. Paroxetine is an exceptionally potent inhibitor, whereas sertraline inhibits to a lesser degree and citalopram and escitalopram are only weak inhibitors. Evidence is conflicting on the success rates of tamoxifen in preventing recurrence of breast cancer when using a concurrent SSRI. For those women who need to begin treatment with an SSRI for depression, citalopram or escitalopram may be the safest choice; however, improvements in flushing are better with venlafaxine and desvenlafaxine, and these appear to be safe choices.

Over-the-counter remedies

A Cochrane systematic review of phytoestrogens included five trials in a meta-analysis, which demonstrated no significant decrease in the frequency of hot flushes (25).

Black cohosh is a native American herb that is thought to behave as a selective oestrogen receptor modulator with mild central oestrogenic effects. A meta-analysis of several short-term and relatively small RCTs comparing black cohosh use with placebo 'revealed a trend towards reducing vasomotor symptoms', but only in cases of mild to moderate symptoms (26). This was particularly notable when hot flushes were associated with sleep and mood disturbances. This was confirmed in another 12-week study of 304 women in addition to improvements in mood, sleep disorders, sexual disorders, and sweating. In contrast, however, the recent Herbal Alternatives for Menopause Trial (HALT) (27) which compared black cohosh to both placebo and oestrogen replacement over 12 months suggested that black cohosh was ineffective in relieving vasomotor symptoms. It is, however, important to exercise caution as there is limited information on its potential to influence breast cancer development or progression.

NICE recommends that, while there is some evidence for the use of black cohosh and isoflavones, it is important to explain to women that there are multiple preparations, these preparations may vary, and their safety is uncertain (2). In addition, interactions with other medicines have been reported.

Vitamin E and evening primrose oil are no better than placebo at reducing the frequency or severity of hot flushes (28, 29).

Alternative therapies

Acupuncture is a popular form of complementary medicine used by women in menopause. It can be defined as the insertion of needles into the skin and underlying tissues at particular sites, known as acupoints, for therapeutic or preventative purposes. A systematic review of six randomized control trials revealed only one with favourable results of acupuncture and this trial was considered too small to generate reliable findings (30).

REFERENCES

1. Harlow SD, Gass M, Hall JE, et al. Executive summary of the Stages of Reproductive Aging Workshop + 10: addressing the unfinished agenda of staging reproductive aging. *Climacteric* 2012;**15**:105–14.

2. National Institute for Health and Care Excellence (NICE). *Menopause: Diagnosis and Management of Menopause.* NICE guideline [NG23]. London: NICE: 2015. Available at: https://www.nice.org.uk/guidance/ng23.

3. Rocca WA, Grossardt BR, de Andrade M, Malkasian GD, Melton LJ 3rd. Survival patterns after oophorectomy in premenopausal women: a population-based cohort study. *Lancet Oncol* 2006;**7**:821–28.

4. Rivera CM, Grossardt BR, Rhodes DJ, et al. Increased cardiovascular mortality after early bilateral oophorectomy. *Menopause* 2009;**16**:15–23.

5. Rivera CM, Grossardt BR, Rhodes DJ, Rocca WA. Increased mortality for neurological and mental diseases following early bilateral oophorectomy. *Neuroepidemiology* 2009;**33**:32–40.

6. European Society for Human Reproduction and Embryology (ESHRE). Management of women with premature ovarian insufficiency. 2015. Available at: https://www.eshre.eu/-/media/sitecore-files/Guidelines/POI/ESHRE-guideline_POI-2015_FINAL_11122015.pdf?la=en&hash=4956225FEC25B0A0752F79EDEAD1A3D4237D1568.

7. Panay N, Kalu E. Management of premature ovarian failure. *Best Pract Res Clin Obstet Gynaecol* 2009;**23**:129–40.

8. van Kasteren YM, Schoemaker J. Premature ovarian failure: a systematic review on therapeutic interventions to restore ovarian function and achieve pregnancy. *Hum Reprod Update* 1999;**5**:483–92.

9. Langrish JP, Mills NL, Bath LE, et al. Cardiovascular effects of physiological and standard sex steroid replacement regimens in premature ovarian failure. *Hypertension* 2009;**53**:805–11.

10. Rossouw JE, Anderson GL, Prentice RL, et al. Risks and benefits of estrogen plus progestin in healthy postmenopausal women: principal results from the Women's Health Initiative randomized control trial. *JAMA* 2002;**288**:321–33.

11. de Villiers TJ, Gass ML, Haines CJ, et al. Global consensus statement on menopausal hormone therapy. *Climacteric* 2013;**16**:203–204.

12. Suckling J, Lethaby A, Kennedy R. Local oestrogen for vaginal atrophy in postmenopausal women. *Cochrane Database Syst Rev* 2006;**4**:CD001500.

13. Sturdee DW, Panay N. Recommendations for the management of postmenopausal vaginal atrophy. *Climacteric* 2010;**13**:509–22.

14. Board of the International Menopause Society, Pines A, Sturdee DW. IMS updated recommendations on postmenopausal hormone therapy. *Climacteric* 2007;**10**:181–94.

15. Le Ray I, Dell'Aniello S, Bonnetain F, Azoulay L, Suissa S. Local estrogen therapy and risk of breast cancer recurrence among hormone-treated patients: a nested case–control study. *Breast Cancer Res Treat* 2012;**135**:603–609.

16. Wills S, Ravipati A, Venuturumilli P, et al. Effects of vaginal estrogens on serum estradiol levels in postmenopausal breast cancer survivors and women at risk of breast cancer taking an aromatase inhibitor or a selective estrogen receptor modulator. *J Oncol Pract* 2012;**8**:144–48.

17. Cody JD, Richardson K, Moehrer B, Hextall A, Glazener CM. Oestrogen therapy for urinary incontinence in post-menopausal women. *Cochrane Database Syst Rev* 2009;**4**:CD001405.

18. Abrams P, Andersson KE, Birder L, et al. Fourth International Consultation on Incontinence Recommendations of the International Scientific Committee: evaluation and treatment of urinary incontinence, pelvic organ prolapse, and fecal incontinence. *Neurourol Urodyn* 2010;**29**:213–40.

19. Compston J, Bowring C, Cooper A, et al. Diagnosis and management of osteoporosis in postmenopausal women and older men in

the UK: National Osteoporosis Guideline Group (NOGG) update 2013. *Maturitas* 2013;**75**:392–96.

20. Writing Group on Osteoporosis for the British Menopause Society Council, Farook Al-Azzawi DB, Hillard T, Rees M, Studd J, Williamson J. Prevention and treatment of osteoporosis in women. BMS Consensus Statements 2015. Available at: https://thebms.org.uk/members/full-consensus-statements/prevention-and-treatment-of-osteoporosis-in-women/ (accessed 26 April 2015).

21. Manson JE, Chlebowski RT, Stefanick ML, et al. Menopausal hormone therapy and health outcomes during the intervention and extended poststopping phases of the Women's Health Initiative randomized trials. *JAMA* 2013;**310**:1353–68.

22. Schierbeck LL, Rejnmark L, Tofteng CL, et al. Effect of hormone replacement therapy on cardiovascular events in recently postmenopausal women: randomised trial. *BMJ* 2012;**345**:e6409.

23. Henderson VW. Action of estrogens in the aging brain: dementia and cognitive aging. *Biochim Biophys Acta* 2010;**1800**:1077–83.

24. Nelson HD, Vesco KK, Haney E, et al. Nonhormonal therapies for menopausal hot flashes: systematic review and meta-analysis. *JAMA* 2006;**295**:2057–71.

25. Lethaby AE, Brown J, Marjoribanks J, Kronenberg F, Roberts H, Eden J. Phytoestrogens for vasomotor menopausal symptoms. *Cochrane Database Syst Rev* 2007;**4**:CD001395.

26. Wong VC, Lim CE, Luo X, Wong WS. Current alternative and complementary therapies used in menopause. *Gynecol Endocrinol* 2009;**25**:166–74.

27. Newton KM, Reed SD, LaCroix AZ, Grothaus LC, Ehrlich K, Guiltinan J. Treatment of vasomotor symptoms of menopause with black cohosh, multibotanicals, soy, hormone therapy, or placebo: a randomized trial. *Ann Intern Med* 2005;**145**:869–79.

28. Barton DL, Loprinzi CL, Quella SK, et al. Prospective evaluation of vitamin E for hot flashes in breast cancer survivors. *J Clin Oncol* 1998;**16**:495–500.

29. Chenoy R, Hussain S, Tayob Y, et al. Effect of oral gamolenic acid from evening primrose oil on menopausal flushing. *BMJ* 1994;**308**:501–503.

30. Lee MS, Shin BC, Ernst E. Acupuncture for treating menopausal hot flushes: a systematic review. *Climacteric* 2009;**12**:16–25.

SECTION 6
Surgical Procedures and Postoperative Care

47

Laparoscopy

Stephanie S. Andriputri, Stephen D. Lyons, and Jason A. Abbott

Bowel preparation prior to laparoscopy

Mechanical bowel preparation (MBP) with preoperative oral or rectal hyperosmotic laxatives prior to intra-abdominal surgery is neither new nor limited to gynaecological surgery. The hypotheses for its use in gynaecological surgery are:

- to improve bowel handling
- to improve visualization
- to decrease risk from faecal contamination if inadvertent bowel injury occurs.

At laparotomy, the bowels may be manually packed or retracted, however this is not feasible at laparoscopic surgery, and bowel manipulation and positioning has been perceived as a major problem (1). Nevertheless, the risk of bowel injury leading to peritoneal contamination and sepsis in laparoscopic gynaecological surgery is minimal, since the risk of injury remains very low (2). There are seven randomized controlled trials (RCTs) from the gynaecological literature that compare MBP with no MBP and the results of these are summarized in **Table 47.1**. Together, these studies report no significant benefit of mechanical bowel preparation at laparoscopy for benign gynaecological conditions.

Further evidence from the colorectal literature has shown similar results for when the bowel is intentionally opened, both in terms of anastomotic leakage and the visualization and handling issues that have been covered in the gynaecological trials. Again, these data collectively suggest that the principles as to why MBP would be used in this setting do not hold true in rigorous, evidence-based assessments with no clinical improvements and significant impacts on patient well-being, and they should not be recommended for routine use at gynaecological laparoscopy (3).

Patient positioning

Correct positioning during laparoscopic surgery is essential to decrease the risk of pressure-related injury to the anaesthetized woman and improve visualization for the surgeon. While the incidence of intraoperative positioning-related nerve injury is low, it carries considerable morbidity and legal implication (8). From a prospective cohort study of 616 patients, the incidence of postoperative peripheral neuropathy was reported to be 1.8%, with a median time to resolution of neuropathic symptoms of 32 days (range 1 day to 6 months), with complete resolution observed in all but one patient (91%) (9).

There is no accepted standard positioning at gynaecological laparoscopy with a comparative evidence base since this would require far too many women given the low incidence of injury and a pragmatic approach is required. This includes the head being straight, the arms being in a physiologically neutral position, with the arms by the side in medial rotation and no more than 90 degrees of abduction (10). The lithotomy position has been described as hip flexion of 80–100 degrees, abduction of 30–45 degrees laterally, with knees flexed to the point that the lower legs are parallel to the body (**Figure 47.1**) (11). The woman's legs should be supported in padded stirrups that may be moved and prevent compression in one area of the foot such as the rigid Allen-type stirrups where foot pronation and internal rotation as well as compression of the common peroneal nerve may lead to substantial neuropathic injuries and do not allow intraoperative changes in leg positioning (12). In a large retrospective review of 198,461 patients in the lithotomy position, nerve injury has been reported to be 1 in 3608 cases (78% common peroneal nerve, 15% sciatic nerve, 7% femoral nerve) (13).

The basis of positioning is to reduce the risk of pressure effects since localized stretch or compression results in ischaemic injury and Schwann cell demyclination. The recovery time is variable with an approximated rate of 1 mm per day (14). Specific nerve injuries have all been reported with the femoral nerve injury affected by excessive hip flexion, abduction, and external rotation and the sciatic nerve affected by knee hyperextension, hip hyperflexion, and external rotation. The upper limbs may also be affected with the brachial plexus affected due to shoulder hyperabduction should the arms be positioned on arm boards intraoperatively. Shoulder braces may lead to nerve compression from the cervical spine and should be avoided, with the surgeon checking the position of limbs prior to beginning surgery and placing additional padding over hands, feet, and arms as needed to reduce risk (15). Increasing procedure duration is associated with increasing nerve injury with an up to 100-fold increase in risk for each additional hour of surgery (13, 16). Periodic repositioning in prolonged procedures is appropriate to avoid sustained pressure on a single segment of the nerve (15).

Table 47.1 Randomized controlled trials on the efficacy of preoperative MBP for gynaecological laparoscopy

First author and year	No. of patients	Techniques studied	Primary study outcomes	Comments
Muzii 2006 (4)	162	MBP vs no MBP	Surgical field exposure, operating time, postoperative complication, postoperative discomfort	More postoperative discomfort with MBP. No significant difference in other outcomes
Lijoi 2009 (5)	83	MBP vs 7-day low-fibre diet	Surgical field exposure, operating time, postoperative complication, length of stay	No significant difference. Low-fibre diet is better tolerated
Won 2013 (1)	308	MBP + 3-day low-fibre diet vs no MBP	Surgical field visualization, bowel handling, patient discomfort	Improved surgical field visualization and bowel handling with MBP, but of negligible clinical significance. Increased patient discomfort with MBP
Siedhoff 2014 (6)	73	MBP vs no MBP	Surgical field visualization, surgical difficulty	No significant difference
Ryan 2015 (7)	78	MBP vs clear fluid diet	Surgical field visualization, bowel handling, ease of operation, gastrointestinal discomfort, patient compliance	No significant difference

The effect of body mass index (BMI) in nerve injury is variable since women with a low BMI are at increased risk due to less adiposity giving inherent padding; however, women with a high BMI are more likely to move during a procedure with greater stretch-related nerve injury and greater care in both groups is recommended (15).

Friedrich Trendelenburg described the tilted, head-down position with elevated legs in the nineteenth century to improve vision at vesicovaginal fistula surgery (17). The steep Trendelenburg position does allow the bowel to move out of the pelvis and into the abdomen and should only be considered once access to the peritoneal cavity is obtained (see later). However, this physical position is associated with

physiological changes that increase systemic vascular resistance and mean arterial pressure, as well as decreased renal perfusion. There is a linear relationship between the peak airway pressure and the degree of Trendelenburg (18). The combination of pneumoperitoneum and head tilt has been shown to increase peak airway pressure and intracranial pressure decrease pulmonary compliance (19). Therefore, pneumoperitoneum, when used in combination with head-down tilt, may elicit a hazardous haemodynamic response in patients with compromised cardiac function (20). Discussion with the anaesthetic team regarding optimal patient positioning at the instigation of and throughout surgery is mandatory. Devices such as bean bags (21)

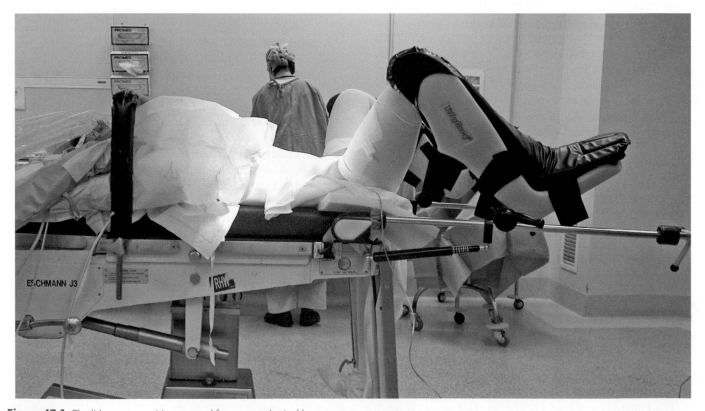

Figure 47.1 The lithotomy position as used for gynaecological laparoscopy.

and non-slip pads are described to reduce the risk of moving once in the Trendelenburg position (22).

Uterine manipulation

Uterine manipulation of any type during laparoscopic surgery allows improved visualization and access to pelvis structures and may change angulation induced by a fixed port placement through the anterior abdominal wall (23) (**Figure 47.2**). Many uterine manipulators are described (24), however little is known about their efficacy (25). Clinical situations such as a pyometra, a small, stenosed or anatomical variant preventing cervical visualization, or suspected intrauterine pregnancy all preclude the use of a uterine manipulator (23). Complications such as uterine and bowel perforation associated with improper placement of a

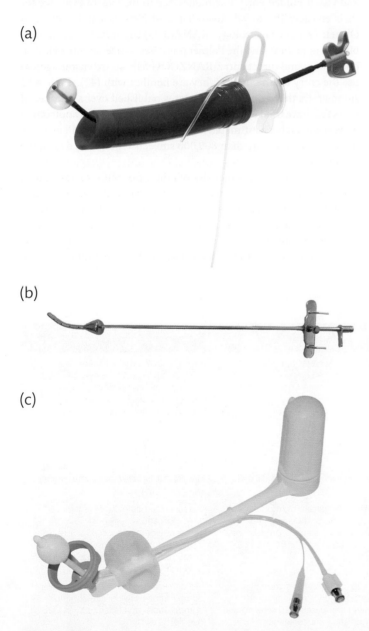

(a)

(b)

(c)

Figure 47.2 A variety of uterine manipulators: (a). ColpotomizOR Tube (b). Spackman cannula (c). ClearView Total.

uterine manipulator are described (26) and care should always be taken with placement. Women with known early endometrial cancer where a manipulator has been used have had no significant difference in lymph-vascular space invasion, positive peritoneal cytology, or tumour recurrence with up to 19 months follow-up period (27–29).

Entry techniques

Entry complications

More than half of major complications associated with laparoscopy occur during entry into the abdomen. While most of these complications are rare, when they do occur, vascular injury and bowel injuries are the most serious and life-threatening and may result in death, with urinary tract injury occurring less commonly and usually with less associated morbidity. Other complications include failed entry and extraperitoneal insufflation (30, 31).

The reported incidence of vascular injury during laparoscopy ranges from 0.02% to 0.5% with up to a 15% mortality rate (30, 31). The distal aorta and the right common iliac artery are the vessels usually involved due to the anatomical relationship to the umbilicus and left-sided approach for the majority of right-dominant handed surgeons. The inferior epigastric vessels may be injured during placement of secondary ports and visualization both during placement and removal of secondary ports is recommended to reduce this risk (31).

The incidence of bowel injury in laparoscopy is 0.04–0.5% with the small bowel accounting for 58% of injuries, the colon 32%, and the stomach 8% of injuries (30–32). (30). Between one-third and one-half of all gastrointestinal injuries occur at the time of entry (30, 31) and unlike vascular injuries that are usually identified intraoperatively, only 30–50% of gastrointestinal injuries are diagnosed intraoperatively, with the remainder diagnosed between 1 and 30 days postoperatively, leading to poorer outcomes (30, 32).

Extraperitoneal insufflation may occur when the insufflating needle is incorrectly placed or when carbon dioxide leaks around the insertion sites into the tissues. This minor complication may lead to extensive extraperitoneal insufflation that could result in failure of entry to the abdomen, visualization difficulties at the time of primary port entry, and subcutaneous emphysema that usually resolves spontaneously and with minimal issue (33).

Types of entry techniques

Laparoscopic entry techniques may be divided into closed entry (using the Veress needle, or direct entry technique), open entry (using the Hasson method), or entry under laparoscopic vision.

Veress needle entry

Developed in 1938, the Veress needle is a common instrument used for peritoneal access in gynaecological surgery (32, 34). It consists of a 2 mm sharp outer needle, with a spring-loaded blunt inner stylet that retracts with tissue resistance through the abdominal wall and rapidly protrudes so the sharp needle is not exposed with loss of tissue resistance into the peritoneal cavity. After entering the peritoneum, carbon dioxide fills the potential space, prior to insertion of the primary trocar with the aim of increasing distance between the anterior abdominal wall and abdominal structures using pressure as a guide (35, 36). This entry method has two blind steps—insertion of the Veress needle, and insertion of the trocar.

The umbilicus is the most widely used entry site for this technique, however Palmer's point, suprapubic, and transfundal approaches are all described. For women with known or suspected periumbilical adhesions, 'Palmer's point' described as being 3 cm below the left costal margin in the midclavicular line may be used as an alternative since adhesions rarely form in this location (37). Palmer's point should not be used in women with previous gastric or splenic surgery, or splenomegaly (38), and an alternate entry method should be considered (39).

Two prospective observational studies have been performed to determine the most reliable test for ensuring correct placement of the Veress needle; both found that the pressure profile test was the most sensitive and specific, when compared with the double click test, aspiration test, and hanging drop test (40, 41).

Direct entry

First described in 1978, direct entry involves an intraumbilical skin incision, followed by blind insertion of the primary trocar without prior insufflation, then inspection by the laparoscope to confirm intraperitoneal placement, prior to gas insufflation (42).

Hasson open entry

Open entry, via the Hasson approach, has no blind steps. The abdominal cavity is entered under direct vision through a small periumbilical incision. A blunt trocar is inserted under direct vision, the laparoscope is then inserted, and pneumoperitoneum established (43).

Other entry techniques

Vision-guided direct entry requires a proprietary trocar and cannula system inserted through the abdominal wall with concurrent laparoscopic vision using downward pressure or a screwing motion following Veress needle insufflation (44, 45). Radially expanding entry utilizes a progressively expanding sleeve over a Veress needle (46).

Comparison of entry techniques

A long-held and often heated debate exists as to which is the safest entry technique and there is no strong evidence that any entry technique is superior in this regard. The Society of Obstetrician and Gynaecologists of Canada and American Congress of Obstetricians and Gynecologists state that practitioners should be proficient in Veress entry, open entry, and direct entry. The United Kingdom Royal College of Obstetricians and Gynaecologists and the French College of Gynaecologists and Obstetricians (CNGOF) similarly acknowledge that Veress, direct, and open entries are considered first-line procedures. CNGOF discourages the use of radially expanding and vision-guided entry techniques due to the lack of evidence for their efficacy. The Royal Australian and New Zealand College of Obstetrics and Gynaecology (RANZCOG) supports the use of umbilical, suprapubic, and the Palmer point Veress needle entry, Hasson open entry, and direct entry. RANZCOG fellows are encouraged to use the entry technique that they are familiar with (47). Table 47.2 summarizes the various meta-analyses published over a number of years that have tried to combine data and report on safety outcomes; however, it has been estimated that RCTs on the subject will never be undertaken with more than 800,000 subjects required to determine an answer (48).

Evidence suggests a higher risk of minor complications and failed entry during Veress placement when compared with Hasson entry (34, 49, 50). However, there is no statistically significant difference in major complications or mortality between the entry methods. It should be noted that these studies include a combination of gynaecological surgery and general surgery, there are limited data on

Table 47.2 Studies comparing entry techniques in laparoscopic surgery

First author and year	Study type	No. of patients	Techniques studied	Principal outcomes	Comments
Molloy 2002 (32)	Meta-analysis	85,350	Direct trocar vs Veress needle	Mortality. Visceral injury. Vascular injury. Delayed diagnosis of complications	Increased risk of bowel injury in open entry compared with Veress and direct trocar. Increased risk of vascular injury in Veress needle group. No significant difference in delayed diagnosis of complications
Merlin 2003 (34)	Systematic review	129,677	Open entry (Hasson) vs closed entry (direct trocar and Veress)	Major complications. Conversion to laparotomy. Minor complications	Trend towards reduced risk of major complications and conversion to open laparotomy in open group (not statistically significant). Fewer minor complications in open entry than closed entry
Ahmad 2012 (49)	Meta-analysis	4,860	Direct trocar vs Veress needle, vs Hasson	Major complications (mortality, visceral injury, vascular injury). Minor complications (preperitoneal insufflation, omental injury). Failed entry	No significant difference in major complications. Lower rate of minor complications in direct entry than Veress. Lower rate of failed entry in Hasson than Veress
Jiang 2012 (50)	Meta-analysis	2940	Direct trocar vs Veress needle	Major complications (mortality, visceral injury, vascular injury). Minor complications (preperitoneal insufflation, subcutaneous emphysema, omental injury). Failed entry	No significant difference in major complications. Higher rate of minor complications and failed entry in Veress needle

patients with extremes of BMI and previous abdominal surgery, and different studies used different Veress techniques (Table 47.2) (47).

Insufflation

Following abdominal entry, gas insufflation (generally using carbon dioxide) lifts the abdominal wall away from the abdominal contents, allowing visualization and space in which to operate. This pneumoperitoneum does result in cardiovascular and respiratory changes relating to increased intra-abdominal pressures and hypercarbia from absorption of carbon dioxide. The increased intra-abdominal pressure may lead to an increase in systemic vascular resistance, increasing afterload and decreasing cardiac output, and the upward diaphragmatic shift decreases the functional residual capacity of the lungs (51, 52). The high solubility of carbon dioxide results in rapid absorption into the circulation and hypercarbia may result in acidosis, decreasing cardiac contractility. Pneumoperitoneum may also compress the renal vasculature and parenchyma resulting in activation of the renin–angiotensin system and renal vasoconstriction (51). The significance of these effects depends on the intra-abdominal pressures achieved, patient positioning, duration of pneumoperitoneum, and the woman's preoperative cardiac and respiratory function (52).

Several prospective studies have been undertaken in the gynaecological setting to determine the effect on cardiorespiratory function at a relatively high intraperitoneal pressure of 25 mm (used commonly at laparoscopic entry) which report no adverse cardiopulmonary events in more than 4000 women having gynaecological surgery with pressures at entry of 25–30 mmHg (35, 53, 54).

Energy sources

Monopolar electrosurgical instruments have been used during laparoscopic procedures since the first half of the twentieth century (55), with the addition of bipolar instruments used for laparoscopic sterilization in 1973 (56). More complex laparoscopic surgeries including laparoscopic cholecystectomy (57) and laparoscopic hysterectomy (58) became both possible and popularized with technological advancements in electrosurgical instrumentation and knowledge.

Adding different effects such as pressure in addition to electrosurgery and ultrasonic has led to new-generation hybrid energy sources designed to provide optimized tissue effects (especially for vessel sealing) with improved safety profiles compared to conventional electrosurgery (59). These instruments are said to be more time efficient by decreasing 'instrument traffic' and to decrease energy source costs by reducing the overall number of surgical instruments (59, 60).

Substantial advantages of using monopolar electrosurgery at laparoscopy are simplicity, availability, and wide range of available tissue effects (55, 59–61). Complex instrumentation with specialist electrosurgical generators is not essential and costs may be minimized with simple instruments. Knowledge of the possibility of stray current injuries that might occur and steps that can be implemented to limit the risk such as the use of active electrode monitoring are essential when utilizing any monopolar electrosurgical instrument at laparoscopy (60, 62–65). All laparoscopic energy sources ultimately generate thermal energy to generate their respective tissue effects. Irrespective of the fact that bipolar, ultrasonic, and laser technologies are not subject to the risk of electrical stray current injuries associated with monopolar electrosurgery, the heat generated by all these modalities has the potential to cause lateral thermal spread injuries (59).

Surgical comparative studies on laparoscopic energy sources often focus on clinical outcomes such as operating time, blood loss, postoperative pain, and complications with new-generation energy sources (i.e. ultrasonic and advanced bipolar devices) reportedly superior to conventional bipolar and monopolar electrosurgery (59). These statistical differences may be of limited clinical value since they may report a significant decrease in blood loss of tens of millilitres—a finding that will have no clinical consequence.

Laboratory-based comparative studies on laparoscopic energy sources have most commonly focused on parameters such as vessel burst pressure, vessel seal time, lateral thermal spread, and smoke plume generation (59, 60). All modern vessel sealing energy sources yield burst pressures in the supraphysiological range (i.e. above mean arterial pressure), therefore any differences observed in burst pressures for individual are probably not clinically significant. The data for lateral thermal spread are inconsistent with no superiority for any particular energy source. Comparative studies on smoke or vapour generation by energy sources generally shows that while all energy sources create a smoke plume, the order of energy sources that produce least to most smoke production is ultrasonic, advanced bipolar, conventional bipolar, and monopolar.

The cost of energy sources may determine the choice of device available and used with both direct and indirect costs to consider (66). Indirect costs include the costs related to time off work, post-discharge care, loss of productivity, etc. Apart the upfront capital cost of the actual device (and generator unit), direct costs include also include ongoing costs such as sterilization of reusable devices, associated disposable equipment, and servicing. In addition, re-admissions due to complications are direct costs. The choice of energy source will depend on consideration of all these factors, with no single energy source appropriate for all laparoscopic procedures. Surgeons will often use a range of instruments depending on their mentors' teaching, their own personal experience, the type of procedure, and the likelihood of distorted anatomy and adhesions (60).

Intraoperative analgesia

The contributory factors to postoperative pain following laparoscopic surgery are discomfort at incision sites, stretching of intra-abdominal cavity, peritoneal inflammation, and dissection of abdominal or pelvic viscera. Therefore, multimodal analgesia is required to address each component of postoperative pain to minimize the use of systemic analgesia as the main source of postoperative pain control due to the potential adverse side effects (67). Regular pain scoring and encouraging patients to ask for analgesia are also important aspects of effective anaesthesia (68).

Overall, multimodal analgesia has been shown to significantly reduce postoperative pain, nausea and vomiting, and total postoperative analgesia requirement, although there is conflicting evidence for the efficacy when comparing individual elements of multimodal analgesia with placebo (Table 47.3). Perhaps what is most important is that a combination of analgesic modalities and locations is of most benefit for women and perhaps it is purely academic as to which one provides the greatest effect when the combination is considered safe and guidelines on the use of local anaesthetics are appropriately followed. Table 47.3 summarizes the data from RCTs regarding the mode of analgesia to minimize postoperative pain.

Port site closure

Port site herniation is a postoperative complication that may lead to small bowel strangulation or incarceration, often requiring emergency intervention and has resulted in deaths when unrecognized (86). The incidence of port site herniation following gynaecological laparoscopy is low and reported to be 0.06–1%, with a size of more than 7 mm and extraumbilical location of ports (particularly lateral) important for subsequent hernia development (87). The risk factors for port site herniation include previous history of port site hernia, postoperative wound infection, poor wound healing, ascites, obesity, connective tissue disorder, and extensive port manipulation (88). Fascial closure should be performed in patients with these risk factors regardless of the port size (63). Closure of a port size less than 5 mm in diameter is generally not required because hernia formation is rare, but it has been reported in the literature. For port sites of at least 7 mm, fascial closure is recommended to reduce the risk

Table 47.3 Randomized controlled trials comparing modes of intraoperative analgesia

First author and year	No. of patients	Mode of analgesia	Principal outcomes	Comments
Benhamou 1994 (69)	25	Intraperitoneal and mesosalpinx local anaesthetic vs placebo	Postoperative pain, analgesia requirement, time to return to normal activities	Less postoperative pain, analgesia requirement and time to return to normal activities in multimodal group
Michaloliakou 1996 (70)	49	Multimodal (port site injection, intramuscular) vs placebo	Postoperative pain, nausea, and readiness for discharge	Significantly less postoperative pain and nausea, faster discharge
Einarsson 2004 (71)	82	Port site injection pre operation vs post operation	Postoperative pain	Less postoperative pain within 1 hour with postoperative infiltration group
Grube 2004 (72)	163	Port site injection pre operation vs placebo	Postoperative pain, analgesia, functional limitation,	No significant difference
Lam 2004 (73)	144	Port site injection pre operation vs post operation vs placebo	Postoperative pain, predischarge analgesia, total analgesia	Less pain in preoperative infiltration group.
Chou 2005 (74)	91	Intraperitoneal instillation postoperatively vs both preoperatively and postoperatively vs placebo	Shoulder tip pain, abdominal visceral pain, abdominal parietal pain, length of stay, postoperative analgesia consumption, side effects	Significant reduction of abdominal visceral pain within 8 hours post operation in preoperative and postoperative instillation of bupivacaine. No significant difference in length of stay
Ghezzi 2005 (75)	170	Preoperative port site injection vs placebo	Postoperative pain and analgesia, time to first analgesic request	No significant difference
Jabbour 2005 (76)	100	Multimodal (intraperitoneal spray, intravenous) vs placebo	Postoperative pain, nausea, vomiting	Significantly reduced postoperative pain and vomiting in multimodal group
Kim 2005 (77)	83	Multimodal (port site injection, intramuscular), vs placebo	Postoperative pain, first analgesia request time	Significantly reduced postoperative time and longer first analgesia request time in multimodal group
Louizos 2005 (78)	214	Port site and intraperitoneal injection vs placebo	Postoperative pain, analgesia, patient satisfaction	Less pain, less analgesia, more patient satisfaction in treatment group
Alessandri 2006 (79)	74	Port site injection vs placebo	Postoperative pain and analgesia time to ambulation, length of stay	Less postoperative pain, analgesia and mobilization. No significant difference in length of stay.
Costello 2010 (67)	66	Multimodal (suppository, port site, intraperitoneal and sub-diaphragmatic local anaesthetic) vs placebo	Postoperative pain, postoperative opioid requirement, nausea, vomiting, sedation, length of stay	Less opioid requirement in multimodal group. No significant difference in other outcomes
Kane 2012 (80)	58	Transversus abdominis plane block post operation vs placebo	Postoperative pain, total analgesia requirement, operating time	Less operating time in treatment group. No other significant differences
Kwon 2012 (81)	40	Topical local anaesthetic vs placebo	Postoperative pain, analgesia requirement, nausea and vomiting, length of stay	Less pain in treatment group. No other significant differences
Manjunath 2012 (82)	196	Intraperitoneal local anaesthetic vs placebo	Postoperative pain, analgesia requirement nausea	Less pain and nausea in treatment group. No significant difference in analgesia requirement
Arden 2013 (83)	157	Intraperitoneal local anaesthetic vs placebo	Postoperative pain, opioid requirement, length of stay, patient satisfaction	No significant differences
Tam 2014 (84)	135	Port site local anaesthetic vs placebo	Postoperative pain	No significant difference
Hotujec 2015 (85)	64	Transversus abdominis block pre operation vs placebo	Postoperative pain, analgesia	No significant difference

of this complication (89, 90). The majority of port site herniation occurs at ports of at least 10 mm although fascial defects of up to 12 mm using the tissue separating plastic trocars may not be at lower risk of this issue (63). It would, however, seem prudent to close the fascia wherever possible.

Fascial closure is the key feature for reducing this complication and the exact technique by which this is achieved is largely up to the surgeon with no clear superiority of one technique or tool over any other (91). Skin closure may be by suture, tissue adhesive with 2-octylcyanoacrylate (Dermabond), and microporous tapes. These latter two options are suggested to approximate superficial wound edges with less tension and maintain the integrity of epidermis, resulting in better cosmesis and fewer early complications such as wound erythema, tenderness, and drainage when compared to suture closure (91, 92).

Postoperative pneumoperitoneum

Postoperative residual pneumoperitoneum remains between a few hours and 24 days, despite the high solubility of carbon dioxide (93). Other sources of residual gas in the subdiaphragmatic region are thought to be water vapour produced by diathermy use and room air. Residual pneumoperitoneum symptoms may mask complications such as bowel perforation, the presentation of which may be of relatively rapid onset or up to a week or more. While the presence of subdiaphragmatic gas in an erect abdominal radiograph is essentially redundant as a diagnostic tool to detect bowel perforation following laparoscopic surgery, the absence of gas may be helpful in excluding bowel perforation (93).

Residual peritoneal gas is associated with postoperative shoulder tip pain that occurs following 35–60% of laparoscopic surgery. Shoulder tip pain is thought to be associated with peritoneal stretching and irritation of the diaphragm and phrenic nerve, secondary to carbon dioxide insufflation (94). There are conflicting data on drains following laparoscopy to remove residual gas and these are summarized in Table 47.4. The use of oral analgesia has been reported to be more cost-effective than peritoneal drainage in

a number of studies (95, 96). Drain complications and the need for a longer hospital stay are the usual reasons for not using them, which is supported by evidence (Table 47.4). Other methods to minimize postoperative shoulder tip pain, such as instillation of normal saline (93, 97, 98), pulmonary recruitment manoeuvre (98, 99), gasless laparoscopy (100), low-pressure laparoscopy (101), or active gas evacuation with aspiration cannula (102), have also been described in the literature but come with issues and complications of their own and have not been assessed in rigorous randomized trials.

The future of laparoscopy

Laparoscopy has come to be the gold standard for many gynaecological techniques such as management of ectopic pregnancy and adnexal surgery. For many newer techniques such as robot-assisted laparoscopy, the comparator is often this minimally invasive approach and throughout the world, women, their doctors, and healthcare institutions have an increasing body of evidence to demonstrate the utility and efficacy of this approach over laparotomy.

It remains to be seen if single incision laparoscopy can produce superior outcomes to current multiport laparoscopy with comparative trials reporting no significant difference in postoperative pain, length of stay, and cosmetic results (106–108). Robotic-assisted laparoscopy is a technological platform with advantages including better proprioception, improved precision with articulating instrumentation, and reduction of the surgeon's hand tremor (109). Disadvantages include increased cost, the lack of tactile feedback to the surgeon, the presence of bulky robotic arms, and the inability to move the surgical table once the robot arms are attached (109). Robotic surgery has been shown to have longer operating times (110–113) and overall higher costs (113–115). There is limited evidence on the relative benefits of robotic surgery at this stage (113). Robotic surgery is designed to assist operation for more challenging cases while keeping the minimally invasive approach, rather than replacing conventional laparoscopy (116). Further high-quality studies are required before the widespread integration of robotic-assisted laparoscopic surgery into the existing gynaecological services (113).

Table 47.4 Studies comparing methods to minimize residual pneumoperitoneum

First author and year	Study type	No. of patients	Methods	Principal outcomes	Comments
Abbott 2001 (95)	RCT	158	Intraperitoneal drain and dummy drain	Postoperative nausea, vomiting, site of pain, analgesic and antiemetic use, analgesic, costs	Significantly more shoulder pain at 4 and 8 hours and more total analgesia requirement in the placebo group. No significant difference in overall pain scores, postoperative nausea and vomiting. The use of simple oral analgesia is more cost effective than the insertion of intraperitoneal drain
Swift 2002 (103)	RCT	67	Non-suction drain vs occluded drain	Postoperative pain, energy level	Significant reduction of shoulder tip pain at 12–72 hours post operation in patent drain group
Shen 2003 (96)	RCT	164	Suction drain vs no drain	Postoperative pain, total analgesic requirement, cost	Significant reduction of total analgesia and shoulder tip pain at 24 and 48 hours in suction drain group. Simple oral analgesia is more cost effective than suction drain
Raymond 2010 (104)	RCT	168	Suction vs non-suction drain	Postoperative pain, nausea, vomiting, total analgesic requirement	No significant difference in all outcomes, but suction drain is significantly more painful on removal
Kerimoglu 2015 (105)	Prospective	111	Non-suction drain vs no drain	Postoperative pain, postoperative complication	No significant difference

REFERENCES

1. Won H, Maley P, Salim S, Rao A, Campbell NT, Abbott JA. Surgical and patient outcomes using mechanical bowel preparation before laparoscopic gynecologic surgery: a randomized controlled trial. *Obstet Gynecol* 2013;**121**:538–46.

2. Yang LC, Arden D, Lee TT, et al. Mechanical bowel preparation for gynecologic laparoscopy: a prospective randomized trial of oral sodium phosphate solution vs. single sodium phosphate enema. *J Minim Invasive Gynecol* 2011;**18**:149–56.

3. Arnold A, Aitchison LP, Abbott J. Preoperative mechanical bowel preparation for abdominal, laparoscopic, and vaginal surgery: a systematic review. *J Minim Invasive Gynecol* 2015;**22**:737–52.

4. Muzii L, Bellati F, Zullo MA, Manci N, Angioli R, Panici PB. Mechanical bowel preparation before gynecologic laparoscopy: a randomized, single-blind, controlled trial. *Fertil Steril* 2006;**85**:689–93.

5. Lijoi D, Ferrero S, Mistrangelo E, et al. Bowel preparation before laparoscopic gynaecological surgery in benign conditions using a 1-week low fibre diet: a surgeon blind, randomized and controlled trial. *Arch Gynecol Obstet* 2009;**280**:713–18.

6. Siedhoff MT, Clark LH, Hobbs KA, Findley AD, Moulder JK, Garrett JM. Mechanical bowel preparation before laparoscopic hysterectomy: a randomized controlled trial. *Obstet Gynecol* 2014;**123**:562–67.

7. Ryan NA, Ng VS, Sangi-Haghpeykar H, Guan X. Evaluating mechanical bowel preparation prior to total laparoscopic hysterectomy. *JSLS* 2015;**19**:e2015.00035.

8. Cheney FW, Domino KB, Caplan RA, Posner KL. Nerve injury associated with anesthesia: a closed claims analysis. *Anesthesiology* 1999;**90**:1062–69.

9. Bohrer JC, Walters MD, Park A, Polston D, Barber MD. Pelvic nerve injury following gynecologic surgery: a prospective cohort study. *Am J Obstet Gynecol* 2009;**201**:531.e1–7.

10. Winfree CJ, Kline DG. Intraoperative positioning nerve injuries. *Surg Neurol* 2005;**63**:5–18.

11. Miller R (ed). *Miller's Anesthesia*. New York: Elsevier Churchill Livingstone; 2007.

12. Akhavan A, Gainsburg DM, Stock JA. Complications associated with patient positioning in urologic surgery. *Urology* 2010;**76**:1309–16.

13. Warner MA, Martin JT, Schroeder DR, Offord KP, Chute CG. Lower-extremity motor neuropathy associated with surgery performed on patients in a lithotomy position. *Anesthesiology* 1994;**81**:6–12.

14. Stewart J. *Focal Peripheral Neuropathies*, 3rd edn. Philadelphia, PA: Lippincott Williams & Wilkins; 2000.

15. Irvin W, Andersen W, Taylor P, Rice L. Minimizing the risk of neurologic injury in gynecologic surgery. *Obstet Gynecol* 2004;**103**:374–82.

16. Koç G, Tazeh NN, Joudi FN, Winfield HN, Tracy CR, Brown JA. Lower extremity neuropathies after robot-assisted laparoscopic prostatectomy on a split-leg table. *J Endourol* 2012;**26**:1026–29.

17. Kompanje EJO, van Genderen M, Ince C. The supine head-down tilt position that was named after the German surgeon Friedrich Trendelenburg. *Eur Surg* 2012;**44**:168–71.

18. Kundra P, Kanna V, Bupathi A, Sudeep K. Evaluation of pelvic wedge for gynaecological laparoscopy. *Anaesthesia* 2008;**63**:1087–91.

19. Gould C, Cull T, Wu YX, Osmundsen B. Blinded measure of Trendelenburg angle in pelvic robotic surgery. *J Minim Invasive Gynecol* 2012;**19**:465–68.

20. Odeberg S, Ljungqvist O, Svenberg T, et al. Haemodynamic effects of pneumoperitoneum and the influence of posture during anaesthesia for laparoscopic surgery. *Acta Anaesthesiol Scand* 1994;**38**:276–83.

21. Suozzi BA, Brazell HD, O'Sullivan DM, Tulikangas PK. A comparison of shoulder pressure among different patient stabilization techniques. *Am J Obstet Gynecol* 2013;**209**:478.e1–5.

22. Ritch JMB, Son M, Wright JD, et al. Evaluation of anti-slide methods to avoid patient shifting during trendelenburg lithotomy position for minimally invasive gynecologic surgery. *J Minim Invasive Gynecol* 2011;**18**:S70.

23. Eltabbakh GH. Uterine manipulation in laparoscopic hysterectomy. In: *The Female Patient*, pp. 18–23. Parsippany, NJ: Quadrant HealthCom Inc; 2010.

24. Mettler L, Nikam YA. A comparative survey of various uterine manipulators used in operative laparoscopy. *Gynecol Surg* 2006;**3**:239–43.

25. van den Haak L, Alleblas C, Nieboer TE, Rhemrev JP, Jansen FW. Efficacy and safety of uterine manipulators in laparoscopic surgery: a review. *Arch Gynecol Obstet* 2015;**292**:1003–11.

26. Akdemir A, Cirpan T. Iatrogenic uterine perforation and bowel penetration using a Hohlmanipulator: a case report. *Int J Surg Case Rep* 2014;**5**:271–73.

27. Lee M, Kim YT, Kim SW, et al. Effects of uterine manipulation on surgical outcomes in laparoscopic management of endometrial cancer: a prospective randomized clinical trial. *Int J Gynecol Cancer* 2013;**23**:372–79.

28. Rakowski JA, Tran TA, Ahmad S, et al. Does a uterine manipulator affect cervical cancer pathology or identification of lymphovascular space involvement? *Gynecol Oncol* 2012;**127**:98–101.

29. Canton-Romero JC, Anaya-Prado R, Rodriguez-Garcia HA, et al. Laparoscopic radical hysterectomy with the use of a modified uterine manipulator for the management of stage IB1 cervix cancer. *J Obstet Gynaecol* 2010;**30**:49–52.

30. Lam A, Kaufman Y, Khong SY, Liew A, Ford S, Condous G. Dealing with complications in laparoscopy. *Best Pract Res Clin Obstet Gynaecol* 2009;**23**:631–46.

31. Philips PA, Amaral JF. Abdominal access complications in laparoscopic surgery. *J Am Coll Surg* 2001;**192**:525–36.

32. Molloy D, Kaloo PD, Cooper M, Nguyen TV. Laparoscopic entry: a literature review and analysis of techniques and complications of primary port entry. *Aust N Z J Obstet Gynaecol* 2002;**42**:246–54.

33. Munro MG. Laparoscopic access: complications, technologies, and techniques. *Curr Opin Obstet Gynecol* 2002;**14**:365–74.

34. Merlin TL, Hiller JE, Maddern GJ, Jamieson GG, Brown AR, Kolbe A. Systematic review of the safety and effectiveness of methods used to establish pneumoperitoneum in laparoscopic surgery. *Br J Surg* 2003;**90**:668–79.

35. Phillips G, Garry R, Kumar C, Reich H. How much gas is required for initial insufflation at laparoscopy? *Gynaecol Endosc* 1999;**8**:369–74.

36. Thomson AJ, Shoukrey MN, Gemmell I, Abbott JA. Standardizing pneumoperitoneum for laparoscopic entry. Time, volume, or pressure: which is best? *J Minim Invasive Gynecol* 2012;**19**:196–200.

37. Granata M, Tsimpanakos I, Moeity F, Magos A. Are we underutilizing Palmer's point entry in gynecologic laparoscopy? *Fertil Steril* 2010;**94**:2716–19.

38. Vilos GA, Ternamian A, Dempster J, Laberge PY, Clinical Practice Gynaecology Committee. Laparoscopic entry: a review of techniques, technologies, and complications. *J Obstet Gynaecol Can* 2007;**29**:433–65.

39. La Chapelle CF, Bemelman WA, Rademaker BM, et al. A multidisciplinary evidence-based guideline for minimally invasive

surgery. Part 1: entry techniques and the pneumoperitoneum. *Gynecol Surg* 2012;**9**:271–82.

40. Yoong W, Saxena S, Mittal M, Stavroulis A, Ogbodo E, Damodaram M. The pressure profile test is more sensitive and specific than Palmer's test in predicting correct placement of the Veress needle. *Eur J Obstet Gynecol Reprod Biol* 2010;**152**:210–13.

41. Teoh B, Sen R, Abbott J. An evaluation of four tests used to ascertain Veres needle placement at closed laparoscopy. *J Minim Invasive Gynecol* 2005;**12**:153–58.

42. Dingfelder JR. Direct laparoscope trocar insertion without prior pneumoperitoneum. *J Reprod Med* 1978;**21**:45–47.

43. Hasson HM. A modified instrument and method for laparoscopy. *Am J Obstet Gynecol* 1971;**110**:886–87.

44. Ternamian AM, Vilos GA, Vilos AG, Abu-Rafea B, Tyrwhitt J, MacLeod NT. Laparoscopic peritoneal entry with the reusable threaded visual cannula. *J Minim Invasive Gynecol* 2010;**17**:461–67.

45. Ternamian AM. Laparoscopy without trocars. *Surg Endosc* 1997;**11**:815–18.

46. Bhoyrul S, Payne J, Steffes B, Swanstrom L, Way LW. A randomized prospective study of radially expanding trocars in laparoscopic surgery. *J Gastrointest Surg* 2000;**4**:392–97.

47. Cuss A, Bhatt M, Abbott J. Coming to terms with the fact that the evidence for laparoscopic entry is as good as it gets. *J Minim Invasive Gynecol* 2015;**22**:332–41.

48. Abbott JA, Garry R. Consensus on the prevention of laparoscopic surgical accidents. *Gynaecol Obstet* 1999;**6**:357–63.

49. Ahmad G, O'Flynn H, Duffy JM, Phillips K, Watson A. Laparoscopic entry techniques. *Cochrane Database Syst Rev* 2012;**2**:CD006583.

50. Jiang X, Anderson C, Schnatz PF The safety of direct trocar versus Veress needle for laparoscopic entry: a meta-analysis of randomized clinical trials. *J Laparoendosc Adv Surg Tech A* 2012;**22**:362–70.

51. Gutt CN, Oniu T, Mehrabi A, et al. Circulatory and respiratory complications of carbon dioxide insufflation. *Dig Surg* 2004;**21**:95–105.

52. O'Malley C, Cunningham AJ. Physiologic changes during laparoscopy. *Anesthesiol Clin North Am* 2001;**19**:1–19.

53. Reich H, Ribeiro SC, Rasmussen C, Rosenberg J, Vidali A. High-pressure trocar insertion technique. *JSLS* 1999;**3**:45–48.

54. Tsaltas J, Pearce S, Lawrence A, Meads A, Mezzatesta J, Nicolson S. Safer laparoscopic trocar entry: it's all about pressure. *Aust N Z J Obstet Gynaecol* 2004;**44**:349–50.

55. Munro MG. Fundamentals of electrosurgery. Part I: principles of radiofrequency energy for surgery. In: Feldman L, Fuchshuber P, Jones DB (eds), *The SAGES Manual on the Fundamental Use of Surgical Energy (FUSE)*, pp. 15–59. New York: Springer; 2012.

56. Rioux JE, Cloutier D. [Tubal sterilization using laparoscopy: presentation of a new bipolar instrument.] *Vie Med Can Fr* 1973;**2**:760–65.

57. Muhe E. [Laparoscopic cholecystectomy—late results.] *Langenbecks Arch Chir Suppl Kongressbd* 1991:416–23.

58. Reich H. Laparoscopic hysterectomy. *Surg Laparosc Endosc* 1992;**2**:85–88.

59. Law KS, Lyons SD. Comparative studies of energy sources in gynecologic laparoscopy. *J Minim Invasive Gynecol* 2013;**20**:308–18.

60. Law KS, Abbott JA, Lyons SD. Energy sources for gynecologic laparoscopic surgery: a review of the literature. *Obstet Gynecol Surv* 2014;**69**:763–76.

61. Voyles CR. The art and science of monopolar electrosurgery. In: Feldman L, Fuchshuber P, Jones DB (eds), *The SAGES Manual on the Fundamental Use of Surgical Energy (FUSE)*, pp. 81–90. New York: Springer; 2012.

62. Brunt ML. Fundamentals of electrosurgery. Part II: thermal injury mechanisms and prevention. In: Feldman L, Fuchshuber P, Jones DB (eds), *The SAGES Manual on the Fundamental Use of Surgical Energy (FUSE)*, pp. 61–80. New York: Springer; 2012.

63. La Chapelle CF, Bemelman WA, Rademaker BM, et al. A multidisciplinary evidence-based guideline for minimally invasive surgery: part 2—laparoscopic port instruments, trocar site closure, and electrosurgical techniques. *Gynecol Surg* 2013;**10**:11–23.

64. Odell RC. Surgical complications specific to monopolar electrosurgical energy: engineering changes that have made electrosurgery safer. *J Minim Invasive Gynecol* 2013;**20**:288–98.

65. Vancaillie TG. Active electrode monitoring. How to prevent unintentional thermal injury associated with monopolar electrosurgery at laparoscopy. *Surg Endosc* 1998;**12**:1009–12.

66. Munro MG. Economics and energy sources. *J Minim Invasive Gynecol* 2013;**20**:319–27.

67. Costello MF, Abbott J, Katz S, Vancaillie T, Wilson S. A prospective, randomized, double-blind, placebo-controlled trial of multimodal intraoperative analgesia for laparoscopic excision of endometriosis. *Fertil Steril* 2010;**94**:436–43.

68. Gibbison B, Kinsella SM. Postoperative analgesia for gynecological laparoscopy. *Saudi J Anaesth* 2009;**3**:70–76.

69. Benhamou D, Narchi P, Mazoit JX, Fernandez H. Postoperative pain after local anesthetics for laparoscopic sterilization. *Obstet Gynecol* 1994;**84**:877–80.

70. Michaloliakou C, Chung F, Sharma S. Preoperative multimodal analgesia facilitates recovery after ambulatory laparoscopic cholecystectomy. *Ancsth Analg* 1996;**82**:44–51.

71. Einarsson JI, Sun J, Orav J, Young AE. Local analgesia in laparoscopy: a randomized trial. *Obstet Gynecol* 2004;**104**:1335–39.

72. Grube JO, Milad MP, Damme-Sorenen J. Preemptive analgesia does not reduce pain or improve postoperative functioning. *JSLS* 2004;**8**:15–18.

73. Lam KW, Pun TC, Ng EH, Wong KS. Efficacy of preemptive analgesia for wound pain after laparoscopic operations in infertile women: a randomised, double-blind and placebo control study. *BJOG* 2004;**111**:340–44.

74. Chou YJ, Ou YC, Lan KC, Jawan B, Chang SY, Kung FT. Preemptive analgesia installation during gynecologic laparoscopy: a randomized trial. *J Minim Invasive Gynecol* 2005;**12**:330–35.

75. Ghezzi F, Cromi A, Bergamini V, et al. Preemptive port site local anesthesia in gynecologic laparoscopy: a randomized, controlled trial. *J Minim Invasive Gynecol* 2005;**12**:210–15.

76. Jabbour-Khoury SI, Dabbous AS, Gerges FJ, Azar MS, Ayoub CM, Khoury GS. Intraperitoneal and intravenous routes for pain relief in laparoscopic cholecystectomy. *JSLS* 2005;**9**:316–21.

77. Kim JH, Lee YS, Shin HW, Chang MS, Park YC, Kim WY. Effect of administration of ketorolac and local anaesthetic infiltration for pain relief after laparoscopic-assisted vaginal hysterectomy. *J Int Med Res* 2005;**33**:372–78.

78. Louizos AA, Hadzilia SJ, Leandros E, Kouroukli IK, Georgiou LG, Bramis JP. Postoperative pain relief after laparoscopic cholecystectomy: a placebo-controlled double-blind randomized trial of preincisional infiltration and intraperitoneal instillation of levobupivacaine 0.25%. *Surg Endosc* 2005;**19**:1503–506.

79. Alessandri F, Lijoi D, Mistrangelo E, Nicoletti A, Ragni N. Effect of presurgical local infiltration of levobupivacaine in the surgical field on postsurgical wound pain in laparoscopic gynecological surgery. *Acta Obstet Gynecol Scand* 2006;**85**:844–49.

80. Kane SM, Garcia-Tomas V, Alejandro-Rodriguez M, Astley B, Pollard RR. Randomized trial of transversus abdominis plane block at total laparoscopic hysterectomy: effect of regional analgesia on quality of recovery. *Am J Obstet Gynecol* 2012;**207**419.e1–5.

81. Kwon YS, Kim JB, Jung HJ, et al. Treatment for postoperative wound pain in gynecologic laparoscopic surgery: topical lidocaine patches. *J Laparoendosc Adv Surg Tech A* 2012;**22**:668–73.

82. Manjunath AP, Chhabra N, Girija S, Nair S. Pain relief in laparoscopic tubal ligation using intraperitoneal lignocaine: a double masked randomized controlled trial. *Eur J Obstet Gynecol Reprod Biol* 2012;**165**:110–14.

83. Arden D, Seifert E, Donnellan N, Guido R, Lee T, Mansuria S. Intraperitoneal instillation of bupivacaine for reduction of postoperative pain after laparoscopic hysterectomy: a double-blind randomized controlled trial. *J Minim Invasive Gynecol* 2013;**20**:620–26.

84. Tam T, Harkins G, Wegrzyniak L, Ehrgood S, Kunselman A, Davies M. Infiltration of bupivacaine local anesthetic to trocar insertion sites after laparoscopy: a randomized, double-blind, stratified, and controlled trial. *J Minim Invasive Gynecol* 2014;**21**:1015–21.

85. Hotujec BT, Spencer RJ, Donnelly MJ, et al. Transversus abdominis plane block in robotic gynecologic oncology: a randomized, placebo-controlled trial. *Gynecol Oncol* 2015;**136**:460–65.

86. Karthik S, Augustine AJ, Shibumon MM, Pai MV. Analysis of laparoscopic port site complications: a descriptive study. *J Minim Access Surg* 2013;**9**:59–64.

87. Magrina JF. Complications of laparoscopic surgery. *Clin Obstet Gynecol* 2002;**45**:469–80.

88. Tonouchi H, Ohmori Y, Kobayashi M, Kusunoki M. Trocar site hernia. *Arch Surg* 2004;**139**:1248–56.

89. Kadar N, Reich H, Liu CY, Manko GF, Gimpelson R. Incisional hernias after major laparoscopic gynecologic procedures. *Am J Obstet Gynecol* 1993;**168**:1493–95.

90. Abbott JA, Phillips AG. Herniation following laparoscopic sterilisation. *Gynae Endosc* 2000;**9**:271–72.

91. Natalin RA, Lima FS, Pinheiro T, et al. The final stage of the laparoscopic procedure: exploring final steps. *Int Braz J Urol* 2012;**38**:4–16.

92. Chen K, Klapper AS, Voige H, Del Priore G. A randomized, controlled study comparing two standardized closure methods of laparoscopic port sites. *JSLS* 2010;**14**:391–94.

93. Thomson AJ, Abbott JA, Lenart M, et al. Assessment of a method to expel intraperitoneal gas after gynecologic laparoscopy. *J Minim Invasive Gynecol* 2005;**12**:125–29.

94. Berberoğlu M, Dilek ON, Ercan F, Kati I, Ozmen M. The effect of CO2 insufflation rate on the postlaparoscopic shoulder pain. *J Laparoendosc Adv Surg Tech A* 1998;**8**:273–77.

95. Abbott J, Hawe J, Srivastava P, Hunter D, Garry R. Intraperitoneal gas drain to reduce pain after laparoscopy: randomized masked trial. *Obstet Gynecol* 2001;**98**:97–100.

96. Shen CC, Wu MP, Lu CH, et al. Effects of closed suction drainage in reducing pain after laparoscopic-assisted vaginal hysterectomy. *J Am Assoc Gynecol Laparosc* 2003;**10**:210–14.

97. Suginami R, Taniguchi F, Suginami H. Prevention of postlaparoscopic shoulder pain by forced evacuation of residual CO. *JSLS* 2009;**13**:56–59.

98. Tsai HW, Wang PH, Yen MS, Chao KC, Hsu TF, Chen YJ. Prevention of postlaparoscopic shoulder and upper abdominal pain: a randomized controlled trial. *Obstet Gynecol* 2013;**121**:526–31.

99. Sharami SH, Sharami MB, Abdollahzadeh M, Keyvan A. Randomised clinical trial of the influence of pulmonary recruitment manoeuvre on reducing shoulder pain after laparoscopy. *J Obstet Gynaecol* 2010;**30**:505–10.

100. Guido RS, Brooks K, McKenzie R, Gruss J, Krohn MA. A randomized, prospective comparison of pain after gasless laparoscopy and traditional laparoscopy. *J Am Assoc Gynecol Laparosc* 1998;**5**:149–53.

101. Bogani G, Uccella S, Cromi A, et al. Low vs. standard pneumoperitoneum pressure during laparoscopic hysterectomy: prospective randomized trial. *J Minim Invasive Gynecol* 2014;**21**:466–71.

102. Leelasuwattanakul N, Bunyavehchevin S, Sriprachittichai P. Active gas aspiration versus simple gas evacuation to reduce shoulder pain after diagnostic laparoscopy: a randomized controlled trial. *J Obstet Gynaecol Res* 2016;**42**:190–94.

103. Swift G, Healey M, Varol N, Maher P, Hill D. A prospective randomised double-blind placebo controlled trial to assess whether gas drains reduce shoulder pain following gynaecological laparoscopy. *Aust N Z J Obstet Gynaecol* 2002;**42**:267–70.

104. Raymond AP, Chan K, Deans R, Bradbury R, Vancaillie TG, Abbott JA. A comparative, single-blind, randomized trial of pain associated with suction or non-suction drains after gynecologic laparoscopy. *J Minim Invasive Gynecol* 2010;**17**:16–20.

105. Kerimoglu OS, Yilmaz SA, Pekin A et al. Effect of drainage on postoperative pain after laparoscopic ovarian cystectomy. *J Obstet Gynaecol* 2015;**35**:287–89.

106. Hoyer-Sorensen C, Vistad I, Ballard K. Is single-port laparoscopy for benign adnexal disease less painful than conventional laparoscopy? A single-center randomized controlled trial. *Fertil Steril* 2012;**98**:973–79.

107. Choi YS, Park JN, Oh YS, Sin KS, Choi J, Eun DS. Single-port vs. conventional multi-port access laparoscopy-assisted vaginal hysterectomy: comparison of surgical outcomes and complications. *Eur J Obstet Gynecol Reprod Biol* 2013;**169**:366–69.

108. Mencaglia L, Mereu L, Carri G, et al. Single port entry – are there any advantages? *Best Pract Res Clin Obstet Gynaecol* 2013;**27**:441–55.

109. Nezhat C, Lewis M, Kotikela S, et al. Robotic versus standard laparoscopy for the treatment of endometriosis. *Fertil Steril* 2010;**94**:2758–60.

110. Gobern JM, Rosemeyer CJ, Barter JF, Steren AJ. Comparison of robotic, laparoscopic, and abdominal myomectomy in a community hospital. *JSLS* 2013;**17**:116–20.

111. Paraiso MF, Ridgeway B, Park AJ, et al. A randomized trial comparing conventional and robotically assisted total laparoscopic hysterectomy. *Am J Obstet Gynecol* 2013;**208**:368.e1–7.

112. Sarlos D, Kots L, Stevanovic N, von Felten S, Schär G. Robotic compared with conventional laparoscopic hysterectomy: a randomized controlled trial. *Obstet Gynecol* 2012;**120**:604–11.

113. Liu H, Lawrie TA, Lu D, Song H, Wang L, Shi G. Robot-assisted surgery in gynaecology. *Cochrane Database Syst Rev* 2014;**12**:CD011422.

114. Pasic RP, Rizzo JA, Fang H, Ross S, Moore M, Gunnarsson C. Comparing robot-assisted with conventional laparoscopic hysterectomy: impact on cost and clinical outcomes. *J Minim Invasive Gynecol* 2010;**17**:730–38.

115. Sarlos D, Kots L, Stevanovic N, Schaer G. Robotic hysterectomy versus conventional laparoscopic hysterectomy: outcome and cost analyses of a matched case-control study. *Eur J Obstet Gynecol Reprod Biol* 2010;**150**:92–96.

116. Smorgick N, Patzkowsky KE, Hoffman MR, Advincula AP, Song AH, As-Sanie S. The increasing use of robot-assisted approach for hysterectomy results in decreasing rates of abdominal hysterectomy and traditional laparoscopic hysterectomy. *Arch Gynecol Obstet* 2014;**289**:101–105.

48

Hysteroscopy

O. A. O'Donovan and Peter J. O'Donovan

Introduction and historical background

The term hysteroscopy comes from the Greek term 'hysteros' meaning uterus and 'scopy' meaning to look and is the cornerstone of modern outpatient endoscopic investigation and treatment in gynaecology (1). Pantaleoni performed the first successful diagnostic and operative hysteroscopy in 1869; he used a modified cystoscope reflecting candle light to examine and treat a polyp in a patient with postmenopausal bleeding (2). This paved the way for urologists and gynaecologists to develop and achieve further advances in endoscopic procedures. Charles David in 1907 was the first to describe a lens system that would allow uterine cavity visualization (3). It was not until 1943 when the combination of a cold light source developed by Fourestier (4) and a rod lens system developed by Hopkins dramatically improved uterine cavity assessment and formed the basis of modern-day gynaecological endoscopy.

Initially hysteroscopy was developed as an inpatient procedure, which was performed under general anaesthetic. Advances in technology, in particular miniaturization of optics, have resulted in both diagnostic and minor operative procedures being performed in the office/outpatient setting (5–8); this has been shown to be safe and acceptable to women. Hysteroscopy is well accepted, convenient, cost-effective, and is seen as a rapid access 'see and treat' solution for several gynaecological disorders (9–11).

Indications for diagnostic hysteroscopy

- *Evaluation of abnormal uterine bleeding*: abnormal uterine bleeding account for 20% of referrals to gynaecologists and 25% of gynaecological procedures in premenstrual women (12). Abnormal uterine bleeding can be subdivided into premenopausal problems, postmenopausal problems, and unscheduled bleeding on hormone replacement therapy or tamoxifen. When combined with pelvic ultrasound scanning and endometrial biopsy, outpatient hysteroscopy is invaluable in the investigation of abnormal uterine bleeding.

- *Diagnosis of focal intrauterine lesions (e.g. polyps and fibroids)*: structural lesions responsible for abnormal bleeding are often at their peak during the perimenopausal period; these include focal lesions such as endometrial polyps and submucosal fibroids. Endometrial cancer is rare between the age of 40 years and its incidence rises steeply between the ages of 45 and 55 (13, 14). Between 5% and 10% of all women with postmenopausal bleeding will have endometrial cancer (15).

- *Investigation and infertility*: the main indication for hysteroscopy is the investigation of infertility is in clarifying intrauterine pathology when an abnormal scan result is obtained, for example, endometrial polyps, submucous fibroids, intrauterine adhesions, or septa.

- *Investigation of recurrent miscarriage*: congenital abnormalities are associated with infertility, there is a high rate of spontaneous miscarriage and preterm labour when these structural abnormalities exist (16, 17). Hysteroscopy is not useful in diagnosing cervical incompetence but can identify cervical adhesions, atresia, and polyps. Cervical incompetence can, however, be suspected when the uterus fails to distend with loss of fluid coming through the cervix.

- *Location and retrieval of a lost intrauterine contraceptive device (IUD)*: a pelvic ultrasound scan will locate the IUD and confirm its presence inside the cavity; if there is any doubt, a plain abdominal X-ray should be ordered. Outpatient hysteroscopy is invaluable in the removal of the IUD; a hysteroscope with an operative channel is used with a grasping forceps inserted into the uterus and either the thread or the IUD itself is grasped with the forceps and the hysteroscope is withdrawn with the IUD.

- *Prior to ablation of the endometrium*: endometrial ablation is designed to treat abnormal uterine bleeding in women with no intrauterine pathology. Preablation hysteroscopy is useful to exclude any unexpected pathology and to rule out endometrial cancer.

- *Assessment for hysteroscopic sterilization*: hysteroscopic sterilization is performed in the outpatient setting and aims to reduce the risks from general anaesthetic, has a shorter recovery time, and aims to be cost-effective; a newer method that aims to achieve this is the Essure system, details of this will be discussed later (15).

Contraindications for operative and diagnostic hysteroscopy

Absolute contraindications

- *Cervical cancer*: hysteroscopy should not be performed in the presence of cervical cancer because of the danger of opening blood or lymphatic vessels and causing systemic dissemination of malignant cells.
- *Heavy uterine bleeding*: hysteroscopy should be avoided during menstruation, because of a theoretical risk of dissemination during endometriosis and mainly because the view is limited and unsatisfactory. Moderate uterine bleeding does not prevent adequate visualization of the uterine cavity.
- *Pelvic inflammatory disease*: due to the danger of causing extended ascending infection and peritonitis.

Relative contraindications

- *Pregnancy*: generally considered a contraindication to hysteroscopy but it may be necessary to perform hysteroscopy to remove an IUD.
- *Recent uterine perforation*: the risk of repeat uterine perforation is considered greater in such cases as the healing process may have left a weak scar.
- *Cervical stenosis*: the risk of uterine perforation is considered greater in such cases; the importance of an experienced operator cannot be overstated.
- *Cardiorespiratory disease*.
- *Uncooperative patient*: although this can be overcome using the vaginoscopic technique

Indications for operative hysteroscopy

Improvements in the design of hysteroscopes have made it possible to carry out operative hysteroscopy in awake patients; other advances include the use of bipolar energy thus making it possible to use normal saline rather than non-ionic distention media (glycine). These advances have made hysteroscopy safer.

- *Targeted biopsy*: suspicious or abnormal-looking focal lesions in the endometrium are best biopsied using a grasping forceps passed down the operating channel.
- *Endocervical and endometrial polypectomy*: polyps in the endocervix can be removed by avulsion or using a large loop excision of the transformation zone if they are sessile. Endometrial polyps are formed by proliferation and hypertrophy of the basal layer of the endometrium, with varying degrees of malignancy (18). At hysteroscopy, they are smooth and soft. They are either sessile or pedunculated; they can be removed using scissors, graspers, or a bipolar electrode. The disadvantage of this latter method is there is no histology. Most experts would recommend that polyps less than 3 cm in diameter can be removed this way.
- *Treatment of submucous fibroids*: submucous fibroids can be removed with the operative hysteroscope. Most experts would recommend that the fibroids should be treated if more than 2 cm in

size, in the inpatient setting. They can be treated using mechanical instruments or ablated using the bipolar spring electrode.

- *Division of intrauterine adhesions*: adhesions are classified as mild, moderate, or severe. Mild adhesions are thin and of recent occurrence, moderate adhesions are thicker and bleed on division. Severe adhesions may be composed of connective tissue and are unlikely to bleed. Division of moderate and severe forms often require general anaesthesia and concomitant laparoscopy and/or intraoperative ultrasound. Usually scissors or a twizzle electrode are used for division under hysteroscopic control. Results following treatment reveal 60–70% pregnancy rates depending on the severity before treatment.
- *Division of uterine septa*: approximately 25% of women with a septate uterus have recurrent pregnancy loss (16). Hysteroscopic division with scissors or a cutting electrode or using the resectoscope under general or regional anaesthesia is generally performed. The operation may need to be carried out under laparoscopic or ultrasound control. Hysteroscopic division offers high success and pregnancy rates of 85–90% have been quoted (19, 20). Generally patients are advised to delay pregnancy for at least 4–7 weeks.
- *Hysteroscopic sterilization*: performed in the outpatient setting, this aims to reduce the risks of general anaesthesia, to have a shorter recovery period, and to be cost effective. Essure consists of a micro-insert, a disposable delivery system which is delivered down a hysteroscope. The micro-insert consists of a stainless steel inner coil, a nitinol and super-elastic outer coil, and polyethylene fibres. The micro-insert is inserted into the fallopian tube and remains anchored across the uterotubal junction. Fibrous tissue grows, anchoring the micro-insert into the fallopian tube and the occlusion results in sterilization. Studies have shown 96% of cases have bilateral occlusion at 6 months and it is 99.8% effective in preventing pregnancy after 3 months of follow-up (21, 22). It can be performed in 15–20 minutes and the bilateral placement rate is 90%; alternative methods of contraception must be used in 3 months after the procedure (23).

Endometrial ablation/resection

Since 1981, patients have been able to choose endometrial ablation as a treatment for heavy periods and over the last 20 years, several endometrial ablation techniques have been introduced. In 1981, Milton Goldrath wrote what is in effect the first description of endometrial ablation, using laser energy to destroy the endometrium in 22 women with menorrhagia (24). Sometime in the mid 1980s, Jacques Hamou, a well-known hysteroscopist from Paris, introduced what has become known as partial endometrial resection into Europe. Hamou popularized endometrial resection as well as hysteroscopic myomectomy in Europe and in 1988 at a meeting held in Oxford he taught the technique to a group of British clinicians. Discussions led to the introduction of the term 'transcervical resection of the endometrium' (TCRE) (25).

Patient selection

Careful patient selection is important. Criteria for offering this type of surgery are summarized in **Table 48.1**.

Table 48.1 Inclusion and exclusion criteria for hysteroscopic endometrial ablation

Inclusion criteria	Exclusion criteria
Abnormal uterine bleeding	Coexisting gynaecological pathology (e.g. uterovaginal prolapse, ovarian pathology, pelvic inflammatory disease, cervical atypia)
No desire for amenorrhoea	Endometrial atypia and cancer
Unsuccessful medical treatment	Submucous fibroids >2 cm
Endometrial biopsy negative for atypia and cancer	Uterus >12 weeks in size
Family complete	Anovulation, endometrial hyperplasia

Techniques of hysteroscopic endometrial ablation

A complete description of the various techniques of endometrial ablation is beyond the scope of this chapter; however, briefly there are two types: electrosurgical and laser methods. Laser methods are no longer widely used as they are both expensive and difficult to learn.

There are two different types of electrosurgical treatment: rollerball endometrial ablation and loop endometrial resection.

Rollerball endometrial ablation

This technique involves using a ball electrode to treat the endometrial lining. It has become popular because of its relative simplicity and cost advantage compared with laser ablation (26, 27).

It is a safe and effective technique, having also the advantage of being quick to perform (28). The safety and efficacy of the technique have been well demonstrated by several studies which have 2-year follow-up on 200 patients, which reported a success rate of 90% and a repeat procedure rate of 4% with 5% of women ultimately undergoing hysterectomy (29).

Rollerball endometrial ablation has the following advantages and disadvantages:

Advantages

- Easier to learn and perform than resection.
- Less risk of uterine perforation, fluid reabsorption, and haemorrhage than endometrial resection.
- Shorter operating time.

Disadvantages

- No endometrial specimen for histology.
- Cannot treat submucous fibroids.
- Use of monopolar energy which is less safe than bipolar energy.

Loop endometrial resection

TCRE is a technique which has also been shown to be an effective and safe method for treating heavy menstrual bleeding (30–32).

The use of the loop-shaped electrode through a monopolar or bipolar continuous flow resectoscope produces efficient resection of the endometrium and underlying superficial myometrium—this provides tissue for histological examination.

Bipolar resectoscopes have been introduced which increases the safety of the procedure with respect to fluid overload as uterine distention with normal saline is associated with less electrolyte disturbance than is the case with electrolyte-free solutions.

The most important principle of loop resection is to only activate the electrode as it is being pulled towards the cervix—this makes accidental perforation of the uterus less likely. TCRE can be combined easily with hysteroscopic myomectomy in women with heavy menstrual bleeding and submucous fibroids.

TCRE is certainly a proven alternative to hysterectomy with high satisfaction rates ranging between 70% and 94% (31).

Endometrial resection has the following advantages/disadvantages:

Advantages

- Provides endometrial tissue for histology.
- Submucous fibroids or polyps can be excised at the same time.
- Suitable if endometrium is thick.

Disadvantages

- It is a skill-dependent technique.
- Greatest risk of uterine perforation.
- Need to use electrolyte-free distention media with monopolar resectoscope.

Prognostic parameters for endometrial ablation

Although endometrial resection or ablation seems to be an effective procedure with high success rates for individual patients, it is recognized that there are certain prognostic parameters which would help to predict outcomes in counselling patients. One should consider pre-existing conditions when counselling patients regarding outcome expectations after an endometrial ablation procedure.

Table 48.2 shows the prognostic factors that have been evaluated and those that were just poorly or never evaluated.

- Adenomyosis: adenomyosis is still not easily diagnosed before treatment but it is related to failure after endometrial ablation (33).
- Sterilization: if the patient was sterilized before endometrial ablation was performed, a higher chance of failure was found (34, 35).

Table 48.2 Prognostic factors that have been evaluated and those that were just poorly or never (PBAC) evaluated for endometrial ablation

Evaluated prognostic values	Poor evaluated values
Sterilization	PBAC
Age	Endometrial thickness
BMI	Adenomyosis
Cavity length (sound length)	
Myomas	
Smoking	
Parity	
Preoperative dysmenorrhoea	

PBAC, Pictorial Blood Loss Assessment Chart.

In all the trials laparoscopic sterilization was performed and there is little known about the effects of hysteroscopic sterilization.

- Age: older age seems to be prognostically favourable for success after endometrial ablation (36–39). Cut-off in the trials was mostly more than 45 years of age.
- Body mass index (BMI): when a woman has a high BMI there is a higher ability for the regeneration of endometrial tissue.
- Cavity length: the longer the cavity length, the more unfavourable the outcomes after ablation (34).
- Smoking: tobacco gives inferior results after endometrial ablation; the relationship between smoking and endometrial ablation is unclear.
- Fibroids: the existence of myomas in the uterus is prognostically unfavourable; the existence of submucous fibroids seems to be correlated with a higher chance of dissatisfaction after endometrial ablation (34, 40).
- Parity: parity of more than five deliveries has a higher chance of reintervention (36, 37).
- Preoperative dysmenorrhoea: the observed instance of failure or reintervention after endometrial ablation is more frequently observed in women with preablation dysmenorrhoea (34, 36–38, 40, 41).

Complications of diagnostic and operative hysteroscopy

What are the established rates of complications associated with hysteroscopic surgery?

Different procedures have different complication rates. There have been numerous large-scale national audits performed (Table 48.3) (42–44). Jansen et al. published a Dutch national audit in 2000, which examined more than 11,000 diagnostic and 2500 operative hysteroscopies. The audit found that there were significantly more complications during operative hysteroscopy compared to diagnostic hysteroscopy. Clinically significant fluid overload occurred in 0.2% of operative hysteroscopies particularly during myomectomy resections. Although uterine perforations occurred during both diagnostic (incidence 0.13%) and operative hysteroscopy (incidence 0.76%) there was no statistically significant difference between entry- and technique-related causes of uterine perforation. Perforations occurred most commonly during dilatation (70%) for diagnostic hysteroscopy. The riskiest operative hysteroscopic procedure was adhesiolysis (risks of complication 4.5%) compared to polypectomy (0.4%). Jansen's publication reported no deaths due to hysteroscopic surgery.

Intraoperative complications

Vasovagal reflex

This commonly occurs when dilating the cervix or passing the hysteroscope. The prevalence of vasovagal reaction (1 in 300 cases) depends on the ability of the endoscopist and on the diameter of the scope.

Cervical trauma

Operative procedures can often be performed without the need to dilate the cervix, especially if the vaginoscopic technique described by Bettocchi et al. is used (45). However, operative hysteroscopy might require cervical dilatation. Trauma can be dealt with using pressure, silver nitrate, or sutures. It is best to avoid overdilating the cervix because this can result in leakage of the distending media of the cervix and around the hysteroscope. Always introduce the hysteroscope under direct vision.

Uterine perforation

Uterine perforation is a rare event; as previously mentioned, the incidence is higher in operative procedures. In a large systematic review of over 25,000 women only 4 cases (1 in 6000 women) of uterine perforation occurred (46). The uterus may be perforated by a dilator, the hysteroscope, or an energy source. Management will depend upon the size, site of perforation, and whether there is a risk of injury to another organ. Perforation occurs more frequently at the level of the fundus, without significant bleeding. Simple perforation rarely causes any further damage and can be treated conservatively by admission, observation, and appropriate broad-spectrum antibiotics. Laparoscopy might be considered to exclude bleeding. Complex perforations might be made with a mechanical or an energy source and therefore can be associated with thermal injury to adjacent structures including bowel or large vessels. However, energy sources used in the outpatient setting are usually bipolar (Versapoint) which reduces energy spread through the tissue during the procedure and hence provides high levels of safety.

It is important to be vigilant during the days after perforation as thermal injury to surrounding organs can present some days after the event due to ischaemic necrosis of thermally compromised tissue.

Haemorrhage

Intra- or postoperative bleeding can be caused by:

- the tenaculum (only used if dilating the cervix)
- uterine perforation
- the procedure.

Management will depend upon the site, severity, and cause of bleeding. Intrauterine bleeding occurring during the procedure

Table 48.3 Large-scale national audits

Year	Author	Number	Perforations (%)	Bleeding (%)	Fluid overload (%)
1995	Scottish Hysteroscopy Audit Group	978	1.1	3.6	0.6
1997	MISTLETOE	10,686	1.5	2.4	1.9
2000	Jansen et al.	2515	1.3	0.16	0.2

should be immediately obvious and can usually be controlled by electrocoagulation. If coagulation fails to control the bleeding, the procedure may have to be abandoned and tamponade performed by inserting a Foley catheter and distending the balloon. The catheter should be left *in situ* for 4–6 hours after which the bleeding nearly always stops.

Complications with distention medium

Gas or liquid distention medium are essential for hysteroscopic surgery in order to keep the uterine wall separated and to obtain a clear view. The use of these media creates complications specific to hysteroscopy. Carbon dioxide has been used for uterine distension during diagnostic hysteroscopy. Deaths have been reported due to carbon dioxide gas embolism. Although fluid media is necessary for hysteroscopic surgery, excessive fluid reabsorption is a relatively uncommon recurrence. The incidence of excessive fluid absorption is 0.1–0.2%. However, the consequences can be very serious, with several death reported due to excessive fluid absorption (47). All types of distention media can result in complications relating to fluid overload. These include dilatational hyponatraemia, and heart failure: this combination can be very dangerous if not recognized and managed appropriately. The transurethral resection syndrome is virtually the same phenomenon that was initially documented by urologists, when performing transurethral resection of the prostate. Istre has shown that absorption of 1 L of 1.5% glycine can reduce serum sodium concentrations in more than 50% of patients who subsequently showed evidence of cerebral oedema on computed tomography scanning (48, 49). Based on these facts, the following risk factors for fluid complications can be identified:

- Large or deep resections of large fibroids.
- Prolonged duration of procedure.
- High pressure used to maintain uterine distension.
- Uterine perforation.
- Anaesthetic used.

Three areas can be focused upon to prevent this complication or at least minimize the risk of permanent damage:

- Attention to the type of media used for performing hysteroscopic surgery.
- Minimization of absorption.
- Recognition and management of the problems promptly.

Delayed complications

- Infection: an incidence of 2:1000 per infection has been reported in over 4000 diagnostic hysteroscopies. Acute pelvic inflammatory disease following hysteroscopic surgery is rare, the diagnosis is made from the classic symptoms and signs and treatment should be by appropriate antibiotics following culture of bloods and vaginal swabs.
- Vaginal discharge: vaginal discharge is common after any ablative procedure and can sometimes be prolonged (2–3 weeks) although it is usually self-limiting. Patients should alert their healthcare provider if the vaginal discharge becomes offensive

or if they develop pyrexia, heavy bleeding, or severe lower abdominal pain.
- Adhesion formation: intrauterine adhesions are common especially after myomectomy when two fibroids are situated on opposing uterine walls; in this case the myomectomy is better performed in stages to prevent adhesion formation. An IUD and 2 months of oral contraception can help prevent adhesion formation following operative hysteroscopy.

Recent developments

New devices for hysteroscopy: imaging systems with readily portable cameras and light sources can be used in examination rooms that are not solely dedicated for hysteroscopy; they enable more flexible use of space.

Endosee

The Endosee device (CooperSurgical) is a hand-held, battery-operated hysteroscopy system that consists of two main parts. The 'HandTower' contains a small (3.5-inch diagonal) touchscreen liquid-crystal display monitor, with video and control electronics and a rechargeable battery. The hysteroscopes are single-use, semi-rigid curved cannulas with a diameter of 3.5 mm and a length of 287 mm. The lens camera and light source are placed at the tip and comprise a digital processing chip. There is a port at the proximal end of the cannula to which can be attached a syringe or inflow tubing for saline irrigation. Results of observational studies using the device for diagnostic hysteroscopy have provided promising preliminary results (50–52).

TELE PACK X LED

The TELE PACK X LED (Karl Storx) although not an entirely new system has been upgraded and now incorporates a new LED light source and a 15-inch LED back light monitor (**Figure 48.1**). In addition, surgical procedures can now be downloaded and recorded via USB ports or on a SD card slot. It remains a portable, all-in-one system, comprising a light source and a monitor, and can be used with all Karl Storz one-chip camera heads and a variety of endoscopes. It is suitable for use in the office setting or operating theatre.

Intrauterine morcellation

Intrauterine morcellation devices with mechanical removal of pathology under direct vision and using normal saline for a distension have been developments that warrant reporting. Smaller devices are now available and from the results of a trial comparing electroresection with hysteroscopic morcellation it seems that the latter is particularly useful for endometrial polypectomy in the outpatient setting in both pre- and postmenopausal women (53). Polyp removal with the morcellator was quicker, less painful, and more likely to be complete than with electrosurgical resection.

Complications are usually self-limiting and consist of vasovagal reactions and a single episode of endometritis. Other pathologies that can be removed with hysteroscopic morcellators include submucosal fibroids and placental remnants as well as adhesions and uterine septa (54–56).

(a)

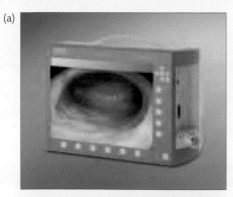

(b)

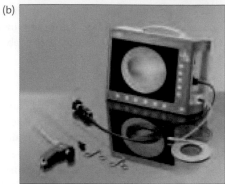

Figure 48.1 (a) TELEPACK X LED; (b) TELEPACK X LED with office hysteroscopy set.

Reproduced from Mencaglia, L., Cavalanti de Albuquerque Neto, L., and Arias Alvarez, R., *Manual of Hysteroscopy*, 2011, with permission from Endo Press.

The relative safety of hysteroscopic morcellators in all settings needs to be confirmed by the assessment of larger patient cohorts. In the meantime, audit of treatment complications and outcomes is required.

Instrumentation and set-up

Setting up a hysteroscopy service

Infrastructure

This involves a multidisciplinary set up. The ability to perform ultrasound scans is important, particularly transvaginal scanning in the same clinic.

Ideal setting

Due to the intimate nature of the procedure, women attending the hysteroscopy clinic are likely to be anxious (57). Outpatient hysteroscopy should be conducted in a well-organized clinic with calm, competent, and experienced doctors and nursing staff. Women should receive appropriate information, providing them with details of the procedure. Background music may act as a complementary adjuvant for anxious patient (58). It is important for patients to be as comfortable as possible and have private changing facilities, a toilet, and refreshments (59). Facilities should be available in the case of unexpected responses, for example, vasovagal responses, with either a bed or recliner accessible.

Equipment

The necessary equipment includes the following:

- Gynaecological couch/chair: positioning the patient comfortably on the examination couch/chair will help the patient to relax during the procedure. It should be possible to manoeuvre the couch if the preference is for an electronically powered modern gynaecological chair. Positioning the patient to perform both diagnostic and operative hysteroscopy is important, particularly in morbidly obese patients. The provision of a good couch helps the operator and also reduces strain on both the arm and hands of the surgeon during both diagnostic and operative procedures.

- Video camera and monitor: it is important to get high-quality images with printing and storage facilities; increasingly both video cameras and monitors are being miniaturized which is helpful in space utilization. Ideally the video camera and monitor should be housed on a single video cart.

- Light source and cable: most hysteroscopes require a cold xenon light source (175 watt). Light cables are easily damaged and require careful handling.

- Pressure cuff for fluid distension medium: generally normal saline is preferred to carbon dioxide as this allows an improved image quality, a quicker procedure, and allows the use of bipolar energy for operative hysteroscopy. There is no significant difference in pain perceived with using either of the distention media for hysteroscopy (60). Normal saline bags 1–3 L should be used, these should be warmed to room temperature. Pressure bags can be used to achieve uterine distention pressure of 80–120 mmHg. A fluid management system is recommended for fibroid resection for a clear view intraoperatively and to accurately monitor fluid balance

- Carbon dioxide insufflator and tubing if using gas distention: if carbon dioxide is used as a distention medium, a carbon dioxide insufflator apparatus is used to achieve a flow rate of 100 mL/min.

- Additional basic instruments: include Cusco Speculum, tenaculum, forceps, sterile cleaning solution, Hegar cervical dilator (1/2 mm onwards).

- Inflow and outflow tubing, dental syringe, local anaesthetic, Pipelle endometrial biopsy sampler, scissors, and silver nitrate sticks.

- Hysteroscope: a range of hysteroscopes, diagnostic and operative, can be used. These vary from rigid diagnostic 3 mm and operative 5 mm.

  - The size of the hysteroscope plays an important role in the acceptance and success of hysteroscopy (61). Randomized control trials compared the effect of size of the outer sheath on pain and success rate of ambulatory hysteroscopy (61–65).

  - Hysteroscopes with an outer sheath diameter of less than 3.5 mm were associated with significantly less intraoperative pain (62–64). Most diagnostic hysteroscope are 30 degrees allowing a thorough inspection of uterine walls, with minimal movement of the shaft. Both diagnostic and operative hysteroscopy clinics should consider investing in more rigid hysteroscopes as the Versapoint bipolar electrode and most miniature mechanical and electrosurgical devices require rigid hysteroscopes with size 4 Fr operative channels.

- Morcellators: the most recent development in operative hysteroscopy is the advent of mechanical miniature hysteroscopic morcellators. There are currently three different products on the market: Truclear, MyoSure, and the Intrauterine Bigatti Shaver.
  - This technology is particularly advantageous for treating multiple endometrial polyps or large polyps. Investing resources in morcellation hysteroscopes can still prove to be cost-effective in terms of the safety, speed, patient acceptability, and complete removal of the polyp/fibroid (66, 67).

Training and accreditation in hysteroscopy

An overview of training and accreditation in hysteroscopy in different countries pointed out the diversity and lack of robust guidelines across Europe. The European Society for Gynaecology Endoscopy has developed training standards for hysteroscopy but these are arbitrary. Since 2010, the United Kingdom Royal College of Obstetricians and Gynaecologists has offered an advanced training skill module for hysteroscopy (diagnostic/operative and outpatient/inpatient) for all senior trainees in obstetrics and gynaecology who wish to train as hysteroscopists. The gynaecologists who choose to train have access to variable training schemes; it is important, however, to attend training in order to perform outcomes. Novel methods of training in endoscopic psychomotor skills have developed such as stimulation training. More recently, advanced virtual reality stimulators have been developed; various studies have evaluated stimulation training, demonstrating improved performance in operative hysteroscopic skills (59, 68–74). HystSim (Virtamed, Symbionic) is a virtual reality stimulator providing realistic stimulation of hysteroscopic scenarios including obscured vision, bleeding control in a variety of modules stimulating diagnostic hysteroscopy, polypectomy, myomectomy, resection, ablation, and more recently hysteroscopic sterilization.

Audit, patient satisfaction, and risk management

Audit is an effective tool to monitor and improve service outcomes. The standards from the Royal College of Obstetricians and Gynaecologists 'Best Practice in Outpatient Hysteroscopy' guideline (59) can be used to audit the performance of individual units. It can be useful to gather outpatient and inpatient hysteroscopy figures to measure throughput and outcomes. Patient satisfaction surveys are important to evaluate the service and to provide insight from the patient's perspective on pain experienced, acceptability, and quality of service. These have a crucial role in maintaining quality.

Risk management is an essential part of patient safety; regular assessment of equipment, infection control, staff training guidelines, and protocols should be undertaken.

Research/current and future developments

Hysteroscopy has developed from a purely diagnostic service to a valuable operative procedure. In addition, more uterine surgeries can now be performed by hysteroscopy in the outpatient setting; endometrial ablation previously only performed by hysteroscopy can now be done without endoscopy. First-generation hysteroscopic treatment of the endometrium does remain an important treatment for women with heavy periods (73). Second-generation known hysteroscopic techniques are popular due to their ease of use and are independent of the surgical skill of the operator.

Outpatient hysteroscopy

Hysteroscopy offers direct visualization of the entire uterine cavity, and provides the possibility of performing the biopsy of suspected lesions that can be missed by dilatation and curettage. It has been demonstrated that dilatation and curettage misses 62% of intra-uterine pathologies (74).

Evidence-based practice

Best practice in outpatient hysteroscopy

The joint guideline from the Royal College of Obstetricians and Gynaecologists and the British Society for Gynaecological Endoscopy (59) recommends the following:

Service provision

- All gynaecology units should provide a dedicated outpatient hysteroscopy service to aid management of women with abnormal uterine bleeding. There are clinical and economic benefits associated with this type of service.
- Outpatient hysteroscopy should be outside of the formal operating theatre setting in an appropriately sized, equipped, and staffed treatment room with adjoining private changing facilities and toilet.
- The healthcare professional should have the necessary skills and expertise to carry out hysteroscopy.
- There should be a nurse chaperone regardless of the gender of the clinician.
- Written patient information should be provided before the appointment and consent for the procedure should be undertaken.

Analgesia

- Routine use of opiate analgesia before outpatient hysteroscopy should be avoided as it may cause adverse effects.
- Women without contraindications should be advised to consider taking standard doses of non-steroidal anti-inflammatory agents around 1 hour before the scheduled outpatient hysteroscopy appointment with the aim of reducing pain in the immediate post-operative period.

Cervical preparation

- Routine cervical preparation before outpatient hysteroscopy should not be used in the absence of any evidence of benefit in terms of reduction of pain, rates of failure, or uterine trauma.

Types of hysteroscope

- Miniature hysteroscopes (2.7 mm with a 3–3.5 mm sheath) should be used for diagnostic outpatient hysteroscopy as they significantly reduce the discomfort experienced by the woman.

- Flexible hysteroscopes are associated with less pain during outpatient hysteroscopy compared with rigid hysteroscopes; however, rigid hysteroscopes may provide better images, fewer failed procedures, quicker examination time, and reduced cost.

Distention medium

- For routine outpatient hysteroscopy, the choice of distention medium between carbon dioxide and normal saline should be left to the discretion of the operator as neither is superior in reducing pain although uterine distention with normal saline appears to reduce the incidence of vasovagal episodes.
- Uterine distention with normal saline allows improved image quality and allows outpatient diagnostic hysteroscopy to be completed more quickly compared with carbon dioxide.

Local anaesthesia and cervical dilatation

- Instillation of local anaesthetic into the cervical canal does not reduce pain during diagnostic outpatient hysteroscopy but may reduce the incidence of vasovagal reactions.
- Topical application of local anaesthetic to the ectocervix should be considered where application of a cervical tenaculum is necessary.
- Application of local anaesthetic into or around the cervix is associated with a reduction of the pain experienced during outpatient diagnostic hysteroscopy. However, it is unclear how clinically significant this reduction in pain is. Consideration should be given to the routine administration of intra- or paracervical local anaesthetic, particularly in postmenopausal women.
- Routine administration of intra- or paracervical local anaesthetic is not indicated to reduce the incidence of vasovagal reactions.

Conscious sedation

- Conscious sedation should not be routinely used in outpatient hysteroscopic procedures as it confers no advantage in terms of pain control and the woman's satisfaction over local anaesthetic.

Vaginoscopy

- Vaginoscopy reduced pain during diagnostic rigid hysteroscopy.

Conclusion

- Hysteroscopy continues to have a well-recognized role in the diagnosis and management of abnormal uterine bleeding.
- Hysteroscopic polypectomy, hysteroscopic submucosal resection of fibroids, and endometrial ablation are safe and effective.
- Prognostic parameters should be taken into account when counselling women who opt for endometrial ablation.
- Important prognostic factors are age (satisfaction increased with age) and preoperative dysmenorrhoea (decreases satisfaction).
- Selection of the right patients is the key to success of ambulatory procedures.

REFERENCES

1. Zacur HA, Murray D. Techniques and instrumentation of operative hysteroscopy. In: Azziz R, Murphy AA (eds), *Practical Manual of Operative Laparoscopy and Hysteroscopy*, pp. 151–65. New York: Springer; 1992.
2. Pantaleoni D. On endoscopic examination of the cavity of the womb. *Med Press Circ* 1869;**8**:26–27.
3. David C. De l'endoscopie de l'uterus après avortement et dans les suites de couches a l'etat pathologique. *Bull Soc Obstet* 1907;Dec.
4. Fourestier M, Gladau A, Vulmiere J. Perfectionments de l'endoscope medicale. *Presse Med* 1943;**5**:46–47.
5. Kremer C, Duffy S, Moroney M. Patient satisfaction with outpatient hysteroscopy versus day case hysteroscopy: randomised controlled trials. *BMJ* 200;**320**:279–82.
6. Clark TJ, Bakour SH, Gupta JK, et al. Evaluation of outpatient hysteroscopy and ultrasonography in the diagnosis of endometrial disease. *Obstet Gynecol* 2002;**99**:1001–1007.
7. Clark TK, Gupta JK. *Handbook of Outpatient Hysteroscopy: A Complete Guide to Diagnosis and Therapy*. Boca Raton, FL: CRC Press; 2005.
8. Clark TJ, Cooper NA, Kremer C. *Best Practice in Outpatient Hysteroscopy*. London: RCOG Press; 2011.
9. Cooper NAM, Clark TJ. Cost effectiveness of diagnostic strategies for the management of abnormal uterine bleeding (heavy menstrual bleeding and post menopausal bleeding): systematic reviews, IPD meta analysis and model based economic evaluation. Available at: http://www.hta.ac.uk/2145 (accessed 27 September 2013).
10. Moawad NS, Santamaria E, Johnson M, et al. Cost effectiveness of office hysteroscopy for abnormal uterine bleeding. *JSLS* 2014;**18**:e2014.00393.
11. Timmermans A, Opmeer BC, Veersema S, Mol BW. Patients' preferences in the evaluation of postmenopausal bleeding. *BJOG* 2007;**114**:1146–49.
12. Hatasaka H. The evaluation of abnormal uterine bleeding. *Clin Obstet Gynecol* 2005;**48**:258–73.
13. Royal College of Obstetricians and Gynaecologists (RCOG). *The Management of Menorrhagia in Secondary Care*. Evidence-based Clinical Guideline No. 5. London: RCOG Press; 1999.
14. Somoye G, Olaitan A, Morcrost A, et al. Age related trends in the incidence of endometrial cancer in South East England 1962–1997. *J Obstet Gynaecol* 2005;**25**:35–38.
15. Goldstein RB, Bree RL, Benson CB, et al. Evaluation of the woman with postmenopausal bleeding: Society of Radiologists in Ultrasound-Sponsored Consensus Conference statement. *J Ultrasound Med* 2001;**20**:1025–36.
16. Royal College of Obstetricians and Gynaecologists (RCOG). *The Management of Recurrent Miscarriage*. Green-top Guideline No. 17. London: RCOG; 2003.
17. Zikopoulos KA, Kolibianakis EM, Platteau P, et al. Live delivery rates in subfertile women with Asherman's syndrome after hysteroscopic adhesiolysis using the resectoscope or the Versapoint system. *Reprod Biomed Online* 2004;**8**:720–25.
18. Bakour SH, Khan KS, Gupta JK. The risk of premalignant and malignant pathology in endometrial polyps. *Obstet Gynecol Surv* 2000;**55**:486–87.
19. Saygili-Yilmaz E, Yildiz S, Erman-Akar M. Reproductive outcome of separate uterus after hysteroscopic metroplasty. *Arch Gynecol Obstet* 2003;**268**:289–92.

20. Homer HA, Li TC, Cooke ID. The separate uterus: a review of management and reproductive outcome. *Fertil Steril* 2000;**73**:1–14.

21. Conceptus, Inc. ESSURE™ System. Available at: http://www.conceptus.com.

22. Food and Drug Administration. Essure. Available at: http://www.fda.gov/cdrh/pdf2/p020014.html.

23. Kerin J, Cooper J, Price T, et al. Hysteroscopic sterilisation using a micro insert device: results of a multicultural phase III study. *Hum Reprod* 2003;**18**:1223–30.

24. Goldrath MH, Fuller TA, Segal S. Laser photovaporization of endometrium for the treatment of menorrhagia. *Am J Obstet Gynecol* 1981;**140**:14–19.

25. Magos AL, Baumann R, Turnbull AC. Transcervical resection of the endometrium in women with menorrhagia. *Br Med J* 1989;**298**:1209–12.

26. Vancaillie TG. Electrocoagulation of the endometrium with the ball end resectoscope. *Obstet Gynecol* 1989;**74**;425–27.

27. Valle RF. Rollerball endometrial ablation in the treatment of menorrhagia. *Baillieres Clin Obstet Gynaecol* 1995;**9**:299–316.

28. Townsend DE, Richart RM, Paskowitz RA, et al. Rollerball coagulation of the endometrium. *Obstet Gynecol* 1990;**76**:310–13.

29. Paskowitz RA. Rollerball ablation of the endometrium. *J Reprod Med* 1995;**40**:333–36.

30. Lethaby A, Hickey M, Garry R. Endometrial destruction techniques for heavy menstrual bleeding. *Cochrane Database Syst Rev* 2005;**4**:CD0015101.

31. O'Connor H, Magos AL. Endometrial resection for menorrhagia. *N Engl J Med* 1996;**335**;151–56.

32. Sutton C. Hysteroscopic surgery. *Best Practice Res Clin Obstet Gynaecol* 2006;**20**;105–37.

33. Mengerink BB, van der Wurff AA, Ter Haar JF, et al. Pijnenborg affect of undiagnosed deep adenomyosis after failed NovaSure endometrial ablation. *J Minim Invasive Gynecol* 2015;**22**:239–44.

34. Peeters JA, Penninx JP, Mol BW, et al. Prognostic factors for the success of endometrial ablation in the treatment of menorrhagia with special reference to previous caesarean section. *Eur J Obstet Gynaecol Reprod Biol* 2013;**167**:100–103.

35. Kreider SE. Endometrial ablation: is tubal ligation a risk factor for hysteroscopy. *J Minim Invasive Gynaecol* 2013;**20**:616–19.

36. El-Nashar SA, Hopkins MR, Creedon DJ, et al. Prediction of treatment outcomes after global endometrial ablation. *Obstet Gynaecol* 2009;**113**:97–106.

37. Madsen AM, El-Nashar SA, Hopkins MR, et al. Endometrial ablation for the treatment of heavy menstrual bleeding in obese women. *Int J Gynaecol Obstet* 2013;**121**:20–23.

38. Thomassee MS, Curlin H. Predicting pelvic pain after endometrial ablation: which preoperative patient characteristics are associated? *J Minm Invasive Gynecol* 2013;**20**:642–47.

39. Longginotti MK, Jacobson GF, Hung YY, et al. Probability of hysteroscopy after endometrial ablation. *Obstet Gynecol* 2008;**112**:1214–20.

40. Smithling KR, Savella G, Raker CA, et al. Preoperative uterine bleeding pattern and risk of endometrial ablation failure. *Am J Obstet Gynaecol* 2014;**211**:556.e1–6.

41. Wishall KM, Price J, Pereira N, et al. Postablation risk factors for pain and subsequent hysterectomy. *Obstet Gynaecol* 2014;**124**:904–10.

42. Overton C, Hargreaves J, Maresh M. A national study of the complications of endometrial destruction for menstrual disorders: the MISTLETOE study. Minimally invasive surgical techniques – laser endothermal or endoresection. *Br J Obstet Gynaecol* 1997;**104**:1351–59.

43. Jansen FW, Vredevoogd CB, Van Ulzen K, et al. Complications of hysteroscopy: a prospective multicentre study. *Obstet Gynaecol* 2000;**96**:266–70.

44. Scottish Hysteroscopy Audit Group. A Scottish audit of hysteroscopic surgery for menorrhagia: complications and follow up. *BJOG* 1995;**102**;249–54.

45. Bettocchi S, Selvaggi L. A vaginoscopic approach to reduce the pain of office hysteroscopy. *J Am Assoc Gyecol Laparosc* 1997;**4**:255–58.

46. Clark TJ, Voit D, Gupta JK, et al. Accuracy of hysteroscopy in the diagnosis of endometrial cancer and hyperplasia: a systematic quantitative review. *JAMA* 2002;**288**:1610–21.

47. Arieff Al, Ayus JC. Endometrial ablation complicated by fatal hyponatraemia encephalopathy. *JAMA* 1993;**270**:1230–32.

48. Istre O, Bjoennes J, Naess R, Hornbaek K, Forman A. Postoperative cerebral oedema after transcervical resection and uterine irrigation with 1.5% glycine. *Lancet* 1994;**344**:1187–89.

49. Istre O, Skajaa K, Schjoensby AP, Forman A. Changes in serum electrolytes after transcervical resection of the endometrium and sub mucous fibroids with the use of glycine 1.5% for uterine irrigation. *Obstet Gynaecol* 1992;**80**:218–22.

50. Harris MS. Experience with EndoSee: a novel hand-held digital hysteroscope for use in diagnostic office hysteroscopy. *J Minim Invasive Gyanecol* 2013;**20**:S67.

51. Munro MG. Pilot evaluation of the Endosee hand held hysteroscopic system for diagnostic hysteroscopy. *J Minim Invasive Gynecol* 2013;**20**:S68.

52. Wortman M. The Endosee hysteroscope: initial experience with a self-contained hand held hysteroscopy system. *J Minim Invasive Gynecol* 2013;**20**:S68.

53. Smith PP, Middelton LJ, Connor ME, et al. Hysteroscopic morcellation compared with electrical resection of endometrial polyps. *Obstet Gynaecol* 2014;**123**:745–51.

54. Hamerlynck TWO, Dietz V, Schoot BS. Clinical implantation of the hysteroscopic morcellator for removal of intrauterine myomas and polyps. *Gynaecol Surgery* 2011;**8**:193–96.

55. Hamerlynck T, Blikkendaal M, Schoot B, et al. An alternative approach for the removal of placental remnants: hysteroscopic morcellation. *J Minim Invasive Gynecol* 2013;**20**:796–802.

56. Simons M, Hamerlynck TW, Abdulkadir L, et al. Hysteroscopic morcellator system can be used for the removal of a uterine septum. *Fertil Steril* 2011;**96**:e118–21.

57. Gupta JK, Clark TJ, More S, et al. Patient anxiety and experiences associated with an outpatient one stop and see and treat hysteroscopy clinic. *Surg Endosc* 2004;**18**:1099–104.

58. Angioli R, De Cicco Nardone C, Plotti F, et al. Use of music to reduce anxiety during office hysteroscopy: prospective randomised control trial. *J Minim Invasive Gynecol* 2014;**21**:454–59.

59. Royal College of Obstetricians and Gynaecologists (RCOG). *Best Practice in Outpatient Hysteroscopy*. Green-top Guideline No. 59. London: RCOG; 2015. Available at: https://www.rcog.org.uk/globalassets/documents/guidelines/gtg59hysteroscopy.pdf.

60. Cooper NA, Smith P, Khan KS, et al. A systematic review of the effect of the distention medium on pain during outpatient hysteroscopy. *Feril Steril* 2011;**95**:264–71.

61. Romani F, Guido M, Morciano A, et al. The use of different size-hysteroscope in office hysteroscopy; our experience. *Arch Gynecol Obstet* 2013;**288**:1355–59.

62. Campo R, Molinas CR, Rombatus L, et al. Prospective multicentre randomized controlled trial to evaluate factors influencing the success rate of office diagnostic hysteroscopy. *Hum Reprod* 2005;**20**:258–63.

63. Giorda G, Scarabelli C, Franceschi S, et al. Feasibility and pain control in outpatient hysteroscopy in postmenopausal women; a randomised trial. *Acta Obstet Gynecol Scand* 2000;**79**:593–97.

64. De Angelis C, Santoro G, Re Me, et al. Office hysteroscopy and compliance: mini hysteroscopy versus traditional hysteroscopy in a randomised trial. *Hum Reprod* 2003;**18**:2441–45.

65. Rullo S, Sorrenti G, Marziali M, et al. Office hysteroscopy comparison of 2.7 and 4mm hysteroscopes for acceptability, feasibility and diagnostic accuracy. *J Reprod Med* 2005;**50**;45–48.

66. Smith PP, Middleton LJ, Connor M, et al. Hysteroscopic morcellation compared with electrical resection of endometrial polyps; a randomised controlled trial. *Obstet Gynecol* 2014;**123**:745–51.

67. Rubino RJ, Lukes AS. Twelve month outcomes for patients undergoing hysteroscopic morellation of uterine polyps and myomas in an office or ambulatory surgical centre. *J Minim Invasive Gynecol* 2015;**22**:285–90.

68. Lim F, Brown I, McColl R, et al. Hysteroscopic stimulator for training and educational purposes. *Conf Proc IEEE Eng Med Biol Soc* 2006;**1**:1513–16.

69. Burchard ER, Lockrow EG, Zahn CM, et al. Simulation training improves resident performance in operative hysteroscopic resection techniques. *Am J Obstet Gynecol* 2007;**197**:e-1–4.

70. Bajka M, Tuchschmind S, Fink D, et al. Establishing construct validity of a new virtual-reality training stimulator for hysteroscopy. *Surg Endosc* 2009;**23**:2026–33.

71. Bajka M, Tuchschmind S, Fink D, et al. Establishing construct validity of a virtual reality training stimulation via a multimetric scoring system. *Surg Endosc* 2010;**24**:79–88.

72. Chudnoff SG, Liu CS, Levie MD, et al. Efficacy of a novel educational curriculum using a simulation laboratory on resident performances of hysteroscopic sterilisation. *Ferti Steril* 2010;**94**:1521–54.

73. Lethaby A, Penninx J, Hickey, et al. Endometrial resection and ablation and techniques for heavy menstrual bleeding. *Cochrane Database Syst Rev* 2013;**8**:CD001501.

74. Bettocchi S, Ceci O, Vicino M, et al. Diagnostic inadequacy of dilatation and curettage. *Feril Steril* 2001;**75**;803–805.

SECTION 7
Benign Disease of the Uterus

49

Benign disease of the uterus

Sahana Gupta and Isaac Manyonda

Endometrial polyps

The endometrial polyp is a common gynaecological lesion associated with abnormal bleeding and infertility. It can also be an asymptomatic incidental finding during imaging. It is a localized overgrowth of the uterine endometrium that can be sessile or polypoid. It usually grows from the fundus towards the internal os and occasionally protrudes through the external os into the vagina.

Aetiology

Age, hypertension, obesity, and tamoxifen use are some of the risk factors (1–3). The causation is likely to be multifactorial. Thus in obese women, while an excess of oestrone may play a role, hypertension may be a confounding factor. There is a 30–60% prevalence of polyps in women using tamoxifen. In women with infertility, the use of gonadotropins may be associated with the development of polyps. Endometrial polyps are also associated with cervical polyps in 24–27% of cases and the association becomes stronger with advancing age and abnormal vaginal bleeding (4). Atypical glandular cells in a cervical smear are also associated with endometrial polyps in 3.4–5% of cases (5). Genetic factors play a role, with altered endometrial proliferation and overgrowth being associated with specific alleles on chromosomes 6 and 12 (6). It has been hypothesized that an excess of endometrial cytokines and metalloproteinases may increase the risk of developing polyps, fibroids, and adenomyosis, the same mediators that are implicated in intrauterine disease associated with infertility. In postmenopausal women there is an excess of growth regulating protein P63, which is also a marker of the reserve cells of the basalis layer. The latter is thought to be the precursor of polyps (7, 8).

While oestrogen and progesterone are key factors in the proliferation and apoptosis of the endometrium, their role in the aetiology and pathophysiology of polyps is controversial. Both hormones appear to contribute to the elongation of the glands, stroma, and spiral arteries that give polyps the characteristic polypoid appearance. In postmenopausal women there is an excess of oestrogen receptors but limited evidence for an excess of progesterone receptors. There also seems to be an excess of these receptors in the glandular epithelium and not the stroma. The timing of the cycle may play a role. Notwithstanding the controversy, there are apparent functional similarities between polyps and normal endometrium with similar functional changes occurring cyclically (9).

Epidemiology

The reported prevalence of polyps is between 7.8% and 34.9% depending on the population studied, the diagnostic tool used, and the definition of polyps. While it is generally thought that polyps are more prevalent in postmenopausal (11.8%) compared to premenopausal women, this could simply reflect the fact that any abnormal bleeding in postmenopausal women will be investigated, which is not the case in premenopausal women (10).

Clinical presentation

Approximately 68% of all women with polyps present with abnormal vaginal bleeding (11) and 6–88% of premenopausal women with polyps have abnormal vaginal bleeding in the form of menorrhagia, intermenstrual bleeding, or postcoital bleeding (11). Endometrial polyps account for 39% of all abnormal vaginal bleeding in premenopausal women and this is thought to be due to stromal congestion leading to venous stasis and apical necrosis.

In contrast, postmenopausal women with polyps are more often symptom free, with approximately 56% presenting with abnormal bleeding (11). Polyps account for only 21–28% of all vaginal bleeding in postmenopausal women (11). In premenopausal women, polyps are associated with infertility (12). This might be due to mechanical obstruction at the tubal ostium or due to a mechanical or biochemical effect on implantation of the developing embryo, possibly due to the excess of intrauterine metalloproteinases and cytokines associated with polyps (7). The incidence of polyps is 3.8–38.5% in primary infertility, 1.8–17% in secondary infertility, and 1.9–24% when combined (12).

Natural history

Polyps can regress spontaneously, with one study reporting a regression rate of 27%, and a correlation between size and regression: polyps smaller than 1 cm are more likely to regress than larger ones (13).

While most polyps are benign, some can become hyperplastic with malignant transformation in 0–12.9% of cases (1). The risk is highest in postmenopausal women with symptoms and low in premenopausal women. There is a significant correlation between age, menopausal status, obesity, hypertension, tamoxifen use, and size of the polyp and incidence of malignant transformation (2). In one study the risk of malignancy was similar in symptomatic and asymptomatic patients, suggesting that polyps should be removed whenever identified (14). Ultrasonography may aid in identification of malignancy with a sensitivity of 67–100% and a specificity of 71–89%. The variation in range is dependent upon the thickness of the endometrium used for further invasive testing.

Diagnosis

Transvaginal ultrasound

On transvaginal ultrasound (TVUS), a polyp typically appears as a hyperechoic lesion with regular contours within the uterine lumen, outlining the endometrial wall on which it rests, surrounded by a hyperechoic halo. Cystic spaces within the polyp corresponding to dilated glands filled with proteinaceous material may be seen, or it may appear as a thickening of the endometrial lining or focal mass within the endometrial cavity. However, such appearances are not pathognomonic of endometrial polyps, since submucosal fibroids can also look similar. To minimize false-positive or false-negative results in the premenopausal woman, TVUS should be performed within the first 10 days of the menstrual cycle.

Compared to hysteroscopy and guided biopsy, studies have reported that TVUS has a sensitivity of 19–96%, specificity of 53–100%, positive predictive value of 75–100%, and negative predictive value of 87–97%. Such a wide variation reflects the poor quality of the studies, and also the inclusion of other conditions such as submucosal fibroids. In a single, large prospective study evaluating the causes of menorrhagia, the sensitivity, specificity, positive predictive value, and negative predictive value of TVS in diagnosing polyps were 86%, 94%, 91%, and 90% respectively (15).

There are limited data to substantiate the use of colour or power Doppler in the diagnosis of malignant change or hyperplasia in a polyp. In one study the specificity and the negative predictive value were claimed to be 95% and 94% respectively for identifying a single large feeding vessel by colour flow Doppler in TVUS (16) whereas others have shown limited value in the diagnosis of endometrial cancer, with no significant difference in histology of polyps depending on their resistive or pulsatility index.

Power Doppler seems to be a more promising technique for the depiction of the vascular network (17) and in one study the sensitivity and specificity were reported to be 87% and 85% respectively in identifying a single large feeding vessel as a marker of an endometrial polyp compared to a network of multiple or scattered vessels for hyperplasia or malignancy (17). However, the study showed this to be more effective for women in whom the polyp was an incidental finding. Ultimately the only way to confirm or exclude malignancy is histological examination following its removal.

Saline infusion sonography

The use of saline infusion sonography (SIS; also referred to as sonohysterography) increases the sonographic contrast helping in the delineation of size, location, and other features of endometrial polyps. Polyps appear as echogenic intracavitary masses with either a broad base or a thin stalk floating in the fluid. This technique is thought to increase diagnostic accuracy and small polyps missed

on grey-scale sonography are picked up on SIS. Differentiating a polyp from a submucosal fibroid can be difficult but examining the echotexture and identifying echogenic endometrium overlying the polyp can be helpful.

A number of studies comparing the diagnostic accuracy of diagnostic hysteroscopy and SIS showed no significant difference between the two (18). When comparing SIS and hysteroscopy with guided biopsy, the sensitivity, specificity, positive predictive value, and negative predictive value were 58–100%, 35–100%, 70–100%, and 83–100% respectively (18).

When compared with hysteroscopy, SIS has the advantage of allowing the assessment of the myometrium and other pelvic organs. It has also been reported to be less painful than diagnostic hysteroscopy when the latter is performed as an outpatient procedure under similar conditions to SIS: both techniques involve insertion of an instrument through the cervix and distending the uterine cavity with fluid. However, these reports are from earlier studies before the advent of present-day hysteroscopes of much smaller diameter (19). The disadvantages of SIS include an inability to give a histological diagnosis, a longer learning curve, and discomfort caused by leakage of fluid or pain by distension with the balloon catheter.

Three-dimensional TVUS and three-dimensional SIS

Three-dimensional (3D) ultrasound can generate multiplanar reconstructed images of the uterus including coronal views and therefore improve the diagnostic accuracy compared to two-dimensional (2D) ultrasound. Three-dimensional SIS includes addition of saline infusion to 3D ultrasound. However, this technique has been shown to improve diagnostic accuracy only slightly and given the greater expense and less frequent availability of 3D SIS, 2D ultrasound with intrauterine contrast will remain the preferred effective and reliable non-invasive method to diagnose polyps.

Histological diagnosis

Blind biopsy

In contemporary practice, blind dilatation and curettage should no longer be used as a diagnostic technique due to its poor sensitivity and negative predictive value compared to hysteroscopy and guided biopsy, which has a specificity and positive predictive value of 100% (20). Use of an endometrial sampler or curette can miss a pedunculated polyp or cause fragmentation of a sessile polyp making histological diagnosis difficult. This is particularly important in postmenopausal women in whom polyps tend to be broad based with an uneven surface covered by atrophic endometrium.

Hysteroscopy with guided biopsy

This is considered the gold standard in the diagnosis of endometrial polyps (21). The ability to diagnose and remove polyps concurrently makes it superior to diagnostic hysteroscopy alone. Despite the growing popularity of outpatient hysteroscopy, most of the diagnostic hysteroscopies are still performed under general anaesthesia, particularly if operative hysteroscopy is required. The evidence supports use of outpatient hysteroscopy for diagnosis with a reported success rate of 92–96% and no difference between premenopausal and postmenopausal women (22). Studies have shown it to be superior both in terms of expense and patient preference.

Flexible hysteroscopy is less painful for patients and allows easier passage through the cervical canal when compared to rigid hysteroscopy, making it more acceptable for office procedures. It is thought to have inferior image quality compared to rigid hysteroscopy as the light and images are transferred through the same fibreoptic bundle. New flexible hysteroscopes with video chips are superior in this respect, although these may be susceptible to breakage, have a limited operative scope, and may be more costly than rigid hysteroscopes. With new, technologically improved narrow scopes, more and more operative hysteroscopies can be performed in the outpatient setting. While smaller endometrial polyps can be removed with minimal patient discomfort, polyps larger than the internal cervical os are best removed under general anaesthesia.

The choice of distension medium is an important consideration for patient comfort and diagnostic accuracy in outpatient settings. Normal saline causes less discomfort and less shoulder tip pain when compared with carbon dioxide and therefore produces images which are clear and reliable. Use of paracervical blocks and intrauterine anaesthesia can also be helpful in outpatient operative hysteroscopy.

Complication rates are low in hysteroscopic polypectomy. When compared to hysteroscopic myomectomy, endometrial ablation, and hysteroscopic adhesiolysis the risks of perforation, cervical laceration, infection, and haemorrhage remain low (23).

Management

The management of polyps is guided by the presence of symptoms, desire for future fertility, risk of malignancy, and operator skills. The options are conservative non-surgical, conservative surgical, and radical surgical.

Conservative non-surgical management

While the removal of polyps is associated with a low risk of complications, it is not a completely risk-free procedure and therefore pre-intervention patient counselling is mandatory. The rate of regression of polyps less than 10 mm in size is 27% over 12 months and the risk of malignancy is very low: such polyps can therefore be managed conservatively in asymptomatic patients (13).

Medical treatment may have some role in the management of polyps. Gonadotropin-releasing hormone (GnRH) agonists have been shown to cause temporary regression of polyps and can be used as a treatment adjunct before polypectomy. However, the cost and side effects of such treatment need to be compared with simple alternative extirpative treatment without the use of such medications. A variety of progesterone preparations including norethisterone, medroxyprogesterone, and tibolone have been used in the context of hormone replacement therapy in postmenopausal women and tibolone, which has the highest androgenic activity, is thought to cause regression of polyps. Hysteroscopic examination at 3 years after treatment revealed a low risk of recurrence after use of these preparations. However, these treatments are not without side effects, and high-quality studies are required to further establish their place.

In a randomized controlled trial of the levonorgestrel-releasing intrauterine system (LNG-IUS) compared with observation, a reduced rate of polyp recurrence was shown in the LNG-IUS group. In a 4.5-year study observation period, eight cases of polyp occurrence were seen in the observation group compared to three in the LNG-IUS group. Out of these three, one woman did not have an IUS inserted and in other two it was taken out after 1 year due to side effects. Reduction in endometrial thickness due to progesterone suppression is thought to contribute to the regression or reduced development of polyps (24).

Conservative surgical treatment

Blind dilatation and curettage has been used as a treatment for endometrial polyps for many years. A survey of practice in the United Kingdom carried out in 2002 showed that 2% of gynaecologists used this technique and 51% used blind curettage after hysteroscopy (21, 25). Evidence suggests that this technique has a high complication rate with a perforation rate of approximately 1 in 100 and an infection rate of approximately 1 in 200 (21). Studies suggest that with blind curettage alone, the rate of polyp removal is only 4% which increases to 41% if a polyp removal forceps is also used. The rate of incomplete removal is also high (26). TVUS-guided polypectomy has been suggested as an alternative in order to improve the rate of removal of polyps, however this has received little enthusiasm (27). Hysteroscopic resection of polyp is safe with a low complication rate, is widely available, and can be performed in the outpatient setting, and therefore should replace blind methods of polyp removal.

Hysteroscopic polypectomy

This is a safe and effective method for polyp removal which allows rapid recovery and can be sometimes be performed in an outpatient setting (28). There are various techniques of polypectomy depending on the type of instrument used. This is dependent on availability, expense, surgical expertise, and also the size and location of polyps. Large and sessile polyps are best removed with a resectoscope, an electrosurgical loop fitted to the hysteroscope, while smaller polyps are best removed either by scissors or polyp forceps under direct hysteroscopic vision (28). Hysteroscopic resection carries more complications, probably due to the greater cervical dilatation required in these cases. However, the polyp recurrence rate is nearly zero after use of the resectoscope compared with about 15% with grasping forceps (28).

Other instruments that may be considered include the bipolar Versapoint, which requires less cervical dilatation and uses normal saline instead of glycine thus reducing the potential risk of postoperative hyponatraemia (11). The hysteroscopic morcellator removes the polyp chips while resecting, thus reducing the operating time, fluid loss, and movement through the cervix. Such techniques are, however, expensive and not readily available and the outcomes are not significantly different from other methods of hysteroscopic removal.

Radical surgical treatment

Hysterectomy is a definitive treatment for endometrial polyps, guaranteeing no recurrence. However, it can only be justified in the presence of other pathology such as symptomatic fibroids, given the significant morbidity associated with such a radical approach.

Outcome of treatment

The outcome of treatment is generally good with reduction or cessation in abnormal vaginal bleeding. The risk of intrauterine adhesion formation after polypectomy is low, as the myometrium is not damaged and the endometrium has excellent regenerative capacity. In women undergoing polypectomy as a treatment of subfertility, reported postoperative pregnancy rates vary between 43% and 80% with improvement seen in both chances of natural and assisted conception (28). In a class 1 study, polypectomy before intrauterine insemination significantly increased subsequent pregnancy rates (29). The rate of pregnancy in the study group was 51%, and of these, 65% had a spontaneous conception before the first intrauterine insemination, whereas all pregnancies in the control group were obtained during the fertility treatment (29). There is a lack of consensus over the size of the polyps that may affect fertility, with data suggesting that removal of a polyp less than 2 cm in size does not improve fertility (30).

Conclusion

Endometrial polyps are a common gynaecological condition whose prevalence increases with age. They are rarely associated with malignancy. They can be associated with both subfertility and abnormal uterine bleeding. Non-invasive techniques such as grey-scale TVUS give a reliable diagnosis and diagnostic enhancement can be achieved by the use of contrast medium. In the management of polyps, hysteroscopic resection is safe and effective and allows histological examination. Blind techniques should be avoided because of the high incidence of incomplete resection and complications such as perforation. Polypectomy is an effective treatment of infertility although evidence from randomized controlled trials to demonstrate improvement in *in vitro* fertilization outcome is still needed. Conservative medical treatment is a viable option pending definitive surgical treatment. Radical surgical treatment such as hysterectomy is unnecessary in the treatment of polyps.

Adenomyosis

Adenomyosis is a common benign uterine pathology that is characterized by the presence of ectopic endometrium within the myometrium. About two-thirds of affected women are symptomatic with dysmenorrhoea and menorrhagia. The two diagnostic tools are good-quality TVUS scanning and magnetic resonance imaging. Treatment remains a challenge and can be either surgical or medical, but the ultimate definitive treatment remains hysterectomy.

Epidemiology

Adenomyosis typically affects multiparous premenopausal women over the age of 30 years (31), but it is also found in nulliparous women, where it may contribute to subfertility.

Pathogenesis

Adenomyosis is often associated with hormone-dependent pelvic lesions such as fibroids, endometrial hyperplasia, and endometriosis. It has been postulated that these other lesions could be cases of 'external' adenomyosis, with connections to deep pelvic endometriosis invading the myometrium from outside inwards. A particular correlation has been found between adenomyosis and lesions of the rectovaginal septum, and it is thought that both adenomyosis and endometriosis are governed by a single pathophysiological/genetic process (32–35). A number of factors appear to promote the development of adenomyosis including multiparity, spontaneous miscarriage, surgical termination of pregnancy, curettage, hysteroscopic resection of the endometrium, myomectomy, caesarean section,

and tamoxifen. A genetic predisposition for adenomyosis has also been proposed (36). Apart from high oestrogen levels, a correlation has also been made between adenomyosis and high levels of human leucocyte antigen 2-type immune response proteins interleukin-18 and leukaemia inhibitory factor, without necessarily implying that there is a causative relationship. Abnormal secretion of interleukin-6 from endometrial stromal cells and overexpression of cyclooxygenase-2 are additional factors implicated in the pathogenesis of adenomyosis. However, the exact mechanisms have yet to be elucidated.

Histology

Adenomyosis is characterized by the presence of ectopic endometrium within the myometrium (with the depth of invasion being at least 2.5 mm below the basal level of the endometrium) that leads to hypertrophy of the smooth muscle. The thickened myometrium is composed of haphazardly distributed hypertrophied muscular trabeculae surrounding the ectopic endometrial tissue. Adenomyosis can be nodular with single or multiple foci scattered in the myometrium or more diffuse with numerous foci affecting the whole of the myometrium. It is often asymmetric, most frequently affecting the posterior uterine corpus (36). There may be superficial lesions, not extending beyond the one-third of the depth of the myometrium, and deep lesions that invade deeper (36). Brownish old haemorrhagic foci corresponding to blood and haemosiderin pigment deposits may be contained within an area of adenomyosis.

Symptoms

One-third of women remain asymptomatic, and these women probably have superficial rather than deep adenomyosis. The remaining two-thirds experience menorrhagia, dysmenorrhoea, and sometimes dyspareunia. On examination, the uterus feels globular and the woman often complains of pain on palpation of the uterus during vaginal examination (36).

What is the role of adenomyosis in infertility?

The association of adenomyosis with subfertility is not fully understood, but up to 14% of women with adenomyosis have been reported to have infertility (37). There are various theories proposed in the pathophysiology: one is that of hypermobility of the uterus which can prevent transfer of spermatozoa to the fallopian tubes, movement of the fertilized ovum, normal implantation of the embryo, and the ability of the trophoblast for effective penetration of the myometrium and thereby effective placentation, or there may be dysfunction of the junctional zone (JZ) (37).

Imaging features

Ultrasonography

The presence of adenomyosis is suggested by the presence of three or more of the following signs:

1. The ectopic dilated endometrial glands in the myometrium appear as subendometrial microcysts, around 2–4 mm in diameter. If the contents are haemorrhagic then there is greater echogenicity (36).
2. There is a non-homogeneous appearance of the myometrium with hyperechoic linear striations, tiny hyperechoic subendometrial nodules, pseudo-nodular hypoechoic zones

with indistinct contours, and a thickened endometrial–myometrial junction. The heterogeneous appearance is due to the presence of heterotopic endometrial tissue and myometrial cell hypertrophy (36).

3. An enlarged uterus with smooth regular contours and asymmetrical hypertrophy of the uterine walls, the posterior wall usually thicker than the anterior wall. This is known as the 'pseudo-widening sign' (38).

4. Lack of visibility of the endometrial–myometrial (junctional) zone. This appearance can mimic endometrial hyperplasia. SIS can be useful in the differential diagnosis, demonstrating so-called pseudo-endometrial thickening (39).

5. Doppler sonography may show linear striations crossing the myometrium within the adenomyotic lesions (36).

6. The corpus uteri is flexed backwards, the fundus of the uterus faces the posterior compartment, and the cervix is directed frontally towards the bladder. This sign called the 'question mark form of the uterus', and has high sensitivity and specificity for adenomyosis (40).

Three-dimensional ultrasound (and magnetic resonance imaging (MRI), see 'MRI for diagnosis of adenomyosis') evaluates the coronal plane of the uterus, allowing visualization of modifications in the JZ. This appears as a hypoechoic halo around the endometrium, whose thickening and integrity can be assessed under 3D ultrasound. It has been reported that when the thickness of the JZ is greater than 8 mm or the difference between thicker and thinner parts is more than 4 mm, adenomyosis is likely (41).

Differential diagnosis on sonography

1. Multiple leiomyoma: localized forms of adenomyosis are more difficult to diagnose as these can mimic fibroids. However, localized adenomyosis has an elliptic form and no calcifications. Colour and power Doppler can help to distinguish these two entities: in adenomyosis the vessels spread through the myometrium, whereas in fibroids they surround the lesion without penetrating it (36).

2. Cystic glandular hypertrophy, frequently caused by medications such as tamoxifen, are more difficult to differentiate from the subendometrial cysts seen in adenomyosis. MRI may prove useful in such cases (36).

3. Endometrial thickening can mimic diffuse adenomyosis, in which case SIS might be useful. This technique uses saline infusion to opacify the subendometrial cysts. It demonstrates continuity of the subendometrial cystic spaces with the endometrial cavity, with the superficial sites remaining in continuity and the deep sites losing continuity.

MRI for diagnosis of adenomyosis

MRI is believed to be the most accurate non-invasive technique for the diagnosis of adenomyosis (sensitivity 78–88%, specificity 67–93%) (42) although recent studies suggest equivalence with TVUS, particularly when 3D TVS is performed (41). TVS is frequently used to screen patients and select those who need to have MRI to confirm the diagnosis.

It is important to be aware that there are pitfalls in the use of MRI to diagnose adenomyosis, due to natural variation in JZ thickness (43). This especially so in the following circumstances:

- Day of the menstrual cycle (the JZ is thickest between day 8 and day 16, and variable during menstruation).
- Ageing and menopause: the JZ thickens up to the time of menopause and then thins and may disappear.
- Pregnancy: the JZ thins and frequently disappears by the third trimester.
- Use of the oral contraceptive pill or GnRH agonists can thin the JZ.
- Myometrial contractions can induce a pseudo-thickening of the JZ.

MRI should therefore be carried out at a time of the cycle when the patient is not menstruating.

Treatment of adenomyosis

Treatment depends on the symptoms and also if fertility is desired. There are various medical and surgical options available (44).

Medical treatment

Oral progestogens such as dydrogesterone can be used to treat premenopausal menometrorrhagia. It causes endometrial atrophy due to its antioestrogen effect and therefore relieves irregular bleeding, dysmenorrhoea, and pain. However, functional signs reappear in 50% of cases in 3–6 months (45).

LNG-IUS (Mirena IUS)

The Mirena IUS is a well-tolerated and effective treatment of menometrorrhagia and can reduce uterine enlargement, pain, and dysmenorrhoea. It might need to be replaced earlier than the 5-year recommended interval due to tachyphylaxis (46).

GnRH agonists

These induce hypo-oestrogenism which in turn leads to reductions in uterine size, JZ thickness, and endometrial deposits that cause dysmenorrhoea. They can also be used for symptom relief for women who do not desire fertility immediately, but who want conservative treatment. They are generally administered for up to 6 months and rarely for up to a year, with add-back oestrogen/gestagen therapy to prevent menopausal symptoms (44). They are also used preoperatively to reduce uterine size prior to hysterectomy or to make resection of adenomyotic lesions easier (44).

Surgical treatment

The age of the patient and whether preservation of fertility is required are the two factors that determine the type of surgery: radical or conservative.

Radical

Radical treatment involves hysterectomy, either total or subtotal, based principally on the condition of the cervix, pouch of Douglas, and rectovaginal septum (44). The decision to remove the adnexa will depend on the presence of endometrioma, deep peritoneal endometriosis, and the age of the patient.

Conservative

This involves local excision of an adenomyotic lesion. This is difficult in terms of preserving fertility because of the ill-defined endometrial–myometrial boundaries (47). Surgery often results in fibrotic scars and suture material in surrounding healthy tissue, which can affect future fertility adversely. Hysteroscopic resection may be performed in women with superficial adenomyosis. However, deep-seated adenomyosis cannot be removed by this intervention. Moreover, conservative surgery is only effective in up to 50% of patients and there are no data on long-term follow-up (48).

More recently, endomyometrial ablation, laparoscopic myometrial electrocoagulation, and excision have been tried as an alternative treatment options for patients with localized adenomyosis. Transcervical endometrial ablation or resection is only possible for patients with submucous or superficial localized adenomyosis (48). However, symptoms may be persistent after use of this approach when the depth of the lesion is greater than 2.5 mm, indicating that there are limitations in treating deep lesions. Although laparoscopic electrosurgical excision can significantly relieve pain, with low rates of complications, a second procedure is often required (49).

Uterine artery embolization

This involves selective embolization of the uterine artery on each side with microarticulate non-calibrated polyvinyl alcohol or calibrated trisacryl alcohol with or without gelatin sponge. On the basis of limited evidence, there seems to be short-term clinical resolution of symptoms particularly menorrhagia, but not pain (50). There seems to be a frequent recurrence of symptoms after 2–3 years and repeat treatment in the form of hysterectomy may be required (51). MRI shows post-treatment changes including reduction in uterine size, decreased JZ thickness, and full or partial infarction of the lesions with non-vascularized areas of low signal intensity on T2-weighted images.

High-intensity focused ultrasound ablation

High-intensity focused ultrasound (HIFU) ablation has been used to treat patients with a variety of malignancies, and can be delivered by ultrasound, magnetic resonance guidance, or more recently and experimentally, by ultrasound. HIFU uses thermal energy to ablate tumours at depth through intact tissue. The fundamental difference to other ablation techniques using coagulation necrosis such as radiofrequency, laser microwave, and cryotherapy is that it does not require the use of applicators to deliver the energy. The advantages are an absence of bleeding or risk of seeding metastasis, and the ability to treat poorly perfused tumours, large volume, or irregular tumours. There are two mechanisms by which HIFU may act on adenomyosis, by coagulation necrosis of the adenomyotic cells or by affecting the blood supply by causing necrosis and embolization in the feeding blood vessels. There have been several case reports using magnetic resonance-guided focused ultrasound surgery (MRgFUS) for the treatment of focal adenomyosis, with satisfactory results (52). However, the high energy levels used may affect tissues in the path of the beam, potentially resulting in inadvertent ablation of the endometrium or the endometrial blood vessels. As the endometrium and the JZ are embryologically a single unit, transient loss of perfusion in the endometrium is inevitable. Compared with other endometrial ablation approaches, which extend several millimetres into the myometrial wall, MRgFUS is less invasive and can safely ablate adenomyosis close to the endometrium or serosal surface. It reduces the uterine volume and width of the myometrial zone and JZ. Patients report amelioration of pain with minimal side effects.

Ultrasound-guided HIFU and more recently the laparoscopic HIFU approach have also been safely and effectively used in the treatment of adenomyosis (53). As a non-invasive approach, HIFU may offer complete ablation of adenomyoma, at a low cost, with less complications, less trauma, and shorter hospital stay. However, high-quality randomized trials are necessary before its introduction into clinical practice.

Conclusion

Adenomyosis is a common benign condition that can cause menorrhagia, dysmenorrhoea, and dyspareunia. Its role in infertility is not fully understood but hypermobility of the uterus and dysfunction of the JZ are thought to play a role. There are two main modalities of diagnosis: TVUS and MRI. With ultrasound it can be difficult to differentiate a leiomyoma from adenomyosis. Medical treatment using progestogens is effective in controlling menorrhagia and pain but symptoms reappear in at least half of the women upon cessation of medication, although the Mirena IUS appears to be more effective. Conservative therapies such as local resection and high-energy ablation are promising, but require further rigorous evaluation. For now, hysterectomy is the only definitive solution.

Uterine fibroids

Introduction

Fibroids are the most common tumour in women of reproductive age (54, 55). Recent years have seen a demographic shift in childbirth trends, with many women delaying starting their families until they reach their third or fourth decade (56, 57). This is the age when fibroids are more prevalent and symptomatic (58, 59). The old adage 'children then fibroids and then hysterectomy' therefore no longer applies to many women, and there is an increasing demand for fertility-preserving treatments for symptomatic uterine fibroids.

The repertoire of uterus-preserving treatments for symptomatic fibroids has increased in recent years. The use of uterine artery embolization (UAE) was first reported over two decades ago (60). The National Institute for Health and Care Excellence (NICE) in the United Kingdom has reviewed its efficacy and recommends UAE as an alternative treatment to hysterectomy and myomectomy (61). Magnetic MRgFUS (62) is another new technique, but its adoption has been slow, partly due to the high infrastructure costs of setting up such a service and because of its limitations in treating large and/or numerous fibroids (63, 64). Pharmaceutical agents continue to be developed. While it was originally introduced as a premyomectomy treatment (65), ulipristal acetate has recently acquired a licence for use as a stand-alone treatment for symptomatic fibroids (66) and is regarded by many as the 'first-in-class' medical therapy for fibroids (67). Despite the emergence of these new treatments for managing symptomatic uterine fibroids, in reality, when the uterus is to be preserved, myomectomy, especially the open abdominal approach, remains the treatment of choice of many gynaecologists.

Incidence, aetiology, and epidemiology of fibroids

Incidence

Although fibroids are undoubtedly the commonest benign tumour in women, their exact incidence is unknown for a variety of reasons including sampling methods, the populations studied, the timing of sampling, and not least because a significant proportion of women with fibroids (often quoted as 50%) are entirely asymptomatic and are not included in studies that identify subjects due to their symptoms. Thus reports, based on clinical diagnosis or diagnostic tests, underestimate the true incidence of fibroids, but nevertheless it is estimated that the lifetime risk of having fibroids for a woman over the age of 45 years is greater than 60% (68). A practical approach is to recognize that fibroids are most prevalent and symptomatic in the third and fourth decade of life, and using round figures, it is estimated that by the age of 50 years up to 50% of white women will have fibroid(s), while the corresponding figure in black women is 60–70% (69). It is highly likely that the prevalence of fibroids is underestimated: the incidence of histological analysis is more than double the clinical incidence, and the incidence increases with increasing age (70).

Aetiology

Despite considerable research, the aetiology of uterine fibroids is unknown. There is no adequate animal model to aid laboratory enquiry. What is well established is that all the cells within a given fibroid originate from a single cell (the monoclonal origin of fibroids) (71, 72)—but what actually causes the transformation from a normal myometrial to a leiomyoma cell remains enigmatic. While it is evident that ovarian steroid hormones promote fibroid growth, there is no evidence for differences in circulating concentrations of these hormones between women with and without fibroids. *In vitro* studies suggest that progesterone rather than oestrogen is the major mitogen for uterine fibroids, and indeed these studies have led to the recent introduction of ulipristal acetate, the first-in-class selective progesterone receptor modulator (SPRM) (see 'Medical treatment of fibroids'). Peptide growth hormones and a range of growth factors are also thought to influence fibroid growth over and above the sex steroids (see 'Pathophysiology of fibroids'). Cytogenetic chromosomal alterations, including translocations, duplications, and deletions have also been found in up to 50% of fibroid tumours. The commonest cytogenetic abnormalities are deletions in chromosome 7, and translocations involving chromosomes 7, 12, and 14 (73–75). Clearly, fibroids are not a single-gene disorder, and this might in part explain the heterogeneity in the phenotype of fibroids between individuals and also between different ethnic groups.

Epidemiology

There is a clear-cut racial disparity in age of onset and number and size of fibroids between black, white, and Asian women (76, 77). The reasons for the racial differences are not known, and while epidemiological factors linked to fibroids are thought to include reproductive factors, sex steroids, and lifestyle/environmental factors in addition to racial origin, the available information should be interpreted with caution. For example, the racial disparity is not reflected in hormonal concentrations or oestrogen receptor expression. In other words, the basis of the racially disparity is not known. The familial predisposition to fibroids is illustrated by a number of observations: female relatives of women with fibroids have a significantly increased risk of developing fibroids; twin pair studies indicate an increased risk of fibroids in monozygotic compared to dizygotic twins (78, 79); and there is a consistent pattern of clinical symptoms, operative findings, and tissue molecular features in families with a prevalence of uterine fibroids compared with those without this prevalence (77). Fibroids are associated with the polycystic ovary syndrome, hypertension, and obesity, while smoking in white (but not black) women appears to be protective (80). There are no dietary factors that have been proven to alter the risk of developing fibroids. Fibroids are commoner in nulliparous women, with the relative risk decreasing with increasing number of term pregnancies. Fibroids initially increase in size in the first trimester of pregnancy and then shrink in size over the next two trimesters. There is therefore an overall relative decrease in uterine fibroid volume during the course of pregnancy (81, 82). The effect of the oral contraceptive pill on the risk of fibroids is unclear, with some studies showing an increased risk, others a decrease, and yet others no association at all.

Pathophysiology of fibroids

The pathophysiology of fibroids is poorly understood. However, it is likely that there is altered smooth muscle cell proliferation in association with disordered angiogenesis (83). When compared with the adjacent myometrium, fibroid vasculature appears to be significantly altered (84–86). A dense vascular rim of tissue surrounds smaller fibroids, but there are fewer blood vessels within the actual fibroid tumour itself (87, 88). The vascular supply within the fibroid tissue increases as the fibroid grows, but does not reach the density of that in the adjacent myometrium. Perhaps due to differences in the levels of angiogenesis promoters and inhibitors within the fibroid tissue, vessels that penetrate the fibroid tissue from the dense perifibroid vascular rim of tissue are abnormally narrow in diameter and lack the normal structure of vessels within the myometrium (89, 90)—it is interesting to speculate that this abnormal and reduced vasculature may render the fibroid tissue prone to ischaemic necrosis after UAE (see 'Radiological treatment of fibroids').

The proliferation of smooth muscle cells also appears to be altered in fibroids compared with adjacent myometrium, and there is an exaggerated response to both progesterone and oestrogen. In addition, a variety of growth factors (IGFs, EGF, bFGF, PDGF, TGF-beta) have differential effects on fibroid cells compared with normal myometrial cells via a variety of mechanisms including alteration of receptor levels and signalling pathways (91–95).

Fundamentally, the importance of understanding the pathophysiology of fibroids is that this will lead to the development of effective intervention strategies. This is exemplified by the recent emergence of SPRMs as potential effective treatments for fibroids (see 'Medical management of symptomatic fibroids').

Clinical presentation of fibroids

While 50% of women with fibroids are asymptomatic (96–98), those who are affected experience significant morbidity and reduced quality of life. Clinical symptoms are varied and include menstrual disturbances (menorrhagia, dysmenorrhoea, and intermenstrual bleeding), pelvic pain unrelated to menstruation, pressure symptoms including bloating, increased urinary frequency and bowel disturbance, compromise of reproductive function including

616

subfertility, early pregnancy loss, and later pregnancy complications such as pain, preterm labour, malpresentations, increased need for caesarean section, and postpartum haemorrhage (99). Large fibroids may distend the abdomen and this may be aesthetically displeasing to many women. Abnormal bleeding occurs in 30% of symptomatic women (100), and with bloating and pelvic discomfort due to mass effect, constitutes the most common symptoms. Black women, who have the highest incidence and tend to have multiple and larger fibroids, also tend to have more symptomatic fibroids at the time of diagnosis (101–103). The prevalence of clinically significant myomas peaks in the perimenopausal years and declines after menopause. It is not known why some fibroids are symptomatic while others are quiescent. The size, number, and location of fibroids undoubtedly determine their clinical behaviour (104, 105), but research has yet to correlate these parameters to the clinical presentation of the fibroids.

Diagnosis and imaging of uterine fibroids

Imaging

Imaging is critical for confirmation of the diagnosis, and is indispensable in guiding decisions on clinical management, especially with the increasing demand for uterus-preserving treatments. Thus the goals of imaging include the exclusion of other pathologies, especially malignancy, and the determination of the number, size, and position of the fibroids and the overall dimensions of the uterus. Imaging may also be used to evaluate the vascular supply to the fibroids, especially when treatments such as UAE are being considered. Considerations when choosing the imaging modality will include individual and global costs of the procedure, and safety aspects if radiation is involved. The current and most frequently used imaging modalities are ultrasound and MRI, while computed tomography is not currently a primary imaging modality for fibroids (106).

Ultrasound

Ultrasound is the most widely used imaging modality as it is relatively cheap, is often part of a routine gynaecological examination, is a rapid procedure, and uses no ionizing radiation and therefore can be used during pregnancy. While both the transabdominal ultrasound (TAUS) and the TVUS approaches may be used, TAUS offers a wide field of view, increased depth of signal penetration, flexibility in transducer movement, and the ability to examine other organs. The TAUS view is more effective than the TVUS approach for the visualization of pedunculated subserosal fibroids extending into the abdominal cavity, and is also more effective when very large fibroids are present (107). During TVUS, the probe is placed in close proximity to the organs of interest, and therefore image resolution is improved compared to the TAUS approach. TVUS provides a better view of the endometrium (108), does not require use of the bladder as an acoustic window, and is not affected by obesity, bowel gas, or a retroverted uterus (108, 109). TVUS is considered reliable, with a high level of interobserver agreement for measurement of uterine size and endometrial thickness (111). The combination of TVUS and TAUS imaging is the most widely used technique for the detection, mapping, and characterization of fibroids (107). TVUS capabilities can be enhanced by the use of hysterosonographic examination (HSE), also known as SIS (110). When used with TVUS, HSE allows identification of endometrial pathology, submucosal myomas, and adhesions (107, 109, 110, 111). The combination of imaging

modalities may also be effective in the evaluation of submucosal myoma location, breadth of attachment, and extent of protrusion into the uterine cavity (113). The use of colour Doppler allows ultrasound assessment of organ vascularity, which may be useful in distinguishing between solid and cystic masses (5, 34), and in the differential diagnosis of adenomyosis.

Ultrasound is not without limitations. The TAUS approach may be less effective in the measurement of uteri larger than 300 mL in total volume (113). Ultrasound may also be less effective when multiple fibroids are present, as the tumours may produce acoustic shadows (108, 113).

Magnetic resonance imaging

This is arguably currently the best imaging technique for fibroids, allowing for precise mapping of the individual fibroid position, including assessment of the depth of submucosal fibroid penetration (39). It is also useful for assessment of very large myomas. MRI is an effective companion to ultrasound in the differential diagnosis of adenomyosis. Use of MRI follow-up may confirm the presence of adenomyosis if low-intensity, poorly demarcated lesions are visualized with ultrasound (114–116). Magnetic resonance angiography (MRA) may be useful in an assessment of the vascularization of the uterus and fibroids. MRA may be helpful in determining the presence of an extrauterine blood supply to fibroids. Evaluation of fibroid vascularity is beneficial when UAE is considered as a uterine-preserving therapy for symptomatic fibroids (117). The main limitation of MRI in the imaging of fibroid disease is the high cost.

Surgical management of symptomatic fibroids

Hysterectomy

Globally, the great majority of symptomatic fibroids continue to be managed surgically, mostly by hysterectomy. Thus, hysterectomy remains the most common major gynaecological operation performed worldwide. About 600,000 hysterectomies are carried out in the United States and 40,000 in England per year (118). Forty per cent of women all over the world will have a hysterectomy by the age of 64 and indications for the majority will be to relieve symptoms due to fibroid disease and improve quality of life. The majority of hysterectomies are carried out abdominally despite evidence that the vaginal route confers many benefits (119). Hysterectomy rates are highest in satisfaction scores compared with other modalities of treatment (120, 121), particularly in the treatment of dysfunctional uterine bleeding, and in the treatment of fibroids it offers a definitive cure with no possibility of recurrence. It is therefore arguably the ideal treatment for a woman whose family is complete, or one who has no desire for future fertility.

The changing demography of childbirth, at least in developed countries such as the United Kingdom, is likely to have a significant impact on the use of hysterectomy to treat fibroid disease. As an increasing number of women are postponing childbirth to the late third and early fourth decade of life, more women wish uterus/fertility-preserving treatments, and developments in assisted reproductive technology using egg donation mean that women can realistically expect to be able to carry a pregnancy in their 50s provided they have managed to retain their uterus (122). Radiological treatments (see later) and myomectomy offer uterus/fertility-preserving options for the treatment of fibroid disease.

Myomectomy

Most myomectomies are still performed by the open abdominal route. Depending on the size, number, and location of the fibroids, this is an operation that requires considerable skill, and may be associated with significant blood loss (123, 124). In skilled hands, this operation benefits many women who often go on to achieve a pregnancy, but it can also compromise the fertility if dense adhesions form, either in the pelvis and/or in the uterine cavity, as a result of the procedure. Much has been written about techniques of open myomectomy, including approaches to the minimization of blood loss and the avoidance of both pelvic and intrauterine adhesions (125–127).

Myomectomy can also be performed by minimal access approaches that include laparoscopic and robotic-assisted procedures. Laparoscopic myomectomy is associated with a lower incidence of adhesions, shorter hospital stay, lower costs, and improved quality of life (128, 129), but requires skills that are not always readily available, and there are limitations on the number and size of fibroids that can be treated by this modality. The costs associated with the use of robotic surgery have led to intense debate concerning the clinical and cost-effectiveness of robotically assisted myomectomy over the laparoscopic approach.

Hysteroscopic myomectomy

There is little debate or controversy concerning the hysteroscopic treatment of submucous fibroids. It is widely accepted that submucous and intracavitary fibroids are a common cause of menorrhagia and intermenstrual bleeding, and can contribute to subfertility and/or miscarriage. In skilled hands, hysteroscopic resection is a relatively simple and safe procedure with proven efficacy in symptom relief (130, 131) and improvement in fertility.

Radiological management of symptomatic fibroids

UAE and MRgFUS are the mainstay radiological treatments of fibroids, but less frequently used modalities include magnetic resonance-guided transvaginal cryotherapy and radiofrequency ablation. In this section, the focus will be on the first two, as the others are rarely used in clinical practice. The indications for both are fibroid-induced severe menorrhagia, dysmenorrhoea, anaemia, and pressure effects on the bladder/bowel. Contraindications to their use include viable pregnancy, suspected malignancy of uterus or ovaries, contrast allergy/renal impairment (UAE), and refusal to accept hysterectomy under any circumstances. Case series of successful pregnancies after both treatments have been published, but there has yet to be a head-to-head comparison between the two, or between either and myomectomy with regard to pregnancy outcomes.

UAE for the treatment of symptomatic uterine fibroids was first reported by Ravina and his colleagues in 1995 (132). The technique involves percutaneous femoral artery puncture with radiologically guided selective catheterization of each uterine artery in turn (133). Embolic particles are then injected until the uterine artery is occluded. While non-spherical polyvinyl alcohol particles were the most commonly used in the early years of the UAE, there are now a range of embolic agents with different properties, although comparative data is scarce (134, 135). There is consensus that complete devascularization of all fibroids is mandatory for effective treatment

(136, 137). While partial devascularization can result in a clinical improvement and volume reduction, there is a higher long-term recurrence rate (138).

The advantages of UAE include the ability for total treatment of the uterus (numbers and size of fibroids are irrelevant), its minimal invasiveness, and the fact that it is performed under local anaesthesia. In addition, it is associated with rapid recovery (2–3 weeks compared with 6–8 weeks for myomectomy), and should new symptomatic fibroids form then the treatment can be repeated (133). There is level 1 evidence to suggest that UAE can achieve similar symptom control as hysterectomy (139, 140, 141), and when compared to hysterectomy, costs are lower with UAE, even when further interventions following UAE are included (142). Hence NICE have approved UAE as an alternative treatment to hysterectomy and myomectomy (143).

Symptom relief after UAE

Symptomatic improvements are often quite dramatic, with some women noticing a reduction in menorrhagia and dysmenorrhoea at the first and certainly by the second menses following treatment. Thus menorrhagia improvement occurs in 85–90% (133) of patients, while improvements in bulk symptoms occur in 70–90% (133). However, women with massive fibroids might find that absolute volume reduction may not live up to their expectation.

Further treatment may be required for recurrent symptoms, and the age of the woman appears to be an important factor. The younger at first treatment, the more likely she is to experience a recurrence, with the risk being 25% over 5 years for patients whose first treatment is when aged less than 40 years, and 10% for patients aged 40–50 years (133).

Outcomes for UAE relative to myomectomy

Research to date suggests that quality of life improvement following UAE is similar to that following myomectomy, while major complications occurred in 3% in association with UAE versus 8% with myomectomy. Reinterventions at 2 years are required in 14% following UAE compared to 3% following myomectomy (144).

Side effects and complications of UAE

These are well documented. The postembolization syndrome is so common that it should perhaps be viewed as an expected side effect of UAE rather than a true complication (133). The syndrome is characterized by low-grade pyrexia, discomfort, and malaise occurring at post-treatment days 3–7, and in the vast majority of cases it settles with conservative measures. True complications include transient amenorrhoea, reported in 5–10% cases, while the incidence of permanent amenorrhoea is related to the patient's age, with reports suggesting an incidence of 7–14% in women over 45 years and 0–3% in younger women. Therefore, a major concern regarding the risk of inadvertent embolization of ovarian vascular supply is the potential negative impact on fertility. Transcervical fibroid expulsion occurs in 0–3%, while endometrial or uterine infection complicates 1–2% of cases. Non-infectious endometritis occurs in 1–2%, and up to 5% of treated women may complain of a chronic vaginal discharge. Fibroid impaction at the cervix can cause significant pain and distress and warrants admission for hysteroscopy and removal of the impacted fibroid (133). Where an UAE service is offered, the potential for complications warrants close collaboration between interventional radiologists and gynaecologists.

Magnetic resonance-guided focused ultrasound surgery

MRgFUS uses focused high-energy ultrasound to sonicate or ablate fibroid tissue. As with conventional diagnostic ultrasound, ultrasound waves pass through the anterior abdominal wall without causing any damage/injury, and significant heat only occurs where the waves converge at the focus (145, 146). Magnetic resonance guidance provides continuous imaging of the fibroid and other vital structures such as bowel, bladder, and sacral nerves (147, 148). Thus, MRgFUS is a truly non-invasive procedure, and research so far has reported significant improvements in clinical symptoms and quality-of-life parameters (149, 150). Complication rates are very low, and women can return to work within a day of treatment, which compares very favourably with 13 days after UAE and a minimum of 6 weeks after abdominal myomectomy or hysterectomy (133). However, MRgFUS is a relative new treatment that warrants further evaluation. It was approved by the United States Food and Drug Administration in 2004, but in the United Kingdom NICE continues to recommend that the procedure be used only in an audit and research setting. MRgFUS is a focal treatment rather than global as with UAE, and volume reduction after treatment is small compared with the mean levels seen after both myomectomy and UAE. Again, because it is a focal treatment, very large fibroids are not amenable to treatment given the time that would be required to achieve sonication of the tumours The use of MRI guidance may be prohibitive in terms of cost compared with UAE and other established treatment modalities (151).

Medical management of symptomatic fibroids

There has long been a need for a medical therapy for the treatment of symptomatic uterine fibroids that is simple, effective, safe, and leads to a resolution of symptoms without affecting fertility. Most of the current medical therapeutic approaches exploit the observations that uterine fibroids have significantly increased concentrations of oestrogen and progesterone receptors compared with normal myometrium (152, 153), and that ovarian steroids influence fibroid growth. Most available therapies are therefore hormonal, or act on the relevant hormones or their receptors to interfere with fibroid growth. Thus GnRH agonists have been used to achieve amenorrhoea and shrink fibroid size in symptomatic women, but their use is restricted due to significant side effects such as bone mineral density loss and vasomotor symptoms. Rebound growth of the fibroids also occurs on cessation of therapy. The authors of this chapter advocate that there is no role for GnRH agonists in the management of fibroid disease because they are not cost-effective (154) and render myomectomy more difficult because they destroy tissue planes (155, 156), increasing rather than reducing perioperative blood loss and operating time. When used before myomectomy they may increase the risk of 'recurrence' because they obscure smaller fibroids that 'recur' when the effects of the GnRH agonists wear off (157–159). Cheaper medications with fewer side effects are also available. Selective oestrogen receptor modulators such as raloxifene have been shown to induce fibroid regression in post- but not premenopausal women, and medical therapies

aiming to antagonize the oestrogen effects on fibroid growth in premenopausal women have not been successful. Conversely, a series of meticulous *in vitro* studies using cultured leiomyoma and normal myometrial cells have led to the development of SPRMs. This class of medications have demonstrated two important effects: firstly that they have a differential impact on the leiomyoma cells versus the normal myometrium, with no negative impact on the latter; and secondly that the SPRMs inhibited leiomyoma cell growth via several mechanisms (160–163). This translational research has led to the emergence of ulipristal acetate as the first-in-class SPRM for clinical use. Given at a 5 mg or 10 mg daily dose, it is highly effective at reducing menstrual blood loss, effecting amenorrhoea in 75% of recipients within 10 days, and has many attributes that arguably render it not only non-inferior but potentially superior to GnRH analogues. Importantly, it has been associated with improved quality of life (164, 165). The original European licence was for pre-myomectomy use of ulipristal acetate to shrink fibroids, to correct anaemia and improve the efficacy of the subsequent myomectomy. More recently, ulipristal acetate has acquired a licence for use as a stand-alone therapy for up to four treatment cycles of 3 months each, interrupted by a month of non-use (166, 167). To date, most of the research on its clinical use has been industry led, and there is a pressing need for researcher-led studies to replicate the findings described previously. Long-term studies are mandatory especially as progesterone receptors are ubiquitous, being found on the breast, bone, heart, brain, and blood cells as well as the genital organs: the impact of long-term use of SPRMs therefore warrants further studies. Moreover, ulipristal acetate has been shown to induce changes in the endometrium of a small proportion of women, changes that are reversible upon cessation of ulipristal acetate, and which have been designated progesterone receptor modulator-associated endometrial changes (168–170) by a panel in a NIH-sponsored workshop. Where ulipristal acetate is used prior to myomectomy, its impact on the surgery itself has yet to be carefully and systematically evaluated.

Conclusion

Fibroids, the most common benign tumour in women, have a major impact on women's quality of life because of the clinical symptoms they cause, and have significant health-cost implications from their treatments. Controversy prevails as to whether they significantly contribute to problems of reproduction such as subfertility, miscarriage, and poor pregnancy outcomes. With women increasingly delaying childbirth until their third and fourth decade of life, when fibroids are more prevalent and symptomatic, a timely and welcome development over the past two decades or so has been the expansion of the repertoire of treatment options available. Interventional radiological treatments, the emergence of effective medical therapies, and the refinement of minimally invasive approaches to myomectomy, accompanied by parallel developments in assisted reproductive technologies, all contribute to an era of increasing choice for women where they can postpone/delay childbirth and yet realistically expect to have successful pregnancy at a later stage in life. However, the exact cause of fibroids remains an enigma, and perhaps because of the benign nature of the tumour, research and funding has not been prioritized on fibroids, and the new treatment options warrant further rigorous evaluation.

REFERENCES

1. Cohen I. Endometrial pathologies associated with postmenopausal tamoxifen treatment. *Gynecol Oncol* 2004;**94**:256–66.
2. Onalan R, Onalan G, Tongue E, Ozdener T, Dogan M, Mollamahmutoglu L. Body mass index is an independent risk factor for the development of endometrial polyps in patients undergoing in-vitro fertilization. *Fertil Steril* 2009;**91**:1056–60.
3. Spiewankiewicz B, Stelmachow J, Sawicki W, Cendrowski K, Kuzlik R. Hysteroscopy in cases of cervical polyps. *Eur J Gynaecol Oncol* 2003;**24**:67–69.
4. Km TJ, Kim HS, Park CT, Park IS, Hong SR, Park JS, et al. Clinical evaluation of follow-up methods and results of atypical glandular cells of undetermined significance (AGUS) detected on cervicovaginal Pap smears. *Gynecol Oncol* 1999;**73**:292–98.
5. Vanni R, Dal Cin P, Marras S, et al. Endometrial polyp: another benign tumor characterized by 12q13–q15 changes. *Cancer Genet Cytogenet* 1993;**68**:32–33.
6. Inagaki N, Ung L, Otani T, Wilkinson D, Lopata A. Uterine cavity matrix metalloproteinases and cytokines in patients with leiomyoma, adenomyosis or endometrial polyp. *Eur J Obstet Gynecol Reproduct Biol* 2003;**111**:197–203.
7. Nogueira AA, Sant'Ana de Almeida EC, Poli Neto OB, Zambelli Ramalho LN, Rosa e Silva JC, Candido dos Reis FJ. Immunohistochemical expression of p63 in endometrial polyps: evidence that a basal cell immunophenotype is maintained. *Menopause* 2006;**13**:826–30.
8. Jakab A, Ovari L, Juhasz B, Birinyi L, Bacsko G, Toth Z. Detection of feeding artery improves the ultrasound diagnosis of endometrial polyps in asymptomatic patients. *Eur J Obstet Gynecol Reproduct Biol* 2005;**119**:103–107.
9. Haimov-Kochman R, Deri-Hasid R, Hamani Y, Voss E. The natural course of endometrial polyps: could they vanish when left untreated? *Fertil Steril* 2009;**92**:828.e11–12.
10. Fabres C, Alam V, Balmaceda J, Zegers-Hochschild F, Mackenna A, Fernandez E. Comparison of ultrasonography and hysteroscopy in the diagnosis of intrauterine lesions in infertile women. *J Am Assoc Gynecol Laparosc* 1998;**5**:375–78.
11. Valle RE. Hysteroscopy for gynecologic diagnosis. *Clin Obstet Gynecol* 1983;**26**:253–76.
12. Shokeir TA, Shalan HM, El-Shafei MM. Significance of endometrial polyps detected hysteroscopically in eumenorrheic infertile women. *J Obstet Gynaecol Res* 2004;**30**:84–89.
13. DeWaay DJ, Syrop CH, Nygaard IE, Davis WA, Van Voorhis BJ. Natural history of uterine polyps and leiomyomata. *Obstet Gynecol* 2002;**100**:3–7.
14. Papadia A, Gerbaldo D, Fulcheri E, et al. The risk of premalignant and malignant pathology in endometrial polyps: should every polyp be resected? *Minerva Ginecologica* 2007;**59**:117–24.
15. Alcazar JL, Castillo G, Minguez JA, Galan MJ. Endometrial blood flow mapping using transvaginal power Doppler sonography in women with postmenopausal bleeding and thickened endometrium. *Ultrasound Obstet Gynecol* 2003;**21**:583–88.
16. Goldstein SR, Monteagudo A, Popiolek D, Mayberry P, Timor-Tritsch I. Evaluation of endometrial polyps. *Am J Obstet Gynecol* 2002;**186**:669–74.
17. De Kroon C. Power Doppler area in the diagnosis of endometrial cancer. *Int J Gynecol Cancer* 2010;**20**:1160–65.
18. Anastasiadis PG, Koutlaki NG, Skaphida PG, Galazios GC, Tsikouras PN, Liberis VA. Endometrial polyps: prevalence, detection, and malignant potential in women with abnormal uterine bleeding. *Eur J Gynaecol Oncol* 2000;**21**:180–83.
19. Exalto N, Stappers C, van Raamsdonk LAM, Emanuel MH. Gel instillation sonohysterography: first experience with a new technique. *Fertil Steril* 2007;**87**:152–55.
20. O'Connell LP, Fries MH, Zeringue E, Brehm W. Triage of abnormal postmenopausal bleeding: a comparison of endometrial biopsy and transvaginal sonohysterography versus fractional curettage with hysteroscopy. *Am J Obstet Gynecol* 1998;**178**:956–61.
21. Clark TJ, Khan KS, Gupta JK. Current practice for the treatment of benign intrauterine polyps: a national questionnaire survey of consultant gynaecologists in UK. *Eur J Obstet Gynecol Reprod Biol* 2002;**103**:65–67.
22. Agostini A, Bretelle F, Cravello L, Maisonneuve AS, Roger V, Blanc B. Acceptance of outpatient flexible hysteroscopy by premenopausal and postmenopausal women. *J Reproduct Med* 2003;**48**:441–43.
23. Jansen FW, Vredevoogd CV, Van Ulzen K, Hermans J, Trimbos JB, Trimbos-Kemper TCM. Complications of hysteroscopy: a prospective, multicenter study. *Obstet Gynecol* 2000;**96**:266–70.
24. Moghal N. Diagnostic value of endometrial curettage in abnormal uterine bleeding – a histopathological study. *J Pak Med Assoc* 1997;**47**:295–99.
25. Lo KW, Yuen PM. The role of outpatient diagnostic hysteroscopy in identifying anatomic pathology and histopathology in the endometrial cavity. *J Am Assoc Gynecol Laparosc* 2000;**7**:381–85.
26. Loffer FD. Hysteroscopy with selective endometrial sampling compared with D&C for abnormal uterine bleeding: the value of a negative hysteroscopic view. *Obstet Gynecol* 1989;**73**:16–20.
27. Lee C, Ben-Nagi J, Ofili-Yebovi D, Yazbek J, Davies A, Jurkovic D. A new method of transvaginal ultrasound guided polypectomy: a feasibility study. *Ultrasound Obstet Gynecol* 2006;**27**:198–201.
28. Preutthipan S, Herabutya Y. Hysteroscopic polypectomy in 240 premenopausal and postmenopausal women. *Fertil Steril* 2005;**83**:705–709.
29. Perez-Medina T, Bajo-Arenas J, Salazar F, et al. Endometrial polyps and their implication in the pregnancy rates of patients undergoing intra-uterine insemination: a prospective, randomized study. *Hum Reprod* 2005;**20**:1632–35.
30. Isikoglu M, Berkkanoglu M, Senturk Z, Coertzee K, Ozgur K. Endometrial polyps smaller than 1.5 cm do not affect ICSI outcome. *Reprod Biomed Online* 2006;**12**:199–204.
31. Matalliotakis IM, Kourtis AI, Panidis DK. Adenomyosis. *Obstet Gynecol Clin North Am* 2003;**30**:63–82.
32. Togashi K, Ozasa H, Konishi I, et al. Enlarged uterus: differentiation between adenomyosis and leiomyoma by MR imaging. *Radiology* 1989;**171**:531–34.
33. Togashi K. Adenomyosis. In: Togashi K (ed), *MRI of the Female Pelvis*, pp. 105–20. Tokyo: Igaku Shoin; 1993.
34. Ota H, Igarashi S, Hatarzawa J, et al. Is adenomyosis an immune disease? *Hum Reprod Update* 1998;**4**:360–67.
35. Byun JY, Kim SE, Choi BG, et al. Diffuse and focal adenomyosis: MR imaging findings. *Radiographics* 1999;**19**:S161–70.
36. Levy G, Dehaene A, Laurent N, et al. An update on adenomyosis. *Diagn Interv Imaging* 2013;**94**:3–25.
37. Valentini AL, Speca S, Gui B, Sogua G, Micco M, Bonomo L. Adenomyosis: from the sign to the diagnosis. Imaging, diagnostic pitfalls and differential diagnosis: a pictorial review. *Radiol Med* 2011;**116**:1267–87.
38. Reves MF, Goldstein RB, Jones KD. Communications of adenomyosis with the endometrial cavity: visualization with saline contrast sonohysterography. *Ultrasound Obstet Gynecol* 2010;**36**:115–19.

39. Lo Monte G, Capobianco G, Piva I, Caserta D, Dessole S, Marci R. Hysterosalpingo contrast sonography (HyCoSy): let's make the point! *Arch Gynecol Obstet* 2015;**291**:19–30.

40. Di Donato N, Seracchioli R. How to evaluate adenomyosis in patients affected by endometriosis? *Minim Invasive Surg* 2014;**2014**:507230.

41. Exacoustos C, Brienza L, Giovanni A, et al. Adenomyosis: three dimensional sonographic findings of the junctional zone and correlation with histology. *Ultrasound Obstet Gynecol* 2011;**37**:471–79.

42. Bazot M, Cortez A, Darai E, et al Ultrasonography compared with magnetic resonance imaging for the diagnosis of adenomyosis: correlation with histopathology. *Hum Reprod* 2001;**16**:2427–33.

43. Taorel P, Laffargue, Dechaud H. Adenomyosis: what imaging modality in the diagnosis and staging? *Gynecol Obstet Fertil* 2004;**32**:976–80.

44. Schweppe KW. The place of dydrogesterone in the treatment of endometriosis and adenomyosis. *Maturitas* 2009;**65**:523–27.

45. He SM, Wei MX, et al. Effect of levonorgestrel-releasing intrauterine system in the treatment of adenomyosis. *Zhonghua Fu Chan Ke Za Zhi* 2005;**40**:536–38.

46. Cho S, Nam A, Kim H, et al. Clinical effects of the levonorgestrel releasing intrauterine device in patients with adenomyosis. *Am J Obst Gynecol* 2008;**198**:373.

47. Keckstein J. Hysteroscopy and adenomyosis. *Contrib Gynecol Obstet* 2000;**20**:41–50.

48. Farquhar C, Brosens I. Medical and surgical management of adenomyosis. *Best Pract Res Clin Obstet Gynecol* 2006;**20**:603–16.

49. Lohle PN, De Vries J, Klazen CA, et al. Uterine artery embolization for symptomatic adenomyosis with or without uterine leiomyomas with the use of calibrated trisacryl gelatin microspheres: midterm clinical and MR imaging follow up. *J Vasc Interv Radiol* 2007;**18**;835–41.

50. Bratby MJ, Walker WJ. Uterine artery embolization for symptomatic adenomyosis: mid-term results. *Eur J Radiol* 2009;**70**:128–32.

51. Kitamura Y, Alison SJ, Jha RC, Spies JB, Flick PA, Ascher SM. MRI of adenomyosis: changes with uterine artery embolization. *AJR Am J Roentgenol* 2006;**186**:855–64.

52. Yoon SW, Kim KA, Cha SH, et al. Successful use of magnetic resonance-guided focused ultrasound surgery to relieve symptoms in a patient with symptomatic focal adenomyosis. *Fertil Steril* 2008;**90**:2018.e13–15.

53. Wang W, Wag YX, Tang J. Safety and efficacy of high intensity focused ultrasound ablation therapy for adenomyosis. *Acad Radiol* 2009;**16**:1416–23.

54. Baird DD, Dunson DB, Hill MC, Cousins D, Schectman JM. High cumulative incidence of uterine leiomyoma in black and white women: ultrasound evidence. *Am J Obstet Gynecol* 2003;**188**:100–107.

55. Laughlin SK, Schroeder JC, Baird DD. New directions in the epidemiology of uterine fibroids. *Semin Reprod Med* 2010;**28**:204–17.

56. Schmidt L, Sobotka T, Bentzen JG, Nyboe Andersen A. ESHRE Reproduction and Society Task Force. Demographic and medical consequences of the postponement of parenthood. *Hum Reprod Update* 2012;**18**:29–43.

57. Office for National Statistics. Births in England in 2013. Available at: http://www.ons.gov.uk/ons/rel/vsob1/birth-summary-tables--england-and-wales/2013/info-births-2013.html.

58. Marshall LM, Spiegelman D, Barbieri RL, et al. Variation in the incidence of uterine leiomyoma among premenopausal women by age and race. *Obstet Gynecol* 1997;**90**:967–73.

59. Okolo S. Incidence, aetiology and epidemiology of uterine fibroids. *Best Pract Res Clin Obstet Gynaecol* 2008;**22**:571–88.

60. Ravina JH, Herbreteau D, Ciraru-Vigneron N, et al. Arterial embolisation to treat uterine myomata. *Lancet* 1995;**346**:671–72.

61. National Institute for Health and Care Excellence. Uterine artery embolisation for fibroids. Interventional procedures guidance [IPG367]. 2010. Available at: https://www.nice.org.uk/guidance/ipg367.

62. Stewart EA, Gedroyc WM, Tempany CM, et al. Focused ultrasound treatment of uterine fibroid tumors: safety and feasibility of a noninvasive thermoablative technique. *Am J Obstet Gynecol* 2003;**189**:48–54.

63. Schlesinger D, Benedict S, Diederich C, Gedroyc W, Klibanov A, Larner J. MR-guided focused ultrasound surgery, present and future. *Med Phys* 2013;**40**:080901.

64. Gizzo S, Saccardi C, Patrelli TS, et al. Magnetic resonance-guided focused ultrasound myomectomy: safety, efficacy, subsequent fertility and quality-of-life improvements, a systematic review. *Reprod Sci* 2014;**21**:465–76.

65. Donnez J, Tatarchuk TF, Bouchard P, et al. Ulipristal acetate versus placebo for fibroid treatment before surgery. *N Engl J Med* 2012;**366**:409–20.

66. Donnez J, Donnez O, Matule D, et al. Long-term medical management of uterine fibroids with ulipristal acetate. *Fertil Steril* 2016;**105**:165–73.e4.

67. Levens ED, Potlog-Nahari C, Armstrong AY, et al. CDB-2914 for uterine leiomyomata treatment: a randomized controlled trial. *Obstet Gynecol* 2008;**111**:1129–36.

68. Day BD, Dunson DB, Hill MC, Cousins D, Schectman JM. High cumulative incidence of uterine leiomyoma in black and white women: ultrasound evidence. *Am J Obstet Gynecol* 2003;**188**:100–107.

69. Marshall LM, Spiegelman D, Barbieri RL, et al. Variation in the incidence of uterine leiomyoma among premenopausal women by age and race. *Obstet Gynecol* 1997;**90**:967–73.

70. Cramer SF, Patel A. The frequency of uterine leiomyomas. *Am J Clin Pathol* 1990;**94**:435–38.

71. Townsend DE, Sparkes RS, Baluda MC, McClelland G. Unicellular histogenesis of uterine leiomyomas as determined by electrophoresis by glucose-6-phosphate dehydrogenase. *Am J Obstet Gynecol* 1970;**107**:1168–73.

72. Hashimoto K, Azuma C, Kamiura S, et al. Clonal determination of uterine leiomyomas by analyzing differential inactivation of the X-chromosome-linked phosphoglycerokinase gene. *Gynecol Obstet Invest* 1995;**40**:204–208.

73. Ozisik YY, Meloni AM, Powell M, Surti U, Sandberg AA. Chromosome 7 biclonality in uterine leiomyoma. *Cancer Genet Cytogenet* 1993;**67**:59–64.

74. Sargent MS, Weremowicz S, Rein MS, Morton CC. Translocations in 7q22 define a critical region in uterine leiomyomata. *Cancer Genet Cytogenet* 1994;**77**:65–68.

75. Andersen J, Barbieri RL. Abnormal gene expression in uterine leiomyomas. *J Soc Gynecol Investig* 1995;**2**:663–72.

76. Okolo SO, Gentry CC, Perrett CW, Maclean AB. Familial prevalence of uterine fibroids is associated with distinct clinical and molecular features. *Hum Reprod* 2005;**20**:2321–24.

77. Kjerulff KH, Langenberg P, Seidman JD, Stolley PD, Guzinski GM. Uterine leiomyomas. Racial differences in severity, symptoms and age at diagnosis. *J Reprod Med* 1996;**41**:483–90.

78. Vikhlyaeva EM, Khodzhaeva ZS, Fantschenko ND. Familial predisposition to uterine leiomyomas. *Int J Gynaecol Obstet* 1995;**51**:127–31.

79. Luoto R, Kaprio J, Rutanen EM, Taipale P, Perola M, Koskenvuo M. Heritability and risk factors of uterine fibroids—the Finnish Twin Cohort study. *Maturitas* 2000;**37**:15–26.

80. Wise LA, Palmer JR, Harlow BL, et al. Reproductive factors, hormonal contraception, and risk of uterine leiomyomata in African-American women: a prospective study. *Am J Epidemiol* 2004;**159**:113–23.

81. Hammoud AO, Asaad R, Berman J, Treadwell MC, Blackwell S, Diamond MP. Volume change of uterine myomas during pregnancy: do myomas really grow? *J Minim Invasive Gynecol* 2006;**13**:386–90.

82. Cooper NP, Okolo S. Fibroids in pregnancy—common but poorly understood. *Obstet Gynecol Surv* 2005;**60**:132–38.

83. Huang SC, Yu CH, Huang RT, et al. Intratumoral blood flow in uterine myoma correlated with a lower tumor size and volume, but not correlated with cell proliferation or angiogenesis. *Obstet Gynecol* 1996;**87**:1019–24.

84. Forssman L. Blood flow in myomatous uteri as measured by intra-arterial ^{133}Xenon. *Acta Obstet Gynecol Scand* 1976;**55**:21–14.

85. Forssman L. Distribution of blood flow in myomatous uteri as measured by locally injected ^{133}Xenon. *Acta Obstet Gynecol Scand* 1976;**55**:101–104.

86. deSouza NM, Williams AD. Uterine arterial embolization for leiomyomas: perfusion and volume changes at MR imaging and relation to clinical outcome. *Radiology* 2002;**222**:367–74.

87. Farrer-Brown G, Beilby JOW, Rowles PM. Microvasculature of the uterus: an injection method of study. *Obstet Gynecol* 1970;**35**:21–30.

88. Farrer-Brown G, Beilby JOW, Tarbit MH. The vasculature patterns in myomatous uteri. *J Obstet Gynaecol Br Comnwlth* 1970;**77**:967–75.

89. Walocha JA, Litwin JA, Miodonski AJ. Vascular system of intramural leiomyomata revealed by corrosion casting and scanning electron microscopy. *Hum Reprod* 2003;**18**:1088–93.

90. Casey R, Rogers PAW, Vollenhoven BJ. An immuohistochemical analysis of fibroid vasculature. *Hum Reprod* 2000;**15**:1469–75.

91. Lee BS, Stewart EA, Sahakian M, et al. Interferon-alpha is a potent inhibitor of basic fibroblast growth factor-stimulated cell proliferation in human uterine cells. *Am J Reprod Immunol* 1998;**40**:19–25.

92. Strawn EY, Novy MJ, Burry KA, et al. Insulin-like growth factor I promotes leiomyoma cell growth in vitro. *Am J Obstet Gynecol* 1995;**172**:1837–44.

93. Swartz CD, Afshari CA, Yu L, et al. Estrogen-induced changes in IGF-I, Myb family and MAP kinase pathway genes in human uterine leiomyoma and normal uterine smooth muscle cell lines. *Mol Hum Reprod* 2005;**11**:411–50.

94. Vollenhoven BJ, Herington AC, Healy DL. Messenger ribonucleic acid expression of the insulin-like growth factors and their binding proteins in uterine fibroids and myometrium. *J Clin Endocrinol Metab* 1993;**76**:1106–10.

95. Gao Z, Matsuo H, Wang Y, et al. Up-regulation by IGF-I of proliferating cell nuclear antigen and Bcl-2 protein expression in human uterine leiomyoma cells. *J Clin Endocrinol Metab* 2001;**86**:5593–99.

96. Parker WH. Etiology, symptomatology, and diagnosis of uterine myomas. *Fertil Steril* 2007;**87**:725–36.

97. Stovall DW. Clinical symptomatology of uterine leiomyomas. *Clin Obstet Gynaecol* 2001;**44**:364–71.

98. Christiansen JK. The facts about fibroids. *Postgrad Med* 1993;**9**:129–37.

99. Gupta S, Jose J, Manyonda IT. Clinical presentation of fibroids. *Best Pract Res Clin Obstet Gynaecol* 2008;**22**:615–26.

100. Lacey CG. Benign disorders of the uterine corpus. In: Pernoll ML (ed), *Current Obstetric and Gynaecologic Diagnosis and Treatment*, 7th edn, pp. 732–38. Norwalk, CN: Appleton & Lange; 1991.

101. Day Baird D, Dunson DB, Hill MC, et al. High cumulative incidence of leiomyoma in black and white women: ultrasound evidence. *Am J Obstet Gynecol* 2003;**188**:100–107.

102. Kjerulff KH, Langenberg P, Seidman JD, et al. Uterine leiomyomas: racial differences in severity, symptoms and age at diagnosis. *J Reprod Med* 1996;**41**:483–90.

103. Marshall LM, Spiegelman D, Barbieri RL, et al. Variation in the incidence of uterine leiomyoma among premenopausal women by age and race. *Obstet Gynecol* 1997;**90**:967–73.

104. Ozumba BC, Megafu UC, Igwegbe AO. Uterine fibroids: clinical presentation and management in a Nigerian teaching hospital. *Ir Med J* 1992;**85**:158–59.

105. Flake GP, Andersen J, Dixon D. Etiology and pathogenesis of uterine leiomyomas: a review. *Environ Health Perspect* 2003;**111**:1037–54.

106. McLucas B. Diagnosis, imaging and anatomical classification of uterine fibroids. *Best Pract Res Clin Obstet Gynaecol* 2008;**22**:627–42.

107. Hurley V. Imaging techniques for fibroid detection. *Bailliere's Clin Obstet Gynaecol* 1998;**12**:213–24.

108. Freimanis MG, Jones AF. Transvaginal ultrasonography. *Radiol Clin North Am* 1992;**30**:955–76.

109. Schiller VL, Grant E. Doppler ultrasonography of the pelvis. *Radiol Clin North Am* 1992;**30**:735–42.

110. Sohaey R, Woodward P. Sonohysterography: technique, endometrial findings, and clinical applications. *Semin Ultrasound CT MR* 1999;**20**:250–58.

111. Dueholm M, Lundorf E, Olesen F. Imaging techniques for evaluation of the uterine cavity and endometrium in premenopausal patients before minimally invasive surgery. *Obstet Gynecol Surv* 2002;**57**:389–403.

112. Dueholm M, Lundorf E, Hansen E, et al. Accuracy of magnetic resonance imaging and transvaginal ultrasonography in the diagnosis, mapping, and measurement of uterine myomas. *Am J Obstet Gynecol* 2002;**186**:409–15.

113. Kugligowska E, Deeds L, Lu K. Pelvic pain: overlooked and underdiagnosed gynecologic conditions. *Radiographics* 2005;**25**:3–20.

114. Spies JB, Ascher SA, Roth AR, et al. Uterine artery embolization for leiomyomata. *Obstet Gynecol* 2001;**98**:29–34.

115. Ascher SM, Arnold LL, Patt RH, et al. Adenomyosis: prospective comparison of MR imaging and transvaginal sonography. *Radiology* 1994;**190**:803–806.

116. Fedele L, Bianchi S, Dorta M, et al. Transvaginal ultrasonography in the differential diagnosis of adenomyoma versus leiomyoma. *Am J Obstet Gynecol* 1992;**167**:603–606.

117. Pelage JP, Cazejust J, Pluot E, et al. Uterine fibroid vascularization and clinical relevance to uterine fibroid embolization. *Radiographics* 2005;**25**:S99–117.

118. Wu JM, Wechter ME, Geller EJ, et al. Hysterectomy rates in the United States, 2003. *Obstet Gynecol* 2007;**110**:1091–95.

119. Wright KN, Jonsdottir GM, Jorgensen S, et al. Costs and outcomes of abdominal, vaginal, laparoscopic and robotic hysterectomies. *JSLS* 2012;**16**:519–24.

120. Thakkar R, Ayers S, Clarkson P, et al. A comparison of outcomes following total or subtotal hysterectomy. *N Engl J Med* 2002;**347**:1318–25.

121. Carlson K, Miller B, Fowler F. The Maine women's health study: outcomes of hysterectomy. *Br J Obstet Gynaecol* 1994;**83**:556–65.

122. Talaulikar VS, Gupta S, Manyonda IT. Pregnancy after complex myomectomy: neither age of patient nor size, number or location of fibroids should be a barrier. *JRSM Short Rep* 2012;**3**:19.

123. Mukhopadhaya N, De Silva C, Manyonda IT. Conventional myomectomy. *Best Pract Res Clin Obstet Gynaecol* 2008;**22**:677–705.

124. Bonney V. A clamp forceps for controlling haemorrhage when performing myomectomy. *Br J Obstet Gynaecol* 1923;**30**:447–49.

125. Ngeh N, Belli AM, Morgan R, Manyonda IT. Pre-myomectomy uterine artery embolization minimizes operative blood loss. *Br J Obstet Gynaecol* 2004;**111**:1139–40.

126. Taylor A, Sharma M, Tsirkas P, et al. Reducing blood loss at open myomectomy using triple tourniquets: a randomized controlled trial. *Br J Obstet Gynaecol* 2005;**112**:340–45.

127. Tsuji S, Takahashi K, Yomo H, et al. Effectiveness of anti-adhesion barriers in preventing adhesions after myomectomy in patients with uterine leiomyoma. *Eur J Obstet Gynecol Reprod Biol* 2005;**123**:244–48.

128. Agdi M, Tulandi T. Endoscopic management of uterine fibroids. *Best Pract Res Clin Obstet Gynaecol* 2008;**22**:707–16.

129. Rosetti A, Sizzi O, Soranna L, et al. Long-term results of laparoscopic myomectomy: recurrence rates in comparison with abdominal myomectomy. *Hum Reprod* 2001;**16**:770–74.

130. Loffer FD. Improving the results of hysteroscopic submucosal myomectomy for menorrhagia by concomitant endometrial ablation. *J Minim Invasive Gynecol* 2005;**12**:254–60.

131. Emmanuel MH, Wamsteker K, Hart AA, et al. Long-term results of hysteroscopic myomectomy for abnormal uterine bleeding. *Obstet Gynecol* 1999;**93**:743–48.

132. Ravina JH, Herbreteau D, Ciraru-Vigneron N, et al. Arterial embolisation to treat uterine myomata. *Lancet* 1995;**346**:671–72.

133. Bratby MJ, Belli A-M. Radiological treatment of symptomatic fibroids. *Best Pract Res Clin Obstet Gynaecol* 2008;**22**:717–34.

134. Chua GC, Wilsher M, Young MP, Manyonda I, Morgan R, Belli AM. Comparison of particle penetration with non-spherical polyvinyl alcohol versus trisacryl gelatin microspheres in women undergoing premyomectomy uterine artery embolization. *Clin Radiol* 2005;**60**:116–22.

135. Pelage JP, Guaou NG, Jha RC, Ascher SM, Spies JB. Uterine fibroid tumors: long-term MR imaging outcome after embolization. *Radiology* 2004;**230**:803–809.

136. Spies JB, Allison S, Flick P, et al. Spherical polyvinyl alcohol versus tris-acryl gelatin microspheres for uterine artery embolization for leiomyomas: results of a limited randomized comparative study. *J Vasc Interv Radiol* 2005;**16**:1431–37.

137. Marret H, Alonso AM, Cottier JP, Tranquart F, Herbreteau D, Body G. Leiomyoma recurrence after uterine artery embolization. *J Vasc Interv Radiol* 2003;**14**:1395–99.

138. Nicholson T. Outcome in patients undergoing unilateral uterine artery embolization for symptomatic fibroids. *Clin Radiol* 2004;**59**:186–91.

139. Volkers NA, Hehenkamp WJ, Birnie E, Ankum WM, Reekers JA. Uterine artery embolization versus hysterectomy in the treatment of symptomatic uterine fibroids: 2 years' outcome from the randomized EMMY trial. *Am J Obstet Gynecol* 2007;**196**:519.e1–11.

140. Hehenkamp WJ, Volkers NA, Donderwinkel PF, et al. Uterine artery embolization versus hysterectomy in the treatment of symptomatic uterine fibroids (EMMY trial): peri- and postprocedural results from a randomized controlled trial. *Am J Obstet Gynecol* 2005;**193**:1618–29.

141. Hehenkamp WJ, Volkers NA, Birnie E, Reekers JA, Ankum WM. Pain and return to daily activities after uterine artery embolization and hysterectomy in the treatment of symptomatic uterine fibroids: results from the randomized EMMY trial. *Cardiovasc Intervent Radiol* 2006;**29**:179–87.

142. Edwards RD, Moss JG, Lumsden MA, et al. Uterine-artery embolization versus surgery for symptomatic uterine fibroids. *N Engl J Med* 2007;**356**:360–70.

143. National Institute for Health and Care Excellence: Uterine artery embolisation for fibroids. Interventional procedures guidance [IPG367]. Available at: https://www.nice.org.uk/guidance/ipg367.

144. Manyonda IT, Bratby M, Horst JS, et al. Uterine artery embolization versus myomectomy: impact on quality of life–results of the FUME (Fibroids of the Uterus: myomectomy versus Embolization) Trial. *Cardiovasc Intervent Radiol.* 2012;**35**:530–36

145. Fruehauf JH, Back W, Eiermann A, et al. High-intensity focused ultrasound for the targeted destruction of uterine tissues: experiences from a pilot study using a mobile HIFU unit. *Arch Gynecol Obstet* 2008;**277**:143–50.

146. Leslie TA, Kennedy JE. High intensity focused ultrasound in the treatment of abdominal and gynaecological diseases. *Int J Hyperthermia* 2007;**23**:173–82.

147. Funaki K, Fukunishi H, Funaki T, Sawada K, Kaji Y, Maruo T. Magnetic resonance-guided focused ultrasound surgery for uterine fibroids: relationship between the therapeutic effects and signal intensity of preexisting T2-weighted magnetic resonance images. *Am J Obstet Gynecol* 2007;**196**:184.e1–6.

148. Gedroyc WM, Anstee A. MR-guided focused ultrasound. *Expert Rev Med Devices* 2007;**4**:539–47.

149. Rabinovici J, Inbar Y, Revel A, et al. Clinical improvement and shrinkage of uterine fibroids after thermal ablation by magnetic resonance-guided focused ultrasound surgery. *Ultrasound Obstet Gynecol* 2007;**30**:771–77.

150. Hindley JT, Law PA, Hickey M, et al. Clinical outcomes following percutaneous magnetic resonance image guided laser ablation of symptomatic uterine fibroids. *Hum Reprod* 2002;**17**:2737–41.

151. Manyonda IT, Gorti M. Costing magnetic resonance-guided focused ultrasound surgery, a new treatment for symptomatic fibroids. *BJOG* 2008;**115**:551–53.

152. Wilson EA, Yang F, Rees ED. Estradiol and progesterone binding in uterine leiomyomata and in normal uterine tissue. *Obstet Gynecol* 1980;**55**:20–24.

153. Tamaya T, Fujimoto J, Okada H. Comparison of cellular levels of steroid receptors in uterine leiomyomas and myometrium. *Acta Gynaecol Scand* 1985;**64**:307–309.

154. Talaulikar VS, Belli A, Manyonda I. GnRH agonists: do they have a place in the modern management of fibroid disease? *J Obstet Gynecol India* 2012;**62**:506–10.

155. Dubuisson JB, Fauconnier A, Fourchotte V, Babaki-Fard K, Coste J, Chapron C. Laparoscopic myomectomy: predicting the risk of conversion to an open procedure. *Human Reprod* 2001;**16**:1726–31.

156. Campo S, Garcea N. Laparoscopic myomectomy in premenopausal women with and without preoperative treatment using gonadotrophin-releasing hormone analogues. *Human Reprod* 1999;**14**:1:44–48

157. Vercellini P, Maddalena S, Giorgi OD, Aimi G, Crosignani PG. Abdominal myomectomy for infertility: a comprehensive review. *Human Reprod* 1998;**13**:873–79.

158. Fauconnier A, Chapron C, Babaki-Fard K, Dubuisson JB. Recurrence of leiomyomata after myomectomy. *Hum Reprod Update* 2000;**6**:595–602.

159. Lethaby A, Vollenhoven B. Fibroids (uterine moyamtosis, leiomyomas). *Clin Evid* 2002;**7**:1666–78.

160. Ohara N, Xu Q, Matsuo H, Maruo T. Progesterone and progesterone receptor modulator in uterine leiomyoma growth. In: Maruo T, Mardon H, Stewart C (eds), *Translational Research in Uterine Biology*. Amsterdam: Elsevier; 2008.

161. Ohara N, Morikawa A, Chen W, et al. Comparative effects of SPRM asoprisnil (J867) on proliferation, apoptosis, and the expression of growth factors in cultured uterine leiomyoma cells and normal myometrial cells. *Reprod Sci* 2007;**14** Suppl 8:20–27.

162. Xu Q, Ohara N, Liu J, et al. Progesterone receptor modulator CDB-2914 induces extracellular matrix metalloproteinase inducer in cultured human uterine leiomyoma cells. *Mol Hum Reprod* 2008;**14**:181–91.

163. Yoshida S, Ohara N, Xu Q, et al. Cell-type specific actions of progesterone receptor modulators in the regulation of uterine leiomyoma growth. *Semin Reprod Med* 2010;**28**:260–73.

164. Donnez J, Tatarchuk TF, Bouchard P, et al. Ulipristal acetate versus placebo for fibroid treatment before surgery. *N Engl J Med* 2012;**366**:409–20.

165. Donnez J, Tomaszewski J, Vázquez F, et al. Ulipristal acetate versus leuprolide acetate for uterine fibroids. *N Engl J Med* 2012;**366**:421–32.

166. Donnez J, Donnez O, Matule D, et al. Long-term medical management of uterine fibroids with ulipristal acetate. *Fertil Steril* 2016;**105**:165–73.e4.

167. Donnez J, Hudecek R, Donnez O, et al. Efficacy and safety of repeated use of ulipristal acetate in uterine fibroids. *Fertil Steril* 2015;**103**:519–27.e3.

168. Spitz IM. Clinical utility of progesterone receptor modulators and their effect on the endometrium. *Curr Opin Obstet Gynecol* 2009;**21**:318–24.

169. Horne FM, Blithe DL. Progesterone receptor modulators and the endometrium: changes and consequences. *Hum Reprod Update* 2007;**13**:567–80.

170. Mutter GL, Bergeron C, Deligdisch L, et al. The spectrum of endometrial pathology induced by progesterone receptor modulators. *Mod Pathol* 2008;**21**:591–98.

SECTION 8
Benign Disease of the Vulva

50

Benign disease of the vulva

Rosalind Simpson and David Nunns

Introduction

Vulval disease has long been a neglected area of research in medicine, resulting in the absence of even basic data such as estimates of disease prevalence. Additionally, it is common for affected individuals to delay seeking medical advice through fear and embarrassment. Current deficiencies in training (1) lead to failure of medical professionals to fully explore vulval symptoms. Women may present to a range of different specialties and making the correct diagnosis may take considerable time. There are unmet training needs for some gynaecologists in the assessment and management of vulval disease including the chronic pain and psychosexual issues that commonly arise so it is important to assess patients and refer difficult patients and non-responders on to a vulval service for a multidisciplinary opinion. Inappropriate treatment is not uncommon.

Survey-based studies indicate that vulval disease is much more prevalent than once thought. In a survey of 79 United Kingdom general practitioners, over half saw more than three patients with vulval disease per month (2) and a United States-based community survey of 303 women reported 18.5% having lower genital tract discomfort lasting longer than 3 months (3).

Vulval disease is important as it causes considerable distress and can affect both physical and psychological and psychosexual well-being (4, 5). Furthermore, certain inflammatory vulval conditions have potential for progression to malignancy. Vulval disease is common in gynaecological practice. This chapter is aimed at the general gynaecologist to enhance knowledge and clinical skills in patient assessment, vulval examination, and treatment.

History taking

A thorough assessment of symptoms can often point to a diagnosis when combined with the clinical examination findings. **Table 50.1** outlines some key questions to ask in the history and why. The impact of the vulval symptoms on function should always be explored. 'How do the symptoms affect you?' or 'What do you miss as a result of the problem?' are helpful questions to ask. A psychosexual history should be investigated if appropriate. Often referral of patients with a vulval problem might reveal sexual pain as the main complaint and secondary psychosexual problems such as vaginismus, avoidance,

phobia of touch, and loss of libido (6). Recognition of this as the significant problem for the patient is important so that treatment can focus on self-management or with a psychosexual counsellor.

Women with vulval pain should have a detailed pain history taken covering the pain's nature, severity, site, and aggravating or relieving factors. Some patients with vulvodynia have pain at other body sites and vulvodynia may be a part of a chronic regional pain syndromes (7). Not infrequently patients may be upset and frustrated which may in part be explained by disjointed care, ineffective treatments, and a lack of understanding of the condition by clinicians.

Vulval examination

A full vulval examination requires good lighting and each part of the vulva should be examined systematically including the mons pubis, inguinal folds, outer and inner labia (majora and minora), clitoris (body and hood), perineum, vestibule, and anus (**Figure 50.1**). Hart's line is the junction between the vestibule and the inner labia and marks a change in epithelium type from mucosal type to stratified squamous. Ideally, digital and speculum examinations should be performed to rule out erosions, mucosal thickening, adhesions, and scarring as these features can be seen in conditions such as erosive lichen planus and lichen sclerosus (8). Digital vaginal examination may be helpful to assess pelvic floor muscle hypertonicity (9).

Dermatological problems of the vulva may be a manifestation of a general skin condition and therefore a complete skin examination should be considered to allow a more complete assessment of disease extent and diagnosis. For example, psoriasis may manifest in 'hidden' sites such as the umbilicus and natal cleft and eczema is found in the skin flexures. Examination of other non-keratinized or mucosal surfaces, including the oral cavity, eyes, and mouth should also be performed as certain conditions such as pemphigus vulgaris, pemphigoid, and erosive lichen planus may affect these regions (10).

Terminology of examination findings

The terms used to describe the appearance of vulval disease are largely synonymous with dermatology terminology. For example:

- *'Erythema'* refers to reddening of the skin, which may be poorly demarcated, as in eczema (**Figure 50.2** demonstrates poorly defined erythema in the context of contact dermatitis) or well

Table 50.1 Vulval history taking

Question	Reasoning
What are the key symptoms and how severe are they? What is the impact on the patient's function?	Important to be clear on the initial symptom. Itch can suggest skin disease or infection. Pain can be secondary to itching from skin damage. Pain as a primary symptom may indicate a pain syndrome. A reduction in symptoms and improvement in function (including sex) are important clinical outcomes
How long has the woman been experiencing symptoms?	Acute symptoms may indicate vulvovaginal thrush or contact dermatitis. Chronic symptoms (more than 6 months) may be due to lichen sclerosus or lichen planus
Are there any other vulval symptoms?	Helps making a diagnosis. For example, vaginal discharge may be caused by infection
What treatments have been tried before?	Inappropriate topical treatments can exacerbate symptoms and potentially cause an irritant reaction. The history should explore 'failed' treatments, e.g. topical steroid type, frequency, duration and amount (under usage with these treatments is common)
How is the patient cleaning the vulval area?	Many women feel unclean and can over-wash leading to skin damage and further irritation
Are there any possible contacts with irritants such as soaps, shampoos, urine, and scented vaginal wipes?	These are potential irritants and can damage the skin potentially causing inflammation. Urine is a potent skin irritant
Are there any other skin conditions present?	For example, eczema (seen elsewhere in the skin flexures) or psoriasis (sometimes hidden as cracking behind the ears, a scaly scalp, or umbilical erythema).
Is there any systemic disease?	Other systemic disease many contribute to treatment outcome, e.g. diabetes, renal failure, anaemia, autoimmune conditions (including family history of autoimmunity), other chronic pain syndromes
Are symptoms stress related?	With lichen simplex and vulvodynia, symptoms are worse at times of stress and acknowledging this can become a part of the treatment plan

demarcated, as in psoriasis (**Figure 50.3**). The presence of erythema usually indicates an underlying inflammatory process. If present in association with pain, infection should be considered.

- *Whitening* of the skin may occur in the presence of a normal epidermis such as in vitiligo, or in conjunction with epidermal change such as in lichen sclerosus.

- *Lichenification* is the term used to describe a leathery thickening of the skin with increased skin markings which occurs in response to persistent rubbing.

- *Scale* is an increase in the dead cells on the surface of the skin. The vulval region is often moist and scale is a less reliable sign than on

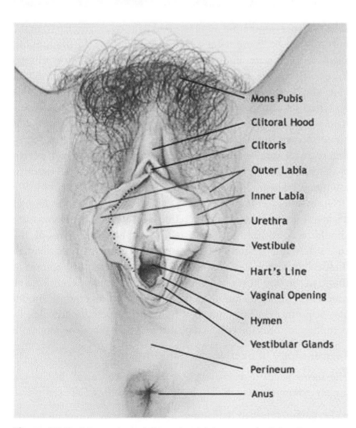

Figure 50.1 Schematic representation of the normal adult vulva.
Courtesy of Dawn Danby and Paul Waggone.

Mons Pubis
Clitoral Hood
Clitoris
Outer Labia
Inner Labia
Urethra
Vestibule
Hart's Line
Vaginal Opening
Hymen
Vestibular Glands
Perineum
Anus

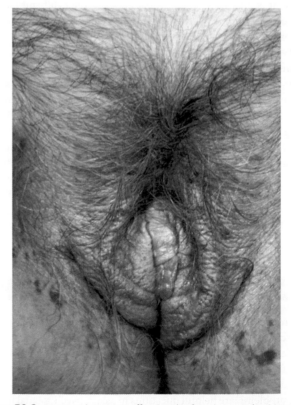

Figure 50.2 Contact dermatitis affecting the female genitalia. Note poorly defined erythema of the genitocrural skin, erosions due to excoriation in the inflamed skin, and white thickening (lichenification) of the labia majora due to scratching.

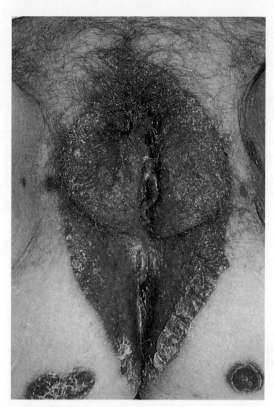

Figure 50.3 Psoriasis affecting the female genitalia. Well-demarcated erythema surrounding the anogenital area with typical psoriatic plaques in surrounding skin. The genital plaque has typical scale in the perianal area, but a lack of scale in the perineal and vulval areas.

Table 50.2 Terminology of lesions that may be seen in the vulval area

Lesion terminology	Description	Example
Fissure	A thin 'hairline' crack in the skin surface. May be due to excessive dryness	Psoriasis and lichen sclerosus
Excoriation	Scratch mark, may be single or multiple	As seen in any itchy skin conditions, e.g. atopic eczema, lichen sclerosus
Erosion	A shallow denuded area due to loss of the epidermis (surface layer of skin)	Erosive lichen planus
Ulcer	Full thickness loss of the epidermis (top layer of skin) ± dermis	Aphthous ulceration
Macule	Flat area of colour change	Vulval melanosis Ecchymosis (subcutaneous purpura) seen in lichen sclerosus
Nodule	Large palpable lesion >0.5 cm in diameter	Squamous cell carcinoma Scabies
Papule	Small palpable lesion <0.5cm in diameter	Genital warts Molluscum contagiosum Seborrhoeic keratosis
Plaque	A palpable flat lesion >0.5 cm in diameter. It may be elevated or may be a thickened area without being visibly raised above the skin surface	Vulval intraepithelial neoplasia Squamous cell carcinoma
Vesicle	Small fluid filled blister <0.5cm in diameter	Bullous pemphigoid

other areas of the skin. It is most reliable on the mons pubis where scale may be a manifestation of psoriasis. On other sites such as the natal cleft, scale and lichenification may result in whiteness and splitting of the skin. This can make common conditions more difficult to diagnose (10).

There are a number of additional terms that are used to describe specific lesions that may be found on the skin, including the vulval area (Table 50.2). The vulval skin surfaces in women with vulvodynia are normal in appearance; however, patients with vestibulodynia, a subgroup of vulvodynia, can have pain on light touch over the vestibule. This phenomenon called *allodynia* is the production of pain by innocuous stimuli by a reduction in the sensory threshold of neurons (11). Patients may also demonstrate *hyperalgesia* which is the exaggerated response to noxious substances through a general increase in the responsiveness of tissues.

Investigations

Vaginal swabs

Microbiological swabs are indicated when the history suggests possible primary or secondary infection with bacterial, candidal, and viral infections. Infection is a common cause for loss of symptom control in inflammatory dermatoses. For example, if a patient with lichen sclerosus appears initially well controlled with potent steroids and then flares, secondary infection with *Candida* should be

considered (12). Occasionally, genital herpes can be a cause of vulval symptoms and a viral culture swab may be necessary. Swabs should ideally be taken before starting antimicrobial therapy.

Vulval biopsy

A vulval biopsy is indicated for (a) asymmetrical pigmented lesions, (b) persistent erosions, (c) indurated or suspicious areas, and (d) when there is poor response to treatment following the initial diagnosis. The site selected for biopsy should be tissue representative of the lesion or area of abnormality. This is usually at the edge of the lesion and should also include some normal tissue. The most central area may be inflamed or necrotic, which will give minimal tissue diagnosis because of the inflammation present. An excisional biopsy can be problematic if the diagnosis is subsequently found to be cancer or vulval intraepithelial neoplasia in that re-excision may be required which can lead to further skin loss that might compromise function. Multiple mapping biopsies are indicated in cases of suspected multifocal disease usually under a general anaesthetic. A 4 mm Keyes punch biopsy is adequate and should ideally be carried out under local anaesthetic at the initial visit. This provides adequate tissue for histology but if direct immunofluorescence is also required, in the case of suspected immunobullous disease, two biopsies are needed. It is important to note that while specimens for histology should be sent in formalin, specimens for direct immunofluorescence must be sent in either normal saline or snap frozen in liquid nitrogen (13).

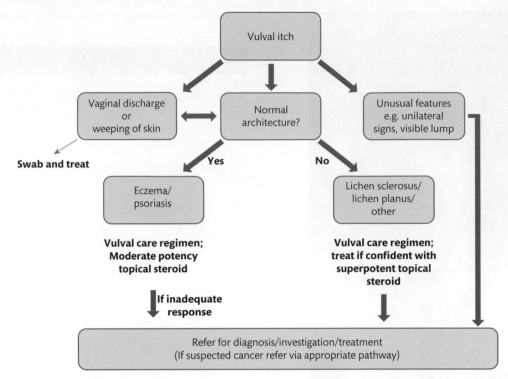

Figure 50.4 Algorithm for the management of vulval itching.

Patch testing

Patch testing by a dermatologist is indicated when allergic contact dermatitis is considered (see 'Contact dermatitis'). Common allergens include topical anaesthetics, fragrances, sodium laurel sulphate, and topical neomycin (14, 15). Allergic contact dermatitis to the adhesive used in sanitary pads may occur and should be considered (16). Since sensitization to topical allergens can occur at any time, it is another reason why symptoms initially well controlled with topical therapies such as steroids can cause a flare-up of symptoms. A clinical history is very important to determine potential sensitizing agents which can then be applied to the skin during the patch testing process.

Inflammatory vulval skin conditions

Vulval itching is often the presenting symptom of a vulval skin condition. The causes can be separated into skin disease (vulval dermatoses), infections, and premalignant/malignant disease. The algorithm outlined in **Figure 50.4** is useful when assessing patients. Many of the conditions outlined in **Table 50.3** require treatment with topical steroids and emollients with a focus on patient education and compliance. The 'Treatment principles for inflammatory vulval skin conditions' section outlines the general principles of these treatments.

Specific inflammatory conditions

The following inflammatory skin conditions are described in detail as they are frequently seen in the vulval clinic and may be encountered by the general gynaecologist in their day-to-day practice.

Lichen sclerosus

Lichen sclerosus is a chronic, inflammatory skin condition that has a predilection for the genital skin in both sexes (**Figure 50.5**). Early-stage disease may be subtle and masked especially if topical steroids have been used prior to referral. Around 15% of patients have extragenital disease. The general management of lichen sclerosus is with superpotent topical steroids and emollients (18). An initial 3-month course of superpotent topical corticosteroids (e.g. clobetasol propionate 0.05%), one finger-tip unit (from the tip of the finger to the first crease) nightly for 4 weeks, alternate nights for 4 weeks, and then twice a week for 4 weeks. A Cochrane review of the management of lichen sclerosus was published in 2011 (19, 20). Seven trials involving 249 patients covering six treatments were included; however, the evidence for optimal treatment was limited. Effective treatments included superpotent (clobetasol propionate 0.05%) and potent mometasone furoate 0.1%) topical steroids. Topical calcineurin inhibitors may have a place in the management of lichen sclerosus and these are usually prescribed under the supervision of a dermatologist. There was no benefit for topical testosterone or progesterone. Further trials are needed to determine the exact steroid potency, frequency, and duration of treatment. The regular usage of emollients should be used to provide a barrier to potential irritants (e.g. urine) and keep the skin hydrated.

There is a high chance of symptom response following the 3-month course, but lichen sclerosus remains a chronic skin disease and the symptoms are likely to recur if the treatment is stopped. Regular use of topical steroids in the long term has been shown to be safe and may reduce the underlying small risk of vulval cancer (see 'The use of topical steroids') (21).

Patients may develop symptomatic skin fissuring at the posterior fourchette. Treatment should involve digital massage of topical

Table 50.3 Summary of the clinical features and treatment of specific skin diseases

Diagnosis	Clinical appearance	Diagnosis	Primary treatment
Lichen sclerosus	• Porcelain white papules and plaques • Ecchymoses (subcutaneous purpura) • Erosions (loss of epidermis) • Fissures • Lichenification (Figure 50.5) • Late signs: loss of anatomy, fusion, adhesions There can be a 'figure-of-eight' appearance to the disease	• Clinically if confident or a vulval biopsy • Consider biopsy if there are indurated or suspicious areas	• Superpotent topical steroid (e.g. clobetasol propionate 0.05%) (see 'Topical steroids and their use in the treatment of vulval skin conditions') • Emollients
Contact dermatitis	• *Irritant form*: poorly defined erythema present where irritant has been applied • *Allergic form*: erythema extends outside of area where allergen has been applied	• Clinical history and examination. • Patch testing if allergic contact dermatitis suspected	• Moderate (e.g. clobetasone butyrate 0.05%) or potent (e.g. mometasone furoate 0.1%) topical steroid (see 'Topical steroids and their use in the treatment of vulval skin conditions') • Emollients • Strict avoidance of irritants/allergens
Seborrhoeic eczema	• Glazed skin in the intralabial sulci	• Clinical examination of other sites: scalp, eyebrows, nasolabial folds for erythema and fine scaling	• Moderate (e.g. clobetasone butyrate 0.05%) or potent (e.g. mometasone furoate 0.1%) topical steroid (see 'Topical steroids and their use in the treatment of vulval skin conditions') • Emollients
Psoriasis	• Classically, well-demarcated, scaly erythematous plaques, but vulval psoriatic plaques are smooth, glossy, and often salmon-pink in colour. Often no scale in vulval creases but surrounding skin may have typical scaly lesions of psoriasis • There is no scarring or loss of anatomy (Figure 50.3).	• Clinical assessment to include examination of 'hidden sites' for other signs of psoriasis, e.g. knees, elbows, umbilicus, scalp, ears, lower back and nails. Biopsy if unsure	• Moderate potency topical steroid as recommended by NICE guidance (17) • As the skin folds can become particularly macerated, there is a chance of secondary bacterial or fungal infection. A combination topical preparation (e.g. clobetasone butyrate 0.05%/oxytetracycline 3%/nystatin) may be helpful • Emollients
Lichen simplex	• Lichenification of the skin with erosions from chronic scratching • Usually no loss of anatomy but can give thick 'leathery' skin • Can be superimposed on other itchy skin disorders such as eczema and lichen sclerosus	• Clinical history and examination	• Superpotent topical steroid (e.g. clobetasol propionate 0.05%) (see 'Topical steroids and their use in the treatment of vulval skin conditions') • Emollient • Once control of symptoms is achieved, moderate-potency topical steroid may be required intermittently • Secondary infection with *Candida* or bacteria is common and may need treatment

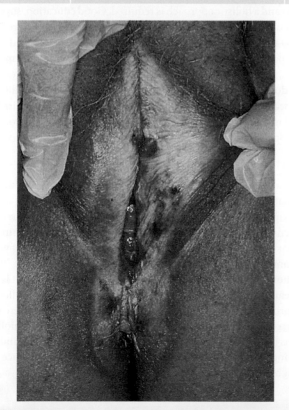

Figure 50.5 Advanced vulval lichen sclerosus. Whiteness, loss of anatomy, ecchymosis seen on the left labia, and scarring over the clitoral hood.

steroid into the fissure on a daily basis. The use of vaginal dilators and a good lubricant should be encouraged to help the scar reforming and help desensitize the area. If these measures do not help then consideration should be given to the use of surgical division or refashioning of the fissure or skin bridge.

There is a small risk of cancer development in lichen sclerosus (<5% risk) (12). Patients should therefore be encouraged to self-exam on a regular (suggested monthly) basis to detect skin cancers. Changes that might indicate premalignant/malignant change include raised lesions, irregular lesions, ulceration, and persistent eroded areas.

Lichen planus

Lichen planus is a autoimmune chronic condition (8). Two main forms of lichen planus may affect the vulval area. '*Classical*' lichen planus outlined in **Table 50.2** is usually very successfully treated with topical steroids and emollients. In contrast, patients with *erosive* lichen planus usually present with pain and burning as erosions occur at the entrance to the vagina and may affect the vaginal mucosal surface. This variant leads to considerable scarring and loss of anatomy (**Figure 50.6**). Erosive lichen planus responds less well to therapy (22) and referral to a vulval specialist is important to optimize disease management. Although the evidence is not as clear cut as with lichen sclerosus, there is probably a small chance of malignant potential in lesions of lichen planus (23). There are currently no specific guidelines for the management of lichen planus; standard

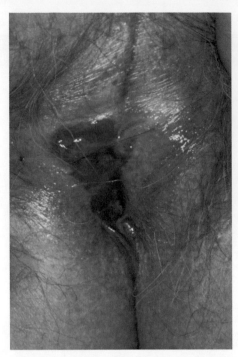

Figure 50.6 Erosive lichen planus. Well-demarcated symmetrical erosions present at the vaginal introitus. Note anatomical changes with loss of the labia minora and clitoral hood, anterior fusion, and narrowing of the vaginal opening.

practice is to use a similar regimen of superpotent topical steroid as for lichen sclerosus and case series evidence supports this (24, 25).

Vulval dermatitis

The terms *dermatitis* and *eczema* are often used interchangeably. There are different types of dermatitis that can affect the vulval area. It is important to note that vulval anatomy is normal with eczematous conditions and scarring does not occur.

Atopic eczema is likely to affect the vulva in conjunction with findings of typical eczema elsewhere. Patients rarely complain of vulval eczema when there is severe eczema elsewhere. However, in a patient who complains of vulval itching and who has a history of atopy, it is worth considering as a diagnosis. Vulval atopic eczema is often seen clinically as intralabial, perianal, and natal cleft erythema. The erythema is often mild. Signs of atopic eczema elsewhere include poorly defined, symmetrical, scaly erythematous areas on the skin creases (especially the antecubital fossae and behind the knees). Small fissures and erosions may be present. The skin is often noticeably dry. Severe eczema is more widespread over the trunk and limbs. Atopic vulvitis is the commonest cause of vulval itch in children.

Contact dermatitis may be either 'irritant' or 'allergic contact'. *Irritant* contact dermatitis is particularly common and may be triggered by soaps, perfumes, medicaments, urine, faeces, and sweat. The barrier function of the skin becomes impaired by local irritants and can subsequently be made worse by continued application of the product. Clinical signs of vulval irritant dermatitis include poorly defined intralabial erythema that occurs anywhere where the irritant has been present. Small fissures and erosions may be present

and lichenification may occur in longstanding disease (15). All of these clinical features are demonstrated in **Figure 50.2**. It is common that fissures become secondarily infected with skin pathogens or *Candida*. It is important to realize this when treatment strategies are implemented. *Allergic contact dermatitis* is less common and around one-fifth of patients with vulval skin conditions having a relevant positive patch test result (15). It can be difficult to distinguish from irritant contact dermatitis clinically, but affected skin usually extends outside of the genital area in 'non-contact' areas. This is because it is an immune-mediated hypersensitivity reaction. The only way to confidently diagnose allergic contact dermatitis is through patch testing (see 'Investigations').

Vulval seborrhoeic eczema is difficult to distinguish from psoriasis. It will often manifest as glazed skin in the interlabial sulci bilaterally. Fine scale and erythema at other affected body sites such as the nasolabial folds, scalp, and eyebrows can aid the diagnosis (26).

Treatment principles for inflammatory vulval skin conditions

There are no core clinical outcome measures for vulval skin disease (24) and suggested clinical outcomes include:

- a reduction in symptoms (e.g. less itch, pain, and fewer flare-ups of symptoms)
- an improvement in function (e.g. sexual function, mobility, and normalizing bladder and bowel function)
- increased confidence in self-management (e.g. management of flare-ups and self-examination).

General principles

Initial principles of management are the same for all vulval skin conditions and a holistic approach is required. Good education, support, and counselling are important with extra time given to address the disease process, discussing general vulval care measures, and managing patient expectations (1). It is useful to provide information leaflets, direct patients to relevant patient-oriented websites, and write down instructions for applying topical agents (see 'Additional resources' for sources of patient information). The use of a mirror or model in the clinic setting is helpful to show patients where to apply their topical treatments.

Correct barrier function

The goal of treatment is to correct barrier function and reduce inflammation. For washing, soap and other routine cleaning agents (e.g. wipes) should be avoided, as they are likely to act as irritants and sensitizing allergens. Irritation from urinary and faecal incontinence need to be addressed as these are a common cause of vulval inflammation and make underlying skin pathology worse. 'Soap substitution' with a bland cream or ointment-based emollient is best for cleansing. The same agent can then be used as an emollient to both provide a barrier to the site and sooth inflamed skin. There is no preferred emollient to use and some can cause irritation. Emollient creams (not ointments) can be placed in the fridge. Patients find this soothing and lowering skin temperature is thought to reduce itch through central inhibitory pathways (27).

The use of topical steroids

Inflammation reduction associated with skin disease (such as in lichen planus, lichen sclerosus, and eczema) is achieved by the use of topical steroids. Topical steroids are often ineffectively used in the vulval area due to concerns from patients and non-specialists about side effects, particularly skin or mucosal atrophy. It is important therefore to use the correct strength of steroid for the necessary length of time on the appropriate body site. Mucosal surfaces such as the vulval vestibule are remarkably resistant to steroid atrophy. In contrast, keratinized surfaces such as the labiocrural folds, perineum, perianal area, and thighs can develop skin thinning and striae (stretch marks) with inappropriate use with potent topical steroids (1). Overuse of topical steroids appears as thinned skin which appears redder and is reversible in the early stages. In the later stages, permanent telangiectasia and striae can develop. Topical calcineurin inhibitors in the vulval region reduce inflammation and do not cause skin atrophy. However, their role is not fully understood and there is a theoretical risk of long-term localized immunosuppression from these agents causing skin cancers (28).

Topical steroids should be used once a day. There is no evidence to suggest that twice-daily application is superior, although twice-daily application has greater potential to cause side effects (29). Ointments are preferable to creams as they contain fewer constituents and therefore have a lower chance of causing irritation/contact allergy. Once control of inflammation and symptoms has been achieved, topical steroids should be reduced to the minimum frequency required to maintain remission. The concept of 'weekend therapy', that is, applying topical steroids on two consecutive days per week, is effective in atopic eczema patients (30) and can be extrapolated to chronic vulval diseases such as lichen sclerosus and lichen planus where long-term maintenance therapy is required. A patient with these conditions will use approximately 30–60 g of topical steroid per year as maintenance therapy (12). Topical steroids should only be used on affected areas to prevent side effects in adjacent skin and the use of a mirror is often helpful to aid application in the correct areas.

Failure to respond to treatment

If a patient fails to respond to appropriate treatment the following should be considered:

1. Poor adherence to prescribed treatment regimen: 'steroid phobia' is a well-recognized problem when treating skin conditions. Many healthcare professionals, including pharmacists, will compound the issue by advising the patient to use sparingly and recommending not to use on 'sensitive areas'. This cautious approach can be detrimental to the patient's treatment plan. The patient should be advised to apply the topical steroid in terms of the finger-tip unit (A finger-tip is from the very end of the finger to the first crease in the finger. It does *not* mean a blob on the fingertip). The number of finger-tip units required is usually one to two but is specifically tailored to the patient depending upon surface area affected by the condition.

2. Inaccurate placement of topical steroid: the patient may be applying the topical treatment to an unaffected area. This is especially common if the patient is elderly and unable to use a mirror to see what they are doing. In clinic the exact location of application should be explained, Diagrams, photographs, or models can be used as an aid.

3. Continued exposure to irritants: urine or faeces, external products such as wipes or non-prescribed topical treatments, and over-washing with water can all contribute towards irritation and ongoing symptoms.

4. An incorrect diagnosis. If adherence and skin care practices are adequate, the diagnosis may be incorrect. An allergic contact dermatitis to topical treatments may have occurred (see 'Patch testing') or there may be premalignant or malignant change in the affected area. If there is any concern, a biopsy should be taken.

The multidisciplinary team

While many patients can respond well to topical treatments, there are many women who have complex needs that can be overlooked. These patients do not tend to follow any agreed clinical pathway, have unmet needs, and require adequate assessment and management (31).

These women require the care of a gynaecologist with a special interest in the management of vulval disease within the context of an appropriate multidisciplinary vulval service. Indications for multidisciplinary input include:

- ongoing symptoms despite appropriate use of topical steroids
- for review of pathology results by a gynaecological pathologist
- associated vulval intraepithelial neoplasia (usual or differentiated type)
- need for patch testing
- for consideration of surgery
- for resolution of ongoing sexual problems.

Other members of a vulval service might include dermatology, genitourinary medicine, physiotherapy, pain management, psychosexual therapy, pathology, and urogynaecology.

Vulval pain conditions

Vulval pain is a frequently encountered complaint. Patients with a pain problem may present to general gynaecologists who may have no special expertise in the diagnosis and management of chronic pain problems. It is important to distinguish those patients with vulval pain syndromes from those who have pain secondary to an active dermatological disease process (e.g. fissures or erosions). Vulvodynia has been defined as 'vulval discomfort, most often described as a burning pain, occurring in the absence of relevant visible findings or a specific, clinically identifiable, neurologic disorder' (32). It is a neuropathic pain syndrome and is analogous to other neuropathic pain syndromes. Patients can be classified by whether pain is *unprovoked* or *provoked*. Patients with *unprovoked* pain may experience spontaneous pain whereas patients with *provoked* pain usually complain of sexual pain and were formerly diagnosed as having 'vestibulitis'. This is incorrect as there is no evidence that vulvodynia is an inflammatory condition and patient with provoked pain should now be diagnosed as '*vestibulodynia*'. Patients can lose confidence in health professionals and can become isolated in their condition through embarrassment and an unwillingness to discuss problems. This can lead to psychological upset. Some patients may have a combination of vulvodynia with another vulval problem, (e.g. irritant dermatitis or thrush) and both conditions may require treatment.

Pain pathophysiology

Acute pain has an important protective function as it limits further harm and encourages healing. This pain is usually inflammatory, is associated with tissue damage or injury, and is self-limiting. If pain persists beyond 6 months, some patients can develop a neuropathic pain cycle as a result of central or peripheral nervous system sensitization. This neuropathic pain is not usually inflammatory and the phenomena of *hyperalgesia* and *allodynia* may or may not be present. It is important to note some patients do not always identify the term 'pain' with neuropathic pain symptoms but can describe a variety of sensations which include burning, stabbing, shooting, aching, and electric shock sensations. Uncommonly, these can include genital arousal states (33).

Vestibulodynia (provoked pain)

Vestibulodynia is a cause of superficial dyspareunia and is characterized by vestibular tenderness on light touch. This excessive sensitivity can be generalized throughout the vestibule or can be more focal, involving the opening of the ducts of the major vestibular glands or the posterior fourchette (34). Women are usually of reproductive age and complain of superficial dyspareunia, tampon intolerance, and pain during gynaecological examinations (35). There is often a delay between the onset of symptoms and receiving a diagnosis, which varies from months to years. As the condition is frequently chronic, a high level of psychological morbidity is common. Some patients are prone to stress and anxiety, which may play a role in developing symptoms (36). Sexual dysfunction is common and frequently reported (37). The vulval skin looks normal and a cotton-tip applicator gently applied can identify allodynia in the area of the vestibule.

Unprovoked vulvodynia

Unlike women with provoked pain, those with unprovoked vulvodynia have more constant neuropathic-type pain in the vulva. Patients can be of all ages (rarely children) and describe intermittent or constant symptoms. Patients may describe tingling or 'electric shock' types symptoms. Superficial dyspareunia is not consistently reported and some experience rectal, perineal, and urethral discomfort. Psychological morbidity is likely to be high as a consequence of chronic pain and there is frequently an impact on function. Clinical examination of the vulva shows no skin changes.

Treatment principles for vulvodynia patients

The management approach to a patient with vulvodynia is similar to a patient with a chronic vulval skin disease with a focus on the same clinical outcomes. As vulvodynia is a chronic pain condition, the treatment options focus on pain modification through pain-modifying drugs, pelvic floor muscle rehabilitation, and psychological and psychosexual support. Many gynaecologists lack the knowledge, skills, and competencies to provide chronic pain management so it is important to refer on to other health professionals if not confident. A gynaecologist should be expected, however, to assess the patients and start basic treatment. The evidence base for the optimal treatment is poor, but the British Society for the Study of Vulval Diseases, a society representing health professionals who have an interest in vulval disease, has produced national guidance on the management based on existing evidence (9). This guidance focuses on stratifying patient care depending on needs and the role of the multidisciplinary team. **Box 50.1** summarizes the principles of managing of vulvodynia (**Figure 50.7**).

Surgery for provoked pain

Surgical excision of the vestibule may be appropriate for a small subgroup of patients with localised provoked pain (vestibulodynia) where there is localised peripheral nerve proliferation. There is evidence to support this treatment (41). The modified vestibulectomy is the procedure of choice for patients with vestibulodynia. It involves excision of a horseshoe-shaped area of the vestibule followed by dissection of the posterior vaginal wall to cover the skin defect. In the largest series, the outcome was pain-free sex in 59%

Box 50.1 Vulvodynia (all types): an outline of treatment strategies which should be combined

Patient education
- An explanation of chronic pain pathways.
- Informal patient support and information through patient organizations such as the Vulval Pain Society (http://www.vulvalpainsociety.org) and the National Vulvodynia Association (http://www.nva.org) can be helpful.

Pain modification treatments
- Pain-modifying drugs (amitriptyline and/or gabapentin) are useful for moderate to severe unprovoked pain. Titrating doses of amitriptyline should be considered (38). Side effects usually settle within 2 weeks.
- Patients who are intolerant of the drugs, have severe pain, or have a decline in function should be referred to a pain management service (nerve blocks, intralesional injections, transcutaneous electrical nerve stimulation, and acupuncture).
- Local anaesthetic gels/ointment prior to sex should be considered. Occasionally, contact dermatitis can develop so they should be used with caution.

Physical therapy
- Pelvic floor muscle hypertonicity may exacerbate the pain cycle (39). Treatment aims to relax and desensitize these muscles. Techniques evidenced in the literature include pelvic floor exercises, use of vaginal dilators, and digital pelvic floor trigger point therapy delivered by a physiotherapist.

Psychological and psychosexual therapy and support
- Basic level psychological support should be given by all health professionals which includes reassurance that there is no underlying medical problem, challenge abnormal beliefs about symptoms, and the role of stress and how it amplifies pain perception
- Some patients require mindfulness/cognitive behavioural therapy self-management or formal referral to a clinical psychologist (39, 40). Figure 50.7 outlines the 'hot-cross bun' connection that can connects thoughts, emotions, physical sensations, and behaviour.

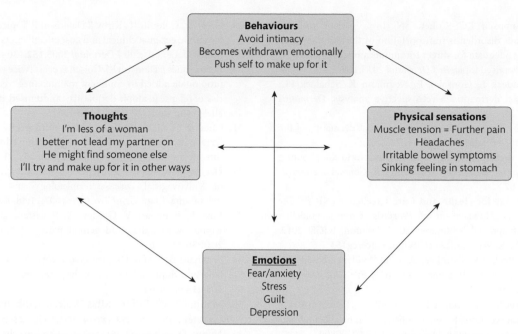

Figure 50.7 A 'hot-cross bun' diagram of how behaviours, thoughts, physical sensation, and emotions may be interlinked in patients with vulvodynia.

with favourable long-term follow-up (41). In a randomized controlled trial, 78 women with vestibulodynia were randomized to one of three arms: group cognitive behavioural therapy (12 weeks' duration), pelvic floor biofeedback therapy (12 weeks duration), and vestibulectomy (42). At 6 months, all patients reported significant improvements in pain scoring. Sexual functioning with surgery had the highest success rates; however, one concern was the high number of participants randomized to surgery who declined to be included in the study. The study supported both non-surgical treatments for vestibulodynia and suggested that patients prefer a behavioural approach to treatment than a surgical one. The clinical community remain divided on the value of surgery to treat this condition.

Conclusion

Vulval skin conditions are common and generally easy to diagnose by an accurate history and examination. Sometimes further investigations such as vulval swabs, patch tests, and biopsies are needed. For patients with unusual clinical features, or who fail to respond to adequate therapy, premalignancy or malignancy should be considered as an alternative diagnosis. Patients with complex or rare disease ideally require a multidisciplinary approach to improve clinical outcomes and improve patient experience through providing a clear explanation of a diagnosis and a treatment plan. The delivery of care should not be restricted to gynaecologists but should involve all health professionals involved with the care of women working within an individual's knowledge, skills, and competencies.

Additional resources

Further information is available online from the following resources:

DermNet NZ—the dermatology resource: http://www.dermnetnz.org.

British Society for the Study of Vulval Disease: http://www.bssvd.org.

International Society for the study of Vulvovaginal Disease: http://www.issvd.org.

National Institute for Health and Care Excellence (NICE)—Clinical Knowledge Summaries: https://cks.nice.org.uk.

REFERENCES

1. Murphy R. Training in the diagnosis and management of vulvovaginal diseases. *J Reprod Med* 2007;**52**:87–92.
2. Nunns D, Mandal D. The chronically symptomatic vulva: prevalence in primary health care. *Genitourin Med* 1996;**72**:343–44.
3. Harlow BL, Wise LA, Stewart EG. Prevalence and predictors of chronic lower genital tract discomfort. *Am J Obstet Gynecol* 2001;**185**:545–50.
4. Hickey S, Bell H. Quality of life in the vulvar clinic: a pilot study. *J Low Genit Tract Dis* 2010;**14**:225–29.
5. Sargeant HA, O'Callaghan FV. The impact of chronic vulval pain on quality of life and psychosocial well-being. *Aust N Z J Obstet Gynaecol* 2007;**47**:235–39.
6. Coulson C, Crowley T. Current thoughts on psychosexual disorders in women. *Obstet Gynaecol* 2007;**9**:217–22.
7. Bair E, Simmons E, Hartung J, Desia K, Maixner W, Zolnoun D. Natural history of comorbid orofacial pain among women with vestibulodynia. *Clin J Pain* 2015;**31**:73–78.
8. McPherson T, Cooper S. Vulval lichen sclerosus and lichen planus. *Dermatol Ther* 2010;**23**:523–32
9. Nunns D, Mandal D, Byrne M, et al. British Society for the Study of Vulval Disease (BSSVD) Guideline Group. Guidelines for the management of vulvodynia. *Br J Dermatol* 2010;**162**:1180–85.
10. Margesson LJ. Overview of treatment of vulvovaginal disease. *Skin Therapy Lett* 2011;**16**:5–7.
11. Hampson JP, Reed BD, Clauw DJ, et al. Augmented central pain processing in vulvodynia. *J Pain* 2013;**14**:579–89.
12. Neill SM, Lewis FM, Tatnall FM, Cox NH. British Association of Dermatologists' guidelines for the management of lichen sclerosus 2010. *Br J Dermatol* 2010;**163**:672–82.

13. Patel AN, Simpson RC, Cohen SN. In a patient with an immunobullous disorder, is transportation of the skin biopsy in normal saline adequate for direct immunofluorescence analysis? A critically appraised topic. *Br J Dermatol* 2013;**169**:6–10.

14. Bhate K, Landeck L, Gonzalez E, Neumann K, Schalock PC. Genital contact dermatitis: a retrospective analysis. *Dermatitis* 2010;**21**:317–20.

15. O'Gorman SM, Torgerson RR Allergic contact dermatitis of the vulva. *Contact Dermatitis* 2013;**24**:64–72.

16. Wujanto L, Wakelin S. Allergic contact dermatitis to colophonium in a sanitary pad-an overlooked allergen? *Contact Dermatitis* 2012;**66**:161–62.

17. National Institute for Health and Care Excellence (NICE). *The Assessment and Management of Psoriasis*. Clinical guideline [CG153], last updated September 2017. London: NICE; 2012. Available at: https://www.nice.org.uk/guidance/cg153.

18. Kirtschig G, Becker K, Günthert A, et al. Evidence-based (S3) guideline on (anogenital) lichen sclerosus. *J Eur Acad Dermatol Venereol* 2015;**29**:e1–43.

19. Cheng S, Kirtschig G, Cooper S, Thornhill M, Leonardi-Bee J, Murphy R. Interventions for erosive lichen planus affecting mucosal sites. *Cochrane Database Syst Rev* 2012;**2**:CD008092.

20. Chi CC, Kirtschig G, Baldo M, Brackenbury F, Lewis F, Wojnarowska F. Topical interventions for genital lichen sclerosus. *Cochrane Database Syst Rev* 2011;**12**:CD008240.

21. Bradford J, Fischer G. Long-term management of vulval lichen sclerosus in adult women. *Aust N Z J Obstet Gynaecol* 2010;**50**:148–52.

22. Simpson RC, Littlewood SM, Cooper SM, et al. Real-life experience of managing vulval erosive lichen planus: a case-based review and U.K. multicentre case note audit. *Br J Dermatol* 2012;**167**:85–91.

23. Simpson RC, Murphy R. Is vulval erosive lichen planus a premalignant condition? *Arch Dermatol* 2012;**148**:1314–16.

24. Simpson RC, Thomas KS, Murphy R. Outcome measures for vulval skin conditions: a systematic review of randomized controlled trials. *Br J Dermatol* 2013;**169**:494–501.

25. Cooper SM, Wojnarowska F. Influence of treatment of erosive lichen planus of the vulva on its prognosis. *Arch Dermatol* 2006;**142**:289–94.

26. Farage MA, Miller KW, Ledger WJ. Determining the cause of vulvovaginal symptoms. *Obstet Gynecol Surv* 2008;**63**:445–64.

27. Carstens E, Jinks SL. Skin cooling attenuates rat dorsal horn neuronal responses to intracutaneous histamine. *Neuroreport* 1998;**9**:4145–49.

28. Thaçi D, Salgo R. Malignancy concerns of topical calcineurin inhibitors for atopic dermatitis: facts and controversies. *Clin Dermatol* 2010;**28**:52–56.

29. Green C, Colquitt JL, Kirby J, Davidson P. Topical corticosteroids for atopic eczema: clinical and cost effectiveness of once-daily vs. more frequent use. *Br J Dermatol* 2005;**152**:130–41.

30. Berth-Jones J, Damstra RJ, Golsch S, et al. Twice weekly fluticasone propionate added to emollient maintenance treatment to reduce risk of relapse in atopic dermatitis: randomised, double blind, parallel group study. *BMJ* 2003;**326**:1367.

31. Cheung ST, Gach JE, Lewis FM. A retrospective study of the referral patterns to a vulval clinic: highlighting educational needs in this subspecialty. *J Obstet Gynaecol* 2006;**26**:435–37.

32. Haefner HK. Report of the International Society for the Study of Vulvovaginal Disease terminology and classification of vulvodynia. *J Low Genit Tract Dis* 2007;**11**:48–49.

33. Pink L, Rancourt V, Gordon A. Persistent genital arousal in women with pelvic and genital pain. *J Obstet Gynaecol Can* 2014;**36**:324–30.

34. Peckham BM, Mak DG, Patterson JJ. Focal vulvitis: a characteristic syndrome and a cause of dyspareunia. *Am J Obstet Gynecol* 1986;**154**:855–64.

35. Marinnoff SC, Turner MLC. Vulvar vestibulitis syndrome: an overview. *Am J Obstet Gynecol* 1991;**165**:1228–33.

36. Nunns D, Mandal D. Psychological and psychosexual aspects of vulval vestibulitis. *Genitourin Med* 1997;**73**:541–44.

37. Rosen NO, Muise A, Bergeron S, Impett EA, Boudreau GK. Approach and avoidance sexual goals in couples with provoked vestibulodynia: associations with sexual, relational, and psychological well-being. *J Sex Med* 2015;**12**:1781–90.

38. Leo RJ, Dewani S. A systematic review of the utility of antidepressant pharmacotherapy in the treatment of vulvodynia pain. *J Sex Med* 2013;**10**:2497–505.

39. Goldfinger C, Pukall CF, Thibault-Gagnon S, McLean L, Chamberlain S. Effectiveness of cognitive-behavioral therapy and physical therapy for provoked vestibulodynia: a randomized pilot study. *J Sex Med* 2016;**13**:88–94.

40. Masheb RM, Kerns RD, Lozano C, et al. A randomized clinical trial for women with vulvodynia: cognitive behavioral therapy vs. supportive psychotherapy. *Pain* 2009;**141**:31–40.

41. Eva LJ, Narain S, Orakwue CO, Luesley DM. Is modified vestibulectomy for localized provoked vulvodynia an effective long-term treatment? A follow-up study. *J Reprod Med* 2008;**53**:435–440.

42. Bergeron S, Bionic YM, Khalife S, et al. A randomised comparison of group cognitive–behavioural therapy, surface electromyographic biofeedback and vestibulectomy in the treatment of dyspareunia resulting from vulvar vestibulitis. *Pain* 2001;**91**:297–306.

SECTION 9
Reproductive Medicine

51

Infertility

Smriti Bhatta and Siladitya Bhattacharya

Introduction

Fertility is the ability to conceive and have children. It involves a complex series of biological events including gamete production, fertilization, implantation, and fetal development necessary to ensure a successful pregnancy and live birth. A number of known and unknown factors can perturb these events and compromise the chance of natural conception. Depending on the underlying factor, the fertility spectrum can range from subfertility, that is, a delay in achieving conception, to sterility, where the chance of treatment-independent conception is nil (1).

In comparison with other mammals, human reproduction is relatively inefficient—as evidenced by the low monthly fecundity rate (the probability of pregnancy in each menstrual cycle). In the absence of any underlying cause for subfertility, it is estimated that around one in five women will become pregnant each cycle, with conception occurring in 84% and 92% over a period of 12 and 24 months, respectively (2). However, the probability of conceiving each month varies significantly among couples and declines with increasing duration of non-conception. These complexities make the task of defining infertility difficult (3) and have led to different ways of describing the condition by clinicians, epidemiologists, and demographers.

Definition

Infertility is defined as a failure to become pregnant over a 12-month period despite exposure to regular, unprotected intercourse (5). This clinical definition is based on anticipated time to pregnancy, measured in months, and represents a prognosis-based approach towards defining the biological potential of a couple (4). It provides practical guidance on when to initiate investigations, that is, at a point in time when 80% of couples could be expected to conceive. However, it does not take into account the age of the female partner and variations in individual prognosis among couples. Crucially, it does not signify sterility (i.e. absolute inability to conceive), and a proportion of couples labelled infertile have the capacity to conceive without treatment.

Some epidemiologists define infertility as a lack of conception after 2 years in women of reproductive age (15–49 years) who are at a risk of becoming pregnant (sexually active, not using contraception) (6). This is similar to the clinical definition apart from the longer duration which results in the exclusion of around 10% of couples who conceive between 12 and 24 months.

For demographic purposes, infertility is described as an inability to become pregnant with a live birth, within 5 years of exposure, based upon a consistent union status, lack of contraceptive use, non-lactation, and continuation of the desire for a child (7). This definition is useful for monitoring fertility trends across different populations and geographical regions but is unhelpful in a clinical context.

Although each of the definitions is relevant in its own context, the inconsistencies between them lead to varying prevalence rates of infertility, making it difficult to estimate the true extent of the problem. This has led to the call for the development of a valid tool for defining infertility based on prognostic factors (8).

Prevalence

Depending on the type of definition used, the estimated overall prevalence of infertility worldwide is 9%, with 56% of those affected choosing to seek medical care (9). In the United Kingdom, it is estimated that infertility affects one in seven heterosexual couples—a rate which is consistent with reports from other European countries (10).

Despite an increase in numbers of couples seeking fertility treatment, the overall prevalence rates for infertility across 190 countries have remained essentially unchanged between 1990 and 2010 (7).

Types of infertility

Table 51.1 discusses types of infertility (11).

Lifestyle factors influencing fertility

Age and fertility

Female age is the most important factor affecting the probability of achieving a conception due to its impact on the quantity and quality

Table 51.1 Types of infertility

Type	Definition	Prevalence (95% CI) 31–50 years age, n = 4466 12 months' duration	Prevalence (95% CI) 31–50 years age, n = 4449 24 months' duration
Primary	Inability to achieve a conception	10.5 (9.5–11.4)	5.9 (5.2–6.6)
Secondary	Inability to conceive after having achieved a pregnancy before	5.3 (4.7–6.0)	2.9 (2.4–3.4)
Primary and secondary	Combination of above	1.7 (1.3–2.0)	0.3 (0.2–0.5)

of the oocyte/follicle pool. Women reach their peak reproductive potential in their 20s. A gradual decline in fertility is observed after the age of 30 which becomes more pronounced after 35 years of age (**Figure 51.1**) (12).

In contrast to gonadal function in women, sperm production in men continues through life. However, sperm quality can deteriorate as men get older which, along with a decrease in sexual activity, is thought to be responsible for reduced fertility in men over the age of 40 years (13).

Body mass index

Obesity can have a huge impact on both male and female fertility. In women, extremes of body weight, including low body mass index (BMI) (<18 kg/m²) or high BMI (>30 kg/m²), can result in hormonal and ovulatory dysfunction. Overweight (BMI ≥25–29.9 kg/m²) and obese (BMI ≥30 kg/m²) women undergoing IVF treatment have a reduced chance of pregnancy (relative risk (RR) 0.84; P = 0.0002) and a higher chance of miscarriage (RR 1.31; P <0.0001) when compared to women with normal BMI (14). Optimization of body weight (loss in obese women or weight gain in women with low BMI) can have a positive impact on fertility.

A number of studies have demonstrated an association between high BMI in men and decrease in semen quality. Overweight and obese men are more likely to have abnormal semen parameters (odds ratio (OR) 1.11; 95% CI 1.01–1.21) when compared to men of normal weight (OR 1.28; 95% CI 1.06–1.55) (15).

Smoking

Cigarette smoking is linked to reduced fertility in both women and men. The OR for risk of infertility in the general population is reported to be 1.6 (95% CI 1.34–1.91) for smokers compared to non-smokers (16).

Women who smoke are reported to have reduced ovarian reserve, ovulation disorders, tubal dysfunction, and altered uterine environment leading to reduced implantation. This can delay the chances of conception in women who actively smoke (OR 1.54; 95% CI 1.19–2.01) or those who are exposed to passive smoking (OR 1.14; 95% CI 0.92–1.42) (17). Smoking also adversely affects the chance of pregnancy following *in vitro* fertilization (IVF) with significantly lower odds of live birth per cycle (OR 0.54; 95% CI 0.30–0.99) (18). The risk of adverse early pregnancy outcomes such as miscarriage and ectopic pregnancy are also higher in smokers (18). Menopause has been reported to occur earlier in women who smoke compared to non-smokers (19).

In men, smoking can affect semen parameters including concentration, motility, and morphology (20). The effect of smoking on sperm DNA integrity has also been observed. Free oxygen radicals and harmful metabolites of the chemicals released from cigarette smoking are thought to be responsible for these changes.

Alcohol

Consumption of alcohol has been reported to compromise fertility (21) but the evidence is conflicting. The proposed underlying mechanism includes an alcohol-induced increase in oestrogen levels resulting in suppression of follicle-stimulating hormone (FSH) levels as well as impaired embryo development and implantation (22). The critical level of alcohol consumption responsible for this effect is unclear. Recently published United Kingdom government guidelines recommend avoiding the use of alcohol when trying for a pregnancy.

Stress

Involuntary childlessness imposes a considerable emotional burden on a couple and this can be worsened by the demands of fertility treatment (23). It is difficult to be certain whether stress causes

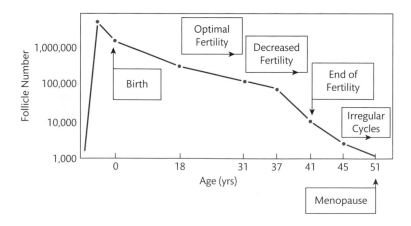

Figure 51.1 Fertility.

Reproduced from te Velde ER, Scheffer GJ, Dorland M, Broekmans FJ, Fauser BC. Developmental and endocrine aspects of normal ovarian aging. *Cell Endocrinol.* 1998 Oct 25; 145(1–2):67–73 with permission from Elsevier.

infertility or is a consequence of the condition and its treatment. Uncertainty surrounding the actual definition of stress and lack of appropriate tools to measure it make it difficult to draw any meaningful conclusions about causality.

Observational studies have shown that psychological stress may impair fertility (24) due to its effects on the hormonal control of the reproductive axis or on the immune system. In males, the effect of stress on erectile dysfunction and ejaculatory problems has been demonstrated.

Caffeine intake

Some studies have shown an association between high levels of caffeine consumption (more than five cups/day) and infertility. The quality of this evidence is weak due to limitations in the recording of caffeine consumed and the presence of other confounding factors such as smoking (25).

History and clinical examination

Couples referred to secondary care should be seen together at the initial clinic visit with sufficient time built into the consultation to allow a comprehensive history and clinical examination.

History

Table 51.2 details the points to be explored during history taking. Length of relationship, sexual history, and duration of infertility are generic questions relevant to the couple while previous pregnancies, relevant medical or surgical history, and social history should be explored individually. In women, menstrual history is important in terms of exploring ovulation status or underlying gynaecological issues.

Clinical examination

General examination

Important components of general examination include checking BMI and baseline blood pressure in addition to a general endocrine

Table 51.2 Points to be explored during history taking

General	Specific female	Specific male
Age	Menstrual history—cycle regularity, frequency and length, amenorrhoea	Vasectomy/reversal
Type of subfertility (primary/secondary)	Previous contraception	Inguinal hernia
Duration	Previous pregnancy if any and outcomes	Testicular trauma/surgery
Conception in past relationship	Sexual/pelvic infections	Sexual infections
Medical disorders/medications and surgical history	Breast problems—lump, galactorrhoea	Varicocoele
Family history	Cervical smear/treatment	Erectile/ejaculatory dysfunction
Social history—occupation, smoking, alcohol intake	Postcoital bleeding/dyspareunia	

assessment of women with irregular cycles. Observation for signs of clinical hyperandrogenism such as acne and body hair distribution is helpful in cases of polycystic ovarian syndrome (PCOS). A history of galactorrhoea necessitates breast examination. A specific history of associated medical conditions should trigger appropriate relevant systemic examination.

Local examination: female partner

A local examination in the female partner should include an abdominal and pelvic examination. The ubiquity of transvaginal ultrasound scanning has meant that this step is often overlooked but abdominal examination can often reveal the presence of large fibroids and ovarian cysts which might otherwise be missed.

Speculum examination

If a history of intermenstrual, postcoital bleeding or vaginal discharge is present, speculum examination should be performed to exclude the presence of infection, polyps, or abnormal appearance of the cervix and lower genital tract. Apart from pelvic masses, bimanual pelvic examination is also helpful in alerting the clinician to the possibility of rectovaginal endometriosis.

Pelvic transvaginal ultrasound

Transvaginal two-dimensional ultrasound of the pelvis is now used routinely for assessment of the uterus including the endometrium and ovaries.

Uterine abnormalities are found in 10–15% of women with subfertility (26) and endometrial polyps followed by submucous fibroids are the most common findings. The size and site of fibroids can be assessed by ultrasound scanning in the majority of cases and further information can be provided by a magnetic resonance imaging (MRI) scan where necessary. Congenital uterine anomalies are more prevalent in women referred for assisted reproductive technology and the most common anomaly is an arcuate uterus seen in around 12% of cases (27). Major congenital uterine anomalies include septate, bicornuate, and unicornuate uteri which have a prevalence of less than 1% (27). Hysterosalpingography (HSG), three-dimensional transvaginal scanning, saline infusion sonography, MRI, and hysteroscopy can all aid in confirming the diagnosis in these cases.

Ultrasound scanning of ovaries is useful for assessing antral follicle count as a marker for ovarian reserve. It also facilitates diagnosis of ovarian cysts, polycystic appearance of the ovary, and gaining information about the accessibility of the ovaries for transvaginal egg retrieval should IVF treatment be necessary.

Local examination: male partner

Examination of the male genitalia is helpful in cases with oligozoospermia or azoospermia. The location and volume of the testicles and any associated lumps should be noted. Reduced testicular volume (<15 mL) can be associated with non-obstructive azoospermia. Palpation of the epididymis and vas deferens helps to exclude absence of vas and epididymal enlargement related to sexual infections or obstruction in the distal sperm transport pathway. Presence of inguinal hernia, varicocoele, or any penile abnormalities such as hypospadias can also be ruled out by careful genital examination.

Investigations

Fertility investigations should be initiated in couples who have been unable to conceive despite attempts to conceive for 12 months. Earlier action should be considered in women over 36 years or in the presence of an obvious cause for infertility such as amenorrhoea (10). The purpose of these tests is to identify the underlying cause (if present) and provide a prognosis for the couple. Initial tests include semen analysis for the male partner and mid-luteal serum progesterone and a rubella screen for the female partner. If these are all normal, the next logical step is to check tubal patency.

Detecting ovulation

A history of regular cycles is usually indicative of ovulation. The biochemical marker commonly used to confirm ovulation is serum progesterone. Levels of serum progesterone rise after ovulation and reach a peak in the mid-luteal phase. In a 28-day cycle, the progesterone peak is usually measured on day 21 and a level equal to or more than 30 nmol/L corresponds with ovulation. Single progesterone measurements have been found be as effective as repeat measurements (28). Anovulatory levels of progesterone based on a single test may not be conclusive as this could be due to inappropriate timing. The correct time for the test is a week prior to the onset of a period, that is, day 23 for a 30-day cycle. In women with amenorrhoea or very irregular cycles, this test is redundant as oligoanovulation can be assumed.

Further tests in women with anovulation/oligo-ovulation

In women with irregular menstrual cycles or those whose serum progesterone measurements have not confirmed ovulation, further hormonal tests can help to identify the underlying cause. As levels of FSH and luteinizing hormone (LH) show cyclical changes, basal levels of these hormones are best measured in the early follicular phase (between day 1 and 5 of a menstrual cycle) to identify the underlying cause (**Figure 51.2**).

Tubal patency assessment

Common diagnostic tests to evaluate patency of the fallopian tubes include HSG (assessment by means of radiography), hysterosalpingo contrast sonography (HyCoSys) (assessment by means of a pelvic ultrasound scan), or a diagnostic laparoscopy and dye test. None of the tests, however, are capable of determining the functional capability of the tubes.

An HSG (**Figure 51.3**) may be offered to the women who are unlikely to have any associated pelvic pathology such as previous pelvic infections, endometriosis, or ovarian cysts. It involves the instillation of a radio-opaque iodine-based dye through the cervix under X-ray guidance to track the flow of dye through the uterine cavity and fallopian tubes with ultimate spill into the peritoneal cavity. Ideally, the procedure should be performed within 1 week following a period or in a cycle where barrier contraceptives are used in order to avoid any chance of pregnancy. Screening for chlamydial infection prior to the procedure can minimize the risk of ascending pelvic infections. Women undergoing HSG can report minor to moderate discomfort and therefore oral analgesics are advisable prior to the procedure. The sensitivity and specificity of HSG compared to laparoscopic assessment of tubal patency is estimated to be 0.94 (95% CI 0.74–0.99) and 0.92 (95% CI 0.87–0.95) respectively (29).

HyCoSy can be used as an alternative to conventional HSG. It is an outpatient ultrasound procedure where a contrast agent such as simple saline or foam is used to delineate the uterine cavity and fallopian tubes. The requirements regarding timing of the procedure during the menstrual cycle, avoiding the risk of pregnancy, and screening for sexual and pelvic infections are similar to HSG. The estimated sensitivity and specificity of HyCoSy as compared to laparoscopic tubal assessment are 0.95 (95% CI 0.78–0.99) and 0.93 (95% CI 0.89–0.96) respectively (29).

Diagnostic laparoscopy and dye test is considered the gold standard for assessment of tubal patency (**Table 51.3**). It is offered as an initial investigation in women with suspected pelvic pathology.

Laparoscopy is usually performed as a day-case procedure under general anaesthetic. Following insufflation of carbon dioxide gas within the abdominal cavity, a laparoscope is introduced, allowing direct inspection of the pelvic organs. Methylene blue dye is then injected through a cervical cannula and the passage of dye is observed through the fallopian tube. Spill of the dye is noted through the fimbrial ends if the tubes are patent.

Laparoscopy also allows assessment of entire pelvic cavity to rule out associated endometriosis or pelvic adhesions comprising the tubal and ovarian function. Additional procedures such as adhesiolysis or ablation of mild endometriosis can be undertaken at the same time.

Male infertility investigations

Semen analysis

Semen analysis is the main tool for evaluating male fertility in routine clinical practice. Men are advised to provide ejaculated samples for analysis after a 2–7-day period of abstinence. Samples produced at home should be submitted to the lab within 1 hour of production as a delay can affect the results. In the presence of abnormal parameters, a minimum of two semen analysis are required 3 months apart (or sooner if the abnormality is severe) for proper interpretation as semen quality can show intra-individual variation. The main parameters of interest during analysis are sperm concentration, motility, and morphology. Computer-assisted semen analysis has replaced the traditional manual counting chambers (haemocytometer and Makler chamber) for measuring sperm concentration and motility. Morphology is assessed by observing the prepared semen film slides which have been air dried and stained.

The World Health Organization (WHO) has provided reference ranges for semen parameters and current values are set at the lower limit of normal (fifth centile), based on data from men with proven fertility (30) (**Table 51.4**).

In clinical practice, the sperm concentration and motility are the important parameters used to determine the likelihood of natural conception. Sperm morphology assessment is dependent on the staining techniques used, shows subjective and inter-laboratory variation, and is difficult to interpret.

With the exception of azoospermia, none of the semen parameters has been shown to reliably predict the true fertility potential of men (31) but serves as a means of identifying a male factor component in an infertile couple (32).

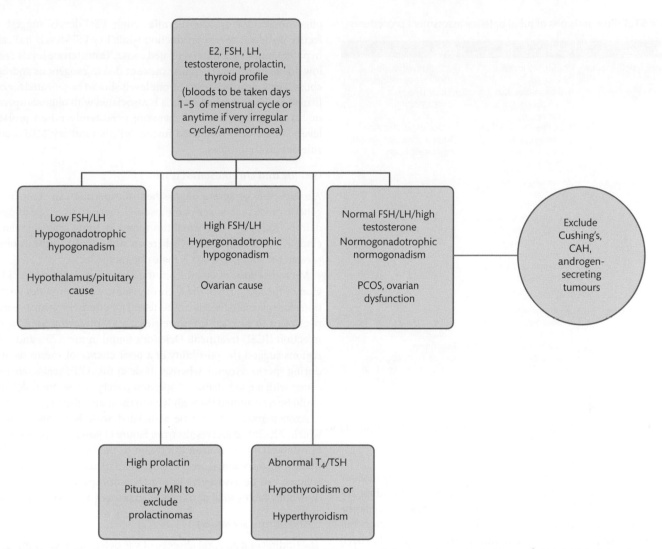

Figure 51.2 Investigations and diagnosis of cause of oligo/anovulation. CAH, congenital adrenal hyperplasia; E2, oestradiol; FSH, follicle-stimulating hormone; LH, luteinizing hormone; MRI, magnetic resonance imaging; PCOS, polycystic ovary syndrome; T₄, thyroxine.

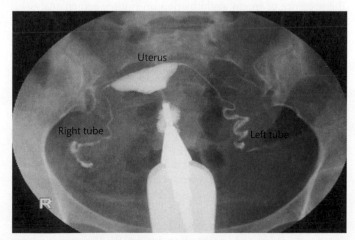

Figure 51.3 Example of a hysterosalpingogram.

Abnormalities in semen analysis

- Oligozoospermia: a sperm count below 15 million/mL is described as oligozoospermia and is often associated with poor sperm motility and morphology. In the majority of cases, the cause of oligozoospermia is unknown (idiopathic). The other known associations are illustrated in **Figure 51.4**.
- Azoospermia: absence of sperm in the semen sample can be due to problems with the sperm production (non-obstructive azoospermia) or the sperm transport (obstructive azoospermia). The causes linked to azoospermia are illustrated in **Figure 51.5**.
- Asthenozoospermia (reduced sperm motility): the WHO grading of sperm motility is from grades a to d implying a range from fast progressively motile to fully immotile sperm. The criteria for normal motility takes into account grade a (swimming fast in a straight line) and grade b (slightly slower moving in a curved line) sperm which should be 32% of the total sperm seen. Motility of the sperm is regulated by calcium pathway and influenced by reactive oxygen species, cell osmolality, and function of the flagellar

Table 51.3 Pros and cons of tubal patency assessment procedures

Test	Pros	Cons
Hysterosalpingogram (HSG)	Minimally invasive Less costly Flushes tubes and relieves minor blockage Can provide additional information about uterine cavity anomalies	Radiation exposure Sensitivity to methylene blue dye Pelvic infection False-positive report in case of tubal spasm Doesn't allow assessment of pelvic cavity
Hysterosalpingo contrast sonography (HyCoSy)	Minimally invasive Avoids radiation exposure Can provide additional information about uterine cavity anomalies Allows assessment of ovaries and other pelvic pathology	Expensive—catheters and contrast foam False positive due to tubal spasm Poor ultrasound views due to bowel gas shadow or high BMI
Laparoscopy and dye test	Definitive test Allows assessment of pelvic cavity and additional procedures as necessary	Invasive Need for general anaesthesia Expensive Risk of injury to blood vessels, bladder, and bowel

components (33). Underlying genetic factors which are poorly understood and lifestyle factors can affect these mechanisms resulting in poor sperm motility (33)

- Teratozoospermia: samples from infertile men are likely to show a higher proportion of abnormally shaped sperm, including abnormalities of the head, acrosome, midpiece, or tail. These may be associated with genetic, lifestyle, and environmental factors but the cause remains unexplained in the majority of cases. It has been proposed that the type of morphological abnormality is more important than the proportion of abnormal forms and a recent study has attempted to establish the reference ranges for morphological abnormalities in population of fertile and infertile men (34).

Further investigations in male factor infertility

Hormonal profile

Measurement of FSH, LH, testosterone, and prolactin may be helpful in identifying the underlying cause in men with significant

Table 51.4 World Health Organization criteria for semen quality

Parameter	Normal value (lower limit of reference range)
Volume	1.5 mL
Concentration (number of sperm per mL of semen)	15 million/mL
Progressive motility (per cent swimming forward)	32%
Morphology (per cent of normal shapes)	4%

Source data from Cooper TG, Noonan E, von Eckardstein S, Auger J, Baker HW, Behre HM, Haugen TB, Kruger T, Wang C, Mbizvo MT, Vogelsong KM. World Health Organization reference values for human semen characteristics. *Reprod Update* 2010;16(3):231–45.

oligozoospermia or azoospermia. High FSH levels suggest defective testicular sperm production while low FSH levels indicate a hypothalamus- or pituitary-related cause. Testosterone levels can be low due to a primary testicular cause or due to exogenous androgen abuse. Early-morning testosterone levels should be repeated for confirmation. Hyperprolactinaemia is associated with oligozoospermia or sexual dysfunction and therefore persistently raised prolactin levels should be investigated further with a pituitary MRI scan to rule out prolactinomas.

Genetic and chromosomal tests

Azoospermia or severe oligoasthenozoospermia can stem from a genetic cause such as sex chromosomal aberrations or specific gene defects. Karyotype abnormalities found in some infertile men include Klinefelter syndrome, where an additional X chromosome is present (47XXY), or a 46XX male phenotype.

Microdeletions of genes from the azoospermia factor (AZF) region of the long arm of the Y chromosome which provides instructions for spermatogenesis can be tested for counselling azoospermic men prior to surgical sperm retrieval and intracytoplasmic sperm injection (ICSI) treatment. Deletions found in the AZFa and AZFb regions suggest the possibility of a poor chance of sperm recovery during sperm retrieval, whereas those in the AZFc region are associated with a good chance of sperm recovery. These microdeletions could be transmitted through ICSI to the male offspring.

Azoospermia can also be associated with Kallman syndrome which is X-linked and results from failure of gonadotropin-releasing hormone (GnRH) neuron migration to the hypothalamus. Ciliary dyskinesia (autosomal recessive dynein deficiency in the sperm flagellum) can be associated with asthenozoospermia and myotonic dystrophy (autosomal dominant) can present as oligozoospermia.

Cystic fibrosis screening

The finding of a bilateral absence of vas deferens on examination of male genitalia should prompt screening for cystic fibrosis. In these cases there is reduced expression or increased mutation in the cystic fibrosis transmembrane regulator gene (*CFTR*) which plays an important role in regulating spermatogenesis.

Antisperm antibodies

The presence of sperm agglutination on routine semen analysis is an indication for antisperm antibody testing. The commonly used techniques are the mixed agglutinin reaction and the immunobead test, which use red blood cells or beads coated with immunoglobulin (Ig)-A/IgG antibodies to detect sperm containing the antisperm antibodies.

Sperm DNA fragmentation

Testing for DNA damage in sperm is not performed routinely and tests report on the percentage of sperm with DNA damage expressed as the sperm DNA fragmentation index (DFI). The damage to sperm DNA can be due to reactive oxygen species or due to an intrinsic defect in the process of spermatogenesis that makes the sperm more prone to damage. DNA fragmentation has been shown to be associated with an increased risk of birth defects, increased miscarriage rates, and reduced fertilization and implantation during IVF. However, evidence regarding this is conflicting. Also, there is a lack of consensus about appropriate cut-off values and effective interventions.

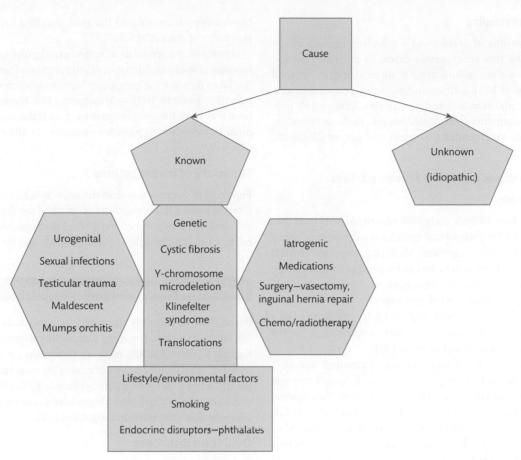

Figure 51.4 Aetiology of male infertility.

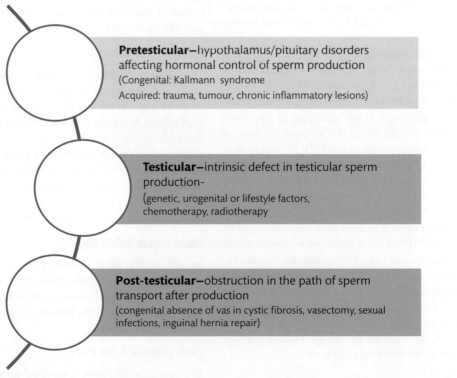

Pretesticular–hypothalamus/pituitary disorders affecting hormonal control of sperm production
(Congenital: Kallmann syndrome
Acquired: trauma, tumour, chronic inflammatory lesions)

Testicular–intrinsic defect in testicular sperm production-
(genetic, urogenital or lifestyle factors, chemotherapy, radiotherapy

Post-testicular–obstruction in the path of sperm transport after production
(congenital absence of vas in cystic fibrosis, vasectomy, sexual infections, inguinal hernia repair)

Figure 51.5 Causes of azoospermia.

Male genital tract imaging

Vasography is a means of assessment for finding the site of obstruction in obstructive azoospermia cases. Its use has gone out of fashion due to better techniques for surgical sperm retrieval and establishment of ICSI. Ultrasound scanning is useful in case of suspected testicular tumours and varicoceles. Venography provides accurate assessment of varicoceles but due to the invasive nature, it is used only for intended treatment and not for diagnostic purposes.

Additional investigations in the female partner

Ovarian reserve tests

The tests in current use include early follicular phase FSH level (between days 1 and 5 of the menstrual cycle), measurement of antral follicle count (AFC), and serum anti-Mullerian hormone (AMH) levels. AFC and AMH are considered to be good predictors of the ovarian response to controlled hyperstimulation used as part of IVF treatment but are poor predictors of pregnancy.

Basal FSH levels in women with regular cycles can be used as a screening test to predict the response to ovarian stimulation but the prediction is accurate only at higher levels (35).

AFC is done by means of transvaginal ultrasound scanning and best done in the follicular phase of cycle. Two-dimensional ultrasonography is used in routine practice but three-dimensional ultrasonography has also been shown to be helpful. Antral follicles of 2–10 mm in diameter are measured to assess AFC. Ultrasound measurements are subject to intra- and inter-observer variability and are operator dependent. Women with an AFC less than four are 8.7 times more likely to have an unsuccessful outcome following IVF (95% CI 2.4–31.7) than women with an AFC of four or more (36). The sensitivity and specificity of AFC to predict cycle cancellation has been found to be 66.7% and 94.7%, respectively (37).

AMH is secreted by the granulosa cells of the antral and preantral follicles in the ovaries and therefore is a good means to assess the reserve of primordial follicle pool. Initiation of follicular recruitment in each cycle is controlled by AMH and levels decline thereafter with age. There is no variation in the levels during a menstrual cycle and therefore the test can be done at any time, which is an advantage compared to FSH. Several studies have reported AMH to be a better marker of ovarian reserve compared to other tests but this has not been fully established. Current clinical application of using AMH is to predict the response to ovarian stimulation in IVF treatment where sensitivity and specificity has been estimated to be 82% and 76% respectively (37). Other scenarios where AMH has been found to be useful are in predicting the age at menopause (38), predicting the ovarian reserve after chemotherapy or surgery, and as a screening test for PCOS. However, technical problems with earlier assays used for measurement of AMH have come to light and newer assays are continuing to evolve with further studies awaited on their reliability and validity. Also, there are no agreed standards regarding the reference ranges from the different assays.

Hysteroscopy

In cases where intrauterine pathology is suspected on pelvic ultrasound scan, assessment of the uterine cavity by means of hysteroscopy is considered the gold standard investigation with a sensitivity of around 98% (39).

Hysteroscopic removals of endometrial polyps, resection of submucosal fibroids, and division of intrauterine adhesions have the potential to increase the pregnancy rates in women with unexplained infertility prior to fertility treatment (40). Hysteroscopy has also been shown to improve pregnancy rates if done prior to IVF treatment in women with previous unsuccessful attempts (RR 1.7; 95% CI 1.5–2.0) (40).

Summary of investigations

Figure 51.6 outlines a systematic approach to investigations in an infertile couple. It is important to consider how the result of each test will contribute to subsequent clinical decision-making and also to balance the benefits against potential costs and invasiveness.

Diagnostic categories in infertility

Based on the previously discussed investigations, infertile couples can be classified into five main diagnostic categories. Male factor infertility accounts for 30% of cases. Ovulation disorders account for 25% and tubal factor for 20% of cases (10) whereas endometriosis is the underlying factor in approximately 2–10%. One in four couples will have unexplained infertility where no obvious cause is found after standard infertility investigations (10).

Ovulation disorders

The hypothalamic–pituitary–ovarian axis orchestrates the process of follicular recruitment and ovulation in each monthly cycle. Disruption of this well-coordinated rhythmic activity can lead to ovulation disorders which have been classified by WHO into three groups (Table 51.5).

Tubal factor infertility

The fallopian tubes play an important role in natural conception by assisting the transport of eggs from the ovaries and providing a site where they can be fertilized by viable sperm. The ciliary action of the endosalpinx helps the migration of the fertilized egg to the uterus for implantation.

Blocked or damaged tubes can result from pelvic inflammatory disease such as that caused by chlamydial infection. Pelvic abscess or infection following on from appendicitis or bowel problems and adhesions related to abdominal/pelvic surgery can also be responsible for tubal damage and subsequent infertility.

Male factor infertility

Impaired sperm production or their transport can result in male infertility. Most cases are idiopathic but known causes include genetic factors, testicular maldescent or trauma, and congenital absence of vas (often related to cystic fibrosis), sexual infections, and iatrogenic causes (Figure 51.4).

Unexplained infertility

In a quarter of all couples, standard tests including semen analysis, serum progesterone to detect ovulation, and tubal patency test are normal and infertility is deemed to be unexplained. A number of putative factors which cannot be diagnosed by the standard tests have

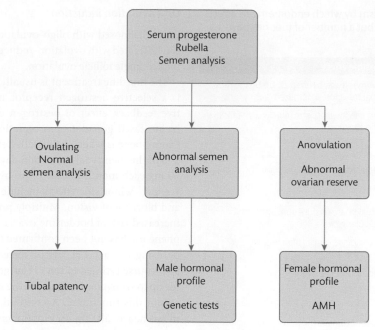

Figure 51.6 Hierarchy of investigations. AMH, anti-Mullerian hormone.

been thought to be linked to this condition, including mild ovulatory dysfunction, compromised tubal transport, suboptimal gamete quality, and immunological causes.

Lack of a specific diagnosis is challenging for the couples but some feel reassured by the fact that, in the absence of an absolute barrier to conception, the chances of spontaneous pregnancy are relatively high (41). The prognosis is better for those with a shorter duration of infertility and younger age of the female partner or where a previous conception has occurred.

Endometriosis

Endometriosis is a common condition that is characterized by presence of endometrial tissue outside the uterine cavity in sites such as the ovarian fossa, pelvic peritoneum, and uterovaginal and rectovaginal folds. Symptoms include pelvic pain, dysmenorrhea, dyspareunia, or heavy bleeding but some women may be totally asymptomatic. Infertile women are six to eight times more likely to have endometriosis (42). The precise mechanism by which endometriosis affects fertility remains to be elucidated (**Table 51.6**) (43) but a number of theories have been proposed. These include an abnormal immune response affecting implantation, pelvic adhesions posing an obstruction to egg pick up after release or transport down the fallopian tube, and increased cytokine levels in the peritoneal and follicular fluid impacting the oocyte quality.

Table 51.5 Ovulation disorders

WHO group	Disorder	Cause	Factors
Group I	Hypogonadotropic hypogonadism	Hypothalamus and pituitary dysfunction	Functional hypothalamic dysfunction—excessive weight loss such as in anorexia nervosa, exercise, stress, drugs, iatrogenic Kallmann syndrome (isolated gonadotropin deficiency and anosmia) Pituitary tumour, pituitary infarct (e.g. Sheehan syndrome) Idiopathic
Group II	Normogonadotropic normogonadism	Ovarian dysfunction	Polycystic ovary syndrome Thyroid dysfunction Hyperprolactinaemia Androgen excess (congenital adrenal hyperplasia, androgen-secreting adrenal and ovarian tumour)
Group III	Hypergonadotropic hypogonadism	Ovarian failure	Iatrogenic (e.g. surgical menopause, after radiotherapy or chemotherapy) Genetic (e.g. Turner syndrome) Autoimmune causes Infection Idiopathic

Source data from World Health Organization. 1975. *The Epidemiology of Infertility*. Report of WHO Scientific Group on the Epidemiology of Infertility. Technical Report Series No. 582. Geneva: World Health Organization.

Table 51.6 The precise mechanism by which endometriosis affects fertility remains to be elucidated but a number of theories have been proposed

Mechanism	Possible effect
Distortion of pelvic anatomy/pelvic adhesions	Ovum release, ovum pick-up by the tube, tubal transport of fertilized egg
Increased concentration of inflammatory markers such as prostaglandins and cytokines in peritoneal fluid	Can effect egg, sperm, embryo, or fallopian tube function
Altered cell-mediated immunity, increased IgA, IgG, and lymphocytes in endometrium	Impaired endometrial receptivity
Endocrine and ovulatory disorders	Luteal phase dysfunction, abnormal follicular growth
Altered progesterone and cytokine in follicular fluid	Poor oocyte quality affecting embryo development
Reduced expression of integrin and enzyme necessary for implantation	Reduced implantation

Source data from Endometriosis and infertility: a committee opinion. The Practice Committee of the American Society for Reproductive Medicine. *Fertility and Sterility*, 2006;86 Suppl 5:S156–60.

Management

The management of subfertile couples starts in primary care with prepregnancy advice on lifestyle measures to optimize BMI and smoking cessation—where appropriate. Information about timing and frequency of intercourse can be helpful for some couples. Preconception folic acid supplementation is recommended to reduce the risk of neural tube defects in the newborn. Existing medical conditions should be treated with input from appropriate specialists and the impact of any regular medication on fertility and pregnancy should be considered. Cervical smears should be up to date and abnormal smears should be managed prior to initiating fertility treatment.

Management of ovulation disorders

WHO group I disorders (hypogonadotropic hypogonadism)

Women with a BMI less than 18 kg/m² with or without a history of an eating disorder can benefit by weight gain towards a normal BMI of 19 kg/m² or above. Women with hypothalamic anovulation can be treated with pulsatile administration of GnRH agonists or gonadotropins to induce ovulation. Intravenous pulsatile administration of GnRH is administered by means of a portable pump and mimics normal cycle physiology resulting in unifollicular ovulation. This is an advantage compared to the use of gonadotropins which can result in multifollicular ovulation, thus increasing the chance of multiple pregnancy and ovarian hyperstimulation. The disadvantage, however, is that the use of a pump can be inconvenient for many women.

WHO group II disorders (PCOS)

Lifestyle modifications in the form of weight loss and structured exercise have been shown to be beneficial in improving the hormonal profile and insulin resistance in obese women with PCOS (44).

Oral ovulation induction

Cases diagnosed with oligo-ovulation or anovulation due to PCOS can be treated with ovulation-induction medications with the aim to induce single follicle ovulation.

The first-line treatment is usually with clomiphene citrate which is a selective oestrogen receptor modulator. It blocks the negative feedback effect of oestrogen on the hypothalamus resulting in increased gonadotropin secretion and induction of ovulation. Clomiphene is taken orally with a starting dose of 50 mg from day 2–3 of the menstrual cycle for 5 days. The dose can be increased by 50 mg each month in case of no ovulation to a maximum dose of 150 mg. Minor side effects include nausea, headache, hot flushes, and blurring of vision. Multiple pregnancies are a major risk. An increased risk of borderline ovarian cancer associated with clomiphene use has not been confirmed (45). Ovulation can be detected by using urinary LH kits or measuring the serum LH level and intercourse is timed to the LH surge. Clomiphene is recommended for up to six ovulatory cycles as the majority of pregnancies are seen within this timeframe. A conception rate of up to 22% per cycle in women ovulating on clomiphene has been reported (46). If a conception doesn't result, further investigations should be carried out to rule out tubal factor. Tamoxifen is an alternative to clomiphene and advised in a dose of 20–40 mg for 5 days starting from day 3 of the cycle. The antioestrogenic effect of tamoxifen is milder than clomiphene and this reduces the effect on cervical mucus. Pregnancy rates have been reported similar to clomiphene (OR 1.00; 95% CI 0.48–2.09) (47).

In women with PCOS, who are not ovulating on clomiphene alone, adding metformin to clomiphene can increase ovulation and pregnancy rates but may not improve livebirth rates (48).

The aromatase inhibitor, letrozole, has also been used for ovulation induction in women with PCOS. It is taken orally starting from day 2–3 of the cycle for 5 days in doses from 2.5 to 7.5 mg daily. The efficacy of letrozole compared to clomiphene in improving the pregnancy and live birth rate has been extensively researched and further studies have been recommended to strengthen the evidence (49). Therefore, letrozole has not yet established its place in routine clinical practice.

Second-line ovulation induction strategies

Women who fail to respond to clomiphene can be offered the second-line option of exogenous gonadotropins or laparoscopic ovarian drilling. The use of gonadotropins is associated with increased chances for multiple pregnancy and hyperstimulation. Ultrasound monitoring is therefore mandatory.

Ovarian diathermy has been shown to reduce testosterone and LH levels with correction of the hormonal imbalance associated with PCOS, resulting in restoration of ovulation. The procedure has been shown in some studies to be as effective as medical treatments, without the risk of hyperstimulation. However, the risks associated with the surgical procedure and general anaesthetic remains. There are also concerns about the long-term effect on ovarian function which can compromise future fertility (50).

WHO group III disorders (ovarian failure)

Women with a diagnosis of ovarian failure need oestrogen supplementation in the form of hormonal replacement therapy or a combined oral pill. Assisted reproduction by means of egg donation is usually necessary for conception.

Hyperprolactinaemia

Raised prolactin levels can decrease the pulsatile secretion of gonadotropin leading to anovulation and subfertility. Dopamine agonists such as bromocriptine, cabergoline, pergolide, quinagolide, and cabergoline have been used to treat hyperprolactinaemia. Cabergoline has the most favourable profile in terms of efficacy and tolerability as well as a long plasma half-life that enables once- or twice-weekly administration. Dopamine agonists are effective in over 80% of cases in normalizing the prolactin levels and reverting anovulation related to hyperprolactinaemia. Side effects include nausea, headache, postural hypotension, and fatigue.

Thyroid dysfunction

Clinical thyroid disorders, subclinical thyroid dysfunction, and thyroid autoimmunity have all been linked to poor outcomes following fertility treatment and pregnancy. The prevalence of positive thyroid peroxidase antibodies is higher in infertile women and can increase the risk of spontaneous miscarriage following IVF treatment (RR 1.99; 95% CI 1.42–2.79; $P < 0.001$) (51). However, the benefits of levothyroxine supplementation in this group of women are unclear and the need for universal screening of all subfertile women for thyroid dysfunction remains debatable (52).

Management of tubal factor infertility

IVF is offered as a first-line treatment for tubal factor infertility. IVF has the advantage of bypassing any problems related to blockage or non-functioning of the fallopian tubes. The success rate of IVF hugely depends on the women's age and the presence of other causes of subfertility can influence it further. To add to this are the financial costs associated with IVF which can be unaffordable for some couples. The numbers of IVF attempts are limited by regulations and success rates have stayed static over the last decade.

Compared to IVF, tubal surgery in suitable cases is relatively inexpensive and can provide unlimited attempts to the couples (53) if other factors are favourable. However, tubal surgery can only restore the anatomical patency of fallopian tubes which is meaningless in case of compromised tubal function. Tubal diseases amenable to surgical correction are previous tubal sterilization, perifimbrial or periovarian adhesions, proximal tubal obstruction, and hydrosalpinges.

The strongest case for tubal surgery is in women with previous sterilization and no other cause for infertility. Microsurgical tubal anastomosis can result in a success rate of up to 70% which is influenced by the duration since the sterilization, type of procedure used, and the tubal length achieved after anastomosis. Shorter duration since the initial operation and tubal length greater than 4 cm are associated with a good prognosis.

The presence of adhesions around the tubes and ovaries can interfere with ovulation or could prove a physical barrier to ovum pick up. Laparoscopic adhesiolysis is commonly considered and success of peritubal adhesiolysis is dependent on the type of adhesion (flimsy or dense), amount of inflammation present, and associated degree of tubal damage. Division of flimsy adhesions is most successful and can improve the conception rate by 60% over 6–12 months (54).

The presence of hydrosalpinx can affect the implantation rates during IVF treatment and this is thought to be due to the effect of embryotoxic factors in the fluid or due to the fluid interfering with the interaction between the embryo and the endometrium. Laparoscopic salpingectomy prior to embarking on IVF treatment has been found to be beneficial in women with hydrosalpinges with higher odds of ongoing pregnancy (Peto OR 2.14; 95% CI 1.23–3.73) and clinical pregnancy rates (Peto OR 2.31; 95% CI 1.48–3.62) (55). Laparoscopic tubal occlusion can be used as an alternative to laparoscopic salpingectomy in women with hydrosalpinges and improvement in pregnancy rates have been noted (55).

Proximal tubal obstruction cases have been traditionally managed by open or laparoscopic tubocornual anastomosis. This has now been superseded by salpingography and transcervical tubal cannulation. Success rates of up to 85% have been observed in achieving a pregnancy following this procedure but the evidence is not supported by trials and the risk of ectopic pregnancy is high at 9%.

Despite the advances in tubal microsurgery, issues remain with technical skills and limited applicability. Moreover, tubal recanalization cannot be effective if the functional capacity of the tubes is compromised. IVF therefore leads the race in tubal factor infertility.

Management of male factor infertility

General advice should include smoking cessation and alcohol intake within recommended limits. Antioxidant supplements may be helpful (OR 4.21; 95% CI 2.08–8.5) in increasing the clinical pregnancy and live birth rate but evidence supporting this is weak (56). Medical treatment options have limited use in the management of male infertility and include cases of azoospermia related to hypogonadotropic hypogonadism, erectile dysfunction, and ejaculatory dysfunction. Surgical techniques are applicable in specific scenarios such as obstructive azoospermia or varicocoeles. Assisted reproduction is the only option in the majority of male infertility cases which offers them the chance of having their own genetic offspring. Management specific to the diagnosis is discussed in the following sections.

Azoospermia

Medical

Azoospermia due to hypogonadotropic hypogonadism can be reversed by GnRH or gonadotropin therapies. Gonadotropins used for inducing spermatogenesis include human chorionic gonadotropin alone or combined with recombinant FSH, urinary FSH, or human menopausal gonadotropins. Restoration of spermatogenesis takes around 6–12 months after initiation of treatment and the overall successful spermatogenesis achieved is 75% (57) with mean sperm concentration obtained of 5.92 (4.72–7.13) and 4.27 (1.80–6.74) million/mL for gonadotropin and GnRH therapy, respectively (57). The success rate is higher in men with lower levels of gonadotropins at the baseline and for those using both human chorionic gonadotropin and FSH (57).

Surgical

Microsurgical reconstruction of vas deferens in the form of vasovasostomy or vasoepididymostomy is a successful treatment option in cases with a previous vasectomy. Patency rate of 60%

and success rates of up to 85% have been reported. These cases also have the option of surgical sperm retrieval if the reconstruction is unsuccessful.

Retrieving sperm surgically for use in IVF/ICSI cycles is advocated in cases of azoospermia. Chances of successful sperm retrieval is higher in cases of obstructive azoospermia (OA) compared to non-obstructive azoospermia (NOA) cases. Sperm can be retrieved from either epididymis or testis. Microsurgical epididymal sperm aspiration (MESA) under general anaesthesia or percutaneous epididymal sperm aspiration (PESA) under local anaesthesia are the commonly used techniques for sperm retrieval from epididymis in men with OA. PESA is a technically simpler procedure not requiring microsurgical training with success rates of up to 84% (58). However, the quantity of sperm retrieved can vary and is much lower than MESA. Testicular sperm extraction techniques include testicular sperm aspiration (TESA), testicular sperm extraction (TESE), or microdissection testicular sperm extraction (microTESE) which are used to retrieve sperm from the testes, both in men with OA who have unsuccessful MESA/PESA and those with NOA. MicroTESE has the advantage of having magnified views of the seminiferous tubules leading to highest rates of sperm extraction and low testicular tissue removal. Choice of sperm retrieval technique depends upon the availability and surgeon preference as the efficacy of one technique over the other is yet to be determined (59)

Transurethral resection of the ejaculatory ducts can be used in postinflammatory obstruction of ejaculatory ducts.

Mild male factor infertility

Intrauterine insemination (IUI) is commonly used for couples where the semen parameters show mild abnormalities compared to standard reference ranges as listed in **Table 51.4**. IUI involves placing a prepared sample of washed motile sperm into the uterus around the time of ovulation in a natural menstrual cycle or in a stimulated cycle. Evidence based on a recent systematic review has found that IUI does not increase the probability of pregnancy when compared to timed intercourse (OR 4.57; 95% CI 0.21–102) (60). Undergoing ovarian stimulation prior to IUI (stimulated IUI) has also not been found to increase the pregnancy rate (OR 1.68; 95% CI 1.00–2.82) or live birth rate (OR 1.34; 95% CI 0.77–2.33) compared to IUI alone (60). IUI is less invasive than IVF and evidence from the same review based on two randomized trials has shown no difference in the live birth rate when comparing IVF versus IUI in cycles with ovarian stimulation (two randomized controlled trials, 86 couples: OR 1.03; 95% CI 0.43–2.45) (60).

Erectile dysfunction

The mainstay of treatment for erectile dysfunction is phosphodiesterase type 5 inhibitors including sildenafil, tadalafil, vardenafil, and avanafil. They act by causing vasodilatation secondary to release of cyclic GMP and administration is through the oral route. Side effects could include changes in vision, sense of smell, vascular tone, or platelet aggregation due to cross-reaction with multiple different phosphodiesterase receptors. Alprostadil is the injectable alternative to the oral medications and at doses of 10–20 mcg induces erections in up to 80% of patients. A surgical approach in the form of microvascular arterial bypass penile revascularization or penile implant is reserved for cases refractory to medical management.

Ejaculatory disorders

Disordered ejaculation can present as premature ejaculation, delayed ejaculation, or anejaculation. A combination of behavioural psychotherapy and serotonin reuptake inhibitors (SSRI) including paroxetine, fluoxetine, sertraline, citalopram, and fluvoxamine are used in the management of premature ejaculation. Dapoxetine is a purpose-built SSRI for on-demand treatment of premature ejaculation as it has a short half-life and can be used 1–3 hours before planned intercourse. Alternative medications prescribed are topical lignocaine, phosphodiesterase inhibitors, or tamsulosin. Psychotherapy is the mainstay of treatment for delayed ejaculation. Anejaculation or retrograde ejaculation is difficult to treat and pharmacological treatment has limited success. Sperm can be recovered from urine in cases of retrograde ejaculation to be used in IVF/ICSI cycle. Electro-ejaculation for sperm recovery could be considered in men with anejaculation due to neurological impairment. The option of surgical sperm retrieval remains if other measures are unsuccessful.

Assisted conception for male factor infertility

The introduction of ICSI technique for fertilization in the early 1990s has revolutionized the management of male infertility cases with very low sperm count and motility as it allows injection of a single sperm per egg to achieve fertilization. The focus is now shifting towards using it in non-male factor infertility despite not being supported by evidence.

The main concerns regarding the ICSI technique are the invasive nature of procedure, lack of an effective method for selecting sperm for injection, and the risk of genetic defects in the offspring. The latter has now been attributed to underlying genetic abnormality in the male partner and the overall health of the babies born following ICSI has been found to be satisfactory.

Management of unexplained infertility

The majority of couples with unexplained infertility can expect to become pregnant without active fertility treatment. An observational Dutch study found that 81% (356/437) of couples with unexplained infertility had an ongoing pregnancy within 5 years of diagnosis, with 74% (263/356) pregnancies being conceived spontaneously (41).

Accurate prediction of the prognosis of natural conception in these couples is useful in counselling and avoiding unnecessary treatment (61). A popular prediction model (62) has identified female age of less than 35 years, duration of infertility less than 2 years, and secondary infertility as good prognostic factors which favour higher odds of spontaneous conception.

Expectant management

Expectant management is recommended as a first-line strategy in couples with a good prognosis for natural conception. Expectant management is cost-effective compared to active treatment (63). The period of expectant management needs to take into account the age of the female partner, duration of fertility, and the couple's preferences. The United Kingdom National Institute for Health and Clinical Excellence guidance suggests waiting for a period of 2 years before moving on to active treatment (10).

Clomiphene citrate

Oral clomiphene citrate therapy has been empirically used for the management of unexplained infertility. It is thought to correct subtle ovulatory dysfunction. Clomiphene has been popular because it is inexpensive compared to other fertility treatments, is non-invasive, and needs less clinical monitoring.

However, studies comparing clomiphene with expectant management have shown a comparable live birth rate (OR 0.79, 95% CI 0.45–1.38) (66) and less cost-effectiveness (63) suggesting no overall benefit with clomiphene use. A Cochrane review has also shown no improvement in pregnancy rates (64).

Intrauterine insemination

IUI is another commonly used management approach which theoretically allows sperm to avoid any hostile cervical factors and increases the number of motile sperm within the upper genital tract around the time of ovulation in a natural or stimulated cycle. IUI in an unstimulated (natural) cycle involves monitoring urinary or serum LH from day 10 to day 12 of the treatment cycle to detect an LH surge. Insemination is performed 20–30 hours after detection of an LH surge. In stimulated cycles, clomiphene or gonadotropins is used to promote ovulation from more than one (ideally two) mature follicles. Human chorionic gonadotropin is administered to trigger ovulation and IUI is scheduled 36–40 hours later.

Unstimulated IUI is not clinically effective (65) or cost-effective (63) when compared to expectant management and may result in lower live birth rates in comparison to stimulated IUI (66). Stimulated IUI has a risk of multiple pregnancy almost similar to IVF with a single embryo transfer or IVF cycles using a low dose of gonadotropins for ovarian stimulation (modified natural cycle IVF) (67).

In vitro fertilization

The rationale of IVF in unexplained infertility is that it is able to bypass known as well as unknown barriers to conception, but it is an invasive and more expensive procedure compared to IUI with a risk of multiple pregnancy and hyperstimulation. A primary strategy of offering IVF straight after a period of expectant management has demonstrated a shorter time to pregnancy and higher per-cycle pregnancy rates compared to treatment with oral agents or gonadotropins in patients with unexplained infertility (68). However, no conclusive difference in the live birth rates have been seen in women undergoing IVF as a primary treatment, when compared to stimulated IUI regardless of whether clomiphene or gonadotropin was used for stimulation (69).

Management of endometriosis

Minimal/mild endometriosis

Medical treatment options for mild and minimal endometriosis include progestogens, combined oral contraceptive pill, danazol, and GnRH agonists. These drugs suppress ovulation and none is effective in terms of improving pregnancy rates when compared to a placebo or expectant management (70). However, they are helpful in alleviating the symptoms of pain. Laparoscopic ablation/excision of minimal to mild endometriosis can increase live birth rates (71). IUI with controlled ovarian stimulation is an alternative option for these women with potential to increase the pregnancy rates compared to expectant management or IUI alone (72).

Ovarian endometriomas

Ovarian endometriomas can be managed surgically by aspiration or cystectomy. The latter has been shown to be associated with increased spontaneous pregnancy rates when compared with aspiration (73). Women with endometriomas should be counselled regarding the risks of reduced ovarian function after surgery and the possible loss of the ovary (72). Surgery should therefore be offered only for symptomatic large endometriomas (>4 cm) or when there is a suspicion of malignancy (74).

Moderate/severe endometriosis

Women with moderate or severe endometriosis are usually considered for laparoscopic excisional surgery to increase the chances of spontaneous conception and improvement in symptoms. Early referral for IVF is considered due to concern about compromised ovarian and tubal function. Hypothalamic–pituitary downregulation for 3–6 months with a GnRH agonist prior to IVF has been shown to increase the odds of clinical pregnancy (75). Pregnancy rates for women with endometriosis-related infertility after IVF are, however, lower than those with tubal factor infertility (OR 0.56; 95% CI 0.44–0.70) (76).

Assisted conception

IVF is the recommended treatment for couples with prolonged unresolved infertility unresponsive to other forms of treatment. The process includes controlled ovarian hyperstimulation, pituitary downregulation, and an ovulation trigger followed by surgical oocyte retrieval. Retrieved eggs are fertilized in the laboratory using sperm from the male partner and cultured in incubators to create embryos which are subsequently transferred to the uterine cavity. Complications associated with IVF include ovarian hyperstimulation syndrome and multiple pregnancies.

Despite technological improvements over time, the live birth rate per fresh IVF cycle is just under 30% (77). The outcome is enhanced by replacement of frozen embryos, where available, and by repeated attempts in women who are able to respond to stimulation. The chance of a live birth after three complete cycles of IVF reaches 42.3% (78). Cumulative live birth rates have been shown to increase to 65.3% (95% CI 64.8–65.8%) by the sixth cycle (77) and up to 83% by the eighth cycle (78). Older women with a longer duration of infertility and no previous pregnancies have a bleaker prognosis. Poor performance over one or more cycles is the main reason for medical advice against continuing further treatment. Psychological distress following unsuccessful attempts and financial pressures are other common reasons for discontinuing treatment.

Summary

Infertility represents a prognosis rather than a diagnosis and encompasses a wide spectrum of situations ranging from delay in conception to sterility. Underlying factors include lifestyle, age, or pathological conditions in either partner. Traditional investigations can help to identify the nature of infertility and inform the choice of treatment but assisted conception remains the intervention of choice in prolonged unresolved infertility. Individualized care, taking into account a couple's chances of natural conception and their physical, emotional, and financial needs, forms the basis of a successful management strategy.

REFERENCES

1. Gnoth C, Godehardt E, Frank-Herrmann P, Friol K, Tigges JG. Definition and prevalence of subfertility and infertility. *Hum Reprod* 2005;**20**:1144–47.

2. Te Velde ER, Eijkemans R, Habbema HD. Variation in couple fecundity and time to pregnancy, an essential concept in human reproduction. *Lancet* 2000;**355**:1928–29.

3. Habbema JDF, Collins J, Leridon H, Evers JLH, Lunenfeld B, teVelde ER. Towards less confusing terminology in reproductive medicine: a proposal. *Hum Reprod* 2004;**19**:1497–501.

4. Joffe M. Time trends in biological fertility in Britain. *Lancet* 2000;**355**:1961–65.

5. Zegers-Hochschild F, Adamson GD, de Mouzon J, et al. International Committee for Monitoring Assisted Reproductive Technology (ICMART) and the World Health Organization (WHO) revised glossary of ART terminology, 2009. *Fertil Steril* 2009;**92**:1520–24.

6. World Health Organization. *The Epidemiology of Infertility. Report of WHO Scientific Group on the Epidemiology of Infertility*. Technical Report Series No. 582. Geneva: World Health Organization; 1975.

7. Mascarenhas MN, Flaxman SR, Boerma T, Vanderpoel S, Stevens GA. National, regional, and global trends in infertility: a systematic analysis of 277 health surveys. *PLoS Med* 2012;**9**:e1001356.

8. Gurunath S, Pandian Z, Anderson Richard A, Bhattacharya S. Defining infertility—a systematic review of prevalence studies. *Hum Reprod Update* 2011;**17**:575–88.

9. Boivin J, Bunting L, Collins JA, Nygren KG. International estimates of infertility prevalence and treatment-seeking: potential need and demand for infertility medical care. *Hum Reprod* 2007;**22**:1506–12.

10. National Institute for Health and Clinical Excellence (NICE). *Fertility: Assessment and Treatment for People with Fertility Problems*. Clinical guideline [CG156], last updated September 2017. London: NICE; 2013.

11. Bhattacharya S, Porter M, Amalraj E, et al. The epidemiology of infertility in the North East of Scotland. *Hum Reprod* 2009;**24**:3096–107.

12. te Velde ER, Scheffer GJ, Dorland M, Broekmans FJ, Fauser BC. Developmental and endocrine aspects of normal ovarian aging. *Cell Endocrinol* 1998;**145**:67–73.

13. Sartorius GA, Nieschlag E. Paternal age and reproduction. *Hum Reprod Update* 2010;**16**:65–79.

14. Rittenberg V, Seshadri S, Sunkara SK, et al. Effect of body mass index on IVF treatment outcome: an updated systematic review and meta-analysis. *Reprod Biomed Online* 2011;**23**:421–39.

15. Sermondade N, Faure C, Fezeu L, et al. BMI in relation to sperm count: an updated systematic review and collaborative meta-analysis. *Hum Reprod Update* 2013;**19**:221–31.

16. Augood C, Duckitt K, Templeton AA. Smoking and female infertility: a systematic review and meta-analysis. *Hum Reprod* 1998;**13**:1532–39.

17. Hull MG, North K, Taylor H, Farrow A, Ford WC. Delayed conception and active and passive smoking. The Avon Longitudinal Study of Pregnancy and Childhood Study Team. *Fertil Steril* 2000;**74**:725–33.

18. Waylen AL, Metwally M, Jones GL, Wilkinson AJ, Ledger WL. Effects of cigarette smoking upon clinical outcomes of assisted reproduction: a meta-analysis. *Hum Reprod Update* 2009;**15**:31–44.

19. Hyland A, Piazza K, Hovey KM, et al. Associations between lifetime tobacco exposure with infertility and age at natural menopause: the Women's Health Initiative Observational Study. *Tob Control* 2016;**25**:706–14.

20. Künzle R, Mueller MD, Hänggi W, Birkhäuser MH, Drescher H, Bersinger NA. Semen quality of male smokers and nonsmokers in infertile couples. *Fertil Steril* 2003;**79**:287–91.

21. Tolstrup JS, Kjaer SK, Holst C, et al. Alcohol use as predictor for infertility in a representative population of Danish women. *Acta Obstet Gynecol Scand* 2003;**82**:744–49.

22. Eggert J, Theobald H, Engfeldt P. Effects of alcohol consumption on female fertility during an 18-year period. *Fertil Steril* 2004;**81**:379–83.

23. Brandes M, van der Steen JO, Bokdam SB, et al. When and why do subfertile couples discontinue their fertility care? A longitudinal cohort study in a secondary care subfertility population. *Hum Reprod* 2009;**24**:3127–35.

24. Lynch CD, Sundaram R, Maisog JM, Sweeney AM, Buck Louis GM. Preconception stress increases the risk of infertility: results from a couple-based prospective cohort study—the LIFE study. *Hum Reprod* 2014;**29**:1067–75.

25. Peck JD, Leviton A, Cowan LD. A review of the epidemiologic evidence concerning the reproductive health effects of caffeine consumption: a 2000–2009 update. *Food Chem Toxicol* 2010;**48**:2549–76.

26. Bosteels J, Kasius J, Weyers S, Broekmans FJ, Mol BW, D'Hooghe TM. Hysteroscopy for treating subfertility associated with suspected major uterine cavity abnormalities. *Cochrane Database Syst Rev* 2015;**2**:CD009461.

27. Jayaprakasan K, Chan YY, Sur S, Deb S, Clewes JS, Raine-Fenning NJ. Prevalence of uterine anomalies and their impact on early pregnancy in women conceiving after assisted reproduction treatment. *Ultrasound Obstet Gynecol* 2011;**37**:727–32.

28. Guermandi E, Vegetti W, Bianchi MM, Uglietti A, Ragni G, Crosignani P. Reliability of ovulation tests in infertile women. *Obstet Gynecol* 2001;**97**:92–96.

29. Maheux-Lacroix S, Boutin A, Moore L, et al. Hysterosalpingo-sonography for diagnosing tubal occlusion in subfertile women: a systematic review with meta-analysis. *Hum Reprod* 2014;**29**:953–63.

30. Cooper TG, Noonan E, von Eckardstein S, et al. World Health Organization reference values for human semen characteristics. *Reprod Update* 2010;**16**:231–45.

31. Guzick DS, Overstreet JW, Factor-Litvak P, et al. Sperm morphology, motility, and concentration in fertile and infertile men. *N Engl J Med* 2001;**345**:1388–93.

32. Silber SJ. The relationship of abnormal semen parameters to male fertility. *Hum Reprod* 1989;**4**:947–53.

33. Pereira R, Sá R, Barros A, Sousa M. Major regulatory mechanisms involved in sperm motility. *Asian J Androl* 2017;**19**:5–14.

34. Auger J, Jouannet P, Eustache F. Another look at human sperm morphology. *Human Reprod* 2016;**31**:10–23.

35. Broekmans FJ, Kwee, J, Hendriks DJ, Mol BW, Lambalk CB. A systematic review of tests predicting ovarian reserve and IVF outcome. *Hum Reprod Update* 2006;**12**:685–718.

36. Gibreel A, Maheshwari A, Bhattacharya S, Johnson NP. Ultrasound tests of ovarian reserve; a systematic review of accuracy in predicting fertility outcomes. *Hum Fertil (Camb)* 2009;**12**:95–106.

37. Broer SL, Dólleman M, Opmeer BC, Fauser BC, Mol BW, Broekmans FJ. AMH and AFC as predictors of excessive response in controlled ovarian hyperstimulation: a meta-analysis. *Hum Reprod Update* 2011;**17**:46–54.

38. Depmann M, Broer SL, van der Schouw YT, et al. Can we predict age at natural menopause using ovarian reserve tests or mother's

age at menopause? A systematic literature review. *Menopause* 2016;**23**:224–32.

39. Bingol B, Gunenc Z, Gedikbasi A, Guner H, Tasdemir S, Tiras B. Comparison of diagnostic accuracy of saline infusion sonohysterography, transvaginal sonography and hysteroscopy. *Obstet Gynaecol* 2011;**31**:54–58.

40. Bosteels J, Weyers S, Puttemans P, et al. The effectiveness of hysteroscopy in improving pregnancy rates in subfertile women without other gynaecological symptoms: a systematic review. *Hum Reprod Update* 2010;**16**:1–11.

41. Brandes M, Hamilton CJ, van der Steen JO, et al. Unexplained infertility: overall ongoing pregnancy rate and mode of conception. *Hum Reprod* 2011;**26**:360–68.

42. Verkauf BS. Incidence, symptoms, and signs of endometriosis in fertile and infertile women. *J Fla Med Assoc* 1987;**74**:671–75.

43. Endometriosis and infertility: a committee opinion. The Practice Committee of the American Society for Reproductive Medicine. *Fertil Steril* 2006;**86** Suppl 6: S156–60.

44. Moran LJ, Hutchison SK, Norman RJ, Teede HJ. Lifestyle changes in women with polycystic ovary syndrome. *Cochrane Database Syst Rev* 2011;**7**:CD007506.

45. Bjørnholt SM, Kjaer SK, Nielsen TS, Jensen A. Risk for borderline ovarian tumours after exposure to fertility drugs: results of a population-based cohort study. *Hum Reprod* 2015;**30**:222–31.

46. Thessaloniki ESHRE/ASRM-Sponsored PCOS Consensus Workshop Group. Consensus on infertility treatment related to polycystic ovary syndrome. *Hum Reprod* 2008;**23**:462–77.

47. Beck JI, Boothroyd C, Proctor M, Farquhar C, Hughes E. Oral anti-oestrogens and medical adjuncts for subfertility associated with anovulation. *Cochrane Database Syst Rev* 2005;**1**:CD002249.

48. Tang T, Lord JM, Norman RJ, Yasmin E, Balen AH. Insulin-sensitising drugs (metformin, rosiglitazone, pioglitazone, D-chiro-inositol) for women with polycystic ovary syndrome, oligo amenorrhoea and subfertility. *Cochrane Database Syst Rev* 2012;**5**:CD003053.

49. Franik S, Kremer JA, Nelen WL, Farquhar C. Aromatase inhibitors for subfertile women with polycystic ovary syndrome. *Cochrane Database Syst Rev* 2014;**2**:CD010287.

50. Farquhar C, Brown J, Marjoribanks J. Laparoscopic drilling by diathermy or laser for ovulation induction in anovulatory polycystic ovary syndrome. *Cochrane Database Syst Rev* 2012;**6**:CD001122.

51. Toulis KA, Goulis DG, Venetis CA, et al. Risk of spontaneous miscarriage in euthyroid women with thyroid autoimmunity undergoing IVF: a meta-analysis. *Eur J Endocrinol* 2010;**162**:643–52.

52. Spencer L, Bubner T, Bain E, Middleton P. Screening and subsequent management for thyroid dysfunction pre-pregnancy and during pregnancy for improving maternal and infant health. *Cochrane Database Syst Rev* 2015;**9**:CD011263.

53. Gomel V. The place of reconstructive tubal surgery in the era of assisted reproductive techniques. *Reprod Biomed Online* 2015;**31**:722–31.

54. Li X, Dong L, Yong S, Wei H. Reproductive outcomes after operative laparoscopy of patients with tubal infertility with or without hydrosalpinx. *Chin Med J* 2014;**127**:593–94.

55. Johnson N, van Voorst S, Sowter MC, Strandell A, Mol BW. Surgical treatment for tubal disease in women due to undergo in vitro fertilisation. *Cochrane Database Syst Rev* 2010;**1**:CD002125.

56. Showell MG, Mackenzie-Proctor R, Brown J, Yazdani A, Stankiewicz MT, Hart RJ. Antioxidants for male subfertility. *Cochrane Database Syst Rev* 2014;**12**:CD007411.

57. Rastrelli G, Corona G, Mannucci E, Maggi M. Factors affecting spermatogenesis upon gonadotropin-replacement therapy: a meta-analytic study. *Andrology* 2014;**2**:794–808.

58. Yafi FA, Zini A. Percutaneous epididymal sperm aspiration for men with obstructive azoospermia: predictors of successful sperm retrieval. *Urology* 2013;**82**:341–44.

59. Van Peperstraten A, Proctor ML, Johnson NP, Philipson G. Techniques for surgical retrieval of sperm prior to ICSI for azoospermia. *Cochrane Database Syst Rev* 2006;**3**:CD002807.

60. Cissen M, Bensdorp A, Cohlen BJ, Repping S, de Bruin JP, van Wely M. Assisted reproductive technologies for male subfertility. *Cochrane Database Syst Rev* 2016;**2**:CD000360.

61. Kersten FA, Hermens RP, Braat DD, et al. Overtreatment in couples with unexplained infertility. *Hum Reprod* 2015;**30**:71–80.

62. Hunault CC, Habbema JD, Eijkemans MJ, et al. Two new prediction rules for spontaneous pregnancy leading to live birth among subfertile couples, based on the synthesis of three previous models. *Hum Reprod* 2004;**19**:2019–26.

63. Wordsworth S, Buchanan J, Mollison J, et al. Clomiphene citrate and intrauterine insemination as first-line treatments for unexplained infertility: are they cost-effective? *Hum Reprod* 2011;**26**:369–75.

64. Hughes E, Brown J, Collins JJ, et al. Clomiphene citrate for unexplained subfertility in women. *Cochrane Database Syst Rev* 2010;**1**:CD000057.

65. Bhattacharya S, Harrild K, Mollison J, et al. Clomifene citrate or unstimulated intrauterine insemination compared with expectant management for unexplained infertility: pragmatic randomised controlled trial. *BMJ* 2008;**337**:a716.

66. Veltman-Verhulst SM, Cohlen BJ, Hughes E, et al. Intrauterine insemination for unexplained subfertility. *Cochrane Database Syst Rev* 2013;**10**:CD001502.

67. Bensdorp AJ, Tjon-Kon-Fat RI, Bossuyt PM, et al. Prevention of multiple pregnancies in couples with unexplained or mild male subfertility: randomised controlled trial of in vitro fertilisation with single embryo transfer or in vitro fertilisation in modified natural cycle compared with intrauterine insemination with controlled ovarian hyperstimulation. *BMJ* 2015;**350**:g7771.

68. Reindollar RH, Regan MM, Neumann PJ, et al. A randomized clinical trial to evaluate optimal treatment for unexplained infertility: the fast track and standard treatment (FASTT) trial. *Fertil Steril* 2010;**94**:888–99.

69. Pandian Z, Gibreel A, Bhattacharya S. In vitro fertilisation for unexplained subfertility. *Cochrane Database Syst Rev* 2015;**11**:CD003357.

70. Hughes E, Brown J, Collins JJ, Farquhar C, Fedorkow DM, Vandekerckhove P. Ovulation suppression for endometriosis. *Cochrane Database Syst Rev* 2007;**3**:CD000155.

71. Jacobson TZ, Duffy JM, Barlow D, Farquhar C, Koninckx PR, Olive D. Laparoscopic surgery for subfertility associated with endometriosis. *Cochrane Database Syst Rev* 2010;**1**:CD001398.

72. Dunselman GA, Vermeulen N, Becker C, et al. ESHRE guideline: management of women with endometriosis. *Hum Reprod* 2014;**29**:400–12.

73. Hart RJ, Hickey M, Maouris P, Buckett W. Excisional surgery versus ablative surgery for ovarian endometriomata. *Cochrane Database Syst Rev* 2008;**2**:CD004992.

74. Garcia-Velasco JA, Somigliana E. Management of endometriomas in women requiring IVF: to touch or not to touch. *Hum Reprod* 2009;**24**:496–501.

75. Sallam HN, Garcia-Velasco JA, Dias S, Arici A. Long-term pituitary down-regulation before in vitro fertilization (IVF) for women with endometriosis. *Cochrane Database Syst Rev* 2006:CD004635.

76. Barnhart K, Dunsmoor-Su R, Coutifaris C. Effect of endometriosis on in vitro fertilization. *Fertil Steril* 2002;**77**:1148–55.

77. Smith AD, Tilling K, Nelson SM, Lawlor DA. Live-birth rate associated with repeat in vitro fertilization treatment cycles. *JAMA* 2015;**314**:2654–62.

78. McLernon DJ, Maheshwari A, Lee AJ, Bhattacharya S. Cumulative live birth rates after one or more complete cycles of IVF: a population-based study of linked cycle data from 178 898 women. *Hum Reprod* 2016;**31**:572–81.

52

Assisted reproduction

William Ledger

Historical perspective

Louise Brown, the first person to be born after conception *in vitro* was delivered by elective caesarean section at Oldham General Hospital in Lancashire, United Kingdom, on 25 July 1978. Her mother was infertile because of tubal blockage, and *in vitro* fertilization (IVF) was developed as a means of bypassing the blocked tube by taking the oocyte from the ovary and replacing the embryo in the uterine cavity. Her pregnancy resulted from collaboration between a pioneering laparoscopic surgeon, Mr Patrick Steptoe, and a Cambridge embryologist and scientist, Professor Robert Edwards. Edwards was awarded the Nobel Prize for Medicine in 2010 for this work (1).

Louise was conceived after over 200 failed attempts at IVF by this group, and after a pregnancy that ended as ectopic conceived after IVF in Melbourne. The principles used in IVF have not changed over the years since her birth although the processes have been refined and improved in numerous ways. The first IVF births followed a laparoscopy performed after the natural luteinizing hormone (LH) surge had been identified using frequent blood sampling. A needle passed transabdominally was guided under laparoscopic control to penetrate the single preovular follicle. Follicular fluid was aspirated and examined microscopically to try to isolate the oocyte. This was placed into culture medium and then incubated with a sample of the partner's sperm. If the egg fertilized, then the resulting embryo would be transferred into the uterine cavity using a transcervical catheter passed under direct vision.

The procedures involved were complex and highly inefficient. Things frequently went wrong at every stage, and the evolution of IVF has revolved around refining and improving the various steps of the IVF pathway. The major developments in assisted reproductive technology (ART) that have improved pregnancy rates, patient acceptability, and safety are outlined in **Table 52.1**.

Since the early days of IVF in the 1980s, the group of IVF-related treatments known as ARTs have resulted in the birth of over 7 million children. Several countries now see more than 3% of all births following ART and ART is globally accessible with major growth of centres in China, India, and South East Asia along with Europe and the United States. ART has become increasingly complex, with many centres now performing intracytoplasmic sperm injection (ICSI) in more than 50% of cycles and increasing numbers of cycles with embryo biopsy for preimplantation genetic diagnosis (PGD)

or preimplantation genetic (aneuploidy) screening (PGS) (2). Many clinicians also use a variety of adjuvant treatments to try and improve oocyte number or quality although the effectiveness of most of these treatments remains unproven.

Who should have *in vitro* fertilization treatment?

Patient selection for ART remains a vexed question that is hotly debated. IVF is costly, carries a small but real risk of harm, and there are anxieties about the long-term health of children born after ART, although these remain largely theoretical. The most significant determinant of success in IVF is the age of the woman so while it may be prudent to promote a conservative policy of access to ART in cases where there is no clear diagnosis for the infertility problem and where the couple are young, a more rapid referral is probably a better option when the woman is approaching or beyond her 35th birthday. There are many powerful social pressures on couples to conceive a child at a certain time in their lives: pressure from younger siblings and friends who are having their children, pressure from parents who wish to be grandparents, and the pressure of the 'biological clock' that is discussed on a daily basis in the popular press. Hence, a consultation concerning ART should always be a negotiation with the couple, respecting their desire to use ART to start their family as quickly as possible while using population-based statistics to help to reach a mutually agreed and medically sensible plan.

Alternative approaches to IVF should always be considered. Many couples have religious or moral objections to the IVF process, particularly if embryo freezing is to be used, and may only consent to an attenuated form of treatment with, for example, fertilization of only one or two oocytes to avoid the possibility of there being supernumerary frozen embryos later. Alternatives that may be applicable to defined diagnostic categories include ovulation induction with oral or injectable agents, ovarian diathermy, intrauterine insemination, or tubal or other reproductive surgery. However, as IVF has become more widely used it has become the dominant form of treatment for most categories of infertility and is a widely used approach to 'unexplained' infertility as it can reveal problems of poor ovarian reserve, failure of sperm to fertilize the oocyte, or poor embryo development that cannot easily be tested outside of an IVF cycle.

Table 52.1 Some significant developments in ART

1980	2017
Natural cycle to obtain one oocyte	Stimulated cycle to obtain multiple oocytes
Multiple blood tests to monitor natural ovulation	Transvaginal ultrasound with minimal blood tests
Lack of control over timing of ovulation	Pituitary downregulation or GnRH antagonist to suppress premature ovulation
Laparoscopic oocyte collection with general anaesthesia	Transvaginal ultrasound-guided egg collection with sedation
Simple culture medium, rudimentary incubators	Stage-specific culture media, sophisticated control of temperature, humidity, gases
Incubation with sperm	Intracytoplasmic sperm injection for male infertility
Embryo transfer 2 days after egg collection	Extended culture to day 5 blastocyst
Operator-blind embryo transfer	Ultrasound-guided embryo transfer
Natural cycle transfer	Luteal support with progestogens or hCG
One attempt, one oocyte	Multiple oocytes allowing for embryo freezing and later replacement of frozen embryo
Multiple embryo transfer, high rates of multiple pregnancy	Single embryo transfer with option for later frozen embryo transfer
Fresh embryo transfer with abnormally stimulated endometrium	'Freeze all' embryo policy with natural cycle transfer for regularly ovulating women
Embryo selection by simple morphological criteria	Video time-lapse and embryo biopsy/ PGS for embryo selection
Significant risk of ovarian hyperstimulation syndrome (OHSS)	GnRH antagonist-controlled superovulation with agonist trigger and 'freeze all' embryos removing risk of severe OHSS

Social changes have led to considerable adjustment in the case mix seen by clinics in the Western world. There has been a widespread trend towards deferring attempts to start a family such that the mean age of the woman at first birth is now over 30 years in many developed countries. This has in turn led to an increase in 'unexplained' infertility caused by poor oocyte quality with an increase in the proportion of aneuploid embryos and also decreases in quality and number of mitochondria in the oocyte. Advancing female age is also associated with an increase in rates of miscarriage and chromosomal abnormality in offspring (3) (**Figure 52.1**). Male infertility has also appeared to increase over the last three decades, possibly mainly due to environmental factors and lifestyle factors such as obesity, smoking, and use of recreational drugs including alcohol (4). The global increase in obesity has also contributed to an increase in the number of women who are found to be anovular with polycystic ovary syndrome (5).

A standard *in vitro* fertilization treatment cycle

Patient selection and workup

Perhaps the most important part of an IVF treatment is the work that takes place before the first injection is given. Patients must have a full understanding of what is planned, including the processes involved, their risks and benefits, the likelihood of pregnancy, and the costs involved. There should be easy access to independent counselling from a trained fertility counsellor and adequate time for reflection and discussion with an accredited clinical specialist before the decision to proceed is taken. The clinician will use markers of ovarian reserve (anti-Mullerian hormone (AMH) and antral follicle count (AFC)) (6, 7) along with patient age and previous history to decide on the dose of follicle-stimulating hormone (FSH) to be used. Various algorithms have been developed to try to optimize FSH dose selection but, to date, they have not gained widespread acceptance.

Ovarian stimulation

Two main types of stimulation protocol are widely used in ART clinics. The older *long protocol* (**Figure 52.2**) was first developed in the late 1980s and involves pretreatment with a gonadotropin-releasing hormone (GnRH) agonist (e.g. buserelin, nafarelin, or leuprolide) (8) given by injection or nasal spray from the mid-luteal phase of

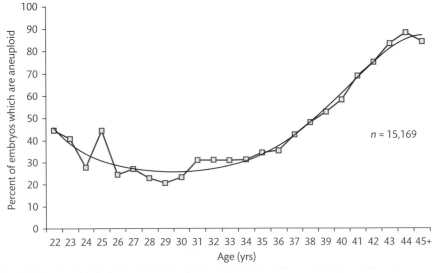

Figure 52.1 Female age and embryonic aneuploidy.

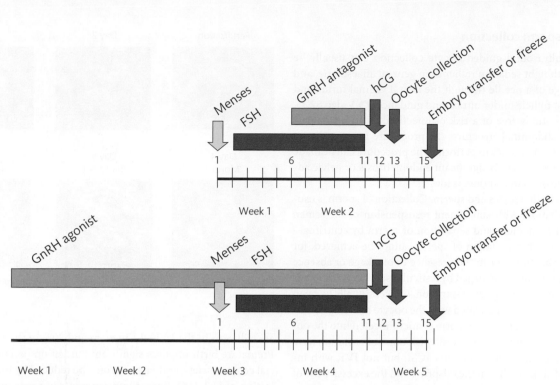

Figure 52.2 Schematic of processes involved in 'long protocol' GnRH antagonist-controlled and GnRH agonist-controlled ovarian stimulation.

the previous menstrual cycle. Initiation of GnRH agonist treatment at this time induces a short-lived increase (flare) in circulating FSH and LH followed by pituitary downregulation with profound suppression of gonadotropin secretion. A normal menstrual bleed follows after a few days, at which point a blood sample is taken to check pituitary downregulation and an ultrasound scan is performed to exclude ovarian cysts and check that the endometrium is thin. This is followed by daily injection of exogenous gonadotropin, either a recombinant FSH (Gonal-F, Puregon) or a urinary derived FSH with LH activity (Menopur, Merional). Both types of gonadotropin preparation seem equally effective at stimulating ovarian follicle growth although the manufacturing companies all claim superiority using different methods of assessment and different studies.

The purpose of ovarian stimulation is to produce multiple ovarian follicles, allowing collection of multiple oocytes. Different women respond very differently to gonadotropin treatment. Some, mainly older women or those with low AMH and AFC levels, require large doses for adequate stimulation whereas others, younger or with signs of polycystic ovary syndrome, are hypersensitive and at risk of ovarian hyperstimulation syndrome even with modest doses. Hence caution must be exercised when prescribing gonadotropins and the ovarian response must be closely monitored during stimulation. Monitoring is carried out both with transvaginal ultrasound and with measurement of oestradiol in serum. Stimulation should result in growth of a cohort of six to ten large follicles with a concomitant increase in serum oestradiol and endometrial thickness on ultrasound scanning. The average duration of stimulation is between 10 and 12 days although this is also variable.

Once a lead follicle diameter of 18–20 mm is reached, a single injection of human chorionic gonadotropin (hCG) 5000–10,000 IU is given: the 'hCG trigger'. This induces final oocyte maturation

with expulsion of the first polar body. Ovulation will occur 38–42 hours later, so a transvaginal ultrasound-guided oocyte collection is scheduled about 36 hours after hCG, allowing collection of mature oocytes (⊙ Video 52.1).

hCG has a half-life of several days (9) and, in the presence of an excessive ovarian response to gonadotropin treatment, can initiate a process of ovarian hyperstimulation. This involves capillary endothelial dysfunction, probably mediated by vascular endothelial growth factor (10), leading to leakage of fluids and small molecules out of the vascular compartment, with ascites, pleural and pericardial effusions, and haemoconcentration. Arterial and venous thrombosis can occur and several deaths from severe ovarian hyperstimulation syndrome (OHSS) have been reported. This has led to a reappraisal of the use of the long protocol for stimulation with high-dose FSH and hCG trigger. Introduction of a new class of GnRH antagonists in the late 1990s allowed the long protocol to be replaced with the *antagonist protocol*. This does not require pretreatment for pituitary downregulation but rather initiates GnRH antagonist treatment on the fifth day of FSH injection (11). Hence, the antagonist protocol is perceived by patients as quicker, with completion of drug treatment within 10–12 days on average. The antagonist protocol is frequently combined with mild stimulation using lower doses of FSH. If there is still excessive follicle growth with high concentrations of oestradiol and risk of OHSS then final oocyte maturation can be induced with a dose of GnRH agonist, an agonist trigger. This releases endogenous LH, mimicking the natural LH surge (12). This approach cannot be used in the long protocol as the pituitary is desensitized to GnRH so no LH would be released. Agonist trigger has almost completely removed risk of OHSS, leading to the concept of the 'OHSS-free clinic' (13), placing safety as of equal importance to efficacy in IVF practice.

Oocyte and sperm collection

Transvaginal ultrasound-guided oocyte collection can usually be carried out with light sedation rather than general anaesthesia, and involves passage of a needle through the lateral vaginal fornix and into the nearest follicle under ultrasound guidance (⊙ Video 52.1). Although not entirely free of a risk of infection, bleeding, or perforation of an abdominal structure, the procedure is low risk and usually takes 15–20 minutes to perform. The procedure can be made more complicated if there is significant endometriosis or pelvic adhesions or if the ovarian response is low.

IVF requires both oocytes and sperm. Collection of sperm is usually by masturbation, with subsequent resuspension of the semen sample in culture medium and separation of sperm by centrifugation. Cases in which ejaculation of sperm cannot be achieved, for example, after vasectomy or in the presence of blockage or absence of the vas deferens, can be managed by testicular sperm extraction or percutaneous epididymal sperm aspiration, or occasionally by open surgery. Sperm are either incubated with the oocyte in a drop of culture medium, for IVF, or a single sperm is microinjected into the oocyte by ICSI if sperm number or motility is poor. Some studies have associated pregnancies conceived after ICSI, but not IVF, with increased risks of abnormality in the offspring and the excessive use of ICSI, particularly for non-male factor infertility, is discouraged (14).

Embryo growth and development

Traditionally, the early division of the embryo has been monitored by removal of the dish containing the embryos from the incubator once per day with analysis of embryo morphology by light microscopy. This disturbs the equilibrium of the embryo, with cooling and loss of oxygenation and buffering. The recent introduction of video time-lapse embryo assessment allows real-time monitoring of embryo growth using a video clip derived from still photographs taken every few minutes by a camera within the incubator (15) (⊙ Video 52.2). This gives a more detailed picture of the development of the embryo, which can be assessed in comparison with optimal developmental stages as a measure of the quality of the embryo. Such an assessment should provide a more rational basis for selection of the best embryo to transfer, although randomized trials demonstrating improvement in live birth rate are still awaited.

In the early days of IVF, the laboratory environment was severely suboptimal for embryo growth and embryos were transferred to the uterine cavity after 2 days, just sufficient time to confirm viability. Early embryo transfer does not allow any assessment of quality, leading to low pregnancy rates per cycle. More recent improvements in culture media and incubators have allowed high rates of embryo development to blastocyst stage, involving 5 days of culture *in vitro* (**Figure 52.3**). Prolonged culture permits a detailed comparison of embryos within one cohort, with selection of the best quality for transfer and for cryopreservation. This policy has dramatically improved success rates and has allowed clinics to reduce the number of embryos transferred per attempt, such that most women under 40 will have a single embryo transfer (SET) in many of the most advanced centres (16). Avoidance of multiple pregnancy, with a fivefold reduction in risk of premature birth and handicap, has become one of the most important targets for ART in the twenty-first century. While multiple pregnancy rates of less than 5% per cycle are reported from Scandinavia and Australia, rates in excess of 10%

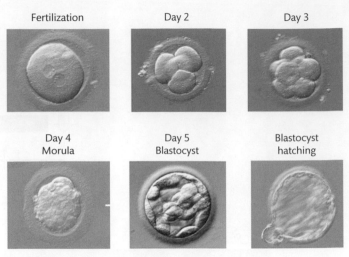

Figure 52.3 Human embryo development from fertilization to blastocyst.

are still seen in the United Kingdom and 30% in the United States. Premature birth imposes significant burden on parents and financial cost to society, and rates can only be reduced by increasing utilization of SET (18). Recent improvements in pregnancy rates after transfer of a single frozen-thawed embryo (19) have given further encouragement to patients to accept a fresh SET, since the cumulative chances of pregnancy with fresh plus frozen embryo transfer are equivalent or better than those seen with fresh transfer of two embryos.

Embryo transfer

A standard embryo transfer involves visualization of the ectocervix using a vaginal speculum followed by insertion of a fine plastic cannula through the cervix to the uterocervical junction. The embryo selected for transfer is then drawn into a narrower flexible transfer catheter. This runs along the outer cannula to pass into the endometrial cavity, at which point the embryo is expelled in a drop of culture medium. The procedure takes a few minutes and is frequently carried out using transabdominal ultrasound to ensure correct catheter placement and to visualize expulsion of the drop of medium containing the embryo (⊙ Video 52.3). Problems can occur when there is cervical stenosis, for example, after previous surgery, and a precycle hysteroscopy and cervical dilation may need to be considered for the next cycle after a difficult transfer.

Transfer of frozen embryos can be performed using a natural or medicated transfer cycle. Most clinics will use the woman's natural cycle if she is regularly ovulating and has good endometrial development on ultrasound scanning. The patient will have monitoring with blood or urine testing for the LH surge and postsurge rise in progesterone, demonstrating that natural ovulation has occurred. Ultrasound is used to confirm development of the corpus luteum and that endometrial thickness is adequate (>6 mm). The day for embryo transfer is then calculated depending on whether the embryo was frozen on day 2, 3, or 5. Transfer technique is as for fresh transfer, but luteal support is not necessary. Women who are anovular or who have poor endometrial development can either use ovulation induction with clomiphene citrate or FSH injection to induce natural ovulation with endometrial development, or can use an artificial cycle with treatment first with oestradiol valerate or oestrogen patch, followed by progestogens.

Luteal phase

Luteal phase support, in the form of either hCG injections or progestogens, is widely used in both long and antagonist protocols. The natural development of the corpus luteum does not occur efficiently after ovarian stimulation and implantation rates after embryo transfer are low if some type of support is not used. Pregnancy rates appear similar whether hCG or progestogens are employed, but hCG injection can worsen symptoms of OHSS so has largely been superseded in modern practice (19). Progestogens are given as a vaginal pessary (Uterogestan), gel (Crinone), or tablet (Endometrin), or by deep intramuscular injection. While many clinics discontinue luteal progestogen when the pregnancy test is positive, others will continue with this support for many weeks. The impact on the likelihood of viable pregnancy of this latter approach is questionable.

Pregnancy testing is by measurement of hCG in serum 10–14 days after embryo transfer. A negative test is followed by cessation of luteal support and by menstruation. It is usual to wait for one further menstrual cycle before beginning stimulation again although some women prefer to carry straight on to another cycle if there has not been ovarian hyperstimulation. A positive test is usually repeated a few days later to monitor the rise in hCG and progesterone, followed by an early pregnancy transvaginal scan at 2–3 weeks after the positive pregnancy test. This first ultrasound scan should demonstrate fetal viability with the presence of a heartbeat, and confirm that the pregnancy is intrauterine (not ectopic) and singleton. Suspicion of miscarriage should trigger further assessment by ultrasonography a few days later rather than early intervention which may inadvertently terminate an early healthy gestation.

Pregnancy management

ART pregnancies are not inherently 'high risk'. Some women will require intensive monitoring in pregnancy following IVF, for example, older women, those with pre-existing medical conditions, and those with multiple pregnancies. However, a healthy singleton pregnancy for a woman under 36 years and previously well can be managed in a shared care system with expectation of a vaginal delivery. Nevertheless, caesarean section rates remain high for IVF pregnancies and many obstetricians treat all such patients with caution.

How to express assisted reproductive technology success rates?

Management of infertility is unusual in medical practice in that it has a binary outcome—the patient is either pregnant or she is not. This should mean that the expression of IVF statistics is simple. However, competition between clinics is frequently intense. Many countries do not provide adequate reimbursement for IVF treatment, with preference for a commercial model of care. Clinics are then judged by potential patients and referring doctors on the basis of their rates of success, leading to distortion of the metrics used for comparison.

Potential IVF patients want to know their chance of having a healthy child from their cycle of treatment. Hence, the best measure of 'success' from a patient perspective is the live birth rate per cycle started. This is defined as the start of FSH injection and takes into account all of the things that can go wrong in an IVF cycle, including failure of the ovaries to respond to stimulation, or overstimulation leading to cycle cancellation, failure of fertilization, failure of implantation, miscarriage, or ectopic pregnancy. This statistic has been championed by the United Kingdom Human Fertilisation and Embryology Authority (http://www.hfea.gov.uk) and forms the basis of their comparative statistics. However, even this can be challenged. As mentioned previously, best practice in IVF may now be use of an antagonist protocol with agonist trigger and freezing of all embryos in order to minimize risk of OHSS. If this approach is followed then the live birth rate per cycle started must include births following transfer of both fresh and frozen embryos derived from the initial stimulation. This 'cumulative conception rate' becomes the most relevant global static but will only be known many months after the start of stimulation, given the delays inherent in utilization of frozen embryos (20). Hence live birth rate per fresh transfer is more often quoted.

Clinics must audit their practice and a number of other markers of success are relevant in this context. The implantation rate—rate of positive pregnancy test per embryo transferred—is the best marker of quality of the embryology laboratory, and clinical pregnancy rate—defined as the rate of observed fetal heart activity on early scan per embryo transferred—is also relevant. However, these measures do not take into account any problems with under- or over-response to stimulation and any statistic quoted with 'per embryo transfer' as the denominator should be viewed with suspicion when clinic success rates are quoted.

New uses for assisted reproductive technology

The process of IVF has allowed clinical scientists to have direct access to the human embryo for the first time. Micromanipulation is now widely used to engineer embryo biopsy to remove one or two cells at day 3 of development or to take a trophectoderm biopsy at the day 5 blastocyst stage. This technology has been applied to develop PGD and PGS. PGD targets a specific mutation that is known to be present within the family undertaking the IVF. Examples include cystic fibrosis, Tay–Sachs disease, thalassaemia, neurofibromatosis, and hundreds of other specific mutations that have a significant effect on the health and life expectancy of the child. PGD can also be applied at chromosomal level for sex selection, for example, to select for female fetuses in the presence of X-linked conditions such as Duchenne muscular dystrophy. Couples undertaking PGD are not necessarily infertile, but rather use the IVF technique to access embryonic DNA to allow exclusion of an affected embryo. Many couples find this approach more ethically acceptable than screening in pregnancy with termination of an affected fetus (21).

Embryonic sex selection is also widely practised for 'family balancing' in some countries, including the United States, although ethical objections are significant and many other countries, including the United Kingdom and Australia, do not permit non-medical sex selection.

PGS involves use of the embryonic tissue to screen for aneuploidy (22). The frequency of aneuploidy increases with advancing female age. An increasing number of women are starting their IVF journey in their late 30s or older, and in theory they should benefit from transfer of an embryo that is known to be euploid. PGS should improve implantation rates, reduce early miscarriage rates, and may circumvent a need for amniocentesis later in pregnancy. However, early work using fluorescent *in situ* hybridization, with screening for abnormalities in only a limited number of chromosomes, was shown in randomized controlled trials to result in lower pregnancy rates than seen in controls (24). Application of methods that assess every chromosome using array comparative genomic hybridization and now 'next-generation' sequencing are giving more promising results but adequately powered, well-designed randomized controlled trials are still needed before this technology is introduced into routine practice.

ART also allows collection of eggs and embryos for elective cryopreservation. The efficiency of cryopreservation has improved dramatically since older slow-freezing methods were replaced by 'snap freezing' or vitrification. The process requires ovarian stimulation and egg collection as in routine IVF, followed either by cryopreservation of oocytes or fertilization and later cryopreservation of embryos. This approach was first developed for use with young women with cancer who were facing chemotherapy or radiotherapy. This treatment would be likely to lead to significant loss of ovarian reserve and later infertility. Storage of eggs or embryos would allow them the chance of having children after successful treatment of their cancer even if their natural ovarian reserve was completely depleted by their treatment. Many pregnancies and births have now been reported in this group of patients and oncofertility preservation is widely practised (24, 25).

The technology of egg freezing is also increasingly being utilized by healthy young women who are anxious about their loss of ovarian reserve before they are in a position to start their family (26). Some have a strong family history of early menopause, while others have left a long-term relationship and are worried because of advancing age. A third group are in a long-term relationship but wish to defer pregnancy for career or family reasons. As IVF becomes safer and more socially acceptable, and as vitrification of oocytes has significantly improved survival and subsequent viability of frozen-thawed oocytes, this approach is being more widely advocated although some fertility specialists remain sceptical about the chances of pregnancy from vitrified oocytes.

Egg freezing has also been widely applied in the creation of 'donor egg banks' (27). These are used by women who have poor or no ovarian reserve, either due to advanced age or premature menopause, and who wish to have a family with donor oocyte. Use of cryopreservation allows for effective screening for infectious diseases since donors can be tested for seroconversion for HIV and hepatitis before the oocytes are released from the bank. Donors are younger women who either wish to donate altruistically or who are paid to donate. While this latter practice is permitted in many jurisdictions, including the United States and many European countries, others, including Australia, permit payment of expenses only. As with children born after sperm donation, modern practice encourages transparency with identification of the donor to the child when he or she

reaches maturity. This allows the child to learn about their biological origins by way of a meeting or meetings with their donor 'parent'.

Next steps

There is no sign that the growth in uptake of ART is slowing. Clinics are opening across the world and national regulatory systems are struggling to keep up with the increasing complexities of treatments, and with cross-border travel to allow couples to access a test or treatment that they desire which is not permitted in their own country. Examples include travel for sex selection, surrogacy, and treatment with donor gametes. Most recently, use of IVF to allow cell nuclear transfer to prevent mitochondrial disorders in the offspring has attracted significant media attention.

As the technology improves, giving couples a high chance of pregnancy from IVF provided that the female partner is not too old, more attention is being paid to safety for both mother and child. Child safety is maximized after SET for avoidance of premature birth and cerebral palsy in multiples. SET is widely practised in Scandinavia and Australia, less so in the United Kingdom, and seldom in the United States and in the developing world. Increasingly, 'segmentation' of the clinic with ovarian stimulation and egg collection being followed by elective 'freeze all' of blastocysts with later transfer in a separate cycle. This almost completely removes the risk of severe OHSS while maintaining good pregnancy rates, provided that the embryo laboratory is capable of delivering high-quality cryopreservation.

Increasing attention is also being paid to quality management and use of Standard Operating Procedures to minimize risk of error in IVF practice. Laboratories now work in a 'clean room' environment with high-grade air quality and minimal exposure of embryos to volatile organic compounds. Such approaches have allowed very large practices, performing in excess of 20,000 IVF cycles per year, to work efficiently in parts of Europe, Japan, and China.

IVF has come a long way since the first faltering steps of the pioneers in the 1970s and 1980s. Perhaps the greatest challenge is for IVF to remain a part of established medical practice instead of becoming a mere money-spinner for large corporate companies. Having a family is one of the most important steps that women and men take in their lives and those who need help to achieve this goal should not be overburdened financially by commercial entities that view IVF purely as a commodity.

REFERENCES

1. Brinsden PR. Thirty years of IVF: the legacy of Patrick Steptoe and Robert Edwards. *Hum Fertil (Camb)* 2009;**12**:137–43.
2. Dyer S, Chambers GM, de Mouzon J, et al. International Committee for Monitoring Assisted Reproductive Technologies world report: Assisted Reproductive Technology 2008, 2009 and 2010. *Hum Reprod* 2016;**31**:1588–609.
3. Franasiak JM, Forman EJ, Hong KH, et al. Aneuploidy across individual chromosomes at the embryonic level in trophectoderm biopsies: changes with patient age and chromosome structure. *J Assist Reprod Genet* 2014;**31**:1501–509.
4. Skakkebaek NE, Rajpert-De Meyts E, Buck Louis GM, et al. Male reproductive disorders and fertility trends: influences of environment and genetic susceptibility. *Physiol Rev* 2016;**96**:55–97.

5. Dumesic DA, Oberfield SA, Stener-Victorin E, et al. Scientific statement on the diagnostic criteria, epidemiology, pathophysiology, and molecular genetics of polycystic ovary syndrome. *Endocr Rev* 2015;**36**:487–525.

6. Tobler KJ, Shoham G, Christianson MS, et al. Use of anti-mullerian hormone for testing ovarian reserve: a survey of 796 infertility clinics worldwide. *J Assist Reprod Genet* 2015;**32**: 1441–48.

7. Li HW, Lee VC, Lau EY, et al. Role of baseline antral follicle count and anti-mullerian hormone in prediction of cumulative live birth in the first in vitro fertilisation cycle: a retrospective cohort analysis. *PLoS One* 2013;**8**:e61095.

8. Rutherford AJ, Subak-Sharpe RJ, Dawson KJ, et al. Improvement of in vitro fertilisation after treatment with buserelin, an agonist of luteinising hormone releasing hormone. *Br Med J (Clin Res Ed)* 1988;**296**:1765–68.

9. Damewood MD, Shen W, Zacur HA, et al. Disappearance of exogenously administered human chorionic gonadotropin. *Fertil Steril* 1989;**52**:398–400.

10. McClure N, Healy DL, Rogers PA, et al. Vascular endothelial growth factor as capillary permeability agent in ovarian hyperstimulation syndrome. *Lancet* 1994;**344**:235–36.

11. Seng SW, Ong KJ, Ledger WL. Gonadotropin-releasing hormone antagonist in in vitro fertilization superovulation. *Womens Health (Lond)* 2006;**2**:881–88.

12. Fauser BC, de Jong D, Olivennes F, et al. Endocrine profiles after triggering of final oocyte maturation with GnRH agonist after cotreatment with the GnRH antagonist ganirelix during ovarian hyperstimulation for in vitro fertilization. *J Clin Endocrinol Metab* 2002;**87**:709–15.

13. Devroey P, Polyzos NP, Blockeel C. An OHSS-free clinic by segmentation of IVF treatment. *Hum Reprod* 2011;**26**:2593–97.

14. Catford SR, McLachlan RI, O'Bryan MK, Halliday JL. Long-term follow-up of intra-cytoplasmic sperm injection-conceived offspring compared with in vitro fertilization-conceived offspring: a systematic review of health outcomes beyond the neonatal period. *Andrology* 2017;**5**:610–21.

15. Wong CC, Loewke KE, Bossert NL et al. Non-invasive imaging of human embryos before embryonic genome activation predicts development to the blastocyst stage. *Nat Biotechnol* 2010;**28**:1115–21.

16. Chambers GM, Wand H, Macaldowie A, et al. Population trends and live birth rates associated with common ART treatment strategies. *Hum Reprod* 2016;**31**:2632–41.

17. hfeaarchive.uksouth.cloudapp.azure.com/www.hfea.gov.uk/10516.html

18. Wong KM, van Wely M, Mol F, Repping S, Mastenbroek S. Fresh versus frozen embryo transfers in assisted reproduction. *Cochrane Database Syst Rev* 2017;**3**:CD011184.

19. van der Linden M, Buckingham K, Farquhar C, Kremer JA, Metwally M. Luteal phase support for assisted reproduction cycles. Cochrane Database Syst Rev 2015;**7**:CD009154.

20. Chambers GM, Paul RC, Harris K, et al. Assisted reproductive technology in Australia and New Zealand: cumulative live birth rates as measures of success. *Med J Aust* 2017;**207**:114–18.

21. Sharpe A, Avery P, Choudhary M. Reproductive outcome following pre-implantation genetic diagnosis (PGD) in the UK. *Hum Fertil (Camb)* 2018;**21**:120–27.

22. Sermon K, Capalbo A, Cohen J, et al. The why, the how and the when of PGS 2.0: current practices and expert opinions of fertility specialists, molecular biologists, and embryologists. *Mol Hum Reprod* 2016;**22**:845–57.

23. Mastenbroek S, Twisk M, van Echten-Arends J, et al. In vitro fertilization with preimplantation genetic screening. *N Engl J Med* 2007;**357**:9–17.

24. Woodruff TK. Oncofertility: a grand collaboration between reproductive medicine and oncology. *Reproduction* 2015;**150**:S1–10.

25. Ataman LM, Rodrigues JK, Marinho RM, et al. Creating a global community of practice for oncofertility. *J Glob Oncol* 2016;**2**:83–96.

26. Birch Petersen K, Hvidman HW, Sylvest R, et al. Family intentions and personal considerations on postponing childbearing in childless cohabiting and single women aged 35–43 seeking fertility assessment and counselling. *Hum Reprod* 2015;**30**:2563–74.

27. Nagy ZP, Chang CC, Shapiro DB, et al. Clinical evaluation of the efficiency of an oocyte donation program using egg cryo-banking. *Fertil Steril* 2009;**92**:520–26.

SECTION 10
Sexual and Reproductive Care

53

Contraception

Zephne M. van der Spuy and Petrus S. Steyn

Introduction

While it is widely agreed that one of the major achievements in women's health in the last millennium has been the availability of safe and effective contraception, there are some 225 million women worldwide with unmet contraceptive needs and this results in about 80 million unintended pregnancies per annum of which about 50% are terminated, often by unsafe abortion. This unmet need is highest among the most vulnerable in society including adolescents, people living with HIV, the poor, and other marginalized groups.

The Millennium Development Goals (MDGs) were formulated following the Millennium Summit in 2000 and MDG 5 aimed at 'Improving maternal health'. This goal specifically dealt with reducing maternal mortality and morbidity by 2015. It was after considerable lobbying by interested parties that in 2007 MDG 5b was included which explicitly presented targets for reproductive health including the contraceptive prevalence rate (1). The MDGs have now been superseded by the 17 Sustainable Development Goals (SDGs) which present the 2030 agenda for a plan of action for 'people, planet and prosperity'. SDG 3 aims to 'ensure healthy lives and promote wellbeing for all at all ages' and it is within this SDG that contraceptive access is mentioned and promoted. Given that effective contraception will prevent unintended pregnancies and significantly impact maternal mortality and morbidity it is concerning that it does not achieve a higher profile (2).

In the Western World, most of the original contraceptive services were male orientated and utilized condoms or coitus interruptus. As new and safe methods for female contraception have become available, these services and technologies have expanded both in industrialized and developing countries. Access to fertility regulation is varied around the world with some notable successes and some unfortunate failures. The commitment of governments in developing countries to fund women's health initiatives is often limited by resources. Darroch and Singh reviewed the trends in contraceptive need and use in developing countries and noted that women who wish to avoid unintended pregnancies and need effective contraception often do not have their requirements adequately addressed within the services available to them (3). There is a considerable literature about the impact of early motherhood on women and their children and it is evident that this puts young women at risk for educational underachievement and prejudices their economic situation (4). This obviously impacts their children and may exacerbate the cycle of deprivation and need. It is therefore essential that good contraceptive services and appropriate counselling are provided to women in all situations. The impact of unintended pregnancy is considerable and affects the lives of both the mother and her children (5, 6).

According to the WHO guideline 'Ensuring human rights in the provision of contraceptive information and services', nine key health and human rights standards should be considered (7). These are outlined in **Box 53.1**. The application of human rights principles to contraceptive service provision is of critical importance and can also be used to identify, reduce, and eliminate barriers to accessing contraception (8).

Contraceptive effectiveness is determined by efficacy (theoretical ability to prevent pregnancy), compliance, continuation, fecundity (ability to conceive), and the timing of coitus. All methods which are offered need to be accessed utilizing these parameters (9) (**Table 53.1**). There is currently a move to classify methods in terms of their duration of effectiveness but this is not yet in place.

The Medical Eligibility Criteria (MEC) for contraceptive use is part of the WHO process for improving the quality of care in contraceptive provision. The fifth edition was published in 2015 and presents current WHO guidance on the safety of various contraceptive methods for use in the context of specific health conditions and characteristics (10). In these guidelines, the safety of each contraceptive method is outlined and several considerations are utilized in the context of both the medical condition and medically relevant characteristics. This very valuable document takes into account whether the contraceptive method worsens the medical condition or creates additional health risks and secondarily whether the medical condition has an effect on the effectiveness of the contraceptive method. The safety of the method should always be weighed against the benefit of preventing unintended pregnancy. The recommendations cover many contraceptive methods and for each condition or characteristic the methods are characterized in one of four numbered categories (11) (**Table 53.2**). Every client should be assessed individually as more than one condition may need to be considered to determine contraceptive eligibility. This document provides valuable information to both clinicians and policymakers and should be regularly accessed.

Box 53.1 Human rights in the provision of contraceptive information and services

1 Non-discrimination
2 Availability
3 Accessibility
4 Acceptability
5 Quality of care
6 Participation
7 Informed decision-making and choice
8 Privacy/confidentiality
9 Accountability

Source data from World Health Organization. *Ensuring Human Rights in the Provision of Contraceptive Information and Services: Guidance and Recommendations.* Geneva: World Health Organization; 2014. http://apps.who.int/iris/bitstream/10665/102539/1/9789241506748_eng.pdf (accessed 10 September 2015).

Table 53.2 WHO Medical Eligibility Criteria categories for contraceptive eligibility

1	A condition for which there is no restriction for the use of the contraceptive method
2	A condition where the advantages of using the method generally outweigh the theoretical or proven risks
3	A condition where the theoretical or proven risks usually outweigh the advantages of using the method
4	A condition which represents an unacceptable health risk if the contraceptive method is used

Source data from World Health Organization. *Medical Eligibility Criteria for Contraceptive Use: A WHO Family Planning Cornerstone* (2015). World Health Organization, 5th edition. http://apps.who.int/iris/bitstream/10665/181468/1/9789241549158_eng.pdf?ua=1 (accessed 26 May 2016).

Table 53.1 Percentage of women experiencing an unintended pregnancy during the first year of typical use and the first year of perfect use of contraception and the percentage continuing use at the end of the first year

Method	Women experiencing an unintended pregnancy within the first year of use		Women continuing use at 1 year (%)
	Typical use (%)	Perfect use (%)	
No method	85	85	
Spermicides	28	18	42
Withdrawal	22	4	46
Fertility awareness methods	24		47
a. Standard days method[a]		5	
b. 2-day method[b]		4	
c. Ovulation method[b]		3	
d. Symptothermal method[b]		0.4	
Condom (male)	18	2	43
Combined pill and progestogen-only pill	9	0.3	67
Combined hormonal patch (Evra)	9	0.3	67
Combined hormonal ring (Nuvaring)	9	0.3	67
Depo medroxyprogesterone acetate, DMPA (Depo-Provera)	6	0.2	56
Cu-IUCD (Copper T)	0.8	0.6	78
LNG-IUS (Mirena)	0.2	0.2	80
Subdermal implant (Implanon)	0.05	0.05	84
Female sterilization	0.5	0.5	100
Male sterilization	0.15	0.1	100

[a] Method involves avoiding intercourse on cycle days 8–19.

[b] The ovulation and 2-day methods are based on evaluation of cervical mucus. The standard days method avoids intercourse on cycle days 8 through 19. The symptothermal method is a double-check method based on evaluation of cervical mucus to determine the first fertile day and evaluation of cervical mucus and temperature to determine the last fertile day.

Source data from Trussell J. Contraceptive efficacy. In: Hatcher RA, Trussell J, Nelson AL, Cates W, Kowal D, Policar M, eds. *Contraceptive Technology*, 20th revised edn, pp. 779–844. New York: Ardent Media; 2011.

There are numerous challenges in providing accessible and appropriate fertility regulation to women around the world. While it has been stated that a women 'cannot die from a pregnancy she does not have', the prevention of unintended pregnancies also impacts perinatal and child mortality. Contraception is central to maternal health and we recognize the needs of developing countries in accessing advances in reproductive health. Health budgets are limited and the newer technologies such as the levonorgestrel-releasing intrauterine system (LNG-IUS) are often unaffordable. The HIV pandemic which has particularly affected Africa has impacted every aspect of healthcare. In providing good contraceptive advice worldwide it must be recognized what the challenges are, what the limitations of provision are due to budgetary constraints, and what is acceptable in different countries and cultures.

Contraceptive options

Hormonal contraceptive methods

Although combined oral contraceptives (COCs) are a popular method of contraception, the effectiveness is dependent on compliance and correct use (11). The COC pill has been used since the 1950s and is currently being prescribed to more than 80 million women. Its efficacy, safety, and acceptability have been meticulously researched through mostly observational studies. COCs consist of two hormones, oestrogen and progestogen. Oestrogen, oestradiol, and mestranol are the only synthetic oestrogens. Mestranol, which is rarely used today, is inactive and needs to be metabolized to ethinyl oestradiol. Lower-dose combined pills contain less than 50 mcg ethinyl oestradiol. A newer addition to the COCs, oestradiol valerate (E2V) is metabolized to oestradiol which is a natural oestrogen (12). Early limited evidence shows that this may lead to fewer changes in lipid metabolism, coagulation factors, and glucose regulation than with ethinyl oestradiol and less oestradiol-related side effects. At this stage, however, contraindications should be the same as with other oestrogens.

Synthetic progestogens are used in hormonal contraceptive methods because potent progestins can be used in very low doses and can be delivered through long-acting delivery systems. They are structurally related to testosterone (19-nortestosterone derivatives, including the estranes and gonanes) and progesterone (17-OH progesterone derivatives or pregnanes, and 19-norprogesterone derivatives or norpregnanes) (13, 14). The main mechanism of action is inhibiting ovulation but these preparations also thicken the cervical mucus rendering it impermeable to sperm penetration. Progestogens are usually combined with oestrogen for better cycle control or used alone as a progestogen-only contraceptive (15).

Recently developed progestogens aim to mimic the benefits of progesterone offering more potent progestational and antioestrogenic actions on the endometrium and with a strong antigonadotropic effect but without any androgenic, oestrogenic, or glucocorticoid receptor interaction to prevent unwanted side effects (13, 14). The effects of available progestogens may differ substantially. This includes the systemic and biochemical impact which is associated with common side effects and some of the risks which have been extensively studied. The common side effects, such as headaches, nausea, dizziness, and breast tenderness, are generally self-limiting and decrease with duration of use (16).

Minor side effects reported by users include irregular, unpredictable bleeding and weight gain. Menstrual abnormalities differ with different COC formulations and regimens and in general occur soon after pill initiation, decreasing from 10–30% in the first month to around 10% by the third (17). Weight gain is often perceived as a side effect of using COCs but evidence shows that weight change is the same for COC and placebo users for low-dose products (18).

Serious adverse events, including venous thromboembolism (VTE), are rare among healthy COC users. The risks and benefits of a contraceptive agent against the consequences of unintended pregnancy should be key in the choice of a method. There is an association with the use of the combined contraceptive pill with an increase in the prevalence of venous thrombosis, pulmonary embolism, and myocardial infarction. The prevalence of VTE (8–10:10,000 women-years exposure) and arterial thrombotic events, including myocardial infarction and stroke (1–4:10,000 woman-years exposure), is very rare among healthy, reproductive-age users of modern COCs (19).

There are considerable non-contraceptive benefits associated with COC use. These include improved cycle control and relief from menstrual symptoms, preventing and reducing acne and hirsutism, improved bone health, and prevention of ovarian and endometrial cancer (19).

Several guidelines and ways to maximize the safety of hormonal contraceptive methods have been developed (11, 20). Countries also adapt these guidelines according to their local needs and produce local tools or guidelines. **Box 53.2** shows an adaptation for South Africa for absolute contraindications (21). Ensuring that patients make an informed choice may also decrease the prescriber's liability in case of complications. All the relevant clinical information to exclude relative and absolute contraindications and the needs of the client should be checked at the first visit. Monophasic COC formulations may be preferred over multiphasic preparations given these offer no clinical advantage and have potential for incorrect use (22). Other advantages of starting with a monophasic pill may be its ease of use, and ease of postponing menstruation when desired by excluding the pill-free interval (23).

When initiating a contraceptive method, guidance, such as the WHO MEC evidence-based recommendations, to help the healthcare provider should be accessed. In addition, a WHO-developed effectiveness chart helps as a counselling tool to advise on the different tiers of contraceptive effectiveness (24) (**Table 53.3**). This table provides a

---

Box 53.2 Absolute contraindications to combined hormonal contraception use (pill, patch ring)/WHO MEC 4: method not to be used

- Smoker (≥15 cigarettes/day), age 35 years or older
- Migraine with aura, any age
- Cardiovascular conditions:
  - Elevated blood pressure levels (systolic >160 mmHg or diastolic >100 mmHg)
  - Current/history of thromboembolic disorders (deep venous thrombosis or pulmonary emboli) or stroke
  - Known thrombogenic mutation
  - Current/history of ischaemic heart disease
  - Current/history of complicated valvular heart disease (pulmonary hypertension, risk of atrial fibrillation, history of subacute bacterial endocarditis)
- Chronic disease/other conditions:
  - Malignant and benign liver tumours (except focal nodular hyperplasia)
  - Active viral hepatitis or severe cirrhosis
  - Diabetes with vascular complication (nephropathy, neuropathy, retinopathy) or more than 20 years' duration
  - Systemic lupus erythematosus with positive or unknown antiphospholipid antibodies
  - Acute porphyria with history of crisis
  - Major surgery with prolonged immobilization

Source data from National Department of Health, Republic of South Africa. *National contraception clinical guidelines.* 2012. Available at: https://www.gov.za/sites/default/files/gcis_document/201409/contraceptionclinicalguidelines28Jan2013-2.pdf.

---

visual aid indicating contraceptive effectiveness per method, enabling better comparison and assists with the subsequent choice.

Transdermal combined contraceptive system

A continuous daily serum level of 20 mcg ethinyl oestradiol and 150 mcg norelgestromin (the primary active metabolite of norgestimate)

Table 53.3 Comparing effectiveness of family planning methods

More effective	First	Implant
Less than one pregnancy per 100 women in 1 year		Vasectomy
		Female sterilization
		IUD (Cu-IUD, LNG-IUS)
	Second	Injectables
		Lactation amenorrhoea method
		Oral contraceptive pill
		Contraceptive patch
		Vaginal ring
	Third	Condoms (male and female)
		Diaphragm
		Sponge
		Fertility awareness-based methods
Less effective	Fourth	Withdrawal
About 30 pregnancies per 100 women in one year		Spermicide

Source data from World Health Organization (WHO). *Comparing Typical Effectiveness of Contraceptive Methods.* Geneva: World Health Organization; 2006. Available at: http://www.fhi.org/nr/shared/enFHI/Resources/EffectivenessChart.pdf.

is delivered transdermally through a 20 cm² adhesive patch. The patch is used once a week for 3 consecutive weeks followed by 1 week of non-use which results in a withdrawal bleed. A benefit is that the compliance and continuation rates are better if compared to the COC pill while the efficacy and side effects are comparable with COC pills.

Combined hormonal vaginal ring

This flexible transparent ring measures 4 mm in cross section and 54 mm in diameter and is administered vaginally releasing 15 mcg ethinyl oestradiol and 120 mcg etonogestrel per day. The contra-indications are the same as for the COC pills. The ring is inserted in the vagina and left there for 3 weeks, after which it is removed for a week during which a withdrawal bleed usually occurs. The effectiveness, continuation, and compliance rates are similar to that of COC pill.

Monthly combined injectables

Several injectable preparations that combine a depo progestogen with an oestrogen are available. There are fewer progestogen-related side effects and menstruation still occurs in more than two-thirds of patients. Failure rates are 0.2–0.4% during the first year of use.

Progestogen-only pill

This method exerts its action mainly through thickening the cervical mucus and in most clients ovulation is not suppressed. The pill should be taken every day at the same time as the effect on the cervical mucus lasts for 22 hours. Progestogen-only pills are usually recommended to lactating patients, in women after the age of 40 years, or when oestrogens are contraindicated.

Progestogen injections

Depot medroxyprogesterone acetate (DMPA) (12-weekly) and norethisterone enanthate (8-weekly) are used in these preparations. DMPA is used widely in several settings. In addition to the main mechanism of action of suppression of ovulation, the cervical mucus is also altered to prevent sperm penetration. Although the theoretical failure rate of this method is very low, continuation rates are poor, mainly due to changes in bleeding patterns.

Adverse effects include irregular bleeding, frequently experienced after the first administration, and amenorrhoea. Weight gain is reported due to an increased appetite. Complaints of headache, loss of libido, and depression are sometimes expressed. There is some concern over the loss of bone density in long-term users which appears to be temporary and the bone mass returns to normal after discontinuation. There are very few absolute contraindications (WHO MEC 4).

Subdermal implants

Several subdermal implants, containing either levonorgestrel (LNG) or etonogestrel are available. These offer a long-acting, reversible contraceptive method (LARC) with the main adverse effects of irregular and prolonged bleeding. The main mechanism of action is preventing ovulation but these preparations also thicken the cervical mucous. Implants are a very effective contraception option compared with combined hormonal contraception and injectables which rely more on consistent and perfect use. Continuation rates

are high and the most common reason for removal of the implant is due to abnormal bleeding patterns.

Emergency contraception

Of the 43.8 million induced abortions in women aged 15–44 in 2005, 49% were judged to be unsafe (25). The aim within clinical service provision is to avoid unsafe abortions through appropriate advice and education. While no emergency contraceptive method offers a 100% guarantee of avoiding pregnancy, emergency contraceptive remains very important as backup for many methods of contraception and for women who have had non-consensual coitus (25). There are many misconceptions about the emergency contraceptive and often inadequate information is provided to both service providers and consumers.

Originally Yuzpe introduced the concept of utilizing ethinyl oestradiol 100 mcg in combination with dl-norgestrel 1 mg within 72 hours of unprotected coitus and repeated after 12 hours (26). This dosage was available through combined contraceptive preparations and there was a rapid acceptance worldwide of this regimen. The success of treatment was dependent on the time of administration after coitus, and probably the stage of the cycle when this was accessed. The main side effects were nausea and vomiting.

Subsequently, the LNG-only pill was investigated for provision of emergency contraception. The original regimen was 0.75 mg administered twice at 12-hourly intervals. The first dose was ideally administered within 24 hours of unprotected coitus. Subsequent research suggested that a single dose was equally effective and had a lower failure rate than the Yuzpe regimen. Currently, a single dose of 1.5 mg LNG is recommended to avoid non-compliance (27).

The copper intrauterine contraceptive device is a very effective method of emergency contraception and has the advantage of offering women efficacy for up to 5 day days after exposure, although earlier use is recommended. In addition it may be utilized as ongoing contraception (28).

Mifepristone is a progesterone receptor modulator and is an effective form of emergency contraception (29). The latest review from the WHO suggested that a dose of 50 mg should be utilized for emergency contraception. The initial study used a much higher dose of mifepristone (600 mg) but it is recognized that lower doses are very effective, although many countries only have access to the 200 mg formulation (30).

Ulipristal acetate, a newer progesterone receptor modulator, has been successfully utilized for emergency contraception with good efficacy. It is proven to be less effective in women with multiple exposures to pregnancy but has a very acceptable side effect profile and is certainly comparable or superior to levonorgestrel. It must be noted that progestogen-only contraception cannot be initiated straight after the use of mifepristone or ulipristal. At present, we could recommend the use of LNG in lower-resource settings and mifepristone or ulipristal acetate in an environment where this is available (31) (**Table 53.4**).

The effectiveness of emergency contraception is dependent on the time of the cycle when it is utilized and this is often not recorded (32). It is regularly debated whether many of the women who receive emergency contraception are actually not at risk of pregnancy which obviously impacts the results of any study and makes assessment of success rates more difficult.

Table 53.4 Methods of emergency contraception

Method	Limits of use after coitus	Side effects
Yuzpe regimen (ethinyl oestradiol + dl-norgestrel)	Up to 72 hours	• Nausea and vomiting • Better methods available
Levonorgestrel (LNG)-only regimen (1.5 mg single dose)	Up to 72 hours	• Less side effects • Better efficacy than Yuzpe • Universal availability
Mifepristone Low dose vs mid dose (25–50 mg) (antiprogestogen)	Up to 120 hours	• Superior to LNG • Menstrual delay • Often only higher dose available
Ulipristal acetate 30 mg (antiprogestogen)	Up to 120 hours	• Superior to LNG • Wider window of efficacy • Not universally available
Copper IUCD (Pre- and postfertilization mechanisms)	Up to 120 hours (can use up to 5 days)	• Universal availability • Ongoing contraceptive method • Most effective emergency contracepion within 120 hours • Can use up to 5 days

Male contraception

The current available male methods of contraception are the condom, withdrawal, and vasectomy, which is regarded as irreversible. Worldwide, male methods are utilized for 10% of contraception use and this rises to 25% in developed countries. The majority of couples utilizing male methods will use condoms which have a high failure rate of 18% in the first year of use (33). There is an unmet need for the development of reversible contraceptive options for men and international surveys have confirmed that many men and women would be willing to utilize new male methods of contraception (34–36).

Considerable research has been undertaken for the development of hormonal male contraception. The use of testosterone to suppress the pulsatile release of gonadotropin-releasing hormone, luteinizing hormone, and follicle-stimulating hormone and thus suppressing endogenous testosterone production and spermatogenesis has informed a number of the early clinical trials. The aim of testosterone administration was to provide suppression of spermatogenesis but maintain secondary sexual characteristics and non-gonadal androgen effects. For contraceptive efficacy, it is necessary to achieve azoospermia or severe oligospermia, (sperm concentration of <1 million/ml) (37). The testosterone-only regimens have considerable delay in initiating suppression of spermatogenesis and often supraphysiological levels of circulating testosterone were necessary to achieve this. Subsequent studies have concentrated on a combination of testosterone with a progestogen. This allows a lower dose of testosterone and enhances the suppression of spermatogenesis with less androgenic side effects. Many different preparations have been utilized and the routes of administration include intramuscular injection, implants, and gels. Ongoing contraceptive research utilizing newer preparations and combinations is in progress (37–39).

There are considerable challenges in the production of effective hormonal contraception and this includes the variability of sperm suppression achieved in men with some 10–15% failing to suppress adequately. There is considerable ethnic variation in response and side effects may include changes in lipid profile and an increase in weight, acne, and male pattern balding.

What has been clearly demonstrated is that with the cessation of treatment there is a complete reversal of the suppression of spermatogenesis. To date, all studies have been conducted on men with normal semen analyses and therefore there is no information about the impact on men with possible subfertile semen parameters. Several studies have compared the addition of a gonadotropin-releasing hormone agonist or antagonist analogue to the testosterone and progestogen combined protocol but showed no significant improvement in suppression. Similarly the use of a 5-alpha reductase inhibitor did not improve the overall impact of the contraceptive regimen (37, 39).

Non-hormonal possibilities for male contraception have also been investigated. These have concentrated on identifying processes in sperm development, maturation, and function which could possibly be targeted with a disruption of fertility. At present, this approach is still largely utilized in animal models. This research has investigated a number of possible testicular targets or targeting sperm motility or sperm–egg fusion (39).

The availability of an effective form of reversible contraception for men would contribute significantly to the provision of adequate contraception for couples. At present, despite the promising research, the widespread availability of male hormonal contraception remains unlikely unless significant additional funding for research becomes available.

The intrauterine device and the intrauterine system

Current intrauterine devices (IUDs) contain either LNG or copper, are extremely safe, highly effective, and long lasting with the added advantage of being reversible (40).

The LNG-IUS constantly releases progestogen locally in the uterine cavity. It is registered for 5 years of use, is very effective, and has a good continuation rate. Common side effects are irregular bleeding, headaches, nausea, and breast tenderness but these usually dissipate after a few months. The device is used as a treatment for idiopathic heavy menstrual bleeding and there is 90% reduction in blood loss after 12 months of use. Non-contraceptive benefits include decreased dysmenorrhoea and improvement of endometriosis symptoms. A smaller LNG-IUS which is effective for 3 years is ideal for the nulliparous woman.

Several copper-containing IUDs are available. The main mechanism of action is on the sperm motility and morphology. The CuT380A is considered to be the gold standard and the effectiveness is less than 2% pregnancies at 5 years (41). The main adverse effects are pain, spotting, light bleeding, and menorrhagia which occur in the initial 3–6 months and usually get better with time.

There are several misconceptions about IUDs, such as causing ectopic pregnancy, infertility, pelvic infection, and contraindicated in teenagers and nulliparous women. The risk of infection which increases during the 20 days after insertion is due to contamination with pre-existing organisms of the cervical canal (42). Women at higher risk of sexually transmitted infections (STIs), as determined by sexual history, should be screened and treated. Routine prophylactic antibiotics, however, do not reduce upper genital tract infection or improve continuation rates (43). The risk of uterine perforation for the IUDs is less than 2 in 1000 and expulsion occurs in 5% of women, usually within the first 3 months after insertion (40).

IUDs can be used in women with HIV and AIDS who are clinically well on antiretrovirals (11). The IUD can also be inserted postpartum and after first- and second-trimester abortion.

Male and female sterilization

Some couples may request permanent contraception and may select either male or female sterilization. Careful counselling is essential and information about LARC methods should be provided. They need to understand that there is sometimes regret after a permanent procedure and that reversal may not be possible or successful. Regret has been expressed in studies of female sterilization in about 7% of women and in 2–6% of men who have a vasectomy. A young age at sterilization is one of the most important factors in predicting regret. Female sterilization remains more common than male sterilization. It is twice as common as vasectomy in industrialized countries, 8 times more common in Asia, and 15 times more common in Latin America and the Caribbean (44). While female permanent contraception is the most popular contraceptive method worldwide its use varies considerably from about 43% of women in Japan but only 1% of women in Zimbabwe (45).

Female sterilization carries an overall failure rate of less than 2%. In the CREST study, the 5-year cumulative failure rate was 1.3% and the 10-year cumulative failure rate was 1.85% (46). There is no evidence of an increase in menstrual dysfunction following sterilization.

Various methods of female sterilization are available and these include laparoscopic techniques such as bipolar and unipolar coagulation, application of the silicone ring (Falope ring), the springclip (Hulka), and the titanium clip (Filshie). An abdominal approach may be used for partial or total salpingectomy or fimbriectomy and the hysteroscopic transcervical approach is utilized to insert micro-inserts (Essure) into the proximal section of each fallopian tube. The failure rate of the different methods varies and is lowest for the Filshie clip and Essure (47–49). Female sterilization can be performed remote from pregnancy, postpartum, or after termination of pregnancy. There is evidence that salpingectomy offers some protection against ovarian carcinoma and this may be considered when deciding on the operative procedure (49).

Vasectomy is more effective, safer, and less invasive than female sterilization, with fewer complications and the failure rate in the first year is 0.15%. Once postvasectomy azoospermia has been confirmed, the failure rate is 1 in 2000. It is essential that couples are counselled about the need for backup contraception after the procedure as this becomes effective after about 3 months when azoospermia has been achieved or there are less than 100,000 non-motile sperm in an ejaculate.

The postoperative complication rate for all forms of sterilization is low at 1–2%. Sometimes couples present requesting reversal of sterilization and it is essential that counselling includes the fact that sterilization is regarded as a permanent form of contraception, that reversal may not be feasible, and it has to be recognized that in many healthcare settings this will not be available (50).

Only those clients who have the capacity to give fully informed consent can agree to permanent contraception. Offering sterilization to intellectually challenged individuals is largely discouraged. With the availability of the very effective LARC methods, it is possible that sterilization may well become a less popular contraceptive option in the future.

Barrier contraception

These contraceptive methods provide a mechanical or chemical barrier to prevent sperm from passing into the uterus and fallopian tubes to fertilize the ovum. It is essential that they are utilized correctly and consistently and couples need to be very aware of the limitations of these contraceptive options. The barrier methods available to our clients include the male and female condoms, spermicides, the cervical cap or vaginal diaphragm, and vaginal sponges (47).

Male condoms are very widely used and are promoted as protection against transmission of HIV and STIs. They provide a physical barrier to prevent sperm from entering the vagina and while their contraceptive efficacy may be limited, their role in transmission of infections is very important. All couples accessing contraception should be counselled on the need and importance of barrier contraception.

Latex condoms provide protection against many STIs but are less effective in preventing infections transmitted by skin-to-skin contact such as herpesvirus and human papillomavirus. Polyurethane condoms have a greater incidence of breakage or slippage during coitus and are definitely inferior in terms of infection protection (51). Lambskin condoms are not recommended for STI prevention as most of the viruses which we wish to avoid such as hepatitis B, herpes simplex virus, and HIV pass through the small pores. In general, latex condoms are considered superior to any of the other available options. Condom use is effective in terms of fertility regulation and perfect use results in a 2% failure rate but typical use has an 18% failure rate.

The female condom is fairly widely available in many low-resource settings. It has a failure rate of 21% with typical use compared with the 5% failure rate with perfect use. Failures occur because of breakage, slippage, misdirection of the condom, and invagination of the condom.

The diaphragm and cervical cap are still used in many countries but are often not available in low-resource settings. The diaphragm provides an intravaginal barrier method which is improved with the use of spermicides. There are several types of diaphragms and the typical success rate of this contraceptive option is 12%. The cervical cap is available in some countries and contributes to the methods of barrier contraception.

There are no non-contraceptive benefits of utilizing barrier contraception and it is advisable that every woman who elects to use this form of contraception is also counselled about emergency contraception and given access to this intervention.

It is recommended that spermicides should be utilized with barrier contraception but there is a concern that the most common preparation (nonoxynol-9 gel) results in lesions in the vagina and possibly increased transmission of the HIV virus (52). The use of vaginal microbicides for reducing HIV infection in women has been extensively reviewed (53). The situation where contraception can be combined with both HIV and STI protection is obviously ideal. An acceptable combination of contraception and spermicides has not yet been developed. This is an area for future research and clinical trials.

At present, we would recommend that any woman who may be exposed to HIV infection or STIs should utilize a modern form of contraception plus barrier contraception. Spermicides are not available in many developing countries where HIV prevalence is high and the concern about HIV transmission militates against their use (54).

Natural contraception

Despite the availability of modern contraceptive methods, natural family planning is still practised by a significant number of couples of reproductive age in most countries. These methods include the fertility awareness-based methods and withdrawal. Pregnancy rates of fertility awareness-based methods with perfect use have ranged between 0.3 and 5.0 per 100 users per year. Unfortunately, with typical use, rates of pregnancy rise considerably and therefore this is not a very effective form of contraception (55).

The methods used include the Billings method which assesses cervical mucus, and the symptothermal method which utilizes temperature changes, cycle length, and also cervical mucus. In addition, the standard days method or the calendar days method which inform a woman of the number of days in which she should avoid coitus based on the length of her cycle have also been utilized. The change of basal body temperature may indicate ovulation has taken place and some couples utilize this. The 2-day method which pays attention only to cervical secretions has also been practised (56).

The lactational amenorrhoea method (LAM) is an important contributor to contraception and is used worldwide. The LAM is only effective when the women is less than 6 months postpartum, is exclusively or nearly exclusively breastfeeding, and is still amenorrhoeic. LAM is 98% effective if used correctly. There are some problems and some contraindications to LAM. Women who are HIV positive have to be very carefully counselled about how they utilize this method. In addition, women with medical conditions utilizing certain medications including cytotoxic therapy and high doses of steroids may not be suitable for this form of contraception (47).

The use of withdrawal is often underestimated by clinicians providing contraceptive advice. It has been estimated that over 10% of Canadian women have utilized this as a contraceptive method and an even higher percentage from the United States have reported using coitus interruptus (47). The effectiveness depends on the willingness of the couple to be consistent in the use of withdrawal with every act of coitus. With typical use the failure rate may be as high as 22%. Abstinence is also being offered as an option for natural family planning but it is limited by the personal circumstances of the couple.

While many clinicians aim to persuade patients to utilize more reliable forms of contraception other than natural contraception, it is important to recognize that for some couples religious or philosophical considerations mean that they do not wish to use modern contraception. In addition, often communities which are perceived as not having access to contraception are in fact utilizing 'natural' or 'traditional' contraceptive methods (57). This to a certain extent reflects the failure of service provision but indicates their need for contraceptive advice. Where possible, couples should be counselled that natural contraception offers no protection against STIs or HIV infection and if barrier methods are acceptable, they should be encouraged to use this together with their traditional or natural contraceptive methods (58).

An overview of long-acting reversible contraception

LARC is a method that requires administration less than once per cycle or month. These methods combine reversibility with high effectiveness because they depend less on compliance or correct use than the short-acting methods such as the COC pills (59, 60). LARC methods include copper IUDs, the LNG-IUS, progestogen-only injectable contraceptives, and progestogen-only subdermal implants.

Benefits of LARC methods include that they are more cost-effective than the COC pill even if only used for 1 year. Studies have reported high satisfaction and continuation rates compared to other contraceptives. These do not include the progestogen-only injectable contraceptives which have a poor continuation rate. The use of LARC methods offers the client an effective, long-acting method which requires limited input from the user.

Special contraceptive needs

Postabortion and postpartum contraception

The provision and easy access of postpartum contraception is not only beneficial for the health of the mothers but also for their children. Adequate spacing between pregnancies prevents a higher risk of prematurity, low birth weight, fetal death, and early neonatal death (61). Maternal health also benefits through lowering of the risk of uterine rupture and uteroplacental bleeding (62). There is still a high unmet need for modern postpartum contraception (63).

Breastfeeding, modern contraceptive methods, sterilization, and emergency contraception should be considered in all cases. The WHO MEC depicts concerns about the theoretical hormonal effects of combined hormonal contraceptives on the suppression of quality and quantity of milk production as well as possible absorption by the infant. There is also an increased risk of thromboembolism postpartum when using COCs or oestrogen-containing contraceptive methods. It is recommended that the earliest date to start is 21 days postpartum if other risk factors for the development of VTE are excluded (63). In 2015, the WHO updated the recommendations which are now more restrictive for oestrogen-containing contraceptives and less restrictive for progestogen-containing methods (Table 53.5)

According to the United Kingdome National Institute for Health and Care Excellence (NICE) guidelines, methods and timing when to start contraception should be discussed within the first week of the birth, and include the provision of contact details for contraceptive advice (64, 65).

The IUD is a LARC method with expulsion rates of 5–15 per 100 woman-years of use when used as a postplacental method immediately after caesarean section. The IUD does not affect breastfeeding and is easy to insert in these women, but appears to be associated with a higher perforation rate (>1 per 100) (66).

Contraception provision after abortion should be discussed with women at the initial assessment and documented. Women should be advised of the greater effectiveness of LARC methods. An IUD is a safe, good method to use after both first- and second-trimester surgical abortions. Sterilization can be safely performed at the time of induced abortion although it may be more likely than interval sterilization to be associated with regret (67).

Table 53.5 Latest recommendations from the WHO MEC fifth edition for hormonal contraception postpartum

Recommendations for combined hormonal contraception (CHC) use among breastfeeding women		
<6 weeks postpartum	Breastfeeding women <6 weeks postpartum should not use CHCs	MEC 4
≥6 weeks to <6 months postpartum	Breastfeeding women ≥6 weeks to <6 months postpartum (primarily breastfeeding) generally should not use CHCs	MEC 3
≥6 months postpartum	Breastfeeding women ≥6 months postpartum can generally use CHCs	MEC 2
Recommendations for CHC use among postpartum women		
<21 days postpartum without other risk factors for venous thromboembolism (VTE)	Women who are <21 days postpartum and do not have other risk factors for VTE generally should not use CHCs	MEC 3
<21 days postpartum with other risk factors for VTE	Women who are <21 days postpartum with other risk factors for VTE should not use CHCs	MEC 4
≥21 days to 42 days postpartum without other risk factors for VTE	Women who are ≥21 days to 42 days postpartum without other risk factors for VTE can generally use CHCs	MEC 2
≥21 days to 42 days postpartum with other risk factors for VTE	Women who are ≥21 days to 42 days postpartum with other risk factors for VTE generally should not use CHCs	MEC 3
>42 days postpartum	Women who are >42 days postpartum can use CHCs without restriction	MEC 1
POC use among breastfeeding women (POCs include progestogen-only pills, implants and injectables)		
<6 weeks postpartum	Breastfeeding women who are <6 weeks postpartum can generally use progestogen-only pills (POPs) and levonorgestrel (LNG) and etonogestrel (ETG) implants	MEC 2
	Breastfeeding women who are <6 weeks postpartum generally should not use progestogen-only injectables (POIs) (DMPA or NET-EN)	MEC 3
≥6 weeks to <6 months postpartum	Breastfeeding women who are ≥6 weeks to <6 months postpartum can use POPs, POIs, and LNG and ETG implants without restriction	MEC 1
≥6 months postpartum	Breastfeeding women who are ≥6 months postpartum can use POPs, POIs, and LNG and ETG implants without restriction	MEC 1

CIC, combined injectable contraceptives; COC, combined oral contraceptive pills; DPMA, depot medroxyprogesterone acetate; ETG, etonogestrel; LNG, levonorgestrel; LNG-IUD, levonorgestrel-releasing intrauterine device; NET-EN, norethisterone enanthate; POC, progestogen-only contraception; POI, progestogen-only injectable; POP, progestogen-only pill.
Source data from World Health Organization. *Medical Eligibility Criteria for Contraceptive Use: A WHO Family Planning Cornerstone* (2015). World Health Organization, 5th edition. http://apps.who.int/iris/bitstream/10665/181468/1/9789241549158_eng.pdf?ua=1 (accessed 26 May 2016).

Contraception for women living with HIV/AIDS

The WHO promotes the provision of effective contraception in HIV-positive women as an important component to prevent mother-to-child-transmission. These recommendations are regularly updated. The guidelines for hormonal contraception and HIV include recommendations for women at high risk of HIV infection, for women living with HIV infection, and women living with HIV using antiretroviral therapy (11, 68).

Women at high risk of HIV infection should have access to most available hormonal contraceptive methods and must be counselled to use male or female condoms consistently in addition to their usual contraceptive method.

Due to the nature of the body of evidence on progestogen-only injectable contraception and risk of HIV acquisition, women using this method should be strongly advised to use condoms, male or female, and take other preventative measures (69).

As new studies with better methodology and newer antiretrovirals develop and are completed, this field is constantly being updated.

The latest recommendations from the WHO MEC and guidance statement are summarized in **Tables 53.6 and 53.7**. The guidance is currently being reviewed and will be on the WHO website available in late 2019.

The adolescent requiring contraception

Adolescence, defined as 10–19 years of age, is a time of physical, sexual, and emotional development and experiences. Adolescents may face pressure to participate in high-risk behaviour, including sexual activity, and have the right to request and receive unbiased contraceptive counselling. They have the right of choice concerning which contraceptive they wish to use. It should be noted that the prescriber should know the legal guidelines of the particular statutory body or bodies where they practise (70).

Most contraceptive methods may be offered to adolescents except permanent methods which are seldom appropriate because of their irreversibility. The adolescent should be advised about the use of a LARC method whenever possible but her choice

Table 53.6 WHO recommendations for use of hormonal contraception for women at high risk of HIV infection and women living with HIV (11, 68)

Women at high risk of HIV infection	Women at high risk of acquiring HIV can use the following hormonal contraceptive methods without restriction: COCs, combined injectable contraceptives (CICs), combined contraceptive patches and rings, POPs, and LNG and ETG implants	(Category 1)
	Women at high risk of acquiring HIV can generally use POIs (DMPA and NET-EN) and LNG-IUDs	(Category 2)
Women living with asymptomatic or mild HIV clinical disease (WHO stage 1 or 2)	Women living with asymptomatic or mild HIV clinical disease (WHO stage 1 or 2) can use the following hormonal contraceptive methods without restriction: COCs, CICs, combined contraceptive patches and rings, POPs, POIs (DMPA and NET-EN), and LNG and ETG implants	(Category 1)
	Women living with asymptomatic or mild HIV clinical disease (WHO stage 1 or 2) can generally use the LNG-IUD	(Category 2)
Women living with severe or advanced HIV clinical disease (WHO stage 3 or 4)	Women living with severe or advanced HIV clinical disease (WHO stage 3 or 4) can use the following hormonal contraceptive methods without restriction: COCs, CICs, combined contraceptive patches and rings, POPs, POIs (DMPA and NET-EN), and LNG and ETG implants	(Category 1)
	Women living with severe or advanced HIV clinical disease (WHO stage 3 or 4) generally should not initiate use of the LNG-IUD until their illness has improved to asymptomatic or mild HIV clinical disease (WHO stage 1 or 2)	(Category 3) (Category 2)
	Women who already have an LNG-IUD inserted and who develop severe or advanced HIV clinical disease need not have their IUD removed	(Category 2 for continuation)

CIC, combined injectable contraceptives; COC, combined oral contraceptive pills; DPMA, depot medroxyprogesterone acetate; ETG, etonogestrel; LNG, levonorgestrel; LNG-IUD, levonorgestrel-releasing intrauterine device; NET-EN, norethisterone enanthate; POI, progestogen-only injectable; POP, progestogen-only pill.
Source data from World Health Organization. Hormonal contraceptive eligibility for women at high risk of HIV Guidance – Recommendations concerning the use of hormonal contraceptive methods by women at high risk of HIV (2017). https://www.who.int/reproductivehealth/publications/family_planning/HC-and-HIV-2017/en/.

of a contraceptive option will determine what method she is given (71, 72).

Sufficient time for consultation should be provided and these clients must be encouraged to return at any time if they experience problems with their contraceptive choice. Young women have been found to be less tolerant of side effects and abandoning contraception will place them at risk of unintended pregnancy. Correct and consistent condom use must be promoted to prevent STIs and dual protection with another effective method of contraception to prevent pregnancy must be encouraged. Adolescents may have specific health concerns or risks which need to be addressed at the first consultation. They should have easy access to emergency contraception.

Sexually active young people are more likely to have short-term sexual relationships with more partners and may have a greater risk

Table 53.7 Women living with HIV using antiretroviral therapy (11)

Nucleoside/nucleotide reverse transcriptase inhibitor (NRTI)	Women taking any NRTI can use all hormonal contraceptive methods without restriction: COCs, CICs, combined contraceptive patches and rings, POPs, POIs (DMPA and NET-EN), and LNG and ETG implants	(Category 1)
	Women taking any NRTI can generally use the LNG-IUD, provided that their HIV clinical disease is asymptomatic or mild (WHO Stage 1 or 2)	(MEC Category 2)
	Women living with severe or advanced HIV clinical disease (WHO stage 3 or 4) and taking any NRTI generally should not initiate use of the LNG-IUD until their illness has improved to asymptomatic or mild HIV clinical disease	(MEC Category 3 for initiation)
	Women taking any NRTI who already have had an LNG-IUD inserted and who develop severe or advanced HIV clinical disease need not have their IUD removed	(MEC Category 2 for continuation)
Non-nucleoside reverse transcriptase inhibitors (NNRTIs)	Women using NNRTIs containing either efavirenz or nevirapine can generally use COCs, CICs, combined contraceptive patches and rings, POPs, NET-EN, and LNG and ETG implants	(MEC Category 2)
	Women using efavirenz or nevirapine can use DMPA without restriction	(MEC Category 1)
	Women taking any NNRTI can generally use the LNG-IUD, provided that their HIV clinical disease is asymptomatic or mild (WHO Stage 1 or 2)	(MEC Category 2)
	Women living with severe or advanced HIV clinical disease (WHO stage 3 or 4) and taking any NNRTI generally should not initiate use of the LNG-IUD until their illness has improved to asymptomatic or mild HIV clinical disease	(MEC Category 3 for initiation)
	Women taking any NNRTI who already have had an LNG-IUD inserted and who develop severe or advanced HIV clinical disease need not have their IUD removed	(MEC Category 2 for continuation)
NNRTIs containing etravirine and rilpivirine	Women using the newer NNRTIs containing etravirine and rilpivirine can use all hormonal contraceptive methods without restriction	(MEC Category 1)

CIC, combined injectable contraceptives; COC, combined oral contraceptive pills; DPMA, depot medroxyprogesterone acetate; ETG, etonogestrel; LNG, levonorgestrel; LNG-IUD, levonorgestrel-releasing intrauterine device; NET-EN, norethisterone enanthate; POI, progestogen-only injectable; POP, progestogen-only pill.
Source data from World Health Organization. *Medical Eligibility Criteria for Contraceptive Use: A WHO Family Planning Cornerstone* (2015). World Health Organization, 5th edition. http://apps.who.int/iris/bitstream/10665/181468/1/9789241549158_eng.pdf?ua=1 (accessed 26 May 2016).

of STIs, including HIV acquisition. In the counselling and other medical advice concerning infection prevention, all victims of non-consensual coitus should be offered postcoital contraception as well as postexposure prophylaxis for HIV acquisition.

Contraception at the end of reproductive life

The contraceptive needs of the perimenopausal woman often do not receive adequate attention. These women are still vulnerable in terms of unintentional conception, are usually still sexually active, and possibly may have a new partner which put them at risk of STIs. Ideally, the contraception they are offered should provide them with health benefits as well as contraceptive protection. A pregnancy which occurs at the end of reproductive life is often unintended and can cause considerable distress and concern. Many women find the choice of termination of pregnancy unacceptable although at the same time they have not planned a pregnancy in their 40s and 50s (45, 73, 74).

When reviewing the contraceptive options for older women, age alone is not a contraindication for most of the contraceptive methods. The current advice, however, is that the combined contraceptive pill and the injectable progestogen options should be stopped at 50 years of age unless there have been earlier contraindications. Factors such as body mass index, medical problems, and risk factors for cardiovascular and hypertensive disease will impact contraceptive options (75). The use of hormonal contraception is also protective in terms of certain cancers (76–78).

The COC can usually be utilized after the age of 50 years in a woman with no additional risk factors and consideration should be given to utilize lower-dose pills (79). Unfortunately these are not universally available and are not supplied in many public health systems in developing countries. Similarly, the other delivery methods such as transdermal patches are not available in low-resource settings (80).

The advantages of the combined contraceptive pill are that this impacts positively on bone metabolism and reduces ovarian and endometrial cancer. Unfortunately there are also considerable risks for thromboembolic disease and arterial disease and there is ongoing concern that combined therapy may impact breast cancer and cervical cancer (81).

Progestogen-only contraception has many routes of administration including oral, subdermal, and intramuscular. Many women have unscheduled bleeding which causes concern and the implications of this therapy need to be carefully discussed with potential users (73, 82).

The copper intrauterine contraceptive device has no systemic impact and in addition has the advantage of offering long-term contraception for the perimenopausal woman. Unfortunately many consumers chose not to use this method, despite the very acceptable efficacy record.

Barrier contraception in the older women may be important as often they are involved in new relationships and protection against human papillomavirus and HIV is needed. Condom difficulty has been reported with older partners who may have erectile dysfunction and the use of the female condom has received variable acceptance. In many countries the diaphragm and the cervical cap are not available and there is considerable concern about the use of spermicides which may increase HIV transmission. Natural contraception is always problematic and while sterilization is appropriate in the older woman, she may find this unacceptable.

Advice on when to stop contraception is important in this age group. At present, it is generally accepted that 1 year after the last menstrual bleed if a woman is 50 years or older is a reasonable time to discontinue contraception. In the younger woman, it is recommended she should continue contraceptive measures for at least 2 years. When a woman reaches 55 years regardless of her menstrual pattern, it is suggested that no contraceptive method needs to be utilized. There may, however, be indications for further investigations of ongoing bleeding. It must be stressed that hormone replacement therapy is not a contraceptive option for older women and the healthcare professional should be aware of the patient's particular needs.

Contraception in women with medical disorders

In the past, medical conditions were often regarded as a contraindication to both contraception and pregnancy. As treatment has improved and management of many medical disorders has been optimized, women who previously would not have considered pregnancy are now requesting contraception and pregnancy management. This involves interdisciplinary consultation and an understanding of the impact of pregnancy on the underlying condition and of the condition on pregnancy.

Pregnancy may trigger cardiovascular disease or escalate underlying problems such as autoimmune disorders (83, 84). It is essential that all healthcare providers are aware of the needs of the woman with medical disorders. In some situations pregnancy is totally contraindicated and the client and her partner need to be appropriately counselled. In many instances, improved medical care will result in stabilization of the patient and the possibility of pregnancy may be considered. It is essential that no pregnancy is unintended, that women are offered appropriate contraception until they desire pregnancy and that this contraceptive advice embraces the particular problems of their condition. In women with significant medical conditions it is essential that postpartum contraception is discussed and adequately implemented (85, 86).

The WHO MEC for contraceptive use offer a valuable resource to healthcare providers who are dealing with patients with medical problems. It is important that we recognize when pregnancy should be best postponed to optimize the medical condition, and when pregnancy is contraindicated as it will impact the mother's survival. Once women with medical disorders have completed their family, permanent or long-acting contraception should be considered (11).

Maternal death through an unintended pregnancy is a tragedy. It impacts not only the mother and her partner but also all the surviving children and results in higher infant and child mortality rates. Ensuring adequate and safe contraceptive provision to women with major medical disorders and ongoing medical input is a cornerstone of good reproductive healthcare.

Conclusion

The unmet need for contraception remains high in many settings. In addition, many women using contraception are not satisfied with their method which potentially puts them at risk for discontinuation without replacement with a more acceptable method, leading to unintended pregnancy.

Addressing unmet need remains a global priority. One of the health targets of the SDGs is to ensure that by 2030 universal access to sexual and reproductive healthcare services, including information and education about contraception, and the integration of reproductive health are incorporated into national strategies and programmes world-wide. The Family Planning 2020 commitment to action pledged to bring modern contraception within reach of an additional 120 million women and girls by the year 2020 and is supported by many funders and national governments. This may well provide the much needed expansion of contraceptive knowledge, accessibility, and use (87).

REFERENCES

1. United Nations. *The Millennium Development Goals Report: 2015*. New York: United Nations; 2015. Available at: http://www.un.org/milleniumgoals/2015_MDG_Report.

2. United Nations. Sustainable development. Available at: http://sustainabledevelopment.un.org.

3. Darroch JE, Singh S. Trends in contraceptive need and use in developing countries in 2005, 2008, 2012: an analysis of national surveys. *Lancet* 2013;**381**:1756–62.

4. Boden JM, Fergusson DM, Horwood LJ. Early motherhood and subsequent life outcomes. *J Child Psychol Psychiatry* 2008;**49**:151–60.

5. Sedgh G, Singh S, Hussain R. Intended and unintended pregnancies worldwide in 2012 and recent trends. *Stud Fam Plann* 2014;**45**:301–14.

6. Vollmer LR, van der Spuy ZM. Contraceptive usage and timing of pregnancy among pregnant teenagers in Cape Town, South Africa. *Int J Gynecol Obstet* 2016;**133**:334–37.

7. World Health Organization (WHO). *Ensuring Human Rights in the Provision of Contraceptive Information and Services: Guidance and Recommendations*. Geneva: WHO; 2014. Available at: http://apps.who.int/iris/bitstream/10665/102539/1/9789241506748_eng.pdf (accessed 10 September 2015).

8. Cottingham J, Germain A, Hunt P. Use of human rights to meet the unmet need for family planning. *Lancet* 2012;**380**:172–80.

9. Trussell J. Contraceptive efficacy. In: Hatcher RA, Trussell J, Nelson AL, Cates W, Dowal D, Policar M (eds), *Contraceptive Technology*, 20th rev edn, pp. 779–844. New York, NY: Argent Media; 2011.

10. World Health Organization. Medical eligibility criteria for contraceptive use, executive summary, 5th edn. 2015. Available at: http://apps.who.int/iris/bitstream/10665/172915/1/WHO_RHR_15.07_eng.pdf?ua=1&ua=1 (accessed 10 September 2015).

11. World Health Organization (WHO). *Medical Eligibility Criteria for Contraceptive Use: A WHO Family Planning Cornerstone*, 5th edn. Geneva: WHO; 2015. Available at: http://apps.who.int/iris/bitstream/10665/181468/1/9789241549158_eng.pdf?ua=1 (accessed 26 May 2016).

12. Meuck AO, Seeger H. Pharmacology of dienogest. *Gynaecol Forum* 2009;**14**:2.

13. Sitruk-Ware R. Pharmacological profile of progestins. *Maturitas* 2008;**61**:151–57.

14. Sitruk-Ware R. New progestagens for contraceptive use. *Hum Reprod Update* 2006;**12**:169–78.

15. Sitruk-Ware R, Nath A. The use of newer progestins for contraception. *Contraception* 2010;**82**:410–17.

16. Coney P, Washenik K, Langley RG, et al. Weight change and adverse event incidence with a low-dose oral contraceptive: two randomized, placebo-controlled trials. *Contraception* 2001;**63**:297–302.

17. Westhoff C, Morroni C, Kerns J, et al. Bleeding patterns after immediate vs. conventional oral contraceptive initiation: a randomized, controlled trial. *Fertil Steril* 2003;**79**:322–29.

18. Gallo M, Lopez L, Grimes D, et al. Combination contraceptives: effects on weight. *Cochrane Database Syst Rev* 2014;**1**:CD003987.

19. Dragoman, Monica V. The combined oral contraceptive pill- recent developments, risks and benefits. *Best Prac Res Clini Obstet Gynaecol* 2014;**28**:825–34.

20. Faculty of Sexual and Reproductive Healthcare of the Royal College of Obstetricians and Gynaecologists (FSRH). *UK Medical Eligibility Criteria for Contraceptive Use (UKMEC 2016)*. London: FSRH; 2016. Available at: https://www.fsrh.org/documents/ukmec-2016/ (accessed 25 May 2016).

21. National Department of Health, Republic of South Africa. National contraception clinical guidelines. 2012. Available at: https://www.gov.za/sites/default/files/gcis_document/201409/contraceptionclinicalguidelines28jan2013-2.pdf.

22. Van Vliet HA, Grimes DA, Helmerhorst FM, et al. Biphasic versus triphasic oral contraceptives for contraception. *Cochrane Database Syst Rev* 2006;**3**:CD003283.

23. Van Vliet HA, Grimes DA, Lopez LM, et al. Triphasic versus monophasic oral contraceptives for contraception. *Cochrane Database Syst Rev* 2006;**11**:CD003553.

24. World Health Organization (WHO). *Comparing Typical Effectiveness of Contraceptive Methods*. Geneva: WHO; 2006. Available at: http://www.fhi.org/nr/shared/enFHI/Resources/EffectivenessChart.pdf.

25. Li HWR, Lo SST, Ho PC. Emergency contraception. *Best Prac Res Clin Obstet Gynaecol* 2014;**28**:835–44.

26. Yuzpe AA, Thurlow HJ, Ramzy I, et al. Post coital contraception: a pilot study. *J Reprod Med* 1974;**13**:53–59.

27. Task Force on Postovulatory Methods of Fertility Regulation. Randomised controlled trial of levonorgestrel versus the Yuzpe regimen of combined oral contraceptives for emergency contraception. *Lancet* 1998;**352**:428–33.

28. Cleland K, Zhu H, Goldstuck N, Cheng L, Trussell J. The efficacy of intrauterine devices for emergency contraception: a systematic review of 35 years of experience. *Human Reprod* 2012;**37**:1994–2000.

29. Hamoda H, Ashok PW, Stalder C, Flett GMN, Kennedy E, Templeton A. A randomized trial of mifepristone (10mg) and levonorgestrel for emergency contraception. *Obstet Gynecol* 2004;**104**:1307–15.

30. Glasier A, Thong KJ, Dewar M, et al. Mifepristone (RU 486) compared with high-dose estrogen and progestogen for emergency contraception: a randomized trial. *N Engl J Med* 1992;**327**:1041–44.

31. Moreau C, Trussell J. Results from pooled phase III studies of ulipristal acetate for emergency contraception. *Contraception* 2012;**86**:673–80.

32. Noé G, Croxatto HB, Salvatierra AM, et al. Contraceptive efficacy of emergency contraception with levonorgestrel given before and after ovulation. *Contraception* 2010;**81**:414–20.

33. Trussell J. Contraceptive failure in the United States. *Contraception* 2011;**83**:397–404.

34. Peterson HB, Darmstadt GL, Bongaarts J, et al. Meeting the unmet need for family planning: now is the time. *Lancet* 2013;**381**;1696–99.

35. Glasier AF, Anakwe R, Everington D, et al. Would women trust their partners to use a male pill? *Hum Reprod* 2000;**15**:646–49.

36. Martin CW, Anderson RA, Cheng L, et al. Potential impact on hormonal male contraception: cross-cultural implications for development of novel preparations. *Hum Reprod* 2000;**15**:637–45.

37. Roth MY, Page ST, Bremner WJ. Male hormonal contraception: looking back and moving forward. *Andrology* 2016;**4**:4–12.

38. Wang C, Festin MPR, Swerdloff RS. Male hormonal contraception: where are we now? *Curr Obstet Gynecol Rep* 2016;**5**:38–47.

39. Chao J, Page ST, Anderson RA. Male contraception. *Best Prac Res Clin Obstet Gynaecol* 2014;**28**:845–57.

40. Faculty of Sexual and Reproductive Healthcare of the Royal College of Obstetricians and Gynaecologists (FSRH). *Intrauterine Contraception*. London: FSRH; 2015.

41. Kulier R, O'Brien P, Helmerhorst FM, Usher-Patel M, d'Arcangues C. Copper containing, framed intrauterine devices for contraception. *Cochrane Database Syst Rev* 2007;7;CD005347.

42. Farley TMM, Rosenberg MJ, Rowe P, Chen JH, Meirik O. Intrauterine devices and inflammatory disease: an international perspective. *Lancet* 1992;**339**:785–88.

43. Grimes DA, Schulz KF. Antibiotic prophylaxis for intrauterine contraceptive device insertion. *Cochrane Database of Syst Rev* 1999;3:CD001327.

44. Pile JM, Barone MA. Demographics of vasectomy – USA and international. *Urol Clin North Am* 2009;**36**:295–305.

45. Hardman SMR, Gebbie AE. The contraceptive needs of the perimenopausal woman. *Best Prac Res Clin Obstet Gynaecol* 2014;**28**:903–15.

46. Peterson HB, Xia Z, Highes JM, Wilcox IS, Tylor LR, Trussell J. The risk of pregnancy after tubal sterilization: findings from the US Collaborative Review of Sterilization. *Am J Obstet Gynecol* 1996;**174**:1611–70.

47. Black A, Guilbert E. Canadian Contraception Consensus (Part 2 of 4) [SOGC Clinical Practice Guideline No 329. November 2015]. *J Obstet Gynaecol Can* 2015;**37**:S1–39.

48. Kovacs GT, Krins AJ. Female sterilizations with Filshie clips: what is the risk of failure? A retrospective survey of 30 000 applications. *J Fam Plann Reprod Health Care* 2002;**28**:34–35.

49. Faculty of Sexual and Reproductive Healthcare of the Royal College of Obstetricians and Gynaecologists (FSRH). Male and female sterilisation summary of recommendations. 2014. Available at: http://www.fsrh.org/pdfs/MaleFemaleSterilisationSummary.pdf (accessed April 2016).

50. Moss C, Isley MM. Sterilization. A review and update. *Obstet Gynecol Clin N Am* 2015;**42**:713–24.

51. Beksinska M, Smit J, Mabude Z, Vijayakumar G, Joanis C. Performance of the Reality polyurethane female condom and a synthetic latex prototype: a randomized crossover trial among South African women. *Contraception* 2006;**73**:386–93.

52. Van Damme L, Ramjee G, Alary M, et al. Effectiveness of COL-1492, a nonoxynol-9 vaginal gel, on HIV-1 transmission in female sex workers: a randomised controlled trial. *Lancet* 2002;**360**:971–77.

53. Obiero J, Murethera PG, Hussey GD, Wiysonge CS. Vaginal microbicides for reducing the risk of sexual acquisition of HIV infection in women: systematic review and meta-analysis. *BMC Infect Dis* 2012;**12**:289.

54. Raymond EG, Trussell J, Weaver MA, Reeves MF. Estimating contraceptive efficacy: the case of spermicides. *Contraception* 2013;**87**:134–37.

55. Freundl G, Sivin I, Batár I. State-of-the-art of non-hormonal methods of contraception. *Eur J Contracept Reprod Health Care* 2010;**15**:113–23.

56. Arévalo M, Jennings V, Sinai I. Efficacy of a new method of family planning: the standard days method. *Contraception* 2002;**65**:333–38.

57. Oosterhoff P, Dkhar B, Albert S. Understanding unmet contraceptive needs among rural Khasi men and women in Meghalaya. *Cult Health Sex* 2015;**17**:1105–18.

58. Grimes DA, Gallo MF, Halpern V, Nanda K, Schulz KF, Lopez LM. Fertility awareness-based methods for contraception. *Cochrane Database Syst Rev* 2004;**4**:CD004860.

59. Winner B, Peipert JF, Qiuhong Z, et al. Effectiveness of long- acting reversible contraception. *N Eng J Med* 2012;**366**:1998–2007.

60. Kluge J, Steyn PS. Long acting reversible contraception. *Obstet Gynaecol Forum* 2010;**20**:21–27.

61. Conde-Agudelo A, Rosas-Bermúdez A, Kafury-Goeta AC. Birth spacing and risk of adverse perinatal outcomes: a meta-analysis. *JAMA* 2006;**295**:1809–23.

62. Conde-Agudelo A, Rosas-Bermúdez A, Kafury-Goeta AC. Effects of birth spacing on maternal health: a systematic review. *Am J Obstet Gynecol* 2007;**196**:297–308.

63. Steyn PS, Goldstuck NM. Postpartum contraception. *Obstet Gynaecol Forum* 2013;**23**:9–13.

64. National Institute for Health and Care Excellence (NICE). *Postnatal Care up to 8 Weeks after Birth*. Clinical guideline [CG37], last updated February 2015. London: NICE; 2006. Available at: https://www.nice.org.uk/guidance/cg37.

65. Royal College of Obstetricians and Gynaecologists (RCOG). *Leading Safe Choices: Best Practice in Postpartum Family Planning*. Best Practice Paper No. 1. London: RCOG; 2015.

66. Goldstuck ND, Steyn PS. Intrauterine contraception after cesarean section and during lactation: a systematic review. *Int J Womens Health* 2013;**5**:811–18.

67. Royal College of Obstetricians and Gynaecologists (RCOG). *Leading Safe Choices: Best Practice in Comprehensive Abortion Care*. Best Practice Paper No. 2. London: RCOG; 2015.

68. World health Organization. Hormonal contraceptive eligibility for women at high risk of HIV Guidance–Recommendations concerning the use of hormonal contraceptive methods by women at high risk of HIV (2017). https://www.who.int/reproductivehealth/publications/family_planning/HC-and-HIV-2017/en/ (accessed 28 July 2019).

69. Polis CB, Curtis KM, Hannaford P, et al. Update on hormonal contraceptive methods and risk of HIV acquisition in women: a systematic review of epidemiological evidence. *AIDS* 2016;**30**(17):2665–83.

70. Steyn PS, Goldstuck ND. Contraceptive needs of the adolescent. *Best Pract Res Clin Obstet Gynaecol* 2014;**28**:891–901.

71. Dodson NA, Gray SN, Burke PJ. Teen pregnancy prevention on a LARC: an update on long- acting reversible contraception for the primary care provider. *Curr Opin Paediatr* 2012;**24**:439–45.

72. McNicholas C, Peipert JF. Long acting reversible contraception for adolescents. *Curr Opin Obstet Gynecol* 2012;**24**:293–98.

73. Lumsden MA, Gebbie A, Holland C. Managing unscheduled bleeding in non-pregnant premenopausal women. *BMJ* 2013;**346**:f3251.

74. Gebbie AE, Glasier A, Sweeting V. Incidence of ovulation in perimenopausal women before and during replacement therapy. *Contraception* 1995;**52**:221–22.

75. Beksinska ME, Smit JA, Kleinschmidt I, Farlay TMM. Assessing menopausal status in women aged 40-49 using depot-medroxyprogesterone acetate, norethisterone enantiate or combined oral contraception. *S Afr Med J* 2011;**101**:131–34.

76. Vessey M, Yeates D. Oral contraceptive use and cancer: final report from the Oxford-Family Planning Association Contraceptive Study. *Contraception* 2013;**88**:678–83.

77. Cibula P, Gompel A, Mueck AO, et al. Hormonal contraception and risk of cancer. *Hum Reprod Update* 2010;**16**:631–50.

78. Wilailak S, Vipupinyo C, Suraseramvong V, et al. Depot medroxyprogesterone acetate and epithelial ovarian cancer: a multicentre case-control study. *BJOG* 2012;**119**:672–77.

79. Blümel JE, Castelo-Branco C, Binfa L, Aparicio R, Mamami L. A scheme of combined oral contraceptives for women more than 40 years old. *Menopause* 2001;**8**:286–89.

80. Faculty of Sexual and Reproductive Healthcare of the Royal College of Obstetricians and Gynaecologists (FSRH). Contraception for women aged over 40 years. 2010. Available at: http://www.fsrh.org/pdfs/ContraceptionOver40July10.pdf (accessed April 2016).

81. Stegeman BH, de Bastos M, Rosendaal FR, et al. Different combined oral contraceptives and the risk of venous thrombosis: systematic review and network meta-analysis. *BMJ* 2013;**347**: fS298.

82. Mansour D, Korver T, Marintcheva-Petrova, Fraser IS. The effects of Implanon® on bleeding patterns. *Eur J Contracept Reprod Health Care* 2008;**13** Suppl 1:13–28.

83. Espey E, Ogburn T, Fotieo D. Contraception: what every internist should know. *Med Clin N Am* 2008;**92**:1037–58.

84. Sliwa K, Anthony J. Late maternal deaths: a neglected responsibility. *Lancet* 2016;**387f**:2072–73.

85. Thorne S, Nelson-Piercy C, MacGregor A, et al. Pregnancy and contraception in heart disease and pulmonary arterial hypertension. *J Fam Plann Reprod Health Care* 2006;**32**:75–81.

86. Folger SG, Curtis KM, Tepper NK, Gaffield ME, Marchbanks PA. Guidance on medical eligibility criteria for contraceptive use: identification of research gaps. *Contraception* 2010;**82**:113–18.

87. Family Planning 2020. Accelerating access. Available at: http://www.familyplanning2020.org/ (accessed 30 May 2016).

54

Termination of pregnancy

Hang Wun Raymond Li and Pak Chung Ho

Introduction

Although effective contraceptive methods are widely available nowadays, contraceptive omissions or failures do occur at times because of various reasons, resulting in unplanned pregnancies. With unplanned pregnancies, women may choose to terminate the pregnancies. Even when pregnancies are planned and wanted, there may be situations such as fetal abnormalities or maternal medical conditions when termination of the pregnancy is indicated. Nonetheless, in many parts of the world, legal restrictions and administrative barriers may deny access to safe abortions. As a result, women with unwanted pregnancies may have to resort to unsafe illegal abortion procedures which can result in significant morbidity or even mortality.

According to the World Health Organization (WHO) definition, unsafe abortion refers to a procedure for terminating an unintended pregnancy carried out by persons lacking the necessary skills and/or in an environment that does not conform to minimal medical standards. It has been estimated that about 43.8 million induced abortions took place worldwide in 2008, out of which 21.5 million were unsafe, and about 13% of all maternal deaths were the result of unsafe abortions. The majority of unsafe abortions happened in developing countries (1, 2). Unsafe abortion is actually an avoidable tragedy. Removal of the various barriers to accessing proper facilities for safe abortion for the women in need, as well as adherence to established evidence-based guidelines, is important to minimize complications.

While the regulations on legal abortions are diverse among different countries, it is unusual, even in countries with restrictive laws on abortions, to prohibit abortions under all circumstances. Most countries would allow abortions to save mothers' lives or when there is a significant fetal abnormality. Physicians should be familiar with the local laws, and make full use of the legal indications to help women obtain legal abortions. It is of paramount importance that every physician should be able to provide the appropriate preliminary counselling in a non-judgemental manner to women who are requesting termination of pregnancy, and to help the women make their informed decision within the provisions of the legal constraints. If a doctor has conscientious objection on ethical or religious grounds to provide counselling or treatment for induced abortions, such a doctor should be obliged to refer the woman to another colleague who, in one's good faith, will be able to provide unbiased counselling.

About two-thirds of major complications from induced abortions are attributable to those performed in the second trimester. As the risk of complications increases with gestation when an abortion is carried out, healthcare facilities should facilitate early assessment of women referred for termination of pregnancy and avoid unnecessary delays as far as possible. Due to the higher risk of serious complications, second-trimester abortions should be carried out in a healthcare facility with access to blood transfusion and emergency laparotomy.

Pre-abortion counselling and assessment

History taking

It is important to explore the circumstances leading to the unintended pregnancy and the reason(s) why contraceptive failure has occurred. A properly taken contraceptive history forms the basis for further education and counselling on proper family planning and safe sex in future. A social history of the woman and preferably that of her partner(s) should be obtained. The menstrual history aids in determining the dating of her gestation. The past obstetric and gynaecological history, sexual history, as well as past medical history need to be noted as these may have relevance to the subsequent management of the pregnancy, be it continued or terminated.

The counselling process

The aim of counselling is to help the woman (or the couple) make an informed decision on the management of the unintended pregnancy. The interview should be conducted in adequate privacy, with confidentiality respected and emphasized. The counsellor should demonstrate an understanding, empathetic, and non-judgemental attitude, with care taken in the counselling process not to imply accusation of the woman being immoral, sexually irresponsible, or to induce guilt feeling. Alternatives to terminating the pregnancy, including continuation of the pregnancy and rearing the child or having the baby adopted, should be discussed. Support from partners and family should be explored, and yet the autonomy of the woman on her final decision should be maintained. Any suggestion that the woman has been a victim of sexual abuse or been coerced to make a decision either way should be tactfully attended to. Social security aids may be explored in cases of financial difficulties. Referral to professional counsellors or social workers may be indicated in case of undue ambivalence or adverse social circumstances being identified.

When the woman or couple makes an informed decision for termination of pregnancy, the decision should be respected. The woman should then be informed of the details of the abortion procedure, including the logistics, treatment method, risks, and long-term complications. A future contraceptive plan needs to be formulated.

Pre-abortion medical assessment and preparation

After an informed decision for induced abortion is made, a careful clinical assessment should be carried out as follows:

1. A proper *medical, drug, and allergy history* should be taken and documented. This may have influence on the choice of the abortion method.

2. A *pregnancy test* should be performed, if not yet done, to confirm pregnancy state.

3. Testing for *haemoglobin level* may be done to exclude pre-existing anaemia, although the evidence is inconsistent as for whether it improves health outcomes (3)

4. Testing for *rhesus type* should be performed in women undergoing medical abortion after 10 weeks of gestation or surgical abortion, in order that rhesus-negative women are given anti-D immunoglobulin prophylaxis postabortion.

5. *Prevention of infective complications*: screening for sexually transmitted infections or empirical antibiotic prophylaxis for sexually transmitted infections should be offered. Postabortion infection is usually caused by pre-existing lower genital tract infection, the risk of which can be significantly reduced either by bacterial screening or administration of antibiotic prophylaxis. Either universal antibiotic prophylaxis, or universal screening and treatment of positive cases (the 'screen-and-treat' approach), or both, can be adopted for prevention of infective complications.

   Various prophylactic antibiotic regimens have been recommended around the world. Although it remains unclear which regimen is the most optimal, it should be one that covers against *Chlamydia trachomatis* and anaerobes. The following regimens are recommended by the United Kingdom Royal College of Obstetricians and Gynaecologists (RCOG) (3):

   - Azithromycin 1 g orally on the day of abortion plus metronidazole 800 mg orally or 1 g rectally prior to or during the abortion procedure, *or*

   - Doxycycline 100 mg orally twice daily for 7 days starting on the day of abortion plus metronidazole 800 mg orally or 1 g rectally prior to or during the abortion procedure, *or*

   - Metronidazole 800 mg orally or 1 g rectally prior to or during the abortion procedure in women who have been tested negative for chlamydial infection.

   The single-dose regimen has the advantage of minimizing compliance problems. There are inconsistent opinions on whether prophylactic antibiotics should be applicable similarly for medical abortion, although the RCOG recommends this regardless of the abortion method in the context of service delivery in the United Kingdom. In the new UK NICE Guideline (2019), metronidazole is not routinely recommended together with another broad-spectrum antibiotic, and antibiotic prophylaxis is only indicated for medical abortion in women with increased risk of sexually transmitted infections. Further research is needed to explore for the best regimen.

While routine universal antibiotic prophylaxis is one acceptable approach, some suggested that the 'screen-and-treat' approach is more economical and appropriate. The RCOG actually recommends screening for *C. trachomatis* for all women undergoing induced abortion (3). Such a 'belt and braces' approach (i.e. combining both universal antibiotic prophylaxis and universal screening), if resources allow, would minimize the possibility of missing the diagnosis of infected women and hence the opportunity of initiating contact tracing and treatment in such cases. Screening for other sexually transmitted infections including HIV should also be considered as appropriate when risk factors are identified in the history.

With regard to treatment, uncomplicated chlamydial infection can be treated with azithromycin 1 g single oral dose or doxycycline 100 mg twice daily for 7 days, whereas bacterial vaginosis can be treated with metronidazole 2 g single oral dose or 400 mg twice daily for 5–7 days (3).

6. *Dating of gestational age*: gestational age should be determined by menstrual history and pelvic examination. A Cochrane review did suggest that routine ultrasonography improves gestational dating in early pregnancy (4), and yet it would add to the costs and may pose a limitation to the delivery of the abortion service, especially in lower-resources settings. Moreover, a small discrepancy may not alter the clinical outcome of treatment (5, 6). Therefore, pre-abortion pelvic ultrasound scanning is not recommended by RCOG as a routine (3), although it should be available for selected cases to ascertain the gestational age, fetal viability, and location of pregnancy when clinically indicated, for instance, when there is significant discrepancy between menstrual date and uterine size or when the woman reports vaginal bleeding or abdominal pain to exclude conditions such as miscarriage, hydatidiform moles, or ectopic pregnancies. When ultrasound scanning is performed, a systematic review (7) considered it acceptable to allow the woman to see the pre-abortion ultrasound image if it is opted for.

7. Women who are indicated for *cervical screening* but have not had one within the recommended interval should be provided with the screening opportunity or be reminded of it.

Abortion methods

First-trimester termination (at or below 12 weeks of gestation)

Both surgical and medical methods are available for termination of first-trimester pregnancies.

Surgical abortion

For surgical abortion, suction evacuation (vacuum aspiration) is performed for gestation under 12 weeks. While electrical vacuum aspiration is the most common method, manual vacuum aspiration is another alternative where the negative pressure is generated by a hand-held syringe attached to the suction curette; the latter is more suitable for earlier gestations. Both electrical vacuum aspiration and manual vacuum aspiration are superior to sharp curettage for surgical abortion (3, 8).

Cervical priming with misoprostol 400 mcg vaginally given 3 hours before operation is recommended to reduce cervical trauma during mechanical dilatation. Such a regimen has been proven effective, although misoprostol is not licensed for such a purpose, and it can result in uterine cramps, bleeding, and unexpected expulsion of the gestational products. A recent study showed that when misoprostol 400 mcg was given sublingually 1 hour before vacuum aspiration, it is still effective in dilating the cervix. The shortened interval will make it easier to organize a day-care abortion service (9). Non-steroidal anti-inflammatory drugs (NSAIDs) can be used for relief of pain encountered during misoprostol cervical priming without reducing its efficacy (10).

Pain control can be achieved by either general anaesthesia or local anaesthesia. Local anaesthesia has the advantage of being less costly, independent of theatre personnel and anaesthetists, and being associated with less anaesthesia-related complications. It can be achieved by paracervical block or topical anaesthetic jelly, and can be coupled with intravenous conscious sedation or Entonox inhalation as an adjunct (8, 11, 12).

Intraoperatively, an aseptic technique should be observed and the cervix should be cleansed with antiseptic before uterine instrumentation (8). A bimanual examination should be performed to assess the size and direction of the uterus. The cervix is dilated gradually to a size, which can allow a suction catheter of a size in millimetres corresponding to the gestational age in weeks. The suction cannula is inserted gently until the fundus of the uterus is reached. Negative pressure is applied and the suction cannula is rotated to evacuate the uterine contents, until a 'gritty' sensation resulting from the clamping down of the emptied uterus around the cannula is felt. Uterotonic medications such as oxytocin should not be routinely used during vacuum aspiration as significant reduction of blood loss was not demonstrated in randomized trials, but may be considered in cases where bleeding is heavy. The procedure should not be completed by sharp curettage. The aspirated tissue should be inspected for the presence of gestational products. When gestational tissue can be visualized, routine histopathological examination of the tissue obtained at abortion is not recommended as it has limited clinical value (13). In case of uncertainty, however, particularly for early abortions before 7 weeks, histopathological examination may be indicated.

Acute complications of surgical abortion include anaesthetic-related complications, vasovagal reaction, cervical and lower genital tract injury, excessive haemorrhage, as well as uterine perforation which can be associated with visceral damage. Delayed surgical complications may include endometritis and pelvic infection, secondary bleeding, retained products of conception, cervical stenosis or incompetence, and Asherman syndrome.

Medical abortion

For medical abortion, the use of mifepristone followed by misoprostol 24–48 hours later is the recommended regimen. Mifepristone is a synthetic compound which blocks the progesterone receptor. Its introduction has revolutionized the method of medical abortions. When used alone, mifepristone can induce first-trimester abortion with an efficacy of only around 60%. However, it can sensitize the myometrium to the action of prostaglandins and their sequential use can achieve abortion with high effectiveness. Misoprostol is a prostaglandin E1 analogue which was initially marketed as a treatment for peptic ulcers, but was subsequently studied widely as an effective agent for abortion treatment. It should be noted, however, that such use is outside the product licence. Compared to other prostaglandin analogues, misoprostol is the superior choice for inducing abortion because it is highly effective, much cheaper, easily available, stable at room temperature, and is active through diverse routes of administration including the oral, vaginal, sublingual, and buccal routes (14).

The regimens recommended by WHO are as follows (8):

- For pregnancies at or below 7 weeks: mifepristone 200 mg, given as a single oral dose, followed 24–48 hours later by a single oral dose of misoprostol 400 mcg.
- For pregnancies between 7 and 9 weeks: mifepristone 200 mg, given as a single oral dose, followed 24–48 hours later by misoprostol 800 mcg as a single vaginal, buccal, or sublingual dose.
- For pregnancies between 9 and 12 weeks: mifepristone 200 mg, given as a single oral dose, followed 36–48 hours later by misoprostol 800 mcg given vaginally, and then up to a maximum of four further doses of misoprostol 400 mcg every 3 hours given through either the vaginal or sublingual (if there is significant vaginal bleeding) route.

It has been shown that vaginal misoprostol is more effective and has a lower incidence of side effects than oral misoprostol when combined with mifepristone in medical abortion, achieving a high complete abortion rate of over 95% (15). Both sublingual and vaginal administration result in similar abortion rates without vaginal bleeding, although the sublingual route produces higher incidence of side effects (16). It has been shown that shortening of the mifepristone–misoprostol interval to 24 hours does not diminish the complete abortion rate (17, 18), and hence can be considered to suit logistic needs.

Since mifepristone is not available in many countries, the use of prostaglandin alone has been studied for medical abortion. When used alone, vaginal misoprostol is more effective than oral misoprostol; it can be administered at 800 mcg up to three doses at 6-, 12-, or 24-hour intervals, and the complete abortion rate varied between 60% and 90% (19). In situations where the vaginal route is not preferred, sublingual misoprostol at 3-hourly frequency is a reasonable alternative, although there can be more side effects (19). Abortion rates are reported at around 80% and 95% by 24 and 48 hours after administration of misoprostol, and failed abortion occurs in about 4–8% of cases for gestations up to 9 weeks.

Depending on the local laws, misoprostol can be administered either as in-patient or out-patient. In the latter case, the patient should be taught to monitor for and report complications, and follow-up care should be arranged to ascertain completeness of abortion.

Women with incomplete abortion can be offered the options of surgical evacuation or a repeat course of misoprostol. Side effects of mifepristone such as heavy bleeding, allergic reaction, and gastrointestinal upset may uncommonly occur. Misoprostol is generally safe and well tolerated, although uterine cramps and bleeding are inevitably encountered, and other common minor side effects may

Table 54.1 Comparison between medical and surgical abortion methods in the first trimester

Medical abortion	Surgical abortion
Usually avoids an invasive procedure; no risk of cervical or uterine injury	More invasive procedure; a small risk of cervical or uterine injury
No anaesthesia is required	Anaesthesia with or without sedation is required
Days to weeks to complete the abortion	Quick procedure, with evacuation accomplished in one go
Complete abortion rate around 95%	Complete abortion rate around 99%
Requires follow-up to ensure completion of abortion if misoprostol alone is used. No routine follow up is required if mifepristone plus misoprostol is used	No routine follow-up is required
Controlled by the women, more autonomy and privacy, may be home based (subject to local laws)	More dependent on healthcare professionals, less autonomy and privacy

include fever, chills, gastrointestinal upset, and diarrhoea, which are transient and self-limiting. NSAIDs can be used for controlling these side effects without affecting the efficacy (20). Paracetamol is not an effective pain relief for abortion. Serious complications such as excessive haemorrhage, anaphylaxis, and septicaemia rarely occur. Once started, termination of pregnancy has to proceed since multiple congenital defects have been reported with misoprostol exposure in early pregnancy (**Table 54.1**), notably the Mobius syndrome, although the absolute risk is only around the order of 1% (21).

Second-trimester termination (beyond 12 weeks of gestation)

Older methods such as intra-amniotic injection of hypertonic saline, urea, or ethacridine lactate is no longer recommended nowadays as these methods are more invasive, less effective than prostaglandins, and associated with a higher incidence of serious complications such as disseminated intravascular coagulopathy. Dilatation and evacuation in the second trimester can be a safe and effective procedure if performed by experienced personnel. The medical method, however, is more commonly adopted for second-trimester abortions. Hysterotomy or hysterectomy are reserved as a surgical abortion method for special circumstances only.

Surgical method (dilatation and evacuation)

It is recommended that dilatation and evacuation (D&E) can be a safe method for second-trimester abortion if it is performed by personnel with appropriate training and experience (3, 8). Preoperative cervical priming is essential. Osmotic dilators such as Lamicel or Dilapan are recommended for the purpose, although misoprostol is an acceptable alternative up to 18 weeks of gestation.

Anaesthesia, aseptic technique, and cervical cleansing with antiseptic are carried out similarly to first-trimester surgical abortions. Careful cervical dilatation up to 12–16 mm is required. Amniotic fluid aspiration followed by evacuation of fetal parts is carried out with a large suction cannula (14–16 mm) aided by forceps. The evacuated products should be inspected to confirm

completeness. Haemorrhage is the most common complication of D&E; uterotonics can be used to control intraoperative bleeding. Other complications may include cervical tear, uterine perforation, incomplete evacuation, and postoperative infection. Continuous ultrasound guidance during the D&E procedure is recommended to reduce the risk of surgical complications such as uterine perforation (3, 8, 22).

Medical method

The medical method using misoprostol with or without mifepristone priming is a widely recommended and adopted means for second-trimester induced abortions. Misoprostol stimulates the uterus to contract, leading eventually to the expulsion of the conceptus, like a 'mini-labour' with durations varying among individuals. Where available, pretreatment with mifepristone can sensitize the uterus to the effect of prostaglandins.

The recommended regimen is oral mifepristone 200 mg followed by vaginal misoprostol 800 mcg (or oral misoprostol 400 mcg) 36–48 hours later, and subsequently vaginal or sublingual misoprostol 400 mcg every 3 hours up to a maximum of four more doses (8). It has been shown that shortening the mifepristone–misoprostol interval to 12–24 hours instead of 36–48 hours resulted in only a slightly longer induction time (misoprostol–abortion interval) by 1–2 hour, but the overall abortion time (mifepristone–abortion interval) would be shorter (23); this is an acceptable alternative to accommodate individual patient or healthcare provider's preference. The effectiveness is significantly lower if mifepristone is given at the same time as misoprostol (24). The average induction–abortion interval with this regimen is around 6 hours, with an abortion rate of 97% within 24 hours.

When mifepristone is not available, vaginal or sublingual misoprostol 400 mcg can be used alone every 3 hours for a maximum of five doses. Compared to when there is mifepristone priming, this has a longer induction–abortion interval (10–15 hours) and lower abortion rate (80–90%) within 24 hours, but is still considered an effective method. In case of significant vaginal bleeding, the vaginal route can be replaced by sublingual or oral routes. Women who fail to abort after 24 hours can be given a second course of misoprostol 12 hours after the last dose, and if it still fails, other prostaglandins or oxytocin can be used. For gestations beyond 20 weeks, the dose or frequency of prostaglandins should be reduced since the uterine sensitivity to prostaglandins increases with advancing gestation (although there is little evidence for the best regimen), and intracardiac injection of potassium chloride to the fetus to achieve fetal demise is also recommended before prostaglandin induction.

The most common side effects related to prostaglandin use include nausea, vomiting, fever, chills, diarrhoea, and occasionally heavy haemorrhage. Infection and allergic reaction are uncommon complications after medical abortion. Uterine rupture is a rare but potentially fatal complication, with an incidence of 0.28% in women with previous caesarean delivery who undergo second-trimester abortion using misoprostol. Analgesia can be provided by NSAIDs without compromising the efficacy of prostaglandins; narcotics can be used if necessary. Oxytocin infusion can be given to aid placental expulsion if not occurring 2 hours after expulsion of the fetus. Surgical evacuation is necessary only if bleeding is severe or placenta is retained.

Postabortion care

Rhesus prophylaxis

Anti-D immunoglobulin should be given to the deltoid muscle to rhesus D-negative women within 72 hours following surgical abortion or medical abortion after 10 weeks of gestation to prevent sensitization. The recommended dose is 250 IU for abortions before 20 weeks, and 500 IU thereafter. After abortions beyond 20 weeks of gestation, the Kleihauer test is recommended to assess the size of fetal–maternal haemorrhage, and if this is more than 4 mL, an additional dose of 125 IU/mL should be given (25). It may be noted that because of lack of good evidence, rhesus testing or anti-D prophylaxis is not recommended for medical abortion before 10 weeks of gestation by the new UK NICE Guideline (2019).

Information to the client

Upon discharge from the abortion facility, the women should be given instructions on the expected side effects and when to seek further medical assessment. This should include symptoms of complications which should necessitate urgent medical attention, as well as symptoms of continued pregnancy for which further management should be sought. A written document stating the treatment procedure received would facilitate the seeking of management from other healthcare providers for any complications arising from the abortion. A plan of future contraception should be discussed and formulated before discharge from the abortion service. Information on long-acting reversible contraceptive methods should be provided.

Postabortion contraception

A full range of contraceptive methods should be available at the abortion service and provided immediately after abortion if applicable. An intrauterine contraceptive device can be inserted immediately after induced abortion as long as continued pregnancy is reasonably excluded; delaying the insertion to a later time has been shown to reduce uptake of the method (26, 27). If the insertion has to be delayed, an effective interim method should be provided. Hormonal contraceptives can be started right after the abortion (28, 29). Female sterilization can be safely performed at the same time following the induced abortion unless there is a serious complication such as sepsis, severe haemorrhage, or genital tract trauma. However, a higher risk of regret and failure may be the result (3, 29).

Follow-up care

Routine follow-up is not mandatory after surgical abortion or medical abortion where mifepristone has been used (3, 8). However, a follow-up visit can be arranged if complete abortion cannot be ascertained, or if the woman has any concern about incomplete abortion or has other issues to discuss with the healthcare personnel.

During the follow-up visit, the healthcare worker needs to assess for complications from the abortion procedure, including symptoms and signs of failed or incomplete abortion and infective complications. An ultrasound scan should not be routinely performed at follow-up. Interventions to manage incomplete abortions should be decided based on clinical signs and symptoms, but not on ultrasound findings. The sonographic presence of intrauterine material correlates poorly with subsequent symptoms of incomplete abortion, and this need not be acted upon if the woman is asymptomatic; most of them can resolve spontaneously without clinical sequelae (30–32). The main indication for a pelvic ultrasound examination is to exclude the possibility of an ongoing pregnancy.

Besides, a proper ongoing contraceptive plan should be reinforced. Compliance and problems with contraceptive use should be assessed. Women engaged in high-risk sexual behaviours should be counselled on safe sex. For those diagnosed with a sexually transmitted infection, proper treatment as well as contact tracing, screening, and/or treatment of partners should be assured. Psychological morbidities such as emotional problems, guilt, or regret, as well as social problems, should be attended to as well.

Conclusion

Contraceptive failures and hence unintended pregnancies do occur even in the modern world. The availability of safe abortion within the legal constraints can help in minimizing the morbidities and mortalities associated with the management of unintended pregnancies. Providers of abortion service should be familiarized with the updated evidence-based guidelines. Induced abortion should never be regarded as a contraceptive method, and proper contraceptive counselling before and after the abortion procedure is essential.

REFERENCES

1. World Health Organization (WHO). *Unsafe Abortion: Global and Regional Estimates of the Incidence of Unsafe Abortion and Associated Mortality in 2008*, 6th edn. Geneva: WHO; 2011.
2. World Health Organization (WHO). *Safe and Unsafe Induced Abortion: Global and Regional Levels in 2008, and Trends during 1995–2008*. Geneva: WHO; 2012.
3. Royal College of Obstetricians and Gynaecologists (RCOG). *The Care of Women Requesting Induced Abortion*. Evidence-based Clinical Guideline No. 7. London: RCOG; 2011.
4. Whitworth M, Bricker L, Neilson JP, Dowswell T. Ultrasound for fetal assessment in early pregnancy. *Cochrane Database Syst Rev* 2010;4:CD007058.
5. Bracken H, Clark W, Lichtenberg ES, et al. Alternatives to routine ultrasound for eligibility assessment prior to early termination of pregnancy with mifepristone–misoprostol. *BJOG* 2011;**118**:17–23.
6. Kaneshiro B, Edelman A, Sneeringer RK, Ponce de Leon RG. Expanding medical abortion: can medical abortion be effectively provided without the routine use of ultrasound? *Contraception* 2011;**83**:194–201.
7. Kulier R, Kapp N. Comprehensive analysis of the use of preprocedure ultrasound for first- and second-trimester abortion. *Contraception* 2011;**83**:30–33.
8. World Health Organization (WHO). *Clinical Practice Handbook for Safe Abortion*. Geneva: WHO; 2014.
9. Sääv I, Kopp Kallner H, Fiala C, Gemzell-Danielsson K. Sublingual versus vaginal misoprostol for cervical dilatation 1 or 3 h prior to surgical abortion: a double-blinded RCT. *Hum Reprod* 2015;**30**:1314–22.
10. Li CFI, Wong CYG, Chan CP, Ho PC. A study of co-treatment of nonsteroidal anti-inflammatory drugs (NSAIDs) with misoprostol for cervical priming before suction termination of first trimester pregnancy. *Contraception* 2003;**67**:101–105.

11. Li HWR, Wong CYG, Lo SST, Fan SYS. Effect of local lignocaine gel application for pain relief during suction termination of first-trimester pregnancy: a randomized controlled trial. *Hum Reprod* 2006;**21**:1461–66.

12. Kan ASY, Ho PC. Pain control in first-trimester suction evacuation. *IPPF Med Bull* 2006;**40**:4.

13. Royal College of Pathologists (RCPath). *Histopathology of Limited or No Clinical Value: Report of a Working Group*, 2nd edn. London: RCPath; 2005.

14. Li HWR, Ng EHY, Ho PC. Clinical applications of misoprostol in gynaecology. *J Paed Obstet Gynaecol* 2010;**36**:81–88.

15. el-Refaey H, Rajasekar D, Abdalla M, Calder L, Templeton A. Induction of abortion with mifepristone (RU 486) and oral or vaginal misoprostol. *N Engl J Med* 1995;**332**:983–87.

16. Tang OS, Chan CC, Ng EH, Lee SW, Ho PC. A prospective, randomized, placebo-controlled trial on the use of mifepristone with sublingual or vaginal misoprostol for medical abortions of less than 9 weeks gestation. *Hum Reprod* 2003;**18**:2315–18.

17. Schaff EA, Fielding SL, Westhoff C, et al. Vaginal misoprostol administered 1, 2, or 3 days after mifepristone for early medical abortion: a randomized trial. *JAMA* 2000;**284**:1948–53.

18. von Hertzen H, Piaggio G, Wojdyla D, et al. Two mifepristone doses and two intervals of misoprostol administration for termination of early pregnancy: a randomised factorial controlled equivalence trial. *BJOG* 2009;**116**:381–89.

19. Faúndes A, Fiala C, Tang OS, Velasco A. Misoprostol for the termination of pregnancy up to 12 completed weeks of pregnancy. *Int J Gynaecol Obstet* 2007;**99** Suppl 2:S172–77.

20. Fiala C, Swahn ML, Stephansson O, Gemzell-Danielsson K. The effect of non-steroidal anti-inflammatory drugs on medical abortion with mifepristone and misoprostol at 13-22 weeks gestation. *Hum Reprod* 2005;**20**:3072–77.

21. Tang OS, Gemzell-Danielsson K, Ho PC. Misoprostol: pharmacokinetic profiles, effects on the uterus and side-effects. *Int J Gynaecol Obstet* 2007;**99** Suppl 2:S160–67.

22. Lee VCY, Ng EHY, Ho PC. Issues in second trimester induced abortion (medical/surgical methods). *Best Pract Res Clin Obstet Gynaecol* 2010;**24**:517–27.

23. Shaw KA, Topp NJ, Shaw JG, Blumenthal PD. Mifepristone-misoprostol dosing interval and effect on induction abortion times: a systematic review. *Obstet Gynecol* 2013;**121**:1335–47.

24. Chai J, Tang OS, Hong QQ, Chen QF, Cheng LN, Ng E, Ho PC. A randomized trial to compare two dosing intervals of misoprostol following mifepristone administration in second trimester medical abortion. *Hum Reprod* 2009;**24**:320–24.

25. Royal College of Obstetricians and Gynaecologists. *The Use of Anti-D Immunoglobulin for Rhesus D Prophylaxis*. London: RCOG; 2011.

26. Stanek AM, Bednarek PH, Nichols MD, Jenson JT, Edelman AB. Barriers associated with the failure to return for intrauterine device insertion following first-trimester abortion. *Contraception* 2009;**79**:216–20.

27. Grimes DA, Lopez LM, Schulz KF, Stanwood NL. Immediate postabortal insertion of intrauterine devices. *Cochrane Database Syst Rev* 2010;**6**:CD001777.

28. Gaffield ME, Kapp N, Ravi A. Use of combined oral contraceptives post abortion. *Contraception* 2009;**80**:355–62.

29. World Health Organization. *Medical Eligibility Criteria for Contraceptive Use*. Geneva: WHO; 2015.

30. McEwing RL, Anderson NG, Meates JB, Allen RB, Phillipson GT, Wells JE. Sonographic appearances of the endometrium after termination of pregnancy in asymptomatic versus symptomatic women. *J Ultrasound Med* 2009;**28**:579–86.

31. Rufener SL, Adusumilli S, Weadock WJ, Caoili E. Sonography of uterine abnormalities in postpartum and postabortion patients: a potential pitfall of interpretation. *J Ultrasound Med* 2008;**27**:343–48.

32. Cheung KW, Ngu SF, Cheung VYT. Sonographic characteristics of the uterus in asymptomatic women after second-trimester medical termination of pregnancy. *J Ultrasound Med* 2015;**34**:611–16.

55

Violence against women and girls

Tonye Wokoma and Stephen Lindow

Definition of violence against women and girls

Violence against women as defined by the United Nations Declaration on the Elimination of Violence against Women (1993) amounts to 'any act of gender-based violence that results in, or is likely to result in, physical, sexual or psychological harm or suffering to women, including threats of such acts, coercion or arbitrary deprivation of liberty, whether occurring in public or in private life' (1). In this definition, violence is given its gender-related status and constructed as a problem which facilitates the enduring subjugation of women in society.

As well as being a violation of individual rights, violence against women and girls prevents them from flourishing and contributing to their families and communities. It thus has an impact on the economic and social well-being of any society. It also holds back progress on international development targets (2).

Violence against women and girls encompasses rape in conflict, female genital mutilation, stalking and harassment, child sexual abuse, 'honour'-based violence, forced marriage, and domestic violence. It has physical, sexual, psychological, and economic consequences.

This chapter examines the health issues relating to violence against women and girls, the steps taken so far to prevent and cater for health implications, and suggests a way forward.

Importance and relevance

Violence against women and girls is a global problem of epidemic proportions affecting many millions of women. It is receiving increasing global recognition and attention resulting in the development of policy both locally within the United Kingdom and globally as a means to tackle the growing problem of violence against women and girls. Past and current studies have provided insight into its causes, types, and corresponding impact.

It is becoming accepted that acts of violence against women are not isolated events but rather form a pattern of behaviour that violates the rights of women and girls, limits their participation in society, and damages their health and well-being (3). It is a major health and human rights issue (4, 5) with sometimes fatal consequences. Serious short- and long-term physical, mental, sexual, and reproductive health problems exist for survivors and for their children, and contribute to high social and economic costs (5).

Recent global prevalence figures indicate that about one in three (35%) of women worldwide have experienced either physical and/or sexual intimate partner violence or non-partner sexual violence in their lifetime. Most of this violence is domestic violence. Worldwide, almost one-third (30%) of women who have been in a relationship report that they have experienced some form of physical and/or sexual violence by their intimate partner. As many as 38% of murders of women globally are committed by an intimate partner. Violence can negatively affect women's physical, mental, sexual, and reproductive health, and may increase vulnerability to human immunodeficiency virus (HIV) (5).

Types of violence against women: who is affected? What is the impact?

Domestic abuse: physical, emotional, and sexual

Definition

Domestic violence and abuse is any incident or pattern of incidents of controlling, coercive, threatening behaviour, violence, or abuse between those aged 16 or over who are, or have been, intimate partners or family members regardless of gender or sexuality. The abuse can encompass, but is not limited to, psychological, physical, sexual, financial, and emotional abuse (5, 6).

At least 4.5 million women (27.1% of women) aged between 16 and 59 experienced domestic abuse in England and Wales in the year ending March 2015. These figures are thought to be an underestimate (7).

Domestic violence cuts across all strata of society regardless of age, ethnicity, religion, social class, and income or where people live (8). However, the variation in the prevalence of violence seen within and between communities, countries, and regions, highlights that violence is not inevitable, and that it can be prevented (3).

Risk factors

Risk factors for domestic violence include:

- female gender
- young women (age group 16–24 years)

- long-term illness or disability with almost double the risk
- substance and alcohol misuse and mental health problems
- women who are separated
- pregnancy and delivery: this is said to offer protection to some women but for others it increases the risk with a strong correlation between postnatal depression and domestic violence and abuse (9, 10).

Signs and symptoms of domestic violence

Women who have experienced partner violence have higher rates of several important health problems and risk behaviours compared to women who have not experienced partner violence: they have 16% greater odds of having a low-birthweight baby; are more than twice as likely to have an induced abortion; are more than twice as likely to experience depression. In some regions, they are 1.5 times more likely to acquire HIV, and 1.6 times more likely to have syphilis, compared to women who do not suffer partner violence (3, 11).

Health conditions associated with domestic violence include asthma, genitourinary symptoms, including frequent bladder or kidney infections, circulatory conditions, cardiovascular disease, fibromyalgia, irritable bowel syndrome, chronic pain syndromes, unexplained central nervous system disorders, unexplained gastrointestinal disorders, joint disease, migraines, and headaches (12).

Other psychological presentations include symptoms of depression, anxiety, post-traumatic stress disorder (PTSD), sleep disorders, suicidal tendencies or self-harming, and alcohol or other substance use (13).

Reproductive problems associated with domestic violence include pelvic pain and sexual dysfunction, adverse reproductive outcomes, including multiple unintended pregnancies or terminations, delayed pregnancy care, miscarriage, premature labour and stillbirth, unexplained vaginal bleeding or sexually transmitted infections, and chronic pain (unexplained) (13). Women who have experienced domestic violence may be more likely to consult their doctors and present with gynaecological problems (14).

Other indicators of domestic violence include traumatic injury, particularly if repeated and with vague or implausible explanations, and repeated health consultations with no clear diagnosis (13).

Adverse mental and physical health outcomes sometimes continue after the violence has ended (15).

Studies globally show that as adults, children who have witnessed violence and abuse are more likely to become involved in a violent and abusive relationship themselves. There is a strong likelihood that this will be a continuing cycle for the next generation with a significant risk of ever-increasing harm to the child's physical, emotional, and social development (16, 17).

Males who have personal experience of childhood emotional abuse and who have witnessed their mother being beaten demonstrate a large increase in the prevalence for them becoming perpetrators of intimate partner violence in studies from Asia and the pacific region. The risk factors, however, vary across different countries (18).

In relationships where there is domestic violence and abuse, children witness about three-quarters of the abusive incidents. About half the children in such families have themselves been badly hit or beaten. Sexual and emotional abuse is also more likely to happen in these families (17).

Personality and behavioural problems among children exposed to violence in the home can take the forms of psychosomatic illnesses, depression, suicidal tendencies, and bed-wetting. Later in life, these children are at greater risk for substance abuse, juvenile pregnancy, and criminal behaviour than those raised in homes without violence.

Management of domestic violence

Healthcare professionals should be trained to recognize indicators of domestic violence and to be able to sensitively enquire about domestic violence and abuse. When domestic violence or abuse is disclosed, care should be individualized and support tailored to suit their individual needs immediately and in the long term with the safety of the women always a priority.

Women with additional support needs should be referred to specialist domestic violence services. Domestic violence specialist services may be able to offer advocacy and support. It also includes housing workers, independent domestic violence advisers, or a multiagency risk assessment conference for high-risk clients (9).

Referrals to other relevant specialist services should be made if there are indications that someone has alcohol or drug misuse or mental health problems.

Screening in healthcare settings increases the identification of women experiencing domestic violence and abuse. Overall, however, rates are low relative to best estimates of prevalence of domestic violence in women seeking healthcare (19). Barriers to routine screening for intimate partner violence are time constraints, a lack of protocols and policies, and departmental philosophies of care that may conflict with intimate partner violence screening recommendations (20). Pregnant women in antenatal settings may be more likely to disclose intimate partner violence when screened. There was no evidence, however, of an effect for other outcomes (referral, re-exposure to violence, health measures, lack of harm arising from screening) (19).

Evidence supporting the effectiveness of routine screening of asymptomatic women in improving health status is lacking. However, identification of domestic violence within specific contexts and provision of targeted interventions may provide health benefits (21). Screening during antenatal care is a situation where the screening and provision of substantive tailored interventions to women who disclose domestic violence may reduce the recurrence of domestic violence and improve maternal and infant outcomes (22, 23).

A randomized controlled trial was performed in 1044 pregnant African American women who were assigned to either an integrated cognitive behavioural intervention or normal care. The intervention was performed at routine antenatal appointments by Masters-level social workers or psychologists and involved specific, evidence-based, interventions for the designated psychobehavioural risks (22). Intimate partner violence was significantly reduced with a halving of the odds of further episodes of minor or severe physical violence during the antenatal or postnatal period. Furthermore, improvements in obstetric outcomes were also seen. These included a significant reduction in very low birthweight (<1.5 kg) and very preterm delivery (<33 weeks) and an increase in gestational age at delivery (38.2 vs 36.9 weeks) between the experimental group receiving cognitive behavioural therapy and the control group receiving standard care. Thus, screening for domestic violence in pregnant women as well as for psychological (e.g. depression) and behavioural risks (e.g. smoking, alcohol abuse, illicit drug use) and providing targeted similar cognitive behavioural intervention appear to provide benefits on rates of recurrent violence and pregnancy outcomes. More than half the women suffering domestic violence in this study reported depression. The authors concluded that addressing domestic violence and depression together may have helped women implement strategies suggested to them to assess risks, consider preventive options, and develop safety plans (22).

Another randomized controlled trial from Hong Kong also lends support to the notion that specific psychobehavioural interventions in pregnancy may help improve maternal outcomes.

In this randomized controlled trial, 110 pregnant women with a history of abuse by their intimate partners were randomized to either empowerment training specially designed for Chinese abused pregnant women or standard care. The trial showed that women receiving empowerment training had significantly higher physical functioning and improved role limitation scores due to physical and emotional problems as measured by the Short-Form (SF)-36 quality of life instrument. Obstetric outcomes were not reported, but there was less postnatal depression recorded in the experimental group. Minor abuse was significantly reduced, although there was no reduction in severe abuse (23).

Thus, evidence to support a strategy of screening and treatment within pregnancy mandates obstetricians, midwives, health service managers, and others involved with caring for pregnant women to implement effective management strategies for domestic violence.

These plans should involve seeing women on their own at some clinic visits with sensitive routine enquiry about domestic violence and appropriate referral for psychobehavioural support.

Rape and sexual assault

Sexual violence is 'any sexual act, attempt to obtain a sexual act, or other act directed against a person's sexuality using coercion, by any person regardless of their relationship to the victim, in any setting. It includes rape, defined as the physically forced or otherwise coerced penetration of the vulva or anus with a penis, other body part or object' (5). Both men and women perpetrate and experience domestic violence and abuse, but it is more common for men to perpetrate violence and abuse against women. This is particularly true for severe and repeated violence and sexual assault (24).

Women who have experienced childhood sexual abuse are more likely than their peers to be in violent relationships, to show a higher rate of obesity, and to suffer financially (25). Studies suggest that sexual victimization in childhood or adolescence increases the likelihood of sexual victimization in adulthood between 2 and 13.7 times (26). In addition, much of the literature shows that women who experience early sexual trauma suffer from symptoms of PTSD and may attempt to 'escape' their pain by using sex or substances (27). These behaviours can, in turn, put people at greater risk.

Past trauma can also desensitize individuals to possible danger in the future. Outcomes can differ depending on whether someone has been abused repeatedly by the same perpetrator, what they call chronic victimization, or attacked multiple times by different people, known as revictimization (28). Physiological changes typical of PTSD may underlie this desensitization. Prolonged exposure to stress and stress-related hormones (primarily cortisol) can lead

to dysregulation of the body's stress response system, called the hypothalamic–pituitary–adrenal axis. Even 10–12 years after experiencing childhood trauma, the women in Noll and Trickett's longitudinal study showed signs, in blood tests, of poor regulation of this system, leaving them less equipped to identify and respond to risky situations (25). Furthermore, chronic exposure to high levels of cortisol caused by stress can leave young people vulnerable to other health problems, including obesity and brain changes that affect memory and cognition (25).

Stalking and harassment

Stalking is relatively common and it is often perpetrated by an intimate partner. It is also poorly understood (29, 30).

It is defined as 'two or more incidents (causing distress, fear or alarm) of obscene or threatening unwanted letters or phone calls, waiting or loitering around home or workplace, following or watching'. Women are more affected than men.

Harassment on the other hand can include 'repeated attempts to impose unwanted communications and contact upon a victim in a manner that could be expected to cause distress or fear in any reasonable person'. In relation to violence against women and girls, it involves attempts to impose explicit and implicit unwanted communications/advances of sexual nature.

The Protection from Harassment Act 1997 in the United Kingdom was introduced because there was limited legal protection for victims who were upset and frightened by a series of disturbing incidents which fell short of being illegal. 'Stalking' was not specifically mentioned in the Act at that time, but it was designed to, and does cover many forms of harassment, including stalking and cyber stalking.

Two new laws were introduced in the United Kingdom in 2012 specific to stalking offences, which fall under the Protection from Harassment Act 1997. This new legislation not only gives the police greater powers of entry to a stalker's property, so that evidence can be gained to corroborate a victim's case, but also supports a victim who is experiencing lesser or more serious stalking behaviour. A person is also guilty of an offence if it is perceived that they are using threatening words, show abusive behaviour, or act in a threatening manner.

A study by Edwards et al. showed that over half of women after termination of an abusive relationship reported stalking behaviours from their abusive ex-partner. This led to greater levels of posttraumatic stress symptomatology (31).

Stalking is a significant risk factor for other forms of partner violence (e.g. psychological, physical, and sexual violence) and the experience of being stalked by a violent partner contributes uniquely to women's perceptions of psychological distress and personal safety (32).

As well as the implications on an individual's social life and finances, stalking and harassment can lead to severe mental and physical health issues such as depression, anxiety, effects of chronic stress such as headaches and hypertension, fatigue from difficulty sleeping, increased use of alcohol, cigarettes, or drugs, anxiety, panic attacks, and agoraphobia (32).

Childhood sexual abuse

Sexual violence against children is a gross violation of children's rights. Yet it is a global reality across all countries and social groups. It has been estimated that between one in ten and one in twenty children have been subjected to child sexual abuse (33–35). One in three children in the United Kingdom who are abused by an adult do not tell anyone (35).

Types of child sexual abuse: contact abuse and non-contact abuse

Contact abuse involves touching activities where an abuser makes physical contact with a child, including penetration. It includes sexual touching of any part of the body (whether the child is wearing clothes or not); rape or penetration by putting an object or body part inside a child's mouth, vagina, or anus; forcing or encouraging a child to take part in sexual activity; making a child take their clothes off; touching someone else's genitals; or masturbating (35).

Non-contact abuse involves non-touching activities, such as grooming, exploitation, persuading children to perform sexual acts over the Internet, and flashing. It includes encouraging a child to watch or hear sexual acts; not taking proper measures to prevent a child being exposed to sexual activities by others; meeting a child following sexual grooming with the intent of abusing them; online abuse including making, viewing, or distributing child abuse images; allowing someone else to make, view, or distribute child abuse images; showing pornography to a child; and sexually exploiting a child for money, power, or status (child exploitation) (35).

Most victims are female, however, male victims may be underrepresented in the literature. For many victims of child sexual abuse in the family environment, abuse begins around age 9. Younger children may experience sexual abuse but they may not have the words to describe or explain their experiences to an adult, and they may not recognize that they are being sexually abused (35).

Victims from some black minority ethnic groups may face additional barriers to getting help, including, for example, a distrust of statutory services, a preference for informal community-based resolution, and the precedence of the 'honour' of the perpetrator and concern for the apparent perceived 'shame' that may be brought to the family and/or community (35).

Children with physical or learning disabilities may not have the capacity to understand or make a verbal disclosure. The symptoms of abuse, for example, inappropriate sexual behaviour, may be attributed to a learning difficulty, rather than the possibility of child sexual abuse in the family (35).

The disclosure or discovery of sexual abuse within a family is likely to have an enormous impact on the victim and their relationship with other family members. Fear, coercion, loyalty to the perpetrator, and/or a desire to protect other family members may prevent a victim of child sexual abuse from telling anyone (35).

Signs and symptoms of child sexual abuse

Children who are sexually abused may stay away from certain people, show sexual behaviour that is inappropriate for their age, and may become sexually active at a young age. Physical symptoms include anal or vaginal soreness, an unusual discharge, sexually transmitted infections, and pregnancy (36).

The child may also display unusual behaviour: be withdrawn, suddenly behaving differently, or be anxious, clingy, or depressed. They can sometimes appear aggressive with difficulties at school, have problems sleeping, and develop eating disorders and bed wetting problems. Obsessive behaviours and nightmares sometimes occur. They may also self-harm and have suicidal thoughts (36).

Several studies show that childhood sexual abuse often leads to long-term mental and physical health problems that continue into adulthood. In a report by Ports et al., it was suggested that adverse childhood experiences including childhood sexual abuse increase the risk of sexual victimization as an adult (37). Childhood sexual abuse may also occur between peers (38).

A study by the NSPCC identified, however, that therapeutic intervention had many beneficial outcomes. These include improved mood, confidence, and being less withdrawn, a reduction in guilt and self-blame, reduced depression, anxiety, and anger, improved sleep patterns, and better understanding of appropriate sexual behaviour (39).

It is argued that the true magnitude of sexual violence is hidden because of its sensitive and illegal nature. Most children and families do not report cases of abuse and exploitation because of stigma, fear, and lack of trust in the authorities. Social tolerance and lack of awareness also contribute to under-reporting (40).

Commercial sexual exploitation

Commercial sexual exploitation includes sexual activities which objectify and harm others (usually women) such as prostitution, phone sex, stripping, Internet sex/chat rooms, pole dancing, lap dancing, peep shows, pornography, trafficking, sex tourism, and 'mail-order brides'.

It legitimizes negative attitudes towards women and is inextricably linked to gender inequality and sexual violence (41). Commercial sexual exploitation can happen to both women and men but women are more commonly affected. Women involved are often on low incomes, are substance abusers, and there is strong evidence that they have experience of other forms of gender-based violence (41).

It is difficult to quantify the numbers of women involved in commercial sexual exploitation, partly because some activities, such as pole dancing, are seen as 'normal' and others, such as trafficking into prostitution, are criminal and therefore hidden (41).

Sex trafficking is a modern-day form of slavery in which a commercial sex act is induced by force, fraud, or coercion, or in which the person induced to perform such an act is under the age of 18 years (42).

The Protocol to Prevent, Suppress and Punish Trafficking in Persons, especially Women and Children is the first international consensus definition of the problem. The Protocol defines 'trafficking in persons' as the recruitment, transportation, transfer, harbouring or receipt of persons, by means of the threat or use of force or other forms of coercion, of abduction, of fraud, of deception, of the abuse of power or of a position of vulnerability, or of the giving or receiving of payments or benefits to achieve the consent of a person having control over another person, for the purpose of exploitation. Exploitation shall include, at a minimum, the exploitation of the prostitution of others or other forms of sexual exploitation, forced labour or services, slavery or practices similar to slavery, servitude, or the removal of organs (43).

Commercial sexual exploitation adversely affects physical, sexual, and mental health and is a serious public health issue. The health impact of commercial sexual exploitation can be profound, both as a result of coping with the consequences of exploitation and because of the greater exposure to violence and other forms of abuse inherent in this activity (41).

Signs found in an individual who has undergone commercial sexual exploitation include substance misuse, headaches, fatigue, dizzy spells, back pain, depression, anxiety, hostility, dissociation and signs of PTSD, suicide ideation, signs of physical assault, rape and sexual assault, HIV infection, sexually transmitted infections, urinary tract infections, and repeated terminations of pregnancy (41).

Other signs of commercial sexual exploitation include difficulty in getting to health services during normal working hours, inability to keep appointments (through drug addiction/intoxication, lack of money to travel to appointments or pay for prescriptions), disclosure of child sexual abuse or domestic abuse, homelessness, or any evidence to suggest control or domination by a partner or pimp (41).

Health workers are again in a unique position to respond to women and girls affected by commercial sexual exploitation. It is important to treat them with dignity and respect. Help can be offered by recognizing possible indicators of abuse, initiating discussion, providing clinical care if necessary, and helping women access safety (41).

It is important to be sensitive to different needs and ensure all patients can access services equally, for example, by providing professional interpreting services (41).

'Honour' crimes

There is no specific offence of 'honour'-based crime. It is an umbrella term to encompass various offences covered by existing legislation. 'Honour'-based violence can be described as a collection of practices which are used to control behaviour within families or other social groups to protect perceived cultural and religious beliefs and/or 'honour'. Such violence can occur when perpetrators perceive that a relative has shamed the family and/or community by breaking their honour code.

'Honour'-based violence is defined as a crime or incident which has or may have been committed to protect or defend the honour of the family and/or community. It may be a form of domestic or sexual violence (44).

Forced marriage

Forced marriage is a term used to describe a situation where one or both people do not (or in cases of people with learning disabilities, cannot) consent to their marriage and pressure or abuse is used. It is recognized in the United Kingdom as a form of violence against women, domestic/child abuse, and a serious abuse of human rights (42).

The pressure put on people to marry against their will can be physical (including threats, actual physical violence, and sexual violence) or emotional and psychological (e.g. when someone is made to feel that they are bringing shame on their family). Financial abuse (taking control of wages or not giving any independent money) can also be a factor (45).

Female genital mutilation/cutting

Female genital mutilation/cutting (FGM/C) is recognized internationally as a violation of the human rights of girls and women (46). United Kingdom laws recognize the problem and the Royal College of Obstetricians and Gynaecologists has issued guidelines to medical professionals. It comprises all procedures that involve partial or total removal of the external female genitalia, or other injury to the female genital organs for non-medical reasons (46).

FGM/C constitutes a form of child abuse and violence against women and girls, and has short-term and long-term physical and psychological consequences. It has no health benefits and harms girls and women in many ways. It involves removing and damaging healthy and normal female genital tissue, and hence interferes with the natural function of girls' and women's bodies (47).

The World Health Organization estimates that 2 million women undergo some form of FGM/C annually (47). Statistics from some developing countries suggest that FGM/C is decreasing with increasing awareness and education. Yet this current progress in FGM/C decline is not sufficient to keep up with the rising population growth. If the current trends continue, the proportion of girls and women undergoing FGM/C will increase significantly over the next 15 years (48).

With increasing migration to Europe and North America, obstetricians and midwives working in these countries have been increasingly exposed to, and asked to care for women who have suffered FGM/C (46).

Much of the behaviour defined as cultural is unnecessary, but for immigrant and refugee communities the maintenance of practices such as FGM/C may be a way of preserving continuity with their past lives. One implication of this is that FGM/C could increase in Western countries with growing immigrant communities.

Female genital mutilation/cutting is classified into four major types (**Table 55.1**) (46):

- Type 1: often referred to as clitoridectomy, this is the partial or total removal of the clitoris and in very rare cases, only the prepuce.
- Type 2: often referred to as excision, this is the partial or total removal of the clitoris and the labia minora with or without excision of the labia majora.
- Type 3: often referred to as infibulation, this is the narrowing of the vaginal opening through the creation of a covering seal. The seal is formed by cutting and repositioning the labia minora, or labia majora, sometimes through stitching, with or without removal of the clitoris (clitoridectomy).
- Type 4: this includes all other harmful procedures to the female genitalia for non-medical purposes, for example, pricking, piercing, incising, scraping, and cauterizing the genital area.

Deinfibulation refers to the practice of opening the sealed vaginal opening in a woman who has been infibulated, which is often necessary for improving physical and psychological health and well-being as well as to allow intercourse or to facilitate childbirth (46).

Table 55.1 Female genital mutilation classification (WHO 1997. Female genital mutilation: a joint WHO/UNICEF/UNFPA statement. World Health Organization).

Type 1	Removal of the clitoris/hood of the clitoris
Type 2	Removal of the clitoris together with partial or total excision of the labia minora with or without excision of the labia majora
Type 3	Removal of the clitoris and labia minora with stitching/narrowing of the vaginal opening—known as infibulation
Type 4	Unclassified. This includes pricking, piercing, or incision of the clitoris and/or labia, stretching of the clitoris and/or labia, cauterization by burning off the clitoris and surrounding tissue, scraping or cutting of the vagina or surrounding tissue

Mental health consequences

The age at which girls undergo FGM/C varies enormously according to the community. The procedure may be carried out when the girl is newborn, during childhood or adolescence, immediately before marriage, or during the first pregnancy. However, the majority of cases of FGM/C are thought to take place between the ages of 5 and 8 years and therefore girls within that age bracket are at a higher risk (47).

There has been relatively little published research that examines the health-related psychological outcomes in black minority ethnic groups. This is also true for health-related attitudes and beliefs. Psychology has a potential to contribute to care and prevention relating to FGM/C. But, perhaps in common with other health professionals, psychological practitioners and researchers in the United Kingdom are relatively uninformed about FGM/C (49).

The time lag between FGM/C (typically in childhood) and the manifestation of psychological or mental health problems in adolescence or adulthood means that women are less likely to make a causal link between any current difficulties to FGM/C (49).

Lockhat suggests that adverse mental health effects are associated with the following factors: severe forms of FGM/C, immediate post-FGM/C complications, chronic health problems and/or loss of fertility secondary to FGM/C, non-consensual circumcision in adolescence or adulthood, and FGM/C as punishment. By contrast, some of the 'mitigating' factors include post-FGM/C affirmation and social support and the absence of complications in the short and long term (50).

Behrendt and Moritz argued that circumcised women showed a significantly higher prevalence of PTSD (30.4%) and other psychiatric syndromes (47.9%) compared to uncircumcised women. PTSD was accompanied by memory problems (51).

It could be claimed that other sources of adversity, such as difficulties relating to cultural transition, poverty, social exclusion, and other socioeconomic factors, provide more salient explanations for mental health difficulties than FGM/C per se. Indeed, for some women, major struggles in the here and now may render unimportant a childhood event that is only vaguely remembered.

Some forms of FGM/C can lead to coital difficulties. While surgical reversal can improve the situation, some women or couples do not wish to undergo reversal and sometimes difficulties are not effectively ameliorated by reversal. For example, as a result of previous experiences of pain during sexual activities, a woman may develop an anxiety response to sexual intercourse or sexual activities in general. Anxiety can hinder arousal mechanisms resulting in vaginal dryness, muscular spasm, and painful intercourse despite an absence of anatomical problems. Education, counselling, and support can be helpful in these situations.

Physical health complications

Women and girls living with FGM/C have experienced a harmful practice and may experience physical health complications as a result of this. These could be short- and/or long-term physical health complications.

Short-term health consequences

- Severe pain: cutting the nerve ends in sensitive genital tissue causes extreme pain. Adequate anaesthesia is rarely used and, when used,

is not always effective. The healing period is also painful. Type 3 FGM/C is a more extensive procedure of longer duration, hence the intensity and duration of pain may be more severe. The healing period is also prolonged.

- Excessive bleeding (haemorrhage): can result if the clitoral artery or other blood vessel is cut during the procedure.
- Shock: can be caused by pain, infection, and/or haemorrhage.
- Infections: may spread after the use of contaminated instruments (e.g. use of same instruments in multiple genital mutilation operations), and during the healing period.
- HIV: the direct association between FGM/C and HIV remains unconfirmed, although the cutting of genital tissues with the same surgical instrument without sterilization could increase the risk for transmission of HIV between girls who undergo female genital mutilation together.
- Urination problems: these may include urinary retention and pain passing urine. This may be due to tissue swelling, pain, or injury to the urethra.
- Death: can be caused by infections, including tetanus and haemorrhage.

Long-term health risks from types 1, 2, and 3 (occurring at any time during life)

- Pain: due to tissue damage and scarring that may result in trapped or unprotected nerve endings.
- Chronic genital infections: with consequent chronic pain, and vaginal discharge and itching. Cysts, abscesses, and genital ulcers may also appear.
- Chronic reproductive tract infections: may cause chronic back and pelvic pain.
- Urinary tract infections: if not treated, such infections can ascend to the kidneys, potentially resulting in renal failure, septicaemia, and death. An increased risk for repeated urinary tract infections is well documented in both girls and adult women.
- Painful urination: due to obstruction and recurrent urinary tract infections.
- Menstrual problems: result from the obstruction of the vaginal opening. This may lead to painful menstruation (dysmenorrhea), irregular menses, and difficulty in passing menstrual blood, particularly among women with FGM/C type 3.
- Keloids: there have been reports of excessive scar tissue formation at the site of the cutting.
- HIV: given that the transmission of HIV is facilitated through trauma of the vaginal epithelium which allows the direct introduction of the virus, it is reasonable to presume that the risk of HIV transmission may be increased due to increased risk for bleeding during intercourse, as a result of FGM/C.
- Female sexual health: removal of, or damage to, highly sensitive genital tissue, especially the clitoris, may affect sexual sensitivity and lead to sexual problems, such as decreased sexual desire and pleasure, pain during sex, difficulty during penetration, decreased lubrication during intercourse, and reduced frequency or absence of orgasm (anorgasmia). Scar formation, pain, and traumatic memories associated with the procedure can also lead to such problems.

- Complications during childbirth: some studies have suggested increased risks of prolonged labour, postpartum haemorrhage, and perineal trauma. Affected women may also have a heightened fear of childbirth (tocophobia). One large World Health Organization study also found an increased risk of caesarean section, increased need for neonatal resuscitation, and risk of stillbirth and early neonatal death (52, 53).

There is an increased risk of adverse health outcomes with increased severity of FGM/C.

It is important for healthcare providers to have a basic understanding of the history, types, and complications related to FGM. Lack of knowledge about the cultural context and clinical best practices can lead to inconsistent care and poor outcomes for women affected by FGM/C.

An aide memoire for discussing FGM/C with patients (54) includes:

- taking a basic history of when and where it was performed
- what community and in what context
- if she has had any treatment
- what beliefs she has around religion and culture
- what are her wishes/thoughts about her daughters undergoing FGM/C
- and if any medical help is required for any symptoms
- any concerns.

A culturally competent, gender and ethically sensitive approach is important to ensure the provision of quality, ethical care for migrant women affected by FGM in host countries (55).

Recognizing a problem and what can be done to help?

Healthcare professionals are well placed to help women and girls who may have experienced violence with the consequences of ill health. It is important that all healthcare providers understand the relationship between exposure to violence and women's ill health, and are able to respond appropriately. One key aspect is to identify opportunities to provide support and link women with other services they need.

Conclusion

More research is needed on various aspects of violence against women and girls especially areas where there is little research such as 'honour'-based violence, forced marriage, and stalking. For domestic violence, screening and intervention for pregnant women in the antenatal period may result in improved obstetric outcomes and reduction in further violence.

REFERENCES

1. United Nations General Assembly. Declaration on the Elimination of Violence against Women, A/RES/48/104, 85th plenary meeting. 1993. Available at: http://www.un.org/documents/ga/res/48/a48r104.htm (accessed 26 February 2016).

2. House of Commons International Development Committee. Violence against women and girls: second report of session 2013–14. Available at: http://www.publications.parliament.uk/pa/cm201314/cmselect/cmintdev/107/107.pdf (accessed 3 January 2016).

3. World Health Organization. Prevalence and health effects of intimate partner violence and non-partner sexual violence. Available at: http://apps.who.int/iris/bitstream/10665/85239/1/9789241564625_eng.pdf?ua=1 (accessed 3 January 2016).

4. World Health Organization. Violence against women and girls. Definition and scope of the problem. Available at: http://www.who.int/gender/violence/v4.pdf (accessed 4 January 2016).

5. World Health Organization. Violence against women. Intimate partner and sexual violence against women. Fact sheet No. 239. Updated January 2016. Available at: http://www.who.int/mediacentre/factsheets/fs239/en/ (accessed 5 February 2016).

6. United Kingdom Home Office. Domestic violence and abuse. Available at: https://www.gov.uk/guidance/domestic-violence-and-abuse (accessed 5 February 2016).

7. Office for National Statistics. Crime Survey England and Wales, 2014–2015. Available at: http://www.ons.gov.uk/peoplepopulationandcommunity/crimeandjustice/compendium/focusonviolentcrimeandsexualoffences/yearendingmarch2015/chapter4intimatepersonalviolenceandpartnerabuse#prevalence-of-intimate-violence-extent (accessed 5 February 2016).

8. Department of Health. *Responding to Domestic Violence: A Handbook for Health Professionals*. London: Department of Health; 2005.

9. National Institute for Health and Care Excellence. Domestic abuse. Available at: http://www.nice.org.uk/guidance/ph50/chapter/1-Recommendations (accessed 5 February 2016).

10. Bazargan-Hejazi S, Kim E, Lin J, Ahmadi A, Khamesi MT, Teruya S. Risk factors associated with different types of intimate partner violence (IPV): an emergency department study. *J Emerg Med* 2014;**47**:710–20.

11. Black MC, Breiding MJ. Adverse health conditions and health risk behaviors associated with intimate partner violence – United States, 2005. *MMWR Morb Mortal Wkly Rep* 2008;**57**:113–17.

12. Centers for Disease Control and Prevention. Intimate partner violence: consequences. 2019. Available at: http://www.cdc.gov/ViolencePrevention/intimatepartnerviolence/consequences.html (accessed 5 January 2016).

13. National Institute for Health and Care Excellence (NICE). *Domestic Violence and Abuse: Multi-Agency Working*. NICE guidelines [PH50]. London: NICE; 2014. Available at: https://www.nice.org.uk/Guidance/PH50 (accessed 7 February 2016).

14. John RR, Johnson JK, Kukreja SS, et al. Domestic violence: prevalence and association with gynaecological symptoms. *BJOG* 2004;**111**:1128–32.

15. Fraser K. *Domestic Violence and Women's Physical Health*. Sydney: Australian Domestic and Family Violence Clearinghouse; 2003. Available at: http://citeseerx.ist.psu.edu/viewdoc/download?doi=10.1.1.564.2861&rep=rep1&type=pdf.

16. United Nations Children's Fund. Behind closed doors: the impact of domestic violence on children. Available at: http://www.unicef.org/protection/files/BehindClosedDoors.pdf (accessed 5 February 2016).

17. Royal College of Psychiatrists. Mental Health and Growing up Factsheet. Domestic violence and abuse - its effects on children: the impact on children and adolescents: information for parents, carers and anyone who works with young people. Available at: http://www.rcpsych.ac.uk/healthadvice/parentsandyouthinfo/parentscarers/domesticviolence.aspx (accessed 7 February 2016).

18. Fulu E, Jewkes R, Roselli T, Garcia-Moreno C. Prevalence of and factors associated with male perpetration of intimate partner violence: findings from the UN Multi-country cross-sectional study on Men and Violence in Asia and the Pacific. *Lancet Glob Health* 2013;**1**:e187–207.

19. O'Doherty L, Hegarty K, Ramsay J, Davidson LL, Feder G, Taft A. Screening women for intimate partner violence in healthcare settings. *Cochrane Database Syst Rev* 2015;**22**;7:CD007007.

20. Hamberger KL, Rhodes K, Brown J. Screening and intervention for intimate partner violence in healthcare settings: creating sustainable system-level programs. *J Womens Health (Larchmt)* 2015;**24**:86–91.

21. Jewkes R. Intimate partner violence: the end of routine screening. *Lancet* 2013;**382**:190–91.

22. Kiely M, El-Mohandes A, El-Khorazaty M, et al. An integrated intervention to reduce intimate partner violence in pregnancy: a randomized controlled trial. *Obstet Gynecol* 2010;**115**:273–83.

23. Tiwari A, Leung WC, Leung TW, et al. A randomised controlled trial of empowerment training for Chinese abused pregnant women in Hong Kong. *BJOG* 2005;**112**:1249–56.

24. National Institute for Health and Care Excellence (NICE). Domestic violence and abuse. Quality standard [QS116]. 2016. Available at: https://www.nice.org.uk/guidance/qs116/resources/domestic-violence-and-abuse-75545301469381 (accessed 7 February 2016).

25. Noll JG, Trickett PK, Putnam FW. A prospective investigation of the impact of childhood sexual abuse on the development of sexuality. *J Consult Clin Psychol* 2003;**71**:575–86.

26. Lalor K, McElvaney R. Child sexual abuse, links to later sexual exploitation/high risk sexual behavior, and prevention/treatment programs. *Trauma Violence Abuse* 2010;**11**:159–77.

27. Subramanian S. Victims of sexual assault in childhood face a higher risk of future abuse. Research is suggesting ways of breaking the cycle. *Sci Am Mind* 2016;**27**:58–61.

28. Matlow RB, DePrince AP. The influence of victimization history on PTSD symptom expression in women exposed to intimate partner violence. *Psychol Trauma* 2013;**5**:241–50.

29. Silverman JG, Raj A, Mucci LA, Hathaway JE. Dating violence against adolescent girls and associated substance use, unhealthy weight control, sexual risk behaviour, pregnancy, and suicidality. *JAMA* 2001;**286**:572–79.

30. Edwards KM, Gidycz CA. Stalking and psychosocial distress following the termination of an abusive dating relationship: a prospective analysis. *Violence Against Women* 2014;**20**:1383–97.

31. Logan T, Walker R. Partner stalking: psychological dominance or "business as usual"? *Trauma Violence Abuse* 2009;**10**:247–70.

32. Edwards KM, Gidycz CA. Stalking and psychosocial distress following the termination of an abusive dating relationship: a prospective analysis. *Violence Against Women* 2014;**20**:1383–97.

33. Logan TK, Cole J. The impact of partner stalking on mental health and protective order outcomes over time. *Violence Vict* 2007;**22**:546–62.

34. United Nations Children's Fund. Sexual violence against children. Available at: http://www.unicef.org/protection/57929_58006.html (accessed 3 January 2016).

35. Children's Commissioner. Inquiry into child sexual abuse in the family environment. Available at: http://www.childrenscommissioner.gov.uk/sites/default/files/publications/Protecting%20children%20from%20harm%20-%20full%20report.pdf (accessed 3 January 2016).

36. NSPCC. Putting the spotlight on sexual abuse. Available at: https://www.nspcc.org.uk/fighting-for-childhood/news-opinion/putting-the-spotlight-on-sexual-abuse/ (accessed 7 February 2016).

37. NSPCC. Signs and symptoms and effects. Available at: https://www.nspcc.org.uk/preventing-abuse/child-abuse-and-neglect/child-sexual-abuse/signs-symptoms-effects (accessed 7 February 2016).

38. Ports KA, Ford DC, Merrick MT. Adverse childhood experiences and sexual victimization in adulthood. *Child Abuse Neglect* 2016;**51**:313–22.

39. Kloppen K, Haugland S, Svedin CG, Mæhle M, Breivik K. Prevalence of child sexual abuse in the Nordic countries: a literature review. *J Child Sex Abus* 2016;**25**:37–55.

40. NSPCC. Letting the future in. Available at: https://www.nspcc.org.uk/globalassets/documents/research-reports/letting-the-future-in-evaluation.pdf (accessed 5 February 2016).

41. United Nations Children's Fund. Sexual violence against children. Available at: http://www.unicef.org/protection/57929_58006.html (accessed 5 February 2016).

42. NHS Health Scotland. National gender-based violence and health programme. Available at: http://www.gbv.scot.nhs.uk/gbv/commercial-sexual-exploitation (accessed 5 February 2016).

43. US Government Office of Trafficking in Persons. Fact sheet: sex trafficking (English). 2012. Available at: http://www.acf.hhs.gov/programs/endtrafficking/resource/fact-sheet-sex-trafficking-english (accessed 5 February 2016).

44. Organization for Security and Co-operation in Europe. Protocol to prevent, suppress and punish trafficking in persons especially women and children supplementing the United Nations Convention against transnational organized crime. Available at: http://www.osce.org/odihr/19223?download=true (accessed 7 February 2016).

45. Crown Prosecution Service. Honour based violence and forced marriage. Available at: http://www.cps.gov.uk/legal/h_to_k/honour_based_violence_and_forced_marriage/#a01 (accessed 7 February 2016).

46. Gov.UK. Law and the justice system – guidance: forced marriage. Available at: https://www.gov.uk/guidance/forced-marriage (accessed 7 February 2016).

47. World Health Organization. Female genital mutilation factsheet. Available at: http://www.who.int/mediacentre/factsheets/fs241/en/ (accessed 7 February 2016).

48. United Nations Children's Fund (UNICEF). *Female Genital Mutilation/Cutting: A Global Concern*. New York: UNICEF; 2016. Available at: http://www.unicef.org/media/files/FGMC_2016_brochure_final_UNICEF_SPREAD.pdf (accessed 10 April 2016).

49. Gov.UK. Female genital mutilation. Available at: https://www.gov.uk/government/uploads/system/uploads/attachment_data/file/380125/MultiAgencyPracticeGuidelinesNov14.pdf http://www.fgmnationalgroup.org/psychological_aspects.htm (accessed 7 February 2016).

50. Lockhat H. *Female Genital Mutilation: Treating the Tears*. London: Middlesex University Press; 2004.

51. Behrendt A, Moritz S. Post traumatic stress disorder and memory problems after female genital mutilation. *Am J Psychiatry* 2005;**162**:1000–1002.

52. Royal College of Obstetricians and Gynaecologists (RCOG). *Female Genital Mutilation and its Management*. Green-top Guideline No. 53. London: RCOG; 2015. Available at: https://www.rcog.org.uk/en/guidelines-research-services/guidelines/gtg53/ (accessed 10 April 2016).

53. WHO Study Group on Female Genital Mutilation and Obstetric Outcome. Female genital mutilation and obstetric outcome: WHO

collaborative prospective study in six African Countries. *Lancet* 2006;**367**:1835–41.

54. Hearst AA, Alexandra M. Molnar female genital cutting: an evidence-based approach to clinical management for the primary care physician. *Mayo Clinic Proc* 2013;**88**:618–29.

55. Vissandjée B, Denetto S, Migliardi P, Proctor J. Female genital cutting (FGC) and the ethics of care: community engagement and cultural sensitivity at the interface of migration experiences. *BMC Int Health Hum Rights* 2014;**14**:13.

SECTION 11

Urogynaecology and Pelvic Floor Disorders

56

Pelvic organ prolapse

Suneetha Rachaneni, Anupreet Dua, and Robert Freeman

Introduction

Pelvic organ prolapse (POP) is a departure from normal sensation, structure, or function, experienced by the woman in reference to the position of her pelvic organs. Symptoms such as the feeling of a bulge, vaginal heaviness, or 'something coming down', are generally worse after long periods of standing or exercise and better when lying supine. Other symptoms include bladder, bowel, and sexual dysfunction. Prolapse may be more prominent with a full bladder and/or rectum and at times of abdominal straining, for example, defecation. POP is not just a problem in older women and represents a health economic challenge for the future due to the costs of surgery, the longer life expectancy, and an increasing demand for a better quality of life.

Epidemiology

Robust epidemiological studies on the natural history, incidence, and prevalence of POP are lacking. A common condition in vaginally parous women, the prevalence rates vary between 40% and 50% on vaginal examination. Though 30% of women in the general population have signs of prolapse, only 8.8% were found to have bothersome prolapse symptoms seeking treatment (1). However, it is not known whether a significant proportion of women 'suffer in silence' and don't seek help.

The prevalence of POP is known to increase with age. It is predicted that by 2050, the number of women suffering from symptomatic prolapse in the United States will increase by 46% (2). In a longitudinal study of parous women with a lifespan of 80 years in the United Kingdom, the lifetime risk of undergoing a surgical procedure was 12% (3). The lifetime risk of a women undergoing surgery due to POP was found to be as high as 19% in Western Australia (4). Similar findings were derived from the Danish national patient registry: the lifetime risk of undergoing POP surgery for an 80-year-old woman was found to be 18.7% (5). With the increase in the ageing population across the world, the disease burden from prolapse is likely to grow much further.

The incidence of POP that required surgical correction following a hysterectomy is 3.6 per 1000 women-years in the United Kingdom (6). The cumulative risk rises to 5% at 15 years after a hysterectomy.

The incidence of POP after a hysterectomy is expected to show a downward trend with fewer hysterectomies being performed for menstrual dysfunction.

Risk factors for prolapse

The aetiology of prolapse may be multifactorial. Possible risk factors include pregnancy, vaginal delivery, connective tissue disorders, denervation or weakness of the pelvic floor, increased body mass index (BMI), smoking, menopause, previous hysterectomy, and chronic increase in intra-abdominal pressure (e.g. chronic straining with constipation).

The risk of POP increases with the number of vaginal deliveries, as depicted in **Table 56.1** (7).

Pathophysiology

The interaction between the pelvic floor muscles and the supportive ligaments was elaborated by DeLancey and Norton as the 'boat in dry dock theory' (8). The boat is analogous to the pelvic organs, the ropes to the ligaments and fasciae, and the water to the supportive layer of the pelvic floor muscles. The connective tissue supports of the cervix and upper vagina maintain the position of the uterus/cervix and upper vagina on the levator plate. When the pelvic floor muscles relax or are damaged, the pelvic organs must be held in place by the ligaments and fasciae alone. If the pelvic floor muscles cannot actively support the organs, the connective tissue will become stretched and damaged.

Three levels of support have been described by DeLancey (**Box 56.1**) (9).

Increases in intra-abdominal pressure compress the vagina against the levator plate rather than through the levator hiatus and prevent pelvic organ descent through the hiatus. Damage to the muscular and/or connective tissue supports of the uterus and vagina include tearing or stretching of the uterosacral and/or cardinal ligaments and/or the levator ani muscle, or neuromuscular damage can occur at vaginal delivery.

During the second stage of labour, voluntary contractions of the abdominal wall and respiratory diaphragm muscles are initiated by

Table 56.1 Risk factors for prolapse

Risk factor	Odds ratio for prolapse (95% CI)
One vaginal delivery	2.8 (1.1–7.2)
Two vaginal deliveries	4.1 (1.8–9.5)
Three vaginal deliveries	5.3 (2.3–12.3)
Irritable bowel syndrome	2.8 (1.7–4.6)
Constipation	2.5 (1.7–3.7)
Poor health status	2.3 (1.1–4.9)
Overweight (BMI 25–30 kg/m²)	2.51 (1.18–5.35)
Obese (BMI >30 kg/m²)	2.56 (1.23–5.35)

the mother to coincide with the peak uterine contraction to drive the fetal head through the levator hiatus. The fetal head stretches the pelvic floor muscles to a significant extent. In a three-dimensional geometric model of the female pelvic floor to predict levator muscle stretch ratios during the second stage of labour, pubococcygeus muscle, the most medial levator ani muscle, had the largest tissue strain with a stretch ratio (tissue length under stretch/original tissue length) of 3.26. Regions of the iliococcygeus, pubococcygeus, and puborectalis muscles reached maximal stretch ratios of 2.73, 2.50, and 2.28, respectively. Tissue stretch ratios were found to be proportional to fetal head size. The use of forceps, anal sphincter tears, and episiotomy increased the odds ratio for levator muscle injury by 14.7-, 8.1-, and 3.1-fold, respectively. Excessive stretch of a striated muscle is a cause of muscle injury: the more mechanical work done on a striated muscle in a lengthening contraction, the higher the risk for stretch-related injury (10, 11).

In a three-dimensional model on nerve stretch injury during childbirth constructed from cadaveric dissection, the inferior rectal nerve was shown to sustain the maximum strain, 15–35%, depending on the degree of perineal descent. The strain in the perineal nerve branch innervating the anal sphincter reached 33%, while the branches innervating the posterior labia and urethral sphincter reached values of 15% and 13%, respectively. The more proximal the nerve fixation point, the greater the nerve strain.

Thus, during the second stage, the nerves innervating the anal sphincter are stretched beyond the 15% strain threshold known to

cause permanent nerve damage, and the degree of perineal descent is shown to influence pudendal nerve strain (12). Partial or complete denervation of pelvic floor musculature and sphincters following childbirth trauma may manifest many years later (following menopause) as pelvic organ descent and/or incontinence (13, 14).

Damage to the connective tissue and/or muscular supports result in distortion of the relationship between uterus/vagina and the levator plate. An increase in intra-abdominal pressure might position the uterus and upper vagina over the levator hiatus and predispose to downward displacement of pelvic organs (9). Damage to level 1 support may result in uterine descent, enterocele, or vault prolapse. Level 2 support damage results in cystocele and rectocele. Damage to level 3 support results in widening of the hiatus and higher-stage POP.

Symptoms of prolapse

A recent joint report from the International Urogynecological Association (IUGA) and International Continence Society (ICS) (15) on the symptoms of POP states that the most common symptom is that of vaginal bulge or 'something coming down' towards or through the vaginal introitus. Other symptoms may include:

- pelvic pressure, heaviness, or dragging in the suprapubic area and/or pelvis
- bleeding, discharge, or infection due to dependent skin ulceration of the prolapse
- splinting/digitation—the need to digitally replace the prolapse or apply manual pressure to the vagina or perineum (splinting), or to the vagina or rectum (digitation) to assist voiding or defecation respectively
- low backache
- lower urinary tract symptoms/overactive bladder, sexual dysfunction (both dyspareunia and psychological due to poor general and genital body image)
- vaginal pain is rarely a symptom of POP.

Symptoms of sexual dysfunction

POP may result in a departure from normal sensation and/or function experienced by a woman during sexual activity:

- Dyspareunia (superficial and deep): persistent or recurrent pain or discomfort associated with attempted or complete vaginal penetration.
- Obstructed intercourse: complaint that vaginal penetration is not possible due to obstruction from the bulge/POP.
- Vaginal laxity: complaint of excessive vaginal laxity.
- Loss of libido due to poor genital body image.

Anorectal dysfunction

- Anal incontinence
- Incomplete emptying of the bowel with digitation
- Faecal urgency
- Rectal prolapse.

Box 56.1 The three levels of support

Level 1 support: the upper part of the vagina adjacent to the cervix is supported by uterosacral and cardinal ligaments.

Level 2 support: this support includes pubocervical fascia anteriorly and the rectovaginal septum posteriorly and is a part of pelvic fascia. This support connects vagina to the lateral pelvic wall through arcus tendinous fascia pelvis.

Level 3 support: anteriorly vagina fuses with the urethra, and is embedded in the connective tissue of the perineal membrane (urogenital diaphragm). Laterally it blends with the margins of the levator ani muscles. Posteriorly it fuses with the perineal body. Urogenital diaphragm forms a platform to support the lower third of the vagina.

Reproduced from DeLancey JO. The anatomy of the pelvic floor. Curr Opin Obstet Gynecol 1994;6(4):313–6 with permission from Wolters Kluwer.

Clinical evaluation of pelvic organ prolapse

POP is a clinical diagnosis classified by symptoms and the degree of anatomical deformity (descent), depending on the site of the defect and the pelvic organs that are involved.

There have been difficulties in designing an objective, reproducible system of grading prolapse. Intra- and interobserver variation on each successive examination can be significantly high leading to confusion. This makes it difficult to compare successive examinations over time in the same woman by the same operator or different operators (16).

The Pelvic Organ Prolapse Quantification system (POP-Q) (17) recommended by the International Consultation on Incontinence (IUGA/ICS) refers to an objective, site-specific system for describing, quantifying, and staging POP in women (15, 18). In this system, specific measurements at nine sites are recorded in a tic-tac-toe grid (**Figure 56.1**). There are six defined points for measurement in the POPQ system—Aa, Ba, C, D, Ap, and Bp—and three other landmarks—gh, tvl, and pb (see caption for **Figure 56.1** for definitions). Each is measured in centimetres above or proximal to the hymen (negative number) or centimetres below or distal to the hymen (positive number) with the plane of the hymen being defined as zero (0). The hymen was selected as the reference point because it is more precisely identified. Pelvic organ prolapse quantification system (POP-Q) provides a standardized tool for documenting, comparing, and communicating clinical findings with proven interobserver and intraobserver reliability (17).

The Baden–Walker Halfway Scoring System is the next most commonly used system. It consists of four grades:

- Grade 0—no prolapse.
- Grade 1–halfway to hymen.
- Grade 2—to hymen.
- Grade 3—halfway past hymen.
- Grade 4—maximum descent.

Although descriptive, some shortcomings exist in the Baden–Walker system. For instance, a strategically placed 1 cm increase in prolapse results in an increase in the assigned stage. It does not provide information on the total vaginal length and the extent of gaping of the genital hiatus. In addition, inter-observer agreement was lower with the Baden–Walker system compared to the POP-Q system (19).

All examinations for POP should be performed with the woman's bladder empty (and if possible an empty rectum too). Fullness of the bladder or rectum has been shown to restrict the degree of descent of the prolapse (20). The choice of the woman's position during examination (e.g. left lateral, supine, standing, or lithotomy) is that which can best demonstrate maximum POP. If the prolapse can't be seen in one position, then examination with the woman standing may be considered. The degree of POP assessed with the patient in the lithotomy position correlates well with assessment performed upright; however, overall there is a higher degree of prolapse with upright examination (21).

The hymen remains the fixed point of reference for prolapse description. The descent of one or more of the anterior vaginal wall, posterior vaginal wall, the uterus (cervix), or the apex of the vagina (vaginal vault or cuff scar after hysterectomy) on maximum Valsalva or coughing needs to be measured. Level of the hymen is taken as a fixed point and descent of pelvic organs is measured in relation to the level of the hymen (**Box 56.2**).

A simplified POP-Q scoring, with the above-mentioned stages 1–4 without inclusion of stage 0, has been described by Swift et al. (22). Higher-stage anterior vaginal wall prolapse will generally involve uterine or vaginal vault/apex (if uterus is absent) descent. Occasionally, there might be anterior enterocele (hernia of peritoneum and possibly abdominal contents) formation after prior reconstructive surgery. Posterior vaginal wall prolapse would usually be due to rectal protrusion into the vagina (rectocele). Higher-stage posterior vaginal wall prolapse after prior hysterectomy will generally involve some vaginal vault (cuff scar) descent and a possible enterocele. Enterocele formation can also occur in the presence of an intact uterus.

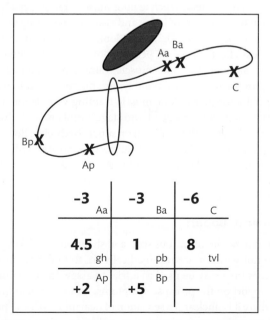

Figure 56.1 POP-Q scoring grid. Aa, point A anterior, Ap, point A posterior, Ba, point B anterior; Bp, point B posterior; C, cervix or vaginal cuff; D, posterior fornix (if cervix is present); gh, genital hiatus; pb, perineal body; tvl, total vaginal length.
Source data from Persu C, Chapple CR, Cauni V, et al. Pelvic Organ Prolapse Quantification System (POP-Q) – a new era in pelvic prolapse staging. *J Med Life* 2011;4(1):75–81.

Box 56.2 POP-Q staging
- Stage 0: no prolapse is demonstrated.
- Stage I: most distal portion of the prolapse is more than 1 cm above the level of the hymen.
- Stage II: most distal portion of the prolapse is 1 cm or less proximal to or distal to the plane of the hymen.
- Stage III: the most distal portion of the prolapse is more than 1 cm below the plane of the hymen but everted at least 2 cm less than the total vaginal length.
- Stage IV: complete eversion of the total length or eversion at least within 2 cm of the total length of the lower genital tract is demonstrated.

Types of prolapse

A significant number of women develop prolapse in multiple compartments due to global pelvic floor weakness. Ageing and menopause are associated with a reduction in muscle force production and fibrosis resulting in pelvic floor dysfunction (23, 24). These symptoms can occur at different timescales, for example, patients can develop prolapse in a new site many years after surgical correction of prolapse in another.

Anterior compartment prolapse

Damage to the apical support of the vagina and/or the anterior vaginal wall might lead to cystocele or uterine descent. Being the most frequent component of the bulge symptoms, anterior compartment prolapse/cystocele accounts for 51% of the vaginal bulge symptoms (7, 25). Symptoms can also include urinary voiding difficulty due to 'kinking' of the urethra and bladder neck by a large cystocele. In some cases surgical correction might expose a weak urethral sphincter resulting in so-called occult incontinence.

Central compartment prolapse

Uterine descent or vault/apical prolapse (in patients with previous hysterectomy) are the components of central compartment prolapse. Overstretching or loss of level 1 support might be the cause.

Vaginal vault prolapse can have coexisting apical enterocele, some degree of high cystocele formation, and high rectocele formation where the pubocervical and rectovaginal fascia have separated (**Figure 56.2**). The peritoneum above the vagina gets stretched and comes in direct contact with the vaginal epithelium creating a true hernia. Herniation of these components might stretch the vaginal wall resulting in loss of rugosity. Consequently, identifying the various components of central compartment prolapse can prove to be difficult during clinical examination.

Posterior compartment prolapse

Rectocele results from herniation of the rectum into the vaginal lumen through a defect in the rectovaginal septum (**Figure 56.3**).

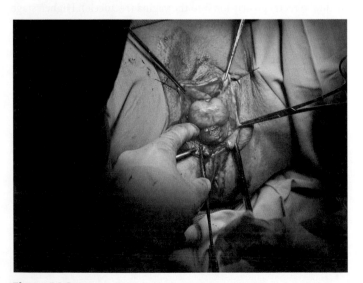

Figure 56.2 Enterocele in the posterior compartment.
Reproduced with permission of Mr S Radley.

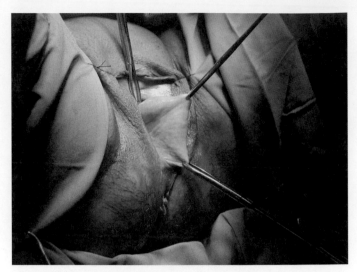

Figure 56.3 Rectocele.
Reproduced with permission of Mr S Radley.

Management of pelvic organ prolapse

The choice of management of POP varies based on the type and severity of symptoms, combinations of the compartments involved, coexisting urinary or bowel symptoms and the risk of developing new ones, and patient factors including general health, BMI and most importantly their expectations from treatment. In addition, the wish to retain sexual function might influence the choice of treatment.

Conservative management

Pelvic floor physiotherapy/pelvic floor muscle training can help improvement of symptoms of bulge and also any coexisting urinary or faecal incontinence (26, 27). In a randomized controlled trial (RCT) on the cost-effectiveness of pelvic floor muscle training versus watchful waiting, pelvic floor muscle training resulted in a significant improvement of pelvic floor symptoms compared to watchful waiting (43% for pelvic floor muscle training vs 14% for watchful waiting) in women with stage 1 and stage 2 prolapse (28). Evidence from the multicentre POPPY Trial on supervised pelvic floor muscle training versus no intervention suggests a greater reduction in patient-reported prolapse symptoms at the end of 1 year. Though there was some reduction in the quantification of prolapse on POP-Q scoring, the difference was not statistically significant (26).

Mechanical support

Rings and pessaries of various sizes and shapes are useful in patients who do not wish, or are not medically fit, to undergo surgery. In some cases they may be used as a trial to assess the effect of pelvic organ support on the prolapse symptoms, for example, in those patients where it is unclear if a sensation of heaviness is due to prolapse or another pathology (e.g. central sensitization). Ring pessaries but not Gelhorn or shelf pessaries, can be used in women who are sexually active. The majority of the women experience resolution of bulge symptoms with nearly 50% reporting improvement in concomitant urinary symptoms. Occult stress incontinence may get unmasked following pessary insertion (21%) resulting in dissatisfaction (29).

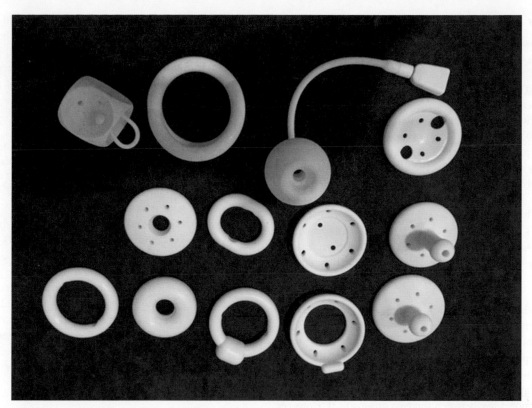

Figure 56.4 Various types of pessaries.

Shelf, Gelhorn, doughnut, and cube pessaries are space occupying and may be used in women who are not sexually active. In a randomized trial comparing pessary use to surgical management of prolapse, no difference was found in subjective outcomes at the end of 1 year of follow-up (30, 31). Patient satisfaction with a pessary after 12 months of use was found to be 59.2%. In women who manage to retain the pessaries, only 28% were found to continue using pessaries at the end of 5 years of follow-up (31, 32). The rationale for discontinuation included failure to retain the pessary, expulsion of the device while performing daily activities, discomfort, a desire for surgery, and an inability or pain during insertion/removal the pessary. Women with enlarged genital hiatus, higher-order vaginal parity, and previous hysterectomy may not be able to retain certain types of pessaries (**Figure 56.4**) (32).

Women who continued to use a pessary for up to 12 months complained of vaginal discharge, infection, and, in certain cases, ulcers in the vaginal epithelium due to contact with the pessary (33). Younger women who had a previous POP surgery and recurrent prolapse had a higher rate of discontinuation of pessary treatment (34).

Minor complications were reported in 12% of the pessary users and included pain, bleeding, ulceration or excoriation, impaction, and constipation during long-term follow-up (32). Rare complications from 'neglected'/forgotten pessaries (i.e. patient is not seen for routine follow-up and pessary change), include fistula (vesicovaginal and rectovaginal), perforation of the vault, and embedment of the pessary with a band of granulation tissue growing on top (35).

Low-dose vaginal oestrogens may alleviate some of these undesirable side effects but data from a RCT on the exact benefit and frequency of use are awaited. One small study showed that women using a non-ring group of pessaries such as Shelf, Gelhorn, and Shaatz using vaginal oestrogens had reduced frequency of ulceration, bleeding, and discharge (36). Conventionally most clinicians replace pessaries every 4–6 months to identify and manage complications with pessary usage. In an IUGA survey, 35% of the members stated that they would change the shelf/Gelhorn pessary every 3 months and 31% changed every 6 months (37).

Surgical management of prolapse

Surgery for prolapse aims to correct the anatomy and relieve symptoms (e.g. the feeling of bulge). In a study by Barber et al., subjective cure (absence of bulge symptoms) occurred in 92.1% (38). An appropriate choice depends on the type of defect, any previous pelvic or prolapse surgery, the woman's age, BMI and fitness for anaesthetic, and the wish to retain vaginal capacity and length for sexual intercourse.

Vaginal hysterectomy

This has been the traditional surgery in women with significant uterine descent who have completed their families with no desire for future fertility. The bladder and rectum are dissected away from the uterus and hysterectomy performed after ligation of pedicles. Support to the vault/apex (e.g. McCall's culdoplasty) is performed by plication of the uterosacral ligaments to the vaginal vault which is then closed. In some cases, sacrospinous fixation (described later) can be added where vault support is suboptimal after the McCall procedure. In a retrospective case–control study of 62 women, comparing sacrospinous ligament fixation and modified McCall culdoplasty during vaginal hysterectomy, sacrospinous ligament fixation was inferior to McCall culdoplasty in terms of operative time, blood loss, and prolapse recurrence (39).

Uterine preservation

In women who wish to retain their uterus, sacrohysteropexy can be performed by an open or laparoscopic approach. Synthetic mesh is used to suspend the uterocervical junction to the sacral promontory or S1. A RCT of 82 women reported subjective failure (consultation within 1 year because of prolapse symptoms) in 39% (16/41) following sacrohysteropexy compared with 12% (5/41) following hysterectomy (40).

A vaginal approach (sacrospinous hysteropexy) to uterine preservation surgery involves attaching the cervix to the sacrospinous ligament (41, 42). Compared with vaginal hysterectomy and prolapse repair, hysteropexy is associated with a shorter operating time, less blood loss, and a faster return to work (41). In a multicentre RCT comparing the outcomes of uterus-sparing vaginal sacrospinous hysteropexy to those of vaginal hysterectomy and uterosacral suspension of the vaginal vault, recurrence of bulge symptoms and reoperation rates were similar at 12 months of follow-up.

Sacrospinous hysteropexy was non-inferior to vaginal hysterectomy/uterosacral suspension of the vaginal vault for anatomical recurrence of the apical compartment with bothersome bulge symptoms or repeat surgery for recurrent apical prolapse at the end of 12 months. Functional outcome, quality of life, complications, hospital stay, measures on postoperative recovery, and sexual functioning did not differ between the two groups (42). However, longer-term follow-up is required before any recommendation can be made regarding which procedure is the best and in which group of patients.

The 'Vault or Uterine prolapse surgery Evaluation' (VUE) study aimed to assess the surgical management of apical compartment prolapse in terms of clinical effectiveness and adverse events; once completed, this will provide valuable information to counsel patients regarding these different surgical options (43).

Vault prolapse

Post-hysterectomy vault prolapse may occur in 11.6% of the women who undergo vaginal hysterectomy for prolapse and 1.8% for benign causes (44). Surgical repair can be performed by an abdominal approach (sacrocolpopexy by laparoscopy or open laparotomy) or vaginally (sacrospinous fixation). In one study, mesh erosion was reported to occur in 3–9% of the cases following open or laparoscopic sacrocolpopexy (45). The United Kingdom National Institute for Health and Care Excellence (NICE) guidance on abdominal surgical techniques for prolapse including sacrohysteropexy and sacrocolpopexy states that these two procedures using mesh have serious and well-recognized complications and need to be carried out where standard arrangements are in place for clinical governance, consent, and audit (46, 47).

Sacrospinous fixation

Transvaginal sacrospinous ligament fixation is a safe and effective technique for apical support without the use of prosthetic materials such as mesh (**Figure 56.5**). Adequate preparation of the pararectal space, dissection up to the sacrospinous ligament, and proper suture positioning through the ligament to suspend the vaginal apex are the key steps. Proximity to the neurovascular pudendal bundle is an important risk factor while taking the sacrospinous

stitch, with complications such as haematoma and chronic buttock pain. Other complications include injury to the bladder or bowel. Uterosacral vault suspension through a vaginal approach has been described by Shull with a 90% success rate. However, the safety of this procedure is limited by an increased risk of ureteric injuries (11%) (48).

Colpocleisis

In women who do not wish to preserve vaginal anatomy for sexual intercourse, colpocleisis is an obliterative surgical procedure for global POP. The entire vaginal epithelium up to 2 cm from the urethral meatus is mobilized by sharp dissection, except for 1 cm from the vault. Similar dissection is needed posteriorly.

The anterior or posterior prolapse will then be reduced by a series of absorbable sutures placed into the fascia (plication) after invaginating the vaginal vault. The procedure is completed by approximating the anterior vaginal epithelium to the posterior vaginal epithelium with interrupted sutures from the vault down to the level of the introitus, leaving a lateral 'tunnel' on each side.

Colpocleisis has the advantage of a short operative time, reduced morbidity, and quicker recovery in elderly patients with several comorbidities. Success rates of 91–100% (49) have been reported with a low regret rate of 4% on 2–5-year follow-up (50).

Sacrocolpopexy

Abdominal sacrocolpopexy is the gold standard procedure to suspend the vault to sacral promontory using synthetic mesh (40). The sacral promontory is approached by dissecting off the peritoneum over the periosteum either laparoscopically or by laparotomy. The vaginal vault is then identified and the bladder is dissected off the anterior vaginal wall. Synthetic mesh is placed between the sacral promontory and vaginal vault using either staples or non-absorbable sutures.

The risks associated with sacrocolpopexy include vaginal mesh exposure (2–5%), *de novo* constipation/obstructive defecatory syndrome (10%), perioperative bladder (1%) or bowel (0.1%) injury, *de novo* dyspareunia (1–3%), pelvic abscess (<1%), spondylodiscitis

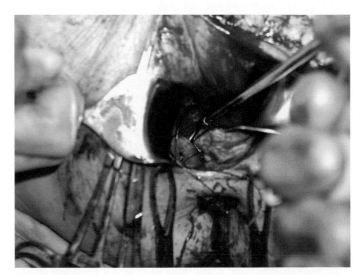

Figure 56.5 Identification of sacrospinous ligament and the use of Miya Hook for sacrospinous ligament fixation.

(<0.1%), visceral (bladder, rectum) mesh exposure (<0.1%) (51), neuropathic pain, and *de novo* urinary incontinence.

The outcomes of sacrocolpopexy performed by an open approach and laparoscopically are clinically equivalent with 90% of women reporting feeling 'much better' symptomatically in the open sacrocolpopexy group and 80% in the laparoscopic group at 1 year of follow-up (52). Current evidence on the safety and efficacy of sacrocolpopexy using mesh for vaginal vault prolapse repair appears adequate to support the use of this procedure provided that appropriate arrangements are in place for clinical governance and audit (40).

Anterior compartment prolapse

Vaginal native tissue repair for cystocele involves dissection of pubocervical fascia from the anterior vaginal wall and plication of the fascia using absorbable sutures. Anterior compartment prolapse is the most common component of vaginal bulge symptoms and the anatomical recurrence rates were reported to be very high at greater than 40% (53, 54). Success after prolapse surgery depends heavily on the criteria that are used to define treatment success. When strict anatomical criteria are used, the success rate will be low (55).

The IUGA/ICS joint report (15) recommends that the following outcomes in women undergoing POP surgery be reported:

- *Subjective*: patient-reported outcomes (particularly the presence or absence of vaginal bulge symptoms), satisfaction, quality of life.
- *Objective*. POP-Q, prolapse grading using other classifications such as the Baden–Walker system.

Given the poor correlation between severity of prolapse and the symptoms women present with, patients' expectations may be met better by getting them to set specific goals for surgical outcomes and comparing them pre- and postoperatively. A qualitative approach using patient satisfaction questionnaires and quality of life questionnaires improve patient satisfaction and overall outcome when treating women with POP (56).

Posterior compartment prolapse

Posterior colporrhaphy has been the most common surgical technique for the repair of posterior compartment defects (e.g. rectocele). Conventional posterior compartment repair techniques involve midline plication of the fascia or repair of the specific site of fascial weakness or defect in the rectovaginal septum. Levator plication during posterior repair is associated with an increased complication rate of dyspareunia (27%) and constipation (33%) and is no longer recommended (57). The transvaginal approach is known to have better outcomes compared to the transrectal approach with respect to bulge symptoms (58). However, uncertainty persists whether obstructive defecation symptoms improve with posterior vaginal repairs.

Bowel symptoms of rectoceles overlap/coexist with those of other pelvic floor, anorectal, and colonic disorders. Vaginal or perineal digitation is thought to be specific to an operatively curable rectocele by some authors, but sometimes even these symptoms are present only when the stool is hard, and may improve with dietary changes. Similarly, the feeling of incomplete emptying may occur from an irritable rectum or a coincident enterocele, sigmoidocoele, or rectal intussusception, despite complete rectal evacuation (59). Women with the descending perineum syndrome may also have difficulty evacuating in the absence of rectocele and may splint their buttocks in order to evacuate (60).

Rectal intussusception develops first as an anterior infolding progressing to an annular infolding of the walls of the rectum; its extension into the anal canal may induce a sensation of incomplete evacuation (61). The presence of rectal intussusception will need a colorectal evaluation as a posterior repair is unlikely to address the symptoms.

Recurrence, reoperation, and further surgery for pelvic organ prolapse following repair

Recurrence following POP surgery was found to be more common in the presence of complete levator avulsion, widened genital hiatus, and higher-order prolapse at index surgery (stages 3–4) (7). Recurrent POP might not always be due to the failure of index surgery. Women who undergo POP surgery are at a 10% lifetime risk of undergoing surgery in a different compartment for their new-onset bulge symptoms.

While the high reoperation rate is commonly quoted, the failure to adjust for both time and variation in operative site reduces the usefulness of the conclusions and might be misleading with regard to the true 'failure rate' of POP surgery. In a study of the follow-up of anterior repair, 12% of women had anatomical recurrence at the end of 3 months. However, the majority of those women were asymptomatic. The reoperation rate was at 3.4% at the end of 50 months of follow-up (62). More recently, several investigators looked specifically at the site-specific recurrence, with reoperation rates ranging from 2.8% to 9.7% (63).

Definition of the terms recurrence/reoperation rates for surgery have been the subject of much debate. Surgery for POP in a new compartment was defined as 'recurrence' which seems inappropriate (53).

In a study by Price et al., 61% of the reoperations for POP were in a different compartment (64). Therefore it is likely that the 'recurrence rate' has been exaggerated due to the variations in definitions used. To ensure uniformity, the IUGA and ICS have issued a joint report on the terminology to be used in reporting surgical outcomes (recurrence/reoperation) of POP in 2012 (65) which are as follows:

Further surgery for POP is a global term for the number of subsequent procedures the patient undergoes, directly or indirectly, relating to the primary surgery. Further surgery per se should not be interpreted as a measure of failure, as the definitions of success and failure will be defined within the context of the individual study.

Further surgery is subdivided into the following:

1. Primary prolapse surgery/different site: a prolapse procedure in a new site/compartment following previous surgery (e.g. anterior repair following previous posterior repair).

2. Repeat surgery: a repeat operation for prolapse arising from the same site. Where combinations of procedures arise, such as new anterior repair plus further posterior repair, these should be reported separately as primary anterior repair and repeat posterior repair.

3. Immediate complications like haemorrhage and medium and long term complications like pain or mesh extrusion.
4. Surgery for non-POP-related conditions: subsequent surgery for stress urinary incontinence or faecal incontinence.

Anterior compartment prolapse has been found to have the highest rates of anatomical recurrence of 40% with native tissue midline plication. Though the use of mesh reduces the recurrence rates, the size of the effect was small and higher rates of complications have been reported (51). Use of delayed absorbable sutures such as polydioxanone has been shown to reduce symptomatic recurrence at the end of 1 year of follow-up compared to rapidly absorbable sutures such as Vicryl or Polysorb, etc. (66). However, longer-term follow-up is required.

Apical prolapse is the most common site for symptomatic recurrence. In a systematic review and meta-analysis comparing mesh sacrocolpopexy to vaginal procedures involving native tissue repairs such as sacrospinous ligament fixation, postoperative durability and anatomic success was found to have a pooled odds ratio of 2.04 (95% confidence interval (CI) 1.12–3.72) at the end of follow-up of 1–2.5 years favouring mesh sacrocolpopexy (67).

Mesh use in pelvic floor surgery

Surgical meshes have been used to repair abdominal hernias, stress urinary incontinence, POP, and colorectal functional disorders. Synthetic and biological meshes have been introduced to reduce the recurrence rates of POP surgery by providing support in patients with no fascia or very poor fascia. The principle of using grafts in reconstructive surgery is to reinforce native tissue. Logically, mesh usage in women with a higher risk of recurrence should result in benefits which outweigh the risks, but there is no evidence thus far. The material must be safe, biologically compatible, and must provide both anatomical and functional results. The ideal material should be chemically and physically inert, noncarcinogenic, mechanically strong while remaining flexible, nonallergenic, non-inflammatory, and non-modifiable by body tissue. None of the meshes so far have satisfied all of these criteria and the ideal mesh is still awaited (68).

Clinical outcome following mesh implantation is influenced by material properties, product design, overall mesh size, route of implantation, patient characteristics, associated procedures (e.g. hysterectomy), and the surgeon's experience (69, 70). Results of the large pragmatic parallel group multicentre RCT from the United Kingdom (PROSPECT study) comparing native tissue, biological (graft trial), and non-absorbable vaginal mesh (mesh trial) usage for anterior or posterior compartment repair surgery did not show any significant difference at the end of 2 years following surgery in the primary outcome of participant-reported prolapse symptoms. Results from the graft trial of the PROSPECT study state that women reporting the feeling of 'something coming down' was higher in the graft (biological mesh) group compared to those who underwent native tissue repairs with a treatment effect size of 1.26 (95% CI 1.01–1.58) and a *P*-value of 0.04 at the end of the 2-year follow-up (71). Mesh complications were seen in 12% of the women in the synthetic mesh arm at the end of the 2-year follow-up (71). Long-term follow-up of these women will shed more light onto the success rates and long-term complication rates.

Mesh in POP surgery has been shown to be associated with complications such as infection, tissue extrusion, mesh exposure, organ perforation, mesh shrinkage, pelvic pain, and sexual dysfunction. Rare, but severe complications, including death, fistula formation, and mesh erosion into adjacent organs, have been reported in the Manufacturer and User Device Experience (MAUDE) database (72, 73). Following complications of mesh, litigation and law suits have resulted in the withdrawal of some mesh products from the market. NICE in its latest guidance on the use of transvaginal mesh in anterior or posterior vaginal wall repairs states that mesh has serious but well-recognized safety concerns and has to be used only in the context of research (74).

Scientific Committee on Emerging and Newly Identified Health Risks opinion

The European Commission has requested the Scientific Committee on Emerging and Newly Identified Health Risks (SCENIHR) to assess the health risks of meshes used in urogynaecology surgery. After a detailed review of evidence, SCENIHR concluded that it is important to consider the overall surface area of material used, the product design, and the properties of the material used. Mesh in POP surgery may be associated with higher morbidity due to the large amount of mesh used compared to that used in the surgical management of stress urinary incontinence. The use of mesh for the treatment of POP should only be considered in complex cases, in particular, after failed primary repair surgery. Mesh exposure rates for vaginal POP surgery with mesh range from 4% to 19% (75).

SCENIHR recommendations:

- The implantation of any mesh for the treatment of POP via the vaginal route should be only considered in complex cases in particular after failed primary repair surgery.
- Due to increased risks associated with the use of synthetic mesh for POP repair via a transvaginal route, this option should only be used when other surgical procedures have already failed or are expected to fail.
- Limiting the amount of mesh for all procedures where possible.
- There is a need for further improvement in the composition and design of synthetic meshes, in particular for POP surgery.
- The introduction of a certification system for surgeons based on existing international guidelines and established in cooperation with the relevant European Surgical Associations.
- Appropriate patient selection and counselling, which is of paramount importance for the optimal outcome for all surgical procedures, particularly for the indications discussed. This should be based on the results of further clinical evidence, which should be collected in a systematic fashion for all of these devices.

Scottish Independent Review of the use, safety and efficacy of transvaginal mesh implants in the treatment of stress urinary incontinence and pelvic organ prolapse in women

Vaginal mesh procedures have been suspended in Scotland from 2015 following a discussion in the parliament amid growing concerns on the safety of these procedures. An independent review has concluded that 'In the surgical treatment of POP, current evidence does not indicate any additional benefit from the use of transvaginal implants (polypropylene mesh or biological graft) over native tissue repair. Transvaginal mesh procedures must not be offered routinely' (68, 76).

Prevention

The effect of education of midwives and obstetricians on childbirth-related trauma with prolonged labour, prolonged active pushing in the second stage of labour, and spontaneous and instrumental vaginal deliveries needs to be studied. Maternal morbidity statistics should include damage to the pelvic floor from vaginal delivery. The role of regular reminders from healthcare professionals to perform pelvic floor exercises in women on a long-term basis to have an impact on pelvic floor health needs to be studied.

Conclusion and recommendations

With increases in ageing populations across the world, the disease burden of POP is set to increase multifold. Strategies to prevent or reduce the incidence of symptomatic POP (reinforcement of the importance of pelvic floor exercises) have to be developed.

Native tissue repairs in anterior and posterior compartments with delayed absorbable sutures are advocated to improve subjective outcomes of POP surgery. In women not wishing to preserve sexual function, obliterative procedures such as colpocleisis have a role in improving patient satisfaction. Long-term outcomes of uterus-preserving surgeries for POP are awaited. Counselling of women undergoing POP surgery should include discussion on its impact on sexual function from shortening and narrowing of the vagina and scarring from surgical repairs.

Though vaginal surgery was the mainstay in the management of POP, abdominal surgery (sacrocolpopexy/sacrohysteropexy) might give better anatomical outcomes compared to vaginal surgery for apical compartment prolapse.

Data on the interventions to prevent or minimize symptomatic POP is lacking. Further insight into the pathology behind development of POP, childbirth related neurological and muscular damage is required. We need to identify women at risk and take measures to reduce pelvic floor trauma in labour or where the risk is high consider caesarean section after discussion with the woman.

REFERENCES

1. MacLennan AH, Taylor AW, Wilson DH, et al. The prevalence of pelvic floor disorders and their relationship to gender, age, parity and mode of delivery. *BJOG* 2000;**107**:1460–70.
2. Wu JM, Hundley AF, Fulton RG, et al. Forecasting the prevalence of pelvic floor disorders in U.S. Women: 2010 to 2050. *Obstet Gynecol* 2009;**114**:1278–83.
3. Abdel-Fattah M, Familusi A, Fielding S, et al. Primary and repeat surgical treatment for female pelvic organ prolapse and incontinence in parous women in the UK: a register linkage study. *BMJ Open* 2011;**1**:e000206.
4. Smith FJ, Holman CD, Moorin RE, et al. Lifetime risk of undergoing surgery for pelvic organ prolapse. *Obstet Gynecol* 2010;**116**:1096–100.
5. Lowenstein E, Ottesen B, Gimbel H. Incidence and lifetime risk of pelvic organ prolapse surgery in Denmark from 1977 to 2009. *Int Urogynecol J* 2015;**26**:49–55.
6. Mant J, Painter R, Vessey M. Epidemiology of genital prolapse: observations from the Oxford Family Planning Association Study. *Br J Obstet Gynaecol* 1997;**104**:579–85.
7. Vergeldt TF, Weemhoff M, IntHout J, et al. Risk factors for pelvic organ prolapse and its recurrence: a systematic review. *Int Urogynecol J* 2015;**26**:1559–573.
8. DeLancey JO. Anatomy and biomechanics of genital prolapse. *Clin Obstet Gynecol* 1993;**36**:897–909.
9. DeLancey JO. The anatomy of the pelvic floor. *Curr Opin Obstet Gynecol* 1994;**6**:313–16.
10. Kearney R, Fitzpatrick M, Brennan S, et al. Levator ani injury in primiparous women with forceps delivery for fetal distress, forceps for second stage arrest, and spontaneous delivery. *Int J Gynaecol Obstet* 2010;**111**:19–22.
11. Kearney R, Miller JM, Ashton-Miller JA, et al. Obstetric factors associated with levator ani muscle injury after vaginal birth. *Obstet Gynecol* 2006;**107**:144–49.
12. Lien KC, Morgan DM, Delancey JO, et al. Pudendal nerve stretch during vaginal birth: a 3D computer simulation. *Am J Obstet Gynecol* 2005;**192**:1669–76.
13. Snooks SJ, Swash M, Henry MM, et al. Risk factors in childbirth causing damage to the pelvic floor innervation. *Int J Colorectal Dis* 1986;**1**:20–24.
14. Snooks SJ, Swash M, Mathers SE, et al. Effect of vaginal delivery on the pelvic floor: a 5-year follow-up. *Br J Surg* 1990;**77**:1358–60.
15. Haylen BT, Maher CF, Barber MD, Camargo S, Dandolu V, Digesu A, Goldman HB, Huser M, Milani AL, Moran PA, Schaer GN, Withagen MI. An International Urogynecological Association (IUGA)/International Continence Society (ICS) joint report on the terminology for female pelvic organ prolapse (POP). *Int Urogynecol J* 2016 Apr;**27**(4):655–84.
16. Swift SE, Barber MD. Pelvic organ prolapse: defining the disease. *Female Pelvic Med Reconstr Surg* 2010;**16**:201–203.
17. Bump RC, Mattiasson A, Bo K, et al. The standardization of terminology of female pelvic organ prolapse and pelvic floor dysfunction. *Am J Obstet Gynecol* 1996;**175**:10–17.
18. Haylen BT, Freeman RM, Lee J, et al. International Urogynecological Association (IUGA)/International Continence Society (ICS) joint terminology and classification of the complications related to native tissue female pelvic floor surgery. *Neurourol Urodyn* 2012;**31**:406–14.
19. Persu C, Chapple CR, Cauni V, et al. Pelvic Organ Prolapse Quantification System (POP-Q)—a new era in pelvic prolapse staging. *J Med Life* 2011;**4**:75–81.
20. Silva WA, Kleeman S, Segal J, et al. Effects of a full bladder and patient positioning on pelvic organ prolapse assessment. *Obstet Gynecol* 2004;**104**:37–41.
21. Barber MD, Lambers A, Visco AG, et al. Effect of patient position on clinical evaluation of pelvic organ prolapse. *Obstet Gynecol* 2000;**96**:18–22.
22. Swift S, Morris S, McKinnie V, et al. Validation of a simplified technique for using the POPQ pelvic organ prolapse classification system. *Int Urogynecol J Pelvic Floor Dysfunct* 2006;**17**:615–20.

23. Alperin M, Cook M, Tuttle LJ, et al. Impact of vaginal parity and aging on the architectural design of pelvic floor muscles. *Am J Obstet Gynecol* 2016;**215**:312.e1–9.

24. Alperin M, Kaddis T, Pichika R, et al. Pregnancy-induced adaptations in intramuscular extracellular matrix of rat pelvic floor muscles. *Am J Obstet Gynecol* 2016;**215**:210.e1–7.

25. Vergeldt TF, van Kuijk SM, Notten KJ, et al. Anatomical cystocele recurrence: development and internal validation of a prediction model. *Obstet Gynecol* 2016;**127**:341–47.

26. Hagen S, Stark D, Glazener C, et al. Individualised pelvic floor muscle training in women with pelvic organ prolapse (POPPY): a multicentre randomised controlled trial. *Lancet* 2014;**383**: 796–806.

27. Piya-Anant M, Therasakvichya S, Leelaphatanadit C, et al. Integrated health research program for the Thai elderly: prevalence of genital prolapse and effectiveness of pelvic floor exercise to prevent worsening of genital prolapse in elderly women. *J Med Assoc Thai* 2003;**86**:509–15.

28. Panman C, Wiegersma M, Kollen BJ, et al. Two-year effects and cost-effectiveness of pelvic floor muscle training in mild pelvic organ prolapse: a randomised controlled trial in primary care. *BJOG* 2017;**124**:511–20.

29. Clemons JL, Aguilar VC, Tillinghast TA, et al. Patient satisfaction and changes in prolapse and urinary symptoms in women who were fitted successfully with a pessary for pelvic organ prolapse. *Am J Obstet Gynecol* 2004;**190**:1025–29.

30. Abdool Z, Thakar R, Sultan AH, et al. Prospective evaluation of outcome of vaginal pessaries versus surgery in women with symptomatic pelvic organ prolapse. *Int Urogynecol J* 2011;**22**:273–78.

31. Lone F, Thakar R, Sultan AH. One-year prospective comparison of vaginal pessaries and surgery for pelvic organ prolapse using the validated ICIQ-VS and ICIQ-UI (SF) questionnaires. *Int Urogynecol J* 2015;**26**:1305–12.

32. Lone F, Thakar R, Sultan AH, et al. A 5-year prospective study of vaginal pessary use for pelvic organ prolapse. *Int J Gynaecol Obstet* 2011;**114**:56–59.

33. Fernando RJ, Thakar R, Sultan AH, et al. Effect of vaginal pessaries on symptoms associated with pelvic organ prolapse. *Obstet Gynecol* 2006;**108**:93–99.

34. de Albuquerque Coelho SC, de Castro EB, Juliato CR. Female pelvic organ prolapse using pessaries: systematic review. *Int Urogynecol J* 2016;**27**:1797–803.

35. Arias BE, Ridgeway B, Barber MD. Complications of neglected vaginal pessaries: case presentation and literature review. *Int Urogynecol J Pelvic Floor Dysfunct* 2008;**19**:1173–78.

36. Bulchandani S, Toozs-Hobson P, Verghese T, et al. Does vaginal estrogen treatment with support pessaries in vaginal prolapse reduce complications? *Post Reprod Health* 2015;**21**:141–45.

37. Khaja A, Freeman RM. How often should shelf/Gellhorn pessaries be changed? A survey of IUGA urogynaecologists. *Int Urogynecol J* 2014;**25**:941–46.

38. Barber MD, Brubaker L, Nygaard I, et al. Defining success after surgery for pelvic organ prolapse. *Obstet Gynecol* 2009;**114**: 600–609.

39. Colombo M, Milani R. Sacrospinous ligament fixation and modified McCall culdoplasty during vaginal hysterectomy for advanced uterovaginal prolapse. *Am J Obstet Gynecol* 1998;**179**:13–20.

40. National Institute for Health and Care Excellence (NICE). *Insertion of Mesh Uterine Suspension Sling (Including Sacrohysteropexy) for Uterine Prolapse Repair*. Interventional procedures guidance [IPG282]. London: NICE; 2009. Available at https://www.nice.org.uk/guidance/ipg282.

41. Ridgeway BM. Does prolapse equal hysterectomy? The role of uterine conservation in women with uterovaginal prolapse. *Am J Obstet Gynecol* 2015;**213**:802–809.

42. Detollenaere RJ, den Boon J, Stekelenburg J, et al. Sacrospinous hysteropexy versus vaginal hysterectomy with suspension of the uterosacral ligaments in women with uterine prolapse stage 2 or higher: multicentre randomised non-inferiority trial. *BMJ* 2015;**351**:h3717.

43. Vault or Uterine Evaluation (VUE) study. Aberdeen: Centre for Healthcare Randomised Trials (CHaRT). Available at: http://w3.abdn.ac.uk/hsru/vue/.

44. Marchionni M, Bracco GL, Checcucci V, et al. True incidence of vaginal vault prolapse. Thirteen years of experience. *J Reprod Med* 1999;**44**:679–84.

45. Ross JW, Preston M. Laparoscopic sacrocolpopexy for severe vaginal vault prolapse: five-year outcome. *J Minim Invasive Gynecol* 2005;**12**:221–26.

46. National Institute for Health and Care Excellence (NICE). *Uterine Suspension using Mesh (Including Sacrohysteropexy) to Repair Uterine Prolapse*. Interventional procedures guidance [IPG584]. London: NICE; 2017. Available at: https://www.nice.org.uk/guidance/ipg584.

47. National Institute for Health and Care Excellence (NICE). *Sacrocolpopexy using Vaginal Mesh to Repair Vaginal Vault Prolapse*. Interventional procedures guidance [IPG583]. London: NICE; 2017. Available at: https://www.nice.org.uk/guidance/ipg583.

48. Spelzini F, Frigerio M, Manodoro S, et al. Modified McCall culdoplasty versus Shull suspension in pelvic prolapse primary repair: a retrospective study. *Int Urogynecol J* 2017;**26**:65–71.

49. FitzGerald MP, Richter HE, Siddique S, et al. Colpocleisis: a review. *Int Urogynecol J Pelvic Floor Dysfunct* 2006;**17**:261–71.

50. Vij M, Bombieri L, Dua A, et al. Long-term follow-up after colpocleisis: regret, bowel, and bladder function. *Int Urogynecol J* 2014;**25**:811–15.

51. Maher C, Feiner B, Baessler K, et al. Surgical management of pelvic organ prolapse in women. *Cochrane Database Syst Rev* 2013;**4**:CD004014.

52. Freeman RM, Pantazis K, Thomson A, et al. A randomised controlled trial of abdominal versus laparoscopic sacrocolpopexy for the treatment of post-hysterectomy vaginal vault prolapse: LAS study. *Int Urogynecol J* 2013;**24**:377–84.

53. Olsen AL, Smith VJ, Bergstrom JO, et al. Epidemiology of surgically managed pelvic organ prolapse and urinary incontinence. *Obstet Gynecol* 1997;**89**:501–506.

54. Weber AM, Walters MD, Piedmonte MR, et al. Anterior colporrhaphy: a randomized trial of three surgical techniques. *Am J Obstet Gynecol* 2001;**185**:1299–304.

55. Chmielewski L, Walters MD, Weber AM, et al. Reanalysis of a randomized trial of 3 techniques of anterior colporrhaphy using clinically relevant definitions of success. *Am J Obstet Gynecol* 2011;**205**:69.e1–8.

56. Srikrishna S, Robinson D, Cardozo L. A longitudinal study of patient and surgeon goal achievement 2 years after surgery following pelvic floor dysfunction surgery. *BJOG* 2010;**117**:1504–11.

57. Kahn MA, Stanton SL. Posterior colporrhaphy: its effects on bowel and sexual function. *Br J Obstet Gynaecol* 1997;**104**:82–86.

58. Kahn MA, Stanton SL. Techniques of rectocele repair and their effects on bowel function. *Int Urogynecol J Pelvic Floor Dysfunct* 1998;**9**:37–47.

59. Klingele CJ, Bharucha AE, Fletcher JG, et al. Pelvic organ prolapse in defecatory disorders. *Obstet Gynecol* 2005;**106**:315–20.

60. Kahn MA, Breitkopf CR, Valley MT, et al. Pelvic Organ Support Study (POSST) and bowel symptoms: straining at stool is associated with perineal and anterior vaginal descent in a general gynecologic population. *Am J Obstet Gynecol* 2005;**192**:1516–22.

61. Tsunoda A, Takahashi T, Ohta T, et al. Anterior intussusception descent during defecation is correlated with the severity of fecal incontinence in patients with rectoanal intussusception. *Tech Coloproctol* 2016;**20**:171–16.

62. Kapoor DS, Freeman RM. Reoperation rate following prolapse surgery. *Am J Obstet Gynecol* 2009;**200**:e15.

63. Diwadkar GB, Barber MD, Feiner B, et al. Complication and reoperation rates after apical vaginal prolapse surgical repair: a systematic review. *Obstet Gynecol* 2009;**113**:367–73.

64. Price N, Slack A, Jwarah E, et al. The incidence of reoperation for surgically treated pelvic organ prolapse: an 11-year experience. *Menopause Int* 2008;**14**:145–48.

65. Toozs-Hobson P, Freeman R, Barber M, et al. An International Urogynecological Association (IUGA)/International Continence Society (ICS) joint report on the terminology for reporting outcomes of surgical procedures for pelvic organ prolapse. *Int Urogynecol J* 2012;**23**:527–35.

66. Bergman I, Soderberg MW, Kjaeldgaard A, et al. Does the choice of suture material matter in anterior and posterior colporrhaphy? *Int Urogynecol J* 2016;**27**:1357–65.

67. Siddiqui NY, Geller EJ, Visco AG. Symptomatic and anatomic 1-year outcomes after robotic and abdominal sacrocolpopexy. *Am J Obstet Gynecol* 2012;**206**:435.e1–5.

68. Scientific Committee on Emerging and Newly Identified Health Risks. Opinion on the safety of surgical meshes used in urogynecological surgery. 2015. Available at: https://ec.europa.eu/health/scientific_committees/emerging/docs/scenihr_o_049.pdf.

69. Huebner M, Hsu Y, Fenner DE. The use of graft materials in vaginal pelvic floor surgery. *Int J Gynaecol Obstet* 2006;**92**:279–88.

70. Maher C, Feiner B, Baessler K, et al. Transvaginal mesh or grafts compared with native tissue repair for vaginal prolapse. *Cochrane Database Syst Rev* 2016;**2**:CD012079.

71. Glazener CM, Breeman S, Elders A, et al. Mesh, graft, or standard repair for women having primary transvaginal anterior or posterior compartment prolapse surgery: two parallel-group, multicentre, randomised, controlled trials (PROSPECT). *Lancet* 2017;**389**:381–92.

72. Glazener CM, Breeman S, Elders A, et al. Mesh, graft, or standard repair for women having primary transvaginal anterior or posterior compartment prolapse surgery: two parallel-group, multicentre, randomised, controlled trials (PROSPECT). *Lancet* 2017;**389**:381–92.

73. Ellington DR, Richter HE. The role of vaginal mesh procedures in pelvic organ prolapse surgery in view of complication risk. *Obstet Gynecol Int* 2013;**2013**:356960.

74. Ellington DR, Richter HE. Indications, contraindications, and complications of mesh in surgical treatment of pelvic organ prolapse. *Clin Obstet Gynecol* 2013;**56**:276–88.

75. National Institute for Health and Care Excellence (NICE). *Transvaginal Mesh Repair of Anterior or Posterior Vaginal Wall Prolapse.* Interventional procedures guidance [IPG599]. London: NICE; 2017. Available at: https://www.nice.org.uk/guidance/ipg599.

76. Milani AL, Vollebregt A, Roovers JP, et al. [The use of mesh in vaginal prolapse]. *Ned Tijdschr Geneeskd* 2013;**157**:A6324.

77. The Scottish Independent Review of the use, safety and efficacy of transvaginal mesh implants in the treatment of stress urinary incontinence and pelvic organ prolapse in women. Final Report. 2017. Available at: http://wwwgovscot/Publications/2015/10/8485/downloads, 2017.

57

Urinary incontinence

Jay Iyer and Ajay Rane

Introduction

According to the most recent definition of the International Continence Society, urinary incontinence (UI), a symptom of impaired storage, is 'the complaint of any involuntary leakage of urine' (1). A condition that primarily affects women, UI is not a lethal condition; however, it significantly affects quality of life. Three types of incontinence are generally distinguished: stress urinary incontinence (SUI), urgency urinary incontinence (UUI), and mixed urinary incontinence (MUI), which associates with the first two (2). Prevalence varies significantly due to variations in definitions and measurement, methodology of data collection, lack of self-reporting, and sampling/non-response issues (3). Age, parity, vaginal childbirth, and body mass index are important factors that affect the prevalence of urinary incontinence. In 2005, the 'Evaluation of the Prevalence of urinary InContinence' (EPIC) study, which was the largest population-based survey of 19,165 individuals, was conducted in five developed countries to assess the prevalence of lower urinary tract symptoms in men and women. Prevalence of overactive bladder (OAB) overall was 11.8%; rates were similar in men and women and increased with age. OAB was more prevalent than all types of UI combined (9.4%) (2). For 2008–2009, the healthcare expenditure in Australia estimated for incontinence (both urinary and faecal) was $201.6 million (not including residential aged care costs) (3). Besides the obvious issue of hygiene, UI results in ramifications that extend to the sufferer's social and sexual life (4).

Anatomy and physiology of the continence apparatus

The female urethra, typically developed by the 12th gestational week from the urogenital sinus, is a 4 cm tubular structure that begins at the bladder neck and terminates at the vaginal vestibule (5). The striated external urethral sphincter (compressor urethrae) is in the distal two-thirds of the urethra (level 5–6) and is composed of type I (slow-twitch) muscle fibres. This sphincter is horseshoe-shaped and is deficient posteriorly. Distally, the sphincter fans out laterally along the inferior border of the pubic rami and is fixed against the anterior vaginal wall. This arrangement is critical for urinary continence. Near the vestibule (level 3–4) lies the urethrovaginal sphincter, which contracts with the bulbospongiosus muscle and tightens the urogenital hiatus. Distally, the female urethra is suspended by the suspensory ligament of the clitoris and the pubovesical ligament. It is this hammock (level 1–2), or sling, of fascial attachments that suspends the urethra beneath the pubis (6) (**Figure 57.1**). The arterial supply to the female urethra comes via the internal pudendal, vaginal, and inferior vesical branches of the vaginal arteries. Venous drainage is via the internal pudendal veins.

The female urethra is a multilayered tube lined by transitional cell epithelium proximally and by non-keratinizing stratified squamous epithelium distally. The highly vascular and oestrogen-dependent submucosa contributes a large percentage of the urethral closing pressure; accordingly, hormone withdrawal can lead to stress incontinence. The urinary bladder has an apex at the anterior end and the fundus as its posteroinferior triangular portion. When completely filled, the bladder can have a capacity of up to 500 mL. The bladder trigone is bounded by the two ureteral orifices and the internal urethral orifice. The bladder neck is where the fundus and the inferolateral surfaces come together, leading into the urethra. At the bladder neck, as opposed to the upper bladder, the detrusor muscle layers—transitional epithelium, lamina propria, and muscularis mucosa—are clearly separable. In females, the inner longitudinal fibres of the bladder neck converge radially to pass downward as the inner longitudinal layer of the urethra. The bladder and urethra are supported by the pubovesical ligament (Table 57.1).

Physiology of micturition

See Figure 57.2 (7).

Classification of urinary incontinence

Urinary incontinence is defined as the complaint of involuntary loss of urine, which could be a urethral or extra-urethral loss (8).

Classification of urinary incontinence:

1. SUI
2. UUI

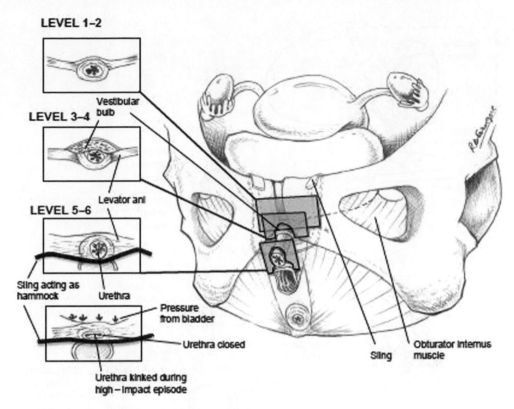

Figure 57.1 Anatomy of the urethra in relation to other pelvic structures.

3. MUI
4. Other:
   a. Transient causes ('DIAPPERS'):
      Delirium
      Infection—urinary
      Atrophic urethritis and vaginitis
      Pharmaceuticals
      Psychologic disorders, especially depression
      Excessive urine output (e.g. from heart failure or hyperglycaemia)
      Restricted mobility
         Stool impaction
   b. Urethral diverticulum
   c. Vesicovaginal fistula
   d. Ectopic urethrae.

In this chapter, we shall be focusing on mainly three types of female urinary incontinence commonly encountered in clinical practice:

- UUI is the complaint of involuntary leakage accompanied by or immediately preceded by urgency.
- SUI is the complaint of involuntary leakage on effort or exertion, or on sneezing or coughing.
- MUI is the complaint of involuntary leakage associated with urgency and also with effort, exertion, sneezing, and coughing (9).

Demographics

UI is a very common symptom, the prevalence of this condition varies between 7% and 55%, with SUI being the most common (40–55%) followed by MUI (25–40%) and UUI (about 10%) (3). The incidence of UI increases with age demonstrating a bimodal distribution with a peak in young women (largely SUI) and postmenopausally around age 70 (MUI and UUI predominate). Racial differences have been noted with UI being commonest in white women and least common in Asian women with an intermediate prevalence in black women. It is not unusual to find a positive family history of UI in the mother or sister(s) (10).

Table 57.1 Efferent pathways and neurotransmitter mechanisms that regulate the lower urinary tract

Parasympathetic postganglionic axons	Acetylcholine	M3 muscarinic receptors	Bladder contraction
Parasympathetic postganglionic nerves		Release ATP nitric oxide	Excite bladder smooth muscle Relax urethral smooth muscle
Sympathetic postganglionic neurons	Noradrenaline	β3-adrenergic receptors	Relax bladder smooth muscle
		Activates α1-adrenergic receptors	Contract urethral smooth muscle
Somatic axons in pudendal nerve	Acetylcholine	Nicotinic cholinergic receptors	Contraction of the external sphincter striated muscle

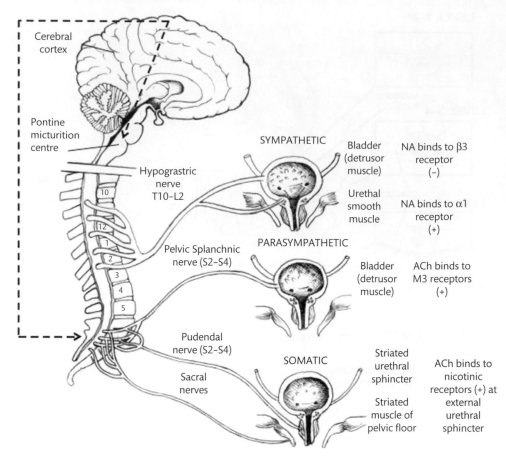

Figure 57.2 Physiological mechanism and basis for pharmacotherapeutics.

Evaluation of female urinary incontinence

A focused history, clinical examination, and urodynamic testing forms the basis of the assessment of a woman suffering from UI. Validated questionnaires such as the Bristol Female Lower Urinary Tract Symptoms (MBFLUTS) questionnaire and bladder diaries are usually administered prior to a consultation, to enable subjective assessment of the effect of symptoms on the patient's quality of life and to gauge its impact on bowel and sexual function.

History taking

History taking is a key element in the assessment of patients with UI and enables the clinician to tentatively categorize patients as having SUI, UUI, or MUI based on their symptoms. History also helps in assessing patients with stand-alone or associated voiding disorders. Typically, symptoms associated with SUI include leak on cough, sneeze, or high-impact physical exertion and occasionally with a change in posture and coital activity. Patients with UUI complain of frequency, nocturia, and urgency with or without incontinence. There may be an overlap of symptoms and occasionally urgency incontinence may be triggered by activities such as coughing and can mimic stress incontinence. Additional MUI is very common finding and it is therefore imperative that management be directed towards the predominant symptom (11). Voiding disorders manifest with symptoms of straining to void, slow and strained stream, misdirected urinary stream, and feeling of incomplete emptying

(12). If, however, the patient complains of continuous leakage and extra-urethral urinary leakage loss, it may indicate urinary fistula and these symptoms need appropriate investigations. Women may complain of pelvic floor symptoms of vaginal or uterocervical prolapse in the form of a bulge at the vaginal introitus, vaginal fullness, double-voiding, needing to digitate the vagina to empty bowels, and sexual dysfunction.

Although pelvic floor disorders are frequently found in women who have delivered vaginally, it is not uncommon to find nulliparous women and those who have had elective caesarean births suffering from symptoms of UI. That being said, obstetric history, in particular the parity, mode of delivery, instrumental deliveries, associated vaginal trauma, and birth weight are some important risk factors. Equally, gynaecological conditions such as large fibroids and ovarian cysts may precipitate UI. The symptoms of UI worsen after menopause. In patients with voiding disorders it is not unusual to have a past surgical history of retropubic continence-enhancing operations such as the Marshall–Marchetti–Krantz or Burch colposuspension. Spinal surgery or complex colorectal surgeries in the past may also be relevant.

Chronic medical conditions, such as diabetes, connective tissue disorders, neurological disorders, in particular Parkinson's disease, multiple sclerosis, spinal cord injuries, and chronic obstructive airway disease should be ruled out. Medications such as diuretics, alpha-blockers, alpha-agonists, and so on may also contribute to lower urinary tract symptoms. Finally, it is important to enquire about the intake of caffeine, alcohol, and carbonated drinks.

Physical examination

A thorough physical examination should follow to elicit positive evidence to support a history of UI. Typically, this involves a general examination to establish body mass index and is followed by abdominal, pelvic, and rectal examinations. A focused neurological examination may be indicated in some patients; however, a quick assessment of sacral segments (S2–S4) is always performed by testing for reflexes such as the bulbocavernosus or the anal 'wink' reflex. Abdominal examination may reveal a mass; more often, abdominal scars may provide clues to previous surgery that may be relevant to the patient's symptoms.

Local genital examination should commence, looking for signs of vaginal atrophy or evidence of maceration of vulval tissues secondary to urinary leakage. Demonstration of urinary leak preferably in the supine and standing positions should follow this and one should look for signs of vaginal/uterocervical prolapse. A large anterior (or occasionally posterior) vaginal prolapse may produce a relative obstruction of the urethra that can impair bladder emptying. Paradoxically, a posterior vaginal wall prolapse may splint the bladder neck and mask SUI; compressing the prolapse may uncover 'occult' incontinence.

Investigations

Urinalysis

Urine microscopy, culture, and sensitivity testing should be performed in all cases to determine if there is any evidence of haematuria, pyuria, glycosuria, or proteinuria. Urinary tract infections and evidence of bladder cancer should be tested for before proceeding with further investigations.

Assessment of residual urine

Measurement of post-void residual urine volume by ultrasonography can test for a bladder-emptying abnormality or incontinence associated with chronic urinary retention. A post-void residual urine volume of 50 mL or less is considered normal and above 200 mL merits further investigation.

Imaging

An ultrasound scan of the urinary tract to demonstrate the anatomy of the kidney, ureter, and bladder should be ordered; a pelvic ultrasound may be ordered to confirm/exclude pelvic pathology such as fibroids or ovarian cysts. Occasionally a computed tomography scan or magnetic resonance imaging may be necessary.

Overview of urodynamics

Urodynamic testing involves an objective assessment of the storage, contractile, and voiding function of the bladder (**Figure 57.3**). In some centres a flexible cystoscopy is also performed. Only the procedure is described here, as a discussion of findings on urodynamics and the pros and cons of this procedure is outside the scope of this chapter.

Uroflowmetry is the first part of urodynamic assessment, and in most centres is done within the privacy of the toilet because the environment within the urodynamics laboratory is not always conducive, and 'stage fright' may affect results. This test requires the patient with her bladder comfortably full to void into a calibrated flowmeter. The recorded parameters during the test include:

- flow rate, which is the volume of urine voided via the urethra per second
- voided volume, which is the total volume expelled via the urethra
- maximum flow rate, which is the maximum measured value of the flow rate
- flow time, which is the time over which measurable flow occurs
- average flow rate, which is the volume voided divided by voiding time.

Based on the patterns elicited, this test is a useful adjunct to diagnosing voiding disorders (13).

Cystometry produces a cystometrogram that demonstrates the pressure–volume relationship of the bladder. This test comprises filling, voiding, and urethral phases, and is designed to reproduce patients' symptoms (i.e. their bladder function in a laboratory environment). Not uncommonly this test may reveal asymptomatic bladder dysfunction; it is also a useful tool to objectively assess postoperative success/failure. The patient's sensation of bladder filling, first desire to void, strong desire to void, urgency/pain are recorded while the cystometrogram plots the corresponding pressures. The test involves the insertion of a urethral catheter (filling catheter typically with an integrated pressure sensitive tip) to measure vesical pressures and a vaginal/rectal catheter to measure the abdominal

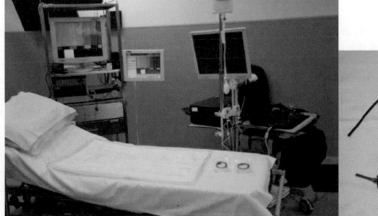
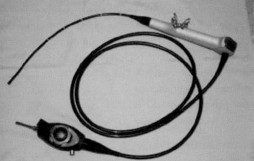

Figure 57.3 Urodynamics and flexible cystoscopy set-up.

pressures. The difference, that is, vesical pressure minus abdominal pressure, gives the detrusor pressure. The detrusor pressure is sometimes measured during voiding; however, its value in detecting obstructive pathology in females is limited. Cystometry is useful for distinguishing SUI from UUI caused by bladder overactivity. It is particularly useful in patients with MUI, where the management, medical or surgical, may be determined on the predominant finding. The final assessment is the measurement of the urethral pressure profile (measured in mmHg) or the Valsalva leak point pressure in cm of H_2O. UPP may be useful in diagnosing a deficiency in urethral function which is proposed as the primary mechanism for SUI. Its role in determining the need for or the type of surgery remains controversial. Patients with low Valsalva leak point pressure/maximum urethral closure pressure are said to have intrinsic sphincter deficiency, as opposed to the majority of patients with SUI who have urethral hypermobility as the primary cause of their leakage (13).

Cystoscopy

Usually an optional evaluation, cystoscopy is routinely offered in some units as a part of urodynamic testing. The procedure is definitely indicated when a patient has microscopic or overt haematuria, has a painful bladder, previous bladder injury, radiation, and previous surgery with mesh or tape. It is also useful if a urethral stricture, urinary fistula, or diverticulum is suspected.

Management of incontinence

Lifestyle modifications and interventions

Lifestyle factors associated with urinary incontinence and stress incontinence in particular, include obesity (an independent risk factor), smoking, heavy lifting, high-impact activity, and constipation. Abdominal adiposity increases intra-abdominal pressure, secondarily increasing intravesicular pressure and urethral mobility, resulting in incontinence. Thus, such patients should be referred for a weight loss programme; studies show that even a 5–10% weight loss resulted in marked improvement of incontinence (14). Obese women who lose significant amounts of weight before surgery may find that weight loss reduces the severity of their symptoms and obviate the need for surgery. At the very least, patients should be encouraged to lose weight preoperatively. A behavioural weight loss intervention should be considered the first-line treatment for overweight and obese women reporting stress incontinence (15). Weight loss and lifestyle interventions may also reduce the prevalence of incontinence in type 2 diabetics who are at increased risk for UI. Women should be encouraged to rationalize their fluid and caffeine intake and to give up smoking; the latter is another independent risk factor for SUI. Chronic constipation may cause pelvic floor muscle damage either directly or indirectly via pudendal nerve damage. These patients are also at a higher risk of recurrence following surgery. Hence dietary modifications such as a higher-fibre diet, laxatives, and stool softeners should be considered.

Non-pharmacological—role of pelvic floor physiotherapy/biofeedback

The mechanisms of action of pelvic floor muscle training (PFMT) are by strength training and counterbalancing. PFMT improves urethral resistance and pelvic visceral support, including urethral support, primarily by increasing the strength of the voluntary pelvic floor muscles. Additionally, voluntary contraction of the PFM precedes the increase in intra-abdominal pressure preventing urinary leakage (16). A focused regimen of PFMT is thought to act by changing the morphology and position of the muscles to enable subconscious contraction similar to continent women (17.) At least 4 months of PFMT are recommended to see tangible results; the improvement in the first 6–8 weeks is mainly caused by neural adaptation which is then followed by muscle hypertrophy, a process that continues over several months (18). PFMT is best administered by a trained physiotherapist and is an excellent first-line treatment for UI. If no improvement is noted after 6 months, the patient should consider alternative management strategies. Biofeedback may be considered in the subset of women who are unable to contract their pelvic floor muscles and therefore are unable to reliably perform PFMT. Biofeedback apparatus such as vaginal cones, manometry, and electromyography are commonly used to assist with PFMT.

Timed or scheduled voiding is a programme developed to increase intervals between voids to attempt to suppress urgency and decrease incontinence episodes. The theory behind pelvic floor muscle retraining for urgency UI is based on the observation that a detrusor contraction can be inhibited by pelvic floor muscle contraction. Increasing the strength of the pelvic floor and ability of an individual to hold a contraction can result in extra time (perhaps just a few more seconds) to reach the toilet and avoid leakage (19).

Pharmacotherapy

Antimuscarinic medications have been used as second-line treatment of OAB symptoms, none is clearly more effective than the others and all have the tendency to cause distressing side effects (20). The clinician should therefore individualize treatment based on product and patient characteristics.

There are five known subtypes of muscarinic receptors within the bladder of which M2 and M3 subtypes predominate. Stimulation of the M2 receptor inhibits relaxation of the detrusor muscle, while activation of M3 receptors results in detrusor contractions (**Figure** 57.2). Antimuscarinic agents (anticholinergics) have been developed to act on these two receptors. Antimuscarinic drugs including trospium, solifenacin, fesoterodine, tolterodine, and oxybutynin reduce the perception of urinary urgency and improve continence. Side effects were commonest with non-selective antimuscarinics such as oxybutynin and least common with solifenacin. Side effects commonly include dry mouth, constipation, and blurred vision. These drugs are contraindicated in patients with narrow-angle glaucoma and also carry the risk of urinary retention and should be used with caution in individuals with chronic open-angle glaucoma. Similarly, these drugs may precipitate urinary retention in patients with bladder neck obstruction. The bladder contains both alpha-adrenergic and beta-adrenergic receptors and stimulation of these receptors can exert some influence on the bladder and urethra. In the past couple of years, mirabegron, a beta-3-adrenergic agonist that acts specifically on the beta-3-adrenoreceptors in the wall of the bladder, has been developed. The drug relaxes the bladder wall during the filling and storage phase of micturition. Mirabegron was found in three separate randomized controlled clinical trials to significantly decrease urinary frequency and incontinence episodes, while significantly increasing bladder capacity (21). Although adverse effects are fewer than anticholinergics, patients may experience side effects such as hypertension, nasopharyngitis, urinary tract infection, and headache. Patients on mirabegron should have their blood pressure monitored and it is contraindicated in patients with uncontrolled hypertension. Anticholinergics have a high rate of discontinuation due to side effects: only 18% of patients continue with antimuscarinic medication after 6 months (21). Thus, pharmacotherapy is useful in cases of OAB but its effectiveness is limited due to side effects resulting in low patient compliance.

Surgeries for incontinence

Overactive bladder

Intradetrusor botulinum toxin

Botulinum toxin is a presynaptic neuromuscular-blocking agent that causes selective and reversible muscle weakness. The effect may last for several months when injected into the detrusor muscles (21): 100–300 units of the toxin, usually of the A subtype, are injected cystoscopically into the detrusor muscle at more than 10–15 different locations sparing the trigone. Postoperative urodynamic assessment usually results in significant increases in cystometric capacity of the bladder secondary to increased bladder wall compliance. There are reduced patient episodes of urgency and urgency incontinence; most patients report a reduction in requirement of antimuscarinic medications, some stopping these altogether. Patient satisfaction rates are high despite the increased incidence of voiding dysfunction and occasional urinary retention, the latter results in some patients needing to self-catheterize intermittently. Intradetrusor botulinum toxin is a safe option both in patients with neurogenic bladders and intractable OAB.

Sacral nerve stimulation

Patients with OAB symptoms refractory to other less invasive methods may be offered sacral neuromodulation. Afferent sacral nerve fibres are activated (typically the S3 segment) which in turn inhibit parasympathetic motor neurons consequently preventing detrusor contractions. The procedure is often two-staged: in the first stage, the electrodes are tested to ascertain if the patient is likely to show an adequate response to stimulation (i.e. reduced number of voids or incontinence episodes). Up to 70% patients show a positive response and go on to have the second stage of the procedure, namely the permanent impulse generator implanted under the skin. Sacral nerve stimulation should be considered in refractory cases of OAB. About 10% of patients show no response and a smaller percentage need removal secondary to infection (21).

Percutaneous tibial nerve stimulation

Percutaneous tibial nerve stimulation (PTNS) is a minimally invasive, outpatient treatment with no major side effects that has been shown to decrease symptoms related to OAB. PTNS involves placing a small needle electrode into the lower inner aspect of either leg near the medial malleolus. The electrode is connected to a stimulator that generates an electrical pulse, which then travels to the sacral nerve plexus via the tibial nerve. Similar to sacral neuromodulation, accessing the posterior tibial nerve stimulates sensory afferent nerves, but PTNS does so in a less invasive manner compared with direct sacral neuromodulation (19).

Augmentation cystoplasty

This involves bivalving a functionally OAB and attaching a segment of intestine, usually ileum or sigmoid, to increase functional capacity and lower the end-filling pressure. Female patients are usually prone to infections in about 30% of cases; additionally, a significant proportion of patients may need to self-catheterize. It involves a major operation and should be used in only a selected group of patients. Advances in tissue engineering may offer a viable alternative to the use of bowel and this operation, as a result, may find a wider application in the future (19).

Suprapubic cystostomy

Intractable cases of OAB, especially patients with significant detrusor sphincter dyssynergia or neurogenic incontinence, who cannot, or find it difficult to void *per urethram*, may need to be offered a urinary diversion procedure such as a suprapubic cystostomy. In this procedure, a suprapubic catheter is inserted into the dome of the bladder usually under cystoscopic guidance. The catheter is then left *in situ* semipermanently. The catheter needs a change every 8–12 weeks, usually in clinic. In some patients it is possible to wean the patient off the catheter after and retrain them to void *per urethram*.

Stress urinary incontinence

- Retropubic bladder neck suspension
- Mid-urethral slings
- Urethral bulking agents (UBAs).

Retropubic bladder neck suspension

Principle: to reduce the hypermobility of the bladder neck thereby improving continence.

The procedure that is most commonly performed in the space of Retzius or the retropubic space is Burch colposuspension. It used to be commonly performed via a transverse suprapubic incision such as a Pfannenstiel; however, for the past 20 years or more the procedure has been done laparoscopically as well. The procedure has lost its 'sheen' since the advent of mid-urethral slings in the 1990s, however it still has a role in women who either do not want a sling, are allergic to mesh, or are having a laparoscopic paravaginal repair for an associated cystocele, or indeed any concomitant laparoscopic procedure. The procedure involves the passage of two or three permanent or delayed absorbable sutures through the endopelvic fascia lateral to the mid urethra and bladder neck and then through the ipsilateral Cooper's (iliopectineal) ligament and tied with gentle tension. Laparoscopic Burch colposuspension has been described using the transperitoneal or extraperitoneal approach. The extraperitoneal approach naturally minimizes the risk of intra-abdominal injury by avoiding intraperitoneal pelvic adhesions and is associated with a shorter learning curve. If patients are undergoing concomitant pelvic surgery, the transperitoneal approach may be more suitable (22); however, it tends to take longer. The advantages of laparoscopic pelvic surgery are better visualization, shorter hospital stay, better cosmetics, less postoperative pain, and faster recovery to normal daily activity. With open Burch colposuspensions, short-term cure rates of 73–92% have been reported; even after 5–10 years, approximately 70% of patients are still continent. With laparoscopic Burch colposuspensions, the short-term cure rates are excellent, nearing 90%; however, the long-term cure rates are lower at about 59–68%. Urinary tract injury both to the bladder and ureter are commoner with laparoscopic Burch, as is the increased incidence of OAB, approximately 3–8% (22). Even in an era dominated by mid-urethral slings, laparoscopic Burch colposuspension does have a niche role in the management of SUI.

Mid-urethral synthetic slings

Principle: to improve continence by enhancing support to the mid urethra.

The hammock theory by DeLancey urethral support is provided by the layers outside the urethra on which it rests (23):

- The anterior vaginal wall
- The endopelvic fascia between the arcus tendineus fascia pelvis on each side
- Pelvic floor muscles (**Figure 57.4**).

When this 'shelf' of tissue is intact, any increase in intra-abdominal pressures causes the urethra to remain shut against it. It is when this shelf is injured during childbirth or atrophied with age and consequent hypo-oestrogenism that urethral hypermobility and/or SUI may result. In fact, in patients with a mid-urethral sling, stress causes a dynamic kinking of the urethra against the resistance provided by the shelf of tissue, thus preventing stress leakage (24).

Since the introduction of mid-urethral slings in the 1995 by Ulmsten based on the 'integral theory of female urinary continence' by Petros and Ulmsten (25), the focus of continence surgery shifted

from the bladder neck to the mid urethra. Procedures for stress incontinence became quicker and less invasive, and at the same time maintained or even exceeded the success rates of previous procedures. Mid-urethral slings have grown in acceptance and popularity to gain a foremost position in SUI surgery.

Retropubic slings The original tension-free vaginal tape (TVT) procedure placed a polypropylene sling at the level of the mid urethra via a 'bottom-to-top' approach. This is still the preferred approach and the GYNECARE TVT EXACT Continence System (Ethicon, USA), is a popular product exemplifying this technique. The trocar attached to the sling is passed from a mid-urethral vaginal incision through the para-urethral tunnels in the endopelvic fascia and the retropubic space to a suprapubic exit point, one on each side of the midline. The 'top-to-bottom' technique was developed in 2001 (26) with the introduction of the Suprapubic Arc system (SPARC, American Medical Systems, Inc., Minnetonka, MN, USA) sling. This technique involves passage of the trocar from a suprapubic incision through all of the above-mentioned layers to a suburethral incision. Regardless of the type of approach, the procedure involves careful identification of mid urethra—a failure to do so may result in the sling being sited close to the bladder neck, predisposing the patient to develop postoperative voiding dysfunction. Most importantly the sling is placed 'tension free': if the sling is placed too tight, there is a potential for postoperative voiding problems that manifest commonly as a failed trial of void, that is, the inability of the patient to pass urine *per urethram* immediately after surgery, or more rarely, as urinary retention or overflow incontinence. Occasionally, the patient needs to return to theatre and the tape may have to be loosened/divided. Interestingly, division of the tape does not lead to failure of

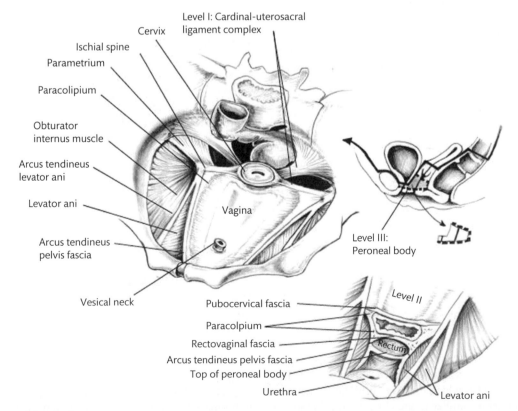

Figure 57.4 DeLancey's levels of support.

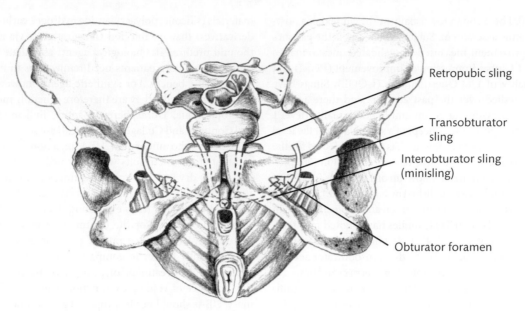

Retropubic sling

Transobturator sling

Interobturator sling (minisling)

Obturator foramen

Figure 57.5 Types of mid-urethral slings and their trajectories.

the procedure as 80% of the patients still remain continent. Hence all patients have a strict 'trial of void' protocol in the first 2–3 hours postoperatively. During this time, patients are given only enough fluid to fill their bladders comfortably enough for them to void spontaneously. A bladder scan is done after voiding to look at residuals. As a rule of thumb, if the patient voids 200–300 mL of urine and has less than this in her bladder on scan, she is deemed to have passed a trial of void. A lot of other factors such as pain, postoperative swelling, associated prolapse surgery, a 'tight sling' (see earlier in this paragraph), and unfamiliar surroundings may impact the patient's ability to void successfully postoperatively. Therefore, patients are given adequate pain relief preferably with anti-inflammatories, prescribed aperients and sent home to more familiar environs. Postoperative voiding difficulty after a mid-urethral sling procedure is an unfortunate but well-known temporary complication of pelvic surgery with an occurrence of approximately 3–10% (27).

Transobturator slings The next generation of mid-urethral slings were the transobturator tape (TOT) slings. The vaginal incision is still very similar to the one described in the previous section and is usually smaller. The double helix needle is inserted through a stab incision in skin overlying the obturator foramen just below the insertion of the adductor longus tendon. The needle is then driven through the obturator fossa to exit via the through the para-urethral tunnels created via the vaginal incision up to the level of inferior pubic ramus. The polypropylene sling is then attached to the needle tip and withdrawn through the track described above to exit at the obturator incision. The original TOT operation was described as an 'outside-in' technique with the tape being passed from the thigh into the vaginal incision (Uratape, PorgesMentor, Le Plessis, Robinson, France & Monarc, AMS, MN, USA). The technique was later modified as an 'inside-out', approach, with a vaginal incision through the obturator foramen and out through the inner thigh as the TVT-Obturator system (TVT-O, Ethicon Inc., Johnson & Johnson, Somerville, NJ, USA) (28). As with the TVT, the sling should be sited in a tension-free manner well away from the bladder neck. Trial of

void protocols are similar. Postoperative voiding dysfunction is lower with TOT when compared to TVT.

Single-incision minislings The latest entrants to the sling 'market' are the single-incision minislings (SIMS). These slings require a vaginal incision similar to the one described previously and involves creation of the para-urethral tunnels to the inferior pubic ramus. The obturator membrane is then 'perforated' with the tip of the scissors to facilitate the passage of the sling needle. The SIMS needle with the polypropylene sling loaded to its tip is inserted via the para-urethral tunnel on the patient's left through the perforation in the obturator membrane and inserted into the obturator internus muscle to which it remains anchored. The procedure is repeated on the patient's right, this time however, the sling is released from the needle only after it is appropriately 'tensioned' under the urethra. Thus the SIMS differs from the TVT and TOT in that it is not 'tension free', in fact, it is quite the opposite. Despite this, the rates of postoperative voiding dysfunction are no different to that with the other two slings.

Type 1, macroporous, monofilament polypropylene mesh is used for all types of slings. The type 1 mesh promotes prompt ingress of fibrous connective tissue and capillaries thus encouraging tissue host ingrowth and integration allowing the mesh to anchor within the tissue. This inflammatory response wanes with time thus reducing the risk of infection (28).

Indications

1. Urodynamic SUI
2. Low-pressure (low maximum urethral closure pressure/Valsalva leak point pressure) SUI (intrinsic sphincter deficiency)
3. (Selected cases) of MUI.

Although the classical indication for slings is patients with urethral hypermobility, slings are also being increasingly used in patients with intrinsic sphincter deficiency who typically get offered UBAs.

Studies comparing TVT, TOT, and SIMS Cure with mid-urethral slings is described in 'objective' or 'subjective' terms. Objective cure is the absence of SUI on a cough test usually in the context of a post-operative urodynamic assessment. Subjective success is the patient's perception of improvement measured via validated questionnaires such as the Patient Global Impression of Improvement (PGI-I) and Incontinence Quality of Life Questionnaire (I-QOL). Slings have been extensively studied over the past 20 years and there are numerous studies that provide a large amount of good quality (level 1 and 2 evidence) that support the concept of a sling placed at the level of the mid urethra. Long-term follow-up has been published for the original TVT procedure with the most recent publication (28) providing level 2 evidence with mean follow-up of 11.5 years (of 77% of patients from the original series published by Nillson et al.), revealing an objective cure was found in 90% of women and subjective cure in 77%, based on the PGI-I. With TOT, studies have quoted mid-term (i.e. 3–5-year) cure rates of 82.4–88.4% (28). High-quality data indicate about a 7–10% failure rate for both the transobturator and the retropubic approaches, with comparable short-term cure rates.

In a 3-year follow-up by Basu and Duckett, there was a significantly higher 3-year failure rate for a SIMS versus a retropubic mid-urethral sling (29). Both procedures had reduced efficacy over time. Another multicentre trial published in 2014 indicated that SIMS has no advantage in terms of safety over TVTs and was found to be less effective than TVTs (30). Other studies, however, indicate otherwise. A meta-analysis published in 2014 showed that there was no evidence of significant differences in patient-reported and objective cure between currently used SIMS and other slings at mid-term follow-up and SIMS were associated with more favourable recovery time (31). A more recent meta-analysis shows no significant difference in the patient-reported cure rate and objective cure rate between SIMS and TOT (32).

Comparison of slings with other procedures for SUI In a high-quality, multicentre randomized controlled trial of TVT versus Burch colposuspension, the authors showed equivalent efficacy of cure for TVT and Burch colposuspension in a 5-year follow-up (33). There was no difference in success in a 1-hour stress pad test (81% vs 90%), stress leakage (63% vs 70%), or satisfaction rates (91% vs 90%). Hospital stay was significantly shorter for the TVT group and there was no difference in the chance of reoperation, although patients who had colposuspension were more likely to require prolapse surgery. TVT was more cost-effective than Burch colposuspension. The Cochrane review found that slings (TVT) had a shorter operating time (35 vs 87 minutes) and shorter hospital stays (34). For open colposuspension versus slings, objective cure rates at 12 months were 79% for synthetic slings versus 82% for colposuspension. For laparoscopic colposuspension versus slings, no significant difference in patient-reported outcomes within 12 months was shown; 80% for slings versus 74% for colposuspension (34).

Urethral bulking agents

UBAs are injectable materials used as a minimally invasive way to treat intrinsic sphincter deficiency by increasing the urethral closure pressure and thus increasing resistance to urinary flow. These agents are also viable alternatives for patients who have failed other options such as slings, who desire a less invasive option, those who pose an anaesthetic risk, those with a fixed scarred urethra, and women of childbearing age who desire more children (35). UBAs are composed of either biological (collagen, autologous fat) or synthetic

materials (silicone, polyacrylamide hydrogel, carbon beads, calcium derivatives) that are injected transurethrally via a cystoscope into the mid urethra. The biological agents assimilate into tissues over time and therefore patients need reinjections to maintain ongoing symptomatic benefit. For synthetic agents, however, reinjection is not often required—they are therefore generally more effective (35). Macroplastique, Durasphere, Coaptite, Bulkamid (all synthetic), and Contigen and Collagen (biological) are some examples of UBAs. In patients who underwent UBA injection with Macroplastique, substantial durable results were obtained during 2 years with 84% of patients dry at 1 year, and two-thirds at 24 months (36). Three studies meeting the inclusion criteria were identified. Three randomized controlled trials evaluating the use of UBAs versus other surgical procedures for the treatment of female SUI showed that the objective recurrence rate of peri- or transurethral injections is significantly higher in comparison with the other surgical procedures in the treatment of primary or recurrent SUI. However, the incidence of voiding dysfunction is lower with UBAs. In summary, UBAs should not be proposed as first-line treatment in those women seeking permanent cure for both primary and recurrent SUI. However, the effectiveness of a procedure should be balanced with its invasiveness and patients' expectations, where UBAs have a definite role (37).

Conclusion

Female UI in an ageing population is a common social and hygienic problem that has a significant economic impact both for the individual and the community as a whole. Making an accurate diagnosis can be difficult and may involve invasive investigations. Conservative methods should be trialled before offering medications and or surgery. Advances in pharmacotherapy, development of improved biomedical products, and minimally invasive surgical techniques have ensured that women suffering from UI have a variety of medical and surgical options available. Patients with UUI can be offered highly specific drugs with fewer side effects. Intravesicular botulinum toxin may be viewed as a panacea for women with intractable UUI unresponsive to medications. Currently, mid-urethral slings are the most commonly used modality for patients with SUI. Laparoscopic Burch colposuspension and UBAs are the alternatives. Unfortunately, the multitude of options currently available to manage the problem of UI is unable to keep pace with the exponentially increasing burden of this disease.

REFERENCES

1. Haylen B, de Ridder D, Freeman R, et al. An international urogynecological association (IUGA)/International Continence Society (ICS) joint report on the terminology for female pelvic floor dysfunction. *Neurourol Urodyn* **2010, 29**:4–20.
2. Cerruto M, DElia C, Aloisi A, Fabrello M, Artibani W. Prevalence, incidence and obstetric factors impact on female urinary incontinence in Europe: a systematic review. *Urol Int* 2013;**90**:1–9.
3. Australian Institute of Health and Welfare (AIHW). *Incontinence in Australia: Prevalence, Experience and Cost 2009*. Bulletin no. 112. Cat. no. AUS 167. Canberra: AIHW; 2012.

4. Sen I, Onaran M, Aksakal N, et al. The impact of urinary incontinence on female sexual function. *Adv Ther* 2006;**23**:999–1008.

5. Brooks JD. Anatomy of the lower urinary tract. In: Wein AJ, Kavoussi LR, Novick AC, Partin AW, Peters CA (eds), *Campbell-Walsh Urology*, 9th edn, pp. 38–77. Philadelphia, PA: Saunders Elsevier; 2007.

6. Park JM. Normal development of the urogenital system. In: Wein AJ, Kavoussi LR, Novick AC, Partin AW, Peters CA (eds), *Campbell-Walsh Urology*, 9th edn, pp. 3121–48. Philadelphia, PA: Saunders Elsevier; 2007.

7. Fowler C, Griffiths D, de Groat W. The neural control of micturition. *Nat Rev Neurosci* 2008;**9**:453–66.

8. Abrams P, Andersson K, Birder L, et al. Fourth international consultation on incontinence recommendations of the International Scientific Committee: evaluation and treatment of urinary incontinence, pelvic organ prolapse, and fecal incontinence. *Neurourol Urodyn* 2010;**29**:213–40.

9. Abdel-Fattah M, Ford J, Lim C, Madhuvrata P. Single-incision mini-slings versus standard midurethral slings in surgical management of female stress urinary incontinence: a meta-analysis of effectiveness and complications. *Eur Urol* 2011;**60**:468–80.

10. Hunskaar S, Burgio K, Diokno A, Herzog A, Hjälmås K, Lapitan M. Epidemiology and natural history of urinary incontinence in women. *Urology* 2003;**62**:16–23.

11. American College of Obstetrics and Gynecologists. Committee Opinion No. 603. *Obstet Gynecol* 2014;**123**:1403–407.

12. Deng D. Urinary incontinence in women. *Med Clin North Am* 2011;**95**:101–109.

13. Zimmern P, Nager CW, Albo M, Fitzgerald MP, McDermott S, Urinary Incontinence Treatment Network. Interrater reliability of filling cystometrogram interpretation in a multicenter study. *J Urol* 2006;**175**:2174–77.

14. Brown J, Wing R, Barrett-Connor E, et al. Lifestyle intervention is associated with lower prevalence of urinary incontinence: the Diabetes Prevention Program. *Diabetes Care* 2006;**29**:385–90.

15. Wing R, West D, Grady D, et al. Effect of weight loss on urinary incontinence in overweight and obese women: results at 12 and 18 months. *J Urol* 2010;**184**:1005–10.

16. Gormley EA. Biofeedback and behavioral therapy for the management of female urinary incontinence. *Urol Clin North Am* 2002;**29**:551–57.

17. Bø K. Pelvic floor muscle training is effective in treatment of female stress urinary incontinence, but how does it work? *J Urol* 2006;**175**:629.

18. Bø K. Pelvic floor muscle training in treatment of female stress urinary incontinence, pelvic organ prolapse and sexual dysfunction. *World J Urol* 2011;**30**:437–43.

19. White N, Iglesia C. Overactive bladder. *Obstet Gynecol Clin North Am* 2016;**43**:59–68.

20. Kaschak Newman D, Wein AJ. *Managing and Treating Urinary Incontinence*, 2nd edn. Baltimore, MD: Health Professions Press, 2009.

21. Wein A, Chapple C. *Overactive Bladder in Clinical Practice*. London: Springer-Verlag; 2012.

22. Prezioso D, Iacono F, Di Lauro G, et al. Stress urinary incontinence: long-term results of laparoscopic Burch colposuspension. *BMC Surg* 2013;**13** Suppl 2:S38.

23. DeLancey J. Structural support of the urethra as it relates to stress urinary incontinence: the hammock hypothesis. *Am J Obstet Gynecol* 1994;**170**:1713–23.

24. DeLancey J. The pathophysiology of stress urinary incontinence in women and its implications for surgical treatment. *World J Urol* 1997;**15**:268–74.

25. Petros P, Ulmsten U. An integral theory of female urinary incontinence. *Acta Obstet Gynecol Scand* 1990;**69**:7–31.

26. Deval B, Levardon M, Samain E, et al. A French multicenter clinical trial of SPARC for stress urinary incontinence. *Eur Urol* 2003;**44**:254–59.

27. Wheeler T, Richter H, Greer W, Bowling C, Redden D, Varner R. Predictors of success with postoperative voiding trials after a mid urethral sling procedure. *J Urol* 2008;**179**:600–604.

28. Fong E, Nitti V. Mid-urethral synthetic slings for female stress urinary incontinence. *BJU Int* 2010;**106**:596–608.

29. Basu M, Duckett J. Three-year results from a randomised trial of a retropubic mid-urethral sling versus the Miniarc single incision sling for stress urinary incontinence. *Int Urogynecol J* 2013;**24**:2059–64.

30. Palomba S, Oppedisano R, Falbo A, et al. Single-incision mini-slings versus retropubic tension-free vaginal tapes: a multicenter clinical trial. *J Minim Invasive Gynecol* 2014;**21**:303–10.

31. Mostafa A, Lim C, Hopper L, Madhuvrata P, Abdel-Fattah M. Single-incision mini-slings versus standard midurethral slings in surgical management of female stress urinary incontinence: an updated systematic review and meta-analysis of effectiveness and complications. *Eur Urol* 2014;**65**:402–27.

32. Zhang P, Fan B, Zhang P, et al. Meta-analysis of female stress urinary incontinence treatments with adjustable single-incision mini-slings and transobturator tension-free vaginal tape surgeries. *BMC Urol* 2015;**15**:64–70.

33. Ward K, Hilton P. A prospective multicenter randomized trial of tension-free vaginal tape and colposuspension for primary urodynamic stress incontinence: two-year follow-up. *Am J Obstet Gynecol* 2004;**190**:324–31.

34. Ogah J, Cody D, Rogerson L. Minimally invasive synthetic suburethral sling operations for stress urinary incontinence in women: a short version Cochrane review. *Neurourol Urodyn* 2011;**30**:284–291.

35. Lee K. Transurethral injection of bulking agent for the treatment of recurrent or persistent female stress urinary incontinence after mid-urethral sling. *UroToday Int J* 2008;**1**:15.

36. Ghoniem G, Corcos J, Comiter C, Westney O, Herschorn S. Durability of urethral bulking agent injection for female stress urinary incontinence: 2-year multicenter study results. *J Urol* 2010;**183**:1444–49.

37. Mock S, Reynolds W. Bulking agents for stress incontinence: are they a real option? *Curr Bladder Dysfunct Rep* 2015;**10**:46–51.

58

Faecal incontinence and anorectal dysfunction

Karen Nugent

Anorectal anatomy

The anatomy of the rectum and anus cannot be studied in isolation. They form part of the pelvic organs and pass through the pelvic diaphragm along with the urethra and the vagina. Injury to any part of the pelvic floor during childbirth may result in dysfunction of one or more pelvic floor organs.

The pelvic diaphragm or levator ani is funnel-shaped and made up of four striated muscles: ileococcygeus, pubococcygeus, coccygeus, and puborectalis. The puborectalis forms a complete sling around the anorectal junction with some fibres blending with the wall of the anal canal. There is evidence that the puborectalis may be a distinct muscle in its own right as its innervations and histology is different from the rest of the levator ani (1). The nerve supply to the levator ani is S4 through the ventral ramus and the perineal branch of the pudendal nerve. The function of the puborectalis is to maintain the angle between the anal canal and rectum—this is important in maintaining continence.

Rectum

The rectum starts at the point where the sigmoid colon loses its mesentery, at the level of the mid sacrum. It is 12–15 cm long and becomes the anus as the tube passes through the pelvic floor. The rectum is covered with peritoneum at its front and sides in its upper third, only the front in its middle third, and not at all in the lower third. The rectum is an extremely distensible chamber and when it is empty the walls collapse—it usually remains empty until just before defecation. The rectum has a variable shape and follows the sacral curve with three lateral flexures and corresponding transverse folds within the rectum (or valves of Houston) (**Figure 58.1**). These valves are thought to support the weight of faecal matter until it is time to defecate. The blood supply of the rectum is a superior rectal branch from the inferior mesenteric artery and middle and inferior rectal arteries from the internal iliac artery. The lymphatic drainage follows the arterial supply. The nerve supply of the rectum consists of a sympathetic component, which follows the branches of the superior rectal artery (from the coeliac plexus), and a parasympathetic supply, which is derived from the second, third, and fourth sacral segments of the spinal cord and passes through the pelvic splanchnic nerves.

Anus

The anal canal is approximately 4–4.5 cm long (2). The proximal 1 cm of the anal canal is lined by columnar epithelium extending down from the rectum. Below this the mucous membrane becomes cuboidal and the lining forms anal valves. Just below the level of the valves there is an abrupt transition to stratified squamous epithelium—the dentate or pectinate line. The squamous epithelium lining the next part of the anal canal is thin and shiny and has no hair or sweat glands. The final 0.5–1 cm of the canal is lined by hair-forming skin. The anal cushions sit in the upper part of the anal canal and help create an airtight seal. These are classically described as being in the 4, 7, and 11 o'clock positions. When these cushions become swollen and symptomatic, they are described as piles or haemorrhoids.

The anal canal is surrounded by muscles. The outermost layer of muscles is the *external sphincter*. This is a somatic voluntary (striated) muscle. Its nerve supply is S3 and S4 via the pudendal nerve and perineal branch of the fourth sacral nerve (3). It is important to remember that the motor fibres of the right and left pudendal nerves have overlapping distributions within the external anal sphincter so that stimulation of the right pudendal nerve causes circumferential contraction of the external anal sphincter. This has clinical implications as damage to one side may leave a functional sphincter but also implantation of a neurostimulator can be unilateral and still result in an improvement of whole anal function.

The *longitudinal muscle* is a direct continuation of the smooth muscle coat of the rectum, reinforced in its upper part by some striated muscle fibres originating from the levator ani muscle. These fibres split into multiple end septa and insert into the skin of the lower part of the anal canal. They provide a supportive mesh but also provide pathways for spread of infection into and from the intersphincteric space. An infection with an intersphincteric gland can spread and when it reaches the skin this may form a fistula track.

During defecation the longitudinal muscle contracts, resulting in eversion of the anal margin, shortening of the canal, and flattening out of the anal cushions, allowing the passageway to open for the passing of stool.

The *internal sphincter* represents the continuation and thickened circular muscle coat of the rectum. This is a non-striated involuntary muscle and is supplied by autonomic nerves.

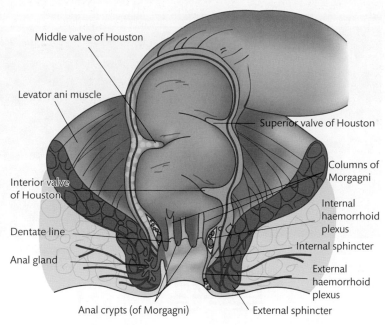

Figure 58.1 Anatomy of the anorectum and pelvic floor.

Anal glands may be found in the submucosa and intersphincteric space (there are normally between zero and ten glands). The glands drain via ducts into the anal sinuses at the level of the dentate line. They secrete mucin and it is thought that they lubricate the anal canal to ease defecation. When the drainage is blocked, abscesses can occur.

Anorectal physiology and function

The *resting pressure* of the anal canal should be high enough to maintain an air and watertight seal during rest and activity. Penninckx et al. (4) estimated that the resting tone was generated by nerve-induced activity of the internal sphincter (45%), myogenic tone of the internal sphincter (10%), tone of the external sphincter (35%), and the anal cushions (15%). These values are difficult to assess and are only estimates. The anal resting pressure is not constant during the day. It exhibits circadian variations and slow waves are seen when measuring the pressure using high-resolution anorectal manometry (HRAM) (**Figure 58.2**).

When the rectum is distended there should be a compensatory relaxation of the internal sphincter muscle. This is known as the rectoanal inhibitory reflex and is mediated by intrinsic nerves as evidenced by the fact that the reflex remains after spinal cord transection. The reflex is probably mediated by nitric oxide and possibly by other non-adrenergic and non-cholinergic neurotransmitters. The reflex is absent in Hirschsprung's disease.

The *squeeze pressure* is mediated by the external sphincter; it can be voluntary, induced by cough or an increase in intra-abdominal pressure, or by digitating the anal canal. At the time of defecation the external sphincter relaxes.

Puborectalis is tonically active and maintains the resting anorectal angle. Further contraction will occur in response to a sudden rise in abdominal pressure and this reduces the anorectal angle further and helps preserve continence.

Measurement

Anorectal physiology

The function of the anus and rectum can be measured using a variety of physiological tests. HRAM can be performed using water-perfused or solid-state catheters. The catheter provides a single pressure, averaged around the circumference at 6 mm intervals, and measures values along the entire length of the anal canal; it is also fitted with an inflatable balloon at the end. Although attempts have been made to define normal resting and squeeze pressures there is considerable overlap between asymptomatic and symptomatic patients. Using HRAM it is possible to measure an average resting pressure, a maximum and sustained squeeze pressure, as well as examining the effect of attempting to expel a balloon filled with water. Rectal volume at first sensation, first urge, and maximum tolerated volume is usually assessed giving some indication as to whether a patient has a hypo-sensate or hyper-sensate rectum. Anal sensation is usually recorded and pudendal nerve latency can also be measured. Anorectal manometry can also be used to identify the very small minority of patients with Hirschsprung's disease. These patients are usually diagnosed in childhood and it is rare to find a patient with Hirschsprung's disease reaching adult life without a prior diagnosis. The rectoanal inhibitory reflex is absent in Hirschsprung's disease. This reflex is elicited by placing the catheter into the anus and inflating a balloon within the rectum with air. There is a reflex decrease in the anal sphincter tone on inflation of the balloon. HRAM is also used in treatment; it is often used to start a biofeedback or retraining programme by showing a patient how to improve their squeeze pressure or method of defecation.

Anal ultrasound

The structure of the anal canal can be visualized using three-dimensional anal ultrasound (**Figure 58.3**). Ultrasound is useful, safe, and well tolerated by patients. Anal ultrasound is the preferred investigation to detect sphincter defects but insertion of the

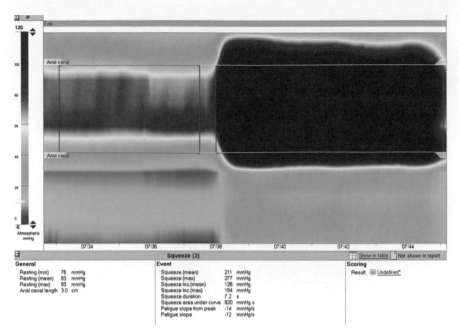

Figure 58.2 High-resolution anorectal manometry.

probe can distort the anal canal. Normal anal sphincter morphology and anal sphincter measurements can also be obtained using transvaginal and transperineal scanning (5).

Proctography

The dynamics of defecation can be assessed radiologically by evacuation proctography or magnetic resonance (MR) proctography (Figure 58.4). These tests assess evacuation after paste or gel has been placed in the rectum to simulate a full rectum. Physiological filling of the rectum would normally occur at or around the time of colonic mass movements and these are not recreated in this laboratory setting. However, at present, these are the best tests available to look for an anatomical abnormality within the pelvic organs on straining. Fluoroscopic proctograms use rectal contrast and contrast may also be placed in the vagina, bladder, and small bowel, helping with better visualization of abnormalities such as an enterocele and rectocele. The patients are then fluoroscopically screened as they sit on the toilet and attempt to evacuate their rectum. MR defecography avoids radiation exposure and is better at visualizing bony landmarks. However, the patient is required to lie in the supine position and expel the gel onto a pad and this sometimes inhibits their normal defecatory push. This test visualizes the uterus, vagina, and anterior compartment as well as the rectum and any potential enterocele. A recent study suggested that MR proctograms may under-report pelvic floor abnormalities especially where there has been poor rectal evacuation (6).

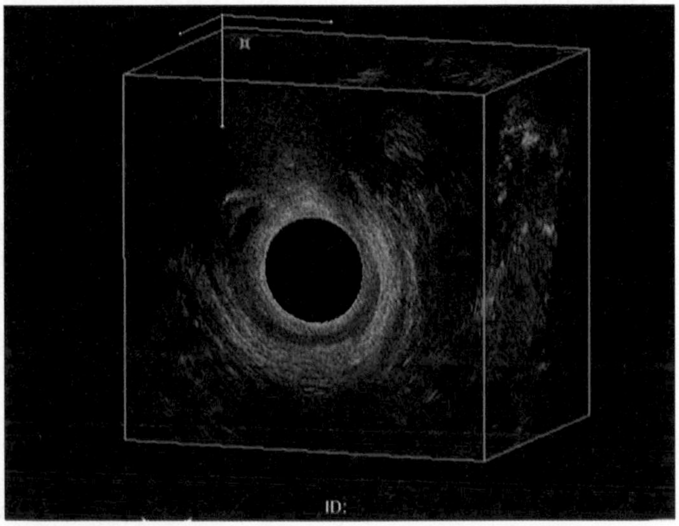

Colon transit studies

The simplest way of studying a colon transit is ingesting a capsule of markers and taking a plain abdominal X-ray after 72 and then 120 hours. The distribution of the markers in the colon provides a crude measure of colonic transit. A normal study should show at least 80–90% of markers are eliminated by 120 hours in the majority of people. The markers have completely disappeared by this day. It is possible to use scintigraphic techniques to study both segmental colonic transit and small bowel transit and to give an idea of the flow of markers through the bowel. Some centres use three different-shaped markers on three different days and take further X-rays during the week.

Maintaining continence and defecation

Continence and normal defecation relies on the complex interaction of the colon (motility and consistency of stools), rectum (sensation, compliance, and anatomy), and the anus (sensation, structure, and function). The overriding complex neurological control is also

Figure 58.3 Three-dimensional anal ultrasonography showing a defect in the external sphincter.

(a)

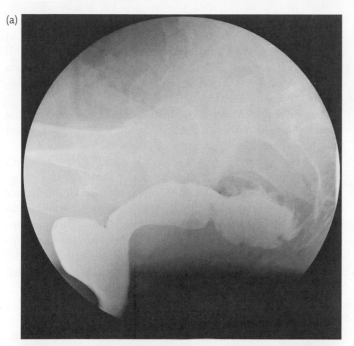

(b)

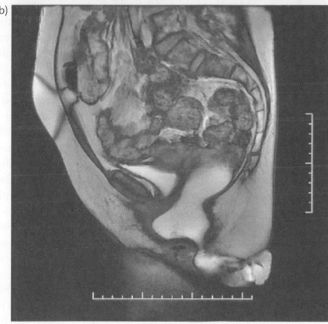

Figure 58.4 (a) Barium proctography. (b) Magnetic resonance proctography.

important. A disorder of any of these may lead to incontinence of faeces.

During the day, several mass movements of the colon occur—these are high-amplitude propagated contractions, which often occur after awakening or meals (7). As the rectum fills, if defecation is convenient, then anal relaxation and increased intrarectal pressure is required for normal defecation. A small amount of straining may be required to initiate defecation. However, excessive straining (particularly using the Valsalva manoeuvre) means pushing against a contracted pelvic floor and is counterproductive. If defecation is not convenient, the urge can be overridden. The rectal contractile response to distension will then subside as the rectum relaxes and

the external sphincter contracts. During the day, as the rectum fills, the anus will relax and sample the contents to ascertain whether it is gas, liquid, or solid.

Faecal incontinence

Definition

Faecal incontinence is the involuntary loss of control of a person's bowels. It can affect over 10% of adults and at least 1–2% of patents will report these as major symptoms. In itself, faecal incontinence is not a disease but a symptom and it is necessary to take a full history and examine a patient to identify any underlying diseases or pathology that may need treatment before focusing on managing incontinence.

The majority of causes of faecal incontinence are acquired. The congenital causes are rare and include imperforate anus, rectal agenesis, and cloacal defects as well as spina bifida. Acquired causes can be divided into anorectal causes—anatomical disruption, neurological causes and age-related causes, or colonic and metabolic causes.

The aim of any treatment for faecal incontinence is to improve the patient's quality of life and give them some control back over their bowel function.

There are three main types of faecal incontinence:

- *Urge incontinence*—when the arrival of stool in the rectum is associated with a rise in rectal pressure and the external anal sphincter is unable to squeeze shut sufficiently to prevent the forcing of the stool out through the anal canal.
- The second type of incontinence is *passive incontinence*. This is usually due to internal sphincter dysfunction which either occurs by direct damage to the muscle or through poor function. This results in symptoms of leakage— the patient is usually unaware of faecal loss until their pad or underwear is stained. It can occur at any time of the day and may be associated with exercise.
- The third type of incontinence is *post-defecatory leakage*. This is when a patient has gone to the toilet, emptied their bowels, and then within the next half hour finds that they have leaked under their underwear. It is often associated with difficulty in cleaning. The aetiology of this is often a rectocele or haemorrhoids and it may be associated with poor rectal emptying; these anatomical problems can be more relatively easily treated.

History and examination

It is essential that anybody presenting with new onset of incontinence has a full history of bowel symptoms taken. This is particularly looking for any of the 'red flag' symptoms associated with bowel cancer. These are change in bowel habit to looser stools and rectal bleeding. Patients with these symptoms should be referred for further investigations. The person presenting with incontinence should be able to describe when the incontinence happens, whether it is associated with the need to go to the toilet (urge incontinence), whether it is associated with walking, whether it happens at a random time (passive incontinence), and the consistency of the motions involved. Incontinence to wind is often a significant issue and may be associated with certain dietary habits. A medication review is essential as certain drugs, for example, metformin, are associated with loosening of the stools and further incontinence.

Examination should include an abdominal examination as well as a visual inspection of the perineum looking for signs of previous episiotomy or tears. A gaping anus will suggest a poor internal anal sphincter. Any anorectal pathology such as fistula or fourth-degree piles should be noted and the patient should be asked to strain to see how much descent of pelvic floor occurs. At the time of straining, assessment of a rectocele and cystocele can be made and this is often easier if the patient is in the lithotomy position in a gynaecological chair. Rectal examination allows the doctor to exclude faecal impaction and overflow and to assess both anal tone and squeeze pressure. It is also useful to be able to place a finger towards the vagina to see whether there is a rectocele and whether the patient has a similar sensation of pocketing as when the finger is placed within the rectocele.

Measuring faecal incontinence

Quantifying the degree of faecal incontinence is important to assess the outcomes of various treatment options. Faecal incontinence can be to solid, liquid, or gas and the impact on quality of life can vary greatly between patients. The Wexner (or Cleveland Clinic) score (**Figure 58.5**) is widely used and scores five domains from 0 to 4 (giving a maximum score of 20). It is generally considered that a score of 9 or more is considered to represent significant incontinence.

The Faecal Incontinence Quality of life questionnaire has 29 items and has good correlation with psychometric evaluation of symptom impact; it is more complicated and time-consuming to complete.

Treatment

Initial bowel management

Many patients with incontinence can be treated with simple aids. Dietary modification to reduce the volume of stool and the softness of the stool can be particularly helpful. There have been two studies which showed considerable impact by lifestyle change on

Cleveland Clinic incontinence score

Type of incontinence	Frequency				
	Never	Rarely	Sometimes	Usually	Always
Solid	0	1	2	3	4
Liquid	0	1	2	3	4
Gas	0	1	2	3	4
Wears pad	0	1	2	3	4
Lifestyle alteration	0	1	2	3	4

Never, 0; rarely, <1/month; sometimes, <1/week, ⩾1/month; usually, <1/day, ⩾1/week; always, ⩾1/day.
0, perfect; 20, complete incontinence.

Figure 58.5 Cleveland Clinic incontinence score.

anal incontinence. The first by Bliss et al. (8) showed that a self-care change of diet or avoidance of certain foods were successful in helping 67% of an elderly mixed cohort of patients presenting with anal incontinence reduce their symptoms. The second study from 2010 (9) showed that lifestyle changes can improve anal incontinence in about a third of the general population.

The most important things within the diet to change are those that result in loose or softer stools; these are foods that contain wheat fibre, pulses, beans, caffeine, and also lactose-containing food.

There are a variety of continence aids that will help patients with faecal incontinence and the newer ones of these are anal plugs. There are two plugs that are available on the National Health Service (NHS) in the United Kingdom. There is, however, little in the way of evidence that these will work except in highly motivated patients. The studies that are published on plugs are relatively poor in terms of methodology. They have limited follow-up and the dropout rates are high. However, continence can be achieved in highly motivated patients with good compliance in up to 37% of people (10, 11).

Medication

One of the mainstays of treatment of faecal incontinence is the use of medication. There are three widely used drugs that control soft or looser stools. Loperamide, a synthetic opioid that does not cross the blood–brain barrier, is the commonest one to be used for faecal incontinence. It has an excellent safety profile and acts directly on the intestine to inhibit peristalsis increasing small intestinal and mouth-to-caecum transit time; this allows more water to be absorbed from the stool. There is some evidence that loperamide may act directly on sphincter tone and resting pressure and may increase rectal perception in healthy subjects. An alternative drug is codeine phosphate, which acts in a similar way to loperamide but crosses the blood–brain barrier and therefore may cause dependency. Finally, Lomotil (diphenoxylate and atropine) is occasionally used; it also crosses the blood–brain barrier and is therefore usually used with a low dose of atropine to prevent over usage. Omar and Alexander published a Cochrane review of medical treatment in 2013 (12). This study identified 16 trials and included 558 participants. There was some limited evidence that antidiarrhoeal drugs may reduce faecal incontinence in patients with liquid stools. The side effects of loperamide such as constipation, abdominal pain, diarrhoea, headache, and nausea were greater than in the placebo group. A liquid form of loperamide (Imodium, paediatric) is available and is widely used by clinicians; it allows titration of symptoms with accuracy to try and reduce volume of stool and minimize side effects. Many patients find this a useful treatment.

Exercises and biofeedback

One of the mainstays of further treatment is pelvic floor exercises, bowel training, and biofeedback. Biofeedback relies on strength training, rectal sensitivity training, and improving coordination of the rectum and anus. In a randomized controlled trial from St Mark's Hospital, Harrow, United Kingdom (13), 171 patients were randomized to four groups. All four groups received patient teaching, emotional support, lifestyle modification, and a programme to explain how to manage both faecal incontinence and urge incontinence. The second group received additional anal sphincter exercises with 50 squeezes a day. The third group had clinic computer biofeedback and the fourth group had in addition to all of these a home biofeedback unit. The results showed that there was no significant difference between the groups; however, all groups had a 50% improvement and the episodes of incontinence throughout the groups reduced from a median of 2 to 0. The incontinence score decreased from 11 to 8.

There are different styles of biofeedback and exercise regimens from sustained squeeze manoeuvres to rapid squeeze manoeuvres and no significant difference has been shown between these different methods. However, what these patients do show is a prolonged improvement in general by having intervention by medical and nursing teams. The Cochrane review from 2012 looking at biofeedback and sphincter exercises reviewed 1525 participants. This suggested that there was not enough evidence to show that any particular method of biofeedback or exercises was better than any other. However, many patients will improve with some form of intervention. The final non-medical way of treating incontinence is to use some form of emptying device. This can be glycerine suppositories, enemas, or water-based systems and many of these are available on the market.

Surgical treatment

There have been a variety of surgical approaches to repair or replace anal sphincters in order to treat faecal incontinence.

Overlapping sphincter repair/sphincteroplasty

For many years the only treatment available for sphincter disruption was an overlapping anterior sphincter repair (**Figure 58.6**). This is done not at the time of the original injury, which usually falls under the remit of the obstetrician, but sometime later after either an occult injury is diagnosed or symptoms have deteriorated from previous surgery. In 2012, the long-term outcomes of the many series within the literature were reviewed (14). The majority of series had mostly obstetric injury patients and the number of patients involved varied from 14 to 191 within each series. The length of follow-up was anything from 5 to 10 years and the results were classified as either excellent or good, fair, or poor. Fair represented minimal improvement or no change whereas poor outcomes included worsening incontinence. Although there was considerable variation across the studies, in the majority the long-term results were that approximately 50% maintained good or excellent results but 50% had fair or poor results. Most of the studies found that there was a poorer outcome with wound infection and older age.

Artificial bowel sphincter

In 1987, John Christenson suggested using the urinary sphincter as an artificial bowel sphincter and over 500 cases have been implanted worldwide. The National Institute for Health and Care Excellence

(NICE) reviewed the use of artificial bowel sphincters and suggested that they may still have a place in patients with significant sphincter disruption or following failure of sacral nerve stimulator and sphincter repair. The Cochrane review in 2010 suggested that the artificial bowel sphincter may be better than conservative treatment but has significant morbidity. This morbidity has been well documented by Paul Lehur's unit in Nantes (15) where in 52 patients followed up for a mean of 5 years over a quarter had their devices explanted due to infection and there was a high rate of revision with over 50% of patients needing some form of revision.

Dynamic graciloplasty

The transposition of the gracilis muscle to reconstruct the anus was first described in 1952 (16); this had relatively poor results and it was not until 1991 when a stimulated dynamic graciloplasty was reported that the procedure started to be adopted by colorectal surgeons (17, 18).

This is an invasive surgical procedure and is reserved for patients who have failed conservative management and do not have a repairable sphincter defect. The procedure involves mobilizing the gracilis muscle, either unilaterally or bilaterally, and wrapping it around the anus, attaching it to the contralateral ischial tuberosity. These procedures are associated with considerable morbidity and mortality and in a small series of 38 patients (19) with a median follow-up of 5 years there were 13 infections and 2 immediate gracilis problems in the short term. In the long-term, 10 patients required 15 procedures to replace pacemaker components and 24 patients suffered from some morbidity in the donor leg including pain, swelling, and paraesthesia. After long-term follow up, 30% had a stoma and although 22 still had a functioning graciloplasty, 13 were incontinent daily, 11 required some form of enema or irrigation to empty, and 64% still had bowel function that adversely affected their daily lives. In view of this, NICE suggested that this procedure was only supported in specialist units and indeed it is no longer available in the United States.

Fenix procedure

A newer procedure to encircle the anal sphincter with titanium wire and magnetic beads has more recently come into practice. It is relatively easily placed in a tunnel in the ischioanal fossa just beneath the levator ani and the number of beads can be measured to fit for each individual patient. The first 35 patients having a Fenix were published in the literature (20). These patients showed an improvement in their Cleveland Clinic Score from 16 to an average of 7.3 with significant improvement in faecal quality of life. There were no intraoperative complications in this series, there were, however,

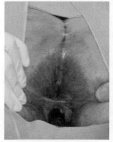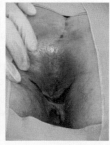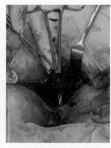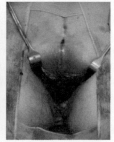

Figure 58.6 Overlapping sphincter repair.

three infections, one device separation problem, two patients had a stoma because of lack of efficacy of the procedure, and one patient had transvaginal erosion.

Other sphincter augmentation methods

Some centres are treating patients with the SECCA system. This is radiofrequency energy delivered to the anal canal that is said to remodel and tighten the collagen. It is done at three to four levels through the anus and some short-term results have suggested an improvement in patients' incontinence scores. However, this is not covered in the NHS and should only be performed in a trial situation.

Anal bulking agents

Over many years surgeons have tried to inject a variety of molecules into the internal anal sphincter or the anal cushions to improve passive leakage by recreating the anal seal. Back in 1993, Teflon was used followed by autologous fat, collagen, silicone, carbon-coated beads, and more recently porcine collagen and hyaluronic acid. Many of these injectables have been associated with complications of granulomas, emboli, and migration of the molecules as well as infection. The studies that have been published show low numbers of patients with short length of follow-up and relatively little improvement in symptoms or incontinence scores. The NICE guidelines from February 2007 suggested that these procedures should only be used in units specializing in assessment and treatment of faecal incontinence and could only be done within a trial or audit.

Sacral neuromodulation

Sacral nerve stimulation (SNS) as a procedure has transformed the treatment of severe faecal incontinence. This was initially described for the treatment of urinary incontinence in 1981 and subsequently for faecal incontinence in 1995. It is now a well-accepted treatment for faecal incontinence for patients with or without a sphincter defect with both good short- and long-term results. Patients are assessed with a bowel diary (**Figure 58.2**) and should be incontinent at least two or three times a week in order to be considered for sacral neuromodulation. The patients complete a bowel diary before intervention but after maximum medical therapy, physiotherapy, and biofeedback and then have a temporary wire placed through the sacrum onto S3 or S4, usually S3 (**Figure 58.7**). If there is a greater than 50% improvement in symptoms, the patient then has a permanent wire placed into the sacrum and attached to a pacemaker battery which is buried in the ipsilateral buttock.

The mechanism of action remains unclear. It is hypothesized that the impulses modulate autonomic and somatic afferent and efferent impulses from the anus and rectum, thereby improving rectal compliance and increasing anal resting pressure (21).

A recent meta-analysis (22) looked at studies published between 1995 and 2008 on SNS for faecal incontinence. Thirty-four studies were included, reporting on 944 patients undergoing peripheral nerve evaluation; 665 then underwent conversion to a permanent SNS. Weekly incontinence episodes and incontinence scores were significantly improved (P <0.001). Results were similar between sphincter intact and impaired subgroups. The complication rate was 15% for permanent SNS, with 3% resulting in permanent explantation.

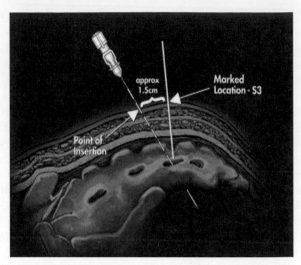

Figure 58.7 Sacral nerve stimulator landmarks.

Posterior tibial nerve stimulation

Peripheral neuromodulation was first described as a method of treating faecal incontinence by Shafik in 2003 (23). As with SNS, the mechanism remains unclear. It is thought that stimulation of the posterior tibial nerve at the ankle may send retrograde stimulation to the sacral nerve. A recent randomized multicentre study investigating posterior tibial nerve stimulation versus sham in patients with faecal incontinence found that 38% of patients in the treatment group and 31% of patients in the sham stimulation group reported a greater than 50% improvement in the number of incontinence episodes (24). This was not significantly different and the treatment is undergoing further evaluation.

End colostomy

This is a disfiguring operation with a significant long-term complication rate. It is reserved for patients who have failed other therapies or for those who are fully informed and understand the implication of long-term stomas. The formation of a stoma is not a specialized procedure and can be performed in a local hospital. However, the patients should be warned that up to a third of patients having these made for incontinence may experience significant issues with leakage from the rectal stump.

Summary

Faecal incontinence has many causes. An accurate history and examination is required to eliminate pathology that requires treatment (e.g. cancer). Simple dietary and lifestyle changes along with medication and exercises may improve patients' quality of life in at least 50% of patients. Those with continuing symptoms should be investigated with anorectal physiology and ultrasound and be examined by a clinician with an understanding of all treatment options available. Patients with a cloacal deformity and/or large sphincter defect may be offered an overlapping sphincter repair. Sacral neuromodulation shows lasting good results in the 75% who show significant improvement with temporary stimulation. There is still a role for an end colostomy in patients with significant faecal incontinence refractory to all other measures.

Constipation and obstructive defecation

Definition

Constipation is an increasing problem in the Western world and it is widely accepted that approximately 50% of adults are constipated at any point in time. Constipation encompasses a multitude of symptoms; the general mental health and social functioning of people with constipation is impaired when compared to health controls. Constipation can mean many things to many people. However, there are well defined criteria such as the Rome II criteria which allow us to compare patients' symptoms and treatment results. The Rome II criteria suggest that constipation can be diagnosed if two or more of the following symptoms have occurred for at least 12 weeks, not necessarily consecutively in the preceding 12 months. Symptoms include straining during more than 25% of bowel movements; lumpy or hard stools for more than 25% of bowel movements; a sensation of incomplete evacuation for more than 25% of bowel movements; a sensation of anorectal blockage for than 25% of bowel movements; and/or the need to use manual manoeuvres to aid defecation for more than 25% of bowel movements. These symptoms along with less than three bowel movements per week result in a diagnosis of constipation.

Constipation can then be categorized into three different types: slow transit constipation, normal transit constipation, and obstructive defecation. Obstructive defecation or difficulty in evacuation is often associated with both normal transit and slow transit constipation.

Prior to a diagnosis of constipation other potential metabolic or physical causes for constipation should be excluded. These include carcinoma or pathology within the colon. Blood tests should be performed to exclude hypothyroidism, hypercalcaemia, and diabetes, all of which may be associated with constipation. A variety of neurological diseases including Parkinson's disease and multiple sclerosis are also associated with constipation.

Once a complete history has been taken, a physical examination has been made, and significant organic pathology has been excluded, there are three main other tests that can be done to evaluate constipation further: colonic transit studies, proctography, and anorectal physiology.

Treatment for constipation

The mainstay of treatment of constipation is use of a variety of laxatives, all of which have different modes of action. There is some evidence that increased physical activity is associated with less constipation and that physical activity may improve quality of life in patients with irritable bowel syndrome. Patients should be encouraged to increase their soluble fibre in their diet, for example, psyllium or ispaghula, as these improve bowel symptoms both in chronic constipation and in irritable bowel syndrome. Although patients treated with bran or psyllium may improve their constipation, approximately 60% of patients will report adverse events including abdominal pain. Patients with chronic abdominal pain may be treated with opiates and this will exacerbate their constipation further. It is essential to wean these patients off their opiates wherever possible.

Laxatives

The next step in the treatment algorithm is to prescribe an osmotic laxative. There are four main types of osmotic agents and these include polyethylene glycol-based solutions (Movicol), magnesium citrate-based products, sodium phosphate-based products, and non-absorbable carbohydrates. These products extract fluid into the intestinal lumen by osmosis and may occasionally cause diarrhoea. However, they are generally well tolerated. The magnesium hydroxide and other salts soften the stool and increase frequency of defecation. The absorption of magnesium is limited and is usually not a significant side effect (patients with renal impairment should be monitored closely). Sodium phosphate-based preparations should not be used long term as they can induce metabolic abnormalities. Lactulose, which is used a lot in general practice, is associated with wind and abdominal pain and a Cochrane review suggested that polyethylene glycol laxatives were superior to lactulose in their effect and in their side effects.

Stimulant laxatives such as bisacodyl and glycerine suppositories and sodium picosulphate and senna are widely used. However, they do cause some gut-related abdominal pain.

Newer agents such as lubiprostone and linaclotide act as secretagogues and increase intestinal chloride secretion by activating channels on the luminal side of the enterocyte. Water secretion follows the ion secretion and it is thought that the secretory affects are why these drugs accelerate small intestine and colonic transit.

Serotonin 5-HT$_4$ receptor agonists induce mucosal secretion by activating submucosal neurons. The agonist most commonly used is prucalopride and this accelerates gastrointestinal and colonic transit in constipation. Side effects include abdominal pain and headaches in the first few days but these wear off rapidly. Much of the work for this drug was done in women and it is approved for use in women in whom laxatives failed to give adequate relief of symptoms.

Biofeedback

If laxative usage fails, patients should be treated with biofeedback-aided pelvic floor training. In patients with a hyposensitive rectum, sensory retraining can be added whereby a patient will learn to recognize weaker signals coming through and then attempt to defecate using abdominal and pelvic floor exercises. Up to two-thirds of patients with defecatory disorder have an improvement of symptoms with biofeedback but these treatments are time-consuming with patients required to attend hospital for five or six training sessions lasting 30–60 minutes each and the defecatory improvement may tail off without regular top-up sessions.

Surgery for constipation

Patients should only be referred for surgery after all non-surgical measures have failed and the symptoms continue to compromise daily life. Constipation is associated with a poorer quality of life but has no mortality associated with it. However, surgery may cause considerable ongoing morbidity and potential mortality.

Subtotal colectomy

Patients with isolated slow-transit constipation who have no evidence of pelvic floor dysfunction or diffuse gastrointestinal dysmotility are occasionally considered for a colectomy and ileorectal anastomosis. It is essential to advise these patients that the primary symptoms of constipation, for example, the infrequent and difficult evacuation, may be eliminated by this surgery, but other symptoms (particularly abdominal pain and bloating) will often persist postoperatively. During surgery, which is now done laparoscopically, the colon is removed to the level of the rectum. It is essential to preserve the presacral nerves and an ileorectal anastomosis should then be performed. Leaving any sigmoid colon or anastomosing the cecum to the rectum reduces the efficacy of this operation. This is not a procedure to be undertaken lightly as most series are associated with high morbidity and readmission rates. In a recent publication from the United States, the authors looked at the admissions for colectomies for constipation in two states from 1998 to 2011 (25). Over 400 patients had been operated during this time. There were no perioperative deaths in this series; however, perioperative complications occurred in 42.7% of the patients and a readmission rate of nearly 30% occurred within the first 30 days. As pointed out in this publication, constipation is a functional disorder that may have a significant impact on quality of life but no true morbidity or mortality. However, a significant number of patients in this series who had been operated on ended up with long-term complications.

Botulinum toxin for pelvic floor dysfunction

Patients who are seen to contract their puborectalis instead of relaxing it at the time of defecation may improve with biofeedback. In the past, the puborectalis muscle has been divided and occasionally botulinum toxin has been injected into puborectalis muscle. The evidence for this is limited and this cannot be recommended at present for managing defecatory disorders.

Stapled transanal resection

The stapled transanal resection (STARR) procedure was developed to try to correct two of the anatomical abnormalities that are seen on defecography associated with constipation. These are rectal intussusception, which is called occult rectal prolapse, and rectoceles (**Figure 58.8a**) The STARR procedure was introduced throughout Europe in the late 2000s and involved excising the redundant rectal mucosa associated with the rectocele and intussusception and reanastomosing using a staple line (Figure 58.8b). Placing a staple line within the rectum/pelvis has resulted in complications. Those reported in the literature include pain, urgency, and bleeding as well as more long-term infective complications such as pelvic sepsis, fistula, and bowel perforation. The long-term results of STARR are also not as good as were initially thought; it is presumed that the anatomical abnormalities that are corrected may actually be caused by the underlying disorder of function rather than causing the symptoms themselves. In general, there are fewer and fewer surgeons performing this procedure.

Lap ventral mesh rectopexy

As the knowledge and technical skills have improved, the procedure of a laparoscopic ventral mesh rectopexy, which was first proposed for external rectal prolapse by D'Hoore et al. (26) has been used more often for patients with rectal evacuatory disorders and rectal intussusception. The benefit of this procedure is an avoidance of posterior rectal mobilization, this preserves the autonomic nerves and hopefully reduces the postoperative complication of constipation seen with posterior rectopexy. The mesh is placed between the rectum and the vagina down to the pelvic floor and sutured onto the rectum and vagina closing the pouch of Douglas. There is a relatively

(a)
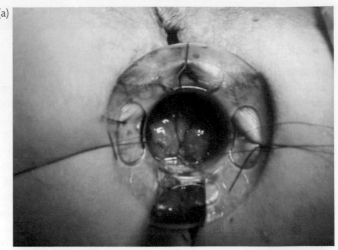

(b)
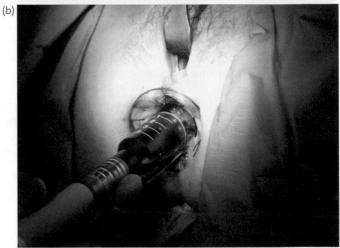

Figure 58.8 (a) Rectal intussusception. (b) STARR procedure resecting the rectal intussusception.

low morbidity rate of 8–10% with this procedure but there are concerns about mesh-related complications which may occur in at least 4.6% of patients (27).

Many of the published studies include patients with full-thickness rectal prolapse and those with internal intussusception and obstructive defecation. A recent study of 100 women with internal rectal prolapse treated with a laparoscopic ventral mesh rectopexy (using a biological mesh) found that constipation was cured in 79% and improved in 92%. Many patients with intussusception suffer from incontinence as well as difficulty in evacuation and the incontinence was improved in 86% of patients (28).

Concerns continue with regard to the potential for mesh erosions using this procedure. A multicentre collaboration looked at 2203 patients undergoing this type of surgery in the United Kingdom. It was a retrospective study, with short and minimal follow-up. Forty-five patients (2%) are known to have had erosions and this almost certainly is an underestimate. Eighteen patients had major morbidity associated with the erosion and the mesh removal (29).

This procedure has potential to help treat patients with intussusception and complex evacuatory disorders but patients should be

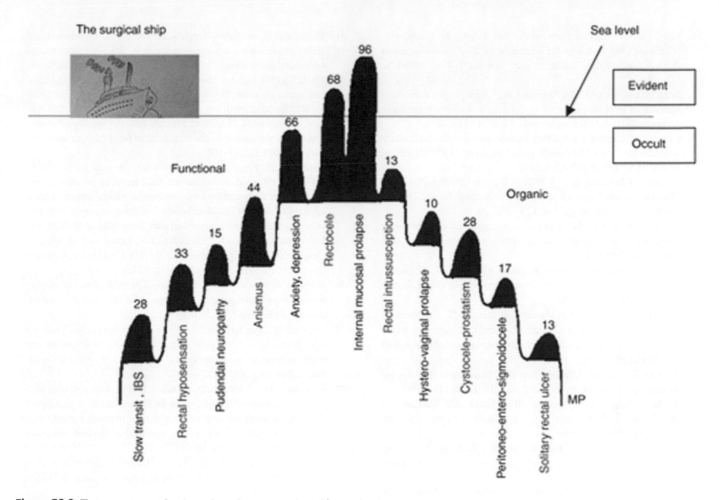

Figure 58.9 There are many other issues in patients presenting with constipation.

carefully counselled as to the potential for complications and major morbidity if the mesh erodes (Montgomery v Lanarkshire Health Board (2015)—a legal ruling).

Summary

The symptoms of constipation occur in a large percentage of the general population. The impact on quality of life when they occur for a long period of time is large. However, patients often have many coexisting other pelvic floor disorders. Pescatori et al. coined the term 'iceberg effect' to explain that while presenting with one symptom or anatomical issue, most patients will have a collection of other problems (30) (**Figure 58.9**).

This study looked at a series of 100 consecutive constipated patients. Although it found that 54% patients had both a rectocele and mucosal prolapse, all 100 patients had at least two further obstructive defecation-related problems. The commonest three issues were anxiety-depression, anismus, and rectal hyposensation (66%, 44%, and 33% respectively). The median number of occult disorders was five (range two to eight). The majority of patients were treated conservatively and only 14% required surgery.

Although there are surgical options available, it is important to treat conservatively and understand the complexity of the other issues involved in patients presenting with constipation.

REFERENCES

1. Cook TA, Mortensen NJ. Colon, rectum, anus, anal sphincters and the pelvic floor. In: Pemberton JH, Swash M, Henry JM (eds), *The Pelvic Floor: Its Function and Disorders*, pp. 61–76. London: Harcourt Publishers; 2002.
2. Bharucha AE. Pelvic floor: anatomy and function. *Neurogastroenterol Motil* 2006;**18**:507–19.
3. Lockhart RD, Fyfe FW, Hamilton GF. *Anatomy of the Human Body*. London: Faber & Faber; 1959.
4. Penninckx F, Lestar B, Kerremans R. The internal anal sphincter: mechanisms of control and its role in maintaining anal continence. *Baillieres Clin Gastroenterol* 1992;**6**:193–214.
5. Abdool Z, Sultan AH, Thakar R. Ultrasound imaging of the anal sphincter complex: a review. *The Br J Radiol* 2012;**85**:865–75.
6. Pilkington SA, Nugent KP, Brenner J, et al. Barium proctography vs magnetic resonance proctography for pelvic floor disorders: a comparative study. *Colorectal Dis* 2012;**14**:1224–30.
7. Bassotti G, Crowell MD, Whitehead WE. Contractile activity of the human colon: lessons from 24 hour studies. *Gut* 1993;**34**:129–33.
8. Bliss DZ, Fischer LR, Savik K. Managing fecal incontinence: self-care practices of older adults. *J Gerontol Nurs* 2005;**31**:35–44.
9. Croswell E, Bliss DZ, Savik K. Diet and eating pattern modifications used by community-living adults to manage their fecal incontinence. *J Wound Ostomy Continence Nurs* 2010;**37**:677–82.

10. Van Winckel M, Van Biervliet S, Van Laecke E, Hoebeke P. Is an anal plug useful in the treatment of fecal incontinence in children with spina bifida or anal atresia? *J Urol* 2006;**176**:342–44.

11. Bond C, Youngson G, MacPherson I, et al. Anal plugs for the management of fecal incontinence in children and adults: a randomized control trial. *J Clin Gastroenterol* 2007;**41**:45–53.

12. Omar MI1, Alexander CE. Drug treatment for faecal incontinence in adults. Cochrane Database Syst Rev 2013;11(6):CD002116. doi:10.1002/14651858.CD002116.pub2.

13. Norton C, Chelvanayagam S, Wilson-Barnett J, Redfern S, Kamm MA. Randomized controlled trial of biofeedback for fecal incontinence. *Gastroenterology* 2003;**125**:1320–29.

14. Glasgow SC, Lowry AC. Long-term outcomes of anal sphincter repair for fecal incontinence: a systematic review. *Dis Colon Rectum.* 2012;**55**:482–90.

15. Wong MT, Meurette G, Wyart V, Glemain P, Lehur PA. The artificial bowel sphincter: a single institution experience over a decade. *Ann Surg* 2011;**254**:951–56.

16. Pickrell KL, Broadbent TR, Masters FW, Metzger JT. Construction of a rectal sphincter and restoration of anal continence by transplanting the gracilis muscle; a report of four cases in children. *Ann Surg* 1952;**135**:853–62.

17. Baeten CG, Konsten J, Spaans F, et al. Dynamic graciloplasty for treatment of faecal incontinence. *Lancet* 1991;**338**:1163–65.

18. Williams NS, Patel J, George BD, Hallan RI, Watkins ES. Development of an electrically stimulated neoanal sphincter. *Lancet* 1991;**338**:1166–69.

19. Thornton MJ, Kennedy ML, Lubowski DZ, King DW. Long-term follow-up of dynamic graciloplasty for faecal incontinence. *Colorectal Dis* 2004;**6**:470–76.

20. Lehur PA, McNevin S, Buntzen S, Mellgren AF, Laurberg S, Madoff RD. Magnetic anal sphincter augmentation for the treatment of fecal incontinence: a preliminary report from a feasibility study. *Dis Colon Rectum* 2010;**53**:1604–610.

21. Michelsen HB, Buntzen S, Krogh K, Laurberg S. Rectal volume tolerability and anal pressures in patients with fecal incontinence treated with sacral nerve stimulation. *Dis Colon Rectum* 2006;**49**:1039–44.

22. Tan E, Ngo NT, Darzi A, Shenouda M, Tekkis PP. Meta-analysis: sacral nerve stimulation versus conservative therapy in the treatment of faecal incontinence. *Int J Colorectal Dis* 2011;**26**:275–94.

23. Shafik A, Ahmed I, El-Sibai O, Mostafa RM. Percutaneous peripheral neuromodulation in the treatment of fecal incontinence. *Eur Surg Res* 2003;**35**:103–107.

24. Knowles CH, Horrocks EJ, Bremner SA, Stevens N, Norton C, O'Connell PR, et al. Percutaneous tibial nerve stimulation versus sham electrical stimulation for the treatment of faecal incontinence in adults (CONFIDeNT): a double-blind, multicentre, pragmatic, parallel-group, randomised controlled trial. *Lancet* 2015;**386**:1640–48.

25. Dudekula A, Huftless S, Bielefeldt K. Colectomy for constipation: time trends and impact based on the US Nationwide Inpatient Sample, 1998-2011. *Aliment Pharmacol Ther* 2015;**42**:1281–93.

26. D'Hoore A, Penninckx F. Laparoscopic ventral recto(colpo)pexy for rectal prolapse: surgical technique and outcome for 109 patients. *Surg Endosc* 2006;**20**:1919–23.

27. Consten EC, van Iersel JJ, Verheijen PM, Broeders IA, Wolthuis AM, D'Hoore A. Long-term outcome after laparoscopic ventral mesh rectopexy: an observational study of 919 consecutive patients. *Ann Surg* 2015;**262**:742–47.

28. Franceschilli L, Varvaras D, Capuano I, et al. Laparoscopic ventral rectopexy using biologic mesh for the treatment of obstructed defaecation syndrome and/or faecal incontinence in patients with internal rectal prolapse: a critical appraisal of the first 100 cases. *Tech Coloproctol* 2015;**19**:209–19.

29. Evans C, Stevenson AR, Sileri P, et al. A multicenter collaboration to assess the safety of laparoscopic ventral rectopexy. *Dis Colon Rectum* 2015;**58**:799–807.

30. Pescatori M, Spyrou M, Pulvirenti d'Urso A. A prospective evaluation of occult disorders in obstructed defecation using the 'iceberg diagram'. *Colorectal Dis* 2006;**8**:785–89.

59

Childbirth trauma

Stergios Doumouchtsis

Introduction

Pelvic floor disorders are strongly associated with childbirth and are more prevalent in parous women. Pelvic floor trauma commonly occurs at the time of the first vaginal childbirth. Conventionally, childbirth trauma refers to perineal and vaginal trauma following delivery and the focus has been on the perineal body and the anal sphincter complex. However, childbirth trauma may involve different aspects of the pelvic floor. Pelvic floor trauma during vaginal childbirth may involve tissue rupture, compression, and stretching, resulting in nerve, muscle, and connective tissue damage. Some women may be more susceptible to pelvic floor trauma than others due to collagen weakness.

Childbirth trauma affects millions of women worldwide. The incidence of perineal trauma is over 91% in nulliparous women and over 70% in multiparous women (1). A clinical diagnosis of obstetric anal sphincter injury (OASIS) is made in between 1% and 11% of women following vaginal delivery (2, 3). Increased training and awareness around OASIS is associated with an increase in the reported incidence (2, 3). Short- and long-term symptoms of childbirth trauma can have a significant effect on daily activities, psychological well-being, sexual function, and overall quality of life.

Classification and types of childbirth trauma

Perineal trauma may occur spontaneously or surgically, in the form of an episiotomy (4). The current classification of perineal trauma according to the Royal College of Obstetricians and Gynaecologists is as follows (3) (**Figure 59.1**):

- First degree: laceration of the vaginal epithelium or perineal skin only (**Figure 59.2**).
- Second degree: involvement of the perineal muscles but not the anal sphincter (**Figure 59.3**).
- Third degree: disruption of the anal sphincter muscles (**Figure 59.4**). This is further subdivided into:
  - 3a: less than 50% thickness of external anal sphincter torn
  - 3b: greater than 50% thickness of external anal sphincter torn
  - 3c: external and internal sphincters torn.

- Fourth degree: a third-degree tear with additional disruption of the anal epithelium (**Figure 59.5**).
- Buttonhole tears are isolated tears of the anal mucosa and the vaginal epithelium without involvement of the anal sphincters.

OASIS encompasses both third- and fourth-degree tears.

Levator ani muscle injuries

The levator ani muscle (LAM) plays a major role in the biomechanical properties of the birth canal and pelvic floor. During labour and delivery, the LAM stretches beyond its limits (5, 6). In passive muscles, a stretch of 50% may cause significant injury, whereas in maximally activated muscles, a stretch of 30% results in injury (7).

The reported incidence of LAM trauma varies widely and has been reported to range between 13% and 26% in women who have a vaginal delivery (8–11). A magnetic resonance imaging (MRI)-based study of the LAM found no defects in nulliparous women (12). In contrast, defects were found in 20% of women after their first vaginal birth. An even greater number of women sustain irreversible distension of the levator hiatus. Acute LAM injuries can be diagnosed clinically by digital examination. MRI, transperineal ultrasound, and transvaginal ultrasound can also be used for diagnosis (13). Levator avulsion can be part of a large vaginal tear and is associated with a twofold risk of significant anterior and apical compartment prolapse, with less effect on posterior compartment prolapse (11).

There are various definitions of LAM injury, according to mode of assessment and imaging modality. According to DeLancey et al., a proposed LAM injury MRI-based classification is as follows:

The left and right muscles are scored separately. A score of 0 is assigned if there is no damage visible on MRI, 1 if less than half of the muscle is missing, 2 if more than half, and 3 if the complete muscle bulk is lost. The total score is sum of both sides, ranging from 0 to 6 and is categorized as follows: 0, normal or no defect; 1–3, minor defect; 4–6 major defect. (14)

Nerve injuries

Pudendal nerve injury can be associated with pelvic floor dysfunction. Nerve compression and stretching during labour and delivery can lead to incontinence. This is reversible in most cases, although in severe cases incontinence may persist (11, 12). The mechanism of denervation injury is similar to nerve injury in patients with

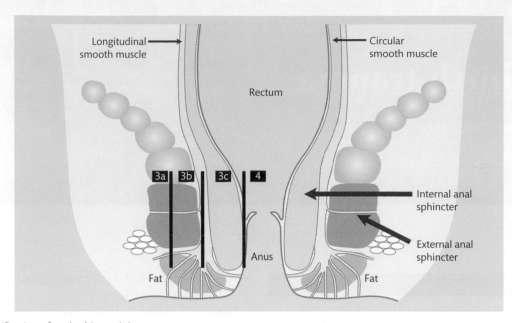

Figure 59.1 Classification of anal sphincter injury.
Reproduced from Cardozo and Staskin (Eds) *Textbook of Female Urology and Urogynecology* 2nd Ed. 2006 Informa Healthcare p1112 with permission from Informa.

chronic constipation (15). It has been associated with the duration of the second stage of labour, size of the baby, and instrumental delivery (16). A study looking at 96 nulliparous women before and after delivery found that vaginal delivery caused partial denervation of the pelvic floor in most women with 80% showing subsequent reinnervation (17).

Connective tissue injuries

During pregnancy, collagen and elastin, components of connective tissue, undergo modifications in order to increase vaginal distensibility and capacity. During labour and delivery, extensive stretching may result in collagen damage. The endopelvic fascia and other connective tissue structures may undergo overstretching, tearing, and detachment from their bony attachments. After delivery, remodelling of the connective tissue takes place, but the new tissue is not as strong as the original (18).

Injuries at the level of the uterine ligaments may result in uterine prolapse. Increases in intra-abdominal pressure generated by

pregnancy itself can cause trauma to these structures, especially in a twin pregnancy, macrosomia, or polyhydramnios. At the level of vaginal apex and posterior compartment, trauma resulting in defects of the pericervical ring and rectovaginal fascia may present as enterocele or high rectocele. The rectovaginal fascia may get overdistended, ruptured, or become detached from the arcus tendineus (19).

Injuries to the pubocervical fascia may result in cystocele or rarely anterior enterocele (8, 19). Loss of support of the vaginal fornices may result in paravaginal defects (20). Injuries to the pubourethral ligaments and pubocervical fascia can be associated with urethrocele, hypermobility of the urethra and bladder neck, and stress urinary incontinence. Direct injury to the urethral sphincter may also cause stress urinary incontinence (8, 19). Trauma to the lower posterior compartment and perineum can result in low rectoceles and perineal tears.

Prolapse is more common in parous compared to nulliparous women (21). Vaginal childbirth, particularly operative vaginal delivery, increases the risk of pelvic organ prolapse (POP) (22, 23). At

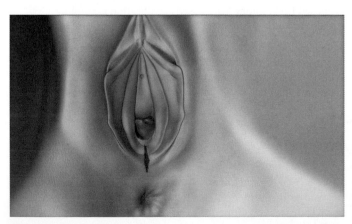

Figure 59.2 First-degree tear.

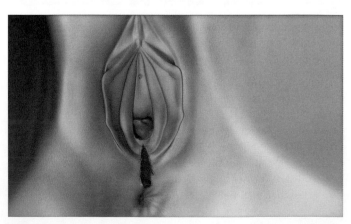

Figure 59.3 Second-degree tear.

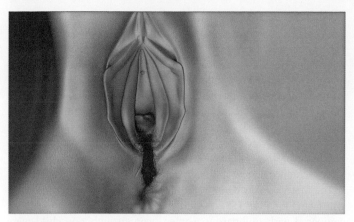

Figure 59.4 Third-degree tear.

6 months postpartum, stage 2 POP was noted in 18% of primiparous Spanish women delivered vaginally compared to 7% of women who delivered by caesarean (24). Similar findings were shown in a multicentre study from the United States (25). No difference in prolapse rates was seen in women delivered by elective caesarean section, compared to those delivered by caesarean after active labour and full cervical dilatation (22). A study of vaginally parous women found that those who had more than one spontaneous laceration were more likely to have prolapse 5–10 years after delivery (23). No increase in POP was found in association with episiotomy.

Pubic bone injuries

Injuries to the pubic bones and symphysis pubis can be evaluated by MRI. An observational study of women who underwent MRI after delivery showed pubic bone fractures in 38% of women at high risk for pelvic floor injury (second stage of labour >150 minutes or <30 minutes, anal sphincter injury, use of forceps, maternal age >35 years, and birth weight >4000 g) and in 13% of women at low risk for pelvic floor injury. Bone marrow oedema in the pubic bones was present in 61% of women (26). Separation of the pubic symphysis at childbirth is uncommon. A review showed an incidence of pubic symphysis diastasis to be 1 in 500 (27).

These injuries can be associated with significant and prolonged pain and disability. Although conservative treatment is sufficient in most cases, invasive orthopaedic treatments are sometimes required.

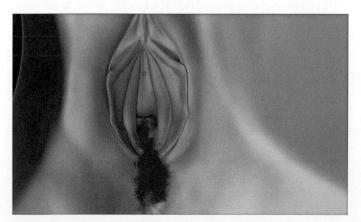

Figure 59.5 Fourth-degree tear.

Epidemiology of perineal trauma

The incidence of perineal trauma varies greatly among different countries. A systematic review from 2008 reported incidences of anal sphincter tears of 0.5% in the United Kingdom, 2.5% in Denmark, and 7% in Canada (4). More recent data from 2013 showed that the incidence of reported third- or fourth-degree perineal tears has tripled from 1.8% to 5.9% from 2000 to 2012 (28). The increasing incidence of OASIS in recent years was also documented in another study of OASIS in a United Kingdom institution, which over a 4-year time period initiated in 2004, showed an incidence of 3.6% (29). Although fourth-degree tears remained constant over the study time period, third-degree tears showed a yearly rise that was more exaggerated in primiparous women.

An increased incidence of OASIS in recent years has been also noted in countries such as Finland, Canada, and China. A comparison of the occurrence of OASIS in Finland took place between 1997–1999 and 2006–2007 (30). Between the two time periods a rise from 0.5% to 1.8% and 0.1% to 0.3% was shown in both primiparous and multiparous women respectively. A study comparing the incidence of OASIS in Sweden and Italy between June 2005 and October 2006 found that Swedish women had a 23 times higher risk than Italian women (31). The incidence was 9.2% in Swedish and 0.4% in Italian women. Gestational age, birth weight, instrumental delivery, and duration of second stage of labour were accountable for the difference.

Data from Nova Scotia showed a twofold increase in OASIS over a 10-year period despite a decline in episiotomy use and instrumental deliveries (32). The number of women experiencing a prolonged second stage of labour increased, however, was not responsible for the twofold rise in severe perineal trauma. It was hypothesized that this increase was due to better recognition of OASIS. The incidence of OASIS in China appears low with an increasing trend. According to a population study it increased from 0.3% in 2011 to 0.38% in 2014 (33).

In contrast to the previously mentioned studies, data from Norway report a decrease in incidence which halved from 4% in 2003–2005 to 1.9% in 2008–2010 (34). This reduction was attributed to a perineal protection training programme that was implemented after an observed increase in OASIS incidence. This programme included interventions such as slowing the delivery of the baby's head, manoeuvres aiming to lower the pressure on the perineum, instructing the women not to push, and training on episiotomy technique.

Management of childbirth in terms of episiotomy rates is also variable with figures of 13% in England, 8% in Netherlands, 25% in the United States, and as high as 99% in Eastern European countries (4).

Another factor that is greatly variable among countries is the number of homebirths with 60% in Netherlands planning to give birth at home (35), whereas in the United Kingdom, only 2.7% of births take place in the home setting (36). The rates of perineal trauma in the hospital setting appear higher even after controlling for instrumental delivery and epidural use (1).

Several explanations have been proposed for the universally increased OASIS incidence in recent years. Many have attributed this to improved diagnosis with emphasis on clinical examination, endoanal ultrasonography, and anal manometry as well as training programmes (37).

The limitation of comparisons between studies as inclusion criteria may differ impacting reported OASIS incidence has also been recognized (38). Another possible reason is the role of maternal age at first birth with many women delaying childbirth. This was supported by a study that demonstrated that levator trauma was increased by 10% for every year of delay of childbirth (39) as well as increased prevalence of stress incontinence in delayed childbearing (40).

Faecal incontinence is common after OASIS, with a prevalence of 16–47% (41–44). Several studies have demonstrated a significant short-term risk of anal incontinence after OASIS (45, 46). The prevalence of postnatal faecal incontinence symptoms 10 months after delivery was 4%. Flatal incontinence was reported in about 29% of women at 9 months after delivery (47).

Risk factors for pelvic floor trauma

Some women are at higher risk of severe childbirth trauma than others. In recent years, attempts have been made to identify and modify risk factors in order to prevent perineal trauma. Of the numerous factors associated with perineal trauma, ethnic origin, nulliparity, and maternal age are considered non modifiable factors. The potentially modifiable risk factors are mainly obstetric: macrosomia, epidural anaesthesia, prolonged second stage of labour, instrumental delivery, and episiotomy.

Maternal risk factors

Ethnicity

A meta-analysis of admittedly heterogeneous studies showed that Asian ethnicity was associated with an increased risk of severe perineal trauma (48). A United States study of maternal morbidity in ethnic groups also found that severe perineal trauma was more likely in Asian women and was the least common complication in non-Hispanic black women (49). Similarly, a study in Californian hospitals found that Asian women had disproportionately high rates of major trauma (50). Interracial marriages, larger babies, gestational diabetes, and increasing body mass index (BMI) were considered responsible for the increased risk in this study. Another study showed that South Asian women have a threefold higher rate of OASIS compared to Australian women (51). However, in this study women were categorized according to the country they were born in.

The variation in perineal trauma rates among different ethnic groups has been attributed to differences in anatomy, skin thickness, and resistance as well as communication challenges. Women may misunderstand instructions during the course of labour and delivery (51). Asian women seem to have a weaker skin, less resistant to stretching (52). A reduced lumbar curvature may result in intra-abdominal forces directed more towards the pelvic floor rather than the anterior abdominal wall (53).

Parity

Nulliparity is a non-disputable risk factor for OASIS. Reduced tissue elasticity seems to play a role. Anal sphincter injuries were associated with nulliparity (odds ratio (OR) 9.8; 95% confidence interval (CI) 3.6–26.2) in a study by Zetterstrom et al. (54). Smith et al. showed that 6.6% of nulliparous and 2.7% of multiparous women sustained

OASIS after vaginal delivery. The incidence of intact perineum was 9.6% and 31.2% in nulliparous and multiparous women, respectively (1). Lower rates of OASIS of 1.7% were found in a study of 20,000 vaginal deliveries with a similar difference in incidence between primiparous women at 2.9% and multiparous at 0.8% (55).

A retrospective cohort study (56) of 20,674 deliveries also concluded that anal sphincter trauma occurred in 16% of women with first vaginal deliveries and 18% with vaginal birth after caesarean section. A meta-analysis by Oberwalder et al. (57) showed a 26.9% incidence of anal sphincter defects in nulliparous women and an 8.5% incidence of new sphincter defects in multiparous women.

The first vaginal delivery seems to have the greatest impact as a risk factor for POP (58). A study by Mant et al. (59) showed that compared with nulliparous women, women with one child were four times more likely and women with two children were 8.4 times more likely to experience POP. Leijonhufvud et al. also showed an increased risk of both stress incontinence and POP with increasing parity (60).

Maternal age

Maternal age has been commonly identified as a risk factor mainly because of the adverse impact of ageing on tissue integrity and elasticity. Maternal age at the time of first delivery seems to have a significant association with pelvic floor trauma (61). Changes in biomechanical properties of the pelvic floor with increasing age may be responsible for the increased pelvic floor injury rates.

Hornemann et al. found maternal age to be the second most important risk factor for severe perineal lacerations (62). However, clear cut-off threshold values for maternal age could not be defined in this study.

Rortveit and Hunskaar (40), however, showed that women 25 years or younger at first birth had a lower risk of incontinence than older women (23% vs 28%; P <0.01). Groutz et al. found that first vaginal delivery at an older age carries an increased risk for postpartum stress urinary incontinence (63).

Smoking

Nulliparous women who smoked throughout pregnancy had a 28% lower risk of OASIS compared to non-smokers (64). Multiparous women also showed comparable findings, although not statistically significant. Nonetheless, the usefulness of these findings is limited, as smoking cannot be recommended due to the other severely adverse outcomes it may cause. These results may be due to the negative effect of smoking on fetal growth (29).

Body mass index

Women with a higher BMI appear less likely to sustain OASIS despite being more likely to have macrosomic babies and instrumental deliveries (65–67). While increasing BMI was correlated with a lower incidence of OASIS, there was an increase in first- and second-degree tears (68). An explanation for the protective effect of higher BMI, although not evidence based, is that the increase in adipose tissue increases the elasticity of the perineum. Also, obese women may have larger perineal bodies.

Obesity was found to be a risk factor for POP in parous women. Dolan et al. (69) reported an almost fourfold increased likelihood of severe stress urinary incontinence in obese women.

Obstetric factors

Instrumental delivery

Instrumental delivery and particularly forceps (41, 70, 71) delivery is an independent risk factor for severe perineal trauma (72). Forceps and vacuum delivery is associated with an increased risk of faecal incontinence by two- to sevenfold (71, 73). Vacuum extraction is generally thought to be less traumatic than forceps. A meta-analysis (74) has implicated both modes of operative delivery, with forceps carrying a greater risk than vacuum. The shanks of the forceps require more space and may cause injury by additional stretching of the introitus and perineum.

Duration of the second stage of labour

A prolonged second stage of labour has been associated with an increased risk of neuromuscular injury. Cheng et al. (75) found that third- or fourth-degree tears were increased when the second stage of labour was prolonged. Maternal exhaustion may necessitate instrumentation, which itself increases the risk of perineal trauma. However, a prolonged second stage of labour does not only result in maternal exhaustion, but sustained pressure on the perineum also predisposes to pelvic floor injury. Prolonged active second stage of labour predisposes to pudendal nerve injury (76).

Episiotomy

Episiotomy is the commonest obstetric procedure; however, there is little evidence to demonstrate any benefit from routine episiotomy. Episiotomy has been shown to double the risk of OASIS when used in non-instrumental deliveries, supporting its restrictive use (77).

Restrictive use of episiotomy seems to reduce perineal and anal sphincter trauma. A Cochrane review showed that compared with routine use, restrictive episiotomy resulted in less severe perineal trauma (relative risk (RR) 0.67; 95% CI 0.49–0.91) (78). The ideal episiotomy rate should be no more than 20–30%. Routine episiotomy did not prevent urinary incontinence at 3 months postpartum according to Klein et al. (79).

There are different types of episiotomy. The most common ones are midline or median and mediolateral episiotomy. Compared to mediolateral episiotomy, median episiotomy increases the risk of anal sphincter injuries (79) (**Figure 59.6**).

Regional anaesthesia

The effect of epidural analgesia on the rates of perineal trauma is complex, due to many confounding factors. Some studies showed protective effects (80) and others harmful effects (81) as well as no effect (82). The harmful effects seen in studies may be a result of its association with instrumental deliveries (83) as after controlling for instrumental delivery, epidural use was no longer a risk factor for perineal trauma (84). Epidural analgesia is used in more nulliparous than parous women. Those with epidural analgesia have a longer second stage of labour, an increased use of augmentation of labour and more use of epidural analgesia with the occipitoposterior position may increase the risk of anal sphincter damage (85, 86). On the other hand, women with epidural analgesia have a higher rate of episiotomy and epidural analgesia results in a more controlled second stage that might reduce the risk (85).

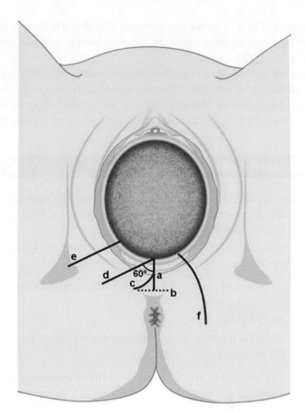

Figure 59.6 Types of episiotomy: (a) midline episiotomy; (b) modified median episiotomy; (c) J-shaped episiotomy; (d) mediolateral episiotomy; (e) lateral episiotomy; (f) radical lateral (Schuchardt incision). Reproduced from Kalis et al. Episiotomy. In: SK Doumouchtsis (Ed) *Childbirth Trauma*, p. 71 (2016) with permission from Springer.

Oxytocin augmentation and birth position

Oxytocin augmentation has been linked with increased perineal trauma and particularly OASIS (87). The lithotomy position has also been associated with increased risk of OASIS irrespective of parity (88). This may be due to increased pressure directed to the anal sphincter during expulsion compared to lateral positions. However, women delivering in the lithotomy position often had other risk factors such as high birthweight, fetal malpresentation, and prolonged labour.

Malpresentation and malposition

In vacuum-assisted deliveries, occipitoposterior position was a significant risk factor for OASIS (OR 4.7; P <0.001) (89). Persistent occipitoposterior position leading to a difficult delivery increases postpartum incontinence (90). Face and brow presentations also increase the risk of incontinence because of the larger presenting diameter.

Fetal factors

Birthweight

Increased birthweight has been shown to increase perineal trauma and subsequently predispose to damage of pelvic floor innervation and stress incontinence (1, 91), with some stating that weight of more than 4000 g has the greatest negative impact on perineal trauma (2).

Increased birthweight is associated with third- and fourth-degree tears, pudendal nerve injury, and significantly weaker anal squeeze pressures (76) and stress incontinence (92, 80). De Leeuw et al. showed a significant correlation between birthweight and third-degree tears (93).

Vaginal birth of macrosomic babies may be associated with disruption of the fascial supports of the pelvic floor and injury to the pelvic and pudendal nerves. Shoulder dystocia and manoeuvres used were also associated with an increased risk of anal sphincter damage (94).

Assessment of perineal trauma

A systematic approach is essential in order to identify the full extent of trauma, the type of the required repair, who should carry out the repair, and where it should take place.

Prior to clinical examination it is important to ensure the following (95):

1. Verbal informed consent for a vaginal and rectal examination.
2. Effective analgesia
3. Adequate lighting
4. Comfortable position of the woman; the lithotomy position is usually necessary.

A clinical examination is undertaken for the assessment of vaginal and perineal tears:

- Parting the labia enables visualization and inspection of the tear. Use of a Sims speculum is helpful to identify the extent and apex of the vaginal tears. The cervix can also be examined for tears if there is clinical suspicion.
- A digital rectal examination is important to assess the integrity of the anal sphincter muscles and rule out buttonhole tears. Anal sphincter injury can still be present with intact perineal skin. The anal sphincter is palpated using the index finger and thumb circumferentially.
- Examination under anaesthesia using pudendal or regional block may be required if complete examination is precluded by discomfort.

Once a tear is diagnosed, repair should be undertaken by a trained healthcare professional in a suitable environment.

Improvements in clinical diagnosis of severe perineal trauma have been documented following standardized training. Improved diagnosis will increase the chances of optimal repair. Third-degree tears repairs undertaken by doctors who have followed a structured training programme appear to result in a lower incidence of persistent sphincter defects (96).

The use of ultrasonography has enabled the accurate visualization of the anal sphincter complex, revealing a high incidence of previously unrecognized occult anal sphincter trauma after delivery. Transvaginal or transperineal ultrasonography and MRI of the pelvis with or without three-dimensional reconstruction are imaging techniques helpful in identifying the types of LAM injuries (97).

Management of perineal trauma

The repair of perineal trauma should be undertaken by an appropriately qualified practitioner as soon as possible after delivery to reduce the risk of bleeding and tissue oedema. Adequate analgesia will enable exposure of the trauma and good visualization without causing additional discomfort to the woman. Local anaesthesia with 1% lidocaine or an epidural top-up are suitable options for uncomplicated tears or episiotomies; however, in cases of severe trauma, significant pain, or bleeding, regional anaesthesia is required. Principles of asepsis, good lighting, and meticulous swab counts should be followed.

For the repair of first- and second-degree tears or perineal skin injuries some practitioners prefer to leave the perineal skin unsutured to heal by secondary intention, as avoiding suture material has been associated with better skin sensation when assessed at 1 year postpartum (98). In two trials on suturing versus non-suturing of first- and second-degree perineal tears (99, 100), there was a similar degree of discomfort with both approaches, but the wound healing appears better after subcuticular closure.

Overall there is no consistent evidence to support one option over the other with regard to healing and recovery, however a Cochrane review concluded that there may be a better feeling of well-being if the wound is left unsutured (101).

Polyglactin 910 (Vicryl, Ethicon) and rapidly absorbable polyglactin 910 material (Vicryl Rapide) are the two most common suture materials used for perineal repair. The tensile strength of Vicryl Rapide is reduced in 10–14 days and it is absorbed in 42 days. Vicryl Rapide is associated with a significant reduction in the need for suture removal up to 3 months postnatally.

Studies have reported less short-term pain and lower resuturing requirements with polyglactin 910 compared to chromic catgut (102). Rapidly absorbed polyglactin is associated with less short-term pain, wound dehiscence, wound infection, and discomfort (103, 104). Comparing standard polyglactin 910 versus rapidly absorbed polyglactin 910, there was no difference in pain at 10 days or dyspareunia at 3 months, but there was a higher requirement for suture removal in the standard polyglactin 910 group (105).

Repair of first- or second-degree tears

- First-degree tears and labial tears can be left unsutured, unless there is significant bleeding or concerns about suboptimal anatomical alignment. In unsutured bilateral labial tears there is a risk of labial adhesions and voiding difficulties.
- The first suture is inserted and tied just above the vaginal apex of the tear to secure haemostasis and optimal anchoring of the suture line.
- The vaginal part of the tear is sutured with a continuous, non-locking technique, which is associated with less pain and dyspareunia compared to interrupted sutures (106).
- The perineal muscles are approximated and sutured with the same continuous suture, aiming to close the dead space and approximate the skin edges as well, which can subsequently be closed without tension. If the muscle tear is deep, a second continuous layer of suturing may be required.
- The perineal skin is closed with a continuous subcuticular suture.
- Episiotomy suturing can be undertaken using this continuous suturing technique (**Figure 59.7**).
- A vaginal and rectal examination is carried out following completion of the suturing, to ensure the repair is complete, restoration of

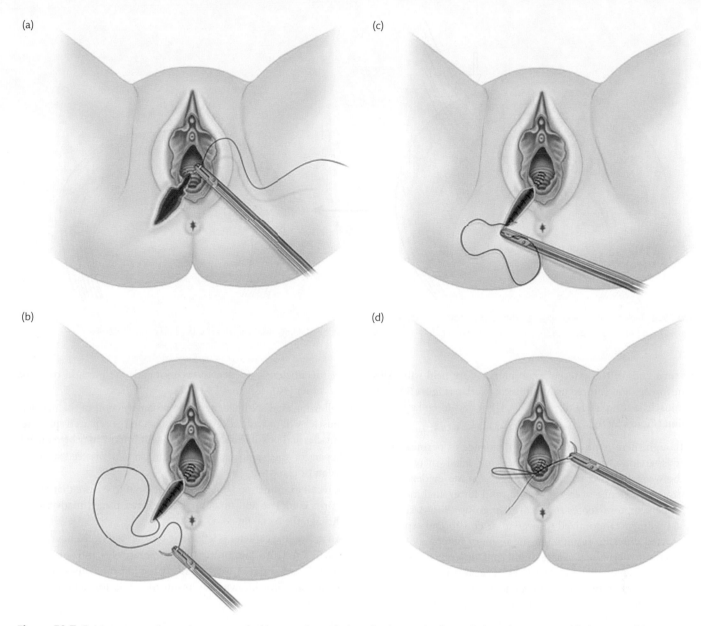

Figure 59.7 Episiotomy repair: continuous non-locking suturing technique for the repair of a mediolateral episiotomy. (a) The apex of the episiotomy is sutured and secured first. Using the same suture, suturing of the vaginal wall follows using a continuous layer. (b) Suturing of perineal muscles. (c) Suturing of perineal skin using subcuticular continuous suture. (d) Knot placement and tying just above the level of hymen.
Reproduced from Kalis et al. Episiotomy In: SK Doumouchtsis (Ed) *Childbirth Trauma*, p. 81 (2016) with permission from Springer.

the anatomy is optimal, and there is no suture material inadvertently placed in the rectal canal.

Repair of third- and fourth-degree tears

Repair of third- and fourth-degree tears should be undertaken by a clinician who has undergone formal training and attained competence in repair of these injuries (3).

Although it is good practice to repair perineal trauma as soon as possible after the delivery, there is no difference in functional outcome if the repair is delayed for a few hours (e.g. because of a lack of trained staff) (107). Repair is best undertaken in the operating theatre with good lighting to achieve optimal exposure and access to the trauma, using aseptic technique, and under regional or general

anaesthesia for muscle relaxation, which allows identification and mobilization of the torn ends of the anal sphincter.

- A buttonhole tear is repaired with two layers of interrupted polyglactin sutures to minimize the risk of a fistula. In the case of gross faecal contamination of the wound, a colorectal surgeon should be called for review and advice.
- In a fourth-degree tear, the anal epithelium is repaired with interrupted 3/0 polyglactin sutures with the suture knots in the anal canal.
- Internal anal sphincter injuries are repaired separately with interrupted sutures using a 3/0 polydioxanone (PDS) or polyglactin suture. Identification and repair of the internal anal sphincter separately is associated with better continence outcomes (108).

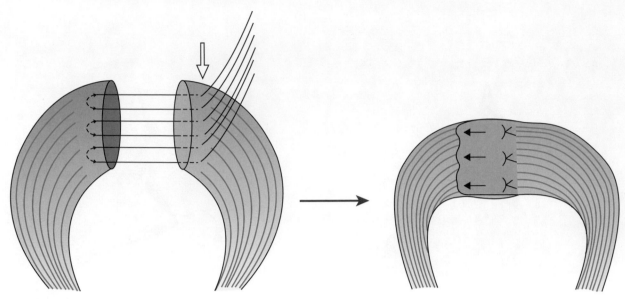

Figure 59.8 Technique of overlapping external anal sphincter repair.
Reproduced from Cardozo and Staskin (Eds) *Textbook of Female Urology and Urogynecology* 2nd Ed. 2006 Informa Healthcare p1117 with permission from Informa.

- The torn ends of the external anal sphincter are held with Allis tissue forceps and sutured using either an overlap (**Figure 59.8**) (if the muscle is completely torn, i.e. 3B/3C) or end-to end approximation (**Figure 59.9**).

  Although there is no difference in incidence of perineal pain, dyspareunia, faecal incontinence, or flatal incontinence between the two techniques, there is some evidence of a lower incidence of faecal urgency and lower anal incontinence symptom scores in the overlap group (90). A study of 64 women randomized to overlap or end-to-end repair reported differing results. For the primary outcome of faecal incontinence, there was a significant difference favouring overlap repair (0% vs 24%) (109). Faecal urgency was also significantly more likely in the end-to-end group. However, the authors of a Cochrane review concluded that there is insufficient evidence to recommend one method over the other (90).

- Following anal sphincter repair, a reconstruction of the perineal muscles will provide additional support to the repaired sphincter muscles and possible risks of subsequent trauma may be reduced.
- Repair of the vagina and perineum should proceed as for a second-degree tear.
- A rectal examination should be carried out to ensure that the repair is complete and no sutures have been placed inadvertently through the rectal mucosa.
- An indwelling catheter is left in the bladder for 12–24 hours.
- Broad-spectrum antibiotics intraoperatively and oral antibiotics for 5–7 days postoperatively are indicated, as wound infection and breakdown may result in fistula formation or anal incontinence.

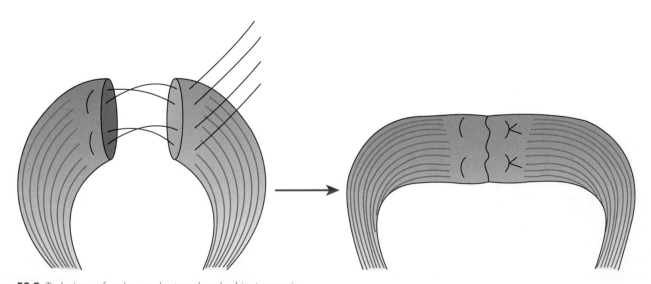

Figure 59.9 Technique of end-to-end external anal sphincter repair.
Reproduced from Cardozo and Staskin (Eds) *Textbook of Female Urology and Urogynecology* 2nd Ed. 2006 Informa Healthcare p1115 with permission from Informa.

- Laxatives are recommended postnatally to avoid constipation, which could disrupt the repair. A stool softener plus a bulking agent for 10 days is recommended, although there is a higher incidence of anal incontinence in the early postnatal period with this regimen compared to stool softeners alone (110).
- Adequate pain relief such as diclofenac suppositories is recommended (111). Constipating analgesics should be avoided.
- Documentation of the extent of the tear and the type of repair, including diagrams, is useful for debriefing the woman and in case of litigation.

Outcomes following OASIS

The reported incidence of anal incontinence following OASIS seems to be lower in more recent studies than in the past, probably due to improvements in training for diagnosis and repair.

In the first 12 months postnatally, symptoms of anal incontinence have been reported in 21–43% of women with OASIS (112, 113). Sonographic evidence of internal anal sphincter injury in the early postnatal period is a significant risk factor for the development of anal incontinence (113). Diagnosis of internal anal sphincter trauma and optimal repair is therefore extremely important. Other independent factors associated with a higher risk of anal incontinence include fourth-degree tears (112) and evidence of persistent sphincter defects. The aetiology of anal incontinence in postnatal women is multifactorial. Anal sphincter defects account for only 45% of cases of anal incontinence (114). Pre-existing anal incontinence and pudendal nerve injury may play a role.

Follow-up after OASIS

Women with OASIS should be reviewed at 6–12 weeks postnatally ideally in a dedicated clinic by a professional with training in perineal trauma, and access to endoanal ultrasound and anal manometry. Endoanal ultrasonography is more accurate than clinical examination for the diagnosis of sphincter defects. There is significant association between sonographic sphincter defects, anal incontinence symptom scores, and low sphincter pressures (115, 116). Sonographic sphincter defects are also predictive of the development of faecal incontinence in later life (117).

Women with mild symptoms such as faecal urgency can usually be managed by dietary modification, constipating agents, and physiotherapy with bowel retraining and biofeedback. Those with more severe incontinence symptoms should be referred to a colorectal surgeon. Counselling on mode of delivery in a future pregnancy should be offered.

Complications of perineal trauma

Postpartum haemorrhage

Vaginal and cervical tears may result in postpartum haemorrhage, which is managed with primary surgical repair and vaginal packing as required. In ongoing bleeding after suturing, pelvic arterial embolization may be considered (118).

Haematomas

Paravaginal (infralevator and supralevator) haematomas

The LAMs divide the paravaginal space into an upper or supralevator fossa and a lower or infralevator fossa (**Figure 59.10**). A paravaginal

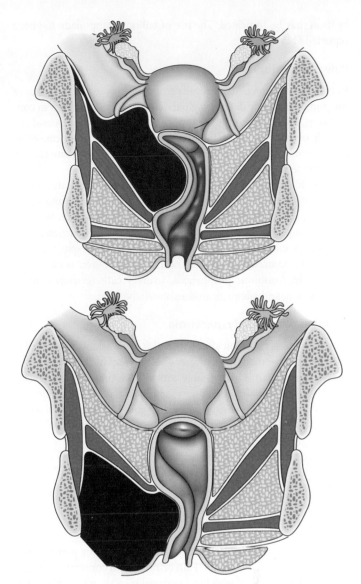

Figure 59.10 (a) Infralevator haematoma. (b) Supralevator haematoma.
Reproduced with permission from Nikolopoulos and Doumouchtsis, *Healing process and complications*. In: SK Doumouchtsis (Ed) *Childbirth Trauma*, p. 201 (2016) with permission from Springer.

haematoma is typically confined to the upper or lower compartment, although massive haemorrhage can extend through the levator barrier.

Haemorrhage into the infralevator space can cause extensive oedema and ecchymosis of the labia, perineum, and lower vagina with severe vulval, vaginal, and perineal pain. Anorectal tenesmus and urinary retention may be caused by extension of the haematoma.

A supralevator haematoma can be palpable as a mass protruding into the vaginal wall potentially causing vaginal or rectal pain and pressure symptoms.

In small infralevator haematomas, ice packs, analgesia, and bladder catheterization may be adequate. Surgical evacuation is indicated in large or expanding haematomas, to prevent tissue ischaemia and necrosis, septicaemia, and further haemorrhage.

Treatment options for supralevator haematomas include conservative measures with vaginal packing for 12–24 hours and haemoglobin monitoring. If bleeding is ongoing, arterial embolization or ligation may be indicated. The use of balloon tamponade has been reported (119).

Vulval haematoma

Vulval haematoma usually results from injuries to the branches of the pudendal artery during vaginal delivery and sometimes in conjunction with episiotomy. Superficial haematomas can extend anteriorly over the mons to the inguinal ligament. Necrosis caused by pressure and rupture of the tissue surrounding the haematoma may lead to external haemorrhage.

Large haematomas usually require exploration in theatre. Initial resuscitation with intravenous fluids may be required, and blood should be sent for haemoglobin, coagulation screen, and crossmatch.

Following a skin incision, the haematoma is evacuated and bleeding points are identified and ligated. The dead space is obliterated with interrupted sutures and the skin incision is closed appropriately. Antibiotic prophylaxis, urinary catheterization, rectal examination, and adequate analgesia are advisable.

Perineal pain and dyspareunia

Perineal pain is common after perineal trauma and was reported to affect 92% of women, resolving in 88% of cases at 2 months (120). In most cases pain is manageable with simple analgesia, however, a small number of women will develop chronic pain. Pain following OASIS can be severe. Severe perineal pain has been observed in 100% of women on day 1 and 91% of women on day 7 following third-degree and fourth-degree tears (121, 122).

Treatment options for perineal pain include oral or rectal analgesia (122). Following primary repair after third- or fourth-degree tears, laxative use will prevent from faecal impaction and possible damage to the recently repaired sphincter muscles. Laxatives result in an earlier and less painful first bowel motion and earlier discharge home (122).

Women who practise perineal massage have lower perineal pain scores than those who do not. Pain refractory to conservative measures may be addressed with local perineal injections with hydrocortisone, Marcaine, and hyaluronidase, which appear well tolerated and lead to a significant improvement in pain scores (123).

Perineal trauma is associated with a decrease in sexual function at 6 months postpartum. Second-degree tears are associated with an 80% increased risk of dyspareunia and third/fourth-degree tears with a 270% increased risk of dyspareunia (124, 125). Dyspareunia is pain that occurs during sexual intercourse, and affects a significant number of women following childbirth—approximately 20% at 3 months postpartum (122, 126). Twenty per cent of women take longer than 6 months before sexual intercourse becomes comfortable. Suboptimal repair of an episiotomy or vaginal tear can also lead to longstanding perineal discomfort and dyspareunia, so attention to anatomy and good surgical technique is important (127).

Dyspareunia secondary to scarring or tightness at the fourchette following suturing is initially treated with dilators and topical oestrogens. Significant scarring and constriction of the introitus may require surgical revision. The appropriate surgical procedure depends on the site and extent of the vaginal constriction, the state of the surrounding tissue, and the overall length and calibre of the vagina. Fenton's procedure, Z-plasty, vaginal incision of constriction ring, vaginal advancement, or placement of free skin graft are reported

techniques (128). Levator muscle spasm can be treated with botulinum toxin injections (129).

Perineal wound infection and breakdown

In one study, one in ten women with a perineal tear that required suturing developed perineal wound infection, defined as the presence of any two of the following markers: perineal pain, wound dehiscence, or purulent vaginal discharge (130). Antepartum risk factors for infection include extremes of maternal age, smoking, poor hygiene, poor nutrition, and pre-existing medical conditions such as diabetes, immunocompromise, severe anaemia and bacterial vaginosis, chlamydia, gonorrhoea, or trichomonas infection. Intrapartum factors include prolonged rupture of membranes, thick meconium, prolonged labour, intrapartum pyrexia, multiple internal examinations, operative vaginal delivery, poor aseptic technique, manual removal of placenta, and retained products. Postpartum factors include delayed or omitted prophylactic antibiotics, suboptimal haemostasis, haematoma, contamination of wound, and residual dead space following repair (131). In cases of second-degree tears, antibiotics are not routinely required. Antibiotic prophylaxis in cases of third/fourth-degree tears results in a lower risk of wound infection (132). Broad-spectrum antibiotics including anaerobic cover are recommended. Most perineal infections resolve with antibiotics and good perineal hygiene.

Perineal wound breakdown can lead to significant morbidity and has an incidence of 0.1–4.6% (133 135). Up to 80% of wound dehiscence cases are secondary to wound infection. There is limited evidence on best practice for the management of perineal wound breakdown. Most practitioners manage these cases conservatively, whereas others offer secondary suturing. A common approach is to allow healing by secondary intention; however, this is a slow process. Resuturing of perineal wound dehiscence within the first 2 weeks following childbirth is another approach and may be associated with less perineal pain during the healing process for up to 6 months after delivery, an improvement of dyspareunia, continuation of exclusive breastfeeding, and increased satisfaction with the aesthetic result of the perineal wound (136). Although there is insufficient evidence to support or refute secondary suturing, the time of presentation and the degree of granulation formation may influence the choice of management.

Labial complications

Spontaneous approximation and healing of labial lacerations may lead to distorted anatomy and dyspareunia. Prevention of labial or clitoral adhesions may be achieved through personal hygiene techniques and instructing women to manually gently separate the labia several times a day while urinating. Oestrogen cream has been used for the management of adhesions of the external genitalia. Surgical correction may be necessary when medical treatment fails (137).

Obstetric fistula

Obstetric fistula, an opening between the vagina and the bladder and/or the rectum, is most frequently caused by unattended prolonged labour, when the pressure of the baby's head against the mother's pelvis causes ischaemia to delicate tissues and necrosis. Obstetric fistula is one of the most severe childbirth injuries that occur when labour is allowed to progress for a long period without timely intervention. More than 2 million women worldwide live with vesicovaginal fistula or recto-vaginal fistula and the majority of them reside in Africa and Asia (138–140).

Prediction and prevention of perineal and pelvic floor trauma

Elective caesarean delivery is the only true primary prevention strategy. Caesarean delivery after the onset of labour is not protective of pelvic floor trauma. The surgical and anaesthetic risks of caesarean section(s) for future pregnancies need to be considered in making an informed decision.

An increased risk of long-term urinary incontinence (141) and surgery for POP and/or stress urinary incontinence (60) following vaginal delivery has been well documented. Caesarean delivery, elective or emergency, seems to provide only partial protection. Eight or nine caesarean sections would need to be performed to avoid one case of urinary incontinence (141).

With regards to POP, women delivered exclusively by caesarean section have a significantly reduced risk of POP in the long term. In a 12-year longitudinal study, women who had all births by caesarean section were the least likely to have prolapse compared with women whose births were all spontaneous vaginal deliveries (OR 0.11; 95% CI 0.03–0.38) (142). As the lifetime risk of undergoing a single operation for POP and urinary incontinence is only 11.1% (143), elective caesarean delivery for prevention of pelvic floor disorders could potentially cause other morbidities to women who would have been delivered vaginally and not have any pelvic floor problems.

Antenatal pelvic floor muscle training

Antenatal pelvic floor muscle training has been shown to reduce the incidence of postnatal stress urinary incontinence in the short term (144–146) but not in the long term (147, 148).

Warm compresses and perineal massage

Antenatal perineal massage can prevent perineal trauma and perineal pain (149). Women practising perineal massage antenatally are less likely to have an episiotomy.

A Cochrane review concluded there is a significant effect of warm compresses and perineal massage during the second stage of labour on reduction of perineal trauma and suturing (150).

Maternal position during delivery

A Cochrane review highlighted possible benefits with upright position in women without epidural anaesthesia, including a very small reduction in the duration of the second stage of labour mainly in primigravid women, and reduction in episiotomy rates and assisted deliveries; however, the authors commented on a possibly increased risk of second-degree tears (151).

A population-based study concluded that the lateral position has a slightly protective effect compared with the sitting position in nulliparous women. An increased risk of OASIS was noted among women in the lithotomy position, irrespective of parity. Squatting and birth seat position were associated with an increased risk among parous women (88).

Instrumental delivery

Women delivered by forceps had more anal sphincter injuries than those delivered by vacuum (74). Compared to vacuum delivery, use of forceps was associated with almost twice the risk of developing faecal incontinence (152).

Perineal support at delivery

A study from Finland suggested that the lower OASIS rate (0.6%) observed there, was a result of the use of perineal support and episiotomy, compared with other Nordic countries (OASIS rates 3.6–4.2%) (153). In Norway, implementation of the 'hands-on' method resulted in a 50% reduction in OASIS rates (34, 154), recommending the use of perineal support as a method of prevention.

Pushing during the second stage

A prolonged second stage with strong voluntary pushes has been implicated in denervation injury (17). A review by Barasinski et al. concluded that the low methodological quality of the studies and the differences between the protocols do not justify a recommendation of a particular pushing technique (155). A Cochrane review of included studies of moderate to low quality suggested that delayed pushing leads to a shortening of the actual time pushing and increase of spontaneous vaginal delivery at the expense of an overall longer duration of the second stage of labour. There was no clear difference in serious perineal trauma and episiotomy (156).

In conclusion, elective caesarean delivery before labour is the only true primary prevention intervention for pelvic floor trauma, but the impact of pregnancy itself on the pelvic floor as well as the risks of a caesarean delivery should be explained and considered during the counselling process. Alternative primary prevention interventions include antenatal pelvic floor exercises and perineal massage. Modifications of obstetric practices such as restrictive use of episiotomy, mediolateral episiotomy when necessary, spontaneous over forceps delivery, vacuum over forceps delivery, and perineal massage in the second stage of labour may result in prevention of pelvic floor trauma. Finally, the choice of mode of delivery in women with previous severe perineal trauma and pelvic floor morbidities may have an impact on risks of recurrence of severe perineal trauma and exposure to or prevention of long-term pelvic floor sequelae. Although the risk of recurrent OASIS is still either similar to the risk of primary OASIS according to Boggs et al. (5.3%) (157) or increased fivefold (7.2%) according to another study (158), a Cochrane review concluded that the effectiveness of interventions for women in subsequent pregnancies following obstetric anal sphincter injury is unknown (159). Jangö et al. recommend that women opting for vaginal delivery after obstetric anal sphincter injury should be informed about the risk of recurrence, which is associated with an increased risk of long-term flatal and faecal incontinence (160). Women with a history of an obstetric anal sphincter injury who are symptomatic or have abnormal endoanal ultrasonography and/or manometry should be offered the option of elective caesarean birth.

REFERENCES

1. Smith LA, Price N, Simonite V, Burns EE. Incidence of and risk factors for perineal trauma: a prospective observational study. *BMC Pregnancy Childbirth* 2013;**13**:59.

2. Dudding TC, Vaizey CJ, Kamm MA. Obstetric anal sphincter injury: incidence, risk factors, and management. *Ann Surg* 2008;**247**:224–37.

3. Royal College of Obstetricians and Gynaecologists (RCOG). *The Management of Third- and Fourth-Degree Perineal Tears*. Greentop Guideline No 29. London: RCOG; 2015.

4. Kettle C, Tohill S. Perineal care. *BMJ Clin Evid* 2008;**2008**:1401.

5. Lien KC, Mooney B, DeLancey JO, Ashton-Miller JA. Levator ani muscle stretch induced by simulated vaginal birth. *Obstet Gynecol* 2004;**103**:31–40.

6. Svabik K, Shek KL, Dietz HP. How much does the levator hiatus have to stretch during childbirth? *BJOG* 2009;**116**:1657–62.

7. Brooks SV, Zerba E, Faulkner JA. Injury to muscle fibres after single stretches of passive and maximally stimulated muscles in mice. *J Physiol* 1995;**488**:459–69.

8. Kearney R, Miller JM, Ashton-Miller JA, DeLancey JO. Obstetric factors associated with levator ani muscle injury after vaginal birth. *Obstet Gynecol* 2006;**107**:144–49.

9. Dietz HP, Gillespie AV, Phadke P. Avulsion of the pubovisceral muscle associated with large vaginal tear after normal vaginal delivery at term. *Aust N Z J Obstet Gynaecol* 2007;**47**:341–44.

10. Dietz HP, Lanzarone V. Levator trauma after vaginal delivery. *Obstet Gynecol* 2005;**106**:707–12.

11. Schwertner-Tiepelmann N, Thakar R, Sultan AH, Tunn R. Obstetric levator ani muscle injuries: current status. *Ultrasound Obstet Gynecol* 2012;**39**:372–83.

12. DeLancey JO, Kearney R, Chou Q, Speights S, Binno S. The appearance of levator ani muscle abnormalities in magnetic resonance images after vaginal delivery. *Obstet Gynecol* 2003;**101**:46–53.

13. Tubaro A, Vodušek DB, Amarenco R, et al. Imaging, neurophysiological testing and other tests. In: Abrams P, Cardozo L, Khoury S, Wein A (eds), pp 509–97. *Incontinence*. Paris: ICUD-EAU; 2013.

14. DeLancey JO, Morgan DM, Fenner DE, et al. Comparison of levator ani muscle defects and function in women with and without pelvic organ prolapse. *Obstet Gynecol* 2007;**109**:295–302.

15. Snooks S.J, Barnes PR, Swash M, Henry MM. Damage to the innervation of the pelvic floor musculature in chronic constipation. *Gastroenterology* 1985;**89**:977–81.

16. Snooks SJ, Swash M, Mathers SE, Henry MM. Effect of vaginal delivery on the pelvic floor: a 5-year follow-up. *Br J Surg* 1990;**77**:1358–60.

17. Allen RE, Hosker GL, Smith AR, Warrell DW. Pelvic floor damage and childbirth: a neurophysiological study. *Br J Obstet Gynaecol* 1990;**97**:770–79.

18. Memon HU, Handa VL. Vaginal childbirth and pelvic floor disorders. *Womens Health (Lond)* 2013;**9**:265–77.

19. Li X, Kruger JA, Nash MP, Nielsen PM. Effects of nonlinear muscle elasticity on pelvic floor mechanics during vaginal childbirth. *J Biomech Eng* 2010;**132**:111010.

20. Cassado-Garriga J, Wong V, Shek K, Dietz HP. Can we identify changes in fascial paravaginal supports after childbirth? *Aust N Z J Obstet Gynaecol* 2015;**55**:70–75.

21. Kudish BI, Iglesia CB, Gutman RE, et al. Risk factors for prolapse development in white, black, and Hispanic Women. *Female Pelvic Med Reconstr Surg* 2011;**17**:80–90.

22. Handa VL, Blomquist JL, Knoepp LR, Hoskey KA, McDermott KC, Muñoz A. Pelvic floor disorders 5-10 years after vaginal or cesarean childbirth. *Obstet Gynecol* 2011;**118**:777–84.

23. Handa VL, Blomquist JL, McDermott KC, Friedman S, Munoz A. Pelvic floor disorders after vaginal birth: effect of episiotomy, perineal laceration, and operative birth. *Obstet Gynecol* 2012;**119**:233–39.

24. Diez-Itza I, Arrue M, Ibanez L, Paredes J, Murgiondo A, Sarasqueta C. Influence of mode of delivery on pelvic organ support 6 months postpartum. *Gynecol Obstet Invest* 2011;**72**:123–29.

25. Handa VL, Nygaard I, Kenton K, et al. Pelvic organ support among primiparous women in the first year after childbirth. *Int Urogynecol J Pelvic Floor Dysfunct* 2009;**20**:1407–11.

26. Brandon C, Jacobson JA, Low LK, Park L, DeLancey J, Miller J. Pubic bone injuries in primiparous women: magnetic resonance imaging in detection and differential diagnosis of structural injury. *Ultrasound Obstet Gynecol* 2012;**39**:444–51.

27. Snow RE, Neubert AG. Peripartum pubic symphysis separation: a case series and review of the literature. *Obstet Gynecol Surv* 1997;**52**:438–43.

28. Gurol-Urganci I, Cromwell DA, Edozien LC, et al. Third- and fourth-degree perineal tears among primiparous women in England between 2000 and 2012: time trends and risk factors. *BJOG* 2013;**120**:1516–25.

29. McPherson KC, Beggs AD, Sultan AH, Thakar R. Can the risk of obstetric anal sphincter injuries (OASIs) be predicted using a risk-scoring system? *BMC Res Notes* 2014;**7**:471.

30. Raisanen S, Vehvilainen-Julkunen K, Gissler M, Heinonen S. The increased incidence of obstetric anal sphincter rupture—an emerging trend in Finland. *Prev Med* 2009;**49**:535–40.

31. Prager M, Andersson KL, Stephansson O, Marchionni M, Marions L. The incidence of obstetric anal sphincter rupture in primiparous women: a comparison between two European delivery settings. *Acta Obstet Gynecol Scand* 2008;**87**:209–15.

32. McLeod NL, Gilmour DT, Joseph KS, Farrell SA, Luther ER. Trends in major risk factors for anal sphincter lacerations: a 10-year study. *J Obstet Gynaecol Can* 2003;**25**:586–93.

33. Tung CW, Cheon WC, Tong WM, Leung HY. Incidence and risk factors of obstetric anal sphincter injuries after various modes of vaginal deliveries in Chinese women. *Chin Med J (Engl)* 2015;**128**:2420–25.

34. Laine K, Skjeldestad FE, Sandvik L, Staff AC. Incidence of obstetric anal sphincter injuries after training to protect the perineum: cohort study. *BMJ Open* 2012;**2**:e001649.

35. de Jonge A, van der Goes BY, Ravelli AC, et al. Perinatal mortality and morbidity in a nationwide cohort of 529,688 low-risk planned home and hospital births. *BJOG* 2009;**116**:1177.

36. Nove A, Berrington A, Matthews Z. Home births in the UK, 1955 to 2006. *Popul Trends* 2008;**133**:20–27.

37. Andrews V, Thakar R, Sultan AH. Structured hands-on training in repair of obstetric anal sphincter injuries (OASIS): an audit of clinical practice. *Int Urogynecol J Pelvic Floor Dysfunct* 2009;**20**:193–99.

38. Abbott D, Atere-Roberts N, Williams A, Oteng-Ntim E, Chappell LC. Obstetric anal sphincter injury. *BMJ* 2010;**341**:c3414.

39. Dietz HP, Simpson JM. Does delayed child-bearing increase the risk of levator injury in labour? *Aust N Z J Obstet Gynaecol* 2007;**47**:491–95.

40. Rortveit G, Hunskaar S. Urinary incontinence and age at the first and last delivery: the Norwegian HUNT/EPINCONT study. *Am J Obstet Gynecol* 2006;**195**:433–38.

41. Combs CA, Robertson PA, Laros RK Jr. Risk factors for third-degree and fourth-degree perineal lacerations in forceps and vacuum deliveries. *Am J Obstet Gynecol* 1990;**163**:100–104.

42. Crawford LA, Quint EH, Pearl ML, DeLancey JO. Incontinence following rupture of the anal sphincter during delivery. *Obstet Gynecol* 1993;**82**:527–31.

43. Henriksen TB, Bek KM, Hedegaard M, Secher NJ. Episiotomy and perineal lesions in spontaneous vaginal deliveries. *Br J Obstet Gynaecol* 1992;**99**:950–54.

44. Walker MP, Farine D, Rolbin SH, Ritchie JW. Epidural anesthesia, episiotomy, and obstetric laceration. *Obstet Gynecol* 1991;**77**:668–71.

45. Bols EM, Hendriks EJ, Berghmans BC, Baeten CG, Nijhuis JG, de Bie RA. A systematic review of etiological factors for postpartum fecal incontinence. *Acta Obstet Gynecol Scand* 2010;**89**:302–14.

46. Borello-France D, Burgio KL, Richter HE, et al. Fecal and urinary incontinence in primiparous women. *Obstet Gynecol* 2006;**108**:863–72.

47. Zetterström JP, Lopez A, Anzen B, Dolk A, Norman M, Mellgren A. Anal incontinence after vaginal delivery: a prospective study in primiparous women. *Br J Obstet Gynaecol* 1999;**106**:324–30.

48. Pergialiotis V, Vlachos D, Protopapas A, Pappa K, Vlachos G. Risk factors for severe perineal lacerations during childbirth. *Int J Gynaecol Obstet* 2014;**125**:6–14.

49. Grobman WA, Bailit JL, Rice MM, et al. Racial and ethnic disparities in maternal morbidity and obstetric care. *Obstet Gynecol* 2015;**125**:1460–67.

50. Guendelman S, Thornton D, Gould J, Hosang N. Obstetric complications during labor and delivery: assessing ethnic differences in California. *Womens Health Issues* 2006;**16**:189–97.

51. Davies-Tuck M, Biro MA, Mockler J, Stewart L, Wallace EM, East C. Maternal Asian ethnicity and the risk of anal sphincter injury. *Acta Obstet Gynecol Scand* 2015;**94**:308–15.

52. Muizzuddin N, Hellemans L, Van Overloop L, Corstjens H, Declercq L, Maes D. Structural and functional differences in barrier properties of African American, Caucasian and East Asian skin. *J Dermatol Sci* 2010;**59**:123–28.

53. Mattox TF, Lucente V, McIntyre P, Miklos JR, Tomezsko J. Abnormal spinal curvature and its relationship to pelvic organ prolapse. *Am J Obstet Gynecol* 2000;**183**:1381–84.

54. Zetterstrom, J, Lopez, A, Anzen, B, Norman, M, Holmstrom, B, Mellgren, A. Anal sphincter tears at vaginal delivery: risk factors and clinical outcome of primary repair. *Obstet Gynecol* 1999;**94**:21–28.

55. Harkin R, Fitzpatrick M, O'Connell PR, O'Herlihy C. Anal sphincter disruption at vaginal delivery: is recurrence predictable? *Eur J Obstet Gynecol Reprod Biol* 2003;**109**:149–52.

56. Lowder JL, Burrows LJ, Krohn MA, Weber AM. Risk factors for primary and subsequent anal sphincter lacerations: a comparison of cohorts by parity and prior mode of delivery. *Am J Obstet Gynecol* 2007;**196**:344.e1–5.

57. Oberwalder M, Connor J, Wexner SD. Meta-analysis to determine the incidence of obstetric anal sphincter damage. *Br J Surg* 2003;**90**:1333–37.

58. Quiroz LH, Munoz A, Shippey SH, Gutman RE, Handa VL. Vaginal parity and pelvic organ prolapse. *J Reprod Med* 2010;**55**:93–98.

59. Mant J, Painter R, Vessey M. Epidemiology of genital prolapse: observations from the Oxford Family Planning Association Study. *Br J Obstet Gynaecol* 1997;**104**:579–85.

60. Leijonhufvud A, Lundholm C, Cnattingius S, Granath F, Andolf E, Altman D. Risks of stress urinary incontinence and pelvic organ prolapse surgery in relation to mode of childbirth. *Am J Obstet Gynecol* 2011;**204**:70.e1–7.

61. Rahmanou P, Caudwell-Hall J, Kamisan Atan I, Dietz HP. The association between maternal age at first delivery and risk of obstetric trauma. *Am J Obstet Gynecol* 2016;**215**:451.e1–7.

62. Hornemann A, Kamischke A, Luedders DW, Beyer DA, Diedrich K, Bohlmann MK. Advanced age is a risk factor for higher grade perineal lacerations during delivery in nulliparous women. *Arch Gynecol Obstet* 2010;**281**:59–64.

63. Groutz A, Helpman L, Gold R, Pauzner D, Lessing JB, Gordon D. First vaginal delivery at an older age: does it carry an extra risk for the development of stress urinary incontinence? *Neurourol Urodyn* 2007;**26**:779–82.

64. Raisanen S, Vehvilainen-Julkunen K, Gissler M, Heinonen S. Smoking during pregnancy is associated with a decreased incidence of obstetric anal sphincter injuries in nulliparous women. *PLoS One* 2012;7:e41014.

65. Kapaya H, Hashim S, Jha S. OASI: a preventable injury? *Eur J Obstet Gynecol Reprod Biol* 2015;**185**:9–12.

66. Voldner N, Froslie KF, Haakstad LA, Bo K, Henriksen T. Birth complications, overweight, and physical inactivity. *Acta Obstet Gynecol Scand* 2009;**88**:550–55.

67. Blomberg M. Maternal body mass index and risk of obstetric anal sphincter injury. *Biomed Res Int* 2014;**2014**:395803.

68. Lindholm ES, Altman D. Risk of obstetric anal sphincter lacerations among obese women. *BJOG* 2013;**120**:1110–15.

69. Dolan LM, Hilton P. Obstetric risk factors and pelvic floor dysfunction 20 years after first delivery. *Int Urogynecol J* 2010;**21**:535–44.

70. MacArthur C, Glazener CM, Wilson PD, et al. Obstetric practice and faecal incontinence three months after delivery. *BJOG* **108**:678–83.

71. Sultan AH, Kamm MA, Hudson CN, Thomas JM, Bartram CI. Anal-sphincter disruption during vaginal delivery. *N Engl J Med* 1993;**329**:1905–11.

72. Hudelist G, Gelle'n J, Singer C, et al. Factors predicting severe perineal trauma during childbirth: role of forceps delivery routinely combined with mediolateral episiotomy. *Am J Obstet Gynecol* 2005;**192**:875–81.

73. Donnelly V, Fynes M, Campbell D, Johnson H, O'Connell PR, O'Herlihy C. Obstetric events leading to anal sphincter damage. *Obstet Gynecol* 1998;**92**:955–61.

74. Eason E, Labrecque M, Wells G, Feldman P. Preventing perineal trauma during childbirth: a systematic review. *Obstet Gynecol* 2000;**95**:464–71.

75. Cheng YW, Hopkins LM, Caughey AB. How long is too long: does a prolonged second stage of labor in nulliparous women affect maternal and neonatal outcomes? *Am J Obstet Gynecol* 2004;**191**:933–38.

76. Sultan AH, Kamm MA, Hudson CN. Pudendal nerve damage during labour: prospective study before and after childbirth. *Br J Obstet Gynaecol* 1994;**101**:22–28.

77. Gerdin E, Sverrisdottir G, Badi A, Carlsson B, Graf W. The role of maternal age and episiotomy in the risk of anal sphincter tears during childbirth. *Aust N Z J Obstet Gynaecol* 2007;**47**:286–90.

78. Carroli G, Mignini L. Episiotomy for vaginal birth. *Cochrane Database Syst Rev* 2009;**1**:CD000081.

79. Klein MC, Gauthier RJ, Jorgensen SH, et al. Does episiotomy prevent perineal trauma and pelvic floor relaxation? *Online J Curr Clin Trials* 1992;Jul 1:Doc 10.

80. Jangö H, Langhoff-Roos J, Rosthoj S, Sakse A. Modifiable risk factors of obstetric anal sphincter injury in primiparous women: a population-based cohort study. *Am J Obstet Gynecol* 2014;**210**:59.e1–6.

81. Naidoo TD, Moodley J. Obstetric perineal injury: risk factors and prevalence in a resource-constrained setting. *Trop Doct* 2015;**45**:252–54.

82. Burrell M, Dilgir S, Patton V, Parkin K, Karantanis E. Risk factors for obstetric anal sphincter injuries and postpartum anal and urinary incontinence: a case-control trial. *Int Urogynecol J* 2015;**26**:383–89.

83. Robinson JN, Norwitz ER, Cohen AP, McElrath TF, Lieberman ES. Epidural analgesia and third- or fourth-degree lacerations in nulliparas. *Obstet Gynecol* 1999;**94**:259–62.

84. Carroll TG, Engelken M, Mosier MC, Nazir N. Epidural analgesia and severe perineal laceration in a community-based obstetric practice. *J Am Board Fam Pract* 2003;**16**:1–6.

85. Bodner-Adler B, Bodner K, Kimberger O, et al. The effect of epidural analgesia on the occurrence of obstetric lacerations and on the neonatal outcome during spontaneous vaginal delivery. *Arch Gynecol Obstet* 2002;**267**:81–84.

86. Albers LL, Migliaccio L, Bedrick EJ, Teaf D, Peralta P. Does epidural analgesia affect the rate of spontaneous obstetric lacerations in normal births? *J Midwifery Womens Health* 2007;**52**:31–36.

87. Drusany Staric K, Bukovec P, Jakopic K, Zdravevski E, Trajkovik V, Lukanovic A. Can we predict obstetric anal sphincter injury? *Eur J Obstet Gynecol Reprod Biol* 2017;**210**:196–200.

88. Elvander C, Ahlberg M, Thies-Lagergren L, Cnattingius S, Stephansson O. Birth position and obstetric anal sphincter injury: a population-based study of 113 000 spontaneous births. *BMC Pregnancy Childbirth* 2015;**15**:252.

89. Rognant S, Benoist G, Creveuil C, Dreyfus M. Obstetrical situations with a high risk of anal sphincter laceration in vacuum-assisted deliveries. *Acta Obstet Gynecol Scand* 2012;**91**:862–68.

90. Fernando RJ, Sultan AH, Kettle C, Thakar R. Methods of repair for obstetric anal sphincter injury. *Cochrane Database Syst Rev* 2013;**12**:CD002866.

91. Wesnes SL, Hannestad Y, Rortveit G. Delivery parameters, neonatal parameters and incidence of urinary incontinence six months postpartum: a cohort study. *Acta Obstet Gynecol Scand* 2017;**96**:1214–22.

92. Goldberg RP, Abramov Y, Botros S, et al. Delivery mode is a major environmental determinant of stress urinary incontinence: results of the Evanston-Northwestern Twin Sisters Study. *Am J Obstet Gynecol* 2005;**193**:2149–53.

93. de Leeuw JW, Struijk PC, Vierhout ME, Wallenburg HC. Risk factors for third degree perineal ruptures during delivery. *BJOG* 2001;**108**:383–87.

94. Gauthaman N, Walters S, Tribe IA, Goldsmith L, Doumouchtsis SK. Shoulder dystocia and associated manoeuvres as risk factors for perineal trauma. *Int Urogynecol J* 2016;**27**:571–77.

95. National Institute for Health and Care Excellence (NICE). *Intrapartum Care: Care of Healthy Women and their Babies during Childbirth*. Clinical Guideline [CG190]. London: NICE; 2014.

96. Andrews V, Thakar R, Sultan AH. Outcome of obstetric anal sphincter injuries (OASIS)—role of structured management. *Int Urogynecol J Pelvic Floor Dysfunct* 2009;**20**:973–78.

97. Wisser J, Schar G, Kurmanavicius J, Huch R, Huch A. Use of 3D ultrasound as a new approach to assess obstetrical trauma to the pelvic floor. *Ultraschall Med* 1999;**20**:15–18.

98. Grant A, Gordon B, Mackrodat C, Fern E, Truesdale A, Ayers S. The Ipswich childbirth study: one year follow up of alternative methods used in perineal repair. *BJOG* 2001;**108**:34–40.

99. Lundquist M, Olsson A, Nissen E, Norman M. Is it necessary to suture all lacerations after a vaginal delivery? *Birth* 2000;**27**:79–85.

100. Fleming VE, Hagen S, Niven C. Does perineal suturing make a difference? The SUNS trial. *BJOG* 2003;**110**:684–89.

101. Elharmeel SM, Chaudhary Y, Tan S, Scheermeyer E, Hanafy A, van Driel ML. Surgical repair of spontaneous perineal tears that occur during childbirth versus no intervention. *Cochrane Database Syst Rev* 2011;**8**:CD008534.

102. Mackrodt C, Gordon B, Fern E, Ayers S, Truesdale A, Grant A. The Ipswich Childbirth Study: 2. A randomised comparison of polyglactin 910 with chromic catgut for postpartum perineal repair. *Br J Obstet Gynaecol* 1998;**105**:441–45.

103. Bharathi A, Reddy DB, Kote GS. A prospective randomized comparative study of vicryl rapide versus chromic catgut for episiotomy repair. *J Clin Diagn Res* 2013;**7**:326–30.

104. Kettle C, Dowswell T, Ismail KM. Absorbable suture materials for primary repair of episiotomy and second degree tears. *Cochrane Database Syst Rev* 2010;**6**:CD000006.

105. Kettle C, Hills RK, Jones P, Darby L, Gray R, Johanson R. Continuous versus interrupted perineal repair with standard or rapidly absorbed sutures after spontaneous vaginal birth: a randomised controlled trial. *Lancet* 2002;**359**:2217–23.

106. Kettle C, Dowswell T, Ismail KM. Continuous and interrupted suturing techniques for repair of episiotomy or second-degree tears. *Cochrane Database Syst Rev* 2012;**11**:CD000947.

107. Nordenstam J, Mellgren A, Altman D, et al. Immediate or delayed repair of obstetric anal sphincter tears-a randomised controlled trial. *BJOG* 2008;**115**:857–65.

108. Norderval S, Oian P, Revhaug A, Vonen B. Anal incontinence after obstetric sphincter tears: outcome of anatomic primary repairs. *Dis Colon Rectum* 2005;**48**:1055–61.

109. Fernando RJ, Sultan AH, Kettle C, Radley S, Jones P, O'Brien PM. Repair techniques for obstetric anal sphincter injuries: a randomized controlled trial. *Obstet Gynecol* 2006;**107**:1261–68.

110. Eogan M, Daly L, Behan M, O'Connell PR, O'Herlihy C. Randomised clinical trial of a laxative alone versus a laxative and a bulking agent after primary repair of obstetric anal sphincter injury. *BJOG* 2007;**114**:736–40.

111. Dodd JM, Hedayati H, Pearce E, Hotham N, Crowther CA. Rectal analgesia for the relief of perineal pain after childbirth: a randomised controlled trial of diclofenac suppositories. *BJOG* 2004;**111**:1059–64.

112. Laine K, Skjeldestad FE, Sanda B, Horne H, Spydslaug A, Staff AC. Prevalence and risk factors for anal incontinence after obstetric anal sphincter rupture. *Acta Obstet Gynecol Scand* 2011;**90**:319–24.

113. Vaccaro C, Clemons JL. Anal sphincter defects and anal incontinence symptoms after repair of obstetric anal sphincter lacerations in primiparous women. *Int Urogynecol J Pelvic Floor Dysfunct* 2088;**19**:1503–508.

114. Abramowitz L, Sobhani I, Ganansia R, et al. Are sphincter defects the cause of anal incontinence after vaginal delivery? Results of a prospective study. *Dis Colon Rectum* 2000;**43**:590–96.

115. Starck M, Bohe M, Valentin L. The extent of endosonographic anal sphincter defects after primary repair of obstetric sphincter tears increases over time and is related to anal incontinence. *Ultrasound Obstet Gynecol* 2006;**27**:188–97.

116. Faltin DL, Boulvain M, Irion O, Bretones S, Stan C, Weil A. Diagnosis of anal sphincter tears by postpartum endosonography to predict fecal incontinence. *Obstet Gynecol* 2000;**95**:643–47.

117. Oberwalder M, Dinnewitzer A, Baig MK, et al. The association between late-onset fecal incontinence and obstetric anal sphincter defects. *Arch Surg* 2004;**139**:429–32.

118. Fargeaudou Y, Soyer P, Morel O, et al. Severe primary postpartum hemorrhage due to genital tract laceration after operative vaginal delivery: successful treatment with transcatheter arterial embolization. *Eur Radiol* 2009;**19**:2197–203.

119. Tattersall M, Braithwaite W. Balloon tamponade for vaginal lacerations causing severe postpartum haemorrhage. *BJOG* 2007;**114**:647–48.

120. Andrews V, Thakar R, Sultan AH, Jones PW. Evaluation of postpartum perineal pain and dyspareunia—a prospective study. *Eur J Obstet Gynecol Reprod Biol* 2008;**137**:152–56.

121. Macarthur AJ, Macarthur C. Incidence, severity, and determinants of perineal pain after vaginal delivery: a prospective cohort study. *Am J Obstet Gynecol* 2004;**191**:1199–204.

122. Fitzpatrick M, O'Herlihy C. Short-term and long-term effects of obstetric anal sphincter injury and their management. *Curr Opin Obstet Gynecol* 2005;**17**:605–10.

123. Doumouchtsis SK, Boama V, Gorti M, Tosson S, Fynes MM. Prospective evaluation of combined local bupivacaine and steroid injections for the management of chronic vaginal and perineal pain. *Arch Gynecol Obstet* 2011;**284**:681–85.

124. Signorello LB, Harlow BL, Chekos AK, Repke JT. Postpartum sexual functioning and its relationship to perineal trauma: a retrospective cohort study of primiparous women. *Am J Obstet Gynecol* 2001;**184**:881–88.

125. Lewis C, Williams AM, Rogers RG. Postpartum anal sphincter lacerations in a population with minimal exposure to episiotomy and operative vaginal delivery. *Int Urogynecol J Pelvic Floor Dysfunct* 2008;**19**:41–45.

126. Connolly A, Thorp J, Pahel L. Effects of pregnancy and childbirth on postpartum sexual function: a longitudinal prospective study. *Int Urogynecol J Pelvic Floor Dysfunct* 2005;**16**:263–67.

127. Phillips C, Monga A. Childbirth and the pelvic floor: 'the gynaecological consequences'. *Reviews in Gynaecological Practice* 2005;**5**:15–22.

128. Vassallo BJ, Karram MM. Management of iatrogenic vaginal constriction. *Obstet Gynecol* 2003;**102**:512–20.

129. Romito S, Bottanelli M, Pellegrini M, Vicentini S, Rizzuto N, Bertolasi L. Botulinum toxin for the treatment of genital pain syndromes. *Gynecol Obstet Invest* 2004;**58**:164–67.

130. Johnson A, Thakar R, Sultan AH. Obstetric perineal wound infection: is there underreporting? *Br J Nurs* 2012;**21**:S28, 30, 32–35.

131. Kamel A, Khaled M. Episiotomy and obstetric perineal wound dehiscence: beyond soreness. *J Obstet Gynaecol* 2014;**34**:215–17.

132. Duggal N, Mercado C, Daniels K, Bujor A, Caughey AB, El-Sayed YY. Antibiotic prophylaxis for prevention of postpartum perineal wound complications: a randomized controlled trial. *Obstet Gynecol* 2008;**111**:1268–73.

133. Ramin SM, Gilstrap LC 3rd. Episiotomy and early repair of dehiscence. *Clin Obstet Gynecol* 1994;**37**:816–23.

134. Williams MK, Chames MC. Risk factors for the breakdown of perineal laceration repair after vaginal delivery. *Am J Obstet Gynecol* 2006;**195**:755–59.

135. Goldaber KG, Wendel PJ, McIntire DD, Wendel GD Jr. Postpartum perineal morbidity after fourth-degree perineal repair. *Am J Obstet Gynecol* 1993;**168**:489–93.

136. Dudley LM, Kettle C, Ismail KM. Secondary suturing compared to non-suturing for broken down perineal wounds following childbirth. *Cochrane Database Syst Rev* 2013;**9**:CD008977.

137. Arkin AE, Chern-Hughes B. Case report: labial fusion postpartum and clinical management of labial lacerations. *J Midwifery Womens Health* 2002;**47**:290–92.

138. Miller S, Lester F, Webster M, Cowan B. Obstetric fistula: a preventable tragedy. *J Midwifery Womens Health* 2005;**50**:286–94.

139. World Health Organization (WHO). *The Prevention and Treatment of Obstetric Fistulae*. Geneva: WHO; 1989.

140. Mselle LT, Kohi TW, Mvungi A, Evjen-Olsen B, Moland KM. Waiting for attention and care: birthing accounts of women in rural Tanzania who developed obstetric fistula as an outcome of labour. *BMC Pregnancy Childbirth* 2011;**11**:75.

141. Gyhagen M, Bullarbo M, Nielsen TF, Milsom I. The prevalence of urinary incontinence 20 years after childbirth: a national cohort study in singleton primiparae after vaginal or caesarean delivery. *BJOG* 2013;**120**:144–51.

142. Glazener C, Elders A, Macarthur C, et al. Childbirth and prolapse: long-term associations with the symptoms and objective measurement of pelvic organ prolapse. *BJOG* 2013;**120**:161–68.

143. Olsen AL, Smith VJ, Bergstrom JO, Colling JC, Clark AL. Epidemiology of surgically managed pelvic organ prolapse and urinary incontinence. *Obstet Gynecol* 1997;**89**:501–506.

144. Sampselle CM, Miller JM, Mims BL, Delancey JO, Ashton-Miller JA, Antonakos CL. Effect of pelvic muscle exercise on transient incontinence during pregnancy and after birth. *Obstet Gynecol* 1998;**91**:406–12.

145. Morkved S, Bo K. Effect of pelvic floor muscle training during pregnancy and after childbirth on prevention and treatment of urinary incontinence: a systematic review. *Br J Sports Med* 2014;**48**:299–310.

146. Reilly ET, Freeman RM, Waterfield MR, Waterfield AE, Steggles P, Pedlar F. Prevention of postpartum stress incontinence in primigravidae with increased bladder neck mobility: a randomised controlled trial of antenatal pelvic floor exercises. *BJOG* 2014;**121** Suppl 7:58–66.

147. Glazener CM, Herbison GP, MacArthur C, Grant A, Wilson PD. Randomised controlled trial of conservative management of postnatal urinary and faecal incontinence: six year follow up. *BMJ* 2005;**330**:337.

148. Agur WI, Steggles P, Waterfield M, Freeman RM. The long-term effectiveness of antenatal pelvic floor muscle training: eight-year follow up of a randomised controlled trial. *BJOG* 2008;**115**:985–90.

149. Beckmann MM, Stock OM. Antenatal perineal massage for reducing perineal trauma. *Cochrane Database Syst Rev* 2013;**4**:CD005123.

150. Aasheim V, Nilsen AB, Lukasse M, Reinar LM. Perineal techniques during the second stage of labour for reducing perineal trauma. *Cochrane Database Syst Rev* 2011;**12**:CD006672.

151. Gupta JK, Sood A, Hofmeyr GJ, Vogel JP. Position in the second stage of labour for women without epidural anaesthesia. *Cochrane Database Syst Rev* 2017;**5**:CD002006.

152. Fitzpatrick M, Behan M, O'Connell PR, O'Herlihy C. Randomised clinical trial to assess anal sphincter function following forceps or vacuum assisted vaginal delivery. *BJOG* 2003;**110**:424–29.

153. Laine K, Gissler M, Pirhonen J. Changing incidence of anal sphincter tears in four Nordic countries through the last decades. *Eur J Obstet Gynecol Reprod Biol* 2009;**146**:71–75.

154. Hals E, Oian P, Pirhonen T, et al. A multicenter interventional program to reduce the incidence of anal sphincter tears. *Obstet Gynecol* 2010;**116**:901–908.

155. Barasinski C, Lemery D, Vendittelli F. Do maternal pushing techniques during labour affect obstetric or neonatal outcomes? *Gynecol Obstet Fertil* 2016;**44**:578–83.

156. Lemos A, Amorim MM, Dornelas de Andrade A, de Souza AI, Cabral Filho JE, Correia JB. Pushing/bearing down methods

for the second stage of labour. *Cochrane Database Syst Rev* 2017;**3**:CD009124.

157. Boggs EW, Berger H, Urquia M, McDermott CD. Recurrence of obstetric third-degree and fourth-degree anal sphincter injuries. *Obstet Gynecol* 2014;**124**:1128–34.

158. Edozien LC, Gurol-Urganci I, Cromwell DA, et al. Impact of third- and fourth-degree perineal tears at first birth on subsequent pregnancy outcomes: a cohort study. *BJOG* 2014;**121**:1695–703.

159. Farrar D, Tuffnell DJ, Ramage C. Interventions for women in subsequent pregnancies following obstetric anal sphincter injury to reduce the risk of recurrent injury and associated harms. *Cochrane Database Syst Rev* 2014;**11**:CD010374.

160. Jangö H, Langhoff-Roos J, Rosthoj S, Sakse A. Recurrent obstetric anal sphincter injury and the risk of long-term anal incontinence. *Am J Obstet Gynecol* 2017;**216**:610.e1–10.

60

Female sexual dysfunction

Ganesh Adaikan

Introduction

According to the World Health Organization, sexual health as a state of physical, emotional, mental, and social well-being in the context of sexuality, excludes the mere absence of disease, dysfunction, or infirmity (1). Thus a woman's sexual function encompasses many areas; the construct of a normal function as a quality of life indicator often but not always conforms to the sexual response cycle, which is an endogenous process contributed by hormonal, vascular, neuronal, and psycho-emotional factors (2). Clinical and scientific evidence abounds about the physiological role of sex steroids viz. oestrogen, testosterone, and also progesterone in facilitating and maintaining the woman's sexual parameters (3). The neurophysiology extends from the central and peripheral nervous systems to the targeted genital structures resulting in coordinated vascular and non-vascular smooth muscle relaxation, to be accompanied by pelvic vasocongestion, vaginal lubrication, and labial and clitoral engorgement. Any detrimental impact on this normal cycle of concerted responses can result in a functional impairment or 'female sexual dysfunction' (FSD) (4). Sexual changes, psychogenic or organic, are common in women at any age; such complaints are frequently accompanied by quality-of-life concerns, varying levels of personal distress, anxiety, depression, and also fertility concerns in younger women. To be diagnosed as a dysfunction, the American Psychiatric Association's *Diagnostic and Statistical Manual of Mental Disorders*, fifth edition (*DSM-5*) necessitates experiencing the disorder about 75–100% of the time (with exception for substance or medication-induced dysfunction), for a duration of approximately 6 months and having significant distress (5). With FSD as a medically diagnosable entity, fewer drugs have met the safety and efficacy criteria for global approval and clinical utility; this is in spite of relentless research efforts by pharmaceutical companies (4, 6, 7). That being so, in an obstetrics and gynaecology (OBGYN) setting, sexual health concerns may commonly surface during a personalized service delivery. In order to appreciate the diverse range of FSD and the extent of its physical, physiological, and psychological implications, it is important to understand the fundamentals as well as the changing paradigms in a woman's sexual functioning.

Essentials of female sexual function

The role of hormone status as the major determinant of women's sexual behaviour has been recognized. While the priming and conditioning of the brain to sexual cues is constituted and maintained by sex steroids, oestrogen and testosterone also facilitate an inherent neurochemical milieu conducive for a facilitated sexual response (8). In studies using animal models, oestrogen and progestin coordinated the proceptive and receptive behaviour; however, the mechanism by which testosterone reinforced the women's sexual function, which is otherwise essentially supported by the female hormones, is somewhat complex. Some scientific inferences are that testosterone may favourably help to modulate the peripheral levels of free oestradiol (E_2) through its preferential binding to sex hormone-binding globulin (SHBG) and/or increase the central/peripheral E_2 levels, which is enabled from its aromatization under the steroid pathway (8, 9).

For the depiction of the progress of sexual events in the female, several models were developed over the years to closely mimic the male sexual response cycle. Nevertheless, the necessary consensus for the transformation of a woman's sexual response is that there is an overriding influence of mind over the body. In the classical representation by Masters and Johnson, which was modified years later by Kaplan, the phases of sexual response progressed from initial excitement and desire, through the plateau and orgasm, to culminate in resolution (10, 11). The recognition of psychological and cognitive factors in the sexual trajectory and the multidimensional nature of the relational factors in women necessitated the inclusion of emotional intimacy into the creation of a circular model (12). Also, multiple physiological accompaniments are imperative for the individual phases of the sexual response, for instance, excitement and arousal generate vascular engorgement, transudation, and vaginal lubrication, albeit the continued excitement may sometimes follow through the remaining phases without a clear distinction. The emotion-centred intimacy in a partnered relationship also dictates the excitement and arousal required for sexual satisfaction and achievement of orgasmic pleasure (4). Similar to men, the suggested mechanism for sexual receptivity in women also includes inherent inclination determined by the feelings of desire, progressing to arousal and orgasm, even in the absence of adequate physical stimulation (13). For a synchronous and combined response, the areas of brain activation have been documented through investigations using functional magnetic resonance imaging (fMRI) at the time of desire and orgasmic responses. Similarly, genital MRI studies have made it possible to visualize the end-organ changes during the progression of an arousal response (9).

In view of the composite nature of a woman's sexual physiology, the desire and/or arousal leading to sexual satiety is not only specific but also variable at different time points. To understand the diversity of the central, peripheral, and genital modulations in the sexual response, it is important to appreciate the interrelated roles of a complex mechanism incorporating the endocrine and neurovascular inputs with the psycho-emotional controls in the limbic system. It is of note that the neocortex is specifically targeted through the sensory inputs (14). The neurochemicals that are differentially modulated in the process include monoamines (dopamine, norepinephrine (noradrenaline), or serotonin/5-hydroxytryptamine (5-HT)), hormone (oxytocin, vasopressin), and neurotropic factors. In the selective conditioning of the brain towards sexual cues, the neurochemical priming appears to facilitate an excitatory rather than an inhibitory response (15). Based on the available information, dopamine, norepinephrine, oxytocin, and melanocortin are involved in the central excitatory system while sexual inhibition is under the modulatory control of serotonin, prolactin, and endogenous opioids or endorphins. The consensus on the trophic effect of sex hormones in the genitals is also indirectly established via the impact of changed endocrine milieu during menopause. Likewise, in younger and premenopausal women, variability in the functional states will be in concert with the cyclical changes in sex steroids. Evidence points to the regulatory involvement of neurochemicals and mediators such as nitric oxide, vasoactive intestinal polypeptide, calcitonin gene-related peptide, substance P, cytokines, and factors at the cellular and molecular levels. The neural dynamics for these second messenger systems are inherent in the autonomic (adrenergic, cholinergic, and non-adrenergic, non-cholinergic) and somatic innervation; the specific sexual stimuli are relayed through the afferent pathways in the pudendal, pelvic, and hypogastric nerves (16). Broadly, to trace the sequence of events, sexual cues initiate sensory, autonomic, and central nervous system activation leading to a cascade of neuromuscular and vasocongestive responses at the end-organ level, both accentuated blood perfusion and transudation contributing to the vaginal lubrication. In the ensuing mechanism, the parasympathetic innervation (sacral anterior and pelvic nerves) sustains and maintains the blood flow, thereby increasing the volume of ultrafiltrate that percolates through the vaginal epithelial cells to coat the mucosal surface. Also, in the adjacent areas, favourable physio-anatomical changes (labial engorgement, trabecular and clitoral smooth muscle relaxation, and vasoperfusion) serve to reinforce the onset of a proactive genital arousal response. The sympathetic nervous system is activated in the final stages of arousal and orgasm to account for the elevated levels of systemic blood pressure and heart rate in women (15, 16). Studies using fMRI and positron emission tomography are also able to document the role of vagal innervation and activation during the orgasmic response in small clinical samples (17).

Genesis of female sexual disorders

Women's sexual problems are widespread, with an incidence variously reported in major studies to range from 25.8% to 91% (4). In a simplistic representation, any impairment of the normal sexual function could result in a form of sexual dysfunction or disorder. Nevertheless, FSD is often multifactorial since a wide number of organic, psychological, emotional, sociocultural, interpersonal, and intrapersonal factors have been causatively documented through systematic approaches. The resulting impairment may primarily affect the qualities of personal life with secondary impacts on the partner-related sexual satisfaction; any accompanying psychological and emotional distress can also impair normal aspects of daily living. In global studies, the psycho-emotional distress impacting quality of life accounted for approximately 22% in women presenting with any type of sexual difficulty. In an age-differentiated survey on the 'prevalence of female sexual problems associated with distress and determinants of treatment seeking' (PRESIDE), quality-of-life changes accounted for 8.9% in women aged 18–44 years, 12.3% in women aged 45–64 years, and 7.4% in women older than 65 years (18, 19). Furthermore, with a potential for negative health outcomes, the sexual disorder can be construed as a contributing factor for the economic burden within the healthcare system.

Epidemiology and classification

Important in the diagnosis of a woman's sexual disorder are a detailed sexual history and any objective measures which can be obtained through validated tools. Prior to the most recent classification by the *DSM-5*, the problems comprised four major categories, viz. disorders of desire, arousal, orgasm, and pain. Through the *DSM-5*, the main divisions of women's sexual dysfunction have been reduced to three groups with a merger of desire and arousal concerns into a unified sexual interest/arousal disorder. As for the pain category, which is including but not limited to vaginismus and dyspareunia, the combined terminology of genitopelvic pain/penetration disorder is a comprehensive description (5). Additionally, a range of stringent requirements are posed to ensure objectivity and to avoid any overdiagnosis of transient sexual problems. As mentioned earlier, they include an occurrence at more than 75% of the time, a minimum duration of 6 months (with an exception for substance or medication-induced disorders), variable levels of severity (mild, moderate, severe), and a criteria checklist for the reported difficulties (9). Based on the tenth revision of the International Statistical Classification of Diseases and Related Health Problems (ICD-10), the broad range of sexual disorders comprise organic and psychological aetiologies for changes in desire, aversion, absence of genital response, orgasmic dysfunction, vaginismus, dyspareunia, excessive sexual drive, other sexual dysfunction not caused by organic disorder or disease, and non-specific sexual dysfunction, not caused by organic disorder or disease (4, 9). That being so, under the umbrella of FSD are primary/secondary aetiologies; psychogenic, organic, or mixed factors; and lifelong/acquired and generalized/situational occurrences. Additionally, the presence (or absence) of significant personal distress is a key factor in order to clinically term a sexual complaint as a form of FSD. With these stringent requirements, the incidence of diagnosable and/or treatable disorder is likely to be lower; for instance, the prevalence of personal distress was 12–15% among 51.2% of women presenting with FSD in population-based surveys (5, 9, 19).

The various subtypes of sexual problems encompassed by the *DSM-5* have important implications in their differential diagnosis. A clinically common presentation in women, irrespective of age, is sexual desire disorder with or without changes in the arousal response. Notwithstanding a harmonious relationship with the partner, lack of desire may impinge on the sensitivity or receptiveness to sexual cues. Sometimes, absent or reduced sexual desire may be the cause or consequence of interpersonal factors in a relationship (7). Backed by large population data, a systematic survey confirmed the prominent role of central desire/arousal in women's sexual functioning. Lack of this essential psychodynamics may manifest in mood disorders and emotional cycles of anger, irritability, frustration, and reduced self-esteem (4, 5, 7).

As mentioned earlier, within the *DSM-5* classification, the hypoactive sexual desire disorder (HSDD) is combined with the female sexual arousal disorder (FSAD) to be diagnosed as a single entity of female sexual interest and arousal disorder (FSIAD), which is then differentiated into lifelong versus acquired and generalized versus situational subtypes compared to normally functional controls. In the absence or presence of a partnered relationship, the terminology also includes any lack of sexual fantasies leading to marked distress or interpersonal difficulty and the incidence of which is not accounted for by any medical, drug-related (prescription or recreational), psychiatric (e.g. depression), or other types of sexual condition (7). The critical point in combining arousal disorder together with changes in desire through the revised *DSM-5* stems from an overlap and limited distinction between the two phases in the cyclic, circular response. However, as a mixed or separate dysfunction, the incidence should be accompanied by a significant level of personal distress (9).

The desire impairment which includes HSDD is a persistent or recurrent lack or absence of sexual fantasies and interest in sexual activity. With a multitude of endogenous and extraneous factors in its causation, HSDD is often complex. Some of the predisposing, precipitating, and maintaining influences for HSDD are low androgen level, hyperprolactinaemia, medical comorbidities, ageing, relational factors, and lifestyle factors (7). Among the coexisting medical conditions, type 2 diabetes mellitus and hypertension and antihypertensive medications used in the treatment have been documented with decreased sexual desire. Concurrent presence of another sexual disorder such as dyspareunia may also secondarily impair desire/arousal. The intensity of sexual desire is a function of sex steroids, which includes oestrogens in women. Therefore, the menopausal transition with attendant vulvovaginal atrophy and dyspareunia would be a factor for declining sexual interest in this age group (20). Sexual problems are a common accompaniment of ageing per se, with a high reported incidence of loss of libido and personal distress in the elderly (2). Any psychiatric manifestation such as depression or anxiety and medications used in their treatment are also likely to adversely affect the desire. Phobic aversion is a variant of desire disorder with a psychological basis stemming from any past sexual abuse/trauma in childhood or puberty (7).

In evidence-based studies, impaired arousal response is correlated with decreased pelvic blood flow and genital lubrication, which is indeed a function of the oestrogen milieu. The empirical data include absence of subjective perceptions of tingling, warmth, and lubrication and objective descriptions of vaginal dryness and lack of genital sensations. In epidemiological studies, the incidence of FSAD ranged from 13% to 24%, increasing significantly with age beyond 50 years (21). Peaking levels of arousal are required for an orgasmic/pleasure perception.

The guidelines for the diagnosis of female orgasmic disorder include marked delay, diminished intensity, or complete lack of the pleasure sensation, in spite of a self-reported state of high sexual arousal/excitement. Orgasmic disorder is well recognized as a common condition with an estimated incidence and prevalence of 24–37% (22). Acquired or sudden-onset anorgasmia is often related to an organic aetiology whereas persistent psychosexual factors may predispose to a lifelong impairment (23).

Normal sexual function is compromised by any type of sexual pain disorder. Various degrees of pain are reported by sexually active women, either singly or in combination with other sexual complaints. The aetiopathogenic source for pain in the genitourinary syndrome of menopause (known earlier as vulvovaginal atrophy) is the underlying structural change; these include thinning of the vaginal epithelium, decrease in the superficial and intermediate cell layers, an increase in the parabasal cell content, and a less acidic vaginal pH (24). In studies, 14–18% of women in the age range of 18–59 years presented with genital pain and/or a penetration difficulty. The two main types of coital pain are distinguishable as dyspareunia, with an organic aetiology, or vaginismus, which is an involuntary retraction/contraction of the pelvic musculature during an attempted penetration (25). A non-coital type of sexual pain is reported by women with provoked vestibulodynia, with a modest prevalence of 8–12% among the vulvovaginal pain disorders. Typically, an acute pain reaction is precipitated in women with provoked vestibulodynia by nonsexual contacts such as gynaecological examination or tampon insertion (26). Studies show that pain disorders inevitably precipitate all other types of sexual problems such as impaired desire/arousal, orgasmic difficulty, and an overall reduction in the frequency of sexual activity or sexual satisfaction. Furthermore, the penetration disorders in women can negatively impact the male partner's sexual capability, with a consequent incidence of psychogenic erectile dysfunction (18, 25, 26).

With a few appropriate questions, the healthcare professional will be able to identify the true nature of the presenting complaint. While much of the evidence supports the role of ovarian sex steroids in the concerted promotion of sexual activity in women, orally administered oestrogens, most commonly used in hormonal contraceptives, have been linked to the incidence and prevalence of sexual disorders in younger women (27). The purported mechanism seems to correlate with elevated levels of SHBG, the transporter for sex hormones binding to testosterone, in view of its preferential affinity for SHBG (28). Nevertheless, the impact of hormonal contraceptives on sexual function is rather ill-defined and the extent of dysfunction remains unclear. While the scientific debate still continues to ascertain whether oestrogen or androgen is the prime modulator for female sexual function, sexual impairments are commonly encountered in women investigated for infertility or endometriosis. Female androgen insufficiency, included in the Princeton consensus, also denotes the existence of a clinical entity with symptoms of loss of desire or libido associated with low testosterone levels in women (8).

Within the OBGYN setting, maternal morbidity related to complications during pregnancy or childbirth is an overriding factor for detrimental changes in sexual health and quality of life (29); notwithstanding any attempts for sexual resumption, the resultant anatomical, physiological, and psychological implications may persist for variable lengths of time. Postpartum depression leading to emotional and sexual difficulties may be an important and often neglected obstetric complication in terms of addressing the couple's intimacy needs (30).

Together with ageing, the stages in the genesis of a sexual disorder in older women may not be easily deducible in view of a number of organic comorbidities impinging on psychological, interpersonal, and sociocultural factors. Studies have consistently demonstrated the gradual and age-related cessation of ovarian function in natural menopause to correlate with accentuated sexual impairment. Supportive evidence also comes from women who underwent bilateral oophorectomy (surgical menopause) for the near-abrupt decline in sexual function, in the context of a pronounced drop in sex steroids (8, 31). The hormonal deficiency state also results in a host of underlying structural and functional changes in the genital organs that reinforce the perceived sexual difficulties. In this predicament, the steroid deprivation has a multisystemic effect, impacting the ageing and physical debility to decrease the qualitative and quantitative measures of sexual health and well-being (8).

Some studies also sought to decipher the association of demographic characteristics, including education and income parity with the woman's sexual activity; while desire disorder was prevalent at mid- and high-income states, other forms of sexual dysfunction were also commonly identified in women from the lower socioeconomic strata or educational levels (32). Furthermore, literature evidence abounds about the association of medical comorbidity with sexual dysfunction in women across all ages (20). Coexisting lower urinary tract symptoms have been shown to interfere with the sexual function to result in desire/arousal disorder, orgasmic problems, and coital as well as non-coital types of genital pain. Incidences of urinary incontinence during intercourse (61.9%) or orgasm (31.7%) also negatively impacted partnered sexual activity and satisfaction (4, 25). Similarly, patients with uterine fibroids or prolapse experienced sexual dissatisfaction. Higher incidences of dysfunction and sexual impairments were accounted for by survivors of gynaecological and genitourinary tumours; likewise, breast cancer is a major risk factor for multiple disorders related to desire/arousal, orgasm and sexual satisfaction (33, 34). Sexual dysfunction frequently coexists with chronic medical conditions such as coronary artery disease, thyroid problems, spinal injury, multiple sclerosis, rheumatoid arthritis, or ankylosing spondylitis (2, 4, 20). Studies variously report the clinical prevalence of sexual impairment in diabetic women as 25–71%. Type 2 diabetes mellitus may contribute to the evident dysfunction through sensory, autonomic neuropathy, vascular insufficiency arising from micro- or macro-angiopathy, and other associated psychogenic factors. Similarly, in women with type 1 diabetes, there was a significant reduction in most domains of sexual function attributable to disease-related metabolic and neurovascular derangements (20, 35). This highlights the importance of physical health for satisfactory sexual well-being and quality of living for women in any age group.

Evaluation, assessment, and diagnosis

For a comprehensive assessment of the presenting sexual complaints, the healthcare providers should attempt to elicit a detailed account of the past, recent, and present sexual history. To break the ice, it may be helpful to include a brief checklist for the sexual concerns within the OBGYN health review (**Table 60.1**). Although about a third of women with distressing sexual concerns are likely to seek professional help, embarrassment may preclude discussion in the rest and a majority also reportedly wait for the healthcare professional to initiate the discussion (1). In the literature, an open dialogue by the health worker minimized stigma and normalized the importance of sexual health while increasing the probability of sharing the delicate sexual history. In conservative societies, women may regard the confines of the OBGYN office as a safe haven for frank disclosure and treatment seeking (6). All these findings reiterate the need for having professionals who are comfortable in initiating these discussions.

Important within the complexity of diagnosing the specific sexual dysfunction is a comprehensive assessment for any coexistent organic or medical condition through relevant screening history. That notwithstanding, a number of psychological, sociocultural, interpersonal factors as also the partner's general and sexual health and relationship difficulties require specific assessment, prior to making a provisional diagnosis. Essentially, the different forms of sexual disorders are distinguishable through a detailed sexual history. Some pertinent information on the type of sexual dysfunction may evolve from the nature of sexual behaviour, safe sex practices, or partner's relationship issues (36) and therefore, the history needs to be viewed as an essential part of the diagnostic algorithm. Albeit difficult in a busy clinical setting, the history should be tailored to help determine the true underlying cause and the level of personal impact of the disorder. Open-ended questions are sometimes vital to gain adequate information; in a patient-centred approach and through rapport creation, the next or follow-up visits may also provide cumulative history for arriving at a diagnosis.

Also in this context, a number of symptom scales or screening tools have been developed over the years and validated through studies to help the clinicians in identifying and differentially diagnosing women's sexual disorders. These instruments are useful to assess the changes in normal functional level and to determine the progress with any administered therapy. Screening tools are routinely used in clinical and academic research as important outcome measures for the qualitative and quantitative impacts. One of

Table 60.1 Female sexual dysfunction: a short screening questionnaire as a reference guide in the initial workup

No.	Question	Yes	No
1	Do you experience interest for sexual activity?		
2	Are you aroused by the foreplay?		
3	Do you normally have adequate lubrication?		
4	Do you ever 'freeze up', making penetration impossible?		
5	Do you generally have orgasm during sex?		
6	Is intercourse always pain-free?		
7	Are you satisfied with your sexual quality of life?		

the earliest examples is the Female Sexual Function Index (FSFI), a self-reporting reference tool of 19 items, used in clinical trials to provide point scores for major sexual domains, viz. desire, arousal, lubrication, orgasm, and sexual satisfaction and it also includes assessment for pain (37). Thus, valuable information can be gathered from detailed medical and OBGYN history, clinical data on physical and psychological health status, and reports from laboratory investigations for any undefined hormonal imbalance, in the systematic process of evaluation, assessment, and diagnosis of FSD.

In summary, the key points in the management algorithm of a woman's sexual problem include a comprehensive medical, sexual, psychological, and sociocultural history, any psychiatric condition such as depression or anxiety, as well as the prescription medication(s) taken for coexistent clinical disorders. Oral contraceptive use needs to be queried for its possible impact on desire/arousal. A physical examination is imperative in cases of genitopelvic/penetration disorders, pelvic trauma, or history suggestive of herpes or lichen sclerosus. Menopausal evidence of vulvovaginal atrophy may cause an effect in dyspareunia, with negative impacts on sexual desire. Independent of age, a detailed genital health assessment will rule out sensory changes of vulval vestibulitis or provoked vulvodynia, involuntary pelvic floor muscle contraction, or pelvic organ prolapse. Since sex steroid hormones are critical for the structural and functional integrity, laboratory investigation for their circulating levels may be sometimes indicated, guided by specific history and/or physical findings. Of equal relevance is the measurement of prolactin levels or thyroid function tests in women with clinical evidence of hyperprolactinaemia or thyroid disease states. In as much as the importance of organic factors is felt in the expression of sexual impairments, women with chronic diseases need to be assessed for the potential impact of the disease process on their sexual health and life quality (4). Conforming to clinical data, in patients with cancer and receiving treatment, the incidence of FSD can be up to 90% after chemotherapy, 9% following surgical intervention, and 3% after radiotherapy (31). Furthermore, premature precipitation of menopause secondary to such therapies can drastically impair the sexual function through multiple mechanisms. Decreased sexual desire/arousal is to be anticipated if the interventions impair sensations in the breast or clitoris. In addition to altered body image, other factors that play an important role in reducing or eliminating sexual interest would include fatigue, debility, and family or relationship demands.

Treatment options: hormonal, non-hormonal, and others

While a number of treatment options are available for male sexual problems, FSD still remains an incompletely managed clinical condition, awaiting the advent of safe and efficacious therapies (38). That being so, the multifactorial dimension of women's sexual disorders also warrants an integrated approach encompassing biopsychosocial within possible pharmacological therapies, subsequent to a detailed diagnostic workup (Table 60.2). In a generic sense, psychosexual education through empowerment and knowledge to improve an understanding of the basic reproductive anatomy, physiology, and aetiopathology forms the essential first step. At this time point, it would be beneficial to make attempts to eliminate any misguided

information or myths, which may be negatively impacting the sexual behaviour. To have a significant sexual outcome, any underlying interpersonal or relationship issues need to be addressed and managed carefully. These measures can be combined with important lifestyle-modifying behaviours of diet, exercise, and control over day-to-day stress and substance use, if any (4, 32).

Systemic hormone therapy is considered in two forms, viz. oestrogen and progesterone for women with an intact uterus or oestrogen alone for those without; the hormone therapy is preferential, used with caution, only in the absence of contraindications and customized to suit individual's needs. Local or vaginal oestrogen as a cream, gel, tablet, or ring is thought of as an equally effective and safer alternative to systemic hormone. However, it must be remembered that, albeit small, variable increases in serum E_2 levels have been reported in studies following local applications. Nevertheless, local hormones have specific usefulness in addressing the clinical signs and symptoms of menopausal genitourinary syndrome (39). Ospemifene, as an oestrogen agonist/antagonist (selective oestrogen receptor modulator/SERM) and approved (by the United States Food and Drug Administration (FDA)) agent for moderate to severe dyspareunia is useful in postmenopausal women. In double-blind, placebo-controlled studies, the vulvovaginal atrophy reversal was founded by an increase in superficial cell content and decreases in parabasal cells and vaginal pH. These functionally relevant improvements in vaginal atrophy not only addressed the genital signs and symptoms but also translated into significant recovery for the other domains in sexual function. Available clinical evidence from short-term follow-up studies thus far is supportive of its safety profile on breast and endometrium, in the absence of changes leading to hyperplasia or uterine bleeding (40). Another agent that may be considered in the treatment of postmenopausal women with vaginal atrophy, dyspareunia, and secondary HSDD is tibolone (41). It is a synthetic hormonal prodrug with oestrogenic and androgenic effects in the body; it is approved and available in many countries and is credited with beneficial effects for loss of libido and overall sexual function.

Apart from those mentioned, several others have been tried as non-specific and off-label drugs in the treatment of women's sexual disorders. Most theories on the purported efficacy of dehydroepiandrosterone (DHEA) are based on its role as a precursor for sex steroids and their actions after conversion in the body. Thus, the potential sequelae of DHEA administration in postmenopausal women would include improvements in sexual desire/arousal on one hand and general well-being on the other. Although data from randomized controlled studies are not forthcoming with the necessary information for its safety and efficacy, a local, intravaginal application of 0.50% DHEA for 12 weeks provided statistically significant improvement in the co-primary parameters of vulvovaginal atrophy in a clinical study (42).

Normally, testosterone is essential in women not only as a major precursor in the oestrogenic steroid pathway but also by virtue of its own androgen receptor-mediated effects in the body. Literature evidence points to an improvement in a number of satisfying sexual events (and concomitant reduction in personal distress) through studies investigating testosterone implants, oral methyl testosterone, or transdermal testosterone. While the transdermal patch is used by surgically menopausal women in some countries for their HSDD, a pharmaceutical attempt to test the efficacy of testosterone gel for

Table 60.2 Female sexual dysfunction: information at a glance

Type of sexual disorder	DSM-5 criteria	Options: approved/off-label/trial/others	Mode of action
Female sexual interest/arousal disorder	Manifested by three of the following: 1. Absent or reduced sexual interest 2. Absent or reduced sexual or erotic thoughts or fantasies 3. No or reduced initiation of sexual activity and unreceptive to partner's attempts to initiate 4. Absent or reduced sexual excitement or pleasure during sexual activity in almost all or all (75–100%) sexual encounters 5. Absent or reduced sexual interest or arousal in response to any internal or external sexual or erotic cues (written, verbal, or visual) 6. Absent or reduced genital or non-genital sensations during sexual activity in almost all or all (75–100%) sexual encounters	Flibanserin	5-HT_{1A} agonist and 5-HT_{2A} antagonist
		Tibolone	Selective tissue oestrogenic activity regulator
		Testosterone	Hormone
		Testosterone + oestrogen	Hormone
		Testosterone + sildenafil	Hormone + PDE5 inhibitor
		Testosterone + buspirone	Hormone + 5-HT_{1A} receptor partial agonist
		DHEA	Hormone precursor
		Bremelanotide	Melanocortin receptor 3,4 agonist
		Bupropion	Dopamine agonist
		PGE1 topical	Direct action through cAMP
Female orgasmic disorder	Presence of either of the following on all or almost all (75–100%) occasions of sexual activity: 1. Marked delay in, marked infrequency of, or absence of orgasm 2. Markedly reduced intensity of orgasmic sensations	Oxytocin	Hormone
		Clitoral vacuum device	External device
		Vibrators and self-stimulators	External device
Genitopelvic pain or penetration disorder	Persistent or recurrent difficulties with one or more of the following: 1. Vaginal penetration during intercourse 2. Marked vulvovaginal or pelvic pain during intercourse or penetration attempts 3. Marked fear or anxiety about vulvovaginal or pelvic pain in anticipation of, during, or because of vaginal penetration 4. Marked tensing or tightening of pelvic floor muscles during attempted vaginal penetration	Oestrogen	Local/systemic hormone
		Oestrogen + progesterone	Hormone
		Oestrogen + testosterone	Hormone
		Ospemifene	Selective oestrogen receptor modulator
		Lignocaine	Local anaesthetic agent
		SSRIs/SNRIs/tricyclic drugs	Serotonergic, antidepressant drugs
		Dilators	Mechanical device
		Vaginal moisturizers and lubricants	Topical restoration
		Vestibulectomy	Surgical option
		Pelvic floor muscle exercises	Physical therapy

SNRIs, serotonin and norepinephrine reuptake inhibitors; SSRIs, selective serotonin reuptake inhibitors.

Source data from Kingsberg SA, Woodard T. Female sexual dysfunction: focus on low desire. *Obstet Gynecol* 2015 Feb;125(2):477–86, Nappi RE, Cucinella L. Advances in pharmacotherapy for treating female sexual dysfunction. *Expert Opin Pharmacother* 2015 Apr;16(6):875–87, and Basson R. Pharmacotherapy for women's sexual dysfunction. *Expert Opin Pharmacother* 2009 Jul;10(10):1631–48.

women was withdrawn at the level of phase III clinical studies. If testosterone is thought of as an off-label option for postmenopausal sexual complaints, due caution for its systemic liabilities especially changes to liver function and breast cancer potential and warnings for virilizing effects viz. acne, hirsutism, voice deepening, and androgenic alopecia need to be in place (8, 13). Lately, studies are ongoing with synergistic combinations of sublingual testosterone with either a phosphodiesterase type 5 (PDE5) inhibitor or a 5-HT_{1A} receptor partial agonist. The former combination is envisaged to improve sensitivity and responsiveness to sexual stimuli while the latter is aimed to overcome any excessive sexual inhibition. Researchers have demonstrated significant improvements in the subjective and objective measures of sexual response in women undergoing these trials and the combinations show unique promise as targeted approaches for the selective types of sexual disorders (43).

Flibanserin is a novel non-hormonal therapy for HSDD; it is a 5-HT_{1A} agonist and 5-HT_{2A} antagonist, with moderate affinity also towards 5-HT_{2B}, 5-HT_{2C}, and dopamine D_4 receptors, which was initially developed as an antidepressant (44). The recognition that flibanserin inhibited the serotoninergic antisexual influence

and concurrently enhanced the dopaminergic prosexual response was the exploited mechanism for its clinical efficacy in HSDD. In large, randomized cohort studies flibanserin significantly increased the number of satisfying sexual events, also particularly in the context of desire, compared to placebo. In approximately less than 10%, nausea, dizziness, fatigue, and somnolence were noted as adverse events related to treatment; any serious hypotension or syncope was precipitated by concurrent alcohol intake. Currently, flibanserin is the only FDA-approved treatment for premenopausal HSDD and clinical trials evaluating its safety and efficacy in postmenopausal HSDD are ongoing (45, 46).

Another centrally acting antidepressant agent, bupropion, which is a combined dopamine, norepinephrine reuptake inhibitor, is also thought to contribute to significant improvements in the key outcome measures of HSDD when tried off-label. Its efficacy is somewhat similar to that of trazodone, which shares its 5-HT receptor antagonism with reuptake inhibition. In the initial years of drug development, clinical studies using the direct-acting dopamine agonist, apomorphine, in the management of desire/arousal disorder yielded variable data on efficacy and tolerability. More recently, bremelanotide, a synthetic agonist of melanocortin 3 and 4 receptors, improved central desire/arousal parameters in controlled studies, with some promise for a therapeutic effect in the combined FSIAD in women (43, 47). In the available literature, the role of PDE5 inhibitors including sildenafil is appreciated only in selective cohorts of organic FSD viz. type 1 diabetes mellitus, spinal cord injury, or multiple sclerosis while in a vast majority of the remaining FSD aetiology, their efficacy was discounted (48). As for the other vasoactive drugs tested, both phentolamine mesylate, an alpha adrenergic agonist, and prostaglandin E_1 failed to provide consistent data for their efficacy in the treatment of FSAD. Several ongoing studies are evaluating the potential efficacy of oxytocin neuropeptide in improving the specific outcome measures for arousal and orgasm, with sufficient preliminary evidence to stimulate further investigation (43).

A significant gap in scientific knowledge exists for the usefulness of nutritional or herbal supplements such as red clover to treat sexual disorders in women (49). Similarly, the only surgical option which is vestibulectomy, removal of painful tissues from the vestibule to treat vulval vestibulitis, has mixed clinical outcomes for patient satisfaction scores (50). Lastly, the drug-induced FSD is an established clinical entity which can benefit from a reduced dosage of the offending agent, change to medications without sexual side effects, or even a brief drug holiday.

Barriers and goals in clinical management

Gynaecologists play a key role in the initial assessment and management of FSD as immediate carers of women's reproductive health. Although measures are available to diagnose and treat the varied types of sexual disorders in women, some specific dimensions such as abuse, violence, trauma, or any associated psychological or psychiatric manifestations may pose considerable challenges, with impacts on patient-related clinical outcomes. At times, the key issues may also stem from unresolved interpersonal factors or partner's sexual dysfunction or the disorder may even be lifelong, necessitating expert referrals. While some traditional or conservative societies preclude masturbation as a form of sexual function, most other cultures often regard a partnered sexual activity to represent emotional well-being and quality of life. Therefore, psychosexual education together with couple counselling may benefit women who are refractory to other management approaches (51). Empirical evidence supports the importance of psychosexual therapy in circumventing the barriers to improve a woman's response to standard interventions, with far-reaching benefits towards couple's sexual health. As mentioned earlier, specific cognitive, behavioural, and lifestyle changes also effectively superimpose on conventional interventions to overcome other obstacles encountered in the process.

Future perspectives in women's sexual healthcare

There are a number of clinical challenges and unmet needs representing women's sexual concerns, essentially due to the multidimensional complexity and minimal availability of therapeutic options.

In contrast to the sexual disorders in males, women's sexual concerns and levels of personal distress are significantly influenced by psycho-emotional factors and major life events and therefore, often no single therapeutic option may suffice. In our attempts to reverse a distressing problem, it is likely that we will encounter difficulties in establishing the clear demarcation among the organic parameters, biopsychosocial triggers, and the evaluated measures of sexual disorders. Nonetheless, healthcare professionals have the duty to look for, identify, and address any and all predisposing, precipitating, and maintaining factors within the holistic context of FSD management. There is no doubt that prospective research and clinical trials are ongoing worldwide to find novel and efficacious treatment options for FSD. Given the overriding modulations by intra- and interpersonal variables, large cohort studies to interpret the cause and effect of changing aspects of life on sexual function in its greater details may be useful to the scientific and clinical community. As in any other medical discipline, identifying and developing preventive measures, including evidence-based education and behavioural approaches to preserve the psychorelational harmony, will be beneficial for a generic sexual well-being.

Conclusion

There are many facets to sexuality in a woman's life and change within normal function or the incidence of a dysfunction has its impact on sexual dynamics at multiple levels. The currently used norm, that is, the presence of personal distress or lack thereof, is a limited indicator of the sexual well-being. Although the importance of an accurate measurement of personal suffering or concern from the disorder is well conceived, the subjective nature of the distress as a symptom and its overlap with individual variations may pose significant challenges. Also, the fundamentals to a woman's involvement in sexual intimacy are complex which includes not only the rewards from the union but also any valid reasons for the avoidance. Therefore, the ultimate goal of healthcare professionals is to deal with the individualistic differences in the patient-centred context while also attempting to fulfil her expectations for an empathetic understanding and management of the presented concerns.

REFERENCES

1. Thackar R. Female sexual dysfunction is an artificial concept driven by commercial interests: against: FSD is a real and complex problem. *BJOG* 2015;**122**:1419.
2. Bruni C, Raja J, Denton CP, Matucci-Cerinic M. The clinical relevance of sexual dysfunction in systemic sclerosis. *Autoimmun Rev* 2015;**14**:1111–115.
3. Wallwiener CW, Wallwiener LM, Seeger H, et al. Are hormonal components of oral contraceptives associated with impaired female sexual function? A questionnaire-based online survey of medical students in Germany, Austria, and Switzerland. *Arch Gynecol Obstet* 2015;**292**:883–90.
4. Khajehei M, Doherty M, Tilley PJ. An update on sexual function and dysfunction in women. *Arch Womens Ment Health* 2015;**18**:423–33.
5. Latif EF, Diamond MP. Arriving at the diagnosis of female sexual dysfunction. *Fertil Steril* 2013;**100**:898–904.

6. Ozaki Y, Nagao K, Saigo R, et al. Sexual problems among Japanese women: data from an online helpline. *Sex Med* 2015 **3**;3:295–301.

7. Kingsberg SA, Woodard T. Female sexual dysfunction: focus on low desire. *Obstet Gynecol* 2015;**125**:477–86.

8. Cappelletti M, Wallen K. Increasing women's sexual desire: the comparative effectiveness of estrogens and androgens. *Horm Behav* 2016;**78**:178–93.

9. Nappi RE, Cucinella L. Advances in pharmacotherapy for treating female sexual dysfunction. *Expert Opin Pharmacother* 2015;**16**:875–87.

10. Masters WH, Johnson VE (eds). *Human Sexual Inadequacy*. Boston, MA: Little Brown; 1970.

11. Kaplan HS (ed). *The New Sex Therapy*. New York: Brunner/Mazel; 1974.

12. Basson R. The female sexual response: a different model. *J Sex Marital Ther* 2000;**26**:51–65.

13. Worsley R, Santoro N, Miller KK, Parish SJ, Davis SR. Hormones and female sexual dysfunction: beyond estrogens and androgens-findings from the fourth International consultation on sexual medicine. *J Sex Med* 2016;**13**:283–90.

14. Bakker J, Brock O. Early oestrogens in shaping reproductive networks: evidence for a potential organisational role of oestradiol in female brain development. *J Neuroendocrinol* 2010;**22**: 728–35.

15. Salonia A, Giraldi A, Chivers ML, et al. Physiology of women's sexual function: basic knowledge and new findings. *J Sex Med* 2010;**7**:2637–660.

16. Graziottin A, Gambini D. Anatomy and physiology of genital organs—women. *Handb Clin Neurol* 2015;**130**:39–60.

17. Komisaruk BR, Whipple B. Functional MRI of the brain during orgasm in women. *Annu Rev Sex Res* 2005;**16**:62–86.

18. Johannes CB, Clayton AH, Odom DM, et al. Distressing sexual problems in United States women revisited: prevalence after accounting for depression. *J Clin Psychiatry* 2009;**70**:1698–706.

19. Mitchell KR, Mercer CH, Ploubidis GB, et al. Sexual function in Britain: findings from the third National Survey of Sexual Attitudes and Lifestyles (Natsal-3). *Lancet* 2013;**382**:1817–29.

20. Valadares AL, Lui-Filho JF, Costa-Paiva L, Pinto-Neto AM. Middle-aged female sexual dysfunction and multimorbidity: a population-based study. *Menopause* 2016;**23**:304–10.

21. Faubion SS, Rullo JE. Sexual dysfunction in women: a practical approach. *Am Fam Physician* 2015;**92**:281–88.

22. Meston CM, Levin RJ, Sipski ML, Hull EM, Heiman JR. Women's orgasm. *Annu Rev Sex Res* 2004;**15**:173–257.

23. Pyke RE, Clayton A. Models vs. Realities in female sexual dysfunction. *J Sex Med* 2015;**12**:1977–78.

24. Portman DJ, Gass ML, Vulvovaginal Atrophy Terminology Consensus Conference Panel. Genitourinary syndrome of menopause: new terminology for vulvovaginal atrophy from the International Society for the Study of Women's Sexual Health and the North American Menopause Society. *J Sex Med* 2014;**11**:2865–72.

25. Wright JJ, O'Connor KM. Female sexual dysfunction. *Med Clin North Am* 2015;**99**:607–28.

26. Boerner KE, Rosen NO. Acceptance of vulvovaginal pain in women with provoked vestibulodynia and their partners: associations with pain, psychological, and sexual adjustment. *J Sex Med* 2015;**12**:1450–62.

27. Wallwiener CW, Wallwiener LM, Seeger H, Mück AO, Bitzer J, Wallwiener M. Prevalence of sexual dysfunction and impact of contraception in female German medical students. *J Sex Med* 2010;**7**:2139–48.

28. Panzer C, Wise S, Fantini G, et al. Impact of oral contraceptives on sex hormone-binding globulin and androgen levels: a retrospective study in women with sexual dysfunction. *J Sex Med* 2006;**3**:104–13.

29. Andreucci CB, Bussadori JC, Pacagnella RC, et al. Sexual life and dysfunction after maternal morbidity: a systematic review. *BMC Pregnancy Childbirth* 2015;**15**:307.

30. Fehniger JE, Brown JS, Creasman JM, et al. Childbirth and female sexual function later in life. *Obstet Gynecol* 2013;**122**:988–97.

31. Lindau ST, Coady D, Kushner D. Female sexual dysfunction: focus on low desire. *Obstet Gynecol* 2015;**125**:1495–96.

32. Stephenson KR, Meston CM. Differentiating components of sexual well-being in women: are sexual satisfaction and sexual distress independent constructs? *J Sex Med* 2010;**7**:2458–68. [Erratum in: *J Sex Med* 2010;**7**:3803.]

33. Boswell EN, Dizon DS. Breast cancer and sexual function. *Transl Androl Urol* 2015;**4**:160–68.

34. Jensen PT, Froeding LP. Pelvic radiotherapy and sexual function in women. *Transl Androl Urol* 2015;**4**:186–205.

35. Bjerggaard M, Charles M, Kristensen E, Lauritzen T, Sandbæk A, Giraldi A. Prevalence of sexual concerns and sexual dysfunction among sexually active and inactive men and women with screen-detected Type 2 diabetes. *Sex Med* 2015;**3**:302–10.

36. Rosen RC, Heiman JR, Long JS, Fisher WA, Sand MS. Men with sexual problems and their partners: findings from the International survey of relationships. *Arch Sex Behav* 2016;**45**:159–73.

37. Wiegel M, Meston C, Rosen R. The female sexual function index (FSFI): cross-validation and development of clinical cutoff scores. *J Sex Marital Ther* 2005;**31**:1–20.

38. Basson R. Pharmacotherapy for women's sexual dysfunction. *Expert Opin Pharmacother* 2009;**10**:1631–48.

39. Santoro N, Worsley R, Miller KK, Parish SJ, Davis SR. Role of estrogens and estrogen-like compounds in female sexual function and dysfunction. *J Sex Med* 2016;**13**:305–16.

40. Constantine G, Graham S, Portman DJ, Rosen RC, Kingsberg SA. Female sexual function improved with ospemifene in postmenopausal women with vulvar and vaginal atrophy: results of a randomized, placebo-controlled trial. *Climacteric* 2015;**18**:226–32.

41. Palacios S, Mejias A. An update on drugs for the treatment of menopausal symptoms. *Expert Opin Pharmacother* 2015;**16**:2437–47.

42. Labrie F, Archer DF, Koltun W, et al. Efficacy of intravaginal dehydroepiandrosterone (DHEA) on moderate to severe dyspareunia and vaginal dryness, symptoms of vulvovaginal atrophy, and of the genitourinary syndrome of menopause. *Menopause* 2016;**23**:243–56.

43. Belkin ZR, Krapf JM, Goldstein AT. Drugs in early clinical development for the treatment of female sexual dysfunction. *Expert Opin Investig Drugs* 2015;**24**:159–67.

44. Robinson K, Cutler JB, Carris NW. First pharmacological therapy for hypoactive sexual desire disorder in premenopausal women: flibanserin. *Ann Pharmacother* 2016;**50**:125–32.

45. Mullard A. FDA approves female sexual dysfunction drug. *Nat Rev Drug Discov* 2015;**14**:669.

46. Dhanuka I, Simon JA. Flibanserin for the treatment of hypoactive sexual desire disorder in premenopausal women. *Expert Opin Pharmacother* 2015;**16**:2523–29.

47. Kingsberg SA, Clayton AH, Pfaus JG. The female sexual response: current models, neurobiological underpinnings and agents currently approved or under investigation for the treatment of hypoactive sexual desire disorder. *CNS Drugs* 2015;**29**:915–33.

48. Gao L, Yang L, Qian S, Li T, Han P, Yuan J. Systematic review and meta-analysis of phosphodiesterase type 5 inhibitors for the treatment of female sexual dysfunction. *Int J Gynaecol Obstet* 2016;**133**:139–45.

49. Adaikan PG, Srilatha B, Wheat AJ. Efficacy of red clover isoflavones in the menopausal rabbit model. *Fertil Steril* 2009;**92**:2008–13.

50. Swanson CL, Rueter JA, Olson JE, Weaver AL, Stanhope CR. Localized provoked vestibulodynia: outcomes after modified vestibulectomy. *J Reprod Med* 2014;**59**:121–26.

51. Srilatha B, Huang Z, Adaikan PG. Sexual activity in midlife women and beyond. *JAMA Intern Med* 2014;**174**:1204–205.

SECTION 12
Gynaecological Oncology

61

Cancer screening and prevention in gynaecology

Lynette Denny and Rengaswamy Sankaranarayan

Introduction

In 1968, the World Health Organization (WHO) published guidelines on the principles and practice of screening for disease, which are often referred to as the 'Wilson and Jungner criteria' (1). These principles are still applicable today (**Box 61.1**).

To quote Wilson and Jungner, 'the central idea of early disease detection and treatment is essentially simple. However, the path to its successful achievement (on the one hand, bringing to treatment those with previously undetected disease, and, on the other, avoiding harm to those persons not in need of treatment) is far from simple, though sometimes it may appear to be deceptively easy'. With the onset of genetic screening, new controversies around screening emerged and in 2008, Andermann et al. (2) synthesized and modified the Wilson criteria (**Box 61.2**).

Screening is a systematic attempt to select those who are at high risk of a specific disease from among apparently healthy individuals (3). The ultimate aim of screening is prevention of disease or to detect disease at an early, curable stage. There are many controversies about screening for cancer, such as the use of prostatic-specific antigen screening for prostate cancer, mammography screening for breast cancer, and debates around current screening for colorectal, lung, and cervical cancers (4).

Various types of screening are described which include the following:

1. Organized mass (population-based) screening: this involves screening of a whole population or a subgroup. It is offered to all, irrespective of the risk status of the individual, with everyone taking part offered the same services, information, and support. The inputs are quality assured and the outcomes are continuously monitored and evaluated (typical of cervical cancer screening programmes in Nordic countries, Netherlands, and the United Kingdom).
2. Opportunistic (sporadic) population screening: refers to health practitioners offering screening tests to those consulting for some other purpose or screening provided in response to request by subjects.
3. High-risk or selective screening among specific populations (e.g. young women with ovarian cancer for *BRCA1* and *BRCA2* gene mutations).
4. Multiphasic screening involves routine use of multiple tests on the same occasion in population screening programmes for the purpose of detecting a disease in preventable or curable stages (e.g. co-testing with cytology and human papillomavirus (HPV) testing for cervical cancer).

Controversies exist with regard to the level of evidence required before screening for a disease is initiated. Even if there is a high level of evidence for efficacy and effectiveness, how the programme should be implemented needs careful consideration, particularly a clear understanding of benefits versus harms, potential or actual. In some countries, mass population screening programmes are implemented and in others, screening is dependent on access to health insurance (5). Screening organized by a healthcare system, as occurs in the United Kingdom, includes personal invitations to screening for eligible individuals and a structured organization for invitation, intervention, and management of screen detected disease, clinical surveillance, and quality assurance—generally known as population-based screening programmes (4). Opportunistic screening usually only refers to a specifically identified group (i.e. people visiting their general practitioners or local pharmacies) and in general is less effective than population-based programmes which are able to achieve a much wider coverage of the target population.

Screening is controversial largely because benefits versus harms are not always clearly defined, there are often vested interests (e.g. fee for service) making screening a business, and the public may be left confused and at the mercy of often untested and biased information (6).

Screening and prevention in gynaecology

Cervical cancer

With this background in mind, this chapter will explore past and current screening activities among women for early detection and prevention of gynaecological cancers, beginning with cervical cancer. There is a well-characterized and strong association between cervical cancer incidence and level of societal development. Approximately 86% of incident cancers and 88% of deaths from cervical cancer are estimated to occur in less developed regions of the world (7). The high incidence of cervical cancer among less educated and socioeconomically disadvantaged women is well documented (8, 9).

Cervical cancer screening and early detection

Cervical cytology testing involves collecting exfoliated cells from the cervix and examining these cells microscopically. The concept of utilizing exfoliated cells to identify women with invasive cervical cancer was introduced by Papanicolaou and Babes in the 1920s (10). Subsequently, Papanicolaou refined his technique and in 1941 he published on the use of conventional cytology to identify invasive cervical cancers and in 1954 published on how to identify and classify cervical cancer precursors (11). In the first paragraph of the

1941 article, the authors comment: 'The death rate from carcinoma of the female genital tract is approximately 32,000 per year in the United States and of this figure, four-fifths or 26,000 deaths may be said to be due to cancer of the uterus. This rate has remained practically constant during the past twenty five years'. What is interesting is that in 2016, the situation in many developing countries is not very different from that in the United States more than 70 years ago. Even in 1941 it was noted that early diagnosis and treatment yielded 'a high percentage of cures in both carcinoma of the fundus and of the cervix'. It was not, however, until the 1960s that cervical cytology began to be used widely in many developed countries as a tool for cervical cancer prevention.

Papanicolaou classified cervical cytology findings into five categories, classes I–V, and focused on how closely the cells resembled truly malignant cells (Table 61.1).

Prior to the implementation of large cervical cytology-based programmes in British Columbia, Canada, and Europe in the 1950s and 1960s, no randomized trials were performed to evaluate the impact of cervical cancer screening on cervical cancer incidence and mortality and all data on the effect of screening came from observational studies. However, the marked reduction in the incidence of and mortality from cervical cancer before and after the introduction of screening programmes in a variety of developed countries was interpreted as strong non-experimental support for organized cervical cancer screening programmes.

The International Agency for Research on Cancer (IARC) conducted a comprehensive analysis of data from several of the largest screening programmes in the world in 1986 and showed that well-organized screening programmes were effective in reducing the incidence of and mortality from cervical cancer (13). In the Nordic countries, following the introduction of nationwide screening in the 1960s, cumulative mortality rates of cervical cancer demonstrated a significant decreasing trend. The greatest decrease was in Iceland (84% from 1965 to 1982) where the screening interval was the shortest and the target age range the widest. The smallest reduction in cumulative mortality (11%) was in Norway where only 5% of the population had been part of organized screening programmes (14). The decreases in Finland, Sweden, and Denmark were 50%, 34%, and 27% respectively. The highest reduction in cervical cancer incidence was in the 30–49-year age group where the focus of screening was the most intense.

In addition, the association between mortality trends and the extent of coverage of the population by organized screening was most pronounced when the proportional reductions in the age-specific rates were related to the target ages of the screening programmes

Table 61.1 Classification of cervical cytology

Class	Description
I	Absence of atypical or abnormal cells
II	Atypical cytology, but no evidence for malignancy
III	Cytology suggestive of, but not conclusive for, malignancy
IV	Cytology strongly suggestive of malignancy
V	Cytology conclusive for malignancy

Source data from Papanicolaou GN. *Atlas of Exfoliative Cytology.* Boston, MA: Commonwealth Fund University Press; 1954.

(15). The age-specific trends indicated that the *target age range* of a screening programme was a more important determinant of risk reduction than the *frequency* of screening within the defined age range. This finding was in agreement with the estimates of the IARC working group, that for interscreen intervals of up to 5 years, the protective effect of organized screening was high throughout the targeted age group (>80%) (16).

It is apparent therefore that the extent to which screening programmes have succeeded or failed to decrease the incidence of and mortality from cervical cancer is largely reflected in (a) the extent of coverage of the population at risk by screening, (b) the target age of women screened, and (c) the reliability of cytology services in that programme (17).

The contrast between Finland, which had an organized screening programme, and Norway, where an equivalent number of smears were performed opportunistically, indicated another important aspect of screening. Even though the difference in the total number of smears taken in the two countries was not great, the reduction in mortality was substantial for all ages in Finland, whereas in Norway, only women aged 30–49 years showed a reduction in mortality rates: even for that age group, the reduction was only half that in Finland. These data suggest that spontaneous or opportunistic screening fails to reach the most at-risk women in the population, that is, middle-aged and older women of high relative risk, and therefore has far less of an impact on the incidence of and mortality from cervical cancer. Other reasons for the failure of opportunistic screening to reduce cervical cancer mortality include suboptimal follow-up and management of women with abnormal smears and the lack of coordinated campaigns of informing and educating women about cervical cancer prevention. This results in women at high risk of disease being excluded from screening.

Mortality from cervical cancer in the United Kingdom fell by 30% after the introduction of screening in the 1960s; however, some of this decrease in mortality was attributed to decreasing rates in older women and could have been a cohort effect unrelated to screening. The need for an effectively managed national programme in the United Kingdom was realized by the mid 1980s, which led to the introduction of a computerized call and recall system for women aged between 20 and 64 years. The invitation-based system, together with target payments for general practitioners, improved population coverage from 40% to 60% in 1989, to 80% in 1992, and to 83% in 1993. In an audit of this programme in 24 self-selected districts in the United Kingdom by Sasieni et al. (18), it was estimated that the number of cases of cervical cancer in the participating districts would have been 57% (95% confidence interval (CI) 28–85%) greater had there had been no screening. Furthermore, they estimated that screening prevented between 1100 and 3900 cases of invasive cervical cancer in the United Kingdom.

Population coverage achieved 80.6% in 2004 in the United Kingdom, but had declined to 77.8% in 2014 (5-year coverage), with the lowest coverage in the age group 25–29 years (19). Forty-seven per cent of women who develop cervical cancer in the United Kingdom have not been screened in the past 5 years or have never been screened in the United Kingdom (20).

Cervical cancer screening programmes

In many developing countries, screening is opportunistic, sporadic, or does not occur at all. In 1986, the WHO estimated that while approximately 40–50% of women in developed countries had been screened in the past 5 years, only 5% of women in developing countries had been screened. In addition, most screening activity in developing countries was limited to women attending primary healthcare, antenatal and family planning clinics in urban areas, with no organized efforts to ensure that high-risk women attended for screening, treatment, and follow-up (21).

While there is a paucity of data on screening programmes and incidence of and mortality from cervical cancer in many developing countries, there have been a number of attempts to establish screening programmes. Some of these programmes have met with marginal success; many, however, have failed to either become established or to have an impact on cervical cancer incidence and mortality. From a developing country perspective, good population-based cancer survival data are not available in the majority of countries, particularly those in Africa, Asia, and Central America. Sankaranarayanan et al. (22), analysed 366,357 cancer cases, including cervical cancer, and nine other sites that were registered from 1990–2001 and followed up until 2003. Only two registries were included from Africa—one from the Gambia and the other from Uganda. The 5-year age-standardized relative survival rate (**Figure 61.1**) for cervical cancer did not exceed 22% in the Gambia and in Uganda the equivalent 5-year survival rate for cervical cancer was 13%. In contrast, in countries such as China, Singapore, South Korea, and Turkey the median relative survival rates were 76–82% for breast cancer and 63–79% for cervical cancer. Gondos et al. (23) evaluated the population-based Cancer Registry of Kampala which collected data on 14 of the commonest types of cancer diagnosed and registered between 1993 and 1997. The 5-year relative survival was 8.3% for patients with colorectal cancer and 17.7% for cervical cancer—the very poor survival most likely reflecting limited access to early detection and treatment.

Gakidou et al. (24) reported on cervical cancer screening from 57 countries across all levels of economic development included in the World Health Surveys, a set of household surveys implemented by the WHO in 2002. In the 30 developing countries surveyed, the population-weighted means of crude and effective coverage of cervical cancer screening were 45% and 19%, respectively. Effective coverage ranged from over 80% in Austria and Luxembourg to 1% or less in Bangladesh, Ethiopia, and Myanmar. In fact, in many countries, the majority of women have never had a pelvic examination—more than 90% of women in Malawi, Ethiopia, and Bangladesh reported never having a pelvic examination, for example.

A key limitation to establishing screening programmes in low-resource settings has been the Pap smear which requires an infrastructure with robust referral structures, reliable quality control, and human and financial resources that are not sustainable in low- and middle-income countries (LMIC). This recognition has prompted a significant paradigm shift in the thinking about cervical cancer prevention in the past 20 years, a shift that took into account the many limitations in low-resource settings as well as the competing health needs (such as infectious diseases, maternal and neonatal morbidity and mortality, human immunodeficiency virus infection (HIV), malaria, tuberculosis, among many others), the impact of war and civil strife on society and its essential structures, environmental challenges, widespread poverty, poor governance, and inadequate state expenditure on healthcare.

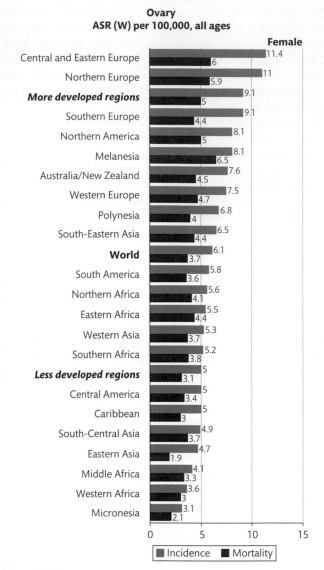

Figure 61.1 Age-standardized relative survival rate per 100,000 women in different regions of the world. ASR (W), age-standardized rate (to world standard population).

Source data from http://globocan.iarc.fr.

Initially attempts were made in India to 'downstage' cervical cancer by simple visual inspection with the naked eye during a genital examination. Later, the application of acetic acid (as is done in colposcopy) was added and called VIA (visual inspection with acetic acid). Many other modalities were tried including cervicography, spectroscopy, and others. Later, molecular testing for HPV DNA was introduced into the menu of options for screening women in both developed and developing countries. New technologies such as liquid-based cytology were designed to improve the accuracy of cervical cytology, which is now approved by the United States Food and Drug Administration.

Screening programmes in developing countries

In India, some attempts to establish screening programmes through hospital or clinic outpatient services and the use of mobile cancer detection clinics have shown a reduction in cervical cancer incidence. Luthra et al. (25) reported on a study in which 38,707 women were initially screened over a 3-year period from 1960 to 1963 and repeat screening was performed on 26,110 women from the same population between 1966 and 1970. The incidence rates of cervical cancer were reduced in the two time periods from 1.7% to 0.63% and the corresponding rates for dysplasia increased from 2.4% to 6.28%.

Subsequently, there have been a number of very successful screening studies conducted in India. Most recently, Shastri et al. (26) reported on a randomized controlled trial in which 75,360 women from ten clusters in the screening group and 76,178 women from ten comparable clusters in the control group were recruited in Mumbai. Women aged 35–64 years were recruited and screened by primary healthcare workers. The screening group received four rounds of cancer education and VIA at 24-month intervals, whereas the control group received one round of cancer education at the time of recruitment. Both groups were actively monitored at 24-month intervals for cervical cancer incidence and mortality. Women who were positive on VIA were referred to the local tertiary hospital where they received repeat VIA, colposcopy, and Pap smears. Those diagnosed with cervical cancer precursors or invasive cancer were treated according to standard protocols.

In the screening group, 89% of women participated and 79.4% complied with the protocol. After 12 years of follow-up, the incidence of invasive cervical cancer was 26.74/100,000 in the screening group and 27.49/100,000 in the control group. There were 67 and 98 cervical cancer deaths in the screening and control groups, respectively. This translated into a 31% reduction in cervical cancer mortality in the screening group compared with the control group (mortality relative risk (RR) 0.69; 95% CI 0.54–0.88; $P = 0.003$).

Parham and colleagues (27) from 2006 to 2013, up-scaled screening services (using VIA) for cervical cancer from 2 to 12 clinics in Lusaka, Zambia through which 102,942 women were screened. The majority (72%) were in the target age range of 25–49 years and 28% were HIV positive. Twenty per cent of women were VIA positive of whom 56.4% were treated with cryotherapy and 44% were referred for histopathological evaluation. Most women received same-day services (including 82% who were VIA negative and 5% undergoing same-visit cryotherapy). Among those referred for histopathological examination 44% had cervical intraepithelial neoplasia grade 2 (CIN 2) or greater. Detection rates for CIN 2+ and cancer were 17 and 7 per 1000 women screened, respectively. This study shows that screening can be performed and up-scaled in remarkably low-resourced settings. This project included many partners and leveraged funding for HIV resources that were provided by a number of organizations such as PEPFAR. The project is yet to report on the ongoing impact on cervical cancer reduction and/or prevention.

In contrast to the two very successful projects previously described, a study conducted by the WHO in six African countries in 2005 encountered many challenges, which are typical of screening programmes in low-resource settings (28). The sites chosen were Madagascar, Malawi, Nigeria, Uganda, United Republic of Tanzania, and Zambia and the study was completed in 2009. During this time period, only 19,579 women were screened from the six countries and overall 10% (n = 1980) were VIA positive and 1.7% (n = 326) had lesions suspicious for cancer. Just under 40% of women underwent screening and treatment on the same day and nearly two-thirds received treatment (cryotherapy) within a week of being screened. Of the women eligible for cryotherapy, 679 (34%) did not undergo the procedure for a range of reasons. Of the 326 women who had cervices suspicious for cancer, there was no information on 230 women and only 96 women were known to be investigated, of whom 79 had cancer and 17 either had no cancer or the outcome was unknown. Overall, 77 or the 326 women with possible cancer (24%) were known to have undergone treatment. By contrast, in the Shastri trial (26), compliance with treatment for invasive cancer was 86.3% in the screening group and 72.3% in the control group.

CONCORD-2

This seminal study (29) analysed individual tumour records from 279 population-based cancer registries in 67 countries for 25.7 million adults aged 15–99 years and 75,000 children from 0 to 14 years diagnosed with cancer during 1995–2009 and followed up to 31 December 2009. Five-year survival from colon, rectal, and breast cancers had increased steadily in most developed countries. For example, for breast cancer, 5-year survival rose to 85% or higher in 17 countries worldwide. Liver and lung cancer remained lethal in all nations with 5-year survivals ranging from 15% (North America) to 7% (Mongolia and Thailand). For cervical cancer, data were available for 602,225 women. The global range in 5-year net survival was very wide, particularly in Africa, Central and South America, and Asia. National estimates of 5-year survival ranged from less than 50% to greater than 70% with marked regional variations and very little improvement in the time periods of 1995–1999 and 2005–2009.

As mentioned earlier, cytology-based screening programmes have either not been initiated or sustained in many developing countries, and in particular in SSA. Research in the past years has focused on evaluating alternative approaches to screening, particularly approaches that use low technology and that can give a result if not immediately, then within a short time period, to enable women to be treated at or shortly after the screening visit. The two tests most studied are VIA and testing for HPV DNA of high-risk types known to have a causal relationship with cervical cancer.

HPV DNA testing

There have been multiple studies on the use of HPV DNA testing for secondary prevention of cervical cancer, in both the developed and developing world. A study that evaluated HPV infection in 10,575 cases of paraffin-embedded samples of histologically confirmed cases of invasive cancer from 38 countries in Europe, North America, central South America, Africa, Asia, and Oceania taken over a 60-year period, found that 85% ($n = 8977$) of the cases were positive for HPV DNA (30). The eight most common types of HPV detected were types 16, 18, 31, 33, 35, 45, 52, and 58 and their combined contribution to the 8977 positive cases was 91%. HPV types 16, 18, and 45 were the three most common types in each type of cervical cancer (squamous cell, adenocarcinoma, and adenosquamous carcinoma) and in the different countries studied. A recent study of HPV types in women with invasive cervical cancer in Africa which involved 570 cases of confirmed invasive cervical cancer from Ghana, Nigeria, and South Africa, found that HPV 16 infection was present in 51.2% of cases and HPV 18 in 17.2% of cases (31). Hence the distribution of HPV 16 and 18 appears to be similar in LMICs to that demonstrated in high-income countries.

Denny et al. (32) randomly assigned 6555 previously unscreened women aged 35–65 years to one of three study arms: (a) HPV and treat, in which all women with a positive HPV DNA test underwent

cryotherapy; (b) visual inspection and treat, in which all women with a positive VIA test underwent cryotherapy; and (c) control, in which further evaluation or treatment was delayed for 6 months. At 36 months there was a sustained decrease in the detection of high-grade cervical cancer precursors in the HPV and treat arm compared to the control arm (1.5% vs 5.6%—difference 4.1%) and the difference in the VIA and treat arm was less at 3.8% compared to 5.6% in the control arm (difference 1.8%). In another randomized controlled trial, Sankararanayanan et al. (33) randomized 131,746 healthy women aged 30–59 years to four groups: (a) screening with HPV, (b) cytological testing, (c) VIA, and (d) standard of care which did not include screening in India at the time. They found that in the HPV testing group the hazard ratio for the detection of advanced cancer was 0.47 (95% CI 0.32–0.69). There was also a statistically significant reduction in the number of deaths from cervical cancer in the HPV group compared to the control group. There were no significant reductions in the numbers of advanced cancers and deaths in the cytological or the VIA group compared to the control group. These data support a programme that utilizes HPV DNA testing and links positive tests to treatment without the intervening steps of colposcopy and histology.

Ronco et al. (34) summarized four randomized controlled trials that used HPV-based screening for cervical cancer compared with cytology-based screening, using cervical cancer precursors as the endpoint in all trials. A total of 176,464 women aged 20–64 years were randomly assigned to HPV-based (experimental arm) or cytology-based (control arm) screening in Sweden, the Netherlands, England, and Italy. Women were followed for a median of 6.5 years and 107 cancers were identified. Detection of cervical cancer was similar between the screening methods during the first 2.5 years of follow-up (RR 0.79; 95% 0.46–1.36) but was significantly lower in the experimental arm thereafter (RR 0.45; 95% 0.25–0.81). The cumulative incidence of cervical cancer in women who had negative tests at entry was 4.6/100,000 and 8.7/100,000 at 3.5 and 5.5 years respectively in the experimental arm, and 15.4/100,000 and 36/100,000 respectively in the control arm. In these four randomized controlled trials, HPV-based screening provided 60–70% greater protection against invasive cervical cancer compared to cytology. The authors asserted that the data supported primary screening with HPV DNA testing with extension of screening intervals to at least 5 years.

There are currently new HPV DNA tests being developed that are not only affordable but can give results within 2.5 hours of screening, almost equivalent to a point-of-care test (35). This approach may enable larger numbers of women to be reached and enable a significant impact on cervical cancer incidence and mortality, particularly if the option of self-testing is included in the screening algorithm (36, 37).

Primary prevention of cervical cancer

Since 2006, two prophylactic HPV vaccines have been available, and each has shown a greater than 90% efficacy in preventing HPV type 16- and type 18-associated high-grade cervical cancer lesions. While both vaccines have been introduced in national immunization programmes (NIPs) in many developed countries, roll out in NIPs in LMICs has been limited. Besides cost, other challenges facing developing countries include the fact that an adolescent health platform does not exist (immunization is included in the care of young children only) and reaching the target population is not easy, the necessity for a cold chain and medical waste management, cultural issues, and reticence to discuss a sexually transmitted infection among others. Despite these challenges, most Latin American middle-income countries have introduced HPV vaccination in their NIPs; on the other hand, only two LMICs in Asia (Bhutan and Malaysia) and five sub-Saharan African countries (Botswana, Lesotho, Rwanda, South Africa, and Uganda) have introduced HPV vaccination in their NIPs as of April 2016.

Ladner et al. (38) reported on 21 HPV vaccination programmes in 14 countries that vaccinated a total of 217,786 girls. All these programmes received vaccine through the Gardasil Access Program that provides HPV vaccine at no cost to help national institutions gain experience in implementing HPV vaccination. Overall, 88.7% of the targeted populations were vaccinated with just over 90% adherence with the three-dose regimen. School-based health clinic-based models predicted high coverage as was management by a non-governmental organization. These programmes convincingly show that it is possible to introduce HPV vaccination into LMICs with a high vaccine uptake and adherence.

On World Cancer Day 2013, Gavi, the Vaccine Alliance, announced that it will provide support for the rollout of HPV vaccination in eight developing countries: Ghana, Kenya, Lao PDR, Madagascar, Malawi, Niger, Sierra Leone, and Tanzania— a price of $4.50 per dose was negotiated. After two rounds of applications, 23 countries have now been approved for Gavi assistance targeting approximately 400,000 girls for HPV vaccination (39). Further, Gavi plans to reach 30 million by 2020 by introducing the vaccine into 40 countries.

Ovarian cancer

Ovarian cancer is a rare gynaecological cancer with an estimated world age-standardized rate of 6.1/100,000, with rates between 9 and 11/100,000 in well-developed regions compared to less than 5/100,000 in less developed regions (40). In 2015, 255,700 women were expected to be diagnosed with ovarian cancer and 163,800 women were estimated to die of it in the world; the corresponding figures for less developed regions were 150,300 and 93,800 respectively. Neither early detection nor screening has been able to reduce mortality from the disease, and the only possible means of reducing mortality is prevention.

Two-thirds of women diagnosed with ovarian cancer are over the age of 55 years and a family history of ovarian or breast cancer in a first-degree relative triples the risk (41). The risk is particularly high among carriers of a BRCA gene mutation with a lifetime risk of 39–46% with BRCA1 mutations and risk of 12–20% with BRCA2 mutations (41, 42). The frequency of BRCA1 and BRCA2 germline mutations in women with ovarian cancer is reported to be between 3% and 27% (43, 44). Germline BRCA mutations are known to be associated with longer survival rates after ovarian cancer diagnosis and a generally favourable response to platin-based therapy (45, 46).

An Australian study recruited 1001 women with non-mucinous ovarian cancer into a population-based case–control study and women were screened for point mutations and large deletions in both genes (47). Survival outcomes and responses to multiple lines of chemotherapy were assessed. Germline mutations were found in 14.1% of patients overall, including 16.6% of serous carcinoma patients (high-grade serous was 22.6%). Of note, 44% had no reported family history of breast or ovarian cancer, and patients carrying mutations had improved rates of progression-free survival and overall survival. In the relapse setting, patients carrying mutations more frequently responded to both platin and non-platin regimens than mutation-negative patients, even those with early relapse post primary treatment. Another important factor to consider in testing for BRCA1/2 mutations is the significant activity of poly (ADP-ribose) polymerase inhibitors in BRCA mutation carriers (48).

Epithelial ovarian cancers have been traditionally divided according to morphological appearance but it now clear that they are a heterogeneous groups of cancers primarily classified by cell type into serous, mucinous, endometrioid, clear cell, transitional, and squamous cell tumours. They are further subdivided into benign, borderline, and malignant carcinomas depending on the degree of cell proliferation, nuclear atypia, and stromal invasion (49). Recently, based on histopathology, immunohistochemistry, and molecular genetic analysis, at least five main types of ovarian cancer are identified: high-grade serous carcinoma (70%), endometrioid carcinoma (10%), clear cell carcinomas (10%), mucinous carcinomas (3%), and low-grade serous carcinoma (<5%) (50). These tumours account for 98% of ovarian carcinomas, can be reproducibly diagnosed on light microscopy, and are inherently different diseases as indicated by differences in epidemiological and genetic risk factors, precursor lesions, patterns of spread, molecular events during oncogenesis, response to chemotherapy, and prognosis (50, 51).

Screening for ovarian cancer

The discovery of cancer antigen 125 (CA125) initiated a sustained effort to identify and use biomarkers to detect ovarian cancer. Transvaginal ultrasound is the other early detection method that has been evaluated widely with CA125 for the early detection of ovarian cancer. Most studies, however, produced disappointing results— even with a specificity of 99% it was evident that as many as 25 surgeries would need to be performed to uncover one case of ovarian cancer (52). Unfortunately, at this moment, there is no reliable early detection test that can detect ovarian cancer in its early stages. There is no convincing evidence to support the introduction of organized screening programmes for ovarian cancer in public health services.

In 2015, Jacobs et al. (53) published data on a trial in which postmenopausal women aged 50–74 from 13 centres in the United Kingdom were recruited. Women were randomly allocated to annual multimodal screening (MMS) with serum CA125 augmented with ultrasound and interpreted with use of the risk of ovarian cancer algorithm, annual transvaginal ultrasound screening (USS) or no screening in a 1:1:2 ratio. The primary outcome was death due to ovarian cancer. A total of 202,638 women were randomized; 50,640 to MMS, 50,639 to USS, and 101,359 to no screening. At a median follow-up of 11.1 years, 1282 cases of ovarian cancer were diagnosed. Of the women diagnosed with ovarian cancer, in the MMS group 0.29% had died of ovarian cancer, 0.30% in the USS group, and 0.34% in the no-screening group. Using the Cox proportional hazards model, a mortality reduction of 15% over 1–14 years was evident in the MMS group and 11% in the USS group. Overall, the reduction in deaths from ovarian cancer in the three groups was not statistically significant, although there was a trend in favour of MMS in years 7–14, if prevalent cases were removed and primary peritoneal cancers were excluded. In an editorial in response to the article, Narod et al. (54) point out that the goal of screening is to prevent death from cancer and that the trial by Jacobs et al. (53) observed a reduction in the annual hazard of dying of ovarian cancer in the short term (the mean follow-up period from diagnosis to death was 2.3 years). They contend that it is necessary to wait for 10–12 years from diagnosis to conclude that an ovarian cancer patient is cured and there are many factors that delay the time from diagnosis to death but do not reduce the absolute numbers of deaths. Whether screening will prevent death from ovarian cancer or delay it by a few years is still too early to tell. Based on all deaths from ovarian/peritoneal cancers over the entire period, the hazard ratio was 0.89 and was not significant ($P = 0.23$).

Prevention of ovarian cancer

There are several ways that the risk of epithelial ovarian cancer may be reduced both in high- and average-risk women; however, much less is known about the means to prevent germ cell and stromal tumours. Studying women with BRCA1 and BRCA2 mutations have provided opportunities to address the feasibility and outcome of prophylactic surgery in the prevention of pelvic serous ovarian carcinoma. Rebbeck et al. (55) identified women with germline disease-associated BRCA1 or BRCA2 mutations who had undergone prophylactic oophorectomy from 11 different institutions. Of 259 subjects who underwent prophylactic oophorectomy, 8 (3.1%) received a diagnosis of ovarian cancer or primary papillary serous peritoneal cancer at or after oophorectomy compared to 58 of 292 matched controls who did not undergo surgery (19.0%). Of the eight cancers in the surgical group, six were stage one ovarian cancers diagnosed at the time of surgery. Neither breast nor ovarian cancer developed in 185 out of 259 subjects who underwent prophylactic oophorectomy.

Crum et al. (56) proposed a model of pelvic serous cancer that is comprised of two distinct pathways of tumour development. The first accepts that Mullerian epithelium is established in the ovary over time in the form of endosalpingiosis, cortical inclusions, or endometriosis. These cells could evolve through metaplasia, or exfoliation of tubal epithelial cells, among other routes, into cancer. These cells could serve as the epithelial source for serous carcinoma. The second pathway Crum et al. (56) propose entails malignant transformation of the distal fallopian tube mucosa, initiating as tubal intraepithelial carcinoma within pre-existing normal-appearing but probably genetically altered epithelium.

Over the last decade, ovarian cancer has been divided into two basic categories that have different aetiologies, molecular pathogenesis, and clinical behaviour. Type 1 tumours are less common, present at a lower stage, and usually arise from a precursor lesion (57). Type 2 tumours present with advanced stage disease and account for the majority of deaths from ovarian cancer (58). There is now evidence to support the proposal that most type 2 ovarian cancers develop from epithelial cells of the fallopian tube, making prophylactic salpingectomy a mode of primary prevention.

Strategies with potential to prevent ovarian, fallopian tube, and peritoneal cancer include the following:

- Oral contraception reduces the risk of both type 1 and 2 ovarian cancer and is considered safe in BRCA1 and BRAC2 mutation carriers (59).
- Tubal ligation both in the general population and high-risk women (60).
- Risk-reducing salpingo-oophorectomy may reduce ovarian cancer by 80% in women with BRCA1 and BRCA2 mutations (55).

- Improved identification and genetic testing of women who are at inherited high risk of ovarian cancer—although the Australian study showed that 44% of women with BRCA1 and BRCA2 gene mutations did not give a family history of ovarian cancer (61).
- Salpingectomy as an alternative strategy to other sterilization techniques to be performed opportunistically at the time of hysterectomy or other pelvic surgery to potentially reduce the incidence as well as death rates from ovarian cancer in the general population, albeit high-quality data on the impact in the general population is lacking as ovarian cancer is a rare disease (62).
- Other risk-reducing strategies include parity and a history of breastfeeding.

Endometrial cancer

Endometrial cancer primarily affects postmenopausal women at an average age of diagnosis in the sixth decade of life. It is the most common invasive gynaecological cancer in developed countries and its incidence in developing countries is increasing. Globally, 345,000 new cases and 82,400 deaths were estimated to occur in 2015. In the United States, 54,900 new cases and 10,200 deaths were estimated to occur in 2015. The number of newly diagnosed cases in Europe in 2012 was 100,000, with an age-standardized incidence rate of 13.6 per 100,000 women (63). In the mid 1970s there was an increased diagnosis of endometrial cancer in the United States of 15,000 cases in excess of the prevailing trend, which was and is attributed to the widespread use of unopposed oestrogen in postmenopausal women. Other risk factors associated with endometrial cancer include:

- obesity
- polycystic ovarian syndrome
- tamoxifen use
- nulliparity
- early menarche
- late menopause
- oestrogen-producing ovarian tumours.

Women with hereditary non-polyposis colorectal cancer (HNPPC/Lynch syndrome) have a markedly increased risk of endometrial cancer compared to women in the general population, ranging from 20% to 60% (64, 65).

There is no evidence that population-based screening has a role in the early detection of endometrial cancer among women at moderate risk and who are asymptomatic. There is no standard or routine test that can be used for detection of endometrial cancer. Screening women for endometrial cancer has only been recommended for women with hereditary Lynch syndrome. Women at risk for endometrial cancer should be educated and strongly advised to report any abnormal symptoms ranging from abnormal bleeding to vaginal discharge and/or pelvic pain.

Factors associated with a decreased risk of endometrial cancer:

- Oral contraception (66).
- Physical activity (67).

Factors associated with an increased risk of endometrial cancer:

- Increased exposure to excess and prolonged endogenous oestrogen, as occurs in women who are obese, experience anovulation secondary to polycystic ovarian syndrome, nulliparity, early menarche, and late menopause (68). Most women with endometrial cancer have an identifiable source of excess oestrogen and typically have a high body mass index, together with other components of the metabolic syndrome, such as diabetes, hyperlipidaemia, and hypertension (69).

- Exogenous exposure to oestrogen as a risk factor for endometrial cancer was first shown in 1975 and subsequently confirmed in other studies leading to the withdrawal of prescribing unopposed oestrogen in women with a uterus. This resulted in a rapid decrease in endometrial cancer incidence (70–72). It is estimated that the use of unopposed oestrogen therapy increases the risk for endometrial cancer 10- to 30-fold if treatment continues for 5 years or more (73).
- Combined oestrogen–progestin replacement therapy. Beral et al. (74) in the Million Women Study, conducted a cohort study in the United Kingdom in women aged 50–64 years and observed a statistically significant decreased risk of endometrial cancer associated with continuous combined oestrogen-progestin therapy compared to never users (RR 0.71; 95% CI, −0.56 to 0.90).
- In other landmark studies, the Women's Health Initiative (WHI) Postmenopausal Hormone therapy trials were launched in 1991 and recruited 161,808 women. The trials had two studies, the oestrogen and progestin (E+P) study of women with a uterus and a group randomized to placebo, and the oestrogen-alone study of women without a uterus and a similar group who were given placebo. Over 100 publications were written from the data collected over a 15-year period, and the findings were dramatic. In the E+P group compared to placebo there was an increase in heart attack, risk of stroke, blood clots, and breast cancer, but a decrease in colorectal cancer and fewer fractures (75).
- In the oestrogen-alone group, compared to placebo there was no difference in risk for heart attack, there was an increased risk of stroke and blood clots, the effect on breast cancer was uncertain, there was no difference in risk for colorectal cancer, but there was a reduced risk of fracture (75).
- In 2013, Manson et al. (76), reported an integrated overview of findings from the two WHI hormone therapy trials with extended post-intervention follow-up in 27,347 postmenopausal women aged 50–79 years enrolled from 40 centres in the United States.
- Overall, the risks of E+P during the intervention phase outweighed the benefits but many of the benefits dissipated in the post-intervention phase. However, cardiovascular disease events remained non-significantly elevated and a *reduction in endometrial cancer emerged.*
- However, overall, the data from both arms of the study did not support the use of E+P or E alone for the prevention of chronic disease.

Early detection of endometrial cancer

All women at menopause should be advised on the risk factors and early symptoms and signs of endometrial cancer and strongly encouraged to report any postmenopausal bleeding, spotting, pain while urinating, and vaginal discharge to their doctor and seek prompt medical attention. Primary care practitioners should reoriented to recognize early symptoms and signs in order to recognize those with suspected endometrial cancers and promptly refer them.

Measuring endometrial thickness by USS and endometrial sampling with cytological testing have been proposed as screening modalities for endometrial cancer. However, there is no evidence to support their role as primary screening modalities for endometrial cancer in asymptomatic postmenopausal women (77). The sensitivity of the Pap test is too low to be suitable for endometrial cancer screening. Although endometrial cancer may be diagnosed following pelvic examination, USS, and biopsy in symptomatic women, there is no evidence that screening by endo- or transvaginal USS and endometrial sampling reduces mortality from endometrial cancer in asymptomatic women. In women with postmenopausal bleeding, the sensitivity of endometrial sampling to detect endometrial cancer and atypical hyperplasia and endometrial disease, including endometrial polyps, is low (78). On the other hand, screening for endometrial cancer among asymptomatic women may be associated with harms due to anxiety, unnecessary biopsies, discomfort, and infections.

Screening for vulval and vaginal cancer

There are no known screening tests for the prevention of either vulval or vaginal cancer; however, greater health awareness may lead to early detection of disease and better clinical outcomes. Both are rare diseases, both have a relationship with HPV 16 infection, and both are more common in women with previous cervical or anal abnormalities.

Two types of vulval cancer are described: basaloid/warty types and keratinizing types. The basaloid warty types are associated with younger women and similar risk factors as for cervical cancer and HPV infection of the cervix. The keratinizing cancers have a low prevalence of HPV infection, occur in older women, and are frequently associated with background lichen sclerosus et atrophicus (79, 80). Over the past decades, the incidence of vulval intraepithelial neoplasia (VIN) and invasive vulval cancer have been increasing, with data emerging from population-based studies (81, 82).

The majority of cancers of the vulva are squamous (>90%). HPV DNA is identified in more than 80% of VIN lesions, whereas 40–50% of invasive vulval cancers have identifiable HPV DNA (83). In 2005, an expert working group was convened by the IARC (84). The group performed a meta-analysis on studies that had done genotyping in intraepithelial and invasive anogenital cancers, specifically for HPV 16. Most studies were performed in Europe and the United States. These studies combined showed HPV prevalence of 84% in VIN with 87.7% in VIN 3 and 40.4% of 1873 vulval cancers. HPV prevalence in vaginal intraepithelial neoplasia (VAIN) was 93.6%, and was 100% in VAIN 1 but 70% in 136 vaginal cancers. Overall prevalence in anal intraepithelial neoplasia (AIN) was 92.7%, 94% of AIN 3 lesions and 84.3% in 955 anal cancers. Other types of HPV were found in all the various lesions; however, over three-quarters of HPV-positive cases were HPV 16 in this analysis.

Conclusion

Screening is more complex than it first appears and requires considerable resources for sustainability and impact. It is critical to identify a health problem that has a significant effect on the selected target population, that can be treated, and to prevent progression to more advanced disease. Benefits versus harms need to be balanced, including costs to the healthcare system and value for money. Cost-effectiveness does not equate to affordability nor does it solve the problem of competing health needs. There is no 'one size fits all', even with cervical cancer screening which has a proven track record of being effective at reducing morbidity and mortality. Compliance with screening programmes is essential for success, and this requires attuned and sensitive messaging that provides true risks and benefits as well as a programme that is acceptable to the screened population.

REFERENCES

1. Wilson JMG, Jungner G. *Principles and Practice of Screening for Disease*. Public Health Papers No. 34. Geneva: World Health Organization; 1968.

2. Andermann A, Blancquaert I, Beauchamp S, Dery V. Revisiting Wilson and Jungner in the genomic age: a review of screening criteria over the past 40 years. *Bull World Health Organ* 2008;**86**:241–320.

3. Cuckle H. Principles of screening. *Obstet Gynaecol* 2004;**6**:21–25.

4. Bretthauer M, Kalager M. Principles, effectiveness and caveats in screening for cancer. *Br J Surg* 2013;**100**:55–65.

5. Trivedi AN, Rakowski W, Ayanian JZ. Effect of cost sharing on mammography in Medicare Health plans. *N Engl J Med* 2008;**358**:3375–83.

6. Jorgensen KJ, Brodersen J, Hartling OJ, Nielsen M, Gotzsche PC. Informed choice requires information about benefits and harms. *J Med Ethics* 2009;**35**:268–69.

7. Arbyn M, Castellesague X, de Sanjose S, et al. World-wide burden of cervical cancer in 2008. *Ann Oncol* 2011;**22**:2675–83.

8. Swaminathan, R, Selvakumaran R, Vinodha J, et al. Education and cancer incidence in a rural population in South India. *Cancer Epidemiol* 2009;**33**:89–93.

9. Prummel MV, Young DW, Candido E, et al. Cervical cancer incidence in Ontario women: differing sociodemographic gradients by morphologic type (adenocarcinoma versus squamous cell). *Int J Gynecol Cancer* 2014;**24**:1341–46.

10. Papanicolaou GN. New cancer diagnosis. In: *Proceedings of the Third Race Betterment Conference*, pp. 528–34. Battle Creek, MI: Race Betterment Foundation; 1928.

11. Papanicolaou GN, Traut HF. The diagnostic value of vaginal smears in carcinoma of the uterus. *Am J Obstet Gynecol* 1941;August:193–206.

12. Papanicolaou GN. *Atlas of Exfoliative Cytology*. Boston, MA: Commonwealth Fund University Press; 1954.

13. IARC Working Group on Cervical Cancer Screening. Summary chapter. In: Hakama M, Miller AB, Day NE (eds), *Screening for Cancer of the Uterine Cervix*, pp. 133–42. Lyon: International Agency for Research on Cancer; 1986.

14. Laara E, Day NE, Hakama M. Trends in mortality from cervical cancer in the Nordic countries: association with organised screening programmes. *Lancet* 1987;**1**:1247–49.

15. IARC Working Group on Evaluation of Cervical Cancer Screening Programmes. Screening for squamous cervical cancer: the duration of low risk after negative result of cervical cytology and its implication for screening policies. *Br Med J* 1986;**293**:659–64.

16. Hakama M, Louhivuori K. A screening programme for cervical cancer that worked. *Cancer Surv* 1988;**17**:403–16.

17. van Oortmarssen GJ, Habbema JD. Cervical cancer screening data from two cohorts in British Columbia. In: Hakama M, Miller AB, Day NE (eds), *Screening for Cancer of the Uterine Cervix*, pp. 47–60. IARC Scientific Publications No. 76. Lyon: International Agency for Research on Cancer; 1986.

18. Sasieni PD, Cuzick J, Lynch-Farmery E, The National Coordinating Network for Cervical Screening Working Group. Estimating the efficacy of screening by auditing smear histories of women with and without cervical cancer. *Br J Cancer* 1996;**73**:1001–1005.

19. Royal College of Obstetricians and Gynaecologists (RCOG). *Progress in Cervical Screening in the UK*. Scientific Impact Paper No.7. London: RCOG; 2016.

20. Herbert A, Anshu CG, Dunsmore H, et al. Invasive cervical cancer audit: why cancers developed in a high risk population with an organised screening programme. *BJOG* 2010;**117**:736–45.

21. Parkin DM. Screening for cervix cancer in developing countries. In: Miller AB, Chamberlain J, Day NE, Hakama M, Prorok PC (eds), *Cancer Screening*, pp 184–98. Cambridge: Cambridge University Press; 1991.

22. Sankaranarayanan R, Swaminathan R, Brenner H, et al. Cancer survival in Africa, Asia and Central America: a population based study. *Lancet Oncol* 2010;**11**:165–73.

23. Gondos A, Brenner H, Wabinga H, Parkin DM. Cancer survival in Kampala, Uganda. *Br J Cancer* 2005;**92**:1808–12.

24. Gakidou E, Nordhagen S, Obermeyer Z. Coverage of cervical cancer screening in 57 countries: low average levels and large inequalities. *PLoS Med* 2008;**5**:e132.

25. Luthra UK, Rengachari R. Organisation of screening programmes in developing countries with reference to screening for cancer of the uterine cervix in India. In: Hakama M, Miller AB, Day NE (eds), *Screening for Cancer of the Uterine Cervix*, pp.273–85. IARC Scientific Publications No. 76. Lyon: International Agency for Research on Cancer; 1986.

26. Shastri SS, Mittra I, Gauravi AM, et al. Effect of VIA screening by primary health workers: randomized controlled study in Mumbai, India. *J Natl Cancer Inst* 2014;**106**:dju009.

27. Parham GP, Mwanahamuntu MH, Kapambwe S, et al. Population-level scale-up of cervical cancer prevention services in a low-resource setting: development, implementation, and evaluation of the Cervical Cancer Prevention Program in Zambia. *PLoS One* 2015;**10**:e0122169.

28. World Health Organization (WHO). *Prevention of Cervical Cancer through Screening Using Visual Inspection with Acetic Acid (VIA) and Treatment with Cryotherapy: A Demonstration Project in Six African countries: Malawi, Madagascar, Nigeria, Uganda, the United Republic of Tanzania, and Zambia*. Geneva: WHO; 2012.

29. Allemani C, Weir HK, Carreira H, et al. Global surveillance of cancer survival 1995–2009: analysis of individual data for 25,676,887 patients from 279 population-based registries in 67 countries (CONCORD-2). *Lancet* 2015;**385**:977–1010.

30. De Sanjose S, Quint WG, Alemany L, et al. Human papillomavirus genotype attribution in invasive cervical cancer: a retrospective cross-sectional worldwide study. *Lancet Oncol* 2010;**11**: 1048–56.

31. Denny L, Adewole I, Anorlu R, et al. Human papillomavirus prevalence and type distribution in invasive cervical cancer in Sub-Saharan Africa. *Int J Cancer* 2013;**134**:1389–98.

32. Denny L, Kuhn L, Hu CC, Tsai WY, Wright TC Jr. Human papillomavirus-based cervical cancer prevention: long-term results of a randomized screening trial. *J Natl Cancer Inst* 2010;**102**:1557–67.

33. Sankaranayanan R, Nene BM, Shastri SS, et al. HPV screening for cervical cancer in rural India. *N Engl J Med* 2009;**360**:1385–94.

34. Ronco G, Dillner J, Elfstrom KM, et al. Efficacy of HPV-based screening for prevention of invasive cervical cancer: follow

up of four European randomised controlled trials. *Lancet* 2014;**383**:524–32.

35. Jeronimo J, Bansil P, Lim J, et al. A multicountry evaluation of careHPV testing, visual inspection with acetic acid, and Papanicolaou testing for the early detection of cervical cancer. *Int J Gynecol Cancer* 2014;**24**:576–84.

36. Kuhn L, Saidu R, Svanholm-Barrie C, et al. HPV testing of self-collected vaginal swabs for cervical cancer prevention in South Africa. Abstract # 60. 4th Annual Symposium on Global Cancer Research. San Francisco, CA, 8 April 2016.

37. Kuhn L, Saidu R, Boa R, et al. Optimizing point-of-care HPV testing for cervical cancer prevention in South Africa. EUROGIN 2016; Saltzburg Austria, 15–18 June 2016.

38. Ladner J, Besson MH, Rodrigues M, Audureau E, Saba J. Performance of 21 HPV vaccination programs implemented in low and middle-income countries, 2009–2013. *BMC Public Health* 2014;**14**:670.

39. Hansen C, Eckert L, Bloem P, Cernuschi T. Gavi HPV programs: application to implementation. *Vaccine (Basel)* 2015;**3**:408–19.

40. International Agency for Research on Cancer. Global Cancer Observatory. Available at: http://globocan.iarc.fr/old/factsheet.asp (accessed 21 June 2016).

41. Rubin SC, Benjamin I, Behbakht K, et al. Clinical and pathological features of ovarian cancer in women with germ-line mutations of BRCA 1. *N Engl J Med* 1996;**335**:1413–16.

42. U.S. Preventive Services Task Force. Genetic risk assessment and BRCA mutation testing for breast and ovarian cancer susceptibility: recommendation statement. *Ann Intern Med* 2005;**143**:355–61.

43. Risch HA, McLaughlin JR, Cole DE, et al. Population BRCA 1 and BRCA 2 mutation frequencies and cancer penetrances: a kin–cohort study in Ontario, Canada. *J Natl Cancer Inst* 2006;**98**:1694–706.

44. Cancer Genome Atlas Research Network. Integrated genomic analyses of ovarian carcinoma. *Nature* 2011;**474**:609–15.

45. Cass I, Baldwin RL, Varkey T, et al. Improved survival in women with BRCA-associated ovarian carcinoma. *Cancer* 2003;**97**:2187–95.

46. Tan DSP, Rothermundt C, Thomas K, et al. 'BRCA-ness syndrome in ovarian cancer: a case-control study describing the clinical features and outcome of patients with epithelial ovarian cancer associated with BRCA 1 and 2 mutations. *J Clin Oncol* 2008;**26**:5530–36.

47. Alsop K, Fereday S, Meldrum C, et al. BRCA mutation frequency and patterns of treatment Response in BRCA mutation-positive women with ovarian cancer: a report from the Australian Ovarian Cancer Study Group. *J Clin Oncol* 2012;**30**:2654–63.

48. McCabe N, Turner NC, Lord CJ, et al. Deficiency in the repair of DNA damage by homologous recombination and sensitivity to poly (ADP-ribose) polymerase inhibition. *Cancer Res* 2006;**66**:8109–115.

49. Prat J. *Pathology of the Ovary*. Philadelphia, PA: Saunders; 2004.

50. Gilks CB, Prat J. Ovarian carcinoma pathology and genetics: recent advances. *Hum Pathol* 2009;**40**:1213–23.

51. Prat J. Ovarian carcinomas: five distinct diseases with different origins, genetic alterations and clinicopathological features. *Virchows Arch* 2012;**460**:237–49.

52. Fields MM, Chevlen E. Ovarian cancer screening: a look at the evidence. *Clin J Oncol Nurs* 2006;**10**:77–81.

53. Jacobs IJ, Menon U, Ryan A, et al. Ovarian Cancer screening and mortality in the UK Collaborative Trial of Ovarian Cancer Screening (UKCTOCS): a randomised controlled trial. *Lancet* 2016;**387**:945–56.

54. Narod S, Sopik V. Should we screen for ovarian cancer? A commentary on the UK Collaborative Trial of Ovarian Cancer Screening (UKCTOCS): a randomised controlled trial. *Gynecol Oncol* 2016;**141**:191–94.

55. Rebbeck TR, Lynch HT, Neuhausen SL, et al. Prophylactic oophorectomy in carriers of BRCA1 or BRCA 2 mutations. *N Engl J Med* 2002;**346**:1616–22.

56. Crum CP, Dropkin R, Kindelberger D, Medeiros F, Miron A, Lee Y. Lessons from BRCA: the tubal fimbria emerges as an origin for pelvic serous cancer. *Clin Med Res* 2006;**5**:35–44.

57. Kurman RJ, Shih IM. Molecular pathogenesis and extraovarian origin of epithelial ovarian cancer—shifting the paradigm. *Hum Path* 2011;**142**:918–31.

58. Bowrell DDL. The genesis and evolution of high-grade serous ovarian cancer. *Nat Rev Cancer* 2010;**31**:161–69.

59. Cibula D, Zikan M, Dusek L, Majek O. Oral contraceptives and risk of ovarian and breast cancers in BRCA mutation carriers: a meta-analysis. *Expert Rev Anticancer Ther* 2011;**11**:1197–207.

60. Cibula D, Widschwendter M, Zikan M, Dusek L. Underlying mechanisms of ovarian cancer risk reduction after tubal ligation. *Acta Obstet Gynecol Scand* 2011;**90**;559–63.

61. Kauff ND, Satagopan JM, Robson ME, et al. Risk-reducing salpingo-oophorectomy in women with a BRCA 1 and BRCA 2 mutation. *N Engl J Med* 2002;**346**:1609–15.

62. McAlpine J, Hanley G, Woo M, et al. Opportunistic salpingectomy: uptake, risks and complications of a regional initiative for ovarian cancer prevention. *Am J Obstet Gynecol* 2014;**210**:471–73.

63. International Agency for Research on Cancer, World Health Organization. GLOBOCAN: estimated incidence, mortality and prevalence of cancer worldwide in 2012. Available at: http://globocan.iarc.fr/Pages/Fact_sheets_population.aspx (accessed 17 May 2015).

64. Watson P, Vasen HF, Mecklin JP, et al. The risk of endometrial cancer in hereditary nonpolyposis colorectal cancer. *Am J Med* 1994;**96**:516–20.

65. Aanio M, Mecklin JP, Aaltonen LA, et al. Life-time risk of different cancers in hereditary non-polyposis colorectal cancer (HNPCC) syndrome. *Int J Cancer* 1995;**64**:430–33.

66. Weiderpass E, Adami HO, Baron JA, et al. Use of oral contraceptives and endometrial cancer risk (Sweden). *Cancer Causes Control* 1999;**10**:277–84.

67. Moradi T, Nyren O, Bergstrom R, et al. Risk for endometrial cancer in relation to occupational physical activity: a nationwide cohort study in Sweden. *Int J Cancer* 1998;**76**:665–70.

68. Lukanova A, Lundin E, Micheli A, et al. Circulating levels of sex steroid hormones and risk of endometrial cancer in postmenopausal women. *Int J Cancer* 2004;**108**:425–32.

69. Esposito K, Chiodini P, Capuano A, et al. Metabolic syndrome and endometrial cancer: a meta-analysis. *Endocrine* 2014;**45**:28–36.

70. Smith DC, Prentice R, Thompson DJ, et al. Association of exogenous estrogen and endometrial cancer. *N Engl J Med* 1975;**292**:1167–70.

71. Antunes CM, Strolley PD, Rosenshein NB, et al. Endometrial cancer and estrogen use. Report of a large case-control study. *N Engl J Med* 1979;**300**:9–13.

72. Austin DF, Roe KM. The decreasing incidence of endometrial cancer: public health implications. *Am J Public Health* 1982;**72**:65–68.

73. Ali AT. Reproductive factors and the risk of endometrial cancer. *Int J Gynecol Cancer* 2014:**24**:384–93.

74. Beral V, Bull D, Reeves G, et al. Endometrial cancer and hormone replacement therapy in the Million Women Study. *Lancet* 2005;**365**:1543–51.

75. National Heart, Lung, and Blood Institute. Women's Health Initiative (WHI). https://www.nhlbi.nih.gov/whi/whi_faq.htm (accessed 17 May 2016).

76. Manson JE, Chlebowski RT, Stefanick ML, et al. Menopausal hormone therapy and health outcomes during the intervention and extended post-stopping phases of the Women's Health Initiative Randomized Trials. *JAMA* 2013;**310**:1353–68.

77. Wolfman W, Leyland N, Heywood M, et al., Asymptomatic endometrial thickening. *J Obster Gynecol Cancer* 2010;**32**:990–99.

78. Van Haneqem N, Prins MM, Bongers MY, et al., The accuracy of endometrial sampling in women with postmenopausal bleeding: a systematic review and meta-analysis. *Eur J Obstet Gynecol Reprod Biol* 2016;**197**:147–55.

79. Van Beurden M, ten Kate FW, Tjong-A-Hung SP, et al. Human papillomavirus DNA in multicentric vulvar intraepithelial neoplasia. *Int J Gynecol Pathol* 1998;**17**:12–16.

80. Rolfe KJ, MacLean AB, Crow JC, Benjamin E, Reid WM, Perrett CW. TP53 mutations in vulval lichen sclerosus adjacent to squamous cell carcinoma of the vulva. *Br J Cancer* 2003;**89**:2249–53.

81. Akhtar-Danesh N, Elit L, Lytwyn A. Trends in incidence and survival of women with invasive vulval cancer in the United States and Canada: a population-based study. *Gynecol Oncol* 2014;**134**:314–18.

82. Baandrup L, Varbo A, Munk C, Johansen C, Frisch M, Kjaer SK. In situ and invasive squamous cell carcinoma of the vulva in Denmark 1978–2007—a nationwide population-based study. *Gynecol Oncol* 2011;**122**:45–49.

83. De Vuyst H, Clifford GM, Nascimento MC, Madeleine MM, Franceschi S. Prevalence and type distribution of human papillomavirus in carcinoma and intraepithelial neoplasia of the vulva, vagina and anus: a meta-analysis. *Int J Cancer* 2009;**124**:1626–36.

84. International Agency for Research on Cancer (IARC). *Human Papillomavirus*. IARC Monographs on the Evaluation of Carcinogenic Risks in Humans, Vol. **90**. Lyon: IARC Press; 2007.

62

Premalignant and malignant disease of the cervix

Walter Prendiville

Introduction

Cervical cancer is a disease of poor and unscreened populations. Globally, it is the fourth most common cancer in women with over half a million new cases and over a quarter of a million deaths per year (1). About 85% of cases occur in less developed regions. In some parts of sub-Saharan Africa, it is the most common cancer in women (**Table 62.1** and **Figure 62.1**).

Aetiology

A number of different risk factors have been identified for cervical cancer and its precursors and these include smoking, early age at first intercourse, nutritional deficiency, chlamydial infection, multiple sexual partners, multiple pregnancies, and long-term use of oral contraceptives (2–6). However, the fundamental and sine qua non causative agent is the persistence of oncogenic human papillomavirus (HPV) in the epithelium of the transformation zone (TZ) and/or adjacent glandular epithelium. The relationship between oncogenic HPV and cervical precancer appears at first paradoxical. Cervical cancer is always associated with oncogenic HPV but oncogenic HPV is a normal and usually transient infection that most normal sexually active women will encounter in early reproductive life. Current thinking is that the oncogenic HPV virus gains entry to the cervical epithelium at the new squamocolumnar junction, possibly associated with minor abrasions and that this allows the virus to access reserve cells underneath the single layer of columnar epithelium.

Screening tests

Systematic high coverage and quality-assured population screening for precursors to cervical cancer is highly effective. This is not surprising given the conditions for an ideal screening test (7) apply very precisely to cervical cancer. The disease has a long precancerous phase, effective screening tests are available and are easily performed, and the disease is common enough to justify the expense of population screening, even in low- and middle-income countries (LMIC) (8). There are effective and low-morbidity preventive treatments of proven value for screen-positive women.

Finally, vaccination is available and effective. Cervical cancer really shouldn't exist.

A positive *diagnostic* test result reveals an abnormality. Advice about management is usually accepted willingly. When a woman receives an abnormal *screening* test result, the expectations and fears that she carries are quite different. Cervical screening tests, whether visual inspection, cervical cytology, or HPV tests, do not give a diagnosis, rather they modify the risk for an individual of developing cervical cancer. The progression to precancer and cancer is slow and is a very uncommon outcome for screen-positive women. The threshold of abnormality at which the risk of cancer outweighs any disadvantage of treatment varies according to patient characteristics and local service considerations. Most clinical guideline documents advise treatment at the high-grade squamous intraepithelial lesion level (HSIL or cervical intraepithelial neoplasia (CIN) 2–3). However, in many countries with established screening programmes, and where low rates of default to follow-up exist, the threshold for treatment may be higher, especially in young women with moderate intraepithelial neoplasia (HSIL-CIN2).

But current screening tests for cervical precancer are neither completely sensitive nor absolutely specific. Oncogenic or high-risk HPV testing is highly sensitive but has poor specificity. Cytology is far more specific but less sensitive (9, 10) and has to be performed relatively frequently. The long natural history of cervical cancer is forgiving of the relatively poor sensitivity of cytology. Molecular biomarkers may soon prove to be cost-effective secondary screening tests.

Visual inspection with acetic acid (VIA) is now the *de facto* primary screening method in many LMICs. Also, a policy of *screen and treat* is gaining popularity as an efficient method of reaching large numbers of women as a once in a lifetime event. However, the specificity of VIA is poor (11). Overtreatment of the majority of VIA-positive women is perceived by many as less of a problem.

VIA (or visual inspection with Lugol's iodine) is inexpensive, simple, and can be carried out by primary care staff trained in a relatively short time. They provide immediate results and may be performed in hospital clinics or in the community. The sensitivity as well as the specificity of visual inspection techniques are highly variable and very reliant on quality-assured training and retraining (12, 13). Of course, these methods only assess the ectocervix and will miss endocervical lesions with consequent poorer performance

Table 62.1 Cervical cancer rates between more and less developed regions

Population	Incidence		Mortality		Prevalance
	Number	ASR (W)	Number	ASR (W)	5-year
World	527624	14.0			
More developed regions	83,078	9.9	35,495	3.3	288,967
Less developed regions	444,546	15.7	230,158	8.1	1,258,194

Source data from Ferlay J, Soerjomataram I, Ervik M, et al. GLOBOCAN 2012 v1.0, IARC CancerBase No. 11. IARC; 2013. Available at: http://globocan.iarc.fr.

in older women. Finally, visual inspection is very unlikely to detect glandular intraepithelial lesions.

HPV DNA testing will probably replace or complement cytology as the primary screening tool in many developed countries for women over 30 years of age (14, 15). Because of the absolute relationship between oncogenic HPV and cervical cancer, its negative predictive value is very high. There are essentially three realms where HPV testing is of proven clinical utility: as a screening tool in women over 30 years, as a triage tool for low-grade abnormalities, and as a follow-up tool for women who have been treated for squamous cervical precancer.

Oncogenic HPV testing as the primary screening tool

Sankaranarayanan and colleagues (16) first demonstrated in a large cluster randomized controlled trial that a single round of HPV testing was superior to cytology or VIA or no screening in reducing the incidence of advanced cervical cancer and of cervical cancer mortality. Four randomized controlled trials of HPV screening versus routine cytological screening in Europe have been undertaken. In these studies, a total of 176,464 women aged 20–64 years were randomly assigned to HPV-based (experimental arm) or cytology-based (control arm) screening in Sweden, the Netherlands, England, and Italy (15). The authors conclude in their summary that 'HPV-based screening provides 60–70% greater protection against invasive cervical carcinomas compared with cytology. Data from large-scale randomized trials support the initiation of HPV-based screening from age 30 years and extension of screening intervals to at least 5 years'. The results of this overview are very convincing.

The biology of cervical intraepithelial neoplasia and cervical cancer

The concept of a continuum, first proposed by Richart (17), has persisted until relatively recently. Greater understanding of the biology of oncogenic HPV has led to a different concept, that is, that there are two different types of HPV infection, the first of which is an innocent and transient infection which may produce mild or low-grade lesions that have limited if any precancerous potential for progression to cancer. This is called a *productive* infection. The key step in the pathogenesis of HPV-linked cancers is the activation of the viral oncogenes *E6* and *E7* in the basal and parabasal cells of the infected epithelium (18–20). These viral genes if expressed in basal or parabasal cells trigger chromosomal instability and major numerical

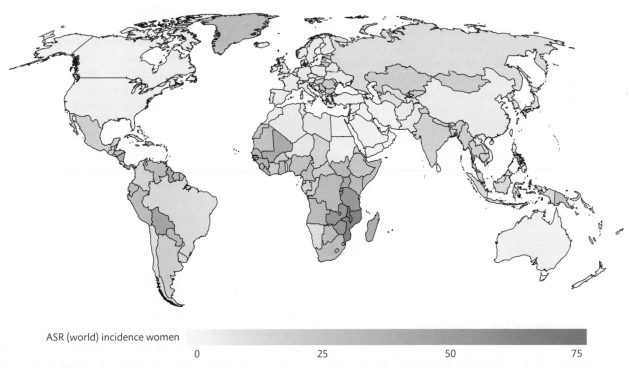

ASR (world) incidence women

0   25   50   75

Figure 62.1 Transformation zone (TZ) types. (a) Diagrammatic representation of a type 1 TZ, which is completely ectocervical, fully visible, and may be small or large. (b) Diagrammatic representation of a type 2 TZ which has an endocervical component but is still fully visible; the ectocervical component may be small or large. (c) Diagrammatic representation of a type 3 TZ which has an endocervical component and the upper limit is not fully visible. The ectocervical component if present may be small or large.

Source data from *Sankaranarayanan International Agency for Research on Cancer (WHO) Lyon, France 2016.*

and structural alterations of the host cell chromosomes. This leads to uneven distribution of the overall DNA content, aneuploidy, and is reflected by shifts of the nuclear staining pattern, the staining intensity. This type of infection is more readily recognized cytologically, colposcopically, and histologically and is called a *transforming* infection (19).

Sometimes, moderate dyskaryosis (at cytology) or moderate dysplasia (at histology) may contain both types of infection and these are difficult to distinguish using cytology or histology. Fortunately, developments in molecular biology have led to specific biomarkers of cell biology that can discriminate between these types where doubt exists.

The assessment of cervical abnormality

Colposcopy is the best means of assessing cervical intraepithelial abnormality. Like most clinical decisions, whether to treat or not is a balance of risks. For low-grade squamous intraepithelial lesions (LSIL) the risk of progression to cancer is probably about 1% whereas for high grade lesions (HSIL-CIN3) it may be as high as 30%. For these two ends of the spectrum the decision to treat or not is relatively easy, HSIL-CIN3 should almost always be treated and LSIL should usually not. The progression rates for HSIL-CIN2 are less well established and there is growing consensus that age should be included in the management equation. Relevant case characteristics will include age, parity, previous treatment, future fertility aspirations, likelihood of default, HPV testing, and any other available biomarker triage test results. Also, the TZ type and size will affect the risk of functional damage to the cervix (Figure 62.2).

Safe treatment will mean a preliminary colposcopic examination by a properly trained colposcopist with adequate documentation of findings in a structured format. It should record the TZ type, the adequacy of the examination and an objective diagnostic score, for example, the Swede score (21) (Table 62.2). If the treatment is excisional then it should be performed under binocular colposcopic guidance to minimize excising excessive or insufficient tissue (22) and of inflicting excessive artefactual damage to the wound or the removed TZ. Treatment should accomplish complete eradication of the TZ and not just the lesion. Whether excising or destroying the TZ, ablation to a depth of 7 mm is considered optimal (23). This is because the deepest gland crypt can contain CIN as low as 4 mm (24) and destroying to 7 mm gives a sufficient degree of safety. A description of how to perform colposcopic examination and treatment is available elsewhere. Practical manuals, image atlases and structured training courses are also available (http://www.ifcpc.org). Colposcopic examination should be undertaken in a systematic way using standard international nomenclature to record findings (25).

Excision or destruction of the transformation zone

Table 62.3 details the different methods of treatment. Where facilities allow, treatment should probably be excisional using electrosurgery (large loop excision of the transformation zone (LLETZ) aka the loop electrosurgical excision procedure (LEEP)). Histological examination allows assessment of the grade of abnormality, the completeness of excision, and the dimensions of the excised tissue calculated. Also, it will sometimes recognize glandular disease where present. Finally, histological examination allows the colposcopist to audit diagnostic acumen both in terms of the diagnosis and the geographical limits of the TZ.

LLETZ should usually be performed in a clinic with access to resuscitation facilities. For high-grade lesions, excision may often be performed at the first visit providing the patient is fully informed, there is no disparity between the referral cytology and the colposcopic assessment, and the TZ is sufficiently small and accessible (i.e. type 1 or shallow type 2 TZ). For every other circumstance there is no urgency about management, providing the risk of default to follow-up attendance is low.

Treatment methods

Destructive therapy

Popular in the United States during the 1970s and 1980s, cryotherapy was introduced into clinical practice by Crisp and colleagues (26) and has been used in many countries for several decades. Where the equipment and gas supply is assured and when the preconditions for destructive therapy (Box 62.1) have been met it is a reasonable choice of therapy. It has few serious complications, and although described as causing relative discomfort it is usually well tolerated without the need for local infiltration so that it may be performed as an outpatient procedure or in a rural clinic. The capital equipment necessary is inexpensive, although the price of gas and the cost of transporting the gas cylinders are quite variable. Cryotherapy gas tanks are large and are heavy (10–15 kg) and thus difficult to transport. They require refilling relatively frequently. At a clinical level, the major disadvantage of cryotherapy, and all destructive techniques, is the lack of tissue to allow histological examination. Finally, cryotherapy treatment takes considerably longer (approximately 15 minutes from start to finish) than thermal coagulation or LLETZ, each of which may be completed in a minute or two, although local anaesthetic infiltration may add a minute to LLETZ. Cryotherapy had become very popular as part of a see-and-treat approach to screening and management in many LMIC in the last decade but difficulties with maintaining a cheap and reliable supply of carbon dioxide has limited its popularity.

Details of standards in cryocautery equipment and how to perform the procedure as well as details of sterilization procedures are contained in the World Health Organization technical specifications document 'Cryosurgical equipment for the treatment of precancerous cervical lesions and prevention of cervical cancer' (27).

Thermal coagulation (aka cold coagulation)

Cold coagulation is a misnomer and should properly be called thermal coagulation. The probe is heated electrically and reaches temperatures of 100–120°C (28). It was named cold coagulation to discriminate it from radical diathermy which reached temperatures of 300°C. The method was introduced to clinical practice by Kurt Semm in Kiel in 1966 and was used widely throughout Europe in the 1970s and 1980s. Much of the published work on cold coagulation came from the United Kingdom, in particular from Ian Duncan's unit in Dundee (28–30). It was not widely used in North America where

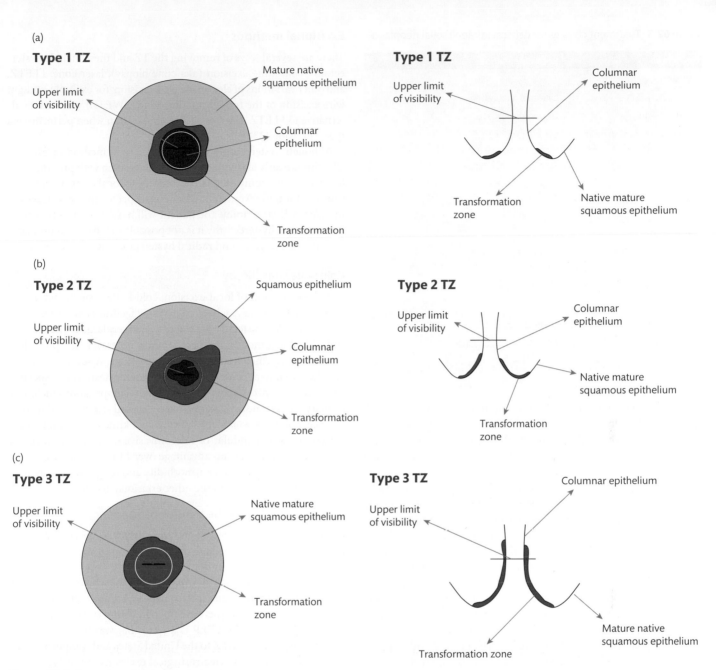

(a)

Type 1 TZ

Upper limit of visibility

Mature native squamous epithelium

Columnar epithelium

Transformation zone

Type 1 TZ

Upper limit of visibility

Columnar epithelium

Transformation zone

Native mature squamous epithelium

(b)

Type 2 TZ

Upper limit of visibility

Squamous epithelium

Columnar epithelium

Transformation zone

Type 2 TZ

Upper limit of visibility

Columnar epithelium

Native mature squamous epithelium

Transformation zone

(c)

Type 3 TZ

Upper limit of visibility

Native mature squamous epithelium

Transformation zone

Type 3 TZ

Upper limit of visibility

Columnar epithelium

Mature native squamous epithelium

Transformation zone

Figure 62.2 Illustration of global cervical cancer rates.
Reproduced with kind permission of Sankaranarayanan International Agency for Research on Cancer (WHO) Lyon, France 2016.

Table 62.2 The Swede score

	0	1	2	Score
Aceto uptake	Zero or transparent	Shady, milky (not transparent not opaque)	Distinct, opaque white	
Margins/surface	Diffuse	Sharp but irregular jagged 'geographical' satellites	Sharp and even difference in surface level including 'cuffling'	
Vessels	Fine, regular	Absent	Coarse or atypical	
Lesion size	<5 mm	5–15 mm or 2 quadrants	>15 mm or 3–4 quadrants or endocervically undefined	
Iodine staining	Brown	Faintly or patchy yellow	Distinct yellow	
			Total score	**Maximum 10**

Reproduced from Strander B, Ellstrom-Andersson A, Franzen S, Milsom I, Radberg T (2005). The performance of a new scoring system for colposcopy in detecting high-grade dysplasia in the uterine cervix. *Acta Obstet Gynecol Scand*. 84(10):1013–1017 with permission from John Wiley and Sons.

Table 62.3 Treatment choices for cervical intraepithelial neoplasia

Technique	Recommendation
Excision	
LLETZ (aka LEEP)	Universal application
Laser excision	Universal application
Straight wire excision (SWETZ) or needle excision (NETZ)	Some type 2 or 3 TZs Glandular disease Suspicion of microinvasion
Hysterectomy	Rarely appropriate
Cold knife conisation	Suspicion of glandular disease or microinvasion
Destruction	
Thermal coagulation	CIN grades 1 and 2 All type 1 TZs Some type 2 TZs No suspicion of cancer, glandular disease, previous treatment, or uncertainty about the grade of abnormality
Laser ablation	As for 'Thermal coagulation'
Cryocautery	As for 'Thermal coagulation'

cryocautery and then laser ablation were the destructive methods of choice. With thermal coagulation the intracellular water reaches boiling point and the cells necrose. It achieves tissue destruction to a depth of 4–7 mm (31). The method fell out of popularity (32) when LLETZ was introduced but is now being reconsidered because of its apparent advantages over cryocautery and because excisional techniques are not considered feasible in remote regions by relatively untrained staff in poorly equipped facilities without the necessary additional resources (e.g. histopathology services and the very occasional need for general anaesthesia). Thermal coagulation has better success rates than cryosurgery, is quicker to perform with similarly low complication rates, and does not require refrigerated gas. The procedure takes less than 2 minutes to complete and is usually performed without either general or local anaesthesia, it appears to be well tolerated. Finally, although the energy is produced electrically, newer thermal coagulation units are battery operated and can provide sufficient battery power for 30 procedures before recharging is necessary.

Box 62.1 Conditions for destructive treatment

- The TZ must be fully visible (i.e. type 1 or 2 TZ) and accessible (type 1 or shallow type 2 TZ).
- The TZ must be small enough to be covered by the destructive method probe.
- Invasive disease must be ruled out.
- There should be no suspicion of glandular disease.
- There should be no disparity between cytology and colposcopy.
- There should not have been a previous treatment of the cervix.
- There should not be upper or lower genital tract infection (relative contraindication).
- The patient should not be pregnant.
- The patient if recently pregnant should be greater than 3 months postpartum.

Excisional methods

There are several ways of removing the TZ and these include hysterectomy, cold knife excision (aka cone biopsy), laser cone, LLETZ, and other variations of electrosurgical excision, for example, straight wire excision of the transformation zone (SWETZ) which is an alternative to LLETZ, laser, or cold knife excision when performing a type 3 excision (33).

Although hysterectomy is widely used as a method of excising CIN this is nearly always inadvisable. For women with precancerous lesions, hysterectomy offers no advantage to local excision of the lesion and for those women in whom unsuspected invasive disease is revealed at hysterectomy, the patient will have been poorly served. After a simple hysterectomy it is not possible to offer the appropriate radiotherapy regimen and radical hysterectomy is also not possible.

Cold knife cone biopsy

The oldest method of local excision, cold knife cone biopsy, is still widely used, especially where colposcopy facilities and or expertise is not available. The technique leaves a relatively large cervical defect and will often remove more tissue than is necessary. The procedure is usually performed under general anaesthesia. A suture or sutures are often used to achieve post-excision haemostasis. It is associated with well-recognized short- and long-term complications including primary and secondary haemorrhage, cervical stenosis, and incompetence. It may be worth considering cold knife excision for a type 3 excisions with glandular or microinvasive disease. But otherwise cold knife excision has no advantage over LLETZ or laser excision and is associated with greater morbidity and long-term pregnancy-related complications than the other excisional techniques (34).

Large loop excision of the transformation zone

LLETZ is the term coined in the early 1980s to describe excision of the TZ using a low-voltage diathermy loop of thin wire usually with blended diathermy under local anaesthetic cover. The term was coined to discriminate it from the small loops which Rene Cartier used for taking biopsies and it is from his technique that LLETZ (aka LEEP) was developed. It was developed in Bristol (United Kingdom) in the early 1980s (35). LEEP is a term that was introduced after the introduction of LLETZ to the United States and was purportedly coined to describe loop electrosurgical excisions of the TZ and for other lower genital tract lesions. In truth, it is identical to LLETZ.

Principles of electrosurgery

Electrosurgery has been used for over a century to both cut and coagulate tissue. The discovery by Faraday that muscle doesn't contract when contacted by very high-frequency alternating current (i.e. >100 kHz) means that it is possible to perform safe passage of electricity through controlled circuits in the human body and to utilize the localized point of contact effect to achieve cutting or coagulation or a combination (blend) of the two. Electrosurgical energy operates at frequencies of over 300 kHz.

The technique is simple and easy to learn, but is best learned *in vitro* using moist ox tongue or some other meat or electroconductive tissue (e.g. Play-Doh).

The technique of LLETZ (aka LEEP) has been described elsewhere (35). After removing the TZ it should be transferred to the attendant who may transect it and pin it to a cork board before immersion in formalin. It is also worth immersing the extirpated TZ in a graduated cylinder of fluid to assess volume (Archimedes' principle). The volume of excision appears to be a reliable prognosticator for future pregnancy-related complications (36–38).

Complications after LLETZ

In the short term, complications after LLETZ are mild. These include light *per vaginal* bleeding, mild discomfort, and a little discharge. The bleeding during the first 2 or 3 weeks is not usually more than at normal menstruation. This is providing the cervix was not inflamed at the time of LLETZ. Severe bleeding or symptoms suggestive of a secondary infection (bleeding greater than that seen during menses, discharge, pain) are uncommon and should precipitate immediate return to the clinic service.

It is entirely biologically plausible that excision of part of a reproductive organ is likely to compromise its function. Since Kyrgiou et al.'s review in 2006 there has been a plethora of publications reporting conflicting evidence about the risk of premature labour after excisional treatment for cervical precancer. The most recent review of the evidence would suggest that removing a small type 1 TZ is associated with an insignificant increase in subsequent pregnancy-related complications whereas removing a large amount of tissue using any method will cause a significant increase in subsequent pregnancy-related complications (34, 36–39).

The type 3 excision

Although type 3 excisions, especially large ones (37), are associated with an increase in the risk of subsequent pregnancy-related complications (primarily premature labour), they are sometimes necessary. Examples would include the type 3 TZ with suspected HSIL, glandular disease, or even suspected microinvasion. Performing a type 3 excision is not as simple as a type 1 excision and may require general anaesthesia, depending on how large and how long the excision needs to be, access to the cervix, and patient compliance. Sometimes a large long loop will be perfectly adequate, sometimes a straight wire excision (SWETZ), although this takes longer (33). Finally some colposcopists (but not the author) prefer to remove the type 3 TZ by way of a 'top hat' technique whereby the TZ is removed in two pieces. After the initial pass removes the ectocervical component, a second and smaller loop removes the upper part of the endocervical TZ.

The evidence from the 29 randomized controlled trials in the Cochrane meta-analysis (40) suggests that there is no overwhelmingly superior surgical technique for eradicating CIN except that cryotherapy appears to be a relatively ineffective treatment of high grade disease.

Follow-up after treatment for cervical intraepithelial neoplasia

Women who have been treated for cervical precancer are much more likely to develop cervical cancer (41). A number of case series of cancer demonstrated that over 50% of cancers occur in women who are lost to follow-up (42) and that this increase in risk lasts for 20 years or more. Involved excision margins at histology is a particular marker and women aged 50 years or older are particularly

at risk of persistent/recurrent disease (42, 43). Post-treatment HPV testing is the most sensitive test, has the best negative predictive values, and is the best test of cure.

Cervical cancer

Pathology

Squamous cell and adenosquamous carcinomas comprise approximately 85% and adenocarcinoma approximately 15% of cervical cancers. Squamous carcinomas are large-cell keratinizing, large-cell non-keratinizing, and small-cell types. Small-cell neuroendocrine type typically behaves like similar disease arising from the bronchus and has a similarly poor prognosis. Adenocarcinomas can be pure or combined with squamous elements—the adenosquamous carcinoma. About 80% of cervical adenocarcinomas are made up of cells of the endocervical type with mucin production. The remaining adenocarcinomas are of endometrioid, clear cell, or intestinal, or a combination of these.

Clinical management

Management of cervical cancer is to determine the stage of the disease and to treat both the primary lesion and other extracervical disease. Cervical cancers spread by direct spread into the cervical stroma, parametrium, and beyond, and by lymphatic metastasis into parametrial, pelvic sidewall, and para-aortic nodes. Blood-borne spread is rare. Among the major factors that influence prognosis are (a) stage, (b) volume, (c) grade of tumour, (d) histological type, (e) lymphatic spread, and (f) vascular invasion. In a large study of patients with clinical disease confined to the cervix, the factors that predicted lymph node metastases and a decrease in disease-free survival were capillary–lymphatic space involvement by tumour, increasing tumour size, and increasing depth of stromal invasion (44, 45). A similar study of 626 patients with locally advanced disease demonstrated that para-aortic and pelvic lymph node status, tumour size, clinical stage, patient age, and performance status were all significant prognostic factors for a reduction in progression-free interval and survival (46). The incidence of para-aortic and pelvic lymph node disease according to stage is illustrated in **Table 62.4** (47–52).

Staging

Women should be fully staged using the International Federation of Gynecology and Obstetrics (FIGO) system (**Box 62.2**). FIGO staging is based largely on clinical assessment. Radiological staging, particularly by magnetic resonance imaging (MRI), allows more accurate determination of local disease spread (53), and also permits assessment of lymph node status. Routine use of imaging enhances the selection of women in whom surgery alone is likely to be curative. MRI has become so accurate at staging disease that formal examination under anaesthetic is no longer required in settings where imaging is routinely practised. In a limited number of pilot studies, positron emission tomography (PET) has demonstrated enhanced accuracy at diagnosing involved lymph nodes, but more robust studies are required. If performed prior to pelvic exenteration a whole-body PET or PET/computed tomography (CT) scan may improve selection of patients and therefore improve survival and reduce morbidity.

Table 62.4 Rate of lymph node involvement according to stage of cervical cancer

Stage	No.	Positive pelvic lymph nodes (%)	Positive para-aortic lymph nodes (%)
IA1 (<1 mm)	23	0	0
IA1 (1–3 mm)	156	0.6	0
IA2 (3–5 mm)	84	4.8	<1
IB	1926	15.9	2.2
IIA	110	24.5	11
IIB	324	31.4	19
III	125	44.8	30
IVA	23	55	40

Source data from references 47–52.

If performed prior to radiotherapy, a whole-body PET or PET/CT scan may change planned radiotherapy fields.

Treatment

Women with cervical cancer should be discussed in expert multidisciplinary forums with specialist surgeons, oncologists, pathologists, radiologists, and specialist nurses. This permits the best possible environment for optimum decision-making. Both surgery and radiotherapy are effective in early-stage disease, whereas locally advanced disease relies on treatment by radiation or chemoradiation. Surgery does provide the advantage of conservation of ovarian function.

Factors that influence the mode of treatment include stage, age, and health status. Radiation can be used for all stages, whereas surgery should only be considered an option for early-disease, stage I and stage IIA. A large randomized trial reported identical 5-year overall and disease-free survival rates when comparing radiation therapy with radical hysterectomy, but women who had surgery and adjuvant radiotherapy suffered significantly higher morbidity than those who had either surgery or radiotherapy alone.

There are clear advantages to surgery in women at low operative risk. Surgery permits conservation of ovarian function in premenopausal women and also reduces the risk of chronic bladder, bowel, and sexual dysfunction associated with radiotherapy. Complications in the hands of skilled surgeons are uncommon. Surgery also permits the assessment of risk factors, such as lymph node status, that will ultimately influence prognosis. Complications of surgery include fistulas (1%), lymphocyst, primary haemorrhage, and bladder injury. Chronic bowel and bladder problems that require medical or surgical intervention occur in up to 8–13% of women (54) due to parasympathetic denervation secondary to surgical clamping at the lateral excision margins. Surgery is commonly done by laparoscopy in modern practice, either by traditional techniques or robotically.

Stage IA disease

Microinvasive disease is one in which neoplastic cells invade from the epithelium to a maximum depth of 5 mm and a maximum horizontal spread of 7 mm. Any invasion beyond these dimensions upstages the disease to stage IB. The identification of early disease allows the selection of a group of women who are not at risk of lymph node disease and can be treated with less aggressive and, importantly, fertility-sparing therapy.

Box 62.2 FIGO staging of carcinoma of the cervix uteri (2019)

Stage I
The carcinoma is strictly confined to the cervix uteri (extension to the corpus should be disregarded)
- IA: invasive carcinoma that can be diagnosed only by microscopy, with maximum depth of invasion <5 mm:[a]
  - IA1: measured stromal invasion <3 mm in depth.
  - IA2: measured stromal invasion ≥3 mm and <5 mm in depth.
- IB: invasive carcinoma with measured deepest invasion ≥5 mm (greater than stage IA), lesion limited to the cervix uteri:[b]
  - IB1: invasive carcinoma ≥5 mm depth of stromal invasion and <2 cm in greatest dimension.
  - IB2: invasive carcinoma ≥2 cm and <4 cm in greatest dimension.
  - IB3: invasive carcinoma ≥4 cm in greatest dimension.

Stage II
The carcinoma invades beyond the uterus, but has not extended onto the lower third of the vagina or to the pelvic wall
- IIA: involvement limited to the upper two-thirds of the vagina without parametrial involvement:
  - IIA1: invasive carcinoma <4 cm in greatest dimension.
  - IIA2: invasive carcinoma ≥4 cm in greatest dimension
- IIB: with parametrial involvement but not up to the pelvic wall.

Stage III
The carcinoma involves the lower third of the vagina and/or extends to the pelvic wall and/or causes hydronephrosis or non-functioning kidney and/or involves pelvic and/or para-aortic lymph nodes.[c]
- IIIA: carcinoma involves the lower third of the vagina, with no extension to the pelvic wall.
- IIIB: extension to the pelvic wall and/or hydronephrosis or non-functioning kidney (unless known to be due to another cause).
- IIIC: involvement of pelvic and/or para-aortic lymph nodes, irrespective of tumour size and extent (with r and p notations):[c]
  - IIIC1: pelvic lymph node metastasis only.
  - IIIC2: para-aortic lymph node metastasis.

Stage IV
The carcinoma has extended beyond the true pelvis or has involved (biopsy proven) the mucosa of the bladder or rectum. A bullous oedema, as such, does not permit a case to be allotted to stage IV.
- IVA: spread of the growth to adjacent organs.
- IVB: spread to distant organs.

[a] Imaging and pathology can be used, when available, to supplement clinical findings with respect to tumour size and extent, in all stages.
[b] The involvement of vascular/lymphatic spaces does not change the staging. The lateral extent of the lesion is no longer considered.
[c] Adding notation of r (imaging) and p (pathology) to indicate the findings that are used to allocate the case to stage IIIC. For example, if imaging indicates pelvic lymph node metastasis, the stage allocation would be stage IIIC1r and, if confirmed by pathological findings, it would be stage IIIc1p. The type of imaging modality or pathology technique used should always be documented. When in doubt, the lower staging should be assigned.

Source data from Bhatla N, Berek JS, Cuello Fredes M, et al. Revised FIGO staging for carcinoma of the cervix uteri. *Int J Gynaecol Obstet* 2019;145:129–35.

Microinvasive disease comprises 20% of invasive cancers. Stage IA1 disease (invasion <3 mm) is rarely associated with lymph node metastases (**Table 62.4**). This disease should be formally diagnosed by cone biopsy or diathermy excision. Knife cone biopsy does not cause any thermal damage, and the extent of disease may be more accurately assessed than on a loop excision specimen. If the disease and any associated intraepithelial neoplasia are removed with clear margins, no further treatment is necessary. If disease is present at the margins, further excision or hysterectomy is required. A simple abdominal total hysterectomy is sufficient, as there is no risk of parametrial involvement. Because invasive disease of less than 3 mm invasion is associated with a very low risk of lymph node disease (Table 62.4), lymphadenectomy is not indicated. Lymphadenectomy should, however, be considered for stage IA2 (invasion 3–5 mm) disease as the rate of node involvement reaches 5%, particularly if the tumour is poorly differentiated.

Stage IB disease

Stage IB is divided into IB1 (≤4 cm diameter) and IB2 (≥4 cm diameter); stage IIA means upper vaginal, but not parametrial involvement.

Surgical therapy for stage IB and IIA tumours 4 cm or less in diameter usually involves radical hysterectomy and pelvic lymphadenectomy. Radical hysterectomy involves removing the tumour with adequate disease-free margins, by means of excising the parametrial tissue around the cervix and upper vagina, with removal of part or all of the cardinal and uterosacral ligaments, depending on the extent of the dissection. More radical dissections are associated with a higher incidence of perioperative morbidity and chronic bladder and bowel dysfunction with no survival advantage (55). Radical hysterectomy can be achieved laparoscopically, reducing the length of in-patient stay, blood loss, and perioperative morbidity and improving patient-reported outcomes.

The lymph node dissection should include obturator, internal, external, and common iliac nodes. The presence of suspicious lymph nodes on preoperative MRI in early-stage disease should dictate chemoradiation as a sole treatment modality. If there is any doubt of the nature of enlarged nodes, laparoscopic biopsy or PET imaging should be considered before the treatment plan is finally decided.

Lymphadenectomy may result in lymphocyst formation. Lymphoedema following pelvic lymphadenectomy can occur, and its incidence increases if adjuvant radiotherapy is given.

In cases in which positive nodes are encountered, there are differing views. Some would advocate abandoning surgery in favour of radical chemoradiation. Others would argue that, if possible, radical surgery should be completed to achieve an adjuvant setting for radiotherapy. If suspicious nodes are identified and confirmed to be diseased at frozen section, it is probably best to remove resectable nodes and treat with chemoradiation, including brachytherapy, which requires the uterus to be *in situ*. Radical surgery followed by radical radiotherapy is associated with increased morbidity.

Adjuvant radiotherapy is normally recommended for women with resected positive pelvic nodes to reduce the risk of recurrence. Patients with 'close' vaginal margins (≤0.5 cm) may also benefit from pelvic irradiation (56).

Indirect evidence from non-randomized studies suggests that radiotherapy can improve pelvic control, but there is no firm evidence of increased survival (55, 57). Careful preoperative radiological imaging reduces the risk of encountering unexpected lymphadenopathy or unexpectedly large tumours, with parametrial invasion.

Because bulky IB2 tumours have a higher risk of positive nodes and close surgical margins, these are now regarded by many as being better treated with chemoradiation as opposed to surgery or radiotherapy alone. Some women with small-volume stage IB disease who wish to conserve their fertility might be suitable for trachelectomy (radical excision of the cervix) combined with either laparoscopic or open lymphadenectomy. The most common approach is a vaginal trachelectomy; however, more recently some surgeons are favouring an abdominal approach facilitating greater excision of the parametrium with this technique. Meta-analyses and large United Kingdom case series based on the vaginal approach have demonstrated recurrence rates of around 4%, and a 70% term delivery rate (58, 59). Some surgeons recommend the insertion of an abdominal isthmic cervical cerclage to reduce the risk of late miscarriage. Indeed, in selected cases of IB1 disease that are just greater than 7 mm in horizontal spread, a large excisional biopsy may be adequate for central control, even though it may need to be combined with lymphadenectomy.

Stage IIB and above

It is not feasible to perform surgery with curative intent in these advanced stages of disease. Radical radiotherapy and chemoradiation are the only modalities of treatment that offer the potential for cure. One randomized trial has suggested that preoperative chemotherapy to shrink disease followed by radical surgery may be superior to radical radiotherapy, but this has not been confirmed (60). It is inevitable that preoperative chemotherapy followed by surgery will still require some women to undergo adjuvant or non-adjuvant radiotherapy that is more likely to result in unacceptable toxicity.

Radical radiotherapy

Radical radiotherapy is indicated for women unfit for surgery, or with bulky stage IB2 disease and more advanced disease. The goals of such treatment are to treat primary disease and to control metastatic pelvic lymph nodes. The radical dose is delivered by external beam and intracavitary treatment (brachytherapy). The standard technique now is of remote after-loading (e.g. using the Selectron). Intracavitary treatment is designed to give high doses locally to the primary site. External beam radiotherapy is designed to treat any pelvic spread. The challenge in administering radiotherapy is in achieving an optimal dose throughout the primary tumour and pelvic sidewall without causing high morbidity. The peripheral field of treatment of intracavitary radiotherapy delivers an insufficient dose to treat the pelvic sidewalls. The dose-limiting normal tissues within the pelvis are the rectum posteriorly, the bladder anteriorly, and any loops of small bowel within the pelvic radiation fields.

Prescribing rules have been devised for determining the precise dose of radiotherapy within the pelvis, and improved planning by CT has enabled more accurate targeting of external beam radiation in particular. An example is the Manchester system. This uses a number of predetermined source sizes and radioactive loadings such that a constant dose rate is delivered to a point A. Point A is defined as a point 2 cm lateral to the central axis of the uterus and 2 cm from the lateral fornix. A second point (B) lying in the same plane 3 cm lateral to point A is used to determine the dose to parametrial tissues. Following the insertion of the sources for each patient, a dose distribution is calculated. The total dose is a product of the dose rate and treatment time. The usual doses delivered are 70–80 Gy to point A and 60 Gy to point B, limiting the bladder and rectal dose to 60 Gy. To achieve this, it is necessary to have adequate packing to keep the bladder and bowel away from the intracavitary source. External beam radiation is usually given 2–3 weeks after intracavitary treatment to allow for involution of the primary disease. External beam radiotherapy is fractionated over 20–30 days' treatment, as this technique allows a cancericidal effect while enabling normal tissue recovery between fractions.

Routine extended field radiotherapy designed to include para-aortic nodes has not been proven to improve survival compared with pelvic radiotherapy alone, and it is associated with significantly more gastrointestinal complications (61). While there does not appear to be significant benefit from extended field irradiation for all cases, para-aortic node irradiation is appropriate in cases of proven para-aortic node involvement as indicated by diagnostic imaging or surgical staging.

Chemoradiation

Five randomized trials from the United States (62–66) have shown an overall survival advantage for cisplatin-based therapy given concurrently with radiation therapy. The patient populations in these studies included women with FIGO stages IB2–IVA cervical cancer treated with primary radiation therapy and women with FIGO stages I–IIA disease found to have poor prognostic factors (metastatic disease in pelvic lymph nodes, parametrial disease, or positive surgical margins) at the time of primary surgery. Although the trials vary somewhat in terms of stage of disease, dose of radiation, and schedule of cisplatin and radiation, they all demonstrate significant survival benefit for this combined approach, the risk of death from cervical cancer being decreased by 30%. These trials reported higher rates of short- and medium-term complications with chemoradiation, and although longer follow-up is required to examine the true morbidity of this treatment regimen, there is now international acceptance that chemoradiation is superior to radiation alone.

Recurrent cancer

Treatment for recurrent cervical cancer depends on the mode of primary therapy and the site of recurrence. Women who have had initial treatment by surgery should be considered for radiotherapy, and those who have had radiotherapy should be considered for exenterative surgery, provided the recurrence is central and there is no evidence of distant recurrence. These women require very careful preoperative assessment and counselling in order to understand the consequences of defunctioning surgery. Exenterative surgery in carefully selected cases can result in 5-year survival rates of 50%. Positive nodes at the time of attempted salvage surgery and positive resection margins are associated with a poor prognosis. Anterior exenteration requires excision of the bladder and most of the vagina en bloc with the recurrence, and posterior exenteration requires excision of the sigmoid rectum with formation of a colostomy. Sometimes a combination of the two is required. This type of surgery should only be undertaken by teams of highly skilled pelvic surgeons. Relapse within 2 years of primary treatment, the presence of hydronephrosis, and symptoms of pain are all associated with poorer outcomes in terms of exenterative surgery.

Palliation of progressive cervical cancer

Chemotherapy is palliative and should be reserved for patients who are not considered curable by the other two treatment modalities. Urinary tract symptoms are particularly common in advanced cervical disease. Ureteric obstruction with subsequent pain, infection, and ultimately impaired renal function are common features.

Mechanical diversion by nephrostomy or ureteric stenting is only usually justified as part of treatment with curative intent. Fistulas can occur in late-stage disease and can cause intolerable symptoms. If there is a prospect of surviving more than 8 weeks, palliative surgery should be offered in order to divert faeces or urine.

In progressive late-stage disease, there is usually ureteric obstruction, which heralds a terminal phase. Pain can be particularly distressing due to infiltration of the lumbosacral nerve plexuses. Meticulous attention to pain control and psychological and emotional support are essential.

REFERENCES

1. Ferlay J, Soerjomataram I, Ervik M, et al. GLOBOCAN 2012 v1.0, IARC CancerBase No. 11. IARC; 2013. Available at: http://globocan.iarc.fr.
2. Bosch FX, Manos MM, Munoz N, et al. Prevalence of human papillomavirus in cervical cancer: a worldwide perspective. International biological study on cervical cancer (IBSCC) Study Group. *J Natl Cancer Inst* 1995;**87**:796–802.
3. Franco EL, Rohan TE, Villa LL. Epidemiologic evidence and human papillomavirus infection as a necessary cause of cervical cancer. *J Natl Cancer Inst* 1999;**91**:506–11.
4. Schiffman M, Brinton LA, Devesa SS, Fraumeni JF Jr. Cervical cancer. In: Schottenfeld D, Fraumeni JF Jr (eds), *Cancer Epidemiology and Prevention*, pp. 1090–116. New York: Oxford University Press; 1996.
5. Walboomers JM, Jacobs MV, Manos MM, et al. Human papillomavirus is a necessary cause of invasive cervical cancer worldwide. *J Pathol* 1999;**189**:12–19.
6. IARC Working Group on the Evaluation of Carcinogenic Risk to Humans. *Human Papillomaviruses.* IARC Monographs on the Evaluation of Carcinogenic Risks to Humans, No. 90. Lyon: International Agency for Research on Cancer; 2007.
7. Wilson JMG, Jungner G. *Principles and Practice of Screening for Disease.* Geneva: World Health Organization; 1968.
8. Prendiville W, Denny L. Cancer of the cervix: early detection and cost effective solutions. *Int J Gynaecol Obstet* 2015;**131** Suppl 1:S28–32.
9. Arbyn M, Rebolj M, De Kok IM, et al. The challenges of organising cervical screening programmes in the 15 old member states of the European Union. *Eur J Cancer* 2009;**45**:2671–78.
10. Nanda K, McCrory DC, Myers ER, et al. Accuracy of the Papanicolaou test in screening for and follow-up of cervical cytologic abnormalities: a systematic review. *Ann Intern Med* 2000;**132**:810–19.
11. Basu P, Mittal S, Banerjee D, et al. Diagnostic accuracy of VIA and HPV detection as primary and sequential screening tests in a cervical cancer screening demonstration project in India. *Int J Cancer* 2015;**137**:859–67.
12. Sankaranarayanan R, Esmy PO, Rajkumar R, et al. Effect of visual screening on cervical cancer incidence and mortality in Tamil Nadu, India: a cluster-randomised trial. *Lancet* 2007;**370**:398–406.
13. Sauvaget C, Fayette JM, Muwonge R, Wesley R, Sankaranarayanan R. Accuracy of visual inspection with acetic acid for cervical cancer screening. *Int J Gynaecol Obstet* 2011;**113**:14–24.
14. Arbyn M, Roelens J, Simoens C, et al. Human papillomavirus testing versus repeat cytology for triage of minor cytological cervical lesions. *Cochrane Database Syst Rev* 2013;**3**:CD008054.
15. Ronco G, Dillner J, Elfstrom KM, et al. Efficacy of HPV-based screening for prevention of invasive cervical cancer: follow-up

of four European randomised controlled trials. *Lancet* 2014;**383**:524–32.

16. Sankaranarayanan R, Nene BM, Shastri SS, et al. HPV screening for cervical cancer in rural India. *N Engl J Med* 2009;**360**:1385–94.

17. Richart RM. Natural history of cervical intraepithelial neoplasia. *Clin Obstet Gynecol* 1968;**5**:748–84.

18. Bergeron C, Ronco G, Reuschenbach M, et al. The clinical impact of using p16(INK4a) immunochemistry in cervical histopathology and cytology: an update of recent developments. *Int J Cancer* 2015;**136**:2741–51.

19. Doorbar J, Quint W, Banks L, et al. The biology and life-cycle of human papillomaviruses. *Vaccine* 2012;**30** Suppl 5:F55–70.

20. Duensing S, Munger K. Mechanisms of genomic instability in human cancer: insights from studies with human papillomavirus oncoproteins. *Int J Cancer* 2004;**109**:157–62.

21. Strander B, Ellstrom-Andersson A, Franzen S, Milsom I, Radberg T. The performance of a new scoring system for colposcopy in detecting high-grade dysplasia in the uterine cervix. *Acta Obstet Gynecol Scand* 2005;**84**:1013–17.

22. Carcopino X, Mancini J, Charpin C, et al. Direct colposcopic vision used with the LLETZ procedure for optimal treatment of CIN: results of joint cohort studies. *Arch Gynecol Obstet* 2013;**288**:1087–94.

23. Shafi MI, Jordan JA, Singer A. The management of cervical intraepithelial neoplasia (squamous). In: Jordan JA, Singer A (eds), *The Cervix*, pp. 462–77. Oxford: Blackwell Publishing; 2006.

24. Anderson MC, Hartley RB. Cervical crypt involvement by intraepithelial neoplasia. *Obstet Gynecol* 1980;**55**:546–50.

25. Bornstein J, Sideri M, Tatti S, Walker P, Prendiville W, Haefner HK. 2011 terminology of the vulva of the International Federation for Cervical Pathology and Colposcopy. *J Low Genit Tract Dis* 2012;**16**:290–95.

26. Crisp WE, Asadourian L, Romberger W. Application of cryosurgery to gynecologic malignancy. *Obstet Gynecol* 1967;**30**:668–73.

27. World Health Organization (WHO). *Cryosurgical Equipment for the Treatment of Precancerous Cervical Lesions and Prevention of Cervical Cancer*. WHO Technical Specifications. Geneva: World Health Organization; 2012.

28. Duncan ID. The Semm cold coagulator in the management of cervical intraepithelial neoplasia. *Clin Obstet Gynecol* 1983;**26**:996–1006.

29. Duncan ID. Destruction of cervical intraepithelial neoplasia at 100°C with the Semm coagulator. In: Heintz APM, Griffiths CT, Trimbos JB (eds), *Surgery in Gynecological Oncology*, pp. 71–85. The Hague: Martinus Nijhoff Publisher; 1984.

30. Gordon HK, Duncan ID. Effective destruction of cervical intraepithelial neoplasia (CIN) 3 at 100 degrees C using the Semm cold coagulator: 14 years experience. *Br J Obstet Gynaecol* 1991;**98**:14–20.

31. Haddad NG, Hussein IY, Blessing K, Kerr-Wilson R, Smart GE. Tissue destruction following cold coagulation of the cervix. *Colposcopy Gynecol Laser Surg* 1988;**4**:23–27.

32. Semple D, Saha A, Maresh M. Colposcopy and treatment of cervical intra-epithelial neoplasia: are national standards achievable? *Br J Obstet Gynaecol* 1999;**106**:351–55.

33. Camargo MJ, Russomano FB, Tristao MA, Huf G, Prendiville W. Large loop versus straight-wire excision of the transformation zone for treatment of cervical intraepithelial neoplasia: a randomised controlled trial of electrosurgical techniques. *BJOG* 2015;**122**:552–57.

34. Arbyn M, Kyrgiou M, Simoens C, et al. Perinatal mortality and other severe adverse pregnancy outcomes associated with treatment of cervical intraepithelial neoplasia: meta-analysis. *BMJ* 2008;**337**:a1284.

35. Prendiville W, Cullimore J, Norman S. Large loop excision of the transformation zone (LLETZ). A new method of management for women with cervical intraepithelial neoplasia. *Br J Obstet Gynaecol* 1989;**96**:1054–60.

36. Castanon A, Landy R, Brocklehurst P, et al. Risk of preterm delivery with increasing depth of excision for cervical intraepithelial neoplasia in England: nested case-control study. *BMJ* 2014;**349**:g6223.

37. Khalid S, Dimitriou E, Conroy R, et al. The thickness and volume of LLETZ specimens can predict the relative risk of pregnancy-related morbidity. *BJOG* 2012;**119**:685–91.

38. Kyrgiou M, Mitra A, Arbyn M, et al. Fertility and early pregnancy outcomes after treatment for cervical intraepithelial neoplasia: systematic review and meta-analysis. *BMJ* 2014;**349**:g6192.

39. Strander B, Adolfsson J. Safety of modern treatment for cervical pre-cancer. *BMJ* 2014;**349**:g6611.

40. Martin-Hirsch PP, Paraskevaidis E, Bryant A, Dickinson HO. Surgery for cervical intraepithelial neoplasia. *Cochrane Database Syst Rev* 2013;**12**:CD001318.

41. Strander B, Andersson-Ellstrom A, Milsom I, Sparen P. Long term risk of invasive cancer after treatment for cervical intraepithelial neoplasia grade 3: population based cohort study. *BMJ* 2007;**335**:1077.

42. Ghaem-Maghami S, Sagi S, Majeed G, Soutter WP. Incomplete excision of cervical intraepithelial neoplasia and risk of treatment failure: a meta-analysis. *Lancet Oncol* 2007;**8**:985–93.

43. Flannelly G, Bolger B, Fawzi H, De Lopes AB, Monaghan JM. Follow up after LLETZ: could schedules be modified according to risk of recurrence? *BJOG* 2001;**108**:1025–30.

44. Delgado G, Bundy BN, Fowler WC, et al. A prospective surgical pathological study of stage I squamous carcinoma of the cervix: a Gynecologic Oncology Group study. *Gynecol Oncol* 1989;**35**:314–20.

45. Zaino RJ, Ward S, Delgado G, et al. Histopathologic predictors of the behavior of surgically treated stage IB squamous cell carcinoma of the cervix. A Gynecologic Oncology Group study. *Cancer* 1992;**69**:1750–58.

46. Stehman FB, Bundy BN, DiSaia PJ, et al. Carcinoma of the cervix treated with radiation therapy. I. A multivariate analysis of prognostic variables in the Gynecologic Oncology Group. *Cancer* 1991;**67**:2776–85.

47. Boyce J, Fruchter R, Nicastri AD, et al. Prognostic factors in stage I carcinoma of the cervix. *Gynecol Oncol* 1981;**12**:154–65.

48. Inoue T, Okumura M. Prognostic significance of parametrial extension in patients with cervical carcinoma stages IB, IIA, and IIB. A study of 628 cases treated by radical hysterectomy and lymphadenectomy with or without postoperative irradiation. *Cancer* 1984;**54**:1714–19.

49. Lohe KJ. Early squamous cell carcinoma of the uterine cervix. *Gynecol Oncol* 1978;**6**:10–30.

50. van Nagell J, Donaldson ES, Wood EG, Parker JC. The significance of vascular invasion and lymphocytic infiltration in invasive cervical cancer. *Cancer* 1978;**41**:228–34.

51. Tinga DJ, Timmer PR, Bouma J, Aalders JG. Prognostic significance of single versus multiple lymph node metastases in cervical carcinoma stage IB. *Gynecol Oncol* 1990;**39**:175–80.

52. Nahhas WA, Sharkey FE, Whitney CW, et al. The prognostic significance of vascular channel involvement and deep stromal penetration in early cervical carcinoma. *Am J Clin Oncol* 1983;**6**:259–64.

53. Scheidler J, Hricak H, Yu KK, et al. Radiological evaluation of lymph node metastases in patients with cervical cancer. A meta-analysis. *J Am Med Assoc* 1997;**278**:1096–101.

54. Landoni F, Maneo A, Colombo A, et al. Randomised study of radical surgery versus radiotherapy for stage IB–IIA cervical cancer. *Lancet* 1997;**350**:535–40.

55. Soisson AP, Soper JT, Clarke Pearson DL, et al. Adjuvant radiotherapy following radical hysterectomy for patients with stage IB and IIA cervical cancer. *Gynecol Oncol* 1990;**37**:390–95.

56. Landoni F, Maneo A, Cormio G, et al. Class II versus class III radical hysterectomy in stage IB–IIA cervical cancer: a prospective randomized study. *Gynecol Oncol* 2001;**80**:3–12.

57. Kinney WK, Alvarez RD, Reid GC, et al. Value of adjuvant whole-pelvis irradiation after Wertheim hysterectomy for early-stage squamous carcinoma of the cervix with pelvic nodal metastasis: a matched-control study. *Gynecol Oncol* 1989;**34**:258–62.

58. Plante M, Renaud MC, Hoskins IA, Roy M. Vaginal radical trachelectomy: a valuable fertility-preserving option in the management of early-stage cervical cancer. A series of 50 pregnancies and review of the literature. *Gynecol Oncol* 2005;**98**:3–10.

59. Shepherd JH, Spencer C, Herod J, Ind TE. Radical vaginal trachelectomy as a fertility-sparing procedure in women with early-stage cervical cancer: cumulative pregnancy rate in a series of 123 women. *BJOG* 2006;**113**:719–24.

60. Sardi JE, Giaroli A, di Paola G, et al. Long-term follow-up of the first randomized trial using neoadjuvant chemotherapy in stage IB squamous carcinoma of the cervix: the final results. *Gynecol Oncol* 1997;**67**:61–69.

61. Haie C, Pejovic MH, Gerbaulet A, et al. Is prophylactic para-aortic irradiation worthwhile in the treatment of advanced cervical carcinoma? Results of a control-led clinical trial of the EORTC radiotherapy group. *Radiother Oncol* 1988;**11**:101–12.

62. Whitney CW, Sause W, Bundy BN, et al. Randomized comparison of fluorouracil plus cisplatin versus hydroxyurea as an adjunct to radiation therapy in stage IIB–IVA carcinoma of the cervix with negative para-aortic lymph nodes: a Gynecologic Oncology Group and Southwest Oncology Group study. *J Clin Oncol* 1999;**17**:1339–48.

63. Morris M, Eifel PJ, Lu J, et al. Pelvic radiation with concurrent chemotherapy compared with pelvic and paraaortic radiation for high-risk cervical cancer. *N Engl J Med* 1999;**340**:1137–43.

64. Rose PG, Bundy BN, Watkins EB, et al. Concurrent cisplatin-based radiotherapy and chemotherapy for locally advanced cervical cancer. *N Engl J Med* 1999;**340**:1144–53.

65. Keys HM, Bundy BN, Stehman FB, et al. Cisplatin, radiation, and adjuvant hysterectomy compared with radiation and adjuvant hysterectomy for bulky stage IB cervical carcinoma. *N Engl J Med* 1999;**340**:1154–61.

66. Peters WA 3rd, Liu PY, Barrett RJ 2nd, et al. Concurrent chemotherapy and pelvic radiation therapy compared with pelvic radiation therapy alone as adjuvant therapy after radical surgery in high-risk early-stage cancer of the cervix. *J Clin Oncol* 2000;**18**:1606–13.

63

Uterine cancer

Nomonde H. Mbatani and Dominic G.D. Richards

Introduction

Uterine cancers (**Figure 63.1**) are the most common female genital cancer in the developed world and the fourth most common malignancy in women. In South Africa and most developing countries it is the second most common genital tract malignancy after cervical carcinoma. While the incidence of uterine cancers is marginally higher in developed countries (5.9 vs 4 per 100,000), the disease-specific mortality rate is higher in developing countries (1).

Uterine cancers include tumours that develop in the endometrium (carcinomas), the endometrial support cells (endometrial stromal sarcomas), and the myometrium (sarcomas) (**Table 63.1**). Endometrial carcinomas represent over 90% of uterine cancers, the incidence of which is increasing and is most likely driven by longer life expectancy, obesity, and a sedentary lifestyle. Most endometrial carcinomas present in postmenopausal women; however, in women with significant risk factors (such as unopposed endogenous oestrogen production as occurs in women with polycystic ovarian syndrome) or a genetic predisposition such as hereditary non-polyposis colorectal cancer (HNPCC)/Lynch 2 syndrome, tumours may present before the age of 40 years.

Sarcomas constitute less than 10% of uterine cancers, the majority of which are leiomyosarcomas. Only 2% of uterine sarcomas originate in the endometrial stromal tissue. Most sarcomas present between the age of 40 and 60 years. For the purpose of this chapter, endometrial carcinomas and sarcomas will be discussed separately.

Endometrial carcinomas

Endometrial carcinomas present at a mean age of 63 years, however 4% of women with endometrial carcinoma are younger than 40, which has significant quality of life implications associated with childbearing and premature menopause related to treatment. Almost all endometrial tumours present with abnormal uterine or postmenopausal bleeding and with prompt intervention they are frequently diagnosed in the early stage and have 5-year survival rates over 95% (2).

Classification of endometrial carcinomas

In 1983, Bokhman classified carcinoma of the endometrium into two distinct groups (3). The first group described a group of tumours that originated in women with metabolic disturbances that include obesity, varying degrees of glucose intolerance, hyperoestrogenism and hyperlipidaemia. These tumours developed in a hyperplastic endometrium, were well to moderately differentiated, were less aggressive, and usually had a favourable prognosis. Tumours in Bokhman's second group were noted to be more aggressive, to have a greater chance of lymphatic spread, have higher recurrence rates, and the prognosis was less favourable than the first group. This dichotomous model has definite limitations due to heterogeneity within the two groups. Fortunately, advances in histological and immunohistochemical assessment of endometrial carcinomas have allowed these tumours to be more appropriately classified into high-risk and low-risk histological subtypes (**Table 63.2**).

The low-risk group incorporates tumours that have progressed through a stage of intraepithelial neoplasia (atypical endometrial hyperplasia) and so have maintained some degree of similarity to the parent tissue exhibiting varying degrees of endometrial gland formation and are thus described as endometrioid. The International Federation of Gynecology and Obstetrics (FIGO) provided a grading system of endometrioid carcinomas in 1988 that classified them into well (grade 1), moderately (grade 2), and poorly (grade 3) differentiated tumours, based on the progressive loss of glandular architecture leading to increasing solid growth patterns, as well as the degree of nuclear atypia. Low-risk tumours include either well-differentiated or moderately differentiated endometrioid cancers and may exhibit genetic alterations including microsatellite instability and mutations in the *PTEN, KRAS*, and beta-catenin genes. They do not exhibit mutations in the *TP53* gene. Poorly differentiated (grade 3) endometrioid carcinomas, while still being endometrioid by definition, bear little resemblance to endometrial glandular tissue. They have a greater chance of lymphatic spread, are more aggressive and often exhibit p53 mutation. For this reason, grade 3 endometrioid cancer is included in the high-risk group of endometrial cancers.

The high-risk groups of tumours, while still originating from glandular epithelium, usually develop in an atrophic endometrium and display morphology that is structurally different from endometrial tissue. This group includes serous carcinomas and clear cell carcinomas. Both these exhibit *TP53* gene mutations and chromosomal instability (4). Two additions to the high-risk group include poorly differentiated (grade 3) endometrioid carcinoma and carcinosarcoma. Carcinosarcoma, which was previously classified

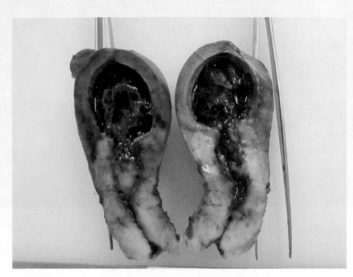

Figure 63.1 Uterine cancer.

as a uterine sarcoma, is now regarded as a carcinoma that has undergone metaplastic sarcomatous differentiation. It is a highly aggressive tumour with its carcinomatous component usually contributing to metastatic spread and is thus included in the high-risk group (5).

The majority of women with endometrial carcinoma have grade 1 and 2 endometrioid tumours and frequently present with early-stage disease and have excellent outcomes. The remaining 10–20% who are diagnosed with carcinomas of high-risk histology usually present in the late sixth and seventh decades. They often have more advanced disease and in over 50% of cases the disease has spread beyond the uterine corpus at the time of diagnosis. Five-year survival rates in this group are significantly poorer and range between 40% and 60%.

Risk factors

Risk factors for developing endometrial cancer can be divided into lifestyle factors, medical conditions, and hereditary factors. Medical conditions which are associated with the development of endometrial cancers are often sequelae of lifestyle factors, which are now becoming more evident in developing countries. Extreme body mass index, diabetes mellitus, hypertension, polycystic ovarian syndrome, early menarche, late menopause, infertility or nulliparity, unopposed oestrogen therapy, postmenopausal use of tamoxifen, oestrogen-secreting tumours, and HNPCC are all associated with

Table 63.1 Uterine malignancies

Glandular Epithelium	Mucinous adenocarcinoma Serous adenocarcinoma Clear cell adenocarcinoma Carcinosarcoma
Supporting Endometrial Stroma/Mesenchymal cells	1. Endometrial stromal sarcoma (previously lLow-grade endometrial stromal sarcoma) 2. Undifferentiated sarcoma (previously high-grade endometrial stromal sarcoma) 3. Adenosarcoma
Myometrium:	Leiomyosarcoma

Table 63.2 Histological subtypes of endometrial carcinoma

Type 1	Type 2
Grade 1 endometrioid adenocarcinoma Grade 2 endometrioid adenocarcinoma	Grade 3 endometrioid adenocarcinoma Serous adenocarcinoma Clear cell adenocarcinoma Carcinosarcoma Undifferentiated carcinoma
Common genetic defects: *KRAS, BRAF, PTEN*, beta-catenin, mismatch repair defects (MMR)	*TP53*

an increased risk. The highest lifestyle-related risk is obesity (relative risk 2.54; 95% confidence interval 2.11–3.06) (6). Women who have inherited a HNPCC gene mutation have a 40–60% lifetime risk of developing endometrial carcinoma and a 9–12% risk of developing ovarian carcinoma due to defects in the DNA mismatch repair genes *MLH1, MSH2, MSH6*, and *PMS2* (7). A recent study has found that young patients with endometriosis have a 40% risk of developing endometrial cancer later on in life, the majority of these being type 1 (8). Pregnancy, use of the combined oral contraceptive pill, and cigarette smoking which either decrease oestrogen or increase progesterone levels have been shown to decrease the risk of endometrial cancer.

Screening for endometrial cancer

Evidence does not support screening for endometrial cancer in a low-risk population as most cases cannot be avoided. There is no standard screening test. Ultrasonographic measurement of the endometrial thickness in low-risk asymptomatic women, may result in unnecessary interventions to sample the endometrium with potential procedure related complications and patient anxiety. To decrease the incidence of disease in the low-risk population, health professionals should rather focus on promoting healthy lifestyle choices, diagnosing and managing manifestations of the metabolic syndrome, and educating patients on the importance of having abnormal uterine or postmenopausal bleeding assessed.

Where tamoxifen is prescribed to postmenopausal women as part of breast cancer treatment, women should be counselled about the risk of endometrial polyps, hyperplasia, and endometrial cancer and that they should report any abnormal bleeding immediately. Tamoxifen has been reported to cause endometrial abnormalities in as many as 39% of women (9). The Mirena intrauterine system (IUS) has been used for endometrial protection. Although studies have not shown significant progesterone-associated risks of breast cancer development and carcinogenesis in breast cancer survivors with the use of Mirena, there are still concerns about oncogenic effects of any progestogens (10–12). Results from a small (*n*= 94) randomized controlled trial by Wong et al. could not demonstrate increased rates of recurrences nor breast cancer-related deaths amongst patients who were offered levonorgestrel as prophylaxis compared to non-users (13). There is no good evidence to support the use of the levonorgestrel IUS (Mirena) as a preventative measure in these women (14).

Women who are deemed high risk for developing endometrial cancer include carriers of the HNPCC mutation, women from families where there is a known mutation or where there is a strong history of colon cancer exhibiting an autosomal dominant penetration. Consensus guidelines from the joint European Societies of Medical Oncology, Gynaecological Oncology, and Radiotherapy and Oncology conference (14) recommend the following:

- Annual surveillance of the endometrium by gynaecological examination, transvaginal ultrasound, and aspiration biopsy starting at 35 years and should continue annually.
- Consider insertion of a levonorgestrel-releasing IUS.
- Prophylactic surgery using a minimally invasive approach should be discussed at the age of 40 years to prevent endometrial and ovarian cancer. The complications associated with surgical procedures as well as the uncertainty about the gains of prophylactic surgery should be discussed with honesty (15).

Endometrial hyperplasia

Endometrial hyperplasia is an abnormal proliferation of the endometrium and is driven by excessive levels of oestrogen, whether exogenous such as unopposed hormone therapy or endogenous from cyclical aromatization of androgens to oestrogens in excessive peripheral adipose tissue found in overweight women. A body mass index greater than 40 kg/m² has been shown to increase the risk of atypical endometrial hyperplasia by 13-fold (9). Abnormal or uterine bleeding is the hallmark of presentation because of an unstable, proliferative endometrial lining. Endometrial sampling should be performed in women who present with abnormal bleeding over the age of 40 years, and in women younger than 40 with significant risk factors for endometrial cancer, including obesity and any suggestion or evidence of a hereditary mutation.

Histologically, endometrial hyperplasia is assessed architecturally as simple (ordered) or complex (disordered), and cytologically as being atypical or not. The most significant finding in the histological report is the presence of atypical cells, irrespective of the architecture as complex atypical hyperplasia is the immediate precursor lesion of endometrial carcinoma. The risk of progression from complex atypical hyperplasia to invasive carcinoma is 29% compared to 8% in simple atypical hyperplasia and less than 3% in non-atypical hyperplasia (16). Atypical hyperplastic endometrium may already harbour a focus of invasive endometrioid carcinoma which may not have been sampled, especially when using blind sampling techniques. Differentiating between atypical hyperplasia and low-grade endometrioid carcinoma is often difficult and the opinion of an experienced gynaecological pathologist may be useful.

Endometrial hyperplasia can be managed medically or with surgery. The choice of method is based on age, comorbid status, desire to retain fertility, and the presence of atypia. It is important to address potential sources of excessive oestrogen including obesity and to exclude oestrogen-secreting ovarian tumours in the management of endometrial hyperplasia.

Management of hyperplasia

Medical treatment

Endometrial hyperplasia without atypia can be managed medically using systemic or local progestins. Oral medroxyprogesterone acetate (10–20 mg daily) or megestrol acetate (160–320 mg daily) can be prescribed in either continuous or cyclical regimes. Response rates with medical therapy are good with positive responses seen after 3 months of treatment and complete response rates usually by 6 months to 1 year. Side effects of progestin therapy include weight gain, oedema, headaches, dizziness, and lack of libido are less common with local progestin therapy. The levonorgestrel-releasing IUS has been proven effective, and even superior, to oral medication in managing hyperplasia with and without atypia (17). Where there is no response to therapy after 6 months, progression to atypical hyperplasia, or unacceptable side effects, surgery should be considered.

Surgical management

In patients who are not medically fit to undergo surgery, progestin therapy must be prescribed (9). Endometrial hyperplasia where atypia is present is best managed by simple hysterectomy using minimally invasive techniques where possible. Bilateral salpingo-oophorectomy should be considered in postmenopausal women. Endometrial ablation and resection may be considered in women with complex non-atypical hyperplasia where medical therapy has failed and hysterectomy carries excessive risk or is against the patient's wishes. However, where atypical hyperplasia is present, ablative techniques are not recommended.

Clinical features of endometrial carcinoma

The most common symptom of endometrial carcinoma is abnormal uterine bleeding. The bleeding may be postmenopausal or in pre- and perimenopausal women it may be intermenstrual or prolonged bleeding. A thorough history, which includes a detailed menstrual history, recent cervical smear results, past and current use of hormone therapy, medical conditions, and family history of cancer and hereditary cancer syndromes must be taken. A full clinical examination should be performed which includes assessment of peripheral lymph node groups, examination of the breasts, abdominal examination, external and speculum examination of the lower genital tract, plus bimanual examination of the upper genital tract. Careful assessment of adnexal masses, uterine size and mobility, nodularity or masses in the pouch of Douglas, and parametrial disease are important to assess possible extrauterine spread and resectability.

Where no obvious cause of bleeding is detected on physical examination, the upper genital tract must be assessed using pelvic ultrasound scanning. Premenopausal women with significant risk factors for endometrial cancer and women over the age of 40 years must undergo histological endometrial assessment. There is no defined upper limit of endometrial thickness in premenopausal women, thus screening using sonographic endometrial thickness is not recommended. However, in premenopausal woman suspicion for hyperplasia or malignancy is increased when the endometrial thickness is greater than 12 mm. Office sampling using a flexible plastic endometrial sampler is adequate. A meta-analysis of sampling devices concluded that the Pipelle was the most sensitive device in detecting endometrial cancer (91–99%) and highly specific (98%) (18). In patients where office sampling is not successful, hysteroscopy is an excellent alternative and offers both visualization of the entire endometrial cavity and allows directed biopsy of any suspicious lesions.

In postmenopausal women, where bleeding is associated with an endometrial thickness greater than 5 mm, endometrial sampling must be performed. In women reporting a single episode of postmenopausal bleeding without significant risk factors, with a normal clinical examination and normal cervical cytology and an endometrial thickness less than 5 mm, sampling is not indicated (19). Studies have investigated the relationship between endometrial thickness and the risk of malignancy. Overall, using a cut-off value of 5 mm to perform endometrial sampling would offer satisfactory sensitivity with a false-negative rate of less than 1% (19). However, repeated episodes of postmenopausal bleeding, even where the endometrial thickness is less than 5 mm, must be histologically assessed as high-risk histological carcinomas develop in an atrophic endometrium (20). In such cases hysteroscopy may better assess an atrophic cavity. One study by Chandavarker et al. reported a diagnosis of either type 1 or type 2 endometrial cancer in 90 out of a total of 250 (36%) patients diagnosed with endometrial cancer, who had a prior endometrial stripe with a thickness not more than 4 mm (21).

Other less common presenting symptoms may include a pelvic mass, lower abdominal pain, and manifestations of metastatic disease including vaginal or vulval tumours or respiratory complaints. Not too infrequently, women may present to other disciplines with venous thromboembolic phenomena and on further investigation an endometrial malignancy may be diagnosed.

Cervical smears that report the presence of atypical glandular cells in an otherwise asymptomatic woman necessitate careful pelvic, colposcopic, and endometrial assessment. The presence of endometrial cells on a cervical smear in asymptomatic postmenopausal women also warrants investigation.

Further investigations following a diagnosis of endometrial cancer

Histological specimens reporting endometrial cancers or atypical hyperplastic endometrium, where possible, should be evaluated by an experienced gynaepathologist. Subtle differences in the continuum between atypical hyperplasia and endometrial cancer as well as the assessment of the grade of differentiation may not always be clear. Appropriate immunohistochemical staining techniques may also be required to differentiate between primary endocervical adenocarcinomas and endometrial adenocarcinomas and between uterine and ovarian serous carcinomas.

Biochemical and radiological preoperative investigations include the following:

- Full blood count.
- Liver function tests, specifically alkaline phosphatase and gamma-glutamyl transferase.
- Urea, electrolytes, and renal function tests.
- Random blood glucose (to exclude undiagnosed diabetes mellitus).
- CA125 (has been shown to correlate with extrauterine spread in high-grade tumour but a consensus opinion is that there is no evidence to support the use of serum tumour markers in endometrial cancer) (14, 22).
- Imaging (dependent on local resources, institutional indications for staging lymphadenectomy, and whether fertility preservation is a treatment goal):
  - Pelvic ultrasound to determine tumour size, assess adnexa, cervical involvement, and depth of tumour invasion into the myometrium.
  - Pelvic magnetic resonance imaging (MRI) to size tumour and assess pelvic spread, myometrial invasion, cervical involvement, and pelvic lymphadenopathy

  - Computed tomography (CT) scan of chest, abdomen, and pelvis to investigate distant metastases to lung and liver, exclude hydronephrosis, assess peritoneal spread, and pelvic, para-aortic, mediastinal, and hilar lymphadenopathy.
  - In low-income countries, a chest X-ray and abdominal ultrasound are often the only available and affordable options.
  - CT-positron emission tomography, where available, has a high specificity but low sensitivity in excluding lymph node disease.

2009 FIGO staging of endometrial carcinoma

Endometrial cancer is staged surgically. In 2009, the Gynecological Oncology Group of FIGO published a revision of the 1988 staging system of endometrial carcinoma. This new system is felt to be a more accurate staging instrument and thus a better prognostic tool than its predecessor (Table 63.3) (23).

Surgical staging includes removal of the uterus and adnexae. A systematic pelvic with or without para-aortic lymphadenectomy should be performed in patients with high-risk tumour features such as grade 3 differentiation, non-endometrioid histology, cervical stromal invasion, lymphovascular system space invasion (LVSI), and where the tumour invades more than 50% of the myometrial thickness.

Cytological examination of peritoneal washings or free abdominal fluid is reported separately and does not upstage the woman. Malignant cells in peritoneal fluid have not been shown to be of prognostic significance (24).

Treatment of endometrioid endometrial cancer

The primary management of endometrial cancer is surgery.

Surgery

Surgery in endometrial cancer aims to remove the primary tumour, to perform comprehensive staging, and, in advanced abdominal disease, to achieve optimal cytoreduction where feasible. Surgery with curative intent may not always be possible where:

- there are patient-related factors such as extreme cachexia, extreme obesity, severe cardiorespiratory compromise, or recent acute pulmonary embolism or venous thromboembolism
- there is unequivocal (cytological or histological) evidence of parenchymal liver or lung metastases as well as lymph node involvement
- clinical or radiological examination suggests that pelvic or abdominal disease is not resectable.

Prior to implementing any form of treatment, each patient must be individualized:

- Fertility desires and surgical menopause in women under the age of 40 years must be discussed (see 'Fertility-sparing options').
- Suitability for surgery must be assessed. Elderly, frail women and women with severe comorbidities may require assessment and optimization by a physician, geriatrician, and anaesthetist.
- The need for systematic lymphadenectomy must be determined. This may be determined by preoperative factors or by intraoperative assessment of the tumour (see 'Lymphadenectomy in endometrial cancer').

Table 63.3 The 2009 FIGO staging of endometrial carcinoma

Stage I	Tumour confined to the corpus uteri
IA	No or less than half myometrial invasion
IB	Invasion equal to or more than half of the myometrium
Stage II	Tumour invades cervical stroma, but does not extend beyond uterus
Stage III	Local and/or regional spread of the tumour
IIIA	Tumour invades the serosa of the corpus uteri and/or adnexae
IIIB	Vaginal and/or parametrial involvement
IIIC	Metastases to pelvic and/or para-aortic lymph nodes
IIIC1	Positive pelvic nodes
IIIC2	Positive para-aortic nodes irrespective of pelvic node status
Stage IV	Tumour invades bladder and/or bowel mucosa, and/or distant metastasis
IVA	Tumour invasion of bladder or rectal mucosa
IVB	Distant metastases, including intra-abdominal metastases and/or inguinal lymph nodes

Source data from 2009 FIGO staging of endometrial carcinoma.

- The extent of surgery must be tailored to each woman. Laparoscopic and vaginal routes may need to be considered. A shorter surgical time and less morbid surgical route may be necessitated by co-morbid disease or cardiorespiratory compromise. Intraoperative limitations in access or visibility due to visceral and abdominal wall adipose tissue may also make the procedure unnecessarily challenging. In certain cases, systematic lymphadenectomy, though indicated, may need to be abandoned.

Conventional surgery should include:

- a midline abdominal incision for non-endometrioid subtypes or where preoperative investigations suggest upper abdominal disease
- careful and bloodless entry to the peritoneal cavity
- peritoneal washings or sampling of free fluid
- abdominal survey exploring the entire peritoneal cavity in a systematic manner looking for tumour deposits and enlarged lymph nodes
- extrafascial hysterectomy with or without a vaginal cuff
- bilateral salpingo-oophorectomy
- removal of all suspicious or enlarged pelvic and para-aortic nodes
- infracolic omentectomy, to be considered in cases with serous histology (14)
- systematic lymphadenectomy, where indicated by institutional policy, based either on preoperative or intraoperative tumour assessment
- a maximal effort at cytoreduction (where feasible) has been shown to improve progression-free and overall survival rates (25).

Further surgical considerations include the following:

- *Obesity* is a major risk factor for endometrial cancer and a lower transverse incision is more suited to patients with clinically early-stage, low-grade disease. This group of patients seldom require systematic lymphadenectomy and rarely have extrapelvic disease. Wound complications, incisional hernias, and complications related to impaired mobility are less.

- *Laparoscopic surgery*: laparoscopy offers great benefit to obese women. It has been extensively researched and is widely used to manage endometrial cancer. For laparoscopy to be an effective alternative, it needs to be as safe and have equivalent oncological outcomes to open surgery. The Gynecologic Oncology Group (GOG) LAP2 trial showed that intraoperative surgical complication rates were similar between the patients who had laparotomy and those who had the laparoscopic approach. The laparoscopic group had significantly less minor postoperative complications and most women were discharged 2 days after surgery (26). A follow-up study of the LAP2 trial and a 2009 meta-analysis of trials comparing open and laparoscopic surgery found that the laparoscopic route did not significantly disadvantage oncological outcomes (27, 28). Retrospective studies have shown robotic surgery to have equivalent oncological outcomes to a laparoscopic approach (29).

- *Routine radical hysterectomy* for overt stage II tumours is not of survival benefit and increases intraoperative and postoperative complications (14). Women with stage II disease will receive adjuvant local radiation and any residual microscopic parametrial disease will be sterilized. Removal of the parametrium should only be considered when there is palpable parametrial spread and radical surgery will achieve clear margins.

- *Synchronous ovarian tumours* are a rare occurrence and more common in younger women. They are frequently of endometrioid histology and to decide whether they are metastatic spread from a primary endometrial tumour or a *de novo* ovarian carcinoma is challenging. In a study of 17 women under 45 years with endometrial cancer, 29.4% had synchronous ovarian tumours compared to 4.6% in women over 45 years (30). In these cases, ovarian preservation is not appropriate. Each tumour site needs to be viewed as an independent cancer and managed with the appropriate surgical and adjuvant therapies.

- A *vaginal approach* should be offered in women fit for anaesthesia, but where abdominal surgery is not safe or achievable. Hysterectomy and bilateral adnexectomy should be possible using this route.

- *Oophorectomy in young women*: there is significant morbidity and mortality associated with removal of ovaries in young women. Not performing bilateral oophorectomy in those under 45 years without a significant hereditary risk and with grade 1 early-stage endometrial disease has not been shown to impact overall survival. Salpingectomy should still be performed (14).

- *Palliative hysterectomy* should be considered, where safe and feasible, in advanced disease to alleviate vaginal bleeding, offensive discharge, and pain. Patients with carcinosarcoma frequently present with distant metastases but also have a rapidly enlarging uterus often with a fungating and necrotic tumour mass protruding through the cervix. In selected patients, quality of life can certainly be improved by removing the uterus.

Lymphadenectomy

The main purpose of lymphadenectomy in endometrial cancer is surgical staging and should be considered in women with intermediate (stage I low-grade tumours with >50% invasion or grade 3 tumours with <50% invasion) or high-risk factors. However, lymphadenectomy also provides important prognostic information and is essential in evaluating the need for adjuvant therapy.

As with all gynaecological cancers, suspicious or enlarged lymph nodes detected at surgery should be removed, or at least sampled if removal is deemed unsafe (i.e. a node densely adherent to a major vessel). Systematic lymphadenectomy is probably the most controversial topic in the management of endometrial cancer. There has been much debate in terms of the indications, extent, and therapeutic and survival benefits of systematic lymphadenectomy.

As the majority of women with endometrial cancer present with early-stage low-grade disease, hysterectomy and bilateral salpingo-oophorectomy is sufficient treatment to achieve cure. Two randomized trials have shown that performing a routine systematic lymphadenectomy on these women offers no survival (31, 32). Such practice is unnecessary and increases intra- and postoperative complication rates. A 2015 European Consensus Conference strongly recommends against performing systematic lymphadenectomy in these women (14). However, the studies on which the current rationale for lymphadenectomy is based have been criticized for a number of reasons including:

- low node yields
- not including or only sampling the para-aortic nodes
- most study participants had early-stage low-risk cancers where lymphadenectomy would not have been of benefit
- a heterogeneous population in terms of tumour characteristics combining endometrioid and non-endometrioid subtypes and grade 1 and 2 with grade 3 tumours
- women were randomized to adjuvant radiotherapy regardless of the results of the lymphadenectomy.

Indications for a lymph node dissection

Systematic lymphadenectomy is performed based on specific indications. These indications try to exclude early-stage low-risk tumours where lymphadenectomy would be of no benefit. The indications have been determined using the results of various trials on endometrial cancer and they may be based on both preoperative and intraoperative factors. Exact indications for systematic lymphadenectomy are often institution dependent and are determined by resources and personal interpretation of controversial and contradicting data (Table 63.4).

Certain intraoperative factors are established using frozen section. This requires the presence of a gynaepathologist in theatre which

may not always be possible, especially in developing countries. As an alternative, intraoperative sectioning of the uterus (preferably in the coronal plane) with visual assessment of the depth of myometrial invasion has been shown to be up to 87% accurate in grade 1 tumours and 65% accurate in grade 2 tumours (33, 34). Where the intraoperative tumour diameter is less than 2 cm, nodal metastases are unlikely (35). This practice may be of benefit where assessing the need for systematic lymphadenectomy via preoperative imaging or frozen section is not always available.

Extent of lymphadenectomy

In women where lymphadenectomy is indicated, there is no doubt of the need for complete resection of all pelvic nodes up to and including the common iliac nodes; however, the need for and extent of para-aortic dissection is controversial.

Complete para-aortic lymphadenectomy significantly increases surgical time, blood loss, surgical incision size, and postoperative complications including a 20% risk of lower limb lymphoedema (36). Women may be obese, frail, and often have significant comorbid conditions and the risk–benefit profile of such extensive surgery needs to be carefully assessed. The single factor that seems most predictive of para-aortic nodal involvement is confirmed pelvic node metastases. Both a Japanese study and one conducted by the Mayo Clinic (United States) have shown nearly 50% of patients with positive pelvic nodes have positive para-aortic nodes, whereas over 95% of patients had negative para-aortic nodes when the pelvic nodes were negative (37, 38). There may be uterine lymph channels that drain directly to the para-aortic nodes at the level of the renal vessels. This is explained by the collateral uterine–ovarian lymphovascular supply and accounts for the small group of women (1.6%) who have para-aortic metastases with negative pelvic nodes, where these positive nodes would be missed by pelvic lymphadenectomy alone (39).

Sentinel node biopsy in endometrial cancer

Following the success of sentinel node biopsy in breast and vulval cancers, sentinel node studies have been performed in endometrial cancer. This practice has the potential to afford every case of endometrial cancer a nodal assessment independent of risk factors. Performing sentinel node biopsy has been shown to detect lymph node metastases in 10% of women who would not usually have undergone systematic lymphadenectomy based on tumour factors (40). Its benefits include less surgical morbidity, specifically lymphoedema, while still providing essential information to stage the disease and tailor adjuvant therapy. There is some controversy about where the dye or fluorescent stain should be injected in endometrial cancer: be it at the cervix, as done when mapping sentinel nodes in early-stage cervical cancer, or via hysteroscopy into the uterine fundus or into the tumour.

Radiotherapy in the management of endometrial cancer

Radiation can be used for a number of indications in endometrial cancer including:

- adjuvant therapy for intermediate or high-risk disease
- primary treatment where surgery is not suitable
- treatment of recurrent disease
- palliation of symptoms including bleeding or symptomatic metastases.

Table 63.4 Indicators for systematic lymphadenectomy

Preoperative	Intraoperative
Assessed using endometrial histology and imaging techniques such as pelvic ultrasound, MRI, or CT	Determined by intraoperative sectioning or frozen section (preferably by an experienced gynaepathologist)
• Non-endometrioid histology • Grade 3 differentiation • Visible cervical involvement • Radiological suggestion of deep myometrial invasion (>50%), cervical stromal invasion, lymphadenopathy >10 mm • Radiological measurement of greatest tumour surface dimension >2 cm (24)	• Upgrade of original grade to grade 3 differentiation • Extrauterine tumour • Non-endometrioid histology • >50% myometrial invasion • Cervical stromal involvement *(Assessing grade of differentiation and myometrial invasion may be difficult on frozen section, especially in the presence of adenomyosis)*

While adjuvant radiotherapy has no significant effect on overall survival it has been shown to increase progression-free survival by reducing pelvic recurrences (32, 41, 42). The need for adjuvant radiotherapy in endometrial cancer is based on specific risk factors in stage I disease but is always indicated in stage II disease and greater.

Adjuvant radiation can be delivered in four forms: vault brachytherapy, external beam pelvic radiation, extended field radiation (to expand the irradiated field to include para-aortic nodes below the renal arteries), and whole abdominal radiation. The vagina is the most common site of recurrence. Vault tumours are difficult to manage surgically but vault brachytherapy and external pelvic radiation are effective and well tolerated adjuvant interventions (41, 43). Whole pelvis irradiation has been shown to be as effective as vaginal vault brachytherapy in reducing tumour recurrence at the vault; however, vaginal brachytherapy is preferred as the total radiation dose is smaller thus reducing radiation-mediated toxicity (42).

Surgery followed by adjuvant pelvic radiation was shown in the ASTEC study to reduce recurrence in the pelvis and at the vault in early-stage disease but demonstrated no improvement in overall survival (32). The findings of the ASTEC study were mirrored in the PORTEC-1 study; however, both studies received much criticism (41). ASTEC had major design faults and the PORTEC-1 study included participants who were considered at low risk of developing recurrent disease.

PORTEC-2 randomized patients with an intermediate-risk profile for local recurrence to either vault brachytherapy or whole pelvis irradiation. No significant difference in vaginal vault recurrence or overall survival was seen in either arm; however, external beam treatment increased long-term morbidity (42). The findings of both PORTEC studies were criticized as lymphadenectomy was not performed in either trial, both were underpowered, and included large numbers of low-risk tumours that had minimal risk of pelvic nodal involvement and recurrence.

In early-stage low-risk tumours (stage I, grade 1–2, <50% myometrial invasion, LVSI negative) vault recurrence is not common and adjuvant radiotherapy is not indicated (14). In stage I disease with high- to intermediate-risk factors (grade 3 endometrioid with <50% myometrial invasion, or grade 1–2 with extensive LVSI) or high-risk factors (grade 3 endometrioid with ≥50% myometrial invasion regardless of LVSI) there is unanimous support in the literature that such cases require adjuvant radiation to decrease local recurrence; this was further supported by the GOG-99 study (44). In stage II disease where the tumour has invaded the cervical stromal tissue, a vaginal brachytherapy boost is often prescribed in addition to external beam radiation. In cases of high–intermediate-risk disease where the nodal status is unknown, adjuvant external beam therapy should be chosen above vault brachytherapy where there is unequivocal LVSI (14).

Primary treatment of endometrial cancer using radiotherapy is reserved for patients not suited to surgery. Radiation is delivered to the uterus using intracavity brachytherapy via a rod or Hayman's pack that is inserted transvaginally into the cavity. Intracavity therapy is usually combined with external beam radiotherapy, however, external radiotherapy may prove problematic as the weight and abdominal girth of certain patients may exceed the limits of the external beam radiation machine.

Chemotherapy in endometrial cancer

Chemotherapy in early-stage endometrial cancer

The role of chemotherapy in early-stage endometrioid endometrial cancer has not been established, however, chemotherapy may be beneficial in patients with early-stage carcinosarcoma. The toxicity of combination chemotherapy and only a marginal increase in overall survival may not justify use of these drugs (45, 46). Ifosfamide-based combination treatment, especially when combined with paclitaxel, has shown more activity in the treatment of advanced stage or recurrent carcinosarcoma (47).

Chemotherapy in advanced-stage disease

The combination of postoperative radiation and chemotherapy seems to give better progression-free and overall survival outcomes compared to either chemotherapy or radiation given as stand-alone treatments (48). Although multiagent chemotherapy is more effective, the cumulative toxicity is not well tolerated (49). In a GOG study, by Randall et al., chemotherapy seemed to offer better progression-free survival in stage III patients, with gross residual disease and endometrioid histology compared to whole abdominal irradiation (50).

Role of targeted therapies

Phosphotidylinositol-3 kinase (PI3K) is mutated in both type 1 and 2 uterine cancers. Current treatments aim at inhibiting this pathway (51).

Targeted therapies such as PI3K/AKT/mammalian/mechanistic target of rapamycin (mTOR) and vascular endothelial growth factor inhibitors are considered in oncological practice to:

- act synergistically with current chemotherapeutic agents
- reduce resistance to chemotherapy
- increase progesterone receptor expression in patients with advanced-stage or recurrent uterine carcinoma resistant to progestogens (52).

Most of these target-based treatments are being tested in phase II studies.

Metformin in endometrial cancer

Metformin is a biguanide that not only counteracts insulin resistance, but has been found to counter proliferative, invasive, and metastatic activity in patients with type 1 endometrial cancer. The antitumour effect of metformin is believed to inhibit the mTOR protein kinase (53).

Fertility-sparing management in endometrial cancer

Increasingly, more women under the age of 40 years are diagnosed with endometrial cancer. Fertility is sometimes a concern at the time of diagnosis. Most of these women are diagnosed with low-risk carcinomas or endometrial hyperplasia, though high-grade (grade 3) endometrioid carcinoma may be found in about 8% of young women (54). A high-stage endometrial cancer diagnosis is also not uncommon. The depth of tumour invasion should be considered before conservative treatment is considered. Dynamic MRI with contrast is more sensitive in assessing depth of tumour infiltration

(55). Hormonal therapy has been used with reasonable resolution of disease. There have also been reports of successful pregnancies after hormonal treatment for endometrial cancer (56). Progression of disease has been observed in 47% of these women. Physicians should have a thorough discussion of possible risks and benefits of the conservative management before embarking on this approach.

Uterine sarcomas

Sarcomas account for 3–7% of all uterine cancers. New FIGO staging systems have been developed for uterine sarcomas.

- *Carcinosarcomas* are now considered and managed as high-grade endometrial carcinomas and no longer form part of uterine sarcomas (5).
- *Leiomyosarcomas* are staged using the new 2009 FIGO system (Table 63.5) (57). They are usually associated with a poor prognosis. Distant spread is common. Tumour size more than 5 cm, epithelioid-type histology, and severe atypia are histological features associated with distant metastasis (58).
- *Adenosarcomas*: adenosarcoma, in contrast to carcinosarcoma, is composed of benign glandular tissue and malignant stromal tissue and has a much better prognosis than carcinosarcoma. Adenosarcoma has its own staging system (Table 63.6). Total hysterectomy and bilateral salpingo-oophorectomy is often sufficient treatment. Deep myometrial invasion is a poor prognostic factor (59).
- *Endometrial stromal tumours*: endometrial stromal cancers are rare and account for less than 1% of uterine tumours. They are classified into two main histological subtypes: endometrial stromal sarcomas and undifferentiated sarcomas. The age of presentation is usually in the fourth and fifth decades and they present in a manner typical of sarcomas including abnormal uterine bleeding, lower abdominal pain, and an abdominal mass.

Endometrial stromal sarcomas are less aggressive than undifferentiated sarcomas but late recurrences are not uncommon. Stage is

Table 63.5 The 2009 FIGO staging of uterine leiomyosarcoma

Stage I	Tumour confined to the corpus uteri
IA	Tumour <5 cm size
IB	Tumour >5 cm size
Stage II	Tumour extends to the pelvis
IIA	Adnexal involvement
IIB	Tumour extends to extrauterine pelvic tissue
Stage III	Tumour involved abdominal tissues (not just protruding into abdomen)
IIIA	
IIIB	1 site
IIIC	>1 site
	Metastases to pelvic and/or para-aortic lymph nodes
Stage IV	Tumour invades bladder and/or rectum, and or distant metastases
IVA	
IVB	Tumour invasion of bladder and/or rectum
	Distant metastases

Source data from FIGO Committee on Gynecologic Oncology. FIGO staging for uterine sarcomas. *Int J Gynecol Oncol* 2009;104:179. doi:10.1016/j.ijgo.2008.12.009.

Table 63.6 The 2009 FIGO staging for uterine endometrial stromal sarcoma and adenosarcoma

Stage I	Tumour confined to the corpus uteri
IA	Tumour confined to the endometrium/endocervix with no myometrial invasion
IB	Less than 50% myometrial invasion
IC	More than half myometrial invasion
Stage II	Tumour extends to the pelvis
IIA	Adnexal involvement
IIB	Tumour extends to extrauterine pelvic tissue
Stage III	Tumour involves abdominal tissues
IIIA	Involves one site
IIIB	More than one site involved
IIIC	Metastases to pelvic and/or para-aortic lymph nodes
Stage IV	Tumour invades bladder and/or rectum, and/or distant metastases
IVA	Tumour invading bladder or rectum
IVB	Distant metastases

Source data from FIGO Committee on Gynecologic Oncology. FIGO staging for uterine sarcomas. *Int J Gynecol Oncol* 2009;104:179. doi:10.1016/j.ijgo.2008.12.009.

the most important risk factor in these with a 90% 5-year survival rate for stage I disease. There is some argument for fertility-sparing management in highly selected women with endometrial stromal sarcoma and definitive surgery should be performed once child-bearing is complete (60).

Undifferentiated sarcomas are highly aggressive tumours with poor survival rates. Sixty per cent of patients present with stage III or IV disease (60).

The mainstay of treatment of both types of stromal sarcoma remains hysterectomy. Bilateral salpingo-oophorectomy is recommended in the endometrial stromal sarcoma group as these tumours often express oestrogen receptors and estrogen replacement therapy post surgery is not advisable (61). The role of adjuvant radiation and chemotherapy in the treatment of endometrial stromal sarcomas has not been established. The use of progestins or aromatase inhibitors may have a place in the treatment of endometrial stromal sarcomas.

Treatment of sarcomas

Surgery in uterine leiomyosarcomas

Lymph node and adnexal involvement are rare in leiomyosarcomas, therefore lymphadenectomy and bilateral salpingo-oophorectomy are not mandatory (62). Restaging surgery in patients with an incidental post-hysterectomy diagnosis of leiomyosarcoma is of no benefit.

Chemotherapy for leiomyosarcomas

The role of chemotherapy in patients with leiomyosarcomas is unclear irrespective of stage (63–65). Distant recurrences still occur in patients with early-stage disease whether they receive chemotherapy or not. Targeted treatments have not demonstrated any improved results as yet (66).

Radiotherapy in the treatment of uterine sarcomas

Establishing the role of radiotherapy in the treatment of uterine sarcomas is difficult as most studies have combined carcinosarcoma and other uterine sarcomas in their analyses. Radiotherapy seems to confer some local control in uterine carcinosarcomas and not in leiomyosarcomas (67).

REFERENCES

1. World Health Organization. GLOBOCAN 2012: estimated cancer incidence, mortality and prevalence worldwide in 2012. 2012. Available at: http://globocan.iarc.fr/Pages/fact_sheets_population.aspx.

2. National Cancer Institute. Endometrial cancer treatment: physician data query (PDQ). 2015. Available at: https://www.cancer.gov/types/uterine/hp/endometrial-treatment-pdq/.

3. Bokhman JV. Two pathogenetic types of endometrial carcinoma. *Gynecol Oncol* 1983;**15**:10–17.

4. Prat J, Gallardo A, Cuatrecasas M, Catasus L. Endometrial carcinoma: pathology and genetics. *Pathology* 2007;**39**:72–87.

5. McCluggage WG. Uterine carcinosarcomas (malignant mixed Mullerian tumours) are metaplastic carcinomas. *Int J Gynecol Cancer* 2002;**12**:687–90.

6. Zhang Y, Liu H, Yang S, et al. Overweight, obesity and endometrial cancer risk: results from a systematic review and meta-analysis. *Int J Biol Markers* 2014;**29**:21–29.

7. Lancaster JM, Powell CB, Chen LM, Richardson DL. Society of Gynecologic Oncology statement on risk assessment for gynecologic cancer predispositions. *Gynecol Oncol* 2015;**136**:3–7.

8. Morgensen J, Kjaer S, Mellemkjaer, Jensen A. Endometriosis and risks for ovarian, endometrial and breast cancers: a nationwide cohort study. *Gynecol Oncol* 2016;**143**:87–92.

9. Chandra V, Kim JJ, Benbrook DM, Dwivedi A, Rai R. Therapeutic options for management of endometrial hyperplasia. *J Gynecol Oncol* 2016;**27**:e8.

10. Dinger J, Bardenheuer, Minh T. Levonorgestrel-releasing and copper intrauterine devices and the risk of breast cancer. *Contraception* 2011;**83**:211–17.

11. Trinh XB, Tjalma WA, Makar AP, Buytaert G, Weyler J, van Dam PA. Use of the levonorgestrel-releasing intrauterine system in breast cancer patients. *Fertil Steril* 2008;**90**:17–22.

12. Backman T, Rauramo I, Jaakkola K, et al. Use of the levonorgestrel-releasing intrauterine system and breast cancer. *Obstet Gynecol* 2005;**106**:813–17.

13. Wong AW, Chan SS, Yeo W, Yu MY, Tam WH. Prophylactic use of levonorgestrel-releasing intrauterine system in women with breast cancer treated with tamoxifen: a randomized controlled trial. *Obstet Gynecol* 2013;**121**:943–50.

14. Colombo N, Creutzberg C, Amant F, et al. ESMO-ESGO-ESTRO consensus conference on endometrial cancer: diagnosis, treatment and follow-up. *Int J Gynecol Cancer* 2016;**26**:2–30.

15. Schmeler KM, Lynch HT, Chen L. Prophylactic surgery to reduce the risk of gynecologic cancers in the Lynch syndrome. *N Engl J Med* 2006;**354**:261–69.

16. Yang Y, Liao Y, Liu X, et al. Prognostic factors of regression and relapse of complex atypical hyperplasia and well-differentiated endometrioid carcinoma with conservative treatment. *Gynecol Oncol* 2015;**139**:419–23.

17. Orbo A, Vereide A, Arnes M, Pettersen I, Straume B. Levonorgestrel-impregnated intrauterine device as treatment for endometrial hyperplasia: a national multicentre randomised trial. *BJOG* 2014;**121**:477–86.

18. Dijkhuizen F, Mol B, Brolman H, Heintz A. The accuracy of endometrial sampling in the diagnosis of patients with endometrial carcinoma and hyperplasia. *Cancer* 2000;**89**:1765–72.

19. Dimitraki M, Tsikouras P, Bouchlariotou S, et al. Clinical evaluation of women with PMB. Is it always necessary an endometrial biopsy to be performed? A review of the literature. *Arch Gynecol Obstet* 2011;**283**:261–66.

20. Wang J, Wieslander C, Hansen G, et al. Thin endometrial echo complex on ultrasound does not reliably exclude type 2 endometrial cancers. *Gynecol Oncol* 2006;**101**:120–25.

21. Chandavarkar U, Kuperman JM, Muderspach LI, et al. Endometrial echocomplex thickness in postmenopausal endometrial cancer. *Gynecol Oncol* 2013;**131**:109–12.

22. Jhang H, Chuang L, Visintainer P, Ramaswamy G. CA 125 levels in the pre-operative assessment of advanced stage uterine cancer. *Am J Obstet Gynecol* 2003;**188**:1195–97.

23. Pecorelli S. Revised FIGO staging for carcinoma of the vulva, cervix, and endometrium. *Int J Gynaecol Obstet* 2010;**108**:176.

24. Takeshima N, Nishida H, Tabata T, et al. Positive peritoneal cytology in endometrial cancer: enhancement of other prognostic indicators. *Gynecol Oncol* 2001;**82**:470–73.

25. Shih K, Yun E, Gardner G, et al. Surgical cytoreduction in stage IV endometrioid endometrial carcinoma. *Gynecol Oncol* 2011;**122**:608–11.

26. Walker J, Piedmonte M, Spirtos N, et al. Laparoscopy compared with laparotomy for comprehensive surgical staging of uterine cancer: Gynecologic Oncology Group Study LAP2. *J Clin Oncol* 2009;**27**:5331–36.

27. Galaal K, Bryant A, Fisher A, et al. Laparoscopy versus laparotomy for the management of early stage endometrial cancer. *Cochrane Database Syst Rev* 2012;**9**:CD006655.

28. Walker J, Piedmonte M, Spirtos N, Eisenkop S, Schlaerth J. Recurrence and survival after random assignment to laparoscopy versus laparotomy for comprehensive surgical staging of uterine cancer: Gynecologic Oncology Group LAP2 Study. *J Clin Oncol* 2012;**30**:695–700.

29. Cardenas-Goicoechea J, Shepard A, Momeni M, et al. Survival analysis of robotic versus traditional laparoscopic surgical staging for endometrial cancer. *Am J Obstet Gynecol* 2014;**210**:160.e1–11.

30. Gitsch G, Hanzal E, Jensen D, Hacker N. Endometrial cancer in premenopausal women 45 years and younger. *Obstet Gynecol* 1995;**85**:504–508.

31. Panici P, Baisile F, Maneschi A, et al. Systematic pelvic lymphadenectomy vs no lymphadenectomy in early-stage endometrial cancer: randomized clinical trial. *J Natl Cancer Inst* 2008;**100**:1707–16.

32. ASTEC study group, Kitchener H, Swart AM, Qian Q, Amos C, Parmar MK. Efficacy of systematic pelvic lymphadenectomy in endometrial cancer (MRC ASTEC trial): a randomised study. *Lancet* 2009;**373**:125–36.

33. Goff B, Rice L. Assessment of depth of myometrial invasion in endometrial adenocarcinoma. *Gynecol Oncol* 1990;**38**:46–48.

34. Franchi M, Ghezzi F, Melpignano M, et al. Clinical value of intraoperative gross examination in endometrial cancer. *Gynecol Oncol* 2000;**76**:357–61.

35. Schink J, Lurain J, Wallemark C, Chmiel J. Tumour size in endometrial cancer: a prognostic factor for lymph node metastasis. *Obstet Gynecol* 1987;**70**:216–19.

36. Ryan M, Stainton MC, Slaytor EK, Jaconelli C, Watts S, Mackenzie P. Aetiology and prevalence of lower limb lymphoedema following

treatment for gynaecological cancer. *Aust N Z J Obstet Gynaecol* 2003;**43**:148–51.

37. Mariani A, Dowdy SC, Cliby WA, et al. Efficacy of systematic lymphadenectomy and adjuvant radiotherapy in node-positive endometrial cancer patients. *Gynecol Oncol* 2006;**101**:200–208.

38. Nomura H, Aoki D, Suzuki N, et al. Analysis of clinico-pathologic factors predicting para-aortic lymph node metastasis in endometrial cancer. *Int J Gynecol Cancer* 2006;**16**:799–804.

39. Abu-Rustum N, Gomez JD, Alektiar KM, et al. The incidence of isolated paraaortic nodal metastases in surgically staged endometrial cancer patients with negative pelvic lymph nodes. *Gynecol Oncol* 2009;**115**:236–38.

40. Ballester M, Dubernard G, Lécuru F, et al. Detection rate and diagnostic accuracy of sentinel-node biopsy in early stage endometrial cancer: a prospective multicenter study (SENTI-ENDO). *Lancet Oncol* 2011;**12**:469–76.

41. Creutzberg CL, van Putten WL, Koper PC, et al. Surgery and postoperative radiotherapy versus surgery alone for patients with stage-1 endometrial carcinoma: multicenter randomised trial. PORTEC study group. Post operative radiation therapy in endometrial carcinoma. *Lancet* 2000;**333**:1404–11.

42. Nout RA, Smit VT, Putter H, et al. Vaginal brachytherapy versus pelvic external beam radiotherapy for patients with endometrial cancer of high-intermediate risk (PORTEC-2): an open-label, non-inferiority, randomised trial. *Lancet* 2010;**375**:816–23.

43. Blake P, Swart AM, Orton J, et al. Adjuvant external beam radiotherapy in the treatment of endometrial cancer (MRC ASTEC and NCIC CTG EN.5 randomised trials): pooled trial results, systematic review, and meta-analysis. *Lancet* 2009;**373**:137–46.

44. Creutzberg CL. GOG-99: ending the controversy regarding pelvic radiotherapy for endometrial carcinoma. *Gynecol Oncol* 2004;**92**:740–43.

45. Sutton G, Kauderer J, Carson LF, et al. Adjuvant ifosfamide and cisplatin in patients with completely resected stage I or II carcinosarcomas (mixed mesodermal tumors) of the uterus: a Gynecologic Oncology Group study. *Gynecol Oncol* 2005;**96**:630–34.

46. Slaughter KN, Rowland M, Bhattacharya R, et al. Integration of adjuvant chemotherapy in first-line management of uterine carcinosarcoma. *Gynecol Oncol* 2015;**137**:97.

47. Galaal K, van der Heijden E, Godfrey K, et al. Adjuvant radiotherapy and/or chemotherapy after surgery for uterine carcinosarcoma. *Cochrane Database Syst Rev* 2013;**2**:CD006812.

48. Secord AA, Havrilesky LJ, Bae-Jump V, et al. The role of multi-modality adjuvant chemotherapy and radiation in women with advanced stage endometrial cancer. *Gynecol Oncol* 2007;**107**:285–91.

49. Fleming GF, Brunetto VL, Cella D, et al. Phase III trial of doxorubicin plus cisplatin with or without paclitaxel plus filgrastim in advanced endometrial carcinoma: a Gynecologic Oncology Group Study. *J Clin Oncol* **22**:2159–66.

50. Randall ME, Filiaci VL, Muss H, et al. Randomized phase III trial of whole-abdominal irradiation versus doxorubicin and cisplatin chemotherapy in advanced endometrial carcinoma: a Gynecologic Oncology Group Study. *J Clin Oncol* 2006;**24**:36–44.

51. Winder A, Yu Y, Unno K, Kim J. The efficacy of an AKT inhibitor for treatment of aggressive endometrial cancer: studied in new models for cancer research. *Gynecol Oncol* 2014;**135**:392.

52. Slomovitz BM, Coleman RL. The PI3K/AKT/mTOR pathway as a therapeutic target in endometrial cancer. *Clin Cancer Res* 2012;**18**:5856–64.

53. Cantrell LA, Zhou C, Mendivil A, et al. Metformin is a potent inhibitor of endometrial cancer cell proliferation—implications for a novel treatment strategy. *Gynecol Oncol* 2010;**116**:92–98.

54. Bandyopadhyay S, Arabi H, Thirabanjasak D, Quddus MR, Lawrence WD, Fehmi RA. Endometrial cancer diagnosed in young patients is not always a low-risk cancer. *Mod Pathol* 2008;**21**:900.

55. Kinkel K, Kaji Y, Yu KK, et al. Radiologic staging in patients with endometrial cancer: a meta-analysis. *Radiology* 1999;**212**:711–18.

56. Ushijima K, Yahata H, Yoshikawa H, et al. Multicenter phase II study of fertility-sparing treatment with medroxyprogesterone acetate for endometrial carcinoma and atypical hyperplasia in young women. *J Clin Oncol* 2007;**25**:2798–803.

57. FIGO Committee on Gynecologic Oncology. FIGO staging for uterine sarcomas. *Int J Gynecol Oncol* 2009;**104**:179.

58. Jones MW, Norris HJ. Clinicopathologic study of 28 uterine leiomyosarcomas with metastasis. *Int J Gynecol Pathol* 1995;**14**:243–49.

59. Prat J, Mbatani NH. Uterine sarcomas. *Int J Gynecol Obstet* **131**:S105–110.

60. Horng H, Wen K, Wang P, et al. Uterine sarcoma. Part II – uterine endometrial stromal sarcoma: the TAG systematic review. *Taiwan J Obstet Gynecol* 2016;**55**:472–79.

61. Chu M, Mor G, Lim C, et al. Low-grade endometrial stromal sarcoma: hormonal aspetcs. *Gynecol Oncol* 2003;**90**:170–76.

62. Major FJ, Blessing JA, Silverberg SG, et al. Prognostic factors in early-stage uterine sarcoma. A Gynecologic Oncology Group study. *Cancer* 1993;**71**:1702–709.

63. Bogani G, Maltese G, Ditto A, et al. Efficacy of adjuvant chemotherapy in early stage uterine leiomyosarcoma: a systematic review and meta-analysis. *Gynecol Oncol* 2016;**143**:443–47.

64. Roque DR, Taylor KN, Palisoul M, et al. Gemcitabine and docetaxel compared to radiation or other chemotherapy regimens as adjuvant treatment for stages I–IV uterine leiomyosarcoma. *Int J Gynecol Cancer* 2016;**26**:505–11.

65. Taylor K, Palisoul M, Rogue DR, et al. Gemcitabine and docetaxel compared to alternative chemotherapy regimens as adjuvant treatment for uterine leiomyosarcoma. *Gynecol Oncol* 2015;**136**:408.

66. Hensley ML, Miller A, O'Malley DM, et al. A randomized phase III trial of gemcitabine + docetaxel + bevacizumab or placebo as first-line treatment for metastatic uterine leiomyosarcoma (uLMS): a Gynecologic Oncology Group study. *Gynecol Oncol* 2014;**133** Suppl 1:3.

67. Reed NS, Mangioni C, Malmstro H, et al. Phase III randomised study to evaluate the role of adjuvant pelvic radiotherapy in the treatment of uterine sarcomas stages I and II: an European Organisation for Research and Treatment of Cancer Gynaecological Cancer Group Study (protocol 55874). *Eur J Cancer* 2008;**44**:808–18.

64

Ovarian, fallopian tube, and peritoneal cancer

Jonathan A. Ledermann and Christina Fotopoulou

Origin, epidemiology, and histological classification

Approximately 90% of malignant cancers of the ovary are epithelial tumours; the remainder are stromal or germ cell tumours. Epithelial ovarian cancer is the commonest cause of death from gynaecological cancer in the developed world. There are approximately 240,000 new cases each year. The approximate lifetime risk of developing the disease is 1.7%, but higher risks are seen in some regions, and in particular in women with a *BRCA* gene mutation who have about a 60% chance of developing ovarian cancer. The median age of onset is 60 years, but it is earlier in women with an inherited predisposition to the disease. The 5-year survival in many countries has improved over the last 30 years, probably due to a combination of better surgery and more effective systemic treatments. Nevertheless, the majority of women present with advanced disease and ultimately die of disease due to the development of resistance to systemic therapies.

The majority of malignant tumours arising from the ovary, fallopian tube, or peritoneum are high-grade serous-type; other histotypes (endometrioid, clear cell, and mucinous) are rarer and have a different biological behaviour. A unifying hypothesis has been proposed in which high-grade tumours (type II) originate from the fimbrial end of the fallopian tube, and may present commonly as ovarian cancer, and less commonly as primary fallopian tube or peritoneal cancers (1). Low-grade epithelial (type I) tumours develop from the ovarian surface and have a distinct molecular profile and different biological behaviour. Stromal tumours are rare and are often localized to the ovary at presentation. Germ cell tumours are a rare subgroup of tumours that present in a younger age group.

Diagnosis and staging

Presentation: screening and initial diagnostics

More than 70% of women with newly diagnosed ovarian cancer present with an advanced (International Federation of Gynecology and Obstetrics (FIGO) stage III or IV) disease. This is due to the biology and clinical behaviour, which typically is associated with locoregional dissemination throughout the peritoneal cavity resulting in symptoms related to the spread of disease. Some women present with symptoms relating to an enlarging pelvic mass, leading to pelvic discomfort and urinary and bowel symptoms but many have a non-specific pattern of symptoms, such as abdominal bloating and distention with pain, and loss of appetite (2).

Management and prognosis are determined by stage at presentation, histological grading, and patients' performance and nutritional status. In most women the underlying cause of the tumour is unknown but previous breast cancer, nulliparity, a history of endometriosis, and long-term use of hormonal replacement therapy are associated with an increased incidence of ovarian cancer. Around 10% of all ovarian cancers, higher in high-grade serous tumours, have a hereditary component with the vast majority being related to mutations of the *BRCA1* and *BRCA2* genes. There is also an association with hereditary non-polyposis colorectal cancer (Lynch syndrome). Prolonged use of combined oral contraceptive medication, high parity, and breastfeeding are associated with a reduced risk, as well as a history of tubal ligation and hysterectomy.

There is no conclusive evidence that screening for sporadic ovarian cancer is associated with a survival benefit. The American Prostate, Lung, Colorectal and Ovarian (PLCO) randomized cancer screening trial using annual cancer antigen 125 (CA125) and transvaginal ultrasound scanning (TVUS) showed no reduction in mortality in asymptomatic postmenopausal women, and false-positive results were associated with complications (3). The United Kingdom Collaborative Trial of Ovarian Cancer Screening (UKCTOCS) trial randomized over 200,000 women to observation alone, multimodal screening (MMS) testing with an algorithm based on serial values of CA125 and follow on TVUS for an abnormal result, or serial TVUS alone. No reduction in mortality was seen in the primary analysis but a possible reduction in mortality after exclusion of prevalent cases after 7 years of follow-up was shown. Long-term data and cost-effectiveness data are still awaited (4).

Women with symptoms suspicious of ovarian cancer should have a serum CA125 measured and a pelvic ultrasound scan. For women with a pelvic mass, a risk of malignancy index (RMI) score of 250 or greater suggests malignancy, and is a helpful diagnostic tool. RMI combines three presurgical features: serum CA125, menopausal status (M), and ultrasound (U) score. The RMI is a product of the U score (score of 1–3), the menopausal status (premenopausal status =1, postmenopausal =3), and the serum CA125 level (IU/mL): RMI = U × M × CA125 (5). A score over 200 indicates a high risk of malignancy. The Risk of Ovarian Malignancy Algorithm (ROMA) is an alternative tool that incorporates human epididymis secretory protein 4 (HE4) and CA125. It appears to be helpful, especially in younger patients, where endometriosis and infections may cause elevation of CA125 levels in the absence of malignant disease (6).

FIGO staging of epithelial ovarian and fallopian tube cancers

The FIGO surgical staging system is most commonly used for ovarian cancer. Recent changes to the FIGO classification (Table 64.1) have been made to take account of the impact of lymph node

Table 64.1 FIGO classification of epithelial ovarian and fallopian tube cancers

FIGO staging 2013	Description
Stage I. Tumour confined to ovaries or fallopian tube(s)	
Stage IA	Tumour limited to one ovary (capsule intact) or fallopian tube; no tumour on ovarian or fallopian tube surface; no malignant cells in the ascites or peritoneal washings
Stage IB	Tumour limited to both ovaries (capsules intact) or fallopian tubes; no tumour on ovarian or fallopian tube surface; no malignant cells in the ascites or peritoneal washings
Stage IC1	Tumour limited to one or both ovaries or fallopian tubes, with surgical spill
Stage IC2	Tumour limited to one or both ovaries or fallopian tubes, with capsule ruptured before surgery or tumour on ovarian or fallopian tube surface
Stage IC3	Tumour limited to one or both ovaries or fallopian tubes, with malignant cells in the ascites or peritoneal washings
Stage II. Tumour involves one or both ovaries or fallopian tubes with pelvic extension (below pelvic brim) or primary peritoneal cancer	
Stage IIA	Extension and/or implants on uterus and/or fallopian tubes and/or ovaries
Stage IIB	Extension to other pelvic intraperitoneal tissues
Stage III. Tumour involves one or both ovaries or fallopian tubes, or primary peritoneal cancer, with cytologically or histologically confirmed spread to the peritoneum outside the pelvis and/or metastasis to the retroperitoneal lymph nodes.	
Stage IIIA1	Positive retroperitoneal lymph nodes only (cytologically or histologically proven)
Stage IIIA1(i)	Metastasis up to 10 mm
Stage IIIA1(ii)	Metastasis more than 10 mm
Stage IIIA2	Microscopic extrapelvic (above the pelvic brim) peritoneal involvement with or without positive retroperitoneal lymph nodes
Stage IIIB	Macroscopic peritoneal metastasis beyond the pelvis up to 2 cm in greatest dimension, with or without metastasis to the retroperitoneal lymph nodes
Stage IIIC	Macroscopic peritoneal metastasis beyond the pelvis more than 2 cm in greatest dimension, with or without metastasis to the retroperitoneal lymph nodes (includes extension of tumour to capsule of liver and spleen without parenchymal involvement of either organ)

involvement and the type of distant metastases. The new staging system differentiates between true distant sites of disease versus a pleural effusion, and iatrogenic rupture of the tumour in early disease is now also included (7).

Imaging modalities and their value in decision-making processes

The management of ovarian cancer is based on a combination of clinical, pathological, biochemical, and radiological factors. Conventional imaging such as computed tomography (CT) and magnetic resonance imaging (MRI) are key staging investigations as they define the extent of disease and identify complicating factors such as renal obstruction or pulmonary emboli that might alter overall management. However, conventional imaging has not yet been shown to predict the operability of advanced ovarian cancer (8). For example, small-volume diffuse disease may be missed on imaging but operability also depends on other factors such as variations in surgical expertise and support facilities. Novel imaging modalities to improve the ability to predict operability, such as diffusion-weighted MRI, are currently being evaluated (9). Routine use of other specialized imaging techniques such as positron emission tomography (PET) CT (**Figure 64.1**) adds little extra information although it is helpful in assessing patients for surgical debulking of relapsed disease, where it may identify thoracic lymph node involvement or more diffuse inoperable disease (10).

Overview of treatment at primary presentation

Surgical staging and treatment of primary epithelial ovarian and fallopian tube cancers

Surgery is the cornerstone of management for early and advanced ovarian cancer. For early ovarian cancer the aim of surgery is to remove the primary tumour and perform adequate staging to exclude occult advanced disease in the omentum and lymph nodes. In advanced stage the aim is maximal tumour reduction, as this has clearly been shown to be associated with a better prognosis. Non-fertility-sparing surgery for disease macroscopically confined to the ovary consists of peritoneal washings or cytology, ideally taken prior to manipulation of the tumour, bilateral salpingo-oophorectomy, hysterectomy, multiple peritoneal biopsies from the paracolic and subdiaphragmatic spaces bilaterally, infragastric omentectomy, and pelvic and bilateral para-aortic lymph node dissection up to the level of the renal vessels. If mucinous carcinoma is suspected, an appendicectomy should be considered. Depending on the histological grade and subtype, up to 30% of the patients with apparently early epithelial ovarian cancer will be upstaged after comprehensive surgical staging (11). The extent of lymph node dissection remains controversial but one prospective randomized trial showed that systematic lymph node dissection compared to sampling in early disease identified an additional 13% of patients (from 9% to 22%) with occult lymph node disease (12). No clear evidence exists to suggest that systematic lymph node dissection is therapeutic and improves survival. In stage IA mucinous cancer, the incidence of lymph node spread is extremely low and there is no value in performing a lymphadenectomy.

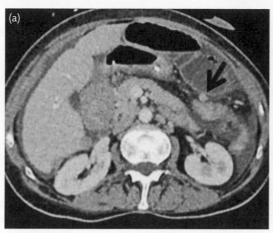
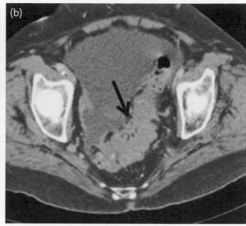

Figure 64.1 False-positive tumour involvement described preoperatively on CT on transverse colon (a); which was intraoperatively part of the omental cake, and of sigmoid colon (b) which was a parasigmoid nodule without affecting the bowel.

Fertility-sparing surgery should be considered and discussed with patients of childbearing age who have early-stage disease, informing patients of the risks and benefits of such an approach. Patients with stage IA and favourable histology, that is, low-grade, mucinous, serous, endometrioid, or mixed histology have been shown to have a lower risk of recurrence after fertility-preserving surgery compared to patients with a higher stage (IC3) or grade, or clear cell histology (13). Retrospective studies showed a risk of 3.5–11% of positive contralateral pelvic lymph nodes in women with unilateral disease despite negative ipsilateral nodes (14, 15). Thus, pelvic lymph node staging should be bilateral.

Total macroscopic tumour clearance of advanced disease has consistently been shown to be associated with a significantly better progression-free survival (PFS) and overall survival (16–18). However, it is unclear if this association is causal or whether resectable tumours intrinsically respond better to chemotherapy and have a more favourable prognosis (19). In a systematic meta-analysis based on 53 studies with 6885 patients overall (period: 1989–1998), Bristow and colleagues (20) showed how the degree of surgical tumour resection influenced the overall survival of patient cohorts. Those with over a 75% rate of 'optimal' cytoreduction (defined as <2 cm residual disease) had a median overall survival of 36.8 months. By contrast, patient cohorts with a maximum tumour reduction rate of less than 25% had a median overall survival of only 23 months. Every 10% reduction in tumour burden was associated with a 6.3% prolongation of median overall survival. In order to achieve total macroscopic tumour clearance of peritoneally disseminated disease, a maximal surgical effort is required, incorporating multivisceral resection techniques such as extensive peritoneal stripping, full-thickness diaphragmatic resection, removal of bulky pelvic and para-aortic lymph nodes, splenectomy, and bowel resection. In a randomised trial the value of systematic lymph node dissection as a therapeutic procedure has been shown not to improve outcome (LION Trial, AGO-OVAR OP.3 (NCT00712218))(21). Increasingly, more extra-abdominal cytoreductive techniques are being applied, including resection of cardiophrenic or paracardiac lymph nodes, pleurectomy, and supraclavicular and axillary lymph node dissection. Surgical expertise and training with continuous feedback of surgical outcome, morbidity, and survival have been proven to be important tools to make extensive surgery safer for the patient (22). There is now a national and international trend towards specialization of such procedures in centres with adequate infrastructure, resources, and training.

Interval debulking surgery after merely a biopsy, or little or low-effort surgical debulking at diagnosis has been shown to improve survival (17), but in situations where maximal effort primary surgery has been undertaken but no total macroscopic tumour clearance could be achieved, there is no survival benefit in interval cytoreductive surgery after three cycles of chemotherapy to clear any remaining disease and it should therefore not be attempted (23). Similarly, a 'second-look' diagnostic laparoscopy or laparotomy after completion of treatment to assess intraperitoneal status should not be routinely performed, except in the context of clinical trials, as its impact on survival has not been demonstrated.

There is internationally ongoing debate as to the best timing of surgery in relation to first-line chemotherapy. Two prospective randomized trials (18, 24) have demonstrated lower surgical morbidity and mortality and equivalent overall survival using a neoadjuvant (primary chemotherapy) approach. The weakness of both studies was, however, that the rate of complete resection was low and operation time, a surrogate marker of surgical effort, was short. Accordingly, it is difficult to adopt neoadjuvant chemotherapy for patients with good performance status who can be rendered tumour free by surgery in specialized centres. A trial comparing neoadjuvant chemotherapy and upfront radical surgery in such centres where surgical quality is established is being planned. There is, however, a significant value of using neoadjuvant chemotherapy in patients with unresectable FIGO IVB disease, low performance status, and significant comorbidities that would make radical debulking surgery impossible.

Systemic treatment of high-grade serous epithelial ovarian, fallopian tube, and peritoneal cancers

Adjuvant therapy for early-stage ovarian cancer

Cytotoxic chemotherapy plays a key role in the treatment of ovarian cancers. Postoperative chemotherapy should be distinguished from adjuvant chemotherapy used to treat some women with FIGO stage I disease. In this group, platinum chemotherapy has been shown in two trials to reduce the recurrence rate and prolong overall survival

(25). However, these trials were done many years ago when the quality of surgical staging was less good, and the studies are likely to have included women with occult FIGO stage III disease. Nevertheless, with a 10-year median follow-up of the ICON1 trial there was in absolute terms a 10% (from 60% to 70%) improvement in recurrence-free survival and a 9% (from 64% to 73%) improvement in overall survival. Patients with high-grade tumours appeared to derive the greatest benefit (26). However, the long-term results of the EORTC ACTION trial still cast doubt on the value of adjuvant chemotherapy as the 10-year follow-up data showed that only patients who had 'suboptimal' surgery benefited from chemotherapy (27).

Chemotherapy for advanced ovarian cancer and recent trial results

Advanced ovarian cancer is one of the most chemosensitive epithelial malignancies and platinum-based therapy has been the mainstay of cytotoxic treatment since the late 1970s. Carboplatin has equivalent activity to cisplatin, but has less neurotoxicity and renal toxicity, and is the key drug used to treat ovarian cancer. The addition of paclitaxel improves tumour response rates, prolongs PFS, and probably increases overall survival (28). Since the late 1990s, the standard of care has been a combination of carboplatin and paclitaxel, given three-weekly for six cycles. The key additional toxicities of paclitaxel are hair loss and peripheral neuropathy. Single-agent carboplatin is used in a minority of women through choice to avoid the additional side effects, or concern about the extra toxicity from paclitaxel. However, carboplatin and pegylated liposomal doxorubicin (PLD) is an alternative combination (29). Over the last 15 years, trials adding additional drugs, either as triplet therapy, sequential doublets, maintenance post carboplatin–paclitaxel, or the use of very high-dose chemotherapy have failed to improve the median PFS. Intraperitoneal delivery is an approach that has been investigated for many years and is discussed in the 'Intraperitoneal chemotherapy and hyperthermic intraperitoneal chemotherapy' section.

Recently, modification of paclitaxel administration, using a weekly (dose-dense) schedule has been shown to increase median PFS from 17.5 to 28.1 months and median overall survival from 62.2 to 100.5 months compared to the three-weekly schedule (30). These data in a Japanese population are provocative and have generated further studies to try and confirm the results. Two trials used a similar design but had key differences to the Japanese study (weekly carboplatin and lower dose of paclitaxel in one, and the addition of bevacizumab in the other) and they failed to confirm a benefit of weekly paclitaxel (31, 32). A third study, ICON8 (NCT01654146), which directly compares the arms in the Japanese trial and has a third arm where both drugs are given weekly has also shown no benefit for weekly paclitaxel (33). Currently, three-weekly carboplatin and paclitaxel remains the standard schedule.

Novel targeted approaches

Targeting the complex molecular pathways responsible for tumour growth is now believed to be the best strategy to improve treatment outcome. Remission of tumours to first-line cytotoxic therapy is not uncommon but eradication is unusual. What happens to tumours from this time until progression is poorly understood, but two main theories predominate: there is evidence that tumour growth is dependent upon angiogenesis and once an antiangiogenic 'switch' or other complex micro-environmental changes occurs, tumour will

regrow (34). Another hypothesis is that tumour growth arrest may be partly under immunological control. Antiangiogenic therapy with a monoclonal antibody, bevacizumab, that targets circulating vascular endothelial growth factor-A (VEGF-A), one of the key ligands driving angiogenic growth, has been shown to result in tumour shrinkage and delayed progression of ovarian cancer. Two key large randomized studies in first-line treatment after surgery, Gynecologic Oncology Group (GOG) 218 and ICON7, showed that median PFS was extended in both trials (by 3.8 and 1.7 months respectively) by giving bevacizumab with chemotherapy and then as maintenance for a year or more (35, 36). There was no difference in overall survival although in a subgroup of women at 'high risk' of recurrence (stage IV; ≥1 cm residual disease stage III, or no surgery) in ICON7, which used half the dose of bevacizumab compared to GOG 218, there was a significant survival benefit favour of bevacizumab (37). The interpretation of the results differed between Europe, where bevacizumab is licensed for use in first-line treatment and the United States, where it was licensed almost 7 years later. Bevacizumab is generally well tolerated; hypertension and proteinuria are the most common adverse effects, and the most serious but rare event is bowel fistula or perforation. It is generally used after surgery although trials in the neoadjuvant setting are in progress. However, the greatest improvement has been in the first-line treatment of advanced BRCA-mutated ovarian cancer where post chemotherapy treatment with olaparib, a PARP inhibitor led to a 70% reduction in the risk of progression (60% patients free of progression at 3 years compared to 27% in the control arm) (38).

Intraperitoneal chemotherapy and hyperthermic intraperitoneal chemotherapy

The concept of using intraperitoneal (IP) chemotherapy remains controversial with conflicting data relating to its efficacy compared to intravenous therapy, and its toxicity. However, randomized clinical trials have consistently favoured an improvement in survival with IP chemotherapy, comprehensively reviewed by Trimble et al. (39). Long-term follow-up of the most recently published trial, GOG 172, demonstrated a survival benefit extending beyond 10 years (40). Cisplatin and paclitaxel are the two drugs usually used. However, because of concerns about toxicity and the complexity of treatment, IP chemotherapy has not been widely adopted. Carboplatin is less toxic and the results of a Japanese trial comparing IP and intravenous carboplatin are awaited (NCT01506856). Uncertainty about the benefit of the IP strategy remains following the recent negative preliminary results from GOG 252, a phase III trial comparing IP and intravenous therapy with the inclusion of bevacizumab (41).

There are even fewer data to support the use of HIPEC (hyperthermic intraperitoneal chemotherapy), a high dose of intraperitoneal chemotherapy under hyperthermic conditions. Most publications are from single centres in a heterogeneous patient population with primary or recurrent disease. Only one randomised trial has supported this approach, so, data should be interpreted with caution (42). Currently, treatment should only be encouraged within the context of trials and several randomized trials are in progress.

Low-grade serous tumours

These represent about 10% of ovarian cancer cases and have a different biological behaviour from the more common high-grade tumours, with slower growth and less frequent spread beyond the ovary. Surgery for primary or recurrent disease is the mainstay of treatment; the role of chemotherapy is less clear. In the absence of randomized trials, therapeutic decisions are based largely on case series. Low-grade serous tumours do respond to platinum-based therapy but less well and frequently than high-grade tumours (43). A large meta-analysis showed a response to platinum-based chemotherapy of approximately 24% in patients with advanced, primary, low-grade ovarian cancer after upfront surgery (44). Chemotherapy, hormone therapy, and observation are all options to consider in women with low-volume residual disease after primary surgery. Even less is known about the activity of cytotoxic drugs for recurrent disease. Inoperable recurrent disease is more chemoresistant; tamoxifen or aromatase inhibitors are often used and bevacizumab may also be active in modifying growth (45–47).

Recently, there has been interest in exploiting mutations in the BRAF and KRAS pathways and the constitutive activation of the MAPK-ERK pathway using inhibitors of MEK. Initial results have shown some activity of these compounds (48) that are now being investigated in randomized trials.

Non-serous tumours

Classification of this group is becoming more complex, particularly for endometrioid tumours, some of which behave more like high-grade serous cancers while others have clear cell components. Pure clear cell tumours represent about 5% of ovarian cancers, but are more common in Japan and the Far East. They respond less well to platinum-based therapies than serous tumours. Many clear cell tumours present with early-stage disease and these have a relatively good prognosis (49, 50). For advanced disease, the outlook is much less good although carboplatin and paclitaxel are usually given. A recent trial comparing this combination with cisplatin and irinotecan failed to show any difference in outcome (51). Future treatment needs to be directed against molecular targets and work to identify these is underway (52). True mucinous tumours of the ovary are rare, and most present at an early stage with a good prognosis. Advanced mucinous cancers carry a poor prognosis. Carboplatin and paclitaxel are often given although there are good reasons to consider drugs such as oxaliplatin and fluoropyrimidine-based therapy that are active in gastrointestinal mucinous tumours. Because of the rarity of these tumours, it has been difficult to complete randomized trials comparing these combinations (53).

Follow-up

With modern surgery and chemotherapy, the majority of patients with advanced ovarian cancer will enter a clinical remission, defined as normalization of the serum CA125 level and resolution of disease on axial imaging (CT or MRI). However, it is known that these indicators have limited sensitivity, and that when a 'second-look' laparotomy was performed after treatment, a significant number of women in remission had residual disease. These operations have now been abandoned, as the outcome of women is not improved by the procedure. Follow-up strategies vary but include regular monitoring of the serum CA125 level and clinical review. There is no evidence that regular imaging by ultrasound or CT scanning, or PET

imaging improves survival. While clear definitions of relapse measured by CA125 levels have been developed (54), there is no evidence from a CA125 follow-up trial that early institution of second-line chemotherapy based on a raised CA125 level leads to an improvement in overall survival (55). In the trial, CA125 levels identified relapse about 4.8 months before clinical relapse. The interpretation of these results has varied, ranging from those who feel that routine CA125 measurement is not worthwhile to those who feel it drives imaging which may identify patients suitable for secondary debulking surgery (see 'Surgical debulking options at relapse'). In routine clinical practice, the CA125 level is commonly checked approximately every 3 months in the first 2 years, and CT scanning is triggered by the CA125 level or symptoms. Follow-up intervals are usually extended beyond 2 years as the majority of relapses will have occurred by this time.

Overview of treatment at relapse

Surgical debulking options at relapse

Despite the established value of cytoreduction in the primary setting, the value of tumour debulking surgery for recurrent epithelial ovarian cancer remains highly controversial. A retrospective analysis of tumour resection in women in first 'platinum-sensitive' recurrence suggested that patients benefit if macroscopic clearance can be achieved. An 'AGO score' was developed, based on performance status, complete resection at primary surgery or early FIGO stage, and the absence of gross ascites at relapse, and it predicted a good outcome in the prospective DESKTOP II trial (56, 57). The scoring system has been used as a basis for the randomized phase III DESKTOP III trial comparing the addition of surgery to chemotherapy for 'platinum-sensitive' recurrent disease. A positive result from this trial could lead to a change in practice with more intensive follow-up to identify patients with potentially resectable disease. A surgical randomization was also included in the GOG 213 trial. There is little evidence to support the use of cytoreductive surgery in the 'platinum-resistant' setting, other than for palliation of bowel obstruction.

Systemic regimens at relapse: current trials and novel/molecular approaches

Relapse of early-stage comprehensively staged FIGO stage I ovarian cancer is uncommon but for all other stages, it occurs in more than 75% of women. Since the 1980s, cisplatin and later carboplatin were the mainstay of therapy or recurrent disease, as these were the most active agents available. During the late 1980s, reports emerged that patients retreated with platinum-based therapy were likely to respond again, depending on the interval from primary therapy. Thus, the terms 'platinum-sensitive' and 'platinum-resistant' relapse were created, based on the probability of responding again if the relapse was less or more than 6 months after the end of primary treatment. The definitions were later modified, somewhat arbitrarily, to subdivide the 'platinum-sensitive' group into a 'partially platinum-sensitive' (relapse interval 6–12 months) and fully 'platinum-sensitive' (relapse interval >12 months). Patients relapsing within 3 months were defined as having 'platinum-refractory' disease. These terms provided a convenient method of categorization for treatment design of clinical trials (58). Not only is much of the literature predicated on these groupings, but regulators and health funders have also often made decisions based on these categories. However, in reality it is clear that resistance is neither absolute in most patients, and is certainly not categorical. Furthermore, the definition was based on response at first relapse and it is less clear how these terms apply to patients who have had several lines of therapy and have been on maintenance regimens. Recently, there has been a move to classify patients according to the treatment interval, as some patients may not have received platinum-based therapy before the most recent relapse.

For most patients the first recurrence will occur more than 6 months after the completion of first-line therapy. Clinical trials combining platinum with either paclitaxel, gemcitabine, or PLD have consistently shown a superior PFS with combination chemotherapy compared to single-agent platinum. It has been harder to demonstrate a benefit in overall survival, but a recent meta-analysis of combination therapy trials supports the use of combination therapy (59). The choice of combination therapy, summarized in Table 64.2, needs to take account of the relative toxicities of the regimen, the side effects experienced during recent treatment, and the likely choices for later-line therapy, particular when tumours become 'platinum resistant'. It is not uncommon for women to receive several lines of therapy; the interval between treatments usually decreases as the degree of chemotherapy (and in particular platinum) resistance increases. Use of non-platinum drugs increases as tumours become resistant, or unmanageable hypersensitivity to platinum occurs. Paclitaxel, PLD, and topotecan are all licensed for use as a single agent in recurrent ovarian cancer and

combinations of non-platinum drugs have not been shown to be superior. Other drugs sometimes used are cyclophosphamide, often continuously in a low dose, etoposide, or gemcitabine. These are usually given as single agents but combinations with platinum (even in the 'platinum-resistant' setting) are sometimes used (Table 64.3). The median PFS following treatment for 'platinum-resistant' ovarian cancer is typically around 3 months and the median overall survival is about 12 months. There is a need to develop better treatments and also to evaluate current treatments carefully, taking account of the control of symptoms, time off chemotherapy, and the patient's quality of life.

Hormone therapy with tamoxifen or letrozole is sometimes used to treat late-stage disease when there are no further options for chemotherapy. Anecdotal and small series report responses to these drugs but for tamoxifen, a systematic review of the literature failed to show any benefit.

Antiangiogenic therapies

Bevacizumab is the antiangiogenic drug that has been most thoroughly explored in recurrent ovarian cancer. In the randomized OCEANS trial, a significant improvement in PFS was seen when bevacizumab was given in combination with carboplatin and gemcitabine, and then as maintenance until progression compared with chemotherapy alone. The median increased from 8.4 to 12.4 months (hazard ratio (HR) 0.484; P <0.0001) without any increase in overall survival (60, 61). A benefit in PFS was also seen in the GOG 213 trial using bevacizumab in combination with carboplatin and paclitaxel (62). In the 'platinum-resistant' setting, the randomized AURELIA trial used an investigator choice of weekly paclitaxel, PLD, or topotecan with or without bevacizumab.

Table 64.2 Randomized trials using drug combinations in 'platinum-sensitive' recurrent ovarian cancer

Combination	Trial	Experimental arm (median PFS in months)	Control arm (median PFS in months)
Carboplatin/paclitaxel	ICON4 Compared to platinum alone	13	10
Carboplatin/gemcitabine	OVAR 2.5 Compared to carboplatin alone	8.6	5.8
Carboplatin/PLD	CALYPSO non-inferiority trial Comparison with carboplatin/paclitaxel	11.3	9.4
Carboplatin/gemcitabine/bevacizumab	OCEANS Addition of bevacizumab to chemotherapy and as maintenance compared to carboplatin/gemcitabine	12.4	8.4
Carboplatin/paclitaxel/bevacizumab	GOG 213 Addition of bevacizumab to chemotherapy and as maintenance	13.8	10.4
Carboplatin-based combination (paclitaxel or gemcitabine) with cediranib	ICON6 Addition of cediranib to chemotherapy and as maintenance	11.0	8.7
Non-platinum combination Trabectedin/PLD	OVA 301 Combination compared to PLD (partially platinum sensitive 6–12-month PFI)	7.4	5.5
Non-platinum combination Weekly paclitaxel and trebananib	TRINOVA 1 Addition of AMG 386 (trebananib) to chemotherapy (includes a partially platinum-sensitive group 6–12-month PFI)	7.4	5.2

PFI, platinum-free interval; PFS, progression-free survival; PLD, pegylated liposomal doxorubicin.

Table 64.3 Chemotherapy drugs used to treat 'platinum-resistant' ovarian cancer (<6 month platinum-free interval)

	Median progression-free survival (months)
Pegylated liposomal doxorubicin (PLD)	3.5
Topotecan	3.4
Weekly paclitaxel	3.9
Weekly paclitaxel + bevacizumab	10.4
PLD + bevacizumab	5.4
Cisplatin and etoposide (<4 month platinum-free interval)	5.0
Weekly carboplatin and paclitaxel	8.0

Entry was restricted to patients with no more than two prior lines of chemotherapy and excluded patients with refractory disease, a history of bowel obstruction, or significant serosal disease on the large bowel. Bevacizumab in conjunction with chemotherapy increased the median PFS from 3.4 to 6.7 months (HR 0.48; P <0.001). Cross-over to bevacizumab on progression was permitted and there was no significant difference in overall survival (63). In this largely symptomatic group of women, bevacizumab increased the tumour response rate from 11.8% to 27.3%. This effect was most marked in patients receiving weekly paclitaxel. Furthermore, a greater number of patients receiving bevacizumab had a more than 15% benefit in abdominal/gastrointestinal symptoms (64). The use of bevacizumab in platinum-resistant ovarian cancer has now received widespread regulatory approval.

Several trials have now reported on the activity of oral VEGF receptor tyrosine kinase inhibitors (VEGFR TKIs) in recurrent ovarian cancer. Trials have been performed with pazopanib, cediranib, and sorafenib in patients with either 'platinum-sensitive' or 'platinum-resistant' disease, and all bar one have shown a similar and significant difference in median PFS; the results are similar to those with bevacizumab, or the angiopoietin antagonist, trebananib (Table 64.2). The pattern of toxicity with oral VEGFR TKIs is different from bevacizumab. Hypertension is more pronounced with VEGFR TKIs and diarrhoea and fatigue are more common and troublesome. None of the oral VEGFR TKIs are currently licensed for use in ovarian cancer, but they are, nevertheless, a potent group of drugs that have considerable potential for further development.

Inhibition of DNA repair

The high response rate of ovarian cancer to platinum-based drugs is largely due to impaired mechanisms to repair cytotoxic-induced DNA damage. Poly(ADP ribose) polymerase (PARP) is activated in response to single-stranded breaks in DNA. Inhibitors of the pathway were initially developed to enhance the effectiveness of DNA-damaging cytotoxic drugs. However, it has been shown that PARP inhibitors are most active in cells that are homozygously deficient in the BRCA1 or BRCA2 genes. These gene products form an essential constituent of the repair proteins required to repair double-stranded breaks of DNA by a process known as homologous recombination repair (HRR) (65). Phase I clinical trials with AZD2281 (olaparib) demonstrated antitumour activity and disease

control in tumours deficient in BRCA protein function. About 15–20% of serous ovarian cancers have either a germline or somatic BRCA gene mutation (66, 67). Clinical trials with olaparib, given as maintenance therapy after platinum-based chemotherapy of recurrent high-grade 'platinum-sensitive' ovarian cancer, demonstrated a significant delay in tumour progression (68). This benefit was greatest in tumours with a germline or somatic BRCA mutation with extension of the median PFS following chemotherapy from 4.3 to 11.2 months (HR 0.18; P <0.0001) (69). Survival was extended and 15% of women with a BRCA mutation remained on the drug for more than 5 years without tumour progression (70). There is emerging evidence that the benefit of maintenance therapy with PARP inhibitors extends to a population without a BRCA mutation that has the phenotypic features of HRR deficiency. Randomized maintenance trials with niraparib and rucaparib, two other PARP inhibitors, in this setting will soon report. A BRCA mutation is the first (genetically determined) predictive marker for a response to a PARP inhibitor.

Olaparib is the first PARP inhibitor to be licensed for maintenance therapy in 'platinum-sensitive' ovarian cancer with a BRCA mutation. Similar trials with niraparib and rucaparib have confirmed the benefit of maintenance therapy post platinum therapy in high grade ovarian cancers, with or without a BRCA mutation. This class of drugs is also active as monotherapy in BRCA mutated ovarian cancer (71). The implication from these results is that all women with high-grade ovarian cancer should undergo BRCA testing. The absence of a family history is not a good negative predictor of a BRCA mutation (72). 'Second-generation' PARP inhibitor studies are now underway, combining the drug with antiangiogenic drugs. There is evidence that this increases the degree of HRR deficiency, and initial trials with olaparib and cediranib have shown promising results, particularly in women without BRCA mutations (73).

Palliation and symptom control

Conservative and systemic management of bowel obstruction

Bowel obstruction and intestinal failure with stasis are common late events in ovarian cancer and can be difficult to manage. Chemotherapy, sometimes supported by total parenteral nutrition, may be used in patients for whom a response is thought to be possible. Extensive tumour dissemination combined by an acute systemic inflammatory immunological response can make any surgical intervention in this setting highly challenging with high morbidity and mortality. When undertaken, surgical procedures include en bloc resections of the involved intestinal package and terminal proximal stomas of the ileum or jejunum, since extensive peritoneal involvement and inflammation makes dissection and formation of anastomoses difficult. The resulting 'short bowel syndrome' can be difficult to manage, and although feasible, prolonged community-based total parenteral nutrition has not been fully assessed. Progress in endoscopic techniques such as placement of intestinal stents and gastrostomies have improved care of patients and have reduced morbidity.

Symptom management and terminal care

Recurrent ascites or pleural effusions can be relieved by drainage. More permanent measures such as pleurodesis or long-term abdominal drainage catheters for recurrent ascites may be helpful. Vomiting and constipation with bowel dysfunction, due to obstruction or more commonly a 'paresis' with stasis due to extensive serosal infiltration, is the most common symptom to manage during end of life care. Medical management of symptoms includes the use of antiemetic and prokinetic drugs, steroids, and octreotide. Careful assessment of fluid and calorie intake is needed and treatment decisions about support need to take account of the disease status, remaining chemotherapy options, and patients' wishes. The success of 'end of life' care, whether at home, in hospital, or in a hospice benefits from the involvement of a multidisciplinary healthcare team that is able to work with the patient to find the most acceptable treatment plan for her.

REFERENCES

1. Kurman RJ, Shih I-M. The origin and pathogenesis of epithelial ovarian cancer: a proposed unifying theory. *Am J Surg Pathol* 2010;**34**:433–43.
2. Goff B. Symptoms associated with ovarian cancer. *Clin Obstet Gynecol* 2012;**55**:36–42.
3. Buys SS, Partridge E, Black A, et al. Effect of screening on ovarian cancer mortality: the Prostate, Lung, Colorectal and Ovarian (PLCO) cancer screening randomized controlled trial. *JAMA* 2011;**305**:2295–303.
4. Jacobs IJ, Menon U, Ryan A, et al. Ovarian cancer screening and mortality in the UK Collaborative Trial of Ovarian Cancer Screening (UKCTOCS): a randomised controlled trial. *Lancet* 2016;**387**:945–56.
5. Jacobs I, Oram D, Fairbanks J, et al. A risk of malignancy index incorporating CA 125, ultrasound and menopausal status for the accurate preoperative diagnosis of ovarian cancer. *Br J Obstet Gynaecol* 1990;**97**:922–29.
6. Dayyani F, Uhlig S, Colson B, et al. Diagnostic performance of risk of ovarian malignancy algorithm against CA125 and HE4 in connection with ovarian cancer: a meta-analysis. *Int J Gynecol Cancer* 2016;**26**:1586–93.
7. Prat J, FIGO Committee on Gynecologic Oncology. Staging classification for cancer of the ovary, fallopian tube, and peritoneum. *Int J Gynaecol Obstet* 2014;**124**:1–5.
8. Nasser S, Lazaridis A, Evangelou M, et al. Correlation of preoperative CT findings with surgical & histological tumor dissemination patterns at cytoreduction for primary advanced and relapsed epithelial ovarian cancer: a retrospective evaluation. *Gynecol Oncol* 2016;**143**:264–69.
9. Fehniger J, Thomas S, Lengyel E, et al. A prospective study evaluating diffusion weighted magnetic resonance imaging (DW-MRI) in the detection of peritoneal carcinomatosis in suspected gynecologic malignancies. *Gynecol Oncol* 2016;**142**:169–75.
10. Mapelli P, Incerti E, Fallanca F, et al. Imaging biomarkers in ovarian cancer: the role of 18F-FDG PET/CT. *Q J Nucl Med Mol Imaging* 2016;**60**:93–102.
11. Garcia-Soto AE, Boren T, Wingo SN, et al. Is comprehensive surgical staging needed for thorough evaluation of early-stage ovarian carcinoma? *Am J Obstet Gynecol* 2012;**206**:242.e1–5.
12. Maggioni A, Benedetti Panici P, Dell'Anna T, et al. Randomised study of systematic lymphadenectomy in patients with epithelial ovarian cancer macroscopically confined to the pelvis. *Br J Cancer* 2006;**95**:699–704.
13. Fruscio R, Corso S, Ceppi L, et al. Conservative management of early-stage epithelial ovarian cancer: results of a large retrospective series. *Ann Oncol* 2013;**24**:138–44.
14. Ditto A, Martinelli F, Reato C, et al. Systematic para-aortic and pelvic lymphadenectomy in early stage epithelial ovarian cancer: a prospective study. *Ann Surg Oncol* 2012;**19**:3849–55.
15. Suzuki M, Ohwada M, Yamada T, et al. Lymph node metastasis in stage I epithelial ovarian cancer. *Gynecol Oncol* 2000;**79**:305–308.
16. du Bois A, Reuss A, Pujade-Lauraine E, et al. Role of surgical outcome as prognostic factor in advanced epithelial ovarian cancer: a combined exploratory analysis of 3 prospectively randomized phase 3 multicenter trials: by the Arbeitsgemeinschaft Gynaekologische Onkologie Studiengruppe Ovarialkarzinom (AGO-OVAR) and the Groupe d'Investigateurs Nationaux Pour les Etudes des Cancers de l'Ovaire (GINECO). *Cancer* 2009;**115**:1234–44.
17. van der Burg ME, van Lent M, Buyse M, et al. The effect of debulking surgery after induction chemotherapy on the prognosis in advanced epithelial ovarian cancer. Gynecological Cancer Cooperative Group of the European Organization for Research and Treatment of Cancer. *N Engl J Med* 1995;**332**:629–34.
18. Vergote I, Tropé CG, Amant F, et al. Neoadjuvant chemotherapy or primary surgery in stage IIIC or IV ovarian cancer. *N Engl J Med* 2010;**363**:943–53.
19. Jayson GC, Kohn EC, Kitchener HC, Ledermann JA. Ovarian cancer. *Lancet* 2014;**384**:1376–88.
20. Bristow RE, Tomacruz RS, Armstrong DK, et al. Survival effect of maximal cytoreductive surgery for advanced ovarian carcinoma during the platinum era: a meta-analysis. *J Clin Oncol* 2002;**20**:1248–59.
21. Harter P, Sehouli J, Lorusso D, et al. A randomized trial of lymphadenectomy in patients with advanced ovarian neoplasms. *N Engl J Med* 2019;**380**(9):822–32.
22. Aletti GD, Gostout BS, Podratz KC, Cliby WA. Ovarian cancer surgical resectability: relative impact of disease, patient status, and surgeon. *Gynecol Oncol* 2006;**100**:33–37.
23. Rose PG, Nerenstone S, Brady MF, et al. Secondary surgical cytoreduction for advanced ovarian carcinoma. *N Engl J Med* 2004;**351**:2489–97.
24. Kehoe S, Hook J, Nankivell M, et al. Primary chemotherapy versus primary surgery for newly diagnosed advanced ovarian cancer (CHORUS): an open-label, randomised, controlled, non-inferiority trial. *Lancet* 2015;**386**:249–57.
25. Trimbos JB, Parmar M, Vergote I, et al. International Collaborative Ovarian Neoplasm trial 1 and Adjuvant ChemoTherapy In Ovarian Neoplasm trial: two parallel randomized phase III trials of adjuvant chemotherapy in patients with early-stage ovarian carcinoma. *J Natl Cancer Inst* 2003;**95**:105–12.
26. Collinson F, Qian W, Fossati R, et al. Optimal treatment of early-stage ovarian cancer. *Ann Oncol* 2014;**25**:1165–71.
27. Trimbos B, Timmers P, Pecorelli S, et al. Surgical staging and treatment of early ovarian cancer: long-term analysis from a randomized trial. *J Natl Cancer Inst* 2010;**102**:982–87.
28. McGuire WP, Hoskins WJ, Brady MF, et al. Cyclophosphamide and cisplatin compared with paclitaxel and cisplatin in patients with stage III and stage IV ovarian cancer. *N Engl J Med* 1996;**334**:1–6.
29. Pignata S, Scambia G, Ferrandina G, et al. Carboplatin plus paclitaxel versus carboplatin plus pegylated liposomal doxorubicin as first-line treatment for patients with ovarian cancer: the MITO-2 randomized phase III trial. *J Clin Oncol* 2011;**29**:3628–35.

30. Katsumata N, Yasuda M, Isonishi S, et al. Long-term results of dose-dense paclitaxel and carboplatin versus conventional paclitaxel and carboplatin for treatment of advanced epithelial ovarian, fallopian tube, or primary peritoneal cancer (JGOG 3016): a randomised, controlled, open-label trial. *Lancet Oncol* 2013;**14**:1020–26.

31. Chan JK, Brady MF, Penson RT, et al. Weekly vs. every-3-week paclitaxel and carboplatin for ovarian cancer. *N Engl J Med* 2016;**374**:738–48.

32. Pignata S, Scambia G, Katsaros D, et al. Carboplatin plus paclitaxel once a week versus every 3 weeks in patients with advanced ovarian cancer (MITO-7): a randomised, multicentre, open-label, phase 3 trial. *Lancet Oncol* 2014;**15**:396–405.

33. Clamp A, McNeish I, Dean A, et al. ICON8: a GCIG phase III randomised trial evaluating weekly dose-dense chemotherapy integration in first-line epithelial ovarian/fallopian tube/primary peritoneal carcinoma (EOC) treatment: results of primary progression-free survival (PFS) analysis. *Ann Oncol* 2017;28(Suppl. 5):abstract 929O_PR.

34. Naumov GN, Bender E, Zurakowski D, et al. A model of human tumor dormancy: an angiogenic switch from the nonangiogenic phenotype. *J Natl Cancer Inst* 2006;**98**:316–25.

35. Burger RA, Brady MF, Bookman MA, et al. Incorporation of bevacizumab in the primary treatment of ovarian cancer. *N Engl J Med* 2011;**365**:2473–83.

36. Perren TJ, Swart AM, Pfisterer J, et al. A phase 3 trial of bevacizumab in ovarian cancer. *N Engl J Med* 2011;**365**:2484–96.

37. Oza A, Perren T, Swart A, et al. ICON7: final overall survival results in the GCIG phase III randomized trial of bevacizumab in women with newly diagnosed ovarian cancer. Abstract 6. Presented at: European Society of Medical Oncology Annual Meeting; Amsterdam, The Netherlands, 30 September 2013.

38. Moore K, Colombo N, Scambia G, Kim B-G, Oaknin A, Friedlander M, et al. Maintenance Olaparib in Patients with Newly Diagnosed Advanced Ovarian Cancer. *N Engl J Med.* 2018 Oct 21;**379**(26):2495–505.

39. Trimble EL, Thompson S, Christian MC, Minasian L. Intraperitoneal chemotherapy for women with epithelial ovarian cancer. *Oncologist* 2008;**13**:403–409.

40. Tewari D, Java JJ, Salani R, et al. Long-term survival advantage and prognostic factors associated with intraperitoneal chemotherapy treatment in advanced ovarian cancer: a gynecologic oncology group study. *J Clin Oncol* 2015;**33**:1460–66.

41. Walker JL, Brady MF, Wenzel L, Fleming GF, Huang HQ, DiSilvestro PA, et al. Randomized Trial of Intravenous Versus Intraperitoneal Chemotherapy Plus Bevacizumab in Advanced Ovarian Carcinoma: An NRG Oncology/Gynecologic Oncology Group Study. *J Clin Oncol* 2019 Jun 1;**37**(16):1380–90.

42. Harter P, du Bois A, Mahner S, et al. Statement of the AGO Kommission Ovar, AGO Study Group, NOGGO, AGO Austria and AGO Switzerland regarding the use of hyperthermic intraperitoneal chemotherapy (HIPEC) in ovarian cancer. *Geburtshilfe Frauenheilkd* 2016;**76**:147–49.

43. Diaz-Padilla I, Malpica AL, Minig L, et al. Ovarian low-grade serous carcinoma: a comprehensive update. *Gynecol Oncol* 2012;**126**:279–85.

44. Grabowski JP, Harter P, Heitz F, et al. Operability and chemotherapy responsiveness in advanced low-grade serous ovarian cancer. An analysis of the AGO Study Group metadatabase. *Gynecol Oncol* 2016;**140**:457–62.

45. Gershenson DM, Sun CC, Bodurka D, et al. Recurrent low-grade serous ovarian carcinoma is relatively chemoresistant. *Gynecol Oncol* 2009;**114**:48–52.

46. Gershenson DM, Sun CC, Iyer RB, et al. Hormonal therapy for recurrent low-grade serous carcinoma of the ovary or peritoneum. *Gynecol Oncol* 2012;**125**:661–66.

47. Grisham RN, Iyer G, Sala E, et al. Bevacizumab shows activity in patients with low-grade serous ovarian and primary peritoneal cancer. *Int J Gynecol Cancer* 2014;**24**:1010–14.

48. Farley J, Brady WE, Vathipadiekal V, et al. Selumetinib in women with recurrent low-grade serous carcinoma of the ovary or peritoneum: an open-label, single-arm, phase 2 study. *Lancet Oncol* 2013;**14**:134–40.

49. Chan JK, Teoh D, Hu JM, et al. Do clear cell ovarian carcinomas have poorer prognosis compared to other epithelial cell types? A study of 1411 clear cell ovarian cancers. *Gynecol Oncol* 2008;**109**:370–76.

50. Tan DSP, Kaye S. Ovarian clear cell adenocarcinoma: a continuing enigma. *J Clin Pathol* 2007;**60**:355–60.

51. Sugiyama T, Okamoto A, Enomoto T, et al. Randomized phase III trial of irinotecan plus cisplatin compared with paclitaxel plus carboplatin as first-line chemotherapy for ovarian clear cell carcinoma: JGOG3017/GCIG Trial. *J Clin Oncol* 2016;**34**:2881–87.

52. Friedlander ML, Russell K, Millis S, et al. Molecular profiling of clear cell ovarian cancers: identifying potential treatment targets for clinical trials. *Int J Gynecol Cancer* 2016;**26**:648–54.

53. Ledermann JA, Luvero D, Shafer A, et al. Gynecologic Cancer InterGroup (GCIG) consensus review for mucinous ovarian carcinoma. *Int J Gynecol Cancer* 2014;**24**:S14–19.

54. Vergote I, Rustin GJ, Eisenhauer EA, et al. Re: new guidelines to evaluate the response to treatment in solid tumors (ovarian cancer). Gynecologic Cancer Intergroup. *J Natl Cancer Inst* 2000;**92**:1534–35.

55. Rustin GJS, van der Burg MEL, Griffin CL, et al. Early versus delayed treatment of relapsed ovarian cancer (MRC OV05/EORTC 55955): a randomised trial. *Lancet* 2010;**376**:1155–63.

56. Harter P, Hahmann M, Lueck HJ, et al. Surgery for recurrent ovarian cancer: role of peritoneal carcinomatosis: exploratory analysis of the DESKTOP I Trial about risk factors, surgical implications, and prognostic value of peritoneal carcinomatosis. *Ann Surg Oncol* 2009;**16**:1324–30.

57. Harter P, Sehouli J, Reuss A, et al. Prospective validation study of a predictive score for operability of recurrent ovarian cancer: the Multicenter Intergroup Study DESKTOP II. A project of the AGO Kommission OVAR, AGO Study Group, NOGGO, AGO-Austria, and MITO. *Int J Gynecol Cancer* 2011;**21**:289–95.

58. Friedlander M, Trimble E, Tinker A, et al. Clinical trials in recurrent ovarian cancer. *Int J Gynecol Cancer* 2011;**21**:771–75.

59. Raja F, Counsel N, Colombo N, et al. Platinum combination chemotherapy versus platinum monotherapy in platinum-sensitive recurrent ovarian cancer: a meta-analysis of randomised trials using individual patients data (IPD). *Ann Oncol* 2012;**23**:982P.

60. Aghajanian C, Goff B, Nycum LR, et al. Final overall survival and safety analysis of OCEANS, a phase 3 trial of chemotherapy with or without bevacizumab in patients with platinum-sensitive recurrent ovarian cancer. *Gynecol Oncol* 2015;**139**:10–16.

61. Aghajanian C, Blank SV, Goff BA, et al. OCEANS: a randomized, double-blind, placebo-controlled phase III trial of chemotherapy with or without bevacizumab in patients with platinum-sensitive recurrent epithelial ovarian, primary peritoneal, or fallopian tube cancer. *J Clin Oncol* 2012;**30**:2039–45.

62. Coleman R, Brady M, Herzog T, et al. A phase III randomized controlled clinical trial of carboplatin and paclitaxel alone or in combination with bevacizumab followed by bevacizumab and secondary cytoreductive surgery in platinum-sensitive, recurrent

ovarian, peritoneal primary and fallopian tube cancer (Gynecologic Oncology Group 0213). *Gynecol Oncol* 2015;**137** Suppl 1:3–4.

63. Pujade Lauraine E, Hilpert F, Weber B, et al. AURELIA: a randomized phase III trial evaluating bevacizumab (BEV) plus chemotherapy (CT) for platinum (PT)-resistant recurrent ovarian cancer (OC). *J Clin Oncol* 2012;**30**:LBA5002.

64. Stockler MR, Hilpert F, Friedlander M, et al. Patient-reported outcome results from the open-label phase III AURELIA trial evaluating bevacizumab-containing therapy for platinum-resistant ovarian cancer. *J Clin Oncol* 2014;**32**:1309–16.

65. Farmer H, McCabe N, Lord CJ, et al. Targeting the DNA repair defect in BRCA mutant cells as a therapeutic strategy. *Nature* 2005;**434**:917–21.

66. Moschetta M, George A, Kaye SB, Banerjee S. BRCA somatic mutations and epigenetic BRCA modifications in serous ovarian cancer. *Ann Oncol* 2016;**27**:1449–55.

67. Ramus SJ, Gayther SA. The contribution of BRCA1 and BRCA2 to ovarian cancer. *Mol Oncol* 2009;**3**:138–50.

68. Ledermann J, Harter P, Gourley C, et al. Olaparib maintenance therapy in platinum-sensitive relapsed ovarian cancer. *N Engl J Med* 2012;**366**:1382–92.

69. Ledermann J, Harter P, Gourley C, et al. Olaparib maintenance therapy in patients with platinum-sensitive relapsed serous ovarian cancer: a preplanned retrospective analysis of outcomes by BRCA status in a randomised phase 2 trial. *Lancet Oncol* 2014;**15**:852–61.

70. Ledermann JA, Harter P, Gourley C, et al. Overall survival in patients with platinum-sensitive recurrent serous ovarian cancer receiving olaparib maintenance monotherapy: an updated analysis from a randomised, placebo-controlled, double-blind, phase 2 trial. *Lancet Oncol* 2016;**17**:1579–89.

71. Mirza MR, Pignata S, Ledermann JA. Latest clinical evidence and further development of PARP inhibitors in ovarian cancer. *Ann Oncol.* 2018 Jun 1;**29**(6):1366–76.

72. Alsop K, Fereday S, Meldrum C, et al. BRCA mutation frequency and patterns of treatment response in BRCA mutation-positive women with ovarian cancer: a report from the Australian Ovarian Cancer Study Group. *J Clin Oncol* 2012;**30**:2654–63.

73. Liu JF, Barry WT, Birrer M, et al. Combination cediranib and olaparib versus olaparib alone for women with recurrent platinum-sensitive ovarian cancer: a randomised phase 2 study. *Lancet Oncol* 2014;**15**:1207–14.

65

Premalignant and malignant disease of the vulva and vagina

Linda Rogers, Maaike Oonk, and Ate van der Zee

Premalignant disease of the vagina

Introduction

Vaginal intraepithelial neoplasia (VAIN) is a rare, premalignant condition of the vagina, which is caused by persistent infection with oncogenic strains of the human papillomavirus (HPV). It occurs either concurrently with intraepithelial neoplasia of other parts of the anogenital tract, or can develop after treatment of cervical lesions or pelvic irradiation (1).

VAIN is much less common than cervical intraepithelial neoplasia (CIN). The incidence is approximately 0.2 per 100,000 women, and it makes up approximately 0.4% of all intraepithelial disease of the lower genital tract (2). It can be difficult to diagnose and treat, due to the proximity of surrounding structures such as the bladder and rectum, and the need to preserve sexual function.

The malignant potential of VAIN is not fully known (3, 4), though the risk of transformation of VAIN to invasive squamous carcinoma has been reported to be 9–10% (Table 65.1) (5).

Epidemiology of vaginal intraepithelial neoplasia

As VAIN is caused by oncogenic HPV infection, one of the commonest sexually transmitted infections, its risk factors include those related to HPV acquisition, such as multiple sexual partners, as well as impaired immunity and cigarette smoking.

VAIN is usually diagnosed at colposcopy for coexisting cervical disease, and is quoted to be present in 1–6% of women with CIN as part of a multifocal field effect of HPV in the lower genital tract (1). Immunocompromised women are more likely to have multifocal lower genital tract neoplasia, and to have VAIN or vulval intraepithelial neoplasia (VIN) without accompanying CIN (6).

VAIN may also be detected on cytology done during follow-up of women who have undergone hysterectomy for persistent CIN or early cervical cancer. The incidence of VAIN in women who have had a hysterectomy for CIN 3, who were followed up for 10 years, has been found to be 0.91% (7).

Women who have had pelvic irradiation are also at risk of developing VAIN (1).

Aetiology of vaginal intraepithelial neoplasia

VAIN is caused by high-risk strains of HPV, particularly HPV 16. HPV is a double-stranded DNA virus which is sexually transmitted and infects the squamous epithelium of the lower genital tract. It can exist in a dormant state, undergo replication, or transform the host DNA, causing uncontrolled cell growth (6).

Presentation of vaginal intraepithelial neoplasia

VAIN is usually asymptomatic, though it may present with symptoms of coexisting vulval or cervical disease, for example, pruritus from warts or VIN, or with postcoital bleeding.

Diagnosis of vaginal intraepithelial neoplasia

Colposcopy of the vagina and staining with Lugol's iodine are necessary in order to diagnose VAIN. Adequate visualization of the entire vagina is essential, as well as biopsy of colposcopically abnormal areas, in order to confirm the diagnosis and exclude invasion. This may need to be done in theatre under anaesthetic. Occult carcinomas have been found in the vaginal vault in 28% of women with VAIN (8).

Management of vaginal intraepithelial neoplasia

There are no standardized guidelines for the treatment of VAIN, and management should be individualized. Treatment options include surgery, radiotherapy (brachytherapy), and medical management. When deciding on a treatment modality, several factors need to be considered: age and comorbidities of the patient, site and extent of disease, preservation of sexual function, patient preference, experience of the treating medical team, and previous treatment modalities (1).

Surgery

Excision

Wide local excision or partial colpectomy is an effective and safe treatment of high-grade VAIN, and has the benefit of providing histological assessment and margin status, though sexual function

Table 65.1 Classification of squamous intraepithelial neoplasia of the vagina

VAIN 1 (warts)	Low-grade squamous intraepithelial lesion (LSIL)
VAIN 2–3	High-grade squamous intraepithelial lesion (HSIL)

can be affected by shortening the vagina (1). Only the vaginal mucosa should be excised, as the risk of recurrence of cancer has not been shown to be affected by excising the underlying fascia or muscle (9). It is crucial to perform colposcopy before the procedure, to identify the extent of disease and ensure adequate excision, and the edges of the lesion can be marked with Lugol's iodine or a marker suture. Submucosal infiltration with local anaesthetic and adrenaline is used to elevate the mucosa, thus helping with dissection (1). Success rates after surgical excision of VAIN are reported to be between 66% and 83% (4, 9).

Vaginectomy

This can be partial or total, and refers to removal of the vaginal mucosa (1). Either a knife or electrocautery loop may be used, though when using diathermy, care must be taken not to injure the bladder or rectum. Upper vaginectomy is the treatment of choice for unifocal VAIN 3 of the vault after hysterectomy, but laser ablation is preferred for multifocal high-grade VAIN (10).

Total vaginectomy and split-thickness skin grafting is occasionally necessary to treat extensive lesions when more conservative therapies have not been successful, though it can have severe complications, such as vesicovaginal and rectovaginal fistulae, and has a severe impact on the patient's psychosexual well-being (1).

Laser

A carbon dioxide laser may be used for both ablation and excision of VAIN. Epithelial destruction to a depth of 1.5 mm is sufficient to destroy the dysplastic epithelium without damaging underlying structures (11). Laser excision has the benefit of providing a specimen for histology, but laser ablation has a minimal impact on psychosexual function, as the anatomy of the vagina is preserved, and is therefore useful in the management of younger women, and for multifocal lesions. However, it cannot be used in the vaginal vault fornices due to the risk of damage to underlying structures (1).

Cavitational ultrasonic surgical aspiration

Where the equipment and expertise are available, this allows selective removal of dysplastic lesions, while preserving the surrounding normal tissue (1).

Brachytherapy

Brachytherapy is internal radiotherapy, where a radiation source is placed close to a lesion, and delivers the required amount of radiation (1). Radiotherapy is not recommended as a first-line treatment for VAIN, due to its early and late side effects, impact on sexual function, and the risk of developing another vaginal malignancy, but can be considered where there has been failure of other treatment options (1).

Medical management

Trichloroacetic acid

This is known to be an effective treatment for HPV lesions of the vulva and cervix, and there has been one study which showed complete remission of all low-grade VAIN lesions following weekly application of 50% trichloroacetic acid (12). The main side effect is vaginal burning.

5-Fluorouracil

This may be used in a dosage of 2 g once weekly for 10–12 weeks (13). It is reported to have varying success rates in treating extensive or multifocal high-grade VAIN, and side effects such as vaginal burning, dyspareunia, ulcers, and discharge are common, and limit its use. It can cause a severe tissue reaction, which may limit colposcopic follow-up for months after treatment (1).

Imiquimod

A topical immune modulator, this is an effective and well-tolerated treatment for low-grade VAIN, and has shown some activity in the treatment of high-grade VAIN (14). It causes a vaginal burning and discomfort, but the dose can be titrated against local side effects and tolerability.

Follow-up of vaginal intraepithelial neoplasia

VAIN has been estimated to progress to cancer in about 9–10% of identified cases (5). It is hoped that very much less of this disease will be seen following HPV vaccination.

The United Kingdom National Health Service Cervical Screening Programme guidelines state that women who have a hysterectomy, and have completely excised CIN, should have vaginal vault cytology at 6 and 18 months after their hysterectomy (15). However, HPV DNA testing may be more effective at detecting VAIN than conventional cytology. Whether vaginal vault smears need to be continued long term after hysterectomy for high-grade CIN or cervical cancer is the subject of ongoing debate (1).

There is no evidence to suggest that there is any benefit from continuing with smears after hysterectomy for benign disease (16).

VAIN recurrence rates after partial vaginectomy, laser ablation, and topical 5-fluorouracil are quoted as 0%, 38% and 59% respectively, with multifocal disease being a major risk factor for recurrence (17). There is no evidence to support a particular duration of follow-up for VAIN, and this may match the duration recommended for CIN.

Premalignant disease of the vulva

Introduction

Squamous carcinoma of the vulva is the most common vulval malignancy, though overall it is a rare tumour, accounting for only 4% of gynaecological malignancies (18). It may arise from two types of VIN, which differ from each other with respect to their aetiology, pathogenesis, and clinical significance (18).

Vulval high grade intra-epithelial lesion (vHSIL) is caused by persistent infection with oncogenic strains of the human papillomavirus (HPV), particularly HPV 16 and 18 (19). The incidence of vHSIL is increasing in young women worldwide due to the increase in HPV infection which has mirrored the HIV pandemic, and may be associated with intraepithelial neoplasia in other areas of the anogenital tract (18). Differentiated VIN (dVIN) occurs in postmenopausal women, and is independent of HPV infection, but may be associated with chronic inflammatory vulval skin disorders such as lichen sclerosus and squamous hyperplasia (18). While vHSIL accounts for 90% of cases of VIN (18), dVIN is significantly more likely to be associated with progression to squamous carcinoma (5.7% vs 33% respectively) (20–22). Besides the role VIN plays in the aetiology of vulval squamous carcinoma, it also causes significant morbidity in terms of symptoms, such as pain, pruritus, and dyspareunia.

Vulval extramammary Paget's disease is a rare intraepithelial adenocarcinoma which accounts for less than 2% of primary vulval tumours (23). It is currently thought that most cases of vulval Paget's disease are a primary intraepidermal neoplasm, with a few being associated with cutaneous sweat gland tumours. It has also been described in association with an underlying adenocarcinoma, such as of the endometrium, endocervix, vagina, Bartholin's gland, urethra, or bladder. It has similar clinical and histological features to other skin neoplasms, such as malignant melanoma and atypical squamous disease (23).

Classification of premalignant vulval lesions

Premalignant vulval lesions have been recognized for nearly 100 years, though the pathological and clinical characteristics of these lesions have been the subject of continuous debate (Table 65.2) (24).

Two different types of VIN were introduced in the 1986 International Society for the Study of Vulval Disease (ISSVD) terminology, and confirmed in 2004, when the ISSVD introduced a two-tier classification of VIN (25). HPV-associated vulval high grade intra-epithelial lesion was made up of high-grade lesions VIN 2–3; lesions which were previously called VIN 1 were categorized under condylomata acuminata. HPV-independent or differentiated VIN is always considered to be a high-grade lesion (25).

In 2012, the ISSVD participated in the introduction of the Lower Anogenital Squamous Terminology (LAST) (Table 65.3) by the American Society for Colposcopy and Cervical Pathology and the College of American Pathologists (26). This terminology is not confined to vulval lesions, but aims to classify all HPV-related lesions of the lower genital tract.

In relation to premalignant vulval lesions, two concerns have been raised about the LAST terminology. Firstly, that as LAST deals only with HPV-related lesions, it does not include dVIN, which accounts for 80% of the burden of invasive cancer, and this omission could lead to dVIN being overlooked by healthcare workers (20, 24). And secondly, that by including vulval low-grade squamous intraepithelial lesion, there is potential for overdiagnosis and overtreatment of benign and occasionally self-limiting lesions (24).

Table 65.2 ISSVD classification of premalignant conditions of the vulva

Squamous intraepithelial neoplasia	VIN	Vulval HSIL Differentiated VIN Unclassified type
Non-squamous intraepithelial neoplasia	Paget's disease Melanocyte tumours	

Table 65.3 Comparison of ISSVD terminologies and Lower Anogenital Squamous Terminology of VIN

ISSVD (1986)	ISSVD (2004)	LAST (2012)
VIN 1	Flat condyloma or HPV effect	Low-grade squamous intraepithelial lesion (LSIL)
VIN 2 and VIN 3	VIN, usual type a) VIN, warty type b) VIN, basaloid type c) VIN, mixed	High-grade squamous intraepithelial lesion (HSIL)
Differentiated VIN	VIN, differentiated type	

Source Bornstein J, Bogliatto F, Haefner H, et al. The 2015 International Society for the Study of Vulvovaginal Disease (ISSVD) terminology of vulvar squamous intraepithelial lesions. *J Low Genit Tract Dis* 2016;**20**:11–14.

Paget's disease may be mammary or extramammary, as well as primary (intraepithelial infiltration by neoplastic cells showing glandular differentiation) or secondary (spread from an underlying adenocarcinoma in a dermal adnexal gland or local organ with contiguous epithelium) (23).

Vulval melanosis is an uncommon, asymptomatic, and benign condition, and has no association with vulval melanoma, though it can be clinically indistinguishable from superficial spreading melanoma. When in doubt, all melanocytic naevi of the vulva require biopsy or excision to exclude malignancy (27).

Epidemiology of premalignant vulval lesions

vHSIL is mainly a condition of younger women, quoted as between 40 and 50 years in the literature (18), though in HIV-infected women, is frequently seen as young as 20–30 years. As it is caused by oncogenic HPV infection, the risk factors for vHSIL include those related to HPV acquisition, such as multiple sexual partners and young age of first intercourse, as well as impaired immunity and cigarette smoking (18).

dVIN is usually found in postmenopausal women, with a mean age of 68 years, and often develops in those with chronic skin conditions such as squamous hyperplasia, lichen sclerosus, and lichen simplex chronicus (18). Vulval Paget's disease is most commonly seen in postmenopausal women (23).

Aetiology of premalignant vulval lesions

vHSIL is caused by integration of high-risk oncogenic HPV DNA into the host genome (18). This leads to thickening of the epidermis, with parakeratosis and hyperkeratosis, loss of cell maturation, increased mitotic figures, pleomorphism, and high nuclear-to-cytoplasmic ratios (28).

Studies show that there is a high prevalence of oncogenic HPV types in the general population, with the lifetime incidence of HPV 16 infection estimated to be more than 50%. Most healthy people's immune systems (in particular the CD4 T cells) are able to clear oncogenic HPV infection before malignancies develop, but those who are infected with HIV, where there is progressive loss of CD4 cells, have an increased prevalence of HPV infection, as well as an increased incidence of HPV-related intraepithelial neoplasia and malignancies (29).

Mutation of the *TP53* gene appears to be implicated in the development of dVIN (30), and studies show identical *TP53* mutations in lichen sclerosus and adjacent squamous carcinomas (31).

Presentation of premalignant vulval lesions

The commonest symptoms caused by premalignancies of the vulva are pruritus, pain, and sexual dysfunction. vHSIL may present as multifocal raised plaques that tend to coalesce, and which may be hyperpigmented (18). Patients may have multifocal lesions in the lower genital tract, particularly if they are immunocompromised. Women with dVIN are often asymptomatic, though may be known to have lichen sclerosus, squamous hyperplasia, or lichen simplex chronicus. They may present with discolouration of the vulval skin, white plaques, as well as red hyperkeratotic lesions (32). Pain and pruritus are present in up to 60% of women (33). Vulval pruritus is also the commonest symptom of women with vulval Paget's disease, and the clinical appearance is similar to mammary Paget's, with an erythematous weeping or crusted lesion with irregular borders (23). An associated tumour may be palpable.

Diagnosis of premalignant vulval lesions

While vulval cancer is uncommon and screening in the general population is not recommended, both patient and clinician delay in diagnosis have been reported more than in any other gynaecological malignancy (34). In one retrospective review of women with vulval cancer, 94% of women had chronic irritation of the vulva, and 85% had abnormal skin around the tumour (35). Inadequate knowledge and medical care contributes to development of these tumours, and appropriate examination of the vulva, referral, and full-thickness biopsy of the vulval skin are vital for identification of preinvasive lesions.

Cervical cytology screening programmes have had an enormous impact on the incidence of cervical cancer, and the use of vulval cytology as a screening test has been examined in a variety of studies. However, unlike in cervical disease, where the preinvasive lesion is not visible to the naked eye and is frequently asymptomatic, vulval cytology has been found to be unreliable when the vulva appears normal, and does not replace the need for biopsy of visible lesions (34).

Similarly, vulvoscopy does not play as central a role in the diagnosis of vulval preinvasive disease as colposcopy does in cervical disease. There is no evidence that it is effective as a screening tool, but it may be useful where early invasion is suspected, and in following up women who have had multiple treatments in the past. It is also important in women who have multicentric disease, in order to examine the cervix and vagina (34).

vHSIL usually presents as a visible lesion, so is identified on examination of the vulva, and during colposcopy for concurrent cervical disease. A biopsy should be taken of all atypical or suspicious areas, to confirm the diagnosis and exclude invasion, which is found in 19–22% of cases of VIN (36). Biopsies can be taken under local anaesthetic in an outpatient setting. The differential diagnosis of vHSIL includes reactive epithelial changes, vulval Paget's disease, and malignant melanoma, and a p16 immunostain is helpful in differentiating between these. In vHSIL lesions, there is a strong band-like pattern of staining with p16 (37). Histologically, vulval Paget's disease has large tumour cells with pale to eosinophilic cytoplasm within the epidermis. When immunohistochemistry is performed, these cells are positive for CK7, CEA, CAM 5.2, and GCDFP-15 (38). Malignant melanoma is positive for melanocytic markers such as HMB-45, S-100, and Melan-A (18).

The histological features of dVIN are subtle, making it difficult to diagnose (18). Five histological criteria are useful in the diagnosis of dVIN: atypical mitosis in the basal layer, basal cell atypia, dyskeratosis, prominent nucleoli, and elongation and anastomosis of the rete ridges (18). Not all dVIN lesions stain positive for p53 (32), and p53 can be positive in up to 80% of lichen sclerosus biopsies, so morphological criteria are more useful in making the diagnosis (18). Due to the previously mentioned diagnostic difficulties, pathology review by an experienced gynaecological pathologist is vital in establishing correct diagnoses in women with vulval premalignancies.

Management of vulval intraepithelial neoplasia

Follow-up of women with VIN is a balancing act between the need for treatment and symptom control, and minimizing morbidity and the risk of developing squamous carcinoma. Untreated VIN presents a far greater risk for malignant transformation than treated disease, with one study showing progression in 3.8% of women who had been treated, versus 87.5% in untreated women (39). VIN is treated in order to relieve symptoms, such as severe pruritus, to exclude invasive disease, and to decrease the risk of developing cancer. Local excision is adequate—it provides a histological specimen, while having the same recurrence rate, but much less effect on sexual function, as simple or radical vulvectomy. Excision also provides higher complete response rates than laser or medical treatments (36).

The consequences of not treating premalignant disease

Untreated, the progression of vHSIL to cancer is low, at about 10–12% (40, 41). The risk of progression is higher in women older than 45 years, and is up to 50-fold higher in immunocompromised women (42, 43). DVIN has a higher progression risk than uVIN (5.7% vs 33% respectively), and the time to progression is shorter (20–22).

Younger women may require more emphasis on the preservation of vulval anatomy and sexual function than older women. Specialist follow-up in multidisciplinary clinics, with access to conservative surgery and reconstruction, as well as psychosexual support, are important in the management of women with vulval premalignant disease (34).

Vulval cancer

Epidemiology and aetiology of vulval cancer

Vulval cancer is the fourth most common gynaecological cancer and accounts for 6–7% of all gynaecological malignancies. The incidence is approximately 2–3/100,000 women per year (44). Vulval cancer is more common in elderly women, with a median age at presentation of approximately 68 years. In the last decades, the incidence of vulval cancer has been slowly increasing (45, 46). This is thought to be related to the ageing of the population and the increasing incidence of VIN (46). Squamous cell carcinoma is the most common type, and accounts for 80–90% of all cases. Malignant melanomas, adenocarcinomas, and basal cell carcinomas are much less common. The initial route of spread is to the inguinofemoral lymph nodes. Haematogenous spread and spread by direct extension also occur, but are much less frequent.

Vulval squamous cell cancer originates following two independent pathways (**Figure 65.1**) (47, 48). The first and most common type occurs in elderly women and is related to the presence of lichen sclerosus and/or differentiated VIN. This type accounts for approximately 80% of all vulval cancers. Studies in differentiated VIN lesions and vulval squamous cell carcinomas indicate that they share identical *TP53* mutations, supporting a pathogenetic connection between them (49). The second type of vulval cancer primarily affects younger women. Persistent infection with high-risk HPV, predominantly HPV 16, is involved in the majority of these cases of vulval cancer. This type of carcinoma is associated with vHSIL. Risk factors include cigarette smoking and immunodeficiency syndromes. The reported proportion of vulval cancers associated with HPV varies widely, ranging from 15% to 79% (47).

Clinical features and diagnosis of vulval cancer

Most patients present with a vulval mass, and often there is a long history of vulval itching, associated with lichen sclerosus. Some patients present with vulval bleeding, discharge, dysuria, or a metastatic mass in the groin. Unfortunately, there is often a delay in diagnosis; patients may feel too embarrassed to visit their general practitioner, which is especially the case in older women (patients' delay). Also doctors may contribute to the delay due to the resemblance of the complaints with more common diagnoses, such as candidal infections, vulval atrophy, or lichen sclerosus (doctors' delay). This delay especially occurs when doctors prescribe medication without proper visual inspection of the vulva.

On physical examination there is a lesion on the vulva that may have a warty or ulcerating appearance (**Figure 65.2**). Several tumour characteristics are important to document, as they may influence primary treatment planning: size of the lesion, uni- or multifocality, and distance to the midline describing whether the tumour encroaches critical midline structures such as the clitoris, anus, or urethra. Distance of the medial margin of tumour to the midline determines whether ipsi- or bilateral lymph drainage to the groins is to be expected and thereby whether groin treatment should be ipsi- or bilateral. Involvement of clitoris, anus, and/or urethra often means

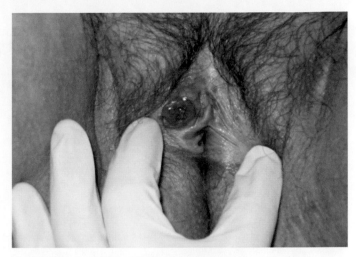

Figure 65.2 Squamous cell carcinoma of the vulva.

that these structures will need to be radically excised together with the primary tumour. Such information is important for treatment planning and for accurate pretreatment counselling of the patient. Palpation of the groins should also be performed, as this is the first site of lymphogenic metastasis.

The diagnosis of vulval cancer is made by an incision biopsy or punch biopsy for histopathological examination. For accurate treatment planning the localization of the primary tumour is important. Excision biopsy should therefore be avoided. In patients with multiple vulval lesions, all lesions should be biopsied separately, with clear mapping of the vulva.

Because vulval cancer is such a rare disease, and outcome of treatment is related to experience of the treating physicians, treatment should be centralized in centres by a multidisciplinary team with adequate experience in the treatment of this disease. Members of the team should include urologists, colorectal surgeons, plastic surgeons, and radiation oncologists.

Staging of vulval cancer

The TNM classification and the International Federation of Gynecology and Obstetrics (FIGO) staging systems are relatively similar and classify vulval cancer on the basis of the size of the tumour (T), whether the cancer has spread to lymph nodes (N), and whether it has spread to distant sites (M). Vulval cancer was clinically staged until 1988. Considering that palpation of the groins is inaccurate in approximately 25% of the patients (50), the FIGO changed to surgicopathological staging of vulval cancer in 1988. This staging provided far better discrimination of survival between stages than the 1970 FIGO clinical staging system (51). In 1994, stage IA was added to the staging system, because of the negligible risk of groin node metastases in tumours with a depth of invasion smaller or equal to 1 mm (52). In 2009, FIGO staging and TNM classification were adjusted in order to allow for better prognostic discrimination between stages and less heterogeneity within stages. The number of lymph node metastases has been shown to have major impact on survival; a 5-year survival of greater than 90% for patients with negative nodes, 75% for patients with one or two positive nodes, 36% for patients with three or four positive nodes, 24% for patients with five or six positive nodes, and 0% for patients with seven or more positive nodes (53). Also, the size of metastases has an

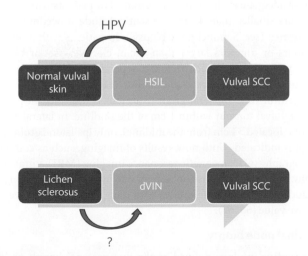

Figure 65.1 The two different pathways for development of vulval cancer. dVIN, differentiated type VIN; HPV, human papillomavirus; SCC, squamous cell cancer; uVIN, HSIL (High-grade squamous intraepithelial lesion).

Table 65.4 FIGO staging of vulval cancer

Stage	Description
Stage I	Tumour confined to the vulva or perineum
	No lymph node metastases
	IA: Lesions ≤2 cm in size, with depth of invasion ≤1 mm
	IB: Lesions >2 cm in size, with depth of invasion >1 mm
Stage II	Tumour of any size with extension to adjacent perineal structures (1/3 lower urethra, 1/3 lower vagina, anus) with negative nodes
Stage III	Tumour of any size with or without extension to adjacent perineal structures (1/3 lower urethra, 1/3 lower vagina, anus), with positive inguinofemoral lymph nodes:
	IIIA: 1 lymph node metastasis (≥5 mm) or 1–2 lymph node metastases (<5 mm)
	IIIB: ≥2 lymph node metastases (≥5 mm) or ≥3 lymph node metastases (<5 mm)
	IIIC: lymph node metastases with extracapsular spread
Stage IV	Tumour invades other regional or distant structures
	IVA: tumour invades any of the following:
	• Upper urethral and/or vaginal mucosa, bladder mucosa, rectal mucosa, or fixed to the pelvic bone
	• Fixed or ulcerated inguinofemoral lymph nodes
	IVB: any distant metastases, including pelvic lymph nodes

Table 65.5 TNM staging classification for vulval cancer

TNM		Description
T = Tumour	T1A	Tumour confined to vulva/perineum, ≤2 cm in size, and depth of invasion ≤1 mm
	T1B	Tumour confined to vulva/perineum, >2 cm in size, or depth of invasion >1 mm
	T2	Tumour involves lower urethra/vagina/anus
	T3	Tumour involves upper urethra/vagina, bladder/rectal mucosa, or pelvic bone
N = Nodes	N0	No lymph nodes involved
	N1a	Lymph node metastases: one or two nodes <5 mm
	N1b	Lymph node metastases: one node ≥5 mm
	N2a	Lymph node metastases: 3 or more nodes <5 mm
	N2b	Lymph node metastases: 2 or more nodes ≥5 mm
	N2c	Presence of extracapsular spread
	N3	Fixed or ulcerated lymph node metastases
M = Metastasis	M0	No distant metastases
	M1	Any distant metastases

impact on survival; 5-year disease-specific survival rates are 90.9% for patients with metastases smaller than 5 mm, 41.6% for those with metastases between 5 and 15 mm, and 20.0% for those with metastases greater than 15 mm (54). Extracapsular tumour growth also negatively influences survival (54, 55). These results led to the incorporation of the number and size of lymph node metastases in the most recent staging system (56). For an overview of the latest vulval cancer TNM and FIGO classifications see **Tables 65.4 and 65.5**.

Management of early-stage vulval cancer

History of surgical treatment

The cornerstone of treatment of vulval cancer patients is surgery. A recent Canadian study on patterns of care in 978 vulval cancer patients showed that 85% had at least one surgical procedure, and approximately 25% received radiotherapy (57). Standard treatment for squamous cell cancer of the vulva has changed dramatically over the last decades. Early in the twentieth century, the 'en bloc' dissection of the vulva and inguinofemoral lymph nodes was introduced (58–60). This radical approach drove out simple local excision in the second half of the last century and became the standard of care for a prolonged period of time. The rationale for this approach was the assumption that prognosis is better after elective inguinofemoral lymphadenectomy compared to surveillance of the groins, despite the fact that only about 30% of patients will have inguinofemoral lymph node metastases. Although highly effective, the morbidity of this treatment was very high. Wound breakdown, infections, and lymphoedema were of great concern and often resulted in prolonged hospitalization. Since then, many modifications of surgery have been proposed in the treatment of vulval cancer patients with the aim of all modifications to reduce morbidity of vulval cancer treatment without compromising survival rates. Steps forward were made with the introduction of inguinofemoral lymphadenectomy through separate groin incisions (61), replacement of radical vulvectomy by wide

local excision (62), abandonment of bilateral lymphadenectomy in lateralized tumours less than 2 cm in size (63, 64), and abandonment of inguinofemoral lymphadenectomy in microinvasive tumours (<1 mm depth of invasion) (52). Due to these modifications, treatment-related morbidity has decreased, but is still significant for patients undergoing inguinofemoral lymphadenectomy. In the short term, wound infections (of the groins 21–39%), lymphoceles (11–40%), and wound breakdown (12.5–39%) (65) cause significant morbidity and prolonged hospital stay and/or frequently cause readmission to the hospital. In the long term, lymphoedema is the most frequent complication, being described in 14–49% of the patients (65).

Currently local excision with a tumour-free margin of 1–2 cm is advised for local treatment. The presence of groin node metastases in vulval cancer is the most important prognostic factor, therefore urging adequate evaluation of the groins. For patients with unifocal tumours smaller than 4 cm, the sentinel node procedure can be performed (see 'Sentinel node biopsy'). In patients with multifocal tumours or tumours larger than 4 cm, elective ipsi- or bilateral inguinofemoral lymphadenectomy, depending on the location of the tumour with respect to the midline (**Figure 65.3**), remains the standard of care. Bilateral groin treatment is indicated in patients with a vulval tumour within 1 cm of the midline. In lateralized tumours (located >1 cm from the midline), only ipsilateral groin treatment is indicated. Until now, results of imaging, such as computed tomography (CT), magnetic resonance imaging (MRI), ultrasonography, and positron emission tomography were not good enough to exclude lymph node metastases with a high enough negative predictive value (66, 67).

Sentinel node biopsy

The sentinel node is defined as the first regional lymph node to which cancer cells are most likely to spread from a primary tumour (**Figure 65.2**). An important benefit of the procedure is that it enables pathological ultrastaging of the first tumour-draining lymph

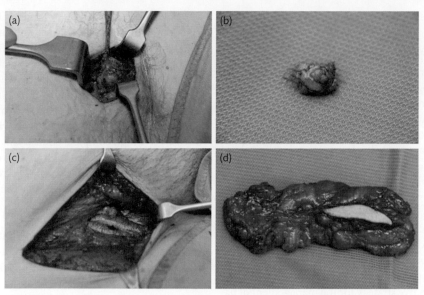

Figure 65.3 The sentinel node procedure versus inguinofemoral lymphadenectomy: (a, b) sentinel node procedure with the removed sentinel lymph node; (c, d) inguinofemoral lymphadenectomy.

node. Pathological ultrastaging consists of multiple sectioning and immunohistochemistry, allowing more accurate examination of the lymph node. Accurate examination of the sentinel node is thought to be crucial since this determines further therapeutic planning. False-negative sentinel node assessment leads to omission of lymphadenectomy, which may lead to tumour outgrowth of metastatic lymph nodes that have been left behind. Especially in vulval cancer missing lymph node metastases is extremely harmful since tumour recurrences in the groin are very hard to treat and often fatal (68).

The first pilot study of the sentinel node procedure (**Figure 65.4**) in vulval cancer was reported in 1994 (69). Subsequently, larger studies (in which the sentinel node procedure always was followed by an inguinofemoral lymphadenectomy) were designed in order to investigate the diagnostic accuracy of the sentinel node

procedure in patients with early-stage vulval cancer. Identification rates were high, especially with the combined procedure (radioactive tracer and blue dye), and false-negative rates were low (70). In 2008, the results of the first large prospective validation study were published. In this study, patients with squamous cell cancers of the vulva less than 4 cm in size and non-suspicious groin nodes at palpation were included. In these patients sentinel node detection was performed using a radioactive tracer and blue dye. When the sentinel node was negative, inguinofemoral lymphadenectomy was omitted. In the course of the study, groin recurrences occurred in a small proportion of vulval cancer patients with multifocal disease. It was hypothesized that lymph flow in these tumours is more complex and not accurately predictable by the sentinel node procedure. This led to a protocol amendment, in which multifocal disease became an exclusion criterion. The study showed that inguinofemoral lymphadenectomy can be safely omitted in patients with a negative sentinel node (2.3% groin recurrences in patients with unifocal vulval cancer) with a 3-year disease-specific survival of 97%. This study also showed a major decrease in treatment-related morbidity after sentinel node dissection compared with inguinofemoral lymphadenectomy (lymphoedema 1.9% vs 25.2%, and recurrent erysipelas 0.4% vs 16.2%) (71). Shortly thereafter, a large accuracy study on sentinel nodes and vulval cancer was published. This study showed similar results on diagnostic accuracy for patients with tumours smaller than 4 cm. Safety could not be evaluated, as all patients underwent sentinel node biopsy, followed by inguinofemoral lymphadenectomy (72). Based on these two large studies, the sentinel node procedure is nowadays recommended in the treatment of early-stage vulval cancer (70). In order to prevent fatal groin recurrences the following criteria should be met:

- Histologically proven primary squamous cell vulval cancer with a depth of invasion greater than 1 mm.
- Tumours less than 4 cm, not involving anus/vagina/urethra.
- Unifocal tumour.
- No clinically suspicious lymph nodes.

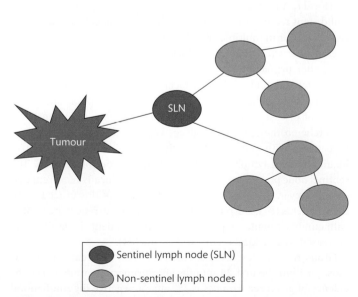

Sentinel lymph node (SLN)

Non-sentinel lymph nodes

Figure 65.4 The concept of the sentinel node procedure.

- Enlarged lymph nodes excluded by preoperative imaging (CT/ultrasonography/MRI).

The size of sentinel node metastases has important prognostic value. Data suggest that 2 mm would be an appropriate cut-off for micrometastases, since prognosis was especially worse for those patients with sentinel node metastases larger than 2 mm. However, there is no cut-off beneath which the chance on additional metastases is that low that inguinofemoral lymphadenectomy can be safely omitted (73). Further data are needed to learn about the clinical significance of these small metastases, and to establish their possible role in clinical decision-making.

Centres that wish to offer the sentinel procedure to their patients should have high enough exposure to guarantee good quality at every step of this multidisciplinary procedure. Only then can fatal groin recurrences be avoided. An exposure of at least ten vulval cancer patients per year is advised to keep experience at a high enough level. Two recent studies showed that sentinel lymph node biopsy is the most cost-effective strategy for the management of patients with early-stage vulval cancer due to lower treatment costs and lower costs due to less long-term complications and its impact on quality of life (74, 75).

Adjuvant radiotherapy

Postoperatively, radiotherapy is indicated for vulval cancer patients with more than one lymph node metastasis, or in the presence of extranodal tumour growth. This policy is based on a study by Homesley et al. in which vulval cancer patients with lymph node metastases at inguinofemoral lymphadenectomy were randomized between pelvic lymph node dissection and postoperative radiotherapy. The results of survival were in favour of the radiation group, and the benefit was most pronounced in those patients who had clinically suspicious or fixed ulcerated groin nodes, or two or more metastatic lymph nodes (76, 77). It seems that adjuvant radiotherapy is not beneficial in patients with only one intranodal lymph node metastasis (78); however, data are conflicting on this subject (79). The addition of chemotherapy as a radiosensitizer might give better treatment outcomes compared to radiotherapy alone (80). Current treatment guidelines are based on data obtained in the 'pre-sentinel node era'. While no one argues the rationale for postoperative radiotherapy in case of two lymph node metastases larger than 2 mm, the evidence for postoperative radiotherapy in case of two sentinel lymph nodes with only isolated tumour cells is at least questionable. Data on this subject in vulval cancer are until now not available.

Management of advanced vulval cancer

Although a formal definition does not exist, vulval cancer is considered to be locoregionally advanced in case of a vulval tumour without distant metastases that is beyond surgical resection with standard (radical) vulvectomy, irrespective of groin node involvement (81). Included in this category are patients with T2 or T3 tumours (Table 65.5). Management in these patients needs to be individualized and requires considerable pretreatment assessment, also taking comorbidity and/or frailty of the patients into account. Therefore, a multidisciplinary setting is needed to optimize treatment planning in this category of patients.

Surgery remains, when possible, the treatment of choice. However, definitive curative surgery in these patients generally is associated with significant morbidity. The surgical treatment options range from radical vulvectomy and bilateral inguinofemoral lymphadenectomy with or without partial resection of the urethra, vagina, or anus to primary pelvic exenteration (81). Plastic reconstructions are often necessary after large vulval excisions.

Considering the often high morbidity associated with upfront surgery (primary or neoadjuvant), chemoradiation might be an alternative. Chemoradiation in patients with locoregionally advanced disease gives high complete clinical and pathological response rates with acceptable toxicity (82, 83). However, in elderly patients in whom comorbidity and frailty may be considerable, the side effects of both treatment options have to be weighed up.

Prognosis and follow-up of vulval cancer

Prognosis of early-stage vulval cancer patients with negative nodes is very good, with a 10-year disease-specific survival of 91%. For early-stage vulval cancer patients with positive nodes, 10-year disease-specific survival is much worse at around 65% (84).

Prognosis is worse for higher FIGO stages. The pooled 5-year overall survival for vulval cancer patients is 65%. For FIGO stages I, II, III and IV, the 5-year overall survival is 84%, 75%, 48% and 9.4%, respectively (85).

The advised follow-up schedule after primary surgical treatment is:

- first visit: 6–8 weeks postoperatively
- first 2 years: every 3 months
- third and fourth year: biannually
- afterwards: annually lifelong.

There is no evidence for the best follow-up schedule. Since local recurrences may occur many years after primary treatment, lifelong follow-up is advised. Regular follow-up is thought to lead to earlier detection, and consequently more effective treatment of local recurrent disease (86). Follow-up visits should include clinical examination of vulva and groins. No standard imaging is advised.

Recurrent disease

Recurrences in vulval cancer can be subdivided according to site: local recurrences (recurrences on the vulva), groin recurrences, and distant recurrences (includes pelvic recurrences). Recurrences can also occur in multiple sites. Local recurrence is a frequent event after primary treatment, and local recurrences can occur many years after primary treatment (84). Local recurrences are treated with curative intent, with wide local excision of the vulval tumour when possible. When surgical excision is not an option due to the extent of disease or the condition of the patients, treatment with radio(chemo)therapy can be given. When local recurrences occur in patients with previously negative sentinel nodes, an elective inguinofemoral lymphadenectomy should be performed too. The sentinel node procedure seems to be feasible in locally recurrent disease; however, there are no data on the safety of this procedure in these patients (87). Despite the fact that local recurrences are treated with curative intent, the prognosis for these patients is significantly decreased when a local recurrence occurs (84).

Groin recurrences are extremely difficult to treat and occur mostly within the first 24 months after primary treatment. The incidence of groin recurrences is 1% after a negative inguinofemoral lymphadenectomy (based on retrospective data), 3% after a negative sentinel node (based on prospective data), and 7% after a negative superficial lymphadenectomy (prospective data) (70). In the case of groin lymph node metastases at the time of primary treatment, groin recurrences are observed in 8–25%, depending on the mode of primary treatment (73, 88). Groin recurrences are preferably treated by lymph node debulking by inguinofemoral lymphadenectomy, followed by radiotherapy. The addition of chemotherapy can be considered in these cases. When debulking surgery is not possible due to the extent of the disease, primary radio(chemo)therapy can be given. Groin recurrences are often fatal, as a very limited number of patients have long-term survival (68).

Patients with distant recurrences cannot be cured. Treatment in these cases should be individualized; treatment options are palliative chemotherapy and/or radiotherapy.

Rare vulval tumours

Vulval melanomas are the second most common vulval malignancy, and account for 5–10% of all vulval malignancies. The biological behaviour of vulval melanoma is similar to that of cutaneous melanoma and therefore it is thought that staging and treatment should follow the same guidelines as for cutaneous melanoma (89, 90). Therefore, surgical treatment consists of wide local excision with a 1 cm margin of normal skin in case of thickness of 1–2 mm or less and a 2 cm margin in case of a thickness of more than 1–2 mm (91). Inguinofemoral lymphadenectomy is not performed as an elective procedure in vulval melanoma, but only in case of suspicious groin nodes. The sentinel node biopsy can also be applied (92), following the same criteria as in cutaneous melanoma (depth of invasion >1 mm, or <1 mm with mitotic rate $\geq 1/mm^2$ or ulceration). Prognosis of vulval melanoma is poor with an overall 5-year survival rate of 27–47% (93, 94). Patients with superficial lesions have an excellent prognosis; however, with increasing depth of invasion, the chances of metastases increase and the prognosis worsens.

Other, even more rare, vulval tumours are Bartholin's gland carcinoma, other adenocarcinomas, basal cell carcinomas, and vulval sarcomas.

Vaginal cancer

Epidemiology and aetiology of vaginal cancer

Primary cancer of the vagina is a rare disease and accounts for only 1–2% of all gynaecological malignancies. The incidence is estimated to be 0.42/100,000 women per year and is increasing with age (95). Median age at diagnosis is 65–70 years. Cases should only be classified as vaginal cancer after exclusion of cervical, urethral, or vulval origin of the disease, as stated by FIGO (96).

The most common histological type is squamous cell carcinomas, accounting for approximately 75% of all vaginal cancers (97). Squamous cell carcinomas can be associated with HPV (98). Suggested risk factors are prior hysterectomy (98, 99), prior vaginal pessary use (due to chronic irritant vaginitis) (100), and finally patients with a history of cervical cancer (presumably because these sites share the same exposure and susceptibility to HPV). However, despite these associations also in these patients, vaginal cancer remains a rare disease, thereby not justifying screening strategies.

Clear cell carcinomas are a rare subtype and are associated with adenosis of the vagina. They usually occur in women below the age of 30 years. Adenosis of the vagina is most commonly seen in women exposed to diethylstilbestrol (DES) *in utero* (101). The drug was prescribed to women between 1948 and 1977 to reduce the risk of miscarriage. Women with DES exposure *in utero* are screened yearly for the presence of adenosis and/or vaginal cancer.

Malignant melanoma can also be located in the vagina. Malignant melanomas of the vagina are very rare. The overall prognosis is poor, as many patients present with deeply infiltrating lesions at the time of diagnosis.

Clinical features and diagnosis of vaginal cancer

The most common symptoms of vaginal cancer are painless vaginal bleeding and/or discharge. In more advanced local disease, urinary problems, tenesmus, constipation, blood in stool, and pelvic pain might be involved, depending on the localization of the vaginal tumour (anterior or posterior wall of vagina, more proximal or distal in vagina). Physical examination may reveal a vaginal mass or ulcer. Diagnosis is confirmed by a biopsy. Primary spread occurs especially to the regional lymph nodes (for tumours in proximal vagina: to the pelvic lymph nodes; in distal vagina: to groin lymph nodes). Frequent sites of distant metastases are lung and liver (98).

Staging of vaginal cancer

Staging is based on clinical criteria. Examination under general anaesthesia is often the best way to get a good impression of the extension of the tumour. Imaging of the thorax and the abdomen with CT should be performed to exclude distant metastases. The current staging system is summarized in **Table 65.6**. MRI has an increasing role in diagnosis, staging, and treatment planning of vaginal cancer (102).

Treatment of vaginal cancer

Treatment of vaginal cancer must be individualized and varies depending on the stage of disease and site of vaginal involvement. In most patients the primary treatment modality is radiotherapy, and can consist of external radiation and brachytherapy. The distal one-third of the vagina drains to the inguinofemoral lymph nodes. When the vaginal tumour is in the distal one-third, these nodes should be involved in the target volume of the radiotherapy as well (103).

Experience with chemoradiation in vaginal cancer is limited. Often for larger tumours, chemotherapy is added, extrapolating the results in cervical cancer that has a similar biology. The rareness of vaginal cancer makes it very hard to ever perform randomized trials on this subject.

Surgery has a limited role in the management of vaginal cancer, because of the radicality required to achieve clear surgical margins. However, in selected cases surgery is possible. For example, patients with a proximal vaginal tumour can be treated like cervical cancer patients with a radical hysterectomy, upper/partial vaginectomy, and pelvic lymphadenectomy. Small early-stage tumours near to the hymen can be treated like vulval cancer, with local excision of the primary tumour combined with inguinofemoral lymphadenectomy.

Table 65.6 FIGO staging of vaginal cancer

Stage	
Stage 0	Carcinoma *in situ*
Stage I	Carcinoma limited to vaginal wall
Stage II	Carcinoma has involved subvaginal tissue but has not extended to the pelvic wall
Stage III	Carcinoma has extended to the pelvic wall
Stage IV	Carcinoma has extended beyond the true pelvis or has involved the musosa of the bladder and/or rectum
Stage IVA Stage IVB	Spread of the growth to adjacent organs Spread to distant organs

Prognosis of vaginal cancer

Overall prognosis of vaginal cancer is poor, which is probably due to the frequent late stage at presentation (96). Vaginal cancer can recur in the vagina, pelvis, or at distant sites. The prognosis of recurrent disease is very poor. In selected cases, a pelvic exenteration may be one option.

Due to the rarity of the disease, patients with vaginal cancer should be referred to a tertiary oncology unit.

REFERENCES

1. Gurumurthy M, Cruickshank ME. Management of vaginal intraepithelial neoplasia. *J Low Genit Tract Dis* 2012;**16**:306–12.
2. Cramer DW, Cutler SJ. Incidence and histopathology of malignancies of the female genital organs in the United States. *Am J Obstet Gynecol* 1974;**118**:443–60.
3. Lenehan PM, Meff F, Lickrish GM. Vaginal intraepithelial neoplasia: biologic aspects and management. *Obstet Gynecol* 1986;**68**:333–37.
4. Rome RM, England PG. Management of vaginal intraepithelial neoplasia: a series of 132 cases with long term follow-up. *Int J Gynecol Cancer* 2000;**10**:382–90.
5. Aho M, Vesterinen E, Meyer B, Purola E, Paavonen J. Natural history of vaginal intraepithelial neoplasia. *Cancer* 1991;**68**:195–97.
6. Abercrombie PD, Korn AP. Lower genital tract neoplasia in women with HIV infection. *Oncology (Williston Park)* 1998;**12**:1735–39.
7. Gemmell J, Holmes DM, Duncan ID. How frequently need vaginal smears be taken after hysterectomy for cervical intraepithelial neoplasia? *Br J Obstet Gynecol* 1990;**97**:58–61.
8. Hoffman DS, DeCesare SL, Roberts WS, Fiorica JV, Finan MA, Cavanagh D. Upper vaginectomy for in situ and occult, superficially invasive carcinoma of the vagina. *Am J Obstet Gynecol* 1992;**166**:30–33.
9. Curtis P, Shepherd JH, Lowe DG, Jobling T. The role of partial colpectomy in the management of persistent vaginal neoplasia after primary treatment. *Br J Obstet Gynecol* 1992;**99**:587–89.
10. Diakomanolis E, Rodolakis A, Boulgaris Z, Blachos G, Michalas S. Treatment of vaginal intraepithelial neoplasia with laser ablation and upper vaginectomy. *Gynecol Obstet Invest* 2002;**54**:17–20.
11. Benedet JL, Wilson PS, Matisic JP. Epidermal thickness measurements in vaginal intraepithelial neoplasia. A basis for optimal CO_2 laser vaporization. *J Reprod Med* 1992;**37**:809–12.
12. Lin H, Huang EY, Chang HY, ChangChien CC. Therapeutic effect of topical applications of trichloracetic acid for vaginal intraepithelial neoplasia after hysterectomy. *Jpn J Clin Oncol* 2005;**35**:651–54.
13. Kirwan P, Naftalin NJ. Topical 5-fluorouracil in the treatment of vaginal intraepithelial neoplasia. *Br J Obstet Gynaecol* 1985;**92**:287–91.
14. Haidopoulos D, Diakomanolis E, Rodolakis A, Voulgaris Z, Vlachos G, Insaklis A. Can local application of imiquimod cream be an alternative mode of therapy for patients with high-grade intraepithelial lesions of the vagina? *Int J Gynecol Cancer* 2005;**15**:898–902.
15. David L, Simon L. *Colposcopy and Programme Management: Guidelines for the NHS Cervical Screening Programme*, 2nd edn. Publication No. 20. London, UK: NHS CSP; 2010.
16. Stokes-Lampard H, Wilson S, Waddell C, Ryan A, Holder R, Kehoe S. Vaginal vault smears after hysterectomy for reasons other than malignancy: a systematic review of the literature. *BJOG* 2006;**113**:1354–65.
17. Dodge JA, Eltabbakh GH, Mount SL, Walker RP, Morgan A. Clinical features and risk of recurrence among patients with vaginal intraepithelial neoplasia. *Gynecol Oncol* 2001;**83**:363–69.
18. Reyes MC, Cooper, K. An update on vulvar intraepithelial neoplasia: terminology and a practical approach to diagnosis. *J Clin Pathol* 2014;**67**:290–94.
19. Van Esch EMG, Dam MCI, Osse MEM, et al. Clinical characteristics associated with development of recurrence and progression in usual-type vulvar intraepithelial neoplasia. *Int J Gynecol Cancer* 2013;**23**:1476–83.
20. Eva LJ, Ganesan R, Chan KK, et al. Differentiated-type vulval intraepithelial neoplasia has a high-risk association with vulval squamous cell carcinoma. *Int J Gynecol Cancer* 2009;**19**:741–44.
21. Eva LJ, Ganesan R, Chan KK, et al. Vulval squamous cell carcinoma occurring on a background of differentiated vulval intraepithelial neoplasia is more likely to recur: a review of 154 cases. *J Reprod Med* 2008;**53**:397–401.
22. Van de Nieuwenhof HP, van Kempen LC, Massuger LF, et al. Differentiated-type vulval intraepithelial neoplasia has a high-risk association with vulval squamous cell carcinoma. *Int J Gynecol Cancer* 2010;**20**:194.
23. Lloyd J, Flanagan AM. Mammary and extramammary Paget's disease. *J Clin Pathol* 2000;**53**:742–49.
24. Bornstein J, Bogliatto F, Haefner H, et al. The 2015 International Society for the Study of Vulvovaginal Disease (ISSVD) terminology of vulvar squamous intraepithelial lesions. *J Low Genit Tract Dis* 2016;**20**:11–14.
25. Sideri M, Jones RW, Wilkinson EJ, et al. Squamous vulvar intraepithelial neoplasia: 2004 modified terminology, ISSVD Vulvar Oncology Subcommittee. *J Reprod Med* 2005;**50**:807–10.
26. Darragh TM, Colgan TJ, Thomas Cox J, et al. Members of the LAST Project Work Groups. The Lower Anogenital Squamous Terminology Standardization project for HPV-associated lesions: background and consensus recommendations from the College of American Pathologists and the American Society for Colposcopy and Cervical Pathology. *Int J Gynecol Pathol* 2013;**32**:76–115.
27. Edwards L. Pigmented vulvar lesions. *Dermatol Ther* 2010;**23**:449–57.
28. Hart WR. Vulvar intraepithelial neoplasia: historical aspects and current status. *Int J Gynecol Pathol* 2001;**20**:16–30.
29. Van der Burg S, Palefsky JM. Human immunodeficiency virus and human papilloma virus—why HPV-induced lesions do not spontaneously resolve and why therapeutic vaccination can be successful. *J Transl Med* 2009;**7**:108.
30. Pinto AP, Miron A, Yassin Y, et al. Differentiated vulvar intraepithelial neoplasia contains Tp53 mutations and is

genetically linked to vulvar squamous cell carcinoma. *Mod Pathol* 2010;**23**:404–12.

31. Rolfe KJ, Maclean AB, Crow JC, et al. TP53 mutations in vulval lichen sclerosus adjacent to squamous cell carcinoma of the vulva. *Br J Cancer* 2003;**89**:2249–53.

32. Del Pino M, Rodriguez-Carunchio L, Ordi J. Pathways of vulvar intraepithelial neoplasia and squamous cell carcinoma. *Histopathology* 2013;**62**:161–75.

33. McNally OM, Mulvany NJ, Pagano R, et al. VIN3: a clinicopathologic review. *Int J Gynecol Cancer* 2002;**12**:490–95.

34. Eva LJ. Screening and follow up of vulval skin disorders. *Best Pract Res Clin Obstet Gynaecol* 2012;**26**:175–88.

35. Jones RW, Joura EA. Analyzing prior clinical events at presentation in 102 women with vulvar carcinoma: evidence of diagnostic delays. *J Reprod Med* 1999;**44**:766–68.

36. Husseinzadeh N, Recinto C. Frequency of invasive cancer in surgically excised vulvar lesions with intraepithelial neoplasia (VIN3). *Gynecol Oncol* 1999;**73**:119–20.

37. Rufforny I, Wilkinson EJ, Liu C, et al. Human papillomavirus infection and p16 (INK4a) protein expression in vulvar intraepithelial neoplasia and invasive squamous cell carcinoma. *J Lower Genit Tract Dis* 2005;**9**:108–13.

38. McCluggage WG. Recent advances in immunohistochemistry in gynaecological pathology. *Histopathology* 2002;**40**:309–26.

39. Jones RW, Rowan D. VIN3: a clinical study of the outcome in 113 cases with relation to the later development of invasive vulvar carcinoma. *Obstet Gynecol* 1994;**84**:741–45.

40. Lawrie TA, Nordin A, Chakrabarti M, Bryant A, Kaushik S, Pepas L. Medical and surgical interventions for the treatment of usual-type vulval intraepithelial neoplasia. *Cochrane Database Syst Rev* 2016;**1**:CD011837.

41. Cruickshank ME, Hay I, Guidelines Committee of the Royal College of Obstetricians and Gynaecologists (RCOG). *The Management of Vulval Skin Disorders*. Green-top Guideline No. 58. London: RCOG; 2011.

42. Jones RW. The natural history of cervical and vulvar intraepithelial neoplasia. *Am J Obstet Gynecol* 2010;**202**:e12–13.

43. Jones RW, Rowan DM, Stewart AW. Vulvar intraepithelial neoplasia: aspects of the natural history and outcome in 405 women. *Obstet Gynecol* 2005;**106**:1319–26.

44. National Cancer Institute. Surveillance, epidemiology, and end results program. Available at: http://seer.cancer.gov/statfacts/html/vulva.html.

45. Akhtar-Danesh N, Elit L, Lytwyn A. Trends in incidence and survival of women with invasive vulvar cancer in the United States and Canada: a population-based study. *Gynecol Oncol* 2014;**134**:314–18.

46. Somoye GO, Mocroft A, Olaitan A. Analysis of the incidence and mortality of vulval cancer in women in South East England 1960-1999. *Arch Gynecol Obstet* 2009;**279**:113–17.

47. Del Pino M, Rodriquez-Carunchio L, Ordi J. Pathways of vulvar intraepithelial neoplasia and squamous cell carcinoma. *Histopathology* 2013;**62**:161–75.

48. Van der Avoort IA, Shirango H, Hoevenaars BM, et al. Vulvar squamous cell carcinoma is a multifactorial disease following two separate and independent pathways. *Int J Gynecol Pathol* 2006;**25**:22–29.

49. Pinto AP, Miron A, Yassin Y, et al. Differentiated vulvar intraepithelial neoplasia contains Tp53 mutations and is genetically linked to vulvar squamous cell carcinoma. *Mod Pathol* 2010;**23**:404–12.

50. Prodratz KC, Symmonds RE, Taylor WF, Williams TJ. Carcinoma of the vulva: analysis of treatment and survival. *Obstet Gynecol* 1983;**61**:63–74.

51. Hopkins MP, Reid GC, Johnston CM, Morley GW. A comparison of staging systems for squamous cell carcinoma of the vulva. *Gynecol Oncol* 1992;**47**:34–37.

52. Hacker NF, Berek JS, Lagasse LD, Nieberg RK, Leuchter RS. Individualization of treatment for stage I squamous cell vulvar carcinoma. *Obstet Gynecol* 1984;**63**:155–62.

53. Homesley HD, Bundy BN, Sedlis A, et al. Assessment of current International Federation of Gynecologic and Obstetrics staging of vulvar carcinoma relative to prognostic factors for survival (A Gynecologic Oncology Group study). *Am J Obstet Gynecol* 1991;**164**:997–1003.

54. Origoni M, Sideri M, Garsia S, Carinelli SG, Ferrari AG. Prognostic value of pathological patterns of lymph node positivity in squamous cell carcinoma of the vulva stage III and IVA FIGO. *Gynecol Oncol* 1992;**45**:313–16.

55. Paladini D, Cross P, Lopes A, Monaghan JM. Prognostic significance of lymph node variables in squamous cell carcinoma of the vulva. *Cancer* 1994;**74**:2491–496.

56. Hacker NF. Revised FIGO staging for carcinoma of the vulva. *Int J Gynecol Obstet* 2009;**105**:105–106.

57. Barbera L, Thomas G, Elit L, et al. Treating vulvar cancer in the new millennium: are patients receiving optimal care? *Gynecol Oncol* 2008;**109**:71–75.

58. Basset A. Traitement chirurgical opératoire de l'épithelioma primitif du clitoris: Indications, technique, résultats. *Rev Chir* 1912;**46**:546–63.

59. Taussig FJ. Cancer of the vulva: an analysis of 155 cases (1911–1940). *Am J Obstet Gynecol* 1949;**40**:764–772.

60. Way S. Carcinoma of the vulva. *Am J Obstet Gynecol* 1960;**79**:692–97.

61. Hacker NF, Leuchter RS, Berek JS, Castaldo TW, Lagasse LD. Radical vulvectomy and bilateral inguinal lymphadenectomy through separate incisions. *Obstet Gynecol* 1981;**58**:574–79.

62. Hacker NF, van der Velden J. Conservative management of early vulvar cancer. *Cancer* 1993;**71**:1673–77.

63. Iversen T, Aas M. Lymph drainage from the vulva. *Gynecol Oncol* 1983;**16**:179–83.

64. Burger MP, Hollema H, Bouma J. The side of groin node metastases in unilateral vulvar carcinoma. *In J Gynecol Cancer* 1996;**6**:318–22.

65. Wills A, Obermair A. A review of complications associated with the surgical treatment of vulvar cancer. *Gynecol Oncol* 2013;**131**:467–79.

66. Selman TJ, Luesley DM, Acheson N, Khan KS, Mann CH. A systematic review of the accuracy of diagnostic tests for inguinal lymph node status in vulvar cancer. *Gynecol Oncol* 2005;**99**:206–14.

67. Oonk MH, Hollema H, de Hullu JA, van der Zee AG. Prediction of lymph node metastases in vulvar cancer: a review. *Int J Gynecol Cancer* 2006;**16**:963–71.

68. Cormio G, Loizzi V, Carriero C, Cazzolla A, Putignano G, Selvaggi L. Groin recurrence in carcinoma of the vulva: management and outcome. *Eur J Cancer Care* 2010;**19**:302–307.

69. Levenback C, Burke TW, Gershenson DM, Morris M, Malpica A, Ross MI. Intraoperative lymphatic mapping for vulvar cancer. *Obstet Gynecol* 1994;**84**:163–67.

70. Covens A, Vella ET, Kennedy EB, Reade CJ, Jimenez W, Le T. Sentinel lymph node biopsy in vulvar cancer: systematic review, meta-analysis and guideline recommendations. *Gynecol Oncol* 2015;**137**:351–61.

71. Van der Zee AG, Oonk MH, de Hullu JA, et al. Sentinel node dissection is safe in the treatment of early-stage vulvar cancer. *J Clin Oncol* 2008;**20**:884–89.

72. Levenback CF, Ali S, Coleman RL, et al. Lymphatic mapping and sentinel lymph node biopsy in women with squamous cell carcinoma of the vulva: a gynecologic oncology group study. *J Clin Oncol* 2012;**30**:3786–91.

73. Oonk MH, van Hemel BM, Hollema H, et al. Size of sentinel-node metastasis and chances of non-sentinel-node involvement and survival in early stage vulvar cancer: results from GROINSS-V, a multicentre observational study. *Lancet Oncol* 2010;**11**:646–52.

74. Erickson BK, Divine LM, Leath CA 3rd, Straughn JM Jr. Cost-effectiveness analysis of sentinel lymph node biopsy in the treatment of early-stage vulvar cancer. *Int J Gynecol Cancer* 2014;**24**:1480–85.

75. McCann GA, Cohn DE, Jewell EL, Havrilesky LJ. Lymphatic mapping and sentinel lymph node dissection compared to complete lymphadenectomy in the management of early-stage vulvar cancer: a cost-utility analysis. *Gynecol Oncol* 2015;**136**:300–304.

76. Homesley HD, Bundy BN, Sedlis A, Adcock L. Radiation therapy versus pelvic node resection for carcinoma of the vulva with positive groin nodes. *Obstet Gynecol* 1986;**68**:733–40.

77. Kunos C, Simpkins F, Gibbons H, Tian C, Homesley H. Radiation therapy compared with pelvic node resection for node-positive vulvar cancer: a randomized controlled trial. *Obstet Gynecol* 2009;**114**:537–46.

78. Fons G, Groenen SM, Oonk MH, et al. Adjuvant radiotherapy in patients with vulvar cancer and one intracapsular lymph node metastasis is not beneficial. *Gynecol Oncol* 2009;**114**:343–45.

79. Woelber L, Eulenburg C, Choschzich M, et al. Prognostic role of lymph node metastases in vulvar cancer and implications for adjuvant treatment. *Int J Gynecol Cancer* 2012;**22**:503–508.

80. Gill BS, Bernard ME, Lin JF, et al. Impact of adjuvant chemotherapy with radiation for node-positive vulvar cancer: a National Cancer Data Base (NSDB) analysis. *Gynecol Oncol* 2015;**137**:365–72.

81. Expert Panel on Radiation Oncology-Gynecology, Kidd E, Moore D, et al. ACR appropriateness criteria management of locoregionally advanced squamous cell carcinoma of the vulva. *Am J Clin Oncol* 2013;**36**:415–22.

82. Van Doorn HC, Ansink A, Verhaar-Langereis M, Stalpers L. Neoadjuvant chemoradiation for advanced primary vulvar cancer. *Cochrane Database Syst Rev* 2006;**3**:CD003752.

83. Moore DH, Ali S, Koh WJ, et al. A phase II trial of radiation therapy and weekly cisplatin chemotherapy for the treatment of locally-advanced squamous cell carcinoma of the vulva: a gynecologic oncology group study. *Gynecol Oncol* 2012;**124**:529–33.

84. Te Grootenhuis NC, van der Zee AG, van Doorn HC, et al. Sentinel nodes in vulvar cancer: long-term follow-up of the Groningen International Study on Sentinel nodes in Vulvar cancer (GROINSS-V) I. *Gynecol Oncol* 2016;**140**:8–14.

85. Zhou J, Shan G. The prognostic role of FIGO stage in patients with vulvar cancer: a systematic review and meta-analysis. *Curr Med Res Opin* 2016;**32**:1121–30.

86. Oonk MH, de Hullu JA, Hollema H, et al. The value of routine follow-up in patients treated for carcinoma of the vulva. *Cancer* 2003;**98**:2624–29.

87. Van Doorn HC, van Beekhuizen HJ, Gaarenstroom KN, et al. Repeat sentinel lymph node procedure in patients with recurrent vulvar squamous cell carcinoma is feasible. *Gynecol Oncol* 2016;**140**:415–19.

88. Nooij LS, Ongkiehong PJ, van Zwet EW, et al. Groin surgery and risk of recurrence in lymph node positive patients with vulvar squamous cell carcinoma. *Gynecol Oncol* 2015;**139**:458–64.

89. Moxley KM, Fader AN, Rose PG, et al. Malignant melanoma of the vulva: an extension of cutaneous melanoma? *Gynecol Oncol* 2011;**122**:612–17.

90. Philips GL, Bundy BN, Okagaki T, Kucera PR, Stehman FB. Malignant melanoma of the vulva treated by radical hemivulvectomy. A prospective study of the Gynecologic Oncology Group. *Cancer* 1994;**73**:2626–32.

91. Sladden MJ, Balch C, Barzilai DA, et al. Surgical excision margins for primary cutaneous melanoma. *Cochrane Database Syst Rev* 2009;**4**:CD004835.

92. Abramova L, Parekh J, Irvin WP Jr, et al. Sentinel node biopsy in vulvar and vaginal melanoma: presentation of six cases and a literature review. *Ann Surg Oncol* 2002;**9**:840–46.

93. Verschraegen CF, Benjapibal M, Supakarapongkul W, et al. Vulvar melanoma at the M.D. Anderson Cancer Center: 25 years later. *Int J Gynecol Cancer* 2001;**11**:359–64.

94. Ragnarsson-Olding BK, Kanter-Lewensohn LR, Lagerlöf B, Nilsson BR, Ringborg UK. Malignant melanoma of the vulva in a nationwide, 25-year study of 219 Swedish females: clinical observations and histopathologic features. *Cancer* 1999;**86**:1273–84.

95. Parkin DM, Bray F, Ferlay J, Pisani P. Global cancer statistics, 2002. *CA Cancer J Clin* 2005;**55**:74–108.

96. Beller U, Benedet JL, Creasman WT, et al. Carcinoma of the vagina. FIGO 26th annual report on the results of treatment in gynecological cancer. *Int J Gynaecol Obstet* 2006;**95** Suppl 1:S29–42.

97. Davis KP, Stanhope CR, Garton GR, Atkinson EJ, O'Brien PC. Invasive vaginal carcinoma: analysis of early-stage disease. *Gynecol Oncol* 1991;**42**:131–36.

98. Daling JR, Madeleine MM, Schwartz SM, et al. A population-based study of squamous cell vaginal cancer: HPV and cofactors. *Gynecol Oncol* 2002;**84**:263–70.

99. Herman JM, Homesley HD, Dignan MB. Is hysterectomy a risk factor for vaginal cancer? *JAMA* 1986;**256**:601–603.

100. Bouma J, Burger MP, Krans M, Hollema H, Pras E. Squamous cell carcinoma of the vagina: a report of 32 cases. *Int J Gynecol Cancer* 1994;**4**:389–94.

101. Herbst AL, Robboy SJ, Scully RE, Poskanzer DC. Clear-cell adenocarcinoma of the vagina and cervix in girls: analysis of 170 registry cases. *Am J Obstet Gynecol* 1974;**119**:713–24.

102. Gardner CS, Sunil J, Klopp AH, et al. Primary vaginal cancer: role of MRI in diagnosis, staging and treatment. *Br J Radiol* 2015;**99**:20150033.

103. Hacker NF, Eifel PJ, van der Velden J. Cancer of the vagina; FIGO cancer report 2015. *Int J Gynecol Obstet* 2015;**131** Suppl 2:S84–87.

66

Gestational trophoblastic disease

Hextan Y.S. Ngan, Karen K.L. Chan, and Siew-Fei Ngu

Introduction

Gestational trophoblastic disease (GTD) arises from an abnormal pregnancy which can subsequently develop into a neoplastic lesion and cancer. The most common abnormal pregnancy preceding GTD is usually benign. Molar pregnancy histologically is classified into partial and complete mole. The malignant histological types include choriocarcinoma, placental site trophoblastic tumour (PSTT), and epithelioid trophoblastic tumour. The presence of abnormal proliferating trophoblastic tissues can be detected by serum human chorionic gonadotropin (hCG) assays. Hence, a disease entity without histology but characterized by a persistently elevated serum hCG concentration after molar or normal pregnancy is named gestational trophoblastic neoplasia (GTN) and forms part of the GTD spectrum where treatment is required. Treatment of the malignant form of GTD is mostly by chemotherapy with good prognosis.

Molar pregnancy

Incidence

Molar pregnancy incidence is decreasing worldwide. It is still more common in South-East Asia (2 per 1000 pregnancies) than Europe and North America (<1 per 1000 pregnancies). A similar decrease was seen in Japan (1) which could be related to a decreasing number of childbirths and an improved economy. The use of ultrasonography early in pregnancy which may have led to early diagnosis and termination of non-viable pregnancies without histology assessment could also result in underestimation of the incidence of molar pregnancy. A decreasing incidence has also been observed in GTN in Korea and Japan (2). For choriocarcinoma, the incidence is difficult to estimate because it is uncommon to have a histological assessment of 'tumour' seen in GTN. The 'tumour' could be invasive or a metastatic mole or choriocarcinoma. Knowing this limitation, the incidence of choriocarcinoma has been reported to be approximately 1–9 in 40,000 pregnancies, and again the incidence rates have been declining.

Presentation

The most common presentation nowadays is abnormal bleeding complicating an early pregnancy and ultrasonographic examination helps to make an early diagnosis (3). Uterine size is variable in relationship to gestation. Hyperemesis gravidarum, hyperthyroidism, bleeding leading to severe anaemia, early-onset severe pre-eclampsia, uterine size larger than dates, bilateral large theca lutein cysts, and pulmonary trophoblastic embolism are rarely seen today as these symptoms and signs tend to be associated with advanced molar pregnancy.

Diagnostic investigations

Ultrasonography is the most useful diagnostic investigation for molar pregnancy. However, the typical snow-storm appearance (**Figure 66.1**) is less commonly seen because of early presentation. Ultrasound features of early molar pregnancy are less typical. It could be an absence of fetal parts, a cystic appearance of the placenta, and a deformed gestational sac similar to a missed miscarriage. In fact, one study showed that the typical sonographic appearance of a first-trimester complete mole is a complex, echogenic, intrauterine mass with many small cystic spaces (**Figure 66.2**) (4). Moreover, 21% and 71% of complete and partial hydatidiform moles respectively could be missed on ultrasonography, especially in early gestational age (5). Hence, histological examination of all gestational products will pick up early molar pregnancy missed by ultrasound examination.

Pathology and cytogenetics

The typical histopathology of molar pregnancy includes hydropic villi and trophoblastic proliferation. The main challenge lies in differentiating between complete mole from partial mole and partial mole from hydropic degeneration of villi in miscarriages (6). Histologically, complete mole has florid cistern formation, trophoblastic proliferation, and an absence of fetal parts (**Figure 66.3**). In partial mole, there is less proliferation and fetal parts or fetal blood cells are present (**Figure 66.4**). Hydropic miscarriage looks very similar to partial mole. Early complete moles may lack florid histological features but have structures such as abnormal budding villous with trophoblast hyperplasia, stromal karyorrhectic debris, and collapsed villous blood vessels. On the other hand, patchy villous hydrops with scattered abnormally shaped irregular villi, trophoblastic pseudoinclusions, and patchy trophoblast hyperplasia are seen in partial moles (7). With the help of a cytomolecular study to identify the origin of the sex chromosomes, an androgenetic diploid complete mole (**Figures 66.5 and 66.6**) (41) or a biparental triploid partial mole can be differentiated from a diploid miscarriage. Using

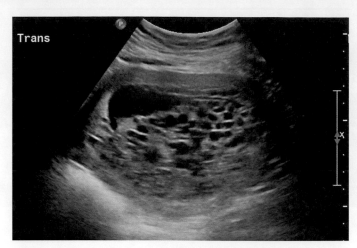

Figure 66.1 Ultrasound image of a molar pregnancy showing a complex echogenic mass containing multiple discrete cystic spaces (snow-storm appearance) in the uterine cavity.

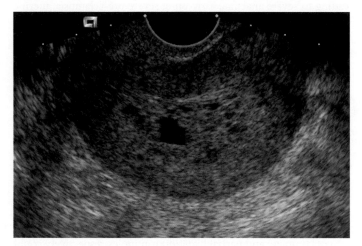

Figure 66.2 Ultrasound image of an early molar pregnancy showing echogenic tissue with numerous cystic vesicles in the uterine cavity.

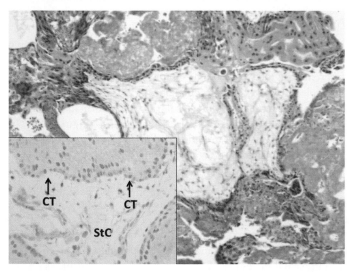

Figure 66.3 Photomicrographs demonstrating complete hydatidiform mole: cytotrophoblasts (CT) and stromal cells (StC) are negative for p57^{KIP2}, encoded by *CDKN1C*, a paternally imprinted gene which is maternally expressed.

Courtesy of Cheung AN, Department of Pathology, The University of Hong Kong.

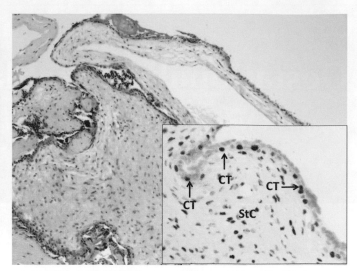

Figure 66.4 Photomicrographs demonstrating partial hydatidiform mole: cytotrophoblasts (CT) and stromal cells (StC) are positive for p57^{KIP2}, encoded by *CDKN1C*, a paternally imprinted gene which is maternally expressed.

Courtesy of Cheung AN, Department of Pathology, The University of Hong Kong.

immunohistochemical staining of p57^{KIP2} (cyclin-dependent kinase inhibitor 1C, encoded by *CDKN1C*) to confirm the presence of maternal genes can exclude complete mole. However, if molar pregnancy still cannot be excluded, it is acceptable to monitor the serum hCG level for at least 6 months or until it becomes normal.

Management of molar pregnancy

The standard treatment is suction evacuation of the uterus. It should be performed by an experienced anaesthetist and gynaecologist because of the risk of bleeding, respiratory complication, and perforation of uterus. To prepare for the heavy bleeding during suction evacuation, it is essential to have venous access with a wide-bore cannula and crossmatched blood readily available. Oxytocics can be used after cervical os dilation and onset of suction curettage with no increase in risk of GTN. As the uterus tends to be soft, the use of intraoperative ultrasound or evacuation by an experienced gynaecologist may reduce the risk of uterine perforation. However, a routine second evacuation is not recommended unless there is a clinical indication such as persistent vaginal bleeding. Termination of pregnancy using medical methods should be avoided except in second-trimester termination of a partial mole with a fetus since it increases the chance of developing GTN (8). Hysterectomy is not indicated for termination of molar pregnancy but can be performed if there is a coexisting indication or life-threatening haemorrhage.

Human chorionic gonadotropin monitoring

Serial serum hCG monitoring following evacuation is essential for early diagnosis of GTN. After evacuation, weekly or biweekly hCG monitoring is performed until the level returns to normal and then it is spaced out to 4 weeks for 6 months. The criteria for a diagnosis of GTN will be discussed later (see 'Diagnosis'). The risk of developing GTN is 0.5–1% after partial mole and 15–20% after complete mole.

Serum hCG assay

The accuracy of serum hCG measurement in monitoring of GTN is affected by the choice of assay method (9). In addition to intact hCG,

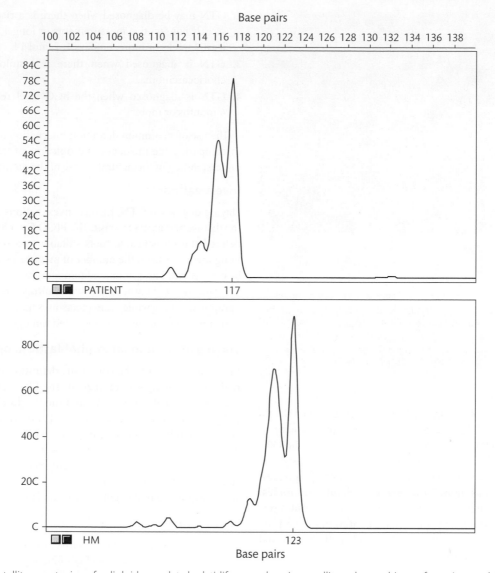

Figure 66.5 Microsatellite genotyping of a diploid complete hydatidiform mole: microsatellite polymorphisms of a patient and the diploid hydatidiform mole (HM). The patient was homozygous for the marker D17S1322, generating an allele of 117 base pairs. The HM also was homozygous for D17S1322, giving rise to an allele of 123 base pairs, which was not found in the maternal DNA and thus was androgenetic.

Reproduced from Cheung AN, Khoo US, Lai CY, Chan KY, Xue WC, Cheng DK et al. Metastatic trophoblastic disease after an initial diagnosis of partial hydatidiform mole: genotyping and chromosome in situ hybridization analysis. *Cancer* 2004;100:1411–17.

patients with GTN also produce nicked hCG, hyperglycosylated hCG, hCG with missing beta-subunit C-terminal segment, and hCG with free beta subunit. Thus, commercially available pregnancy test kits which often measure only total hCG are not suitable and may lead to false-negative results thus either missing the diagnosis or leading to inadequate treatment.

False-positive serum hCG

False-positive serum hCG is due to the presence of heterophilic antibodies in sera. This can explain the 'phantom hCG' when serum hCG levels are persistently raised in the absence of GTN (10). It could be differentiated by a negative urine hCG assay or by a serial dilution assay where the levels do not follow the dilution factor.

Central registry

Ideally, all women with a molar pregnancy should be registered with a central registry to facilitate central hCG assay, monitoring,

and management. Especially in countries with decreasing incidence, pooling of expertise and resources would ensure better quality of patient care. Early diagnosis and proper management of postmolar GTN has a high cure rate.

Contraception after molar pregnancy

A reliable contraceptive method is advised to allow monitoring of serum hCG after a molar pregnancy without the interference of a normal pregnancy. The combined oral contraceptive pill can be used immediately after termination of a molar pregnancy (11) or after hCG has returned to normal (12). Termination of pregnancy is not indicated if pregnancy occurs during surveillance after the hCG has declined to normal levels.

Recurrent molar pregnancy

The risk of having another molar pregnancy after a complete mole is around 1% but women with two complete moles have

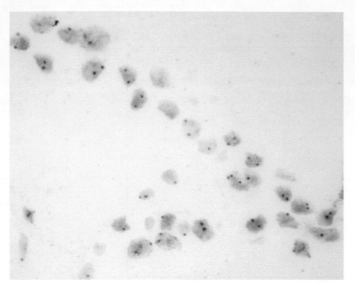

Figure 66.6 Chromosome *in situ* hybridization of a diploid complete hydatidiform mole: two hybridization signals, as detected by DNA probes for chromosome 16, were found in the majority of nuclei.

Reproduced from Cheung AN, Khoo US, Lai CY, Chan KY, Xue WC, Cheng DK et al. Metastatic trophoblastic disease after an initial diagnosis of partial hydatidiform mole: genotyping and chromosome in situ hybridization analysis. *Cancer* 2004;100:1411–17.

a one in four risk of another mole (13) and have a higher risk of persistent GTN (14). The risk of further molar pregnancies in women with a partial mole was only slightly increased (1 in 350). Women should be reassured that the majority of women have a normal pregnancy and delivery following a molar pregnancy. A small proportion has 'familial recurrent hydatidiform moles', which is a rare autosomal recessive disorder caused by mutations in the *NLRP7* (NLR family, pyrin domain containing 7) and the *KHDC3L* (KH domain containing 3-like, subcortical maternal complex member) genes.

Mole with coexisting normal twin

Rarely, molar pregnancy is found on ultrasonography together with a normal twin pregnancy. Although the risk of spontaneous miscarriage is high, about 40% achieve live births. There is no increase in the risk of developing GTN (15). Thus, pregnancy need not be terminated after confirming normal karyotype and an otherwise normal pregnancy.

Gestational trophoblastic neoplasia

Diagnosis

Historically, different countries have used different criteria in the diagnosis of GTN which result in a wide range of quoted incidence, from 8% in the United Kingdom to 20% in the United States. Consensus criteria were reached by the International Federation of Gynecology and Obstetrics (FIGO) in 2000 (16) and this is now used internationally to diagnose GTN:

1. GTN may be diagnosed when the plateau of hCG lasts for four measurements over a period of 3 weeks or longer, that is, for days 1, 7, 14, and 21.

2. GTN may be diagnosed when there is a rise in hCG for three weekly consecutive measurements or longer, over a period of at least 2 weeks or more, on days 1, 7, and 14.

3. GTN is diagnosed when there is histological diagnosis of choriocarcinoma.

4. GTN is diagnosed when the hCG level remains elevated for 6 months or more.

The use of a common definition internationally would be helpful in comparing the incidence and outcome of treatment and in the understanding of the natural course of the disease.

Investigations

Having diagnosed GTN, further investigations are needed to stage the disease and assess the risk. The FIGO Oncology Committee also defined the investigative tools suitable to assess metastases (16). Lung metastases and the number of metastases should be evaluated by chest X-ray. Lung computed tomography can be used if available. Liver metastases may be diagnosed by ultrasound or computed tomography scanning while brain metastases may be diagnosed by magnetic resonance imaging or computed tomography scanning.

Staging of gestational trophoblastic neoplasia

In conjunction with the consensus definition of GTN, FIGO also revised the staging system in 2000. The FIGO 2000 staging include the stage of the disease (I–IV) and the World Health Organization (WHO) risk score (**Table 66.1**) (16). Those with a risk score of 7 or above would be classified as high risk while those with a risk score of 6 or below would be classified as low risk (16). Comparison of the FIGO 1992 staging, the WHO scoring system, and the FIGO 2000 staging systems showed comparable results though fewer patients were categorized in the high-risk group (17).

Treatment

Since GTN is highly chemosensitive, the mainstay of treatment is chemotherapy. The choice of chemotherapy depends on the risk.

Low-risk GTN

Methotrexate with or without folinic acid rescue has been the most commonly used first-line regimen for low-risk disease while actinomycin D is an effective alternative (**Table 66.2**). In recent years, randomized controlled trials were carried out comparing methotrexate with actinomycin D. Overall, actinomycin D has higher primary cure rates with no significance difference in side effects, although side effects data were too heterogeneous to be conclusive (18). Once the hCG level has normalized, three cycles of consolidation chemotherapy is associated with about a 50% lower recurrence rate compared to two cycles (19). Other single agents known to be effective include etoposide and 5-fluorouracil. For patients resistant to methotrexate, a change of chemotherapy would be able to salvage almost all patients. Patients with serum hCG levels below 300 IU/L can change to actinomycin D while those with hCG levels above 300 IU/L would require combination chemotherapy as for high-risk disease (20). With appropriate management, the overall survival rate in low-risk disease approaches 100%.

High-risk GTN

Combination chemotherapy is required for high-risk disease. The earliest combinations include MAC (methotrexate, actinomycin

Table 66.1 FIGO 2000 gestational trophoblastic neoplasia staging and classification

FIGO anatomical staging	
Stage I	Disease confined to the uterus
Stage II	GTN extends outside of the uterus, but is limited to the genital structures (adnexa, vagina, broad ligament)
Stage III	GTN extends to the lungs, with or without known genital tract involvement
Stage IV	All other metastatic sites

Modified WHO prognostic scoring system as adapted by FIGO				
Scores	**0**	**1**	**2**	**4**
Age (years)	<40	≥40	–	–
Antecedent pregnancy	Mole	Abortion	Term	–
Interval from index pregnancy (months)	<4	4–6	7–12	≥13
Pretreatment serum hCG (IU/L)	$<10^3$	10^3–$<10^4$	10^4–$<10^5$	$≥10^5$
Largest tumour size including uterus (cm)	–	3–4	≥5	–
Site of metastases	Lung	Spleen, kidney	Gastrointestinal	Brain, liver
Number of metastases	–	1–4	5–8	>8
Previous failed chemotherapy	–	–	Single drugs	2 or more drugs

Source data from FIGO Oncology Committee. FIGO staging for gestational trophoblastic neoplasia 2000. *Int J Gynaecol Obstet* 2002;77:285–87.

Table 66.2 Low-risk GTN treatment—single-agent chemotherapy

Chemotherapy agents	Common regimens
Methotrexate	*5-day regimen*
	0.4 mg/kg/day (max. 25 mg) for 5 days IM or IV, repeat cycle every 2 weeks
	8-day alternating regimen
	1 mg/kg IM on day 1, 3, 5 and 7 plus folinic acid 15 mg PO 30 hours after each methotrexate dose on days 2, 4, 6 and 8, repeat cycle every 2 weeks
	Weekly regimen
	30–50 mg/m² weekly IM
	100 mg/m² IV bolus, then 200 mg/m² IV infusion over 12 hours plus folinic acid 15 mg IM or PO every 12 hours for 4 doses, initiate 24 hours after start of methotrexate, repeat cycle every 2 weeks
Actinomycin D	*5-day regimen*
	12 mcg/kg/day or 0.5 mg/day for 5 days IV bolus, repeat cycle every 2 weeks
	Pulsed actinomycin D
	1.25 mg/m² IV bolus every 2 weeks

IM, intramuscular; IV, intravenous; PO, orally.

Table 66.3 High-risk GTN treatment—multiple-agent chemotherapy

EMA-CO given every 2 weeks	Day 1	Actinomycin D 0.5 mg IV bolus Etoposide 100 mg/m² over 30 minutes Methotrexate 100 mg/m² IV bolus and then 200 mg/m² IV infusion over 12 hours
	Day 2	Actinomycin D 0.5 mg IV bolus Etoposide 100 mg/m² over 30 minutes Folinic acid 15 mg IV or PO every 12 hours for 4 doses, initiate 24 hours after start of methotrexate
	Day 8	Vincristine 0.8 mg/m² IV bolus (max. 2 mg) Cyclophosphamide 600 mg/m² IV over 30 minutes

IV, intravenous; PO, orally.

D, and cyclophosphamide), CHAMOMA (cyclophosphamide, hydroxyurea, actinomycin D, methotrexate, vincristine, melphalan, and doxorubicin), or its modified regimen without melphalan and doxorubicin, CHAMOC (cyclophosphamide, hydroxyurea, actinomycin D, methotrexate, and vincristine). After etoposide was found to be very effective, EMA-CO (etoposide, methotrexate, and actinomycin D alternating weekly with cyclophosphamide and vincristine) (Table 66.3) has become the most widely used regimen worldwide (21). Up until now, there has been no randomized controlled trial comparing EMA-CO with other regimens (22). For those with very high hCG levels or extensive metastases, starting with low-dose etoposide and cisplatin (EP) for the first 1–3 weeks can reduce the risk of major complications such as a metabolic catastrophe or haemorrhage (23).

Ultra-high-risk GTN and resistant disease

The majority of patients will respond to first-line chemotherapy as mentioned previously. However, those with very high FIGO risk scores (>12), and liver, brain, or multiple metastases have a high risk of drug resistance (24). About 20% of high-risk patients may require second-line salvage chemotherapy (25). Second-line chemotherapy such as EP-EMA (EP alternating weekly with EMA) or TE/TP (Taxol and etoposide alternating two-weekly with Taxol and cisplatin) regimens can salvage over 70% of patients (Table 66.4) (26). Other regimens such as MBE (methotrexate, bleomycin, etoposide) and BEP (bleomycin, etoposide, cisplatin) have also been used with reasonable outcomes (27, 28). Due to the rarity of the disease, it is difficult to carry out sufficiently powered randomized studies to evaluate the best regimen in these situations. In patients with brain metastasis, high-dosage methotrexate which can cross the blood–brain barrier or intrathecal methotrexate in addition to intravenous chemotherapy may offer a better outcome (29).

Adjunctive treatment to chemotherapy

Surgery

GTN is highly responsive to chemotherapy and surgery is not necessary in most cases. Although hysterectomy in older women with low-risk non-metastatic disease with no fertility wish was reported to reduce by one cycle the amount of chemotherapy required (30),

Table 66.4 Ultra-high-risk and recurrent GTN treatment

	Chemotherapy regimens	
GTN resistant to EMA-CO or recurrence	EP-EMA given every 2 weeks	
	Day 1	Etoposide 150 mg/m² IV over 1 hour
		Cisplatin 75 mg/m² IV infusion over 12 hours
		Posthydration
	Day 8	Actinomycin D 0.5 mg IV bolus
		Etoposide 100 mg/m² IV over 1 hour
		Methotrexate 100 mg/m² IV bolus and then 200 mg/m² IV infusion over 12 hours
		Folinic acid 15 mg IV or PO every 12 hours for 4 doses, initiate 24 hours after start of methotrexate
GTN with brain metastases	EMA-CO with high-dose methotrexate (1000 mg/m² IV infusion over 24 hours)	
Alternate combination chemotherapy	TE/TP (Taxol, etoposide/Taxol, cisplatin)	
	MAC (methotrexate, actinomycin D, cyclophosphamide)	
	BEP (bleomycin, etoposide, cisplatin)	
	MBE (methotrexate, bleomycin, etoposide)	
	FAEV (floxuridine, actinomycin D, etoposide, vincristine)	
	FA (5-fluorouracil, actinomycin D)	

this is not a common clinical practice since most patients present in the reproductive age and the risk of hysterectomy needs to be balanced against the risk of one additional cycle of chemotherapy. Surgery is usually reserved for isolated chemoresistant tumour or life-threatening complications. Pulmonary lobectomy for isolated drug-resistant lung metastasis is the commonest surgery for resistant disease (31). However, it is important to realize that residual lung lesions on imaging may still be seen after hCG has normalized. hCG would be a more accurate reflection of disease status and no treatment is required as long as hCG remains normal during monitoring. Hysterectomy for resistant uterine lesions is also indicated. On histological examination, the lesion may turn out to be a PSTT, which is known to be more chemoresistant than invasive moles. Uncontrolled haemorrhage is one of the commonest life-threatening complications associated with GTN. Hysterectomy can be performed for uncontrolled vaginal bleeding and craniotomy may be performed for an intracranial bleed to relieve intracranial pressure. Laparotomy may be required for an intra-abdominal bleed from liver metastasis, but it is often difficult to control the bleeding. Arterial embolization may offer an alternative to surgery in some of these situations such as in patients with heavy vaginal bleeding but who would like to preserve fertility and in those with internal organ bleeding (32, 33).

Radiotherapy

Radiotherapy has a relatively limited role in GTN. It can reduce tumour size and vascularity and hence decrease the chance of complications. In patients with brain metastases with a high risk of bleeding, whole-brain irradiation, together with craniotomy and combination chemotherapy (EP-EMA or EMA-CO) was reported to give the best outcome (34). Irradiation of large hepatic metastases may decrease the chance of spontaneous hepatic rupture and bleeding (35).

Follow-up after treatment

Most GTN recur within the first year after treatment, therefore, close monitoring with serum hCG (similar to postmolar pregnancy) is required. Women should be advised not to conceive for the first 12 months after treatment since hCG levels would be high during pregnancy and hCG would lose its role as a disease marker, leading to a delay in the diagnosis of recurrence. Moreover, repeat mole and increased pregnancy complications such as miscarriage or still-birth have been reported if the pregnancy is within 6 months after treatment (36). However, the chance of relapse was not found to be increased in these patients compared to those who were not pregnant during the 12 months of surveillance (37). The reproductive performance and outcome of the offspring after treatment of GTN showed no difference from the normal population (38).

Placental site trophoblastic tumour

PSTT is even rarer than choriocarcinoma. PSTT occurs in the reproductive age group and typically presents with non-specific symptoms of abnormal vaginal bleeding or amenorrhoea. Although tumour load with PSTT is not reflected by hCG, free beta hCG is a reliable marker for PSTT especially in conditions where there is uncertainty about whether the patient has choriocarcinoma (high proportion of hyperglycosylated hCG) or PSTT (high proportion of free beta hCG) (39). Histologically, PSTT is composed predominantly of intermediate trophoblast, and chorionic villi are typically not seen. The monotonous population of implantation site intermediate trophoblast usually has significant cytological atypia and scattered mitotic figures (**Figure 66.7**). The trophoblastic tumour cells infiltrate the myometrium, and there is prominent lymphatic and vascular invasion. PSTT is less chemosensitive than choriocarcinoma. Hysterectomy is the main mode of treatment in most cases.

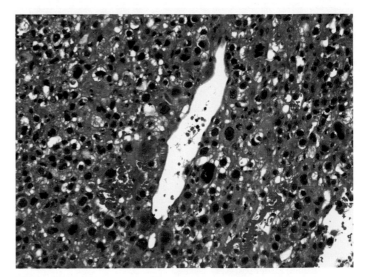

Figure 66.7 Photomicrographs demonstrating placental site trophoblastic tumour where a monotonous population of implantation site intermediate trophoblasts with significant cytological atypia and scattered mitotic figures are found.
Courtesy of Cheung AN, Department of Pathology, The University of Hong Kong.

However, fertility-preserving management such as uterine curettage, hysteroscopic resection, and chemotherapy may be considered in young patients with limited myometrial involvement. Fertility preservation is not appropriate for diffuse lesions. EP-EMA is the most commonly used chemotherapy. An interval from the antecedent pregnancy of more than 48 months seems to be the most significant adverse prognostic factor (40).

Epithelioid trophoblastic tumour

Epithelioid trophoblastic tumour arises from the chorionic-type intermediate trophoblast. Occasionally, epithelioid trophoblastic tumour can coexist with choriocarcinoma or PSTT. Most epithelioid trophoblastic tumours affect women of reproductive age and present with abnormal vaginal bleeding or amenorrhoea. The serum hCG level is usually slightly raised. Similar to PSTT, epithelioid trophoblastic tumour is mainly treated by hysterectomy because it is relatively chemo-insensitive.

Format for reporting to FIGO Annual Report

In order to stage and allot a risk factor score, a patient's diagnosis is allocated to a stage as represented by a Roman numeral: I, II, III, and IV. This is then separated by a colon from the sum of all the actual risk factor scores expressed in Arabic numerals, for example, stage II:4, stage IV:9. This stage and score will be allotted for each patient.

REFERENCES

1. Matsui H, Iitsuka Y, Yamazawa K, Tanaka N, Seki K, Sekiya S. Changes in the incidence of molar pregnancies. A population-based study in Chiba Prefecture and Japan between 1974 and 2000. *Hum Reprod* 2003;**18**:172–75.
2. Martin BH, Kim JH. Changes in gestational trophoblastic tumors over four decades. A Korean experience. *J Reprod Med* 1998;**43**:60–68.
3. Soto-Wright V, Bernstein M, Goldstein DP, Berkowitz RS. The changing clinical presentation of complete molar pregnancy. *Obstet Gynecol* 1995;**86**:775–79.
4. Benson CB, Genest DR, Bernstein MR, Soto-Wright V, Goldstein DP, Berkowitz RS. Sonographic appearance of first trimester complete hydatidiform moles. *Ultrasound Obstet Gynecol* 2000;**16**:188–91.
5. Fowler DJ, Lindsay I, Seckl MJ, Sebire NJ. Routine pre-evacuation ultrasound diagnosis of hydatidiform mole: experience of more than 1000 cases from a regional referral center. *Ultrasound Obstet Gynecol* 2006;**27**:56–60.
6. Paradinas FJ, Browne P, Fisher RA, Foskett M, Bagshawe KD, Newlands E. A clinical, histopathological and flow cytometric study of 149 complete moles, 146 partial moles and 107 non-molar hydropic abortions. *Histopathology* 1996;**28**:101–10.
7. Sebire NJ, Fisher RA, Rees HC. Histopathological diagnosis of partial and complete hydatidiform mole in the first trimester of pregnancy. *Pediatr Dev Pathol* 2003;**6**:69–77.
8. Tidy JA, Gillespie AM, Bright N, Radstone CR, Coleman RE, Hancock BW. Gestational trophoblastic disease: a study of mode of evacuation and subsequent need for treatment with chemotherapy. *Gynecol Oncol* 2000;**78**:309–12.

9. Cole LA, Butler S. Detection of hCG in trophoblastic disease. The USA hCG reference service experience. *J Reprod Med* 2002;**7**:433–44.
10. Cole LA. Phantom hCG and phantom choriocarcinoma. *Gynecol Oncol* 1998;**71**:325–29.
11. Costa HL, Doyle P. Influence of oral contraceptives in the development of post-molar trophoblastic neoplasia—a systematic review. *Gynecol Oncol* 2006;**100**:579–85.
12. Royal College of Obstetricians and Gynaecologists (RCOG). *The Management of Gestational Trophoblastic Disease*, Green-top Guideline No. 38. London: RCOG; 2010.
13. Eagles N, Sebire NJ, Short D, Savage PM, Seckl MJ, Fisher RA. Risk of recurrent molar pregnancies following complete and partial hydatidiform moles. *Hum Reprod* 2015;**30**:2055–63.
14. Parazzini F, Mangili G, Belloni C, La Vecchia C, Liati P, Marabini R. The problem of identification of prognostic factors for persistent trophoblastic disease. *Gynecol Oncol* 1988;**30**:57–62.
15. Sebire NJ, Foskett M, Paradinas FJ, et al. Outcome of twin pregnancies with complete hydatidiform mole and healthy co-twin. *Lancet* 2002;**359**:2165–66.
16. FIGO Oncology Committee. FIGO staging for gestational trophoblastic neoplasia 2000. *Int J Gynaecol Obstet* 2002;**77**:285–87.
17. Hancock BW, Welch EM, Gillespie AM, Newlands ES. A retrospective comparison of current and proposed staging and scoring systems for persistent gestational trophoblastic disease. *Int J Gynecol Cancer* 2000;**10**:318–22.
18. Alazzam M, Tidy J, Hancock BW, Osborne R, Lawrie TA. First-line chemotherapy in low-risk gestational trophoblastic neoplasia. *Cochrane Database Syst Rev* 2012;**7**:CD007102.
19. Lybol C, Sweep FC, Harvey R, et al. Relapse rates after two versus three consolidation courses of methotrexate in the treatment of low-risk gestational trophoblastic neoplasia. *Gynecol Oncol* 2012;**125**:576–79.
20. Sita-Lumsden A, Short D, Lindsay I, et al. Treatment outcomes for 618 women with gestational trophoblastic tumours following a molar pregnancy at the Charing Cross Hospital, 2000–2009. *Br J Cancer* 2012;**107**:1810–14.
21. Bower M, Newlands ES, Holden L, et al. EMA/CO for high-risk gestational trophoblastic tumors: results from a cohort of 272 patients. *J Clin Oncol* 1997;**15**:2636–43.
22. Deng L, Zhang J, Wu T, Lawrie TA. Combination chemotherapy for primary treatment of high-risk gestational trophoblastic tumour. *Cochrane Database Syst Rev* 2013;**1**:CD005196.
23. Alifrangis C, Agarwal R, Short D, et al. EMA/CO for high-risk gestational trophoblastic neoplasia: good outcomes with induction low-dose etoposide-cisplatin and genetic analysis. *J Clin Oncol* 2013;**31**:280–86.
24. Seckl MJ, Sebire NJ, Berkowitz RS. Gestational trophoblastic disease. *Lancet* 2010;**376**:717–29.
25. Powles T, Savage PM, Stebbing J, et al. A comparison of patients with relapsed and chemo-refractory gestational trophoblastic neoplasia. *Br J Cancer* 2007;**96**:732–37.
26. Newlands ES, Mulholland PJ, Holden L, Seckl MJ, Rustin GJ. Etoposide and cisplatin/etoposide, methotrexate, and actinomycin D (EMA) chemotherapy for patients with high-risk gestational trophoblastic tumors refractory to EMA/cyclophosphamide and vincristine chemotherapy and patients presenting with metastatic placental site trophoblastic tumors. *J Clin Oncol* 2000;**18**:854–59.
27. Ngan HY, Tam KF, Lam KW, Chan KK. Methotrexate, bleomycin, and etoposide in the treatment of gestational trophoblastic neoplasia. *Obstet Gynecol* 2006;**107**:1012–17.

28. Song SQ, Wang C, Zhang GN, et al. BEP for high-risk gestational trophoblastic tumor: results from a cohort of 45 patients. *Eur J Gynaecol Oncol* 2015;**36**:726–29.

29. Newlands ES, Holden L, Seckl MJ, McNeish I, Strickland S, Rustin GJ. Management of brain metastases in patients with high-risk gestational trophoblastic tumors. *J Reprod Med* 2002;**47**:465–71.

30. Suzuka K, Matsui H, Iitsuka Y, Yamazawa K, Seki K, Sekiya S. Adjuvant hysterectomy in low-risk gestational trophoblastic disease. *Obstet Gynecol* 2001;**97**:431–34.

31. Jones WB, Romain K, Erlandson RA, Burt ME, Lewis JL Jr. Thoracotomy in the management of gestational choriocarcinoma. A clinicopathologic study. *Cancer* 1993;**72**:2175–81.

32. McGrath S, Harding V, Lim AK, Burfitt N, Seckl MJ, Savage P. Embolization of uterine arteriovenous malformations in patients with gestational trophoblastic tumors: a review of patients at Charing Cross Hospital, 2000–2009. *J Reprod Med* 2012;**57**:319–24.

33. Keepanasseril A, Suri V, Prasad GR, et al. Management of massive hemorrhage in patients with gestational trophoblastic neoplasia by angiographic embolization: a safer alternative. *J Reprod Med* 2011;**56**:235–40.

34. Piura E, Piura B. Brain metastases from gestational trophoblastic neoplasia: review of pertinent literature. *Eur J Gynaecol Oncol* 2014;**35**:359–67.

35. Barnard DE, Woodward KT, Yancy SG, Weed JC Jr, Hammond CB. Hepatic metastases of choriocarcinoma: a report of 15 patients. *Gynecol Oncol* 1986;**25**:73–85.

36. Matsui H, Iitsuka Y, Suzuka K, et al. Risk of abnormal pregnancy completing chemotherapy for gestational trophoblastic tumor. *Gynecol Oncol* 2003;**88**:104–107.

37. Blagden SP, Foskett MA, Fisher RA, et al. The effect of early pregnancy following chemotherapy on disease relapse and foetal outcome in women treated for gestational trophoblastic tumours. *Br J Cancer* 2002;**86**:26–30.

38. Woolas RP, Bower M, Newlands ES, Seckl M, Short D, Holden L. Influence of chemotherapy for gestational trophoblastic disease on subsequent pregnancy outcome. *Br J Obstet Gynaecol* 1998;**105**:1032–35.

39. Cole LA, Khanlian SA, Muller CY, Giddings A, Kohorn E, Berkowitz R. Gestational trophoblastic diseases: 3. Human chorionic gonadotropin-free beta-subunit, a reliable marker of placental site trophoblastic tumors. *Gynecol Oncol* 2006;**102**:160–64.

40. Schmid P, Nagai Y, Agarwal R, et al. Prognostic markers and long-term outcome of placental-site trophoblastic tumours: a retrospective observational study. *Lancet* 2009;**374**:48–55.

41. Cheung AN, Khoo US, Lai CY, et al. Metastatic trophoblastic disease after an initial diagnosis of partial hydatidiform mole: genotyping and chromosome *in situ* hybridization analysis. *Cancer* 2004;**100**:1411–17.

Chemotherapy and biological, targeted, and immune therapies in gynaecological cancers

Stephanie Lheureux and Amit M. Oza

Introduction

Current treatment paradigms are based on understanding cancer biology and its influence on the aetiology, development, and growth of cancer. This has also shaped therapeutic strategy with evidence-based integration of surgery, radiation, and systemic therapies in solid tumour and haematological malignancies (1). There is a complex interplay between genomic, immune, and proteomic disturbances in the development and behaviour of cancer (1). Cancer is the culmination of a variety of insults to the genome—some heritable in nature and therefore transmittable between generations; while others are non-heritable or somatic, and as such are found only in tumour tissue. The coordinated evasion of highly sensitive immune surveillance, and the reprogramming of cellular signalling, protein expression/production, and resetting of the local tumour microenvironment have all been shown to contribute to the development and evolution of disease. Understanding these elementary biological processes—and vulnerabilities when these go awry—can be exploited to improve precision with systemic therapies and are the identified hallmarks or roadmap for contemporary anticancer drug development (2, 3). Improved understanding of these biological hallmarks of cancer have heralded the era of precision or targeted therapy in oncology. In gynaecological malignancies, the advances and clinical adoption of targeted therapies now mean that precision medicine is achievable as an appropriate standard in diseases such as high-grade serous epithelial ovarian cancer (EOC) (**Figure 67.1**). New standards of care are beginning to be established, with targeted agents complementing chemotherapy. Improvement in outcome has to be meaningful, with validated outcomes which include overall survival and progression-free survival in randomized trials for the majority of new agents, but also can include meaningful improvement in response in others (4). In addition, for non-curative therapy, there is increased awareness and appropriate assessment of quality of life and symptoms with development of tools to track patient-reported outcomes (4).

Gynaecological cancers affect any organs of the reproductive tract and may arise in the peritoneum, ovaries, fallopian tubes, uterus, cervix, vagina, and vulva. Cancers of the cervix, endometrium, and ovary have a major global impact in terms of incidence and mortality (GLOBOCAN 2012 data (available at http://gco.iarc.fr/)). There is a very large spectrum of gynaecological malignancies, including epithelial as well as non-epithelial tumours, which range in incidence from common to extremely rare. Understanding risk, development, and disease biology will allow for the development of treatment strategies to prevent, detect early, and treat cancers more effectively.

Systemic therapy

The goals of systemic therapy are context dependent and can be broadly categorized into improving likelihood of cure, controlling disease, and palliation of active disease. Systemic therapy to improve cure is generally through treatment administered before or after locoregional therapy (surgery or radiation) and is termed neoadjuvant or adjuvant. The choice of systemic therapy, schedule, frequency, sequence, and combinations has and continues to be refined with prospective clinical trials with, in general, gradual improvements in cancer control. Implementation and changes in standard of care therapy requires rigor in assessment and validation of impact. Standard of care chemotherapy guidelines for neoadjuvant, adjuvant, and palliative treatment are currently used across the world and refined through meta-analyses, consensus conferences, and evidence-based reviews such as those by the Cochrane collaboration, the National Institute for Health and Care Excellence (NICE) in the United Kingdom (https://www.nice.org.uk/), Cancer Care Ontario (https://www.cancercare.on.ca/), British Columbia Cancer Agency (http://www.bccancer.bc.ca/), and the National Comprehensive Cancer Network (NCCN) (https://www.nccn.org/). These provide a rich repository of validated and updated information, including the evidentiary analyses for recommendations, and should be foundations of treatment decisions. This chapter will focus on current approaches to precision medicine in gynaecological

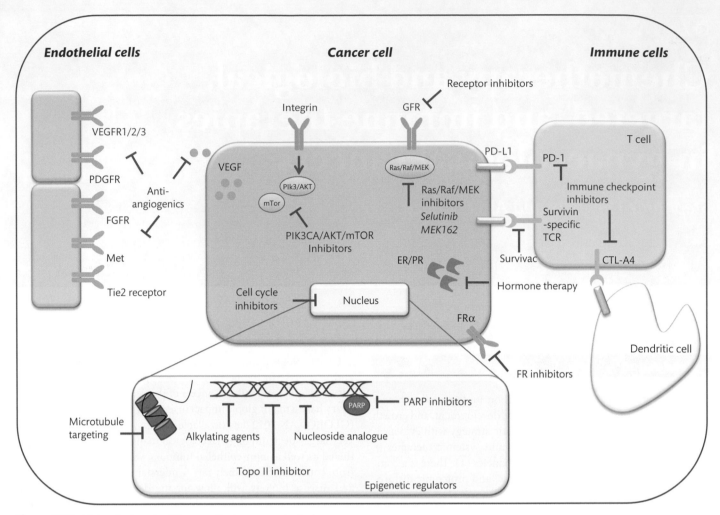

Figure 67.1 Molecular targets of therapeutics in gynaecological cancer.

cancers, with an overview of recent trials which have led to approvals for targeted agents, as well as ones presently underway. It will also include a matrix approach integrating tumour biology, targets, and target-specific therapy.

Improvements in the understanding of cancer biology have facilitated the advent of target-directed precision therapies that are driven by tumour origin, biological subtype, and molecular characterization. The earliest target-directed therapy in gynaecological cancers was hormonal therapy. The backbone of systemic chemotherapy for the past four decades has been with platinum compounds. More recently, identification of tumour vulnerabilities has been exploited to direct therapy. Contemporary examples of tumour vulnerabilities includes an increasingly deeper understanding of cell cycle properties and the DNA repair pathway, and these constitute specific targets for the development of novel therapies. Poly(ADP ribose) polymerase (PARP) inhibitor treatment, has been approved in women with platinum sensitive high-grade serous ovarian cancer (HGSOC) with confirmed *BRCA1/2* mutations. Targeting the microenvironment is a rapidly developing area of research, based on tumour-specific neoangiogenesis capacity and more recently, the role of immune cells and complex cellular interactions that have been effectively leveraged for anticancer-directed treatment. Bevacizumab, a recombinant humanized monoclonal antibody directed against the

vascular endothelial growth factor (VEGF), a proangiogenic cytokine, has also been approved in ovarian and cervical cancers.

The deregulation of different pathways, such as PI3K, HER, or MAPK, needs further investigation to define the clinical impact and the specific subgroup of patients who may have benefit from these therapies. For example, targeting PI3K/AKT/mTOR and the angiogenic pathways in endometrial cancer have been associated with intriguing clinical activity, but balancing this with toxicity has challenged clinical development. Presently, hormonal therapy remains the only approved 'targeted' therapy in endometrial cancer. Overcoming hormone resistance is an active area of investigation. Vulval and vaginal cancers are rare entities and the level of evidence for treatment modalities remains poor and tends to be adapted from cervical cancer. As such, clinical trials are needed in these cancers, as well as rare tumours, to truly define future therapy. Given the heterogeneity of the gynaecological disease, novel hypotheses are under investigation and include stem cell-like population, the role of tumour metabolism, and epigenetic modulation.

Gynaecological malignancies can be subdivided into multiple subtypes of cancer, which individually have distinct behaviour and response patterns to standard and targeted therapy. Well-designed translational clinical trials that analyse response, define the appropriate treatment schedule or combination, explore, and eventually validate potential predictive biomarkers help stratify gynaecological cancers based on behaviour and response to therapy. This necessitates defining biomarkers that are integral, integrated, or exploratory, alongside rigor in trial conduct. Importantly, this also requires collaboration and long-term follow-up for efficacy as well as safety data to achieve meaningful improvement in the prognosis of women with gynaecological cancers.

Systemic therapy in gynaecological malignancies

Epithelial ovarian cancer

EOC is the most common type of ovarian cancer and comprises five histological subtypes: high- and low-grade serous, mucinous, clear cell, and endometrioid, each with distinct pathological morphology and predicted clinical outcome (**Figure 67.1**). Treatment algorithms have clumped all subtypes of ovarian cancer for many years, but were largely driven by the clinical behaviour of the most frequent subtype, high-grade serous. It has been only within the last few years that subtype-specific treatments are being considered. As a consequence, level 1 evidence for rare subtypes remains elusive and recommendations have been based on expert opinion and consensus statements.

Following surgery, systemic treatment with a DNA-damaging agent (cisplatin or carboplatin) in combination with a taxane (paclitaxel) for six cycles has remained the mainstay of treatment for several decades in the first-line setting. The defined number of cycles was established initially, like most other indications for chemotherapy, on the concept of log-cell kill from the Skipper–Schobel–Wilcox and Goldie–Coldman models of cell growth kinetics and validated by lack of improvement in overall survival by increasing the number of cycles. Chemotherapy primarily damages rapidly proliferating cells and thus, is effective only in that proportion of tumour cells within the cell growth cycle. Following first-line therapy, duration of progression-free interval identifies likelihood of successful rechallenge to platinum agents and this has led to a simple and internationally used treatment algorithm. Specifically, disease recurrence less than 3 months from completion of therapy is *refractory* and highly resistant; recurrence within 6 months is considered *resistant*; and greater than 6 months as *sensitive* to rechallenge with platinum agents. For platinum-resistant disease, subsequent treatment with alternate single-agent chemotherapies is an option, albeit with modest activity, and includes weekly paclitaxel, liposomal doxorubicin, or gemcitabine.

First-line chemotherapy after surgery

The outcome in women who receive chemotherapy after surgery is dependent on the effectiveness of surgery and the presence or absence of residual disease. The most commonly used systemic therapy regimen post surgery has been with a combination of carboplatin and paclitaxel and this has been accepted as the standard of care (5). Carboplatin is administered at a dose based on renal clearance, calculated as the area under the curve (AUC) of six (6), and paclitaxel at a dose of 175mg/m² over 3 hours (6). This regimen, derived from well-conducted randomized clinical trials was extensively compared with other variations which assessed alternate platinums, taxanes, and combinations (three or more chemotherapy drugs vs. two), but has emerged as the best tolerated regimen. Ovarian cancer consensus

guidelines by the Gynecologic Cancer InterGroup (GCIG) have also validated the use of this regimen as the control arm for future clinical trials. The most common schedule of administration is every 3 weeks, with prior confirmation of haematological and biochemistry parameters, particularly renal function. Recent studies have investigated the potential role of dose-dense chemotherapy using a weekly paclitaxel regimen (7). Given the features of ovarian cancer evolution and peritoneal extension, intraperitoneal chemotherapy has been explored after optimal debulking surgery to potentially increase overall survival and progression-free survival from advanced ovarian cancer (8).

Neoadjuvant chemotherapy

The timing of chemotherapy in relation to surgery has been the subject of intense investigation and debate over the past 20 years. The initial paradigm of surgery followed by chemotherapy was challenged as there were many patients who either were not surgical candidates or had disease that was very extensive and not debulkable. In this setting, chemotherapy was seen to be an effective way of controlling disease given the likelihood of response and allowed a second opportunity for surgery after an 'interval'. This alternate sequence of chemotherapy followed by surgery and completion chemotherapy has gained considerable traction and has been shown to be effective in two prospective randomized clinical trials (9, 10) that are landmark studies in defining treatment sequence. However, there remain important questions and challenges mainly based on patient selection, such as the question of best sequence if patients can be debulked at outset that will be addressed in a planned randomized trial being led by the AGO group. It is also intriguing that disease biology and not simply surgical skill may in fact be very important in determining debulkability (11).

Maintenance therapy

Given the 'relapse–response' pattern with shorter disease-free intervals with each subsequent line of therapy, a maintenance approach with well-tolerated chronic therapy to keep disease under control has been developed. For maintenance therapy to be acceptable, it has to improve outcome for patients, without significantly compromising quality of life. For HGSOC, incorporating complementary mechanisms of action beside standalone chemotherapy such as targeting angiogenesis and deficiencies in the homologous recombination repair pathway have been successful strategies.

Antiangiogenics in ovarian cancer

Tumour-associated angiogenesis and targeting the microenvironment has been an effective strategy. The advent of antiangiogenics heralded an important era in ovarian cancer therapy. Ovarian cancer is very dependent on angiogenesis for growth and has shown important prognostic reliance on microvessel density. Ovarian cancer is a disease which produces excessive amounts of VEGF leading to the hallmarks of disease such as capillary leakiness and ascites. Early studies with bevacizumab, a humanized monoclonal antibody against VEGF, showed single-agent activity and symptoms benefit with control of ascites. Early studies were also challenging due to complications related to bowel perforation and fistulization, related to bowel involvement with disease. Antiangiogenesis has since been extensively incorporated in therapy in different settings—first line for high-risk patients and the platinum-sensitive and platinum-resistance setting in combination with chemotherapy and followed by maintenance therapy (12).

In a first-line setting, the Gynecologic Oncology Group (GOG) 218 (13) and ICON7 (14) provided evidence for improvement of disease control and progression-free survival with the addition of bevacizumab to carboplatin and paclitaxel. Both these studies demonstrated that progression-free survival was significantly improved with the addition of bevacizumab concurrently with carboplatin and paclitaxel chemotherapy, followed by maintenance bevacizumab. The doses of bevacizumab used in the two trials were different—7.5 mg/kg in ICON7 and 15 mg/kg in GOG 218, with some differences in duration of maintenance period. ICON7 further demonstrated that the benefit is greatest in women with high risk of recurrence defined by suboptimally debulked stage III/IV or non-operated patients (15). In this setting, addition of bevacizumab may improve median overall survival by 9.4 months. This has now led to the approval of bevacizumab for treatment of women with advanced ovarian cancer in a first-line setting. In the platinum-sensitive (OCEANS study) and -resistant recurrence setting (AURELIA), two phase III trials with bevacizumab prescribed until disease progression or intolerance, a significant benefit for maintenance on disease control rate was shown (16, 17). The benefit of adding and/or continuing an antiangiogenic agent has also been validated in other settings such as platinum-sensitive recurrent disease, and platinum-resistant disease with bevacizumab, as well as proof of principle activity with other antiangiogenics such as AMG386, pazopanib, and cediranib (18, 19). Bevacizumab has received regulatory approval for ovarian cancer in a first-line setting, as well recurrent disease and is currently the most widely used antiangiogenic added to chemotherapy around the world.

PARP inhibitors

DNA repair defects consistent with homologous recombination repair dysfunction are referred to as the 'BRCAness phenotype'. Two randomized phase II trials testing the PARP inhibitor olaparib as maintenance therapy—prescribed as long as patients were benefiting from therapy—have demonstrated a marked improvement in progression-free survival for recurrent platinum-sensitive HGSOC patients, particularly for those patients with *BRCA1/2* mutations (20, 21). Based on disease vulnerability, olaparib, a PARP inhibitor treatment has been approved following response to platinum-based chemotherapy in *BRCA1/2*-mutated ovarian cancer. Several randomized phase III trials confirmed the benefit of PARP inhibitor in high grade serous ovarian cancer with BRCA1/2 mutations and beyond (ref: PMID:31099893) This existing treatment strategy in ovarian cancer has been largely driven by activity in HGSOC but response to cytotoxic chemotherapy varies according to the histological subtypes (22). Patients with HGSOC and *BRCA1/2* mutation have been described as more sensitive to standard chemotherapy; while chemoresistance has been reported in low-grade serous, mucinous, and clear cell ovarian cancer.

Non-epithelial ovarian cancers

Non-EOCs which include sex cord-stromal and other such as germ cell are categorized as rare and treatment guidelines have been extrapolated from EOC, but are not based on level 1 evidence (23). Given the rarity of this disease type, expert gynaecological pathology review is essential for diagnosis. Consensus guidelines by the GCIG form an excellent repository of information on therapy and management, and should be referred to.

Endometrial cancer

Endometrial cancer is the fifth most common female cancer globally, accounting for 4.8% of all cancers (GLOBOCAN 2012). Contrary to ovarian cancer, the majority of endometrial cancer patients present with operable early-stage disease with 5-year survival of approximately 80%. Optimizing adjuvant therapy, usually carboplatin and paclitaxel particularly in high- and intermediate-risk patients, is currently an active area of research. Adjuvant radiotherapy is currently the standard of care for the International Federation of Gynecology and Obstetrics (FIGO) stages IB to II with intermediate risk of relapse. Many advocate chemotherapy for those with stage III disease or poor prognostic histology based on GOG 122 (24) and confirmed in other studies (25). The role of chemotherapy in addition to radiotherapy for high-risk, higher stage, and poor prognostic histology is being further investigated in the phase III studies PORTEC3, GOG 249, and GOG 258. For patients inoperable at presentation or diagnosed with metastatic or recurrent disease, treatment options are limited. The most active agents in chemotherapy-naive endometrial cancer patients are platinum, taxanes, and anthracyclines with response rates of 20–30% (26). The first-line regimen is often based on carboplatin and paclitaxel. Prior radiation potentially complicates delivery by compromising penetrance and impacting bone marrow reserve. Triplet regimens have demonstrated a superior response rate at the cost of increasing toxicity (27). Results are expected from GOG 209 shortly, but preliminary data suggest that doublet therapy (carboplatin/paclitaxel) is similar to triplet. Response rates after first-line chemotherapy are disappointing. Various agents have been tested in a number of small phase II trials (28). The majority of monotherapy trials have shown minimal activity with response rates varying from 0% to 12% including; doxorubicin or weekly paclitaxel is usually used in this situation.

Endometrial cancer has been divided into type I (endometrioid) and II (serous, clear cell, and carcinosarcoma) subtypes reflecting their grade and aggressiveness. Type I tumours expressing oestrogen (ER) or progesterone (PR) receptors may be indicative of slow growth and favourable survival (29). A significant proportion of endometrial cancers, particularly the type I subtype, express ER or PR and thus make hormonal therapies an attractive therapeutic option. Progestins remain the main hormone treatment available; however, other agents include tamoxifen (a selective oestrogen receptor modulator), gonadotropin-releasing hormone agonists, and aromatase inhibitors (29) are commonly used sequentially. Recent data showed potential benefit of immune therapy in the subgroup of patients diagnosed with recurrent Microsatellite Instability-High (MSI) endometrial cancer (ref: PMID: 30787022).

Cervical cancer

The fourth most common female cancer worldwide, cervical cancer has the fourth highest mortality rate among cancers in women (GLOBOCAN 2012). The leading risk factor for disease is human papillomavirus (HPV) infection (30–33); specifically, subtypes 16 and 18, which have been associated with high-grade dysplasia and cancer, and confer an 11–16.9 times increased risk of development of high-grade cervical intraepithelial neoplasia (CIN) (34–36). Routine screening for cytological dysplasia includes the Papanicolou (Pap) test with a growing body of evidence to show the incorporation of HPV DNA testing for higher likelihood of detecting early disease (37). Two histological subgroups have been described, the

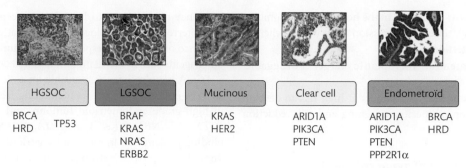

HGSOC	LGSOC	Mucinous	Clear cell	Endometroïd
BRCA HRD TP53	BRAF KRAS NRAS ERBB2	KRAS HER2	ARID1A PIK3CA PTEN	ARID1A BRCA PIK3CA HRD PTEN PPP2R1α

Figure 67.2 Epithelial ovarian cancer histological subtypes.

most common being squamous cell carcinoma and cervical adeno-carcinoma (**Figure 67.2**).

Early-stage cervical cancer is managed either by surgery (for those diagnosed with FIGO stage IA/B1 disease) or by a combination of low-dose platinum chemotherapy administered concurrently with radiotherapy followed by intracavitary brachytherapy. The evidence for this came from several randomized clinical trials of radiation therapy versus chemotherapy/radiation, led by the National Cancer Institute (United States), cooperative groups such as the GOG, and the Southwest Oncology Group (38). The National Cancer Institute released a clinical alert in the late 1990s, which set the new standard as chemotherapy in combination with radiation therapy (39, 40). Patients diagnosed with metastatic disease or recurrence after initial treatment have poor outcomes with 5-year survival rates between 5% and 15%. In this setting any treatment is palliative and first-line systemic therapy is based on cisplatin doublet combination.

In the GOG 204 trial, the four-arm study compared cisplatin in combination with paclitaxel, vinorelbine, gemcitabine, or topotecan (41). Outcomes were similar in all arms with a non-significant trend in favour of cisplatin/paclitaxel (overall survival at 12.9 months compared to the other three arms 10–10.3 months) and similar overall response rates. In a further randomized phase III clinical trial conducted by the Japanese GOG (JGOG) carboplatin in combination with paclitaxel was found to be non-inferior to cisplatin/paclitaxel (42). Besides standard chemotherapy, bevacizumab was assessed in combination in a large randomized phase III trial (GOG 240). The addition of bevacizumab to chemotherapy increased the objective response rate from 36% to 48% (*P* = 0.008) and the overall survival benefit compared to a standard regimen (overall survival increased from 13.3 to 17 months) (43). A significant improvement in progression-free survival was also seen (8.2 vs 5.9 months; hazard ratio for disease progression 0.67; 95% confidence interval 0.54–0.82). Bevacizumab was associated with a reasonable toxicity profile. The side effects were consistent with those previously known to be associated with bevacizumab, and included hypertension, febrile neutropenia, and thromboembolism, or formation of blood clots. Specifically, treatment with bevacizumab was associated with more grade 3–4 bleeding, thrombosis/embolism, and gastrointestinal fistula (8.6%). This overall survival improvement has led to the United States Food and Drug Administration-approved anti-VEGF agent, bevacizumab, for the treatment of advanced stage, persistent, or recurrent cervical cancer in combination with chemotherapy. No biomarkers of response were identified. At the time of relapse, there is no standard of care second-line options. In June 2018, Pembrolizumab, a programmed death-1 (PD-1) inhibitor has

been granted approval by the FDA for the treatment of patients with advanced, PD-L1+ cervical cancer progressing after chemotherapy (ref: PMID:30943124)

Rare malignancies—vagina and vulval

The incidence of vaginal and vulval cancers is low rendering these particularly rare diseases. Published NCCN guidelines for vulval cancer suggest chemotherapy for advanced, recurrent/metastatic disease with cisplatin, or cisplatin in combination with vinorelbine or paclitaxel (44). There is no standard chemotherapy for vulval cancer, and reports describing the use of this modality in the setting of metastatic or recurrent disease are anecdotal. Working from regimens used for anal or cervical squamous cell cancers, chemotherapy has been studied in combination with radiation in the neoadjuvant setting or as primary therapy in advanced disease. Chemotherapy regimens have included various combinations of 5-fluorouracil (5-FU), cisplatin, mitomycin-C, or bleomycin.

Taken together, response rates remain low in the majority of gynaecological cancers and as such, an increasing trend in histological subtype specific and molecular basis of clinical trials is in motion.

Precision medicine—approaches to targeted therapy

Understanding tumour biology, identifying mutations and genomic abnormalities, and elucidating their role in cancer pathogenesis have important implications in the optimal clinical management of patients. Disease biology influences tumour behaviour and this information can potentially be harnessed to plan therapy in a number of ways:

1. Potential roles as prognostic or predictive factors. A predictive role is best exemplified when a genomic or proteomic alteration represents a biomarker of response or resistance to a specific target therapy.

   The advent of genomic medicine has laid the foundation for predictive and prognostic markers. As a result, there is increasing use of these markers within the treatment planning of women with gynaecological cancers. Prognostic markers are clinical or biological characteristics that assist in estimating the likely outcome of untreated patients as well as the likelihood of disease recurrence. Predictive biomarkers are biological elements that can help predict likelihood of response to a specific treatment or describe how it contributes to increased risks of developing disease. Again, in gynaecological cancers these include mutations in DNA repair genes or mutations in the homologous recombination repair pathway; time to progression from the last chemotherapy; or HPV infection.

2. Identify novel potential therapeutic target ('druggable' mutations).

3. Identify individuals or family members at high risk to develop cancer and activation of specific screening and risk reduction strategies.

Molecular characteristics of gynaecological malignancies

Tumour-specific targets in gynaecological malignancies

The Cancer Genome Atlas Research Network (TCGA) has been responsible for important genomic data that have accelerated molecularly driven research in high-grade serous ovarian and endometrial cancers. Findings from the TCGA in HGSOC illustrate the catalogue of mutations detected such as the universal mutation of *TP53* in all tumours (96%); homologous recombination deficiency in almost half of tumours analysed; as well as the low prevalence but statistically recurrent somatic mutations in *NF1, BRCA1, BRCA2, RB1*, and *CDK12*; 113 significant focal DNA copy number aberrations; and promoter methylation events involving 168 genes (45) (**Figure 67.3**). TCGA findings and results published from subsequent studies clearly demonstrate that HGSOC is inherently genomically unstable and not characterized by a solitary driver mutation that is druggable. Furthermore, the frequency of mutations to homologous recombination pathways—also referred to as homologous recombination deficiency—and the influence on treatment response to platinum compounds as well as other agents such as PARP inhibitors is well documented (46).

TCGA has also been responsible for a similar in-depth examination of endometrial cancers identifying frequent *TP53* mutations in high-grade endometrioid tumours and frequent mutations in *PTEN, CTNNB1, PIK3CA, ARID1A, KRAS*, and ARID5B DNA-binding protein (47) in most endometrioid tumours (**Figure 67.3**). The data also provide a strong rationale for a reclassification of these cancers into four distinct subtype—*POLE* ultramutated, microsatellite instability hypermutated, copy-number low and high—that may have clinical impacts at the time of postsurgical adjuvant treatment (47). Indeed, patients diagnosed with *POLE* ultramutated tumour have generally very good outcome. Additional investigations are needed to interpret the functionality of these observed genomic alterations and whether this can translate into therapeutic targets that could improve treatment outcomes (**Figure 67.4**).

Contemporary investigations into the molecular landscape of clear cell cancer and low-grade serous (LGSOC) ovarian cancers have also been published. Clear cell ovarian carcinomas harbour defects in *PTEN* (approximately 10% of cases), *PIK3CA* (approximately 50% of cases), roughly 50% of cases harbour *ARID1A* mutations, a minority harbour *PPP2R1A* mutations (48), and lastly, roughly 33% exhibit amplification of chr20q13.2 and do not typically harbour Wnt-activating *CTNNB1* mutations (49). Comprising 5–10% of

Gynaecological cancer mutations											
Mutations	Ovarian						Endometrial			Cervix	Vulvo-vaginal
	HGS	LGS	Mucinous	Clear cell	Endo-metroid	Sex cord-stromal	Endo-metroid	Serous	Carcino-sarcoma		
TP53	●							●	●		○
BRCA1/2	●										
Rb1	●							●			
KRAS		●	●				○		●	○	
BRAF		●									
ERBB3		●									
PTEN				●	●		○				
PIK3CA				●	●		○	○	○	○	
CTNNB1					●		○				
EGFR										○	
ARID1A				●	●						

Figure 67.3 Common mutations according to gynaecological cancer subtypes. HGS, high-grade serous; LGS, low-grade serous.

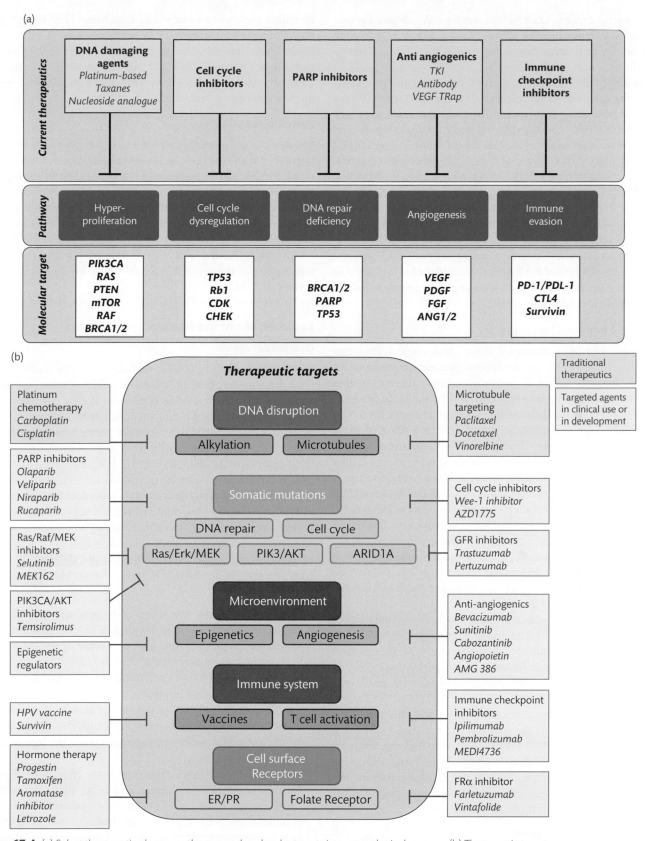

Figure 67.4 (a) Select therapeutic classes, pathways, and molecular targets in gynaecological cancers. (b) Therapeutic targets.

serous ovarian cancers, LGSOC tumours have documented prevalence of *KRAS* mutations (35–57% of cases) as well as mutations in *BRAF* during early-stage disease but rare in the advanced setting (50, 51).

Pathogenic HPV infection is the most important and potentially preventable causative factor in cervical cancer and responsible for more than 95% of cervical cancers. The molecular landscape of the disease was recently updated (52) and study findings show several mutations such as recurrent E322K substitutions in the *MAPK1* gene (8%), inactivating mutations in the *HLA-B* gene (9%), and mutations in *EP300* (16%), *FBXW7* (15%), *NFE2L2* (4%), *TP53* (5%), and *ERBB2* (6%) genes in primary squamous cell carcinomas, as well as somatic *ELF3* (13%) and *CBFB* (8%) gene mutations in 24 adenocarcinomas. In cervical cancer, mutations in *TP53*, PI3K pathway, and *KRAS* are found with some different patterns between squamous carcinoma and adenocarcinoma. Furthermore, study gene expression data suggest that HPV integration into the host cell genome is a common mechanism for overexpression of target genes, and potential drivers of carcinogenesis (52).

Spatial and temporal heterogeneity

Therapeutic resistance remains a clinical and research challenge which has to be overcome to improve effectiveness of precision targeted therapies. There is significant genetic diversity within and between common tumours (53) which builds on recognition of morphological heterogeneity within tumours (54). This spatial and temporal heterogeneity may arise as a result of either random genetic drift or as a result of phenotypic advantage selected from a particular environment (55, 56). Ovarian cancers exhibit branched patterns of evolution, whereby several subclones grow out driving disease progression and manifest as intratumoural heterogeneity (54). Treatment may also induce selection pressure for intratumoural driver mutations or between tumours. This means that tumours develop new patterns of resistance and emphasize the need for repeat assessment of patient samples throughout disease to accurately profile and understand tumour genomic architecture (54). Heterogeneity between primary and metastatic lesions impacts the efficacy of subsequent therapy.

Spatial heterogeneity within HGSOC has been elegantly shown by several groups (57, 58). The degree of genomic diversity is evident within primary untreated tumours exhibited by extensive intratumoural variations in mutation, copy number, and gene expression profiles, with key driver alterations in genes present in only a subset of samples (e.g. *PI3KCA*, *CTNNB1*, *NF1*) (57). *TP53* mutation is the most prevalent abnormality in HGSOC and essentially defines the disease, and is the only somatic mutation consistently present in all samples (57). Taken together, spatial and temporal heterogeneity in gynaecological cancers must be considered during treatment selection and throughout disease. Clinically relevant biomarkers may differ between primary and metastatic disease as has been shown in other cancers (59, 60).

Inherent and acquired resistance

Inherent and acquired forms of resistance impact treatment course whether in the upfront or advanced setting. Despite the lack of classical driver mutations in gynaecological cancers, frequently mutated genes exist within each subtype. The mutational landscape of gynaecological cancers is varied with several driver-like mutations

identified; the current most widely cited being *TP53* in high-grade serous cancers, mutations in DNA repair genes *BRCA1/2*, as well as homologous recombination repair pathway genes (45). Disease recurrence in a previously radiated area, commonly used in the treatment of gynaecological cancers, may also have acquired specific mechanisms of drug resistance.

Germline mutations

Mutations in germ cells are referred to as germline since these mutations occur in cells responsible for creating gametes and as such, mutations that can be passed on to offspring (61). With respect to gynaecological malignancies, well-documented mutations in heritable genes are those in *BRCA1/2* and loss of DNA mismatch repair in Lynch syndrome. Mutations in these genes have also been suggested to contribute to several other malignancies such as prostate, pancreatic, and stomach cancers (62). Germline mutations in the DNA repair pathway beyond *BRCA1/2* are under investigation, such as *RAD51* or *PABL2*.

Key aberrations in gynaecological cancers

Ovarian cancer

EOC encompasses five distinct diseases, each with individual patterns of epidemiological and genetic risk factors, precursor lesions, patterns of spread, and molecular events during oncogenesis, response to chemotherapy, and prognosis (63). Low-grade serous ovarian tumours (LGSOC) commonly arise from precursor lesions and clear cell potentially from endometriosis. Conversely, *TP53* mutations are ubiquitous in HGSOC; whereas mutations in *BRCA1/2* and the homologous recombination repair pathway genes are key drivers in carcinogenesis (45). Beyond *BRCA1/2* mutations in HGSOC, there are no validated predictive genetic biomarkers, though work is ongoing to evaluate the impact on outcome based on patterns of homologous recombination deficiency, loss of heterozygosity, and somatic mutations. The five different EOC subtypes are defined by particular molecular profiles that correlate with outcome:

- HGSOC is a disease characterized by genomic instability and ubiquitous *TP53* mutations, frequent deficiency in homologous recombination pathway, and high prevalence of copy number alterations with few recurrent mutations.

- LGSOC harbours a *KRAS* mutation in 20–40% while only 5% have a *BRAF* mutation. This implicates the MAPK signalling pathway as a key node in LGSOC—in fact, 80% of LGSOC have activation of the MAPK pathway (64). Although, at this stage, there remains insufficient data to use this mutation as a predictive biomarker for a treatment decision.

- Mucinous ovarian cancer is a rare entity characterized by resistant disease and low response rate to platinum/paclitaxel chemotherapy. Based on the analogy with gastrointestinal cancer, oxaliplatin and 5-FU chemotherapy has been used with modest activity. Approximately 60% of cases show a *KRAS* mutation and the presence of a *KRAS* mutation predicts resistance to anti-EGFR treatment, as already demonstrated in gastrointestinal cancer (65). HER2 is amplified in about 15–20% of cases and anti-HER2 agents may be active in this subgroup of patients but no data from clinical trials are available.

- Clear cell ovarian cancer is also associated with a low response to platinum-based chemotherapy. Molecular profiling of this disease is characterized by the lack of BRCA1/2 mutations as well as a high frequency of PI3K/AKT/mTOR pathway alterations (40–50%) (66). Interestingly, it has been documented that roughly 50% of clear cell ovarian cancer cases harbour mutations in the ARID1A gene (48).

- Endometrioid EOC is characterized by mutations in the beta-catenin and PTEN genes, as well as the tumour suppressor genes PIK3CA and ARID1A. Functional loss of PTEN through mutations in the PI3K/AKT/mTOR pathways has been the subject of considerable therapeutic research, with some promising results (67). Endometrioid ovarian cancer has histological and molecular aspects similar to endometrial adenocarcinoma.

Endometrial cancer

Findings from TCGA have helped illustrate the genomic landscape of this disease. In total, the collaborative analysed 373 endometrial carcinomas using array- and sequencing-based technologies. Data show uterine serous tumours and approximately 25% of high-grade endometrioid tumours harbour extensive copy number alterations, few DNA methylation changes, low ER/PR levels, and frequent TP53 mutations (47). Most endometrioid tumours had few copy number alterations or TP53 mutations; and findings also highlight frequent mutations in PTEN, CTNNB1, PIK3CA, ARID1A, and KRAS, as well as novel mutations in the SWI/SNF chromatin remodelling complex gene ARID5B. Interestingly, a subset of endometrioid tumours analysed had a markedly increased transversion mutation frequency and newly identified hotspot mutations in POLE. As a result, a novel classification system which has prognostic value has been devised to include four categories: POLE ultramutated, microsatellite instability hypermutated, copy-number low, and copy-number high (47). Ongoing studies are evaluating the predictive value of this classification with targeted and immunological therapies.

Cervical cancer

While HPV infection contributes significantly to the development of cervical cancer, several genes have been documented to play a role in the development of disease. Involvement of TP53 gene mutations are documented related to HPV molecular transformation—HPVE6 gene-stimulated degradation interferes with p53 function (68). The HPV oncoproteins E5, E6, and E7 are the primary viral factors responsible for initiation and progression of cervical cancer. E6, E7, and to a lesser extent E5 play key roles in upregulating angiogenesis through the VEGF pathway through their effects on p53 degradation, hypoxia-inducible factor-1α (HIF-1α), and inactivation of retinoblastoma protein (pRb). PIK3CA, STK11, KRAS, EGFR, NOL7, CDKN2A, PTEN, and binding protein p300 (EP300) genes have all been documented in the Cervical Cancer Gene Database, as well as the National Human Genome Research Institute, the National Cancer Institute, the COSMIC Database and TGCA (68–70).

Other cancers–vaginal and vulval cancers

The aetiology of vulval squamous cell carcinoma (VSCC) includes high-risk HPV-dependent infection manifesting with usual vulval intraepithelial neoplasia (VIN) as a precursor lesion, and an HPV-independent route associated with differentiated VIN, lichen sclerosus (a chronic dermatosis associated with autoimmune diseases), and genetic alterations such as TP53 mutations (71). As reported recently by Trietsch et al. (2015), a review of current literature confirms the hypothesis that HPV and TP53 mutations play almost separate, but key roles in the carcinogenesis of VSCC. Study findings go on to suggest that in the small number of articles with survival data available, tumours harbouring a mutation, which are most often HPV-independent VSCC, have a worse prognosis than VSCC without (epi)genetic changes (71). Other mutations described in VSCC and its precursor lesions include PTEN and CDKN2A gene mutations (72, 73). In a study of 107 formalin-fixed, paraffin-embedded primary surgically treated tissues from patients with VSCC, Sanger sequencing and mass spectrometry revealed somatic mutations in 62% of samples (74). In addition to HPV infection and TP53 mutations, CDKN2A(p16), HRAS, and PIK3CA mutations were frequently seen in HPV-negative patients (74). Interestingly, patients with somatic mutations, especially HRAS, have significantly worse prognosis than those patients lacking these changes (74).

Potential druggable mutations

TP53 mutations

The tumour suppressor gene TP53 (MIM#191117) is responsible for the production of p53 protein, which is charged with regulating cell division and death; and thus regarded as the guardian of the genome (75). During times of cellular stress such as DNA damage, hypoxia, oncogene activation, or/and nutrient deprivation, p53 functions as a transcription factor that is activated and leads to cell cycle arrest, apoptosis, and metabolic adaptation (76). While non-heritable or somatic mutations in p53 are one of the most frequent alterations in cancer (77), germline mutations in TP53 have been documented (77). Germline mutations in TP53 are responsible for the rare Li–Fraumeni syndrome, a familial clustering of early-onset tumours including sarcomas, breast, brain, and adrenal cortical carcinomas (78, 79). Direct and indirect approaches are under investigation to target p53 alterations in gynaecological cancers.

BRCA1/2 mutations

With respect to gynaecological cancers, heritable or germline mutations in BRCA1 or -2 increase the lifetime risk of developing breast and ovarian cancers. Published findings show that while the lifetime risk of developing ovarian cancer is low in the general population, risk increases to between 40% and 60% for BRCA1 and 11–27% for BRCA2 germline mutation carriers, respectively (80). In all ovarian cancer, these particular mutations are associated with 10–15% of cases and in HGSOC, almost 20% of cases (81). Importantly, this includes women with HGSOC who do not have a family history of either breast or ovarian cancer. As such, NCCN guidelines suggest germline testing for BRCA1/2 germline mutation is made available for all HGSOC diagnoses.

Over the last several years, there are increasing data showing the benefits of targeting pathways necessary for maintaining/safeguarding DNA integrity, including BRCA1 and BRCA2 (82). Clinically, germline BRCA1/2 mutation has been shown to be predictive of sensitivity to platinum (83) as well as to agents targeting impairments in DNA repair pathways—typically conferred by BRCA mutations—as evidenced by recent approval of PARP inhibitors, such as olaparib, responsible for blocking a major DNA repair enzyme. Mechanistically, these agents operate via the parallel endorsement of

DNA double-stranded breaks and interference of double-stranded break repair by PARP protein inhibition (84, 85) that collectively results in cell death. Germline and tumour testing for *BRCA1/2* mutations gives important information to clinicians regarding the potential predictive benefit of PARP inhibitors in women with ovarian cancer and has led to the subsequent approval of these agents. Together, this is a successful example of targeted therapy development that showcases how understanding germline and somatic mutations, and their function, enables the strategic targeting of these vulnerabilities and leads to effective therapeutic agents.

Homologous recombination deficiency

There are numerous genes involved in homologous recombination repair pathways that also contribute to disease including *ATM, CHEK2, BARD1, BRIP1, Mre11, RAD50, NBS1, RAD51C, RAD51D,* and *PALB2* (86). Other alterations affecting homologous recombination repair include amplification of *EMSY* (8%), deletion/mutation of *PTEN* (7%), hypermethylation of *RAD51C* (3%), mutation of *ATM* or *ATR* (2%), or mutation of other homologous recombination genes (5%). These are suggested to have the phenotype of 'BRCAness' in serous cancers and are predicted to behave like *BRCA*-deficient tumours despite normal germline *BRCA1* and *BRCA2* genes (86, 87). These patients may also benefit from PARP inhibitors.

An autosomal dominant, inherited cancer-susceptibility syndrome in women with endometrial cancer, Lynch syndrome (LS) has also been found to harbour defects in DNA repair in *MLH1*, mutS homolog 2 (*MSH2*), *MSH6*, PMS1 homolog 2 (*PMS2*) (a mutations of DNA mismatch repair system component) genes, and others (88). Similar to HGSOC, *BRCA1/2* germline history is insufficient to identify affected women and as such, changes in disease screening are gaining momentum. In addition to clinical criteria, immunohistochemistry is universally used to screen for impairments in mismatch repair genes with a high sensitivity, which is followed by subsequent mutation testing for microsatellite instability (89). It has been hypothesized that these patients are more likely to respond to immunotherapy and prospective trials are ongoing to assess this question.

Targeting somatic mutations

DNA repair

BRCA1/2 and homologous repair deficiency

PARP inhibitors are a new class of agents developed and refined for clinical use over the last several years. Cancer cells with homologous repair deficiency are not able to repair double-stranded DNA breaks and if PARP is inhibited, the single-stranded breaks also cannot be repaired, which leads to cell death. This mechanism or concept is known as synthetic lethality. Olaparib, the first developed PARP inhibitor, has been approved in the United States as monotherapy for *BRCA1/2*-mutated patients that have received three or more lines of the treatment and as maintenance therapy in patient with relapse platinum-sensitive HGSOC and more recently after the first line therapy for women diagnosed with BRCA1/2 mutation HGSOC. Several other PARP inhibitors have been approved since.

PARP inhibitors have shown activity in different trials as monotherapy or as maintenance, in *BRCA* mutated women but also in *BRCA* wild-type patients, leading to the definition of a special

subgroup of HGSOC patients with a 'BRCAness' phenotype similar to *BRCA*-mutated patients (higher platinum sensitivity and benefit from PARP inhibitor treatment). Other trials are ongoing with different PARP inhibitors such as rucaparib, niraparib, and veliparib to address the benefit of this targeted therapy beyond *BRCA1/2* mutation.

CDK12 (a member of cyclin-kinase protein family) is mutated in 3% of HGSOC and its activity is important for homologous recombination. When *CDK12* is not active, depletion in HR enzymes occurs and reduction in *BRCA* expression has been observed. Cells harbouring a mutation in the *CDK12* gene could be more sensitive to cisplatin and PARP-inhibitor, representing an interesting new therapeutic option.

The cell cycle

DNA repair pathways have cell cycle specificity, especially within the G2/M checkpoint (90). Agents targeting CHK1/2 and WEE-1 kinases have minimal single-agent activity in the absence of p53, or more likely, p53 and second (so far undefined) mutations. Efficacy is much greater when examined in a defined p53 mutant background in which the G1/S checkpoint is aberrant and also in combination. There is a subset of patients with ovarian cancer with wild-type *BRCA1/2* function and cyclin E amplification and overexpression.

TP53

Somatic mutations in *TP53* are the most documented mutations contributing to cancer and a defining characteristic of HGSOC (45) as well as in endometrial carcinomas (47). The majority of *TP53* mutations are missense and cause single amino acid changes at many different positions and as such, vary in their structural impact (77). These typically result in high levels of dysfunctional p53 protein (91) and efforts remain underway to devise novel therapies targeting these proteins. Alternatively, in cervical cancers that have low mutation rates, p53 is inactivated by an alternate mechanism; specifically, it is targeted for degradation by HPV E6 (77, 92). Future studies are warranted to determine the precise manner in which p53 proteins or *TP53* somatic mutations can be leveraged to devise novel therapies in gynaecological cancers.

KRAS/BRAF/MAPK pathway

Between 40% and 60% of LGSOCs have a *RAS* mutation (93). *RAS* is a family of different oncogenes and the most relevant are *KRAS, NRAS,* and *HRAS* and point mutations are frequently detected in codons 12, 13, and 61. Activating mutations in *KRAS, NRAS,* or *BRAF* promote tumourigenesis through a constitutive activation of the MAPK/ERK (mitogen-activated protein kinase/extracellular-signal-regulated kinase) pathway. MAPK inhibition with anti-MEK agents is being investigated. Further research is necessary to analyse the possible prognostic or predictive role of these mutations in order to select patients that may benefit from this treatment or define which tumours could be resistant to a specific drug.

PIK3CA/AKT/mTOR pathway

Aberrant activation of PI3K induces phosphorylation of AKT that subsequently activates mTOR. mTOR promotes cell proliferations and angiogenesis. Different mechanisms contribute to activate this pathway such as receptor tyrosine kinase activation or amplification, mutation, or silencing of negative regulators and activation or amplification of downstream kinase.

Approximately 70% of ovarian cancers are associated with activation of PI3K signalling, with a higher incidence in clear cell ovarian cancer and endometrial cancer. This activation may occur following mutation or amplification in one of the two subunits of PI3K (PIK3CA (12%) or PIK3R1 (3.8%)), AKT1 (2%), AKT2 (13.3%), or mTOR or through loss of function of PTEN that in normal cells acts as an inhibitor of the PI3K pathway (94). In HGSOC, activation of PI3K cascade is rare (<5%) but is more frequent in clear cell ovarian cancer and endometrioid ovarian cancer. Loss of PTEN is present in 40% of clear cell ovarian cancer.

Different clinical trials exploring the activity of PI3K, AKT and mTOR inhibitors are ongoing as a single agent or in combination with chemotherapy. Agents targeting this pathway have shown interesting activity in gynaecological cancers, starting with mTOR inhibitors; however, the ability to predict outcome based on somatic mutations in the pathway genes has been challenging, perhaps due to a redundancy of molecular pathways to allow cells to survive. As a consequence, combination studies are underway to understand and overcome resistance, such as combinations of PI3K inhibitors and RAS/RAF/MEK inhibitors, with potential synergy in blocking an overactive pathway but also limited by toxicity.

ARID1A

ARID1A encodes the protein BAF250α, a core subunit of SWI/SNF that acts by inhibiting cancer cell development. Mutations of this gene have been found in 46–57% of clear cell ovarian cancer, 30% of endometrioid ovarian cancer, and 40% of uterine endometrioid carcinoma and loss of ARID1A expression is common in endometriosis (48, 95). Currently a specific treatment targeting ARID1A has not been identified, as usually happens with loss-of-function mutations; however, a study by Bitler et al. has shown that inducing synthetic lethality by way of inhibiting EZF2 (enhancer of zeste homology 2) in ARID1A-mutated patients results in clear cell ovarian cancer growth inhibition (96).

Targeting the microenvironment

Angiogenesis inhibition

Angiogenesis is required for cancer cell proliferation. Various mediators of angiogenesis have been reported, including VEGF. Hypoxia and the mechanisms that mediate hypoxic response are key drivers of physiological angiogenesis. Under hypoxic conditions expression of HIF-1α is induced in endothelial cells, resulting in VEGF-A, and vascular endothelial growth factor receptor 2 (VEGFR-2) expression. Targeted therapy against angiogenesis using bevacizumab, a humanized VEGF-neutralizing monoclonal antibody, improved the median progression-free survival rate in advanced ovarian cancer and the overall survival in cervical cancer (97). These two indications have been approved in gynaecological cancers. Despite several positive phase II trials with progression-free survival improvement, no antiangiogenetic has been approved in endometrial cancer. A crucial first step is to determine potential markers of response.

Epigenetic modulation

Epigenetics is a field that focuses on the study of heritable changes which do not result from changes in the DNA sequence,

including DNA methylation. These are divided into histone acetylation, deacetylation, and methylation events carried out by histone acetyltransferases, histone deacetylases, and histone methyltransferases, respectively. Aberrant methylation of CpG islands which are found in close proximity to gene transcription initiation sites and are normally methylated has been linked to tumour initiation and progression. Because of their involvement in tumourigenesis, the biology of these changes is now being investigated so that its potential in the treatment of ovarian cancer is fully understood.

Immunotherapy

The ability of cancer cells to evade immune destruction has become recognized as one of the hallmarks of cancer. This has paved the way for the development of novel therapeutic agents that can enhance activation of antitumour immune responses or reverse immunosuppressive mechanisms through which tumours escape immune-mediated rejection (98).

Vaccines

The most notable example of this approach is vaccination for HPV which is now approved for the prevention of cervical cancer.

The identification of unique differentiation proteins expressed in gynaecological cancer has led to the exploration of various vaccination approaches, including simple vaccine preparations consisting of specific peptides and proteins, as well as more complex strategies, such as engineered cellular vaccines, dendritic cell vaccines, virus-vectored vaccines, and oncolytic viruses. The majority of studies have explored the cancer-testis antigens (e.g. NY-ESO-1) and proteins known to be overexpressed in EOC (e.g. p53, survivin, and MUC1). Although many studies have demonstrated induction of an immune response to the vaccines, very few have demonstrated clinical benefit. It is likely that these strategies are insufficient to overcome immune tolerance to self-antigens and to result in efficient activation of antigen-specific T cells, although they may prove to be valuable in combination with other therapies or be used in a different treatment schedule.

Therapies to enhance T-cell activation

The survival, proliferation, and activation of T cells are controlled by a variety of factors, including cytokines and a range of immunostimulatory and inhibitory receptors. Identification of the co-stimulatory and co-inhibitory receptors that regulate T-cell activation has led to the development of antibodies that target these receptors. Targeting such receptors, an approach termed 'immune checkpoint blockade', has demonstrated activity in preclinical cancer models and in clinical trials. In particular, antibodies targeting the inhibitory receptors cytotoxic T-lymphocyte-associated antigen 4 (CTLA-4) and programmed death 1 (PD-1), as well as the PD-1 ligand (PD-L1), are the agents of this type that are most advanced in clinical development. Given the potential interest in gynaecological cancers, these strategies are being actively assessed. Indeed, tumour infiltrating lymphocyte (TIL) counts and peritumoural lymphocytes have been described as independent predictors for microsatellite instability high-status group in endometrial cancers (99). Moreover, the presence of TILs appears to be an independent prognostic factor (100). TIL infiltration and the presence of CD8 at diagnosis of ovarian cancer have been also described to be predictive of clinical outcomes in ovarian cancers.

Another approach under investigation is the adoptive cell therapies which rely on the infusion of large numbers of autologous tumour-reactive T cells that have been isolated from tumours and expanded *in vitro*.

Targeting cell surface receptors

Hormones

Hormonal therapy remains the sole approved targeted therapy in endometrial cancer. A significant proportion of endometrial cancer—in particular, type I tumours—express ER or PR, described to be predictors of favourable survival and rendering hormonal therapy an attractive therapeutic strategy. Current investigations are ongoing to understand mechanisms of resistance to hormonal therapies and the potential interest of combination therapies.

Folate

Several publications report that folate receptor alpha (FRα) is an attractive candidate for targeted biological therapy of ovarian cancer and potentially endometrial cancers (101–103). Indeed, approximately 90% of EOC express FRα and its expression correlates with stage and grade of malignancies (104). In contrast, FRα has a low expression on the apical surface of most normal cells (105). This difference in expression leads to high tumour-to-normal ratios and makes FRα a very attractive target for therapeutic and imaging purpose (106).

Combination approaches

Incorporating a novel targeted or immunological therapy into a therapeutic algorithm requires careful thought related to the current evidence-based standard of care. Therefore, early-phase studies are investigating strategies to combine as well as sequence novel agents in conjunction with chemotherapy, radiation, or other targeted agents. These early studies need to integrate strong translational studies to understand mechanisms of response and resistance that will guide future drug development to optimize treatment for our patients with a balance between drug activity and toxicity. Early examples of the efficacy of this approach have emerged from combinations incorporating antiangiogenics such as bevacizumab and cediranib as well as subsequent sequential use as a single agent.

The ability to develop combinations is inherently related to the potential for synergy as well toxicity—PARP inhibitors have been more challenging to combine with chemotherapy because of overlapping haematological toxicity, but proven to be synergistic in sequence (21, 107). Many studies are currently evaluating evidence-informed combinations which will be evaluated in prospective trials.

Summary and conclusion

Systemic therapy in gynaecological cancer is being reshaped as a result of an evolving understanding of the biology of cancer development, progression, and resistance. This also allows for the constant re-evaluation of long-established therapeutic platforms and paradigms as a means of challenging not only dogma, but also to separate treatments that are standard but ineffective, and to retain therapies that are effective and evidence informed. It is requisite to base treatment decisions that directly impact patients upon sound evidence from well-designed clinical trials, and shy away from logical but unsubstantiated therapies. This is an area of rapid change with tremendous promise for development of precision therapeutics, and the reader should assess updated information from validated national and international peer-reviewed guidelines on therapy to appropriately incorporated targeted agents into standard therapy (e.g. GCIG, NICE, NCCN).

REFERENCES

1. DeVita VT Jr, Chu E. A history of cancer chemotherapy. *Cancer Res* 2008;**68**:8643–53.
2. Hanahan D, Weinberg RA. Hallmarks of cancer: the next generation. *Cell* 2011;**144**:646–74.
3. Hanahan D, Weinberg RA. The hallmarks of cancer. *Cell* 2000;**100**:57–70.
4. Stuart GC, Kitchener H, Bacon M, et al. 2010 Gynecologic Cancer InterGroup (GCIG) consensus statement on clinical trials in ovarian cancer: report from the Fourth Ovarian Cancer Consensus Conference. *Int J Gynecol Cancer* 2011;**21**:750–55.
5. McGuire WP, Hoskins WJ, Brady MF, et al. Cyclophosphamide and cisplatin compared with paclitaxel and cisplatin in patients with stage III and stage IV ovarian cancer. *N Engl J Med* 1996;**334**:1–6.
6. Eisenhauer EA, ten Bokkel Huinink WW, Swenerton KD, et al. European-Canadian randomized trial of paclitaxel in relapsed ovarian cancer: high-dose versus low-dose and long versus short infusion. *J Clin Oncol* 1994;**12**:2654–66.
7. Kumar A, Hoskins PJ, Tinker AV. Dose-dense paclitaxel in advanced ovarian cancer. *Clin Oncol (R Coll Radiol)* 2015;**27**:40–47.
8. Jaaback K, Johnson N, Lawrie TA. Intraperitoneal chemotherapy for the initial management of primary epithelial ovarian cancer. *Cochrane Database Syst Rev* 2016;**1**:CD005340.
9. Vergote I, Tropé CG, Amant F, et al. Neoadjuvant chemotherapy or primary surgery in stage IIIC or IV ovarian cancer. *N Engl J Med* 2010;**363**:943–53.
10. Kehoe S, Hook J, Nankivell M, et al. Primary chemotherapy versus primary surgery for newly diagnosed advanced ovarian cancer (CHORUS): an open-label, randomised, controlled, non-inferiority trial. *Lancet* 2015;**386**:249–57.
11. Riester M, Wei W, Waldron L, et al. Risk prediction for late-stage ovarian cancer by meta-analysis of 1525 patient samples. *J Natl Cancer Inst* 2014;**106**:dju048.
12. Colombo N, Conte PF, Pignata S, Raspagliesi F, Scambia G. Bevacizumab in ovarian cancer: focus on clinical data and future perspectives. *Crit Rev Oncol Hematol* 2016;**97**:335–48.
13. Burger RA, Brady MF, Bookman MA, et al. Incorporation of bevacizumab in the primary treatment of ovarian cancer. *N Engl J Med* 2011;**365**:2473–83.
14. Perren TJ, Swart AM, Pfisterer J, et al. A phase 3 trial of bevacizumab in ovarian cancer. *N Engl J Med* 2011;**365**:2484–96. [Erratum in: *N Engl J Med* 2012;366:284.]
15. Oza AM, Cook AD, Pfisterer J, et al. Standard chemotherapy with or without bevacizumab for women with newly diagnosed ovarian cancer (ICON7): overall survival results of a phase 3 randomised trial. *Lancet Oncol* 2015;**16**:928–36.
16. Aghajanian C, Blank SV, Goff BA, et al. OCEANS: a randomized, double-blind, placebo-controlled phase III trial of chemotherapy with or without bevacizumab in patients with platinum-sensitive

recurrent epithelial ovarian, primary peritoneal, or fallopian tube cancer. *J Clin Oncol* 2012;**30**:2039–45.

17. Pujade-Lauraine E, Hilpert F, Weber B, et al. Bevacizumab combined with chemotherapy for platinum-resistant recurrent ovarian cancer: the AURELIA open-label randomized phase III trial. *J Clin Oncol* 2014;**32**:1302–308. [Erratum in: *J Clin Oncol* 2014;32:4025.]

18. du Bois A, Floquet A, Kim JW, et al. Incorporation of pazopanib in maintenance therapy of ovarian cancer. *J Clin Oncol* 2014;**32**:3374–82.

19. Ledermann JA, Embleton AC, Raja F, et al. Cediranib in patients with relapsed platinum-sensitive ovarian cancer (ICON6): a randomised, double-blind, placebo-controlled phase 3 trial. *Lancet* 2016;**387**:1066–74. [Erratum in: *Lancet* 2016;387:1722.]

20. Ledermann J, Harter P, Gourley C, et al. Olaparib maintenance therapy in patients with platinum-sensitive relapsed serous ovarian cancer: a preplanned retrospective analysis of outcomes by BRCA status in a randomized phase 2 trial. *Lancet Oncol* 2014;**15**:852–61. [Erratum in: *Lancet Oncol* 2015;16:e158.]

21. Oza AM, Cibula D, Benzaquen AO, et al. Olaparib combined with chemotherapy for recurrent platinum-sensitive ovarian cancer: a randomized phase 2 trial. *Lancet Oncol* 2015;**16**:87–97. [Erratum in: *Lancet Oncol* 2015;16:e6, e55.]

22. Lheureux S, Karakasis K, Kohn EC, Oza AM. Ovarian cancer treatment: the end of empiricism? *Cancer* 2015;**121**:3203–11.

23. Colombo N, Peiretti M, Castiglione M, ESMO Guidelines Working Group. Non-epithelial ovarian cancer: ESMO clinical recommendations for diagnosis, treatment and follow-up. *Ann Oncol* 2009;**20** Suppl 4:24–26.

24. Randall ME, Filiaci VL, Muss H, et al. Randomized phase III trial of whole-abdominal irradiation versus doxorubicin and cisplatin chemotherapy in advanced endometrial carcinoma: a Gynecologic Oncology Group Study. *J Clin Oncol* 2006;**24**:36–44.

25. Hogberg T, Signorelli M, de Oliveira CF, et al. Sequential adjuvant chemotherapy and radiotherapy in endometrial cancer—results from two randomised studies. *Eur J Cancer* 2010;**46**:2422–31.

26. Hoskins PJ, Swenerton KD, Pike JA, et al. Paclitaxel and carboplatin, alone or with irradiation, in advanced or recurrent endometrial cancer: a phase II study. *J Clin Oncol* 2001;**19**:4048–53.

27. Fleming GF, Brunetto VL, Cella D, et al. Phase III trial of doxorubicin plus cisplatin with or without paclitaxel plus filgrastim in advanced endometrial carcinoma: a Gynecologic Oncology Group Study. *J Clin Oncol* 2004;**22**:2159–66.

28. Lheureux S, Wilson M, Mackay HJ. Recent and current phase II clinical trials in endometrial cancer: review of the state of art. *Expert Opin Investig Drugs* 2014;**23**:773–92.

29. Lheureux S, Oza AM. Endometrial cancer-targeted therapies myth or reality? Review of current targeted treatments. *Eur J Cancer* 2016;**59**:99–108.

30. Muñoz N, Bosch FX, Chichareon S, et al. A multinational case-control study on the risk of cervical cancer linked to 25 HPV types: which are the high-risk types? In: Castellsagué X, Bosch FX, de Sanjosé S, Moreno V, Ribes J (eds), *International Papillomavirus Conference—Program and Abstracts Book*, p. 125. Barcelona: International Papillomavirus Conference; 2000.

31. Schiffman M, Castle PE, Jeronimo J, Rodriguez AC, Wacholder S. Human papillomavirus and cervical cancer. *Lancet* 2007;**370**:890–907.

32. Trottier H, Franco EL. The epidemiology of genital human papillomavirus infection. *Vaccine* 2006;**24** Suppl 1:S1–15.

33. Ault KA. Epidemiology and natural history of human papillomavirus infections in the female genital tract. *Infect Dis Obstet Gynecol* 2006;**2006** Suppl:40470.

34. Brisson J, Morin C, Fortier M, et al. Risk factors for cervical intraepithelial neoplasia: differences between low- and high-grade lesions. *Am J Epidemiol* 1994;**140**:700–10.

35. Koutsky LA, Holmes KK, Critchlow CW, et al. A cohort study of the risk of cervical intraepithelial neoplasia grade 2 or 3 in relation to papillomavirus infection. *N Engl J Med* 1992;**327**:1272–78.

36. Schiffman MH, Bauer HM, Hoover RN, et al. Epidemiologic evidence showing that human papillomavirus infection causes most cervical intraepithelial neoplasia. *J Natl Cancer Inst* 1993;**85**:958–64.

37. Moyer VA, U.S. Preventive Services Task Force. Screening for cervical cancer: U.S. Preventive Services Task Force recommendation statement. *Ann Intern Med* 2012;**156**:880–91, W312. [Erratum in: *Ann Intern Med* 2013;158:852.]

38. Whitney CW, Sause W, Bundy BN, et al. Randomized comparison of fluorouracil plus cisplatin versus hydroxyurea as an adjunct to radiation therapy in stage IIB-IVA carcinoma of the cervix with negative para-aortic lymph nodes: a Gynecologic Oncology Group and Southwest Oncology Group study. *J Clin Oncol* 1999;**17**:1339–48.

39. Trimble E, Gius D, Harlan LC. Impact of NCI announcement upon use of chemoradiation for women with cervical cancer. *J Clin Oncol* 2007;**25**:283s.

40. McNeil C. New standard of care for cervical cancer sets stage for next questions. *J Natl Cancer Inst* 1999;**91**:500–501.

41. Monk BJ, Sill MW, McMeekin DS, et al. Phase III trial of four cisplatin-containing doublet combinations in stage IVB, recurrent, or persistent cervical carcinoma: a Gynecologic Oncology Group study. *J Clin Oncol* 2009;**27**:4649–55.

42. Kitagawa R, Katsumata N, Shibata T, et al. Paclitaxel plus carboplatin versus paclitaxel plus cisplatin in metastatic or recurrent cervical cancer: the open-label randomized phase III trial JCOG0505. *J Clin Oncol* 2015;**33**:2129–35.

43. Tewari KS, Sill MW, Long HJ 3rd, et al. Improved survival with bevacizumab in advanced cervical cancer. *N Engl J Med* 2014;**370**:734–43.

44. Greer BE, Koh WJ. New NCCN guidelines for vulvar cancer. *J Natl Compr Canc Netw* 2016;**14** Suppl 5:656–58.

45. Cancer Genome Atlas Research Network. Integrated genomic analyses of ovarian carcinoma. *Nature* 2011;**474**:609–15. [Erratum in: *Nature* 2012;490:298.]

46. Ledermann JA. PARP inhibitors in ovarian cancer. *Ann Oncol* 2016;**27** Suppl 1:i40–44.

47. Cancer Genome Atlas Research Network, Kandoth C, Schultz N, et al. Integrated genomic characterization of endometrial carcinoma. *Nature* 2013;**497**:67–73. [Erratum in: *Nature* 2013;500:242.]

48. Wiegand KC, Shah SP, Al-Agha OM, et al. ARID1A mutations in endometriosis-associated ovarian carcinomas. *N Engl J Med* 2010;**363**:1532–43.

49. Hollis RL, Gourley C. Genetic and molecular changes in ovarian cancer. *Cancer Biol Med* 2016;**13**:236–47.

50. Grisham RN. Low-grade serous carcinoma of the ovary. *Oncology (Williston Park)* 2016;**30**:650–52.

51. Singer G, Oldt R 3rd, Cohen Y, et al. Mutations in BRAF and KRAS characterize the development of low-grade ovarian serous carcinoma. *J Natl Cancer Inst* 2003;**95**:484–86.

52. Ojesina AI, Lichtenstein L, Freeman SS, et al. Landscape of genomic alterations in cervical carcinomas. *Nature* 2014;**506**:371–75 (PMID: 28112728).

53. Fisher R, Pusztai L, Swanton C. Cancer heterogeneity: implications for targeted therapeutics. *Br J Cancer* 2013;**108**:479–85.

54. Hiley C, de Bruin EC, McGranahan N, Swanton C. Deciphering intratumor heterogeneity and temporal acquisition of driver events to refine precision medicine. *Genome Biol* 2014;**15**:453.

55. Burrell RA, McGranahan N, Bartek J, Swanton C. The causes and consequences of genetic heterogeneity in cancer evolution. *Nature* 2013;**501**:338–45.

56. Greaves M, Maley CC. Clonal evolution in cancer. *Nature* 2012;**481**:306–13.

57. Bashashati A, Ha G, Tone A, et al. Distinct evolutionary trajectories of primary high-grade serous ovarian cancers revealed through spatial mutational profiling. *J Pathol* 2013;**231**:21–34.

58. Schwarz RF, Ng CK, Cooke SL, et al. Spatial and temporal heterogeneity in high-grade serous ovarian cancer: a phylogenetic analysis. *PLoS Med* 2015;**12**:e1001789.

59. Yachida S, Jones S, Bozic I, et al. Distant metastasis occurs late during the genetic evolution of pancreatic cancer. *Nature* 2010;**467**:1114–17.

60. Gerlinger M, Rowan AJ, Horswell S, et al. Intratumor heterogeneity and branched evolution revealed by multiregion sequencing. *N Engl J Med* 2012;**366**:883–92. [Erratum in: *N Engl J Med* 2012;367:976.]

61. Griffiths AJF, Miller JH, Suzuki DT, et al. Somatic versus germinal mutation. In: *An Introduction to Genetic Analysis*, 7th edn. New York: W.H. Freeman; 2000. Available at: http://www.ncbi.nlm.nih.gov/books/NBK21894/.

62. Cavanagh H, Rogers KM. The role of BRCA1 and BRCA2 mutations in prostate, pancreatic and stomach cancers. *Hered Cancer Clin Pract* 2015;**13**:16.

63. Prat J. Ovarian carcinomas: five distinct diseases with different origins, genetic alterations, and clinicopathological features. *Virchows Arch* 2012;**460**:237–49.

64. Hsu CY, Bristow R, Cha MS, et al. Characterization of active mitogen-activated protein kinase in ovarian serous carcinomas. *Clin Cancer Res* 2004;**10**:6432–36.

65. McAlpine JN, Wiegand KC, Vang R, et al. HER2 overexpression and amplification is present in a subset of ovarian mucinous carcinomas and can be targeted with trastuzumab therapy. *BMC Cancer* 2009;**9**:433.

66. Friedlander ML, Russell K, Millis S, Gatalica Z, Bender R, Voss A. Molecular profiling of clear cell ovarian cancers: identifying potential treatment targets for clinical trials. *Int J Gynecol Cancer* 2016;**26**:648–54.

67. Catasús L, Bussaglia E, Rodrguez I, et al. Molecular genetic alterations in endometrioid carcinomas of the ovary: similar frequency of beta-catenin abnormalities but lower rate of microsatellite instability and PTEN alterations than in uterine endometrioid carcinomas. *Hum Pathol* 2004;**35**:1360–68.

68. Husain RS, Ramakrishnan V. Global variation of human papillomavirus genotypes and selected genes involved in cervical malignancies. *Ann Glob Health* 2015;**81**:675–83.

69. Agarwal SM, Raghav D, Singh H, Raghava GP. CCDB: a curated database of genes involved in cervix cancer. *Nucleic Acids Res* 2011;**39**(Database issue):D975–79.

70. Forbes SA, Bindal N, Bamford S, et al. COSMIC: mining complete cancer genomes in the Catalogue of Somatic Mutations in Cancer. *Nucleic Acids Res* 2011;**39**(Database issue):D945–50.

71. Trietsch MD, Nooij LS, Gaarenstroom KN, van Poelgeest MI. Genetic and epigenetic changes in vulvar squamous cell carcinoma and its precursor lesions: a review of the current literature. *Gynecol Oncol* 2015;**136**:143–57.

72. Holway AH, Rieger-Christ KM, Miner WR, et al. Somatic mutation of PTEN in vulvar cancer. *Clin Cancer Res* 2000;**6**:3228–35.

73. Soufir N, Queille S, Liboutet M, et al. Inactivation of the CDKN2A and the p53 tumour suppressor genes in external genital carcinomas and their precursors. *Br J Dermatol* 2007;**156**:448–53.

74. Trietsch MD, Spaans VM, ter Haar NT, et al. CDKN2A (p16) and HRAS are frequently mutated in vulvar squamous cell carcinoma. *Gynecol Oncol* 2014;**135**:149–55.

75. Surget S, Khoury MP, Bourdon JC. Uncovering the role of p53 splice variants in human malignancy: a clinical perspective. *Onco Targets Ther* 2013;**7**:57–68.

76. Hong B, van den Heuvel AP, Prabhu VV, Zhang S, El-Deiry WS. Targeting tumor suppressor p53 for cancer therapy: strategies, challenges and opportunities. *Curr Drug Targets* 2014;**15**:80–89.

77. Olivier M, Hollstein M, Hainaut P. TP53 mutations in human cancers: origins, consequences, and clinical use. *Cold Spring Harb Perspect Biol* 2010;**2**:a001008.

78. Li FP, Fraumeni JF Jr, Mulvihill JJ, et al. A cancer family syndrome in twenty-four kindreds. *Cancer Res* 1988;**48**:5358–62.

79. Malkin D, Li FP, Strong LC, et al. Germ line p53 mutations in a familial syndrome of breast cancer, sarcomas, and other neoplasms. *Science* 1990;**250**:1233–38. [Erratum in: *Science* 1993; 259:878.]

80. Chen S, Parmigiani G. Meta-analysis of BRCA1 and BRCA2 penetrance. *J Clin Oncol* 2007;**25**:1329–33.

81. Alsop K, Fereday S, Meldrum C, et al. BRCA mutation frequency and patterns of treatment response in BRCA mutation-positive women with ovarian cancer: a report from the Australian Ovarian Cancer Study Group. *J Clin Oncol* 2012;**30**:2654–663. [Erratum in: *J Clin Oncol* 2012;30:4180.]

82. McCabe N, Turner NC, Lord CJ, et al. Deficiency in the repair of DNA damage by homologous recombination and sensitivity to poly(ADP-ribose) polymerase inhibition. *Cancer Res* 2006;**66**:8109–115.

83. Pennington KP, Walsh T, Harrell MI, et al. Germline and somatic mutations in homologous recombination genes predict platinum response and survival in ovarian, fallopian tube, and peritoneal carcinomas. *Clin Cancer Res* 2014;**20**:764–75.

84. Ashworth A. A synthetic lethal therapeutic approach: poly(ADP) ribose polymerase inhibitors for the treatment of cancers deficient in DNA double-strand break repair. *J Clin Oncol* 2008;**26**:3785–90.

85. Farmer H, McCabe N, Lord CJ, et al. Targeting the DNA repair defect in BRCA mutant cells as a therapeutic strategy. *Nature* 2005;**434**:917–21.

86. Walsh CS. Two decades beyond BRCA1/2: homologous recombination, hereditary cancer risk and a target for ovarian cancer therapy. *Gynecol Oncol* 2015;**137**:343–50.

87. Turner N, Tutt A, Ashworth A. Hallmarks of 'BRCAness' in sporadic cancers. *Nat Rev Cancer* 2004;**4**:814–19.

88. McAlpine JN, Temkin SM, Mackay HJ. Endometrial cancer: not your grandmother's cancer. *Cancer* 2016;**122**:2787–98.

89. Erten MZ, Fernandez LP, Ng HK, et al. Universal versus targeted screening for Lynch syndrome: comparing ascertainment and costs based on clinical experience. *Dig Dis Sci* 2016;**61**:2887–95.

90. Kristeleit RS, Miller RE, Kohn EC. Gynecologic cancers: emerging novel strategies for targeting DNA repair deficiency. *Am Soc Clin Oncol Educ Book* 2016;**35**:e259–68.

91. Bykov VJ, Wiman KG. Mutant p53 reactivation by small molecules makes its way to the clinic. *FEBS Lett* 2014;**588**:2622–27.

92. Tommasino M, Accardi R, Caldeira S, et al. The role of TP53 in cervical carcinogenesis. *Hum Mutat* 2003;**21**:307–12.

93. Fujiwara K, McAlpine JN, Lheureux S, Matsumura N, Oza AM. Paradigm shift in the management strategy for epithelial ovarian cancer. *Am Soc Clin Oncol Educ Book* 2016;**35**:e247–57.

94. Salvesen HB, Werner HM, Krakstad C. PI3K pathway in gynecologic malignancies. *Am Soc Clin Oncol Educ Book* 2013. doi: 10.1200/EdBook_AM.2013.33.e218.

95. Jones S, Wang TL, Shih IM, et al. Frequent mutations of chromatin remodeling gene ARID1A in ovarian clear cell carcinoma. *Science* 2010;**330**:228–31.

96. Bitler BG, Aird KM, Garipov A, et al. Synthetic lethality by targeting EZH2 methyltransferase activity in ARID1A-mutated cancers. *Nat Med* 2015;**21**:231–38.

97. Sonoda K. Molecular biology of gynecological cancer. *Oncol Lett* 2016;**11**:16–22.

98. Bourla AB, Zamarin D. Immunotherapy: new strategies for the treatment of gynecologic malignancies. *Oncology (Williston Park)* 2016;**30**:59–66, 69.

99. Oku H, Hase S. Studies on the substrate specificity of neutral alpha-mannosidase purified from Japanese quail oviduct by using sugar chains from glycoproteins. *J Biochem* 1991;**110**:982–89.

100. de Jong RA, Leffers N, Boezen HM, et al. Presence of tumor-infiltrating lymphocytes is an independent prognostic factor in type I and II endometrial cancer. *Gynecol Oncol* 2009;**114**:105–10.

101. Salazar MD, Ratnam M. The folate receptor: what does it promise in tissue-targeted therapeutics? *Cancer Metastasis Rev* 2007;**26**:141–52.

102. Reddy JA, Allagadda VM, Leamon CP. Targeting therapeutic and imaging agents to folate receptor positive tumors. *Curr Pharm Biotechnol* 2005;**6**:131–50.

103. Kalli KR, Oberg AL, Keeney GL, et al. Folate receptor alpha as a tumor target in epithelial ovarian cancer. *Gynecol Oncol* 2008;**108**:619–26.

104. Toffoli G, Russo A, Gallo A, et al. Expression of folate binding protein as a prognostic factor for response to platinum-containing chemotherapy and survival in human ovarian cancer. *Int J Cancer* 1998;**79**:121–26.

105. Markert S, Lassmann S, Gabriel B, et al. Alpha-folate receptor expression in epithelial ovarian carcinoma and non-neoplastic ovarian tissue. *Anticancer Res* 2008;**28**:3567–72.

106. Walters CL, Arend RC, Armstrong DK, Naumann RW, Alvarez RD. Folate and folate receptor alpha antagonists mechanism of action in ovarian cancer. *Gynecol Oncol* 2013;**131**:493–98.

107. Ledermann J, Harter P, Gourley C, et al. Olaparib maintenance therapy in platinum-sensitive relapsed ovarian cancer. *N Engl J Med* 2012;**366**:1382–92.

Radiation therapy in the management of gynaecological cancer

Anthony Fyles, Anuja Jhingran, David Gaffney, Dustin Boothe, Marco Carlone, and Tim Craig

Basic principles of radiotherapy

External beam radiation

Therapeutic applications for radiation therapy followed quickly from the discovery of X-rays by Roentgen in 1895 (1). The first radiation treatment is credited to Grubbe, who reported the external beam treatment of breast cancer in 1896 (2). Application to gynaecological cancers was almost immediate (3).

However, the limited penetrating ability of the low-energy radiation of early X-ray tubes and isotopes was a major limitation. Therefore, treating targets deep within the pelvis required simultaneously delivering a high dose to the skin, often with substantial toxicity. These features limited the application of external beam radiation therapy, where the beam originates outside of the patient. Consequently, brachytherapy and near-contact external beam therapy (4) were preferred for gynaecological cancer until the advent of cobalt-60.

Isotopes versus linear accelerators

Radiative cobalt-60 releases 1.17 and 1.33 mega-electron volt gamma rays and was the first source of a penetrating beam of megavoltage photons with a high dose rate, long half-life, and reasonable cost. This led to cobalt-60 machines becoming the most widely utilized treatment machine from the 1950s to 1970s (5). Radar research during World War II dramatically improved microwave technology. Linear accelerator-based machines (linacs) applied these advances to use microwaves to accelerate electrons onto a tungsten target and emit a fraction of their kinetic energy as mega-electron volt energy X-rays. The emitted X-rays are collimated into a beam and directed towards the patient. Advantages of linacs over cobalt-60 include higher dose rates, sharper beam edges, higher energies, and simplified radiation protection.

Typical modern linac configurations include 6–18 MV X-rays, a multileaf collimator that can dynamically shape the beam aperture with a 5 mm resolution, mechanical accuracy of about 1 mm, and integrated volumetric imaging devices. These features allow delivery techniques, such as intensity-modulated radiation therapy (IMRT), where differential beam intensities are created, and image-guided radiation therapy (IGRT) to image the patient and adjust the targeting immediately prior to radiation delivery.

Simulation

The simulation stage of radiation treatment planning acquired its name from the historical use of machines called 'simulators' that reproduced the linac geometry. This allowed simple treatment geometries to be simulated and two-dimensional (2D) radiographs of the patient in the planned position could be acquired (7). Today's 'computed tomography (CT) simulator' is a diagnostic CT scanner used to acquire images of the patient in the treatment position. These images are transferred to a treatment planning computer system to create a treatment plan. Tumours and relevant anatomy in gynaecological cancers may be better visualized on magnetic resonance imaging (MRI) or positron emission tomography (PET) (8, 9) and these images can be 'fused' in the treatment planning system and used for visualization during planning.

Treatment planning: two- versus three-dimensional

Classical (also known as 2D or conventional) and modern 3D treatment planning share the concepts of using imaging to define target volumes, setting beam parameters to irradiate targets and avoid healthy tissue, and making accurate dose calculations; however, different technologies are used.

Target definition in classical treatment planning used radiographs to define a rectangular target area. Current planning involves careful 'contouring' of images, where the radiation oncologist draws the tumour volumes and normal tissues to be avoided on the images acquired during simulation. At the end of this process, a 3D model of the patient anatomy has been constructed.

Contouring is crucially important for the quality of the treatment plan, since it will influence all future planning steps. In recognition of the importance of this step, guidelines have been created to promote accurate and consistent contours between different institutions

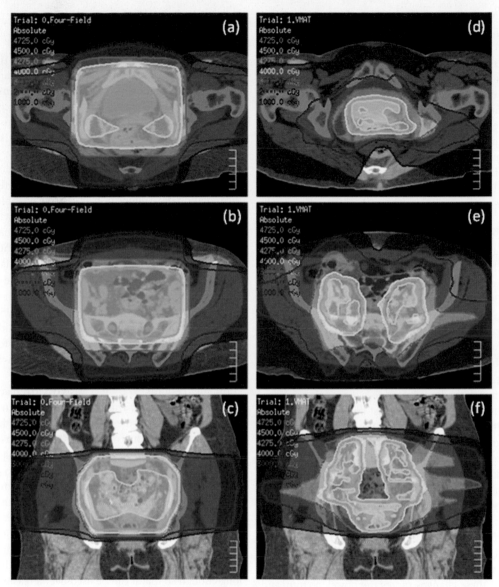

Figure 68.1 Axial CT image and dose (colourwash) illustrating a typical conventional four-field box and intensity-modulated radiation therapy treatment at the level of vagina (a, d), pelvic lymph nodes (b, e), and coronal view (c, f).

and radiation oncologists, with several dedicated solely to gynaecological cancers (10–13).

The contoured model of the patient is used to design a personalized treatment plan. The goal is always to plan a high, therapeutic target dose while minimizing normal tissue toxicity. However, modern techniques differ substantially from conventional 2D approaches.

Two classic techniques for gynaecological cancers are the 'parallel-opposed pair' and 'four-field box' (**Figure 68.1**). The parallel-opposed pair technique uses two beams, one entering from the anterior and one posterior. The resulting dose distribution is a relatively uniform column of dose from the anterior to posterior of the patient. The four-field box technique uses four beams, with one entering though each of the anterior, left, posterior, and right directions. The resulting dose features a uniform box-shaped high-dose region at the intersection of the beams, and is frequently used to irradiate a primary tumour and pelvic lymph nodes. These classic techniques are still used, albeit with modern planning tools. However, they have limited ability to shape the dose distribution, and a consequence of a column or box-shaped high-dose volume is that the rectum, bladder, sigmoid, and small bowel are also treated to the prescription dose.

IMRT is a revolutionary technology that uses varying intensity patterns created by dynamic multileaf collimator motion (14–17). The planner will specify objectives (e.g. a minimum dose for the target, maximum doses for normal tissue), and an optimization algorithm determines the intensity patterns that most closely achieve the objectives. The result is high-dose regions that very closely conform to even irregularly shaped target volumes while minimizing the dose to healthy tissues.

A planning study of the use of IMRT in gynaecological cancer indicated it could substantially reduce the dose to small bowel, rectum, and bladder in postoperative cervix and endometrial cancers (18).

A clinical study followed, demonstrating favourable acute (19) and chronic toxicity (20). A phase 2 Radiation Therapy Oncology Group study (RTOG 0418) demonstrated that multi-institutional studies are feasible and the single-institution experiences of toxicity reduction could be replicated (21, 22). A randomized trial (RTOG 1203, NCT01672892) of conventional treatment versus IMRT in this population has confirmed these results.

IMRT has also been applied to locally advanced vulval carcinoma to avoid the high skin, gastrointestinal, and haematological toxicities associated with conventional 2D approaches. A comparison of conventional and IMRT plans demonstrated sparing of small bowel, rectum, and bladder, good disease control, and low rates of toxicity (23).

Image-guided radiotherapy

IGRT refers to real-time daily acquisition of patient images in the treatment position and adjustment prior to delivering radiation. Cone-beam computed tomography, the most common volumetric IGRT technology (24), integrates a modified CT scanner into the treatment machine. The acquired image is compared with the reference CT image acquired during the simulation, and the adjustment required to match the two images is calculated and performed remotely using a robotic treatment couch. This approach can position an easily identifiable target with an error of less than 2 mm. However, integration with the linac introduces some compromises, as cone-beam CT images have poor contrast compared with diagnostic CT images. In addition to ensuring the patient is correctly targeted, daily imaging demonstrates substantial variations in the positions of the uterus, cervix, vagina, bladder, rectum, and small bowel from day to day during a typical treatment (25–28). This has generated interest in adaptive radiation therapy. Adaptive radiation therapy uses imaging from the first few treatments to personalize and adapt treatment. In gynaecological cancers, adaptive radiation therapy may be useful when variations in uterus position and tumour regression exist. CT and MRI have demonstrated that cervical tumour volumes shrink dramatically over 5 weeks of treatment (29), and adapting to these changes spares the bowel, rectum, and bladder (30).

Another novel approach uses MRI with deformable image registration to map and accumulate the dose to mobile and deforming organs during treatment (31, 32). This accumulated dose can be used to trigger one or more replanning events to ensure targets are appropriately treated (33).

Future directions

X-ray-producing linacs are by far the most common treatment machine today; however, there is interest in other radiation types. Protons beams feature a peak dose at depth, then stop completely. Proton planning has shown this could be exploited to better spare bone marrow, bowel, and kidneys compared to IMRT (34, 35).

Carbon ion beam facilities are rare and extremely expensive; however, they produce complex DNA damage that should counteract the adverse effect of hypoxia within the cervical cancers, which is prognostic of a poor response (36, 37). A report of locally advanced cervical cancer patients treated with carbon ions was unable to demonstrate differences in disease-specific survival for oxic or hypoxic tumours, supporting this hypothesis (38).

Brachytherapy

Isotopes

Brachytherapy for gynaecological cancers has its origins very close to the isolation of radium-226 (^{226}Ra) by Marie Curie. Within a decade of the isolation of ^{226}Ra, treatment techniques for many cancers had been developed (39), including gynaecological cancers.

Radium was very useful for initial therapies using radiation; however, it suffers from several physical characteristics, which make it non-ideal as a radionuclide for brachytherapy. Its mean and maximum energies are large, which makes the dose deposition area larger than ideal, where the overarching goal of the therapy is to keep the radiation dose deposition as close as possible to the targeted lesion. In addition, the production of radon gas as the first product of its radioactive decay is problematic since this can lead to problems in containing the radioactive material, and is thus a radiation safety hazard. Finally, the long half-life of 1622 years is also undesirable in that once the radionuclide is isolated, it must be managed and safely stored for a significant time. The advent of high-energy accelerators and nuclear reactors between the 1930s and 1950s allowed the production of non-naturally occurring radionuclides, many of which have more favourable properties than ^{226}Ra for therapeutic purposes. With these new radionuclides, radium was gradually phased out of clinical use by the end of the 1980s.

Initially, cesium-137 (^{137}Cs) was used to replace ^{226}Ra in gynaecological brachytherapy. This radionuclide has a mean photon energy of 660 keV and a half-life of 30.2 years. Although this is an improvement from ^{226}Ra, this radionuclide suffers from a poor specific activity (the number of disintegrations per mass), thus the source size for ^{137}Cs needs to be quite large in order to produce a dose rate suitable for clinical procedures. Today, most gynaecological brachytherapy is done using iridium-192 (^{192}Ir), which has a mean photon energy of 380 keV, a very high specific activity, and a half-life of 74.2 days, making it a very good radionuclide for brachytherapy. In particular, radiation protection issues are minimized with a half-life that is short enough to simplify disposal of the radionuclide, but long enough so that it can be used over a reasonable period of time in the clinic.

Applicators

Due to the rapid fall-off of dose of the brachytherapy sources, very consistent and reproducible brachytherapy source positions are required in order to reproduce the desired therapeutic effect of brachytherapy. In addition, to better control the overall dose delivered (which depends on the dwell time of the radionuclide sources), it is desirable to use a device which is first placed without sources being loaded, in order to determine the localization of the source positions, allowing the sources to subsequently be quickly inserted and removed when treatment is finished.

In the early days of brachytherapy, inconsistent positioning of sources and other dosimetric problems led to an inconsistently delivered dose, which had a negative effect on the perception of the treatment technique. In order to address this, and to provide tools for clinicians to be able to achieve a more uniform level of implant, certain brachytherapy insertion 'systems' were developed. These 'systems' provided rules for source positioning and significantly improved the consistency of the clinical outcomes. In gynaecology, the

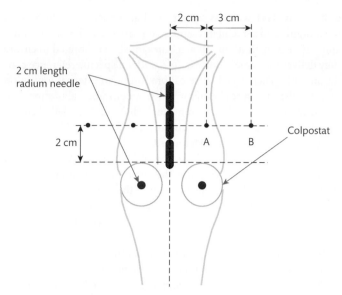

Figure 68.2 Illustration of the Manchester system. Radium needles 2 cm in length were inserted in the uterus (up to three) and in the vaginal fornixes. Dose was prescribed at point A, which is 2 cm lateral to the intrauterine needles and 2 cm superior to the surface of the colpostats, which are assumed to be flush with the vaginal mucosa. Point B, which is 3 cm lateral to point A, represents lateral dose fall off and dose to obturator lymph nodes.

'Stockholm' and 'Paris' systems prescribed a manner for inserting tubes of ^{226}Ra into the uterus and vagina, both spatially and temporally (dose rate and number of insertions), in order to provide a dose coverage that could be tailored to the clinical presentation of the disease. The space distribution of the Paris system combined with the temporal placement of sources was combined into what became known as the 'Manchester' system. Initially, this system used flexible tubing to place intrauterine sources and sources adjacent to the cervix. This involved inserting 2 cm long ^{226}Ra sources (1.5 cm active length), either 1, 2, or 3 into the uterus (called the uterine tandem) and two separate 2 cm long source perpendicular to the intrauterine sources, in cylindrical applicators called colpostats inserted in the vaginal fornices. Finally, to allow consistent reporting of dose to the disease treated, specific dose calculation points were described, known as points A and B. Point A is specified as 2 cm lateral to the central intrauterine tandem and 2 cm superior to the mucous membrane of lateral vaginal fornix. This point is meant to represent the coverage dose to the cervix. Point B is taken as 3 cm lateral to point A, and represents the lateral dose drop off, and as well was considered to be representative of dose to the obturator nodes (**Figure 68.2**). Finally, the Manchester system also specified how to calculate the dose received at specific points in order to represent the dose to the bladder and rectum, which are the normal healthy tissues to which doses are to be minimized.

The Henschke applicators were developed in the 1960s and 1970s, and were specifically designed to give a dose distribution consistent with the Manchester system, but to be used specifically with ^{137}Cs. The design consists of a central intrauterine tandem and two colpostats/ovoids. The separation of the colpostats could be adjusted to provide adequate lateral dose coverage. Finally, tungsten shielding was available for both the bladder and rectum as well as for the ovoids to reduce normal tissue dose if required.

The Fletcher–Suit (and later Delclos) applicators were similar to the Henschke applicator, in that it used a central tandem and two ovoid-type applicators and mimics the Manchester system. The ovoid design, however, was adjusted specifically to allow for remote afterloading, as opposed to manual loading of sources. With automated source placement, care was taken in the Fletcher–Suit–Delclos design to minimize friction in source movement, which can lead to stuck sources, and are a major risk of afterloader techniques.

Another commonly used applicator is the tandem and vaginal ring, which also allows the use of interstitial catheters inserted through the ring into parametrial tumour extension. Although requiring image-guided techniques (see 'Image guidance'), this optimizes the dose to the residual tumour while also reducing the dose to the bladder and rectum (40).

Remote afterloading

The practice of brachytherapy necessarily involves placement of radioactive sources in patients in order to provide a therapeutic benefit. The radiation action on cancer cells also affects normal healthy tissues, including those of the clinical staff. By using suitable shielding, and by keeping the distance to the sources large (using forceps) and exposure times low, doses to the attending physician, therapists, and nurses can be kept quite low for an individual treatment. However, the cumulative exposure of the staff over multiple patient treatments can lead to a large lifetime radiation dose. For this reason, technology was developed through the 1970s in order to automate the placement of radioactive source without the need for manual placement. This work was led by the Nucletron Corporation, who developed the Selectron remote afterloader (RAL), which was marketed in the early 1980s.

The Selectron RAL was specifically designed for cervical brachytherapy, and implemented a Manchester type of source loading using ^{137}Cs. The unit utilized a source selector, which could choose between an active source and a non-radioactive spacer. By adjusting the sequence of active source and non-active spacer, the Selectron could generate a variable pattern of radioactivity, and hence dose distribution. The unit utilized air pressure to push sources from the inner source 'safe' out to the Fletcher-type applicator, and suction to retrieve the sources when the treatment is completed. The unit was limited by the large ^{137}Cs source size (2.5 mm spheres), resulting in a large applicator which was only useful for gynaecological brachytherapy, limiting its use and thus marketability as a generalized brachytherapy device. With the higher specific activity of ^{192}Ir, modern brachytherapy RALs now have much smaller sources (<1 mm diameter) utilizing a single source (as opposed to a bank of sources), which is welded to a stainless steel cable. The source can then be 'stepped' through the target treatment volume to generate the desired dose distribution. With smaller source dimensions, generalized brachytherapy techniques are now available for a wide array of disease sites, not just gynaecological cancers.

Current RALs have other advantages as the degree of dose modulation is considerably higher than for caesium, due to the small size, but also the lower photon energy of the iridium spectra. Finally, the very high specific activity of iridium allows for considerably higher dose rates permitting treatment delivery in times in the order of minutes, as opposed to days. This also introduces new problems since the biological effect of radiation is dose-rate dependent.

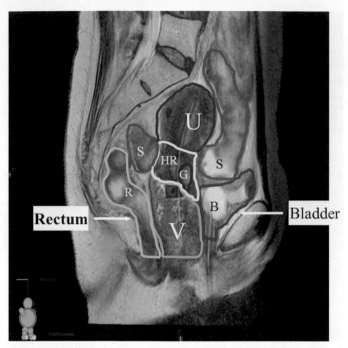

Figure 68.3 Sagittal MRI with intrauterine applicator and Foley catheter in bladder, illustrating high-risk (HR) clinical target volume, gross tumour volume (G), uterus (U), sigmoid (S), and vagina (V) with packing.

Image guidance

The correct placement of the brachytherapy applicator relative to the targeted disease area is critical to the success of the treatment. A poorly placed applicator is problematic because not only will the tumour receive less dose than required, but the normal healthy tissues will receive an unnecessary dose. Imaging is an important component of the brachytherapy applicator placement procedure, which verifies correct placement of the device. Originally, 2D planar X-ray imaging was used to define the applicator placement in relation to the target area, which could be defined using radio-opaque clips inserted into the cervix; and contrast used to define the bladder and rectal dose points.

Currently, 3D CT imaging is the method of choice for defining applicator positions. However, recent evidence (41) has shown that magnetic resonance-based imaging is the current standard for the definition of tumour volumes, including areas of suspected clinical extension. Also, the modern method of reporting doses to both the target and normal tissues is to report the integrated dose to a volume of tissue, as opposed to point doses. Thus, MRI is the imaging modality of choice, where T2-weighted imaging has been shown to be useful in defining target volumes as well as the normal tissues, namely the bladder, rectum, sigmoid, and small bowel (**Figure 68.3**). In addition, involved lymph nodes can be readily identified with MRI, thus allowing an accurate determination of their doses from brachytherapy.

Physics/biology

Radiation dosimetry

Modern linacs deliver a specified amount of X-ray energy with high accuracy and precision. Absorbed dose is defined as the energy absorbed per unit mass, and has the International System of Units (SI)

unit of gray (Gy), which is equal to 1 J/kg. For radiation doses to be meaningful, and to facilitate comparison between different machines and different institutions, all machines must be calibrated to ensure they deliver the same absorbed dose under a specific reference condition. This is achieved by the calibration of an internal ionization monitor that measures 'monitor units'. A common calibration is to adjust the output of the machine such that 1 cGy is delivered per monitor unit at a depth of 1.5 cm in water for a 6 MV X-ray beam with 10 × 10 cm field size. Methods to perform this calibration are described in protocols developed by the American Association of Physicists in Medicine (42) and the International Atomic Energy Association (43). These protocols require the use of dosimeters calibrated at a national or accredited dosimetry standards laboratory, ensuring that the dose is delivered and reported consistently around the world.

The performance of linacs is maintained by routine quality assurance activities. Guidance documents from the American Association of Physicists in Medicine, for example, describe a detailed list of radiation safety features, dosimetry parameters, mechanical function, and imaging tests that are variously performed on a daily, weekly, monthly, and annual basis. A well-maintained modern machine can typically be expected to deliver the intended dose with an accuracy of 2%, and have a total mechanical accuracy of about 1 mm.

Radiation protection

While the irradiation of the patient is intentional, specific, and intended to be beneficial, any dose to others is undesirable and should be maintained as low as reasonably achievable. Limits on the permitted dose to the public and staff in a radiotherapy facility are specified nationally; however, most countries apply limits based on recommendations of the International Commission on Radiation Protection (44). Radiation protection conventionally uses the SI unit of sievert (Sv), which is the dose multiplied by a radiation effectiveness factor and an organ weighting factor. Grays, the unit of absorbed dose, and sieverts are numerically equivalent for whole-body exposure to X-rays (where the weighting factors are both equal to 1.0). In this formalism, occupational exposure is limited to 20 mSv/year (using a 5-year average) and 1 mSv/year for the public.

These limits are achieved through well-educated qualified staff and stringent facility design. The walls, door, ceiling, and floors of the room containing a linac are constructed considering the materials to be used, occupancy of adjacent spaces by staff or the public, and machine features such as maximum energy and anticipated workload. The shielding required can be substantial, and a common treatment room design that satisfies International Commission on Radiation Protection requirements uses walls constructed of 2.5 m of solid concrete.

Cervix cancer

Introduction

In many developing countries, cancer of the cervix is the second most common cancer and cause of cancer deaths in women, in part due to limited access to cervical cancer screening and prevention programmes.

Staging

Staging of cervix cancer using the International Federation of Gynecology and Obstetrics (FIGO) system is largely defined by physical examination and limited imaging. In practice, many centres will utilize combinations of CT, MRI, and PET imaging to better define the extent of the primary tumour, and nodal and distant metastases. The FIGO staging system is shown in Chapter 62 (Box 62.2).

Role for concurrent chemotherapy and radiation

Based on a series of five randomized trials reported in 1999, which demonstrated improved survival and acceptable toxicity, concurrent weekly cisplatin in five courses (at a dose of 40 mg/m²) and radiotherapy has become the standard of care in cervix cancer (45).

Role for radiotherapy by stage

Decisions regarding optimal treatment for early-stage disease are critically dependent on a multidisciplinary discussion between gynaecological, radiation, and medical oncologists, with input from gynaecological imaging and pathology. Definitive chemoradiotherapy is curative in women with cervix cancer, in part due to the combination of external bean radiation with intracavitary brachytherapy, delivering a high local dose to the tumour while sparing normal tissues (46); and in part due to the increased radiosensitivity and better outcomes associated with human papillomavirus-related tumours, including other human papillomavirus-related sites such as oropharynx (47, 48).

Early-stage disease (stages IB2–IIA)

For women with a low risk of unrecognized local invasion or nodal metastases (IB1 without lymphovascular or deep cervical invasion), radical hysterectomy and lymph node staging is the standard of care or radical trachelectomy for those wishing to preserve fertility). With larger stage IB2 tumours where the likelihood of requiring postoperative radiotherapy is intermediate to high (i.e. 20% or greater), a single treatment approach using chemoradiation is favoured to avoid the additional toxicity of combining surgery and radiotherapy (49, 50). Long-term pelvic control and survival is seen in 70–85% (49). Typical treatment includes external beam pelvic radiotherapy (45 Gy in 25 daily fractions over 5 weeks) plus concurrent weekly cisplatin chemotherapy, followed by intracavitary brachytherapy.

Advanced disease (stages IIB–IVA)

Bulky and advanced disease with parametrial/sidewall or nodal involvement is optimally treated with pelvic with or without para-aortic nodal chemoradiotherapy followed by brachytherapy (51). External beam pelvic radiotherapy (45–50 Gy) plus concurrent cisplatin chemotherapy, followed by intracavitary brachytherapy results in progression-free and overall survival in 65–70%, depending on stage (52).

Locally advanced/metastatic cervix cancer

Patients with locally advanced or metastatic disease are assessed for suitable palliative treatment, which may include combinations of chemotherapy, radiation, or no active treatment until symptoms arise. Locally recurrent tumours may be suitable for retreatment with radiation to deal with pain and bleeding (53).

External beam radiotherapy

Treatment planning for external beam radiotherapy typically involves 3D imaging such as CT and MRI to define the extent of primary tumour and nodes (see earlier text). The clinical target volume includes the primary cervical tumour, upper vagina, parametria, and pelvic lymph nodes including the external and internal iliac and presacral lymph nodes. In patients with involved pelvic nodes, the clinical target volume may be expanded to include common iliac nodes, and those with common iliac involvement may require treatment of the next echelon para-aortic lymph nodes.

Treatment techniques typically consist of four coplanar pelvic radiation fields (anterior, posterior, and right and left lateral) (Figure 68.1). The use of high-energy photons (6–18 MV) maximizes dose to tumour while sparing skin and superficial normal tissue. A pelvic dose of 45 Gy in 25 fractions of 1.8 Gy daily over 5 weeks is sufficient to treat microscopic nodal disease, and results in significant tumour regression starting in weeks 3–4 in most patients, thereby optimizing brachytherapy dosimetry. Alternately, a dose of 50.4 Gy in 28 daily fractions may be used for bulky primary or node-positive patients. If para-aortic nodes are involved, they receive 40–45 Gy in 20–25 fractions. An important component includes shields to reduce the bowel, bladder, and femoral head dose.

Postoperative radiotherapy

External beam chemoradiation therapy is recommended for high-risk features following modified radical hysterectomy and pelvic lymph node dissection including close or positive surgical resection margins, the presence of capillary lymphatic invasion, and positive pelvic lymph nodes. Randomized studies have shown improved outcomes, particularly with adenocarcinomas, with low rates of serious toxicity (54). External beam pelvic radiation therapy encompasses the upper vagina, parametria, central pelvic tissues, and lymph nodes, using a four-field arrangement or IMRT technique (see 'Basic principles of radiotherapy').

Brachytherapy

Intrauterine tandem applicator with vaginal colpostats or ring using high-dose rate afterloading brachytherapy is used during or following external radiotherapy. Increasingly, brachytherapy is being planned using MRI guidance to optimize the dose to the residual tumour while sparing normal tissue (referred to as organs at risk) such as the bladder and the rectum (Figure 68.3). Guidelines developed by the GEC-ESTRO group have standardized target volume and normal organ definition (41). Typical doses are 28–30 Gy in four to five fractions (36–40 Gy low-dose rate equivalent) of high-dose rate brachytherapy in the third to fifth week of external beam radiotherapy, depending on tumour response.

Follow-up care

This involves clinic visits for assessment including pelvic exam every 3–4 months for 2 years after completing treatment, then every 6 months to 5 years. Follow-up PET-CT or MRI pelvis is done at 3–6 months after completing treatment to confirm tumour eradication. Cervical/vaginal cytology is performed at the discretion of the oncologist beginning 1 year after completing radiotherapy in order to avoid false-positive results due to radiation effects.

Vaginal dilators are recommended for 6 months after the completion of brachytherapy to prevent vaginal stenosis. Some patients may require ongoing use of dilators. Hormone replacement therapy may be considered for patients who were premenopausal prior to treatment.

Uterine cancer

Role for radiotherapy by stage

Despite decades of study, the role of adjuvant therapy in the treatment of endometrial cancer has been difficult to define. Radiotherapy has been shown to reduce the risk of local recurrence but its effects on survival remains unclear. Several factors contribute to the uncertainty of the role of radiotherapy, including the overall failure rate which is only 15% in all newly diagnosed endometrial cancer confined to the uterus treated with surgery, resulting in a very small improvement in prognosis with the addition of any further therapy. Additional factors include biased retrospective studies and randomized studies that included many low-risk patients who would not benefit from any further therapy. Therefore, the decision to treat with adjuvant therapy, including radiotherapy, is based on the understanding of the risk factors of recurrence, natural history of disease, the interpretation of data, and the risk of complications in each individual case.

Stage I

Stage I disease includes all disease confined to the endometrium. This stage is further subcategorized based on risk factors including age, size of tumour, lymphovascular space invasion (LVSI), depth of invasion into the myometrium, grade, and histological subtypes. The low-risk category includes patients with grade 1 or 2 tumours and less than 50% myometrial invasion with no LVSI. These patients have a 90% cure rate with surgery alone and do not need further adjuvant therapy.

The intermediate-risk group includes patients with grade 1/ 2 tumours with greater than 50% myometrial invasion, grade 3 less than 50% myometrial invasion, or a combinations of factors including age, depth of invasion, grade 1/2, size, and LVSI. Three randomized studies (55–57) evaluated the role of adjuvant pelvic radiotherapy and found improvement in local control but no improvement in overall survival with the addition of radiotherapy in intermediate-risk patients. The patients who did not receive adjuvant radiotherapy recurred most commonly at the apex of the vagina. Therefore, the Postoperative Radiation Therapy in Endometrial Carcinoma (PORTEC)-2 trial randomized this intermediate-risk group of patients to pelvic radiotherapy versus vaginal cuff brachytherapy alone (58). No difference in local control or overall survival between the two arms was found but as expected there were more gastrointestinal and genitourinary toxicities in the arm that received pelvic radiotherapy, and the conclusion was that patients with intermediate-risk disease should be treated with vaginal brachytherapy alone.

The high-risk group includes grade 3, deeply invasive disease (>50% invasion) or grade 2, deeply invasive disease with other risk factors including LVSI and older age. This group of patients has a 14–42% risk of recurrence. The Gynecologic Oncology Group

(GOG)-99 study subgroup analysis of patients in this high-risk group had a 2-year incidence of recurrence of 27% and a slight but non-significant benefit in survival with the addition of pelvic radiotherapy (57). Creutzberg did a separate analysis of stage IB, grade 3 endometrial carcinomas and found that this high-risk group of patients had a 14% risk of recurrence and a 31% risk of distant metastases (59). This group is best treated with pelvic radiotherapy but as seen in the earlier discussion has a high risk of distant metastases and questions arise whether they would benefit from systemic chemotherapy as well.

Stage II

Patients with stage II disease have invasion into the cervical stroma, typically found pathologically following simple hysterectomy. Most of these patients are treated with adjuvant pelvic radiotherapy including vaginal brachytherapy. However, if the cervical invasion is known upfront and is clinically evident by physical exam, these patients can be treated with either radical hysterectomy followed by either pelvic radiotherapy or vaginal brachytherapy depending on pathological risk factors, or preoperative pelvic radiotherapy and brachytherapy followed by a simple hysterectomy in 4–6 weeks.

Stage III

Stage III is a very broad and heterogeneous category with respect to disease spread, patterns of failure, and treatment outcomes. Stage IIIA involves spread to adnexa, and stage IIIC to regional nodes, typically requiring adjuvant therapy (see Table 63.3 in Chapter 63). Stage IIIB involves spread to vagina or parametria, which is sometimes inoperable (see 'Radiation therapy alone for medically or surgically inoperable disease'). Five-year recurrence-free survival for patients in stage III therefore ranges from 25% to 90%, depending on pathological findings.

Controversy and questions remain on the best adjuvant treatment for patients with this stage of disease. Several retrospective studies have shown that adjuvant radiotherapy for node-positive disease results in excellent local control and survival and pelvic recurrences range from 19% to 50% in patients who are receiving chemotherapy for node-positive disease (60, 61).

An older GOG randomized study compared whole abdominal radiation therapy to chemotherapy in stage III and IV endometrial carcinoma and found that patients who received chemotherapy had a significant improvement in disease-free survival compared to patients who received whole abdominal radiation therapy (62). There was more toxicity in the chemotherapy arm, and despite receiving chemotherapy patients had a 40–50% recurrence rate with stage III disease. A more recent Italian study randomized patients with high-risk factors, including patients with stage III disease, to chemotherapy or tailored radiation therapy (63). There was similar overall survival in the two arms but radiotherapy delayed local relapses and chemotherapy delayed metastases. Overall, the authors felt that the combination of chemotherapy and radiation may be a better treatment. Hogberg et al. published results of two randomized studies in high-risk endometrial carcinoma including stage III patients and compared radiotherapy alone to radiotherapy plus chemotherapy and found that patients who received the combination treatment had better progression-free survival than patients who received radiotherapy alone (63).

Two ongoing randomized trials of concurrent and adjuvant chemotherapy and radiotherapy (PORTEC-3 and GOG-258) will help define the treatment for patients with stage III disease; however, currently stage IIIC disease should include radiotherapy plus chemotherapy for improvement of local control and distant metastases (65).

Radiation therapy alone for medically or surgically inoperable disease

Even though surgery is the primary treatment for early-stage disease, patients who are at a high risk for complications after surgery can be treated with radiotherapy alone. Disease-specific survival rates of 75–85% and local recurrence rates of 10–20% have been reported for patients with clinical stage I or II endometrial carcinoma treated with radiotherapy alone. Prognosis is correlated with clinical stage and histological grade (66). Brachytherapy alone yields excellent local control in most patients with grade 1 tumours. Patients with large uterine cavities, cervical involvement, or grade 2 or 3 tumours should be considered for a course of external beam radiation before brachytherapy to treat regional nodes at risk.

Recurrent disease

The most common site of recurrence as mentioned earlier is the vaginal cuff—the region of the hysterectomy scar in the apical vagina. Recurrences also may occur suburethrally in the distal vagina but are less common than the apical vagina. Patients with isolated vaginal recurrences after hysterectomy have a 5-year local control rate of 40–80% and 5-year survival rates of 30–80% when treated with curative radiation therapy, consisting of a combination of external beam radiation therapy and brachytherapy (67, 68).

Radiotherapy volumes

Pelvic radiotherapy may be delivered using a four-field technique or using IMRT to a dose of 45–50.4 Gy. The areas that are targeted are the pelvic nodes including external iliac, internal iliac, obturator, and common iliac nodes as well as the vaginal cuff and the parametrial region. The advantage of IMRT is that it may reduce long-term toxicity of pelvic radiotherapy, especially gastrointestinal toxicity. A recent randomized study (RTOG 1203 TIME-C trial) confirmed that IMRT is superior to 3D conformal therapy. If there are positive nodes, especially para-aortic nodes, then fields may extend to include the para-aortic region up to T-12 or at least above the renal vessels. When extended fields are treated, the majority of physicians will use IMRT to reduce the dose to the kidneys, spinal cord, and small bowel. Controversy remains on whether adding vaginal brachytherapy to pelvic radiotherapy has any benefit, but presently for patients with stage II disease, vaginal brachytherapy is added to pelvic radiotherapy.

Vaginal brachytherapy usually targets the upper one-third to one-half of the vagina. The dose is delivered using high-dose rate brachytherapy and is given completely on an outpatient basis. Doses range from 7 Gy to 5 mm depth for three fractions to 6 Gy to the vaginal surface for five fractions when give as a solo treatment. There really is no circumstance where the whole length of the vagina should be treated.

Rare tumours

Vaginal cancer

Role for radiotherapy by stage

Vaginal cancer represents only 3% of gynaecological cancers, and given its rarity management is based largely on single-institution experience and consensus guidelines (69).

Early stage

Stage 1 cancer limited to the vagina can often be managed by resection or partial vaginectomy with postoperative radiation or chemoradiotherapy for high-risk features such as positive margins or nodes. However, in stage 2 disease involving the paravaginal tissues or bulkier stage 1 tumours where resection may result in significant vaginal morbidity, the option for primary radiotherapy should be considered. Single-institution series have demonstrated 40–90% 5-year disease-specific survivals with radiotherapy (70, 71).

Advanced stage

Surgical treatment of advanced or node-positive vaginal cancer is limited by the extent of surgery required (total vaginectomy or exenteration) or the need for chemoradiation if nodes are positive. Chemoradiation using weekly cisplatin is increasingly considered the standard of care for both locally advanced and early disease, based in large part on the experience in cervix cancer. Limited data with chemoradiation in vaginal cancer supports this approach (72). For these reasons, chemoradiation is preferred as an organ-sparing approach.

Radiation doses and volumes are similar to those used for cervix cancer (see earlier sections), with the exception that lower-third vaginal tumours often require treatment of the inguinal nodes (similar to vulval cancer (see later sections)).

Adjuvant therapy

Adjuvant radiation/chemoradiotherapy is associated with 5-year survival rates of 69–100% in stage I/II disease (73). Neoadjuvant chemotherapy has been used prior to surgery in stage II with complete response rates of 27% (74), although similar approaches in cervical cancer are under investigation (75).

Brachytherapy

As with cervix cancer, brachytherapy plays a critical role in the management of vaginal cancers. Vaginal brachytherapy alone may be used in superficial stage I tumours with excellent results (70, 71). In stage II, the combination of external beam and brachytherapy appears to result in better outcomes (76).

Vulval cancer

Role for radiotherapy by stage

Early stage

Early-stage vulval cancer includes FIGO stages I and II (node-negative tumours limited to the vulva with limited extension to adjacent perineal structures). The mainstay treatment for early-stage vulval cancer is surgical resection, with adjuvant radiation utilized for those patients with high-risk pathological features. Definitive radiotherapy for early-stage disease is limited to those patients who are not surgical candidates.

Advanced stage

Advanced-stage vulval cancer includes node-positive disease and/or extensive invasion into adjacent perineal structures (FIGO stages III and IV). For those without distant metastases, radiotherapy can be delivered either as an adjuvant treatment following surgical resection or as a definitive modality. To achieve optimal results, definitive radiotherapy is often combined with chemotherapy (see 'Definitive radiotherapy'). Radiotherapy among patients with distant metastatic disease is reserved for palliative purposes only, either to the primary or distant sites of disease.

Adjuvant versus definitive radiotherapy

Adjuvant radiotherapy

Surgical pathology of the primary site dictates the indication for adjuvant radiotherapy in the node-negative patient. Heaps et al. analysed surgical pathological variables associated with local recurrence following radical vulvectomy, revealing patients with margins less than 8 mm were at a significantly increased risk of local recurrence (77). Subsequently, Faul et al. showed that patients with close (<8 mm) or positive margins receiving adjuvant radiotherapy experienced a significant decrease in local failure, 58% versus 16% (78). Adjuvant radiotherapy may also be considered in patients with widely clear margins if a combination of the following is present: depth of invasion greater than 9 mm, tumour thickness greater than 1 cm, lymphovascular invasion, or greater than ten mitosis per high-power field.

Adjuvant radiotherapy has been shown to benefit those with multiple positive inguinal lymph nodes. GOG-37 evaluated the role of postoperative nodal irradiation in women with node-positive vulval cancer. The 6-year cause-specific survival was 71% versus 49% favouring the radiotherapy group, with an overall survival advantage being limited to patients with N2–N3 disease or with two or more positive groin nodes (79).

Definitive radiotherapy

In locally advanced vulval carcinomas, radiation has been utilized as a definitive modality, particularly when combined with chemotherapy. Support of this approach comes from two neoadjuvant trials showing a large proportion achieving complete clinical and/or pathological response. The first GOG neoadjuvant trial evaluated split course radiochemotherapy to 47.6 Gy in patients with locally advanced T3 or T4 disease requiring an extensive resection. Following chemoradiotherapy, 46.5% had a clinical complete response and only 2.8% of patients had residual unresectable disease (80). The second GOG neoadjuvant trial used 57.6 Gy with weekly cisplatin, and 64% of patients had a complete clinical response, and 49% had a complete pathological response to combined modality treatment (81).

Radiotherapy volumes

Treatment volumes in vulval cancer are individualized based on the clinical circumstance. The primary site, whether treated definitively or in the adjuvant setting, should include an extended margin encompassing adjacent perineal skin. When nodal radiotherapy is

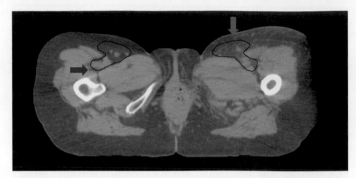

Figure 68.4 CT-based inguinal lymph node volumes. The posterior border should not extend beyond the deep margin of inguinal vessels (red arrow). The anterior border should allow for significant skin sparing, unless gross disease or skin involvement is present (blue arrow).

indicated, treatment volumes include the lower pelvic nodes and bilateral inguinal nodes. The superior extent of coverage should include one nodal echelon cephalad to the level of clinical involvement. The caudal extent of coverage extends to cover the inguinal lymph nodes down to the saphenous vein, or lesser trochanter (82). CT-guided planning is used to assess the coverage of the lower pelvic and inguinal lymph nodes (**Figure 68.4**). Daily fractions are generally 1.8 Gy to a dose of 45–54 Gy in the absence of gross disease. Positive margins should be treated to 54–64 Gy, and gross disease should generally be treated to 60–66 Gy. Extracapsular extension or clinically positive lymph nodes should be boosted to 50–66 Gy depending on the volume of disease. Critical normal tissues include the femoral heads/necks, small bowel, rectum, bladder, and anus. In 3D radiotherapy, a common technique is to use a large anterior photon field in conjunction with a small posterior photon field to exclude the femurs. IMRT has been used in the treatment of vulval cancer to limit normal tissue toxicities with good outcomes (23).

Ovarian cancer

Although not a rare tumour per se, ovarian cancer is now rarely treated with radiation, apart from palliative treatment to deal with recurrent inoperable symptomatic pelvic masses causing pain and bleeding.

However, there may be a role for radiotherapy in patients with rarer subtypes of ovarian cancer (clear cell and endometrioid), who tend to present with pelvic-confined disease and have lower response rates to chemotherapy. Retrospective studies show that the addition of radiotherapy to adjuvant chemotherapy (carboplatin–paclitaxel) leads to improvements in disease-free survival for patients with stage IC (cytological positivity/unknown or surface involvement) and stage II disease (83–85). The radiotherapy techniques used at that time consisted of whole abdominal-pelvic radiotherapy; however, abdominal relapses were uncommon so pelvic radiotherapy is currently used. Future clinical trials may clarify the roles of chemotherapy and radiation in these histologies (86).

REFERENCES

1. Rontgen WG. Ueber eine neue Art von Strahlen. Sitzungsberichte der physikalisch-medicinischen Gesellschaft zu Wurzberg, 1895. *Sitzung* 1895;**30**:132–31.

2. Grubbe EH. Priority in the therapeutic use of X-rays. *Radiology* 1933;**21**:156–62.

3. Allen CW. *Radiotherapy, Photography and Radium High Frequency Currents*. London: Kimpton; 1905.

4. Lederman M. The early history of radiotherapy: 1895–1939. *IJROBP* 1981;**7**:639–48.

5. Robison RF. The race for megavoltage. *Acta Oncol* 1995;**34**:1055–74.

6. Leksell L. Stereotactic radiosurgery. *J Neurol Neurosurg Psychiatry* 1983;**46**:797–803.

7. Farmer F, Fowler J, Haggith JW. Megavoltage treatment planning and the use of zeroradiography. *Br J Radiol* 1963;**36**:426–35.

8. Haie-Meder C, Mazeron R, Magne N. Clinical evidence on PET-CT for radiation therapy planning in cervix and endometrial cancer. *Radiother Oncol* 2010;**96**:351–55.

9. Xu-Welliver M, Yuh W, Fielding J, et al. Imaging across the life span: innovations in imaging and therapy for gynecologic cancer. *Radiographics* 2014;**34**:1062–81.

10. Small W, Mell L, Anderson P, et al. Consensus guidelines for delineation of clinical target volume for intensity-modulated pelvic radiotherapy in postoperative treatment of endometrial and cervical cancer. *Radiother Oncol* 2008;**71**:428–34.

11. Lim K, Small W, Portelance L, et al. Consensus guidelines for delineation of clinical target volume for intensity-modulated pelvic radiotherapy for the definitive treatment of cervix cancer. *Radiother Oncol* 2011;**79**:348–55.

12. Lim K, Erikson B, Jurgenliemk-Schultz I, et al. Variability in clinical target volume delineation for intensity modulated radiation therapy in 3 challenging cervix cancer scenarios. *Pract Radiat Oncol* 2015;**5**:e557–65.

13. Gay H, Barthold H, O'Meara E, et al. Pelvic normal tissue contouring guidelines for radiation therapy: a Radiation Therapy Oncology Group Consensus Panel Atlas. *Radiother Oncol* 2012;**83**:e353–62.

14. Peacock CM. A system for planning and rotational delivery of intensity-modulated fields. *Int J Imag Sys Tech* 1995;**6**:56–65.

15. Webb S. Optimisation of conformal radiotherapy dose distribution by simulated annealing. *Phys Med Biol* 1989:**34**:1349.

16. Brahme A. Design principles and clinical possibilities with a new generation of radiation therapy equipment: a review. *Acta Oncol* 1987;**26**:403–12.

17. Bortfeld T, Kahler D, Waldron T, Boyer A. X-ray field compensation with multileaf collimators. *Radiother Oncol* 1994;**28**:723–30.

18. Roeske J, Lujan A, Rotmensch J, Waggoner S, Yamada D, Mundt A. Intensity-modulated whole pelvic radiation therapy in patients with gynecologic malignancies. *Radiother Oncol* 2000;**48**:1613–21.

19. Mundt A, Lujan A, Rotmensch J, et al. Intensity-modulated whole pelvic radiotherapy in women with gynecologic malignancies. *Radiother Oncol* 2002;**52**:1330–37.

20. Mundt A, Mell L, Roeske J. Preliminary analysis of chronic gastrointestinal toxicity in gynecology patients treated with intensity-modulated whole pelvic radiation therapy. *Radiother Oncol* 2003;**56**:1354–60.

21. Jhingran A, Winter K, Portelance L, et al. A phase II study of intensity modulated radiation therapy to the pelvis for postoperative patients with endometrial carcinoma: Radiation Therapy Oncology Group Trial 0418. *Radiother Oncol* 2012;**84**:e23–28.

22. Klopp A, Moughan J, Portelance L, et al. Hematologic toxicity in RTOG 0418: a phase 2 study of postoperative IMRT for gynecologic cancer. *Radiother Oncol* 2013;**86**:83–90.

23. Beriwal S, Heron D, Kim H, et al. Intensity-modulated radiotherapy for the treatment of vulvar carcinoma: a comparative dosimetric study with early clinical outcome. *Radiother Oncol* 2006;**64**:1395–400.

24. Jaffray D, Drake D. A radiographic and tomographic imaging system integrated into a medical linear accelerator for localization of bone and soft-tissue targets. *Radiother Oncol* 1999;**45**:773–89.

25. Taylor A, Powell M. An assessment of interfractional uterine and cervical motion: implications for radiotherapy target volume definition in gynaecological cancer. *Radiother Oncol* 2008;**88**:250–57.

26. Langerak T, Mens J, Quint S, et al. Cervix motion in 50 cervical cancer patients assessed by daily cone beam computed tomographic imaging of a new type of marker. *Radiother Oncol* 2015;**93**:532–39.

27. Van de Bunt L, van der Heide U, Ketelaars M, de Kort G, Jurgenliemk-Schulz I. Conventional, conformal, and intensity-modulated radiation therapy treatment planning of external beam radiotherapy for cervical cancer: the impact of tumor regression. *Radiother Oncol* 2006;**64**:189–96.

28. Chan P, Dinniwell R, Haider M, et al. Inter- and intrafractional tumor and organ movement in patients with cervical cancer undergoing radiotherapy: a cinematic-mri point-of-interest study. *Radiother Oncol* 2008;**70**:1507–15.

29. Beadle B, Jhingran A, Salehpour M, Sam M, Iyer R, Eifel P. Cervix regression and motion during the course of external beam chemoradiation for cervical cancer. *Radiother Oncol* 2009;**73**:235–41.

30. Kerkhof E, Raaymakers B, van der Heide U, van de Bunt L, Jurgenliemk-Schultz I, Lagendijk J. Online MRI guidance for healthy tissue sparing in patients with cervical cancer: an IMRT planning study. *Radiother Oncol* 2008;**88**:241–49.

31. Oh S, Stewart J, Moseley J, et al. Hybrid adaptive radiotherapy with on-line MRI in cervix cancer IMRT. *Radiother Oncol* 2014;**110**:323–28.

32. Stewart J, Lim K, Kelly V, et al. Automated weekly replanning for intensity-modulated radiotherapy of cervix cancer. *Radiother Oncol* 2010;**78**:350–58.

33. Lim K, Stewart J, Kelly V, et al. Dosimetrically triggered adaptive intensity modulated radiation therapy for cervical cancer. *Int J Radiat Oncol Biol Phys* 2014;**90**:147–54.

34. Song W, Huh S, Liang Y, et al. Dosimetric comparison study between intensity modulated radiation therapy and three-dimensional conformal proton therapy for pelvic bone marrow sparing in the treatment of cervical cancer. *J Applied Clin Med Phys* 2010;**11**:83–92.

35. Milby A, Both S, Ingram M, Lin L. Dosimetric comparison of combined intensity-modulated radiotherapy (IMRT) and proton therapy versus IMRT alone for pelvic and para-aortic radiotherapy in gynecologic malignancies. *Int J Radiat Oncol Biol Phys* 2012;**82**:e477–84.

16. Fyles A, Milosevic M, Hedley D, et al. Tumor hypoxia has independent predictor impact only in patients with node-negative cervix cancer. *J Clin Oncol* 2002;**20**:680–87.

37. Fyles A, Milosevic M, Wong R, et al. Oxygenation predicts radiation response and survival in patients with cervix cancer. *Radiother Oncol* 1998;**48**:149–56.

38. Nakano T, Suzuki Y, Ohno T, et al. Carbon beam therapy overcomes the radiation resistance of uterine cervical cancer originating from hypoxia. *Clin Can Res* 2006;**12**:2185.

39. Janeway HH, Baringer BS, Failla G. *Radium Therapy in Cancer at the Memorial Hospital*. New York: Paul Hoeber Publishers; 1917.

40. Fokdal L, et al. Image guided adaptive brachytherapy with combined intracavitary and interstitial technique improves the therapeutic ratio in locally advanced cervical cancer: analysis from the retroEMBRACE study. *Radiother Oncol* 2016;**120**:434–40.

41. Haie-Meder C, Pötter R, Van Limbergen E, et al. Recommendations from Gynaecological (GYN) GEC-ESTRO Working Group (I): concepts and terms in 3D image based 3D treatment planning

in cervix cancer brachytherapy with emphasis on MRI assessment of GTV and CTV. *Radiother Oncol* 2005;**74**:235–45.

42. Almond P, Biggs P, Coursey B, et al. AAPM's TG-51 protocol for clinical reference dosimetry of high-energy photon and electron beams. *Med Phys* 1999;**26**:1847–70.

43. International Atomic Energy Agency (IAEA). *Absorbed Dose Determination in External Beam Radiotherapy*. Technical Report Series No. 398. Vienna: IAEA; 2000.

44. Valentin J (ed). The 2007 Recommendations of the International Commission on Radiological Protection. ICRP Publication 103. *Ann ICRP* 2007;**37**:1–332.

45. Chemoradiotherapy for Cervical Cancer Meta-analysis Collaboration (CCCMAC). Reducing uncertainties about the effects of chemoradiotherapy for cervical cancer: individual patient data meta-analysis. *Cochrane Database Syst Rev* 2010;**1**:CD008285.

46. Han K, Milosevic M, Fyles A, Pintilie M, Viswanathan AN. Trends in the utilization of brachytherapy in cervical cancer in the United States. *Radiother Oncol* 2013;**87**:111–19.

47. Mirghani H, Amen F, Tao Y, Deutsch E, Levy A. Increased radiosensitivity of HPV-positive head and neck cancers: molecular basis and therapeutic perspectives. *Cancer Treat Rev* 2015;**41**:844–52.

48. Petrelli F, Sarti E, Barni S. Predictive value of human papillomavirus in oropharyngeal carcinoma treated with radiotherapy: an updated systematic review and meta-analysis of 30 trials. *Head Neck* 2014;**36**:750–59.

49. Small W Jr, Strauss JB, Jhingran A, et al. ACR Appropriateness Criteria® definitive therapy for early-stage cervical cancer. *Am J Clin Oncol* 2012;**35**:399–405.

50. Kokka F, Bryant A, Brockbank E, Powell M, Oram D. Hysterectomy with radiotherapy or chemotherapy or both for women with locally advanced cervical cancer. *Cochrane Database Syst Rev* 2015;**4**:CD010260.

51. Gaffney DK, Erickson-Wittmann BA, Jhingran A, et al. ACR Appropriateness Criteria® on Advanced Cervical Cancer Expert Panel on Radiation Oncology-Gynecology. *Radiother Oncol* 2011;**81**:609–14.

52. DiSilvestro PA, Ali S, Craighead PS, et al. Phase III randomized trial of weekly cisplatin and irradiation versus cisplatin and tirapazamine and irradiation in stages IB2, IIA, IIB, IIIB, and IVA cervical carcinoma limited to the pelvis: a Gynecologic Oncology Group study. *J Clin Oncol* 2014;**32**:458–64.

53. Croke J, Leung E, Fyles A. Gynecological malignancies. In: Nieder C, Langendijk J (eds), *Re-Irradiation: New Frontiers*, pp. 267–280. Heidelberg: Springer; 2011.

54. Rogers L, Siu SS, Luesley D, Bryant A, Dickinson HO. Radiotherapy and chemoradiation after surgery for early cervical cancer *Cochrane Database Syst Rev* 2012;**5**:CD007583.

55. Aalders J, Abeler V, Kostad P, et al. Postoperative external irradiation and prognositc parameters in stage I endometrial carcinoma. *Obstet Gynecol* 1980;**56**:419–27.

56. Creutzberg CL, Van Putten WL, Koper PC, et al. Surgery and post-operative radiotherapy versus surgery alone for patients with stage-1 endometrial carcinoma: multicentre randomized trial. PORTEC study group. *Lancet* 2000;**355**:1404–11.

57. Keys, HM, Roberts JA, Brunetto VL, et al. A phase III trial of surgery with or without adjunctive external pelvic radiation therapy in intermediate risk endometrial adenocarcinoma: a Gynecologic Oncology Group study. *Gynecol Oncol* 2004;**92**:744–51.

58. Nout RA, Smit VT, Putter H, et al. Vaginal brachytherapy versus pelvic external beam radiotherapy for patients with endometrial cancer of high-intermediate risk (PORTEC-2): an open-label, non-inferiority, randomised trial. *Lancet* 2010;**375**:816–23.

59. Creutzberg CL, Wim LJ, Van Putten CC, et al. Outcome of high-risk stage IC, grade 3, compared with stage I endometrial carcinoma patients: the Postoperative Radiation Therapy in Endometrial Carcinoma trial. *J Clin Oncol* 2004:**22**:1234–41.

60. Randall ME, Filiaci VL, Muss H, et al. Randomized phase III trial of whole -abdominal irradiation versus doxorubicin and cisplatin chemotherapy in advanced endometrial carcinoma: a Gynecologic Oncology Group study. *J Clin Oncol* 2006;**24**:36–44.

61. Klopp AH, Jhingran A, Ramondetta L, et al. Node-positive adenocarcinoma of the endometrium: outcome and patterns of recurrence with and without external beam irradiation. *Gynecol Oncol* 2009;**115**:6–11.

62. Mundt AJ, McBride R, Rotmensch J, et al. Significant pelvic recurrence in high-risk pathologic stage I-IV endometrial carcinoma patients after adjuvant chemotherapy alone: implications for adjuvant radiation therapy. *Radiother Oncol* 2001;**50**:1145–53.

63. Maggi R, Lissoni A, Spina F, et al. Adjuvant chemotherapy vs radiotherapy in high-risk endometrial carcinoma: results of a randomized trial. *Br J Cancer* 2006;**95**:266–71.

64. Hogberg T, Signorelli M, de Oliveira CF, et al. Sequential adjuvant chemotherapy and radiotherapy in endometrial cancer-results from two randomized studies. *Eur J Cancer* 2010;**46**: 2422–31.

65. Klopp A, Smith BD, Alektiar K, et al. The role of post-operative radiation therapy for endometrial cancer: executive summary of an American Society for Radiation Oncology evidence based guideline. *Pract Radiat Oncol* 2014:**4**:137–44.

66. Rouanet P, Dubois JB, Gely S, et al. Exclusive radiation therapy in endometrial carcinoma. *Radiother Oncol* 1993;**26**:223–28.

67. Lin, LL, Grigsby PW, Powell MA, Mutch DG. Definitive radiotherapy in the management of isolated vaginal recurrences of endometrial cancer. *Radiother Oncol* 2005;**63**:500–504.

68. Jhingran A, Burke TW, Eifel PJ. Definitive radiotherapy for patients with isolated vaginal recurrence of endometrial carcinoma after hysterectomy. *Radiother Oncol* 2003;**56**:1366–72.

69. Lee LJ, Jhingran A, Kidd E, et al. ACR appropriateness Criteria management of vaginal cancer. *Oncology (Williston Park)* 2013;**27**:1166–73.

70. Frank SJ, Jhingran A, Levenback C, Eifel PJ. Definitive radiation therapy for squamous cell carcinoma of the vagina. *Radiother Oncol* 2005;**62**:138–47.

71. Kirkbride P, Fyles A, Rawlings GA, et al. Carcinoma of the vagina—experience at the Princess Margaret Hospital (1974–1989). *Gynecol Oncol* 1995;**56**:435–43.

72. Samant R, Lau B, Choan E, Le T, Tam T. Primary vaginal cancer treated with concurrent chemoradiation using cis-platinum. *Radiother Oncol* 2007;**69**:746–50.

73. Otton GR, Nicklin JL, Dickie GJ, et al. Early-stage vaginal carcinoma—an analysis of 70 patients. *Int J Gynecol Cancer* 2004;**14**:304–10.

74. Benedetti Panici P, Bellati F, Plotti F, et al. Neoadjuvant chemotherapy followed by radical surgery in patients affected by vaginal carcinoma. *Gynecol Oncol* 2008;**111**:307–11.

75. Rydzewska L, Tierney J, Vale CL, Symonds PR. Neoadjuvant chemotherapy plus surgery versus surgery for cervical cancer. *Cochrane Database Syst Rev* 2012;**12**:CD007406.

76. Perez CA, Grigsby PW, Garipagaoglu M, Mutch DG, Lockett MA. Factors affecting long-term outcome of irradiation in carcinoma of the vagina. *Radiother Oncol* 1999;**44**:37–45.

77. Heaps JM, Fu YS, Montz FJ, Hacker NF, Berek JS. Surgical-pathologic variables predictive of local recurrence in squamous cell carcinoma of the vulva. *Gynecol Oncol* 1990;**38**:309–14.

78. Faul CM, Mirmow D, Huang Q, Gerszten K, Day R, Jones MW. Adjuvant radiation for vulvar carcinoma: improved local control. *Int J Radiat Oncol Biol Phys* 1997;**38**:381–89.

79. Kunos C, Simpkins F, Gibbons H, Tian C, Homesley H. Radiation therapy compared with pelvic node resection for node-positive vulvar cancer: a randomized controlled trial. *Obstet Gynecol* 2009;**114**:537–46.

80. Moore DH, Thomas GM, Montana GS, Saxer A, Gallup DG, Olt G. Preoperative chemoradiation for advanced vulvar cancer: a phase II study of the Gynecologic Oncology Group. *Int J Radiat Oncol Biol Phys* 1998;**42**:79–85.

81. Moore DH, Ali S, Koh WJ, et al. A phase II trial of radiation therapy and weekly cisplatin chemotherapy for the treatment of locally-advanced squamous cell carcinoma of the vulva: a gynecologic oncology group study. *Gynecol Oncol* 2012;**124**:529–33.

82. Gaffney DK, King B, Viswanathan AN, et al. Consensus recommendations for radiotherapy contouring and treatment of vulvar carcinoma. *Int J Radiat Oncol Biol Phys* 2016;**95**:1191–200.

83. Hoskins PJ, Le N, Gilks B, et al. Low-stage ovarian clear cell carcinoma: population-based outcomes in British Columbia, Canada, with evidence for a survival benefit as a result of irradiation. *J Clin Oncol* 2012;**30**:1656–62.

84. Kumar A, Le N, Tinker AV, Santos JL, Parsons C, Hoskins PJ. Early-stage endometrioid ovarian carcinoma: population-based outcomes in British Columbia. *Int J Gynecol Cancer* 2014;**24**:1401–405.

85. Swenerton KD, Santos JL, Gilks CB, et al. Histotype predicts the curative potential of radiotherapy: the example of ovarian cancers. *Ann Oncol* 2011;**22**:341–47.

86. Thomas G. Revisiting the role of radiation treatment for non-serous subtypes of epithelial ovarian cancer. Presented at the American Society of Clinical Oncology. Meeting, 1 June 2013. Available at: https://meetinglibrary.asco.org/record/79711/edbook.

Palliative care

Joanna M. Cain and Shelley M. Kibel

Overview of palliative care

What is palliative care?

Palliative care is an integrated approach that focuses on quality of life of patients and their families facing the problems associated with life threatening illness, through the prevention and relief of suffering by means of early identification and treatment of pain and other problems, physical, psychosocial, and spiritual' (1). This embraces the concept that quality care is embedded not only in individual health, but also the environment and setting of care and touches the domains included in the previous World Health Organization (WHO) definition. Palliative care focuses caregivers on the important goals of medicine—alleviating pain and suffering (at all levels), improving the experience of daily living, supporting psychological transitions with changing physical abilities, and advancing the patient's and family's understanding of the nature of the disease facing an individual and the outcomes (2). With that in mind, it represents a basic tenet of care for all patients, particularly those with diseases that lead to significant loss of quality of life and function. While this chapter focuses more on oncological palliative care, the tenets of palliative care and the research about symptom management can extend to the care of women with chronic conditions such as chronic pelvic pain, severe endometriosis, interstitial cystitis, untreatable pelvic prolapse, and other conditions. Palliative care, then, can be a focus for fatal and non-fatal diseases, and can and should be provided to address diminished quality-of-life issues as a part of ongoing treatment of a disease process, not just at the end of life.

The therapeutic relationship

At the basis of the therapeutic relationship are trust and a reliable presence. It is essential that patients are able to trust that their physicians, nurses, and team will continue to care for their needs or advocate for what they need and not reject them as a patient even if there is no longer the possibility of a cure: this is in and of itself therapeutic. Communication with patients and families and coordination of care are other cornerstones of the therapeutic relationship that underpins palliative care. Listening to patient's wishes, concerns, and making sure they are heard as a unique individual facing unique problems that we—their caregivers—are united in addressing, is the basis of setting therapeutic goals. Care for the dying or those

dealing with chronic issues challenges healthcare givers to review their attitudes, communication styles, and beliefs. It also challenges healthcare givers to identify the areas where they may not have the most expertise and engage the interprofessional teams and experts who are needed to provide palliative care for their patients, even if it means they are no longer the primary health provider.

In general, healthcare givers, particularly physicians, have not had the training to provide optimal palliative care although the evidence for efficacy and cost-effectiveness is well established (3, 4). Given the general lack of adequate numbers of palliative care specialists even in well-resourced settings, there is an obligation owed to patients for healthcare workers to be knowledgeable and informed in order to assure high-quality care of patients in need of palliative care.

Interdisciplinary care

Effective palliative care requires a team—usually a doctor, nurse, social worker, and others as needed, including dieticians, occupational therapists, physical therapists, and therapeutic massage. Use of the creative arts and music, spiritual support, psychologists, pain specialists, and disease experts should all be added to the mix of carers. Different communities use different healthcare providers, such as traditional healers, herbalists, acupuncture, and Ayurvedic medicine (among many others), and relationships with these diverse groups of healers should be pursued and respected. Not all settings will have all the elements that are needed, but the broader the perspectives and support that can be brought to bear, the better the ultimate palliation of symptoms and support for quality of life. Incorporating psychologists and spiritual care in particular helps address the family's as well as the patient's needs and the needs of the team itself to find meaning in the process of transcending suffering through palliative care including the process of dying.

Pain control

Trade-offs

Pain is the most frequent symptom for cancer patients and distressing to all, including caregivers. Caregivers often make assumptions about what the goal of pain control is for a patient, without engaging the patient in that discussion. Patients may give different weights to the trade-offs that come with options for pain control. Some may be willing to tolerate a little more pain in order to be more active with family, or may be intolerant of a loss of sensation or loss of bladder or bowel function that might come with complete resolution of pain with blocks or other forms of pain management. The patient's goal for pain control needs to be discussed at multiple intervals as pain changes with the advance of disease or changing activity. Goals may change as patients achieve the time they needed or the psychological or spiritual resolution desired and no longer want the same clarity of mentation. So specific conversations that clarify the level of pain control desired, the level of alertness, and choices about which side effects are acceptable or not are the basis of developing a pain control plan for each individual patient.

Baseline pain management

We know that pain can be controlled in the majority (>90%) of patients (5). Pain control does not mean that all pain can be removed in most circumstances, but rather its intensity and the subsequent disruption of quality of life can be reduced to tolerable and acceptable levels. In addition, well-trained patients can self-manage their pain with good control (6). Every setting—home, hospital, and hospice—should have systems of care that involve patients and families in reassessing and adjusting pain management as conditions change (7).

Ongoing chronic pain management

The basis of a pain plan depends on assessment of the source and type of pain and targeting the therapy to this type. Assessment requires understanding type, acuity, inciting and diminishing factors, and physical, mental, and contextual status associated with the pain. The goal is to tailor the management to the type of pain with particular attention to whether the source is neuropathic, pressure/mechanical (ascites, fixed position), inflammatory, pressure related, or infiltrating nerve endings. This might lead to a combination approach with targeted radiation (for a bone metastasis), anxiolytics, anti-inflammatory, massage, or physical therapy as part of the pain management package. Each patient will need a different constellation of approaches.

The basis of pain management still rests with the WHO pain ladder, starting with non-narcotic therapies at the base and moving to narcotic medications if the pain is not adequately controlled. For cancer pain, and particularly end of life care, establishing a satisfactory around-the-clock base relief system with attention to known side effects from the onset (constipation, somnolence, nausea) is key to success. While controlled-release morphine is the most common base control narcotic used, oxycodone or oxymorphone have also been used with near equal efficacy and side effects (8). Short-acting oral morphine is the cheapest and most widely used opioid worldwide. If a base level of pain control is not achieved with significant progressive cancer pain, and there is availability of advanced localized therapy such as implantable drug delivery systems or nerve blocks for highly localized pain (9), these may address the pain without sedation, constipation, or even fatigue. However, the trade-off may be numbness or loss of function including mobility depending on the area required for the spinal block or implant. The use of epidural and peripheral nerve blocks at the end of life can enhance analgesia, reduce or deescalate the use of opiates, and still can allow for care at home or in a hospice (10). However, globally, these are either not available or cost prohibitive in many settings.

Broadening availability of oral, subcutaneous, transdermal, and sublingual narcotic options allows good-quality home-based analgesia. Intravenous or intramuscular injections are best avoided if home-based therapy is being implemented. Home-based therapy has other challenges including the need for a caregiver who can carry out pain assessment, how pain assessment is performed, compliance with the regimen, and issues of hesitance to report pain and lack of education (11). The availability of in-home hospice support, free standing hospice support, or respite care in whatever setting allows for refinement or escalation of therapy for pain management at times of change in symptoms, as well as education and support of family and caregivers. Community-based or hospital-based hospice settings themselves vary widely and standards for ongoing evaluation of the quality of care and improving care should be part of their structure (12).

Acute pain and rescue management

Breakthrough pain requires analysis of the cause before deciding on an approach. For example, breakthrough pain caused by anxiety will require different management from that caused by disease progression. An escalation in pain may also be due to hyperalgesia associated with the opioid itself which may require switching to another derivative or switching the base management drug (13). This is a rare issue but if the pain is beyond the pre-existing pain and is diffuse in a way that seems out of proportion with the underlying issue, it is worth considering.

Breakthrough pain is best dealt with by rapid-onset formulations of narcotics. However, in some patients with morphine tolerance, consideration of other narcotics for management of recalcitrant breakthrough pain may be needed, such as the use of fentanyl in an intravenous, transdermal, or subcutaneous formulation (14).

Escalation of pain with surgery

It is important to understand that management of pain around surgery has a different quality with patients already on significant doses of narcotics to accomplish baseline control of pain. Use of blocks or indwelling epidurals for the local area of surgery or addition of other narcotics to maintain pain control, often in the same pattern as breakthrough pain management, may be needed. However, if the surgery results in reduction of the source of the original pain (e.g. reducing ascites or reducing bowel or ureteral obstruction) then adjustment of pain control postoperatively may require reductions in the baseline doses. If this is the case, the potential for symptoms of withdrawal must be considered and factored in as well.

Musculoskeletal pain management

Bone metastases have specific potential therapies for pain management that should be considered when this is the primary source of pain. Local radiation therapy has long been recognized as effective in palliation of bone pain, with up to 80% receiving relief and up to 50% complete relief from this pain (15). Even a single 8 Gy dose has been shown to provide pain relief equal to longer courses of palliative care, although retreatment is more likely (16). Additionally, bisphosphonates may have a role for pain relief if radiation therapy is not adequate or available and pain medicine is not adequate for therapy, although the impact is not as great as radiation therapy (17).

Issues from lack of movement/being bed-bound

Musculoskeletal sources of pain can often be more effectively treated by consideration of issues related to lack of movement and positioning. Passive bed physical therapy and massage may often restore circulation and relieve pressure on joints and muscles and provide significant symptom improvement. Additionally, the use of cold or warm compresses can lead to muscle relaxation with concurrent improvement of symptoms.

Management of gastrointestinal symptoms

Loss of appetite

Loss of appetite or anorexia is common during treatment for cancer and at the end of life. The treatment always depends on causative factors and the overall distress the symptom is causing the patient. During cancer treatment, effective antiemetic medication can prevent loss of appetite associated with mild nausea. However, the symptom of loss of appetite has other drivers such as opioid-related suppression of appetite, gastric dysfunction, constipation, and simply disease progression. Options to just treat the symptom are generally a progesterone or a glucocorticoid, both of which have limited efficacy (18).

The difficult issue for end of life palliative care is the social and cultural meaning attached to eating and feeding the sick that can make it difficult for patients and families to accept that lack of hydration or reduction in eating is normal in the course of the transition to death. Provision of hydration or other forms of intravenous nutrition does not change the outcome or the quality of life (19).

Discussions with the patient and family about hydration and nutrition form an important part of understanding the process of dying and should be part of the care offered. Sometimes judicious use of intravenous solutions with dextrose, or subcutaneous saline, can be helpful if the patient and family cannot overcome their beliefs and the distraction of their concern about failing to feed their loved one is keeping them from focusing on each other and the other tasks of transitioning to death.

Constipation

Constipation can be a major source of discomfort and nausea, and active management is warranted for prevention, as long as there is no underlying bowel obstruction. The most common source of constipation for women receiving palliative care is from other drug use, primarily opioid use for pain control. Disorders of electrolytes (magnesium, potassium, and calcium) also contribute and depending on general status might warrant treatment. Finally, lack of motility due to ascites and tumour studding of the bowel may also contribute.

Generally, stimulant therapy with senna or bisacodyl should be started concurrently with opioid use and additional agents added as needed to manage constipation. In the setting of palliative care where hydration is limited, the use of bulking agents such as psyllium or methylcellulose should be limited as they require hydration for efficacy. Non-absorbed laxatives such as lactulose can be added to find an ongoing balance. Enemas are also helpful, depending on the type of constipation and location. In some cases of severe and disabling opioid-related constipation, the use of an opioid receptor antagonist such as naloxone or newer peripheral mu opioid receptor antagonists (which are still under study) that will not counteract the benefits of pain control may be warranted (20, 21).

Nausea and vomiting

Nausea and vomiting are common end of life and palliative challenges in women with gynaecological cancers. There are mechanical, metabolic, as well as pharmacological aetiologies for this. With ovarian cancer, gastroparesis, large and small bowel involvement, as well as frank obstruction may cause significant nausea. With cervical cancer, nausea may be more derived from large bowel, anal, or sigmoid obstruction. If there is a clearly distinct area of obstruction and the patient is otherwise stable, a surgery with limited risk (e.g. loop colostomy) and limited recovery needs may offer palliative relief. Unfortunately, there are often multiple areas of involvement which make surgical options unacceptable. Colostomies or ileostomies should be considered as a preventative measure while the patient is well enough or to palliate conditions such as rectovaginal or vesicovaginal fistula where a diversionary procedure is likely to bring a significant relief of symptoms without too much morbidity. However, some patients may not find them acceptable under any circumstances. Other options if available may include gastric percutaneous drainage systems placed with endoscopic or surgical approaches or gastrointestinal stents in rare circumstances.

Nausea due to opioids is usually short lived and avoided by using antiemetics such as metoclopramide at the initiation of therapy. Pharmacological management for pain with opioids and other medications can add to the symptoms and as more pain medications or nausea medications are added, the resulting constipation further complicates the picture. Seeking a balance and an optimal plan for management of bowel function along with other symptoms is highly individual and needs frequent revision and tailoring to changes in patient status. Standard treatments exist for most sources of nausea and vomiting such as metoclopramide for gastroparesis, octreotide and glucocorticoids for bowel obstruction symptoms, relieving pressure symptoms with ascites with a port or repeated paracenteses (22), haloperidol for hepatic dysfunction and other metabolic disturbances, and cyclizine for brain metastases. Antiemetics used for nausea should work around the clock and, like a pain management strategy, have a strategy for breakthrough nausea and vomiting that allows for escalation of therapy.

Faecal incontinence and fistula management

The uncontrolled leakage of bowel contents occurs with faecal incontinence and enterocutaneous and enterovaginal fistulas in women with gynaecological malignancies. In the palliative care setting, where no further surgical intervention is appropriate, the introduction of suction-based or negative pressure wound management systems has allowed for better control of enterocutaneous fistulas and limited the skin exposure to the often highly caustic material. Lacking access to these approaches, ostomy management with ostomy bags and careful skin protection can limit skin breakdown and pain but can be difficult with high output small bowel enterocutaneous fistulas (23).

Enterovaginal fistulas are perhaps the hardest to treat as there is no firm surface on which to place a negative pressure or ostomy bag device and the area is too moist to allow for durable seals. Variations of devices based on a vaginal diaphragm model have been trialled over decades with generally poor management because of the pelvic distortion due to the cancer and/or treatment (surgery and radiation) as well as the other challenges. The best approach is an aggressive approach to skin management in the perineum with skin protective gels and creams applied after gentle cleansing and drying. Often topical lidocaine or other analgesic creams or burn creams (e.g. silver-based creams) can assist in relieving pain from these fistulae.

Faecal incontinence as a result of other treatments where the gastrointestinal system is intact can be treated with diet as well as loperamide and psyllium with nearly equal efficacy (24).

Management of urinary tract symptoms

Vesicovaginal or ureterovaginal fistulae

The classic management of these fistulae have included diversion to bowel conduits or complicated repairs, neither of which is appropriate in palliative care settings with gynaecological cancers. Options include the use of urethral catheters or percutaneous nephrostomies (25). Of these, the preferred management would be a urethral catheter if it is able to functionally manage output and eliminate most of the vaginal discharge.

Urinary retention

While both indwelling catheters and repeated catheterization may treat retention, practically the less management that is required in palliative end of life care the better. Hence, indwelling catheters are the most commonly used technique for relief of symptoms from retention. For individuals with cancer blocking the urethra (e.g. vulvovaginal cancers), consideration of a suprapubic catheter placement are warranted as a urethral catheter may be both difficult to place and also cause unwanted additional bleeding and local pain. It is important to note that while indwelling catheters are accompanied by colonization of the bladder, suppressive antibiotics are not indicated and even treatment for true infections should be based on symptoms.

Ureteral obstruction and renal failure

Acute and chronic ureteral obstruction leading to renal failure is common in late-stage gynaecological malignancies. While these can mechanically be relieved with ureteral stents or percutaneous nephrostomies, the benefit of relief and improvement of renal function needs to be considered in the context of their disease progress and overall comfort. Chronic renal failure and uraemia add symptoms that can increase the burden of symptoms to be palliated, for example, increased neuropathy, sensory changes and obtundation, increased musculoskeletal cramping and even seizures, fluid retention, and nausea with abnormal electrolytes. The benefit and risks of an intervention have to be weighed against the anticipated survival of individual patients. If it is a few weeks, there is little benefit from relief of the obstruction during that small window, and potential harm with enhanced pain sensation. Furthermore, dialysis is rarely warranted even for other acute causes of renal failure without obstruction. The only exception would be an acute, reversible event in a patient for whom a single episode of dialysis might treat the underlying renal injury and who would benefit symptomatically from that relief.

Urinary tract infections (acute, chronic)

Urinary tract infections (UTIs) can be secondary to many of the entities previously discussed—retention, obstruction, fistula, as well as prior history and other comorbidities. When to treat in the palliative care setting is an important question and revolves around comfort and goals of care. If the patient is having symptoms directly referable to a UTI, then a simple dipstick can confirm the source of the new pain symptoms and antibiotic therapy considered if it will improve pain and overall quality of life. If a woman has an asymptomatic UTI found in the course of other activities, it should not be treated—just as it should not be treated in older women with no other symptoms (26).

Pelvic bleeding and symptoms

Pelvic bleeding can be a major source of anxiety for the patient and her family. Fears of 'letting her bleed to death' or not knowing any way to manage a haemorrhage if it occurs can overwhelm patients and care givers. In fact, one option for pelvic bleeding in the setting of end of life palliative care is local management (pads) alone if it is low volume. Heavy or repeated bleeding can be limited with a short course of antihaemorrhagic medication, such as tranexamic acid. Other interventions for major haemorrhage depend on the goals of treatment and overall quality of life and survival if the haemorrhage is treated. These discussions can be very difficult as the very human fear of bleeding doesn't disappear simply with the horizon to death being close. Local pelvic packing with haemostatic agents is always a consideration particularly if it might be both effective and short in duration given the pelvic pressure and associated pain. If, however, bleeding is not relieved with this, is causing significant quality of life issues, and the time to death is likely to be prolonged, consideration for pelvic vessel embolization is an option. Finally, high-dose, short-interval radiation for palliation of bleeding can be attempted even in the setting of prior pelvic radiation (given that the long-term effects of radiation are not a consideration).

Respiratory symptoms

Respiratory symptoms may be related to a cancer or due to concurrent illness such as asthma or chronic obstructive airways disease. In the palliative situation, in-depth investigations of the aetiology are often not appropriate or available. Accurate history and examination are the cornerstones of diagnosis which is essential in order to identify the cause and whether there are reversible factors. Common symptoms are cough, breathlessness, and chest pain.

It is important to look at all symptoms holistically, in the current context before instituting treatment.

Key questions are:

1. What is the most likely diagnosis?
2. What investigations are needed and what is the risk of these investigations?
3. What treatment is needed and what is the risk?
4. What is the prognosis?
5. How frail is the patient?
6. Will treatment improve quality of life or prolong suffering?

Solutions must constantly balance and re-evaluate risks and bene-fits and involve the patient and family in decision-making.

Thromboembolic disease with pulmonary emboli is a par-ticular example of the importance of balancing risks and benefits. Anticoagulation will improve symptoms and prevent recurrence but at what cost? They increase the risk of bleeding, especially where wounds are present. Regular monitoring might be inconvenient or impossible and a drain on resources, especially in resource-poor communities. Low-molecular-weight heparin (Clexane) is more convenient but often unaffordable. Is treatment likely to prolong life or prolong suffering? Ventilation/perfusion or computed tom-ography pulmonary angiography scans for diagnosis of pulmonary emboli might not be available, or indicated.

Treatment

Treatment includes four elements: general management, treatment of reversible factors, disease-directed treatment (e.g. radiation), and management of symptoms.

General measures may be very effective and should not be under-estimated. They include reassurance, building trust, a fan, sitting up-right, open windows, and 'calm, positive approach … adjustments to patient's life style and expectations' (27).

Reversible factors and specific treatment measures are listed in Table 69.1.

Cough

Cough is often the most distressing symptom for patients, causing exhaustion and insomnia, and adding to the pain. While the first response may be to suppress cough, the underlying cause should sought first—if it is secondary to aspiration or reflux, simple ele-vation of the head of the bed and perhaps the addition of a proton pump inhibitor or a H_2 receptor antagonist may resolve the problem. Drugs such as an angiotensin-converting enzyme inhibitor may add to the symptoms and need to be stopped. Underlying asthma may need bronchodilators. Finally, cough due to failure to clear ac-cumulating secretions might benefit from expectorants (guaifen-esin, acetylcysteine) to make the cough more effective in clearing airways. If there is no treatable source underlying the cough, then management with cough suppression (codeine, dextromethorphan) is warranted.

Skin/wound care and lymphoedema

Pressure wounds are the most common wound management issue in palliative care. Prevention is a vital part of overall care. Good skin care and meticulous attention to pressure areas with regular turning and massage are imperative.

Skin breakdown/discharge

Disease and radiotherapy can lead to skin breakdown. This is aggra-vated by discharge or incontinence and good skin care is essential to prevent and minimize problems. Discharge is common with ad-vanced gynaecological malignancy and might be offensive and very distressing. Regular, gentle washing with saline or vinegar water can minimize odour. The skin should be dabbed dry to avoid excoriation and maceration. Patients may become fixated on the problem which may cause embarrassment and shame leading to psychological

Table 69.1 Underlying factors which may be reversible or require specific treatment

Underlying factors	Specific treatment
Breathlessness	
	Low dose opioids—2–4-hrly
	Oxygen—may relieve symptoms even if not hypoxic, reassuring
Bronchospasm	Bronchodilators—preferably by nebulization or spacer
Pleural effusion	Pleural aspiration ± pleurodesis
Lung metastases	Radiotherapy/chemotherapy
Lymphangitis carcinomatosis	Corticosteroids—betamethasone 12–18 mg or equivalent
Superior vena caval obstruction	Corticosteroids—betamethasone 12–18 mg or equivalent
	Radiotherapy/chemotherapy/stent
Infection/pneumonia	Antibiotics/corticosteroids (short course)
Heart failure	Diuretics, inotropes
Pericardial effusion	Refer to specialist/may need open drainage
Dying/bronchial secretions (terminal breathlessness)	Hyoscine butylbromide intramuscular injection or subcutaneously (20 mg as soon as symptom occurs)/can be repeated or given by continuous subcutaneous infusion
Anaemia	Consider transfusion/iron/erythropoietin
Anxiety	Non-pharmacological treatment + anxiolytics
	Short-acting lorazepam for panic/long-acting diazepam for persistent anxiety
Cough	
Dry	Suppressants—codeine or morphine
Wet	Do not suppress
	Secretions can be loosened with saline nebulization or N-acetylcysteine
Haemoptysis	Tranexamic acid (Cyklokapron) or radiotherapy, if fit enough.
	Prepare the family but be careful not to increase fear
Acute chest pain	
Pulmonary embolus/ deep vein thrombosis	Consider pros and cons of anticoagulation—warfarin or low-molecular-weight heparin
Acute myocardial infarction	Refer if indicated

Source data from Watson M, Lucas C, Hoy A, Wells J (eds). Respiratory symptoms. In: *Oxford Handbook of Palliative Care*, 2nd edn, pp. 363–79. Oxford: Oxford University Press; 2009.

problems. Barrier creams (zinc oxide, Cavilon, Fissan paste, Friars Balsam) are useful to protect the skin and prevent breakdown. Other suggestions for management of fistulae may help with skin care for pressure ulcers and vice versa.

Care of open wounds

As well as causing pain, discharge, odour, and bleeding, wounds are a visual reminder of the disease and add to psychological distress. They may significantly limit mobility and need adjustment of life-style. In advanced cancer, wounds may be large, infected, and bleed easily, particularly if there is a cutaneous metastasis present (28, 29).

Table 69.2 Inexpensive alternatives for wound care

To prevent adhesion	Petroleum jelly-based gauze
Infection control	Glycerine and ichthammol
Wet areas	Corn starch (Maizena)
To facilitate adhesion	Friars' Balsam
Superficial small wounds	Mercurochrome
Good for drying	Gentian violet
Minor bleeding	Gauze soaked in adrenaline 1:1000
Odour	Oil of peppermint (1 or 2 drops applied to the top of the wound dressing)

Wounds should be cleaned gently but thoroughly with normal saline to prevent infection and control odours. Spray dressings with saline before removing. A spray bottle and a hand shower are useful. Antiseptics should generally be avoided except under special circumstances where their use might advance comfort and reduce pain. Povidone iodine is useful in drying out necrotic tissue and hydrogen peroxide 3% can assist in debridement but both may cause damage to normal cells so long-term use is not viable. Dressing changes can be particularly difficult, so wetting the dressing with saline before removal as well as judicious use of topical analgesics, short-acting analgesics, and relaxation techniques may all aid in making this less painful.

Control odour in the room with incense, deodorizing substances (fabric softener, cat litter, charcoal), and air freshener machines.

Dressing changes should be limited. There are a large number of dressings now available. However, simple is usually best and most cost-effective (Table 69.2). Cost, comfort, availability, and appearance need to be taken into account. Simple petroleum jelly-based gauze will prevent adhesion which can add to discomfort and cause bleeding. 'Selecting the proper dressing will control pain, absorb exudates, and lessen the number of dressing changes' (29). Dressings will also limit exposure to flies in the global context which can lead to maggot infestation.

Antibiotics should be reserved for skin infections which are advancing. Choices are determined by local sensitivities and availability and include flucloxacillin, co-amoxiclav, trimethoprim, and erythromycin and metronidazole for anaerobic infection. Topical metronidazole (powder, creams, gel, intravenous solution) is excellent at reducing odour and can be applied weekly or daily if necessary.

Debridement, surgical or autolytic (e.g. honey), may be necessary to prevent infection (29) and surgical excision or debulking may be helpful in some situations.

Radiotherapy is helpful in shrinking the size of the wound and limiting bleeding.

Oedema

Oedema may be generalized (due to hypoalbuminaemia, or cardiac or renal failure), or localized lymphoedema. Good skin care is imperative. Localized lymphoedema due to obstruction of lymphatics is common with pelvic disease and may be due to the disease itself or after radiotherapy. Compression, mobilization, and massage may help. Lymphoedema massage is a specialized technique that family members can learn so that it can be done on a daily basis. It can improve comfort even if lymphoedema cannot be relieved. Wrapping the limb with elastic bandages or compression stockings after massage or after reduction with reclining may assist in prevention. Elevation of the feet or the foot of the bed is helpful.

Generalized oedema needs pharmacological treatment of the underlying cause of extracellular fluid accumulation and includes diuretics, such as spironolactone, thiazides or loop diuretics.

Oedema may be associated with ascites which may be assisted by paracentesis and diuretics if causing discomfort from either the ascites or the dependent oedema.

Psychological issues: concerns and management

People with gynaecological cancer as well as those with chronic pelvic diseases may be prone to issues with role identity, sexual and body image, depression and anxiety, agitation, and confusion. In addition, with a life-limiting illness they need to deal with dying and grief.

Role identity

Women rarely have single roles, and with terminal illness, many of these identities are lost. Women often have a strong identity with being the mother and primary care giver for the family. It is a painful struggle to give this up and allow others to attend to their needs and look after them. Women may have to give up identities as career women, artists, or other roles that require a level of activity and engagement they can no longer sustain. Together with this, they may lose their income, support, and social network. Loss of income may be an overriding worry as well as the burden they might place financially and socially on their families. The inability to fulfil a role as a sexual partner can be a painful loss in a relationship. Failure to fulfil these roles as well as an inability to fulfil hoped-for roles, such as grandmother or mother, take a deep toll. Women and their supporters have to deal with many simultaneous losses that add to their grief and to a sense of loss of value. All of these are worthy of addressing to find ways to empower and support the woman as she adjusts to new circumstances.

Sexual problems and body image concerns

Cancer can be very disfiguring. Problems can relate to the underlying disease or long-term scarring. External manifestations bring the cancer to the surface, while hidden disease might be associated with considerable shame. It should not be assumed that patients with advanced illness do not have sexual needs and the desire for intimacy. Sexuality is an integral part of the way women see themselves and is intricately linked with the experience of pleasure and joy.

Frequent sexual concerns of patients with cancer are discharge, 'loss of interest in sexual activity, difficulty becoming sexually aroused, pain with sexual activity, changes in orgasmic response and concern about incontinence' (30). Vaginal dryness, atrophy, and anatomical changes after surgery or radiotherapy may be problematic (31, 32).

Illness, generally, causes fatigue and decreased libido. However, with gynaecological disease there are specific problems. If the topic is not intentionally and sensitively opened it is very easy to overlook this important aspect of life. Simply put, 'We don't ask!' (33). Instead, healthcare workers often make assumptions such as 'sexual health is not important when one has cancer' or that 'prognosis is too poor for the patient to care' or 'I don't have time for this' (30). Unless the healthcare practitioner intentionally opens the discussion, the patient may be reluctant or too embarrassed to bring up the subject. Gynaecological cancer survivors may have high rates of sexual inactivity and sexual dysfunction (34). Many of these problems can be addressed and improved (35).

Treatment

In the palliative care setting, treatment for sexual dysfunction (Table 69.3) still follows the same tenets as general treatment. Simple questions that are open ended can lead to an important discussion. Simply raising the question of whether a woman is sexually active and what has changed with her treatment and disease progression may be enough to open the door. Further exploring what needs are not being met and normalizing sexuality as part of life and even end of life can allow some problem-solving to occur. The use of vaginal dilators for stenosis and scarring from treatment, lubricants, and even oestrogen all may assist in overcoming issues related to treatment or disease.

Depression and anxiety

These are important symptoms which need to be identified and treated aggressively (36). They may significantly impact quality of life and may aggravate all the other physical symptoms. A key clinical task is to distinguish true depression from normal sadness as a response to loss and disease progression. For one, support and listening may be adequate, but for true depression, more may be needed. Medication can play an important part but is not a substitute for good supportive care, clear compassionate communication, counselling, and free expression of feelings. Relaxation techniques, breathing, mindfulness, mediation, and complementary therapy are helpful.

Antidepressants, such as amitriptyline, venlafaxine, and duloxetine, are useful for neuropathic pain and selective serotonin reuptake inhibitors for panic as well as depression. Citalopram is safest if hepatic impairment is present. The goal with palliative care is to avoid polypharmacy and to aim to have as few medications as possible with the lowest side effect profile, while taking into account metastatic disease and the risk of hepatic and renal failure. The

Table 69.3 Sexual dysfunction contributors

Low desire/ arousal	• Fatigue, depression, anxiety • Body image • Partner anxiety or conflict • Changes in levels of sex hormones • Medications • Comorbidities—physical and psychological and pain
Physiological issues	• Pain • Treatment related (e.g. vaginal radiation, post chemotherapy, aromatase inhibitors) vaginal dryness • Menopausal/low oestrogen, vaginal/vulval atrophy
Orgasm issues	• Surgical, tumour, or radiation damage to nerve supply • Antidepressant use

Source data from Ramondetta L. Challenges in the treatment of sexual function in patients with gynecological cancers. Presentation given at AORTIC conference 2015, Marrakesh, Morocco.

decision when to start pharmacological treatment may be difficult but an important guide is to ask if mood is interfering with quality of life, sleep, or treatment decisions. If support and other options have not resolved this, and particularly if treatment might also assist with pain control, then medication should be started. Prognosis should be considered before commencing treatment.

Agitation and confusion

Agitation with confusion needs to be distinguished from anxiety and panic as it requires different treatment. It may be part of underlying delirium but occasionally true psychosis may be triggered, especially if there is pre-existing psychiatric illness. If delirium is suspected, exclude infection, especially urinary tract, hypercalcaemia and other metabolic disturbance, renal and hepatic failure, and brain metastases. All of these may have specific therapies that can reverse the symptoms quickly.

Agitation may also occur at the end of life, especially when there is a prior history of behavioural problems, substance abuse, drug withdrawal, or psychiatric illness or if there are many unresolved issues and a sense of panic about addressing them before death.

Treatment must first address reversible factors. Then non-pharmacological measures, antipsychotics (haloperidol is safe in low doses and safe in hepatic impairment), and anxiolytics (lorazepam by mouth or IMI) can be used. Corticosteroids are useful for brain metastases but they should be used with caution because they may aggravate the mental disturbance.

Hypercalcaemia is more common with bone metastases—and may first have symptoms of persistent nausea, thirst, altered mood, confusion, worsening pain, and constipation before agitation. Hydration and bisphosphonates can help although gauging the benefit versus the time to death is important before starting such therapy.

Dying

Discussions about death and dying are generally avoided by both patients and healthcare workers. In some cultures, it is totally taboo. However, if we are to deal effectively with the end of life we need to develop the skills to explore feelings, beliefs, fantasies, and practical issues. Discussions about legal aspects for end of life such as drawing up a will and an advanced directive ('living will') are ideal opportunities to open the discussion. Timing this discussion requires sensitivity but is essential and should not be delayed until death is approaching. Ideally, the status of disease and the implications for the patient have been part of an ongoing discussion that will allow for this to be an extension of ongoing discussions rather than a new discussion. For example, a discussion which can begin with 'I know that we hoped that this treatment would stabilize disease and give you more time, however our exam today shows that it has progressed' opens the door more effectively to a 'What comes now that we are not going to treat the disease?' question. Such continuity allows for many opportunities over the course of a disease to have discussions about what is important or not important to the patient and family with respect to her dying process. To have such discussions, however, requires healthcare practitioners to address their own fears about death and dying in order to effectively cope with the challenges being faced by their patients and families.

There is a role for health professionals to provide significant support beyond palliative care for symptoms. Even nearing death, there may be things to look forward to and goals to achieve. It might be a chance to reach closure with individuals or a chance to see one last school play, a graduation, a major birthday, or meet a new grandchild. Having a discussion that focuses on goals the patient hopes to achieve and the symptom management required to achieve those goals, can provide closure and healing for families, patients, and caregivers alike.

Spiritual management: issues and concerns

The international palliative care community makes a clear distinction between religious and spiritual care while acknowledging the need for both. There is considerable overlap between psychological and spiritual needs and these are best seen as a continuum of psychospiritual needs. 'Spirituality is the aspect of humanity that refers to the way individuals seek and express meaning and purpose, and the way they experience their connectedness to the moment, to self, to others, to nature and to the significant or sacred' (37).

Spiritual care is 'Care that is designed to offer a person an opportunity to explore values, ideals, meaning and purpose'. It addresses common human questions such as:

- Who am I?
- Where do I come from?
- Why am I here?
- Where is the meaning and purpose in my life?

In addition, it may also address the value of a transcendent 'enduring reality' and 'the non-material aspects of life' (38, 39).

Religious care addresses the same issues within the framework of organized religion, particular to that individual patient, and may include significant rituals, such as last rites or communion.

Both religious and spiritual care need to be acknowledged and incorporated at every stage of the illness. The basis of both is compassion.

At times spiritual, religious, and cultural beliefs may be in conflict with medical care being offered, causing conflict or impeding effective management. Fixed beliefs may block the open exploration of death and dying as this is taboo in many cultures and religions. Unrealistic beliefs in alternative therapies can seriously hamper effective palliative care. Sometimes beliefs are put forward as a reason for avoiding discussions and denying the status of disease even when the belief system may be misrepresented in doing so. Gently examining this with the patient or an influential family member or even a spiritual or religious guide can assist in dealing with the present and making plans for the future.

Denial can be both a protection and an impediment and cannot be forcefully confronted. The goal of counselling is to develop realistic hope, at the patient's pace. Unrealistic hopes and denial by the patient and/or the family may block treatment and lead to unnecessary suffering. Ask questions (40) in order to understand the individual. Being seen as a unique person and being treated with care and love brings true comfort and spiritual healing.

Bringing things back to practical realities allows hope to develop—being supported and being pain free, comfortable, and safe. Look for achievable goals and expectations in the conversation and plan

Table 69.4 The FICA spiritual assessment tool—an acronym to remember what to ask in a spiritual history

F: Faith or belief	What is your faith or belief? What gives your life meaning?
I: Importance and Influence	What is important to you? What importance does your spirituality have in your life? Have your beliefs influenced your behaviour during this illness? What role do your beliefs play in your understanding of healing?
C: Community	Are you part of a faith community as a member of a group? Is this of support to you and how? Is there a person or group of people you really love or who are important to you?
A: Address	How would you like me to address these issues in your healthcare?

Source data from Puchalski C, Ferrell BR, 2010. *Making Health Care Whole: Integrating Spirituality into Patient Care.* West Conshohocken, PA: Templeton Press.

ahead appropriately. Try to enable and empower in every way, to help people make the best of the possible in this impossible, irreversible situation.

Spiritual care includes counselling, non-verbal support, and complementary therapy. There are tools to help in assessing and discussing this area (Table 69.4). The aim is to help people express their fears and find meaning in their lives and in their illness. It allows people to come to a place of acceptance and peace by acknowledging what was and working through the fears of the present and future.

Social considerations

Recognizing end of life and providing preferences

The palliative care patient cannot be considered without taking into account the family unit, the home, and the community in which they reside. Families vary enormously in their resilience, their ability to cope, and their resources. Including a social worker in the palliative care team is imperative. Patients and their families generally underestimate how seriously ill the patient is and overestimate the role that treatments, including chemotherapy or other cancer-directed therapies, might have in prolonging life or reducing suffering (41).

Management of hospice care at home, hospice, and hospital

The majority of people express a wish to die at home, although in many countries, the majority actually dies in hospital. Access to hospice services can assist in bridging the gap. In the United Kingdom, the Gold Standards Framework sets out a framework for improving services. The goals are to enable patients to 'die well', supported and symptom free. The cornerstone of good community care is communication—between the patient and healthcare providers, and within the network of healthcare providers involved (42). The palliative care team can assist in identifying available resources within the family and within the community and empower the family to use them, taking into account the patient's wishes.

In-patient hospice facilities are increasingly reserved for short-term care (usually 2 weeks) comprising symptom control and family respite. Less commonly, patients prefer to die in hospice. If available, hospices provide a far more, gentle, supportive environment than do hospitals where the focus is on curative treatment. Hospitals, too, are starting to incorporate palliative care approaches, even into casualty departments and intensive care units (43).

There is some evidence even in the hospital-centric medical cultures, such as in the United States, that the value and importance of palliative home care, particularly for end of life care, is gaining ground. Medicare data from 1999 to 2013 do show that total hospitalizations and inpatient expenditures are decreasing in the last 6 months of life (44).

Environmental considerations

Hospice is generally regarded as an attitude rather than a place and the principles of palliative care can be applied in almost any environment. Wherever possible, a nursing sister or care worker should visit the patient in their own home. Often people nearing the end of life like peace and quiet but others prefer the hustle and bustle of everyday life. Other considerations are stairs, hospital beds, commodes, and other nursing aids. Hospital beds make nursing of bed-bound patients considerably easier.

Hospital or hospice admission may be required if there are too many or too few people in the home, if the environment is totally unsuitable, or if the needs of the patient are beyond the scope of the family. If hospice or hospital admission is necessary, the aim would be to make the environment as homely and peaceful as possible with family presence and involvement encouraged.

Family/caregiver needs and supports

There is a wide range of grief needs in family members after the death of the patient. For most, the grief goes through standard phases and can be managed with familial and individual support. However, it is worth noting that there is an entity of 'complicated grief' defined as a 'persistent complex bereavement disorder … consistent with the notion that complicated grief is a stressor-related condition' (45). This entity should be suspected if the family member shows new cognitive or functional impairments, has difficulty accepting or adapting to the loss over time, and even suicidal ideation. Treatment requires more than simple support and referral for therapy should be considered (46).

Caring for a terminally ill patient can be a drawn-out and exhausting process, physically and emotionally. Caregivers will need to be actively supported, individually or in groups, and encouraged to receive help and care for themselves. In addition, healthcare workers need to be encouraged to attend to their own wellness needs.

Despite the many challenges, a time spent facing a life-limiting illness can be a time of healing. Patients and those close to them can be assisted to express their feelings of loss and love. The four important messages of 'I love you', 'Thank you', 'Sorry', and 'Goodbye' can bring peaceful closure and heal relationships in a deep and meaningful way (47). It might take time to reach this point with sincerity, but the journey is deeply rewarding for patients, families, and caregivers. Support for the family should not end at the death of patients. Bereavement support should be offered and extended to the family members (48) and to the professional caregivers who also need support in order to continue to care maximally for patients with life-limiting illness and facing the end of their lives.

Summary

It is clear that many patients and their families have preferences for deaths at home or in a hospice. Palliative care can help avoid hospital and particularly the intensive care unit for end of life cancer care (49). While the growth of hospice and palliative care as a specialty has advanced care considerably, many women and their families do not have access to these specialists and still need compassionate, knowledgeable care from their primary care and gynaecological oncology care givers, whether primary or secondary members of their care team. 'We are left to help the dying using the qualities we value in care for the living, such as empathy and respect for patients' preferences and goals' (50). These are attributes that every health professional can call on to assist in palliative and hospice care.

REFERENCES

1. World Health Organization. WHO definition of palliative care. Available at: http://www.who.int/cancer/palliative/definition/en.
2. Kelley AS, Morrison RS. Palliative care for the seriously ill. *N Engl J Med* 2015;**373**:747–55.
3. Rabow M, Kvale E, Barbour L, et al. Moving upstream: a review of the evidence of the impact of outpatient palliative care. *J Palliat Med* 2013;**16**:1540–49.
4. Smith S, Brick A, O'Hara S, Normand C. Evidence on the cost and cost effectiveness of palliative care: a literature review. *Palliat Med* 2014;**28**:130–50.
5. Meuser T. Symptoms during cancer pain treatment following WHO guidelines: a longitudinal follow up study of symptom prevalence, severity, and etiology. *Pain* 2001;**93**:247–57.
6. Jahn P, Kuss O, Schmidt H, et al. Improvement of pain related self-management for cancer patients through a modular transitional nursing intervention: a cluster-randomized multicenter trial. *Pain* 2014;**155**:746–54.
7. Gordon DB, Dahl JL, Miaskowski C, et al. American pain society recommendations for improving the quality of acute and cancer pain management. *Arch Intern Med* 2005;**165**:1574–80.
8. Schmidt-Hansen M, Bennett MI, Hilgart J. Oxycodone for cancer pain in adult patients. *JAMA* 2015;**314**:1282–83.
9. Smith TJ, Staats PS, Deer T, et al. Randomized clinical trial on an implantable drug delivery system compared with comprehensive medical management for refractory cancer pain: impact on pain, drug related toxicity, and survival. *J Clin Oncol* 2002;**20**:4040–49.
10. Anghelescu DL, Faughnan LG, Baker JN, Yang J, Kane JR. Use of epidural and peripheral nerve blocks at the end of life in children and young adults with cancer: the collaboration between a pain service and a palliative care service. *Ped Anesthesia* 2010;**20**:1070–77.
11. Oliver DP, Wittenberg-Lyles E, Demiris G, Washington K, Porock D, Day M. Barriers to pain management: caregiver perceptions and pain talk by hospice interdisciplinary teams. *J Pain Symptom Manage* 2008;**36**:374–82.
12. Herr K, Titler M, Fine P, et al. Assessing and treating pain in hospices: current state of evidence based practices. *J Pain Symptom Manage* 2010;**39**:803–19.

13. Angst MS, Clark JD. Opioid induced hyperalgesia: a qualitative systematic review. *Anesthesiology* 2006;**80**:319–24.

14. Hwang IC, Bruera E, Park SM. Use of intravenous fentanyl against morphine tolerance in breakthrough cancer pain: a case series and literature review. *Am J Hospice Palliat Med* 2014;**31**:109–11.

15. Bates T. A review of local radiotherapy in the treatment of bone metastases and cord compression. *Int J Radiat Oncol Biol Phys* 1992;**23**:217–21.

16. Hartsell WF, Scott CB, Bruner DW, et al. Randomized trial of short versus long-course radiotherapy for palliation of painful bone metastases. *J Natl Cancer Inst* 2005;**97**:798–804.

17. Wong RKS, Wiffen PJ. Bisphosphonates for the relief of pain secondary to bone metastases. *Cochrane Database Syst Rev* 2002;**2**:CD002068.

18. Dy AM, Apostol CC. Evidence-based approaches to other symptoms in advanced cancer. *Cancer J* 2010;**16**:507–13.

19. Bruera E, Hui D, Dalal S, et al. Parenteral hydration in patients with advanced cancer: a multicenter, double-blind, placebo controlled randomized trial. *J Clin Oncol* 2013;**31**:11–18.

20. Ford AC, Brenner DM, Schoenfeld PS. Efficacy of pharmacological therapies for the treatment of opioid-induced constipation: systematic review and meta-analysis. *Am J Gastroenterol* 2013;**108**:1566–74.

21. Wrald A. Constipation advances in diagnosis and treatment. *JAMA* 2016;**315**:185–95.

22. Blinderman CD, Billings JA. Comfort care for patients dying in the hospital. *N Engl J Med* 2015;**373**:2549–61.

23. Brindle CT, Blankenship J. Management of complex abdominal wounds with small bowel fistulae. *J Wound Ostomy Continence Nurs* 2009;**36**:396–403.

24. Markland AD, Burgio KL, Whitehead WE, et al. Loperamide versus psyllium fiber for treatment of fecal incontinence: the fecal incontinence prescription management (FIRM) randomized clinical trial. *Dis Colon Rectum* 2015;**58**:983–89.

25. Gupta D, Sanjeev Kumar Sharma, Khurana H, Mishra S, Bhatnagar S. Long term silicone urinary catheter is a simpler alternative to radical bilateral percutaneous nephrostomy for palliation of malignant vesicouterine fistula. *Am J Hosp Palliat Care* 2009;**26**:66–67.

26. Mody L, Juthani-Mehat M. Urinary tract infections in older women: a clinical review. *JAMA* 2014;**311**:844–54.

27. Watson M, Lucas C, Hoy A, Wells J (eds). Respiratory symptoms. In: *Oxford Handbook of Palliative Care*, 2nd edn, pp. 363–79. Oxford: Oxford University Press; 2009.

28. Watson M, Lucas C, Hoy A, Wells J (eds). Skin problems in palliative care. In: *Oxford Handbook of Palliative Care*, 2nd edn, pp. 381–84. Oxford: Oxford University Press; 2009.

29. Alvarez OM, Kalinski C, Nusbaum J, et al. Incorporating wound healing strategies to improve palliation (symptom management) in patients with chronic wounds. *J Palliat Med* 2007;**10**:1161–89.

30. Ramondetta L. *Challenges in the Treatment of Sexual Function in Patients with Gynecological Cancers*. Presentation given at AORTIC 2015 Conference, Marrakesh, Morocco, 18–22 November 2015.

31. Carter J, Stabile C, Seidel B, et al. Baseline characteristics and concerns of female cancer patients/survivors seeking treatment at a female sexual medicine program. *Support Care Cancer* 2015;**23**:2255–65.

32. Grimm D, Hasenburg A, Eulenburg C, et al. Sexual activity and function in patients with gynecological malignancies after completed treatment. *Int J Gynecol Cancer* 2015;**25**:1134–41.

33. Dizon DS, Suzin D, McIlvenna S. Sexual health as a survivorship issue for female cancer survivors. *Oncologist* 2014;**19**:202–10.

34. Bradford A, Fellman B, Urbauer D, et al. Assessment of sexual activity and dysfunction in medically underserved women with gynecologic cancers. *Gynecol Oncol* 2015;**139**:134–40.

35. Lindau ST, Gavrilova N, Anderson D. Sexual morbidity in very long-term survivors of vaginal and cervical cancer: a comparison to national norms. *Gyncol Oncol* 2007;**106**:413–18.

36. Hospice Palliative Care Association of South Africa. Clinical guidelines for palliative care. 2012. Available at: https://hpca.co.za/download/hpca-clinical-guidelines-2012/.

37. Puchalski C, Ferrell BR. *Making Health Care Whole: Integrating Spirituality into Patient Care*. West Conshohocken, PA: Templeton Press; 2010.

38. Canadian Virtual Hospice. Glossary. Available at: http://www.virtualhospice.ca/en_US/Main+Site+Navigation/Zoom+Navigation/Glossary/S/Spiritual+care.aspx.

39. Twycross R. *Introducing Palliative Care*. 4th edn. Johannesburg: University of the Witwatersrand; 2003.

40. Gawande A. *Being Mortal: Medicine and What Matters in the End*. New York: Metropolitan Books, Holt, Henry & Company; 2014.

41. Weeks JC, Cook EF, O'Day SJ, et al. Relationship between cancer patients' predictions of prognosis and their treatment preferences. *JAMA* 1998;**279**:1709–14.

42. Watson M, Lucas C, Hoy A, Wells J (eds). Palliative care in the home. In: *Oxford Handbook of Palliative Care*, 2nd edn, pp. 858–77. Oxford: Oxford University Press; 2009.

43. Heaney M, Foot C, Freeman WD, Fraser J. Ethical issues in withholding and withdrawing life-prolonging medical treatment in the ICU. *Curr Anaesth Crit Care* 2009;**18**:277–83.

44. Krumholz HM, Nuti SV, Downing NS, Normand SL, Wang Y. Mortality, hospitalizations, and expenditures for the Medicare population aged 65 and older, 1999–2013. *JAMA* 2015;**314**:355–65.

45. Simon NM. Is complicated grief a post loss stress disorder? *Depress Anxiety* 2012;**29**:541–44.

46. Simon NM. Increasing support for the treatment of complicated grief in adults of all ages. *JAMA Psychiatry* 2014;**71**:1287–95.

47. Watson M, Lucas C, Hoy A, Wells J (eds). Social work. In: *Oxford Handbook of Palliative Care*, 2nd edn, pp. 886. Oxford: Oxford University Press; 2009.

48. Simon NM. Increasing support for the treatment of complicated grief in adults of all ages. *JAMA* 2015;**313**:2172–73.

49. Wright AA, Keating NL, Ayanian JZ, et al. Family perspectives on aggressive cancer care near the end of life. *JAMA* 2016;**315**:284–92.

50. Rosenbaum L. Falling together—empathetic care for the dying. *N Engl J Med* 2016;**374**;**6**:587–90.

Pathology of tumours of the female genital tract

Jaime Prat

Introduction

Pathology reports include not only histopathological diagnoses but also specific information relating to prognosis and treatment; thus, pathologists must have sufficient familiarity with the staging classification and management of gynaecological cancers to assure that their reports communicate clinically relevant information. On the other hand, full understanding of the pathology report by the gynaecologist requires familiarity with the terminology used in gynaecological pathology. This chapter summarizes the pathological features of the most common gynaecological tumours.

Vulva

Malignant tumours and premalignant conditions

Squamous cell carcinoma

Carcinoma of the vulva accounts for 3% of all female genital cancers and occurs mainly in women aged over 60 years. Squamous cell carcinoma is the most common type (86%). These tumours are divided into two groups: keratinizing squamous cell carcinomas unrelated to human papillomavirus (HPV) (>70% of cases), and warty and basaloid carcinomas, which are strongly associated with high-risk HPV (<25% of cases), mainly HPV16 (1, 2).

Aetiological factors and precursor lesions

Keratinizing squamous carcinomas frequently develop in older women (mean age 76 years), sometimes in the context of long-standing lichen sclerosus. The precursor lesion is referred to as differentiated vulval intraepithelial neoplasia dVIN or VIN simplex (**Figure 70.1a**), which carries a high risk of cancer development. In contrast, the less common HPV-associated warty and basaloid carcinomas develop from a precursor lesion called squamous intraepithelial lesion (SIL) VIN comprising a spectrum of alterations ranging from low-grade SIL VIN (VIN1) to high-grade SIL VIN (VIN 2–3) (**Figure 70.1b**). Recent proposals from both the International Society for the Study of Vulvovaginal Disease (ISVVD) and the College of American Pathologists (CAP)/American Society for Colposcopy and Cervical Pathology (ASCCP) have recommended replacement of the older three-tiered system (VIN 1–3) used to describe these lesions with a two-tiered system. HPV-associated SIL VIN lesions have a low risk of progression to invasive carcinomas (approximately 6%), except in older or immunosuppressed women (1, 2).

Pathology

SIL VIN may be single or multiple, and macular, papular, or plaque-like. Histological grades are labelled low-grade SIL VIN I, corresponding to mild dysplasia, and high-grade SIL (VIN 2–3) corresponding to, moderate, and severe dysplasia, respectively. However, high-grade SIL (VIN 3)—which includes squamous cell carcinoma *in situ* (CIS)—is by far the most common.

Keratinizing squamous cell carcinomas usually follow differentiated VIN (VIN simplex). Most tumours are exophytic but some may be ulcerative. Microscopically, the tumour is composed of invasive nests of malignant squamous epithelium with central keratin pearls (**Figure 70.2**). The tumours grow slowly, extending to contiguous skin, vagina, and rectum. They metastasize initially to superficial inguinal lymph nodes, and then to deep inguinal, femoral, and pelvic lymph nodes (1, 2).

Clinical features

Prognosis correlates with stage of disease and lymph node status. The number of inguinal lymph nodes with metastases is the most important single factor. The International Federation of Gynecology and Obstetrics (FIGO) staging of vulval cancer defines tumors of any size limited to the vulva as Stage I carcinomas; tumors extending to adjacent perineal structures (lower one-third of the urethra, lower one-third of the vagina, or anus) as Stage II; tumors with positive inguinofemoral lymph nodes as Stage III; and tumors invading the upper two-thirds of the urethra, upper two-thirds of the vagina, distal structures, or distant metastasis as Stage IV. Tumor grade and number, size, and location of lymph node metastases determine survival. Well-differentiated tumors have a better mean survival, approaching 90% if nodes are negative. Two-thirds of women with inguinal node metastases survive 5 years, but only one-fourth of those with pelvic node metastases live that long (1).

(a)

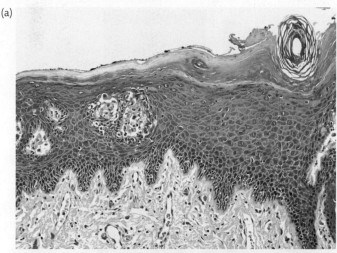

(b)

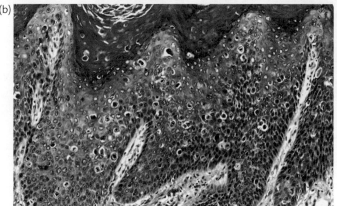

Figure 70.1 Vulval intraepithelial neoplasia (VIN). (a) Well-differentiated (simplex) type. The atypia is accentuated in the basal and parabasal layers. There is striking epithelial maturation in the superficial layers. (b) HPV-related undifferentiated (classic) VIN. Beneath a hyperkeratotic surface the epithelial cells are atypical. There are numerous mitoses.

Verrucous carcinoma

Vulval verrucous carcinoma is a distinct variety of squamous cell carcinoma that manifests as a large fungating mass resembling a giant condyloma acuminatum. HPV, usually type 6 or 11, is commonly identified. The tumour invades with broad tongues. Verrucous

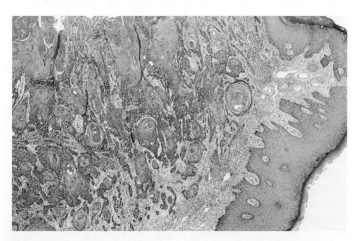

Figure 70.2 Keratinizing squamous cell carcinoma of the vulva. Nests of neoplastic squamous cells, some with keratin pearls, are evident.

carcinomas rarely metastasize. Wide local surgical excision is the treatment of choice.

Basal cell carcinoma

Basal cell carcinomas of the vulva are identical to their counterparts in the skin. They are not associated with HPV, rarely metastasize, and are usually cured by surgical excision.

Malignant melanoma

Although uncommon, malignant melanoma is the second most frequent cancer of the vulva (5%). It occurs in the sixth and seventh decades but occasionally is found in younger women. It is highly aggressive, and the prognosis is poor.

Extramammary Paget's disease

The disorder usually occurs on the labia majora in older women. The lesion is large, red, moist, and sharply demarcated. The origin of the diagnostic cells (Paget cells) is controversial: they may arise in the epidermis or epidermally derived adnexal structures.

Intraepidermal Paget's disease may have been present for many years and is often far more extensive throughout the epidermis than preoperative biopsies indicate. Unlike Paget's disease of the breast, which is almost always associated with underlying duct carcinoma, extramammary Paget's disease is only rarely associated with carcinoma of the skin adnexa. Metastases rarely occur, so treatment requires only wide local excision or simple vulvectomy (1, 2).

Vagina

Malignant tumours of the vagina

Primary malignant tumours of the vagina are uncommon, constituting about 2% of all genital tract tumours. Most (80%) vaginal malignancies represent metastatic spread. Tumours confined to the vagina are usually treated by radical hysterectomy and vaginectomy. Squamous cell carcinomas account for over 90% of primary vaginal malignancies. Prognosis is related to the extent of spread of the tumour at the time of its discovery. The 5-year survival rate for tumours confined to the vagina (stage I) is 80%, whereas it is only 20% for those with extensive spread (stages III/IV) (1).

Embryonal rhabdomyosarcoma (sarcoma botryoides)

Embryonal rhabdomyosarcoma occurs almost exclusively in girls under 4 years old. It arises in the lamina propria of the vagina and consists of primitive spindle rhabdomyoblasts, some of which show cross-striations. Tumours less than 3 cm in greatest dimension tend to be localized and may be cured by wide excision and chemotherapy. Larger tumours have often spread to adjacent structures, regional lymph nodes, or distant sites. Even in advanced cases, half of patients survive with radical surgery and chemotherapy (1, 2).

Cervix

Squamous cell neoplasia

Cytological screening in high-resource countries decreased cervical carcinoma by 50% to 85%; however, worldwide, cervical cancer remains the fourth most common cancer in women.

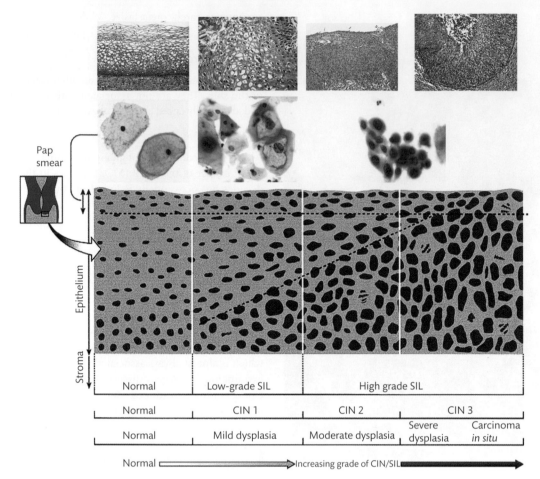

Figure 70.3 Inter-relations of naming systems in precursor cervical lesions. This chart integrates multiple aspects of the disease. It illustrates the changes in progressively more abnormal disease states and provides translation terminology for the dysplasia/carcinoma *in situ* (CIS) system, cervical intraepithelial neoplasia (CIN) system, and the Bethesda system. The scheme also illustrates the corresponding cytological smear resulting from exfoliation of the most superficial cells as well as the equivalent histopathological lesions (top row). SIL, squamous intraepithelial lesion.

Cervical squamous intraepithelial neoplasia (SIL)

Cervical squamous intraepithelial neoplasia SIL (CIN) is a spectrum of intraepithelial changes that begins with minimal atypia and progresses through stages of greater intraepithelial abnormalities to invasive squamous cell carcinoma. The terms CIN, dysplasia, CIS, and squamous intraepithelial lesion are commonly used interchangeably (1, 2) (**Figure 70.3**).

Epidemiology and molecular pathogenesis

HPV infection leads to CIN and cervical cancer. Low-grade SIL (CIN 1) is a permissive infection (i.e. HPV is episomal, freely replicates, and thereby causes cell death). Huge numbers of virus must accumulate in the cytoplasm before being visible as a koilocyte (**Figure 70.3**). In most cases of higher-grade SIL (CIN 2–3), viral DNA integrates into the cell genome. Proteins encoded by the *E6* and *E7* genes of HPV 16 respectively bind and inactivate p53 and Rb proteins, thereby invalidating their tumour suppressor functions. After HPV integrates into host DNA, copies of the whole virus do not accumulate and koilocytes are absent in many cases of high-grade dysplasia and all invasive cancers. Cells in high-grade CIN usually contain HPV types 16, 18, 31, 33, 35, 39, 45, 51, 52, 56, 58, 59, and 68. HPV types 16 and 18 are found in 70% of invasive cancers; the other high-risk types account for another 25% (4).

Pathology

SIL (CIN) is nearly always a disease of metaplastic squamous epithelium in the transformation zone. The normal process by which cervical squamous epithelium matures is disturbed in CIN, as evidenced morphologically by changes in cellularity, differentiation, polarity, nuclear features, and mitotic activity. High-grade SIL (CIN 3) is synonymous with severe dysplasia and CIS. The sequence of histological changes from low-grade SIL (CIN 1) to high-grade SIL (CIN 2–3) is shown in **Figure 70.3** (1, 2).

Clinical features

The mean age at which women develop SIL (CIN) is 24–27 years for low-grade SIL (CIN 1) and CIN 2, and 35–42 years for CIN 3. Based on morphological criteria, half of cases of CIN 1 regress, 10% progress to high-grade SIL (CIN 3), and less than 2% become invasive cancer. The average time for all grades of dysplasia to progress to high-grade SIL (CIN 3) is about 10 years. At least 20% of cases of high-grade SIL (CIN 3) progress to invasive carcinoma in that time (1).

When SIL (CIN) is discovered, colposcopy, together with a Schiller test, delineates the extent of the lesion and indicates the areas to be biopsied. Diagnostic endocervical curettage also helps to determine the extent of endocervical involvement. Women with low-grade SIL

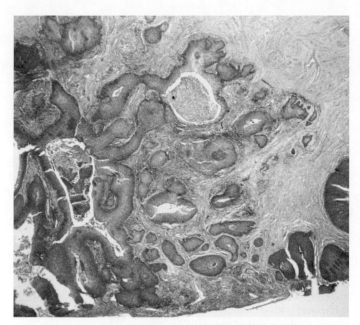

Figure 70.4 Microinvasive squamous cell carcinoma. The tumour invades 5 mm deep and 4 mm wide. This tumour is stage IA2 according to FIGO's classification.

(CIN 1) are often followed conservatively (i.e. repeated Pap smears plus close follow-up). High-grade lesions are treated according to the extent of disease. The loop electrosurgical excision procedure, cervical conization (removal of a cone of tissue around the external os), cryosurgery, and (rarely) hysterectomy may be performed (1).

Microinvasive (superficially invasive) squamous cell carcinoma

This is the earliest stage (IA) of invasive cervical cancer. In this setting, stromal invasion usually arises from overlying SIL (CIN) (Figure 70.4). Staging of microinvasive disease is based on width and depth of invasion, defined as follows:

- Invasion less than 3 mm (stage IA1) or 5 mm (stage IA2) below the basement membrane.

The earliest invasive changes ('early stromal invasion') appear as tiny irregular epithelial buds emanating from the base of high-grade SIL (CIN 3) lesions. These small (<1 mm) tongues of neoplastic epithelial cells do not affect the prognosis of high-grade SIL (CIN 3) lesions; hence, both can be treated similarly with conservative surgery. In the 2009 International Federation of Gynecology and Obstetrics (FIGO) classification, early stromal invasion was excluded from stage IA1. Some gynaecological oncologists further limit microinvasive carcinoma to tumours lacking lymphovascular invasion. Stage IA2 tumours are associated with lymph node metastases in about 8% of cases whereas those that invade up to 3 mm (stage IA1) have only a 1–2% risk of lymph node metastases. Conization or simple hysterectomy generally cures microinvasive cancers less than 3 mm deep (1–3).

Invasive squamous cell carcinoma

Pathology

Early stages of cervical cancer are often poorly defined lesions or nodular and exophytic masses. If the tumour is within the

endocervical canal, it can be an endophytic mass, which can infiltrate the stroma and cause diffuse cervical enlargement. Most tumours are non-keratinizing, with solid nests of large malignant squamous cells and no more than individual cell keratinization. Most remaining cancers show nests of keratinized cells in concentric whorls, so-called keratin pearls.

Cervical cancer spreads by direct extension, through lymphatic vessels and only rarely by the haematogenous route. Local extension into surrounding tissues (parametrium) results in ureteral compression (stage IIIB); the corresponding clinical complications are hydroureter, hydronephrosis, and renal failure secondary to ureteric obstruction—the most common cause of death (50% of patients). Bladder and rectal involvement (stage IVA) may lead to fistula formation. Metastases to regional lymph nodes involve paracervical, hypogastric, and external iliac nodes. Overall, tumour growth and spread are relatively slow, since the average age for patients with high-grade SIL (CIN 3) is 35–40 years; for stage IA carcinoma, 43 years; and for stage IV, 57 years (1–3).

Clinical features

HPV testing is the most reliable screening test for detecting cervical cancer, and is supplanting cytology in some screening algorithms in women aged over 25 years. Co-testing with HPV testing and cytology is also recommended in women aged over 30 years. Where HPV testing is not available, the Pap smear remains the most commonly used screening test, but quality assurance is a vital component of such screening programs.

The clinical stage of cervical cancer is the best predictor of survival. Overall 5-year survival is 60%, and by each stage it is as follows: I, 90%; II, 75%; III, 35%; and IV, 10%. About 15% of patients develop recurrences on the vaginal wall, bladder, pelvis, or rectum within 2 years of therapy. Radical hysterectomy is favoured for localized tumour, especially in younger women; radiation therapy, chemotherapy, or combinations of the two are used for more advanced tumours (1–3).

Endocervical adenocarcinoma

This tumour makes up 20% of cervical cancers. The incidence of cervical adenocarcinoma has increased recently, with a mean age of 56 years at presentation. Most tumours are of the endocervical cell (mucinous) type. These tumours are often associated with adenocarcinoma *in situ* and are frequently infected with HPV types 16 and 18 (1, 2).

Adenocarcinoma *in situ* generally arises by the squamocolumnar junction and extends into the endocervical canal. Associated high-grade squamous cell CIN occurs in 40% of cases of adenocarcinoma *in situ*. Invasive adenocarcinoma typically presents as a polypoid or papillary mass. Adenocarcinoma of the endocervix spreads by local invasion and lymphatic metastases, but overall survival is somewhat worse than for squamous carcinoma.

Corpus uteri

Endometrial hyperplasia

Endometrial hyperplasia forms a morphological continuum of abnormal proliferation ranging from focal glandular crowding or simple hyperplasia to well-differentiated adenocarcinoma.

Pathology

The 2014 World Health Organization (WHO) scheme distinguishes only two categories of endometrial hyperplasia: (1) hyperplasia without atypia; and (2) atypical hyperplasia/endometrial intraepithelial neoplasia (EIN) (1, 2).

Hyperplasia without atypia

This is an exaggerated proliferation of glands of irregular size and shape with increase in the gland-to-stroma ratio compared with proliferative endometrium, but without significant nuclear atypia. Hyperplasia without atypia is the result of unopposed oestrogenic stimulation. Progression to endometrial carcinoma occurs in 1–3% of women with hyperplasia without atypia

Atypical hyperplasia/endometrial intraepithelial neoplasia

This lesion shows marked glandular crowding, often as back-to-back glands, with little intervening stroma and cytological atypia. Epithelial cell nuclei are large and hyperchromatic with prominent nucleoli. One-quarter to one-third of these women will be diagnosed with endometrioid carcinoma at immediate hysterectomy or during the first year of follow-up. (2).

EIN refers to a monoclonal neoplastic growth of genetically altered cells with a greatly increased risk of becoming the endometrioid type of endometrial adenocarcinoma. The main diagnostic criterion of EIN is that the gland area exceeds that of the stroma (volume percentage stroma <55%). Atypical hyperplasia/EIN contains many of the genetic changes seen in endometrioid endometrial carcinoma, that is, microsatellite instability, and *PTEN, KRAS,* and *CTNNB1* (beta-catenin) mutation (1, 2).

Clinical features

Hysterectomy is usually the therapy of choice if a woman does not want more children. Women who want more children or those with high operative risks may be treated with progestins.

Endometrial adenocarcinoma

Endometrial carcinoma is the sixth most frequent cancer diagnosed in women globally with an age-standardized incidence rate of 8.2 per 100,000. It is the fourth most common cancer in women in industrialized countries and the most common gynaecological cancer. Three-quarters of women with endometrial cancer are postmenopausal. The median age at diagnosis is 63 years (1, 2).

Endometrial carcinoma is classified into two different types (**Figure 70.5** and **Table 70.1**). Type I tumours (**Figure 70.5a**) (about 80%), endometrioid carcinomas, are often preceded by endometrial hyperplasia or EIN and are associated with oestrogenic stimulation. They occur mainly in pre- or perimenopausal women and are associated with obesity, hyperlipidaemia, anovulation, infertility, and late menopause. Typically, most endometrioid carcinomas are confined to the uterus and follow a favourable course. In contrast, type II tumours (**Figure 70.5b**) (about 10%) are non-endometrioid, largely serous carcinomas, arising occasionally in endometrial polyps. Type II tumours are not associated with oestrogen stimulation or hyperplasia, readily invade myometrium and vascular spaces, and are highly lethal (1).

Endometrial cancer is the most common extracolonic cancer in women with hereditary non-polyposis colon cancer syndrome, a defect in DNA mismatch repair that is also associated with breast and ovarian cancers (5).

Molecular pathogenesis

A dualistic model of endometrial carcinogenesis has been proposed. According to this model, normal endometrial cells transform into endometrioid carcinoma through replication errors, so-called microsatellite instability (**Figure 70.5e**) and subsequent accumulation of mutations in oncogenes and tumour suppressor genes. For non-endometrioid carcinomas, alterations of p53 (Figures 70.5f and 70.5g) and loss of heterozygosity on several chromosomes drive malignant transformation (5).

Five main molecular alterations have been described in type I endometrioid carcinomas: microsatellite instability (25–30% of cases) (**Figure 70.5e**); *PTEN* mutations (30–60%); *PIK3CA* mutations (26–39%); *ARID1A* mutations (20%); *K-RAS* mutations (10–30%); and *CTNNB1* (beta-catenin) mutations with nuclear protein accumulation (25–38%). In contrast, most type II non-endometrioid carcinomas have p53 mutations (**Figure 70.5g**), Her-2/*neu* amplification, and loss of heterozygosity on several chromosomes. Non-endometrioid carcinomas may also derive from endometrioid carcinoma with microsatellite instability through tumour progression and subsequent p53 mutations (5).

The Cancer Genome Atlas (TCGA) has conducted the most comprehensive genomic analysis of endometrial carcinomas reported to date (8). TCGA has expanded the dualistic classification of endometrial carcinoma (types I and II) to four distinct molecular subgroups: (1) an ultramutated *POLE* subgroup; (2) a hypermutated microsatellite unstable subgroup; (3) a copy-number low/microsatellite stable subgroup; and (4) and a copy-number high/serous-like subgroup. Even if overlapping of the molecular genetic findings makes it still difficult to separate significant prognostic categories, *POLE* mutations predict favourable prognosis, particularly in high-grade tumours. Patients with endometrioid tumours that are serous-like at the molecular level might benefit from treatments that are typically used for serous carcinomas (6).

Pathology

Endometrioid adenocarcinoma of the endometrium

This type of endometrial cancer is composed entirely of glandular cells and is the most common histological variant (80–85%) (**Figure 70.5c**). The FIGO system divides this tumour into three grades on the basis of the ratio of glandular to solid elements, the latter signifying poorer differentiation. Less common histological variants include endometrioid adenocarcinoma with squamous differentiation and the mucinous and secretory types, both associated with good prognosis (1–3).

Non-endometrioid endometrial carcinomas

They are aggressive as a group, and histological grading is not clinically useful, all cases being considered high grade:

- Serous adenocarcinoma histologically resembles, and behaves like, high-grade serous adenocarcinoma of the ovary (Figure 70.5d). It often shows transtubal spread to peritoneal surfaces. An intraepithelial form has been termed 'serous endometrial intraepithelial carcinoma' (serous EIC), not to be confused with EIN, described earlier. Patients with this type of tumour need to be staged and treated as if they had ovarian cancer.
- Clear cell adenocarcinoma is a tumour of older women. It contains large cells with abundant cytoplasmic glycogen ('clear cells')

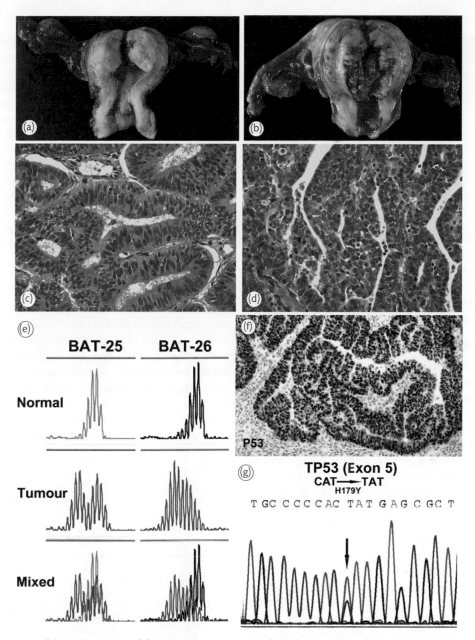

Figure 70.5 Adenocarcinoma of the endometrium. (a) Endometrioid carcinoma (type I). Polypoid endometrial tumour with only superficial myometrial invasion. (b) Serous (non-endometrioid) carcinoma (type II). Large haemorrhagic and necrotic tumour with deeper myometrial invasion. (c) Well-differentiated (grade 1) endometrioid adenocarcinoma. The neoplastic glands resemble normal endometrial glands. (d) Serous (non-endometrioid) carcinoma exhibiting stratification of markedly atypical tumour cells with numerous mitoses. (e) Endometrioid carcinoma. MLH1 inactivation by promoter hypermethylation is the most common cause of the microsatellite instability (MI) phenotype in endometrioid endometrial carcinoma. Progressive accumulation of alterations secondary to MI affects important regulatory genes, and promotes carcinogenesis. (f) Serous (non-endometrioid) carcinoma usually shows a strong p53 overexpression as a result of TP53 mutation (g).

or cells with bulbous nuclei that line glandular lumina ('hobnail cells'). Clear cell carcinomas have poor prognosis.

- Carcinosarcoma (malignant mixed mesodermal tumour): in this highly malignant tumour, pleomorphic epithelial cells intermingle with areas showing mesenchymal differentiation. These mixed neoplasms are derived from a common clone thought to be of epithelial origin. Overall 5-year survival is 25% (1, 2).

Clinical features

Unlike cervical cancer, endometrial cancer may spread directly to para-aortic lymph nodes, thereby skipping pelvic nodes. Patients with advanced cancers may also develop pulmonary metastases (40% of cases with metastases).

Women with well-differentiated cancers confined to the endometrium are usually treated by simple hysterectomy. Postoperative radiation is considered if (1) the tumour is poorly differentiated or non-endometrioid in type; (2) the myometrium is deeply invaded; (3) the cervix is involved; or (4) the lymph nodes contain metastases.

Survival in endometrial carcinoma is related to multiple factors: (1) stage, histotype, and, for endometrioid tumours, grade; (2) age; and (3) other risk factors, such as progesterone receptor activity, depth of myometrial invasion, and extent of lymphovascular

Table 70.1 Clinicopathological features of endometrial carcinoma

	Type I: endometrioid carcinoma	Type II: serous carcinoma
Age	Pre- and perimenopausal	Postmenopausal
Unopposed oestrogen	Present	Absent
Hyperplasia precursor	Present	Absent
Grade	Low	High
Myometrial invasion	Superficial	Deep
Growth behaviour	Stable	Progressive
Genetic alterations	Microsatellite instability, *PTEN, PIK3CA*, β-catenin	*TP53* mutations, loss of heterozygosity

invasion (7). Actuarial survival of all patients with endometrial cancer following treatment is 80% after 2 years, decreasing to 65% after 10 years. Tumours that have penetrated the myometrium or invaded lymphatics are more likely to have spread beyond the uterus. Endometrial cancers involving the cervix have a poorer prognosis. Spread outside the uterus entails the worst outlook (3, 7).

Endometrial sarcomas

Currently, endometrial sarcomas are classified into three categories: (a) low-grade endometrial stromal sarcoma (LGESS); (b) high-grade endometrial stromal sarcoma (HGESS); and (c) undifferentiated endometrial sarcoma (UES) (2). LGESSs represent less than 2% of uterine cancers. They may be polypoid or may diffusely invade the myometrium. The tumour cells resemble endometrial stromal cells in the proliferative phase. Nuclear atypia may be minimal to severe and mitotic activity may be restrained. Expression of CD10 and oestrogen and progesterone receptors helps confirm the diagnosis. The most common cytogenetic abnormality of LGESS is a recurrent translocation involving chromosomes 7 and 17 t(7;17)(p15;q21) which results in a fusion between *JAZF1* and *SUZ12* genes (formerly designated as JJAZ1) (1, 2).

The recently re-established HGESS has features intermediate between LGESSs and undifferentiated sarcomas. It may appear as intracavitary polypoid or a mural mass. Microscopically, it consists predominantly of high-grade round-cells which are sometimes associated with a low-grade spindle cell component usually fibromyxoid. Mitotic activity is very striking and typically greater than ten per 10 high power fields (HPF). Necrosis is usually present. HGESS typically harbours the *YWHAE–FAM22* genetic fusion as a result of t(10;17)(q22;p13) (1, 2).

Higher-grade poorly differentiated sarcomas originating in the endometrium are designated as undifferentiated endometrial sarcoma (1, 2).

Clinical features

Many years may elapse before LGESSs recur clinically, and metastases may occur even if the original tumour was confined to the uterus at initial surgery. Recurrences usually involve the pelvis first, followed by lung metastases. Prolonged survival and even cure are feasible, despite metastases. By contrast, UESs recur early, generally with widespread metastases. In comparison to patients with LGESSs, those with HGESSs and UES, have earlier and more frequent recurrences (often <1 year) and are more likely to die of disease. LGESSs can be successfully treated with surgery and progestin therapy, with an expectation of 90% survival 10 years after diagnosis (1, 2).

Uterine adenosarcoma

Uterine (Mullerian) adenosarcoma is a distinctive low-grade tumour with benign glandular epithelium and malignant stroma. It should be distinguished from carcinosarcoma, in which both epithelial and stromal elements are malignant and which is highly aggressive. One-quarter of patients with adenosarcoma, particularly cases with myometrial invasion and sarcomatous overgrowth, eventually succumb to local recurrence or metastatic spread (1, 2).

Leiomyosarcoma

Leiomyosarcoma is a malignancy of smooth muscle origin whose incidence is only 1/1000 that of leiomyoma. It accounts for 2% of uterine malignancies. Its pathogenesis is uncertain. Women with leiomyosarcomas are on average more than a decade older (age >50 years) than those with leiomyomas, and the malignant tumours are larger (10–15 cm vs 3–5 cm) (1, 2).

Pathology

Leiomyosarcoma should be suspected if an apparent leiomyoma is soft, shows areas of necrosis on gross examination, or has irregular borders (invasion of adjacent myometrium). Mitotic activity (ten or more mitoses per 10 HPFs), nuclear atypia, and geographic necrosis are the best diagnostic criteria (Figures 70.6a and 70.6b). Myxoid and epithelioid leiomyosarcomas may contain only five mitoses per

(a)
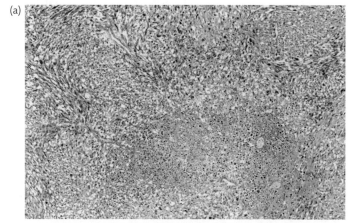

(b)
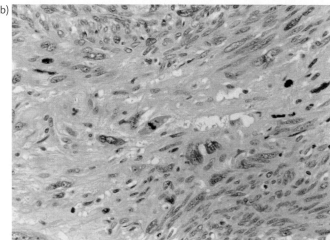

Figure 70.6 Leiomyosarcoma of the uterus. (a) A zone of coagulative tumour necrosis appears demarcated from the viable tumour. (b) The tumour shows considerable nuclear atypia and abundant mitotic activity.

10 HPFs. Size is important as tumours less than 5 cm in diameter almost never recur.

Most leiomyosarcomas are large and are advanced when detected. They are usually fatal despite combinations of surgery, radiation therapy, and chemotherapy. Five-year survival is about 25% (1, 2).

Fallopian tube

Tumours of the fallopian tube are rare. Most primary malignancies are adenocarcinomas, with peak incidence among women aged 50–60 years. Recent observations suggest that some cases of high-grade serous carcinoma of the ovary (see later paragraphs) may arise from the fimbriated end of the fallopian tube. Tubal carcinomas behave similarly to ovarian carcinoma and frequently appear as a solid mass in the wall of a grossly dilated tube, but may sometimes only be identified upon microscopic examination. The tumour is bilateral in 25% of cases. Prognosis is poor, as the disease is almost always detected at advanced stage (1, 2).

Risk reducing salpingo-oophorectomy

An increasingly common indication for salpingectomy is prophylactic for patients who have *BRCA1/2* gene mutations, a personal history of breast cancer, or strong family history of breast and/or tubo-ovarian cancer. Typically the specimen is grossly unremarkable, however these fallopian tubes, along with the corresponding ovaries, should be submitted entirely for histological examination (1, 2).

Ovary

Ovarian tumours

There are many types of ovarian tumours including benign, borderline, and malignant types. About two-thirds occur in women of reproductive age. Approximately 80% of ovarian tumours are benign. Almost 90% of malignant and borderline tumours are diagnosed after the age of 40 years (1, 8).

Ovarian tumours are classified by the cell type of origin. Most are common epithelial tumours (approximately 60%). Other important groups are germ cell tumours (30%), sex cord/stromal tumours (8%), and tumours metastatic to the ovary. Common epithelial tumours account for about 90% of ovarian malignancies, high-grade serous adenocarcinoma being the most common (70%).

Ovarian cancer is the second most frequent gynaecological malignancy after endometrial cancer and carries a higher mortality rate than all other female genital cancers combined. As it is difficult to detect early in its evolution when it is still curable, over three-quarters of patients already have extraovarian tumour spread to the pelvis or abdomen at the time of diagnosis (1, 8).

Epithelial tumours

Tumours of common epithelial origin can be broadly classified, according to cell proliferation, degree of nuclear atypia, and presence or absence of stromal invasion: (1) benign, (2) of borderline malignancy, and (3) carcinoma.

Common epithelial neoplasms most commonly affect nulliparous women and occur least frequently in women in whom ovulation has been suppressed (e.g. by pregnancy or oral contraceptives). Whereas

the lifetime risk for developing ovarian cancer in the general population is 1.6%, women with one first-degree relative with ovarian cancer have a 5% risk. Also, women with a family history of ovarian carcinoma are at greater risk for breast cancer and vice versa. Defects in repair genes implicated in hereditary breast cancers, *BRCA1* and *BRCA2*, are incriminated in familial ovarian cancers as well. As for endometrial carcinoma, women with hereditary non-polyposis colon cancer (HNPCC) are also at greater risk for ovarian cancer (1, 8).

Epithelial ovarian tumours are primarily classified according to cell type into serous, mucinous, endometrioid, clear cell, transitional, and squamous cell tumours (1, 2, 8). However, none of these cells are found in the normal ovary and their development has long been attributed to Mullerian 'neometaplasia' of the ovarian surface epithelium (mesothelium). During embryonic life, the coelomic cavity is lined by mesothelium which also covers the gonadal ridge. The same mesothelial lining gives rise to Mullerian ducts, from which the fallopian tubes, uterus, and vagina arise. Thus, the tumour cells would resemble morphologically the epithelia of the fallopian tube, endometrium, or endocervix (1, 8). Recently, it has been hypothesized that cytokeratin 7-positive embryonic/stem cells would give rise to immunophenotypically distinct neoplastic progeny (9) which would support the old concept of 'Mullerian neometaplasia'. Besides the mesothelial origin, there is now compelling evidence that a number of what have been thought to be primary ovarian cancers actually originate in other pelvic organs and involve the ovary secondarily. It has been shown that some high-grade serous carcinomas arise from precursor epithelial lesions in the distal fimbriated end of the fallopian tube, whereas endometrioid and clear cell carcinomas originate from ovarian endometriosis (8).

Borderline tumours

Borderline tumours show epithelial proliferation greater than that seen in their benign counterparts and variable nuclear atypia; however, in contrast to carcinomas, there is absence of stromal invasion, and their prognosis is much better than that of carcinomas.

Serous borderline tumours generally occur in women aged 20–50 years (average, 46 years). Serous tumours are more commonly bilateral (34%) than mucinous ones (6%) or other types. The tumours vary in size, although mucinous tumours may be gigantic. Serous borderline tumours have one or more cysts lined to varying extents by papillary projections, ranging from fine and exuberant to grape-like clusters. These structures show (1) epithelial stratification, (2) moderate nuclear atypia, and (3) mitotic activity. By definition, the presence of more than focal microinvasion (i.e. discrete nests of epithelial cells <3 mm into the ovarian stroma) identifies a tumour as low-grade serous carcinoma (LGSC), rather than a borderline tumour (1, 2).

Despite the lack of ovarian stromal invasion, serous borderline tumours, particularly those with exophytic growth, can implant on peritoneal surfaces and, rarely (about 10% of peritoneal implants), progress to LGSC and invade the underlying tissues. Histopathologically, invasive peritoneal implants and LGSC are identical lesions only distinguished by the timing of the disease and the volume of the tumour. Whereas invasive implants are early superficial lesions of microscopic or small macroscopic size (≤1–2 cm), LGSC frequently presents as bulky disease (peritoneal carcinomatosis) (1, 2, 8).

Surgical cure is almost always possible if the serous borderline tumour is confined to the ovaries. Even if it has spread to the pelvis or abdomen, 90% of patients are alive after 5 years. Although there is a significant rate of late recurrence, the tumours rarely recur beyond 10 years. Late progression to LGSC has been reported in approximately 7% of cases (1, 2, 7). After fertility-sparing surgery, mucinous borderline tumours may 'recur' as carcinomas in the contralateral ovary; however, such tumours should be considered independent primary tumours (10, 11).

Malignant epithelial tumours (carcinomas)

Carcinomas of the ovary are most common in women aged 40–60 years, and are rare under the age of 35 years. Based on light microscopy and molecular genetics, ovarian carcinomas are classified into five main subtypes, which, in descending order of frequency, are high-grade serous carcinomas (>70%), endometrioid carcinomas (10%), clear cell carcinomas (10%), mucinous carcinomas (3–4%), and LGSCs (<5%) (8) (Table 70.2). These subtypes, which account for 98% of ovarian carcinomas, can be reproducibly diagnosed and are inherently different diseases, as indicated by differences in epidemiological and genetic risk factors, precursor lesions, patterns of spread, molecular events during oncogenesis, responses to chemotherapy, and outcomes. With progress towards subtype-specific management of ovarian cancer, accurate subtype assignment is becoming increasingly important.

Serous carcinomas

Molecular pathogenesis

Low-grade and high-grade serous carcinomas are fundamentally different tumours. Whereas low-grade tumours are frequently associated with serous borderline tumours and have mutations of *KRAS* or *BRAF* oncogenes, high-grade serous carcinomas lack ovarian precursor lesions and have a high frequency of mutations in *TP53*, but not in *KRAS* or *BRAF*. Interestingly, carcinomas arising in patients with germline *BRCA1* or *BRCA2* mutations (hereditary ovarian cancers) are almost invariably the high-grade serous type and commonly have *TP53* mutations. An undetermined number of *BRCA1*- or *BRCA2*-related tumours arise from the epithelium of the

fimbriated end of the fallopian tube, suggesting that at least some sporadic high-grade ovarian and 'primary' peritoneal serous carcinomas may actually develop from the distal fallopian tube and 'spill over' onto the adjacent tissues (Table 70.2) (1, 8).

Pathology

High-grade serous carcinomas are the most common ovarian cancers and most patients present with advanced stage disease (approximately 80%). Two-thirds of serous cancers with extraovarian spread are bilateral. They are predominantly solid masses, usually with necrosis and haemorrhage and typically show obvious stromal invasion. Most tumours have a high nuclear grade with highly cellular papillae and solid areas (Figure 70.7a). The mitotic rate is very high. Psammoma bodies are often present (1, 2, 8).

LGSCs show irregular stromal invasion by small, tight nests of tumour cells within variable desmoplasia. The uniformity of the nuclei is the principal criterion for distinguishing low- and high-grade serous carcinomas (Figure 70.7b). LGSCs rarely progress to high-grade tumours (1, 2, 8).

Mucinous carcinoma

Molecular pathogenesis

Mucinous ovarian tumours are often heterogeneous. Benign, borderline, non-invasive, and invasive carcinoma components may coexist within the same tumour. Such a morphological continuum suggests that tumour progression occurs from cystadenoma and borderline tumour to non-invasive, microinvasive, and invasive carcinomas. This hypothesis is supported by *KRAS* mutations in mucinous tumours: 56% of cystadenomas and 85% of carcinomas express mutated *KRAS*, with borderline tumours being intermediate (Table 70.2) (1, 8).

Pathology

Mucinous carcinomas are usually large, unilateral, multilocular cystic masses containing mucinous fluid. They often exhibit papillary architecture (Figure 70.7c). Since benign and malignant components may coexist within a single specimen, these tumours should be sampled extensively. Mucinous tumours are bilateral in only 5%

Table 70.2 Main types of ovarian carcinoma

	High-grade serous	Low-grade serous	Mucinous	Endometrioid	Clear cell
Usual stage at diagnosis	Advanced	Early or advanced	Early	Early	Early
Presumed tissue of origin/ precursor lesion	Tubal metaplasia in inclusions of ovarian surface epithelium or fallopian tube	Serous borderline tumour	Adenoma–borderline– carcinoma sequence; teratoma	Endometriosis, adenofibroma	Endometriosis, adenofibroma
Genetic risk	BRCA1/2	?	?	HNPCC	?
Significant molecular abnormalities	p53 and pRb pathways	*BRAF* or *KRAS*	*KRAS*	*PTEN* β-catenin *ARID1A* *PIK3CA* *K-RAS* Microsatellite instability	*HNF1B* *ARID1A* *PIC3CA*
Proliferation	High	Low	Intermediate	Low	Low
Response to primary chemotherapy	80%	26–28%	15%	?	15%
Prognosis	Poor	Favourable	Favourable	Favourable	Intermediate

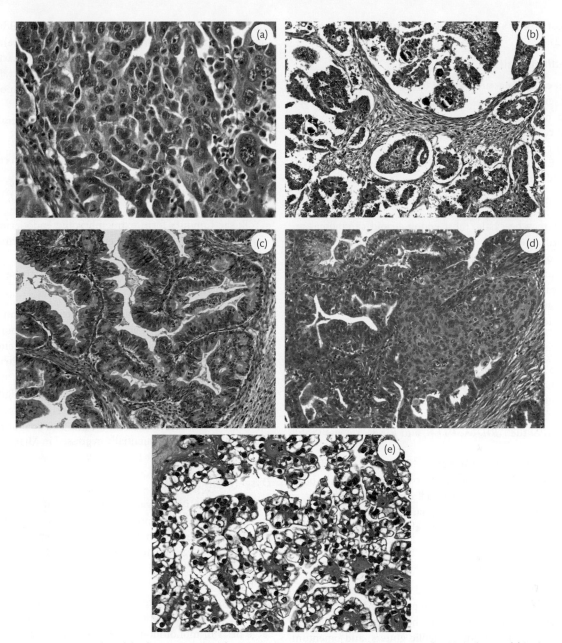

Figure 70.7 Representative examples of the five main types of ovarian carcinoma, which together account for 98% of cases: (a) high-grade serous carcinoma; (b) low-grade serous carcinoma; (c) mucinous carcinoma; (d) endometrioid carcinoma; and (e) clear cell carcinoma.

of the cases; thus, finding bilateral or unilateral mucinous tumours smaller than 10 cm should raise suspicion of metastases from a mucinous carcinoma elsewhere (e.g. gastrointestinal tract).

The category of mucinous borderline tumour with intraepithelial carcinoma is reserved for tumours that lack architectural features of invasive carcinoma but, focally, show unequivocally malignant cells lining glandular spaces. Mucinous borderline tumours with intraepithelial carcinoma have a very low likelihood of recurrence (1, 2, 8).

Mucinous carcinomas showing expansile or confluent glandular growth appear to have a more favourable prognosis than mucinous carcinomas with destructive stromal invasion. The combination of extensive infiltrative stromal invasion, high nuclear grade, and tumour rupture should be considered a strong predictor of recurrence for stage I mucinous carcinomas (1, 2, 8).

Pseudomyxoma peritonei is a clinical condition of abundant gelatinous or mucinous ascites in the peritoneum, fibrous adhesions, and frequently mucinous tumours involving the ovaries. The appendix is also involved by a similar mucinous tumour in 60% of the cases and appears normal in the remaining 40%. Current data suggest that in most cases the ovarian tumours are metastases from the appendiceal lesions (1, 2).

Endometrioid carcinoma

Endometrioid carcinoma histologically resembles its uterine counterpart (**Figure 70.7**d), may have areas of squamous differentiation, and is second only to serous carcinoma in frequency. It accounts for 10% of all ovarian cancers. These tumours occur most commonly after menopause. Up to half of these cancers are bilateral and, at diagnosis, most tumours are either confined to the ovary or within the pelvis (1, 2).

Molecular pathogenesis

Endometrioid carcinomas are thought to arise by malignant transformation of endometriosis, and not from ovarian surface epithelium. The most common genetic abnormalities in sporadic endometrioid carcinoma of the ovary are somatic mutations of the *ARID1A*, beta-catenin (*CTNNB1*), and *PTEN* genes and microsatellite instability. Endometrioid borderline tumours also have *CTNNB1* mutations (Table 70.2) (8).

Pathology

Although they may be cystic, most endometrioid carcinomas are largely solid with areas of necrosis. These tumours are graded like their uterine counterparts. Between 15% and 20% of patients also harbour a uterine endometrioid carcinoma. Strong data suggest that most of these cases arise independently, although some may be metastases from one or the other. This distinction has important prognostic implications (1, 2).

Clear cell carcinoma

This enigmatic ovarian cancer is closely related to endometrioid adenocarcinoma, and often occurs in association with endometriosis. It constitutes 5–10% of all ovarian cancers usually occurring after menopause. The most common genetic abnormalities are somatic mutations of the *ARID1A, PTEN,* and *PIK3CA* genes (Table 70.2) (1, 8).

Although patients typically present with stage I or II disease, clear cell carcinomas have a poor prognosis compared with other low-stage ovarian carcinomas. Clear cell carcinomas of the ovary resemble their counterparts in the vagina, cervix, and corpus; they show sheets or tubules of malignant cells with clear cytoplasm (Figure 70.7e).

Clinical features

By the time ovarian cancers are diagnosed, many have metastasized to (i.e. implanted on) the surfaces of the pelvis, abdominal organs, or bladder. Ovarian tumours have a tendency to implant in the peritoneal cavity on the diaphragm, paracolic gutters, and omentum. Lymphatic spread is preferentially to para-aortic lymph nodes near the origin of the renal arteries and to a lesser extent to external iliac (pelvic) or inguinal lymph nodes (1, 2).

Survival for patients with malignant ovarian tumours is generally poor. The most important prognostic index is the surgical stage of the tumour at the time it is detected (12). Overall, 5-year survival is only 35%. Prognostic indices for epithelial tumours also include histological type (grade) and the size of the residual neoplasm.

Surgery, which removes the primary tumour, establishes the diagnosis, and determines the extent of spread, is the mainstay of therapy. The peritoneal surfaces, omentum, liver, subdiaphragmatic recesses, and all abdominal regions must be visualized, and as much metastatic tumour removed as possible. Adjuvant chemotherapy is used to treat distant occult sites of tumour spread.

Germ cell tumours

Tumours derived from germ cells make up one-quarter of ovarian tumours. In adult women, ovarian germ cell tumours are virtually all benign (mature cystic teratoma or dermoid cyst), but in children

and young adults, they are largely cancerous. In children, germ cell tumours are the most common ovarian cancer (60%); they are rare after menopause. Rarely, germ cell tumours may arise from pre-existing somatic neoplasms of the female genital tract. In these cases, the teratoid tumours derive most likely from a pluripotent stem cell population of somatic neoplasms (1, 2).

Neoplastic germ cells may differentiate along several lines producing the following tumours:

- Dysgerminomas are composed of neoplastic germ cells, similar to oogonia of fetal ovaries
- Teratomas differentiate towards somatic (embryonic or adult) tissues.
- Yolk sac tumours form extraembryonic endoderm and mesenchyme and, less frequently, embryonic endodermal derivatives (intestine and liver).
- Choriocarcinomas feature cells similar to those covering the placental villi.

Malignant germ cell tumours in women older than 40 years usually result from transformation of one of the components of a benign cystic teratoma. Malignant germ cell tumours tend to be highly aggressive; however, with current chemotherapy, survival rates for many exceed 80% (1, 2).

Recent stem cell research has provided several highly diagnostic pluripotency markers, including transcription factors (SALL4, LIN28, OCT3/4, and SOX2) and cytoplasmic/membranous proteins (glypican-3) that are sequentially expressed in MGCTs according to their differentiation stage (1, 2).

Dysgerminoma

Dysgerminoma is the ovarian counterpart of testicular seminoma, and is composed of primordial germ cells. It accounts for less than 2% of ovarian cancers in all women. Most patients are between 10 and 30 years of age. The tumours are bilateral in about 15% of cases.

Pathology

Dysgerminomas are often large and firm and have a bosselated external surface. The cut surface is soft and fleshy. They contain large nests of monotonously uniform tumour cells that have clear glycogen-filled cytoplasm and irregularly flattened central nuclei. Fibrous septa containing lymphocytes traverse the tumour (1, 2).

Dysgerminomas are treated surgically; 5-year survival for patients with a stage I tumour approaches 100%. As the tumour is highly radiosensitive and also responsive to chemotherapy, even for higher-stage tumours 5-year survival rates still exceed 80%.

Teratoma

Teratoma is a tumour of germ cell origin that differentiates towards somatic structures. Most teratomas contain tissues from at least two, and usually all three, embryonic layers. Immature teratomas contain elements derived from the three germ layers. However, unlike mature cystic teratomas, immature teratomas contain embryonal tissues. These tumours account for 20% of malignant tumours in women under the age of 20. Microscopically, they show multiple components such as immature neural tissue (neuroepithelial rosettes and glia), glands, and other structures found in mature cystic teratomas. Grading is based on the amount of immature tissue present. Survival correlates with tumour grade (1, 2).

Yolk sac tumour

Yolk sac tumours are highly malignant neoplasms in women under the age of 30 years that histologically resemble the endoderm and mesenchyme of the primitive yolk sac (extra-embryonal) and embryonal somatic tissues (intestine and liver). They are typically large, with extensive necrosis and haemorrhage. The most common histotype is the reticular form. Schiller–Duval bodies are characteristic. They consist of papillae that protrude into spaces lined by tumour cells, resembling the glomerular spaces. The papillae are covered by a mantle of embryonal cells and contain a fibrovascular core and a central blood vessel.

Yolk sac tumours secrete alpha-fetoprotein. Detection of alpha-fetoprotein in the blood is useful for diagnosis and for monitoring the effectiveness of therapy. Once uniformly fatal, 5-year survival with chemotherapy for stage I yolk sac tumours exceeds 80% (1, 2).

Choriocarcinoma

Choriocarcinoma of the ovary is a rare tumour that mimics the epithelial covering of placental villi, namely, cytotrophoblast and syncytiotrophoblast. The pregnancy test is positive and the elevated serum level of human chorionic gonadotropin (hCG) may lead to precocious sexual development in young girls or menstrual abnormalities in older patients.

Sex cord/stromal tumours

These represent 10% of ovarian tumours, vary from benign to low-grade malignant, and may differentiate towards female (granulosa and theca cells) or male (Sertoli and Leydig cells) structures (1, 2).

Granulosa cell tumour

Granulosa cell tumours are the prototypical functional neoplasms of the ovary associated with oestrogen secretion. They should be considered low-grade malignancies because of their potential for local spread and the rare occurrence of distant metastases.

Most granulosa cell tumours occur after menopause (adult form) and are unusual before puberty. A juvenile form occurs in children and young women and has distinct clinical and pathological features (hyperoestrinism and precocious puberty).

Pathology

Adult-type granulosa cell tumours are large and focally cystic to solid. The cut surface shows yellow areas, due to lipid-rich luteinized granulosa cells, white zones of stroma, and focal haemorrhages. Random nuclear arrangement about a central degenerative space (Call–Exner bodies) gives a characteristic follicular pattern. Tumour cells secrete alpha-inhibin, a protein that suppresses pituitary release of follicle-stimulating hormone. Besides alpha-inhibin, calretinin and FOXL2 are the most important positive immunoreactions (1, 2).

Clinical features

Three-quarters of granulosa cell tumours secrete oestrogens. Thus, endometrial hyperplasia is a common presenting sign. Endometrial adenocarcinoma may develop if a functioning granulosa cell tumour remains undetected. At diagnosis, 90% of granulosa cell tumours are within the ovary (stage I). Over 90% of these patients survive 10 years. Tumours that have extended into the pelvis and lower abdomen have a poorer prognosis. Late recurrence after surgical removal is not uncommon after 5–10 years and is usually fatal (1, 2).

Sertoli–Leydig cell tumours

Ovarian Sertoli–Leydig cell tumours are rare androgen-secreting mesenchymal neoplasms of low malignant potential that resemble embryonic testis. Tumour cells typically secrete weak androgens (dehydroepiandrosterone). Sertoli–Leydig cell tumours occur at all ages but are most common in young women of childbearing age. They vary from well to poorly differentiated and some have heterologous elements (e.g. mucinous glands and, rarely, even skeletal muscle and cartilage).

Nearly half of all patients with Sertoli–Leydig cell tumours exhibit signs of virilization. Initial signs are often defeminization, manifested as breast atrophy, amenorrhea, and loss of hip fat. Once the tumour is removed, these signs disappear or at least lessen. Well-differentiated tumours are virtually always cured by surgical resection, but poorly differentiated ones may metastasize (1, 2).

Steroid cell tumour

Steroid cell tumours of the ovary, also called lipid cell tumours, are composed of cells that resemble lutein cells, Leydig cells, and adrenal cortical cells. Most steroid cell tumours are hormonally active, usually with androgenic manifestations.

Tumours metastatic to the ovary

About 3% of cancers found in the ovaries arise elsewhere, mostly in the large intestine, breast, endometrium, and stomach, in descending order. These tumours vary from microscopic lesions to large masses. Metastatic tumours large enough to cause symptoms originate most often in the colon.

Krukenberg tumours are metastases to the ovary, composed of nests of mucin-filled 'signet-ring' cells in a cellular stroma derived from the ovary. The stomach is the primary site in 75% of cases and most of the rest are from the colon (1, 2).

Bilateral ovarian involvement and multinodularity suggest a metastatic carcinoma, and both ovaries are grossly involved in 75% of cases.

Gestational trophoblastic disease

The term gestational trophoblastic disease is a spectrum of disorders with abnormal trophoblast proliferation and maturation, as well as neoplasms derived from trophoblast (see Chapter 66).

Complete hydatidiform mole

Complete hydatidiform mole is a placenta with grossly swollen chorionic villi, resembling bunches of grapes, and showing varying degrees of trophoblastic proliferation. Villi are enlarged, often exceeding 5 mm in diameter.

Molecular pathogenesis and aetiological factors

Complete mole results from fertilization of an empty ovum that lacks functional maternal DNA. Most commonly, a haploid (23,X) set of paternal chromosomes introduced by monospermy duplicates to 46,XX, but dispermic 46,XX and 46,XY moles also occur. Moles characteristically lack maternal chromosomes. Paternally imprinted genes, such as *p57* (also known as *CDKN1C*), in which only the maternal allele is expressed, are not expressed in villous trophoblasts of androgenetic-derived complete moles. Since the embryo dies at a very early stage, before placental circulation has developed, few chorionic villi develop blood vessels and fetal parts are absent. Women with a prior hydatidiform mole have a 20-fold greater risk of a subsequent molar pregnancy than the general population (1, 2).

Pathology

Microscopically, many individual villi have cisternae. Trophoblast is hyperplastic and composed of syncytiotrophoblast, cytotrophoblast, and intermediate trophoblast. Considerable cellular atypia is present.

Clinical features

Serum hCG levels are markedly elevated, and increase rapidly. Complications of complete mole include uterine haemorrhage, disseminated intravascular coagulation, uterine perforation, and trophoblastic embolism. The most important complication is development of choriocarcinoma, which occurs in about 2% of patients.

Treatment consists of suction curettage of the uterus under ultrasound guidance and an oxytocic infusion and subsequent monitoring of serum hCG levels. Up to 20% of patients require adjuvant chemotherapy for persistent disease, and a 100% cure rate is expected even under these circumstances.

Invasive hydatidiform mole

The villi of a hydatidiform mole may only enter the superficial myometrium or they may invade the uterus, and even the broad ligament. They tend to enter dilated venous channels of the myometrium and one-third spread to distant sites, mostly the lungs. Uterine perforation is a major complication, but occurs in only a minority of cases (1, 2).

Gestational choriocarcinoma

Choriocarcinoma occurs in 1 of 160,000 normal gestations, 1 of 15,000 spontaneous abortions, 1 of 5000 ectopic pregnancies, and 1 of 40 complete molar pregnancies. Unlike most other cancers, choriocarcinomas lack intrinsic tumour vasculature. Thus, the tumours are typically necrotic and haemorrhagic and viable tumour is confined to the rim of the neoplasm. There is a dimorphic population of cytotrophoblast and syncytiotrophoblast, with varying degrees of intermediate trophoblast. hCG is localized to the syncytiotrophoblastic element. By definition, tumours containing any villous structures, even if metastatic, are considered hydatidiform mole and not choriocarcinoma (1, 2).

Choriocarcinoma invades mainly through venous sinuses in the myometrium. It metastasizes widely via the bloodstream, especially to lungs (over 90%), brain, gastrointestinal tract, liver, and vagina. With current chemotherapy, recognition of risk factors (high hCG levels and prolonged interval since antecedent pregnancy), and early treatment, most patients are cured.

Placental site trophoblastic tumour

Placental site trophoblastic tumours are the least common trophoblastic tumours, and are mainly composed of intermediate trophoblastic cells. Mononuclear and multinuclear trophoblast may be present as sheets of cells interspersed among myometrial cells. No chorionic villi are seen. Placental site trophoblastic tumour is distinguished from choriocarcinoma by its monomorphic (intermediate) trophoblastic proliferation, unlike the dimorphic pattern of trophoblast in choriocarcinoma. Most trophoblastic cells express human placental lactogen, but a few express hCG (1, 2).

Placental site trophoblastic tumour must be excised completely (hysterectomy) to prevent local recurrence. It sometimes metastasizes and may be fatal. Large tumours and mitotic indices of more than five mitoses/10 HPFs are associated with worse prognosis.

REFERENCES

1. Mutter GL, Prat J (eds). *Pathology of the Female Reproductive Tract*, 3rd edn. Edinburgh: Churchill Livingstone; 2014.
2. Kurman RJ, Carcangiu ML, Herrington CS, Young RH (eds). *WHO Classification of Tumours of Female Reproductive Organs*, 4th edn. Lyon: IARC; 2014.
3. Mutch DG. The new FIGO staging system for cancers of the vulva, cervix, endometrium and sarcomas. *Gynecol Oncol* 2009;**115**:325–28.
4. Stoler MH. Human papillomaviruses and cervical neoplasia: a model for carcinogenesis. *Int J Gynecol Pathol* 2000;**19**:16–28.
5. Matias-Guiu X, Prat J. Molecular pathology of endometrial carcinoma. *Histopathology* 2013;**62**:111–23.
6. The Cancer Genome Atlas Research Network, Kandoth C, Schultz N, et al. Integrated genomic characterization of endometrial carcinoma. *Nature* 2013;**497**:67–73.
7. Prat J. Prognostic parameters of endometrial carcinoma. *Hum Pathol* 2004;**35**:649–62.
8. Prat J. Ovarian carcinomas: five distinct diseases with different origins, genetic alterations, and clinicopathological features. *Virchows Arch* 2012;**460**:237–49.
9. Crum CP, Herfs M, Ning G, et al. Through the glass darkly: intraepithelial neoplasia, top-down differentiation, and the road to ovarian cancer. *J Pathol* 2013;**231**:402–12.
10. Uzan C, Nikpayam M, Ribassin-Majed L, et al. Influence of histological subtypes on the risk of an invasive recurrence in a large series of stage I borderline ovarian tumor including 191 conservative treatments. *Ann Oncol* 2014;**25**:1312–19.
11. Prat J. The results of conservative (fertility-sparing) treatment in borderline ovarian tumors vary depending on age and histological type. *Ann Oncol* 2014;**25**:1255–58.
12. Prat J; FIGO Committee on Gynecologic Oncology. Staging classification for cancer of the ovary, fallopian tube, and peritoneum. *Int J Gynaecol Obstet* 2014;**124**:1–5.

71

Premalignant disease of the genital tract in pregnancy

Andy Nordin and Manas Chakrabarti

Introduction

The age of women at the time of delivery of their first child has been steadily increasing in the developed world for several generations. In the United States, the average age of first-time mothers increased by 3.6 years from 21.4 years in 1970 to 25.0 years in 2006 (1). Globally, the use of modern contraception methods has risen slightly, from 54% in 1990 to 57.4% in 2014. There remains inequality in the access to contraception in the developing world, with access remaining low in sub-Saharan Africa, and teenage pregnancy remains a major international public health problem. However, increasing contraceptive use in many parts of the developing world, especially in Asia and Latin America, enables women to delay childbirth, leading to a relative rise in the maternal age of first pregnancy (2).

As women extend their reproductive lives into their 30s and 40s, more pregnancies will be complicated by comorbidities of premalignant diseases of the genital tract. National cervical screening programmes are generally initiated at the age of 20 or 25 years, and in many countries opportunistic screening is performed during antenatal visits. It is therefore essential that clinicians understand the natural history, risk of progression to malignancy, and pregnancy implications of premalignant disease of the genital tract, in order to guide patients through difficult management decisions regarding treatment options.

Cervical intraepithelial neoplasia

Introduction: precancerous changes of cervix in pregnancy

Most of the precancerous lesions of the cervix occur in women of childbearing age. The mean age of incidence of precancerous changes of cervix requiring treatment is 30 years (3). The incidence of high-grade cervical intraepithelial neoplasia (CIN3) is four times higher at the age of 40 than at the age of 70 (4). In countries without a population-based cervical screening programme, many obstetricians, family doctors, and midwives take opportunistic cervical cytology samples at the time of the booking antenatal consultation.

Consequently, it is common to diagnose precancerous lesions during pregnancy. Many expectant mothers are anxious regarding the potential for fetal and pregnancy complications during pregnancy, and the news of a diagnosis of a precancerous condition heightens these anxieties.

Generally, clinicians and their patients need to decide between conservative management until after delivery or treatment during pregnancy, both of which can cause significant psychological morbidity. The overall risk of progression of CIN3 to invasive carcinoma is uncertain, but the limited observational data available suggests that it may be in the region of 30–50%. A retrospective observational study of 143 women in New Zealand with high-grade CIN managed conservatively showed a cumulative incidence of invasive cancer of the cervix or vaginal vault of 31.3% (95% confidence interval (CI) 22.7–42.3) at 30 years, and 50.3% (95% CI 37.3–64.9) in the subset of 92 such women who had persistent disease within 24 months (5). It is stated that the rate at which invasive cancer develops from CIN is usually slow, measured in years and perhaps decades (6). However, a meta-analysis of the published literature showed a small risk of progression of high-grade cervical cytology to invasive cancer over 24 months of 1.44% (95% CI 0–3.95%) (7). Quality data generally regarding the risk of progression and time to progression of cervical cancer in pregnancy is lacking. Interpretation of data is complicated by the possibility of occult microinvasive disease present at the time of initial presentation, which is only revealed on histology following excisional treatment after the puerperium in cases managed conservatively throughout pregnancy. However, it has been estimated that the risk of progression from high-grade preinvasive disease to carcinoma during pregnancy is likely to be low, in the order of 0.4% (8). Notwithstanding the low risk of malignant transformation, many patients experience anxieties about deferring treatment of known high-grade CIN until after the puerperium due to the risk of evolving cervical cancer.

Pregnancy and pathogenesis of CIN and cervical cancer

CIN arises from the transformation zone, where columnar epithelium transforms through a normal process called metaplasia into squamous epithelium. Dysplasia is the pathological process which distorts this process, under the impact of oncogenic 'high-risk' human papillomavirus (HPV) infection. Squamous metaplasia accelerates during puberty and most importantly during first pregnancy. The impact of first pregnancy on the transformation zone and the increased vulnerability to dysplasia appears to be greater in very young women, leading to AN increased risk of high-grade CIN and invasive cancer. Pooled data worldwide suggest the relative risk for developing cervical cancer in later life women with the first full-term pregnancy at age less than 17 years compared with 25 years or older is 1.77 (95% CI 1.42–2.23) (9).

Cervical cytology in pregnancy

Indication

In countries such as the United Kingdom with national cervical cancer screening programmes with effective call/recall systems, routine cervical cytology samples are generally avoided in pregnancy (10). However, in many countries pregnancy is thought to be an excellent opportunity to screen not only for precancerous cells in the cervix but also for various sexually transmitted infections. The benefit of opportunistic cervical cytology sampling is limited in a screened population, but can prove effective in reducing the incidence of cervical cancer in an otherwise unscreened cohort (11, 12).

Pitfalls

Performing a cytology sample in early pregnancy is safe, with no apparent risk to the pregnancy. However, cytological interpretation can be challenging and in some cases can cause confusion and a dilemma both for patients and clinicians. The pathologist must be informed if the sample is taken from a pregnant woman. Since 1960, a number of researchers have investigated unique pregnancy-related changes on cervical cytology samples in an effort to reduce diagnostic errors.

The cervix undergoes both glandular and stromal changes during pregnancy, similar to those occurring in the endometrium (13). The glandular epithelium frequently everts onto the ectocervix to form a glandular ectropion, caused by pregnancy-related hormonal effects, and subsequently the acidic vaginal milieu precipitates extensive squamous metaplasia. Immature metaplastic cells in a large quantity can be misinterpreted on cervical cytology as high-grade precancerous change.

Sloughed off decidual cells can be mistaken for high- or low-grade CIN as they acquire orangeophilic cytoplasm and pyknotic nuclei in the process of degeneration (14). Hyperplastic and hypertrophic endocervical glands with Arias-Stella type changes can mimic atypical glandular cells of uncertain significance (15, 16). The recommended investigations in non-pregnant patients of endocervical curetting and endometrial biopsy for atypical glandular cells are absolutely contraindicated in the pregnant population (17). Therefore, this has the potential of giving rise to anxiety for the entire duration of the pregnancy, before the changes can be effectively investigated after the puerperium. Transrectal ultrasound and diagnostic conization during pregnancy have been considered in these circumstances. However, the transrectal ultrasound has low sensitivity for small volume endocervical pathology in pregnancy, and conization is associated with significant pregnancy risks and cervical haemorrhage risk, and therefore neither are considered routine clinical practice (18, 19).

Colposcopy in pregnancy

Indication

Under most circumstances, colposcopy in pregnancy is performed to exclude invasive malignancy in order to safely defer treatment of high-grade CIN until after the natural completion of the pregnancy. The indications for colposcopy are the same as in non-pregnant patients, except that the follow-up colposcopy after adequate excisional treatment of CIN lesions can be deferred until completion of the postpartum period (10). Performing colposcopy is safe in pregnancy but the interpretation of findings is challenging because of varied pregnancy-induced changes of the cervix. Beyond 20 weeks' gestation, it is advisable to use corrective measures for the colposcopy couch to prevent gravid uterus-induced supine hypotension.

Pitfalls

Increased oestrogen levels in pregnancy increase the volume of the cervix, and cause pronounced eversion of the columnar epithelium leading to a glandular ectropion (20). When the upper limit of the transformation zone is hidden within the endocervical canal in early pregnancy, this frequently changes during the course of pregnancy leading to adequate colposcopy with full visualization of the transformation zone by the third trimester. However, during the second half of pregnancy the more relaxed vaginal walls and abundant cervical mucous can obscure visualization. Third-trimester colposcopy is more technically challenging and is best avoided where possible. The cervix appears vascular and oedematous, often with a blue discolouration of the squamous epithelium and florid glandular ectropion with contact bleeding, leading to inaccurate colposcopic suspicion of significant cervical pathology. It is easy to under- or overestimate the severity of the lesions during pregnancy. Proliferation and dilatation of cervical surface vessels progressively increase with pregnancy and lesions can appear higher grade colposcopically than revealed on histology. Decidualization of cervical stroma can mimic high-grade lesions with dense acetowhite plaques and spidery superficial blood vessels. Normal capillaries can develop decidualized stroma, which can appear acetowhite ('starry sky' appearance) (8). Conversely, colposcopists may falsely downgrade lesions as cervical oedema can reduce the intensity of acetowhite epithelial changes. With a high-grade intraepithelial lesion, signs of invasion are easily missed. Colposcopists are reluctant to take diagnostic biopsies due to the risk of haemorrhage, and an experienced colposcopist is required to interpret these changes clinically.

Management of CIN in pregnancy

In view of the difficulties and limitations of colposcopy in pregnancy, it is prudent to repeat colposcopy examination for the initial assessment of cervical cytology abnormalities 12 weeks following delivery, even if high-grade CIN is not detected. CIN1 in early pregnancy should be managed with initial conservative management. A significantly higher tendency of regression of CIN1 lesions in pregnancy compared with non-pregnant controls has been reported (69% vs 48.7%; $P = 0.03$) (21). The United Kingdom National Health Service Cervical Screening Programme recommends that if CIN2 or -3 is suspected, repeat colposcopy is recommended at the end of the second trimester, to exclude progression to invasive carcinoma. If the pregnancy has already advanced beyond the second trimester, colposcopy can be deferred until 3 months following delivery (22).

Providing colposcopy during pregnancy suggests stable disease, treatment can safely be deferred until after the natural completion of pregnancy.

Excisional treatment is rarely performed by most colposcopists during pregnancy, balancing the apparent low risk of progression to invasive disease with the potential for disruption to the pregnancy and the risk of haemorrhage. There is little evidence to quantify the risk of excisional or ablative treatment precipitating miscarriage. The risk of miscarriage and severe bleeding is likely to be small in the first trimester and some colposcopists advocate treatment of high-grade CIN if it presents very early in pregnancy. However, due to the apparent very low-risk of progression to cancer during the course of the pregnancy, most advocate conservative management. The risk of significant bleeding is generally small from diagnostic cervical biopsy and this can be performed safely in early pregnancy to confirm the diagnosis, and should always be performed if there is any suspicion of invasive carcinoma. Most colposcopists would only consider biopsy of the cervix beyond the end of the first trimester if cervical cancer is suspected.

If biopsy is indicated, sharp biopsy forceps should be used to reduce tearing damage to the vascular cervix. The pregnant cervix should not be biopsied without adequate recourse to means of haemostasis. Monsel's paste and silver nitrate should available, but both are caustic and can cause considerable slough if used for prolonged period on a pregnant cervix. Gelatine paste, oxidized regenerated collagen, microfibrillar collagen, or a thrombin-soaked gelatine sponge can be applied for haemostasis with or without vaginal packing if significant bleeding is encountered (8).

Particularly during pregnancy, cervical punch biopsy can miss invasive disease. If there is suspicion of an invasive carcinoma, a diagnostic wedge or diathermy loop biopsy should be considered, potentially during examination under anaesthesia. In keeping with other surgical procedures during pregnancy, the cumulative maternal and fetal risks may be lowest if the general anaesthesia procedure is performed during the second trimester. If carcinoma is confirmed in the first trimester, termination of pregnancy may be considered, while carcinoma diagnosed during the second trimester may be managed by expediting delivery once adequate fetal maturity has been achieved (23). Cases have been reported performing radical trachelectomy during pregnancy with preservation of the uterus (24) and utilizing chemotherapy during late pregnancy to manage the cancer while the pregnancy progresses (25). Investigation with magnetic resonance imaging can be performed during pregnancy, and depending on the stage, a Wertheim's hysterectomy caesarean section can be planned for delivery in conjunction with the obstetrics and neonatology teams (23).

Mode of delivery

It has been hypothesized that vaginal delivery will lead to extensive remodelling of the cervix, allowing a higher chance of spontaneous regression of precancerous lesions compared to caesarean section delivery (26). However, other authors suggest that mode of delivery is not a significant risk factor for either progression or regression of precancerous lesions (27).

There is concern regarding the vertical transmission of high-risk subtypes of HPV during vaginal delivery, posing a theoretical risk of conditions including recurrent respiratory papillomatosis. However, respiratory papillomatosis is most commonly caused by HPV subtypes 6 or 11, associated with benign genital warts, while high-grade CIN is most commonly associated with HPV 16 or 18 (28). It has been estimated that the risk of a child contracting recurrent respiratory papillomatosis from a mother who has active condylomata and delivers vaginally is approximately 1 in 400, and the maternal and fetal risks associated with caesarean section likely outweigh the small fetal risk of HPV transmission during vaginal delivery (29).

Therefore, the evidence suggests that the route of delivery of pregnant women with precancerous lesions of the cervix should be based on standard obstetric parameters.

Puerperium

Observational studies suggest that there is a trend of natural regression of severity of cervical precancerous changes through pregnancy and the puerperium (30–33). However, it is not clear if this relates to the extensive remodelling and inflammation that occurs in the cervix during pregnancy and the postpartum period, or because of the natural history of HPV infection. Both colposcopic and cytological assessments may be difficult during the immediate postpartum period because of the relative hypo-oestrogenic state. It is therefore advisable to defer assessment for at least 8–10 weeks following delivery, to allow involution of the cervix. In the United Kingdom, a 12-week interval is recommended (22). Cases of abnormal cervical cytology tests undergoing colposcopy during pregnancy should be reassessed with another colposcopy regardless of the findings during pregnancy. Colposcopists should be aware that compared to antenatal observations, lesions may appear smaller and more centrally located in the cervix after the puerperium (17).

Effect of excisional treatment on subsequent pregnancy

On fertility

It has been suggested that destruction and removal of part of the mucous-producing glands of the endocervix can interfere with fertility and a healthy pregnancy (34). Additionally, authors have proposed that cicatrization of the cervix after excisional treatment leads to cervical stenosis which may compromise fertility (35). Studies to evaluate such risks are difficult to conduct as there are many variables and confounding factors including social, clinical, psychological, and lifestyle issues. A large Finnish study involving follow-up of over 250,000 women-years did not report any negative effect on fertility (36). However, a United States-based study evaluating 152 treated women and 1172 untreated women, suggested an increased risk of subfertility with prolonged (>1 year) time to conceive (37). A systematic review and meta-analysis found no conclusive evidence to suggest that fertility is affected adversely by excisional treatment (38).

On pregnancy and preterm birth

First trimester

The rate of first-trimester miscarriage is not significantly different between women treated for CIN and untreated women. The rate of termination of pregnancy and ectopic pregnancy were found to be higher in treated women. The reason for this is unclear but may relate to lifestyle factors and sexual behaviours of the group of women studied, power of the studies analysed, or publication bias (38).

Second trimester

A meta-analysis identified a significantly higher rate of second-trimester miscarriage in women previously treated for CIN compared to the cohort without a history of CIN (relative risk 2.60; 95% CI 1.45–4.67). It is unclear if this is related to cervical weakness, ascending infection due to possible dysfunction of the mucous plug, or the method of excisional treatment (38). Analyses are complex, as the increased risk of adverse pregnancy outcomes such as second-trimester miscarriage may not be attributable solely to the treatment itself, but to common risk factors that predispose to both precancerous cervical conditions and these obstetric complications. Data pertaining to valid control groups are difficult to capture. Additionally, treatment modalities are likely to have varying impacts on the cervix, and the impact on the cervix for any given modality may vary from operator to operator.

Third trimester

Meta-analyses published in 2006 and 2008 suggested adverse third-trimester obstetric outcomes in women who underwent excisional treatment of CIN (39, 40). Cold knife conization had the greatest increased risk of preterm delivery, low birthweight, and caesarean section. The most prevalent excisional treatment (large loop excision of the transformation zone (LLETZ)) was also associated with a significant increase in premature delivery. However, extreme preterm birth (<32 weeks) was associated with cold knife conization but not LLETZ. Perhaps most importantly, there was no difference seen in perinatal mortality between women previously treated for CIN and untreated women.

A meta-analysis in 2015 included 20,832 women who gave birth after treatment for CIN before pregnancy, 52 women who gave birth after treatment for CIN during pregnancy, 64,237 women with CIN who gave birth before treatment, and 8,902,865 women who gave birth without CIN. Compared to women with untreated CIN, women treated for CIN before or during pregnancy had a significantly higher risk of preterm birth (<37 weeks) (odds ratio (OR) 1.7; 95% CI 1.0–2.7). Women treated for CIN before pregnancy had no significant difference in the rate of premature birth to women with CIN where treatment was delayed until after pregnancy (OR 1.4; 95% CI 0.85–2.3). Women treated during pregnancy had a clearly increased risk for premature delivery (OR 6.5; 95% CI 1.1–37), and premature rupture of membranes (OR 1.8; 95% CI 1.4–2.2) (41). These data support the policy of deferral of treatment of high-grade CIN until the puerperium.

While these systematic reviews have established an association between excisional treatments for CIN and premature delivery, the cause remains uncertain. An association between diagnosis of high-grade CIN and other factors predisposing for premature delivery such as smoking is hypothesized. Additionally, anatomical changes following cervical treatment, cicatrization of cervix, and alteration of cervical mucous and flora may predispose to prematurity. It has also been proposed that the pathophysiology of CIN could be contributory (42). The dose–effect relationship of cervical tissue excised appears relevant, with greater cervical stromal excision increasing the subsequent cervical deficit and prematurity risk (43).

A meta-analysis in 2008 suggested that ablative treatments are not associated with increased perinatal mortality (40). LLETZ has superseded ablative treatment in Western countries because it allows confirmation of clearance of disease and full histological examination, but many studies show that both are equally effective (44). Analysis is ongoing to explore the safety and validity of ablative techniques with satisfactory colposcopy in women with reproductive wishes, to minimize the potential impact on future pregnancies (45). Patients who intend to have a further pregnancy should undergo documented and well-informed counselling regarding potential risks and benefits before any excisional treatment is performed.

Vulval intraepithelial neoplasia in pregnancy

Vulval intraepithelial neoplasia (VIN) is a term used for precancerous skin conditions affecting the vulva. There are two distinct types, a type associated with HPV infection (usual type or uVIN) and a rarer form related to chronic inflammatory skin conditions such as lichen sclerosis (differentiated or dVIN). High-grade uVIN (VIN2 and VIN3) is also known as high-grade squamous intraepithelial lesion (HSIL) (46).

uVIN is increasingly a problem of younger women and its incidence increased fourfold from 1973 to 2000 (47, 48). VIN causes symptoms in approximately 80% of cases, including pain, soreness, pruritus, and psychosexual dysfunction. Symptoms can be severe and protracted, causing a significant impact on quality of life. Disease can be unifocal or multifocal. Spontaneous regression of high-grade uVIN is uncommon in older women, but authors have suggested spontaneous regression occurs in pregnancy in approximately 40% of cases and less commonly in non-pregnant women under the age of 35 years (49).

Treatment is historically surgical, involving excision of involved vulval skin with a narrow surgical margin. Various medical treatments have been studied in small trials and case series, with current evidence suggesting that topical imiquimod is an effective treatment for high-grade uVIN with the potential for complete clearance of disease in 40–60% of cases (46). The risk of progression to cancer is uncertain, but large case series suggests that it is in the region of 16% if high-grade uVIN is untreated, and approximately 4% where disease has been previously treated surgically, usually associated with multifocal disease (50).

It is therefore often a dilemma whether uVIN should to be treated during pregnancy. Unifocal, high-grade VIN can usually be excised during the second trimester with acceptable morbidity, providing the lesion is relatively small and does not involve the important structures of the clitoris, urethra, or perianal region. Data on the use of medical treatments during pregnancy is sparse, and imiquimod and other topical medical treatments such as 5-flurouracil, cidofovir, bleomycin and dinitrochlorobenzene are contraindicated in pregnancy (46). The United States Food and Drug Administarion classifies the use of imiquimod during pregnancy as a class 'C' medication, where animal reproduction studies have shown an adverse effect on the fetus and there are no adequate and well-controlled studies in humans (51).

It is not known if imiquimod is excreted via breast milk after vulval application, and therefore caution should be observed regarding its use by nursing mothers.

Premalignant disease of the uterus

Endometrial cancer is the commonest gynaecological malignancy in the Western world, and the incidence increased in the United Kingdom by 43% between 1993–1995 and 2007–2009 (52). Endometrial hyperplasia is a precursor for endometrial cancer (53). The increasing obesity epidemic is the main factor behind the rising incidence of this disease, as obesity, diabetes, and hypertension are important risk factors. In younger women, polycystic ovarian syndrome (PCOS) is an additional recognized risk factor, due to prolonged unopposed oestrogen exposure of the endometrium. Women with PCOS are three times more likely to develop endometrial cancer than women without PCOS (54). While unopposed endogenous oestrogen is the main risk factor, other factors including infection, immunosuppression, insulin resistance, glutathione-S-transferase and progesterone resistance can be instrumental (55–57).

Endometrial hyperplasia should be suspected in premenopausal women with risk factors who present with abnormal vaginal bleeding. United Kingdom guidelines published in 2014 concluded that endometrial hyperplasia is unlikely where the endometrial thickness measures less than 7 mm on transvaginal ultrasound scan. Endometrial biopsy and usually hysteroscopy are indicated in women with persistent symptoms, and women with complex endometrial hyperplasia with atypia should be counselled regarding the possibility of occult malignant disease (58).

Young women with endometrial hyperplasia who wish to preserve fertility are managed with progesterone, and require monitoring with endometrial biopsy to assess response to treatment. The levonorgestrel-releasing intrauterine system (Mirena®) or continuous oral progesterone should be used for a minimum of 6 months for the management of hyperplasia without atypia, with longer treatment planned for women with atypical hyperplasia. While on progesterone treatment, women treated for atypical hyperplasia should undergo endometrial biopsy every 3 months to exclude progression to invasive cancer (59). Disease regression should be demonstrated on at least one endometrial sample before women attempt to conceive, and it is advised that women with endometrial hyperplasia who wish to conceive are referred to a fertility specialist to discuss the options for attempting conception. Assisted reproduction may be considered as it is associated with a higher live birth rate and it may also prevent relapse of hyperplasia, compared with women who attempt natural conception. Regression of endometrial hyperplasia prior to attempting conception is associated with higher implantation and clinical pregnancy rates (60).

Due to high circulating endogenous progesterone levels in pregnancy, endometrial hyperplasia is unlikely to progress during pregnancy. Endometrial biopsy during pregnancy is clearly contraindicated, but repeat biopsy is recommended after the puerperium. Once fertility is no longer required, hysterectomy should be offered in view of the high risk of disease relapse. Following pregnancy, evidence of histological disease regression should be confirmed by a minimum of two consecutive negative endometrial biopsies, and long-term follow-up with an endometrial biopsy every 6–12 months is recommended until a hysterectomy is performed (61).

REFERENCES

1. Mathews TJ, Hamilton BE. *Delayed Childbearing: More Women are Having their First Child Later in Life.* NCHS data brief, No. 21. Hyattsville, MD: National Center for Health Statistics; 2009.
2. World Health Organization. Family planning/contraception. Fact sheet No. 351. Updated May 2015. Available at: http://www.who.int/mediacentre/factsheets/fs351/en/ (accessed 22 March 2016).
3. Royal College of Obstetricians and Gynaecologists (RCOG). *Obstetric Impact of Treatment for Cervical Intraepithelial Neoplasia.* Scientific Impact Paper No. 21. London: RCOG; 2010.
4. Nauth HF. *Gynecologic Cytology.* Stuttgart: Thieme; 2007.
5. McCredie MR, Sharples KJ, Paul C, et al. Natural history of cervical neoplasia and risk of invasive cancer in women with cervical intraepithelial neoplasia 3: a retrospective cohort study. *Lancet Oncol* 2008;**9**:425–34.
6. National Cancer Institute. Cervical Cancer Screening–Health Professional Version (PDQ®). Available at: http://www.cancer.gov/types/cervical/hp/cervical-screening-pdq#link/_248_toc (accessed 22 March 2016).
7. Melnikow J, Nuovo J, Willan AR, Chan BK, Howell LP. Natural history of cervical squamous intraepithelial lesions: a meta-analysis. *Obstet Gynecol* 1998;**92**:727–35.
8. McIntyre-Seltman K, Lesnock J. Cervical cancer screening in pregnancy. *Obstet Gynecol Clin North Am* 2008;**35**:645–58.
9. International Collaboration of Epidemiological Studies of Cervical Cancer. Cervical carcinoma and reproductive factors: Collaborative reanalysis of individual data on 16,563 women with cervical carcinoma and 33,542 women without cervical carcinoma from 25 epidemiological studies. *Int J Cancer* 2006;**119**:1108–24.
10. Royal College of Obstetricians and Gynaecologists (RCOG). Cervical smears and pregnancy. Available at: https://www.rcog.org.uk/globalassets/documents/patients/patient-information-leaflets/pregnancy/cervical-smears-and-pregnancy.pdf (accessed 22 March 2016).
11. Saslow D, Castle P, Myers E, et al. American Cancer Society, American Society for Colposcopy and Cervical Pathology, and American Society for Clinical Pathology screening guidelines for the prevention and early detection of cervical cancer. *CA Cancer J Clin* 2012;**62**:147–72.
12. Saslow D, Herschel WL, Waldman J, et al. American Cancer Society, American Society for Colposcopy and Cervical Pathology, and American Society for Clinical Pathology screening guidelines for the prevention and early detection of cervical cancer. *J Low Genit Tract Dis* 2012;**16**:175–204.
13. Michael CW, Esfahani FM. Pregnancy-related changes: a retrospective review of 278 cervical smears. *Diagn Cytopathol* 1997;**17**:99–107.
14. Arias-Stella J. A topographic study of uterine epithelial atypia associated with chorionic tissue: demonstration of alteration in the endocervix. *Cancer* 1959;**12**:782–90.
15. Murad TM, Tehart K, Flint A. Atypical cells in pregnancy and postpartum smears. *Acta Cytol* 1981;**25**:623–30.
16. Shrago SS. The Arias-Stella reaction; a case report of a cytologic presentation. *Acta Cytol* 1977;**21**:310–13.
17. Sellors JW, Sankaranarayanan R. *Colposcopy and Treatment of Cervical Intraepithelial Neoplasia: A Beginners' Manual.* Lyon: International Agency for Research on Cancer; 2003.
18. Slama J, Freitag P, Dundr P, et al. Outcomes of pregnant patients with Pap smears classified as atypical glandular cells. *Cytopathology* 2012;**23**:383–88.

19. Freeman-Wang T, Walker P. Colposcopy in special circumstances: pregnancy, immunocompromise, including HIV and transplants, adolescence and menopause. *Clin Obstet Gynecol* 2011;**25**:653–65.

20. Coppleson M, Pixley E, Reid BL. *Colposcopy: A Scientific Approach to the Cervix, Vagina and Vulva in Health and Disease*, 3rd edn. Springfield, IL: Thomas; 1986.

21. Serati M, Uccella S, Laterza RM. Natural history of cervical intraepithelial neoplasia during pregnancy. *Acta Obstet Gynecol Scand* 2008;**87**:1296–300.

22. Tidy J. *Colposcopy and Programme Management*, 3rd ed. London: Public Health England; 2016.

23. Han SN, Mhallem Gziri M, Van Calsteren K, Amant F. Cervical cancer in pregnant women: treat, wait or interrupt? Assessment of current clinical guidelines, innovations and controversies *Ther Adv Med Oncol* 2013;**5**:211–19.

24. Ungár L, Smith JR, Pálfalvi L, Del Priore G. Abdominal radical trachelectomy during pregnancy to preserve pregnancy and fertility. *Obstet Gynecol* 2006;**108**:811–14.

25. da Fonseca AJ, Dalla-Benetta AC, Ferreira LP, Martins CR, Lins CD. Neoadjuvant chemotherapy followed by radical surgery in pregnant patient with invasive cervical cancer: case report and literature review. *Rev Bras Ginecol Obstet* 2011;**33**:43–48.

26. Siristatidis C, Vitoratos N, Michailidis E, et al. The role of the mode of delivery in the alteration of intrapartum pathological cervical cytologic findings during the postpartum period. *Eur J Gynaecol Oncol* 2002;**23**:358–60.

27. Cubo-Abert M, Centeno-Mediavilla C, Franco-Zabala P, et al. Risk factors for progression or persistence of squamous intraepithelial lesions diagnosed during pregnancy. *J Low Genit Tract Dis* 2012;**16**:34–38.

28. Larson DA, Derkay CS. Epidemiology of recurrent respiratory papillomatosis. *APMIS* 2010;**118**:450–54.

29. Silverberg MJ, Thorsen P, Lindeberg H, Grant LA, Shah KV. Condyloma in pregnancy is strongly predictive of juvenile-onset recurrent respiratory papillomatosis. *Obstet Gynecol* 2003;**101**:645–52.

30. Paraskevaidis E, Koliopoulos G, Kalantaridou S, et al. Management and evolution of cervical intraepithelial neoplasia during pregnancy and postpartum. *Eur J Obstet Gynecol Reprod Biol* 2002;**104**:67–69.

31. Jain AG, Higgins RV, Boyle MJ. Management of low-grade squamous intraepithelial lesions during pregnancy. *Am J Obstet Gynecol* 1997;**177**:298–302.

32. Palle C, Bangsboll S, Andreasson B. Cervical intraepithelial neoplasia in pregnancy. *Acta Obstet Gynecol Scand* 2000;**79**:306–10.

33. Benedet JL, Selke PA, Nickerson KG. Colposcopic evaluation of abnormal Papanicolaou smears in pregnancy. *Am J Obstet Gynecol* 1987;**157**:932–37.

34. Kennedy S, Robinson J, Hallam N. LLETZ and infertility. *Br J Obstetr Gynaecol* 1993;**100**:965.

35. Luesley DM, McCrum A, Terry PB, et al. Complications of cone biopsy related to the dimensions of the cone and the influence of prior colposcopic assessment. *Br J Obstetr Gynaecol* 1985;**92**:158–64.

36. Kalliala I, Anttila A, Dyba T, Hakulinen T, Halttunen M, Nieminen P. Pregnancy incidence and outcome among patients with cervical intraepithelial neoplasia: a retrospective cohort study. *Br J Obstetr Gynaecol* 2012;**119**:227–35.

37. Spracklen CN, Harland KK, Stegmann BJ, Saftlas AF. Cervical surgery for cervical intraepithelial neoplasia and prolonged time to conception of a live birth: a case-control study. *Br J Obstetr Gynaecol* 2013;**120**:960–65.

38. Kyrgiou M, Mitra A, Arbyn M, et al. Fertility and early pregnancy outcomes after treatment for cervical intraepithelial neoplasia: systematic review and meta-analysis *BMJ* 2014;**349**: g6192.

39. Kyrgiou M, Koliopoulos G, Martin-Hirsch P, Arbyn M, Prendiville W, Paraskevaidis E. Obstetric outcomes after conservative treatment for intraepithelial or early invasive cervical lesions: systematic review and meta-analysis *Lancet* 2006;**367**:489–98.

40. Arbyn M, Kyrgiou M, Simoens C, et al. Perinatal mortality and other severe adverse pregnancy outcomes associated with treatment of cervical intraepithelial neoplasia: meta-analysis. *BMJ* 2008;**337**:a1284.

41. Danhof NA, Kamphuis EI, Limpens J, van Lonkhuijzen LR, Pajkrt E, Mol BW. The risk of preterm birth of treated versus untreated cervical intraepithelial neoplasia (CIN): a systematic review and meta-analysis. *Eur J Obstet Gynecol Reprod Biol* 2015;**188**:24–33.

42. Castanon A, Brocklehurst P, Evans H, et al. Risk of preterm birth after treatment for cervical intraepithelial neoplasia among women attending colposcopy in England: retrospective-prospective cohort study. *BMJ* 2012;**345**:e5174.

43. Founta C, Arbyn M, Valasoulis G, et al. Proportion of excision and cervical healing after large loop excision of the transformation zone for cervical intraepithelial neoplasia. *BJOG* 2010;**117**:1468–74.

44. Martin-Hirsch PL, Paraskevaidis E, Kitchener H. Surgery for cervical intraepithelial neoplasia. *Cochrane Database Syst Rev* 2000;**2**:CD001318.

45. Paraskevaidis E, Kyrgiou M, Martin-Hirsch P. Have we dismissed ablative treatment too soon in colposcopy practice? *BJOG* 2007;**114**:3–4.

46. Pepas L, Kaushik S, Nordin A, Bryant A, Lawrie TA. Medical interventions for high-grade vulval intraepithelial neoplasia. *Cochrane Database Syst Rev* 2015;**8**:CD007924.

47. Joura EA, Losch A, Haider-Angeler MG, et al. Trends in vulvar neoplasia. Increasing incidence of vulvar intraepithelial neoplasia and squamous cell carcinoma of the vulva in young women. *J Reprod Med* 2000;**45**:613–15.

48. Judson PL, Habermann EB, Baxter NN, Durham SB, Virnig BA. Trends in the incidence of invasive and in situ vulvar carcinoma. *Obstet Gynecol* 2006;**107**:1018–22.

49. Seters MV. *Vulvar Intraepithelial Neoplasia: New Concepts and Strategy*. Thesis, Erasmus University, Rotterdam, The Netherlands; 2008.

50. Jones RW, Rowan DR, Stewart AW. Vulvar intraepithelial neoplasia. Aspects of the natural history and outcome in 405 women. *Obstet Gynecol* 2005;**106**:1319–26.

51. Food and Drug Administration. Highlights of prescribing information Aldara* (imiquimod). 2010. Available at: http://www.accessdata.fda.gov/drugsatfda_docs/label/2010/020723s022lbl.pdf (accessed 22 March 2016).

52. Public Health England Knowledge and Intelligence Team for East Midlands. *Outline of Uterine Cancer in the United Kingdom: Incidence, Mortality and Survival. Gynaecological Cancer SSCRG.* London: National Cancer Intelligence Network UK; 2013.

53. Kurman RJ, Kaminski PF, Norris HJ. The behavior of endometrial hyperplasia. A long-term study of "untreated" hyperplasia in 170 patients. *Cancer* 1985;**56**:403–12.

54. Haoula Z, Salman M, Atiomo W. Evaluating the association between endometrial cancer and polycystic ovary syndrome. *Hum Reprod* 2012;**27**:1327–331.

55. Bobrowska K, Kamiński P, Cyganek A, et al. High rate of endometrial hyperplasia in renal transplanted women. *Transplant Proc* 2006;**38**:177–79.

56. Hardiman P, Pillay O, Atiomo W. Polycystic ovary syndrome and endometrial carcinoma. *Lancet* 2003;**361**:1810–12.

57. Atiomo W, Khalid S, Parameshweran S, Houda M, Layfield R. Proteomic biomarkers for the diagnosis and risk stratification of polycystic ovary syndrome: a systematic review. *BJOG* 2009;**116**:137–43.

58. Royal College of Obstetricians and Gynaecologists (RCOG). *Long-term Consequences of Polycystic Ovary Syndrome*. Green-top Guideline No. 33. London: RCOG; 2014.

59. American College of Obstetricians and Gynecologists, Society of Gynecologic Oncology. Practice Bulletin No. 149: Endometrial cancer. *Obstet Gynecol* 2015;**125**:1006–26.

60. Gallos ID, Yap J, Rajkhowa M, Luesley DM, Coomarasamy A, Gupta JK. Regression, relapse, and live birth rates with fertility-sparing therapy for endometrial cancer and atypical complex endometrial hyperplasia: a systematic review and metaanalysis. *Am J Obstet Gynecol* 2012;**207**:266.e1–12.

61. Royal College of Obstetricians and Gynaecologists (RCOG). *Management of Endometrial Hyperplasia*. Green-top Guideline No. 67, RCOG/BSGE Joint Guideline. London: RCOG; 2016.

72

Cancer in pregnancy

Matthys Hendrik Botha

Introduction

For some women, the happiest time in their lives is complicated by the scariest events in their lives. Cancer in pregnancy is generally a rare occurrence but it is a shocking concept that, at a time when advice is to avoid coffee, wine, and some cheese for a healthy baby, you may need X-rays and even chemo- or radiotherapy for diagnosis and treatment of cancer. The incidence of invasive cancer in pregnancy is about 1:1000 to 1:2000 pregnancies (1). About 3500 new cases are diagnosed during pregnancy in the United States every year. Breast cancer is the most common pregnancy-associated malignancy and 7–15% of all breast cancers in premenopausal women occur during pregnancy. There is some evidence that there is an increase in incidence of pregnancy-associated breast cancer with one large cohort study from Sweden, reporting an increase from 16 to 37 per 100,000 deliveries from 1963 to 2002 (2). Of the reported cancers, breast cancer is by far the most common at 46%, followed by haematological malignancies, dermatological malignancies, cervical cancer, brain tumours, and ovarian tumours (3).

Recent observations from Belgium seem to suggest that a pregnant patient should not have a poorer outcome of their cancer management when they are cared for by a multidisciplinary team with necessary input from obstetricians, oncologists, surgeons, paediatricians, and pharmacologists (4). Oncological treatment is possible during pregnancy, often without significantly endangering fetal safety.

Diagnosis and staging of cancer during pregnancy

Many symptoms associated with malignancy might also be experienced during normal pregnancy. These include nausea and vomiting, bowel discomfort and pain, anaemia, chronic tiredness, and lethargy. Patients often hesitate to contact their caregiver when they discover a worrying symptom for fear of bad news, especially during a pregnancy because of their concern that the diagnosis and treatment of the disease will jeopardize the health of their baby. Physicians also fail to focus on other health aspects in the presence of a pregnancy. This leads to a delayed diagnosis.

Histological specimens should be interpreted with caution during pregnancy and the pathologist should be informed about the pregnant state. The interpretation of tissue biopsies may be difficult in the presence of pregnancy hormones which may cause significant changes in normal and pathological tissues.

Imaging investigations

In physics, electromagnetic energy is broadly categorized into ionizing and non-ionizing energy. Ionizing radiation ionizes matter by detaching electrons from atoms or molecules. These energy sources may directly cause mutations due to DNA or RNA damage. In general, fetal exposure of more than 5–10 centigray (cGy) should be avoided. In contrast, non-ionizing energy as it is used in medical diagnostics does not usually pose a direct (deterministic) or indirect (stochastic) risk and it is often safely used in pregnancy. Non-ionizing energy may produce some heat in tissues. Examples of non-ionizing radio waves or sound waves include magnetic resonance imaging (MRI) and ultrasonography.

The ionizing radiation effects on the mother and fetus can be categorized into deterministic and stochastic effects. Deterministic effects are dose dependent and cause cellular damage with loss of organ development or function. Stochastic effects are usually associated with low-dose ionizing radiation and have a longer-term random element to it, causing genomic damage, which over time may lead to secondary cancers. In a workup for a patient with a malignancy, the aim is to determine whether a solid tumour has progressed to systemic spread by means of careful imaging investigations. Fetal radiation exposure remains a concern due to possible teratogenic effects of radiation exposure. The so-called ALARA ('as low as reasonably achievable') principle should be used when radiation exposure is considered in a pregnant patient (5). A threshold dose for the deterministic effects is generally regarded as 100 milligray (mGy) to a fetus. Any dose above this may lead to congenital malformations, intellectual disability, and even fetal death.

The American Association of Physicists in Medicine recommends that adequate shielding is necessary for the use of X-rays and computed tomography (CT) investigations (**Table 72.1**).

MRI is usually considered to be safe during pregnancy. However, the use of gadolinium is not recommended. Gadolinium is regarded

Table 72.1 Fetal irradiation dose for different diagnostic tests

Diagnostic test	Fetal irradiation dose (mGy)
Chest X-ray	0.0006
Abdominal X-ray	1.5–2.6
Computed tomography (CT) chest	0.1–13
CT abdomen	8–30
Positron emission tomography (PET)	1.1–2.43

by the United States Food and Drug Administration as a category C drug. Category C means that animal studies have shown adverse fetal effects and there are no adequate and well-controlled studies in humans. Potential benefits may warrant use of the drug in pregnant women despite potential risks because it crosses the placenta. In some reported studies there were no adverse effects on fetal development after inadvertent administration of gadolinium.

Ultrasound is generally regarded as safe in pregnancy. The 'Essential Steps in the Management of Obstetric Emergencies' (ESMOE) training programme states in clinical practice guidelines in 2010 that there is also a theoretical risk of fetal heating and possible cavitation with the use of MRI and it should best be avoided during the first trimester.

Radiotherapy during pregnancy

Radiotherapy in a pregnant patient should be carefully planned and discussed with the radiation oncologist and the radiophysicist in order to minimize direct and indirect sources of radiation to the fetus. The fetal dose should not exceed 100 mGy. The specific risk of radiotherapy is associated with fetal gestation at the time of radiotherapy (Table 72.2).

Even with proper shielding there is still the concern of so-called scatter and leakage radiation. Risks can be minimized by adequate shielding. Shielding of the uterus, especially in advanced pregnancy, can become quite challenging due to the heavy materials used for shielding. It may need to be adapted to gestational age and the size of the uterus. Some obstetric experts advise regular clinical and ultrasound examinations to determine the lie of the fetus to get the

Table 72.2 Risks of radiotherapy to fetus during pregnancy

Gestational age (weeks)	Risk
Preimplantation (1)	Lethality
Organogenesis (2–7)	Lethality, gross malformations, growth retardation, sterility, cataracts, other neuropathology, malignant disease
Early fetal (8–15)	Lethality, gross malformations, growth retardation, intellectual disability, sterility, cataracts, malignant disease
Mid fetal (16–25)	Gross malformations, growth retardation, intellectual disability, sterility, cataracts, malignant disease
Late fetal (>25)	Growth retardation, sterility, cataracts, malignant disease

position of the fetal head out of the potential field of radiotherapy, for example, in the case of chest radiotherapy, the fetus should be in the cephalic position and external cephalic version may be necessary.

Surgery during pregnancy

There is ample published evidence about safe surgery during pregnancy. However, oncological surgery is less well described. The important outcome measures that need to be considered include:

- optimal oncological and surgical outcome
- maternal well-being
- fetal well-being.

Optimal oncological and surgical outcome

Most oncological surgery during pregnancy is outside the abdominal cavity and can usually be performed without serious risk to the developing child. Laparotomy for intra-abdominal tumours is complicated by an enlarged uterus and access to the pouch of Douglas may be impossible in advanced pregnancy. The use of laparoscopy during pregnancy has become more accepted in recent times with a lot of experience being gained in many centres around the world. The precautions during laparoscopic surgery include open laparoscopic entry and using lower intra-abdominal pressures of less than 15 mmHg. Preferably the surgeon performing the procedure should be a skilled laparoscopic surgeon with experience in operating on pregnant patients.

Maternal well-being

Anaesthetic considerations for pregnant patients are well known. Important changes in respiratory function mean that preoxygenation is absolutely essential. Doses for anaesthetic agents may need to be adjusted for the metabolic state of pregnant physiology. Other considerations include a high risk for thromboembolic events during pregnancy and in cancer cases, which necessitate the use of prophylaxis in the form of low-molecular-weight or unfractionated heparin.

Fetal well-being

Fetal oxygen supply is dependent on effective maternal ventilation and even short periods of maternal hypoventilation can lead to fetal distress. In more advanced pregnancies and long surgical procedures, it is prudent to monitor the fetus with continuous cardiotocography (CTG) in theatre. In first-trimester pregnancies, it is adequate to check the fetal heart with fetal Doppler preoperatively and postoperatively. Preventing premature labour or miscarriage may be achieved by administering non-steroidal anti-inflammatory drugs (NSAIDs) but it needs to be kept in mind that in the third trimester, NSAIDs may lead to the closing of the ductus arteriosus (7). Tocolytic agents are generally used perioperatively to prevent preterm labour. Postoperative care is not dissimilar from non-pregnant patients; however, considerations for safe analgesia include omitting NSAIDs in the third trimester. Antiemetics are essential due to an already increased risk for nausea and vomiting.

Chemotherapy during pregnancy

Major advances have been achieved with chemotherapy use in pregnancy over the last few decades. After the first trimester, which is the most important in organogenesis of the fetus, most chemotherapeutic agents can be used with relative safety. The transplacental transport of chemotherapeutic agents differ widely, with some agents such as paclitaxel crossing the placenta at a low rate, anthracyclines crossing at an intermediate rate, and carboplatin crossing at a high rate (8, 9). Although some of these agents cross the placenta, the relatively high concentration after 12–14 weeks of pregnancy seems to do little harm to the developing fetus. Certain agents are completely contraindicated including trastuzumab (Herceptin) because of the binding of Her-2 receptors to the kidneys in the fetus, resulting in oligo- or anhydramnios and fetal lung hypoplasia. The antifolates such as methotrexate are also contraindicated.

The risk of congenital malformation is directly linked to the gestational age and before 12 weeks there is a risk for abnormalities of the eyes, ears, and blood systems while the risk decreases significantly after complete organogenesis.

Chemotherapy may cause a significant reduction in blood production leading to, among other abnormalities, low platelet counts and a risk for overwhelming infection. When chemotherapy is used, the timing of delivery should be planned carefully. Elective delivery should not be planned within 3 weeks after chemotherapy. For this reason, chemotherapy should not be administered after 37 weeks of gestation due to the risk of spontaneous onset of labour.

Recent work on long-term follow-up of children born to mothers receiving chemotherapy during pregnancy does not indicate an increased risk for congenital abnormalities or mental delay. The number of children with long-term follow-up is still small and the data should be interpreted with caution. Potential risks include a concern for cardiac function in children exposed to anthracyclines during the fetal period. Anthracyclines are commonly used for breast cancer treatment and have a direct effect on cardiac function. In a follow-up study on 17 children, no changes in electrocardiography or echocardiography could be found after the use of anthracyclines.

Organ-specific management

Preinvasive cervical cancer

High-grade squamous intraepithelial lesions on cytology need to be referred to colposcopy to exclude invasive tumours. Colposcopy can be quite challenging during pregnancy due to increased vascularity and an increase in genital oedema (10). In case of a visible tumour, a superficial cone biopsy ('coin biopsy') can be performed. The risk for bleeding is increased in a pregnant patient due to vascularity. It may be necessary to repeat the colposcopy at 12-weekly intervals if an abnormality is found distant from term. Definitive treatment in the absence of an invasive tumour is usually delayed until after delivery. A biopsy can be performed by loop excision or by an old-fashioned cold knife method. The term 'coin biopsy' is sometimes used in pregnancy to highlight the fact that the incision should not be deep enough to cause damage to the fetal membranes. This should be performed in a theatre with adequate anaesthesia. Prophylactic cerclage may be an option both for the prevention of premature labour and for the management of operative bleeding.

Invasive cervical cancer

Cervical cancer remains one of the most common malignancies in pregnancy. A conservative approach is only appropriate if the patient has a firm desire to continue with the pregnancy (11). Some patients and their care givers opt for 'watchful waiting' due to the risks of therapy in pregnancy.

Uterus-conserving surgery is appropriate only in highly selected cases. A wide cone biopsy or a modified radical trachelectomy have been performed in pregnancy but outcomes so far have not been universally good due to significant bleeding during the procedures (12). Laparoscopic extraperitoneal or open lymphadenectomy has been described in small series for patients at less than 25 weeks' gestation (13). The pathological information about nodal status may influence management but imaging with MRI to determine nodal status is more widely used. Immediate, definitive treatment, regardless of gestational age, is generally appropriate in the following settings:

- Documented lymph node metastases
- Progression of disease during the pregnancy
- Patient choice to terminate the pregnancy (14).

Where the decision is made to sacrifice the pregnancy before 24 weeks' gestation and in patients with International Federation of Gynecology and Obstetrics (FIGO) stage IA2–IIa and where surgery is possible, a radical hysterectomy and pelvic node dissection with the fetus *in situ* is the most common treatment pathway. After 24 weeks and viability, surgical treatment is usually delayed until 32–34 weeks at which time a classical caesarean section plus radical hysterectomy and pelvic lymphadenectomy is performed. This approach requires individualization and will be influenced by tumour size, patient's wishes, etc.

In more advanced stages where radiotherapy is indicated, the management of the termination of the pregnancy is dependent on the gestation. Before 12 weeks of gestation, radiotherapy can be given without removal of the fetus but often the patient prefers to start chemoradiation after medical termination of pregnancy. Between 12 to 24 weeks, hysterotomy is generally performed followed by chemoradiation 7–14 days later. This includes external beam therapy and high-dose intracavitary brachytherapy.

Chemotherapy is often used in a neoadjuvant approach until such time that definitive surgery or radiotherapy can be performed (15). Caesarean section is the preferred choice for delivery of the baby in the presence of bulky tumours. Vaginal delivery risks the possibility of catastrophic bleeding and implant metastases in vaginal tears or episiotomy scars. In locally advanced tumours, it is recommended that a lower segment transverse caesarean section is best avoided due to the risk of cutting or tearing into tumour tissue. A classical incision will minimize blood loss and avoid the large tumour vessels.

Ovarian cancer

Ovarian masses are often found incidentally during pregnancy ultrasonography. Most of these are benign and care should be individualized based on ultrasound and clinical features. Risks include torsion, rupture, and bleeding. Laparoscopic removal is relatively contraindicated in masses suspicious of malignancy.

Invasive epithelial ovarian cancer is exceedingly rare in pregnancy but proper surgical management remains the cornerstone of treatment. Proper surgical staging is often very difficult due to a lack of good exposure, especially the pouch of Douglas. Neoadjuvant chemotherapy is usually administered and completion surgery can be delayed until after the delivery of the baby.

Endometrial cancer associated with pregnancy is rare and is usually only diagnosed in postpartum patients with persistent vaginal bleeding. Other gynaecological cancers include vulval cancer where surgery is certainly possible. Each case should be individually managed. For very large, advanced-stage disease, abdominal delivery is preferred due to a risk of bleeding if the tumour is stretched or torn during vaginal birth.

Breast cancer

Normal pregnancy is associated with many physiological changes that affect the density and nodularity of the breast tissue. It is often difficult for patients and clinicians to determine abnormal, pathological breast masses from normal physiological changes. For this reason, the diagnosis of breast cancer is often delayed during pregnancy. It is estimated that approximately 1:3000 pregnancies will be complicated by breast cancer (16).

The diagnostic accuracy of mammography in pregnancy is generally low and the information gained from a mammogram is difficult to interpret due to the density of breast tissue in young, pregnant women. Fortunately, the risk of radiation to the fetus is low, especially when shielding is used for the uterus. Ultrasound examination of the breast is the preferred method and guided biopsies will often confirm the diagnosis.

The majority of breast tumours diagnosed in pregnancy are high-grade, infiltrating ductal carcinomas with lymphovascular space invasion. Up to 70% are oestrogen and progesterone receptor negative and nearly 70% will have lymph node involvement at the time of diagnosis (16).

Surgery, which may include mastectomy, lymphadenectomy, or lumpectomy, can be performed safely during pregnancy. Sentinel lymph node biopsies may also be used because the risk of radiation from technetium sulphur colloid is very low according to the National Council on Radiation Protection and Measurement (17). Blue dyes such as lymphazurin and methylene blue are best avoided due to the risk of fetal abnormalities.

Commonly used chemotherapeutic agents include 5-fluorourasil, doxorubicin, and cyclophosphamide, which have all been used safely during the second and third trimesters of pregnancy. Methotrexate should be avoided. Tamoxifen and Herceptin have both been associated with fetal complications and should therefore not be used during pregnancy.

The management of breast cancer should be individualized in a multidisciplinary team environment.

Placental and fetal involvement

Metastatic disease to the placenta and to the fetus is fortunately quite rare. The most likely tumours to metastasize to the placenta include melanomas and haematological malignancies. In all cases where malignant spread is possible, the placenta should be submitted for careful histological evaluation. The fetus should be examined carefully at birth and at regular intervals after birth to look for any signs of metastatic disease.

Patient support

The diagnosis and management of cancer in pregnancy is usually extremely stressful for the patient and her family. Support services in many oncology units provide patient and family support.

Research

Recently, the International Network on Cancer, Infertility and Pregnancy was launched by a group of the European Society of Gynaecological Oncology. The primary objective is to establish an international registry on cancer during pregnancy and fertility preservation during cancer treatment. The group has already improved our understanding of the most important aspects of management.

REFERENCES

1. Cardonick E, Dougherty R, Grana G, Gilmandyar D, Ghaffar S, Usmani A. Breast cancer during pregnancy: maternal and fetal outcomes. *Cancer J* 2010;**16**:76–82.
2. Andersson TM, Johansson AL, Hsieh CC, Cnattingius S, Lambe M. Increasing incidence of pregnancy-associated breast cancer in Sweden. *Obstet Gynecol* 2009;**114**:568–72.
3. Van Calsteren K, Heyns L, De Smet F, et al. Cancer during pregnancy: an analysis of 215 patients emphasizing the obstetrical and the neonatal outcomes. *J Clin Oncol* 2010;**28**:683–89.
4. Amant F, Han SN, Gziri MM, Vandenbroucke T, Verheecke M, Van Calsteren K. Management of cancer in pregnancy. *Best Pract Res Clin Obstet Gynaecol* 2015;**29**:741–53.
5. Groen RS, Bae JY, Lim KJ. Fear of the unknown: ionizing radiation exposure during pregnancy. *Am J Obstet Gynecol* 2012;**206**:456–62.
6. Stovall M, Blackwell CR, Cundiff J, et al. Fetal dose from radiotherapy with photon beams: report of AAPM Radiation Therapy Committee Task Group No. 36. *Med Phys* 1995;**22**:63–82.
7. Koren G, Florescu A, Costei AM, Boskovic R, Moretti ME. Nonsteroidal antiinflammatory drugs during third trimester and the risk of premature closure of the ductus arteriosus: a meta-analysis. *Ann Pharmacother* 2006;**40**:824–29.
8. Van Calsteren K, Verbesselt R, Beijnen J, et al. Transplacental transfer of anthracyclines, vinblastine, and 4-hydroxy-cyclophosphamide in a baboon model. *Gynecol Oncol* 2010;**119**:594–600.
9. Calsteren KV, Verbesselt R, Devlieger R, et al. Transplacental transfer of paclitaxel, docetaxel, carboplatin, and trastuzumab in a baboon model. *Int J Gynecol Cancer* 2010;**20**:1456–464.
10. Hunter MI, Monk BJ, Tewari KS. Cervical neoplasia in pregnancy. Part 1: screening and management of preinvasive disease. *Am J Obstet Gynecol* 2008;**199**:3–9.
11. Hunter MI, Tewari K, Monk BJ. Cervical neoplasia in pregnancy. Part 2: current treatment of invasive disease. *Am J Obstet Gynecol* 2008;**199**:10–18.

12. Căpîlna ME, Szabo B, Becsi J, Ioanid N, Moldovan B. Radical trachelectomy performed during pregnancy: a review of the literature. *Int J Gynecol Cancer* 2016;**26**:758–62.

13. Vercellino GF, Koehler C, Erdemoglu E, et al. Laparoscopic pelvic lymphadenectomy in 32 pregnant patients with cervical cancer: rationale, description of the technique, and outcome. *Int J Gynecol Cancer* 2014;**24**:364–71.

14. Amant F, Halaska MJ, Fumagalli M, et al. Gynecologic cancers in pregnancy: guidelines of a second international consensus meeting. *Int J Gynecol Cancer* 2014;**24**:394–403.

15. van Vliet W, van Loon AJ, ten Hoor KA, Boonstra H. Cervical carcinoma during pregnancy: outcome of planned delay in treatment. *Eur J Obstet Gynecol Reprod Biol* 1998;**79**:153–57.

16. Dietz JR, Partridge AH, Gemignani ML, Javid SH, Kuerer HM. Breast cancer management updates: young and older, pregnant, or male. *Ann Surg Oncol* 2015;**22**:3219–24.

17. Spanheimer PM, Graham MM, Sugg SL, Scott-Conner CE, Weigel RJ. Measurement of uterine radiation exposure from lymphoscintigraphy indicates safety of sentinel lymph node biopsy during pregnancy. *Ann Surg Oncol* 2009;**16**:1143–47.

Index